Physical Rehabilitation:

Assessment and Treatment

Physical Rehabilitation:
Assessment and Treatment

Fourth Edition

SUSAN B. O'SULLIVAN, EdD, PT
Professor
Department of Physical Therapy
University of Massachusetts Lowell
Lowell, Massachusetts

THOMAS J. SCHMITZ, PhD, PT
Associate Professor
Division of Physical Therapy
Long Island University
Brooklyn Campus
New York, New York

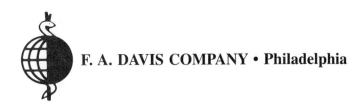
F. A. DAVIS COMPANY • Philadelphia

F. A. Davis Company
1915 Arch Street
Philadelphia, PA 19103

Copyright © 2001 by F. A. Davis Company

Printed in the United States of America
Last digit indicates print number: 10 9 8 7 6 5

Publisher: Jean-François Vilain
Developmental Editor: Michael Schnee
Cover Designer: Louis J. Forgione

As new scientific information becomes available through basic and clinical research, recommended treatments and drug therapies undergo changes. The author(s) and publisher have done everything possible to make this book accurate, up to date, and in accord with accepted standards at the time of publication. The authors, editors, and publisher are not responsible for errors or omissions or for consequences from application of the book, and make no warranty, expressed or implied, in regard to the contents of the book. Any practice described in this book should be applied by the reader in accordance with the professional standards of care used in regard to the unique circumstances that may apply in each situation. The reader is advised always to check product information (package inserts) for changes and new information regarding dose and contraindications before administering any drug. Caution is especially urged when using new or infrequently ordered drugs.

Library of Congress Cataloging-in-Publication Data

Physical rehabilitation : assessment and treatment / [edited by] Susan
B. O'Sullivan, Thomas J. Schmitz. — 4th ed.
    p. ; cm.
   Includes bibliographical references and index.
   ISBN 0-8036-0533-1 (alk. paper)
  1. Physical therapy.
   [DNLM: 1. Physical Therapy—methods. 2. Disability Evaluation. WB
460 P57763 2000] I. O'Sullivan, Susan B. II. Schmitz, Thomas J. III.
O'Sullivan, Susan B. Physical rehabilitation.
  RM700 .O88 2000
  615.8′2—dc21
                                       00-031700

Preface

We have been gratified at the wide acceptance of *Physical Rehabilitation: Assessment and Treatment* by both physical therapy faculty and students. Designed as a comprehensive text on the rehabilitation management of adult patients, it also serves as a valuable reference for practicing physical therapists as well as for other rehabilitation professionals. This fourth edition recognizes the continuing growth of the field and strives to integrate current research in basic and clinical sciences with physical therapy assessment and treatment procedures. It also integrates the American Physical Therapy Association's Guide to Physical Therapist Practice.

The conceptual basis of *Physical Rehabilitation: Assessment and Treatment* is established at the outset with three chapters examining clinical decision making, psychosocial concomitants to disability and rehabilitation, and the influence of values on patient care. Thus, the reader is directed early on to develop an understanding of the whole patient and to build effective problem-solving skills. Chapters 4 through 12 focus on procedures used in assessment of patients with physical impairments and disabilities. Chapters 13 and 14 outline general treatment strategies for improving motor control and motor learning and gait. Subsequent chapters, 15 through 30, examine common conditions encountered in general clinical practice together with appropriate examination and intervention strategies. New to the fourth edition is a chapter on vestibular rehabilitation (Chapter 25). Content on special rehabilitation topics includes: prosthetics (Chapter 20), orthotics (Chapter 31), the prescriptive wheelchair (Chapter 32), and biofeedback (Chapter 33).

This fourth edition has benefited from the input of numerous readers who have used this text in either an academic or a clinical setting. In response to their constructive feedback, we have attempted to expand and update content, correct errors, rectify omissions, and delete material as deemed appropriate.

We continue to utilize a format designed to facilitate and reinforce the learning of key concepts. To that end, each chapter of *Physical Rehabilitation: Assessment and Treatment* includes an initial set of learning objectives, chapter outline, an introduction and summary, study questions for self-assessment, glossary, and extensive references. In addition, supplemental reading lists and resources are provided for further investigation of the theories and intervention strategies presented. New to the fourth edition is the addition of clinical case studies with each chapter with suggested answers presented in an appendix. Numerous photographs and illustrations have been included to reinforce the concepts and techniques presented in the text. Summary tables, sample assessment tools, and treatment protocols are provided to assist the learner in organizing information.

We recognize the primary strength of this text comes from the input provided by our talented contributors. These individuals are recognized authorities from different clinical specialty areas with unique perspectives, knowledge, and skills. Their integration of current research and clinical experience has immeasurably strengthened this text.

Because physical therapy is a growing profession with frequent and often rapid advances, we will always consider this book a "work in progress." With this in mind, we welcome the continuing suggestions for improvement from our colleagues and students.

Susan B. O'Sullivan
Thomas J. Schmitz

Acknowledgments

A project of this scope would not be possible without the valuable contributions of many individuals throughout the development of its four editions. We extend our gratitude to all our contributing authors. This text is reflective of their collective talent, expertise, and commitment to physical therapy education. Our gratitude, too, goes to the various individuals who have reviewed portions of the manuscript during various stages of development. Their constructive comments greatly enhanced the contents of each edition. Our grateful thanks go also to those individuals who contributed their time, energy, and talent to the completion of the photographs and to those individuals whose photographs appear throughout the text. Finally, our thanks go to our students whose enthusiasm for learning continues to challenge and inspire us.

Appreciation is extended to Jean-Francois Vilain, Publisher, F.A. Davis Company, for his continued encouragement, support, and commitment to excellence in expanding physical therapy literature. Thanks are also extended to Sharon Lee, Developmental Editor, and Jack Brandt, Illustration Specialist, and Sam Rondinelli, Assissant Director of Editing, Design and Production.

Contributors

Adrienne Falk Bergen, PT
Seating Specialist
Dynamic Medical Equipment, Ltd.
Westbury, New York

Carol M. Davis, EdD, PT
Associate Professor
Division of Physical Therapy
Department of Orthopaedics and Rehabilitation
University of Miami
Coral Gables, Florida

Joan E. Edelstein, MA, PT
Associate Professor of Clinical Physical Therapy
Director, Program in Physical Therapy
Columbia University
New York, New York

Timothy L. Fagerson, MCSP, PT, MS
Orthopaedic Physical Therapy Services, Inc.
Wellesley Hills, Massachusetts

George D. Fulk, MS, PT
ACCE and Assistant Professor
Notre Dame College
Manchester, New Hampshire

Aaron S. Geller, MD
Associate Medical Director
Health South Rehabilitation Hospital
Concord, New Hampshire

Kate Grimes, MS, PT, CCS
Massachusetts General Hospital
Institute of Health Professions
Boston, Massachusetts

Andrew A. Guccione, PhD, PT, FAPTA
Senior Vice President
Division of Practice and Research
American Physical Therapy Association
Alexandria, Virginia

Barbara J. Headley, MS, PT
President
Innovative Systems for Rehabilitation
Boulder, Colorado

Susan J. Herdman, PhD, PT
Professor and Director of Vestibular Rehabilitation
Department of Otolaryngology
University of Miami
School of Medicine
Coral Gables, Florida

C. Alan Knight, PT, CWS
Section Chief, Physical Therapy
Department of Rehabilitation Services
Louisiana State University Medical Center
Shreveport, Louisiana

David Krebs, PhD, PT
Professor and Director
MGH Biomotion Laboratory
Graduate Program in Physical Therapy
Massachusetts General Hospital
Institute of Health Professions
Boston, Massachusetts

Aaron Lieberman, DSW
Associate Professor
Wurzweler School of Social Work
Yeshiva University
Diplomate
American Academy of Social Work
American Academy of Pain Management
Administrative Director
Psychological Consulting Associates
New York, New York

Bilha Reichberg Lieberman, RN, MS, MSW
Fellow
American Orthopsychiatric Association
American Academy of Pain Management
Clinical Member
American Association of Marriage and Family
    Therapists
Clinical Director
Psychological and Consulting Associates
New York, New York

Morris B. Lieberman, PhD
Professor
Long Island University
Diplomate in Behavioral Medicine
International Academy of Behavioral Medicine
Diplomate
American Academy of Pain Management
Director, Psychological Service
Psychological and Consulting Associates
New York, New York

Bella J. May, EdD, PT, FAPTA
Professor Emerita
Department of Physical Therapy
Medical College of Georgia
President
BMJ Enterprises, PC
Augusta, Georgia

Marion A. Minor, PhD, PT
Associate Professor
Department of Physical Therapy
School of Health Related Professions
University of Missouri–Columbia
Columbia, Missouri

Cynthia Clair Norkin, EdD, PT
Cataumet, Massachusetts

Susan B. O'Sullivan, EdD, PT
Professor
Department of Physical Therapy
College of Health Professions
University of Massachusetts Lowell
Lowell, Massachusetts

Leslie Gross Portney, PhD, PT
Assistant Professor and Director
Professional Program in Physical Therapy
MGH Institute of Health Professions
Boston, Massachusetts

Reginald L. Richard, MS, PT
Burn Clinical Specialist
Miami Valley Hospital Regional Adult Burn Center
Physical Therapy Department
Dayton, Ohio

Serge H. Roy, ScD, PT
Research Associate Professor
Neuromuscular Research Center and
Sargent College of Health and Rehabilitation Sciences
Boston University
Boston, Massachusetts

Martha Taylor Sarno, MA, MD (Hon)
Professor
Clinical Rehabilitation Medicine
New York University School of Medicine
Director
Speech-Language Pathology Department
Rusk Institute of Rehabilitation Medicine
New York University Medical Center
New York, New York

Michael C. Schubert, MSPT
Department of Physical Therapy
Department of Orthopaedics and Rehabilitation
University of Miami
Coral Gables, Florida

Thomas J. Schmitz, PhD, PT
Associate Professor
Division of Physical Therapy
Long Island University
Brooklyn Campus
New York, New York

Marlys J. Staley, MS, PT
Burn and Wound Care Consultant
Pleasant Plain, Ohio

Julie Ann Starr, MS, PT, CCS
Clinical Associate Professor
Department of Physical Therapy
Sargent College of Health and Rehabilitation Services
Boston University
Boston, Massachusetts

Carolyn Unsworth, PhD, OTR
School of Occupational Therapy
La Trobe University
Bundoora, Victoria
Australia

D. Joyce White, DSc, PT
Associate Professor
Department of Physical Therapy
College of Health Professions
University of Massachusetts Lowell
Lowell, Massachusetts

Contents

Clinical Decision Making 1
Planning Effective Treatments

Susan B. O'Sullivan

LEARNING OBJECTIVES

1. Describe the key steps in the clinical decision making process.
2. Define the major responsibilities of the physical therapist in planning effective treatments.
3. Identify potential problems that could adversely affect the physical therapist's clinical reasoning.
4. Analyze and interpret patient/client data, formulate realistic goals and outcomes, and develop a plan of care when presented with a clinical case study.

PROCESS OF CLINICAL DECISION MAKING

Clinical decision making involves a series of interrelated steps that enable the physical therapist to plan an effective treatment compatible with the needs and **goals** of the **patient** or **client** and members of the health care team. These steps include (1) examination of the patient, (2) evaluation of the data and identification of problems, (3) determination of the diagnosis, (4) determination of the prognosis and plan of care (POC), (5) implementation of the POC, and (6) reexamination of the patient and evaluation of treatment **outcomes** (Fig. 1-1).[1] Important components of skilled decision making include adequate knowledge base and experience, cognitive processing strategies, self-monitoring strategies, and communication and teaching skills. Effective documentation is required for communication among the rehabilitation team members and timely reimbursement of services.

STEP 1. Examine the Patient

This step involves identifying and defining the patient's problem(s) and the resources available to determine appropriate intervention. It consists of three components: patient history, a review of relevant systems, and tests and measures.[1] Assessment begins with patient referral or initial entry, and continues as an ongoing process throughout the course of rehabilitation. Reexaminations allow therapists to evaluate progress and modify **interventions** as appropriate.

HISTORY

Information about the patient's past history and current health status is obtained from a review of the medical record and interviews. The medical record provides detailed reports from members of the health care team; processing these reports requires an understanding of disease processes,

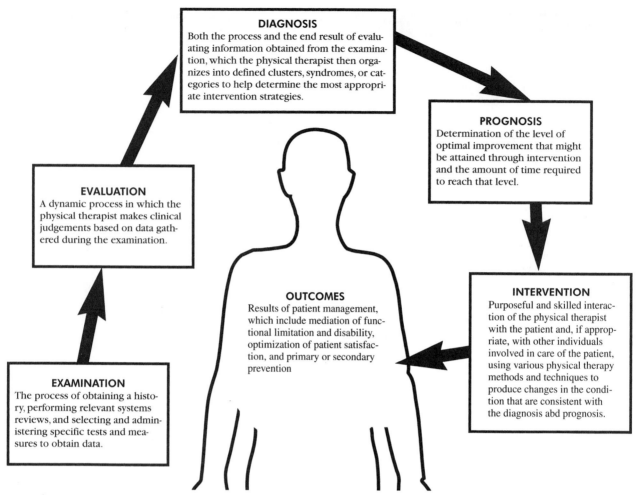

Figure 1-1. Elements of patient management leading to optimal outcomes. (From APTA Guide for Physical Therapist Practice,[1] pp 1–4, with permission.)

medical terminology, differential diagnosis using laboratory and other diagnostic tests, and medical management. The use of resource material or professional consultation can assist the novice clinician. The types of data that may be generated from a patient history are presented in Figure 1-2.

The interview is an important tool used to obtain information directly from the patient, family, significant others, caregivers, and other interested persons. Data that should be obtained include the patient's primary complaint, the history of the present illness or injury, knowledge of the medical condition, personal goals and expectations, and motivation. Information should be obtained about premorbid life-style, including health habits, exercise likes and dislikes, and frequency and intensity of regular activity. Pertinent information about the patient's family or caregiver situation and home and work environments also should be gathered. The therapist should be sensitive to differences in culture and ethnicity that may influence how the patient responds during the interview or examination process. For example, different beliefs and attitudes toward health care may

influence how cooperative the patient is. During the interview, the therapist should listen carefully to what the patient says. The patient should be observed for any physical manifestations that reveal emotional context (e.g., slumped body posture, grimacing facial expression, poor eye contact, etc.). Finally, the interview should be used to establish rapport, effective communication, and mutual trust. Patient cooperation serves to make the therapist's observations more valid and becomes crucial to the success of any rehabilitation program.

SYSTEMS REVIEW

The use of screening or brief examinations allows the therapist to quickly scan the body systems: cardiopulmonary, integumentary, musculoskeletal, and neuromuscular. The data generated relates to specific anatomical and physiological dysfunction. Screening examinations indicate areas of deficit where more detailed assessments and interventions are warranted. They also allow the therapist to determine if the patient's problems are outside the scope of physical therapy. Thus, the patient who presents with signs and symptoms of a significant medical condition would be referred for consultation. During a systems review, preliminary data concerning affect, cognition, communication ability, and learning style can also be obtained.

TESTS AND MEASURES

More definitive assessments are used to provide objective data to accurately determine the degree of specific function and dysfunction (e.g., manual muscle test, range of motion [ROM] test, oxygen

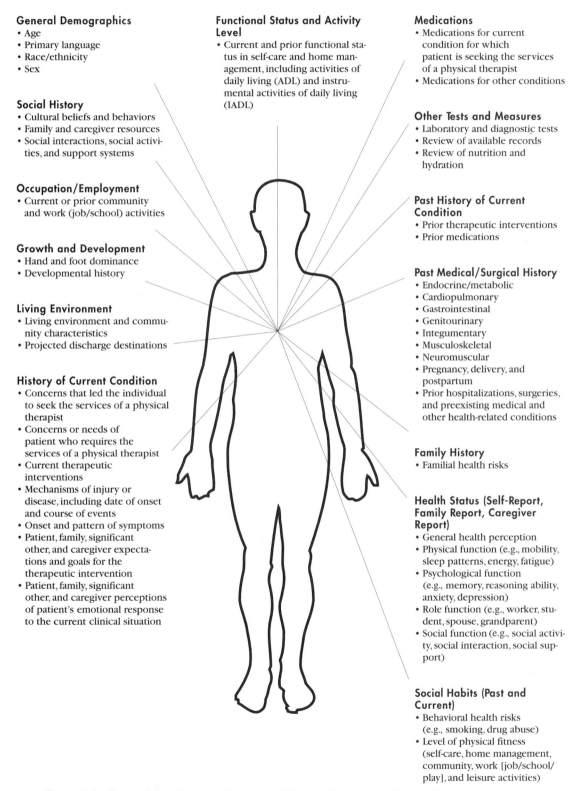

General Demographics
• Age
• Primary language
• Race/ethnicity
• Sex

Social History
• Cultural beliefs and behaviors
• Family and caregiver resources
• Social interactions, social activities, and support systems

Occupation/Employment
• Current or prior community and work (job/school) activities

Growth and Development
• Hand and foot dominance
• Developmental history

Living Environment
• Living environment and community characteristics
• Projected discharge destinations

History of Current Condition
• Concerns that led the individual to seek the services of a physical therapist
• Concerns or needs of patient who requires the services of a physical therapist
• Current therapeutic interventions
• Mechanisms of injury or disease, including date of onset and course of events
• Onset and pattern of symptoms
• Patient, family, significant other, and caregiver expectations and goals for the therapeutic intervention
• Patient, family, significant other, and caregiver perceptions of patient's emotional response to the current clinical situation

Functional Status and Activity Level
• Current and prior functional status in self-care and home management, including activities of daily living (ADL) and instrumental activities of daily living (IADL)

Medications
• Medications for current condition for which patient is seeking the services of a physical therapist
• Medications for other conditions

Other Tests and Measures
• Laboratory and diagnostic tests
• Review of available records
• Review of nutrition and hydration

Past History of Current Condition
• Prior therapeutic interventions
• Prior medications

Past Medical/Surgical History
• Endocrine/metabolic
• Cardiopulmonary
• Gastrointestinal
• Genitourinary
• Integumentary
• Musculoskeletal
• Neuromuscular
• Pregnancy, delivery, and postpartum
• Prior hospitalizations, surgeries, and preexisting medical and other health-related conditions

Family History
• Familial health risks

Health Status (Self-Report, Family Report, Caregiver Report)
• General health perception
• Physical function (e.g., mobility, sleep patterns, energy, fatigue)
• Psychological function (e.g., memory, reasoning ability, anxiety, depression)
• Role function (e.g., worker, student, spouse, grandparent)
• Social function (e.g., social activity, social interaction, social support)

Social Habits (Past and Current)
• Behavioral health risks (e.g., smoking, drug abuse)
• Level of physical fitness (self-care, home management, community, work [job/school/play], and leisure activities)

Figure 1-2. Types of data that may be generated from patient history. (From APTA Guide for Physical Therapist Practice,[1] pp 1–6, with permission.)

consumption, etc.). Adequate training and skill in performing specific tests and measures are crucial in ensuring both validity and reliability of the tests. Failure to correctly perform a procedure can lead to the gathering of inaccurate data and the formation of an inappropriate plan of care. Later chapters will focus on specific assessment procedures and will discuss issues of validity and reliability. The use of a standardized assessment protocol (e.g., stroke assessment instrument) can facilitate the evaluation process but may not always be appropriate for each individual patient. The therapist needs to carefully review the unique problems of the patient to determine the appropriateness and responsiveness of an instrument. Therapists should resist the tendency to gather excessive and extraneous data under the mistaken belief that more information is better. Unnecessary data will only confuse the picture, rendering clinical decision making more difficult and unnecessarily raising the cost of care. If problems arise that are not initially identified in the history or systems review, or if the data obtained are inconsistent, additional tests or measures may be indicated. Consultation with an experienced thera-

pist can provide an important means to clarify inconsistencies and determine the appropriateness of specific tests and measures. Box 1–1 presents a summary of the tests and measures commonly performed by the physical therapist and the types of data obtained.

STEP 2. Evaluate the Data and Identify Problems

Data gathered from the initial examination must then be analyzed and organized. Physical therapists must consider a number of factors when evaluating data, including the level of impairments, the degree of functional loss, the patient's overall health and physical function, availability of social support systems, living environment, and potential discharge destination. Multisystem involvement, severe impairment or functional loss, extended time of involvement (chronicity), comorbid conditions, and overall instability of the patient are important parameters that increase the difficulty and shape the decision making process.[1]

Box 1–1 MODEL DEFINITION OF PHYSICAL THERAPY FOR STATE PRACTICE ACTS[a]

Physical therapy, which is the care and services provided by or under the direction and supervision of a physical therapist, includes:

1. **Examining** (history, systems review, and tests and measures) individuals with impairment, functional limitation, and disability or other health-related conditions to determine a diagnosis, prognosis, and intervention; tests and measures may include the following:
   - Aerobic capacity and endurance
   - Anthropometric characteristics
   - Arousal, mentation, and cognition
   - Assistive and adaptive devices
   - Community and work (job/school/play) integration or reintegration
   - Cranial nerve integrity
   - Environmental, home, and work (job/school/play) barriers
   - Ergonomics and body mechanics
   - Gait, locomotion, and balance
   - Integumentary integrity
   - Joint integrity and mobility
   - Motor function
   - Muscle performance
   - Neuromotor development and sensory integration
   - Orthotic, protective, and supportive devices
   - Pain
   - Posture
   - Prosthetic requirements
   - Range of motion
   - Reflex integrity
   - Self-care and home management
   - Sensory integrity
   - Ventilation, respiration, and circulation

2. **Alleviating impairment and functional limitation** by designing, implementing, and modifying therapeutic interventions that may include, but are not limited to:
   - Coordination, communication, and documentation
   - Patient-related instruction
   - Therapeutic exercise (including aerobic conditioning)
   - Functional training in self-care and home management (including activities of daily living and instrumental activities of daily living)
   - Functional training in community and work (job/school/play) integration or reintegration activities (including instrumental activities of daily living, work hardening, and work conditioning)
   - Manual therapy techniques (including mobilization and manipulation)
   - Prescription, application, and, as appropriate, fabrication of assistive, adaptive, orthotic, protective, supportive, and prosthetic devices and equipment
   - Airway clearance techniques
   - Wound management
   - Electrotherapeutic modalities
   - Physical agents and mechanical modalities

3. **Preventing injury, impairment, functional limitation, and disability**, including the promotion and maintenance of fitness, health, and quality of life in all age populations

4. **Engaging in consultation, education, and research**

---

[a]Direct interventions, which begin with "Therapeutic exercise," are listed in order of preferred usage. *From:* American Physical Therapy Association, *Guide to Physical Therapy Practice.*[1] APTA, Alexandria, VA, 1999, p 1–2, with permission.

DISABLEMENT TERMINOLOGY

Terminology of the World Health Organization's International Classification of Impairments, Disabilities, and Handicaps (ICIDH)[2] can be used to categorize clinical observations systematically. *Impairments (direct)* are the result of pathology (disease or insult) and consist of the specific alterations in anatomical, physiological, or psychological structures or functions. For a patient with stroke, examples of impairments that are the direct result of pathology might include sensory loss, paresis, dyspraxia, and hemianopsia. Schenkman and Butler[3,4] expanded on this classification system with the addition of categories of indirect and composite impairments. *Indirect impairments* are sequelae or secondary conditions that occur as a result of the primary disabling condition. They are clinical manifestations of expanding multisystem dysfunction and result from prolonged inactivity, ineffective management, or lack of rehabilitation intervention. Commonly encountered indirect impairments include disuse atrophy, contracture, pressure sores, urinary tract infections, pneumonia, and depression. *Composite impairments* refer to those impairments that have multiple underlying causes, resulting from both direct and indirect causes. Faulty postural control and balance are examples of impairments that can have both direct and indirect causes. Clinical decision making can be facilitated by the identification and classification of impairments into direct, indirect, and composite categories.

According to the ICIDH, a *disability* is an inability to perform an activity in the manner or range considered normal for that individual, and results from an impairment. Four main categories of function are defined: (1) physical, (2) mental, (3) social, and (4) emotional. *Handicap* is the ICIDH term used to describe the social disadvantage that results when an impairment or disability prevents an individual from fulfilling his or her normal role. An inability to return to work or participate in community activities because of an inaccessible environment are examples of handicaps (societal limitations) that might affect the patient with stroke. Nagi[5,6] offered a variation in this disablement scheme. He suggested using the term functional limitation to bridge the gap between impairments and disabilities. *Functional limitation* is defined as restrictions in performance at the level of the whole person. Common functional limitations that might affect the person with stroke include limitations in the performance of locomotor tasks (gait), other basic mobility tasks (transfers), basic activities of daily living (BADLs; dressing, feeding, bathing), or instrumental activities of daily living (IADLs; housecleaning, preparing meals, shopping, telephoning, managing finances, etc.). Thus performance of the physical action, activity, or task is impaired. Nagi then used the term disability to refer to societal functioning rather than individual functioning. He defined disability as an inability to engage in specific societal roles that are age-, sex-, and gender-specific in a particular context and physical environ-ment. Thus the individual is unable to assume societal roles such as working, parenting, going to school, attending church or other group activities, or participating in leisure activities (sports, recreation, trips, etc.).

The American Physical Therapy Association (APTA), in the *Guide to Physical Therapist Practice*[1] as well as other professional bodies (National Advisory Board on Medical Rehabilitation Research,[7] the Institute of Medicine[8]) have adopted a terminology framework that utilizes both the ICIDH and the Nagi recommendations (Box 1–2). The terms impairment (from the ICIDH model), and functional limitation and disability (from the Nagi model) are used as a basis to provide services to patients. Clinical examples and applications of this terminology for decision making of patients with orthopedic and neurological dysfunction are present in the physical therapy literature.[4,10–12]

Data obtained from functional assessments allow the therapist to determine functional limitations and disabilities. The level of performance is typically rated from complete independence to modified dependence to complete dependence. Figure 1-3 presents the Functional Independence Measure (FIM) levels of function and their scores.[9] This instrument is used in approximately 50 percent of the rehabilitation facilities in the United States and is discussed more fully in Chapter 11 Functional

---

Box 1–2 DISABLEMENT TERMINOLOGY

Disability: inability to engage in age-specific, gender-related, or sex-specific roles in a particular social context and physical.

Disablement: impact of pathology or insult on the functioning of specific body systems, on human performance, and on functioning in necessary, usual, and desired roles in society.

Risk factors: behaviors, attributes, or environmental influences that increase the chance of developing impairments, functional limitations, or disability when an individual demonstrates an active pathology.

Buffers: actions or interventions the individual makes to resist the development of impairments, functional limitations, or disability.

Handicap: social disadvantage for a given individual of an impairment, functional limitation, or disability.

Impairment (direct): any loss or abnormality of physiologic, psychological, or anatomic structure or function; the natural consequence of pathology or disease.

Indirect impairments: sequelae or secondary complications occurring in systems other than the system affected by the original pathology or insult; the clinical manifestations of expanding multisystem dysfunction.

Composite impairment: an impairment whose underlying cause includes both direct and indirect effects of the original pathology or insult.

Functional limitation: restriction of the ability to perform, at the level of the whole person, a physical action, activity, or task in an efficient, typically expected, or competent manner.

From American Physical Therapy Association: Guide to Physical Therapist Practice. APTA, Alexandria, VA, 1999, p ix, with permission.

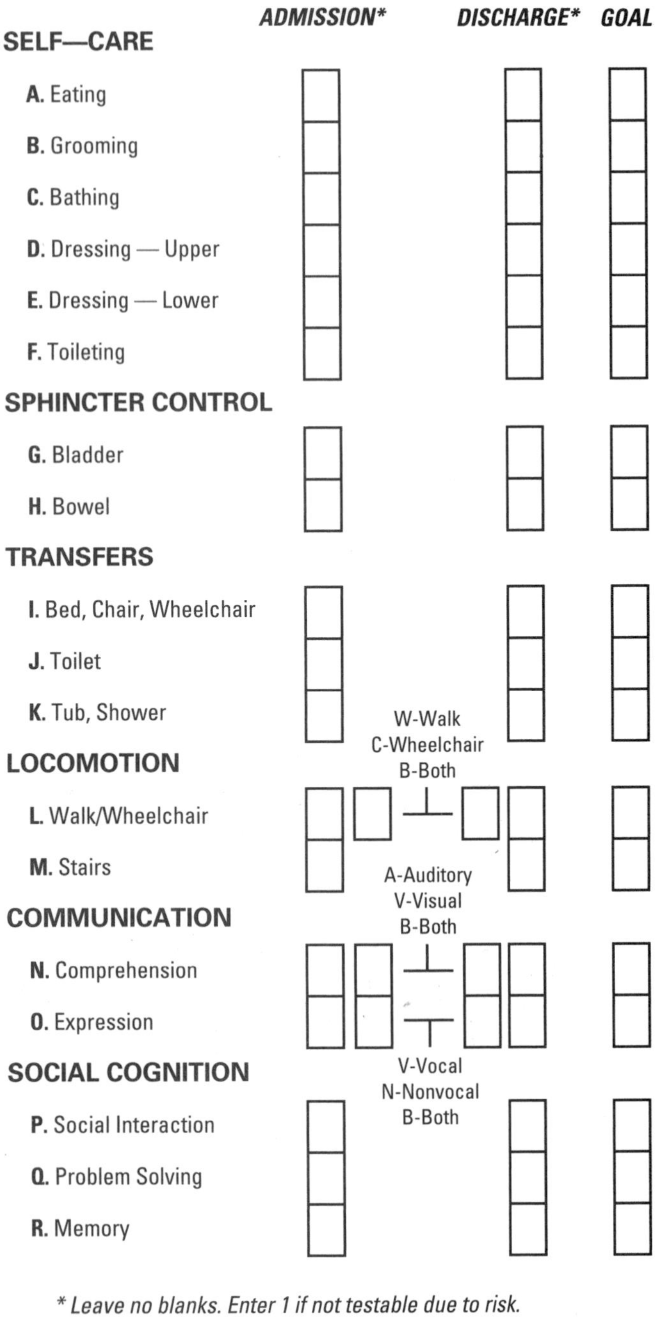

	ADMISSION*	DISCHARGE*	GOAL

SELF—CARE

A. Eating

B. Grooming

C. Bathing

D. Dressing — Upper

E. Dressing — Lower

F. Toileting

SPHINCTER CONTROL

G. Bladder

H. Bowel

TRANSFERS

I. Bed, Chair, Wheelchair

J. Toilet

K. Tub, Shower

LOCOMOTION

W-Walk
C-Wheelchair
B-Both

L. Walk/Wheelchair

M. Stairs

COMMUNICATION

A-Auditory
V-Visual
B-Both

N. Comprehension

O. Expression

V-Vocal
N-Nonvocal
B-Both

SOCIAL COGNITION

P. Social Interaction

Q. Problem Solving

R. Memory

Leave no blanks. Enter 1 if not testable due to risk.

FIM LEVELS

No Helper
   7 Complete Independence (Timely, Safety)
   6 Modified Independence (Device)

Helper — Modified Dependence
   5 Supervision (Subject = 100%)
   4 Minimal Assistance (Subject = 75% or more)
   3 Moderate Assistance (Subject = 50% or more)

Helper — Complete Dependence
   2 Maximal Assistance (Subject = 25% or more)
   1 Total Assistance or not testable (Subject less than 25%)

Figure 1-3. UDS$_{MR}$^{SM} FIM^{SM} instrument. (Reprinted with permission of the Uniform Data System for Medical Rehabilitation, a division of U B Foundation Activities, Inc. [UDS$_{MR}$^{SM}]. Copyright 1996. Guide for the Uniform Data Set for Medical Rehabilitation [including the FIM^{SM} instrument], Version 5.0. Buffalo, NY: State University of New York at Buffalo, 1996.)

Assessments. Jette[13] suggests disablement risk factors, and buffers should be evaluated. He defines *disablement risk factors* as behaviors, attributes, or environmental influences that increase the chances of developing impairments, functional limitations, or disability when an individual demonstrates an active pathology. For example, an individual may demonstrate predisposing characteristics (negative affect, psychosocial instability), demographics (limited financial/health resources, limited education), social and life-style factors (inadequate family support, disengaged life-style), or restrictive environment (numerous architectural barriers). *Buffers*, on the other hand, are defined as the actions or interventions the individual makes to resist the development of impairments, functional limitations, or disability. For example, an individual may adopt behaviors (positive attitudes, prayer, meditation) or helping strategies (use of adaptive equipment, peer support groups). Sometimes the strategies adopted are ineffective, leading to increased disablement (e.g., increased alcohol use).

Impairments and disabilities must be analyzed to identify causal relationships. For example, shoulder pain in the patient with hemiplegia may be due to several factors, including hypotonicity and immobility (direct impairments) or soft tissue damage (an indirect impairment). Determining which of these factors is the primary cause of the problem is a difficult yet critical step in determining appropriate treatment interventions and resolving the patient's pain. Impairments may not be related to the patient's functional limitations or lead to disability. A plan of care that focuses on these impairments is not likely to achieve successful clinical outcomes. Rather, the major focus of treatment should be on producing meaningful changes in the person's function. Functional outcomes of independence in ambulation or daily activities, return to work, or participation in recreational activities are far more important to the patient.[14] An improvement in **quality of life** and a sense of total well-being that encompasses both physical and psychosocial aspects of the patient's life must become the major emphasis of treatment. Finally, not all impairments can be remediated by physical therapy. Some impairments are permanent, the direct result of unrelenting pathology, such as progressive dementia in Alzheimer's disease. Therapists need to recognize the scope of physical therapy intervention. In this example, a primary emphasis on reducing the number and severity of indirect impairments and functional limitations is far more appropriate.

The generation of an **asset** list is also an important part of the clinical decision making process. The therapist analyzes the assessment data and determines patient strengths (nonimpairments) and abilities. These are areas that can be reinforced and emphasized during therapy, providing the patient with the opportunity for positive reinforcement and success. For example, the same patient with stroke may have intact communication skills, cognitive skills, and good function of the uninvolved extremities. Assets can also include supportive and knowledgeable family members/caregivers, and an appropriate living environment. Improved motivation and compliance are the natural outcomes of reinforcement of patient assets.

STEP 3. Determine the Diagnosis

The development of a classification scheme of diagnostic categories unique to physical therapy is a natural outcome of organization, interpretation, and evaluation of data. **Diagnosis** is defined as a "label encompassing a cluster of signs and symptoms, syndromes, or categories."[1] The use of diagnostic categories clarifies the body of knowledge in physical therapy and the role of physical therapists in the health care system. It assists the therapist in determining an effective POC and in selecting appropriate interventions.[12,15-19] As the availability of direct access to physical therapy services continues to expand, use of diagnostic categories can facilitate successful reimbursement particularly when linked to functional outcomes.

The APTA has affirmed the use of physical therapy diagnoses in its publication, *Guide to Physical Therapist Practice*.[1] The specific diagnoses included in this document represent the collaborative efforts of experienced physical therapists who have detailed the broad categories of problems commonly seen by physical therapists within the scope of their knowledge, experience, and expertise. Expert consensus was used to develop the guidelines. The primary focus of the diagnostic categories in this document is at the level of impairment and functional limitations, a more appropriate level to guide physical therapy interventions than the medical diagnosis. The term *pathokinesiologic* has been used by some therapists to refer to diagnostic labels at this level.[15] Therapists unable to determine an identifiable diagnosis when referring to the *Guide to Physical Therapist Practice* will need to plan interventions based on the specific deficits identified. Therapists will also need to refer to other professional disciplines as appropriate. For example, the patient with stroke may present with unilateral neglect, necessitating a referral for occupational therapy services.

STEP 4. Determine the Prognosis and Plan of Care

The term **prognosis** refers to "the predicted optimal level of improvement in function and amount of time needed to reach that level."[1] An accurate prognosis may be determined at the onset of treatment for some patients. For other, more complicated diagnoses such as the patient with severe traumatic brain injury, a prognosis or prediction of levels of improvement can only be determined at various increments during the course of rehabilitation. Knowledge of recovery patterns (stage of disorder) is sometimes useful to guide decision making. The amount of time needed to reach optimal recovery is an important determination, one that is required by Medicare and other insurance providers. Predicting optimal levels of recovery and time frames can be very difficult for the inexperienced therapist. Use of experienced, senior staff as resources and mentors can facilitate this step in the decision making process. The *Guide to Physical Therapist Practice* should also be consulted.

The **plan of care (POC)** outlines anticipated patient management. The therapist must integrate data obtained from the patient history and examination to determine the diagnosis, prognosis, and appropriate interventions. It is challenging, requiring skills in the interpretation and integration of data, and clinical reasoning. Essential components of the POC include (1) goals and outcomes, (2) specific interventions to be used, (3) duration and frequency of the interventions, and (4) criteria for discharge.[1]

An important first step in the development of the POC is the determination of anticipated goals and outcomes. *Goals* refer to the remediation of impairments, to whatever extent possible. *Outcomes* refer to the remediation of functional limitations and disability, and the optimization of health status and patient satisfaction.[1]

Involving the patient in determining goals and outcomes is critical in ensuring patient compliance. Many rehabilitation plans have failed miserably simply because the patient did not see the relevance of the professionals' goals or outcomes. The patient may have established a very different set of personal goals and expectations. Payton et al.[20] address this issue in an excellent reference entitled *Patient Participation in Program Planning: A Manual for Therapists*, which provides suggestions for promoting the mutual planning process. The authors suggest asking the patient such questions as:
- What are your concerns?
- What is your greatest concern?
- What do you want to see happen?
- What would make you feel that you are making progress?
- What are your goals?
- What is your first goal?

The therapist can then use this information to generate goal and outcome statements that truly reflect patient needs and expectations.

Outcomes define the patient's expected level of functional performance at the end of physical therapy. Anticipated outcomes are discussed in rehabilitation team meetings to ensure consensus and support of outcomes by all team members. The attainment of anticipated outcomes will later become the focus of the discharge summary. Outcome statements should specify:
1. Who will perform the behavior (or aspect of care); for example, patient, family, or caregiver?
2. What is the specific functional task or behavior the person will demonstrate?

3. Under what conditions the behavior will be performed; for example, what help is needed to accomplish the behavior: level of independence, assistance, or supervision involved; the type of assistive device or other equipment needed; the type of environment required (controlled or closed, open)?

4. How will outcome be measured; for example, what is the expected level of functional performance at the time of discharge; or in instances of long-term care, what is the expected level of functional performance attained in a specific time frame, generally 2 to 3 months? The following are examples of outcome statements:
   1. The patient will be independent and safe in ambulation using an ankle-foot orthosis and a quad cane on level surfaces for unlimited distances and for all daily activities.
   2. The patient will require close supervision in wheelchair propulsion for limited distances (up to 75 feet) and minimum assistance of one person in all transfer activities.
   3. The patient will demonstrate functional independence in basic activities of daily living (BADLs) with minimal set up and equipment (use of a reacher).
   4. The patient and family will demonstrate enhanced decision making skills regarding the health of the patient and use of health care resources.

Goals define the anticipated remediation of impairments, the outcomes of treatment. The therapist reviews the list of impairments, prioritizes them, and develops goals designed to achieve the anticipated outcomes. The written goal includes the same four elements as outcome statements, although they do not generally have the same functional emphasis. **Short-term goals (STGs)** specify a short time span (generally 2 to 3 weeks) or a specific number of treatments. **Long-term goals (LTGs)** may extend over a longer time frame (e.g., more than 3 weeks). The following are examples of goal statements:

1. The patient will increase strength in shoulder depressor muscles and elbow extensor muscles in both upper extremities from good to normal within 2 weeks.
2. The patient will increase ROM 10 degrees in knee extension bilaterally to within normal limits within 2 weeks.
3. The patient will be independent in the application of lower extremity orthoses within 1 week.
4. The patient will perform sit-to-stand transfers from wheelchair to standing with crutches and moderate assistance of one person within 2 weeks.
5. The patient will maintain static balance in sitting with centered, symmetrical weight-bearing and no upper extremity support for up to 5 minutes within 4 weeks.
6. The patient will ambulate with bilateral knee-ankle orthoses in parallel bars using a swing-through gait and supervision for 25 feet within 3 weeks.
7. The patient and family will recognize personal

and environmental factors associated with falls during ambulation within 3 weeks.

Each treatment plan has multiple goals. Goals may be linked to the successful attainment of more than one outcome. For example, attaining ROM in dorsiflexion is critical to the functional outcome of independence in transfers and ambulation. The successful attainment of an outcome is also dependent on achieving a number of different goals. For example, independent ambulation (the outcome) is dependent on increasing strength, ROM, and balance skills. In formulating a POC, the therapist needs to accurately identify the relationship between goals and outcomes and to sequence them appropriately.

The next step is to determine the interventions that can be used to achieve the goals and outcomes. *Interventions* include (1) the skilled and purposeful interactions between the physical therapist and patient, family, caregiver, or other appropriate individuals, and (2) the various different procedures and techniques included in the practice of physical therapy (see Box 1–1). Prerequisite to accomplishing interventions include skill in coordination, communication, and documentation, and skills in patient-related instruction, and providing direct interventions.[1]

Case management requires that therapists be able to communicate effectively with all members of the rehabilitation team, directly or indirectly. For example, the therapist communicates at case conferences, team meetings, or rounds. Therapists are also responsible for coordinating care at many different levels. For example, for early transfer training to be effective, consistency is important. Thus the therapist needs to communicate effectively with the occupational therapist, nurse, family, and other interested persons about the specifics of the approach being used. Coordination with the patient and family for discharge planning is another example. The therapist delegates appropriate aspects of treatment to physical therapy assistants or aides. Decisions must also be made concerning effective time management.

Patient-related instruction is a critical component of successful rehabilitation. Therapists provide direct one-on-one instruction for patients, clients, families, caregivers, and other interested persons. They can provide interventions such as group discussions or classes, or instruction through printed or audiovisual materials. Educational interventions are directed toward ensuring an understanding of the patient's condition, POC, and the expected course in rehabilitation. In addition, interventions are directed toward ensuring a successful transition in returning home, to work, or resumption of social activities in the community.[1] In an era of managed care and time-based allocation of services, patient-related instruction is increasingly important in ensuring optimal care and successful rehabilitation. For example, instruction in a home exercise program (HEP) allows the patient to follow through on many of the interventions begun in the rehabilitation setting.

Direct interventions include a wide variety of procedures and techniques practiced by the physical therapist, including therapeutic exercise, functional training, manual therapy, modalities, and so forth. Many of these interventions are the focus of later chapters of this textbook. Interventions are chosen on the basis of the data obtained, the diagnosis, prognosis, and anticipated goals and outcomes. It is important to identify all possible interventions early in the process, to carefully weigh those alternatives, and then to decide on those interventions that have the best probability of success. Narrowly adhering to one treatment approach reduces the available options and may limit or preclude success. Use of a protocol (e.g., predetermined exercises for the patient with hip fracture) standardizes care but may not meet the individual needs of the patient. Henry[21] points out that protocols foster a separation of evaluation findings from the selection of treatments. In addition, an overdependence on the use of protocols may be reflective of a therapist's difficulty in problem solving.

Watts[22] suggests that clinical judgement "is clearly an elegant mixture of art and science." Professional consultation with expert clinicians is an effective means of helping the inexperienced therapist sort through the complex issues involved in decision making, especially when complicating factors intervene. For example, a consultation would be beneficial for decision making with a patient who is chronically ill, has multiple comorbidities or complications, impaired cognition, inadequate social supports, and/or severe functional limitations or disability.

A general outline of the treatment plan is constructed. Schema can assist the therapist in organizing knowledge. One such example is the frequency-intensity-time-type **(FITT) equation** to prescribe exercise. An estimate is made of the

- Frequency: number of times per day or week treatment will be given
- Intensity: number of repetitions or activities
- Time: duration of the treatment session
- Type of exercise: specific physical therapy interventions

Specific treatment procedures may then be described. Another schema identifies the specific components of a therapeutic exercise intervention.[23] For example, the components of an exercise procedure can be delineated by:

- A description of the activity: the specific posture and movement
- The technique to be used: mode of therapist intervention (guided, assisted, or resisted movement), or specific technique
- Other required elements: verbal commands, equipment, and so forth

An example of this schema for the patient with stroke with poor dynamic sitting balance is: sitting, weight-shifting (position/activity), active-assisted reaching (mode of intervention), and verbal cueing and assisted stabilization of the affected upper extremity (required elements).

The therapist should ideally choose procedures that accomplish more than one goal and should sequence the procedures effectively to address key problems first. Procedures should also be sequenced to achieve optimum motivational effects, interspacing the more difficult or uncomfortable procedures with easier ones. The therapist should include tasks that ensure success during the treatment session and, whenever possible, should end each session on a positive note. This helps the patient retain a positive feeling of success and look forward to the next treatment. The POC should also include a statement regarding potential discharge plans, including equipment needs and plans for a home visit and/or modifications.

STEP 5. Implement the Plan of Care

The therapist must take into account a number of factors in structuring an effective treatment session. The treatment area should be properly arranged to respect the patient's privacy, with adequate draping and positioning. The environment should be structured to reduce distractions and focus attention on the task at hand. In applying exercise procedures the therapist should consider good body mechanics, effective use of gravity and position, and correct application of techniques and modalities. Any equipment should be gathered prior to treatment and be in good working order. All safety precautions must be observed.

The patient's pretreatment level of function or initial state should be carefully assessed. General state organization of the central nervous system and homeostatic balance of the somatic and autonomic systems are important determinants of how a patient may respond to treatment. Stockmeyer[24] points out that a wide range of influences, from emotional to cognitive to organic, may affect how a patient reacts to a particular treatment. Patients with altered homeostatic mechanisms (high or low arousal) can be expected to react to treatment in unpredictable ways. Responses to treatment should be carefully monitored throughout the course of rehabilitation, and treatment modifications implemented as soon as needed to ensure successful performance. Therapists develop the "art of clinical practice" by learning to adjust their input (voice commands, manual contacts, and so forth) in response to the patient's movements.[22] Treatment thus becomes a dynamic and interactive process between patient and therapist. Shaping of behavior can be further enhanced by careful orientation to the purpose of the tasks and how they meet the patient's needs, thereby ensuring optimal cooperation and motivation.

STEP 6. Reexamine the Patient and Evaluate Treatment Outcomes

This last step is ongoing and involves continuous reexamination of the patient and efficacy of treatment. The patient's abilities are evaluated in terms of the specific goals and outcomes set forth in the treatment plan. A determination is made as to whether the goals and outcomes are reasonable given the patient's diagnosis and progress made. If the patient attains the desired level of competence for the stated outcomes, discharge is considered. If the patient fails to achieve the stated goals or outcomes, the therapist must determine why. Were the goals and outcomes realistic given the database? Were the interventions selected at an appropriate level to challenge the patient, or were they too easy or too difficult? Was the patient sufficiently motivated? Were intervening and constraining factors (disablement risk factors) identified? If the interventions were not appropriate, additional information is sought, goals modified, and different treatment alternatives selected. A revision in the plan of care is also indicated if the patient progresses more rapidly or slowly than expected. Each modification must be evaluated in terms of its overall effect on the POC. Thus the plan becomes a fluid statement of how the patient is progressing and where he or she is going. Its overall success depends on the therapist's ongoing clinical decision making skills and on engaging the patient's cooperation and motivation. The level of patient and family satisfaction is an important outcome requiring assessment. Dissatisfaction is frequently the result of failure to fully involve patient and family in the clinical decision making process or to keep them fully informed.

In his text on clinical decision making, Wolf[25] cautions against empiricism, that is, continuing to use a treatment simply because it has worked in the past. Rather therapists should strive to develop a concrete database through research on which the validity of treatment can be substantiated. Expansion of the body of knowledge with the continued development of sound theories of action enhances continued professional development and is the responsibility of every therapist.

Discharge planning is initiated early in the rehabilitation process during the data collection phase and intensifies as goals and functional outcomes are close to being reached. Discharge planning may also be initiated if the patient refuses further treatment, or becomes medically or psychologically unstable. If the patient is discharged before outcomes are reached, the reasons for discontinuation of services must be carefully documented. Components of effective discharge planning include (1) evaluation and modification of the home environment for the patient returning home, (2) patient, family, or caregiver education, (3) plans for appropriate follow-up care or referral, and (4) instruction in a HEP.

CLINICAL DECISION MAKING: EXPERT VERSUS NOVICE

Inherent to the therapist's success in clinical decision making are an appropriate knowledge base and experience, cognitive processing strategies, self-monitoring strategies, communication and teaching skills, and documentation. Research delineating the dimensions of expert decision making in physical therapy is accumulating[26–30] and provides a useful framework for discussion of these elements. This information has important implications for novice therapists and for educators involved in teaching clinical decision making.

Knowledge Base and Experience

Decision making is influenced by knowledge and experience. Skilled individuals are able to organize and shape their knowledge into a usable format.[31] Specific clinical patterns or conditions are organized and stored based on past experiences and retrieved for comparison when current cases are in evidence. This pattern recognition and use of procedural knowledge allows for effective clinical decision making. The novice therapist, on the other hand, may collect similar data, but is unable to organize and categorize the information. Simple memorization of data and use of book-learned, declarative knowledge does not allow the novice to recognize meaningful relationships and generate hypotheses within a realistic time frame. Organization of knowledge is specific and highly dependent upon the mastery of a particular content area.[26–29] Content domains in physical therapy take the form of the specialty areas (orthopedic, neurological, pediatric, etc.). As expertise increases, master clinicians increase in their abilities to categorize information, improving in both mastery of depth and complexity of content. Jensen et al.[27] found that master clinicians demonstrated increased confidence in evaluating patients and in using well-developed schema for interpreting data and predicting outcomes. The novice therapists collected data but did not always recognize important data. They also tended to rigidly adhere to an evaluation or treatment framework whereas the expert group could easily refocus if a different direction was indicated.

Cognitive Processing Styles

The individual who utilizes a **receptive data-gathering style** generally suspends judgement until all possible data are gathered. The data are analyzed individually and collectively before a final determination is made of how to organize and use them. These same individuals are likely to adopt a **systematic processing style,** in which a methodical step-by-step approach is used, completing one step before progressing to the next. Contrasting styles are perceptive and **intuitive.** The individual who utilizes a **perceptive data-gathering style** will seek and respond to ongoing cues and patterns, defining and organizing problems early. Information processing is largely *intuitive.* Thus these clinicians are able to respond to a large number of stimuli as they occur and consider initiation of early treatment options.[26,30] Research suggests that styles may differ by expert group. May and Dennis[26] and Jensen et al.[27] found that clinicians with expertise in orthopedics tended to utilize a receptive/systematic style, generating a hypothesis only after all the data were collected. A methodical, ordered search of data was used. Embrey et al.[28] found that pediatric expert clinicians tended to utilize a perceptive data-gathering style and process information intuitively. Thus they responded rapidly to cues and patterns (movement scripts) and changes that occurred within the treatment session. Psychosocial sensitivity was a key factor in directing the experienced pediatric clinicians during the physical therapy sessions. Novice therapists were less responsive to the psychosocial needs of the children and kept their attention focused on procedural matters. May and Dennis[26] reported that practitioners experienced in cardiopulmonary and neurological physical therapy also tended to respond more favorably to the perceptive/intuitive style. Thus the differences noted in terms of the types of cognitive strategies reported appear to be evoked by specific problem structure and domain.

FORMAL DECISION MAKING

Rothstein and Echternach[32,33] proposed a **hypothesis-oriented algorithm for clinicians (HOAC)** for use by physical therapists. This model uses a systematic, step-by-step approach that includes initial data collection, generation of a problem statement, establishment of goals, examination, formation of working hypotheses, reevaluation of goals, establishment of a treatment plan, implementation, and reevaluation. The reader will recognize similarities to the steps previously discussed. The determination of a hypothesis focuses the therapist's attention on consideration of either referral to an appropriate practitioner or continuation with treatment. An algorithm is used to outline the decision process and includes a series of yes/no responses that plot the decisions made (Fig. 1-4).

Decision analysis[25,34,35] is a widely adopted approach used in medical education. It considers choice in the face of uncertainty, allowing the decision maker to integrate variables and calculate relevant probabilities and outcomes. The key steps in decision analysis are to (1) define or structure the decision problem, (2) define successful and unsuccessful outcomes, (3) determine alternative approaches and their consequences, (4) estimate and analyze probabilities, (5) estimate costs in terms of tangible and intangible resources, and (6) select a preferred strategy. Decision analysis recognizes a series of choices, the timing of these choices, the key uncertainties or risks, and the potential benefits of each strategy. Thus, the final decision best represents a realistic balance between the necessary resources and expected outcomes. The generation of a **decision tree** or flow diagram allows components of the decision process to be displayed in a sequence that embodies both temporal and logical structure

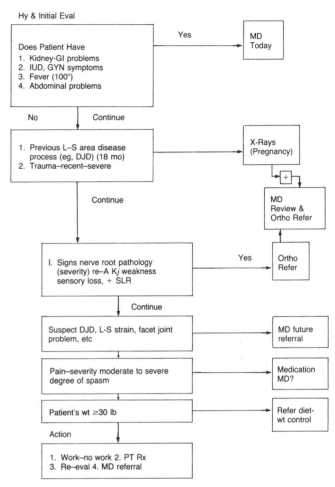

Figure 1-4. Low back pain algorithm (*top*) and review of systems (*bottom*). (From Echternach, J, and Rothstein, J,[33] p 564, with permission.)

(Fig. 1-5). Statistical probabilities of various possible outcomes, when known, are entered at appropriate points. Decision trees serve to highlight various different strategies without, as Weinstein et al.[35] point out, losing sight of the whole problem.

There are drawbacks to using formal decision analysis in physical therapy. Human limitations exist related to memory and information processing, a problem that has been reduced with the availability of computerized decision support tools. These tools are becoming available for medical education.[36,37] In physical therapy, there are currently

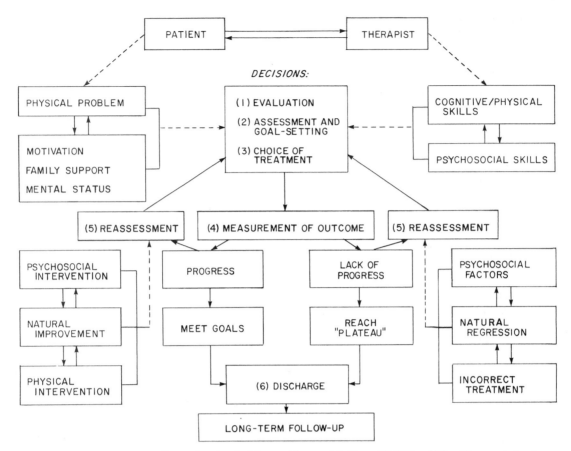

Figure 1-5. Flow chart illustrating the decision making model. (From Wolf,[25] p 172, with permission.)

limited, reliable, standardized databases of outcomes on which to base decisions. Watts[22] states that this is a time-consuming method, and should be used selectively. Formal decision analyses is also impractical for the generation of rapid, within-treatment session decisions, for example, as required in the practice of pediatrics.[28]

Self-Monitoring Strategies

Important differences exist between expert versus novice clinicians in the area of self-monitoring. Expert clinicians were found to frequently and effectively utilize self-assessment to modify and redefine clinical decisions.[27,28] This reflective aspect of practice resulted in improved improvisational performance, the actions that occur when therapists are actually treating patients. They were better able to control the treatment situation (i.e., constant interruptions, the demands of many scheduled patients, multiple tasks, etc.), and the time allotted. Conversely, novice therapists demonstrated self-monitoring, but were less able to utilize the information effectively to control the environment. They reacted more to external stimuli and the confusion of competing demands and were less able to offer alternate intervention strategies. Self-monitoring was viewed as a positive experience by the experts

twice as often as by novice therapists, an indication that the inexperienced therapists were sensitive to their limitations. Embrey et al.[28] suggest that novices may benefit from a period of active mentoring by expert clinicians early in clinical practice.

Communication and Teaching Skills

Expert clinicians were able to maintain focus on the patient as evidenced in their verbal and non-verbal communications. They were able to provide hands-on assessment and treatment while interacting socially with their patients. This smooth interplay was responsive to the needs of each individual patient. Conversely, novice therapists were more structured by the demands of completing evaluations or interventions. Their focus was more on the mechanics of treatment rather than on the psychosocial needs of the patient.[27,28] Pediatric expert clinicians were able to consistently end each therapy session with a positive activity, frequently chosen by the children. Strong emotional bonding was evident. Novice pediatric therapists were less consistent in attention to the psychosocial needs of their patients.[28] Effective communication provides an open dialogue and enhances cooperation and understanding. Communication needs to be modified for patients of different ages, cultural backgrounds, language and educational levels, and for patients with impairments in communication or cognition.

Expert clinicians recognized the importance of teaching, relying on teaching as an essential clinical skill. They affirmed the importance of teaching in assisting patients to assume control over their own health care. In an era of cost containment and limited services, this is an important value and one that is essential for ensuring successful long-term outcomes. Novice therapists, on the other hand, demonstrated greater interest in mastering hands-on skills and in ensuring the success of their treatments.[27]

DOCUMENTATION

Guidelines for Physical Therapy Documentation

Documentation is an essential requirement for timely reimbursement of services and communication among the rehabilitation team members. Written documentation is formally done at the time of admission and discharge, and at periodic intervals during the course of rehabilitation. The format and timing of notes will vary according to the regulatory requirements specified by institutional policy and third party payers. Data included in the medical record should be meaningful (important, not just nice to have), complete and accurate (valid and reliable), timely (recorded promptly), and systematic (regularly recorded).[39] All handwritten entries should be in ink, legible, and signed. Charting errors should be corrected by a single line through the error with initialing and dating directly above the error. Electronic entries should comply with appropriate provisions for security and confidentiality.

According to APTA Guidelines, documentation should include[1]:

1. Appropriate identification of the patient's full name and the provider's name
2. The manner in which physical therapy services are initiated (i.e., referral, direct access)
3. Results of the history and initial examination
4. Results of evaluation, and diagnosis
5. The POC including goals, outcomes, and interventions
6. Results of interventions or services provided, including patient status, progress, or regression
7. Reexamination and reevaluation
8. Summation at the conclusion of care (discharge note)

Only acceptable medical terminology should be used. Confusing abbreviations should be avoided. Generally, a facility will have an approved list of abbreviations. Physical therapists should ensure that notes are understandable to all who read and use the medical record.

Problem-Oriented Medical Record

In the **problem-oriented medical record (POMR)**, originally developed by Weed,[38] has been adopted by many institutions. The patient–treatment process is divided into four phases:

- Phase 1: Formation of a database, including history, physical examination, and laboratory and other assessment results.
- Phase 2: Identification of a specific problem list from the interpretation of the database, including specific impairment of function (physical, psychological, social, and vocational) resulting from the disease process or from secondary impairments.
- Phase 3: Identification of a specific treatment plan for each of the problems described; evaluative and progress notes are included for each problem.
- Phase 4: Assessment of the effectiveness of each of the plans and subsequent changes in these plans as a result of patient progress.

Each member of the health care team records his or her findings and plans, according to the specific phases. Progress notes are written in the *s*ubjective, *o*bjective, *a*ssessment, *p*lan **(SOAP) format.**[39] Subjective findings are what the patient and his or her family report. Objective findings are what the therapist observes, tests, or measures. The assessment includes professional judgements about the subjective and/or objective findings, formulated into both long- and short-term goals. The plan includes both general and specific aspects of treatment. The POMR thus highlights the relationship of the database to the treatment plan and allows the specific patient problems to become the central focus of planning. Computerization of the POMR is available to store vast amounts of data and relate them to a range of possible diagnoses and available management options.[36,37]

SUMMARY

An organized process of clinical decision making allows the therapist to systematically plan effective treatments. The steps identified in this process include (1) examining the patient, and collecting data through history, systems review, and tests and measures; (2) evaluating the data and identifying problems; (3) determining the diagnosis; (4) determining the prognosis and plan of care; (5) implementing the plan of care; and (6) reexamining the patient and evaluating treatment outcomes. Inherent to the therapist's success in this process are an appropriate knowledge base and experience, cognitive processing strategies, self-monitoring strategies, and communication and teaching skills. Documentation is an essential requirement for effective communication among the rehabilitation team members and for timely reimbursement of services.

QUESTIONS FOR REVIEW

1. Identify the key steps and required elements in the clinical decision making process.

2. Differentiate between impairments, functional limitations, and disability.

3. Define and give an example of direct, indirect, and composite impairments.

4. In evaluating treatment outcomes, why might a patient fail to reach the stated outcome? What are risk factors for disablement?

5. What are the advantages and disadvantages of formal systems for decision analysis?

6. What are the four components of the SOAP format of written documentation?

CASE STUDY

PRESENT HISTORY: The patient is a 78 year-old woman who tripped and fell at home ascending the stairs outside the front door. She was admitted to the hospital after sustaining a transcervical, intracapsular fracture of the right femur. The patient had an open reduction internal fixation (ORIF) procedure to reduce and pin the fracture.

PAST MEDICAL HISTORY: Patient is a very thin woman (98 pounds) with long-standing problems with osteoporosis (on medication x 8 years). She has a history of falls, 3 in the last year alone. Approximately 3 years ago she had a myocardial infarction, and presented with third-degree heart block, requiring implantation of a permanent pacemaker. She underwent cataract surgery with implantation 2 years ago; the left eye is scheduled for similar surgery.

MEDICAL DIAGNOSES INCLUDE: CAD, HTN, mitral valve prolapse, s/p permanent heart pacer, s/p right cataract with implant, osteoporosis (moderate to severe in the spine, hips, and pelvis), osteoarthritis with mild pain in right knee, s/p left elbow fracture (1 year ago), left ankle fracture (2 years ago), urinary stress incontinence.

MEDICATIONS

Calcitonin 50 U q sun & wed

Estrogen patch 0.05 mg to skin q sun & wed

Atenolol 24 mg po qd

MVI with Fe tab po qd

Metamucil tbs prn po qd, Colace 100 mg po bid

Tylenol #3 tab prn/mild pain

SOCIAL SUPPORT/ENVIRONMENT

Patient was recently widowed from her husband of 48 years. She has two sons and one daughter and four grandchildren, all of whom live within an hour's distance. One of her children visits every weekend. She has a rambunctious black Labrador puppy that is 8 months old and was given to her "for company" at the time her husband died. She was walking the dog at the time of the accident. She is a retired schoolteacher. She is an active participant in a garden club, which meets twice a month and in weekly events at the local senior center. Previously she was driving her car for all community activities.

She lives alone in a large old New England farmhouse. Her home has an entry with four stairs and no rail. Inside she has 14 rooms on 2 floors. The downstairs living area has a step down into the family room with no rail. There are 14 stairs to the second floor with rails on either side. The upstairs sleeping area is cluttered with large, heavy furniture. The second floor bathroom is small, with a high old tub and pedestal feet and a lip. There is no added equipment.

PHYSICAL THERAPY ASSESSMENT

1. **Mental Status:** alert and oriented x 3
   pleasant, cooperative, articulate
   no apparent memory deficits
   good problem solving and safety awareness
   re hip precautions

2. **Cardiopulmonary Status:** pulse 74; BP 110/75
   endurance: good; min. SOB with 20 min. of activity

3. **Sensation:** wears glasses
   hearing WFL
   depth perception impaired
   sensation BLEs intact

4. **Skin:** incision is healed and well approximated
   wears bilateral TEDs q am x 6 wks

5. **ROM:** LLE, BUEs: WFL
   affected RLE:
   Flex 0 to 85°
   Ext NT
   Abd 0 to 20°
   Add NT
   IR, ER NT
   right knee and ankle WFL

6. **Strength:** LLE, BUEs: WFL
   affected RLE:
   hip flex NT
   hip ext NT
   hip abd NT
   knee ext 4/5
   ankle DF 4/5, PF 4/5

7. **Posture:** flexed, stooped posture: moderate kyphosis, flexed hips and knees
   1/2" leg length difference; uses wedge when sitting
   mild resting head tremor

8. **Balance:** Sitting balance: WFL
   Standing balance:
   eyes open: good; leans slightly to left side
   eyes closed: unsteady, begins to fall
   sternal nudge: unsteady, begins to fall
   Arises from chair without help, some initial unsteadiness;
   sitting down: safe, smooth motion
   Uses 2-inch foam cushions to elevate seat of kitchen chair and living room chair

9. **Functional Mobility:** patient was completely I before her fall
   results of functional assessment:
   I bed mobility
   I transfers; unable to do tub transfers at present
   I ambulation with standard walker x 200 feet on level surfaces
       partial weight-bearing right hip
       increased flexion of knees and dorsal spine
   I one flight of stairs with rail and SBQC
10. **ADLs:** I dressing; requires min. assist of home health aide for sponge baths
    requires moderate assistance of home health aide for homemaker services
11. **Patient Is Highly Motivated:** "I want to get my life back together, get my dog home again so I can take care of him."

PRIMARY INSURANCE
Medicare

Guiding Questions

1. Identify and categorize the patient's impairments into direct, indirect, and composite.
2. Identify her functional limitations, disabilities, and assets.
3. What are your concerns regarding potential disablement risk factors?
4. What is her prognosis?
5. Write two outcome and two goal statements for her plan of care.
6. Identify two treatment interventions you might include in her plan of care. What precautions should you observe?
7. What assessments will you use to determine successful attainment of outcomes?

REFERENCES

1. American Physical Therapy Association: Guide to Physical Therapist Practice. APTA, Alexandria, VA, 1999.
2. World Health Organization: International Classification of Impairments, Disabilities, and Handicaps. WHO, Geneva, Switzerland, 1980.
3. Schenkman, M, and Butler, R: A model for multisystem evaluation, interpretation, and treatment of individuals with neurologic dysfunction. Phys Ther 69:538, 1989.
4. Schenkman, M, and Butler, R: A model for multisystem evaluation and treatment of individuals with Parkinson's disease. Phys Ther 69:932, 1989.
5. Nagi, S: Disability and Rehabilitation. Ohio State Univ. Pr., Columbus, 1969.
6. Nagi, S: Disability concepts revisited: Implications for prevention. In Pope, A, and Tarlov, A (eds): Disability in America: Toward a National Agenda for Prevention. Washington, DC, National Academy Press, 1991, p 309.
7. National Advisory Board on Medical Rehabilitation Research: Draft V: Report and Plan for Medicare Rehabilitation Research. National Institutes of Health, Bethesda, MD, 1992.
8. Defining Primary Care: An Interim Report. Institute of Medicine, National Academy Press, Washington, DC, 1995.
9. Guide for the Uniform Data Set for Medical Rehabilitation (including the FIM instrument), Version 5.0. State University of New York, Buffalo, 1996.
10. Harris, B, and Dyrek, D: A model of orthopaedic dysfunction for clinical decision making in physical therapy practice. Phys Ther 69:548, 1989.
11. Wagstaff, S: The use of the International Classification of Impairments, Disabilities and Handicaps in Rehabilitation. Physiotherapy 68:233, 1982.
12. Guccione, A: Physical therapy diagnosis and the relationship between impairments and function. Phys Ther 71:499, 1991.
13. Jette, AM: Physical disablement concepts for physical therapy research and practice. Phys Ther 74:380, 1994.
14. Rothstein, J: Disability and our identity. Phys Ther 74:375, 1994.
15. Sahrmann, S: Diagnosis by the physical therapists prerequisite for treatment. Phys Ther 68:1703, 1988.
16. Rose, S: Diagnosis: Defining the term. Phys Ther 69:162, 1989.
17. Jette, A: Diagnosis and classification by physical therapists: A special communication. Phys Ther 69:967, 1989.
18. Behr, D, et al: Diagnosis enhances, not impedes boundaries of physical therapy practice. J Orthop Sports Phys Ther 13:218, 1991.
19. Dekker, J, et al: Diagnosis and treatment in physical therapy: An investigation of their relationship. Phys Ther 73:568, 1993.
20. Payton, O, et al: Patient Participation in Program Planning: A Manual for Therapists. FA Davis, Philadelphia, 1990.
21. Henry, J: Identifying problems in clinical problem solving. Phys Ther 65:1071, 1985.
22. Watts, N: Decision analysis: A tool for improving physical therapy education. In Wolf, S (ed): Clinical Decision Making in Physical Therapy. FA Davis, Philadelphia, 1985, p 8.
23. Sullivan, P, and Markos, P: Clinical Decision Making in Therapeutic Exercise. Appleton & Lange, East Norwalk, CN, 1995.
24. Stockmeyer, S: Clinical decision making based on homeostatic concepts. In Wolf, S (ed): Clinical Decision Making in Physical Therapy. FA Davis, Philadelphia, 1985, p 79.
25. Wolf, S: Clinical Decision Making in Physical Therapy. FA Davis, Philadelphia, 1985.
26. May, BJ, and Dennis, JK: Expert decision making in physical therapy: A survey of practitioners. Phys Ther 71:190, 1991.
27. Jensen, GM, et al: Attribute dimensions that distinguish master and novice physical therapy clinicians in orthopedic settings. Phys Ther 72:711, 1992.
28. Embrey, DG, et al: Clinical decision making by experienced and inexperienced pediatric physical therapists for children with diplegic cerebral palsy. Phys Ther 76:20, 1996.
29. Riolo, L: Skill differences in novice and expert clinicians in neurologic physical therapy. Neurology Report 20:60, 1996.
30. Payton, O: Clinical reasoning process in physical therapy. Phys Ther 65:924, 1985.
31. Glaser, R: Education and thinking: The role of knowledge. Am Psychol 39:93, 1984.
32. Rothstein, JM, and Echternach, JL: Hypothesis-oriented algorithm for clinicians: A method for evaluation and treatment planning. Phys Ther 66:1388, 1986.
33. Rothstein, JM, and Echternach, JL: Hypothesis-oriented algorithms. Phys Ther 69:559, 1989.
34. Raiffa, H: Decision Analysis: Introductory Lectures on Choices under Uncertainty. Addison-Wesley, Reading, MS, 1968.
35. Weinstein, M, et al: Clinical Decision Analysis. Saunders, Philadelphia, 1980.
36. Weed, LL, and Zimny, NJ: The problem-oriented system, problem-knowledge coupling, and clinical decision making. Phys Ther 69:656, 1989.
37. Weed, LL: Knowledge Coupling: New Premises and New Tools for Medical Care and Education. Springer-Verlag, New York, 1991.

38. Weed, LL: Medical Records, Medical Education and Patient Care. The Press of Case Western Reserve Univ., Cleveland, 1969.

39. Kettenbach, G: Writing S.O.A.P. Notes. FA Davis, Philadelphia, 1990.

GLOSSARY

Asset: An individual's strengths (nonimpairments) and abilities that can be used for reinforcement and emphasis during therapy; also includes supportive social structure and environment.

Client: An individual who is not necessarily sick or injured, but who can benefit from a physical therapist's consultation, professional advice, or prevention services.[1]

Clinical decision making: A complex process of analytical thinking enacted within the context of patient treatment.

Cognitive processing styles

  Systematic processing style: A step-by-step approach to clinical decision making; the solution to each problem is dependent on information obtained in the preceding step.

  Intuitive: An approach that keeps the total problem in focus during assessment and considers treatment alternatives simultaneously.

Data-gathering styles

  Receptive data-gathering style: Judgement is suspended until all possible data are gathered.

  Perceptive data-gathering style: As data are being gathered, judgements are being made based on cues and patterns perceived.

Decision analysis: A systematic approach to decision making under conditions of uncertainty. Decision analysis focuses on structuring and diagramming the problem over time, the management alternatives and consequences, the uncertainties, and the preferences of the decision makers.

Decision tree: A flow diagram that allows the components of the decision analysis process to be displayed in a sequence that embodies both temporal and logical structure.

Diagnosis: A label encompassing a cluster of signs and symptoms, syndromes, or categories.

FITT equation: A general formula for outlining a treatment plan, including frequency, intensity, time, and type of therapeutic intervention.

Goals: The remediation of impairments. Goals specify (1) who will perform the behavior, (2) what the specific behavior is, (3) under what conditions the behavior will be performed, and (4) how the outcome will be measured.

  Short-term goals: (STGs) Reflect a limited time span, generally 2 to 3 weeks.

  Long-term goals (LTGs): Reflect a time span longer than 3 weeks.

  Outcomes: The remediation of functional limitations, prevention of disability, and optimization of health status and patient satisfaction.

Hypothesis-oriented algorithm for clinicians (HOAC): A systematic, step-by-step approach of initial data collection, generation of a problem statement, establishment of goals, examination, formation of working hypotheses, reevaluation of goals, establishment of a treatment plan, implementation, and reevaluation.

Interventions: The skilled and purposeful interactions between the physical therapist and patient, family, caregiver, or other appropriate individuals, and the various different procedures and techniques included in the practice of physical therapy.

Patient: An individual who is the recipient of physical therapy care and direct intervention.[1]

Plan of care (POC): The delineation of the physical therapy diagnosis, prognosis, treatment goals and outcomes, interventions, and discharge plans.

Problem-oriented medical record (POMR): An organized approach to the patient–treatment process characterized by four phases: (1) formation of a database, (2) identification of a specific problem list, (3) identification of a specific treatment plan, and (4) evaluation of the effectiveness of treatment plans.

Prognosis: The predicted optimal level of improvement in function and amount of time needed to reach that level.

Quality of life: A sense of total well-being that encompasses both physical and psychosocial aspects of an individual's life.

SOAP format (subjective, objective, assessment, plan): Progress note format utilized in the POMR; delineation is made among subjective findings, objective findings, assessment results, and plan of care.

APPENDIX A

Suggested Answers to Case Study Guiding Questions

1. Identify and categorize the patient's impairments into direct, indirect, and composite.

DIRECT	INDIRECT	COMPOSITE
dec. ROM RLE	dec. standing	postural kyphosis
dec. strength RLE	balance: static and	dec. endurance
½ inch leg length diff.	dynamic	

2. Identify her functional limitations, disabilities, and assets.

FUNCTIONAL LIMITATIONS

Modified independence (walker) in ambulation

Modified independence (SBQC) in elevation activities (stairs)

Modified dependence (min. assist) in BADLs (bathing)

Modified dependence (mod. assist) in IADLs (homemaking)

Safety issues: hx of frequent falls

DISABILITIES

Unable to participate in previous level of social activities (garden club, senior center)

ASSETS

Previous level of independence

Cooperative and motivated

Good problem solving and safety awareness

3. What are your concerns regarding potential disablement risk factors?

Patient demonstrates an advanced level of osteoporosis, postural changes, impaired balance, and visual impairments that result in a loss of depth perception. She is at moderate risk for falls. She lives alone and currently depends on home health aides (weekly) and family (weekends) to assist her.

Her endurance is decreased. The status of her osteoporosis puts her at increased risk for failure of the internal fixation device and fracture.

4. What is her prognosis?

Patient will return to previous level of functional independence in the home and community.

5. Write two outcomes and two goal statements for her plan of care.

OUTCOMES:

Patient will be independent and safe with cane on all surfaces and stairs within 6 weeks.

Patient will be independent and safe in all ADLs within 6 weeks.

GOALS:

Patient will increase strength in R knee extension to N within 3 weeks.

Patient will demonstrate safe and appropriate balance reactions for all functional activities within 6 weeks.

6. Identify two treatment interventions you might include in her plan of care. What precautions should you observe?

GAIT TRAINING: PWB to FWB; walker to SBQC to straight cane;

supervised to independent

HOME EXERCISE PLAN (HEP):

Bilateral exercises for:

hip extensors, abductors, hip flexors (involved hip: active–assisted and active exercises to light resistance)

knee extensors, knee flexors

ankle dorsiflexors, plantarflexors

Postural reeducation: corner stretches,

sitting exercises: trunk extension, head and neck retraction

7. What assessments will you use to determine the successful attainment of outcomes?

FUNCTIONAL ASSESSMENT

Tinetti's Performance Oriented Mobility Assessment

PRECAUTIONS: No hip adduction, internal rotation, flexion beyond 90°

2

Psychosocial Concomitants to Disability and Rehabilitation

Aaron Lieberman
Morris B. Lieberman
Bilha Reichberg Lieberman

LEARNING OBJECTIVES

1. Recognize the impact of psychological functioning and social interaction on health, disease, accident proneness, and adjustment to illness and physical trauma.
2. Recognize the physical cause of disability as but one factor among a myriad of other contributory aspects of disability.
3. Identify the psychological impact of disablement on the patient.
4. Identify the importance of self-concept, motivation, emotions, drive, and values, and their effect on disability and its outcome.
5. Identify the role played by cognition, perception, and premorbid personality structures on disability and its outcome.
6. Identify the stages of psychological adjustment to loss and disability outcome.
7. Recognize the warning signs of possible post-traumatic stress disorder.
8. Describe the general adaptation syndrome, its aims, uses, and potential dangerous side effects.
9. Identify the contributions of mental health professionals and rehabilitation clinicians in enhancing psychosocial adjustment.
10. Identify crisis points in the rehabilitation process.
11. Recognize the potential warning behavior and signs of poor adjustment warranting a mental health consult.
12. Describe general approaches and practices potentially helpful in promoting adjustment to loss and disability.
13. Recognize the importance of psychosocial adjustment, without which rehabilitation cannot be successful.

In recent years, there have been significant ongoing empirical, didactic, and experiential findings that have expanded our understanding of psychosocial issues. These advances have contributed to our knowledge base and have simultaneously highlighted the significance of the psychosocial concomitants to rehabilitation. It is particularly gratifying to note that the "mind-body" link has been generating increasing recognition and attention in all fields and disciplines involved in physical rehabilitation. A comprehensive offering of the state-of-the art of physical rehabilitation cannot limit itself solely to the administration of physical therapy intervention without addressing the emotional partnership of the body total. There is now an ever-growing body of evidence that indicates, in no uncertain terms, that the psychological state of patients (their mood, perceptions, expectations, and resulting response patterns), strongly shape their response to their physical condition, their motivation to work with the physical therapist, their ability to follow through on home care, and even their interactions with the therapist during treatment sessions. This chapter will introduce these constructs and the supporting empirical findings. The chapter will also present a brief practical guide for the health care practitioner which can serve as a broad outline of possible psychologically based patient responses which can interfere with rehabilitation. The chapter will present some general strategies for interaction with patients, and suggest circumstances where it may be advisable to seek mental health consultation, all in the service of attaining positive outcomes. The materials presented should be of value to all health care professionals involved with rehabilitation.

Similarly, this presentation of psychosocial aspects of rehabilitation refrains from elaborating on specific populations, such as the special considerations involved with pediatric or geriatric populations, among others. Likewise, the emphasis of this chapter is on physical disability and rehabilitation.

DISABILITY AND ADJUSTMENT

Disability can be likened to the proverbial iceberg; the onlooker can only see its tip, while the iceberg itself contains more hidden aspects than revealed on the surface. An expression of physical pain, the lack of sensory input or output, a missing or dysfunctional limb or structure, and other such reflections of loss are just the surface structure of physical disability. Yet, these are the major domains that traditionally have been addressed when dealing with physical disability.

Experience, as well as a growing body of research, reveal that these surface domains can often be misleading, in and of themselves, as indices of the extent of damage or the patients' experience of the disablement. Research and optimal practice very clearly demonstrate the large role that psychosocial factors play in mitigating the extent of a disability,

the treatment process itself, the length of treatment and the adequacy of treatment outcomes. Kennedy et al.,[1] for example, corroborate other research findings demonstrating that organic factors (such as the extent or level of injury, age of onset, etc.) are, in themselves, not predictive of long-term adjustment. Others[2] have found no correlation between the degree of disfigurement and the level of adjustment, whereas other significant research has found that premorbid functioning is a strong predictor of the long-term disruption of a disablement.[3] There is evidence that the patients' perception of changes in health may influence the recovery process in either direction.[4] This information, together with an understanding that moderate to severe psychiatric disturbances are common during rehabilitation,[5] will emphasize the crucial importance of understanding and considering psychosocial factors in the provision of rehabilitation services. The lack of awareness of this larger framework and of the psychosocial factors involved can easily undermine treatment goals and outcomes. It can also bewilder the physical therapist in regard to unexpected mood shifts, motivation shifts, hostility, sabotaging behaviors and/or medically unsupported somatic complaints, or complaints of exaggerated pain or difficulties in either extreme. There are a growing number of researchers, such as Watts,[6] who advocate for a universally applied proactive mental health intervention for all trauma and rehabilitation patients based on the findings of poor or prolonged outcome in rehabilitation efforts without such involvement.

One illustration of the impact of these factors is the large body of empirical findings suggesting that even the perception of pain is a very subjective experience. Even if one takes into account great individual discrepancies regarding pain tolerance (such as individual levels of pain thresholds, cultural differences, and culturally induced gender differences involved in shaping the level and manner of the expression of pain or discomfort) we still find that individual psychosocial factors impinge upon the individual sensation and expression of pain. Research has found that negative thought patterns as well as illness-focused strategies can result in a higher tendency to report pain as compared to the results of having a positive outlook and active coping strategies.[7] We do know that outlook and strategies can be shifted, leading others[8] to empirically demonstrate that certain therapeutic modalities can improve pain coping strategies and ameliorate the impact of pain expression and pain tolerance on treatment interventions and rehabilitation. The specific issue of pain aside for the moment, it is documented that more than half of all visits to primary care physicians can be attributed to psychosocial problems presented as somatic complaints, thus further reinforcing the complex mind-body connection, even in the general population.[9] There is a large body of research focused on the concept of the "sick role," a culturally supported role of helplessness and dependency, which can sometimes explain overly dependent behaviors in our patients and their resistance to improved functioning and independence. Being "sick" can involve a **secondary gain,** which promotes maintaining the disability status.

At best, our understanding of what a disabled individual might feel about the state he or she is in can only be an approximation of the individual's unique **perceptions** or feelings. It is all of those uniquely combined thoughts and feelings that the individual has gathered during a lifetime of personal experience that shape and impinge on that individual's perceived state as a result of the **disablement.** The factors that shape individual reactions include the set of values, directions, and prohibitions taken on by the individual. These then combine with **innate,** conditioned, and acquired drives, needs, experiences, pleasures, and pains in creating an individual with a unique perceptual mode and cognitive base. It is through this that the individual has learned to see the self and the surrounding world. The resultant **self-image,** whether conscious or unconscious, creates a set of values and expectations by which one measures oneself and one's worth. It becomes the compass with which one steers life, relationships, and structures the goals and foundations of one's individualized world.

Through this process, a unique way of **coping** and functioning emerges, which becomes the **style of coping** through which one recognizes himself or herself. Then suddenly, or gradually, depending on the nature and extent of a disablement, that lifelong foundation and the structure of that "self" becomes damaged and weakened by the impact of the disability; often to the point of total collapse. The disabling condition, as well as the perception of it, disrupts the structure, the "persona" which, through years of shaping and conditioning, became the essence of one's selfhood. That sense of self, that unique individual identity, is severely challenged or altogether altered. Current life situation as well as future plans, goals, and expectations are impacted, and the patient must confront and work through these painful alterations. To do so, patients can only rely on whatever tools (adaptive or maladaptive), they have at their disposal, their premorbid level of personality stability and functioning, their unique set of coping strategies, as well as the stage of life and the stage of identity formation they find themselves in at the time of the disablement. All of these factors can then either be compounded negatively or facilitated by the impact of their socioenvironmental situation.

Self-Concept

Self-concept and its interrelationship with, and impact on, the above constructs is a complex yet important factor in adjustment. There is much evidence to suggest that a positive self-concept acts as a buffer against the impact of a disability and the rehabilitation process.[10] Findings suggest that par-

ticular aspects of self-concept are seemingly more determinative[11] than a general construct of self-concept. Low self-concept was found to be a primary correlate of behavior problems[12] and to have a negative impact on adjustment,[13] whereas positive perception as an effective problem solver predicted positive adjustment.[14] There is little doubt that self-concept also has an impact on coping and coping outcome. It is important to note that although coping is a dynamic, changing process, positive and problem-focused coping strategies have been found to be palliative in adjustment and positive long-term outcomes in rehabilitation.[7,15–20] There are, indeed, findings that provide no evidence that coping is so strongly palliative,[21,22] but there are a plethora of strong findings that do support this notion. Kennedy at al.[23] hold that coping strategy is more important than other cognitive and behavioral styles as a crucial factor in the rehabilitation process. Disability upsets the rules and changes the individual's roles. The relative independence and ability to perform the essential tasks of living are jeopardized, if not gone, even if only perceived as such. The ability to give and take love, care, affection, and support are diminished or lost. The desire to give or take these feelings may even be diminished or lost and the ability to open up or to trust others has been shown empirically to also be diminished or lost. The relative financial stability and security may just vaporize into thin air.

Intellectually, we the "healers" can understand the trauma; with our ability to empathize we may even feel some of it. We may associate our patient's suffering with recollections of some past pain or loss we may have personally experienced. The therapist, working toward the goal of rehabilitating a patient, needs to be cognizant of the possibility that **adjustment** to the actual functional disability may not be the most difficult adjustment for the patient. The individual will most likely have a more difficult task adjusting to the new perceptions about themselves and the societal attitudes toward their disability. These factors and the individual's reactions to the new situation will most likely impact the overall adjustment, the rehabilitation process, and its outcome. Ignoring this probability might allow for a serious level of interference with and/or complicate the therapeutic outcome. An awareness of these issues can prevent or minimize their interference and enable the clinician to mobilize these very same factors in the service of the rehabilitative effort. What follows is an attempt to suggest some practical guidelines, which should enhance the therapeutic impact.

ADAPTATION: A SURVIVAL STRATEGY

Living is a constant, ongoing adjustment and **adaptation** process, encompassing different levels of the organism and its life space. This process is active at the physiological, physical, psychological, and social levels of one's functioning. Although there are indeed significant differences among these aspects of functioning, one should keep in mind that they are but a part of a unitary entity that functions as an integrated whole. Any separation between levels and parts of an individual's system is an artificial convenience, because no part within the person is independent from the rest of that individual. **Psychological adjustment** is likewise part and parcel of adjustment in general rather than an independent entity. The same holds true for each and every component that comprises the many aspects of a dynamic, interactive, and ongoing process of an individual's adaptation to the internal physiological processes and the external surrounding reality that make up one's total life space. This life space includes, among others:

1. The body total with its various genetic, electrochemical, hormonal, and neurological configurations.
2. Its innate instinctual drives as well as conditioned mental mechanisms.
3. Its sociocultural, spiritual, and ethnic belief and value system within the socioeconomic realities of the time and place within which one interacts.
4. The historical/mythological, philosophical/ideological, or even imagined/delusional image that one feels and is influenced by.

NATURE AND NURTURE

As we grow and age, various sets of expectations change and evolve. The *nature* or direction of these changes are species specific and depend on individual, genetically inherited developmental capacities, **proscribed roles,** and the individual's ethnic and social status. Other aspects, such as the prevailing political/ideological climate, religious beliefs, the historical period (with its economic and technological systems), and family idiosyncrasies and structure, are among the contributing factors to the individual's adaptive and adjusting style. They are part of the mold from which the unique individual emerges. They create a specific style of adaptive (or **maladaptive**) functioning, and **personality structure,** through which the individual negotiates the surrounding environment. As that self evolves it combines and channels innate drives and needs with learned or reinforced behaviors and values. Because coping is a constant learning process, which is affected by a variety of social and environmental influences, the uniqueness of individual **coping styles** is to be expected, as is the variability in coping effectiveness.

The individual's interaction with the internal and external reality therefore can be seen as selective, subjective, and idiosyncratic. It can be seen as the sum total of an interactional history of one's **nature and nurture.** The chronology of this interactional history includes the genetic evolution that is species specific, and the cultural and environmental forces that shape the world into which the individual was born. This then shapes the individual's unique subjective perception of the world and of the self. It likewise shapes an intricate **mental defense** and adaptation system resulting in a unique response repertoire. This adjustment process is therefore an ongoing re-learning experience that constantly readjusts the response style. An individual's adjustments will depend on the developed "ego" (or self) and its defense structure. It will also depend on the relative strength and/or vulnerability of the ego, the adjustment style adopted, and the perceived impinging stimulus of the moment. Catering to these often conflicting needs requires the balancing of internal and external resources. We will call this balancing act "coping," even though many other names are used to describe the same concept. Coping is a combination of innate and learned behaviors, which are utilized to deal with the demands of internal and external conditions. It is an active process aimed at creating a state of biological and psychological equilibrium. The attempt to bring about such a balance and satisfy or mediate between internal and external pressures is what adjustment is all about. This is an ongoing process without which life would be difficult, if not impossible. The lack of such fluidity is detrimental and maladaptive for any individual.

Coping may at times differ from accepted values or inner needs resulting in a failure to serve the best interest of the individual. When this occurs, it will most likely be termed **"deviant"** in the first instance and "maladaptive" in the second. Maladaptive adjustment might develop as the result of faulty perception, learned rejection of the self, misguided values, or misinterpretations of reality. Deviant coping strategies might be due to justified or unjustified disagreement and open rejection of the accepted values of the individual's environment. Whether adaptive or maladaptive, the coping response of an individual is part of an adaptation process that aims toward survival, even though the coping responses may be contrary to this goal.

In summary, psychological adjustment is an intricate, interactive, and complicated process. It represents the consciously perceived self as well as unconscious motivations, emotions, drives, values, and perceptual functioning. Psychological adjustment is of paramount importance in any consideration of what an individual "is all about." It includes the need to maintain and develop a **self-identity** within a biological and social structure of which one is part. The psychological adjustment of an individual is crucial to what is meaningful in life for that individual. This adjustment can significantly enhance the utilization of one's resources for rehabilitation from a functional disability.

REACTION TO DISABLEMENT AS AN ADJUSTMENT PROCESS

For the purpose of differentiation between objective loss of function and the ensuing subjective state, we have chosen to call the objective and actual loss a disablement. Thus the loss of a leg is, within this context, a disablement; the ensuing way the individual copes with such a loss will be presented as the disability. Accordingly, we will consider an individual's reaction to injury, illness, or loss of function an adjustment process that contributes to, or results in, the ensuing physical disability. Disability can therefore be considered an adjustment process to a disruptive event that impinged on, and interrupted the, "normal mode" of functioning of that individual. This implies that when an individual is confronted with a disablement, various adjustments are attempted in order to cope with the newly created situation. The elicited response to the disablement may encompass most, if not all, levels of the individual's functioning. This would include, among others, the vegetative process, the autonomic nervous system and cortical, hormonal, and autoimmune response, as well as intra- and interpersonal reactions. Above all, the response to disablement and rehabilitation would depend on what the disabling condition means to that specific, affected individual. The ensuing disability is therefore seen as the interaction of the actual disablement and the individual's adjustment process, with the latter hinging on the factors enumerated above. The level of a disability can therefore be severe or mild relative to the disablement depending on the adjustment strategies of the client.

The response thus triggered by the various aspects of one's functioning and coping style might optimize, or conversely, minimize rehabilitative efforts. Accepting the resultant objective limitations, developing compensatory functioning, and adapting to a different mode of life and different societal roles (which are called for by the newly created conditions) will usually be adaptive. Unwarranted retreats to lower-level functioning, isolation, rejection of oneself, loss of self-appreciation, or even an escape into nihilism or death would obviously be considered maladaptive. For some individuals who experienced coping difficulties prior to a disablement, disability may be utilized as an escape from responsibility and/or a tool for manipulations. In others, it may bring about further deterioration or its opposite, an opportunity to turn a stagnant life around. Engel[24] reports that in some instances of emotionally dysfunctional individuals, disability may contribute positively to their overall adjustment. Moos[25] sees in such findings a provocative challenge. He claims that most researchers tend to accentuate the negative reactions to disability obscuring any positive compensations some individuals are able to tap when faced with a disabling condition. Ehrenteil[26] also stresses the possible positive reaction to disability and suggests that disability may have an ego-integrative role. For example, a doctoral student of ours utilized her crippling neurological disease as a chance to change her premorbid, mundane life as a secretary, into a professional one. Becoming wheelchair bound and dependent on unemployment and disability income enabled her to pursue doctoral-

level study in psychology, a dream that could not be realized while being in good health and self supporting. She, for one, gladly found a positive way to integrate and convert the disability to a new life and a professional career.

At the other extreme, we can recall another student who, experiencing a moderate disablement due to a vehicular accident, withdrew into herself, developed a set of severe phobias, became socially isolated, dependent upon welfare financing, and eventually moved from misuse of her prescription medications to sustained cocaine addiction. Conversely, the authors recall a social acquaintance, an established periodontist who lost functioning in one arm. Acquaintances would bemoan the situation and, behind his back, whisper concerns as to how he would afford to raise his three young children. After stabilization of the disablement, this periodontist utilized his vast knowledge and experience to share his expertise with others, and now travels the country providing advanced lectures and seminars to periodontists. He reports that this change of life-style not only allows him to maintain an identity as a functioning periodontist, but affords a previously unimagined level of economic stability, increased time available to spend with his family, and extensive opportunity to travel.

SUBJECTIVITY OF DISABILITY

A person's disability or handicap is to a significant extent directly related to the degree that one perceives the handicapping condition. The extent of a disability will increase if the focus is on deficiencies rather than assets. Likewise, the length of treatment and the lack of patient compliance and follow through with the treatment regimen will also be negatively impacted by a problem-focused orientation and an inability to alter initial perceptions and adapt to changed realities. Much of such focusing depends on the premorbid make-up of an individual, his or her coping repertoire, and the cultural perception of the disabling situation. The outcome of this will result in an adjustment to the disablement. It is our task as clinicians to assist our patients in making an adjustment to their disablement that is favorable and to prevent an unfavorable adaptation to their condition.

As health care practitioners, we should realize the significance of our impact on our patient's adaptive adjustment, which extends beyond the direct physical interventions we administer. Instilling positive emotional input and negating maladaptive ones will catapult the rehabilitation efforts toward positive adaptation of our patients. This will promote a more positive perception and assist our patients to find meaning to their life regardless of their disablement.

Adjustments are attempts to develop a fit between two or more variables. In living organisms adjustment usually implies adapting for the sake of survival, although under certain circumstances individual survival is sacrificed for the survival of the species. The same holds true for humans.

To effectively serve the complicated survival needs of our species, human beings have developed various mental mechanisms, called **ego defense** or **defense mechanisms,** that assist us in this task. These mechanisms are used to alleviate the pressures and conflicting demands encountered in our trip through life. There are many such mechanisms. The reader is encouraged to survey the literature: discussion of these mechanisms is beyond the scope of this chapter. Even though aimed at survival, the pressures and conflicts are often such that individuals utilize these defenses for the sake of alleviating pressures at the cost of what is indeed best for survival. To accomplish this the individual will turn a blind eye to the encountered reality. These defense mechanisms will invariably create faulty perceptions, which will trigger behaviors that may alleviate the pressures felt, sometimes also at the cost of what is in the best interest of survival. The individual creates these faulty perceptions, and resorts to them, to alleviate the pressures, all the while denying or being unaware of their inappropriateness.

Our aim as clinicians is to prevent maladaptive adjustment. We will usually consider the acceptance of a life spent in a wheelchair for an individual who has the capacity to learn to ambulate independently, as maladaptive adjustment. Yet we must realize that the choice is still an adjustment, which may indeed be the best choice from that person's point of perception if not from a realistic point of view. As stated, the terms adjustment, coping, and adaptation are given to value interpretation and do not, in themselves, imply a positive outcome. For the purpose of convenience, we will use the term "maladaptive" for faulty adaptation and the term "adaptive" for its opposite.

When a maladaptive response is the result of faulty reality testing, value judgements, misinformation, or defective neuronal brain activity it becomes the province of "responsible others" to enable that individual to shift to a more appropriate and adaptive one. Parents, spouses, teachers, clinicians and at times, society, will take on the role of the "responsible other." Yet, who really knows best? We have to respect the individual's rights to make personal life decisions unless there is objective evidence that their judgemental faculties are significantly diminished. But let us always ensure that our own information is correct and that our own judgement is not clouded. We carry a professional obligation to make every conceivable effort to understand the individual's covert reasons for his or her functioning before passing judgement as to its appropriateness. This takes special skills, objectivity, and an ability to put our own values and interests aside. If we do not do this, then it is our judgement that may be in need of correction.

The adjustment process has been discussed owing to its significance in the rehabilitation process. Most of life's adjustments become routine and almost automatic. Nonroutine but expected events can have considerable impact, whereas those that are unexpected and disruptive can have catastrophic impact, at times, out of proportion to the actual damage sustained. Adjustment to disability is an encompassing one, which denotes an ongoing, fluid process of adjustments and readjustments at all levels of one's functioning. It can be seen as a chain reaction because each adjustment causes changes and is followed by other reactions. In addition, it interacts with all levels of the person and the environment. The need to adjust to an immediate disruption of homeostatic balance during a traumatic injury is different in its intensity and urgency than the adjustment needs that arise afterward.

ADJUSTMENT TO DISABLEMENT

Among the factors contributing to disability adjustment are the extent of the injury or illness; the onset mode; the prognosis of the physical aspect of the disability; the central processing of the brain when affected; the social, medical, psychological, and economic support systems; and the subjective perception of the situation as well as the **premorbid** coping capacity of the patient. Also of significance is the realistic degree of interference the disability may have on the vocational and personal mode of life of the given individual. A loss of one finger should objectively have little effect on a professional singer but will most likely bring an end to much more than just the career of a concert pianist. Good psychological adjustment may catapult an individual into becoming successful, whereas a bad adjustment might cripple the same individual for life.

Adjustment is typically more dramatic during a major disabling condition and is therefore the focus of this discussion. Remember that what makes a condition major or minor is subjective. Even minor physical conditions are major to most of their owners. What is discussed here is applicable to most patients in need of physical rehabilitation.

Pain and reaction to injury are subjective and individualistic and not in direct proportion to the actual extent of injury. The difference in the adjustment need is rather due to personal perception. We would obviously expect an injury that ceases to impact realistically on the injured within a relatively short period, or does not require any special attention or changes in one's functioning, to leave little, if any, scars. When the subjective reaction to a disablement is disproportionate to the level of actual damage, it can be assumed that the response is most likely triggered by some emotional factor and/or personality structure rather than the precipitating injury or illness.

Successful adjustment would imply the restoration or some approximation to the premorbid condition of the function and compensation for the loss by use of other assets. We have previously implied that disability of physical functioning is usually accompanied by disruptions of psychological and social functioning. Compensating the physical loss by itself does not necessarily bring with it a correction of the other losses a patient experiences. Ignoring those other subjective, perceived losses may interfere with physical rehabilitation, increase the level of the functional disability, and even contribute toward creating additional ailments.

Psychological adjustment to injury or disablement can be divided into the three phases. The first is the period immediately following the injury or disablement; this is followed by the second phase, which lasts until a relatively stable adjustment has been made. The third period is the one where a relative equilibrium has been reached either by a return to premorbid functioning to the extent possible, or by having reached a level of relative optimal functioning and coping in view of the nature of the disablement. For the purpose of our discussion we will refer to these as the **traumatic reaction period (or stage),** the **posttraumatic adjustment period,** and the **stabilization period,** respectively.

Even though the first step in aiding an individual suffering an injury or illness can be initiated during the acute stage, rehabilitation intervention is usually initiated after the traumatic reaction period. Most of our emphasis will be on the second phase of the disablement, during which rehabilitation interventions are usually at their peak. During the third phase, the stabilization period, the patient may still need, and will most likely benefit from, the guidance of the clinical team as he or she settles into a relatively stabilized or adjusted state.

THE TRAUMATIC REACTION AND THE GENERAL ADAPTATION SYNDROME

During a catastrophic event, whether due to accident or acute severe illness, an individual's response will, of necessity, be primarily at the physiological level, possibly overshadowing the concomitant emotional reaction. When a body perceives itself to be in danger it will trigger its own physiological emergency responses. Likewise, the medical emergency team will occupy itself with the immediate life-saving attempts aimed at physical survival. Psychological adjustment would most likely be extreme but not as discernible or noticeable until a later time, and will therefore not be catered to.

When the trauma is of a lesser level or the physical disablement has a gradual onset, as happens during a progressive illness, the psychological reaction may be the one most affected or noticeable. In either case, an interactive feedback loop will establish itself between the physiological and emotional functioning of the individual as a result of the ensuing **stress reaction.**

During a perceived or real catastrophic reaction an organism would most likely respond with what Selye[27] termed the **general adaptation syndrome (GAS).** Selye described GAS as an organism's defensive adaptation attempt, which expresses itself through physiological and emotional interactions of responses aimed at dealing with such emergencies. During GAS there is a physiochemical chain reaction, whereby a peptide called corticotropin-releasing factor (CRF) is secreted to stimulate secretion of a hormonal release of adrenocorticotropic hormone (ACTH). The ACTH sets into motion an increase of specific physiological activity aimed at maximizing the body's defense capacity while minimizing the utilization of physiological activities that are not essential during the emergency period. Although such corticosteroid increase is serving the defensive stance, its inhibitory effect on other body needs, such as the production of insulin and calcium, is undesirable in the long run. Studies have shown that injection of a CRF antagonist reduces the sense of anxiety in stress.[28] When such inhibition is prolonged, additional undesirable effects such as hypertension, digestive problems, and interference with the immune system will result. Selye has documented the devastating effect a prolonged GAS response has on human mental and physical functioning. Theorell et al.[29] have documented the occurrence of resultant illnesses long after the stress-producing event was over.

Situations that activate the sympathetic system through repeated alarms, traumas, or chronic stress may alter synaptic transmission and lead to anxiety and depression of normal bodily functions. It should be noted that the physiological and psychological interaction to stress is not limited to catastrophic conditions. An extensive body of research shows stress reactions to be present in individuals under conditions that would hardly affect the average person. Everyday life frustrations, internal and external conflict situations, and changes in life conditions are major causes of stress reaction, which may have a devastating effect on a person's functioning and health. The physical therapist should be cognizant of the fact that even though a patient's objective emergency situation is over, stress reaction still looms and may easily rear its head.

The above is not intended to minimize or rule out individual perception in regard to stress. The word "stress" generally has a negative connotation regarding its impact on the individual. Stress, however, can be more accurately described as either **distress,** conveying the negative impact of any particular stressor, or **eustress,** referring to the ability to convert a particular stressor to energize or motivate, all depending on the individual's attitude and perception of the stressor. A ready example can be found as one looks around a classroom to note that the stress of an impending final examination causes one student to become focused on study habits while another displays the overt symptoms of anxiety, panic, and lowered functioning sometimes to the point of "mental freezing," thereby not being able to respond on a test even though having the correct answer to the problem.

Accordingly, the stress reaction is not limited to the traumatic reaction period or the primary injury or illness. As awareness of the trauma increases, frustration is experienced. All activities that were previously performed almost automatically and effortlessly, become difficult and often impossible tasks to perform. These become compounded with readjustment needs of daily life activities and a new and usually lower self-image. Guilt feelings and/or blame are interlaced with anger toward the real or imagined causal agents of the condition of the disablement. This extra load of stress may lead to a chronic stress level, which will interfere with rehabilitation efforts.

POSTTRAUMATIC ADJUSTMENT

The posttraumatic period is usually the time during which much, if not most, of the rehabilitative intervention takes place; it is also the period during which the psychological effects of the traumatic experience are mostly felt by the patient. Mann and Gold[30] claim that the psychological problems after injury are as disabling as the physical ones, and found this to be even more pronounced when the physical injury was less evident. It seems as if most of the psychological defenses and reactions that took a secondary place during the initial traumatic period start emerging as the physical injury is diminished. These repressed reactions seem to interact with a growing awareness of the effects of the disablement creating perceptions, fears, anxieties, and behaviors that the rehabilitation team must confront, be aware of, and address. Of particular interest to the rehabilitation team at this stage is the emergence of the **posttraumatic stress disorder (PTSD)**. Knowledge of this secondary disorder and its prevalence will assist the therapist in understanding the patient's reactions and feelings at this stage of rehabilitation. The importance of this awareness is underscored by the findings of Epstein,[31] which indicate that avoidant symptoms of PTSD can interfere with diagnosis of PTSD and its impact can be overlooked altogether. PTSD has recently received increased attention as a common psychological response to a wide variety of traumatic experiences and will be explored later in this chapter.

STABILIZATION PERIOD

The stabilization period is the third and last phase of the disability. During this phase the role of the clinical team is usually phased out or minimized as the patient enters into a relatively adjusted and balanced state of living. It should be noted, however, that adjustment or stabilization are relative terms and do not imply a return to premorbid or optimal adaptation. Stabilization or adaptation indicates a comparative balanced fit of one's functioning within the "world" and can be either adaptive or maladaptive. For example, in a highly publicized case reported in *The New York Times* (October 7, 1987), an individual weighing over 1000 pounds was

described. This individual's total life was confined to a prone, bedridden position for over a decade as a result of the weight, which precluded any mobility. The disability was reportedly due to an enormous appetite. This individual adjusted to the love for food and modified his life to the ensuing body weight. The enormous body weight and size limited his capacity to carry himself or even to exit through the door, which became too narrow for his size. He reportedly was content with the confined condition created by his eating habit. It can be said that this bedridden, immobilized person was living a stabilized and adjusted life; adjusted to an imprisoned state and without any activity except the incessant food intake, staring at television, and getting attention from his care-taking relatives. This is a severe case of maladaptation, but nevertheless an adjusted and stabilized one.

The above case illustrates the importance of the quality the stabilization period assumes. It is during this latter period that an individual may accept a given quality and value of the life the disablement affords, the optimization of which should be a goal worthy of our clinical interventions. Likewise it is during the stabilization period that life again can become meaningful or meaningless for the given individual. Being alert to all the needs of the patient as well as to the signs and symptoms of maladaptation during the posttraumatic adjustment period is therefore vital. This emphasizes the need for an integrated holistic approach, which must essentially include the psychosocial aspect of disability as well as the physical one.

This points to a primary goal of this chapter, which is to alert the physical therapist to the emotional wounds that illness and injury create. It points to the importance of interacting with the other rehabilitation team members in meeting the needs of the patient as an integrated human being.

THE ROLE OF COGNITION

One of the psychological factors that exerts a major impact on an individual's rehabilitative functioning is cognitive make-up. In present day, psychology **cognition** is regarded as one of the most significant factors in determining an individual's way of dealing with the world. Dollard and Miller[32] claimed that cognition and motives are the major determinants of individual functioning. Subsequent psychological research seems to confirm this view, considering emotions and stress as the result of the individual's cognitive functioning. This view has since been supported by numerous studies, and indicates the important role played by one's perception in dealing with the situations with which an individual is confronted.[33-36] Selye[37] emphasizes that it is not what happens to you that matters, but how you take it.

Accordingly, the traumatic severity of a noxious stimulus hinges, to a great degree, on the individual's perception of an event, and the subjective value assigned to the factors that it affects. Likewise, the ability to cope with the situation as perceived is significantly dependent on the individual's perception of his or her coping ability and on the actual resources available. This indicates that an individual's perception of a given situation, and the ability to cope with it effectively, is significantly determined by his or her psychological make-up. Thus, the choice of any adjustment toward loss of function and illness is dictated from within the personal world of an individual's belief and value system and the ensuing perception it creates. Faulty reality appraisal and/or misguided coping strategies will create maladaptation. Conversely, confidence in one's resources and a positive set of values will help overcome disability through actualizing untapped and/or dormant assets. Experience shows that identical physical or physiological damage will result in different levels of disability when affecting different individuals.[38]

SUBJECTIVITY OF PHYSICAL DISABILITY

It becomes clear that the rehabilitation team's understanding of the psychological adjustment of a given patient is paramount. The seasoned therapist knows that an amputated limb is not a discarded anatomical part but rather an inseparable part of the patient even after its loss. The individual will not only feel phantom sensation in the lost limb but may also perceive life as worthless without it regardless of the actual and objective significance of the loss and its physical effect. The prosthesis replacing a limb may quite effectively enable physical ambulation but fail its owner emotionally. Without that limb the patient may feel impotent, worthless, estranged, punished, guilty, unloved, frightened, and/or crippled even though physical functioning has been restored.

It is doubtful that an individual having lost some essential function or an anatomical part will not lose part of the psychological self. The lack of a visible catastrophic response to such a loss would most likely indicate a defensive stance rather than a positive, healthy adjustment. Thus the rehabilitation team will fail such a patient by ignoring the meaning of the lost anatomical part or by exclusively addressing treatment to the physical dysfunction.

It is imperative to consider a patient's psychological make-up as a major prognostic determinant. One cannot isolate the physical body from the totality of the person and expect to treat it successfully. Of no less importance is the effect one's psychological functioning can have on the disabling condition itself. For a better understanding of the interaction between psychological functioning and physical disability we will attempt to differentiate between the contributing causative factors of the disability and the disability itself.

INTERACTION OF CAUSAL AND AFFECTED FACTORS IN DISABILITY

Traditionally the causative factor of physical disablement is considered to be any external or internal agent that disrupts an individual's physical or physiological functioning (direct impairment). Examples include a foreign body intrusion, an ingested poison or microorganism that causes organ damage, a degenerative disease or genetic flaw that destroys or interferes with body functions, and other such physiochemical assaults. The ensuing psychological response state would therefore be appropriately termed an indirect or secondary impairment and a complicating or contributing factor to the disability.

Accordingly, disability is the end result of both primary and secondary impairments, which shape the response of the individual. It follows that disability is not necessarily in direct proportion to the physical damage, but rather represents the end result of the synergistic effect of the physical loss and the individual's perception and mental attitude toward this loss. Just like pain, disability is very much the result of the subjectivity of the experiencing individual. This does not imply that the physical loss itself is dependent on the mental state of the individual, but rather that the extent of the disability hinges on that state. Likewise, a positive mental outlook will not negate a disablement but will most likely improve chances of healing. A limb will not regrow by wishing for it or by having a positive mental attitude; however, without the latter, the chance of a prosthesis replacing the lost limb and improving function will significantly diminish.

PSYCHOLOGICAL FACTORS IN PHYSICAL DISABILITY

The psychological and medical literature is replete with evidence indicating the presence of emotional factors and emotional disruption as primary contributors to accidents and debilitating disease.[39–41] Moreover, Freud demonstrated the undeniable role psychological factors play in the development of disease.[42]

One of the earlier theories to consider emotions as the cause of illness was the psychosomatic model presented by Alexander.[39] Not until the publication of the contributions of Hughlins et al.[43] was the psychosomatic model accepted by classical medicine. These discoveries brought an awareness of the unity of the organism and the mind-body relationship.

The psychosomatic theory posits that physical illness may be secondary to an emotional condition and should be treated as such when appropriate. Neglect of the psychological causal agent will result in a continuation of its malevolent effect and interfere with rehabilitation interventions. This theory suggests that the disablement, whether due to accident or illness, may at times have psychopathologic origins.

In the previous discussion of Selye's GAS, we mentioned the interaction of perception and cognitive functioning with the physiological reactions. It follows that faulty perception and cognition resulting in stress will expose one to increased risks of injury and illness.[44,45] Of considerable importance to the physical therapist is an awareness of the role that mental functioning plays in reinforcing physical illness and injury and at times even in their creation. Such beliefs are shared by most psychological theories and are increasingly accepted by medical science. Psychodynamic theorists and practitioners consider much of physical disease and accidental injury as the outcome of repressed, displaced, or somatosized mental energy.[46] Freud[46] posited the idea of *thanatos*, described as a destructive, inborn drive, needed for survival. Freud believed that under certain psychopathologic conditions this drive turns toward the self and may express itself in conscious suicidal attempts and/or in unconscious self-destructive behaviors.

The *Diagnostic and Statistical Manual*, fourth edition, of the American Psychiatric Association[47] provides a special diagnostic category for the psychological factors affecting physical conditions. The predominant symptomatology of "psychological factors affecting physical conditions" (DSM-IV code 316.00) is described in the **DSM-IV** manual as any physical condition or disorder which has been triggered by a psychosocial **stressor.**

The manual further states that the physical disturbance will eventually remit after the stressor ceases or may be replaced by a different type of adaptation. The way psychopathology contributes to physical ailments and accidents is obviously dependent on the type of emotional disturbance that exists. A brief overview of how psychopathologic factors might affect disability will be presented.

During psychotic functioning when lack of reality testing and/or states of confusion are prevalent, risk of accidents and disease states are increased. Similarly, emotionally troubled individuals may be preoccupied with their problems and/or exhaust their capacity for coping with life to a degree that will interfere with alertness and their ability to properly take care of their own safety and health.

Some emotional disorders and personality types find their expression in dangerous behaviors such as aggression against others and the self, or in impulsive behaviors, which may result in serious injury. These disorders would include the sociopathic, the antisocial, the impulsive, and the inadequate personality types, as well as pyromaniacs, psychotics, and depressed patients. An individual's compliance with rehabilitative efforts would likewise be hindered by their emotional state. Under such circumstances, the physical dysfunctions are an indirect outcome of the emotional state.

STRESS AND DISEASE

Stress has been defined as a state induced by a stimulus that manifests itself by virtue of one's cognitive interpretation.[36,48] The stimulus itself is considered a stressor. Accordingly, a stressor is any stimulus that evokes stress, whereas stress reactions are the observable consequences of the stressor. Various types of neuroses and certain personality problems run an above-average risk of falling prey to somatic or stress-induced physical illness because stress constantly accompanies many of these conditions. Constant stress is not limited to those suffering from emotional dysfunction. All of us are at times given to stressful situations. We have discussed how the prolongation of stress will eventually create physical as well as emotional dysfunction resulting in illness. Research links stress to a variety of medical, social, and psychological dysfunctions,[49,50] and has shown stress inoculation as palliative.[51]

We will present stress from an adaptation point of view. The stress response, similar to other adaptation mechanisms, is also aimed at survival. This response is an attempt to deal with a real or imagined impinging stimulus perceived as a threat to the self or one's homeostatic balance. The stress response consists of the mobilization of the body's resources to ward off the perceived danger. An appropriate analogy can be found in the mobilization of a nation's military and civilian resources against a perceived "enemy threat," which may or may not exist. By shifting its peacetime manpower and productivity toward the "war effort," a nation attempts to strengthen its defensive and aggressive powers at the cost of diminished peaceful and everyday maintenance of the country. If prolonged, such a state of affairs may impoverish the nation to the point of collapse, rebellion, and/or a weakened condition, which may indeed bring about its dissolution. An appropriate analogy can be seen in the dissolution of the Soviet Union, which concentrated most of its resources on military build-up to the point of economic collapse. This situation eventually brought about the actual collapse of the political system that the "defensive" stance aimed to preserve. Mobilization for defense, although taxing, is an appropriate response in face of realistic danger. When stress is the result of prolonged or repetitive faulty perception, the resulting exhaustion of limited resources may indeed endanger survival, which the stress reaction attempted to preserve.

An imaginary perceived danger will create a genuine stress situation just as a real danger would. Because falsely perceived danger is not based in reality, it does not end by changes in reality and tends to linger. Prolonged stress will endanger survival by depriving resources needed for the "peaceful" life of the individual. Woolfolk and Lehrer[49] illustrate this as follows: "The individual is not a passive recipient in stressful transactions between the person and the environment, but . . . [is an active interacting participant who may even] . . . generate stress through maladaptive beliefs, attitudes and patterns of action."

Others similarly postulate that the appraisal of an event by its perception, rather than the reality of circumstances, creates the cause of stress and conclude that one's cognitive appraisal of a problem will determine the ensuing coping pattern.[52–54] This development in cognitive psychology was instrumental in a gradual movement from normative research to an emphasis on individual differences.

Lazarus[55] and Serban[56] considered stress a cause of pathologic modes of adaptation to impairment of human functioning and cognitive and behavioral disturbances. For the sake of rehabilitative intervention, it is important to realize the interaction of personal characteristics with the external situation a patient is faced with, or feels faced with. The stress level can be considered the outcome of a reciprocal interaction between the individual and the environment. Such interaction plays a significant role in any strategy the individual utilizes to manage the world and him- or herself. Faulty coping will result in an abundance of stressors, which diminishes one's coping ability. Because much of what constitutes a stressor depends on one's perceptual functioning, psychological and emotional guidance and support may diminish the amount of stressors perceived and falsely created. Such support from the therapeutic environment would most likely result in improved adaptation to one's **life events,** which would encompass those major changes that confront the newly disabled individual.

Much of the literature on stress and coping in general has identified major life events as stressors. Life events refer to major changes in life-style, status, **role,** or situation. This view is consistent with the notion that stress, though individually mediated, is to some degree environmentally based and/or exacerbated by environmental and social conditions. Various life event measures have been developed and are used in assessing potential environmental stress. One of the better known and used assessment instruments is the **Holmes-Rahe Social Re-adjustment Rating Scale** (Appendix A), which quantifies the effects of life changes on stress and health.[57] Such measures of life events assume a relatively global impact, and take into account only those items listed. Although there is justified validity in such an approach, there exist potentially more sensitive and valid measures, one of which is the "Hassles Scale."

The **Hassles scale** (Appendix B) developed by Kanner et al.[58] is increasingly recognized in recent literature. This scale requires subjects to identify the irritating and frustrating demands of everyday transactions with the environment. This approach takes into account the individual's perception, or cognitive mediation, of events felt to pose a threat. It is consistent with the theoretical assumption that struggle with chronic difficulties may tax coping abilities and lead to greater difficulties in attempting

to manage events encountered in daily life. Empirical evidence indicates a more direct association and a greater predictability of health and emotional outcome through measuring one's daily hassles. It has long been established that major alterations in social circumstances can produce deleterious effects on mental and physical well-being.[59]

Considering the enormous changes in many aspects of one's functioning when disability strikes, patients are more likely to expect an increase in daily hassles and a relative increase in the amount of stressors confronting them. Dealing with life becomes more taxing when disabling circumstances block one's coping style, resulting in a greater gap of the person's fit within his or her world and contributes more stress to an already overstressed situation. This becomes even more profound when one of the aspects in need of adjusting is the core of the self, the self-image.

In our introduction, the evolving "self" was shown to be part of a unitary integrated life. Part of that self-image is the body as well as the roles one plays within one's world. These roles can be profoundly affected by disablement. A brief review of the implications of these inevitable changes to the self-image will help the physical therapist gain a better understanding of the disabled patient.

Role and status changes, as part of our developmental growth are expected and accepted. In our early life we start a process of maturation, become more independent, and gradually evolve into the various roles that life experience brings about. These changes are rather rapid during the early stages in life and slow down as the years pass. Even though most of these changes are biosocially guided and anticipated, they still become stressors as evidenced by the Rahe-Holmes study. It should therefore be of no surprise that unanticipated events, generated by disruptive accidental occurrences rather than by one's natural biological and social flow, will assume a much higher stress level. Berger[60] states that the ensuing emotional devastation can assume a dangerous proportion. Such a situation will often even lead to emotional suicide, a triggering of a slow kind of physical self-destruction or actual suicide.

Durkheim,[59] the "father of sociology" and one of the first to conduct a scientific study of suicide, stated that one of the major factors in suicide is the discrepancy between the expected and the achieved. We can indeed see that it is not so much the condition people are in but where they think they ought to be that shapes their disappointments. It follows that the more an individual expects out of life the more he or she will experience disappointment when such expectations are cut short by a traumatic event. It seems that a child who has not built up expectations of independence can find it easier to adapt to a disability than a person who achieved, or was about to achieve, independent status. A **congenital** disability or one that develops gradually may not be as emotionally devastating as one that disrupts prior expectations that may have been realistic in the premorbid state but become unachievable when disablement strikes. It is clear that the type of onset and the stage of life which a person with a disability is in will have important implications.

ROLE THEORY

Role theory appears to have significant predictive value in explaining human interaction. Berger[61] notes that "Role Theory, when pursued to its logical conclusions, does far more than provide us with a convenient shorthand for the description of various social activities. It gives us . . . a view of man based on his existence in society." Berger defines role as "a typified response to a typified expectation." A **role** then, analogous to that of an actor in a play, is the "part" played by an individual during interaction with another individual playing another part.

These related parts have in them a **script,** which defines the general behaviors, feelings, and acts belonging to each "part." Labovitz[62] correctly expands the notion that roles are both the collection of rights and duties and the behavior attached to a position. It is the "pattern according to which the individual is to act in the particular situation." Simply put, a role is a specified cluster of behaviors and expectations attached to each distinct, identified relationship to another person or persons. Some example of roles are male, female, athlete, patient, brother, wife, professor, policeman, and so forth. Each role carries certain expectations of behavior such as dress, attitude, and the like, each of these becoming a part of the individual's make-up and identity. Each individual takes on or is assigned many different roles in the course of a lifetime, which are enacted individually or simultaneously. Roles provide the individual with an identity, predictability in social intercourse, and parameters of behavioral expectations, both his or hers and that of others. Roles help society and the individual put order and predictability of expectations from others in his or her world and in personal interactions by delimiting and defining how each individual must behave.

A role, then, is a script for behavioral limits and responsibilities in social interaction and a social artifact with analogous roles differing from culture to culture. It is, however, a powerful and important artifact in that it defines and prescribes status, social behavioral and interactional patterns, social identity vis-à-vis self and others, and organizes and adds predictability to daily life. Roles are shaped and defined by the culture or society and have internal and interrelated meanings and relationships to each other within the culture that defines them. Role theory holds that these roles are not innate, but are rather conditioned and learned. They are social manifestations and are defined socially. As McCandless[63] notes, "through implicit and explicit codes, most of which have a moral, or right-wrong overtone, societies set up standards of behavior for their members." From the point of view of the individual, learning or fulfilling a role, whether ascribed or attained, is largely an unconscious, unreflective process. The powerful impact of this process on the individual lies in its unconscious nature. "The role forms, shapes, patterns both action and actor."[61] Accepting the role of "female," which is difficult not to accept, because it is an **ascribed role,** implies accepting the identity of a female, the behaviors, dress, activities, preferences, and feelings of a female. Roles, as Berger[61] notes, "Carry with them both certain actions and the emotions and attitudes which belong to these actions."[61]Mead,[64] a progenitor of role theory, asserted that the genesis of the self is the same event as the individual's discovery of society. In discovering and defining oneself, the individual is representing one's society in oneself, and is the reflection of how society shaped and defined the individual. This notion seems analogous to Cooley's **"looking glass self,"** whereby the child begins to define him or herself and develops his or her identity from the way others treat and interact with the child.[65]

Many proponents of role theory, such as Goffman[66] and Blumer,[67] view self-identity as developing in a negotiation process that takes place with two or more people as they establish their social roles. The **self and self-identity** are derived from the social roles assumed through the evaluative and comparative process to others in the social and interactive universe. One's self is defined primarily in regard to one's roles.

All this illustrates the significance of roles and what a role change might mean to an individual. We also referred to what an individual might be going through after having sustained a severe loss of function and relative independence, change of lifestyle and self-image, social interaction, financial and vocational upheaval, and body comfort. How then does one adjust to these upsetting changes?

Obviously such adjustment will be quite individualistic and is affected by any or all of the following: preexisting coping style and conditions, the responsibility or blame one feels about the illness or injury, the value a person sets on the self and the meaning of the loss, the reality of the conditions that have changed as a result of the situation, the messages received from within and without, the support/rejection balance of circumstances, and the functioning capacity of the body and mind.

ADJUSTMENT AS A FUNCTION OF ROLE, SOCIETAL VALUES AND SELF-IMAGE

Labovitz,[68] in discussing the interrelation between roles, self-identity, self-perception, and the way they either aid or interfere with adjustment, states that "It is largely through the process of 'role taking' that one's self-identity (or personality) develops . . . it is assumed that self-identity, self-image, or personality emerge from socialization . . . ."

It can be assumed that any change of status as

well as any change in abilities or physical attributes bring with them an impact in this interactional negotiating process. Through this process we constantly adjust our own view of ourselves and internalize the positive or negative value messages we receive from these interactions.

This process is not fully determinative and depends on how these messages are filtered through our own perceptions. However, these changes in the responses of others interact with changes in ourselves in the negotiating processes of social interactions. This ever-changing interaction process constantly adjusts and shapes our view and the modes of interactions with our surrounding world as well as the fit between it and ourselves.

Messages of assurance and support enable forward positive movement toward stable and vital adjustment. Studies have shown that even drastic and encompassing disablement can be incorporated as part of a self-image that is positive, adjusted, and stable. Weinberg[69] found that 50 percent of those disabled early in life would chose not to revert to their pre-disabled state. The need to reestablish self-identity with a change in physical appearance or abilities can work against lifelong patterns and developed images as well as internalized societal values. In western society, the image of disablement most often carries a negative value. Livneh[70] classified the sources of the negative values as follows: sociocultural conditioning, childhood influences, psychodynamic mechanisms, disability as a punishment for sin; anxiety-provoking unstructured situations, aesthetic aversion, threats to body image integrity, minority group comparability, disability as a reminder of death, as well as prejudice inviting behaviors. Indeed, the disabled tend to view themselves as different in both psychological as well as physical dimensions. In a study about the introjection of societies' negative views by the disabled, Weinberg and Asher[71] found no difference when comparing the view toward the disabled between the able-bodied and the disabled themselves. Identical findings were also reported by Gokhales[72] and others. Wright[73] tells us that positive life attitudes will not thrive when the focus is on the disabling aspects of a disability.

Constructive views within a coping framework can be an excellent venue for providing positive attitudes. The ability to see the person as a whole with particular strengths and weaknesses, particular attributes of which the disablement is only one factor is a more realistic and constructive approach. Although such a message may seem implicit to the physical therapist, the need to verbally reinforce and restate this viewpoint to the patient and the family facilitates cooperation and positive adjustment.

SOCIAL SUPPORT

The psychosocial perspective would hold that the extent of a disability is, in large part, dependent on the nature and extent of the physical and social resources available to those afflicted. Evidence abounds suggesting that social support plays a strong preventative and palliative role in a wide range of physical and medical conditions.[74–82] The physical therapist will have a strong impact on physical resources such as adaptive equipment and environmental devices to smooth out life for the patient with a disability. The therapist should also be cognizant of and encourage the social supports available to the patient. Social support is defined as the availability of other persons in the environment who can potentially offer either instrumental or emotive support such as financial or material help, a listening ear, advice, or encouragement. Mackelprang and Hepworth[83] state that the availability of social support exerts a direct impact on the speed and adequacy of adjustment and the overall happiness and quality of life. Similar findings are reported by Flaherty,[84] Dean et al.[85] Gallo,[86] Maddox,[87] MacMahon and Pugh,[88] Schultz and Moore,[89] Maguire,[90] Ward et al.[91] Quam,[92] and Clark.[93] These studies confirm the palliative benefit that a social support network exerts on the recovery and adjustment process as well as its potential impact upon patient management.

Crisp[94] reports that perceived levels of social support, among other factors, were predictive of higher levels of psychological adjustment to disabling conditions. Rintala et al.[95] found that the amount of social support was directly related to a sense of life satisfaction and sense of well-being in patients with spinal cord injury. Hardy et al.[96] and Kaplan[97] both found that high social support was predictive of return to vocational functioning after rehabilitation.

Social support not only mediates the impact of a disability and hastens positive adjustment as noted above, it also mediates some of the other psychological reactions stemming from a trauma or disability. Research suggests that events disrupting expectations of life or life activities are strongly associated with depression, regardless of the extent of disruption or the extent of the disability.[98–102] In fact, some researchers, such as Kishi et al.[103] have asserted that failure of recovery from depression stemming from disability may originate from lack of adequate social support. As with other psychological factors, it is the appraisal of the event or appraisal of the extent of impact that appears to be most determinative of the level of depression. For example, Langer[104] reports that patient self-ratings of disability were more predictive of depression than other ratings. Other reports have shown that severity of depression was not related to the severity of the illness or disability.[105] Regardless, social support is shown to have a mediating effect on depression.[106] Considering that withdrawal[107] and depression are some of the commonly found and generally expected initial reactions of a patient to his or her condition and that social exposure is likewise diminished with the advent of a disabling condition, it becomes clear that the beneficial effect of social support has to be part and parcel of treatment planning. This area holds important implications for the physical therapist because social support can be used to enhance treatment interventions and promote patient compliance.

STAGES OF ADJUSTMENT

Depending on the interactive intensity of all the above factors, adjustment will be relatively rapid or prolonged, adaptive or maladaptive. The literature reviewed indicates the prevalence of a stage type of emotional adjustment to physical traumatization. The described stages seem to indicate that after the initial stage of shock and anxiety reaction, most individuals go into a **denial stage,** which may last from several days to weeks. During this stage the individual may believe that the loss will be restored or may not even exist. Repression, daydreaming, or fantasy are other expressions of this stage.

Denial may at times mask depression or anxiety, which are believed to be an expected outcome of the condition the patient is in. When denial eventually lifts, the third reaction stage of grief **(grief reaction stage)** may exhibit itself in forms such as depression and/or mourning and might become complicated by exaggerated self-blame, which may or may not be realistic. The symptoms of this grief reaction will be similar to those found in the mourning following the loss of a loved one. The grief reaction, as is true in mourning reaction, needs to be resolved by the patient in order to move on with life. Anger **(anger reaction stage) and hostility,** the fourth reaction stage, usually assumes the form of projections or externalization of blame, anger, and hostility. Negativism, rebelliousness, opposition, and noncompliance are other forms of expressing this anger. Resolution of this stage should preferably culminate in an eventual **adaptive reconciliation (acceptance)** with the newly created reality. Conversely, the patient may instead end up in a maladaptive retreat and **regression.**

These stages of adjustment are within the realm of expected reactions that help the individual deal with the severity of the situation in which they find themselves. Siller[108] considers such reactions essential for the process of living through the traumatic period and working through a reconstitution of a personality structure. Accordingly, unbearable affects are "displaced, delayed or disguised suggesting a clinical picture of their absence." These are obvious generalizations, but can be used as general guidelines within the context of the unique aspects of each individual case. Although the stages might be quite similar, the content of individual reactions may differ significantly from person to person. As is true for the rest of the population, individuals with disabilities are different from each other in their personal preferences. Whereas some patients may feel vulnerable and ashamed about their helplessness and dependency, others will feel secure and may even savor the care provided. Some will show resiliency while others will not.

POSTTRAUMATIC STRESS AND EMOTIONAL COMPLICATIONS

Apart from the less common lapses into a severe psychotic state, a more common psychopathologic reaction is either **acute stress disorder (ASD),** or posttraumatic stress disorder (PTSD). Both are specific forms, or subsets, of "Anxiety Disorders." *The Diagnostic Statistical Manual of Mental Disorders* is the authoritative reference and criteria guide for mental health diagnosis, and differentiates between both disorders in terms of the duration of the disorder and its symptoms. ASD involves symptoms that must range in duration between 2 days to 4 weeks, whereas PTSD is differentiated as "acute PTSD" if the symptoms last less than 3 months, and as "Chronic PTSD" with the persistence of symptoms for 3 months or longer. Both ASD and PTSD, however, must result from exposure to a traumatic event, and PTSD can be qualified with the term "With Delayed Onset," if symptoms first occur at least half a year after the traumatic event. Research notes that PTSD is an expected outcome for a certain percentage of patients experiencing even mild traumas.[109–112] Others, such as Schreiber and Galai[113] report that it is the secondary stressors that are more predictive of PTSD; others highlight the complexity or subjectivity of PTSD.[114,115]

Among the symptoms exhibited are one or more of the following: re-experiencing the traumatic event; numbing of responsiveness to, or reduced involvement with, the external world; and/or a variety of autonomic, **dysphoria,** or cognitive symptoms. The re-experiencing of the event is described as recurrent, painful, **intrusive recollections,** dreams and nightmares, and on rare occasions dissociative-like states during which the individual may act as if reliving the actual traumatic event. This may take only several minutes but may last hours and even days.

It is worth reemphasizing at this point that the rehabilitation team may be prone to thinking about stress as the concept relates to physical systems. There are stressors that will undoubtedly affect everyone (e.g., immersion into extremely cold water). The severity of the effect depends on objective factors such as the temperature of the water and the duration of immersion and will be mitigated by the physical health and capacity of the person immersed. Yet when we consider circumstances that involve emotions, such as anxiety, helplessness, or fear, the range of potential impact of mediating factors becomes exponential. Remember, these latter situations are dependent on perception, experience, temperament, and all the other factors that can allow an identical situation to overwhelm one person to the point of psychological and social dysfunction and another person to make adjustments and continue in stride. An example of this can be noticed in the "polar bears," a group of people who voluntarily enter the icy water of Coney Island Beach on New Year's Day, and others who accidentally fall through the ice on the same beach.

Although in both cases the physical stress to the body may be similar, there is no emotional stress in the first case but probably a severe one in the second.

The numbing of responsiveness, also called psychic **numbing or emotional anesthesia,** is expressed by complaints of feeling detached or estranged from others, a loss of ability or interest in previously enjoyable activities, or the lack of any emotions or feelings. The other possible symptoms are excessive autonomic arousal, hyperalertness, exaggerated startle response, and difficulty falling asleep. Also listed in DSM-IV are other symptoms, such as sleep interruption, recurrent nightmares, impairment of memory, concentration or task completion ability, and survival guilt in those cases were others were also affected during a catastrophic event. Horowitz[116] describes the latter two symptoms as the intrusive and the denial states, respectively. The first is a super-alert type of reaction expressed in anticipatory anxiety, excessive alertness, and constant scanning to a point of perceiving things that are not there (hallucinations). The denial reaction is in direct contrast to the first in that it exhibits itself in a diminution of responsiveness to the condition.

Additional associated features that should alert the physical therapist to the presence of PTSD are increased irritability, hostile behavior, constant tension, and somatic stress symptom. Other emotional reactions specific to sudden onset of a disabling condition are brief reactive psychoses immediately following the event. The emotional turmoil and the delusions exhibited may diminish after several hours or may last several weeks. Modlin[117] found that about one-third of the patients with trauma he assessed exhibited a chronic type of **free-floating anxiety,** concentration and memory difficulties, nightmares and muscle tension, and sexual and social difficulties. These are the typical posttraumatic psychopathologies found among the patients whose disability was due to a catastrophic or sudden onset. Many disabilities are more gradual or anticipated as a result of an expected outcome of illness. Patients with such conditions may also succumb to similar emotional disruptions and dysfunctions. Because their condition progresses at a slower pace the adjustment requirements are not as intense. But like the proverbial straw that breaks the camel's back, a point may be reached that tips the balance. Such balance loss may be triggered indirectly or by issues other than the disability, such as a spouse who can no longer bear the engendered difficulties, or a boss who will not accept the productivity loss or other such conditions. The outcome may result in an emotional avalanche that is no less devastating in its effect than a sudden accident. Whether sudden or gradual, the loss can, and will, leave psychological wounds and scars on the individual. We all have our breaking point and a limitation of personal resources. At periods when stress becomes more than the individual's coping repertoire is capable of dealing with, the fluidity of adaptive capacity may be overtaxed, resulting in a variety of maladaptive responses, even in individuals who would otherwise be able to cope more appropriately. This is certainly true in disablement. The aforementioned reaction stages the patient goes through do not always ward off the severe onslaught of the trauma, pain, dramatic life changes, or losses experienced. Instead of the positive attempts at an eventual reconstruction of personality, faulty coping, severe depression, regression, and even psychosis or suicide may ensue.

Other severe forms of psychopathology may gradually develop after the trauma and sometimes appear right at the beginning. These pathologic reactions would predominantly fall within the depressive and anxiety disorder categories. Less debilitating reactions, but still affecting every aspect of life, would include phobic avoidance, **lability,** guilt, addictions, and other self-defeating behaviors as well as suicide attempts. Any signs of severe reaction or inappropriate lack of reaction should be indicators of a need to consult the mental health professional.

Similarly any protraction over periods beyond that which is considered typical for mourning, anger, depression, anxiety, withdrawal, and other such behaviors should not be ignored. Prolonged depression will usually indicate a process depression that is more serious than what may be called a reactive depression, which can be expected to appear during times of emotional upset. Lack of rehabilitative progress in patients expected to do better is a marker that should not be ignored. Other signs to look for include an increase in alcohol intake or smoking, accident proneness, suicidal ideation, and excessive use of tranquilizers, sedatives, and other drugs, as well as changes in sleep and food patterns. A breakdown of cognitive functioning, confusion, disorientation, illogical thinking, lack of reality testing, childlike dependencies, and/or exaggerated fears are all danger signals that require immediate attention.

Most of these described reactions are usually ignored and are mistakenly considered to be minor problems or stay unnoticed altogether. The visible absence of emotional problems is no guarantee of their absence, neither should minor problems be considered as such unless clinically confirmed.

Because PTSD is a specific diagnostic entity, it is not the responsibility of the rehabilitation team to determine a diagnosis or to treat the syndrome. This is, of course, true for any psychological or emotional difficulty. In all cases, however, the rehabilitation team members should have an awareness of the salient clinical features to determine the need for a mental health consultation. It should be clear at this point that some degree of emotional reactivity is to be expected from almost everyone requiring physical therapy expertise and services. The difference between a natural, expected response and a pathologic response requiring immediate attention is often a difference in the degree of the response, the duration of the response pattern, and frequently of the specific type of response. There are some response patterns that, by their very nature, would clearly trigger the physical therapist to seek consultation, while others can perhaps be difficult to gauge regarding their seriousness or meaning without further investigation. Armed with certain knowledge, the physical therapist may be able to recognize, address, and mitigate common emotional responses. An overview of suggested practices to deal with these responses will be presented later in the chapter. Box 2–1 summarizes some of the prominent behavioral indices that are found as features of PTSD to be used as a guide to the rehabilitation team as to behaviors which should trigger concern of PTSD and of the need for a mental health consult.

Locus of Control

There is yet another, related construct that the rehabilitation team may find of value in mitigating some of the behaviors identified in Table 2–1, in promoting positive rehabilitation outcomes, and in facilitating patient engagement and compliance in the treatment regimen. This is the broad concept of locus of control. Although this construct has generated vast amounts of research and theory with wide implications both as a mediating agent and as a treatment issue, we will highlight its relevance within the context of a rehabilitation setting. **Locus of control** generally refers to the perception held by an individual of the level of influence that individual has, regarding the events of life, or a specific event. It is loosely tied to the distinction made in labeling a person as either inwardly or outwardly directed and has significant influence on such issues as how much control over one's life and life events one feels to possess. This clearly has significant ramifications in shaping feelings such as helplessness, hopeless-

ness, or lethargy and withdrawal versus feelings of optimism, empowerment, and ability to take responsibility for one's life, situation, health, or rehabilitation. Classic studies by Weiss[118–120] have demonstrated that primates exposed to electric shocks over which they had no control, forewarning, or ability to mitigate developed ulcers and other symptoms of physical stress as well as a plethora of anxiety responses, bizarre behaviors, and lethargy. Other primates, given some ability to mitigate or anticipate the shocks, exhibited no such symptoms. Other studies have demonstrated the counterpart in human functioning.[121–123] Other researchers, such as Seligman[124] and Selye,[37,125,126] have contributed to a deeper understanding of these issues. Studies with humans revealed better coping abilities, diminution of deleterious effects, quicker recoveries, increased motivation, hope, energy, and a greater proactive stance when the held perception involved a sense of influence on the experience, its process, or outcome.

Although a patient's perception of locus of control serves as a mediating factor influencing the response to the onset of the disability, the utility of this construct is greatest for the physical therapist during treatment itself. The patient's perception of his or her role and influence in the treatment process can readily be influenced by the therapist in most cases. Accordingly the therapist can empower the patient through education and clarification of the nature of the situation, giving the patient an understanding of his or her part in shaping the outcome. Including the patient in all phases of goal setting and treatment planning may, at first blush, appear to be a time-consuming activity of little obvious benefit. However, it does have great benefit in the long run. Involving the patient in planning serves to reinforce and shape whatever perception of appropriate control the patient may have in shaping his or her life. It also engenders a greater level of engagement with the therapist and with the overall treatment, enhances the probability of optimum treatment outcome, and may reduce the time for which skilled intervention is needed.

PHYSICAL REHABILITATION AND EMOTIONAL FUNCTIONING

It is imperative that the rehabilitation team be alert to the implication of emotional disorders and the adjustment process. The team should be able to differentiate between those emotional reactions expected as a result of a given illness or injury and the appearance of a severe process of pathology. Such an awareness can have significant implications for the rehabilitation process and the future survival of the patient. In dealing with disabling trauma and disease the physical therapist stands out as the front line clinician in the rehabilitative effort. The patient will usually spend more time and be more intimately involved with a particular therapist than with most other health professionals.

Consequently the therapist is more apt to notice

> ### Box 2–1 WARNING SIGNS OF POSSIBLE POSTTRAUMATIC STRESS DISORDER (PTSD)
>
> **Any one of the following behaviors:**
>   I. Recurrent, intrusive recollection of traumatic event
> II. Intrusive and distressing dreams of event
> III. Disassociative states (behaving as if reliving event)
>   A. Can last from a few seconds to a few minutes
> IV. Amnesia of events
>
> **More than one of the following:**
>   I. Psychic numbing
>   A. Lack of interest in social or physical environment or activities
>   B. Significantly lowered participation in social or physical environment or activities
> II. Unable to feel emotions (intimacy, love, sexuality, anger, etc.)
> III. Disturbed sleep patterns
> IV. Hypervigilance
>   V. Exaggerated startle response
> VI. On-going level of irritability
> VII. Heightened difficulty with concentration

and effect changes in the emotional problems of a given patient. The therapist who is alert to the psychological dynamics of adjustment, maladjustment, and how they interact with each other and within the rehabilitative effort, can be expected to have a healing effect beyond that of the physical interventions administered. In many instances the effect of such alertness to the emotional state of the patient will enhance his or her satisfactory life adjustment through the maximization of dormant potentials. Accordingly rehabilitation should be considered as much more than the physical restoration, replacement, or acceptance of physical loss. Trieshman[127] deems rehabilitation a process "of learning to live with one's disability in one's own environment." We add here that such learning should include the utilization and shifting of one's premorbid, underutilized, or unrealized potentials. As aptly stated by Trieshman, the learning process dynamic is one "That starts at the moment of injury and continues for the remainder of the person's life."

There is no definable end point that can be labeled "rehabilitated" or "adjusted" because, as with all people in all areas of life, people with disabilities are continually learning to adapt to their environment. Like everyone else, the person with a disability has to be able to gain some rewards and fulfillment to "continue to endure the fatigue and frustration that life with a physical disability may include."[127]

STABILIZATION AND REINTEGRATION

It becomes imperative that the physical and medical treatment goals and outcomes contain the restoration of the secondary, emotional impairment created by the trauma of the physical disability. Restoration of physical function, activities of daily living (ADL) training, and vocational retraining alone will go only so far and no more. Even successful psychotherapy within the walls of the hospital will not ensure successful reintegration back to the premorbid environment. Until the hospitalized patient is prepared for reintegration to outside life, discharge may be counterproductive. The patient as well as his or her family have to be prepared for the social, emotional, sexual, and financial adjustments they will have to face within their respective home arrangements and community environment. Until then, rehabilitation should not be considered complete. The changes from the **patient role** to the giving up on that role can be as devastating as the original change to patient role; this may result in significant levels of depression, anxiety, and lack of social integration as exhibited in the studies by Berk and Feibel[128] and Udin and Keith.[129] Most of what was discussed so far addressed the posttraumatic adjustment period during which the major involvement of rehabilitation takes place. The stabilization period was described as the third and final stage, during which the patient is expected to enter into a relatively adjusted and stabilized state of living. As stated previously, adjustment and stabilization do not imply beneficial adaptation. Stabilization therefore indicates a balanced fit of one's functioning within one's world regardless of whether it is adaptive or maladaptive.

All of this points to the importance that the quality of the stabilization period takes on. It is this latter period during which the patient is experiencing the quality, and even the value, of the life toward which our clinical efforts are aimed. It is easy to lose sight of the fact that, in some respects, the operational period within which the rehabilitation team is exerting efforts can be compared to or is analogous with the gestation period of pregnancy. It is the preparation for the life after birth when life takes on its real meaning. Likewise, it is the stabilization period following the posttraumatic adjustment when life again becomes meaningful (or meaningless) with the rehabilitation team members acting as the "midwife" whose input can indeed make a difference.

Being alert to all the needs of the patient as well as to the signs and symptoms of maladaptation during the posttraumatic adjustment period is therefore vital for a good "delivery." It points again to the need for an integrated holistic approach, the focus of which has to include the psychosocial aspects of disability together with the physical rehabilitation interventions. This chapter aims to alert clinicians to all that the wounds, illness and injury open up. Interacting with the other members of the clinical team becomes therefore paramount for the clinician regardless of one's specialty. Close communication and collaboration among all rehabilitation team members is paramount to achieving optimal patient outcomes.

INTERACTIVE CLINICAL TEAM APPROACH

Having considered the enormity of the problem and the uniqueness of each case, it becomes clear that rehabilitation demands a clear understanding of premorbid life-style and desired patient outcomes. Insight into a patient's background, status, spiritual and cultural values, the perception of the handicapping condition by the patient, as well as the patient's philosophy of life will enhance the physical therapist's capacity as a healer. Above all, skills in observing and listening to what the patient says, either in words, expressions, joking, or crying, are important in this process. A patient's interaction with others and any differences exhibited depending on whether these interactions occur with other patients, staff, or friends and family are the clues the therapist has to be alert to.

Collecting all this data and becoming familiar with the scientific findings about human psychosocial functioning will help develop the needed tools to enhance therapeutic efforts. It will enable turning emotional disruptions around and put these in the service of the rehabilitation process.

To this end a cooperative effort among the many clinical disciplines in the rehabilitative effort is essential. Integration of the physical therapy interventions with those of the other health professionals, combined with an awareness of each profession's boundaries and limitations, will engender team work and give the patient a better chance for maximizing compensatory functioning within his or her place in the world. This will be a place adjusted to the reality of the new circumstances imposed by the disability.

This underscores the importance of the team approach of clinicians from the various disciplines. Rehabilitation is an encompassing term that includes many disciplines and techniques, each one of which specializes in different aspects of the rehabilitative effort yet shares many aspects of the rehabilitation process. It may therefore be tempting for one therapist to let the other therapists "do their thing" while the other one does his or hers. The return of physical functioning can seldom, if ever, succeed unless the emotional aspects of the patient's functioning are considered or enhanced and psychological techniques incorporated into the treatment.

This is not to say that a therapist should go beyond the boundaries of one's profession or specialization when treating patients. The psychologist should not do physical therapy nor should the physical therapist treat or diagnose emotional illness; but the utilization of some psychological techniques and an alertness to emotional problems have to be considered to optimize physical therapeutic intervention.

The interactive team approach can enhance rehabilitation work by sharing each other's expertise in a cooperative effort. The mental health professional can hardly be effective without the input from the rehabilitation team and their perspectives from patient observations. In return, the mental health worker can help the rehabilitation effort through evaluation of the patient's intellectual capacity, motivation, and emotional functioning.

The mental health professional can advise about patient management and the use of psychological techniques for direct or indirect intervention of problem patients and problems with patients. Likewise, the mental health professional can provide and assist in the utilization of specific techniques for stress and pain management. Another area that some members of the mental health team are specialized in is discharge planning, family therapy, and the use and enhancement of social and natural support networks.

EVALUATION AND PSYCHOLOGICAL TESTING

A thorough evaluation of the patient's psychological and social functioning can significantly contribute to a better understanding of needs, fears, anxieties, and capacities that may be utilized in the rehabilitative effort. It may guide the therapeutic effort toward a more rapid and appropriate recovery

effort and may prevent unnecessary, frustrating attempts toward less realistic goals. The importance of psychological and cognitive assessment is exemplified by a case in which gait training was attempted with a patient who was cognitively limited. That patient, once able to ambulate after a cerebrovascular accident (CVA), walked across a stairway as if it was a regular flat floor. The broken hip would have been prevented if cognitive functioning had been assessed prior to gait training. Proper evaluation of psychological rehabilitative capacity will minimize the frustration and any eventual loss of motivation shared by the patient, the family, and the staff when rehabilitative efforts are exerted beyond the capacity of the patient.

Such assessment has been proven to furnish essential information about the patient's emotional adjustment to the disablement, assets and liabilities, personality structure, and perceptual-motor and cognitive functioning. These can then be utilized to better understand coping barriers and behavioral difficulties, and in the development of strategies for dealing with overt or covert interpersonal and intrapersonal difficulties. Beals and Hickman[130] showed that psychological assessment of readiness to return to work for individuals with back injury was more predictive than that of physician reports. Psychoneurological testing such as the Halstead-Reitan Neuropsychological Battery has been shown to detect brain damage better than electroencephalography, x-rays, brain scan, or neurological evaluations.[131] Tsushima and Wedding[132] found the Halstead-Reitan Neuropsychological Battery to be as accurate as that of a computerized axial tomography (CAT) scan. These authors also found **neuropsychological assessment** more sensitive in detecting subtle brain damage than clinical medical assessment.

Subtle damage may have no gross medical implications but should prove of great importance for rehabilitation because it may seriously interfere with the patient's learning capacity. Psychological assessment is especially helpful in assessing subjective symptomatology, hypochondriasis, or malingering and can be especially useful when dealing with such complaints as pain, headaches, or vertigo. Such assessments require the specialized expertise of the psychologist and neuropsychologist. Psychologists, psychiatrists, clinical social workers, occupational therapists, and counselors also specialize in other assessment methods that can reveal personality and social problem areas, educational potential, and vocational and learning capacity. These assessments are geared toward individual patient needs. Although not inclusive, Box 2–2 highlights the major areas of consideration in a mental health assessment. These mental health assessments are limited to what the authors consider most significant for the process of rehabilitation. The derived findings of these assessments can direct the rehabilitative efforts toward the areas that can most benefit from therapeutic intervention.

Box 2–2 MAJOR AREAS OF CONSIDERATION IN A MENTAL HEALTH ASSESSMENT

1. Present and premorbid intellectual, emotional and coping functioning.
2. Present and premorbid psychopathologies and personality structure and diagnosis of levels of depression, anxiety, and other mental disabilities.
3. Evaluation of suicidal, decompensation, and other risks.
4. Degree of organicity and cognitive disability and its relationship to the patient's rehabilitative capacity.
5. Symbolic meaning of the disability and loss, and the compensatory reserves that can be elicited.
6. Frustration tolerance, motivation, and secondary gain interference.
7. Pain, stress, and tolerance evaluation.
8. Assessment of vocational interests and background, and present functioning capacity.
9. Sexual attitudes and dysfunction.
10. Assessment of the present and pre-morbid family structure and interaction, social and economic status and the natural support network (environmental support systems).

DISABILITY AND MENTAL HEALTH PRACTICE

Within the constraints of this discussion we will highlight some intervention methods aimed at overcoming psychological disruptions, maladaptive defense mechanisms, and the enhancement of motivation toward recovery. Apart from direct intervention, the mental health clinician can consult and assist the rehabilitation team in the utilization of psychological and behavior-modification principles available for patient management and the rehabilitation effort. The results of psychosocial assessment can highlight strengths that should be optimized and weaknesses that should be corrected or compensated for. In order to maximize the benefits that can be derived from the mental health team it is important to realize the different specializations that make it up. A brief description of each of the mental health disciplines is given in Box 2–3. Within these professions there are multiple subspecialties. These include neuropsychology, neuropsychiatry, psychoanalysis, **behavioral medicine,** behavior modification, forensic psychiatry and psychology, geriatrics, group therapy, family and marital therapy, sex therapy, stress and pain reduction, **biofeedback,** and hypnotherapy.

Mental health clinicians can render significant help in dealing with special problems (e.g., discharge planning and the use of environmental support groups, which have been proven to be invaluable in mainstreaming patients back to a comparatively integrated life). The significance of self-help groups as a most effective resource for reintegration into society has been documented by Lieberman and Borman.[133]

Another area of great concern is the sexual functioning or the lack of it during disability. This is an area beyond the scope of this writing. Of necessity we have left out all issues relating to the family of the disabled individual, including their own reactions to the disability and its victim. According to Hartman et al.,[134] these reactions encompass a broad range of human feelings. We can only touch on this as well as on the other important areas mental health workers deal with, such as family and marital therapy. These can play a major role in the rehabilitative effort and their techniques can be utilized directly by patients and family members, or through their counsel, indirectly.

Crisis Points in the Rehabilitative Process

At an earlier point, we presented the adjustment process and the stages or periods each individual intrinsically moves through as adjustment to disability takes place. It should now be clear that the adjustment process is influenced and shaped by the interplay of both internal and external factors. The provision of service can also be seen to have its

---

Box 2–3 THE MENTAL HEALTH TEAM

1. The psychiatrist is a medically trained physician specializing in mental disorders and their treatment.
2. The psychologist has a doctorate in one of the psychological specialties. The individuals most involved in the rehabilitation process are: the clinical psychologist specifically trained in diagnostic assessment and treatment of personality and emotional dysfunctions. Additional specialization would include neuropsychology and **behavioral medicine** as well as health and counseling psychology. For certain patient populations the role of child psychology as well as school, educational or industrial psychology can assume great importance.
3. The clinical, psychiatric, and social case workers (social workers), are trained in the assessment and intervention of environmental, social, and family dysfunction and their interaction with the individual's adjustment and functioning.
4. The occupational therapist is trained in assessment of psychosocial and cognitive function. Emphasis is on relationships between deficits in these areas and associated functional impairments.
5. Counselors and/or counseling psychologists are also trained practitioners who deal with the social emotional state of the patient through either verbal therapies or behavioral modalities, individually or in groups. Counselors can focus on emotional adjustment issues and interpersonal issues when the level of pathological reaction is mild or moderate.
6. Other therapists, such as speech language and pathologists, art therapists, dance and movement therapists, vocational counselors, rehabilitation counselors, psychiatric nurses, and pastoral counselors specialize in their distinctive support areas.

own structure and process. Regardless of where one receives health services in this country, treatment often might involve the various phases from acute hospitalization, to inpatient rehabilitation, discharge, outpatient or clinic care, and finally to reintegration into general life. Each of these treatment points present the patient with an externally imposed identity (e.g., inpatient), an imposed, universal external reality (ward living, dependence on nurses, removal/isolation from outside world, etc.). The process and structure of treatment that we superimpose presents its own stress points and its own reality as an almost universal or common impingement on psychosocial adjustment. Because these experiences are common enough, it behooves us to consider their impact on the adjustment process.

Each new phase of treatment or therapy has its own meaning for the patient, presents its unique set of challenges to cope with, face, or overcome, and presents often a physical and social environment unique to that phase. These realities both require accommodation as well as shape accommodation and adjustment. Admission to an acute care facility or initial hospitalization generally occurs during the initial stages of accommodation. The reality of this environment can often give further impetus and added meaning to the patient's initial sense of the significance of their personal crises and feelings of loss, depression, and helplessness. Conversely, this experience can also be utilized by the patient to focus on themselves without the impingement of day-to-day concerns and allows safely taking time to grieve and to adjust. Such an environment often can help to break down or mitigate initial denial as growing awareness of their environment and of their circumstance or permanence of the disability or illness imposes its unavoidable reality.

During the inpatient experience, and occasionally even on an outpatient basis, the changing status of other patients often present as crises and adjustment periods. New admittance, death, or discharge of other patients on the ward or in treatment can easily precipitate a personal crisis or imposed adjustment. This can occur whether or not a personal relationship had been formed with the other patient. A new admittance can very easily trigger personal recollections, concerns, and/or a reengagement with their own denial or avoidance issues. Discharge or death engenders reappraisal of the patient's own mortality and danger and raises questions about their own rehabilitation potentialities, degree of disablement, any one of which can present and does impose a crisis in adjustment. Other, less obvious triggering points include staff tension, family disputes or reactions, and even family opinions about treatment or goals.

The patient's own discharge and/or termination from service can be seen as another crisis point. This event, however anticipated, generally raises a questioning of the patient regarding capacity to function outside the protective environment of the treatment facility. This event often also serves to reinforce the reality of the disablement, however mild or severe, and also serves to raise and reintroduce the feelings, thoughts, fears, and anxieties experienced around the initial disablement. Discharge often raises awareness of the loss of security and safety of the hospital environment and of the support and care of the staff there. Although it is a cliché, it is nonetheless true that change, great or small, is difficult for most of us. Leaving a protective and supportive environment is difficult under any circumstance, as for example, evidenced by the universally recognized problem college freshmen experience upon leaving home for the first time or their return to the postcollege world after getting their degree. While hospitalized, it is easier to deny both the severity of one's disability or even one's differentness than when interacting with the general population. Upon discharge the patient is unconditionally forced to confront the physical and social otherness in the nonhospitalized population and the stigma or difficulties engendered therein. This universal point of crisis commonly can result in the development of obstacles to discharge such as reinjury, falls, regression, new complications, and the like. These can be conscious or unconscious, as can be other sabotage attempts and/or a sudden, inexplicable increase of complaints of pain or of inability to function.

The rehabilitation worker should be aware of the above crisis points but generally needs to be cognizant of our overriding assertion that the environmental impact on psychosocial adjustment includes the realities of the structure and the process of treatment imposed upon patients. We have listed some traditional treatment impacts, but future treatment trends will also impose their own imprint on the adjustment process. There are some new trends that may have profound impact on patient adjustment. These current trends include a push for abbreviated hospitalization, emphasis on accelerated treatment procedures, brief or short-term treatment, and a generally increasing shift toward outpatient rather than inpatient treatment where possible, warranted or dictated by insurance companies or other financial dictates. Although increased efficiency and efficacy are laudable goals that the authors support, care must be taken in judging the readiness of the patient for discharge as well as for each new phase of treatment. This becomes particularly important considering their impact on adjustment. Psychosocial adjustment must be considered alongside the physical adjustment. Premature discharge and abbreviated treatment protocols may present additional emotional adjustment issues that need to be assessed and considered by the entire treatment team. Natural responses such as initial denial, depression, mourning, and the overall emotional adjustment to physical disability cannot be abbreviated or forestalled, and require their own process over time.

Deciding on a Mental Health Consult: Behaviors Indicating Adjustment Problems

As the physical therapist interacts with the patient, there will undoubtedly be times when concern is raised in the mind of the therapist as to the patient's reactions and their potential meaning regarding adjustment. Some reactions will be clear and will prompt the therapist to seek a consultation with the mental health team, whereas others, probably most reactions, will appear to be ambiguous as to their meaning or importance. Although it is impossible to note all of the potential warning signs of poor adjustment, some general pointers are offered. Table 2–1 identifies patient reactions that should receive attention from the physical therapist.

While examining the table, it is advisable to keep in mind as a general rule that the disturbance noted must produce clinically significant distress and/or significant impairment of personal and interpersonal functioning. If unsure, it might always be safer to err in favor of being overly concerned. Be sure to note whether the behaviors and underlying verbalizations are a one-time occurrence, situationally determined, transient, or persist over time.

As described, certain emotional responses are normal and expected whereas others require professional mental health intervention. We can always expect to note some signs of depression and grieving, for example. Some patients will have their coping response overwhelmed at the outset due to the interplay between the perceived or real severity of their state and their premorbid psychological state. Others may deteriorate over time as coping

Table 2–1 PATIENT BEHAVIORS WARRANTING A MENTAL HEALTH CONSULT

Regression	Regression involves reverting to earlier, more immature patterns of functioning. This may be more commonly observed in children but might be observed in adults as well. For example, children may revert back to sucking their thumb, or may appear to have lost their toilet training skills, etc. Regression in adults may generally be seen in lost skills and abilities and/or even in the extreme behavior of reverting to taking a fetal position.
Disorientation	Disorientation is confusion as to time, place, activity, self-identity, or identity of others. Occasional, transient disorientation is not wholly uncommon in the average person, yet persistence in frequency or duration of occurrence is cause for assessment and intervention. Any more extreme confused behaviors and thought processes need to be carefully examined.
Delusional thinking	Delusional thinking refers to faulty and mistaken beliefs and, although related to inaccurate interpretation of environment, is distinguished by the persistence of this belief system. This can run the gamut from delusions of grandeur or of persecution, to delusions about the nature and scope of a disability. These delusions hold up and persist in the face of contrary information.
Inaccurate interpretation of environment	This is the broadest category in this list, but fortunately is also the most readily understood category. Clearly when a patient significantly misinterprets and misunderstands the objective situation and reality about them, it is probably most readily noted by non-mental health practitioners in its many expressions. This should draw attention and intervention, not only in its extreme form of a psychotic break, but also in its minor form of small, repeated episodes of misinterpretations.
Inappropriate affect	Affect refers to the mood state displayed by the patient, where feelings such as joy, sadness, fear, and so forth are reflected in body language, facial expression, and verbalizations. Inappropriate affect can be seen in an affective expression alien to the situation; for example, demonstrating and expressing joy upon hearing bad news. It also refers to a split between displayed affect and verbalization; for example, the verbal expression of mourning and condolence offered while smiling brightly and jumping for joy.
Hypo- or hypervigilance	Hypovigilance can be noted in a patient being oblivious to his or her surroundings and the events around them, socially, as well as physically. Hypervigilance refers to an intense focus and alertness to social and physical surrounds. Each of these have different ramifications and meaning to the mental health team. Suffice it to say that a consult is suggested as either extreme is approached.
Mood swings	We all experience changes in mood, yet hopefully, most of the time these changes are relatively appropriate reactions to external determinants, such as the receipt of news and information or to changing occurrences and circumstances in our environment. Although changeable, moods are generally persistent and stable. When mood shifts either to extremes and/or with some frequency, it suggests either instability or that mood is being driven predominantly by internal rather than external factors.
Self-destructive behaviors	Any self-destructive behavior, particularly ones that persist, are cause for serious concern. Self-destructive behaviors can run the gamut from subtle, difficult to detect signs to very clear and frightening overt signs. Subtle signs can include noncompliance with treatment regimen, poor self-maintenance activities such as not eating, overeating, diminishment of personal care, and hygiene, or carelessness in negotiating the environment. Clearer signs can include self-inflicted wounds and suicidal ideation and expressions. This important issue is covered in greater depth at a later point.
Normal behaviors taken to extremes	Normal human behavior enjoys a wide latitude of response repertoire before drawing attention as being out of expected bounds. This latitude must usually be extended further when dealing with someone undergoing a more extreme, traumatic, or stressful experience. Someone confronted with a disability would be expected to naturally focus their attention, concerns, and anxiety around this issue. The level of focus on a left leg given by someone preparing to have that leg amputated would be considered obsessive in a healthy ambulatory person, yet normal here. Care in judgement is required by the clinician when determining behavior expressions. That said, issues such as obsessiveness, extreme distractibility, immobilization in the face of routine decisions, and unexpected egocentricity or self-denigration may require a consult. An overly compliant patient, an extremely calm patient, as well as an overly contentious, argumentative, or extremely anxious or hysterical patient also requires concern. Any response (verbal or behavioral) that appears unwarranted to the stimuli should draw attention. Overreactions in opposite directions or any behavior which appears to be at an extreme, using reasonable judgement, deserves attention.

strategies fail them. Others may adjust positively to their new condition and integrate their identity into an appropriate functional, full, objectively realistic participation in all aspects of life. Lack of appropriate affect after a disablement (e.g., acting as if nothing happened) should raise a red flag. Adjustment to disability includes adjustment to these psychological factors as well.

SUGGESTIONS FOR REHABILITATIVE INTERVENTION

We have further delineated some important issues and offer a list of potential signs that might suggest inappropriate and pathologic response patterns that should alert the therapist to seek consultation. The list provided in Table 2–2 is not meant to be fully inclusive or determinative, but again, as hallmarks for further consideration. Judgement and care is required and it is also important to bear in mind that even mild expressions of any of the behaviors suggesting pathologic response patterns can become chronic or pathologic over time (Table 2–2).

As we have seen, human reactions, response patterns, and the adaptation process are variable and individualistic. Each patient must ideally be addressed as an individual and the physical therapy regimen must consider and adjust to individual characteristics, responses, and needs. It is therefore impractical to cover all the possible responses and situations with a list of applicable and inclusive practice principles. There are, however, certain general practice principles or approaches we might suggest. These might be derived from the literature as applicable and potentially helpful to the majority of patients as these set a general atmosphere of communication and cooperation toward joint goals of a positive outcome. Some of these are undoubtedly familiar to the physical therapist as simply good practice. We wish, however, to present the rationale from a psychosocial perspective as to the potential impact of these practices. The mental health practitioner, as the expert, should be consulted and looked to for guidance and the mental health practitioner will provide the expertise to help shape and influence the nature of the patient-therapist relationship, its norms, atmosphere, and nuance of interaction. The patient has his or her part in shaping the nature of the relationship as well. The more compliant the patient, often the more influence the physical therapist may have in shaping the nature of the relationship. It is incumbent upon all rehabilitation team members to consciously utilize this opportunity for positive ends. We can sometimes forget the powerful influence we have in setting the tone of this interaction. The very structure and atmosphere of service delivery, the personality and type of communica-

Table 2–2 BEHAVIORS SUGGESTING PATHOLOGIC RESPONSE PATTERNS

Grieving	Depression	Damaged Self-Esteem	Heightened Possibility for Suicide	Heightened Possibility for Violence
Grieving for actual or perceived impairment of functioning or actual loss is normal and expected, but the following might serve as clues to a more severe reaction: Denial of problem or its severity Exaggeration or idealizing the loss Obsession with the past or the preloss state Obsession with guilt related to loss Regression Difficulty with concentration Loss of interest in activities and events Lability of mood Inability to discuss loss Fear of being left alone Acting out behaviors (tantrums, suicidal gestures, promiscuity) Angry stance	Flat affect (showing little emotion) Very low energy levels Manic energy and behavior Psychomotor retardation (slowing down of movement and action) Ruminating about negative thoughts Change in eating and sleeping patterns (insomnia or hypersomnia) Regression Social withdrawal Self-destructive behaviors Loss of interest in environment, people, and events Self-blame and self-criticism	Isolation from social sphere Self-destructive behavior Inability to sustain eye contact Inability to accept praise Judgemental attitude Self-deprecating and self-critical Unwarranted pessimism Unconcern for appearance Unconcern for personal safety	Depression Giving away possessions Hoarding/hiding medications or potential weapons Writing suicide note Updating will Verbalizing loneliness or hopelessness Statements regarding benefit of release of pain, absence, etc. Intrusiveness of such thoughts	Low threshold for anger Depression High anxiety state Motoric agitation Self-mutilation Oversensitive Argumentative Inability to express feelings Fears of abandonment Highly dependent Disassociative states

tion given by the practitioner all have strong influence on patient participation and response to your efforts.

Optimizing Patient Involvement

To the degree possible, the patient should be involved as fully as possible in his or her own treatment. This includes involvement in goal setting and treatment planning as well as in ongoing assessment of progress. This is, of course, dependent on clear explanation and communication with the patients as to their situation, realistic physical therapy treatments, potential outcomes, and so forth. Doing so will serve to empower the patient and allow for increased motivation and participation in treatment regimen and follow through. This should engender a heightened engagement in cooperation and trust with the therapist. Patients' sense of enhanced control and ability (locus of control) will also increase and hopefully mitigate the sense of helplessness and sense of responsibility for the outcome.

Maintain Optimistic but Realistic Outlook

The physical therapist must be honest and realistic in all communication with the patient. Expected rehabilitation outcomes, however meager, can be presented as positive goals. It is important to encourage and remind the patient of all success and progress, however small, however obvious, so as to instill hope, increase motivation, and encourage continued struggle against the disability.

Limit Use of Jargon and Labels

Labeling a patient's behaviors or approach is often self-defeating in that it is a generalization highlighting just one aspect of the patient and promotes a rigidity of perception that misses the reality that no one is truly one characterization. Rather, a stance in which the therapist is receptive and open will encourage listening and communication. Real listening will reveal the patient's concerns and issues. Clear and articulate communication is not always easy but is compounded when emotion (i.e., anxiety), import, unfamiliarity of topic or situation, or power discrepancies impinge on the dialogue, as they most always do under therapist patient situations and make true communication more difficult. Hearing the patient's real communication can calm the patient and offers a sense of input and control to their rehabilitation efforts. Perhaps as important, it often mediates first impressions received by the physical therapist.

Enforce Independence and Self-Reliance

It may sometimes appear easier to do for the patients than to have the patients do for themselves, particularly when many patients will likely encourage this. Enforcing self-reliance and independence whenever feasible fosters engagement and responsibility on the part of the patient. Not doing so fosters helplessness and dependency and slows progress in the long term.

Rehabilitation Team Members' Self-Awareness

Finally, and perhaps most importantly, being aware of and in touch with your own feelings, motivations, and reactions can be crucial to understanding patient response and adjustment difficulties. It also raises awareness of actions on the patient's part, or your part, which interfere with progress. It is natural to sometimes react or respond to others because they consciously or unconsciously remind one of someone else, such as a sibling, parent, or past significant other. The resulting behavior, whether positive or negative, obviates the characteristics or needs of the person these behaviors are directed toward because they often have little to do with that person. We can therefore become overprotective or, at the other extreme, give short shrift to a patient without realizing that this behavior on our part is both unfair and not helpful to this individual. Awareness of our own responses and reactions allows us to appropriately and realistically engage with the people before us and allows us an awareness of the feelings and responses their behavior raises in us. This objective awareness is the first step in an appropriate response to and understanding of the rehabilitation effort.

SUMMARY

Psychological and social adjustment to illness and physical trauma is a uniquely personal experience, dependent on innate and acquired characteristics as well as the many environmental factors impinging on an individual. The interplay between the physical damage and the physiological resources with the emotional self are but part of the determining forces affecting the outcome of illness or injury. Social pressures versus social support systems are an important force to be considered. These pressures can facilitate or hinder the treatment effort and the eventual outcome of rehabilitation. The personality structure that has evolved during a lifetime of innate and external conditioning, the acquired input of values and roles, and the individual's coping capacity are part of what the rehabilitation specialist must consider beyond the techniques available for treatment. Furthermore, the social milieu surrounding the patient—the hospital, family, finances, bias, sexual needs and pressures, and other available support systems—are all factors that shape successful recovery.

An important factor the rehabilitation team is constantly confronted with is the patient's personality. The understanding of the uniqueness of each and every individual becomes therefore mandatory. The knowledge that personality structure is the sum total of lifelong experience and a conglomeration of a very unique temperament, perceptual selectivity, set of ego defenses, and a perceptual structure of the self and the world, clarifies the idiosyncratic nature of individuals.

These then shape an individual's adaptive or maladaptive process. Coping skills combine both innate and learned adaptive behaviors and allow an individual to balance internal and external resources in the presence of conflicting biologic, psychological, and social needs. Ultimately, coping responses allow for survival of the individual, even though the outcome may be contrary to what seems best for the individual. Thus psychological adjustment is an intricate interactive process incorporating body mechanism and the external world, conscious perceptions of self as well as unconscious perceptions, motivation, emotions, drive, and values.

Reactions to disability are influenced by the extent of the injury, or illness, its mode of onset, prognosis, affected brain mechanisms, support systems, and subjective perceptions. The latter (subjective perception) is one of the major forces shaping the form the disability takes on, as well as being highly determinative of the adjustment and return of function.

The initial reaction to a catastrophic event or illness is primarily physiological (GAS) as the general adaptation syndrome. During the posttraumatic period, the psychological aspect of functioning assumes major importance. Such a response is defined as an attempt to cope with a real or imagined stimulus—a stressor—which is perceived as a threat to one's self or one's homeostatic balance.

The disabled person is more likely to experience increases in the amount of daily stressors. Role and status changes are also important parts of the disablement experience.

Adjustment may be rapid or prolonged, adaptive or maladaptive. Stages in the process of adjustment to loss and disability have been identified. Initial shock or anxiety is followed by progression through stages of denial, depression, and anger. The end result of this process may be the final acceptance of the newly created reality or, instead, a maladaptive retreat and regression. Adjustment may also be characterized by posttraumatic stress syndrome or other pathology. Therapists need to recognize their characteristic danger signs.

The physical therapist who considers these factors and makes them part of the methods and techniques of treatment intervention can indeed enhance the chances for recuperation. It would be an insurmountable task for a rehabilitation team member to become specialized in all areas significant to a patient. An ever-expanding knowledge base has clearly been influential in development of the number of health disciplines and specializations. Yet there is a dire need that every one of those specialists become cognizant of the rudiments of those areas that impinge on one's effectiveness. Such knowledge can only improve the understanding of a patient's level of cooperation, compliance, and attitude toward rehabilitation. The psychological dynamic of adjustment can be facilitated by an interactive team approach in which the contribution of all members is maximized. Rehabilitation should not be considered completed unless the patient and family are prepared for the social, emotional, and sexual adjustment they will have to face when the patient returns to home and community.

QUESTIONS FOR REVIEW

1. How does the general adaptation syndrome serve the body during a catastrophic event and at what cost?

2. Describe how an individual's attempt to best serve his or her survival needs may result in maladaptation.

3. In what conscious or unconscious ways might a disablement serve the needs of an individual to the degree that he or she might prefer to stay disabled?

4. Describe the difference in the needs for intervention comparing the traumatic reaction phase and the posttraumatic adjustment period.

5. Explain the meaning of psychic numbing and give the reasons for its development.

6. What is the importance of the role one plays in life in regard to disability?

7. Name five stages of adjustment to loss or disablement.

8. What are some of the features that should alert the physical therapist to the presence of posttraumatic stress disorder?

9. Describe the role of perception in the formation of a disability.

10. How can emotional factors create a disability?

11. Name some of the contributions of the various different mental health clinicians toward physical rehabilitation.

12. What are some of the major areas of consideration in a mental health assessment?

13. Identify potential crisis points in the rehabilitation process and describe some of the possible triggering points.

14. Identify and describe three potential patient behaviors that warrant a mental health consult.

15. Describe how you would recognize when the normal reactions of grieving and depression have become pathologic.

16. Describe how you can optimize patient involvement in the rehabilitation process and promote self-reliance.

17. At what point can one consider the rehabilitation process complete?

CASE STUDY

A young woman, whom for the sake of confidentiality we will call Mary, had been involved in an automobile accident where she sustained a serious spinal cord injury. She subsequently became hemiplegic as a result of the accident and was confined to a wheelchair. Mary was a 24 year-old single woman at the time of the accident. She was employed as a factory worker and was therefore completely self-supporting, though at levels not much above subsistence. Mary was a high school graduate living in a one-bedroom basement rental. Social contacts consisted primarily of a small number of acquaintances and sparse contact with her family of origin.

Mary was physically stabilized during the period immediately following the accident. Throughout, while receiving intensive medical intervention and all required medical procedures, she reacted essentially as a compliant and passive recipient. She did not draw special attention from either the medical team nor the rehabilitation team until it was noticed that her rehabilitation was not progressing as expected. The goals became modest, yet realistic, in that not much could be done for her except to teach her to function in a wheelchair and accept her condition. She was not disruptive and was therefore not referred for psychological intervention. Rehabilitation team goals were basic. These were to teach Mary self-help and self-care skills appropriate to her condition so as to enable continued self-sufficiency in daily life skills. Further goals consisted of teaching Mary to transport herself into and out of the wheelchair and to develop and improve body strength and mobility to accomplish all of the above tasks. The team reported that Mary was quite sad-looking, and followed all instructions without complaint. She appeared to be cooperative but it became apparent over time that she was clearly going through the motions without much effort, motivation, or results. The rehabilitation team was coming close to the conclusion that Mary was destined to end her life bedridden, or at best, having the ability to use a wheelchair yet remaining dependent for many of her ADL needs and dependent on public support for the rest of her life.

Guiding Questions

1. Having read the chapter, list some possible psychosocial issues requiring further exploration: what factors are interfering with Mary's recovery (physical and/or psychosocial factors)?

2. Is the patient inner or outer directed? How might the physical therapist utilize this knowledge/information in the service of treatment?

3. List potential social resources the physical therapist might draw on in treating or motivating Mary.

REFERENCES

1. Kennedy, P, et al: Childhood onset of spinal cord injury: Self-esteem and self-perception. British Journal of Clinical Psychology 34:581, 1995.
2. Sheerin, D, et al: Psychological adjustment in children with port-wine stains and prominent ears. J Am Acad Child Adolesc Psychiatry 34:1637, 1995.
3. Wade, S, et al: Assessing the effects of traumatic brain injury on family functioning: Conceptual and methodological issues. J Pediatr Psychol 20:737, 1995.
4. Wilcox, VL, et al: Self-rated health and physical disability in elderly survivors of a major medical event. J Gerontol B Psychol Sci Soc Sci 51B:S96, 1996.
5. Gleckman, AD, and Brill, S: The impact of brain injury on family functioning: Implications for subacute rehabilitation programs. Brain Inj 9:385, 1995.
6. Watts, R: Trauma counseling and rehabilitation. J Appl Rehab Counseling 28:8, 1997.
7. Gil, KM, et al: Coping strategies and laboratory pain in children with sickle cell disease. Ann Behav Med 19:22, 1997.
8. Phillips, M-E, et al: Work-related posttraumatic stress disorder: Use of exposure therapy in work simulation activities. Am J Occup Ther 51:696, 1997.
9. Wickramasekera, I, et al: Applied psychophysiology: A bridge between the biomedical model and the biopsychosocial model in family medicine. Professional Psychology Research and Practice 27:221, 1996.
10. Tam, SF: Pre-training self concept and computer skills learning outcomes of Hong Kong Chinese with physical disability. Journal of Psychology in the Orient 37:185, 1996.
11. King, GA, et al: Self-evaluation and self-concept of adolescents with physical disabilities. Am J Occup Ther 47:132, 1993.
12. Winkelman, M, and Shapiro, J: Psychosocial adaptation of orthopedically disabled Mexican children and their siblings. Journal of Development and Physical Disabilities 6:55, 1994.
13. Vargo, JW: Some psychological effects of physical disability. Am J Occup Ther 32:31, 1978.
14. Elliot, TR, et al: Problem solving appraisal and psychological adjustment following spinal cord injury. Cognitive Therapy and Research 15:387, 1991.
15. Weastbrook, M, and McIlwain, D: Living with the late effects of disability: A five-year follow-up survey of coping among post-polio survivors. Australian Occupational Therapy Journal 43:60, 1996.
16. Miller, D, et al: Psychological distress and well-being in advanced cancer: The effects of optimism and coping. Journal of Clinical Psychology in Medical Settings 3:115, 1996.
17. Hanson, SJ, et al: The relationship of personality characteristics, life stress, and coping resources to athletic injury. Journal of Sport and Exercise Psychology 14:262, 1992.
18. Dorland, S, and Hattie, J: Coping and repetitive strain injury. Australian Journal of Psychology 44:45, 1992.
19. Bermond, B, et al: Spinal cord lesions: Coping and mood states. Clin Rehabil 1:111, 1987.
20. Phillips, ME, et al: Work related traumatic stress disorder: Use of exposure therapy in simulation activities. Am J Occup Ther 8:696, 1997.
21. Hanson, S, et al: The relationship between coping and adjustment after spinal cord injury: A five-year follow-up study. Rehabilitation Psychology 38:41, 1993.

22. Mitchley, N, et al: Burden and coping among the relatives and caregivers of brain injured survivors. Clin Rehabil 10:3, 1996.

23. Kennedy, P, et al: Traumatic spinal cord injury and psychological impact: A cross-sectional analysis of coping strategies. Br J Clin Psychol 34:627, 1995.

24. Engel, GL: Guilt, pain and success. Psychosom Med 24:37, 1962.

25. Moos, RH: Coping with Physical Illness. Plenum, New York, 1977.

26. Ehrentheil, Otto F: Common medical disorders rarely found in psychotic patients. Archives of Neurology and Psychiatry - Chicago, 1957; 77:178–186.

27. Selye, H: The general adaptation syndrome and the disease of adaptation. J Clin Endocrinol Metab 6:117, 1946.

28. Heinrichs, SC, et al: Anti-stress action of a corticotropin-releasing factor antagonist on behavioral reactivity to stressors of varying type and intensity. Neuropsychopharmacology 11:179, 1994.

29. Theorell, T, et al: "Person Under Train" incidents: Medical consequences for subway drivers. Psychosom Med 54:480, 1992.

30. Mann, AM, and Gold, EM: Psychological sequelae of accident injury: A medico-legal quagmire. Canadian Medical Association Journal 95:1359, 1966.

31. Epstein, RS: Avoidant symptoms cloaking the diagnosis of PTSD in patients with severe accidental injury. J Trauma Stress 6:451, 1993.

32. Dollard, J, and Miller, NE: Personality and Psychotherapy: An Analysis in Terms of Learning, Thinking and Culture. McGraw-Hill, New York, 1950.

33. Ellis, A: Humanistic Psychology: The Rational-Emotive Approach. New York, Julian, 1973.

34. Lazarus, R: Psychological Stress and the Coping Process. McGraw-Hill, New York, 1966.

35. Malmo, RB: Overview. In Greenfield, N, and Sternbach, R (eds): Handbook of Psychophysiology. Holt, Rinehart & Winston, New York, 1972.

36. Kirtz, S, and Moos, RH: Physiological effects of social environments. Psychosom Med 36:96, 1974.

37. Selye, H: Stress. In: Health and Disease. Butterworth, Reading, MA, 1976.

38. Bourestom, N, and Howard, M: Personality characteristics of three personality groups. Arch Phys Med Rehabil 46:626, 1965.

39. Alexander, F: Studies in Psychosomatic Medicine. Ronald Press, New York, 1948.

40. Alexander F: Psychosomatic Medicine: Its Principles and Applications. Norton, New York, 1950.

41. Engel, GL, and Schmale, S: Psychoanalytic theory of somatic disorder: Conversion, specificity, and the disease onset situation. J Am Psychoanal Assoc 15:344, 1967.

42. Wittkower, ED, et al: A global survey of psychosomatic medicine. International Journal of Psychiatry 7:576–591, 1969.

43. Dunbar, F: Emotions and Bodily Changes, ed 3. Columbia Univ. Pr., New York, 1947.

44. Henry, JP, and Stephens, P: Stress, Health and the Social Environment. Springer, New York, 1977.

45. Eisler, R, and Polak, P: Social stress and psychiatric disorder. Journal of Mental and Nervous Disease 153:227, 1971.

46. Freud, S: Civilization and its discontent. In: The Standard Edition of the Complete Psychological Works of Sigmund Freud, Vol 21. 1930, p 64. NY: J. Cape and H. Smith Publishers.

47. American Psychiatric Association: Diagnostic and Statistical Manual of Mental disorders, ed 4. American Psychiatric Association, Washington, DC, 1994.

48. Ellis, A: Humanistic Psychology: The Rational-Emotive Approach. Julian, New York, 1973.

49. Woolfolk, RL, and Lehrer, PM: Principles and Practice of Stress Management. The Guilford Press, New York, 1984.

50. Kirtz, S, and Moos, RH: Physiological effects of social environments. Psychosom Med 36:96, 1974.

51. Ross, MJ, and Berger RS: Effects of stress inoculation training on athletes' postsurgical pain and rehabilitation after orthopedic injury. J Consult Clin Psychol 64:406, 1996.

52. Lazarus, RS: Patterns for Adjustment. McGraw-Hill, New York, 1976.

53. Malmo, RB: Overview. In Greenfield, N, and Sternbach, R (eds): Handbook of Psychophysiology. Holt, Rinehart and Winston, New York, 1972.

54. Lazarus, RS: Psychological Stress and the Coping Process. McGraw-Hill, New York, 1966.

55. Lazarus, RS: The concept of stress and disease. In Levi, L (ed): Society, Stress and Disease, Vol 1. Oxford Univ. Pr., London, 1971.

56. Serban, G: Stress in schizophrenics and normals. Br J Psychiatry 126:397, 1975.

57. Holmes, T, and Rahe, R: The Social Readjustment Scale. J Psychosom Res 11:213, 1967.

58. Kanner, AD, et al: Comparison of two modes of stress management: Daily hassles and uplifts versus major life events. J Behav Med 4:1, 1981.

59. Durkheim, E: Suicide. Free Press, Glenkove, IL, 1951.

60. Berger, PL: Invitation To Sociology: A Humanistic Perspective. Anchor Books, New York, 1963.

61. Berger, PL: Invitation To Sociology: A Humanistic Perspective. Anchor Books, New York, 1963.

62. Labovitz, S: An Introduction to Sociological Concepts. Wiley, New York, 1977, p 95.

63. MacCandless, BR: The socialization process. In Seidman, JM (ed): The Child: A Book of Readings. Holt, Rinehart and Winston, New York, 1969, p 42.

64. Mead, GH: Mind, Self, & Society. University of Chicago Press, Chicago, 1934.

65. Cooley, CH: Human Nature and the Social Order, rev ed. Scribner's, New York, 1922.

66. Goffman, E: The Presentation of Self in Everyday Life. Double-Day Anchor, New York, 1959.

67. Blumer, H: Symbolic Interactionism: Perspective and Method. Prentice-Hall, Englewood Cliffs, NJ, 1969.

68. Labovitz, S: An Introduction to Sociological Concepts, New York, John Wiley and Sons, 1977, p 98.

69. Weinberg, N: Physically disabled people assess the quality of their lives. Rehabilitation Literature 42:12, 1984.

70. Livneh, H: On the origins of negative attitudes toward people with disabilities. Rehabilitation Literature 43:338, 1982.

71. Weinberg, N, and Asher, N: The effect of physical disability on self perception. Rehabilitation Counseling Bulletin 20:15, 1976.

72. Gokhale, SD: Dynamics of attitude change. International Social Work 28:31, 1985.

73. Wright, BA: Developing constructive views of life with a disability. Rehabilitation Literature 41:274, 1980.

74. Kotchick, BA, et al: The role of parental and extra familial social support in the psychosocial adjustment of children with a chronically ill father. Behav Modif 21:409, 1997.

75. Ormel, J, et al: Chronic medical conditions and mental health in older people: Disability and psychosocial resources mediate specific mental health effects. Psychol Med 27:1065, 1997.

76. McColl, MA, and Skinner, H: Assessing inter- and intra-personal resources: Social support and coping among adults with a disability. Disabil Rehabil 17:24, 1995.

77. McColl, MA, et al: Structural relationship between social support and coping. Soc Sci Med 41:395, 1995.

78. Elliot, TR, et al: Social relationships and psychosocial impairment of persons with spinal cord injury. Psychology and Health 7:1, 1992.

79. Elliot, TR, et al: Assertiveness, social support and psychological adjustment following spinal cord injury. Behav Res Ther 29:485, 1991.

80. Kaplan, SP: Social support, emotional distress, and vocational outcomes among persons with brain injuries. Rehabilitation Counseling Bulletin 34:16, 1990.

81. Wong, DFK, and Kwok, SL: Difficulties and patterns of social support of mature college students in Hong Kong: Implications for student guidance and counseling services. British Journal of Guidance and Counseling 25:377, 1997.

82. Varni, JW, and Setoguchi, Y: Effects of parental adjustment on the adaptation of children with congenital or acquired limb deficiencies. J Dev Behav Pediatr 14:13, 1993.

83. Mackelprang, RW, and Hepworth, DH: Ecological factors in rehabilitation of patients with severe spinal cord injuries. Soc Work Health Care 13:23, 1987.

84. Flaherty, J: The role of social support in the functioning of patients with unipolar depression. Am J Psychiatry 140:473, 1983.

85. Dean, A, et al: The epidemiological significance of social support systems on depression. Research in Community and Mental Health 2:77, 1981.

86. Gallo, F: Social support networks and the health of elderly persons. Social Work Research and Abstracts 20:13, 1984.

87. Maddox, G: Persistence of life-style among the elderly: A longitudinal study of patterns of social activity in relation to life satisfaction. In Neugarten, B (ed): Middle Age and Aging. University of Chicago Press, Chicago, 1968, p 181.

88. MacMahon, B, and Pugh, TF: Epidemiology: Principles and Method. Little, Brown, Boston, 1970.

89. Schultz, NR, and Moore, D: Lankiness: Correlates, attributes, and coping among older adults. Personality and Social Psychology Bulletin 10:75, 1984.

90. Maguire, G: An exploratory study of the relationship of valued activities to the life satisfaction of elderly persons. Occupational Therapy Journal of Research 3:164, 1983.

91. Ward, RA, et al: Informal networks and knowledge of services for older persons. J Gerontol 39:216, 1984.

92. Quam, J: Older women and informal supports: Impact on prevention. Prevention and Human Services 3:119, 1983.

93. Clark, A: Personal and social resources as correlates of coping behavior among the aged. Psychol Rep 51:577, 1982.

94. Crisp, R: The long term adjustment of persons with spinal cord injury. Australian Psychologist 27:43, 1992.

95. Rintala, DH, et al: Social support and the well-being of persons with spinal cord injury living in the community. Rehabilitation Psychology 37:155, 1992.

96. Hardy, C, et al: The role of social support in the life stress/injury relationship. Sport Psychologist 5:128, 1991.

97. Kaplan, SP: Psychosocial adjustment three years after traumatic brain injury. Clinical Neuropsychologist 5:360, 1991.

98. Zeiss, AN, et al: Relationship of physical disease and functional impairment to depression in older people. Psychol Aging 11:572, 1996.

99. Lachmann, FM, and Beebe, B: Trauma, interpretation and self-state transformations. Psychoanalysis and Contemporary Thought 20:269, 1997.

100. Brewer, BW: Self-identity and specific vulnerability to depressed mood. J Pers 61:343, 1993.

101. Jorge, RE, et al: Comparison between acute and delayed onset depression following traumatic brain injury. J Neuropsychiatry Clin Neurosci 5:43, 1993.

102. Boekamp, JR, et al: Depression following a spinal cord injury. Int J Psychiatry Med 26:329, 1996.

103. Kishi, Y, et al: Prospective longitudinal study of depression following spinal cord injury. J Neuropsychiatry Clin Neurosci 6:237, 1994.

104. Langer, K: Depression and physical disability: Relationship of self-rated and observer-rated disability to depression. Neuropsychiatry Neuropsychol Behav Neurol 8:271, 1995.

105. Silverstone, PH, et al: The prevalence of major depressive disorder and low self-esteem in medical inpatients. Can J Psychiatry 41:67, 1996.

106. Zea, MC, et al: The influence of social support and active coping on depression among African Americans and Latinos with disabilities. Rehabilitation Psychology 41:225, 1996.

107. Leach, LR, et al: Family functioning, social support and depression after traumatic brain injury. Brain Inj 8:599, 1994.

108. Siller, J: Psychological situation of the disabled with spinal cord injuries. Rehabilitation Literature 30:290, 1969.

109. Wright, JC, and Telford, R: Psychological problems following minor head injury: A prospective study. Br J Clin Psychol 35:399, 1996.

110. Mayou, RA, and Smith, KA: Posttraumatic symptoms following medical illness and treatment. J Psychosom Res 43:121, 1997.

111. Epstein, RS: Avoidant symptoms cloaking the diagnosis of Posttraumatic Stress Disorder in patients with severe accidental injury. J Trauma Stress 6:451, 1993.

112. Bryant, RA, and Harvey, AG: Avoidant coping style and PTS following motor vehicle accidents. Behav Res Ther 33:631, 1995.

113. Schreiber, S, and Galai, GT: Uncontrolled pain following physical injury as the core trauma in the PTSD. Pain 54:107, 1993.

114. Perry, SW, et al: Predictors of PTSD after burn injury. Am J Psychiatry 149:931, 1992.

115. Sbordone, RJ, and Liter, JC: Mild Traumatic Brain Injury does not produce PTSD. Brain Inj 9:405, 1995.

116. Horowitz, MJ: Stress-response syndromes: Posttraumatic and adjustment disorders. In Cooper, AM, et al (eds): The Personality Disorders and Neuroses. Lippincott, Philadelphia, 1986, p 409.

117. Modlin, HC: The post-accident and anxiety syndrome: The psychosocial aspects. Am J Psychiatry 123:1008, 1967.

118. Weiss, JM: Effects of coping response on stress. Journal of Comparative and Physiological Psychology 65:251, 1968.

119. Weiss, JM: Effects of coping behavior in different warning signal conditions on stress pathology in rats. Journal of Comparative and Physiological Psychology 77:1, 1971.

120. Weiss, JM: Effects of coping behavior with and without feedback signal on stress pathology in rats. Journal of Comparative and Physiological Psychology 77:20, 1971.

121. Rodin, J: Managing the stress of aging: The role of control and coping. In Levine, S, and Ursin, H (eds): Coping and Health. Plenum, New York, 1980, p 171.

122. Halmhuber, NL, and Paris, SG: Perceptions of competence and control and the use of coping strategies by children with disabilities. Learning Disability Quarterly 16:93, 1993.

123. Craig, AR, et al: The influence of spinal cord injury on coping styles and self perceptions two years after the injury. Aust N Z J Psychiatry 28:307, 1994.

124. Seligman, MEP: Helplessness. Freeman, San Francisco, 1975.

125. Selye, H: The Stress of Life. McGraw-Hill, New York, 1956.

126. Selye, H: Stress Without Distress. Lippincott, Philadelphia, 1974.

127. Trieshman, RB: Spinal Cord Injuries: Psychological, Social and Vocational Adjustment. Pergamon, Elmsford, NY, 1980.

128. Berk, S, and Feibel, J: The unmet psychological and family needs of stroke survivors. Paper presented at The American Congress of Rehabilitation Medicine, New Orleans, November 1978. In Trieshman, RB: Spinal Injuries: Psychological, Social and Vocational Adjustment. Pergamon, Elmsford, NY, 1980.

129. Udin, H, and Keith, R: Patients' daily activities after discharge from a rehabilitation hospital. Paper Presented at American Congress of Rehabilitation Medicine, New Orleans, November 1978. In Trieshman, RB: Spinal Injuries: Psychological, Social and Vocational Adjustment. Pergamon, Elmsford, NY, 1980.

130. Beals, RK, and Hickman, NW: Industrial injuries of the back and extremities. J Bone Joint Surg 54A:1593, 1972.

131. Filskov, SB, and Goldstein, SG: Diagnostic validity of The Halstead-Reitan Neuropsychological Battery. Journal of Consulting and Clinical Psychology 42:382, 1974.

132. Tsushima, WT, and Wedding, D: A comparison of The Halstead-Reitan Neuropsychological Battery and computerized tomography in the identification of brain disorder. American Journal of Nervous and Mental Disease 167:704, 1979.

133. Lieberman, M, and Borman L: Self Help Groups For Coping With Crises. Jossey-Bass, San Francisco, 1979.

134. Hartman, C, et al: The neglected and forgotten sexual partner of the physically disabled. Soc Work 28:370, 1983.

SUPPLEMENTAL READINGS

Adamson, JD, and Schmale, AH Jr: Object loss, giving up, and the object of psychiatric disease. Psychonomic Medicine 27:557, 1965.

Ader, R (ed): Psychoneuroimmunology. Academic, New York, 1981.

Alexander, F: Studies in Psychosomatic Medicine. Ronald Press, New York, 1948.

Alexander F: Psychosomatic Medicine: Its Principles and Applications. Norton, New York, 1950.

American Psychiatric Association: Diagnostic and Statistical Manual of Mental Disorders. American Psychiatric Association, Washington, DC, 1987.

Anderson, TR, and Cale, TM: Sexual counseling of the physically disabled. Postgrad Med 58:117, 1975.

Beals, RK, and Hickman, NW: Industrial injuries of the back and extremities. J Bone Joint Surg 54A:1593, 1972.

Berger, PL: Invitation to Sociology: A Humanistic Perspective. Anchor Books, New York, 1963.

Berk, S, and Feibel, J: The unmet psychological and family needs of stroke survivors. Paper presented at The American Congress of Rehabilitation Medicine, New Orleans, 1980.

Blumer, H: Symbolic Interactionism: Perspective and Method. Prentice-Hall, Englewood Cliffs, NJ, 1969.

Bourestom, N, and Howard, M: Personality characteristics of three personality groups. Arch Phys Med Rehabil 46:626, 1965.

Brown, MR, et al (eds): Stress: Neurobiology and Neuroendocronology. Marcel Dekker, New York, 1990.

Burstein, A: Posttraumatic stress disorder in victims of motor vehicle accidents. Hospital and Community Psychiatry 40:295, 1989.

Cannon, WB: Bodily Changes in Pain, Hunger, Fear and Rage. Charles T. Branford Co., Boston, MA, 1950.

Chigier, E: Sexual Adjustment of the handicapped. Proceeding Preview of the 12th World Congress of Rehabilitation International, Sydney, Australia, 1972.

Chigier, E (ed): Sex and the Disabled. The Israel Rehabilitation Annual, 1977.

Clark, A: Personal and social resources as correlates of coping behavior among the aged. Psychol Rep 51:577, 1982.

Cook, R: Sex education program service model for the multi-handicapped adult. Rehabilitation Literature 35:264, 1974.

Cooley, CH: Human Nature and the Social Order, rev ed. Scribner's, New York, 1922.

Costella, CG: The adaptive function of depression. Canada's Mental Health 25:20, 1977.

Davidson, LM, and Baum, A: Chronic stress and posttraumatic stress disorders. Journal of Consulting and Clinical Psychology 54:303, 1986.

Dean, A, et al: The epidemological significance of social support systems on depression. Research in Community and Mental Health 2:77, 1981.

Dollard, J, and Miller, NE: Personality and Psychotherapy: An Analysis in Terms of Learning, Thinking and Culture. McGraw-Hill, New York, 1950.

Dunbar, F: Emotions and Bodily Changes ed 3. Columbia Univ. Pr., New York, 1947.

Durkheim, E: Suicide. Free Press, Glenkove, IL, 1951.

Ehrentheil, Otto F.: Common medical disorders rarely found in psychotic patients. Archives of Neurology and Psychiatry. Chicago, 1957; 77:178-186.

Eisenberg, MG, and Falconer, J: Current trends in sex education programming for the physically disabled: Some guidelines for implementation and evaluation. Sexual Disabilities 1:6, 1978.

Eisler, R, and Polak, P: Social stress and psychiatric disorder. Journal of Mental and Nervous Disease 153:227, 1971.

Elliot, TR, et al: Social relationships and psychosocial impairment of persons with spinal cord injury. Psychology and Health 7:55, 1992.

Elliot, TR, et al: Assertiveness, social support and psychological adjustment following spinal cord injury. Behav Res Ther 29:485, 1991.

Ellis, A: Humanistic Psychology: The Rational-Emotive Approach. Julian, New York, 1973.

Engel, GL, and Schmale, S: Psychoanalytic theory of somatic disorder: Conversion, specificity, and the disease onset situation. J Am Psychoanal Assoc 15:344, 1967.

Engel, GL: Guilt, pain and success. Psychosom Med 24:37, 1962.

Filskov, SB, and Goldstein, SG: Diagnostic validity of The Halstead-Reitan Neuropsychological Battery. Journal of Consulting and Clinical Psychology 42:382, 1974.

Flaherty, J: The role of social support in the functioning of patients with unipolar depression. Am J Psychiatry 140:473, 1983.

Ford, AB, and Orfirer, AP: Sexual behavior and the chronically ill patient. Medical Aspects of Human Sexuality 1:51, 1967.

Freud, S: Civilization and its discontent. In: The standard edition of The Complete Psychological Works of Sigmund Freud, Vol 21. 1930, p 64. Boston: J. Cape and H. Smith Publishers.

Gallo, F: Social support networks and the health of elderly persons. Social Work Research and Abstracts, 20:13, 1984.

Goffman, E: The Presentation of Self in Everyday Life. Double-Day Anchor, New York, 1959.

Gokhale, SD: Dynamics of attitude change. International Social Work 28:31, 1985.

Goodwin, DW, and Guze, SB: Psychiatric Diagnosis, ed 5. Oxford Univ. Pr., New York, 1996.

Hardy, C, et al: The role of social support in the life stress/injury relationship. Sport Psychologist 5:128, 1991.

Hartman, C, et al: The neglected and forgotten sexual partner of the physically disabled. Soc Work 28:370, 1983.

Heinrichs, SC, et al: Anti-stress action of a corticotropin-releasing factor antagonist on behavioral reactivity to stressors of varying type and intensity, Neuropsychopharmacology 11:179, 1994.

Henry, JP, and Stephens P: Stress, Health and the Social Environment. Springer, New York, 1977.

Holmes, T, and Rahe, R: The social readjustment scale. J Psychosom Res 11:213, 1967.

Horowitz, MJ: Stress-response syndromes: posttraumatic and adjustment disorders. In Cooper, AM, et al (eds): The Personality Disorders and Neuroses. Lippincott, Philadelphia, 1986, p 409.

Kaplan, SP: Psychosocial adjustment three years after traumatic brain injury. Clinical Neuropsychologist 4:360, 1991.

Kaplan, SP: Social support, emotional distress, and vocational outcomes among persons with brain injuries. Rehabilitation Counseling Bulletin 34:16, 1990.

Kanner, AD, et al: Comparison of two modes of stress management; daily hassles and uplifts versus major life events. J Behav Med 4:1, 1981.

Kirtz, S, and Moos, RH: Physiological effects of social environments. Psychosom Med 36:96, 1974.

Kotchick, BA, et al: The role of parental and extrafamilial social support in the psychosocial adjustment of children with a chronically ill father. Behav Modif 21:409, 1997.

Krantz, DS, and Glass, D.C.: Personality, behavior patterns, and physical illness: Conceptual and methodological issues. In Gentry, DW (ed): Behavioral Medicine. Guilford Press, New York, 1984.

Labovitz, S: An Introduction to Sociological Concepts. Wiley, New York, 1977.

Lazarus, RS: Patterns for Adjustment. McGraw-Hill, New York, 1976.

Lazarus, RS: Psychological Stress and the Coping Process. McGraw-Hill, New York, 1966.

Lazarus, RS: The concept of stress and disease. In Levi, L (ed): Society, Stress and Disease, Vol 1. Oxford Univ. Pr., London, 1971.

Lazarus, RS, and Folkman, S: Coping and adaptation. In Gentry, DW (ed): Behavioral Medicine. Guilford Press, New York, 1984.

Lieberman, MA: Adaptive process in late life. In Datan, N, and Ginsberg, LH (eds): Life-span Developmental Psychology. Academic Press, New York, 1975.

Lieberman, M, and Borman L: Self Help Groups For Coping With Crises. Jossey-Bass, San Francisco, 1979.

Livneh, H: On the origins of negative attitudes toward people with disabilities. Rehabilitation Literature 43:338, 1982.

McColl, MA, and Skinner, H: Assessing inter- and intrapersonal resources: Social support and coping among adults with a disability. Disabil Rehabil 17:24, 1995.

McColl, M, et al: Structural relationship between social support and coping. Soc Sci Med 41:395, 1995.

Mackelprang, RW, and Hepworth, DH: Ecological factors in rehabilitation of patients with severe spinal cord injuries. Social Work in Health Care 13:23, 1987.

MacCandless, BR: The socialization process. In Seidman, JM (ed): The Child: A Book of Readings. Holt, Rinehart & Winston, New York, 1969, p 42.

MacMahon, B, and Pugh, TF: Epidemiology: Principles and Method. Little, Brown, Boston, 1970.

Mcfarlane, AC: The phenomenology of posttraumatic stress disorders following a natural disaster. The Journal of Nervous and Mental Disease 176:22, 1988.

Madakasira, S, and O'Brien, KF: Acute posttraumatic stress disorder in victims of natural disaster. The Journal of Nervous and Mental Disease 175:286, 1987.

Maddox, G: Persistence of life-style among the elderly: A longitudinal study of patterns of social activity in relation to life satisfaction. In Neugarten, B (ed): Middle Age and Aging. University of Chicago Press, Chicago, 1968, p 181.

Maguire, G: An exploratory study of the relationship of valued activities to the life satisfaction of elderly persons. Occupational Therapy Journal of Research 3:164, 1983.

Malmo, RB: Overview. In Greenfield, N, and Sternbach, R (eds): Handbook of Psychophysiology. Holt, Rinehart & Winston, New York, 1972.

Mann, AM, and Gold, EM: Psychological sequelae of accident injury: A medico-legal quagmire. Canadian Medical Association Journal 95:1359, 1966.

Mead GH: Mind, Self, and Society. University of Chicago Press, Chicago, 1934.

Menninger, K: The Vital Balance: The Life Process in Mental Health and Illness. Vikings, New York, 1963.

Modlin, HC: The post-accident and anxiety syndrome: The psychosocial aspects. Am J Psychiatry 123:1008, 1967.

Moos, RH: Coping with Physical Illness. Plenum, New York, 1977.

Ormel, J, Kempen, et al: Chronic medical conditions and mental health in older people: Disability and psychosocial resources mediate specific mental health effects. Psychol Med 27:1065, 1997.

Patrick, GD: Comparison of novice and veteran wheelchair athletes' self-concept and acceptance of disability. Rehabilitation Counseling Bulletin 27:186, 1984.

Platt, J, and Husband, SD: Posttraumatic stress disorder and the motor vehicle accident victim. American Journal of Forensic Psychology 5:35, 1987.

Plutchik, R, and Kellerman, H, (eds): Theories of Emotion. Academic Press, New York, 1980.

Quam, J: Older women and informal supports: Impact on prevention. Prevention and Human Services 3:119, 1983.

Rintala, DH, et al: Social support and the well-being of persons with spinal cord injury living in the community. Rehabilitation Psychology 37:155, 1992.

Rodin, J: Managing the stress of aging: The role of control and coping. In Levine, S, and Seligman, H: Helplessness. Freeman, San Francisco, 1975.

Russell, RA: Concepts of adjustment to disability: An overview. Rehabilitation Literature 42:330, 1981.

Shuchter, S, and Zisook, S: Psychological reactions to the PSA crash. International Journal of Psychiatry in Medicine 14:293, 1984.

Schulz, R, and Decker, S: Long-term adjustment to physical disability. J Pers Soc Psychol 48:1162, 1985.

Schultz, NR, and Moore, D: Loneliness; correlates, attributes, and coping among older adults. Personality and Social Psychology Bulletin 10:75, 1984.

Schweitzer, NJ: Coping with stigma: An integrated approach to counseling physically disabled persons. Rehabilitation Counseling Bulletin 25:204, 1982.

Selye, H: The Stress of Life. McGraw-Hill, New York, 1956.

Selye, H: The general adaptation syndrome and the disease of adaptation. J Clin Endocrinol Metab 6:117, 1946.

Selye, H: Stress in Health and Disease. Butterworth, Reading, MA, 1976.

Serban, G: Stress in schizophrenics and normals. Br J Psychiatry 126:397, 1975.

Sigelman, CK, et al: Disability and the concept of life functions. Rehabilitation Counseling Bulletin 23:103, 1979.

Siller, J: Psychological situation of the disabled with spinal cord injuries. Rehabilitation Literature 30:290, 1969.

Sloan P: Posttraumatic stress in survivors of an airplane crash-landing: A clinical and exploratory research intervention. J Trauma Stress 1:211, 1988.

Syme, LS: Sociocultural factors in disease etiology. In Gentry, DW (ed): Behavioral Medicine, Guilford Press, New York, 1984.

Theorell, T, et al: "Person under train" incidents: Medical Consequences for Subway Drivers. Psychosom Med 54:480, 1992.

Thorn-Gray, BE, and Kern, LH: Sexual dysfunction associated with physical disability: A treatment guide for the rehabilitation practitioner. Rehabilitation Literature 44:138, 1983.

Trieshman, RB: Spinal Injuries: Psychological, Social and Vocational Adjustment. Pergamon, Elmsford, NY, 1980.

Tsushima, WT, and Wedding, D: A comparison of The Halstead-Reitan neuropsychological battery and computerized tomography in the identification of brain disorder. American Journal of Nervous and Mental Disease 167:704, 1979.

Udin, H, and Keith, R: Patients' daily activities after discharge from a rehabilitation hospital. Paper Presented at American Congress of Rehabilitation Medicine, New Orleans, November 1978. In Trieshman, RB (ed): Spinal Injuries: Psychological, Social and Vocational Adjustment. Pergamon, Elmsford, NY, 1980.

Ursin (ed): Coping and Health. Plenum, New York, 1980, p 171.

Versluys, HP: Physical rehabilitation and family dynamics. Rehabilitation Literature 41:58, 1980.

Ward, RA, et al: Informal networks and knowledge of services for older persons. J Gerontol 39:216, 1984.

Watts, R: Trauma counseling and rehabilitation. Journal of Applied Rehabilitation Counseling 28:8, 1997.

Weiss, JM: Effects of Coping response on stress. Journal of Comparative and Physiological Psychology 65:251, 1968.

Weiss, JM: Effects of coping behavior in different warning signal conditions on stress pathology in rats. Journal of Comparative and Physiological Psychology 77:1, 1971.

Weiss, JM: Effects of coping behavior with and without feedback signal on stress pathology in rats. Journal of Comparative and Physiological Psychology 77:20, 1971.

Weinberg, N: Physically disabled people assess the quality of their lives. Rehabilitation Literature 42:12, 1984.

Weinberg-Asher, N: The effect of physical disability on self-perception. Rehabilitation Counseling Bulletin 20:15, 1976.

Wittkower, ED, et al: A global survey of psychosomatic medicine. International Journal of Psychiatry 7:576, 1969.

Wollff, HG, and Itace, CC (eds): Life Stress and Bodily Disease. Williams & Wilkins, Baltimore, 1950.

Woolfolk, RL, and Lehrer, PM: Principles and Practice of Stress Management. Guilford Press, New York, 1984.

Wright, BA: Value laden beliefs and principles for rehabilitation. Rehabilitation Literature 42:266, 1981.

Wright, BA: Developing constructive views of life with a disability. Rehabilitation Literature 41: 274, 1980.

Yudofsky, SC, and Hales, RE: The American Psychiatric Press Textbook of Neuropsychiatry. American Psychiatric Press, Washington DC, 1997.

Zeitlin, S, and Williamson, GG: Coping characteristics of disabled and non-disabled young children. Am J Orthopsychiatry 60:404, 1990.

GLOSSARY

Acute stress disorder (ASD): A diagnostic subset of "stress disorders" generally indicating a sudden onset of relatively short duration. According to DSM-IV criteria, symptoms must range in duration between 2 days and 4 weeks, as opposed to a chronic stress disorder, which has a prolonged duration of symptomology.

Adaptation (adaptive): The ongoing, active process through which an individual adjusts to changing environmental life situations.

Adaptive reconciliation (acceptance): The fifth and final reaction stage of adjustment to physical disablement or loss. During this stage, the loss is no longer considered an obstacle to be overcome but as one of many personal characteristics; approaches to meeting personal needs with respect to realities of the life situation have been reconciled. In some instances acceptance is failed and the patient may instead end up in a maladaptive retreat and regression.

Adjustment: Alignment of one's inner needs with the realities of personal capabilities, and/or environment; may be adaptive or maladaptive.

Anger reaction stage (and hostility): The fourth emotional reaction stage of adjustment to physical disablement or loss manifested by animosity, negativism, rebelliousness, opposition, antagonism, and noncompliance.

Ascribed role: Implies the identity that one is born into, such as gender, and requires accepting the behaviors, dress, activities, preferences, feelings, and all that society accepts or decrees for that identity.

Behavioral medicine: A subspecialty in mental health that addresses the interaction of psychological factors with those of medical intervention and the disease process.

Biofeedback: A method of treatment and diagnostics that utilizes the measurements of physiological reactions through instrumentation to increase patient awareness and control of those reactions.

Cognition: The process by which an organism becomes knowledgeable. It is influenced by one's personality characteristics, emotional factors, and subjectivity. It is one of the most significant factors in determining an individual's way of dealing with one's world.

Congenital: A condition that an individual is born with; not necessarily genetic.

Coping: The process through which individuals deal with the variety of social and environmental factors encountered in life.

Coping style: An individual, evolved response repertoire that is relatively solidified and predictable.

Defense mechanisms: See *ego defense*.

Denial: An ego defense mechanism that is utilized to deny an unacceptable reality.

Denial stage: The second reaction stage of psychological adjustment to physical disablement or loss; an unconscious defense mechanism in which existence of unpleasant realities is blocked from conscious awareness.

Deviant: A term used to describe an individual's coping that is contrary to environmental standards.

Disability: Within this writing, the term is used to describe a reduction or loss of function that is directly or indirectly due to a real or imagined incapacity to function.

Disablement: Within this writing, the term is used to describe the actual, objective loss of function as a result of illness or accident.

Distress: A term denoting a negative perception or response to a stressor whereby the stressor becomes immobilizing, overwhelming, and so forth, initiating a sympathetic physiological stress response on the individual. Also see *stress reaction*, *eustress*.

DSM-IV: The revised fourth edition of the *Diagnostic Statistical Manual* of The American Psychiatric Association, which is the accepted manual for categorizing emotional disorders and their diagnostic indicators.

Dysphoria: Exaggerated feelings of depression; may be accompanied by anxiety.

Ego defense: Also called *defense mechanism*. The ego utilizes unconscious defense mechanisms to protect itself from real or imagined dangers, pressures, and conflicting demands through a process by which unpleasant realities are blocked from conscious awareness. Among these defensive mechanisms are rationalizations, projection, overcompensation, reaction formation, repression, and perceptual distortion.

Eustress: A term denoting a positive perception or response to a stressor whereby the stressor is seen as, or becomes, enervating or motivating, rather than overwhelming or negative. Also see *stressor*, *stress reaction*, *distress*.

Free-floating anxiety: A psychodynamic construct denoting generalized feelings of anxiety whereby the individual is unable to state or locate the source, cause, or reason for such feelings. The anxiety is not attached to a source or event (a specific feared object, such as an elevator, heights, and such, or a specific event, such as a job interview, or examination, and so forth).

General adaptation syndrome (GAS): An organism's immediate reaction to an extreme catastrophe; a defensive adaptation response aimed at dealing with real or perceived emergency situations.

Grief reaction stage: The third emotional reaction stage of adjustment to physical disablement or loss. It is distinguished by mental suffering, sorrow, and regret, and might become complicated by exaggerated self-blame which may or may not be realistic. The grief reaction, as is true in mourning reaction, needs to be resolved by the patient in order to move on with life.

Hassles scale: An instrument measuring the irritating and frustrating demands of everyday transactions an individual feels faced with.

Holmes-Rahe Social Readjustment Rating Scale: One of the better known and used assessment instruments that quantifies the effects of life changes on stress and health.

Innate: Characteristics determined by heredity.

Intrusive recollections: The experiencing of dreams and nightmares about disturbing events of the past; often experienced during the PTSD stage.

Lability: Emotional instability manifested by alterations or fluctuations in emotional state.

Life events: A term used to describe those major changes in an individual's life and considered to be a source of stress.

Locus of control: A construct attributed to Seligman (see references) that distinguishes the degree or location of attributed responsibility for one's situation or life events as well as the perception of the degree of control one is able to exert on life events or one's situation. For example, a person might have a strong "internal" locus of control, indicating the perception or belief that the person can indeed influence or change his or her life situation. "External" locus of control denotes the degree to which one feels that outside events—the social or physical environment—are determinative. Locus of control influences the degree of helplessness, or empowerment felt by the individual.

Looking glass self: A term suggested by Cooley whereby a child begins to define him- or herself and develops his or her identity from the way others treat and interact with the child.

Maladaptive: A term used to describe coping that is contrary to an individual's own best interest or survival; usually the result of faulty perception, learned rejection of the self, misguided values, or misinterpretations of reality.

Mental defense: Same as *ego defense mechanisms*, or *defense mechanisms*.

Nature and nurture: The first term describes inherited characteristics; while the second is reserved for those attributes developed as a result of environmental input.

Neuropsychological assessment: An evaluation system utilizing the measurement of behavioral and psychological expressions that seem to reveal subtle brain damage that may not be revealed by other neurological instruments.

Numbing or psychic numbing (emotional anesthesia): Feelings of being detached or estranged from others, a loss of ability or interest in previously enjoyable activities, or the lack of any emotions or feelings.

Patient role: According to role theory an individual will tend to grow into this role when becoming a patient; usually a painful transition that, once adjusted to, may create difficulties in returning to the premorbid role.

Perceptions: Response repertoire through which the individual combines information input with his or her personality structure.

Personality structure: The characteristics of a given individual and the respective internalized ideology, value system, and the behavioral tendencies one has accumulated.

Posttraumatic adjustment period: The second reaction stage of adjustment to physical disablement or loss; this is usually the time during which psychological effects of the traumatic experience are mostly felt by the patient.

Posttraumatic Stress Disorder (PTSD): Psychopathologic reaction to a traumatic event; symptoms exhibited may include re-experiencing the traumatic event; numbing of responsiveness to, or reduced involvement with, the external world; and/or a variety of autonomic, dysphoric, or cognitive symptoms.

Premorbid: The functioning and conditions of a patient prior to the present pathologic state; a reference point of the level of loss and deterioration.

Proscribed roles: The ethnic and social status roles one is born into.

Psychological adjustment: The intricate interactive process dictated by the conscious and unconscious motivations, emotions, drives, values, and perceptual functioning.

Regression: A return or retreat to a former state; a defense mechanism to illness or life frustration; characterized by appearance of less mature behaviors, which were successful during earlier periods of the individual's life.

Role: A specified cluster of behaviors and expectations attached to each distinct, identified, relationship to another person or persons; typified response to a typified expectation or as a part played by an individual in interaction with other individuals.

Script: A term within role theory that defines the general behaviors, feelings, and acts belonging to each part of the various roles an individual plays out in life.

Secondary gain: A concept that suggests that illness or disablement, regardless of severity, might also carry with it some secondary benefit to the person affected. Secondary gain should always be considered, especially in cases where the disablement or illness persists beyond the normal or typical time frame or where resistance to treatment or sabotage is suspected. This concept is useful in suggesting why some patients might tenaciously hold on to their condition. Some examples of secondary gain might include the gaining of sympathy, attention, or the ability to shirk responsibilities as a result of a disablement or illness.

Self and self-identity: Derived from the social roles assumed through the evaluative and comparative process vis-à-vis others in the social and interactive universe.

Self-image: A term used to describe the individual's self-perception as a part of a unitary integrated life-space. Part of that self-image is the body as well as the roles one plays within one's world.

Stabilization period: The final stage of psychological adjustment to injury or disablement characterized by a return to either a stable life adjustment to the condition or a return to premorbid functioning. See *traumatic reaction period, posttraumatic adjustment period.*

Stress reaction: The observable consequences of the stressor; accompanied by sympathetic signs and symptoms such as palpitations, cold sweat, faint feelings, dilated pupils, pallor, fear, and a host of other complaints.

Stressor: Any stimulus that evokes stress.

Style of coping: A unique style of coping and functioning characteristic of an individual's personality and developed during a lifetime.

Traumatic reaction period (or stage): The first emotional reaction stage of adjustment to physical disablement or loss; characterized by disbelief, tension, and an inability to acknowledge that the traumatic event took place.

APPENDIX A

Holmes-Rahe Social Readjustment Scale

Rank	Life Event	Mean Value	Rank	Life Event	Mean Value
1	Death of spouse	100	23	Son or daughter leaving home	29
2	Divorce	73	24	Trouble with in-laws	29
3	Marital separation	65	25	Outstanding personal achievement	28
4	Jail term	63	26	Wife begin or stop work	26
5	Death of close family member	63	27	Begin or end school	26
6	Personal injury or illness	53	28	Change in living conditions	25
7	Marriage	50	29	Revision of personal habits	24
8	Fired at work	47	30	Trouble with boss	23
9	Marital reconciliation	45	31	Change in work hours or conditions	20
10	Retirement	45	32	Change in residence	20
11	Change in health of family member	44	33	Change in schools	20
12	Pregnancy	40	34	Change in recreation	19
13	Sex difficulties	39	35	Change in church activities	19
14	Gain of new family member	39	36	Change in social activities	18
15	Business readjustment	39	37	Mortgage or loan less than $10,000	17
16	Change in financial state	38	38	Change in sleeping habits	16
17	Death of close friend	37	39	Change in number of family get-togethers	15
18	Change to different line of work	36	40	Change in eating habits	15
19	Change in number of arguments with spouse	35	41	Vacation	13
20	Mortgage over $10,000	31	42	Christmas	12
21	Foreclosure of mortgage or loan	30	43	Minor violations of the law	11
22	Change in responsibilities at work	29			

From Holmes and Rahe, with permission.[57]

APPENDIX B

The Hassles Scale

Directions: Hassles are irritants that can range from minor annoyances to fairly major pressures, problems, or difficulties. They can occur few or many times.

Listed in the center of the following pages are a number of ways in which a person can feel hassled. First, circle the hassles that have happened to you *in the past month.* Then look at the numbers on the right of the items you circled. Indicate by circling a 1, 2, or 3 how *severe* each of the *circled* hassles has been for you in the past month. If a hassle did not occur in the last month, do *not* circle it.

	Severity		
Hassles	1. Somewhat Severe	2. Moderately Severe	3. Extremely Severe
(1) Misplacing or losing things	1	2	3
(2) Troublesome neighbors	1	2	3
(3) Social obligations	1	2	3
(4) Inconsiderate smokers	1	2	3
(5) Troubling thoughts about your future	1	2	3
(6) Thoughts about death	1	2	3
(7) Health of a family member	1	2	3
(8) Not enough money for clothing	1	2	3
(9) Not enough money for housing	1	2	3
(10) Concerns about owing money	1	2	3
(11) Concerns about getting credit	1	2	3
(12) Concerns about money for emergencies	1	2	3
(13) Someone owes you money	1	2	3
(14) Financial responsibility for someone who does not live with you	1	2	3
(15) Cutting down on electricity, water, etc.	1	2	3
(16) Smoking too much	1	2	3
(17) Use of alcohol	1	2	3
(18) Personal use of drugs	1	2	3
(19) Too many responsibilities	1	2	3
(20) Decisions about having children	1	2	3
(21) Non-family members living in your house	1	2	3
(22) Care for pet	1	2	3
(23) Planning meals	1	2	3
(24) Concerned about the meaning of life	1	2	3
(25) Trouble relaxing	1	2	3
(26) Trouble making decisions	1	2	3
(27) Problems getting along with fellow workers	1	2	3
(28) Customers or clients give you a hard time	1	2	3
(29) Home maintenance (inside)	1	2	3
(30) Concerns about job security	1	2	3
(31) Concerns about retirement	1	2	3
(32) Laid-off or out of work	1	2	3
(33) Do not like current work duties	1	2	3
(34) Do not like fellow workers	1	2	3
(35) Not enough money for basic necessities	1	2	3
(36) Not enough money for food	1	2	3
(37) Too many interruptions	1	2	3
(38) Unexpected company	1	2	3
(39) Too much time on hands	1	2	3
(40) Having to wait	1	2	3
(41) Concerns about accidents	1	2	3
(42) Being lonely	1	2	3
(43) Not enough money for health care	1	2	3
(44) Fear of confrontation	1	2	3
(45) Financial security	1	2	3
(46) Silly practical mistakes	1	2	3
(47) Inability to express yourself	1	2	3
(48) Physical illness	1	2	3
(49) Side effects of medication	1	2	3
(50) Concerns about medical treatment	1	2	3
(51) Physical appearance	1	2	3
(52) Fear of rejection	1	2	3
(53) Difficulties with getting pregnant	1	2	3
(54) Sexual problems that result from physical problems	1	2	3
(55) Sexual problems other than those resulting from physical problems	1	2	3

Hassles	Severity		
	1. Somewhat Severe	2. Moderately Severe	3. Extremely Severe
(56) Concerns about health in general	1	2	3
(57) Not seeing enough people	1	2	3
(58) Friends or relatives too far away	1	2	3
(59) Preparing meals	1	2	3
(60) Wasting time	1	2	3
(61) Auto maintenance	1	2	3
(62) Filling out forms	1	2	3
(63) Neighborhood deterioration	1	2	3
(64) Financing children's education	1	2	3
(65) Problems with employees	1	2	3
(66) Problems on job due to being a woman or man	1	2	3
(67) Declining physical abilities	1	2	3
(68) Being exploited	1	2	3
(69) Concerns about bodily functions	1	2	3
(70) Rising prices of common goods	1	2	3
(71) Not getting enough rest	1	2	3
(72) Not getting enough sleep	1	2	3
(73) Problems with aging parents	1	2	3
(74) Problems with your children	1	2	3
(75) Problems with persons younger than yourself	1	2	3
(76) Problems with your lover	1	2	3
(77) Difficulties seeing or hearing	1	2	3
(78) Overloaded with family responsibilities	1	2	3
(79) Too many things to do	1	2	3
(80) Unchallenging work	1	2	3
(81) Concerns about meeting high standards	1	2	3
(82) Financial dealings with friends or acquaintances	1	2	3
(83) Job dissatisfactions	1	2	3
(84) Worries about decisions to change jobs	1	2	3
(85) Trouble with reading, writing, or spelling abilities	1	2	3
(86) Too many meetings	1	2	3
(87) Problems with divorce or separation	1	2	3
(88) Trouble with arithmetic skills	1	2	3
(89) Gossip	1	2	3
(90) Legal problems	1	2	3
(91) Concerns about weight	1	2	3
(92) Not enough time to do the things you need to do	1	2	3
(93) Television	1	2	3
(94) Not enough personal energy	1	2	3
(95) Concerns about inner conflicts	1	2	3
(96) Feel conflicted over what to do	1	2	3
(97) Regrets over past decisions	1	2	3
(98) Menstrual (period) problems	1	2	3
(99) The weather	1	2	3
(100) Nightmares	1	2	3
(101) Concerns about getting ahead	1	2	3
(102) Hassles from boss or supervisor	1	2	3
(103) Difficulties with friends	1	2	3
(104) Not enough time for family	1	2	3
(105) Transportation problems	1	2	3
(106) Not enough money for transportation	1	2	3
(107) Not enough money for entertainment and recreation	1	2	3
(108) Shopping	1	2	3
(109) Prejudice and discrimination from others	1	2	3
(110) Property, investments, or taxes	1	2	3
(111) Not enough time for entertainment and recreation	1	2	3
(112) Yardwork or outside home maintenance	1	2	3
(113) Concerns about news events	1	2	3
(114) Noise	1	2	3
(115) Crime	1	2	3
(116) Traffic	1	2	3
(117) Pollution	1	2	3

HAVE WE MISSED ANY OF YOUR HASSLES? IF
SO, WRITE THEM IN BELOW.

(118) _____

ONE MORE THING: HAS THERE BEEN A
CHANGE IN YOUR LIFE THAT AFFECTED
HOW YOU ANSWERED THIS SCALE? IF SO,
TELL US WHAT IT WAS.

From Kanner, et al.[58] with permission.

APPENDIX C

Suggested Answers to Case Study Guiding Questions

Questions

1. Having read the chapter, list some possible psychosocial issues requiring further exploration: what factors are interfering with Mary's recovery (physical and/or psychosocial factors)?

ANSWER: The clinical problem list from a physical therapy perspective is rather straightforward in Mary's case. It becomes clear, however, on careful exploration of this case study that the impediments to maximum functioning for Mary lie within issues of motivation, self-image, isolation, and depression. Mary presents with a premorbid history of not living up to her potential and not having been able to maximize her resources. She is a high school graduate working in a menial, low-paying position who has not demonstrated any ability to rally her strength, determination, or will to pursue a betterment of her life, intellectually, economically, or socially. This is clear, not only from the life situation she presents with but also in her passive response to the current medical crisis. We can initially hypothesize from the information given in the case study that the passivity expressed might stem from any one, or a combination of the following:

1. Depression, stemming from either a negative turn in her life situation as a result of the accident or from a continuation of a premorbid depressive stance. Making a distinction as to whether the possible depression is of an acute or chronic nature, although crucial to the treating mental health worker, is of little practical import to the physical therapist. In either case, aside from a referral to the mental health team, the physical therapist can continually put forth realistic, yet supportive, reminders of Mary's condition and the potential for improved functioning. In doing so, the physical therapist, without giving false hope, can make expectations more reality-based and less onerous than the often typical perception in a depressive state where situations are often assessed in their most extreme negative potentiality. Support, a caring stance, and a relationship based on trust and reliability can often go a long way in helping to mitigate a depressive episode. Depression is a possible factor in all such cases and some of the telltale signs include negative attitude, hopelessness, helplessness, and changes in eating and sleeping patterns as well as a significant diminution of energy and motivation.

2. Self-image is a very real factor suggested by the above case study in that one's perception of one's self and/or self-worth are often tied into issues of motivation and often a perception of deserving any disaster coming our way. Self-deprecating statements, though not deterministic, often suggest a low self-image (or sometimes, an overinflated one) and can sometimes be mitigated by the physical therapist in both action and words through demonstration of support, the effort to work with the patient, and realistically correcting unrealistic self assessments by the patient.

3. Isolation is also a factor to be dealt with in Mary's case. The case study suggests that Mary has led an apparently socially isolated premorbid life-style. Social supports, particularly emotive supports, are both palliative and preventive factors to accidents and disability. To the degree that the physical therapist can offer support and to the degree that Mary can be encouraged to increase a connection to others might prove helpful. The physical therapist might encourage interaction with other patients, schedule Mary in treatment sessions with other patients, or otherwise attempt to join her with a rehabilitation group or partner, reconnect with family, and so forth.

These are just some of the more blatant psychosocial factors to be considered by the physical therapist. You will not be called on to provide treatment for these factors, yet an increasing awareness of these issues will prompt timely and appropriate referral to the mental health team. Awareness will also allow modifications to your approach and interactions with the patient which, when used expediently, may aid and hasten the rehabilitation effort.

To further the information presented in the initial case study presented, Mary was initially approached due to the belief on the part of the authors, that even noncomplaining or nondisruptive patients could benefit from psychotherapeutic intervention. She was approached in an attempt to facilitate a conversation. Her responses were concrete and shallow, and she was distant but superficially cooperative. It took many attempts to have her open up a little and talk about some uneventful "safe" parts of her life. After further attempts she related that although she had dreams and aspirations during her high school years, these were eventually felt to be overwhelmed. She stopped expecting much out of her life, having been born poor, not being able to "become someone with any merit." She hinted at the thinking process underlying her response to the recent disablement by explaining that working in a factory, and having been unable to have children, she exclaimed "so what did I lose being here?" It was clear that she gave up, prompted, in part, by premorbid feelings that her life was worthless, a fear only reinforced by the accident. Her premorbid perception seemed to indicate that her feelings of failure were due to some discrepancy between dreams and ambitions, which she felt were beyond her ability to achieve. Being born in poverty and having to work is an accepted way of life by a great percentage of the population who still find life meaningful. It is usually disruptive only when an individual does not accept the limitations of life's conditions due to unfulfilled striving.

The authors are of a unified mind, based on experience with rehabilitation patients, that behaviors exhibited by such patients are usually an expression of their unique interpretation of the condition they find themselves in as it relates to the perceived disruption of their premorbid world. To better understand this behavior, it becomes imperative to assess and investigate a patient's unique premorbid world and its effect on the many aspects of life and the individual's perception and idiosyncratic interpretation of all the involved factors. Thus the premorbid world of the patient is the womb from which the ensuing, newly created self-image emerges, which drives the individual's perception. This then is a major factor as to how one deals with his or her inner and outer world. Once these factors become clearer to the therapist, the observed odd behaviors of the patient can be better understood and dealt with more effectively.

Perception, being a major tool through which one tackles life, itself becomes the tool through which the therapist can elicit changes in the patient's functioning. Understanding or experiencing the extreme effect of any disablement, it becomes quite clear as to how much more the resulting trauma affects the ensuing world of an individual than almost any other life event in nondisabled patients.

These then are the general issues we may identify broadly from the presented case. For those interested in further detail about these issues in the treatment of Mary, we include a brief synopsis of these issues for Mary.

Continued supportive prodding revealed that Mary was an excellent student during her public school period. She was praised by her teachers who told her that with her academic facility she could become a productive professional. Her ambitions were heightened and she began to envision a future as a career woman. In her perception, poverty and the need to support herself without the requisite skills closed the doors on her dream. She claimed to have lost her self-confidence to a degree that she accepted a low-level factory job instead of trying to look for something more fulfilling and lucrative. The accident only confirmed her lack of any hope and actually seemed to enable her to shift her feelings of failure from the self to the outside factor, the accident. In her case, as it happens sometimes, her becoming disabled took away some of her feelings of guilt and even of helplessness due to the fact that now others will take care of her.

2. Is the patient inner or outer directed? How might the physical therapist utilize this knowledge/information in the service of treatment?

ANSWER: It would appear that Mary's premorbid feelings of failure are due to the discrepancy between her achievements and her expectations as described in addressing the previous question. Whatever the genesis, it is clear by both her passive stance to rehabilitation and her history of settling for whatever comes her way in life that she is indeed outer directed. Her unwillingness to act in a determined, planned, or proactive manner, in her social situation, family interactions, educational attainment, or her career, all attest to this stance. This stance can be mitigated to some degree by the physical therapist's approach to Mary on many levels. On one level, the message might be verbalized and reinforced that the outcome of any rehabilitation effort is dependent, in large part, on her active participation in goal setting, treatment cooperation, and the effort she brings to the process. If goals and activities can be broken down into small concrete steps, such a message might become acceptable to Mary and any success in this endeavor may pave the way to a broader generalization of a more active, deterministic, and inner-directed stance.

Therapeutic work with Mary proceeded with the understanding that her disablement had helped her negate the premorbid self-blame but had to retain the feeling of the wide discrepancy between the expected and the achieved to some degree. This latter was tapped into to present and reinforce an exploration of the need to change her perception to one where she can recognize her ability to impact and alter life circumstances. Specifically, the following messages were presented:

- Her intellectual capacities were not affected by the disability.
- Although her situation took an unfortunate turn, the accident and resulting disability may open the road to a good turn and a positive change in her life.
- The financial conditions that prevented previous academic achievement have changed due to her new circumstance and may pave the way for her to pursue goals previously perceived as unobtainable; she is now free from the preoccupation with making a living.

3. List potential social resources the physical therapist might draw on in treating or motivating Mary.

ANSWER: Given the extremely strong empirical evidence on the palliative nature of social support systems, this becomes an important area to address, and certainly any effort to strengthen such resources can be seen as positive. There are usually some resources to build on, even for someone as socially isolated as Mary. However strained or tenuous family relations may appear to be, such

Continued on following page

ties can often be strengthened under circumstances of medical involvement. If cooperation is obtainable, involving the family in the rehabilitation may be feasible if the patient is agreeable. At minimum, this can involve including family members in discussions about the condition, the goals, and even the activities of rehabilitation. Connections between the patient and other patients or group sessions may facilitate both formal and informal bonds, which might be supportive. Alerting the patient to groups, organizations, or other possible supports is often a very easy and very direct act that a physical therapist might make. If possible and warranted, setting up a mentoring situation where more advanced patients might offer guidance, direction, or support to newly admitted patients may prove beneficial to both parties.

Conclusion to Case Study

Because Mary was an actual case, let us conclude our chapter with a summation of the work done with Mary and the outcome of the rehabilitation and mental health efforts she had received.

As therapy proceeded, an attempt was made to clarify Mary's perceptions and desires. At one point we started playing the game of "if you can start life over again and take your pick of what you want to have" and of "if you had three wishes." It was revealed that in high school, during some study of human behavior she became fascinated with the human mind and the study of psychology and hoped to go to college and become a psychologist. Financially, this was out of the question and she felt that she had to settle for a menial job.

Without going into details of the many hours of work with Mary, she started realizing that, as a result of the disablement and the unoccupied time she increasingly found onerous, her impossible dream might be realized now that she is disabled. She cannot work or support herself, she will have the free time, and because her academic ambitions are in an area unaffected by her physical condition, she might try to realize her dream. Needless to say that once she was able to visualize her previously unreachable dream as coming within her grasp, Mary became active in applying for scholarships and admissions to college. She eventually majored in psychology and later went on to become a certified clinical social worker, devoting her life to counseling people with handicaps from her wheelchair.

Influence of Values on Patient Care

3

Foundation for Decision Making

Carol M. Davis

LEARNING OBJECTIVES

1. Identify what a value is and how it directs human behavior.
2. Recognize how humans acquire values.
3. Identify how values influence the choices of patients, clients, and health professionals.
4. Distinguish between value-directed behavior that enhances healing and value-directed behavior that is likely to interfere with healing.
5. Clarify examples of ethical distress that accompany health care provided by managed care organizations.
6. Learn a special clinical reasoning process to aid in resolving ethical dilemmas.

INTRODUCTION

Initially, one might question the logic of including a chapter on values in a text related to management of adult rehabilitation patients. The fact is that the entire book is devoted to educating the reader about the proper decisions to make in the rehabilitation process. Values play a critical role in most decision making, and to omit this aspect of decision making would be unwise.

Providing an operating definition of a *value* poses something of a challenge. Many interpretations have been made, and several authors have provided a variety of definitions.[1-5] For the purposes of this chapter, a **value** is defined as an inner force that provides the standards by which patterns of choice are made. For example, if people value the safety of their lives, among other acts, they will probably choose to wear a seat belt while driving or riding in an automobile. That choice is guided by the importance they place on their safety, or by their value of safety.

Because values are internal and difficult to measure, they have not been studied as vigorously as other aspects of human behavior. One cannot see a value; one can only feel it working. Values play a particularly important role in influencing our choices. The importance of this influence is emphasized when one considers that *knowing* the right thing to do and *doing* it are two separate phenomena. The first has to do with knowledge or cognition, the second with values or attitudes. This text is aimed at teaching the "knowing" aspect; this chapter, however, is devoted to elucidating the value aspect in choosing.

Most choices are value based; some decisions seem more difficult to make than others. Difficulty may arise when the therapist must resolve a values dilemma, when two seemingly equal goals or choices compete with one another. Difficulty also may arise when the therapist's values conflict with the values of the patient, the patient's family, colleagues, the larger health care system, and/or society. This chapter further defines values, describes how we acquire our values, and illustrates the influence values have on decisions. In addition, the influence that patient's values have on therapist's decisions is explored; examples of common difficult decisions in rehabilitation are provided. The **ethical distress** that can occur when providing care while working with a for-profit-business or managed care organization is explored. Value issues inherent in the process of delegating care to supportive staff as the role of the physical therapist becomes further refined as a diagnostician are also explored. Finally, the role communication plays in the process of making difficult choices is discussed.

PROCESS OF DECISION MAKING

How choices are made is different from *what* choices are made. The latter can be viewed as the answer or the solution; the former describes a process. Decision making or choosing in rehabilitation is sometimes composed of nothing more than a reactive, instinctive stimulus-response effort, or haphazard trial-and-error guessing. But more often, making the right decision, choosing the best alternative, results from professionally educated problem solving. One type of problem solving in health care is termed **clinical reasoning.** Even before the therapist first sees a patient, the process of clinical reasoning begins. Upon reviewing patient information, hypotheses are generated and various questions are asked in sequence to assess the patient's problem fully and, inevitably, to decide on the diagnosis that will guide physical therapy treatment, usually at the level of impairment. Further reasoning results in a decision about the most appropriate treatment for this particular person at this point in time, ideally as verified by evidence in the literature.

The greater part of professional education in health care is devoted to developing good clinical reasoners. The best instructors bravely refuse to give the "right" answer and encourage students to learn the process of discovery. In this way, students rise above the technical level of training. They are encouraged to become professionals capable of responding to complex patient situations by carefully reading the literature, questioning, touching, testing, and listening with the "third ear" to what is said as well as to what is left unsaid.

Problem solving is fundamental to our daily lives as human beings. We often do not realize we are problem solving because the process is so habitual, so subconscious. Just deciding what to have for breakfast can involve an intricate multi-step process:

What shall I have for breakfast?
What's in the kitchen?
Cereal, eggs, bacon, pancakes, juice, toast.
How hungry am I?
Starved!
How much time do I have?
Thirty minutes.
What did the scale say?
Five pounds over.
That does it; juice and dry toast!

The answer to this problem solving process was based on identifying the importance of one value over others. The fact that the scale revealed 5 excess pounds became a determining factor for making the final choice. Another person might have made the same choice but for a different reason:

How much time do I have?
5 minutes.
No time to eat! I'll have toast and juice and eat it on the way!

Most choices result from prioritizing values. The more we know about our values, the more we learn and understand our science, and the more we know about the facts of the situation, the easier it is to make a decision that seems best.[1]

Deciding what to eat for breakfast is a decision making process of a different sort than deciding whether a patient is a good candidate to receive an above-knee prosthesis. The differences are important. The first, what to eat, is a personal choice; the second, whether to recommend a prosthesis, is a professional decision. The first is a choice that bears little consequence for the chooser if the less-than-best decision is made. However, the decision about the prosthesis has profound consequence for another person if the less-than-best decision is made. The first example, what to eat for breakfast, is more accurately viewed as a value preference or a **non-moral value** choice; the prosthesis decision is made up largely of several moral- and value-laden decisions. **Moral values,** such as justice, honesty, compassion, and integrity, all reflect a way of relating to human beings; thus moral values carry more importance than value preferences, because humans are more important than food, or music, or what we wear.[2,6]

When we study to become professionals, part of the professional socialization process involves the adoption of values that usually overlap with our personal values. At times, however, they might conflict with them. Professional responsibility, we learn, requires that we put the patient's needs before our own and act in ways that show we deserve the patient's trust.[7,8] Let us take a closer look at what a value is and how we obtain our personal and professional values.

VALUES AND VALUING

A value cannot be seen directly, and it cannot be measured. Values are constructs (moral schemes) that are made up of beliefs, emotions, and attitudes about what is best and what is not good.[3] We can view values only indirectly by asking a person what he or she values, or even more important, by watching another person's behavior. Values are reflected in our actions, especially the pattern of our actions over a period of time. Thus one might say, "I value honesty," but we might wonder how much when he or she knowingly cheats on income tax returns. Another value obviously has priority over honesty for this person.

Values, at times, cooperate and, at times, conflict with each other. A dilemma exists when we have difficulty choosing which value should have priority. For example, respect for life is the central value for advocates of a woman's right to choose abortion as well as for those opposed to abortion. The difference in opinion and belief of these two groups is not over the value of life, but the importance of the mother's life over the fetus' life above all considerations; the reproductive freedom advocates claim the primacy of the mother's choice for the quality of her life and resist outside interference with her right to choose.[6] Resolving dilemmas involves a special form of clinical reasoning that will be explained later.

People are not born with values, but they are born with instincts and needs. Values are acquired from those who socialize us, primarily parents and family, and, for many, religion. The initial learning of values takes the form of "following the rules" that parents believe will minimize personal pain and conflict, maximize pleasure and meaning, and promote harmony and peace in the home.

Adolescents, as a part of natural maturation, test the values of the home by breaking rules and trying forbidden behaviors. This process marks the beginning of a transformation in which value-based rules followed to avoid punishment become internalized and, upon reflection, are adopted as one's own. Most people end up with a very similar set of values to that of their parents. However, for some, the difference in the way they prioritize their values causes a distancing between themselves and certain family members. One example of children prioritizing their values differently from their parents is the son or daughter who is the first in four generations not to study law.

The values of health professionals take on a different priority from the values of people in other careers whose primary satisfaction in work comes not from helping people directly but largely from working with ideas or inanimate objects. Likewise, although physical therapists as a group seem to display a consistent set of values, it might be conjectured that one of the key differences that distinguishes profoundly different specialists—for example, sports physical therapists who care for those who are well but injured, from those devoted to caring for seriously ill brain-injured patients—is the way which the specialist prioritizes values. The sports physical therapist expresses different interests and focuses professional goals on a population with needs very different from those of brain-injured patients. The different choices made in preferred patient populations may stem from different values as well as different needs and interests.[6]

We make our most meaningful choices based on what attracts us and leads us to growth and self-fulfillment, a life of pleasure and meaning.[3] Being aware of our values helps us to make informed and consistent choices that lead to personal and professional satisfaction. This is part of the process physical therapists undergo as they search out a specialty area of interest following their first few years in clinical practice.

CODE OF ETHICS

The set of moral norms adopted by a professional group to direct value-laden choices in a way consistent with professional responsibility is termed a **code of ethics** (Box 3–1). Most codes of ethics of the professions are composed of statements that have at their core one of four value principles, **autonomy, beneficence,** non-maleficence, and **justice,** and three rules that follow from these four principles, veracity, **confidentiality,** privacy, and **fidelity**[9] (Box 3–2). One might follow their code without

---

Box 3–1 CODE OF ETHICS OF THE AMERICAN PHYSICAL THERAPY ASSOCIATION

Preamble
This Code of Ethics sets forth ethical principles for the physical therapy profession. Members of this profession are responsible for maintaining and promoting ethical practice. This Code of Ethics, adopted by the American Physical Therapy Association, shall be binding on physical therapists who are members of the Association.

Principle 1
Physical therapists respect the rights and dignity of all individuals.

Principle 2
Physical therapists comply with the laws and regulations governing the practice of physical therapy.

Principle 3
Physical therapists accept responsibility for the exercise of sound judgement.

Principle 4
Physical therapists maintain and promote high standards in the provision of physical therapy services.

Principle 5
Physical therapists seek remuneration for their services that is deserved and reasonable.

Principle 6
Physical therapists provide accurate information to the consumer about the profession and the services they provide.

Principle 7
Physical therapists accept the responsibility to protect the public and the profession from unethical, incompetent, or illegal acts.

Principle 8
Physical therapists participate in efforts to address the health needs of the public.

Adopted by the House of Delegates
June 1981
Amended June 1987

(From the American Physical Therapy Association, with permission.)

Box 3–2 MORAL PRINCIPLES AND RULES THAT FORM THE FOUNDATIONS OF HEALTH CARE ETHICS[9]

Principles

1. **Autonomy**
   The patient's right to choose for one's life, and to voice that choice for as long as possible.
2. **Beneficence**
   Doing what is best for one's patient. Contrasts with paternalism or patronizing. Beneficence is a moral obligation of all health care practitioners. We must act with beneficence when we are aware of the facts and the patient is at significant risk of harm or loss and our action is needed to prevent that harm or loss. We must act with beneficence if the benefit to the patient outweighs the potential harm to the health care practitioner.
3. **Non-maleficence**
   Do no harm. Do not injure, disable, or kill a person, or undermine a person's reputation, property, or privacy.
4. **Justice**
   Fairness
   Distributive—equal distribution to all members of a group
   Compensatory—making up for past injustice (affirmative action)
   Procedural—first come, first served, alphabetical order, and so forth

Ethical Rules that Follow these Principles

1. **Veracity**—Tell the truth, do not lie.
   From the principles of autonomy and beneficence. Key ethical issue is how much of the truth to tell in view of beneficence.
2. **Confidentiality and Privacy**
   From the principle of beneficence.
   Health care practitioners are morally obliged to keep confident all information concerning patients even if not requested specifically, except when to do so would bring harm to innocent people or to the patient. Patients have the right to keep private any information not relevant to their care.
3. **Fidelity**
   From the principle of beneficence.
   Health care practitioner's actions and treatments will remain faithful to their patient and to their colleagues, even when they disagree with their colleagues.

---

internalizing it, just as small children follow the "rules of the house." For the code of ethics to function as a set of professional values, one must reflect on it and decide that it, indeed, forms a values complex around which one is willing to organize professional choices. Thus, as was previously stated, reflection is necessary to the internalization of values to make them truly one's own.[3–5] The choices that then follow this internalization are likely to be consistent with one's basic beliefs, show coherence, be authentic or genuine, and be adequate to the task of decision making. Those who make the smoothest transitions into professional practice are likely to be those whose personal values and priorities significantly overlap with the values inherent in their chosen professional practice. Given that one's basic human survival needs are met, the more one reflects on one's choices and on which choices result in a good and meaningful life, the more one is apt to experience consistent reward from opportunities.[3]

THE VALUES OF PATIENTS AS A FACTOR IN CARE

Patients come to physical therapy as whole persons in need of professional help and guidance. All people can be viewed as possessing four quadrants of need that comprise the whole: the physical, the intellectual, the emotional, and the spiritual (Fig. 3-1).[6] It could be said that a more meaningful and peaceful life results when choices are made that respond equally to the demands of all four quadrants of need. Central to the work of Carl Jung is the belief that a healthy personality results from obtaining a *balance* between thinking and feeling and between intuition and sensation.[10]

Patients come to physical therapy at various stages in their lives and with a unique history of having made thousands of choices. Over time the therapist comes to realize that some patients display a life pattern of meaningful, consistent, well thought-out choices; others reveal a life of capricious, noncentered, unorganized value-based behavior. Often patients' risky choices have directly or indirectly brought them to therapy; for example, the young patient with quadriplegia who drove into a tree while drunk. Many patient problems in movement and function that are encountered in rehabilitation are not the result of "fate," but result from a lifetime of choices that placed other values and needs at a higher priority than physical health, or than the prevention of illness and injury. The more physical therapists become aware of how much control people actually have over their state of wellness and health, the more difficult it becomes for some therapists to remain nonjudgemental about their patients. It is exceedingly difficult for some clinicians, for example, to remain nonjudgemental while treating a chronic smoker for emphysema or a tremendously obese patient for hip and knee joint problems.[11]

It is important, however, to remember that we are morally and ethically bound to give the highest quality of care as free from judgement and bias as possible to all patients. This is where balance in all four of our quadrants helps us (see Fig. 3-1). If our needs are being met in all four areas (physical, intellectual, emotional, and spiritual), we feel less frustrated and irritated by personal stress and can remain centered and better able to remain nonjudgemental and can set more adequate boundaries with compassion. Patients, with all their frailties can be seen as separate from us, doing the best for themselves that they can.[6]

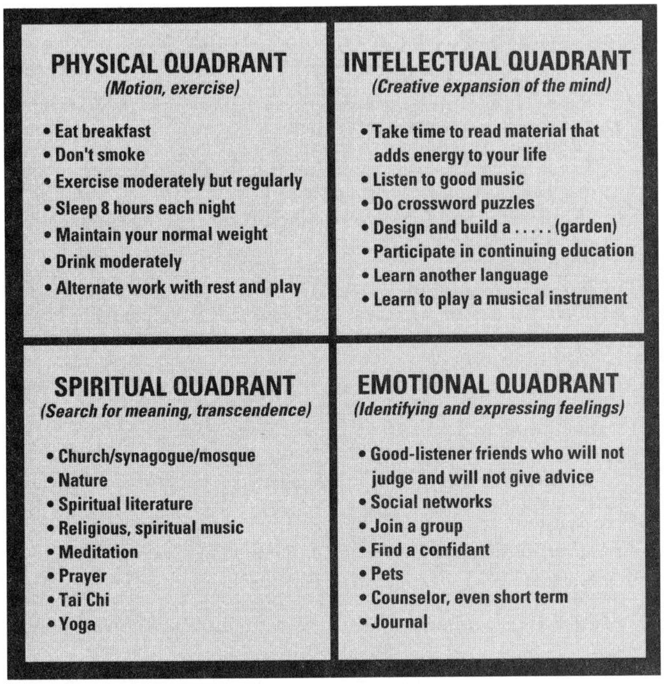

PHYSICAL QUADRANT
(Motion, exercise)

- Eat breakfast
- Don't smoke
- Exercise moderately but regularly
- Sleep 8 hours each night
- Maintain your normal weight
- Drink moderately
- Alternate work with rest and play

INTELLECTUAL QUADRANT
(Creative expansion of the mind)

- Take time to read material that adds energy to your life
- Listen to good music
- Do crossword puzzles
- Design and build a . . . . . (garden)
- Participate in continuing education
- Learn another language
- Learn to play a musical instrument

SPIRITUAL QUADRANT
(Search for meaning, transcendence)

- Church/synagogue/mosque
- Nature
- Spiritual literature
- Religious, spiritual music
- Meditation
- Prayer
- Tai Chi
- Yoga

EMOTIONAL QUADRANT
(Identifying and expressing feelings)

- Good-listener friends who will not judge and will not give advice
- Social networks
- Join a group
- Find a confidant
- Pets
- Counselor, even short term
- Journal

Figure 3-1. Four quadrants of need and function: How to meet needs in each and strive for balance.

When a reflex wave of judgement and criticism starts to make its way into the conversation with a patient, it helps to breathe deeply, center yourself, and adopt the value-neutral attitude of *curiosity*. Remember none of us can literally put ourselves into the shoes of our patients, so as soon as we think we know better, and are ready to admonish our patients, it is better to stop, breathe, and say, "I'm *curious*. What made you decide to do that?" And then be quiet and listen to try to understand free of judgement.

To be "centered" is to experience one's energy concentrated in the middle and balanced so that no one quadrant's needs predominate (see Fig. 3-1). When we feel centered, we feel balanced, just as the balanced karate expert stands with his or her weight so distributed that blows coming in any direction can be absorbed and pushed away without loss of balance. If, for example, our emotional needs are not being met, we often feel unbalanced or uncentered. We either spend energy repressing or expressing energy in the stress of loneliness, neediness for attention, or irritability. On the other hand, when our four quadrants are equally attended to, we feel centered and thus can feel the whole in every part. Centered energy and consciousness then allow us to free our attention away from our needs and toward the patient's needs, and we can be therapeutically present to the other.

When we need nothing more than to assist our patients in healing, whatever they choose to do can be viewed with greater objectivity. When we, ourselves, "need" our patients to get better, to thank us, to praise us, to acknowledge our skill and intellect because those common human emotional needs are not being met outside the clinic, we are more likely

to judge our patients when they fail to meet our needs.[6]

THE INFLUENCE OF VALUES ON THE PRIMARY GOAL OF PATIENT CARE

When a feeling of criticism and negative judgement of a patient occurs within health practitioners, we must be aware of it and consciously work not to let it affect our behavior. The primary goal of health practitioners is to help *all* people recover or maintain their health so they may function at the highest, most independent, most autonomous level possible day to day. If the primary goal is to achieve optimal health and healing, certain values seem to promote that goal more than others. One way to ascertain values that promote health and healing is to describe behavior between a therapist and patient that does the very opposite, or that interferes with health and healing. Putting yourself in the place of the patient, what therapist behaviors would *interfere* with your progress toward getting well or healing? Table 3–1 presents a sample list of very obvious behaviors that would detract from a patient's ability to function optimally in a therapeutic setting. Also included are a list of possible negative values that might underlie each of these behaviors.[11]

Behaviors and underlying values that *facilitate* healing might be described as the exact opposite of those that detract from healing[11] (Table 3–2). These therapist behaviors, it seems, would obviously help restore a patient's hope, promote progress toward recovery, and assist with achieving the highest possible level of independent function.

Many of us who would read the list of negative behaviors (see Table 3–1) that detract from healing would respond, "I'd never behave in such a way with my patients!" But, in fact, a huge gap exists between knowing the right thing to do, wanting to do it, and actually doing it.

Essential to a "therapeutic use of self" is the capacity to feel **compassion** for those who suffer. Compassion is quite different from **pity,** where a person feels sorry for those who are less fortunate. The compassion of the mature health professional is fueled by imagination, or the ability to envision what is possible from the other person's perspective.[6,12] Imaginative understanding involves **self-transposal** (a cognitive attempt to put one's self in the place of another) at the least and **empathy** (a complex type of **identification** with another's experience) at the most.[6] As healers, therapists must not block but, rather, must allow empathy to occur, a momentary "crossing over" into the patient's frame of reference. Thus, compassion is a very personal, intimate experience that is built on "trust, honesty, and the time and willingness to listen."[12]

Let us examine some patient care situations that require professional choice that may result in a less-than-optimal prioritizing of our professional and personal values.

VALUES THAT DETRACT FROM THE HEALING PROCESS

Therapist Behaviors that Interfere or Detract from the Healing Process	Negative Values that Might Underlie Each Behavior
1. Acting cool or aloof, obviously paying more attention to other patients.	1. a. Prejudice: to prejudge or to classify a person as belonging to a larger group and thus to believe things about that person that one believed about the larger group. b. **Indifference:** lack of interest or concern: aloofness, detachment.
2. Overly criticizing you (the patient) so that you feel as if nothing you do is right.	2. a. **Prejudice.** b. **Perfectionism:** the doctrine that the perfection of moral character is a person's highest good and that freedom from imperfection is attainable. c. Lack of flexibility.
3. Treating you as an object rather than as a person with feelings of pain, worry, and insecurity.	3. **Depersonalization:** to detract from an individual's uniqueness: to fail to honor a person's individuality.
4. Treating you as if you were a child, incapable of really understanding anything that is said.	4. **Patronizing:** to adopt an air of condescension.
5. Being unable or unwilling to help you in your exercises; leaving you alone most of the time.	5. a. Indifference. b. Prejudice.
6. Making fun of you in your presence and behind your back.	6. Depersonalization.
7. Telling others things you have shared in confidence.	7. Breaking confidentiality; not keeping another person's trust private and secret.
8. Not letting you work on your own.	8. Fostering dependence.
9. More often than not guessing about what is best for you. Admitting he or she "is not sure" what to do, but "let us not let that stop us."	9. Failure to recognize and to act on one's limits of knowledge.
10. Always fitting you in as if everything else in the therapist's life is more important than you are.	10. Placing self-interest over patient's needs.

VALUE-LADEN SITUATIONS IN REHABILITATION

What would you do, and *why*, if this situation happened to you? Joyce, a 22-year-old college student was referred to physical therapy following surgical removal of her left leg owing to osteogenic sarcoma. Other than generalized weakness from chemotherapy, surgery, and bed rest and incisional pain and soreness, she was in "good health" on her arrival to the rehabilitation center.

You have been treating her for several weeks, having begun therapy from her admission to the rehabilitation center. Preoperative training was given

Table 3–2 THERAPIST BEHAVIORS AND POSSIBLE UNDERLYING VALUES THAT FACILITATE THE HEALING PROCESS

Therapist Behaviors that Facilitate or Promote the Healing Process	Positive Values that Might Underlie Each Behavior
1. Offering you (the patient) the same amount of attention offered other patients, so it balances out from day to day.	1. Justice: the quality of impartiality or fairness.
2. Accepting your weaknesses along with your strengths and verbally reinforcing the desired behaviors.	2. Unconditional positive regard; acceptance.
3. Always treating you as a person with feelings and being sensitive to those feelings each day.	3. a. Respect: the act of giving particular attention to a person; worthy of high regard. b. Compassion: sympathetic consciousness of another's situation and the desire to be of effective help in relieving a painful situation.
4. Explaining things at your level, not oversimplifying or making things too complex.	4. a. Respect. b. Accurate and sensitive communication.
5. Always reachable yet never fostering dependence; encouraging independent activity.	5. a. Autonomy: a quality or state of self-governance; independence. b. Dignity: the quality of being worthy, honored, esteemed; to have distinction as a person.
6. Never using humor inappropriately, never laughing *at* you, but encouraging you to be able to laugh, sometimes even at yourself.	6. Appropriate humor, nondefensive humor.
7. Always keeping your confidence.	7. Confidentiality: keeping another person's trust private and secret.
8. Fostering your own independent activity without letting you feel stranded.	8. Autonomy.
9. Realizing when he or she needs the advice of someone else and asking for help in a timely fashion.	9. Recognizing the limits to one's knowledge, knowing when to get help or to refer; honesty.
10. Making you feel special, cherished, and unique; showing individual concern for you and your progress.	10. a. Compassion. b. Sensitivity to your uniqueness.

in the acute setting. You have assisted her with preprosthetic training, strengthening, prosthetic training and acceptance, and gait training. She has been progressing well.

Joyce is intelligent and inquisitive, yet somewhat stubborn. Two weeks before discharge you notice an increasing tendency on her part to be careless and to take unnecessary risks, like hopping on one foot rather than donning her prosthesis. In addition, she admits to thinking that her daily strengthening exercises are stupid and that, after discharge, she may just throw the prosthesis away and depend on a wheelchair. Even crutches are too much bother.

You feel confused and frustrated. You have invested a great deal of energy into the successful rehabilitation of this person and her behavior at this point seems ignorant and manipulative. Her refusal to cooperate with your suggestions angers you; you feel that her basic laziness in requesting a wheelchair existence represents settling for a quality of life that is less than optimal and selfish. You feel as if you have failed to help her realize her full adult potential. You feel overstressed with the demands of your work.

Once the patient care day has begun, therapists seldom find or take the time to reflect on the larger issues, those that hover on the fringe of the work consciousness. Instead, therapists tend to focus on the immediate situation in front of them, quickly gathering data and problem solving as they go. Joyce's growing problem of reluctance could be viewed as a peripheral issue at first, one the therapist hoped would pass without needing to be confronted. But as her discharge date comes closer, the therapist is forced to respond to what appears to be regressive behavior.

The therapist's responses may reveal one or more of several thoughts and feelings. Especially when under stress, one may become impatient and angry and lecture Joyce to "grow up." The therapist may feel personal failure and frustration and, in a condescending way, let her know he or she expected far more reward for the efforts placed in her successful rehabilitation. These are often reactive, automatic, emotion-based responses based on a value of, or need for, spontaneous honesty and the right to express feelings regardless of the impact that expression may have on others. The therapist is unhappy and wants the situation to change but does not know how to change it, so the therapist displays poor impulse control and aggressively "lets off steam."

As "human" as this choice may seem, more mature behavior is required of health professionals. No longer may we claim the luxury of spontaneous outburst, for the impact of the therapists' outbursts rarely solves value-based problems and often creates larger ones. Obviously, this is not conducive to healing.

On reflection, one realizes that Joyce's regressive behavior may likely reveal inner conflict, fear, and/or depression. From Joyce's point of view, it is not difficult to come to some understanding that a person under these circumstances might be afraid and might see a safer existence in a wheelchair. Stopping to breathe, and then acting on the value of compassion, funded by empathy and self-transposal, elevates the problem-solving process from reaction to a professional choice to sit down and to discuss this issue comprehensively with Joyce, referring her to the social worker for psychological support and counseling, if necessary.

Nonjudgemental concern and understanding are foundations of healing. In addition, health professionals caring for adults must accept that occasionally they will encounter a patient who is unwilling to cooperate with their suggestions and who resists their attempts to offer therapeutic care and advice. With the value of patient autonomy in mind, the professional's role is not to assume a paternalistic stance indicating "I know what's better for you than you do," but instead to outline as clearly, creatively, and accurately as possible the predictable results of the choices the patient is making. Patients must have control over their own lives to the greatest extent possible.[6,7] But in the end, we cannot and should not force patients to undergo treatment when they have simply refused. It is their autonomous right to refuse care and we must honor that.

These guidelines exist in their purest sense when therapists are treating adult patients who are not suffering from confusion, mental or intellectual disorders, or significant depression. With children or adults who do suffer the conditions mentioned, therapists must aim for the greatest extent of autonomous choice possible and focus appropriate attention on parents and family care givers.

RESOLVING ETHICAL OR MORAL DILEMMAS IN PRACTICE

A special kind of clinical reasoning is required when one confronts a true moral or **ethical dilemma.** In the presence of an ethical dilemma, when the best action eludes us, it helps to reflect in a systematic way, and then consult with a fellow professional or someone skilled in dilemma resolution (Box 3–3).[6] In resolving moral or ethical dilemmas in health care, the best decision usually results only when the facts or context of the situation are delineated as clearly and as precisely as possible. Whether you decide to resolve the dilemma *teleologically* (deciding what the best outcome would be [for the greatest number, for example]) or *deontologically* (weighing the two or more values that seem to be fighting with each other, and deciding which is the "higher" or "more moral" action in this particular case with these particular facts), the best decision can only be made with careful thought. Box 3–3 outlines a process of reasoning that can guide you in resolving ethical dilemmas in your practice. You should be able to justify your final decision by explaining both your ethical reasoning process and your conscious weighing of one value over another in this situation. A

Box 3–3 SOLVING THE ETHICAL DILEMMA[6]

Ethical dilemmas occur when two or more ethical principles conflict with each other in a given situation and it is unclear what the best or highest moral action would be. This problem solving process can be applied in the search for the best alternative.

1. **Gather all of the facts** that can be known about the situation.
2. **Decide which ethical principles or rules are involved,** such as beneficence, autonomy, nonmaleficence, justice, confidentiality, veracity, or fidelity. Is self-interest a factor on the part of the health professional?
3. **Clarify your professional duties** in this situation; for example, do no harm, obey the law, tell the truth, stand up for one's colleagues even when you disagree. Do the Code of Ethics and Guide to Professional Conduct speak to this particular issue?
4. **Describe the general nature of the outcome that would be most desired, or the consequences of a poor action.** What seems to be most important of all in this situation?
5. **Describe the practical features** of this situation. What are the disputed facts? Does the law instruct here? What are the wishes of the people involved? What about resources available? What is the main risk here? How certain can we be of the truth and the completeness of the facts that are known? What are the predominant values of the people involved?

When all of the pertinent aspects that go into this particular decision are laid out before you, then **you must use your discernment to decide which action is the highest moral alternative.** Most often simply asking, "What is best for my patient?" is the simplest route. But there are times when beneficence is not the best alternative, when it can be shown that others would suffer by acting on what is best for your patient. Self-interest, acting on what benefits you before considering the needs of your patient, is almost never a justifiable moral choice. Exceptions might be argued for a professional who must act on behalf of his or her child, parent, or spouse in an emergency situation, for example.

---

well-reasoned moral decision is always a combination of one's personal values system (discernment) guided by one's professional values or the values of health care.

Let's take a rather simple example that would be familiar in physical therapy. A 90 year-old man had recently had a revision of his trans-tibial amputation to an trans-femoral amputation. The surgeon requested the physical therapist teach the patient exercises for home, but not to prepare him for a new above-knee prosthesis because the literature indicated that his age prohibited a successful outcome with an above-knee prosthesis. The physical therapist knew the patient well, and disagreed with the physician's decision. The patient had exercised all his life and had excellent cardiopulmonary fitness. Can you identify the values at war with each other in this dilemma? The dilemma was between benefi-

cence and autonomy (the patient clearly hoped to get a new limb), and fidelity to the physician colleague. After discussing this with a supervisor, and with the supervisor's support, the therapist rigged a pylon. This allowed the patient to successfully begin ambulation. The therapist invited the surgeon to watch the patient in the parallel bars, and based on this new information, the surgeon facilitated the process of securing a new limb.

REACTIVE VERSUS PROACTIVE DECISION MAKING

Reactive care, characterized by on-the-spot problem solving and decision making, is an unavoidable part of rehabilitation. However, the greater the number of our decisions that are based on reaction rather than on proaction or well thought-out alternatives, the more idiosyncratic, inconsistent, and erratic our behavior will seem. It was suggested that to stop, breathe, and center is a useful way to avoid reactive judgement. Stopping to breathe will help bring about more proactive decisions, rather than reactive ones. Part of professional responsibility is to anticipate possible problems and to think through alternatives in advance. Likewise, the more that therapists base their decisions on scientific evidence and the more that they reflect on the values behind alternative choices, the more apt they are to experience consistent, scientific-based decisions reflective of the highest professional care. These decisions are inevitably more conducive to healing.

VALUE DECISIONS AND MANAGED CARE

Corporate health care, managed competition, capitation, and prepaid health organizations (PPOs) in many cases have been limiting patient access to physical and occupational therapists, and limiting the therapists' choice of and duration of reimbursed treatments. Under managed care, physical therapists have both professional obligations to treat patients and may have contractual obligations to managed care organizations (MCOs). It is important that health care professionals be able to carefully analyze their patients' needs and use sound moral reasoning and ethical dilemma resolution skills to decide on appropriate care when there is a shortage of professional care available, or when there is inadequate reimbursement for needed care.

Remember that until recently, managed care corporations had no moral obligations to their clients, the patients. Managed care is a business only. In the eyes of the law, MCOs do not practice health care. The primary duty of the health care professional is always to the patient, and secondarily to the business contract. This can result in *ethical distress* when you know the best thing to do, but are prohibited from doing it by the organization within which you practice.[13] For example, if under capitation agreement, the MCO provides coverage for only six visits and the goals set with the patient at the initial examination cannot be met in such a short time, the health care professional can be held liable for abandonment if his or her response is to discharge the patient short of the agreed upon goals with the comment, "Your MCO told me I had to stop care." *Business cannot dictate to a health professional when to discontinue treatment.*[13] MCOs do not tell professionals when to stop care, but simply when they will no longer pay for care. Professionals are obligated to provide needed care. Likewise, professionals have the right to maintain an adequate financial base of practice, and thus should seek private reimbursement or other reimbursement from the patient, and work diligently to reverse inadequate payment decisions by lobbying insurance groups and by conducting and publishing the research needed to show reasonable time frames for efficacious care.

Case law now indicates that the court's expectations are for the professional to carry out the duty to continue to serve the patient pro bono, or without compensation.[13] Thus each practice needs to develop a policy or guide outlining how it will determine the incidents and limits of pro bono care, and beyond that, the care of the patient who cannot pay but requires treatment should be transferred to colleagues who have pro bono capacity at that time.[13]

When health care as a service is managed as if it were a business, where profit is the primary reason for its existence, a conflict is bound to emerge. The foundational ethic of business is *buyer beware*. Business exists to make a profit, and will go to great lengths to convince the consumer that they need what business is selling. On the other hand, the professions were created to provide a service to those in need, and thus the foundational ethic of the professions is, *primum non nocere*, above all, do no harm.[8] It is easy to see how these foundational ethical principles are fundamentally at war with each other.

We have seen the concept of facilitating the *healing of the whole patient or client* all but disappear from health care in the United States. Business executives with their eyes on the bottom line dictating to health care professionals *who they can treat, for how long, and what is reasonable to charge*, strip health professionals of their ethical foundations. The very definition of a profession's autonomy requires that professionals are the only ones who can make those judgements, and they are morally obligated to make them free from interference, not with profit or self-interest in mind, but with service for those in need.[8]

It is important that health professionals stay current with local, state, and federal guidelines on health care practice and reimbursement, and learn how to identify and resolve the ethical dilemmas that result in these unstable times. Some predict that the negative impact of business on health care will become even more restrictive to providing quality care before improvements begin. But benefits have occurred as a result of this shift toward managed care. The current trend has resulted in greater cost containment, which is absolutely necessary, as well as a greater shift of the burden of care to patients and their families. This has resulted in more responsibility on the part of patients for their own health, and for prevention and maintenance of their own care.[6]

Above and beyond all trends and reimbursement mechanisms, when the interests of the patient and the professional collide, always remember that beneficence and autonomy ethically must outweigh self-interest[8] (see Box 3–2). If professionals were engaged only in business, there would be no dilemma. But health care professionals are bound by codes of ethics of service, not profit, that mandate advocacy for patients who come to them because they have both the education and the commitment to help them. To use patients for our own benefit beyond service literally destroys the profession.[8]

VALUES INHERENT IN DELEGATING TO SUPPORTIVE PERSONNEL

A majority of states now provide direct access to the services of physical therapists. As the profession of physical therapy advances to assume more autonomous responsibility for the prevention, diagnosis, and management of problems within the movement system, the role of the professional becomes more centered on diagnosis and planning for appropriate treatment, and health and community education. In day-to-day patient care it is becoming more important to delegate treatment to others who are qualified to carry out care at less expense to the patient. What values and principles can guide us so that we know when we can delegate safely and wisely? Watts[14] suggests that there is a way to make these decisions based on task analysis and recognition of the qualifications of various supportive personnel involved in patient care. In patient care circumstances where the predictability of consequences of action are certain, the stability of the situation indicates that change is unlikely to occur rapidly, the basic indicators of treatment are readily observable and nonambiguous, and the criticality of methods used is not severe, it is likely that care can be safely delegated to an assistant or family member. The values behind appropriate and cost-effective delegation of care are beneficence, non-maleficence, and justice. Many times physical therapists continue with treatment of a patient that could be carried out by a physical therapist assistant, while other patients wait to be examined and evaluated to begin care. This is an example of breaking the moral principle of distributive justice. Beneficence, or doing good for the patient, can be action. The physical therapist is the only professional who can examine and diagnose patients, and then plan treatment based on that diagnosis. To continue carrying out care that can be rendered by others, or that the patient can carry out in a home program, while making patients wait to be examined violates the moral principle of distributive justice.[15]

VALUE DECISIONS IN TRIAGE SITUATIONS

Triage situations always pull forth value priorities. A decision as simple as who to see first of three new inpatient referrals requires a value-based choice. What factors seem important in making the decision among these three new patients?

1. An 80 year-old, frail elderly woman with osteoporosis admitted following surgery to repair a fractured hip. Room 300.
2. A 30 year-old man with severe low back pain secondary to possible herniated disk. Room 201.
3. A 53 year-old woman who had a mild heart attack three weeks ago, admitted for cardiac rehabilitation. Room 302.

How would you decide, at 8 AM, which of these three patients to see first? What facts seem to make a difference? The patient's age? His or her location in the hospital (closest versus farthest away from where you are now)? Your existing patient load and schedule? Your subconscious or conscious aversion to certain patients, such as those with low back pain, worker's compensation patients, or elderly patients? If our primary goal in rehabilitation is to help patients recover their health so that they might function at the highest, most independent level possible, how can we use this goal to help direct our choices?

Putting the patient's needs first by way of autonomy and beneficence seems to be critical to this decision. The therapist's choice should not be based solely on personal convenience or self-interest. What additional facts are needed?[1,6] Putting oneself in the place of the patient, one comes to realize that the existence of certain factors calls forth our immediate attention. One factor that readily comes to mind that demands our immediate consideration is responding to patients in pain. Pain can totally consume one's attention and will take immediate priority in our choices. Responding first to patients in severe discomfort seems very important in sequencing the order of treatments. The therapist needs to find out which of these three individuals may have had a difficult night and is most in need of attention for relief of pain.

SUMMARY

Professional rehabilitative care requires problem solving that is proactive, based on scientific data or is evidence based, and demonstrates a consistent, conscious value of choosing behavior that is conducive to healing. Clinicians must become "informed reasoners"[2] who have systematically gathered the facts, have recognized potential choices and values dilemmas, and have taken the time to weigh which choice is most conducive to the healing process.

Central to this process is the courage to confront seemingly peripheral factors that therapists are tempted to hope will go away. Likewise central to this process is the willingness to put oneself in the place of the patient. Pellegrino[16] cautions us not to be so egocentric as to treat others simply as we would like to be treated. Instead, he suggests that the Golden Rule of health care should be to *give each patient the opportunity to tell you what his or her needs or wants are, as you would want them to give you.*

Finally, sensitive and accurate communication is required. In health, people feel alive by their connectedness to the world, and in illness they feel cut off, fragmented, and uninterested in the world. As healers, the therapist's role then becomes one of entering the patient's context of meaning. By using human-to-human skills of listening accurately to words and feelings; by communicating trust, truth, **respect,** interest, and caring; by explaining in ways that are relevant and intelligible to the patient; and by being sensitive to the patient's values, the therapist facilitates the patient's hope and strong belief that he or she is the patient's advocate in the world. In other words, the therapist helps the patient do what is necessary to feel once more alive in the world, connected, and hopeful of recovery to a meaningful life. Even in the face of chronic debilitating disease, terminal illness, or irreversible paralysis, there is a sense that the therapist can help patients feel reconnected to the possibility of a life with meaning.

The behaviors that enhance the therapeutic moment flow out of placing the person and his or her meaning of what is wrong central to any and all attempts to offer help. Behaviors that emerge from valuing a patient's humanity—sensitive and accurate listening, respect, trust, compassion, and problem solving, to name a few—work to reinforce autonomy and **dignity** and to restore a patient's hope and personal control of his or her life as therapists simultaneously apply their scientific knowledge and skill.[11] This is what is required of health care professionals in day-to-day patient care. To do less is to render less than compassionate, professional help. Reflecting, coming to know with greater confidence the best or right thing to do, and consistently doing it, results in a professional life of growth and meaning. These actions, one by one, weave a cloak of integrity that supports the professional mantle of responsibility that health professionals accept at their graduation. And thus not only do we grow as individuals, our profession grows and we are better able to contribute to the meaningful growth of our patients and of our society.

QUESTIONS FOR REVIEW

1. A person's values are difficult to identify. How can one know what a person values?

2. How are values related to behavior?

3. A belief is not a value, but beliefs direct our values. If a person believes fairness is good, what values can you predict the individual will hold?

4. What is the difference between a moral and a nonmoral value?

5. What four values make up most codes of ethics in the professions?

6. Give an example of a nonmoral value choice and a moral value choice.

7. What is the difference between behavior that agrees with a code of ethics and behavior that is value based?

8. What is our obligation as health professionals when a patient of sound mind refuses to take our suggestions and recommendations for healing?

9. What role does communication play in making value-based decisions in rehabilitation?

10. What is our obligation to the patient when his or her insurance no longer covers our care and the agreed upon goals have not been met?

CASE STUDY

You are a physical therapist specializing in hand therapy and have been working for 5 years. You have decided that the time is right to establish a practice of your own, and you have spent considerable time cultivating referrals from local orthopedists. Unfortunately, your practice is still in the red, and you have not been able to pay yourself a salary, yet. Managed care has shifted your referral base to more primary care physicians who hesitate to refer for specialty care.

One patient, for whom you created a wrist and hand splint, begins to regain function sooner than expected. You call the referring physician, and orthopedist who refers most of your patients to you, to inform him that you need to remove the splint, because it is actually hindering the healing process. The physician is on vacation, and you are unable to reach his colleague covering for him. So after a thorough examination, you remove the splint, give the patient precise instructions for a home exercise program, and ask him to return for physical therapy three times a week for 3 weeks. You send a copy of your notes to the vacationing physician.

When the physician returns to the office, he reads your correspondence and immediately calls you and says, "Who gave you the authority to remove the splint from this patient's hand? I want you to call the patient and tell him that you made a mistake, and put that splint back on and send him to me immediately. I will remove it if I feel it should come off." He then bangs the phone down in your ear.

Guiding Questions

What do you do? (Box 3–3 can serve as a guide to your problem solving.)

1. List the facts affecting this situation.

2. Identify the arms of the dilemma and values at war with each other (ethical principles involved).

   On the one hand: On the other hand:

3. List your professional duties.

4. List the practical features that impact this situation.

5. Come to a final decision that you can justify because you are acting on the higher value in this situation.

This case also appears in Davis, CM: When the interests of PT and patient collide: Habits of thought. PT Magazine January:71, 1995.

REFERENCES

1. Purtilo, RB, and Cassel, CK: Ethical Dimensions in the Health Professions. Saunders, Philadelphia, 1981.
2. Wehlage, G, and Lockword, AL: Moral relativism and values education. In Purpel, D, and Ryan, K (eds): Moral Education: It Comes with the Territory. McCutchen, Berkeley, CA, 1976.
3. Morrill, RL: Teaching Values in College. Jossey-Bass, San Francisco, 1980.
4. Beck, C: A philosophical view of values and value education. In Hennessy, T (ed): Values and Moral Development. Paulist Press, New York, 1976.
5. Raths, LE, et al: Values and Teaching. Charles E. Merrill, Columbus, Ohio, 1966.
6. Davis, CM: Patient Practitioner Interaction: An Experiential Manual for Developing the Art of Health Care, ed 3. SLACK, Inc., Thorofare, NJ, 1998.
7. Pellegrino, ED: What is a profession? J Allied Health 12:161, 1983.
8. Pellegrino, ER: Altruism, self interest and medical ethics. In Mapes, TA, and Zembang, JS (eds): Biomedical Ethics, ed 3. McGraw-Hill, New York, 1991.
9. Beauchamp, TL, and Childress, JF: Principles of Biomedical Ethics, ed 3. Oxford Univ. Pr., New York, 1989.
10. Jung, CG: The Structure and Dynamics of the Psyche. Pantheon, New York, 1960.
11. Davis, CM: The influence of values on patient care. In Payton, OD (ed): Psychosocial Aspects of Clinical Practice. Churchill Livingston, New York, 1986, p 119.
12. Pence, GE: Can compassion be taught? J Med Ethics 9:189, 1983.
13. Scott, R: Challenges in professional ethics. Symposium of Annual Scientific Meeting, American Physical Therapy Association, June, 1997, San Diego, CA.
14. Watts N: Task analysis and division of responsibility in physical therapy. Phys Ther 51:23, 1971.
15. Pellegrino, ED: Personal communication, March, 1995.
16. Pellegrino, ED, and Tomasma, D.C.: A Philosophical Basis of Medical Practice. Oxford Univ. Pr., New York, 1981.

SUPPLEMENTAL READINGS

Caplan, A: Moral Matters/Ethical Issues in Medicine and the Life Sciences. Wiley, New York, 1995.

Clancy, CM, and Brody, H: Managed care. Jekyll or Hyde? JAMA 273:338, 1995.

Curtin, LL: Why good people do bad things. Nursing Management 27:63, 1996.

Palermo, BJ: Capitation on trial. California Medicine 7:25, 1996.

Rodwin, MA: Medicine, Money and Morals. Oxford Univ. Pr., New York, 1993.

Scott, R: Professional Ethics: A Guide for Rehabilitation Professionals. Mosby, St. Louis, MO, 1998.

Zwerner, AR: Capitation empowers doctors. California Medicine 7:29, 1996.

GLOSSARY

Association: Strong feelings of identification with another person.

Autonomy: A quality of state of self-governance or independence. The patient's right to choose for their life, and to voice that choice for as long as possible.

Beneficence: Doing what is best for the patient.

Clinical reasoning: A problem-solving process based on identifying the importance of one value over others; process of prioritizing values in formulating a response to a situation.

Code of ethics: A set of moral norms adopted by a professional group to direct value-laden choices in a way consistent with professional responsibility.

Compassion: Sympathetic consciousness of another's situation and the desire to alleviate pain or suffering.

Confidentiality: Keeping another person's trust private and secret, whether requested or not.

Depersonalization: To detract from an individual's dignity or worth; failure to honor a person's uniqueness.

Dignity: The quality of being worthy, honored, esteemed; to have distinction as a person.

Empathy: A three-stage process that includes: (1) identification with another's experience or situation, (2) a shared experience with another person, and (3) a reclaiming of one's individuality separate from the shared moment.

Ethical dilemma: A conflict of values where each value action is seen to be equally bad or good, and to act on one value cancels out the other so that you can't have it "both ways."

Ethical distress: A conflict of duties when one knows the best or right thing to do, but is prohibited from doing it by some structure or process, for example, organizational policy.

Fidelity: Being faithful to one's patients, to one's colleagues and to one's profession, even when one disagrees.

Identification: Close personal association with another person leading to a feeling of sameness.

Indifference: Lack of interest or concern. Aloofness. Detachment.

Justice: The quality of impartiality or fairness.

Moral values: Values that dictate how one interacts with or treats another human being, which reflect a person's basic uniqueness, dignity, and worth.

Nonmoral values: Values that do not reflect on how one treats another person but reflects esthetic, political, intellectual, personal, or social choices.

Patronizing: To adopt an air of condescension.

Perfectionism: The doctrine that the perfection of moral character is a person's highest good and that freedom from imperfection is attainable.

Pity: Sympathetic heartfelt sorrow; shared feeling wherein the individual pitied is deemed "less than" the one pitying.

Prejudice: To prejudge or to classify a person as belonging to a larger group and thus to believe things about that person that one believes about the larger group.

Respect: The act of giving particular attention to a person; worthy of high regard.

Self-transposal: The attempt to put oneself cognitively in the place of the other; to "walk in another person's shoes."

Sympathy: Feeling at one with another's feelings.

Value: An inner force that provides the standards by which patterns of choice are made.

APPENDIX

Suggested Answers to Case Study Guiding Questions

Remember, in ethics we strive for the *best* (versus the *right*) answer according to established normative biomedical ethical reasoning, depending on our perceptions of the facts of the situation at the time.

1. List the facts affecting this situation.

ANSWER: (1) You (PT) made the splint. (2) The splint is interfering with healing (above all do no harm). (3) The patient trusts you; there is an ongoing patient/practitioner relationship built on trust. (4) You are in charge of this patient's rehabilitation. (5) You do not want to alienate the referring physician or lose the trust of your patient. (6) The patient also has an ongoing relationship of trust with his physician that is valuable and to be honored and not interfered with (fidelity to colleagues).

2. Identify the arms of the dilemma and values at war with each other (ethical principles involved).

ANSWER:

On the one hand:
- beneficence
- non-maleficence
- veracity
- autonomy of the clinician (PT)

On the other hand:
- fidelity to the referring physician
- self-interest (Keeping your practice viable)

3. List your professional duties.

ANSWER
- Tell the truth.
- Educate the referring physician as to the science and clinical reasoning behind your decision.
- Do nothing to harm the relationship of the patient with you *or with his physician.*

4. List the practical features that impact this situation.

ANSWER
- Loss of this physician's referrals may contribute to the financial failure of your new practice.
- You want a better relationship with this physician than appears now.
- The physician just may have information bearing on this case that is not known to you that may make it clearer to you why he is so adamantly opposed to what you have determined to be your best action for the patient.

5. Come to a final decision that you can justify because you are acting on the higher value in this situation.

ANSWER: Above all, you cannot harm your patient, and you do have to do what you determine

is clinically best for him at this time. You may argue that removing the splint for the time it takes for the patient to return to the referring physician will not really "harm" him, but you must also remember that there is potential for harm of your relationship with the patient if you do exactly what the physician requires of you. Your highest value here is *beneficence*, doing what you determine is clinically best for the patient. But if you act carefully, you can also help sustain the patient's relationship with his physician (*fidelity*) and respectfully disagree with the physician (*autonomy of the physical therapist*). What you do not want to do is simply blindly obey the physician's angry command "because he told you to do it and he's the doctor." Your code of ethics prohibits acting in ways that are not in the patient's best interest except when to do so would bring harm to others. Therefore, I suggest that this plan would be a "best" plan, but you may come up with other ideas that improve on this answer, depending on how you read the situation.

1. First, you must converse further with the referring physician. Show him relevant science and written material that sustains your decision. Respectfully request his rationale for his decision. The physician must explain to you, as a professional colleague, why he wanted the splint retained until he evaluated the patient before you act against your best clinical decision. This relationship needs some repair, and it probably is going to be up to you to initiate that action, whether you feel this disagreement is caused by you or not.

2. Do not lie to your patient. It is not ethical to say, "I made a mistake," as the physician requires, because that is not your truth. Instead, you might tell your patient that you and the physician have different points of view about the removal of the splint, and that you are communicating further. In the meantime, the physician wants to see the patient with the splint on. You would like the patient to see the physician as soon as possible.

3. It may be true that without this physician's referrals, your practice would suffer, and then your professional contribution to the community would be severely diminished, but doing exactly as the referring physician demands, at this point, is not ethically justified. Keeping your business going is an important goal, but when the needs of the patient collide with your need to keep your business going, then you must recognize this is a conflict of self-interest with beneficence. Your professional ethics prohibit you from putting your own needs before your patient's.

Vital Signs 4

Thomas J. Schmitz

LEARNING OBJECTIVES

1. Identify the rationale for including vital sign measures in patient examination data.
2. Explain the importance of monitoring vital signs in establishing a database of patient information.
3. Recognize the importance of monitoring vital signs as a method of assessing physiological response to selected treatment interventions.
4. Describe the common techniques for monitoring temperature, respiration, blood pressure, and pulse palpation.
5. Identify normal and abnormal values or ranges for each vital sign.
6. Describe the normative variations in vital signs and the factors that influence these changes.
7. Describe methods for recording data obtained from monitoring vital signs.

INTRODUCTION

The Guide to Physical Therapist Practice includes assessment of standard **vital signs** (e.g., blood pressure, heart rate, respiratory rate) and pulse palpation among the examination procedures recommended for many diagnostic groups.[1] Vital signs, also referred to as *cardinal signs*, provide quantitative measures of both cardiovascular and respiratory function. These signs are important indicators of the body's physiological status and reflect the function of internal organs. Variations in vital signs are a clear indicator that some change in the patient's physiological status has occurred. Taken at rest, during, and after exercise these measures also provide important data on aerobic capacity and endurance.[1] Together with other examination data, vital sign measures assist the physical therapist in formulating clinical judgements for:
1. Determining diagnosis and prognosis.
2. Designing the plan of care (identification of goals and outcomes, and selection of specific interventions).

3. Evaluating the effectiveness of selected interventions in achieving *goals* (remediation of impairments).
4. Evaluating the effectiveness of selected interventions in achieving *outcomes* (minimization of functional limitation and disability, optimization of health status, prevention of disability, and optimization of patient satisfaction).

In assessing vital signs it is important to note that *normal* values are specific to an individual. Although average or normative ranges have been established (Table 4–1), some individuals will typically or *normally* display higher or lower values than those represented by these normative figures. This addresses the importance of monitoring vital signs as a serial process. Vital sign measurements yield the most useful information when performed and recorded at *periodic intervals over time* as opposed to a one-time assessment. This type of serial recording allows changes in patient status or response to treatment to be monitored over time as well as indicating an acute change in physiological status at a specific point in time.

Table 4–1 NORMATIVE VITAL SIGN VALUES BY AGE. TEMPERATURE VALUES ARE GIVEN IN BOTH FAHRENHEIT AND CELSIUS SCALES

Age	Temperature (° F)	Temperature (° C)	Pulse Rate (beats per minute)	Respiratory Rate (breaths per minute)	Blood Pressure (mmHg)
Newborn	98.6–99.8	37–37.6	100–190	30–50	systolic: 50–52 diastolic: 25–30 mean: 35–40
3 years	98.5–99.5	36.9–37.5	80–125	20–30	systolic: 78–114 diastolic: 46–78
10 years	97.5–98.6	36.4–37	70–110	16–22	systolic: 90–120 diastolic: 56–84
16 years	97.6–98.8	36.4–37.1	55–100	15–20	systolic: 104–120 diastolic: 60–84
Adult	96.8–99.5	36–37.5	60–90	12–20	systolic: 95–140 diastolic: 60–90
Older adult	96.5–97.5	35.9–36.3	60–90	15–22	systolic: 140–160 diastolic: 70–90

From Fitzgerald,[5] p 39, with permission.

ALTERATIONS IN VITAL SIGN DATA

Overview of Influential Variables

Several life-style patterns (modifiable) and patient characteristics (nonmodifiable) are influential in altering vital sign measures. Life-style patterns include, but are not limited to, caffeine intake, tobacco use, diet, alcohol consumption, response to stress, obesity, level of physical activity, medications, and use of illegal drugs.[2] Patient characteristics include hormonal status, age, gender, and family history. Other variables that affect vital sign measures include time of day, time of the month (menstrual cycle), general health status, and pain. Data on these areas should be collected during history taking and, if modifiable, addressed during patient education interventions. Specific factors influencing individual vital sign measures will be addressed in greater detail later in the chapter.

Culture and Ethnicity

As with any physical therapy examination procedure, the influence of cultural and ethnicity can vary from having a subtle to marked impact on vital signs measures. For example, a patient who appears anxious or hostile during a vital signs assessment may be displaying a standard response to stress shared by others who have a deep-seated distrust of American health care practices. This situation would clearly affect the accuracy of the vital sign measures.

Culture refers to an integration of learned behaviors (not biologically inherited) characteristic of a society. Ethnicity is defined as an affiliation with a group of people who share a common cultural origin or background, or common racial, national, religious, linguistic, or cultural characteristics.[3] Recent demographic changes in the United States have created greater societal diversity and heightened the need for health care providers to address these issues during examination and treatment interventions. Culture and ethnicity directly impact the values, beliefs, and attitudes held by an individual toward health care.[4] Metzgar[3] and Fitzgerald[5] offer the following general suggestions for interaction with a culturally diverse patient population:

- Stereotypes should be avoided. Although a patient may share characteristics with others of the same culture, each patient will also have unique, individual differences.
- Respect cultural inferences and individual differences in beliefs and attitudes toward health care.
- Focus on developing the patient's trust and rapport.
- Remain aware that one's own personal values and beliefs may distort the assessment of a patient from a different background.
- Be cautious not to interpret ethnic or cultural preferences in dress, manner, and physical appearance for abnormal behavior or psychological disorder.

For additional information on the impact of cultural diversity in health care the reader is referred to the work of Spector,[4] Purnell and Paulanka,[6] Lynch and Hanson,[7] and Galanati.[8]

PATIENT OBSERVATION

Prior to a formal assessment of vital signs, careful systematic observation of the patient can reveal important preliminary data. Observation alone will not provide definitive diagnostic information; however, when combined with data from vital sign measures, it will provide important clues for directing further examination procedures. Lewis[2] offers the following general strategies to guide the therapist's observations:

- Signs of immediate patient distress or discomfort are typically evident by observation of facial expressions, use of accessory muscles for breathing, an irregular breathing pattern, and frequent positional changes.
- Clues about nutritional status may be indicated by obesity or the presence of **cachexia** (state of

ill health, appearance of malnutrition, and wasting; associated with many chronic diseases).

- Skin color changes will indicate if **cyanosis** is present. Color changes in the mucous membranes are associated with **central cyanosis.** These membranes are normally pink and shiny irrespective of skin color. Central cyanosis is indicative of marked arterial desaturation. **Peripheral cyanosis** is observed by skin color changes in the earlobes, nose, lips, and toes. It is usually transient, occurs secondary to vasoconstriciton, and is typically relieved by warming the area.
- The skin should be observed for changes in texture and hair growth. Patients with diabetes mellitus or atherosclerosis will typically lack hair growth on the legs and display thickening of the nails of the fingers and toes. Skin texture also varies with age and poor nutritional status.
- **Diaphoresis** (profuse perspiration) of the skin is usually indicative that the body is working to compensate for a reduced cardiac output. It is associated with a variety of diagnostic categories including myocardial infarction, **hypotension,** and shock.
- Abnormal sitting postures may be indicative of pain or structural abnormalities of the pectoral or vertebral regions which may interfere with respiratory patterns.
- Use of accessory muscles of breathing may be indicative of cardiac or pulmonary impairments.
- Peripheral observations of the extremities should include the presence of edema or **clubbing** (a gradual development of bulbous swelling at the distal fingers and toes accompanied by a loss of the normal angle between the nailbed and the skin). Peripheral edema is typically associated with right heart failure or venous insufficiency. Clubbing is associated with diagnoses imposing long-standing hypoxia and cyanosis such as congenital heart defects and pulmonary disorders.

During this initial observation, use of well-structured, impairment-specific questions will assist development of an initial database of patient information. Depending on individual patient needs, data may be gathered from the patient, family member, or caregiver. Box 4–1 presents a sample of clinical indicators that typically warrant monitoring of vital signs. Below each clinical indicator are sample guiding statements or questions designed to facilitate history taking during initial observation of the patient. Associated tests, and vital sign measures of most immediate interest are also included.

MEASURING VITAL SIGNS

Temperature

Body temperature represents a balance between the heat produced or acquired by the body and the amount lost. Because humans are warm-blooded, or **homoiothermic,** body temperature remains relatively constant, despite changes in the external environment. This is in contrast to cold-blooded, or **poikilothermic,** animals (such as reptiles) in which body temperature varies with that of their environment.

The Thermoregulatory System

The purpose of the thermoregulatory system is to maintain a relatively constant internal body temperature. This system monitors and acts to maintain temperatures that are optimal for normal cellular and vital organ function. The thermoregulatory system consists of three primary components: the thermoreceptors, the regulating center, and the effector organs (Fig. 4-1).[9–11]

THERMORECEPTORS

The thermoreceptors provide input to the temperature-regulating center located in the hypothalamus. The regulating center is dependent on information from thermoreceptors to achieve constant temperatures. Once this information reaches the regulatory center, it is compared with a "set point" standard or optimal temperature value. Depending on the contrast between the "set" value and incoming information, mechanisms may be activated either to conserve or to dissipate heat.[10]

Afferent temperature input is provided to the regulating center by both *peripheral* and *central* thermoreceptors. The peripheral receptors, composed primarily of free nerve endings, have a high distribution in the skin (cutaneous thermoreceptors). They are also located in the abdominal organs and nervous system.[9,10] Thermoreceptors may also be present in other deep structures not yet identified.[10] The cutaneous thermoreceptors demonstrate a larger distribution of cold to warmth receptors and are sensitive to rapid changes in temperature.[11] Signals from these receptors enter the spinal cord through afferent nerves and travel to the hypothalamus via the lateral spinothalamic tract.

The central thermoreceptors are located in the hypothalamus and are sensitive to temperature changes in blood perfusing the hypothalamus. These cells also can initiate responses to either conserve or dissipate heat. They are particularly sensitive to core temperature changes and monitoring body warmth.[11]

REGULATING CENTER

The temperature-regulating center of the body is located in the hypothalamus. The hypothalamus functions to coordinate the heat production and loss processes, much like a thermostat, ensuring an essentially constant and stable body temperature. By influencing the effector organs, the hypothalamus achieves a relatively precise balance between heat production and heat loss. In a healthy individual, the hypothalamic thermostat is set and carefully maintained at $98.6° \pm 1.8°F$ ($37° \pm 1°C$).[11] In situations in which input from thermoreceptors

---

Box 4–1 SAMPLE OF CLINICAL INDICATORS THAT TYPICALLY WARRANT DETERMINATION OF VITAL SIGN MEASURES

Below each clinical indicator are sample guiding statements or questions designed to facilitate history taking during initial observation of the patient prior to, or during, gathering of vital sign data. If warranted by the clinical indicator, specific areas of needed observation and vital sign measures *beyond the standard* are noted.

Clinical indicator
Dyspnea (shortness of breath, breathlessness, uncomfortable awareness of one's sensation of breathlessness).

Sample statements or questions
- Obtain a description of the dyspnea.
- What provokes it?
- What alleviates it?
- Does the dyspnea have a sudden or gradual onset?
- Does position affect it?
- Does time of day affect it?
- Review medications patient is taking.

Clinical indicator
Fatigue (weakness) and syncope.

Sample statements or questions
- Obtain a description of the fatigue (weakness) and syncope.
- What provokes the onset?
- What alleviates the fatigue and syncope?
- Review medications patient is taking.

Clinical indicator
Chest pain (discomfort).

Sample statements or questions
- Obtain a description of the chest discomfort.
- Where is the discomfort located?
- Identify the severity of the discomfort on a scale of 1 to 10.
- What provokes the discomfort?
- What alleviates it?
- Has the discomfort occurred before?
- Does rest stop the discomfort?
- Does the discomfort radiate (move) in any direction?
- Is the discomfort sudden or gradual in onset?
- Review medications patient is taking.

Clinical indicator
Irregular heartbeat (palpitations).

Sample statements or questions and specific vital sign measure
- Obtain a description of the palpitations.

- Identify heart rhythm.
- Does the patient sense skipped beats or experience a sensation that the heart is racing?
- What provokes and alleviates the irregular heartbeat?
- Review medications the patient is taking.

Clinical indicator
Cyanosis.

Areas of needed observation
- Central cyanosis: observed by inspecting the mucous membranes; indicates a shunting of deoxygenated blood to the arterial circulation.
- Peripheral cyanosis: observed by assessing the extremities; associated with a vasoconstriction in response to cold and is usually not a serious clinical manifestation.

Clinical indicator
Intermittent claudication (leg pain that occurs with activity or rest).

Sample statements or questions and specific vital sign measures
- Obtain a description of the leg pain.
- Locate site of pain.
- Assess femoral, popliteal, and pedal pulses.
- Assess skin color and temperature of legs.
- What provokes the pain?
- What alleviates the pain?
- Assess severity of the pain on a scale of 1 to 10.
- Assess quality of the pain.
- Review medications the patient is taking.

Clinical indicator
Pedal edema (swelling of the feet and lower legs).

Areas of needed observation and specific vital sign measures
- Assess femoral, popliteal, and pedal pulses.
- Assess skin condition and color.
- Observe edema. Note the extent of edema in the tissue (i.e., from toes to ankle). To determine pitting edema, gently touch edematous tissue. In 15-second intervals, observe how long it takes the skin to return to a normal state. A time interval of 0 to 15 seconds is 1+ edema, 16 to 30 seconds is 2+ edema, 31 to 45 seconds is 3+ edema, and greater than 46 seconds is 4+ edema. Pitting edema can also be assessed by depth using a small ruler such that 1+ edema = 2 mm depth, 2+ edema = 4 mm depth, 3+ edema = 6 mm depth, and 4+ edema = 8 mm or greater depth.

Adapted from Lewis,[2] with permission.

---

indicates a drop in temperature below the "set" value, mechanisms are activated to conserve heat. Conversely, a rise in temperature will activate mechanisms to dissipate heat. Mechanisms to dissipate heat are particularly important during strenuous exercise. Figure 4-2 summarizes the primary physiological adjustments during heat acclimation (the physiological adaptations that improve tolerance to heat) to exercise or increases in environmental temperature. These responses are activated through hypothalamic control over the effector organs. Input to the effector organs is transmitted through nervous pathways of both the somatic and autonomic nervous systems.[9–11]

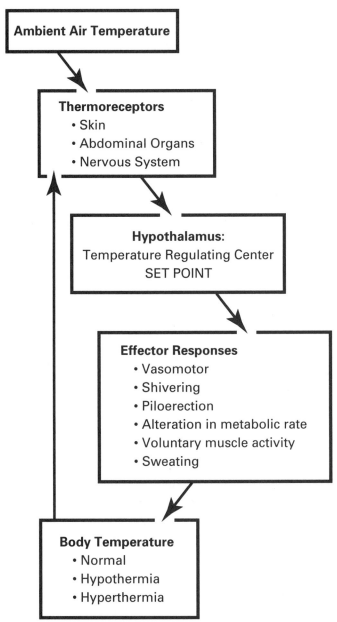

Figure 4-1. Thermoregulatory responses. The thermoreceptors provide input regarding changes in body temperature, which signal the preoptic nucleus of the hypothalamus. This physiological thermostat compares incoming signals of actual body temperature with the set point value. If body temperature is lower than the set point value, heat gain mechanisms are implemented. If body temperature is higher than the set point value, heat loss mechanisms are implemented.[9–11]

EFFECTOR ORGANS

The effector organs respond to both increases and decreases in temperature. The primary effector systems include vascular, metabolic, skeletal muscle (shivering) responses, and sweating. These effector systems function either to increase or to dissipate body heat.

CONSERVATION AND PRODUCTION OF BODY HEAT

When body temperature is lowered, mechanisms are activated to conserve heat and increase heat production. Following are descriptions of heat conservation and production mechanisms.

Vasoconstriction of Blood Vessels

The hypothalamus activates sympathetic nerves, an action that results in vasoconstriction of cutaneous vessels throughout the body. This significantly reduces the lumen of the vessels and decreases blood flow near the surface of the skin where the blood would normally be cooled. Thus the amount of heat lost to the environment is decreased.

Decrease in or Abolition of Sweat Gland Activity

To reduce or to prevent heat loss by evaporation, sweat gland activity is diminished. Sweating is totally abolished with cooling of the hypothalamic thermostat below approximately 98.6°F (37°C).[10,11]

Cutis Anserina or Piloerection

Also a response to cooling of the hypothalamus, this heat conservation mechanism is commonly described as "gooseflesh." The term *piloerection* means "hairs standing on end." Although of less significance in man, in lower mammals with greater hair covering, this mechanism functions to trap a layer of insulating air near the skin and decrease heat loss.

The body also responds to decreased temperature with several mechanisms designed to produce heat. These mechanisms are activated when the body thermostat falls below approximately 98.6°F (37°C).[10] Following are descriptions of heat production mechanisms.

Shivering

The primary motor center for shivering is located in the posterior hypothalamus. This area is activated by cold signals from the skin and spinal cord. In response to cold, impulses from the hypothalamus activate the efferent somatic nervous system causing increased tone of skeletal muscles. As the tone gradually increases to a certain threshold level, shivering (involuntary muscle contraction) is initiated and heat is produced. This reflex shivering can be at least partially inhibited through conscious cortical control.[10]

Hormonal Regulation

The function of hormonal influence in thermal regulation is to increase cellular metabolism, which subsequently increases body heat. Increased metabolism occurs through circulation of two hormones from the adrenal medulla: *norepinephrine* and *epinephrine*. Circulating levels of these hormones, however, are of greater significance in maintaining body temperature in infants than in adults. Heat production by these hormones can be increased in an infant by as much as 100 percent, as opposed to 10 to 15 percent in an adult.[10]

A second form of hormonal regulation involves increased output of thyroxine by the thyroid gland. Thyroxine increases the rate of cellular metabolism throughout the body. This response, however, occurs

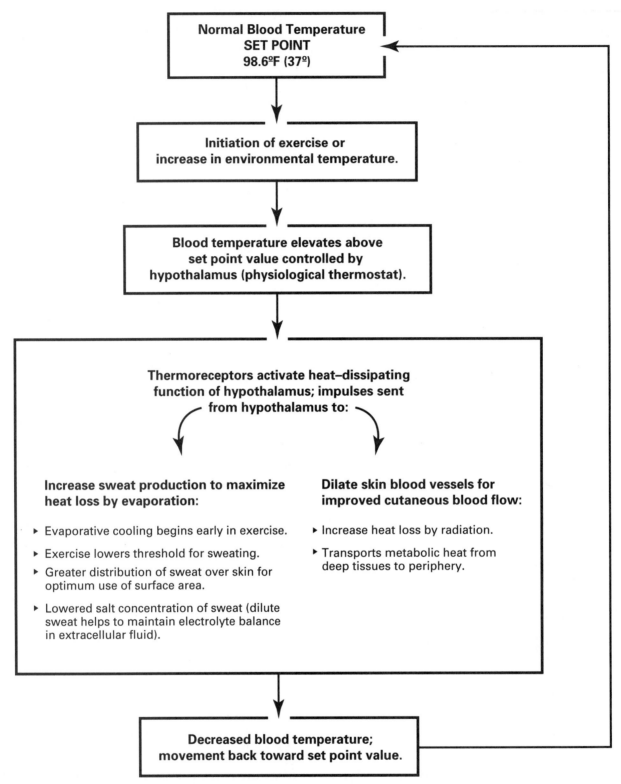

Figure 4-2. Physiological adjustments during heat acclimation. Increased body temperature activities heat dissipation to maintain normal body temperature.

only as a result of prolonged cooling, and heat production is not immediate.[11] The thyroid gland requires several weeks to hypertrophy before increased demands for thyroxine can be achieved.

LOSS OF BODY HEAT

Excess heat is dissipated from the body through four primary methods: radiation, conduction, convection, and evaporation.

Radiation is the transfer of heat by electromagnetic waves from one object to another. This heat transfer occurs through the air between objects that are not in direct contact. Heat is lost to surrounding objects that are colder than the body (e.g., loss of heat to a wall or surrounding room objects). As depicted in Fig. 4-3, a person without clothing in a room maintained at normal temperature loses approximately 60 percent of total heat loss to radiation.[10]

Conduction is the transfer of heat from one object to another through a liquid, solid, or gas. This type of heat transfer requires direct molecular contact between two objects, as when a person is sitting on a cold surface, or when heat is lost in a cool swimming pool. Heat is also lost by conduction to air.

Convection is the transfer of heat by movement of air or liquid (water). This form of heat loss is accomplished secondary to conduction. Once the heat is conducted to the air, the air is then moved away from the body by convection currents. Use of a fan or a cool breeze provides convection currents. Heat loss by convection is most effective when the air or liquid surrounding the body is continually moved away and replaced.

Evaporation is the conversion of a liquid to a vapor. This form of heat loss occurs on a continual basis through the respiratory tract and through perspiration from the skin. Evaporation provides the major mechanism of heat loss during heavy exercise. Profuse sweating provides a significant cooling effect on the skin as it evaporates. In addition, this cooling of the skin functions to further cool the blood as it is shunted from internal structures to cutaneous areas.

ABNORMALITIES IN BODY TEMPERATURE

Increased Body Temperature

An elevation in body temperature is generally believed to assist the body in fighting disease or infection. **Pyrexia** is the elevation of normal body temperature, more commonly referred to as **fever.** **Hyperpyrexia** and **hyperthermia** are terms that describe an extremely high fever, generally above 106°F (41.1°C).[12] The primary clinical manifestations of hyperthermia are presented by body system in Table 4–2.

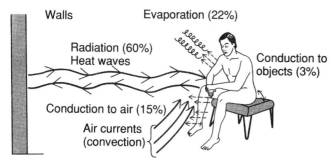

Figure 4-3. Mechanisms of heat dissipation from body. (From Guyton, et al.,[10] p 576, with permission.)

Table 4–2 PRIMARY CLINICAL MANIFESTATIONS OF HYPERTHERMIA PRESENTED BY BODY SYSTEM

System	Effects
Cardiovascular	Heart rate may increase by 8.5 beats/min for each 33.8°F (1°C) rise in temperature during fever, and up to 25 beats/min in other forms of hyperthermia. Decreased perfusion and high metabolic rate promote metabolic acidosis.
Nervous	Febrile seizures occur in 2–4% of young children with high temperatures. Hypoxia and decreased perfusion result in sleepiness and confusion in lower-grade fevers and in delirium, stupor, or coma in extreme hyperthermia.
Respiratory	Increased metabolic rate and activation of heat loss mechanisms induces hypoxia and respiratory alkalosis.
Renal	Increased metabolic rate and dehydration promote electrolyte imbalances and accumulation of metabolic wastes in the blood (azotemia). Thermal injury to muscle may cause rhabdomyolysis (release of myoglobin), which obstructs renal tubules.
Hematologic	Dehydration results in hemoconcentration. Disseminated intravascular coagulation can occur secondary to tissue injury.

From Hansen,[9] p 223, with permission.

Pyrexia occurs when the "set" value of the hypothalamic thermostat rises. This elevation is caused by the influence of **pyrogens** (fever producing substance). Pyrogens are secreted primarily from toxic bacteria or are released from degenerating body tissue.[10] The effects of these pyrogens result in fever during illness. As a result of the new, higher thermostat value, the body responds by activating its heat conservation and production mechanisms. These mechanisms raise body temperature to the new, higher value over a period of several hours. Thus a fever, or **febrile** state, is produced.

The clinical signs and symptoms of a fever vary with the level of disturbance of the thermoregulatory center, and with the specific stage of the fever (onset, course, or termination). These signs and symptoms may include general malaise, headache, increased pulse and respiratory rate, chills, piloerection, shivering, loss of appetite **(anorexia),** pale skin that later becomes flushed and hot to the touch, nausea, irritability, restlessness, constipation, sweating, thirst, coated tongue, decreased urinary output, weakness, and insomnia.[9,13] With higher elevations in temperature (hyperpyrexia), disorientation, confusion, convulsions, or coma may occur. These latter symptoms are more common in children under the age of 5 years and are believed to be related to the immaturity of the nervous system.

Three specific stages have been identified describing the course of a fever:

1. Invasion or *onset* is the period from either gradual or sudden rise until the maximum temperature is reached.

2. Fastigium or *stadium* (course) is the point of highest elevation of the fever. Once maximum temperature is reached, it remains relatively stable.
3. *Difervescence* (termination) identifies the period during which the fever subsides and temperatures move toward normal. This drop in temperature can occur suddenly (crisis) or gradually (lysis).

Lowered Body Temperature

Exposure to extreme cold produces a lowered body temperature called **hypothermia.** With prolonged exposure to cold there is a decrease in metabolic rate, and body temperature gradually falls. As cooling of the brain occurs, there is a depression of the thermoregulatory center. The function of the thermoregulatory center becomes seriously impaired when body temperature falls below approximately 94°F (34.4°C) and is completely lost with temperatures below 85°F (29.4°C).[10] The body's heat regulatory and protection mechanism is therefore lost. Symptoms of hypothermia include decreased pulse and respiratory rates, cold and pale skin, cyanosis, decreased cutaneous sensation, depression of mental and muscular responses, and drowsiness, which may eventually lead to coma. If left untreated, the progression of these symptoms may lead to death. The primary clinical manifestations of hypothermia are presented by body system in Table 4–3.

Factors Influencing Body Temperature

A statistical average or normal temperature of 98.6°F (37°C) taken orally has been established for body temperature in an adult population. However, body temperature is most accurately presented as a range. A range of values is more representative of normal body temperature because certain everyday circumstances (e.g., time of day) or activities (e.g., exercise) influence the body's temperature. In addition, some individuals typically run a *slightly higher* or *lower* body temperature than the statistical average. Therefore, deviations from the average will be apparent from individual to individual, as well as between measures taken from a single subject under varying circumstances.

Time of Day. The term **circadian rhythm** describes a 24-hour cycle of normal variations in body temperature. Certain predictable and regular changes in temperature occur on a daily basis. Body temperature tends to be lowest in the early morning hours, between 4 and 6 AM, and highest in the late afternoon and early evening hours, between 4 and 8 PM. These regular changes in body temperature are influenced significantly by both digestive processes and the level of skeletal muscle activity. For individuals who work at night, this pattern is usually inverted.[9–11]

Age. Compared with adults, infants demonstrate a higher normal temperature because of the immaturity of the thermoregulatory system (see Table 4–1). Infants are particularly susceptible to environmental temperature changes, and their body temperature will fluctuate accordingly. Young children also average higher normal temperatures because of the heat production associated with increased metabolic rate and high physical activity levels. Elderly populations tend to demonstrate lower than average body temperatures. Lower temperatures in elderly

Table 4–3 PRIMARY CLINICAL MANIFESTATIONS OF HYPOTHERMIA PRESENTED BY BODY SYSTEM

System	Effects
Cardiovascular	Decreased perfusion results from increased blood viscosity and denaturation of serum proteins.
	Vasoconstriction further decreases peripheral perfusion, promoting injury of peripheral tissues with freezing (frostbite). Lactic acidosis develops.
	First **tachycardia** then **bradycardia** is the typical cardiac rhythm.
	Decreased cardiac perfusion produces electrocardiographic changes, including Osborne (J) waves following the QRS complex, and lengthening of the PR, QRS, and QT intervals. Blood pressure drops.
	Atrial and ventricular dysrhythmias are induced by myocardial hypoxia. Asystole occurs at temperatures below 82.4°F (28°C).
Nervous	Hypothalamic heat gain mechanisms are activated early, including vasoconstriction, shivering, and increased metabolic rate.
	Shivering stops with moderate hypothermia as muscles stiffen. Stupor and coma occur with reduced cerebral perfusion.
	Pupils become nonreactive, and reflexes disappear. Response to pain decreases.
	Electroencephalogram may be flat with severe hypothermia.
Respiratory	Respiratory rate is initially increased but soon decreases as oxygen consumption declines. Arterial blood gas values obtained from hypothermic patients are unreliable.
	A 50% decrease in CO_2 production occurs with a decrease of 46.4°F (8°C) in temperature.
	Bronchorrhea and cough suppression are apparent at first, followed by pulmonary edema.
	Hypothermia shifts the oxyhemoglobin dissociation curve to the left, decreasing oxygen delivery to tissues.
Renal	Cold-induced diuresis occurs. Renal acid excretion is impaired. Glycosuria and electrolyte imbalances develop.
Hematologic	Hematocrit increases 2% for each 33.8°F (1°C) decline in temperature, contributing to hypercoagulability.
	Cold directly inhibits the clotting cascade.
	Production of thromboxane B_2 by platelets declines, and thrombocytopenia results from bone marrow suppression and hepatic sequestration.

From Hansen,[9] p 227, with permission.

populations are associated with a variety of factors, including lower metabolic rates, decreased subcutaneous tissue mass (which normally insulates the body against heat loss), decreased physical activity levels, and inadequate diet.

Emotions. Extremes in emotions will increase body temperature due to increased glandular secretions and a subsequent increase in metabolic rate.

Exercise. The effects of exercise on body temperature are an important consideration for physical therapists. Strenuous exercise significantly increases body temperature because of increased metabolic rate. Active muscle contractions are an important and potent source of heat production. During exercise, body temperature increases are proportional to the relative intensity of the workload. Vigorous exercise can increase the metabolic rate by as much as 20 to 25 times that of the basal level.[11]

Menstrual Cycle. Increased levels of progesterone during ovulation cause body temperature to rise 0.5° to 0.9°F (0.3° to 0.5°C). This slight elevation is maintained until just prior to the initiation of menstruation, at which time it returns to normal levels.

Pregnancy. Because of increased metabolic activity, body temperature remains elevated approximately 0.9°F (0.5°C). Temperature returns to normal after parturition.

External Environment. Generally, warm weather tends to increase body temperature, and cold weather decreases body temperature. Environmental conditions influence the body's ability to maintain constant temperatures. For example, in hot, humid environments the effectiveness of evaporative cooling is severely diminished because the air is already heavily moisture laden. Other forms of heat dissipation are also dependent on environmental factors such as movement of air currents (convection). Clothing also can be an important external consideration because it can function both to conserve and to facilitate release of body heat. The amount and type of clothing is important. To dissipate heat, absorbent, loose-fitting, light-colored clothing is most effective. To conserve heat, several layers of lightweight clothing to trap air and to insulate the body are recommended.

Location of Measurement. Rectal temperatures are from 0.5° to 0.9°F (0.3° to 0.5°C) higher than oral temperatures; axillary temperatures are approximately 1.1°F (0.6°C) lower than oral temperatures.

Ingestion of Warm or Cold Foods. Oral temperatures will be affected by oral intake, including smoking. Patients should refrain from smoking or eating for at least 15 minutes (preferably 30 minutes) prior to an oral temperature reading.

ASSESSING BODY TEMPERATURE
Types of Thermometers

Electronic Thermometers. This type of thermometer provides a rapid (several second), highly accurate measure of body temperature.[5] Standard oral electronic thermometers consist of a portable battery operated unit, an attached probe, and plastic disposable probe covers (Fig. 4-4). The units provide a flashed, digital display of body temperature, or a stationary scale and needle marker display. An important advantage of these thermometers is the low chance of cross-infection, inasmuch as the probe covers are used only once.

Hand-held electronic oral thermometers are also commercially available. These units are typically about 6 inches in length with a tapered design (Fig. 4-5). One end of the device is narrow and serves as the probe. The opposite end is broad and houses the battery. These thermometers also provide a flashed, digital display of body temperature. Some models allow use with disposable covers.

Electronic thermometers are also available that measure body temperature from the external ear (Fig. 4-6). These battery-operated hand-held units include an ear probe (with disposable covers) and provide a rapid, digital readout of body temperature. Other types of electronic thermometers include both earlobe clips and finger sleeve or clip sensors. Nipple-shaped pacifier designs are also available for monitoring oral temperatures of infants.

Clinical Glass Thermometer. Traditionally, temperatures have been taken by a glass thermometer, which consists of a glass tube with a bulbous tip filled with mercury. Once the bulb is in contact with body heat, the mercury expands and rises in the glass column to register body temperature. Reflux of mercury down the tube is prevented by a narrowing of the base. The device must be shaken vigorously to return the mercury to the bulb before the next use.

Glass thermometers are calibrated in either (or both) Celsius and Fahrenheit scales. The range is from approximately 93° to 108°F (34° to 42.2°C), with slight variations among different manufacturers. The calibrations are in degrees and tenths of a

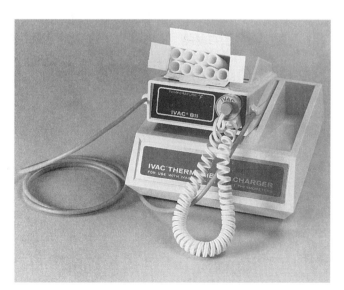

Figure 4-4. Standard electronic oral thermometer. Components include a battery-powered unit with a digital display, a probe, and disposable probe covers. (Courtesy of IVAC Corporation, San Diego, CA.)

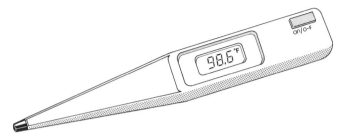

Figure 4-5. Hand-held electronic oral thermometer.

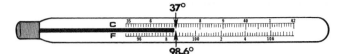

A. Blunt end.

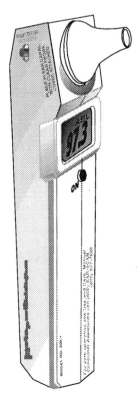

B. Elongated end.   C. Rounded end.

Figure 4-7. Clinical glass thermometer, illustrating the three shapes of bulbous ends. The blunt end (A) can be used for both oral and rectal temperatures. The elongated end (B) is for oral measures, and the rounded end (C) is for rectal measures. (From Saperstein, AB and Frazier, MA: The Assessment of Vital Signs. In Saperstein, AB and Frazier, MA (eds): Introduction to Nursing Practice. FA Davis, Philadelphia, 1980, p 456, with permission.)

degree. As such, each long line represents a full degree and each short line indicates 0.1 degrees on the Celsius thermometer and 0.2 degrees on the Fahrenheit thermometer. When recording temperatures it is common practice to round the fractions of degrees to the nearest whole number.

There are three different shapes of bulbous ends on glass thermometers, depending on their intended use (Fig. 4-7). A blunt tip can be used for either oral or rectal temperatures. The elongated end is for oral or axillary measures, and the rounded tip is for rectal measures.

Chemical Thermometers. These instruments are used in a similar fashion to a clinical glass thermometer because they are placed under the tongue. They consist of a series of calibrated dots impregnated with a temperature-sensitive chemical. After removal, the dots are examined for color changes to determine the temperature reading. They are disposed of after use.

Temperature-Sensitive Tape. Heat-sensitive tape or disks respond to body temperature by changing color. They are frequently used with pediatric patients. The forehead and abdomen are common placement sites. The temperature readings are nonspecific and are usually confirmed with a more precise measure if deviations are noted.

Procedure for Assessing Body Temperature

For purposes of establishing baseline data and assessing response to treatment, physical therapists generally use oral monitoring. However, in situations in which oral temperatures may be contraindicated and an electronic unit with an alternative sensor is unavailable, an axillary measure may be substituted. Both procedures will be described.

Electronic Thermometer for Assessing Oral Temperature
  A. Wash hands.
  B. Assemble equipment.
    1. An electronic thermometer unit.
    2. Disposable probe cover.
    3. Worksheet and pen or pencil to record collected data.
  C. Procedure
    1. Explain procedure and rationale in terms appropriate to the patient's understanding.
    2. Assure patient comfort.
    3. Turn on power unit (some units require a warm-up period).
    4. Place disposable cover over probe.
    5. Ask patient to open mouth, and place the covered probe at the posterior base of the tongue to the right or left of the frenulum. Instruct patient to close the lips (not teeth) around the probe and hold it in place.
    6. Electronic thermometer probes should be left in place following manufacturer's instructions for that particular unit (frequently between 10 and 45 seconds).
    7. Remove probe and dispose of cover.
    8. Temperature reading is obtained from digital readout or scale.
    9. Record results.

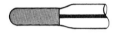

Figure 4-6. Hand-held electronic external ear thermometer.

Clinical Glass Thermometer for Assessing Oral Temperature

A. Wash hands.
B. Assemble equipment.
1. An oral thermometer.
2. Soft tissue to wipe thermometer.
3. Worksheet and pen or pencil to record collected data.
C. Procedure
1. Explain procedure and rationale in terms appropriate to the patient's understanding.
2. Assure patient comfort.
3. The thermometer should be held firmly between the thumb and forefinger at the end opposite the bulb.
4. If the thermometer has been soaked in a disinfectant solution, rinse under cold water.
5. Dry the thermometer using a clean tissue, wiping from the bulb toward the fingers in a rotating fashion.
6. Hold the thermometer at eye level and rotate until the column of mercury is clearly visible. Note the level of the column.
7. If necessary, shake the thermometer until the mercury is below 95°F (35°C). While holding the thermometer securely, use quick, downward motions of the wrist, which will effectively lower the column.
8. Ask patient to open mouth, and place thermometer at the posterior base of the tongue to the right or left of the frenulum. Instruct patient to close the lips (not teeth) around thermometer to hold it in place.
9. Leave the clinical glass thermometer in place for 7 to 8 minutes. It should be noted that considerable discrepancy exists in the literature regarding the length of time the thermometer should be left in place. Times vary from 5 to 10 minutes.
10. Remove the thermometer.
11. Using a clean tissue, wipe the thermometer away from the fingers in a rotating fashion.
12. Hold the thermometer at eye level, rotate until the mercury is clearly visible, and read the highest point on the scale to which the mercury has risen.
13. Record results.
14. Return the thermometer to an appropriate area for disinfecting.

Assessing Axillary Temperature. Although less accurate, axillary temperatures are used when oral temperatures are contraindicated and an electronic unit with an alternative sensor is unavailable. Contraindications for taking an oral temperature might include **dyspnea,** surgical procedures involving the mouth or throat, very young children, and delirious or irrational patients. In these circumstances axillary measures are considered safer. Axillary temperatures are approximately 1.1°F (0.6°C) lower than oral temperatures. The following procedure should be used.

A. Wash hands.
B. Assemble equipment.
1. An oral clinical glass thermometer is usually used.
2. Soft tissue to wipe thermometer.
3. A towel to dry axillary region (moisture will conduct heat).
4. Worksheet and pen or pencil to record collected data.
C. Procedure
1. Follow procedure, steps 1 through 7, for assessing oral temperature with a clinical glass thermometer.
2. Expose axillary region. If any moisture is present, the area should be gently towel dried with a patting motion (vigorous rubbing will increase temperature of the area).
3. Place the thermometer in the axillary region between the trunk and upper arm (Fig. 4-8). The patient's arm should be placed tightly across the chest to keep the thermometer in place (asking the patient to move his or her hand toward the opposite shoulder is often a useful direction). If the patient is disoriented or very young, the thermometer must be held in place.
4. Leave thermometer in place for 10 minutes.
5. Remove thermometer.
6. Using a clean tissue, wipe the thermometer away from the fingers in a rotating fashion.
7. Holding the thermometer at eye level, rotate it until the mercury is clearly visible, and read the highest point on the scale to which the mercury has risen.
8. Record results. Generally, a temperature reading is assumed an oral measure unless otherwise noted. An axillary temperature is designated by a circled A after the temperature (e.g., 95°F Ⓐ). Similarly, a circled R indicates a rectal measure (e.g., 99°F Ⓡ).
9. Return the thermometer to appropriate area for disinfecting.

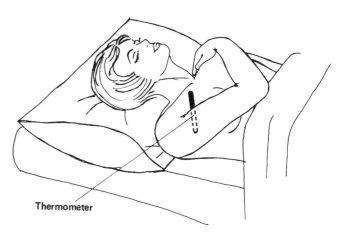

Figure 4-8. Positioning for monitoring axillary temperature.

PULSE

The **pulse** is the wave of blood in the artery created by contraction of the left ventricle during the cardiac cycle (one complete cycle of cardiac muscle contraction and relaxation). With each contraction, blood is pumped into an already full aorta. The inherent elasticity of the aortic walls allows expansion and acceptance of the new supply. The blood is then forced out and surges through the systemic arteries. It is this wave or surge of blood that is felt as the pulse.

Pressure changes in the large arteries during the cardiac cycle are reflected in the normal arterial waveform (Fig. 4-9 [top]). The lowest point of pressure occurs during ventricular **diastole;** the highest point occurs during ventricular **systole** (peak ejection). The notch on the descending slope of the pulse wave represents closure of the aortic valve and is not palpable.[14] A healthy adult heart beats an average of 70 times per minute, a rate that provides continuous circulation of approximately 5 to 6 liters of blood through the body. The pulse can be palpated wherever a superficial artery can be stabilized over a bony surface. In monitoring the pulse, specific attention is directed toward assessing three parameters: rate, rhythm, and volume.

Rate

The *rate* is the number of beats per minute. A pulse range of 60 to 90 beats per minute is considered normal for an adult. However, multiple factors will influence the pulse rate including age, sex, emotional status, and physical activity level. Body size and build also influence pulse rate.[11,14] Tall, thin individuals generally have a slower pulse rate than those who are obese or have stout frames.

Rhythm

The *rhythm* describes the intervals between beats. In a healthy individual, the rhythm is regular or constant and indicates the time intervals between beats are essentially equal.

Volume

The *volume* (force) refers to the amount of blood pushed through the artery during each ventricular contraction. The quantity (volume) of blood within the vessel produces the force of the pulse. Normally, the force of each beat is equal. With a higher blood volume, the force of the pulse is greater and with lower volumes it is weaker. The volume is assessed by how easily the pulse can be obliterated. With lower volumes, the pulse is *small*, is easily obliterated, and termed **weak** or **thready.** With an increased volume the pulse is *large*, difficult to obliterate, and is termed a **bounding** (or full) pulse; a feeling of high tension is noted.

Several other important terms are used to describe variations in pulse.[2,12,14] **Bigeminal** pulse is an increased arterial pulse having two beats (double systolic peak). **Pulsus alterans (alternating pulse)** is marked by a fluctuation in amplitude between beats (weak and a strong) with minimal change in overall rhythm. The term bigeminal is used to describe an abnormality in pulse rhythm. A normal pulse beat is followed by a premature beat of diminished amplitude. A **paradoxical pulse (pulsus paradoxus)** is a decreased amplitude of the pressure wave detected during quiet inspiration with a return to full amplitude on expiration; it is often associated with obstructive lung disease. Figure 4-9 provides a schematic illustration of normal (top) and common alterations in arterial pulse waveforms.

In addition to rate, rhythm, and volume, the quality or feel of the arterial wall should be assessed. Typically, a vessel will feel smooth, elastic, soft, flexible, and relatively straight. With advancing age, vessels may demonstrate sclerotic changes. These changes frequently cause the vessels to feel twisted, hard, or cordlike with decreased elasticity and smoothness.

Factors Influencing Pulse

Essentially, any factor that alters the metabolic rate will also influence heart rate. Several factors are of particular importance when considering pulse rate.

Age. Fetal pulse rates average 120 to 160 beats per minute. The pulse rates for a newborn range between 100 and 190, with an average of 120 beats per minute. Pulse rate gradually decreases with age until it stabilizes in adulthood (see Table 4–1). The average adult pulse rate is generally considered to be between 60 and 90 beats per minute; however, much wider variations, from 50 to 100 beats per minute, are considered within a normal range for adults.

Gender. Men and boys typically have slightly lower pulse rates than women and girls.

Emotions. Responses to a variety of emotions (e.g., grief, fear, anxiety, or pain) activate the sympathetic nervous system, with a resultant increase in pulse rate.

Exercise. Oxygen demands of skeletal muscles are significantly increased during physical activity. At rest, only 20 to 25 percent of the available muscle capillaries are open.[10,11] During vigorous exercise, extensive vasodilation causes all capillaries to open. The heart rate increases to provide additional blood flow to muscles and to meet the increased oxygen requirement. For physical therapists, monitoring a patient's pulse rate is an important method of assessing response to exercise. Typically, the pulse rate will increase as a function of the intensity of the activity. A linear relationship exists between pulse rate and intensity of workload. To use the pulse rate effectively, both the patient's resting and predicted maximal heart rates must be determined. Maximum heart rate values are determined by a maximal graded exercise test whenever possible or by using the formula for age-adjusted heart rate. Maximum heart rate (HR_{max}) equals 220 minus age (see Chapter 16: Coronary Artery Disease). Generally, pulse rates during a 15- to 30-minute therapeutic exercise program for a healthy individual should not

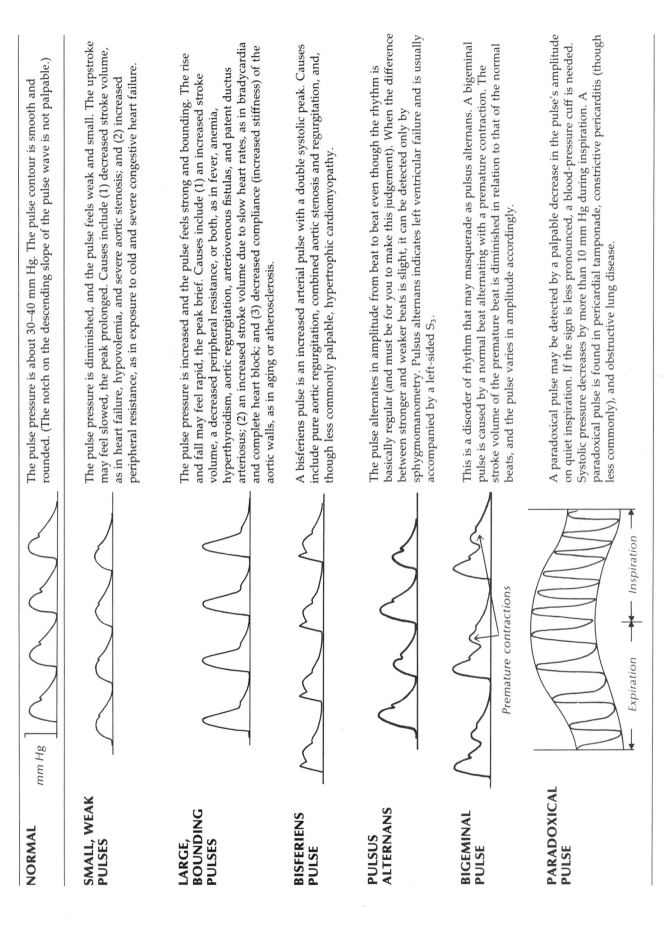

NORMAL — mm Hg

The pulse pressure is about 30–40 mm Hg. The pulse contour is smooth and rounded. (The notch on the descending slope of the pulse wave is not palpable.)

SMALL, WEAK PULSES

The pulse pressure is diminished, and the pulse feels weak and small. The upstroke may feel slowed, the peak prolonged. Causes include (1) decreased stroke volume, as in heart failure, hypovolemia, and severe aortic stenosis; and (2) increased peripheral resistance, as in exposure to cold and severe congestive heart failure.

LARGE, BOUNDING PULSES

The pulse pressure is increased and the pulse feels strong and bounding. The rise and fall may feel rapid, the peak brief. Causes include (1) an increased stroke volume, a decreased peripheral resistance, or both, as in fever, anemia, hyperthyroidism, aortic regurgitation, arteriovenous fistulas, and patent ductus arteriosus; (2) an increased stroke volume due to slow heart rates, as in bradycardia and complete heart block; and (3) decreased compliance (increased stiffness) of the aortic walls, as in aging or atherosclerosis.

BISFERIENS PULSE

A bisferiens pulse is an increased arterial pulse with a double systolic peak. Causes include pure aortic regurgitation, combined aortic stenosis and regurgitation, and, though less commonly palpable, hypertrophic cardiomyopathy.

PULSUS ALTERNANS

The pulse alternates in amplitude from beat to beat even though the rhythm is basically regular (and must be for you to make this judgement). When the difference between stronger and weaker beats is slight, it can be detected only by sphygmomanometry. Pulsus alternans indicates left ventricular failure and is usually accompanied by a left-sided S$_3$.

BIGEMINAL PULSE

This is a disorder of rhythm that may masquerade as pulsus alternans. A bigeminal pulse is caused by a normal beat alternating with a premature contraction. The stroke volume of the premature beat is diminished in relation to that of the normal beats, and the pulse varies in amplitude accordingly.

Premature contractions

PARADOXICAL PULSE

A paradoxical pulse may be detected by a palpable decrease in the pulse's amplitude on quiet inspiration. If the sign is less pronounced, a blood-pressure cuff is needed. Systolic pressure decreases by more than 10 mm Hg during inspiration. A paradoxical pulse is found in pericardial tamponade, constrictive pericarditis (though less commonly), and obstructive lung disease.

Expiration — *Inspiration*

Figure 4-9. Normal (*top*) and abnormal pulses, as reflected in the arterial waveforms. (From Bates,[14] p 308, with permission.)

exceed 60 to 90 percent of predicted HR_{max}. A lower exercise intensity is indicated for individuals with a very low fitness level.[11]

In assessing pulse rate response to exercise, level of aerobic fitness also must be considered. Both resting and submaximal exercise heart rates are typically lower in trained individuals. In response to an identical exercise intensity, a sedentary person's heart rate will demonstrate greater acceleration when compared with a trained individual. Although the metabolic requirements of an activity are the same, the lower heart rate response in a trained individual occurs as a result of a more efficient (increased) stroke volume. The linear relationship between pulse rate and workload exists for both trained and untrained individuals. However, the rate of rise will differ. When compared with a sedentary person, the trained individual will achieve a higher work output and greater oxygen consumption before reaching a specified submaximal heart rate. Beta-blocking agents decrease both resting heart rate and heart rate response to exercise.[11]

Systemic or Local Heat. During periods of fever, the heart rate will increase. The body will attempt to dissipate heat by vasodilation of peripheral vessels. Heart rate will increase to shunt blood flow to cutaneous areas for cooling. Local applications of thermal modalities (such as a hot pack) may also elevate heart rate to provide increased circulation to cutaneous areas secondary to arteriolar and capillary dilation.

Assessing the Pulse

A peripheral pulse can be monitored at a variety of sites on the body. Superficial arteries located over a bony surface are easiest to palpate and are referred to as "pulse points." These pulse sites, their locations, and some common indications for use are described. Pulse locations are illustrated in Fig. 4-10.

- **Temporal**: superior and lateral to the outer canthus of the eye; used when the radial pulse is inaccessible.
- **Carotid**: on either side of the anterior neck below the earlobe and between the sternocleidomastoid muscle and the trachea, used in cardiac arrest, in infants, and to monitor blood flow to brain.
- **Brachial**: medial aspect of the antecubital fossa; used to monitor blood pressure.
- **Radial**: radial aspect of the wrist at the base of the thumb; easily accessible; used for routine pulse monitoring.
- **Femoral**: inguinal region; used in cardiac arrest and to monitor lower extremity circulation.
- **Popliteal**: behind the knee (usually easier to palpate with slight knee flexion); used to monitor lower extremity circulation and blood pressure.
- **Pedal (dorsalis pedal)**: dorsal, medial aspect of foot; used to monitor lower extremity circulation.

In addition to the peripheral sites, the apical pulse may be monitored by auscultation (listening), using a stethoscope directly over the apex of the heart.

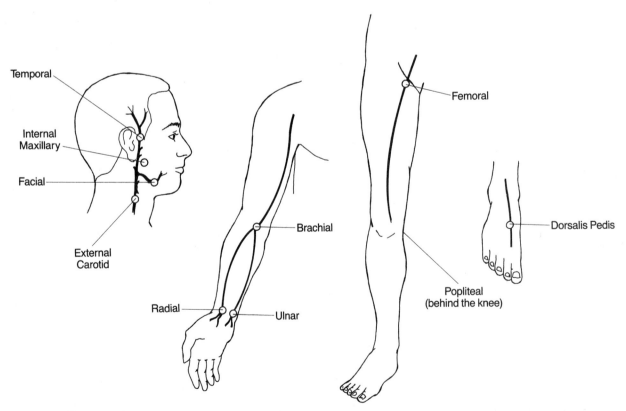

Figure 4-10. Common sites for monitoring peripheral pulses. Site selection will be influenced by patient condition and reasons for monitoring pulse.

Apical pulses are used when other sites are inaccessible (e.g., medical or surgical contraindications) or difficult to locate and palpate, such as in newborns and some patients with cardiac involvement.

Procedures for Assessing Pulse. A site should be selected that will not cause discomfort and consequently alter the pulse rate. Additionally, site location will be influenced by the specific diagnosis or the reason(s) for pulse monitoring. Peripheral pulses are monitored by palpation, using the tips of the first three fingers. Pulse rates obtained from the apex of the heart require use of a stethoscope.

Assessing Peripheral Pulses
A. Wash hands.
B. Assemble equipment.
  1. A watch with a second hand.
  2. Worksheet and pen or pencil to record collected data.
C. Procedure
  1. Explain procedure and rationale to patient in terms appropriate to his or her understanding.
  2. Assure patient comfort.
  3. Select the pulse point to be monitored.
  4. Place the first three fingers squarely and firmly over the pulse site; use only enough pressure to feel the pulse accurately (if the pressure is too great it will occlude the artery).
  5. Count the pulse for 30 seconds and multiply by 2; if any irregularities are noted, a full 60-second count should be taken; note the rhythm, volume, and quality or feel of the vessel.
  6. Record results.

Assessing Apical Pulse
A. Wash hands.
B. Assemble equipment.
  1. A stethoscope.
  2. Antiseptic wipes for cleaning earpieces and diaphragm of stethoscope before and after use.
  3. A watch with a second hand.
  4. Worksheet and pen or pencil to record collected data.
C. Procedure
  1. Explain procedure and rationale to patient in terms appropriate to his or her understanding.
  2. Assure patient comfort.
  3. Use antiseptic wipe to clean the earpieces and diaphragm of the stethoscope.
  4. Locate the site where pulse will be monitored; the apical pulse is located approximately 3.5 inches (8.9 cm) to the left of the midsternum, in the fifth intercostal space, within an inch of the midclavicular line drawn parallel to the sternum. These landmarks are guides to locating the apical pulse. In some individuals a stronger pulse may be noted by altering placement of the stethoscope (e.g., placement in the fourth or sixth intercostal space).
  5. Warm the diaphragm of the stethoscope in the palm of hand.
  6. Place stethoscope in ears so that the ear attachments are tilted forward when viewed at eye level.
  7. Place diaphragm of the stethoscope over the apex of heart. Count the pulse for 60 seconds; the pulse will be heard as a "lubb-dubb." The "lubb" represents closure of the atrioventricular (tricuspid and mitral) valves. The "dubb" represents closure of the semilunar (aortic and pulmonic) valves.
  8. Record results.

If the same examiner is using the stethoscope again, it is not necessary to clean the earpieces; the diaphragm should always be cleaned.

Assessing the Apical-Radial Pulse. Typically, the apical and radial pulse values are the same. However, in some situations (e.g., cardiac disease or vascular occlusion) blood pumped from the left ventricle may not be reaching the peripheral site or may be producing a weak or imperceptible pulse. The apical pulse in such cases would be stronger than the radial.

To monitor the apical-radial pulse, two examiners are needed to simultaneously monitor each of the pulses for 60 seconds. The results from the two assessments are then compared. The difference between the two counts is called the **pulse deficit.** This type of monitoring provides additional information regarding the status of the cardiovascular system.

Electronic Pulse Monitoring. Electronic pulsemeters (Fig. 4-11) use sensors to detect the pulse. Pulsemeters have gained expanded use in prescribed exercise and training programs because they provide a practical, accurate method of continual pulse monitoring. The devices consist of small, battery-operated units that can be strapped to the patient's wrist or waist, or bracketed to a piece of exercise equipment. Most units incorporate a lead wire with a distal sensor. The sensors are typically housed in a finger sleeve, earlobe clip, or chest strap attachment. The sensors transmit heart rate information back to the monitors. Many of the units allow programming target heart rate zones and storage of exercise information over a variable number of entries. Some of the newer units can transfer exercise information directly to a computer for storage and later analysis. This provides a permanent record and serial data on exercise performance.

Some pulsemeters are equipped with more than one type of sensor. This feature allows selection of a sensor appropriate to the activity (e.g., an earlobe clip or chest strap would be preferable to a finger sleeve for monitoring an activity that involved upper extremity movement). Pulse values are provided by a digital display or stationary scale and needle marker.

Some pulsemeters provide wireless transmission from chest sensor strap to a wristwatch display. Other units provide pulse values by placing the thumb firmly against a flat metal sensor. Various

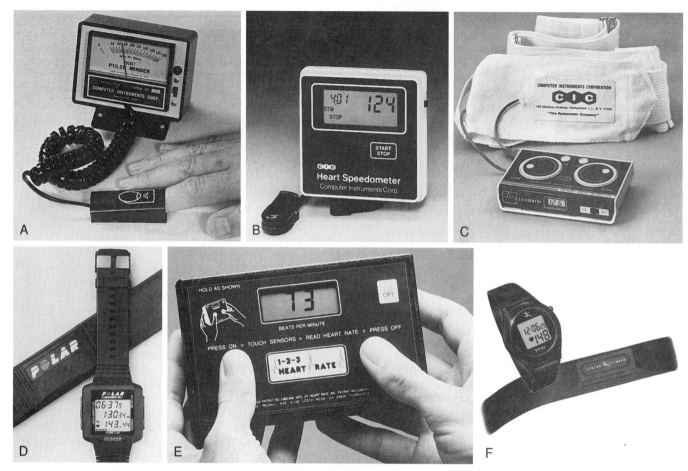

Figure 4-11. Sample models of electronic pulsemeters. (*A*) Stationary scale and needle marker readout with finger sleeve sensor. (*B*) Earlobe clip sensor with digital display. (*C*) Chest strap sensor with digital display. (*D*) Wireless chest strap sensor with wristwatch display. (Courtesy of Computer Instruments Corporation, Port Washington, NY.). (*E*) Touch sensor (thumbs in contact with sensors) with digital display (Courtesy of Heart Rate Incorporated, Costa Mesa, CA.) (*F*) A second example of a wireless chest strap sensor and wristwatch display, featuring a low-profile design (Courtesy of Vision Fitness, Lake Mills, WI).

additional options are available on these units and differ with the model and manufacturer. Among the more common features are the ability to preset the upper and lower limits of the pulse rate for a specific activity and an auditory signal when pulse values move outside the target range.

Leger and Thivierge[15] examined the validity of 13 commercially available heart rate monitors by comparing findings with electrocardiogram (ECG) readings. A high correlation ($r = 0.93$) was found between ECG readings and heart rate values obtained with conventional chest electrodes. Lower correlations were obtained using other types of electrodes (such as those used in finger sleeve and wrist monitors). Findings from this study suggest some unconventional electrodes (e.g., photocell) will yield unreliable results and are inadequate for clinical use.

RESPIRATION

The primary function of respiration is to supply the body with oxygen for metabolic activity and to remove carbon dioxide. The respiratory system, consisting of a series of branching tubes, brings atmospheric oxygen into contact with the gas ex-

change membrane of the lungs in the alveoli. Oxygen is then transported throughout the body via the cardiovascular system.

The Respiratory System

The entire pathway that transports air from the environment extends from the mouth and nose down to the alveolar sacs. Figure 4-12 illustrates an overview of the respiratory system. The upper respiratory airways include the nose, mouth, pharynx, and larynx. Air enters the body by way of the nose and mouth and is then moved to the pharynx, where it is warmed, filtered, and humidified. The pharynx serves as a common pathway for both air and food. Inspired air is then moved to the larynx, which contains the epiglottis, vocal cords, and cartilaginous structures. The anatomical arrangement of the larynx and pharyngeal muscles provide the critical function of protecting the lungs from entry of foreign particles as well as assisting with phonation (production of vocal sounds) and coughing, which is the primary physiological mechanism for clearing the airways. The **laryngopharynx** is the area where solid and liquid food intake is separated

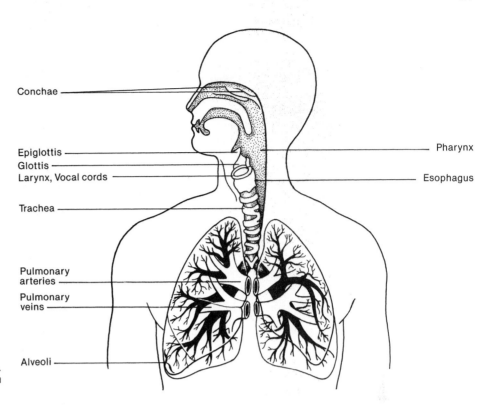

Conchae

Epiglottis
Glottis
Larynx, Vocal cords

Trachea

Pulmonary
arteries

Pulmonary
veins

Alveoli

Pharynx

Esophagus

Figure 4-12. The respiratory pathways. (From Guyton and Hall,[10] p 316, with permission.)

from inspired air. It is also the site of bifurcation into the larynx and esophagus. The pharyngeal muscles close the glottis during swallowing to protect the lungs from aspiration. If a foreign body passes the glottis and enters the tracheobronchial tree, the cough reflex is initiated to clear the air passage. Immediately below the thyroid cartilage of the larynx ("Adam's apple") is the site for emergency opening to the tracheal air pathway.[10,16,17]

The trachea is approximately 4 to 5 inches (11 to 13 cm) long and continues from the cartilaginous structures of the neck into the thorax. At the level of the carina (Fig. 4-13) the trachea divides into two mainstem bronchi. (The carina contains the majority of cough receptors and is located approximately between the sternum and manubrium at the second intercostal space.) The right and left mainstem bronchi are asymmetrical in size and shape (see Fig. 4-13) and continue into the lower respiratory tract further subdividing into the respiratory bronchioles where gas exchange begins. However, gas exchange primarily occurs in the alveolar ducts and the large surface area provided by the alveoli. The bronchioles, alveolar ducts, and alveoli (alveolar sacs) comprise the functional zones of the respiratory tract for air exchange (Fig. 4-14). The airways do not contribute to air exchange and comprise *the anatomical dead space.*[10,16–19]

Inspiration. Inspiration is initiated by contraction of the diaphragm and intercostal muscles. During contraction of these muscles, the diaphragm moves downward and the intercostals lift the ribs and sternum up and outward. The thoracic cavity is thus increased in size and allows for lung expansion.

Expiration. During relaxed breathing, expiration is essentially a passive process. Once the respiratory muscles relax, the thorax returns to its resting position, and the lungs recoil. This ability to recoil occurs because of the inherent elastic properties of the lungs.

Regulatory Mechanisms. Regulation of respiratory function is a complex process. It involves multiple components of both neural and chemical control and is closely integrated with the cardiovascular system. Breathing is controlled by the *respiratory center*, which lies bilaterally in the pons and medulla. The respiratory muscles are controlled by motor nerves whose cell bodies are located in this area. This respiratory center provides control of both the rate and the depth of breathing in response to the metabolic needs of the body.[20,21]

Both *central* and *peripheral* chemoreceptors influence respiration. *Central* chemoreceptors located in the respiratory center are sensitive to changes in either carbon dioxide or hydrogen ion levels of arterial blood. An increase in either carbon dioxide levels or hydrogen ions will stimulate breathing.[10,16] *Peripheral* chemoreceptors are located at the bifurcation of the carotid arteries (carotid bodies) and in the arch of the aorta (aortic bodies). These receptors are sensitive to the partial pressure of oxygen (Pao_2) in the arterial blood. When Pao_2 levels in arterial blood drop, afferent impulses carry this information to the respiratory center. Motor neurons to the respiratory muscles are stimulated to increase **tidal volume** (amount of air exchanged with each breath) or, with very low oxygen levels, to also increase the respiratory rate. These peripheral chemoreceptors

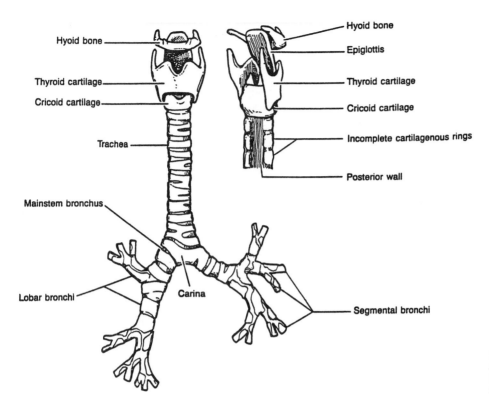

Figure 4-13. Structure of cartilaginous airways, including the trachea and major bronchi. (From Henderson,[17] p 388, with permission.)

cause an increase in respiration only when Pao_2 levels fall to approximately 60 mmHg (from a normal level of about 90 to 100 mmHg). This is because the receptors are sensitive only to Pao_2 levels in plasma and not to the total oxygen in blood.[20,21]

Respiration also is influenced by a protective stretch mechanism called the *Hering-Breuer reflex*. Stretch receptors throughout the walls of the lungs monitor the amount of entering air. When overstretched, these receptors send impulses to the respiratory center to inhibit further inhalation. Impulses stop at the end of expiration so that another inspiration can be initiated.[10,18] Respiration is also stimulated by vigorous movements of joints and muscle (exercise) and is strongly influenced by voluntary cortical control.

Factors Influencing Respiration. Multiple factors can alter normal, relaxed, effortless respiration. As with temperature and pulse, any influence that increases the metabolic rate also will increase the respiratory rate. Increased metabolism and subsequent demand for oxygen will stimulate increased respiration. Conversely, as metabolic demands diminish, respirations also will decrease. Several influencing factors are of particular importance when assessing respiration. These include age, body size, stature, exercise, and body position.

Age. The respiratory rate of a newborn is between 30 and 50 breaths per minute. The rate gradually slows until adulthood, when it ranges between 12 and 20 breaths per minute. In elderly individuals the respiratory rate increases owing to decreased elas-

ticity of the lungs and decreased efficiency of gas exchange (see Table 4-1).[5]

Body Size and Stature. Men generally have a larger vital capacity than women; adults larger than adolescents and children. Tall, thin individuals generally have a larger vital capacity than stout or obese individuals.

Exercise. Respiratory rate and depth will increase with exercise as a result of increased oxygen consumption and carbon dioxide production.

Body Position. The supine position can significantly affect respiration and predispose the patient to stasis of fluids. The two influential factors are compression of the chest against the supporting surface and increased volume of intrathoracic blood.[17] Both of these factors will limit normal lung expansion. In addition to the above-mentioned factors, respiration also may be affected by drug intake, certain disease states, and the patient's emotional status.

Parameters of Respiratory Assessment. In assessing respiration, four parameters are considered: rate, depth, rhythm, and character. The *rate* is the number of breaths per minute. Either inspirations or expirations should be counted, but not both. The normal adult respiratory rate (RR) is 12 to 20 per minute. The rate should be counted for 30 seconds and multiplied by two. If any irregularities are noted, a full 60-second count is indicated.

The *depth* of respiration refers to the amount (volume) of air exchanged with each breath. Normally, the depth of respirations are the same, producing a relatively even, uniform movement of

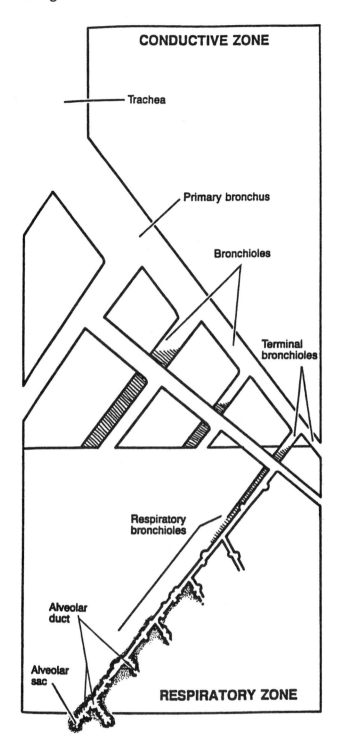

CONDUCTIVE ZONE

Trachea

Primary bronchus

Bronchioles

Terminal bronchioles

Respiratory bronchioles

Alveolar duct

Alveolar sac

RESPIRATORY ZONE

Figure 4-14. Schematic illustration of the functional zones of the respiratory tract. The top area from the trachea to the terminal bronchioles is called the "conductive zone" because these airways transport (conduct) inhaled air to and from the respiratory zone. The bottom area of the illustration represents the areas where air exchange takes place. The air exchange occurs in progressively increasing increments in the respiratory bronchioles, alveolar ducts, and alveolar sacs. Collectively these areas constitute the "respiratory zone." (From Henderson,[17] p 389, with permission.)

less than normal.[19] With deep respirations, a large volume of air is exchanged; with shallow respirations, a small amount of air is exchanged, with minimal lung expansion or chest wall movement.

The *rhythm* refers to the regularity of inspirations and expirations. Normally, there is an even time interval between respirations. The respiratory rhythm is described as regular or **irregular.**

The *character* of respirations refers to deviations from normal, quiet, effortless breathing. Two important deviations that alter the character of breathing are the amount of effort required and the sound produced during respiration.

Difficult or labored breathing is called **dyspnea.** Patients with dyspnea require increased, noticeable effort to breathe. This is frequently evident by increased activity noted in accessory respiratory muscles such as the intercostals and abdominals. Use of these muscles helps to increase effectiveness of respiration. The intercostals assist in raising the ribs to expand the thoracic cavity; the abdominals assist function of the diaphragm. Additional muscles that may provide accessory functions in respiration are the sternocleidomastoid, pectoralis major and minor, scalene, and the subclavius.

The sound of breathing is also important in assessing the character of respirations. Following, several relevant terms related to respiratory sounds are described:

- **Wheezing:** a whistling sound produced by air passing through a narrowed airway such as a bronchi or bronchiole; the sound is often compared to the whistling produced when stretching the neck of a balloon and allowing air to escape slowly through the narrowed passageway; it may be heard on both inspiration and expiration but is more prominent on expiration; apparent in patients with emphysema and asthma.
- **Stridor:** a harsh, high-pitched crowing sound that occurs with upper airway obstructions caused by narrowing of the glottis or trachea; apparent in patients with tracheal stenosisole or presence of a foreign object.
- **Crackles** (historically called rales): rattling or bubbling sounds that occur owing to secretions in the air passages of the respiratory tract; the sound is often compared to that of rustling a cellophane bag. Crackles may be heard with the ear but are most accurately assessed by use of a stethoscope; apparent in patients with congestive heart failure (CHF).
- **Sigh:** a deep inspiration followed by a prolonged, audible expiration; occasional sighs are normal and function to expand alveoli. Frequent sighs are abnormal and may be indicative of emotional stress.
- **Stertorous:** a snoring sound owing to secretions in the trachea and large bronchi.

Respiratory Patterns. Data from assessing rate, rhythm, and depth allows the therapist to determine the *pattern* of respiration. Not all patient assessment data will indicate a distinct pattern of respiration. However, several patterns occur with sufficient

the chest. The normal adult tidal volume is approximately 500 mL of air. The depth of respiration is assessed by observation of chest movements. It is usually described as deep or shallow, depending on whether the amount of air exchanged is greater or frequency that uniform terminology has developed for their identification. Common respiratory patterns are presented in Fig. 4-15.

Assessing Respiration. Because respiration is under both voluntary (cortical) and involuntary control, it is important that the patient is unaware that respiration is being assessed. Once aware of the assessment, usual breathing characteristics may be altered. Therefore, it is often recommended that respirations be observed immediately after taking the pulse. After monitoring the pulse, the fingers can remain in place at the pulse site, and respiration can be assessed. With the use of this technique the patient's conscious attention will not be drawn to the breathing pattern. Ideally, respiration should be assessed with the chest exposed. If this is not possible, or if respirations cannot be easily observed through clothing, maintain fingers on the radial pulse site and place the patient's arm across the chest. This will allow limited palpation without drawing conscious input from the patient.

Procedure for Assessing Respiration

A. Wash hands.
B. Assemble equipment.
   1. A watch with a second hand.
   2. Worksheet and pen or pencil to record collected data.
C. Procedure
   1. Assure patient comfort.
   2. Expose chest area if possible; if area cannot be exposed and respirations are not readily observable, place patient's arm across chest and keep your fingers positioned as if continuing to monitor the radial pulse.
   3. Count the respirations (either inspirations or expirations, but not both) for 30 seconds and multiply by two; if any irregularities are noted, count for a full 60 seconds.
   4. Observe the depth, rhythm, character, and pattern of respiration.
   5. Return clothing if chest has been exposed.
   6. Record results.

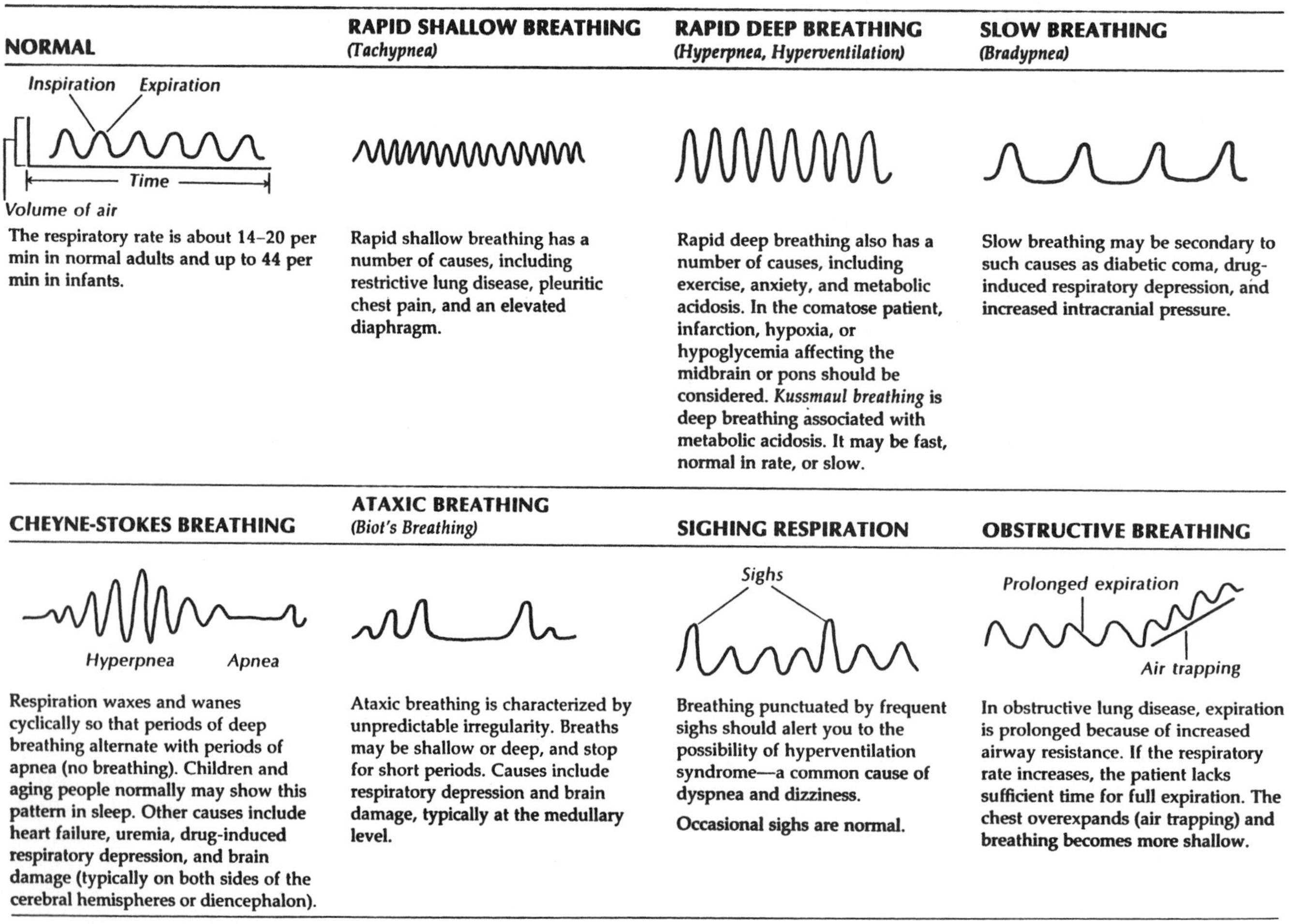

NORMAL	**RAPID SHALLOW BREATHING** *(Tachypnea)*	**RAPID DEEP BREATHING** *(Hyperpnea, Hyperventilation)*	**SLOW BREATHING** *(Bradypnea)*
The respiratory rate is about 14–20 per min in normal adults and up to 44 per min in infants.	Rapid shallow breathing has a number of causes, including restrictive lung disease, pleuritic chest pain, and an elevated diaphragm.	Rapid deep breathing also has a number of causes, including exercise, anxiety, and metabolic acidosis. In the comatose patient, infarction, hypoxia, or hypoglycemia affecting the midbrain or pons should be considered. *Kussmaul breathing* is deep breathing associated with metabolic acidosis. It may be fast, normal in rate, or slow.	Slow breathing may be secondary to such causes as diabetic coma, drug-induced respiratory depression, and increased intracranial pressure.

CHEYNE-STOKES BREATHING	**ATAXIC BREATHING** *(Biot's Breathing)*	**SIGHING RESPIRATION**	**OBSTRUCTIVE BREATHING**
Respiration waxes and wanes cyclically so that periods of deep breathing alternate with periods of apnea (no breathing). Children and aging people normally may show this pattern in sleep. Other causes include heart failure, uremia, drug-induced respiratory depression, and brain damage (typically on both sides of the cerebral hemispheres or diencephalon).	Ataxic breathing is characterized by unpredictable irregularity. Breaths may be shallow or deep, and stop for short periods. Causes include respiratory depression and brain damage, typically at the medullary level.	Breathing punctuated by frequent sighs should alert you to the possibility of hyperventilation syndrome—a common cause of dyspnea and dizziness. Occasional sighs are normal.	In obstructive lung disease, expiration is prolonged because of increased airway resistance. If the respiratory rate increases, the patient lacks sufficient time for full expiration. The chest overexpands (air trapping) and breathing becomes more shallow.

Figure 4-15. Normal (*top left*) and abnormal respiratory patterns. When assessing respiratory patterns, consider rate, rhythm, and depth of the patient's breathing. Describe what is seen in these terms. Note that below each descriptor of abnormal breathing pattern are more traditional terms, such as tachypnea, hyperpnea, and hyperventilation. It is important to understand what these traditional terms mean. However, for purposes of documentation, simpler descriptions (such as "rapid, shallow breathing") are recommended. (Adapted from Bates,[14] p 256, with permission.)

BLOOD PRESSURE

Blood pressure refers to the force the blood exerts against a vessel wall. Because liquid flows only from a higher to a lower pressure, the pressure is highest in the arteries, lower in the capillaries, and lowest in veins.[10,11] Inasmuch as the heart is an intermittent pulsatile pump, pressure is measured at both the highest and lowest points of the pulse. These points are represented by the systolic (ventricular contraction) and diastolic (ventricular relaxation) pressures. The **systolic pressure** is the highest pressure exerted by the blood against the arterial walls. The **diastolic pressure** (which is constantly present) is the lowest pressure. The difference between the two pressures is called the **pulse pressure.**

Regulatory Mechanisms

The *vasomotor center* is located bilaterally in the lower pons and upper medulla. It transmits impulses through sympathetic nerves to all vessels of the body. The vasomotor center is tonically active, producing a slow, continual firing in all vasoconstrictor nerve fibers. It is this slow, continual firing that maintains a partial state of contraction of the blood vessels and provides normal *vasomotor tone*.[10] The vasomotor center assists in providing the stable arterial pressure required to maintain blood flow to body tissue and organs. This occurs because of its close connection to the cardiac controlling center in the medulla (because changes in cardiac output will influence blood pressure). Additionally, the vasomotor and cardiac controlling centers require input from afferent receptors.

Afferent Receptors

Input regarding blood pressure is provided primarily by *baroreceptors* and *chemoreceptors*. The *baroreceptors* (pressoreceptors) are stimulated by stretch of the vessel wall from alterations in pressure. These receptors have a high concentration in the walls of the internal carotid arteries above the carotid bifurcation and in the walls of the arch of the aorta. The areas where baroreceptors are located in the carotid arteries are called *carotid sinuses* and monitor blood pressure to the brain. Their locations on the aortic arch are called *aortic sinuses* and are responsible for monitoring blood pressure throughout the body.

In response to an increase in blood pressure the baroreceptor input to the vasomotor center results in an inhibition of the vasoconstrictor center of the medulla and excitation of the vagal center.[10] This results in a decreased heart rate, decreased force of cardiac contraction, and vasodilation, with a subsequent drop in blood pressure. The baroreceptor input during a lowering of blood pressure would produce the opposite effects.

The *chemoreceptors* are stimulated by reduced arterial oxygen concentrations, increases in carbon dioxide tension, and increased hydrogen ion concentrations.[22] These receptors lie close to the baroreceptors. Those located in the carotid artery are called *carotid bodies*, and on the aortic arch they are termed *aortic bodies*. Impulses from these receptors travel to the brain (cardioregulatory and vasomotor centers) via afferent pathways in the vagus and glossopharyngeal nerves. Efferent impulses from these centers, in response to alterations in blood pressure, will alter heart rate, strength of cardiac contractions, and size of blood vessels.[22]

Factors That Influence Blood Pressure

Many factors influence pressure. As with all vital signs, blood pressure is represented by a range of normal values and will yield the most useful data when monitored over a period of time. Several important factors that should be considered when assessing blood pressure include blood volume, diameter and elasticity of arteries, cardiac output, age, exercise, and arm position.

Blood Volume. The amount of circulating blood in the body directly affects pressure. Blood loss (e.g., hemorrhage) will cause pressure to drop, and can result in hypovolemic shock. Conversely, an increased blood volume (e.g., blood transfusion) will cause the pressure to rise.

Diameter or Elasticity of Arteries. The size (diameter) of the vessel lumen will provide either increased peripheral resistance (vasoconstriction) or decreased resistance (vasodilation) to cardiac output. The elasticity of the vessel wall also influences resistance. Normally the expansion and recoil properties of the arterial walls provide a continuous, smooth flow of blood into the capillaries and veins between heartbeats. With age, these properties are diminished. Thus, there is a higher resistance to blood flow with resultant increase in systolic pressure. Because the flexibility and recoil properties are diminished, there is a lower diastolic pressure.

Cardiac Output. When increased amounts of blood are pumped into the arteries, the walls of the vessels distend, resulting in a higher blood pressure. With lower cardiac output, less blood is pushed into the vessel, and there is a subsequent drop in pressure.

Age. Blood pressure varies with age (see Table 4-1). It normally rises gradually after birth and reaches a peak during puberty. By late adolescence (18 to 19 years), adult blood pressure is reached. The normal, average adult blood pressure is usually considered 120/80 mmHg (the top number indicates systolic pressure; the bottom, diastolic pressure). The rise in blood pressure values for older adults is primarily because of the degenerative effects of arteriosclerosis. Small arteries and arterioles lose their elasticity, the walls of the vessels become thick and hard, and the lumen gradually narrows and may eventually become blocked. This primarily affects the systolic pressure and accounts for the isolated high systolic pressure seen frequently in elderly individuals.[23]

Exercise. Physical activity will increase cardiac output, with a consequent linear increase in blood pressure. Greater increases are noted in systolic pressure owing to proportional changes in pressure gradient of peripheral vessels during vasodilation. Blood pressure increases are proportional to the intensity of the workload.

Valsalva Maneuver. The **Valsalva maneuver** is an attempt to exhale forcibly with the glottis, nose, and mouth closed. It causes an increase in intrathoracic pressure with an accompanying collapse of the veins of the chest wall. There is a subsequent decrease in blood flow to the heart, a decreased venous return, and a drop in arterial blood pressure. This maneuver serves to internally stabilize the abdominal and chest wall during periods of rapid and maximum exertion such as lifting a heavy object. When the breath is released, the intrathoracic pressure decreases and venous return is suddenly reestablished. This produces a marked increase in heart rate and arterial blood pressure. This rapid rise in arterial pressure causes vagal slowing of the heart rate **(bradycardia).** Although the Valsalva maneuver can temporarily enhance muscle function via the internal stabilization, it has a direct undesirable effect by increasing blood pressure (BP) and should be avoided by individuals with cardiac impairment.[11]

Postural (Orthostatic) Hypotension. Associated with prolonged immobility and bed rest, **postural (othostatic) hypotension** is a sudden drop in blood pressure that typically occurs when a patient moves to a standing or sitting posture (although it may occur in any position). The positional change causes a gravitational blood pooling in the lower extremity veins. Venous return and cardiac output are reduced with a resultant cerebral hypoperfusion. This triggers an episode of light-headedness or loss of consciousness. In response to positional changes under normal circumstances, blood pressure is maintained by reflex vasoconstriction (baroreceptors), which increases heart rate. After a period of inactivity, postural hypotension should be anticipated and requires a gradual acclimation to the upright position until normal reflex control returns. Other predisposing factors for postural hypotension include exercise, drugs such as antihypertensives and vasodilators, reduction in baroreceptor response with aging, the Valsalva maneuver, and **hypovolemia** (abnormally low volume of circulating blood).[23,24]

Arm Position. Blood pressure may vary as much as 20 mmHg by altering arm position. For consistency of measures, the patient should be sitting with the arm in a horizontal, supported position at heart level. If patient condition or the type of activity precludes these positions, alterations should be carefully documented. As with other vital signs, factors such as fear, anxiety, or emotional stress also will cause an increase in blood pressure.

Other Risk Factors. Although the exact etiology is not known, high blood pressure is also associated with high sodium intake,[10] obesity,[10] and race[25] (occurs 2 to 3 times more frequently in individuals from African-American descent).

Assessing Blood Pressure

Equipment. The equipment required for taking blood pressure includes a *blood pressure cuff*, a *sphygmomanometer*, and a *stethoscope* (Fig. 4-16). The blood pressure cuff is an airtight, flat rubber bladder that can be inflated with air. The bladder is covered with cloth that extends beyond the length of the bladder. There are two tubes that extend from the cuff. One is attached to a rubber bulb that has a valve used to maintain or to release air from the cuff. The second tube is attached to a manometer (portion of sphygmomanometer that registers the pressure reading).

Blood pressure cuffs are secured on the patient's extremity by Velcro. Some older models use snaps, or hooks, and some are simply wrapped to keep them in place. They come in a variety of sizes. Obtaining a cuff of appropriate size is important. The cuff should cover approximately one-half to two-thirds of the patient's upper arm or leg and should be long enough to encircle the limb. Cuffs that are too narrow will show inaccurately high readings, and cuffs that are too wide, inaccurately low. Generally, the cuff width should be 20 percent wider than the diameter of the limb. A typical adult cuff width is 4.5 to 5.5 inches (12 to 14 cm) with a bladder length of 9 inches (23 cm).

The sphygmomanometer registers the blood pressure reading. There are two types: *aneroid manometers* and *mercury manometers* (see Fig. 4-16). The aneroid manometer registers the blood pressure by way of a circular calibrated dial and needle. The mercury manometer registers blood pressure on a mercury-filled calibrated cylinder. At the uppermost portion of the mercury column is a convex curve called the *meniscus*. A reading is obtained by viewing the meniscus at *eye level*. If not observed directly at eye level, an inaccurate reading will be obtained.

The stethoscope is used to listen to the sounds over the artery as pressure is released from the cuff. It includes an amplifying mechanism (diaphragm) and earpieces connected by rubber tubing. There are two types of diaphragms: a *bell-shaped* and a *flat disk* shape. Stethoscopes may have a single type of diaphragm or a combination of the two (see Fig. 4-16). The bell-shaped diaphragms are generally recommended for assessing blood pressure. By a combination of listening through the stethoscope and watching the manometer, the blood pressure reading is obtained.

Electronic sphygmomanometers are also commercially available. They contain a microphone and transducer built into the cuff. Thus the need for a stethoscope is eliminated. A flashing light or audible "beep" indicates both the systolic and diastolic pressures. Some electronic units also have a built-in paper printer to provide a hard copy of data (Fig. 4-17).

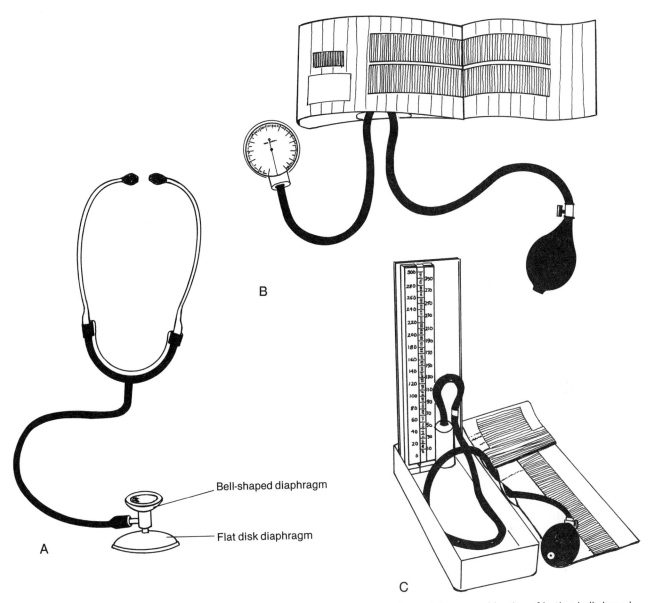

Figure 4-16. Blood pressure equipment includes (*A*) a stethoscope (this stethoscope has a combination of both a bell-shaped and a flat disk diaphragm) and either (*B*) an aneroid manometer and cuff or (*C*) mercury manometer and cuff.

Korotkoff's Sounds. When assessing blood pressure, a series of sounds are heard through the stethoscope called **Korotkoff's sounds.** Initially when pressure is applied in the cuff, the blood flow is occluded and no sound is heard through the stethoscope. As the pressure is gradually released, a series of five phases or sounds have been identified.

- **Phase 1:** The first clear, faint, rhythmic tapping sound that gradually increases in intensity; period when blood initially flows through the artery; systolic pressure.
- **Phase 2:** A murmur or swishing sound is heard.
- **Phase 3:** Sounds become crisp and louder.
- **Phase 4:** Sound is distinct, abrupt muffling; soft blowing quality; first diastolic pressure.
- **Phase 5:** Sounds disappear; second diastolic pressure.

Controversy exists as to the point of true diastolic pressure (phase 4 versus phase 5). The American Heart Association recommends use of the fifth phase as the most accurate index of diastolic pressure in adult populations.[26] Recording only one diastolic pressure (phase 5) is common practice in most clinical settings. For example, a blood pressure reading with a systolic pressure of 120 and a second diastolic reading of 76 would be recorded as 120/76. In facilities where both diastolic pressures are routinely documented, three numbers are recorded. For example, a systolic pressure of 120, a first diastolic reading of 80 and a second of 76 would be recorded as 120/80/76.

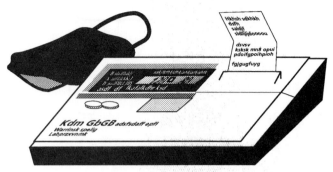

Figure 4-17. Electronic blood pressure unit with built-in paper printer and digital display.

Procedure for Assessing Blood Pressure

A primary consideration in assessing blood pressure is that it should be done in a minimal amount of time. The blood pressure cuff acts as a tourniquet. As such, venous pooling and considerable discomfort to the patient will occur if the cuff is left in place too long.

The brachial artery is the most common site for blood pressure monitoring and an assessment at this site will be described in detail. A description for monitoring lower extremity blood pressure is also presented.

Assessing Brachial Artery Pressure
A. Wash hands.
B. Assemble equipment.
1. A stethoscope.
2. A sphygmomanometer with a blood pressure cuff (size of cuff should be appropriate for size of extremity).
3. Antiseptic wipes for cleaning earpieces and diaphragm of stethoscope before and after use.
4. Worksheet and pen and pencil to record collected data.
C. Procedure
1. Explain procedure and rationale to patient in terms appropriate to his or her understanding.
2. Assist the patient to the desired position (the sitting position is recommended); assure patient comfort.
3. Expose the arm, and place at heart level with the elbow extended.
4. Wrap the blood pressure cuff around the arm approximately 1 to 2 inches (2.5 to 5 cm) above the antecubital fossa; the center of cuff should be in line with the brachial artery (Fig. 4-18).
5. Check that the sphygmomanometer registers zero.
6. Use an antiseptic wipe to clean the earpieces and diaphragm of the stethoscope.
7. Place the earpieces of the stethoscope (tilting forward) into ears; the tubes of the stethoscope should not be crossed and should hang freely.
8. Locate and palpate the brachial artery in the antecubital fossa; place the diaphragm

of the stethoscope over the artery (see Fig. 4-18).
9. Close the valve of the blood pressure cuff (turn clockwise).
10. Pump the blood pressure cuff until the manometer registers approximately 20 mmHg above the anticipated systolic pressure.
11. Release the valve carefully, allowing air out slowly; air should be released at a rate of 2 to 3 mmHg per heartbeat.
12. Watch the manometer closely and note the point at which the first sound is heard (a mercury manometer must be viewed at eye level); this is the point where blood first begins to flow through the artery and represents the systolic pressure; deflections in the dial or column of mercury will now be noted.
13. Continue to release air carefully. Note the point on the manometer when the sound first becomes muffled; this is the first diastolic pressure.
14. Continue to release air gradually.
15. Note the point on the manometer when the sound disappears and deflection

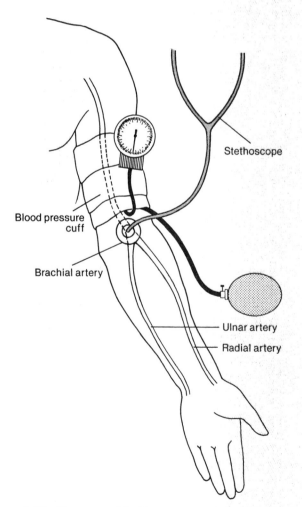

Figure 4-18. Placement of the blood pressure cuff and stethoscope for monitoring brachial artery pressure.

ceases; this is recorded as the second diastolic pressure.

16. Allow remainder of air to release quickly.
17. If the same examiner is using the stethoscope again, it is not necessary to clean the earpieces; however, the diaphragm of the stethoscope should always be cleaned between patients.
18. Record results.

Assessing Popliteal (Thigh) Pressure. Lower extremity readings are indicated in situations in which comparisons between the upper and lower extremities is warranted, such as peripheral vascular disease. They also are used when upper extremity pressures are contraindicated, such as following trauma or surgery. Essentially, the procedure is the same as that for assessing pressure at the brachial artery, with the following variations:

1. The patient is placed in a prone position with slight knee flexion.
2. The popliteal artery is used to monitor pressure; in comparison with the brachial artery, the popliteal artery usually yields higher systolic and lower diastolic values.
3. A wide cuff is used (approximately 17 inches [43 cm]). This is placed around the lower third of the thigh. The center of the cuff should be in line with the popliteal artery.

Recording Results. For purposes of physical therapy documentation, many therapists include vital signs data directly within the narrative format of their note. The most important element in

recording this information is that it allows easy comparison from one entry to the next. The date, time of day, patient position, examiner's name, and equipment used should all be clearly indicated. For example, assume a vital signs assessment provided the following data: Temperature: 98.9°F, taken orally; a pulse of 84 beats per minute (bpm) with fluctuations between weak and strong beats; a respiratory rate of 16 per minute with a regular rhythm and unlabored quality, and a blood pressure reading of 122/84 mmHg in sitting and 120/86 mmHg standing. A sample format for including these data as a component of narrative documentation is presented in Box 4–2.

Traditionally, nursing personnel have used graph sheets to record vital sign information. For the therapist practicing in a facility where such forms are used, they will be useful in providing recent vital sign data. Familiarity with the specific recording system is important. Several methods are used; they generally include some variation of open and closed circles, connecting lines, and/or color codes. A sample of a vital sign clinical record sheet is presented in Figure 4-19. Modifications of this type of form also may be useful for documenting response to physical therapy treatment.

SUMMARY

Values obtained from monitoring vital signs provide the physical therapist with important informa-

---

Box 4–2 SAMPLE FORMAT FOR DOCUMENTING VITAL SIGN ASSESSMENT FINDINGS WITHIN A PHYSICAL THERAPY NARRATIVE REPORT. THE MOST IMPORTANT ELEMENT IN DEVELOPING A FORM IS THE ABILITY TO EASILY COMPARE ENTRIES FROM ONE ASSESSMENT TO THE NEXT.

Patient Name:

Date: (examination date) **Time:** (time of day of examination) **Position:** sitting; BP sitting and standing. **PT:** (therapist's name) **Equipment:** PT Dept. electronic thermometer (ID# 06); stethoscope (ID# 21); mercury manometer (ID# 22).	**Date:** **Time:** **Position:** **PT:** **Equipment:**
T: 98.9° F. **HR:** 84/minute, alternating quality. **RR:** 16/minute, regular, deep, unlabored. **BP:** 122/84 mmHg sitting; 120/86 standing.	**T:** **HR:** **RR:** **BP:**
Date: **Time:** **Position:** **PT:** **Equipment:**	**Date:** **Time:** **Position:** **PT:** **Equipment:**
T: **HR:** **RR:** **BP:**	**T:** **HR:** **RR:** **BP:**

Abbreviations: T, temperature; HR, heart rate (pulse); RR, respiratory rate; BP, blood pressure.

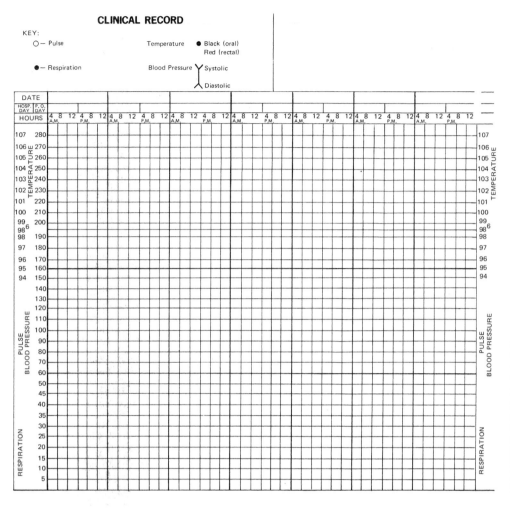

CLINICAL RECORD

KEY:
○ — Pulse

Temperature ● Black (oral)
Red (rectal)

● — Respiration

Blood Pressure ⅄ Systolic

∀ Diastolic

Figure 4-19. Sample vital sign clinical record sheet. Note the coding key, which indicates use of open circles for the pulse, closed circles for respiration, color codes for temperature (black for oral and red for rectal), and a line entry (upright and inverted "Y" shapes) for blood pressure. (From Saperstein, AB, and Frazier, MA: The assessment of vital signs. In Saperstein, AB, and Frazier, MA: (eds): Introduction to Nursing Practice. FA Davis, Philadelphia, 1980, p 483, with permission.)

tion about the patient's physiological status. Results from these measures assist in establishing and maintaining a database of values for an individual patient. They also assist in formulating clinical judgements for determining the diagnosis and prognosis, designing plan of care, and establishing and evaluating effectiveness of selected treatment interventions.

The procedure for assessing each vital sign has been presented. Because multiple factors influence vital signs, the most useful data are obtained when measures are taken at periodic intervals rather than at a one-time assessment. This will allow changes in patient status or response to treatment to be monitored over time, as well as indicate an acute change in status at a specific point in time.

For purposes of physical therapy documentation, vital signs data are typically included within the narrative format of the note. Use of a graph to record this information may prove a useful adjunct to the physical therapy record. Regardless of the system of documentation selected, of critical importance is that it allow easy comparison of serial entries over time.

QUESTIONS FOR REVIEW

1. Identify the reasons for monitoring vital signs.

2. Prior to a vital signs assessment, what preliminary data can be obtained by a careful systematic observation of the patient?

3. Why are vital sign values more significant when monitored as a serial process rather than as a one-time assessment?

4. Describe the primary mechanisms by which the body conserves and produces heat; differentiate the four primary heat loss mechanisms: radiation, conduction, convection, and evaporation.

5. Describe the procedure for assessing axillary temperatures using a standard clinical glass thermometer.

6. Define pulse rate, rhythm, and volume.

7. What factors influence the pulse?

8. Describe the procedure for assessing both radial and apical pulses.

9. What parameters are addressed during a respiratory assessment? Define each.

10. What factors will influence respiration?

11. Describe the Valsalva maneuver. Identify its influence on heart rate (HR) and blood pressure (BP) during and after the maneuver.

12. Describe the procedure for assessing respiration.

13. What factors influence blood pressure?

14. What are the five phases of Korotkoff's sounds?

15. What changes will be noted in blood pressure readings if an inappropriate size cuff is used?

16. Describe the procedure for assessing blood pressure using a stethoscope and sphygmomanometer.

CASE STUDY

EMERGENCY ROOM ADMISSION: A 24 year-old male was separated from his skiing group due to an unexpected and violent snowstorm. The situation was complicated by his being in an unfamiliar area without electronic communication. A 2-day helicopter search located him after approximately 48 hours of exposure to temperatures which ranged between 10° and 20°F. The emergency team initiated intravenous fluid replacement (to help restore fluid and electrolyte balance) en route to the hospital.

History: As reported by his parents, medical history is unremarkable except for the usual childhood diseases. He had recently relocated to the area because of a desire to be a competitive skier (an activity he has enjoyed all his life). He works as an accountant for a local investment firm.

Admitting Diagnosis: Hypothermia and frostbite of the toes, thumb, and index and middle fingers, bilaterally.

Blood Pressure: Systolic pressure is 45 mmHg; diastolic not perceptible.

Pulse: Decreased rate, small, weak carotid pulse (12 bpm); peripheral pulses not perceptible.

Respiratory Rate: 6 breaths per minute; respirations are barely perceptible.

Temperature: 82°F ®.

Cognition: Depressed, unresponsive.

Deep Tendon Reflexes: Absent.

Cutaneous Sensation: Unresponsive to all sensory modalities, including pain.

Skin Observation: Marked skin color changes; bluish gray appearance of earlobes, lips, fingers, and toes.

Physical Therapy: The patient is now in the Intensive Care Unit (ICU) and a referral has been made to physical therapy requesting "examination and treatment."

Guiding Questions

1. Describe the body system responses to hypothermia as presented by the clinical features of the case.

2. Considering this patient is unresponsive and cyanotic, what would be the most appropriate pulse to monitor? Provide a brief rationale for your answer.

3. The function of the thermoregulatory center becomes seriously impaired when body temperature falls below approximately _____ and is completely lost with temperatures below _____ .

4. Extremes in environmental temperature have a large impact on the body's ability to maintain constant temperatures. What type of clothing can best assist in protecting the body from low environmental temperatures?

REFERENCES

1. American Physical Therapy Association: Guide to physical therapist practice. Phys Ther 77:11, 1997.

2. Lewis, PS: Cardiovascular Assessment. In Ruppert, SD, et al (eds): Dolan's Critical Care Nursing: Clinical Nursing Through the Nursing Process, ed 2. FA Davis, Philadelphia, 1991, p 151.

3. Metzgar, ED: The Health History. In Morton, PG (ed): Health Assessment, ed 2. FA Davis, Philadelphia, 1995, p 3.

4. Spector, RE: Cultural Diversity in Health and Illness, ed 4. Appleton & Lange, Stamford, CT, 1996.

5. Fitzgerald, MA: Nursing Health Assessment: Concepts and Activities. FA Davis, Philadelphia, 1995.

6. Purnell, LD, and Paulanka, BJ (eds): Transcultural Health Care. FA Davis, Philadelphia, 1998.

7. Lynch, EW, and Hanson, MJ (eds): Developing Cross-Cultural Competence: A Guide for Working with Young Children and Their Families. Brookes Publishing, Baltimore, 1992.

8. Galanti, G: Caring for Patients from Different Cultures. Univ. of Pennsylvania Pr., Philadelphia, 1991.

9. Hansen, M: Pathophysiology: Foundations of Disease and Clinical Intervention. Saunders, Philadelphia, 1998.

10. Guyton, AC, and Hall, JE: Human Physiology and Mechanisms of Disease, ed 6. Saunders, Philadelphia, 1997.

11. McArdle, WD, et al: Exercise Physiology: Energy, Nutrition, and Human Performance. Lea & Febiger, Philadelphia, 1991.

12. Thomas, CL (ed): Taber's Cyclopedic Medical Dictionary, ed 18. FA Davis, Philadelphia, 1997.

13. Goodman, CC: Infectious Disease. In Goodman, CC, and Boissonnault, WG (eds): Pathology: Implications for the Physical Therapist. Saunders, Philadelphia, 1998, p 124.

14. Bates, B: A Guide to Physical Examination and History Taking, ed 5. Lippincott, Philadelphia, 1991.

15. Leger, L, and Thivierge, M: Heart rate monitors: Validity, stability, and functionality. Physician Sports Med 16:143, 1988.

16. Schuman, L: Respiratory Function. In Copstead, LC (ed): Perspectives on Pathophysiology. Saunders, Philadelphia, 1995, p 428.

17. Henderson, BS: Anatomy and Physiology of the Respiratory System. In Ruppert, SD, et al (eds): Dolan's Critical Care Nursing: Clinical Management Through the Nursing Process, ed 2. FA Davis, Philadelphia, 1996, p 387.

18. Brannon, JF, et al: Cardiopulmonary Rehabilitation: Basic Theory and Application, ed 3. FA Davis, Philadelphia, 1998.

19. Jones, TL: Respiratory Assessment: Clinical History and Physical Examination. In Ruppert, SD, et al (eds): Dolan's

Critical Care Nursing: Clinical Management Through the Nursing Process, ed 2. FA Davis, Philadelphia, 1996, p 421.

20. Goodman, CC: The Respiratory System. In Goodman, CC, and Boissonnault, WG (eds): Pathology: Implications for the Physical Therapist. WB Saunders, Philadelphia, 1998, p 399.
21. Dean, E, and Hobson, L: Cardiopulmonary Anatomy. In Frownfelter, D, and Dean, E (eds): Principles and Practice of Cardiopulmonary Physical Therapy, ed 3. Mosby, New York, 1996.
22. Ford, PJ: Anatomy of the Cardiovascular System. In Price, SA, and Wilson, LM (eds): Pathophysiology: Clinical Con-

cepts of Disease Processes, ed 4. McGraw-Hill, New York, 1992, p 371.
23. Gould, BE: Pathophysiology for the Health Related Professions. Saunders, Philadelphia, 1997.
24. Goodman, CC: The Cardiovascular System. In Goodman, CC, and Boissonnault, WG (eds): Pathology: Implications for the Physical Therapist. Saunders, Philadelphia, 1998, p 263.
25. American Heart Association: 1993 Heart and Stroke Facts. Dallas, American Heart Association, 1993.
26. Frolich, ED, et al: Recommendations for Human Blood Pressure Determination by sphygmomanometers. Dallas, American Heart Association, 1987.

SUPPLEMENTAL READINGS

Arrants, J: Hypertension and cardiovascular risk. Heart Lung 23:118, 1994.

Blumenthal, JA, et al: Do exercise and weight loss reduce blood pressure in patients with mild hypertension? N C Med J 56:92, 1995.

Brody, GM: Hyperthermia and hypothermia in the elderly. Clin Geriatr Med 10:213, 1994.

Chen, HI, and Kuo, CS: Relationship between respiratory muscle function and age, sex, and other factors. J Appl Physiol 66:943, 1989.

Cunha, BA: The clinical significance of fever patterns. Infect Dis Clin North Am 10:33, 1996.

Danzl, DF, and Pozos, RS: Accidental hypothermia. N Engl J Med 331:1756, 1994.

Fletcher, EC: The relationship between systemic hypertension and obstructive sleep apnea: Facts and theory. Am J Med 98:118, 1995.

Gentillelo, LM: Advances in the management of hypothermia. Surg Clin North Am 75:243, 1995.

Gift, AG, and Cahill, CA: Psychophysiologic aspects of dyspnea in chronic obstructive pulmonary disease: A pilot study. Heart Lung 19:252, 1990.

Gorney, DA: Arterial blood pressure measurement technique. AACN Clinical Issues in Critical Care 4:66, 1993.

Harchelroad, F: Acute thermoregulatory disorders. Clin Geriatr Med 9:621, 1993.

Kaplan, NM: The treatment of hypertension in women. Arch Intern Med 155:563, 1995.

Lee-Chiong, TL, and Stitt, JT: Accidental hypothermia: When thermoregulation is overwhelmed. Postgrad Med 99:77, 1996.

Lee-Chiong, TL, and Stitt, JT: Heatstroke and other heat-related illness: The maladies of summer. Postgrad Med 98:26, 1995.

Manolio, TA, et al: Trends in pharmacologic management of hypertension in the United States. Arch Intern Med 155:829, 1995.

McCord, M, and Cronin-Stubbs, D: Operationalizing dyspnea: Focus on measurement. Heart Lung 21:167, 1992.

Mortin, L, and Khahil, H: How much reduced hemoglobin is necessary to generate central cyanosis? Chest 97:182, 1990.

Norman, DC, and Yoshikawa, TT: Fever in the elderly. Infect Dis Clin North Am 10:93, 1996.

Prisant, LM, et al: Hypertensive heart disease: How does blood pressure affect left ventricular mass? Postgrad Med 95:59, 1994.

Ross, J, and Dean, E: Integrating physiologic principles into the comprehensive management of cardiopulmonary dysfunction. Phys Ther 69:255, 1989.

Simon, HB: Hyperthermia. N Engl J Med 329:305, 1994.

Sulzbach, LM: Measurement of pulsus paradoxus. Focus on Critical Care 16:142, 1989.

GLOSSARY

Anorexia: Loss of appetite.

Apnea: Absence of respirations, usually temporary in duration.

Blood pressure: Tension exerted by the blood on the walls of a vessel.

Bradycardia: Abnormally slow (low) pulse rate; below approximately 50 beats per minute.

Bradypnea: Decreased respiratory rate; less than 10 breaths per minute.

Cachexia: State of ill health; appearance of malnutrition, and wasting; associated with many chronic diseases.

Circadian rhythm: Variations in vital sign values that occur on a regular and predictable 24-hour cycle.

Clubbing: Bulbous swelling of the distal fingers and toes which develops slowly over a period of time; loss of the normal angle between the nailbed and the skin; associated with diagnoses imposing long-standing hypoxia and cyanosis such as congenital heart defects and pulmonary disorders.

Crackles (historically called rales): Rattling or bubbling sounds that occur owing to secretions in the air passages of the respiratory tract; the sound is often compared to that of rustling a cellophane

bag. Crackles may be heard with the ear but are most accurately assessed by use of a stethoscope.

Cyanosis, types of

Central cyanosis: Dusky, bluish, gray, or dark purple color changes in the mucous membranes (which are normally pink and shiny irrespective of skin color); indicative of marked arterial desaturation.

Peripheral cyanosis: Bluish, gray, or dark purple tinge of the skin of the earlobes, nose, lips, or toes; it is usually transient, occurs secondary to vasoconstriction, and is typically relieved by warming the area.

Diaphoresis: Profuse perspiration.

Diastole: Period of relaxation of the ventricles of the heart; the muscle fibers lengthen and the heart dilates.

Diastolic pressure: The pressure of the blood during relaxation (diastole) of the ventricles.

Dyspnea: Difficult or labored breathing, sometimes accompanied by pain; normal occurrence following vigorous physical activity.

Fever: Elevated body temperature.

Febrile: Pertaining to a fever; state of elevated body temperature.

Homoiotherm (homoiothermic): An animal whose body temperature remains relatively constant regardless of the temperature of the external environment; a warm-blooded animal.

Hyperpyrexia: Extremely high fever; temperature reading of 106°F (41.1°C) or greater.

Hypertension: Higher than normal blood pressure.

Hyperthermia: Extremely high fever; temperature reading of 106°F (41.1°C) or greater.

Hyperventilation: Increase in the rate and depth of respiration.

Hypopnea: Abnormal decrease in both rate and depth of respiration.

Hypotension: Lower than normal blood pressure.

Hypothermia: Body temperature below average normal range.

Hypoventilation: Decrease in the rate and depth of respiration.

Hypovolemia: Abnormally low volume of circulating blood.

Korotkoff's sounds: The series of sounds heard through the stethoscope when assessing blood pressure. Initially when pressure is applied in the cuff, the blood flow is occluded and no sound is heard through the stethoscope. As the pressure is gradually released, a series of five phases or sounds have been identified.

Phase 1: The first clear, faint, rhythmic tapping sound that gradually increases in intensity; period when blood initially flows through the artery; systolic pressure.

Phase 2: A murmur or swishing sound is heard.

Phase 3: Sounds become crisp and louder.

Phase 4: Sound is distinct, abrupt muffling; soft blowing quality; first diastolic pressure.

Phase 5: Sounds disappear; second diastolic pressure.

Laryngopharynx: Anatomical area which marks the opening into the larynx and esophagus; area where solid and liquid food intake is separated from inspired air.

Orthopnea: Difficulty breathing in positions other than upright sitting and standing.

Poikilotherm (poikilothermic): An animal whose body temperature varies with that of the external environment; a coldblooded animal.

Postural (orthostatic) hypotension: A sudden drop in blood pressure; typically occurs with movement to an upright posture after prolonged inactivity and bed rest; gravitational pooling of blood in the lower extremities occurs with resultant cerebral hypoperfusion; triggers an episode of light-headedness or loss of consciousness.

Pulse, common terms used to describe

Alternating (pulsus alterans): Fluctuation between a weak and a strong beat.

Bigeminal: Two regular pulse beats followed by a long pause.

Bounding: A pulse that is difficult to obliterate; usually owing to high blood volume within a vessel; artery has a feeling of tension on palpation (synonym: full, high-tension).

Intermittent: Pulse that occasionally skips a beat.

Irregular: Pulse that varies in both force and rate.

Paradoxical (pulsus paradoxus): Decreased amplitude of the pressure wave with inspiration and return to full amplitude on expiration.

Thready: Fine and barely perceptible pulse; easily obliterated (synonym: filiform, weak).

Weak: Fine and barely perceptible pulse; easily obliterated (synonym: filiform, thready).

Pulse deficit: The difference between the apical and radial pulses.

Pulse pressure: The difference between the diastolic and systolic pressures.

Pyrexia: Increased body temperature; fever.

Pyrogens: Fever-producing substances.

Sigh: A deep inspiration followed by a prolonged, audible expiration; occasional sighs are normal and function to expand alveoli. Frequent sighs are abnormal and may be indicative of emotional stress.

Stertorous: A snoring sound owing to secretions in the trachea and large bronchi.

Stridor: A harsh, high-pitched crowing sound that occurs with upper airway obstructions caused by narrowing of the glottis or trachea (e.g., tracheal stenosis, presence of a foreign object).

Systole: Period during which the ventricles of the heart are contracting.

Systolic pressure: The pressure of the blood during contraction (systole) of the ventricles.

Tachycardia: Abnormally rapid (high) pulse rate; over approximately 100 beats per minute.

Tachypnea: Increased respiratory rate; greater than 24 breaths per minute.

Tidal volume: Volume or amount of air exchanged with a single breath.

Vital signs: The signs of life; that is, pulse, body temperature, respiration, and blood pressure (synonym: cardinal signs).

Valsalva maneuver: An attempt to exhale forcibly with the glottis, nose, and mouth closed; causes increased intrathoracic pressure, slowing of the pulse, decreased return of blood to the heart, and increased venous pressure.

Wheezing: A whistling sound produced by air passing through a narrowed airway such as a bronchi or bronchiole; it may be heard on both inspiration and expiration but is more prominent on expiration; apparent in patients with emphysema and asthma.

APPENDIX

Suggested Answers to Case Study Guiding Questions

1. Describe the body system responses to hypothermia as presented by the clinical features of the case.

ANSWER: The patient's exposure to such extreme environmental conditions for a 48-hour period caused the thermoregulatory center to essentially shut down. The patient lost all normal heat regulatory and protection mechanisms. This caused a decrease in metabolic rate as his body temperature gradually dropped. As cooling of the brain occurred, reduced cerebral perfusion caused a depression in cognitive function.

Respiratory rate diminished as oxygen consumption dropped which decreased profusion of peripheral tissues. Increased blood viscosity and vasoconstriction further impaired peripheral perfusion to the extremities. These factors contributed to the lack of cutaneous sensation and peripheral cyanosis, which led to tissue damage from freezing (frostbite). Once the shivering mechanism was lost, the skeletal muscles became stiff with loss of deep tendon reflexes. Decreased cardiac profusion resulted in a decreased stroke volume. The combined effects of a diminished stroke volume, increased blood viscosity, and peripheral vasoconstriction all contributed to the alterations noted in pulse pressure and blood pressure.

2. Considering this patient is unresponsive and cyanotic, what would be the most appropriate pulse to monitor?

ANSWER: The carotid pulse. The peripheral resistance (increased blood viscosity and vasoconstriction) would preclude obtaining an accurate pulse value from a peripheral site. In addition, monitoring the carotid pulse would provide important information about blood flow to the brain.

3. The function of the thermoregulatory center becomes seriously impaired when body temperature falls below approximately 94°F (34.4°C) and is completely lost with temperatures below 85°F (29.4°C).

4. Extremes in environmental temperature have a large impact on the body's ability to maintain constant temperatures. What type of clothing can best assist in protecting the body from low environmental temperatures?

ANSWER: Clothing is an important consideration because it can function to conserve body heat. The optimum approach for conserving heat is the use of several layers of lightweight clothing to trap air and help insulate the body.

Musculoskeletal 5 Assessment

D. Joyce White

LEARNING OBJECTIVES

1. Identify the purposes of performing a musculoskeletal assessment.
2. Describe the components of a musculoskeletal assessment.
3. Identify questions that should be included in a patient interview.
4. Describe the procedures used to selectively test types of tissues in a musculoskeletal assessment.
5. Identify additional assessment procedures that often compliment a musculoskeletal assessment.
6. Using the case study examples, apply clinical decision making skills in evaluating musculoskeletal assessment data.

The musculoskeletal system includes bones, muscles with their related tendons and synovial sheaths, bursa, and joint structures such as cartilage, menisci, capsules, and ligaments. Acute injuries or chronic conditions that disrupt the anatomy or physiology of musculoskeletal tissues can greatly affect a patient's function by causing impairments such as pain, inflammation, structural deformity, restricted joint movement, joint instability, and muscle weakness. Examples of diagnoses that result in direct impairment of the musculoskeletal system include fracture, rheumatoid arthritis, osteoarthritis, joint dislocation, tendinitis, bursitis, muscle strain/rupture, and ligament sprain/rupture.

Many pathological conditions that initially affect other body systems such as the neurological, cardiovascular, or pulmonary systems can result in secondary or what is referred to as indirect impairment of the musculoskeletal system. This often occurs when patients' activities are restricted by the condition—perhaps they are confined for a period of time to a bed or wheelchair, or move the upper or lower extremities in an inefficient or stressful pattern. Diagnoses that can cause indirect impairments of the musculoskeletal system included traumatic brain injury, cerebral vascular accident, cerebral palsy, spinal and peripheral nerve injury, burns, and myocardial infarction, just to name a few. From these few examples of diagnoses that cause direct and indirect musculoskeletal impairments, it can be appreciated how often physical therapists and other health professionals need to assess the musculoskeletal system. Musculoskeletal assessment is almost always a major component of an initial examination of a patient.

This chapter will discuss the purposes of performing a musculoskeletal assessment and provide a general framework for conducting an assessment. Other texts are available that provide detailed musculoskeletal testing procedures of specific body regions.[1-3] This chapter will emphasize the principles and components of a musculoskeletal assessment, and how to organize and integrate the assessment with those of other body systems.

PURPOSE

Evaluation of data from the musculoskeletal examination contributes to establishing a diagnosis and prognosis, setting goals and outcomes, and developing and implementing a plan of care. Musculoskeletal assessment is also an important component of evaluating treatment outcome both periodically during the treatment process and at the conclusion of therapy.

The purposes of performing a musculoskeletal assessment include the following:

1. To determine the presence or absence of impairment involving muscles, bones, and related joint structures; to determine baseline status.
2. To identify the specific tissues that are causing the impairment.
3. To help formulate appropriate therapeutic goals, outcomes, and interventions.
4. To determine orthotic and adaptive equipment necessary for functional ability in daily, occupational, and recreational activities.
5. To assess the effectiveness of rehabilitation, medical or surgical management.
6. To motivate the patient.

EXAMINATION PROCEDURES

Patient History and Interview

Prior to beginning the physical examination it is important to gain as much information as possible about the patient's current condition and past medical history. This information will help to direct and focus examination to an area and system of the body. Information on symptoms and functional ability will help to establish a baseline against which to judge treatment effectiveness. It will also enable the examination and treatment of the patient to be conducted safely.

Typically, most of this information is obtained by interviewing the patient. However, utilizing other information sources can be very efficient and provide objectivity and details to supplement an interview. If the patient is hospitalized in an acute care or rehabilitation setting, the medical records, including admission reports, progress notes, medication sheets, surgical summaries, body imaging reports, and laboratory test results should be available and sought out. Referral summaries from previous medical care settings, which review prior treatment approaches and discuss functional status, may also be included. Other members of the health care team can be consulted for their input.

Outpatients often arrive with just a general diagnosis from a referring physician, or may have been self-referred. In such cases it will be helpful to ask the patient to complete a medical history form prior to starting the examination process. A medical history form should include space for the patient to note the chief problem and date of onset, diagnostic tests performed for the current problem, name and date of all surgeries, all medications currently being taken, a checklist of common medical conditions the patient may have experienced, brief family medical history, patient's age, occupation, and life-style questions pertaining to smoking, alcohol use, and exercise. An example of a medical history form is shown in Fig. 5-1. A thorough understanding of the patient's background is critical for safe examination and treatment. For example, a history of a myocardial infarction would cause the examiner to limit and more closely monitor the patient during muscle performance testing. A history of diabetes mellitus would cause the examiner to suspect and test for a compromised peripheral vascular and peripheral nervous systems, and possibly avoid the use of heat modalities during treatment. Even though a patient may complete a medical history form, it is important for the therapist to review and clarify the information with the patient. Sometimes important medical background is inadvertently forgotten as the patient focuses on current problems. Verbally reviewing the information with the patient may jog the patient's memory.

After reviewing the information gained from medical records, other health care providers, and the patient-completed medical history form, the examiner is ready to begin the patient interview. Ideally, the patient interview should be conducted in a quiet, well-lit room that offers a measure of privacy. To encourage good communication, the examiner and patient should be at a similar eye level, facing each other, with a comfortable space between them—about 3 feet apart is customary in the United States. The patient should have the examiner's undivided attention; telephone calls and other interruptions should be avoided. The examiner may wish to have paper and pen available to record particular dates and information that is easily forgotten, but the interview should flow as an active conversation not a dictation session. Repeated practice greatly improves the examiner's ability to listen, direct the interview, and establish a positive working relationship with the patient.

Over the course of the interview the examiner needs to gain information about the patient's current complaints including onset, location, type and behavior of symptoms, current medications, previous treatments, secondary medical problems, and medical history. The patient's age and gender should be noted; some conditions are more common in particular age groups and genders. Often, detailed information about a patient's occupation, recreational activities, and social/living situation are required to understand the cause of the impairments, functional limitations, and to develop a relevant plan of care that focuses on the patient's goals. Open-ended, objective questions that do not lead to biased answers should be asked. However, the examiner will need to guide the interview to keep it focused on pertinent information and concluded in a timely manner. All questions should use lay rather than medical terminology so the questions are easily understood by the patient. The examiner should ask one question at a time and be sure to obtain a response before proceeding to other questions. Follow-up inquiries will be needed to clarify initial answers. It is important for the examiner to keep an open mind during the interview and not rush to conclusions about the patient's symptoms and diagnosis.

The following sequence is suggested as a way of organizing the interview. Similar information on

The purpose of this questionnaire is to assist us in providing you with quality care by obtaining a better understanding of your total health status. This questionnaire is part of your confidential medical record.

NAME: _____   DATE: _____

CHIEF PROBLEM OR COMPLAINT: _____

REFERRING MD: _____   DATE OF NEXT MD VISIT: _____

MEDICATIONS: Please list *all* medications currently being taken, along with the dosage, if known, and frequency.

1. _____   4. _____

2. _____   5. _____

3. _____   6. _____

SURGERY: Please list *all* surgeries and approximate date.

1. _____   DATE: _____

2. _____   DATE: _____

3. _____   DATE: _____

4. _____   DATE: _____

DIAGNOSTIC TESTS: Please check tests for current problem only.

X-rays: _____   CT Scan: _____   MRI: _____   Bone Scan: _____

EMG: _____   Blood Test: _____   Myelogram: _____   Others: _____

OCCUPATION: _____

LIFE STYLE: Non Smoker: _____ Smoke _____/day

No Alcohol: _____ Alcohol _____/day or _____/week

No Exercise: _____ Exercise _____/day or _____/week

FAMILY HISTORY: Mother, Father, siblings: Alive and healthy: _____

If deceased, cause of death: _____

Figure 5-1. An example of a medical history recording form. (Courtesy of North Andover Physical Therapy Associates, North Andover, MA.)   *Continued.*

DO YOU HAVE, OR HAVE YOU HAD, ANY OF THE FOLLOWING: Please check *All* that apply.

___ High blood pressure
___ Heart problems
___ Heart palpitations, murmur
___ Chest pain

___ Shortness of breath
___ Coughing

___ Difficulty sleeping lying flat
___ Lung problems
___ Asthma
___ Allergies

___ Ulcers
___ Recent weight gain or loss
___ Nausea, vomiting
___ Bowel or bladder changes
___ Loss of appetite

___ Sexual dysfunction
___ Abnormal or painful menstruation
___ Pelvic inflammatory disease
___ Currently pregnant
___ Date of last mammogram:_____

___ Blood in urine
___ Incontinence

___ Seizures
___ Head trauma
___ Paralysis
___ Loss of consciousness
___ Headaches

___ Numbness or tingling
___ Dizziness
___ Balance problems

___ Arthritis

___ Hot or cold intolerance
___ Diabetes
___ Low blood sugar
___ Thyroid problems

___ Tumors ___ Cancer
___ Bleeding or bruising
___ Dialysis
___ Blood transfusion

___ Rashes
___ Scars
___ Changes in hair or nails

___ Wear eye glasses, contacts
___ Changes in vision
___ Blurred or double vision

___ Difficulty swallowing
___ Ear pain
___ Vocal changes
___ Ringing in ears

___ Dentures
___ Major dental work
___ Difficulty eating

___ Varicose veins
___ Muscle cramps
___ Joint or muscle pain

___ Psychiatric or psychological care

___ Fractures (broken bones)
      Where?_____
___ Problem requiring orthopedic shoes
___ Hip or ankle problem
___ Unusual illness as child

Please check if you have ever been in a motor vehicle accident _____

Figure 5-1. *Continued.*

general patient interviewing, that includes slight variations in format, can be found in texts by Talley and O'Connor,[4] Hertling and Kessler,[1] and Paris.[5]

1. *Opening Question*. The interview should begin with a general question such as "What brings you to physical therapy today?" or "What seems to be the problem?" If the patient is hospitalized the question needs to be rephrased to avoid having the patient retell his or her recent medical history to every health care provider. "I see from your medical chart that you fractured your hip and underwent a surgical repair yesterday. Is that what happened?" The patient should be given the opportunity to present the story. After several minutes when the patient has concluded his or her statement, it is appropriate to say "That's good. Now I have an idea of the problem. I have some other questions I need to ask to help me understand your problem better." Depending on the information provided by the patient, some of the following questions will need to be asked.

2. *Onset of symptoms.* "How did this pain (. . . swelling, limitation, problem, etc.) begin?" The examiner needs to know if the onset was sudden—caused by trauma such as a fall, blow, or skiing or automobile accident. Specific information about the patient's body position at the time of trauma and the mechanism of injury will help to identify the structures involved. If the onset was more gradual or insidious, a systemic condition or chronic biomechanical problem may be more likely. A congenital onset is also a possibility.

3. *Location of the symptoms.* "Where is your pain? Can you point to the location?" A body chart (Fig. 5-2) can help document the location of symptoms. Often the location of the symptoms coincides with the location of the lesion. This is more likely if the lesion is in superficial and distal tissues. For example, a lesion in a superficial tendon near the ankle will usually cause pain to be perceived over the tendon site. Lesions in deeper, more proximal tissues often refer pain distally following sclerotome patterns (Fig. 5-3). This referred pain may be perceived as originating from any or all tissues innervated by the same segmental spinal level as the lesion. For example, pain due to osteoarthritis of the hip is often felt in the anterior groin and thigh along sclerotome L2 and L3.

"Has the pain changed in location? Spread to other areas? Become more focused?" Pain that is spreading usually indicates a worsening condition, while more focused symptoms

indicate improvement. Changes in symptoms in relationship to varying body positions, activities, and treatments should be noted.

4. *Quality of the symptoms.* "How severe is the pain? Is the pain sharp? dull? throbbing?" A simple yet effective approach is to ask the patient to rate his or her pain from 0 (no pain) to 10 (most severe pain imaginable) as seen in Fig. 5-4. A visual analog scale (Fig. 5-5) or thermometer pain scale (Fig. 5-6) can also be used if preferred. A checklist of adjectives like that found in the McGill-Melzack Pain Questionnaire[6] can clarify symptoms further (Fig. 5-7). The adjectives used to describe pain may have diagnostic implications. Dull, aching pain may indicate muscle or joint lesions. Numbness, tingling, shooting pain, or burning sensations may indicate nervous system involvement. Deep, throbbing pain, or coolness in a body region may indicate vascular problems. Weakness, clumsiness, or incoordination may suggest muscle and possibly peripheral or central nervous system dysfunction.

5. *Behavior of the symptoms.* "What makes your symptoms increase? Decrease?" Pain from overuse syndromes such as tendinitis will decrease with rest, whereas joint stiffness caused by osteoarthritis may increase following rest. If a patient reports that the sitting position reduces back pain, then the therapist will likely have more success in relieving the pain using back flexion exercises rather than extension exercises. Musculoskeletal conditions have typical patterns of varying symptoms. Symptoms that do not vary with a change in activity or body position are rarely due to musculoskeletal lesions, and in fact are a "red flag" for more serious conditions such as space-occupying tumors and pathologies involving internal organs. Often patients will report that "nothing helps the pain." This statement should be fully explored with follow-up questions such as "Is your pain better or worse in the morning when you wake up from sleeping? Does your pain vary if you sleep on your back versus on your stomach?"

6. *Behavior of the symptoms over the last 48 hours.* It is important to understand the behavior of the symptoms over the past few days, not just now. Sometimes symptoms suddenly worsen or disappear at the time of the physical examination. A more accurate picture of the situation is told if the time frame is over 48 hours. "Are the symptoms getting better, worse, or staying the same?" The answer to this question will help the examiner judge the effectiveness of future treatment. If the patient's pain has been steadily worsening over the last 48 hours and treatment stabilizes the pain, then the treatment may be judged as helpful. However, if

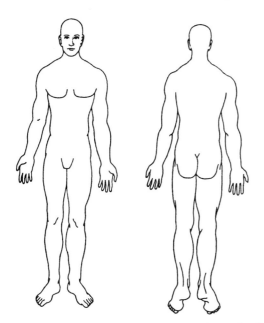

Figure 5-2. This body chart can supplement the patient's verbal description of the location of the pain. (From Dyrek,[8] p 74, with permission.)

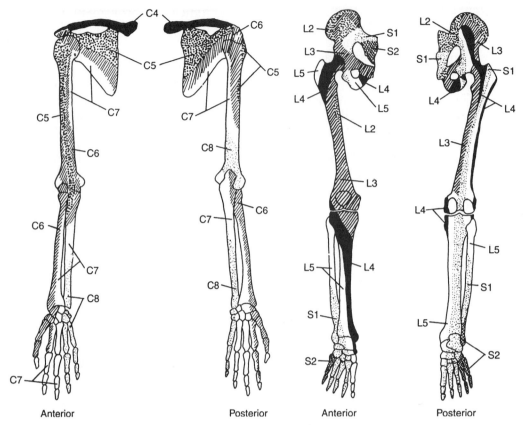

Figure 5-3. Sclerotomes. (From Hertling and Kessler,[1] p 52, with permission.)

the patient reports that the pain has been steadily improving over the last 48 hours and treatment stabilizes the pain, then the treatment may be judged as detrimental.

7. *Previous care.* "What previous care has been sought for the problem? Who else (physician, therapist, chiropractor, etc.) has treated the problem? What tests and treatments did they perform? What have you done to relieve the problem?" From these and similar questions all previous exercises, physical modalities, manual treatments, medications, injections,

Circle the number below which best represents the intensity of your pain today.

0	1	2	3	4	5	6	7	8	9	10
		Minimal			**Moderate**				**Severe**	

Circle the number below which best represents the intensity of your pain today.

0	1	2	3	4	5	6	7	8	9	10
No Pain									**Worst Pain Imaginable**	

Figure 5-4. Two types of numerical pain rating scales.

On the line provided below please mark where the intensity of your pain is today.

No pain   **Most severe**
                                           Pain imaginable

Figure 5-5. Visual analog pain rating scale. The line is usually 3.9 in (10 cm) in length. The patient's mark is measured from the left (no pain) end of the scale and is recorded in centimeters.

orthotics, and surgical procedures should be delineated. The answers to these questions help the examiner to decide if further medical referrals are needed and to focus on the most effective treatment for the condition. For example, a patient who fell 3 days ago is experiencing severe ankle pain and swelling. The patient borrowed a friend's crutches and has

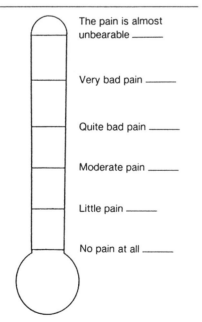

Pain Rating Scale

Instructions:

   Below is a thermometer with various grades of pain on it from "No Pain at all" to "The pain is almost unbearable." Put a × by the words that describe your pain best. Mark how bad your pain is AT THIS MOMENT IN TIME.

The pain is almost unbearable _____

Very bad pain _____

Quite bad pain _____

Moderate pain _____

Little pain _____

No pain at all _____

Figure 5-6. Thermometer pain rating scale. (From Brodie, DJ, et al: Evaluation of low back pain by patient questionnaires and therapist assessment. J Orthop Sport Phys Ther 11:528, 1990, with permission.)

Look carefully at the twenty groups of words. If any word in any group applies to *your* pain, please circle that word — but do not circle more than *one word in any one group* — so you must choose the *most suitable word* in that group.
   In groups that do not apply to your pain, there is no need to circle *any* word — just leave them as they are.

Group 1	*Group 2*	*Group 3*	*Group 4*	*Group 5*
Flickering	Jumping	Pricking	Sharp	Pinching
Quivering	Flashing	Boring	Gritting	Pressing
Pulsing	Shooting	Drilling	Lacerating	Gnawing
Throbbing		Stabbing		Cramping
Beating		Lancinating		Crushing
Pounding				
Group 6	*Group 7*	*Group 8*	*Group 9*	*Group 10*
Tugging	Hot	Tingling	Dull	Tender
Pulling	Burning	Itching	Sore	Taut
Wrenching	Scalding	Smarting	Hurting	Rasping
	Searing	Stinging	Aching	Splitting
			Heavy	
Group 11	*Group 12*	*Group 13*	*Group 14*	*Group 15*
Tiring	Sickening	Fearful	Punishing	Wretched
Exhausting	Suffocating	Frightful	Gruelling	Blinding
		Terrifying	Cruel	
			Vicious	
			Killing	
Group 16	*Group 17*	*Group 18*	*Group 19*	*Group 20*
Annoying	Spreading	Tight	Cool	Nagging
Troublesome	Radiating	Numb	Cold	Nauseating
Miserable	Penetrating	Drawing	Freezing	Agonizing
Intense	Piercing	Squeezing		Dreadful
Unbearable		Tearing		Torturing

Figure 5-7. The McGill Melnack Pain Questionnaire. Patients are asked to underline not more than one word from any or all of the 20 groups which best describe their pain. The simplest scoring methods involve (1) total number of words underlined, and (2) intensity, measured by allotting score 1 to the first word in any group, 1 to the second, and so on. The first 10 groups of words are somatic (describing what the pain feels like), 11–15 are affective, 16 is evaluative, and 17–20 miscellaneous. (From Wells, PE, et al: Pain Management in Physical Therapy. Appleton & Lange, Norwalk, CT, p 14, with permission.)

been self-treating the ankle with ice and elevation. The therapist would want to have the patient examined by a physician and have radiographs taken to rule out a fracture, if this has not already occurred, prior to beginning physical therapy. In another scenario, if a patient has been treated previously by two physical therapists with ultrasound and had no improvement, then other treatments should be considered.

8. *Specific medical history.* "Has this problem occurred before? How was it treated? How did it resolve?" Many musculoskeletal problems tend to recur with continued occupational, recreational, and daily activities if underlying biomechanical abnormalities, weaknesses, joint laxity, or tightness remain. Information about previous successful and unsuccessful treatments can help in treatment planning for the current problem.

9. *Past medical history.* A brief history should be obtained about medical problems and prior surgeries involving other body regions and systems. Conditions involving the cardiac, respiratory, neurological, vascular, metabolic, endocrine, gastrointestinal, genital urinary, visual, and dermatological systems should be noted. Having a patient complete a medical history form prior to the interview and exam-

ination is an efficient means of obtaining this information, but the information should also be verified during the interview. Examiners also need to be aware of other conditions that mimic signs and symptoms often attributable to the musculoskeletal system. For example, inflammation of the gallbladder may result in right shoulder pain. However, shoulder pain related to cholecystitis typically will not increase with shoulder movements or resisted isometric testing of shoulder musculature, as would be the case in musculoskeletal conditions. Patients with cholecystitis would likely have additional symptoms such as upper abdominal discomfort, bloating, belching, nausea, and intolerance of fried foods. Knowledge of systemic human pathology is needed to recognize conditions requiring additional physician assessment and intervention. Boissennault[7] has written a helpful text to assist physical therapists in screening for medical conditions.

10. *Medications.* The type, frequency, dose, and effect of medications the patient is taking should be noted. The examiner should recognize that use of analgesic or anti-inflammatory medications may reduce the level of symptoms during the examination.[8] Changes in use of these medications may make it difficult to assess the effects of physical therapy treatment. Prolonged use of corticosteroids is associated with osteopenia and reduced tensile strength of ligaments. The therapist may need to limit manual force applied through the lever of a long bone shaft to prevent a fracture or ligament tear. The use of anticoagulants may make the patient susceptible to contusions and hemarthrosis.

These patients should be closely monitored for bruising and joint swelling. The amount of force used in exercise and manual therapies may need to be reduced.

11. *Occupational, recreational, and social history including functional status.* Questions in this area might include: "What type of work do you do in and outside of the home? How has this problem affected your ability to perform your job? care for your children? play golf? dress? bathe?" and so forth. Particular occupational and recreational activities may contribute to the problem or interfere with recovery. Figure 5-8 presents questions that can be used to quantify the effects of the problem on function. Strategies and assistive devices may need to be explored to allow the completion of necessary tasks. Medical insurance companies often make treatment reimbursement decisions based on a patient's functional status as related to the medical problem.

"Do you have stairs to climb to get into your house? to reach the bedroom? bathroom?" Home architecture will determine whether a patient dependent on ambulating with a walker, crutches, or cane needs instruction in stair activities prior to returning home. The condition of floors, size of halls and doorways, placement of furniture, and bathroom facilities will need to be assessed for a patient using a wheelchair. Information on environmental assessment of the home, workplace, and community can be found in Chapter 12.

"Do you live alone?" It is helpful to understand the patient's living situation to determine if others are available to assist in exercise programs, ambulation, and transfer

What percentage of your normal <u>work</u> activities are you able to perform?

0%   10%   20%   30%   40%   50%   60%   70%   80%   90%   100%

What percentage of your normal <u>home</u> activities are you able to perform?

0%   10%   20%   30%   40%   50%   60%   70%   80%   90%   100%

What percentage of your normal <u>recreational</u> activities are you able to perform?

0%   10%   20%   30%   40%   50%   60%   70%   80%   90%   100%

Figure 5-8. Questions used to rate a patient's function.

activities. Some patients have responsibility for the care of children, elderly parents, or a disabled spouse or sibling. These responsibilities may need to be restructured to allow time for rest and recovery.

"Do you use tobacco products? Alcohol? Recreational drugs?" Cigarette smoking has been associated with decreased bone density,[9,10] greater spinal disk degeneration,[11] increased low back pain,[12,13] and increased upper and lower extremity musculoskeletal disorders.[14–16] Use of alcohol and recreational drugs can lead to risk-taking behaviors resulting in increased injuries. Examiners may wish to advise a patient to reduce the use of these substances and refer the patient to appropriate social services or self-help organizations for counseling.

12. *Patient's treatment goals and anticipated time frame of recovery.* "What do you hope the outcome of this therapy will be? When do you anticipate returning home? to work? playing football?" and so forth. These questions enable the examiner and patient to discuss and determine mutually agreeable treatment goals. The examiner should not presume to know what issues are important to the patient. Answers to these questions help the examiner to assess whether the patient has realistic expectations or will need further patient education concerning his or her condition and typical recovery. For example, an elderly patient who suffered a fractured hip yesterday and is currently hospitalized may expect to remain in the acute care hospital until she can independently ambulate and care for herself in 2 weeks. More realistic goals given current health insurance practices may need to be discussed, such as discharge from the hospital in 3 or 4 days to a rehabilitation or extended care facility for further nursing care, physical and occupational therapy; or discharge home with home health aides, and visiting nurses, and physical and occupational therapy.

13. *Concluding question.* When the examiner has finished obtaining the above information, one final question needs to be asked. "Is there anything else you wish to tell me?"[5] Most likely the patient will respond by saying that he or she has no further information to offer and believe you understand the problem clearly. But, sometimes a patient may take this opportunity to clarify a previous point or share a concern that is adding stress to his or her life. Without this open-ended question at the conclusion of the interview, important information that may impact treatment and recovery may be lost.

The information elicited with the questions listed above will need to be supplemented with additional questions based on the specific region of the body being examined and suspected etiologies. The examiner needs extensive background in the areas of anatomy, kinesiology, pathokinesiology, physiology, and pathophysiology, as well as the physical presentation and progression of musculoskeletal conditions to interview the patient adequately.

Vital Signs

If a patient's medical record or interview suggests a compromised cardiovascular system, heart rate, blood pressure, and respiratory rate should be assessed prior to beginning other physical examination procedures (see Chapter 4: Assessment of Vital Signs). Patients getting out of bed for the first time following prolonged bed rest or recent surgery should have vital signs taken to establish baseline function prior to movement.

Mental Status

The patient's orientation to person, place, and time as well as general arousal state, cognitive, and communication abilities should be noted. If deficits in these areas are present the examination may need to be modified to gain accurate information. The use of simple words, concise instructions, and task demonstrations may be helpful. Distractions in the environment should be kept to a minimum. Communication difficulties may be improved through the use of foreign language interpreters, gestures, drawings, and language boards. Changes in medications and access to natural light via windows and skylights may improve patient arousal and orientation to time. Depending on the type of deficit, the patient may benefit from an assessment by a neurologist, neuropsychologist, speech-language pathologist, and/or occupational therapist.

Observation/Inspection

Observation begins with the examiner's first contact with the patient, whether at bedside in the case of hospitalized patients, or in the waiting room for outpatients. The patient's general posture and ability to perform functional tasks—change bed position, transfer from sitting to standing, ambulate to the examining room—provides information as to the patient's severity of symptoms, willingness to move, range of joint motion, and muscle strength. This information, although cursory, helps to focus and individualize the physical examination. For example, a patient with a shoulder disorder who uses the upper extremity to push off from a chair during transfers, stands with level bilateral shoulder height, and has an alternating arm swing during gait, would be expected to have milder symptoms, tolerate a more extensive examination, and have a greater range of motion and muscle function than a patient who stands with an elevated scapula and protectively cradles the upper extremity during transfers and gait. If functional difficulties and gait abnormalities are noted, detailed functional and gait assessments would be performed later in the examination.

To continue the physical examination and inspect specific areas of the body, the patient must be suitably dressed. Observation of the shoulders, elbows, or spine will require males to remove their shirt and females to wear only a bra or loose "Johnny" that can be draped to expose the upper extremity and back. To observe the lower extremities, patients should undress from the waist down, wearing only shorts.

Once the patient is in the privacy of an examining room and appropriately undressed, the examiner begins a careful inspection of the body region implicated in the interview as well as biomechanically related areas. The lower extremities and lumbar region, being intricately involved in weight-bearing activities should be inspected as a functional unit. Likewise, conditions involving the shoulder require the examination of the cervical and thoracic regions, and vice versa. Visual inspection should focus on bone, soft tissue structures, and the skin and nails. The examiner should view the body region anteriorly, posteriorly, and laterally. Often palpation, which is discussed in the next section, is combined with observation.

Bone shafts and joints are judged against normative models as well as for symmetry, comparing one side of the body to the other. Contour and alignment should be considered. Common causes of changes in bone contour include acute fractures, callus formations following healed fractures, congenital variations, bone hyperplasia at tendon insertions, and arthritis. Alignment differences can be due to the above conditions as well as muscle tightness, muscle weakness, ligament laxity, and joint dislocation.

Often a gross postural screening is performed to assist in assessing alignment. From an anterior view both eyes, shoulders (acromion processes), iliac crests, anterior superior iliac spines, greater trochanters of the femur, patella, and ankle malleoli should be horizontally level. Waist angles should be symmetrical. Patella and feet should face anteriorly. Laterally the line of gravity should bisect the external auditory meatus, acromion process, greater trochanter, lie just posterior to the patella and approximately 2 inches anterior to the lateral malleolus (Fig. 5-9).[17] The cervical and lumbar spine should exhibit moderate lordotic curves, and the thoracic spine, a moderate kyphotic curve. Posteriorly the ear lobes, shoulders, inferior angles of the scapula, iliac crests, posterior superior iliac spines, greater trochanters, buttock and knee creases, and malleoli should be level. The spine should be straight, with the medial borders of the scapula equidistant from the spine bilaterally. Varus and valgus deformities of the knee and calcaneus should be noted.

The size and contour of soft tissue structures should be inspected and compared bilaterally. An increase in size may indicate soft tissue edema, joint effusion, or muscle hypertrophy. A decrease in size

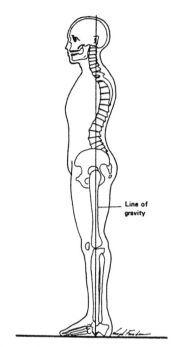

Figure 5-9. The location of the line of gravity from the lateral view. (From Norkin and Levangie,[17] p 426, with permission.)

often indicates muscle atrophy. A loss of soft tissue continuity can suggest a muscle rupture. Cysts, rheumatoid nodules, ganglia, and gouty tophi can all change soft tissue contour. *Clubbing*, a rounded increase in soft tissue in distal fingers and toes, is believed to be caused by chronic hypoxemia and is typically associated with cardiovascular diseases, respiratory diseases, or neurovascular abnormalities.[4] Skin color and texture provide important clues to pathological conditions. *Cyanosis*, a blue discoloration of the skin and nail bed, indicates a lack of oxygen and excessive carbon dioxide in superficial blood vessels.[4] Inspection of the tongue for cyanosis helps determine if the poor perfusion is due to central or peripheral causes. *Pallor* is noted with a decrease in blood flow or blood hemoglobin—for example, in situations such as peripheral vasoconstriction, shock, internal bleeding, and anemia. *Erythema*, a localized redness, usually indicates increased blood flow and inflammation. Generalized redness can suggest fever, sunburn, or carbon monoxide poisoning. Yellow skin tone may be due to increased carotene intake, or liver disease. Brown, highly pigmented, hairy areas sometimes overlay bony defects such as spina bifida. Open wounds should be measured and diagrammed in patient records. New scars will be red, and older scars will be white in color. Skin tissue thickenings such as *calluses* can indicate chronic overloading and stress. Thin, glossy skin with decreased elasticity and hair loss is often found with peripheral nerve lesions or neurovascular disorders.

Palpation

It is suggested that palpation immediately follow or be integrated with observation, and occur prior to other testing procedures. Often these other procedures will aggravate the patient's condition, making it more difficult to localize tenderness if palpation is performed later. The information gained from palpation will also help direct the examiner to choose additional, appropriate testing procedures.

Palpation requires detailed knowledge of anatomy and a systematic approach. All structures on one body surface should be palpated before proceeding to another surface. For example, all structures on the anterior surface of the patient should be palpated before beginning to palpate structures on the posterior surface. The uninvolved side is examined first to acquaint the patient to the procedure and can serve as a normative model for comparison. The examiner should develop a system of moving from superior to inferior structures, medial to lateral, or superior and inferior from a joint line. The choice of system is important, and being consistent and thorough is critical. Bone, soft tissue structures, and the skin will need to be palpated by varying the examiner's tactile pressure. Light tactile pressure allows palpation of superficial tissues like the skin, whereas more pressure is needed to palpate deeper structures like bone. Usually the fingertips are used for palpation, but large, deeper structures such as the greater trochanter of the femur or borders of the scapula are easier to locate using the entire surface of the hand. Rolling the skin and soft tissue between the fingertips and thumb helps the examiner judge myofascial mobility. Changes in skin temperature may be easier to detect using the posterior surface of the examiner's hand. When moving from one area to another the examiner's hand should stay in firm contact with the skin whenever possible to prevent a tickling sensation. The fingers should not "crawl" or "walk" across the skin.

During palpation the examiner is seeking feedback from the patient to help localize painful structures. Some lesions in deep or proximal structures will refer symptoms to other body areas, but localized tenderness often helps to implicate particular structures. Localized skin temperature can be noted: cool temperatures suggest reduced circulation, whereas warmth indicates increased circulation and often inflammation. Skin and soft tissue density and extensibility should be examined. Often muscle spasms and adhesions in skin and connective tissue can be found with palpation. The quality (amplitude) of peripheral pulses will provide gross information on arterial blood supply. Bilateral edema in the ankles and legs that forms pits with tactile pressure (termed *pitting edema*) can indicate cardiac failure, liver, or renal conditions. Unilateral pitting edema can be found with obstruction of returning circulation.

Anthropometric Characteristics

Abnormalities noted during observation and palpation may be further documented with anthropometric measurements. Limb lengths are measured from one bony landmark to another and compared bilaterally. For example, true leg length is measured from the anterior superior iliac spine to the medial or lateral malleolus. Circumference measurements help substantiate joint effusion, edema, and muscle hypertrophy and atrophy. Typically, these measurements are taken at specified distances above and below a bony landmark so they can be reproduced during reassessment of a patient's status. If measurements are needed of the hands or feet, these distal extremities can be submerged in containers of water and the volume of water displacement noted.

Range of Motion

Joints and their related structures are assessed by performing various active and passive joint motions. Joint motion is a necessary component of most functional tasks. Studies have identified the range of motion needed to ambulate on level surfaces, descend stairs, rise from a chair, put on a shirt, eat with a spoon, and many other activities.[18-21] Careful examination of joint motion for range of motion (ROM), end-feel, effect on symptoms, and pattern of limitation help identify and quantify impairments causing functional disabilities, and determine the structures that need focused treatment.

ACTIVE RANGE OF MOTION

The assessment of joint motion begins by testing **active range of motion (AROM).** Active motion is the unassisted voluntary movement of a joint. The patient is asked to move a body part through the osteokinematic motions at the involved and other biomechanically related joints. **Osteokinematics** refers to the gross angular motions of the shafts of bones. These motions are described as occurring in the three cardinal planes of the body: flexion and extension in the sagittal plane, abduction and adduction in the frontal plane, and medial and lateral rotation in the transverse plane. For example, in an assessment of the hip the patient would be asked to move the hip into flexion, extension, abduction, adduction, and medial and lateral rotation. Often flexion and extension of the knee, as well as flexion, extension, rotation, and lateral flexion of the lumbar spine are tested, as knee and spine motions will impact hip function. Some examiners prefer to have the patient move in functional, combined motions rather than straight plane motions. For example, a patient would be asked to reach his or her hand behind the head to test shoulder abduction and medial rotation simultaneously rather than perform isolated, individual motions.

Active motion is a good screening procedure to further focus the physical examination. The amount, quality, and pattern of motion, as well as the occurrence of pain and crepitus should be noted. Often active ROM is visually estimated, but if more objective and accurate measurements are needed, a goniometer should be used. Normal ROM varies among individuals and is influenced by factors such as age,[22–26] gender,[26–28] and measurement methods.[29,30] Ideally, to determine if a ROM is impaired, the ROM should be compared with values obtained with the same measurement methods from people of the same age and gender. Studies that provide normative values by age and gender have been summarized by Norkin and White.[31] However, when particular values are not available, the examiner must compare ROM values to those of the patient's contralateral extremity or to average adult values available from the American Academy of Orthopedic Surgeons,[32] American Medical Association,[33] and other sources.[22,34,35] If the patient can complete active ROM easily, without pain or other symptoms, then further passive testing of that motion is usually unnecessary.

If, however, the amount of active motion is less than normal the examiner will not be able to isolate the cause without further testing. Capsule, ligament, muscle and soft tissue tightness, joint surface abnormalities, and muscle weakness are all capable of causing limited active ROM. Pain during active ROM may be due to the contracting, stretching, or pinching of contractile tissues such as muscles, tendons, and their attachments to bone; or due to the stretching or pinching of noncontractile tissues such as ligaments, joint capsules, and bursa.[36] Variations in the quality and pattern of active motion can result from central and peripheral nervous system disorders and metabolic conditions, in addition to disorders involving musculoskeletal structures. So, although active motion is an effective screening procedure, positive findings require a variety of additional tests to identify the underlying etiology and thus enable an effective treatment.

PASSIVE RANGE OF MOTION

Passive motions are movements performed by the examiner without the assistance of the patient. The term **passive range of motion (PROM)** typically refers to the amount of osteokinematic motion, the rotary motion of shafts of bone in relationship to each other that occur in the cardinal planes of the body. Normally, passive ROM is slightly greater than active ROM because joints have a small amount of motion at the end of the range that is not under voluntary control. This additional range helps to protect joint structures by allowing the joint to absorb extrinsic forces. Passive ROM is examined not only for amount of motion, but also for the motion's effect on symptoms, end-feel, and pattern of limitation.

Passive range of osteokinematic motions depends on the integrity of joint surfaces and the extensibility of the joint capsule, ligaments, muscles, tendons, and soft tissue. Limitations in passive ROM may be due to bone or joint abnormalities or tightness of these structures. Because the examiner provides the muscle force needed to perform passive ROM, rather than the patient, passive ROM (unlike active ROM) does not depend on the patient's muscle strength and coordination.

Pain during passive ROM is often due to moving, stretching, or pinching noncontractile structures. Pain occurring at the end of passive ROM may be due to stretching contractile structures, as well as noncontractile structures. Pain during passive ROM is not due to the active shortening (contracting) of muscle and the resulting pull on tendon and bone attachments. By comparing which motions (active versus passive) cause pain, and noting the location of the pain, the examiner can begin to determine which injured tissues are involved.

For example, on examination a patient is found to have limited and painful active knee flexion. This pain and limitation may be due to a lesion in the hamstring muscles (including tendons and bone attachments), the quadriceps muscles (including patella tendon and bone attachments), tibiofemoral and patellofemoral joint surfaces, meniscus, joint capsule, collateral and cruciate ligaments, or various anterior and posterior bursa. If the patient had similar pain and limitation during passive ROM, the quadriceps muscles, tibiofemoral and patellofemoral joint surfaces, meniscus, joint capsule, collateral and cruciate ligaments, or various anterior bursa could be involved. The hamstring muscles would not be implicated as these structures are put on slack and relieved of tension during passive knee flexion. Careful consideration of patient history, observation and palpation findings, and the results of additional tests such as end-feel assessment, capsular versus **noncapsular** joint limitation **patterns,** accessory joint motion tests, and ligament stress tests will help to isolate the involved structures. These additional tests are discussed later in this chapter. If, however, passive knee flexion ROM were now normal and painfree as compared to painful during active flexion, a lesion in the hamstring muscles would be likely. The performance of resisted isometric muscle contractions would be used to confirm a lesion in the hamstring muscles.

In the clinical setting, passive ROM is usually measured with universal goniometers (Fig. 5-10) or to a lesser extent with inclinometers, tape measures, and flexible rulers. Visual estimates should not be used because they are less accurate than measurements taken with universal goniometers.[37,38] Both the beginning and the end of the motion are measured and recorded so as to clearly indicate the range of motion. Using the most common notation system, the 0- to 180-degree system, all motions except rotation begin in anatomical position at 0 degrees and progress toward 180 degrees. For example, a motion that begins at 0 degrees and ends at 135 degrees would be recorded as 0 to 135 degrees. A ROM that does not start with 0 degrees or ends prematurely indicates joint **hypomobility.** Joint **hypermobility** at the beginning of the range is noted by the inclusion of a zero (the normal starting position) between the starting and ending measurements. Hypermobility at the end of the ROM is denoted with an excessive ending measurement as compared to normal values. Measurement results are incorporated

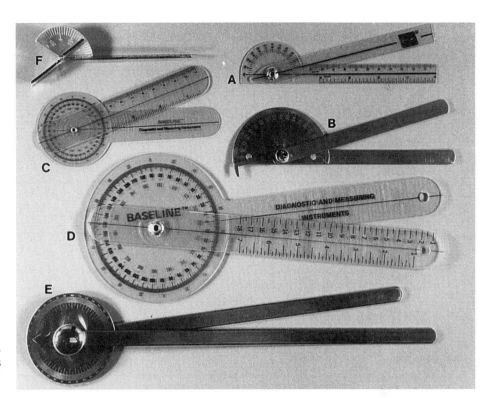

Figure 5-10. A variety of metal and plastic universal gonimeters in different sizes and shapes. (From Norkin and White,[31] p 17, with permission.)

into narrative reports or recorded on specialized forms (Fig. 5-11). Texts such as Norkin and White's *Measurement of Joint Motion*[31] and Clarkson and Gilewich's *Musculoskeletal Assessment*[39] provide detailed descriptions of goniometric measurement procedures.

ROM measurements taken with a universal goniometer of the extremity joints generally have good to excellent reliability. Reliability does vary depending on the joint and motion being measured. ROM measurements of upper extremity joints have been found to be more reliable than measurements of the lower extremity[29,40,41] and spine.[42–44] In an often quoted study, Boone et al.[40] found the average standard deviation between measurements made on the same subjects by different testers to be 4.2 degrees for upper extremity motions and 5.2 degrees for lower extremity motions. These differences in reliability have been attributed to difficulties in measuring complex as compared to simple hinged joints, in palpating bony landmarks, and in moving heavy body parts.[40,45] The use of standardized positions, stabilization of the body part proximal to the joint being tested, bony landmarks to align the goniometer, and the same examiner rather than multiple examiners for repeated testing all help to improve the validity and reliability of goniometric measurements.[29,30,38]

End-feel

The end of each motion at each joint is limited from further movement by particular anatomical structures. The type of structure that limits a joint motion has a characteristic feel, which may be detected by the examiner performing the passive ROM. This feeling, which is experienced by the examiner as resistance, or a barrier to further motion, is called the **end-feel.** Cyriax,[36] Kaltenborn,[46] and Paris[47] have described a variety of normal (physiological) and abnormal (pathological) end-feels. A summary of the types of end-feels has been adapted from the work of these authors.[31] Normal end-feels are generally described as *soft, firm,* or *hard* (Table 5–1). A soft end-feel has a gradual increase in resistance as muscle, skin, and subcutaneous tissues are compressed between body parts.[48] A firm end-feel has a more abrupt increase in resistance as compared to a soft end-feel. Firm end-feels include varying amounts of creep (or give), depending on whether the barrier to the end of the motion is the stretching of muscle, capsule, or ligament tissue. The firm end-feel with the most creep would be the rubbery resistance offered by the stretch of muscle tissue, and the least amount of creep would be provided by the stretch of ligament tissue. The firm end-feel created by the stretch of a joint capsule usually has a moderate amount of creep. A hard end-feel is abrupt; there is an immediate stoppage to movement as when bone contacts bone.

End-feels are considered to be abnormal when they occur sooner or later in the ROM than is typical, or if they are not the type of end-feel that is normally found for that motion and joint. Many pathological end-feels have been described, but most can be categorized as variations of soft, firm, and hard end-feels (Table 5–2). An abnormal end-feel that cannot be categorized as soft, firm, or hard, is an *empty end-feel*. This term describes the inability of the examiner to detect any anatomical barrier to

RANGE OF MOTION RECORD - UPPER EXTREMITY

NAME									
		Left					Right		
				Examiner					
				Date					
				Shoulder					
				Flexion					
				Extension					
				Abduction					
				Medial Rotation					
				Lateral Rotation					
				Comments:					
				Elbow and Forearm					
				Flexion					
				Supination					
				Pronation					
				Comments:					
				Wrist					
				Flexion					
				Extension					
				Ulnar Deviation					
				Radial Deviation					
				Comments:					

Figure 5-11. Range of motion recording form for the upper extremity. (From Norkin and White,[31] p 229, with permission.)

the end of the ROM. Rather, the patient through verbal nor nonverbal cues indicates that no further motion should occur, usually due to pain.

The ability to determine the type of end-feel is important in helping the examiner identify the limiting structures and choose a focused and effective treatment. Developing this ability takes practice and sensitivity. Passive ROM, particularly toward the end of the motion, must be performed slowly and carefully. Secure stabilization of the bone proximal to the joint being tested is critical to prevent multiple joints and structures from moving and interfering with assessment of the end-feel.

Capsular Patterns of Restricted Motion

Cyriax[36] initially described characteristic patterns of restricted joint ROM due to diffuse, intra-articular inflammation involving the entire joint capsule. These patterns of restricted motion, which usually involve multiple motions at a joint, are called

Table 5–1 NORMAL END-FEELS

End-feel	Structure	Example
Soft	Soft tissue approximation	Knee flexion (contact between soft tissue of posterior leg and posterior thigh)
Firm	Muscular stretch	Hip flexion with the knee straight (passive elastic tension of hamstring muscles)
	Capsular stretch	Extension of metacarpophalangeal joints of fingers (tension in the anterior capsule)
	Ligamentous stretch	Forearm supination (tension in the palmar radioulnar ligament of the inferior radioulnar joint, interosseous membrane, oblique cord)
Hard	Bone contacting bone	Elbow extension (contact between the olecranon process of the ulna and the olecranon fossa of the humerus)

From Norkin and White,[31] p 9, with permission.

capsular patterns. The restrictions do not involve the loss of a fixed number of degrees, but rather the loss of a proportion of one motion relative to another. Capsular patterns vary from joint to joint. Table 5–3 presents common capsular patterns as described by Cyriax[36] and Kaltenborn.[46] Although examiners have been using capsular patterns in clinical decision making for many years, studies are needed to test the hypotheses regarding the cause of capsular patterns and to determine the capsular pattern for each joint.[49]

Hertling and Kessler,[1] expanding on Cyriax's work, have suggested that capsular patterns are due to one of two general situations: (1) joint effusion or

Table 5–2 ABNORMAL END-FEELS

End-feel		Examples
Soft	Occurs sooner or later in the ROM than is usual, or in a joint that normally has a firm or hard end-feel. Feels boggy.	Soft tissue edema Synovitis
Firm	Occurs sooner or later in the ROM than is usual, or in a joint that normally has a soft or hard end-feel.	Increased muscular tonus Capsular, muscular, ligamentous shortening
Hard	Occurs sooner or later in the ROM than is usual, or in a joint that normally has a soft or firm end-feel. A bony grating or bony block is felt.	Chondromalacia Osteoarthritis Loose bodies in joint Myositis ossificans Fracture
Empty	No real end-feel because pain prevents reaching end of ROM. No resistance is felt except for patient's protective muscle splinting or muscle spasm.	Acute joint inflammation Bursitis Abscess Fracture Psychogenic disorder

From Norkin and White,[31] p 9, with permission.

Table 5–3 CAPSULAR PATTERNS OF EXTREMITY JOINTS

Shoulder (glenohumeral joint)	Maximum loss of external rotation Moderate loss of abduction Minimum loss of internal rotation
Elbow complex	Flexion loss is greater than extension loss
Forearm	Full and painless Equally restricted in pronation and supination in presence of elbow restrictions
Wrist	Equal restrictions in flexion and extension
Hand	
Carpometacarpal joint I	Abduction and extension restriction
Carpometacarpal joints II–V	Equally restricted in all directions
Upper extremity digits	Flexion loss is greater than extension loss
Hip	Maximum loss of internal rotation, flexion, abduction Minimal loss of extension
Knee (tibiofemoral joint)	Flexion loss is greater than extension loss
Ankle (talocrural joint)	Plantarflexion loss is greater than extension loss
Subtalar joint	Restricted varus motion
Midtarsal joint	Restricted dorsiflexion, plantarflexion, abduction, and medial rotation
Lower extremity digits	
Metatarsalphalangeal joint I	Extension loss is greater than flexion
Metatarsalphalangeal joints II–V	Variable, tend toward flexion restriction
Interphalangeal joints	Tend toward extension restriction

From Dyrek,[8] p 72, with permission. Capsular patterns are from Cyriax[36] and Kaltenborn.[46]

synovial inflammation, and (2) relative capsular fibrosis. Joint effusion or synovial inflammation cause a capsular pattern of limitation by distending the entire joint capsule, causing the joint to maintain a position that allows the greatest intra-articular volume. Pain triggered by stretching the capsule, and muscle spasms that protect the capsule from further stretch, inhibit movement and cause a capsular pattern of restricted motion. The other general situation that causes capsular patterns is relative capsular fibrosis, seen in the resolution of acute capsular inflammation, chronic low-grade capsular inflammation, and immobilization of a joint. These conditions cause a decrease in the extensibility of the entire capsule from an increase in collagen content of the capsule relative to the mucopolysaccharide content, or from internal changes in the collagen tissue.

To plan an effective treatment, the examiner must determine whether the capsular pattern is caused by joint effusion/synovial inflammation or capsular fibrosis. If joint effusion or synovial inflammation is present, treatment methods need to focus on resolving the acute inflammation typically with rest, cold modalities, compression, elevation and joint mobilization using grade 1 sustained and grade 1 and 2 oscillations, gentle ROM exercise, and anti-inflammatory medications. Capsular fibrosis, a more chronic condition, will usually benefit from heat modalities, joint mobilization using grade 3 sustained stretch and grade 3 and 4 oscillations, passive stretching procedures, and more vigorous ROM exercises. Patient history, observation, palpation, and careful assessment of end-feels will help determine the cause of the capsular pattern.

Noncapsular Patterns of Restricted Motion

Restricted passive ROM that is not proportioned similarly to a capsular pattern is called a **noncapsular pattern** of restricted motion.[1,36] Noncapsular patterns usually involve only one or two motions of a joint, in contrast to capsular patterns, which involve all or most motions of a joint. Noncapsular patterns are caused by conditions involving structures other than the entire joint capsule. Internal joint derangement, adhesion of a part of a joint capsule, and extracapsular lesions such as ligament shortening, muscle strain, and muscle shortening are examples of conditions that can result in noncapsular patterns. For instance, shortening of the iliopsoas muscle will result in the noncapsular pattern of limited passive hip extension; the passive range of other hip motions will not be affected. This is in contrast to the capsular pattern of the hip caused by diffuse joint effusion or capsular fibrosis, in which there is loss of passive internal rotation, flexion, and abduction.

The sole recognition of a noncapsular pattern is not enough to direct appropriate treatment. Information gained from the patient history, observation, palpation, active and passive ROM, end-feels, resisted isometric muscle tests, joint mobility tests, and special tests must be integrated to determine the most likely cause of the noncapsular pattern. For example, both chronic shortening and acute strain of the iliopsoas muscle may result in a noncapsular pattern of limited passive hip extension. However, they will present differently in terms of patient history, pain during active and passive ROM, end-feel, and resisted isometric muscle tests, and will require different treatment approaches.

Accessory Joint Motions

If passive ROM is found to be limited or painful, a musculoskeletal examination will also need to include an assessment of arthrokinematic motions. **Arthrokinematics** refers to the motion of joint surfaces. These motions, usually called **accessory** or **joint play motions,** are used to assess joint mobility and integrity. MacConaill and Basmajian[50] describe accessory joint motions as slides (or glides), spins, and rolls. A **slide (glide)** is a translatory motion of one surface sliding over another. A **roll** is a rotary motion similar to the bottom of a rocking chair rolling over the floor. A **spin** is a rotary motion around a fixed point or axis.

Accessory motions usually occur in combination with each other and result in angular movement of the bone shaft, or osteokinematic motion. Kaltenborn[46] refers to the combination of translatory glide and the rotary motion of rolling as **roll-gliding.** The combination of a roll and glide allows for increased ROM by postponing the joint compression and separation that would occur at either side of the joint during a pure rolling motion. The direction of the rolling and gliding components of roll-gliding depends on whether a concave or convex joint surface is moving. If a concave joint surface is moving, the gliding component occurs in the same direction as the rolling or angular movement of the shaft of the bone (Fig. 5-12). For example, during flexion of the knee, the shaft of the tibia moves dorsally while the joint surface of the tibia also moves dorsally. If, instead, a convex joint surface is moving, the gliding component occurs in the direction opposite to the rolling or angular movement of the shaft of the bone. As an example, during abduction of the glenohumeral joint, the shaft of the humerus moves cranially, while the joint surface of the humerus moves caudally. In the human body, roll-gliding is by far the most frequently occurring arthrokinematic motion, although there are several instances of pure spin motions. An example of a spin joint motion would be supination and pronation of the radius at the humeroradial joint.

Normal arthrokinematic (accessory) motions are necessary for full and symptom-free osteokinematic motions. The careful examination of accessory motions helps to more specifically locate and treat the source of impaired osteokinematic motions. Assessory motions cannot be performed actively by the patient because these motions are not under voluntary control. Rather, they are tested passively by the examiner. The accessory motions most commonly tested are translatory motions: glides that are paral-

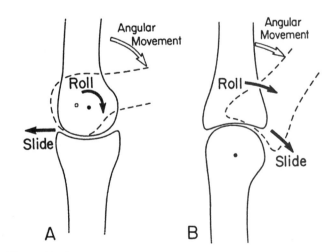

Figure 5-12. Diagrammatic representation of the concave-convex rule. (*A*) If the joint surface of the moving bone is convex, sliding is in the opposite direction of the angular movement of the bone. (*B*) If the joint surface of the moving bone is concave, sliding is in the same direction as the angular movement of the bone. (From Kisner and Colby,[51] p 187, with permission.)

lel to the joint surfaces, and **distractions** and **compressions** that are perpendicular to the joint surfaces. Texts by Kaltenborn,[46] Kisner and Colby,[51] and Hertling and Kessler[1] describe specific testing and treatment techniques that focus on accessory motions—usually under the topic of **joint mobilization.** Careful attention must be given to general patient positioning, specific joint positioning, relaxation of surrounding muscles, stabilization of one joint surface, and mobilization of the other joint surface.

Accessory joint motions are examined for amount of motion, effect on symptoms, and end-feel. The ranges of accessory motions are very small and cannot be measured with goniometers or standard rulers. Rather, they are typically compared to the same motion on the contralateral side of the patient's body, or compared to the examiner's past experience in testing people of similar age and gender as the patient. Accessory motions are assigned a joint play mobility grade of 0 to 6 (Table 5–4).[46] These mobility grades have implications for treatment[1,52]:

- Grades 0 and 6: Joint mobilization is not indicated. Surgery should be considered.
- Grades 1 and 2: Joint mobilization to increase the extensibility of joint structures is indicated. Heat modalities prior to mobilization and ROM exercises after mobilization should be considered.
- Grades 4 and 5: Joint mobilization to increase joint extensibility is not indicated. Taping, bracing, strengthening exercises, and education regarding posture, and positions to be avoided, should be considered.

The testing of accessory motions puts stress on specific anatomical structures. A change in symptoms during the performance of an accessory motion helps to implicate particular structures. Distraction stresses the entire joint capsule and numerous ligaments surrounding and supporting the joint. Glides more specifically stress a part of the joint capsule and particular ligaments, depending on the direction of the glide and joint. Compression applies force to intracapsular structures such as meniscus, bone, cartilage, and projections of the synovial lining of the joint capsule into the joint space. Accessory motions are of such a small magnitude that they do not stress surrounding muscles. Angular changes in joint position that typically occur during osteokinematic ROM movements more effectively change the length of muscle tissue.

Normal and abnormal end-feels noted during passive accessory motions are characterized as soft, firm, and hard. Similar to end-feels noted during passive osteokinematic motions, they help to determine the limiting structures and appropriate treatment.

Muscle Performance

Muscle performance is the ability of a muscle to do work.[53] **Linear work** is defined as force multiplied by distance, while **rotational work** is defined as torque (force multiplied by perpendicular distance from the axis of rotation) by arc of movement. Usually during a musculoskeletal assessment, a component of muscle performance—muscle strength—is tested. **Muscle strength,** as described in the *Guide to Physical Therapy Practice,*[53] is the force exerted by a muscle or group of muscles to overcome a resistance in one maximal effort. Clinical methods of assessing muscle strength include manual muscle testing, hand-held dynamometry, and isokinetic dynamometry. Depending on the patient, other characteristics related to muscle performance may also be tested. **Muscle power** is work produced per unit of time, or the product of strength and speed. **Muscle endurance** is the ability of the muscle to contract repeatedly over time. In addition to these quantitative measures, the patient's qualitative response in terms of changes in pain during resisted isometric testing is important in identifying musculotendinous lesions.

RESISTED ISOMETRIC TESTING

During the performance of active and passive ROM testing a patient may complain of pain. The patient history, location of pain, and the pattern of painful motions may suggest a lesion in contractile tissues such as muscle, tendons and their insertions into bone, or involvement of inert tissues such as the joint surfaces, joint capsule, or ligaments. Resisted isometric testing can be used to further clarify which type of tissue, contractile or inert, is involved. *Increased pain* during a resisted isometric contraction, caused by shortening of the muscle and pulling on the tendon, helps to confirm the involvement of contractile tissues. Sometimes more pain is felt when the contraction is released and lengthening occurs; this would still be considered a positive finding for a lesion in contractile tissues. The *lack of pain* during resisted isometric testing, pain noted with limited accessory joint motions, a capsular pattern of joint restriction, or particular end-feels during passive ROM and accessory joint motions help to confirm the involvement of inert tissues. For example, bicipital tendinitis would be painful during resisted isometric testing of elbow flexion and shoulder flexion. An adhesive capsulitis of the glenohumeral joint would be painless during these same maneuvers.

Table 5–4 ACCESSORY JOINT MOTION GRADES

Grade	Joint Status
0	Ankylosed
1	Considerable hypomobility
2	Slight hypomobility
3	Normal
4	Slight hypermobility
5	Considerable hypermobility
6	Unstable

Adapted from Wadsworth, CT: Manual Examination and Treatment of the Spine and Extremities. Williams & Wilkins, Baltimore, 1988, p 13, with permission.

Resisted isometric testing must be performed carefully to stress particular contractile tissue while avoiding stress to surrounding inert tissue. The examiner should place the patient's joint in a position midway through the ROM, so that minimal tension is put on inert structures. The body part proximal to the joint being tested must be well stabilized by the examiner to allow the patient to relax and avoid extraneous muscle substitutions. Then the patient is asked to hold this position while the examiner gradually applies resistance. Joint movement is strictly avoided. Although some compression of articular surfaces will occur during the isometric contraction, this does not usually present a problem in interpreting the results. However, a bursa located deep to the musculotendinous tissue will also be compressed. Although bursae are not considered to be connective tissue, pain will be felt during the isometric contraction if the bursa is inflamed. Fortunately, treatment for a bursitis is similar to treatment for musculotendinous strains and inflammation.

In addition to determining the absence or presence of pain during the resisted isometric testing, the examiner should also note the strength of the muscle contraction. If weakness is found, more extensive testing of muscle strength should be performed utilizing manual muscle testing or dynamometers. Muscle weakness may be due to many causes, including pathologies involving upper motor neurons, peripheral nerves, neuromuscular junctions, muscles, and tendons. Pain, fatigue, and disuse atrophy can also cause weakness. The pattern of muscle weakness will help to identify the site of the pathology and direct treatment. The patient history and the results of sensory, coordination, motor control, cardiopulmonary, and electromyography testing will also clarify findings.

Cyriax[36] and others[1,2] have suggested using the results of resisted isometric testing to determine the type of pathology. The strength of the muscle contraction as well as its effect on pain are used to categorize the findings (Table 5–5). A study by Franklin et al[54] indicates that the conditions related to the finding of "weak and painful" need to be expanded to include not only serious pathologies, but relatively minor muscle damage such as that induced by eccentric isokinetic exercise.

MANUAL MUSCLE TESTING

Manual muscle testing (MMT) was developed by Wright and Lovett in 1912[55,56] as a means of testing and grading muscle strength based on gravity and manually applied resistance. Others have described various MMT methods,[57–59] but the two methods most frequently used in the United States are those presented by Daniels and Worthingham,[60] and Kendall et al.[61] Both methods, based on the work by Wright and Lovett, use arc of motion, gravity, and manually applied resistance by the examiner to test and determine muscle grades. Generally, the patient is positioned so that the muscle or muscle group

Table 5–5 RESULTS OF RESISTED ISOMETRIC TESTING

Findings	Possible Pathologies
Strong and painless	There is no lesion or neurological deficit involving the tested muscle and tendon.
Strong and painful	There is a minor lesion of the tested muscle or tendon.
Weak and painless	There is a disorder of the nervous system, neuromuscular junction, or a complete rupture of the tested muscle or tendon, or disuse atrophy.
Weak and painful	There is a serious, painful pathology such as a fracture or neoplasm. Other possibilities include an acute inflammatory process that inhibits muscle contraction, or a partial rupture of the tested muscle or tendon.

being tested has to hold or move against the resistance of gravity. If this is well tolerated, the examiner applies manual resistance gradually to the distal end of the body part in which the muscle inserts, and in a direction opposite to the torque produced by the muscle(s) being tested. In recent editions, both methods recommend applying manual resistance in the form of a **break test** in which the patient holds a joint position until the examiner gradually overpowers the patient and an eccentric contraction begins to occur. Both methods suggest that the break test occur at the end of the range of motion when testing one-joint muscles, and at mid-range when testing two-joint muscles. In the case of weaker muscles that cannot hold or move well against gravity, the patient is repositioned and attempts to move the body part through a gravity-minimized (horizontal) plane of motion. During all testing, stabilization of the body part on which the muscle originates and careful avoidance of substitution by other muscle groups are emphasized. Results can be noted in a narrative report or on standardized recording forms (Fig. 5–13).

Although there are many similarities, there are some differences between these two popular MMT methods. Kendall et al.[61] propose to examine individual muscles insofar as practical, whereas Daniels and Worthingham[60] examine muscle groups that perform particular joint motions. Some testing positions are similar but others vary between the two methods, with Daniels and Worthingham providing more instruction and emphasis on gravity-minimized positioning for weaker muscle groups. Daniels and Worthingham recommend that the patient move through the arc of motion when testing both against gravity or with gravity minimized. Kendall et al. have the patient move through an arc of motion only when testing with gravity minimized; otherwise the patient is positioned against gravity and asked to hold the position. Both methods use a grading system based on the work of Lovett with categories of Normal, Good, Fair, Poor, Trace, and Zero. However, Kendall et al. suggest a 0 to 100 percent or a 0 to 10 scale; Daniels and

DOCUMENTATION OF MUSCLE EXAMINATION

LEFT				RIGHT		
3	2	1	Date of Examination Examiner's Name	1	2	3
			NECK			
			Capital extension			
			Cervical extension			
			Combined extension (capital plus cervical)			
			Capital flexion			
			Cervical flexion			
			Combined flexion (capital plus cervical)			
			Combined flexion and rotation (Sternocleidomastoid)			
			Cervical rotation			
			TRUNK			
			Extension—Lumbar			
			Extension—Thoracic			
			Pelvic elevation			
			Flexion			
			Rotation			
			Diaphragm strength			
			Maximal inspiration less full expiration (indirect intercostal test) (inches)			
			Cough (indirect forced expiration) (F, WF, NF, O)			
			UPPER EXTREMITY			
			Scapular abduction and upward rotation			
			Scapular elevation			
			Scapular adduction			
			Scapular adduction and downward rotation			
			Shoulder flexion			
			Shoulder extension			
			Shoulder scaption			
			Shoulder abduction			
			Shoulder horizontal abduction			
			Shoulder horizontal adduction			
			Shoulder external rotation			
			Shoulder internal rotation			
			Elbow flexion			
			Elbow extension			
			Forearm supination			
			Forearm pronation			
			Wrist flexion			
			Wrist extension			
			Finger metacarpophalangeal flexion			
			Finger proximal interphalangeal flexion			
			Finger distal interphalangeal flexion			
			Finger metacarpophalangeal extension			
			Finger abduction			
			Finger adduction			
			Thumb metacarpophalangeal flexion			
			Thumb interphalangeal flexion			

*After Hislop and Montgomery

Figure 5-13. An example of a manual muscle testing recording form. (From Hislop and Montgomery,[60] p 7, with permission.)

Worthingham suggest a 0 to 5 scale (Table 5–6). If numerical scoring is used, it is important to clarify which scale is being used by noting the score followed by a slash indicating the maximal value of the scale. For example, a grade of Fair strength should be noted as $^5/_{10}$ if using a 0 to 10 scale, or $^3/_5$ if using a 0 to 5 scale. Clinicians should also remember that these numerical scales indicate ordinal data only the intervals between the numbers do not represent equal units of measure. Sharrard,[62] counting alpha motor neurons in spinal cords of individuals with poliomyelitis at the time of autopsy, found that muscles previously receiving a grade of Good had 50 percent of their innervated motor neurons, while muscles assessed as Fair had only 15 percent of their motor neurons. Beasley[63] noted that patients with poliomyelitis were graded as having Good, Fair, and Poor knee extension when they had on average only 43, 9, and 3 percent of the knee extension force of normal subjects, respectively.

The results of studies on intertester reliability of MMT vary widely, but some generalizations can be noted. Studies[64–67] report complete agreement between testers who examine the same patient to be low, ranging from 28 to 75 percent. Agreement between testers within plus or minus half a grade is better, ranging from 50 to 97 percent. Agreement between testers within plus or minus one full grade is high, ranging from 89 to 100 percent. Standardization of testing positions, stabilization, and grading criteria resulted in higher agreement between testers. Similar to many testing procedures, intratester reliability was found to be slightly higher than intertester reliability.

To improve reliability, grading definitions modified from Daniels and Worthingham,[60] Kendall et al.,[61] and Hines[68] are presented with specific criteria in Table 5–6. Although grades Zero through Fair are based on objective criteria, grade Fair+ through Normal depend on the examiner's subjective opinion of what is minimal, moderate, and maximal resistance. A Normal grade is typically equated with the average strength for that muscle given the patient's age, gender, and body size. It should be kept in mind that there is considerable variability in the amount of resistance normal muscles can take; that is, large muscles in the lower extremity will normally take considerably more resistance than small muscles of the hand. The application of resistance throughout the arc of motion (**make test** or **active resistance test**) in addition to resistance at only one point in the arc of motion (break test) may help in judging a muscle's strength. Although more costly and time consuming than MMT, hand-held or isokinetic dynamometers can be used to improve objectivity and sensitivity when needed.

HAND-HELD DYNAMOMETRY

Hand-held dynamometers are portable devices, placed between the examiner's hand and the patient's body, that measure mechanical force. Patients are typically asked to push against the examiner in a maximal isometric contraction (make test), or hold a position until the examiner overpowers the muscle producing an eccentric contraction (break test). The force measured by the dynamometer will vary depending on the method of applying the resistance, the patient's body position in relationship to gravity, joint angle, dynamometer placement on the patient (lever arm), stabilization, and the examiner's strength.[69,70] Normative values for particular muscle groups by patient age and gender have been established, but clinicians must be careful to replicate the study's methods to ensure appropriate comparisons.[71–74] Many authors report testing most muscle groups in supine, except for knee flexors and extensors, which were tested in sitting. In both positions, a gravity-neutral position in mid-range of motion was usually used, with the dynamometer held perpendicular to the tested limb segment. For patients with unilateral conditions, it may be helpful to compare results to the uninvolved extremity. Andrews et al.[71] found no statistically significant difference between the dominant and nondominant lower extremities using a hand-held dynamometer, but did find a difference between the dominant and

Table 5–6 MANUAL MUSCLE TESTING GRADES

Grades				Criteria
Normal	N	5	10	Full available ROM, against gravity, strong manual resistance
Good Plus	G+	5–	9	Full available ROM, against gravity, nearly strong manual resistance
Good	G	4	8	Full available ROM, against gravity, moderate manual resistance
Good Minus	G–	4–	7	Full available ROM, against gravity, nearly moderate manual resistance
Fair Plus	F+	3+	6	Full available ROM, against gravity, slight manual resistance
Fair	F	3	5	Full available ROM, against gravity, no resistance
Fair Minus	F–	3–	4	At least 50% of ROM, against gravity, no resistance
Poor Plus	P+	2+	3	Full available ROM, gravity minimized, slight manual resistance
Poor	P	2	2	Full available ROM, gravity minimized, no resistance
Poor Minus	P–	2–	1	At least 50% of ROM, gravity minimized, no resistance
Trace Plus	T+	1+		Minimal observable motion (less than 50% ROM), gravity minimized, no resistance
Trace	T	1	T	No observable motion, palpable muscle contraction, no resistance
Zero	0	0	0	No observable or palpable muscle contraction

nondominant upper extremities. In general, differences were between 0 and 4.5 pounds or between 0 and 11.2 percent of the average forces generated.

Depending on the study, hand-held dynamometers have demonstrated good to excellent intratester reliability, and poor to excellent intertester reliability.[71,75-80] Reliability seems to be better when testing the upper extremities than when testing the lower extremities and trunk.[75,80] Agree et al.[75] found the standard deviation of the repeated measurements expressed as a percent of the mean force measurements (coefficient of variation of replication) to be 5.1 to 8.3 percent for the upper extremity muscle groups, and 11.3 to 17.8 percent for the lower extremity muscle groups. Researchers believe some of the error in using hand-held dynamometers is due to off-center loading of the dynamometer, difficulties in positioning and stabilization, and limitations in the strength and experience of the examiners.[70,75]

ISOKINETIC DYNAMOMETRY

Isokinetic dynamometers are stationary, electromechanical devices that control the velocity of a moving body segment by resisting the patient's effort so that the body segment cannot accelerate beyond the preset angular velocity. For example, the velocity of a Cybex II Isokinetic Dynamometer can be set from 0 to 300 degrees per second, and the resistance, measured in the form of **torque,** can be monitored from 0 to 448 newton meters.[81] Speeds of 60, 120, and 180 degrees per second are commonly tested in relatively sedentary patients, and faster speeds may be warranted in athletes. Isokinetic dynamometers can be used to measure the torque produced during isometric contractions (if the velocity is set to 0 degrees per second), concentric contractions, and in some models eccentric contractions. Isokinetic dynamometers, although expensive and cumbersome, are especially helpful in examining the performance of large, relatively strong muscle groups. In such situations manual muscle testing and hand-held dynamometers are often insensitive to muscle performance abnormalities.[63,70] Muscle groups acting at the knee, back, and to a lesser extent the elbow and shoulder are the ones most frequently tested with isokinetic devices.

Isokinetic dynamometers measure torque and ROM as a function of time. Muscle performance characteristics most often noted are peak (maximal) torque, and less frequently peak torque/body weight (nm/Kg), and average torque. Work measurements can be derived from the angular displacement and torque values. Power, which is work per unit time, can be determined. Endurance (muscle fatigue) can also be measured. One common method of measuring endurance is to note the time required for peak torque to drop by a certain percentage (e.g., 50 percent). Peak torque ratios of reciprocal (agonist-antagonist) muscle groups such as the hamstrings/quadriceps and external/internal rotators of the shoulder have been noted. However, careful corrections for the weight of the limb (gravity effects) are necessary to arrive at an accurate relationship.[82-84] If gravity corrections are not utilized, the muscles assisted by gravity will exhibit erroneously higher torque values, whereas the muscles that resist gravity will exhibit erroneously lower torque values.

It has been suggested that submaximal patient effort can be detected by the increased variability of repeated measures of peak torque, average torque, and slope to peak torque in isometric and concentric contractions.[85-87] However, research in this area has produced conflicting findings and demonstrated large errors in classifying effort into maximal and submaximal categories.[83,88-90] Many factors such as patient pain, fear, fatigue, damp settings, preload forces, mechanical artifact, and acceleration and deceleration rampings can affect the variability of torque measurements. The use of isokinetic dynamometer records to form clinical opinions of patient effort is not advised until further research is conducted.

To ensure the validity of isokinetic dynamometry measurements, calibration of the equipment is necessary and should be performed each day of testing, at the same speed and damp setting to be used during testing.[83] Proper alignment of joint axis and machine axis, stabilization of proximal body parts, and gravity correction are needed. Several practice trials of the motion to acquaint the patient with the equipment and testing protocol is helpful, and at least three maximal test repetitions should be performed to establish stable measurements.[91] Examiners should realize that torque values will vary with changes in velocity settings, type of muscle contractions (isometric, concentric, eccentric), joint angle, patient position, lever arm length, test trials, rest intervals, patient feedback, and preload, damp, and ramping machine settings. These factors must be kept constant in order to use repeat testing to judge patient progress. Keating and Matyas,[92] Rothstein,[83] and Davies[93] have presented excellent reviews of factors to improve the validity and reliability of isokinetic testing. Peak torque and work measurements have shown good to excellent reliability for concentric contractions, and poor to good reliability for eccentric contractions.[91,94-98] Reciprocal (agonist-antagonist) ratios have shown less reliability than peak torque measurements.[99]

Normative data, when available, can provide a reference for evaluating and interpreting patient data.[100-108] However, comparisons with published data are appropriate only when identical procedures are used and tested populations are similar. Patient age, weight, gender, and athletic participation can affect values.[92] Out of necessity, the involved extremity is often compared to the contralateral extremity. Studies have found no statistically significant difference between dominant and nondominant sides in torque measurements for muscles surrounding the knee joint,[109-111] whereas differences have been found for muscles surrounding the shoulder joint.[112,113] A difference of at least 10 percent in torque values between opposing sides of the body has been suggested as an indicator of impairment.[114,115] However, others have noted frequent findings of imbalances of more than 10 percent in healthy populations[104,109] and 10 percent differences in repeated measurements.[96] Further research is needed to establish the magnitude of difference between opposite limbs that indicates impairment.[92]

Special Tests

After completing the patient interview, observation, palpation, and assessment of ROM, accessory motions, and muscle performance, the examiner may suspect the nature of the pathology. Special tests, designed to focus on specific conditions in a particular region of the body, may be helpful in confirming the diagnosis. An examiner would ordinarily choose to perform only those tests indicated by previous findings and relevant to the area of the body being examined. False positive and false negative results are possible. However, a positive test finding in conjunction with other aspects of the examination would be highly suggestive of the pathology. There are many special tests discussed in texts by Hoppenfeld,[34] Caillet,[116] and Magee.[2]

One category of special tests assesses the integrity of ligaments in supporting a joint. These *ligamentous instability tests,* also called ligament stress tests, are performed by the examiner on a relaxed, passive patient. These maneuvers are often similar to accessory joint motion tests. Results should be compared with those from the uninvolved, contralateral joint. The amount of laxity is usually graded from I to IV (Table 5–7).[117] Although these tests focus on ligament integrity, capsular integrity as well as dynamic muscle support may influence the results. Examples of ligamentous instability tests include the Lachman test, posterior draw test, and varus and valgus stress tests at the knee. In addition to ligament instability tests, there are more general tests that assess joint subluxation and dislocation. These tests are often called **apprehension tests** because the patient is placed in a vulnerable joint position while monitored for apprehension.

The length of muscles that cross and act at one joint are usually assessed in the process of testing passive ROM. However, some muscles cross and act at two or more joints. Some special tests examine the length of these muscles. The Thomas Test,[61] which assesses the length of one and two joint hip flexors; the Ober test,[61] which focuses on the length of the tensor fascia lata; and the Bunnel-Littler

test,[34] which assesses the role of the lumbricales, interossei, extensor digitorum, and joint capsule in limited flexion of the proximal interphalangeal joints of the hand, are examples of special muscle length tests.

Numerous special tests assess for common conditions affecting the integrity of muscle and tendon structures. These tests typically stretch or contract the inflamed or injured muscle, resulting in pain if the tests are positive. For example, the Finkelstein Test[34] assesses inflammation of the tendons of the abductor pollicis longus and extensor pollicis brevis by stretching these structures. The tennis elbow test[34] has the patient isometrically contract the extensor carpi radialis muscles against manual resistance. Often the examiner will have previously noted pain, limitation, and possibly weakness during ROM and muscle performance; special tests are used to clarify these earlier findings.

Another category of special tests reproduces the symptoms caused by compression of peripheral nerves or diminished blood flow. For example, the test for carpal tunnel syndrome places the wrist in full flexion for 60 to 90 seconds to reproduce the numbness and tingling caused by compression of the median nerve by the transverse carpal.[116] Homan's sign utilizes ankle dorsiflexion, knee extension, and deep palpation to elicit calf pain caused by deep vein thrombophlebitis.[34]

Additional Testing

Depending on assessment findings, other procedures may be indicated. Many of these additional assessment procedures are discussed in detail in other chapters of this book. For example, patient complaints of paresthesia or difficulty in muscle performance often indicate neurological involvement that calls for testing of superficial and proprioceptive sensations (see Chapter 6: Sensory Assessment), reflexes and motor tone (see Chapter 8: Motor Control Assessment), coordination (see Chapter 7: Coordination Assessment), or nerve conduction velocity (see Chapter 9: Electromyography and Nerve Conduction Velocity Tests). These tests, in conjunction with muscle performance results, help to identify conditions affecting peripheral nerves, spinal nerve roots, and the central nervous system. Examiners must distinguish peripheral nerve versus nerve root patterns of sensory and motor innervation. References on manual muscles testing, such as those by Kendall,[61] and Hislop and Montgomery[60] provide extensive information on innervation patterns. Figure 5-14 presents muscle testing recording forms that are helpful in recognizing impaired innervation patterns. Myotomes and deep tendon reflexes that are often assessed as part of a musculoskeletal assessment are shown in Tables 5–8 and 5–9. Upper motor neuron lesions usually result in hyperreflexia, whereas lower motor neuron lesions involving the spinal nerve root or peripheral nerves usually cause hyporeflexia when testing deep tendon reflexes.

Table 5–7 GRADING OF LIGAMENTOUS INSTABILITY TESTS

Grades	Amount of Movement
I	0–5 mm
II	6–10 mm
III	11–15 mm
IV	>15 mm

SPINAL NERVE AND MUSCLE CHART
NECK, DIAPHRAGM AND UPPER EXTREMITY

Name _____   Date _____

KEY →
- D. = Dorsal Prim. Ramus
- V. = Vent. Prim. Ramus
- P.R. = Plexus Root
- S.T. = Superior Trunk
- P. = Posterior Cord
- L. = Lateral Cord
- M. = Medial Cord

	MUSCLE	Cervical (T.)	Cervical (V.)	Cervical (V.)	Phrenic (V.)	Long. Thor. (P.R.)	Dor. Scap (P.R.)	N. to Subcl. (S.T.)	Suprascap (S.T.)	U. Subscap. (P.)	Thoracodor (P.)	L. Subscap. (P.)	Lat. Pect. (L.)	Med. Pect. (M.)	Axillary (P.)	Musculocu. (L.)	Radial (P.)	Median (L.M.)	Ulnar (M.)	C1	C2	C3	C4	C5	C6	C7	C8	T1
		1-8	1-8	1-4	3,4,5	5,6,7,(8)	4,5	5,6	4,5,6	(4),5,6,(7)	(5),6,7,8	5,6,(7)	5,6,7	(6),7,8	5,6	(4),5,6,7	5,6,7,8	5,6,7,8	7,8									
	HEAD & NECK EXTENSORS	●																		1	2	3	4	5	6	7	8	1
Cervical nerves	INFRAHYOID MUSCLES		●																	1	2	3						
	RECTUS CAP ANT. & LAT.		●																	1	2							
	LONGUS CAPITIS		●																	1	2	3	(4)					
	LONGUS COLLI	●																			2	3	4	5	6	(7)		
	LEVATOR SCAPULAE		●		●																	3	4	5					
	SCALENI (A. M. P.)	●																				3	4	5	6	7	8	
	STERNOCLEIDOMASTOID		●																	(1)	2	3						
	TRAPEZIUS (U. M. L.)		●																		2	3	4					
	DIAPHRAGM			●																		3	4	5				
Brachial Plexus — Root	SERRATUS ANTERIOR					●																		5	6	7	8	
	RHOMBOIDS MAJ & MIN						●																	4	5			
Trunk	SUBCLAVIUS							●																5	6			
	SUPRASPINATUS								●															4	5	6		
	INFRASPINATUS								●															(4)	5	6		
P Cord	SUBSCAPULARIS									●		●													5	6	7	
	LATISSIMUS DORSI										●														6	7	8	
L	TERES MAJOR											●													5	6	7	
M&L	PECTORALIS MAJ (UPPER)												●												6	7	8	1
	PECTORALIS MAJ (LOWER)												●	●											(6)	7	8	1
	PECTORALIS MINOR													●											6	7	8	1
Axil.	TERES MINOR														●										5	6		
	DELTOID														●										5	6		
Musculo-cutan.	CORACOBRACHIALIS															●										6	7	
	BICEPS															●									5	6		
	BRACHIALIS															●									5	6		
Radial	TRICEPS																●									6	7	8	1
	ANCONEUS																●										7	8	
Lat. M	BRACHIALIS (SMALL PART)																●								5	6		
	BRACHIORADIALIS																●								5	6		
	EXT CARPI RAD L																●								5	6	7	8
	EXT CARPI RAD B																●									6	7	(8)
	SUPINATOR																●								5	6	(7)	
Post Inter	EXT DIGITORUM																●									6	7	8
	EXT DIGITI MINIMI																●									6	7	8
	EXT CARPI ULNARIS																●									6	7	8
	ABD POLLICIS LONGUS																●									6	7	8
	EXT POLLICIS BREVIS																●									6	7	8
	EXT POLLICIS LONGUS																●									6	7	8
	EXT INDICIS																●										6	7	8
Median	PRONATOR TERES																	●								6	7	8
	FLEX CARPI RADIALIS																	●								(6)	7	8	1
	PALMARIS LONGUS																	●									7	8	1
	FLEX DIGIT SUPERFICIALIS																	●									7	8	1
A Inter	FLEX DIGIT PROF I & II																	●								(6)	7	8	1
	FLEX POLLICIS LONGUS																	●								(6)	7	8	1
	PRONATOR QUADRATUS																	●									6	7	8	1
	ABD POLLICIS BREVIS																	●									6	7	8	1
	OPPONENS POLLICIS																	●									6	7	8	1
	FLEX POLL BREV (SUP. H)																	●								(6)	7	8	1
	LUMBRICALES I & II																	●										7	8	1
Ulnar	FLEX CARPI ULNARIS																		●								7	8	1
	FLEX DIGIT. PROF. III & IV																		●								(7)	8	1
	PALMARIS BREVIS																		●								(7)	8	1
	ABD DIGITI MINIMI																		●								(7)	8	1
	OPPONENS DIGITI MINIMI																		●								(7)	8	1
	FLEX DIGITI MINIMI																		●								(7)	8	1
	PALMAR INTEROSSEI																		●									8	1
	DORSAL INTEROSSEI																		●									8	1
	LUMBRICALES III & IV																		●								(7)	8	1
	ADDUCTOR POLLICIS																		●									8	1
	FLEX POLL BREV. (DEEP H.)																		●									8	1

SENSORY

Dermatomes redrawn from Keegan and Garrett Anat Rec 102. 409. 437. 1948
Cutaneous Distribution of peripheral nerves redrawn from Gray's Anatomy of the Human Body. 28th ed

Figure 5-14. A manual muscle testing recording form that aids in determining the site or level of a nerve lesion. (From Kendall, McCreary, and Provance,[61] p 393, with permission.)

Table 5–8 MYOTOMES

Upper Quarter Myotomes		
Level	**Action to Be Tested**	**Muscle**
C5	Shoulder abduction	Deltoid
C5, C6	Elbow flexion	Biceps
C7	Elbow extension	Triceps
C8	Ulnar deviation	Flexor carpi ulnaris
		Extensor carpi ulnaris
T1	Digit abduction/adduction	Interossei

Lower Quarter Myotomes		
Level	**Action to Be Tested**	**Muscle**
L2, L3	Hip flexion	Iliopsoas
L3, L4	Knee extension	Quadriceps
L5	Ankle dorsiflexion	Anterior tibialis
	Extension of great toe	Extensor hallucis longus
S1	Plantarflexion	Gastrocnemius

From Dyrek,[8] p 76, with permission.

Impairments in ROM, accessory joint motions, and motor performance may impact on daily living, occupational, and recreational activities. In such cases the assessment of gait (see Chapter 10: Gait Analysis), functional abilities (see Chapter 11: Functional Assessment), and environmental surroundings (see Chapter 12: Environmental Assessment) are often appropriate. Sometimes assessment findings indicate the need for additional testing by other health professionals such as physician specialists, psychologists, speech-language pathologists, and occupational therapists.

EVALUATION OF FINDINGS

At the conclusion of the musculoskeletal assessment, all pertinent historical, subjective, and physical findings are evaluated to establish a diagnosis upon which to base treatment. A *diagnosis* has been defined as a label encompassing a cluster of signs and symptoms, syndromes, or categories.[53] If possible, the specific tissues causing the impairments should be identified so that treatment can be focused and effective. The examiner must have a thorough

Table 5–9 DEEP TENDON REFLEXES

	Root Level	Muscle	Peripheral Nerve
Upper quarter:	C5–6	Biceps	Musculocutaneous
	C5–6	Brachioradialis	Radial
	C7	Triceps	Radial
Lower quarter:	L3–4	Quadriceps	Femoral
	S1	Gastrocnemius	Sciatic (tibial)

The degree of reflex activity is graded on a 0 to 4 scale. Grades are awarded based on a predicted response and comparison of responses between body halves.

0 = no reflex response
1 = minimal response
2 = moderate response }
3 = brisk, strong response } normal range
4 = clonus

From Dyrek,[8] p 76, with permission.

understanding of the pathologies commonly affecting the body segment under consideration.[8] The symptoms and clinical manifestations of these pathologies must be known for comparison to the current assessment finding. Sometimes the evaluation process does not yield an identifiable diagnosis; not all patients present with textbook-perfect symptoms. In such cases, a provisional diagnosis and the alleviation of symptoms and impairments become the basis for treatment. In other instances the evaluation may indicate the presence of two or more conditions. The examiner will then prioritize and focus initially on the condition causing the most serious impairments, functional limitations, and disability.

The evaluation should clearly determine the baseline for the patient's symptoms, impairments, functional limitations, and disabilities. This information becomes the basis of the clinical problem list and guides development of goals (remediation of impairments) and outcomes (remediation of functional limitations and disability). The results of future assessments can be compared to this baseline to evaluate the effectiveness of treatment.

In addition to establishing a diagnosis and baseline, the evaluation of findings should ascertain etiological factors. Unless the underlying causes of the condition are recognized and treated, chronic problems can be expected.[1] The examiner must direct attention to not only the specifically involved tissues, but must think more broadly of physiological units of function and biomechanics. For example, a patient with a sprain of the medial collateral ligament of the knee may initially respond well to treatment consisting of compression ace wrapping, ice, elevation, reduced activity, and a protective non-weight bearing crutch gait. However, if the condition is partially due to abnormal foot pronation, the resumption of normal weight-bearing activities may cause reinjury unless the alignment of the foot and leg is improved with orthotics. Similarly, a patient with tendinitis of the supraspinatus muscle may react well to rest, modalities applied to the tendon, and gentle glenohumeral ROM exercises, but often also requires eventual strengthening of the rotator cuff, trapezius, and serratus anterior muscles, as well as lengthening of the posterior and inferior glenohumeral capsule to restore normal scapulohumeral rhythm and prevent recurrent subacromial impingement of the supraspinatus tendon.

Other information that impacts on the prognosis and course of treatment can be determined during the evaluation process. The mode and mechanism of onset must be established. Was the onset sudden, gradually acquired, or congenital? Generally, the prognosis is better for a condition caused by a well-defined event than for a congenital condition or one with an insidious, gradual onset. The mode and mechanism of onset also provide clues to prevent reoccurring episodes of the injury or condition.

Finally, an analysis of the assessment findings

should establish the stage of the patient's condition. The stage, whether acute, subacute, or chronic, can indicate how well the patient will tolerate mechanical loads such as those imposed by daily activities or by a therapist during treatment.[8] The **acute stage** is usually defined as occurring up to the first 48 to 72 hours after onset. The **subacute stage** may continue up to 2 weeks to several months after onset. Typically, conditions are considered **chronic** after 3 to 6 months. Another way of defining the stages, which is probably more relevant to treatment planning, focuses on tissue inflammation and the repair process.[1] Conditions in an acute inflammation stage will show signs and symptoms of inflammation associated with hyperemia, increased capillary permeability with protein and plasma leakage, and an influx of granulocytes and other defensive cells. These signs and symptoms include swelling, elevated skin temperature at the lesion site, and pain at rest that worsens with ROM and resisted isometric contractions that even minimally stress the involved tissues. The chronic inflammation stage produces signs and symptoms associated with attempts at tissue repair, including an increase in the number of fibrocytes and the presence of granulation tissue. The patient will now have minimal or no swelling and elevated temperature at the lesion site; pain tends to occur only at the extremes of ROM when the end-feel is reached, or with a moderate to maximal amount of isometric resistance. Tissues in an acute stage will often not tolerate mechanical loading from daily, recreational, occupational, or therapeutic activities. The force, frequency, and duration of treatment procedures must be monitored closely so as not to increase inflammation and worsen the condition. In contrast, tissues in the **chronic stage** will usually tolerate and require treatment procedures involving more mechanical loading, frequency, and duration to effect positive changes in the tissues. The stage of the condition also adds prognostic information. Typically, an acute condition will show more spontaneous improvement over a shorter period of time than a chronic condition. A chronic condition usually requires a longer period of treatment to effect a smaller improvement in status.

SUMMARY

The musculoskeletal assessment provides important information concerning the status of bones, articular cartilage, joint capsules, ligaments, and muscles. The assessment process begins with a review of the patient's medical records and a detailed interview. Careful observation, palpation, ROM, accessory joint motion, and muscle performance tests are typically performed. Depending on the findings, special tests particular to the body region being examined may need to be included. Assessment of the peripheral and central nervous system, gait, functional ability, and the environment are often required. At the conclusion of this process, all assessment findings must be evaluated to determine the diagnosis, baseline status, etiological factors, mode of onset, and stage (acute, subacute, or chronic) of the condition. At this point the prognosis, treatment outcomes, rehabilitation outcomes, and plan of care can be developed.

QUESTIONS FOR REVIEW

1. Identify the components of an assessment for musculoskeletal disorders. Describe the best sequence of performing these procedures. Provide a rationale for your selection.

2. What information should be obtained during a patient interview? Why is this information important?

3. What are the three types of normal end-feels? What types of tissue contribute to these end-feels?

4. Provide an example of a capsular and a noncapsular pattern of restriction at a joint of your choice. What would cause these two different patterns?

5. Compare and contrast osteokinematic and arthrokinematic motions. Give three examples of each type of motion. How are they integrated in a typical synovial joint in which the moving joint surface is concave? convex?

6. What are the differences between muscle performance, strength, endurance, work, and power?

7. Discuss the implications of a finding of pain versus no pain, and strength versus weakness during the performance of resisted isometric testing.

8. Describe the criteria for the manual muscle testing grades of Zero, Poor, Fair, Good, and Normal. Compare and contrast the criteria for the grades of Poor minus, Poor, and Poor plus.

9. What are the advantages and disadvantages of using manual muscle testing, hand-held dynamometers, and isokinetic dynamometers to assess muscle strength?

10. What summary information should be determined from the evaluation of the musculoskeletal assessment findings to develop a clinical problem list, goals, outcomes, prognosis, and plan of care?

CASE STUDIES

Case Study 1

A 45 year-old man enters the outpatient physical therapy department with a complaint of right shoulder pain of 1 week duration. The pain began Monday morning following a weekend of scraping and painting his house. The patient describes his pain as aching and troublesome; his pain is a 6 on a pain scale of 0 to 10. He reports that he is married, and having difficulty in home maintenance activities such as lawn mowing. He is able to perform only 30 percent of his normal home and recreational activities. The examiner decides to conduct a musculoskeletal assessment.

While palpating the shoulder region, the examiner notes increased tenderness and skin temperature in the region of the bicipital groove of the right anterior shoulder. Active ROM of the right shoulder reveals increased pain and some limitations in ROM during shoulder flexion, abduction, and extension; all other active motions are pain free and within normal ROM limits. Passive shoulder motions are pain free with normal ROM, except for shoulder extension, which is limited and causes an increase in pain toward the end of motion.

Guiding Questions

1. What are the purposes of a musculoskeletal assessment?

2. What additional information does the examiner need to gather during the interview?

3. What is a capsular pattern of limitation? Does this patient have a capsular pattern of limitation for the glenohumeral joint?

4. The examiner suspects the presence of bicipital tendinitis. Do the findings during testing of active and passive ROM support this diagnosis? Explain.

5. What additional tests should be performed during the physical examination that will selectively examine contractile tissue and help to support or repudiate the diagnosis of bicipital tendinitis? Provide a rationale for your selection.

Case Study 2

A 14 year-old girl is referred for outpatient physical therapy 12 weeks after sustaining midshaft fractures of her left tibia and fibula from a bicycle accident. Her long leg cast was removed yesterday.

The fracture is reported to be well healed. The patient reports her left knee and ankle are stiff and painful when she tries to bend them. She also describes her left leg as weak. At this time she is ambulating with two crutches, weight-bearing as tolerated, with hopes of progressing off the crutches as soon as possible.

Guiding Questions

1. The examiner notes on observation that the patient's left thigh and calf appear to be thinner than the right. How can the examiner objectively assess and document this observation? Why might the patient's left leg be thinner than the right?

2. The examiner assesses passive ROM for left knee flexion and finds it to be 10 to 70 degrees. The end-feel for left knee flexion is firm. What is an end-feel? What are the three general types of normal end-feels? What tissues could be causing a firm end-feel for knee flexion in this patient?

3. What accessory joint motion should be assessed given the limitation in passive knee flexion ROM? Apply the concave-convex rules for determining the direction of the glide given the shape of the joint surfaces. The examiner found the accessory joint motion to be very hypomobile. What grade should the accessory joint motion be given?

4. The examiner conducts a manual muscle test of the left lower extremity. What three factors are important in determining manual muscle testing grades? What would be the criteria for a manual muscle testing grade of fair?

5. In addition to observing, palpating, and testing active ROM, passive ROM, accessory joint motions, and muscle performance, what other testing procedures would be important to include in the examination of this patient?

REFERENCES

1. Hertling, D, and Kessler, RM: Management of Common Musculoskeletal Disorders: Physical Therapy Principles and Methods, ed 3. Lippincott, Philadelphia, 1996.
2. Magee, DJ: Orthopedic Physical Assessment, ed 2. Saunders, Philadelphia, 1992.
3. Tomberlin, JP, and Saunders, HD: Evaluation, Treatment, and Prevention of Musculoskeletal Disorders, Vol 2, ed 3. Saunders Group, Minnesota, 1994.
4. Talley, N, and O'Connor, S: Clinical Examination: A Guide to Physical Diagnosis. Williams & Wilkins, Baltimore, 1988.
5. Paris, SV: The Spine. Course notes, Boston, MA, 1976.
6. Melzack, R: The McGill pain questionnaire: Major properties and scoring methods. Pain 1:277, 1975.
7. Boissonnault, WG: Examination in Physical Therapy Practice: Screening for Medical Disease. Churchill Livingstone, New York, 1991.
8. Dyrek, DA: Assessment and Treatment Planning Strategies for Musculoskeletal Deficits. In O'Sullivan, SB, and Schmitz, TJ (eds): Physical Rehabilitation: Assessment and Treatment, ed 3. FA Davis, Philadelphia, 1994.
9. Slemenda, CW, et al: Long-term bone loss in men: Effects of genetic and environmental factors. Ann Intern Med 117: 286, 1992.
10. Hopper, JL, and Seeman, E: The bone density of female twins discordant for tobacco use. N Engl J Med 330:387, 1994.
11. Battie, MC, et al: Smoking and lumbar intervertebral disc degeneration: An MRI study of identical twins. Spine 16:1016, 1991.
12. Deyo, RA, and Bass, JE: Lifestyle and low-back pain: The influence of smoking and obesity. Spine 14:501, 1989.
13. Heliovaara, M, et al: Determinants of sciatica and low-back pain. Spine 16:608, 1991.
14. Boshuizen, JC, et al: Do smokers get more back pain? Spine 18:35, 1993.
15. Ekberg, K, et al: Case-control study of risk factors for disease in the neck and shoulder area. Occup Environ Med 51:262, 1994.
16. Brage, S, and Bjerkedal, T: Musculoskeletal pain and smoking in Norway. J Epidemiol Community Health 50:166, 1996.

17. Norkin, CC, and Levangie, PK: Joint Structure and Function: A Comprehensive Analysis, ed 2. FA Davis, Philadelphia, 1992.
18. Morrey, BF, et al: A biomechanical study of normal functional elbow motion. J Bone Joint Surg Am 63:872, 1981.
19. Safee-Rad, R, et al: Normal functional range of motion of upper limb joints during performance of three feeding activities. Arch Phys Med Rehabil 71:505, 1990.
20. Professional Staff Association, Rancho Los Amigos Medical Center: Observational Gait Analysis Handbook. Ranchos Los Amigos Medical Center, Downey, CA, 1989.
21. Livingston, LA, et al: Stairclimbing kinematics on stairs of differing dimensions. Arch Phys Med Rehabil 72:398, 1991.
22. Boone, DC, and Azen, SP: Normal range of motion of joints in male subjects. J Bone Joint Surg Am 61:756, 1979.
23. Wanatabe, H, et al: The range of joint motions of the extremities in healthy Japanese people: The difference according to age. Cited in Walker, JM: Musculoskeletal development: A review. Phys Ther 71:878, 1991.
24. Walker, JM, et al: Active mobility of the extremities in older subjects. Phys Ther 64:919, 1984.
25. Roach, KE, and Miles, TP: Normal hip and knee active range of motion: The relationship to age. Phys Ther 71:656, 1991.
26. Allander, E, et al: Normal range of joint movement in shoulder, hip, wrist and thumb with special reference to side: A comparison between two populations. Int J Epidemiol 3:253, 1974.
27. Beighton, P, et al: Articular mobility in an African population. Ann Rheum Dis 32:23, 1973.
28. Fairbank, JCT, et al: Quantitative measurements of joint mobility in adolescents. Ann Rheum Dis 43:288, 1984.
29. Rothstein, JM, et al: Goniometric reliability in a clinical setting: Elbow and knee measurements. Phys Ther 63:1611, 1983.
30. Ekstrand, J, et al: Lower extremity goniometric measurements: A study to determine their reliability. Arch Phys Med Rehabil 63:171, 1982.
31. Norkin, CC, and White, DJ: Measurement of Joint Motion: A Guide to Goniometry, ed 2. FA Davis, Philadelphia, 1995.
32. American Academy of Orthopaedic Surgeons: Joint Motion: A Method of Measuring and Recording. AAOS, Chicago, 1965.
33. American Medical Association: Guide to the Evaluation of Permanent Impairment, ed 3. AMA, Milwaukee, 1990.
34. Hoppenfeld, S: Physical Examination of the Spine and Extremities. Appleton-Century-Crofts, New York, 1976.
35. Kapandji, IA: Physiology of the Joints, vols 1 and 2, ed 2. Churchill Livingstone, London, 1970.
36. Cyriax, JH, and Cyriax, PJ: Illustrated Manual of Orthopaedic Medicine. Butterworths, London, 1983.
37. Low, JL: The reliability of joint measurement. Physiotherapy 62:227, 1976.
38. Watkins, MA, et al: Reliability of goniometric measurements and visual estimates of knee range of motion obtained in a clinical setting. Phys Ther 71:90, 1991.
39. Clarkson, HM, and Gilewich, GB: Musculoskeletal Assessment: Joint Range of Motion and Manual Muscle Strength. Williams & Wilkins, Baltimore, 1989.
40. Boone, DC, et al: Reliability of goniometric measurements. Phys Ther 58:1355, 1978.
41. Pandya, S, et al: Reliability of goniometric measurements in patients with Duchenne muscular dystrophy. Phys Ther 65:1339, 1985.
42. Tucci, SM, et al: Cervical motion assessment: A new, simple and accurate method. Arch Phys Med Rehabil 67:225, 1986.
43. Youdas, JW, et al: Reliability of measurements of cervical spine range of motion: Comparison of three methods. Phys Ther 71:2, 1991.
44. Fitzgerald, GK, et al: Objective assessment with establishment of normal values for lumbar spine range of motion. Phys Ther 63:1776, 1983.
45. Gajdosik, RL, and Bohannon, RW: Clinical measurement of range of motion: Review of goniometry emphasizing reliability and validity. Phys Ther 67:1867, 1987.
46. Kaltenborn, FM: Mobilization of the Extremity Joints: Examination and Basic Treatment Techniques, ed 3. Olaf Norlis Bokhandel, Oslo, 1980.
47. Paris, S: Extremity Dysfunction and Mobilization. Institute Press, Atlanta, 1980.
48. Riddle, DL: Measurement of accessory motion: critical issues and related concepts. Phys Ther 72:865, 1992.
49. Hayes, KW, et al: An examination of Cyriax's passive motion tests with patients having osteoarthritis of the knee. Phys Ther 74:697, 1994.
50. MacConaill, MA, and Basmajian, JV: Muscles and Movement: A Basis for Human Kinesiology, ed 2. Robert E Krieger, New York, 1977.
51. Kisner, C, and Colby, LA: Therapeutic Exercise: Foundations and Techniques, ed 3. FA Davis, Philadelphia, 1996.
52. Edmond SL: Manipulations and Mobilization: Extremity and Spinal Techniques. CV Mosby, St. Louis, 1993.
53. Guide to physical therapy practice. Phys Ther 77:1177, 1997.
54. Franklin, ME, et al: Assessment of exercise-induced minor muscle lesions: The accuracy of Cyriax's diagnosis by selective tension paradigm. J Orthop Sports Phys Ther 24:122, 1996.
55. Wright W: Muscle training in the treatment of infantile paralysis. Boston Med Surg J 167:567, 1912.
56. Lovett, R: Treatment of Infantile Paralysis. Blakiston's Son & Co., Philadelphia, 1917.
57. Lowman, CL: Muscle strength testing. The Physical Therapy Review 20:69–71, 1940.
58. Stewart, HS: Physiotherapy: Therapy and Clinical Application. Paul B. Hoeber, New York, 1925.
59. Legg, AT, and Merrill, J: Physical Therapy in Infantile Paralysis. In Mock (ed): Principles and Practice of Physical Therapy, Vol 2. WF Prior, Hagerstown, MD, 1932.
60. Hislop, HJ, and Montgomery, J: Daniels and Worthingham's Muscle Testing: Techniques of Manual Examination, ed 6. Saunders, Philadelphia, 1995.
61. Kendall, FP, et al: Muscles Testing and Function, ed 4. Williams and Wilkins, Baltimore, MD, 1993.
62. Sharrard, WJW: Muscle recovery in poliomyelitis. J Bone Joint Surg Br 37:63, 1955.
63. Beasley, WC: Quantitative muscle testing: Principles and application to research and clinical services. Arch Phys Med Rehabil 42:398, 1961.
64. Frese, E, et al: Clinical reliability of manual muscle testing: Middle trapezius and gluteus medius muscles. Phys Ther 67:1072, 1987.
65. Silver, M, et al: Further standardization of manual muscle test for clinical study: Applied in chronic renal disease. Phys Ther 50:1456, 1970.
66. Iddings, DM, et al: Muscle testing: Part 2. Reliability in clinical use. The Physical Therapy Review 41:249, 1961.
67. Lilienfeld, AM, et al: A study of the reproducibility of muscle testing and certain other aspects of muscle scoring. Physical Therapy Reviews 34:279, 1954.
68. Hines, TF: Manual Muscle Examination. In Licht, S, and Johnson, EW (eds): Therapeutic Exercise, ed 2. Waverly Press, Baltimore, MD, 1965.
69. Smidt, GL, and Rodger, MW: Factors contributing to the regulation and clinical assessment of muscular strength. Phys Ther 62:1283, 1982.
70. Mulroy, SJ, et al: The ability of male and female clinicians to effectively test knee extension strength using manual muscle testing. J Orthop Sport Phys Ther 26:192, 1997.
71. Andrews, AW, et al: Normative values for isometric muscle force measurements obtained with hand-held dynamometers. Phys Ther 76:248, 1996.
72. Bohannon, RW: Upper extremity strength and strength relationships among young women. J Orthop Sport Phys Ther 8:128, 1986.
73. Backman, E, et al: Isometric muscle force and anthropometric values in normal children aged between 3.5 and 15 years. Scand J Rehabil Med 21:105, 1985.
74. Van der Ploeg, RJO, et al: Hand-held myometry: Reference values. J Neurol Neurosurg Psychiatry 54:244, 1991.
75. Agre, JC, et al: Strength testing with a portable dynamome-

ter: Reliability for upper and lower extremities. Arch Phys Med Rehabil 68:454, 1987.

76. Reinking, MF, et al: Assessment of quadriceps muscle performance by hand-held, isometric, and isokinetic dynamometry in patients with knee dysfunction. J Orthop Sport Phys Ther 24:154, 1996.

77. Bohannon, RW: Test-retest reliability of hand-held dynamometry during a single session of strength assessment. Phys Ther 6:206, 1986.

78. Bohannon, RW, and Andrews, AW: Interrater reliability of hand-held dynamometry. Phys Ther 67:931, 1987.

79. Riddle, DL, et al: Intrasession and intersession reliability of hand-held dynamometer measurements taken on brain-damaged patients. Phys Ther 69:182, 1989.

80. Moreland, J, et al: Interrater reliability of six tests of trunk muscle function and endurance. J Orthop Sport Phys Ther 26:200, 1997.

81. Isolated Joint Testing and Exercise: A Handbook for Using the Cybex II and U.B.X.T. Cybex, Ronkonkoma, NY, 1981.

82. Keating, JL, and Matyas, TA: Method-related variations in estimates of gravity correction values using electromechanical dynamometry: A knee extension study. J Orthop Sports Phys Ther 24:142, 1996.

83. Rothstein, JM, et al: Clinical uses of isokinetic measurements: Critical issues. Phys Ther 67:1840, 1987.

84. Winter, DA, et al: Errors in the use of isokinetic dynamometers. Eur J Appl Physiol 46:397, 1981.

85. Lin, PC, et al: Detection of submaximal effort in isometric and isokinetic knee extension tests. J Orthop Sports Phys Ther 24:19, 1996.

86. Bohannon, RW: Differentiation of maximal from submaximal static elbow flexor efforts by measurement variability. Am J Phys Med Rehabil 66:213, 1987.

87. Kishino, ND, et al: Quantification of lumbar function. Spine 10:921, 1985.

88. Robinson, ME, et al: Variability of isometric and isotonic leg exercise: Utility for detection of submaximal efforts. Journal of Occupational Rehabilitation 4:163, 1994.

89. Murray, MP, et al: Maximum isometric knee flexor and extensor contractions: Normal patterns of torque versus time. Phys Ther 57:637, 1977.

90. Hazard, RG, et al: Lifting capacity: Indices of subject effort. Spine 17:1065, 1992.

91. Johnson, J, and Siegel, D: Reliability of an isokinetic movement of the knee extensors. Research Quarterly 49:88, 1978.

92. Keating, JL, and Matyas, TA: The influence of subject and test design on dynamometric measurements of extremity muscles. Phys Ther 76:866, 1996.

93. Davies, GJ, et al: Assessment of strength. In Malone, TR, et al (eds): Orthopedic and Sports Physical Therapy, ed 3. Mosby, St. Louis, 1997.

94. Mawdsley, RH, and Knapik, JJ: Comparison of isokinetic measurements with test repetitions. Phys Ther 62:169, 1982.

95. Farrel, M, and Richards, J: Analysis of the reliability and validity of the isokinetic communicator exercise device. Med Sci Sports Exerc 18:44, 1986.

96. Thorstensson, A, et al: Force-velocity relations and fiber composition in human knee extensor muscles. J Appl Physiol 40:12, 1976.

97. Tredinnick, TJ, and Duncan, PW: Reliability of measurements of concentric and eccentric isokinetic loading. Phys Ther 68:656, 1988.

98. Molnar, GE, et al: Reliability of quantitative strength measurements in children. Arch Phys Med Rehabil 60:218, 1979.

99. Kramer, JF, and Ng, LR: Static and dynamic strength of the shoulder rotators in healthy, 45 to 75 year-old men and women. J Orthop Sports Phys Ther 24:11, 1996.

100. Cahalan, TD, et al: Quantitative measurements of hip strength in different age groups. Clin Orthop 246:136, 1989.

101. Falkel, J: Plantar-flexor strength testing using the Cybex isokinetic dynamometer. Phys Ther 58:847, 1978.

102. Highenboten, CL, et al: Concentric and eccentric torque comparisons for knee extension and flexion in young adult males and females using the kinetic communicator. Am J Sports Med 16:234, 1988.

103. Smith, SS, et al: Quantification of lumbar function, part I: Isometric and multispeed isokinetic trunk strength measures in sagittal and axial planes in normal subjects. Spine 10:757, 1985.

104. Goslin, B, and Charteris, J: Isokinetic dynamometry: Normative data for clinical use in lower extremity (knee) cases. Scand J Rehabil Med 11:105, 1979.

105. Watkins, M, and Harris, B: Evaluation of isokinetic muscle performance. Clin Sports Med 2:37, 1983.

106. Weltman, A, et al: Measurement of isokinetic strength in prepubertal males. J Orthop Sports Phys Ther 9:345, 1988.

107. Murray, MP, et al: Strength of isometric and isokinetic contractions: Knee muscles of men aged 20 to 86. Phys Ther 60:412, 1980.

108. Holmes, JR, and Alkerink, GJ: Isokinetic strength characteristics of the quadriceps femoris and hamstring muscles in high school students. Phys Ther 64:914, 1984.

109. Grace, TG, et al: Isokinetic muscle imbalance and knee-joint injuries. J Bone Joint Surg Am 66:734, 1984.

110. Hageman, PR, et al: Effects of speed and limb dominance on eccentric and concentric isokinetic testing of the knee. J Orthop Sports Phys Ther 10:59, 1988.

111. Lucca, JA, and Kline, KK: Effects of upper and lower limb preference on torque production in the knee flexors and extensors. J Orthop Sports Phys Ther 11:202, 1989.

112. Hinton, RY: Isokinetic evaluation of shoulder rotational strength in high-school baseball pitchers. Am J Sports Med 16:274, 1988.

113. Perrin, DH, et al: Bilateral isokinetic peak torque, torque acceleration energy, power, and work relationships in athletes and nonathletes. J Orthop Sports Phy Ther 9:184, 1987.

114. Mira, AJ, et al: A critical analysis of quadriceps function after femoral shaft fracture in adults. J Bone Joint Surg Am 62:61, 1980.

115. LoPresti, C, et al: Quadriceps insufficiency following repair of the anterior cruciate ligament. J Orthop Sports Phys Ther 9:245, 1988.

116. Caillet, R: Soft Tissue Pain and Disability. FA Davis, Philadelphia, 1977.

117. Paulos, LE: Knee and leg: Soft-tissue trauma. In American Academy of Orthopedic Surgeons: Orthopedic Knowledge Update 2, 1987.

SUPPLEMENTAL READINGS

Casanov, JS (ed): Clinical Assessment Recommendations, ed 2. American Society of Hand Therapists, Chicago, 1992.

Clark, RC, and Bonfiglio, M (eds): Orthopaedics: Essentials of Diagnosis and Treatment. Churchill Livingstone, New York, 1994.

Cookson, JC, and Kent, BE: Orthopedic manual therapy: An overview. Part I. Phys Ther 59:136, 1979.

Corrigan, B, and Maitland, GD: Practical Orthopaedic Medicine. Butterworths, Boston, 1983.

Cyriax J: Textbook of Orthopaedic Medicine: Diagnosis of Soft Tissue Lesions, ed 8. Bailliere Tindall, London, 1982.

Goodman, CC, and Snyder, TEK: Differential Diagnosis in Physical Therapy. Saunders, Philadelphia, 1995.

Hartley, A: Practical Joint Assessment: Upper Quadrant, ed 2. Mosby, St. Louis, 1995.

Hartley, A: Practical Joint Assessment: Lower Quadrant, ed 2. Mosby, St. Louis, 1995.

Kelley, MJ, and Clark, WA: Orthopedic Therapy of the Shoulder. Lippincott, Philadelphia, 1995.

Lehmkuhl, LD, and Smith, LK: Brunstrom's Clinical Kinesiology, ed 4. FA Davis, Philadelphia, 1983.

Malone, TR, et al (eds): Orthopedic and Sports Physical Therapy, ed 3. Mosby, St. Louis, 1997.

Minor, MAD, and Minor, SD: Patient Evaluation Methods for the Health Professional. Reston Publishing Co., Reston, VA, 1985.

Moffroid, M: Principles of isokinetic instrumentation. In O'Sullivan, S (ed): Topics in Physical Therapy. American Physical Therapy Association, Alexandria, VA, 1990.

Palmer, ML, and Epler, M: Clinical Assessment Procedures in Physical Therapy. Lippincott, Philadelphia, 1990.

Richardson, JK, and Iglarsh, ZA: Clinical Orthopaedic Physical Therapy. Saunders, Philadelphia, 1994.

Rothstein, JM (ed): Measurement in Physical Therapy. Churchill Livingstone, New York, 1985.

Salter, RB: Textbook of Disorders and Injuries of the Musculoskeletal System, ed 3. Williams & Wilkins, Baltimore, 1999.

Soderberg, GL: Kinesiology: Application to Pathological Motion. Williams & Wilkins, Baltimore, 1986.

Starkey, C, and Ryan, J: Evaluation of Orthopedic and Athletic Injuries. FA Davis, Philadelphia, 1996.

Tan, JC: Practical Manual of Physical Medicine and Rehabilitation. Mosby, St. Louis, 1998.

Tubiana, R, et al: Examination of the Hand and Wrist. Mosby, St. Louis, 1996.

Wadsworth, CT: Manual Examination and Treatment of the Spine and Extremities. Williams & Wilkins, Baltimore, 1988.

Wells, PE, et al (eds): Pain Management in Physical Therapy. Appleton & Lange, Norwalk, CT, 1988.

GLOSSARY

Accessory (joint play) motions: Motions between adjacent joint surfaces that occur when a bone moves through a range of motion. These motions are not under voluntary control. Includes slides (glides), distractions, compressions, rolls, and spins.

Active range of motion (AROM): The amount of joint motion obtained with unassisted voluntary joint motion.

Acute stage: The first 48 to 72 hours following the onset of an injury; usually characterized by tissue inflammation associated with hyperemia.

Apprehension test: A test in which a patient's joint is placed in a vulnerable position for subluxation or dislocation. The test is positive if the patient becomes apprehensive.

Arthrokinematics: Refers to the motion of adjacent joint surfaces that occurs when a bone moves through a range of motion.

Break test: A method of applying resistance during manual muscle testing or hand-held dynamometry in which the patient holds a joint position until the examiner gradually overpowers the patient and an eccentric contraction begins to occur.

Capsular pattern: A characteristic pattern of restricted passive osteokinematic motion, usually involving more than one motion at a joint. Indicates intra-articular joint inflammation or capsular fibrosis.

Chronic stage: Time span beyond 3 to 6 months following the onset of a condition; characterized by the body's attempt at tissue repair.

Compression: The approximation of joint surfaces.

End-feel: The tissue resistance experienced by the examiner when over pressure is applied at the end of a range of motion or accessory motion.

Distraction: The linear separation of joint surfaces.

Hand-held dynamometer: A portable testing device that is placed between the patient's body part and the examiner's hand that measures mechanical force.

Hypermobility: Excessive joint motion.

Hypomobility: Restricted joint motion.

Isokinetic dynamometer: A testing and exercise device that controls the velocity of a limb movement, keeping it at a constant rate while offering accommodating resistance throughout the range of motion.

Joint mobilization: Passive therapeutic techniques applied specifically to joint structures that utilize arthrokinematic motions to increase or maintain joint play and range of motion or to treat pain.

Joint play (accessory) motions: Motions that occur between joint surfaces that accompany osteokinematic motions, but are not under voluntary control. Includes slides (glides), distractions, compressions, rolls, and spins. Joint play can also refer to the distensibility of the joint capsule and ligaments that allow joint motion to occur.

Linear work: Force multiplied by distance.

Make test (active resistance test): A method of applying resistance during manual muscle testing in which the patient moves through an arc of motion against the examiner's resistance. In hand-held dynamometry, the term has also been used to indicate a patient's performance of a maximal isometric contraction against the examiner's resistance.

Muscle endurance: The ability of a muscle to contract repeatedly over time.

Muscle performance: The ability of a muscle to do work (force × distance).

Muscle power: Work produced per unit of time.

Muscle strength: The force exerted by a muscle to overcome a resistance in one maximal effort.

Noncapsular pattern: A restriction of passive osteokinematic motion that is not proportioned similar to a capsular pattern. Indicates a cause other than intra-articular inflammation or capsular fibrosis.

Osteokinematics: Refers to the gross, angular motions of bones around a joint axis, such as flexion, extension, abduction, adduction, or rotation.

Passive range of motion (PROM): The amount of joint motion available when an examiner moves the joint through the range without assistance from the patient.

Roll: An angular motion between two surfaces, similar to the bottom of a rocking chair rolling over the floor. New points on one surface come into contact with new points on the other surface.

Roll-gliding: The combination of a roll and glide. As a roll occurs between two surfaces, one surface slides on the other.

Rotational work: Torque multiplied by the arc of movement.

Slide (glide): The translatory (linear) motion of one surface sliding over another surface. The same point on one surface comes into contact with new points on the other surface.

Spin: The rotation of a surface around a stationary axis. The same point on the moving surface creates an arc of a circle as the surface moves.

Subacute stage: The time period between the acute and chronic stages of a condition; considered to begin by 72 hours after injury and continuing for as long as several months.

Torque: Force multiplied by perpendicular distance from the axis of rotation

APPENDIX

Suggested Answers to Case Study Guiding Questions

CASE STUDY 1

1. What are the purposes of such a musculoskeletal assessment?

ANSWER
- Determine presence or absence of impairment; establish a baseline of function.
- Identify the specific tissues causing the impairment and establish a diagnosis.
- Help formulate therapeutic goals, outcomes, and interventions.
- Determine if orthotic and adaptive equipment is needed for functional tasks.
- Information gathered at this time will be compared to future findings to assess the effectiveness of treatment.
- Motivate the patient.

2. What additional information does the examiner need to gather during the interview?

ANSWER: Location of pain, behavior of pain—what makes it better/worse, behavior of pain in last 48 hours, previous care, specific medical history, past medical history, medications, more specific information on occupational and recreational activities, patient's treatment goals and anticipated time frame of recovery.

3. What is a capsular pattern of limitation? Does this patient have a capsular pattern of limitation for the glenohumeral joint?

ANSWER: A capsular pattern is a characteristic pattern of restricted passive osteokinematic motion, usually involving more than one motion at a joint. The capsular pattern for the glenohumeral joint is maximal loss of external rotation, moderate loss of abduction, and minimal loss of internal rotation. This patient does not have a capsular pattern of limitation.

4. The examiner suspects the presence of bicipital tendinitis. Do the findings during testing of active and passive ROM support this diagnosis? Explain.

ANSWER: Yes. Active ROM in shoulder flexion and abduction will require the active contraction of the biceps muscle and thus put tension on the biceps tendon, causing pain. Active ROM and passive ROM in shoulder extension will be painful and limited because these motions will stretch the biceps tendon.

5. What additional tests should be performed during the physical examination that will selectively examine contractile tissue and help to support or repudiate the diagnosis of bicipital tendinitis? Provide a rationale for your selection.

ANSWER: Resisted isometric testing should be used to isolate the involvement of contractile tissues (muscle, tendon and bone insertion of tendon) from noncontractile tissues (joint surfaces, capsule, ligaments). The examiner should resist shoulder flexion and elbow flexion without allowing movement of those joints.

CASE STUDY 2

1. The examiner notes on observation that the patient's left thigh and calf appear to be thinner than the right. How can the examiner objectively assess and document this observation? Why might the patient's left leg be thinner than the right?

ANSWER: Circumference measurements should be taken of the patient's left and right lower extremities, for example at 12, 8, 4, and 0 inches above and below both knees. The left lower extremity is probably thinner than the right due to muscle atrophy caused by immobility for 12 weeks within the cast.

2. What is an end-feel? What are the three general types of normal end-feels? What tissues could be causing a firm end-feel for knee flexion in this patient?

ANSWER: An end-feel is the tissue resistance experienced by the examiner when over pressure is applied at the end of a range of motion or accessory motion. The three types of normal end-feels are soft, firm, and hard. The firm end-feel could be caused by tightness (shortening) of the quadriceps muscles, patella ligament, anterior joint capsule of the knee, and/or cruciate ligaments.

3. What accessory joint motion should be assessed given the limitation in passive knee flexion ROM? The examiner found the accessory joint motion to be very hypomobile. What grade should the accessory joint motion be given?

ANSWER: The superior articular surface of the tibia is concave and will glide in a posterior direction (the same direction as the shaft of the tibia) during knee flexion. Therefore, a posterior glide of the tibia should be assessed. A very hypomobile joint would be given a grade of 1.

4. What three factors are important in determining manual muscle testing grades? What would be the criteria for a manual muscle testing grade of Fair?

ANSWER: The three factors are arc of motion, amount of resistance provided by gravity, and amount of resistance applied manually by the examiner. A manual muscle testing grade of Fair would require that the patient move the joint through the full arc of available motion, in a position so the motion is against gravity, with no additional manual resistance applied by the examiner.

5. In addition to observing, palpating, and testing active ROM, passive ROM, assessory joint motions, and muscle performance, what other testing procedures would be important to include in the evaluation of this patient?

ANSWER: Assessment of gait, functional abilities, and sensation should be made.

Thomas J. Schmitz

LEARNING OBJECTIVES

1. Understand the purpose(s) of performing a sensory examination.
2. Understand the relationship between preliminary mental status screening tests and tests for sensory integrity.
3. Describe the classification and function of the receptor mechanisms involved in the perception of sensation.
4. Identify the spinal pathways that mediate sensation.
5. Understand the general guidelines for completing a sensory assessment.
6. Describe the testing protocol for each sensory modality.
7. Using the case study example, apply clinical decision making skills to application of sensory assessment data.

SENSORY INTEGRITY

Sensory integrity is the ability to organize and use sensory information. *Sensory testing* examines sensory integrity by determining the patient's ability to interpret and discriminate among incoming sensory information. Sensory testing is based on the premise that within the intact human system, sensory information is taken in from the body and the environment, the central nervous system (CNS) then processes and integrates the information for use in planning and organizing behavior. This premise is more aptly termed a **theoretical construct** (a concept that represents an *unobservable* event). We cannot *directly* observe CNS processing, integration of sensory information, or the motor planning process. However, our current knowledge of CNS function and motor behavior provides evidence that these unobservable events do occur. We *can* observe impairments in motor behavior, but can only *hypothesize* that they truly result from faulty sensory integration mechanisms.[1]

The scope of sensory integrity provided in *The Guide to Physical Therapist Practice*[2] includes peripheral sensory processing (e.g., sensitivity to touch); cortical sensory processing (e.g., **two-point and sharp/dull discrimination**); **proprioception,** which includes position sense and the awareness of the joints at rest; and **kinesthesia,** which is the awareness of movement. (*Note:* Perception is also included within the definition of sensory integrity[2] and is presented in detail in Chapter 29).

CLINICAL IMPLICATIONS

Diagnostic Groups

Sensory impairments can impose significant functional limitations for the patient and may be associated with any disease or trauma affecting the nervous system. These impairments can result from dysfunction at any point within the sensory system, from the receptor or the peripheral nerve, to the spinal cord nuclei, sensory tracts, brainstem, thalamus, or sensory cortex.[3] Examples of diagnostic categories that generally demonstrate some level of sensory impairment include disease or injury to the peripheral nerves, nerve roots, or spinal cord, burns, cerebrovascular accident, arthritis, multiple sclerosis, fractures, and brain trauma or disease. This list, which is not all-inclusive, indicates the wide variety of diagnostic groups that may present with some element of sensory deficit and the importance of a thorough knowledge of techniques for testing sensation. The clinical indications for testing sensory integrity are cited in *The Guide to Physical Therapist Practice.*[2] Sensory integrity tests and measures are appropriate in the presence of one or more of the following impairments or functional limitations:

- Edema, lymphedema, or effusion
- Impaired gait, locomotion, and balance
- Impaired joint integrity and mobility
- Impaired motor function (motor control and motor learning)
- Impaired muscle performance (strength, power, endurance)
- Impaired neuromotor development and sensory integration
- Impaired reflex integrity
- Impaired posture
- Impaired ventilation, respiration (gas exchange), and circulation
- Pain

PATTERNS OF SENSORY LOSS

The actual pattern of sensory loss varies considerably. Peripheral nerve injuries present sensory loss, which parallels the distribution of the nerve and corresponds to the dermatome pattern of innervation. Evidence of both sensory and motor loss is typically indicative of root involvement. With peripheral neuropathy, sensory loss is often an early presenting symptom ("glove and stocking" distribution). CNS lesions may produce significant sensory impairments characterized by diffuse distribution (e.g., head, trunk, and limbs). Sensory loss can result in significant motor dysfunction (sensory ataxia), impairment of fine motor control, and motor learning as well as present a significant threat of injury to anesthetic limbs.

Age-Related Sensory Changes

Alterations in sensory function occur with normal aging. Decreased acuity of many sensations occur and are considered a characteristic finding with aging.[4] The exact morphology of diminished sensation with age has not been clearly established. However, several neurological changes have been identified and suggest potential explanations.

Over the lifespan neurons are replaced at a declining rate and this accounts for decline of average weight of the brain with aging. Other changes in the brain include degeneration of neurons with presence of replacement gliosis, lipid accumulation in the neurons, loss of myelin sheath, and development of neurofibrils (masses of small, tangled fibrils) and plaques on the cells.[5,6] There is also a decrease in the number of enzymes responsible for dopamine and norepinepherine synthesis,[7] as well as depletion of the neuronal dendrites in the aging brain.[6,8]

Several authors have reported a gradual reduction in conduction velocity of sensory nerves with advancing age, and this may be reflective of a loss of sensory axons.[9,10] Others have found no significant change in conduction velocity with age.[11] A reduction in the number of Meissner's corpuscles[12] has been found. These corpuscles, responsible for touch detection, are limited to hairless areas and become sparse, take on an irregular distribution, and vary in size and shape with age.[13] Age-related changes in morphology and decreased concentrations of Pacinian corpuscles, responsive to rapid tissue movement (e.g., vibration), have also been reported.[14] Merkel disks, also touch receptors, have not yet been associated with any significant age-related changes.[14]

Degeneration of some myelinated fibers of the spinal cord[15] and a decrease in distance between the nodes of Ranvier in peripheral nerves have also been associated with advancing age.[16,17] This later finding may be related to a slowing of saltatory conduction identified by some authors.[5,9] Other peripheral nerve findings indicate a gradual reduction of fibers in cranial nerves and spinal nerve roots. This reduction appears preferential to large fibers; loss has been reported in the sciatic, anterior tibialis, and sural nerves and has not been identified in more superficial nerves.[18,19]

Documented changes in sensory integrity with aging include changes in response to tactile[20] and vibratory stimuli,[21] decreased two-point discrimination,[22] decreased kinesthetic awareness,[23] and minimal alterations in the perception of pain.[24] These changes frequently appear in the presence of age-related visual or hearing losses that impair compensatory capabilities. In addition, some medications may further influence the distortion of sensory input.[4] This combination of sensory changes may pose a variety of functional limitations for the elderly individual such as postural instability, exaggerated body sway, balance problems, wide-based gait, diminished fine motor coordination, tendency to drop items held in the hand, and difficulty in recognizing body positions in space.[25]

TYPES AND USE OF DATA GENERATED

The close relationship between sensory input and motor output makes knowledge of sensory integrity critical to sound clinical judgement in establishing the diagnosis and prognosis and developing a plan of care. Sensory impairments interfere with acquisition of new motor skills because motor learning is highly dependent on sensory information and feedback. For example, a patient who has decreased awareness of where a limb is in space may be unable to execute appropriate motor responses to accomplish a task. Data from the sensory assessment assists the therapist in determining the source of deficits in motor performance (e.g., sensory ataxia). These data may also provide a partial explanation for the functional limitation and will help guide selection of an appropriate treatment strategy and safety precautions (anesthetic limbs are at high risk for injury).

Sensory testing is typically a component of the physical therapy examination process.[2] Because sensory impairments will influence motor performance, testing is completed prior to tests that involve elements of active motor function (such as manual muscle testing, active range of motion, functional assessments, etc.). Sensory tests are also an important component of periodic reexamination to determine the effectiveness of the plan of care. The purpose of performing a sensory examination is to determine the integrity of sensory processes as abnormalities are a frequent indicator of pathology.[2] Data generated from sensory tests typically includes[2]:

- Accuracy of cortical perceptions (e.g., tactile recognition of objects, recognition of symbols drawn on the skin, and ability to localize touch sensations)
- Joint position sense
- Perception of movement in the extremities
- Superficial sensory capabilities

Together with findings from other tests and measures, the data generated can be used to formulate clinical judgements to (1) establish a diagnosis and prognosis, (2) determine anticipated goals and desired outcomes, and (3) select, apply, or modify direct interventions.

AROUSAL, ATTENTION, ORIENTATION, AND COGNITION

Accuracy of data from sensory integrity tests relies on the patient's ability to respond to application of multiple cutaneous stimuli. Use of several easily administered preliminary tests will provide sufficient data to determine the patient's ability to concentrate on, and respond to, the battery of sensory test items. The areas tested include: arousal level, attention span, orientation, and cognition.[26,30]

A necessary first step is to determine the patient's arousal level for participation in the test protocol. **Arousal** is the physiological readiness of the human system for activity.[2] It is assessed by using traditionally accepted key terms and definitions to describe the patient's level of consciousness. These terms include alert, lethargic, obtunded, stupor, and coma. The terms represent a continuum of physiologic readiness for activity and are defined as follows[26]:

1. *Alert.* Patient is awake and attentive to normal levels of stimulation. Interactions with the therapist are normal and appropriate.

2. *Lethargic.* Patient appears drowsy and may fall asleep if not stimulated in some way. Interactions with the therapist may get sidetracked. Patient may have difficulty in focusing or maintaining attention on a question or task.

3. *Obtunded.* Patient is difficult to arouse from a somnolent state and is frequently confused when awake. Repeated stimulation is required to maintain consciousness. Interactions with therapist may be largely unproductive.

4. *Stupor* (semicoma). Patient responds only to strong, generally noxious stimuli and returns to the unconscious state when stimulation is stopped. When aroused, patient is unable to interact with the therapist.

5. *Coma* (deep coma). patient cannot be aroused by any type of stimulation. Reflex motor responses may or may not be seen.

Reliable information on the integrity of the sensory system can be obtained from patients who are alert. Reliability is proportionally reduced in patients with lethargy and nonexistent in patients who are obtunded, stuporous, or comatose.

Attention is awareness of the environment or responsiveness to a stimulus or task without being distracted by other stimuli.[2,26,28] Attention can be assessed by asking the patient to repeat a progressively more challenging list of items. These repetition tasks can begin with two or three items and gradually progress to longer lists. For example, the patient might be asked to repeat a series of numbers, letters, or words. Another approach to assessing attention is to ask the patient to spell words backwards (e.g., book, fork, bottle, garden). The task can be made more challenging by using progressively longer words. Individuals with a high attention span will be able to perform the task. Attention deficits will be apparent when the order of letters is confused.[26]

Orientation refers to the patient's awareness of time, person, and place. In medical record documentation the results of this mental status test are often abbreviated "oriented x 3" referring to the three parameters of time, person, and place. If a patient is not fully oriented to one or more domains, the notation would read, "oriented x 2 (time)" or "oriented x 1 (time, place)." With partial orientation entries, it is customary to include the *domains of disorientation* within parentheses. Box 6–1 presents sample questions for assessment of orientation.[26,27,28]

Cognition is defined as the process of knowing and includes both awareness and judgement.[2] Nolan[26] suggests three areas for testing cognition-dependent functions: (1) fund of knowledge; (2) calculation ability; and (3) proverb interpretation. **Fund of knowledge** is defined as the sum total of an individual's learning and experience in life. This will be highly variable and different for each patient. Detailed information about premorbid knowledge base is often not available. However, a number of general categories of information can be used to test

---

Box 6–1 SAMPLE QUESTIONS FOR ASSESSMENT OF ORIENTATION

A series of simple questions is posed to the patient. The questions are designed to assess the patient's understanding of recognition of who he or she is, location including the present facility (the name of hospital or clinic), the present time, and the passage of time.

Person
- What is your name?
- Do you have a middle name?
- How old are you?
- When were you born?

Place
- Do you know where you are right now?
- What kind of a place is this?
- Do you know what city and state we are in?
- What city or town do you live in?
- What is your address at home?

Time
- What is today's date?
- What day of the week is it?
- What time is it?
- Is it morning or afternoon?
- What season is it?
- What year is it?
- How long have you been here?

From Nolan,[26] p 26, with permission.

---

this cognitive function. Sample questions might include[26]:
- Who became president after Kennedy was shot?
- Who is the current vice president of the United States?
- Which is more—a gallon or a liter?
- In what country is the Great Pyramid?
- What would you add to your food to make it sweeter?
- In what state would you find the city of Boston?
- From where do the space shuttles take off?
- What are the elements that make up water and salt?
- Can you name a car made by general motors?
- Who is Charles Dickens?

Calculation ability assesses foundational mathematical abilities.[26,28] Two associated terms are **acalculia** (inability to calculate) and **dyscalculia** (difficulty in accomplishing calculations).[26] This cognitive test can be administered either verbally or in written format. The patient is asked to mentally perform a series of calculations when provided with mathematical problems. The test should be initiated with simple problems and progressed to the more difficult. Adding and subtracting are generally easier than multiplication and division. An alternative approach is to provide written mathematical problems and ask the patient to fill in the answer (e.g., $4 + 4 = \underline{\hphantom{00}}$; $10 + 22 = \underline{\hphantom{00}}$; $46 - 8 = \underline{\hphantom{00}}$; $13 - 7 = \underline{\hphantom{00}}$; $4 \times 3 = \underline{\hphantom{00}}$; $6 \times 6 = \underline{\hphantom{00}}$ etc.).

Proverb interpretation tests the patient's ability to interpret use of words outside of their usual context or meaning. This is a sophisticated cognitive function. During testing the patient should be asked to describe in his or her own words the meaning of the proverb. Several sample proverbs are[26,28]:
- People who live in glass houses should not throw stones.
- A rolling stone gathers no moss.
- A stitch in time save nine.
- The early bird catches the worm.
- The dog that trots about finds the bone.
- The empty wagon makes the most noise.
- Every cloud has a silver lining.

MEMORY, HEARING, AND VISUAL ACUITY

Also related to the ability to respond during sensory testing is the status of the patient's memory and hearing function as well as visual acuity.

Memory. Both long- and short-term memory should be assessed. Impairments of short-term memory will be the most disruptive to collecting sensory information owing to patient difficulties in remembering and following directions. Long-term (remote) memory can be assessed by requesting information on date and place of birth, number of siblings, date of marriage, what schools were attended, historical facts, and so forth. Short-term memory can be addressed by verbally providing the patient with a series of words or numbers. For example, a series of words might include "car, book, cup"; use of numbers could include a seven-digit list; a short sentence could also be used to test short-term memory. The sequence should be repeated immediately by the patient to ensure understanding of the task. Individuals with normal memory function should be able to recall the list 5 minutes[28] later and at least two of the items from the list after 30 minutes.[26]

Hearing. A gross assessment of hearing can be made by observing the patient's response to conversation. Note should be made of how alterations in voice volume and tone influence patient response.

Visual Acuity. A gross visual assessment can be made by use of a standard Snellen chart mounted on the wall or visual acuity cards for use at bedside. If the patient uses corrective lens, they should be worn during testing. Visual acuity is typically recorded at 20 feet from the Snellen chart (standard eye chart). This distance (20 feet) is then placed over the size of the type the individual is able to read comfortably. For example, on a continuum of visual acuity 20/20 is considered excellent and 20/200 is considered poor acuity.[28]

Peripheral field vision can be assessed by sitting directly in front of the patient with outstretched arms. The index fingers should be extended and gradually brought toward the midline of the patient's face. The patient is asked to identify when the therapist's approaching finger is first seen. Differences between right and left visual field should be noted carefully. Depth perception may be grossly checked by holding two pencils or fingers (one behind the other) directly in front of the patient. The patient is asked to identify the foreground object.

Because tests of sensory integrity require a verbal response to the stimulus, patients with arousal, attention, orientation, cognitive, or short-term memory impairments generally cannot be accurately tested. However, impairments in vision, hearing, or speech will not adversely affect test results if appropriate adaptations are made in providing instructions and indicating responses (e.g., signally with either one or two fingers during tests for two-point discrimination, pointing to an area of stimulus contact, mimicking joint position sense or awareness of movement with the contralateral extremity or object identification by selecting from a group of items during tests for stereognosis).

CLASSIFICATION OF THE SENSORY SYSTEM

Several different schemes have been proposed for categorizing the sensory system. Among the more common is classification by the type (or location) of *receptors* and the *spinal pathway* mediating information to higher centers.

Receptors

The three divisions of sensory receptors include those that mediate the (1) superficial, (2) deep, and (3) combined (cortical) sensations.[28]

1. *Superficial Sensation.* **Exteroceptors** are responsible for the superficial sensations.[29] They receive stimuli from the external environment via the skin and subcutaneous tissue. Exteroceptors are responsible for the perception of pain, temperature, light touch, and pressure.[28–30]
2. *Deep Sensation.* **Proprioceptors** are responsible for the deep sensations. These receptors receive stimuli from muscles, tendons, ligaments, joints, and fascia,[27] and are responsible for position sense and awareness of joints at rest,[2] movement awareness **(kinesthesia),** and vibration.[31]
3. *Combined Cortical Sensations.* The combination of both the superficial and deep sensory mechanisms makes up the third category of combined sensations. These sensations require information from both the exteroceptive and proprioceptive receptors, as well as intact function of cortical sensory association areas. The cortical combined sensations include stereognosis, two-point discrimination, barognosis, graphesthesia, tactile localization, recognition of texture, and double simultaneous stimulation.[3,31,32]

Spinal Pathways

Sensations also have been classified according to the system by which they are mediated to higher centers. Sensations are mediated by either the *anterolateral spinothalamic system* or the *dorsal column-medial lemniscal system.*[27–32]

ANTEROLATERAL SPINOTHALAMIC

This system initiates self-protective reactions and responds to stimuli that are potentially harmful in nature. It contains slow-conducting fibers of small diameter, some of which are unmyelinated.[27] The system is concerned with transmission of thermal and nociceptive information,[3] and mediates pain, temperature, crudely localized touch,[3,32] tickle, itch, and sexual sensations.[33]

DORSAL COLUMN-MEDIAL LEMNISCAL SYSTEM

The dorsal column is the system involved with responses to more discriminative sensations. It contains fast-conducting fibers of large diameter with greater myelination.[27,31,32] This system mediates the sensations of discriminative touch and pressure sensations, vibration, movement, position sense, and awareness of joints at rest.[3,31,32] The two systems are interdependent and integrated so as to function together.

Design and Function of Sensory Receptors

The sensory receptors frequently are divided according to their structural design and the type of stimulus to which they preferentially respond. These divisions include: (1) *mechanoreceptors*, which respond to mechanical deformation of the receptor or surrounding area; (2) *thermoreceptors*, which respond to changes in temperature; (3) *nociceptors*, which respond to noxious stimuli and result in the perception of pain; (4) *chemoreceptors*, which respond to chemical substances and are responsible for taste, smell, oxygen levels in arterial blood, carbon dioxide concentration, and osmolality (concentration gradient) of body fluids; and (5) *photic (electromagnetic) receptors*, which respond to light within the visible spectrum.[3,29–31,33]

The perception of pain is not limited to stimuli received from nociceptors, because other types of receptors and nerve fibers contribute to this sensation. High intensities of stimuli to any type of receptor may be perceived as pain (e.g., extreme heat or cold, and high-intensity mechanical deformation).

TYPES OF SENSORY RECEPTORS

The general classification of sensory receptors is presented in Box 6–2.[27,32–34] Note that this list also includes the receptors responsible for electromagnetic (visual) and chemical stimuli.

Cutaneous Receptors

Cutaneous sensory receptors are located at the terminal portion of the afferent fiber. These include free nerve endings, hair follicle endings, Merkel's disks, Ruffini endings, Krause's end-bulbs, Meissner's corpuscles, and Pacinian corpuscles. The den-

Box 6–2 CLASSIFICATION OF SENSORY RECEPTORS

I. Mechanoreceptors
   A. Cutaneous sensory receptors
      1. Free nerve endings
      2. Hair follicle endings
      3. Merkel's disks
      4. Ruffini endings
      5. Krause's end-bulbs
      6. Meissner's corpuscles
      7. Pacinian corpuscles
II. Deep sensory receptors
   A. Muscle receptors
      1. Muscle spindles
      2. Golgi tendon organs
      3. Free nerve endings
      4. Pacinian corpuscles
   B. Joint receptors
      1. Golgi-type endings
      2. Free nerve endings
      3. Ruffini endings
      4. Paciniform endings
III. Thermoreceptors
   A. Cold
      1. Cold receptors
   B. Warmth
      2. Warmth receptors
VI. Nocioceptors
   A. Pain
      1. Free nerve endings
      2. Extremes of stimuli[a]
V. Electromagnetic receptors
   A. Vision
      1. Rods
      2. Cones
V. Chemoreceptors
   A. Taste
      1. Receptors of taste buds
   B. Smell
      1. Receptors of olfactory nerves in olfactory epithelium
   C. Arterial oxygen
      1. Receptors of aortic and carotid bodies
   D. Osmolality
      1. Probably neurons of supraoptic nuclei
   E. Blood CO_2
      1. Receptors in or on surface of medulla and in aortic and carotid bodies
   F. Blood glucose, amino acids, fatty acids
      1. Receptors in hypothalamus

Adapted from Waxman and deGroot,[27] p 204, Fitzgerald,[32] p 86, Guyton and Hall,[33] p 376, and Fredericks[35] p 78.

[a]Extremes of stimuli to other sensory receptors will be perceived as pain.

sity of these sensory receptors varies for different areas of the body. For example, there are many more tactile receptors in the fingertips than in the back. These areas of higher receptor density correspondingly display a higher cortical representation in somatic sensory area I.[33] Receptor density is a particularly important consideration in interpreting the results of a sensory assessment for a given body surface. Figure 6-1 illustrates the cutaneous sensory receptors and their respective locations within the various layers of skin.

1. *Free nerve endings*. These receptors are found throughout the body. Stimulation of free nerve endings result in the perception of pain, temperature, touch, pressure, tickle, and itch sensations.[27,33]
2. *Hair follicle endings*. At the base of each hair follicle a free nerve ending is entwined. The combination of the hair follicle and its nerve provides a sensitive receptor. These receptors are sensitive to mechanical movement and touch.[3]
3. *Merkel's disks*. These receptors are located below the epidermis in hairy and glabrous skin. They are sensitive to low-intensity touch, as well as to the velocity of touch. They provide for the ability to perceive continuous contact of objects against the skin and are believed to play an important role in both two-point discrimination and localization of touch.[33,34]
4. *Ruffini endings*. Located in the deeper layers of the dermis, these encapsulated endings are involved with the perception of touch and pressure. They are particularly important in signaling continuous states of skin deformation.[28]
5. *Krause's end-bulb*. These receptors are located in the dermis. They are believed to have a contributing role in the perception of touch and pressure.[33]

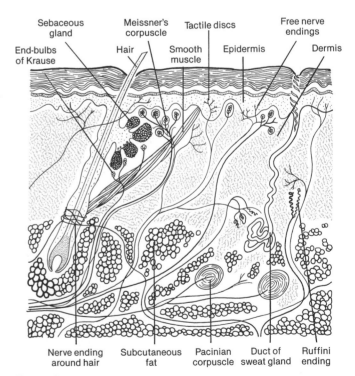

Figure 6-1. The cutaneous sensory receptors and their respective locations within the various layers of skin (epidermis, dermis, and the subcutaneous layer). From Gardner, E: Fundamentals of Neurology: A Psychophysiologic Approach, ed 6. WB Saunders, Philadelphia, 1975, p 222, with permission.

6. *Meissner's corpuscles.* Located in the dermis, these encapsulated nerve endings contain many nerve filaments within the capsule. They are in high concentration in the fingertips, lips, and toes, areas that require high levels of discrimination. These receptors play an important role in discriminative touch and the recognition of texture.[31–34]

7. *Pacinian corpuscles.* These receptors are located in the subcutaneous tissue layer of the skin and in deep tissues of the body (including tendons and soft tissues around joints). They are stimulated by rapid movement of tissue and are quickly adapting. They play a significant role in the perception of deep touch and vibration.[29,31,33]

Deep Sensory Receptors

The deep sensory receptors are located in muscles, tendons, and joints.[27,31,32] They include both muscle and joint receptors. They are concerned primarily with posture, position sense, proprioception, muscle tone, and speed and direction of movement. The deep sensory receptors include the muscle spindle, Golgi tendon organs, free nerve endings, pacinian corpuscles, and joint receptors.

Muscle Receptors

1. *Muscle spindles.* The muscle spindle fibers (intrafusal fibers) lie in a parallel arrangement to the muscle fibers (extrafusal fibers). They monitor changes in muscle length as well as velocity of these changes. The muscle spindle plays a vital role in position and movement sense and in motor learning.

2. *Golgi tendon organs.* These receptors are located in series at both the proximal and distal tendinous insertions of the muscle. The Golgi tendon organs function to monitor tension within the muscle. They also provide a protective mechanism by preventing structural damage to the muscle in situations of extreme tension. This is accomplished by inhibition of the contracting muscle and facilitation of the antagonist.

3. *Free nerve endings.* These receptors are within the fascia of the muscle. They are believed to respond to pain and pressure.

4. *Pacinian corpuscles.* Located within the fascia of the muscle, these receptors respond to vibratory stimuli and deep pressure.

Joint Receptors

1. *Golgi-type endings.* These receptors are located in the ligaments, and function to detect the rate of joint movement.

2. *Free nerve endings.* Found in the joint capsule and ligaments, these receptors are believed to respond to pain and crude awareness of joint motion.

3. *Ruffini endings.* Located in the joint capsule and ligaments, Ruffini endings are responsible for the direction and velocity of joint movement.

4. *Paciniform endings.* These receptors are found in the joint capsule and primarily monitor rapid joint movements.

TRANSMISSION OF SENSORY SIGNALS

Somatic sensory information enters the spinal cord through the dorsal roots. Sensory signals are then carried to higher centers via ascending pathways from one of two systems: *the anterolateral spinothalamic system* or the *dorsal column-medial lemniscal system.*

Anterolateral Spinothalamic System

The spinothalamic tracts are diffuse pathways concerned with nondiscriminative sensations such as pain, temperature, tickle, itch, and sexual sensations. This system is activated primarily by mechanoreceptors, thermoreceptors, and nociceptors, and is composed of afferent fibers that are small and slowly conducting. Sensory signals transmitted by this system do not require discrete localization of signal source or precise gradations in intensity.

After originating in the dorsal roots, the fibers of the spinothalamic system cross to the opposite anterolateral segment of the white matter (Fig. 6-2) and ascend diffusely in the anterior and lateral white columns. They demonstrate a diffuse pattern of termination at all levels of the lower brainstem as well as at the thalamus.[3,28,32]

Compared with the dorsal column-medial lemniscal system, the anterolateral spinothalamic pathways make up a cruder, more primitive system. The spinothalamic tracts are capable of transmitting a wide variety of sensory modalities. However, their diffuse pattern of termination results in only crude abilities to localize the source of a stimulus on the body surface, and poor intensity discrimination.[27]

The three major tracts of the spinothalamic system include the (1) *anterior (ventral) spinothalamic tract,* which carries the sensations of crudely localized touch and pressure; (2) the *lateral spinothalamic tract,* which carries pain and temperature; and (3) the *spinoreticular tract,* which is involved with diffuse pain sensations.[27]

Dorsal Column-medial Lemniscal System

This system is responsible for the transmission of discriminative sensations received from specialized mechanoreceptors. Sensory modalities that require fine gradations of intensity and precise localization on the body surface are mediated by this system. Sensations transmitted by the dorsal column-medial lemniscal pathway include discriminative touch, **stereognosis,** tactile pressure, **barognosis, graphesthesia,** recognition of texture, kinesthesia, **two-point discrimination,** proprioception, and vibration.[3,27,32]

This system is composed of large, rapidly conducting fibers. After entering the dorsal column the fibers ascend to the medulla and synapse with the

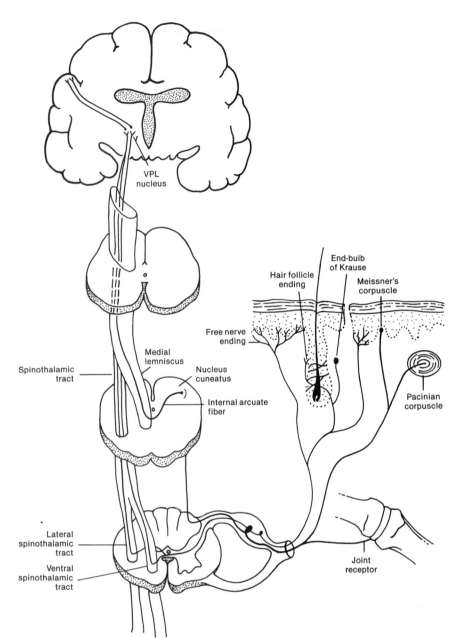

Figure 6-2. Cutaneous receptors and major spinal pathways mediating sensations. The afferent fibers conveying the superficial sensations are small, slow conducting, and travel by way of the spinothalamic tracts. The afferent fibers conveying the discriminative sensations are larger, faster conducting, and travel by way of the dorsal-lemniscus pathway. Branches for reflexes, pain, and temperature have been omitted. (From Brown, DR: Neurosciences for Allied Health Therapies. CV Mosby, St. Louis, 1980, p 222, with permission.)

dorsal column nuclei (nuclei gracilis and cuneatus). From here they cross to the opposite side and pass up to the thalamus through bilateral pathways called the *medial lemnisci*. Each medial lemniscus terminates in the ventral posterolateral thalamus. From the thalamus, third-order neurons project to the somatic sensory cortex. Projection to sensory association areas in cortex allows for the perception and interpretation of the combined cortical sensations (see Fig. 6-2).[27,33,34] Table 6–1 presents a comparison of the most salient features of each ascending fiber system.

SENSORY EXAMINATION PROTOCOL

The examination protocol includes the initial patient screening tests for mental status (arousal,

attention, orientation, cognition and memory), vision and hearing acuity (addressed earlier in this chapter); preparation of the testing environment; patient preparation and instruction; implementation of the tests; and documentation of findings.

For each sensory test, the following data will be generated:

1. The type of sensation tested
2. The quantity of involvement or body surface areas affected
3. The degree or severity of involvement (e.g., absent, impaired, or delayed responses)
4. Localization of the exact boundaries of the sensory impairment
5. The patient's subjective feelings about changes in sensation
6. The functional outcomes of sensory loss (e.g., injury to anesthetic limbs)

Table 6–1 SENSATION: ASCENDING FIBER SYSTEMS

System	Type of Sensation	Afferent Fibers	Origin	Termination
Spinothalamic	Nondiscriminative (e.g., pain, temperature); crude localization	Small, slowly conducting	Skin	From dorsal roots (horn), cross in spinal cord, second order neurons project to lower brainstem and thalamus.
Lemniscal	Discriminative (e.g., stereognosis, two-point discrimination); precise localization	Large, rapidly conducting	Skin, joints, tendons	From dorsal column nuclei; second-order neurons project to contralateral thalamus (cross in medulla); third-order neurons project to sensory cortex.

Preparation of the Testing Environment

The sensory examination should be administered in a quiet, well-lighted treatment area. Depending on the number of body areas to be tested, either a sitting or recumbent position may be used. If full body testing is indicated, both prone and supine positions will be required and use of a treatment table is recommended to allow assessment of each side of the body.

EQUIPMENT

To perform a sensory assessment the following equipment and materials are required:

1. A large-headed or safety pin or a large paper clip that has one segment bent open (providing one sharp and one dull end). The sharp end of the instrument should not be sharp enough to risk puncturing the skin. If a large-headed or safety pin is used, the sharp end may be made more blunt by a light sanding.
2. Two test tubes with stoppers.
3. A camel hair brush, a piece of cotton, or a tissue.
4. A variety of small commonly used articles such as a comb, fork, paper clip, key, coin, pencil, and so forth.
5. An aesthesiometer or an electrocardiogram (ECG) caliper[36] with the tips sanded to blunt the ends[37] and a small ruler. The aesthesiometer is a small hand-held instrument designed for measuring two-point discrimination. It consists of a small ruler with two moveable (sliding) brass tips coated with vinyl. Some instruments also have a third tip allowing ease of alternating from two-points to a single point of contact during testing.
6. A series of small weights of the same dimension but representing graduated increments in weight.
7. Samples of fabrics of various textures such as cotton, wool, or silk (approximately 4 × 4 inches [10 × 10 cm]).
8. Tuning fork and earphones (to reduce auditory clues).

PATIENT PREPARATION AND INSTRUCTION

Patient instruction prior to the sensory examination is an important consideration. A full explanation of the purpose of the testing should be provided. The patient also should be informed that his or her cooperation is necessary to obtain accurate test results. It is of considerable importance that the patient be instructed not to guess if he or she is uncertain of the correct response.

During the assessment, the patient should be in a comfortable, relaxed position. Preferably, the tests should be performed when the patient is well rested. Considering the high level of concentration required, it is not surprising that fatigue has been noted to affect results of some sensory tests adversely.[36] A "trial run" or demonstration of each test should be performed just prior to actual administration. This will orient the patient to the sensation being tested, what to anticipate, and what type of response is required.

Some method of occluding the patient's vision during the testing should be used (vision should not be occluded during the explanation and demonstration). Visual input is prevented because it may allow for compensation of a sensory deficit and thus decrease the accuracy of test results. The traditional methods of occluding vision are by use of a blindfold (a small folded towel can be used effectively) or by asking the patient to keep the eyes closed. These methods are practical in most instances. However, in situations of CNS dysfunction, a patient may become anxious[38] or disoriented[39] if vision is occluded for a long period of time. In these situations a small screen[38,39] or folder[38] can be used as a visual barrier may be preferable to restrict visual input. Whatever method is used, it should be removed between the tests while directions and demonstrations are provided.

Implementation of Tests and Documentation of Findings

The superficial (exteroceptive) sensations are usually assessed first, inasmuch as they consist of more primitive responses, followed by the deep (proprioceptive), and then the combined cortical sensations. If a test indicates impairment of the superficial responses, some impairment of the more discriminative (deep and combined) sensations also will be noted and may be a contraindication to further testing (e.g., lack of touch sensation would be a contraindication for testing stereognosis). The primary mode of sensation must be sufficiently intact to permit meaningul testing of cortical sensory function.

Knowledge of peripheral nerve innervation (Fig. 6-3) and the sensory nerve segmental (dermatome) supply is required for making sound, accurate diagnostic and prognostic judgements. The **dermatomes** (Fig. 6-4) are the cutaneous areas that correspond to the spinal segments providing their innervation. Dermatome charts do not represent discrete boundaries because some overlap of innervation exists at the borders of adjacent dermatomes. However, peripheral nerve innervation and dermatome charts (see Figs. 6-3 and 6-4) are useful references during testing, and they provide a guide for recording results.

Sensory tests are typically performed in a distal to proximal direction. This progression will conserve time, particularly when dealing with localized lesions involving a single extremity, where deficits tend to be more severe distally. It is generally not necessary to test every segment of each dermatome; testing general body areas is sufficient. However,

once a deficit area is noted, testing must become more discrete and the exact boundaries of the impairment should be identified. A skin pencil may be useful to mark the boundaries of sensory change directly. This information should be transferred later to a sensory assessment form, graphically presented on a dermatome chart, and peripheral nerve involvement identified (Fig. 6-5). This form will then be entered in the medical record.

Most often the dermatome charts are completed using a color code (i.e., each color represents a different sensation). The colors used to plot each sensation are then coded by the examiner directly on the assessment form (see Fig. 6-5). In many instances hatch marks of varying density are used to represent gradations in sensory impairment (i.e., the closer together, the greater the sensory impairment). With this method, a completely colored-in area indicates no response to a given sensation. With varied or "spotty" sensory loss it is not uncommon that more than one dermatome chart is required to completely depict all test findings. With use of several dermatome charts, the sensation represented should appear in bold print at the top of each page.

During testing, the application of stimuli should be applied in a random, unpredictable manner with variation in timing.[39] This will improve accuracy of the test results by avoiding a consistent pattern of application, which might provide the patient with "clues" to the correct response. During application

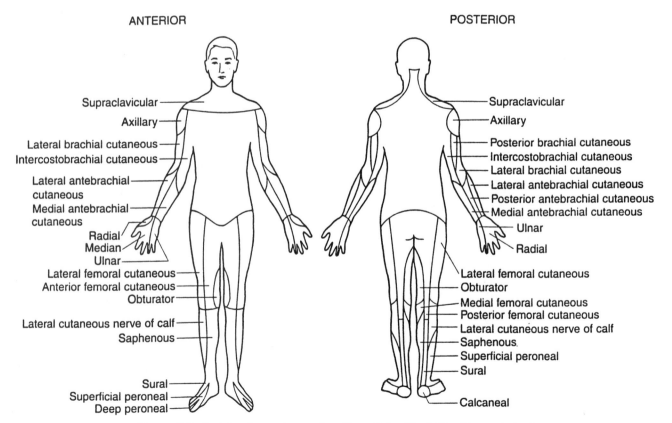

Figure 6-3. Peripheral nerve innervation. (From Nolan,[26] p 168, with permission.)

ANTERIOR POSTERIOR

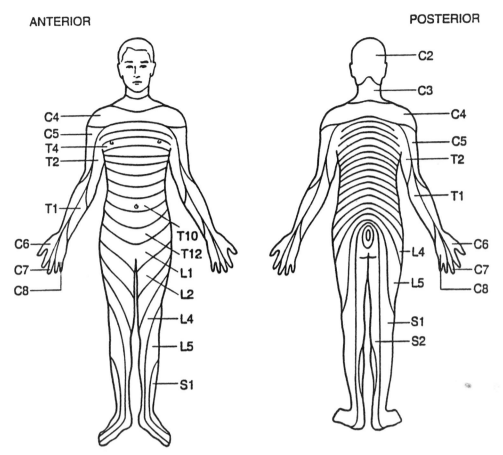

Figure 6-4. The dermatome chart represents the cutaneous areas supplied by a single dorsal root and its ganglia. (From Nolan,[26] p 167, with permission.)

of stimuli, consideration must be given also to skin condition. Scar tissue or callused areas are generally less sensitive and will demonstrate a diminished response to sensory stimuli.

The following sections present the individual sensory tests. The tests are subdivided for superficial, deep, and combined cortical sensations. Table 6–2 provides the terminology used to describe common sensory deficits.

SUPERFICIAL SENSATIONS
Pain
Test. The sharp end of a large-headed or safety pin, or reshaped paperclip is used (the segment pulled away from the body of the paper clip provides a sharp end). The instrument should be carefully cleaned before administering the test and disposed of immediately afterward. The sharp point is applied to the patient's skin (sharp end of pin or paper clip). To avoid summation of impulses, the stimuli should not be applied too close to each other or in rapid succession. To maintain a uniform pressure with each successive application of stimuli, the pin or reshaped paper clip should be held firmly and the fingers allowed to "slide" down the pin or paper clip once in contact with the skin. This will avoid the chance of gradually increasing pressure during application. The instrument used to test pain per-

ception should be sharp enough to deflect the skin, but not puncture it.

Response. The patient is asked to verbally indicate when a stimulus is felt. All areas of the body should be tested.

Temperature
Test. Two test tubes with stoppers are required for this assessment; one should be filled with warm water and the other with crushed ice. Ideal temperatures for cold are between 41°F (5°C) and 50°F (10°C) and for warmth, between 104°F (40°C) and 113°F (45°C). Caution should be exercised to remain within these ranges, because exceeding these temperatures may elicit a pain response and consequently inaccurate test results. The test tubes are randomly placed in contact with the skin area to be tested. All skin surfaces should be tested.

Response. The patient is asked to indicate when a stimulus is felt and to reply "warm," "cold," or "unable to tell."

It should be noted that clinical usefulness of thermal testing may be problematic. Nolan[36] points out that the tests are extremely difficult to duplicate on a day-to-day basis because of rapid changes in temperature once the test tubes are exposed to room air. Although it is a simple test to perform, assessing changes over time is not practical unless a method

This form provides a record of the type, severity, and location of the sensory impairment(s). It should be used in conjunction with additional dermatome sheets, if needed, to graphically outline the exact boundaries of the impairment. The designations P and D may be added to the grading key to indicate either a proximal (P) or a distal (D) location of the impairment on the limb or body part. The dermatome chart should be color coded and filled in using varying density hatch mark (higher density for more severe the impairment). Please also indicate the color code used for documenting the data (a different color should be used for superficial, deep, and combined sensations). Separate notation should be made for assessment of the face. Abnormal responses should be briefly described in the comments section.

Name: _____ Date: _____
Examiner: _____

Key to Grading*
1. Intact: normal, accurate response
2. Decreased: delayed response
3. Exaggerated: increased sensitivity or awareness of the stimulus after it has ceased
4. Inaccurate: inappropriate perception of a given stimulus
5. Absent: No response
6. Inconsistent or ambiguous: response inadequate to assess sensory function accurately

Sensations	Upper Extremity		Lower Extremity		Trunk	
	Right	Left	Right	Left	Right	Left
Superficial						
Pain						
Temperature						
Light touch						
Pressure						
Deep (Proprioceptive)						
Movement sense			NA	NA	NA	NA
Position sense			NA	NA	NA	NA
Vibration						
Combined (Cortical)						
Sharp/dull discrimination						
Tactile localization						
Two-point discrimination						
Bilateral simultaneous stimulation						
Stereognosis			NA	NA	NA	NA
Barognosis			NA	NA	NA	NA
Graphesthesia			NA	NA	NA	NA
Recognition of texture						

Color Code:
Superficial _____
Deep _____
Combined _____

Peripheral Nerve Involvement: _____

Comments:

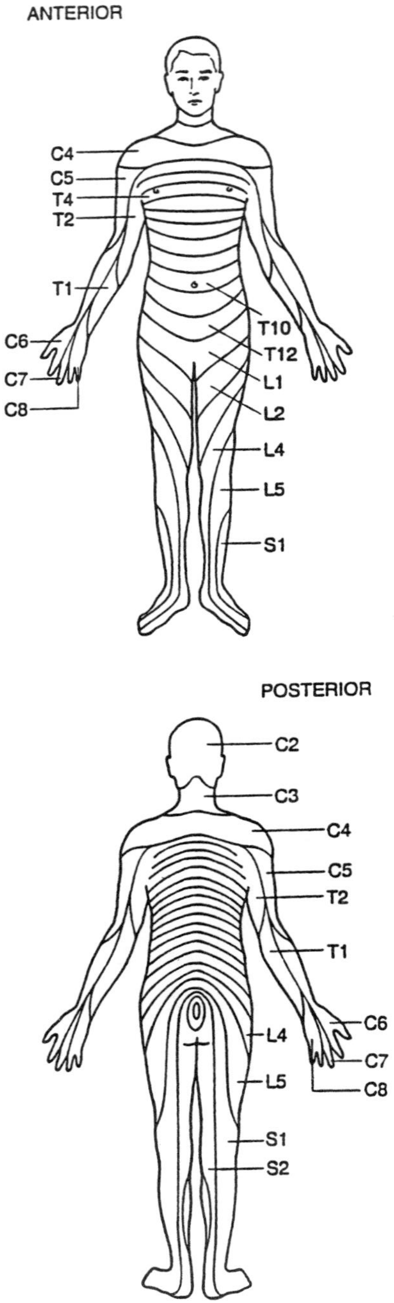

Figure 6-5. Sensory assessment documentation form.

144

Table 6–2 TERMINOLOGY DESCRIBING COMMON SENSORY IMPAIRMENTS

Abarognosis	Inability to recognize weight
Allesthesia	Sensation experienced at a site remote from point of stimulation
Allodynia	Pain produced by a non-noxious stimulus (e.g., touch)
Analgesia	Complete loss of pain sensitivity
Astereognosis	Inability to recognize the form and shape of objects by touch (synonym: tactile agnosia)
Atopognosia	Inability to localize a sensation
Causalagia	Painful, burning sensations, usually along the distribution of a nerve
Dysesthesia	Touch sensation experienced as pain
Hypalgesia	Decreased sensitivity to pain
Hyperalgesia	Increased sensitivity to pain
Hyperesthesia	Increased sensitivity to sensory stimuli
Hypesthesia	Decreased sensitivity to sensory stimuli
Pallanesthesia	Loss or absence of sensibility to vibration
Paresthesia	Abnormal sensation such as numbness, prickling, or tingling, without apparent cause
Thalamic syndrome	Vascular lesion of the thalamus resulting in sensory disturbances and partial or complete paralysis of one side of the body, associated with severe, boring-type pain. Sensory stimuli may produce an exaggerated, prolonged, or painful response
Thermanalgesia	Inability to perceive heat
Thermanesthesia	Inability to perceive sensations of heat and cold
Thermhyperesthesia	Increased sensitivity to temperature
Thermhypesthesia	Decreased temperature sensibility
Thigmanesthesia	Loss of light touch sensibility

of monitoring the temperature of the test tubes is used.[36]

Light Touch

Test. For this test a camel-hair brush, piece of cotton, or tissue is used. The area to be tested is lightly touched or stroked.

Response. The patient is asked to indicate when he or she recognizes that a stimulus has been applied by responding "yes" or "now."

Pressure

Test. The therapist's thumb or fingertip is used to apply a firm pressure on the skin surface. This pressure should be firm enough to indent the skin[38,39] and to stimulate the deep receptors.[39] This test can also be administered using the thumb and fingers to squeeze the Achilles tendon.[26]

Response. The patient is asked to indicate when he or she recognizes that a stimulus has been applied by responding "yes" or "now."

DEEP SENSATIONS

The deep sensations include **kinesthesia, proprioception,** and **vibration.** Kinesthesia is the awareness of movement. Proprioception includes position sense and the awareness joints at rest.[2] Vibration refers to the ability to perceive a rapidly oscillating or vibratory stimuli. Although these sensations are closely related, they should be assessed individually.

Kinesthesia

Test. This test examines *awareness of movement.* The extremity or joint(s) to be assessed is moved passively through a relatively small range of motion. Small increments in range of motion are used as joint receptors fire at specific points throughout the range. The therapist should identify the range of motion being assessed (e.g., initial, mid-, or terminal range). As discussed, a trial run or demonstration of the procedure should be performed prior to actual testing. This will ensure that the patient and the therapist agree on terms to describe the direction of movements.

Response. The patient is asked to indicate verbally the direction of movement while the extremity is in *motion.* The patient is asked to describe the direction and range of movement in terms previously discussed with the therapist ("up," "down," "in," "out," etc.). The patient may also respond by simultaneously duplicating the movement with the opposite extremity. This second approach, however, is usually impractical with proximal lower extremity joints, owing to potential stress on the low back. During testing, movement of larger joints is usually discerned more quickly than that of smaller joints. The therapist's grip should remain constant and minimal (finger-tip grip over bony prominences), to reduce tactile stimulation.

Proprioception

Test. This test examines *joint position sense* and *the awareness joints at rest.* The extremity or joint(s) to be assessed is moved through a range of motion and held in a static position. Again, small increments in range of motion are used. The words selected to identify the range of motion examined should be identified to the patient during the practice trial (e.g., initial, mid-, or terminal range). As with kinesthesia, caution should be used with hand placements to avoid excessive tactile stimulation.

Response. While the extremity or joint(s) under assessment is held in a static position by the therapist, the patient is asked to describe the position verbally or to duplicate the position of the extremity or joint(s) with the contralateral extremity.

Vibration

Test. This test requires a tuning fork that vibrates at 128Hz.[26] The ability to perceive a vibratory stimulus is tested by placing the base of a vibrating tuning fork on a bony prominence (such as the sternum, elbow, or ankle). If intact, the patient will perceive the vibration. If there is impairment, the patient will be unable to distinguish between a vibrating and nonvibrating tuning fork. Therefore, there should be a random application of vibrating and nonvibrating stimuli. Earphones may be used for this test procedure to reduce auditory clues from the vibrating fork. It should be noted that the tuning fork provides only a gross assessment of the ability to perceive vibrating stimuli; the frequency of vibration cannot be held constant during the test procedure.

Response. The patient is asked to respond by verbally identifying the stimulus as vibrating or nonvibrating each time the base of the fork is placed in contact with a bony prominence.

COMBINED CORTICAL SENSATIONS
Tactile Object Recognition (Stereognosis)

Test. Testing for tactile object recognition requires use of items of differing size and shape. A variety of small, easily obtainable and culturally familiar objects can be used. These objects may include keys, coins, combs, safety pins, pencils, and so forth. The patient is given a single object, allowed to manipulate the object, and then asked to identify the item verbally. The patient should be allowed to handle several sample test items during the explanation and demonstration of the procedure.

Response. The patient is asked to name the object verbally. For patients with speech impairments the item can be selected from a group after each test.

Tactile Localization

Test. This test assesses the ability to localize touch sensation on the skin. Using a fingertip, the therapist touches different skin surfaces. After each application of a stimulus the patient is given time to respond.

Response. The patient is asked to identify the location of the stimuli by pointing to the area or by verbal description. The patient's eyes may be open during the response component of this test. Tactile localization may be tested separately or included with other tests.[39] The distance between the application of the stimulus and the site indicated by the patient can be measured and recorded. Accuracy of localization over different parts of the body may be compared to determine the relative sensitivity of different areas.

Two-Point Discrimination

Test. This test assesses the ability to perceive two points applied to the skin simultaneously. It is a measure of the smallest distance between two stimuli (applied simultaneously and with equal pressure) that can still be perceived as two distinct stimuli.[36] This assessment is among the most practical and easily duplicated test for cutaneous sensation. Two-point discrimination has been the subject of a series of studies by Nolan.[41–43] The purpose of his research was to establish normative data on two-point discrimination for young adults. His sample consisted of 43 college students ranging in age from 20 to 24 years. Values from Nolan's studies are presented in Table 6–3 for the upper extremity, Table 6–4 for the lower extremity, and Table 6–5 for the face and trunk. These findings are consistent with earlier, less extensive studies on two-point

Table 6–3 TWO-POINT DISCRIMINATION VALUES FOR THE UPPER EXTREMITIES OF HEALTHY SUBJECTS 20 TO 24 YEARS OF AGE (N = 43)

Skin Region	$\overline{X}$ (mm)	s
Upper—lateral arm	42.4	14.0
Lower—lateral arm	37.8	13.1
Mid—medial arm	45.4	15.5
Mid—posterior arm	39.8	12.3
Mid—lateral forearm	35.9	11.6
Mid—medial forearm	31.5	8.9
Mid—posterior forearm	30.7	8.2
Over first dorsal interosseous muscle	21.0	5.6
Palmar surface—distal phalanx, thumb	2.6	0.6
Palmar surface—distal phalanx, long finger	2.6	0.7
Palmar surface—distal phalanx, little finger	2.5	0.7

From Nolan,[43] with permission of the American Physical Therapy Association.

discrimination in the upper limb.[40,44] Normative values are extremely useful in interpreting test results from sensory assessments, as well as from other types of assessments. However, the results from these studies[41–43] must be used cautiously, inasmuch as they relate to a specific population. They should not be generalized for interpreting data from older or younger patients.

Several instruments have been described for use in measuring two-point discrimination. These include a reshaped paper clip,[45] a Boley gauge,[37] an aesthesiometer,[36,39] and an ECG caliper. The ECG caliper (a compass-type device) has been identified as a particularly practical, inexpensive, and easily obtained tool for measuring two-point discrimination.[36] Prior to use for two-point discrimination testing, the tips of the ECG caliper should be lightly sanded to form blunt ends.[37] This will ensure that the tactile stimulus will not be perceived as painful.

During the test procedure the two tips of the instrument are applied to the skin simultaneously. With each successive application, the two tips are gradually brought closer together until the stimuli are perceived as one. The smallest distance between the stimuli that is still perceived as two distinct points is measured with a ruler and recorded. To

Table 6–4 TWO-POINT DISCRIMINATION VALUES FOR THE LOWER EXTREMITIES OF HEALTHY SUBJECTS 20 TO 24 YEARS OF AGE (N = 43)

Skin Region	$\overline{X}$ (mm)	s
Proximal—anterior thigh	40.1	14.7
Distal—anterior thigh	23.2	9.3
Mid—lateral thigh	42.5	15.9
Mid—medial thigh	38.5	12.4
Mid—posterior thigh	42.2	15.9
Proximal—lateral leg	37.7	13.0
Distal—lateral leg[a]	41.6	13.0
Medial leg	43.6	13.5
Tip of great toe	6.6	1.8
Over 1–2 metatarsal interspace	23.9	6.3
Over 5th metatarsal	22.2	8.6

From Nolan,[41] with permission of the American Physical Therapy Association.

[a]n = 41.

Table 6–5 TWO-POINT DISCRIMINATION VALUES FOR THE FACE AND TRUNK OF HEALTHY SUBJECTS 20 TO 24 YEARS OF AGE (N = 43)

Skin Region	X̄ (mm)	s
Over eyebrow	14.9	4.2
Cheek	11.9	3.2
Over lateral mandible	10.4	2.2
Lateral neck	35.2	9.8
Medial to acromion process	51.1	14.0
Lateral to nipple	45.7	12.7[a]
Lateral to umbilicus	36.4	7.3[b]
Over iliac crest	44.9	10.1[c]
Lateral to C7 spine	55.4	20.0[b]
Over inferior angle of scapula	52.2	12.6[b]
Lateral to L3 spine	49.9	12.7[b]

From Nolan,[42] with permission of the American Physical Therapy Association.
[a]n = 26.
[b]n = 42.
[c]n = 33.

increase the validity of the test, it is appropriate to alternate the application of two stimuli with the random application of only a single stimulus. It is also important to consider that perception of two-point discrimination varies considerably for different individuals and body parts, being most refined in the distal upper extremities. In testing for two-point discrimination, both intraindividual[41] and interindividual[41–43] variations in perception of the stimulus must be considered.

Response. The patient is asked to identify the perception of "one" or "two" stimuli.

Double Simultaneous Stimulation (DSS)

Test. The test examines the ability to perceive a simultaneous touch stimulus on opposite sides of the body; proximally and distally on a single extremity; or proximally and distally on one side of the body. The therapist simultaneously (and with equal pressure) (1) touches identical locations on opposite sides of the body, (2) touches proximally and distally on opposite sides of the body, and (3) touches proximal and distal locations on the same side of the body. The term *extinction phenomena* is used to describe a situation in which only the proximal stimulus is perceived, with "extinction" of the distal.

Response. The patient verbally states when he or she perceives a touch stimulus and the number of stimuli felt.

Several additional tests for the combined (cortical) sensations include recognition of weight (barognosis), traced finger identification (graphesthesia), and recognition of texture. However, these tests are usually not performed if stereognosis and two-point discrimination are found to be intact.

Recognition of Weight (Barognosis)

Test. To assess recognition of weight, a series of small objects of the same size but of graduated weight is used. The therapist may choose to place a series of different weights in the same hand one at a time, or to place a different weight in each hand simultaneously.

Response. The patient is asked to identify the comparative weight of objects in a series (i.e., to compare the relative weight of the object with the previous one); or when the objects are placed in both hands simultaneously the patient is asked to compare the weight of the two objects. The patient responds by indicating that the object is "heavier" or "lighter."

Traced Figure Identification (Graphesthesia)

Test. The recognition of letters, numbers, or designs traced on the skin is assessed by the use of the eraser end of a pencil. A series or combination of letters, numbers, or designs is traced on the palm of the patient's hand. During the practice trial, agreement should be reached about the orientation of the tracings. (For example, the bottom of the traced figures will always be oriented toward the base of the patient's hand.) Between each separate drawing the palm should be gently wiped with a soft cloth to clearly indicate a change in figures to the patient. This test is also a useful substitute for stereognosis when paralysis prevents grasping an object.

Response. The patient is asked to identify verbally the figures drawn on the skin. For patients with speech deficits the figures can be selected (pointed to) from a series of line drawings.

Recognition of Texture

Test. This test examines the ability to differentiate among various textures. Suitable textures may include cotton, wool, or silk. The items are placed individually in the patient's hand. The patient is allowed to manipulate the sample texture.

Response. The patient is asked to identify the individual textures as they are placed in the hand. They may be identified by name (e.g., silk, cotton) or by texture (e.g., rough, smooth).

Reliability of Sensory Testing

As with all examination procedures, the reliability of sensory testing is an important consideration for physical therapists. Currently, there are few systematic reports of data collection related to the reliability of sensory tests. In a study by Kent,[40] the upper limbs of 50 adult patients with hemiplegia were tested for sensory and motor deficits. Three sensory tests were administered and then repeated by the same examiner within 1 to 7 days. Results revealed a high reliability for both stereognosis ($r = 0.97$) and position sense ($r = 0.90$). A lower reliability was reported for two-point discrimination, with correlation coefficients ranging from 0.59 to 0.82, depending on the body area tested.

Although limited published data are available related to reliability measures, several approaches can be used to improve this aspect of the tests. These include (1) use of consistent guidelines for completing the tests; (2) administration of the tests by trained, skillful examiners; and (3) subsequent retests performed by the same individual. It also should be noted that the reliability of sensory tests will be further influenced by the patient's understanding of the test procedure and the patient's ability to communicate results.

Additional research related to standardization of testing protocols, development of quantitative approaches to collecting information, and establishment of additional normative data for various age groups will improve the reliability, validity, and future clinical application of test results.

SOMATOSENSORY SYSTEM

Interpretation and analysis of sensory information occurs in the sensory association areas of the cortex (see Fig. 6-6A). This process of assessing information provides meaning to environmental and peripheral sensory input. The somatosensory cortex is divided into three main divisions: the primary (SI) and secondary (SII) areas, and the posterior parietal cortex. These higher level somatosensory processing areas integrate cognitive and perceptual information in preparation for a motor response.[46,47]

Animal models have provided considerable insight into the function of the cortical association areas. Complete removal of area SI of the somatosensory system produces deficits in position sense and the ability to determine the size, texture, and shape of objects. Temperature and pain perception are diminished but not abolished. Owing to reliance on input from SI, removal of SII results in severe impairment of the perception of both shape and texture of objects. Animal models have also shown reduced ability to learn new discriminative tasks, which are based on the shape of an object. Insult to the posterior parietal cortex presents profound impairments in attending to sensory input from the contralateral side of the body.[46]

The sensory homunculus is a useful reference tool for gross localization of impairment within the sensory cortex. Although it has been criticized as an overly simplified view of the somatosensory system, it also provides insight into the relative density of sensory innervation for different parts of the body (see Fig. 6–6B). Note that the cortical areas for the trunk and back are small, implying a reduced role in sensory perception and lower receptor density. In contrast, relatively large areas represent the lips, face, and fingers. This distortion in size of body parts is representative of differences in innervation density. The areas with

Table 6–6 FUNCTIONAL COMPONENTS OF THE CRANIAL NERVES

Number	Name	Components	Function
I	Olfactory	Afferent	Olfaction (smell)
II	Optic	Afferent	Vision
III	Oculomotor	Efferent	
		Somatic	Elevates eyelid
		Visceral	Turns eye up, down, in
			Constricts pupil
			Accommodates lens
IV	Trochlear	Efferent (somatic)	Turns the adducted eye down and causes intorsion of eye
V	Trigeminal	Mixed	
		Afferent	Sensation from face
			Sensation from cornea
			Sensation from anterior tongue
		Efferent	Muscles of mastication
			Dampens sound (tensor tympani)
VI	Abducens	Efferent (somatic)	Turns eye out
VII	Facial	Mixed	
		Afferent	Taste from anterior tongue
		Efferent (somatic)	Muscles of facial expression
			Dampens sound (stapedius)
		Efferent (visceral)	Tearing (lacrimal gland)
			Salivation (submandibular and sublingual glands)
VIII	Vestibulocochlear	Afferent	Balance (semicircular canals, utricle, saccule)
			Hearing (organ of Corti)
IX	Glossopharyngeal	Mixed	
		Afferent	Taste from posterior tongue
			Sensation from posterior tongue
			Sensation from oropharynx
		Efferent	Salivation (parotid gland)
X	Vagus	Mixed	
		Afferent	Thoracic and abdominal viscera
		Efferent	Muscles of larynx and pharynx
			Decreases heart rate
			Increases GI motility
XI	Spinal accessory	Efferent	Head movements (sternocleidomastoid and trapezius)
XII	Hypoglossal	Efferent	Tongue movements and shape

From Nolan,[26] p 44, with permission.
GI, gastrointestinal.

greater cortical representation perceive finer gradations of sensory stimuli. Given the paucity of normative values for sensory testing, the homunculus can guide interpretation of results by indicating body areas that typically respond to discrete gradations of sensation versus those which normally provide only crude localization.[46]

CRANIAL NERVE SCREENING

Screening tests for the cranial nerves provide the physical therapist with information about location of dysfunction within the brainstem as well as which cranial nerves require an in-depth examination.[2] Data generated may include function of muscles innervated by the cranial nerves; visual, auditory, sensory, and gag reflex integrity; perception of taste; swallowing characteristics; eye movements; and constriction and dilation patterns of the pupils.[2]

Screening tests are guided by their specific function (e.g., taste, smell, visual acuity). Table 6–6 provides a summary of the functional components of the cranial nerves. Box 6–3 presents screening tests for each cranial nerve. Deficits noted in response to a screening test indicate a detailed assessment of function is warranted.

Box 6–3 SCREENING TESTS FOR CRANIAL NERVES[26,28]

Cranial nerve I: Assess olfactory acuity using non-noxious odors such as lemon oil, coffee, cloves or tobacco.

Cranial nerve II: Examine visual acuity using a Snell chart; both central and peripheral vision are tested.

Cranial nerves III, IV, and VI: Determine equality and size of pupils; reaction to light; presence of strabismus (loss of ocular alignment); ability of eyes to follow a moving target without head movement; presence of ptosis of eyelid.

Cranial nerve V: Sensory tests of face (sharp/dull discrimination, light touch); open and close jaw against resistance; jaw jerk reflex.

Cranial nerve VII: Assess any asymmetry of face at rest and during voluntary contraction.

Cranial nerve VIII: Test auditory acuity using a vibrating tuning fork (Weber test) placed on vertex of skull or forehead, patient indicates on which side the tone is louder; rub fingers together at a distance and gradually bring toward patient, note distance when first heard; alter volume of conversation; Rinne test (air versus bone conduction) vibrating tuning fork place on mastoid process, then near external ear canal, note hearing acuity.

Cranial nerve IX: Assess taste on posterior one-third of tongue; assess gag reflex.

Cranial nerve X: Assess swallowing; observe uvula and soft palate for any asymmetry (tongue depressor).

Cranial nerve XI: Assess strength of the sternocleidomastoid and trapezius muscles.

Cranial nerve XII: With tongue protruded, assess ability to move tongue rapidly from side-to-side.

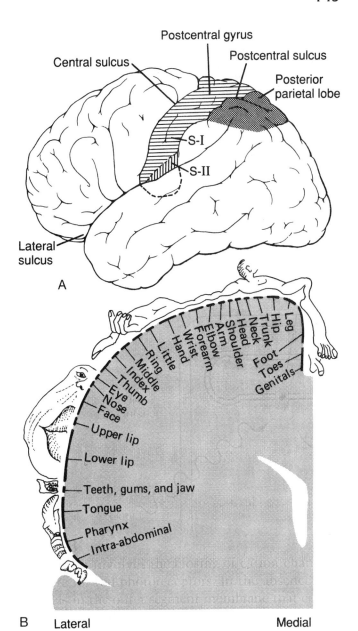

Figure 6-6. (*A*) The somatosensory cortex has three main divisions: The primary (SI) and secondary (SII) areas, and the posterior parietal lobe. (*B*) The sensory homunculus. Areas of the body used for tactile discrimination are represented by large areas of cortical tissue, such as the lips, tongue, and fingers. Areas with reduced cortical representation, such as the trunk, are reflective of body parts with lesser roles in sensory perception. (From Kandel, ER, Schwartz, JH and Jessel, TM: Principles of Neural Science (ed. 3) Appleton and Lange, Norwalk, CT, 1991 with permission,[46] pp 368 and 372.

SENSORY INTEGRITY WITHIN THE CONTEXT OF TREATMENT

Learning a motor behavior is dependent on the patient's ability to take in sensory information from the body and the environment (sensory intake), process it (sensory integration), and use it to plan and organize behavior (output). When patients experience impairment in processing sensory intake, deficits occur in planning and organizing behavior. This produces behaviors that may interfere with successful motor learning and motor function.

The plan of care designed for a patient with impaired sensation is typically guided by one of two approaches, the *Sensory Integration Approach* and the *Compensatory Approach*. The physical therapist's selection of a treatment model is based on a complete data set of information from all examinations together with the established prognosis and diagnosis. The treatment approach depicted in Fig. 6-7 is based largely on the Sensory Integration Model developed by Ayers.[48–53] The basic premise of this approach is that specific treatment techniques can enhance sensory integration (CNS processing) with a resultant change in motor performance.

Using the Sensory Integration Approach, data obtained from sensory testing assist the physical therapist in developing a plan of care to enhance opportunities for *controlled* sensory intake within a framework of meaningful functional skills (see Chapter 13). During treatment, the patient is provided guided practice in planning and organizing motor behaviors using both *intrinsic* feedback (from the movement itself) and *augmented* feedback (cues planned by the therapist). This approach is designed to improve the ability of the CNS to process and integrate information and promote motor learning.[1] The reader is referred to the work of Ayers[48–53] and Fisher et al.[1] for a detailed presentation of both the theory and practice of the Sensory Integration Model.

The Compensatory Approach is a more traditional intervention that focuses on patient education to accommodate to the limitations imposed by the sensory deficit. The therapist's role is to assist the patient in achieving optimum functional capacity, minimizing functional limitations, protecting anesthetic limbs, and creating appropriate environmental adaptations to enhance safety and function. Guided by this approach, the therapist instructs the patient in practical strategies such as testing bath water with a thermometer or body part with intact sensation before entering; not going barefoot; regularly checking insensitive skin areas for cuts or bruises (particularly important for patients with diabetes); adaptations can include: substituting vision for absent tactile cues when carrying objects; wearing heat-resistant gloves when working in the kitchen; using a rolling cart in kitchen or other work space to transport items from one area to another; and arranging kitchen supplies to eliminate need for access to storage areas directly over the stove.

SUMMARY

Sensory tests provide important information related to the integrity of the sensory system. Results from these tests assist in making clinical judgements about diagnosis, prognosis, and establishing goals and outcomes. The data also assist in determining the plan of care. Periodic repetition of the sensory tests assists in determining progress toward achieving anticipated goals and desired outcomes.

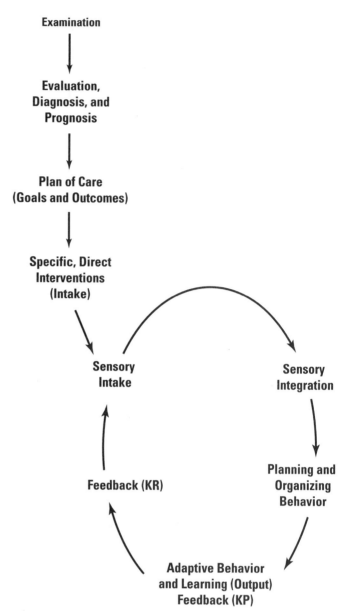

Figure 6-7. Elements of patient management for sensory impairment. KP refers to knowledge of performance (feedback about the quality of movement produced) and KR refers to knowledge of result (feedback about the end result or outcome of the movement). (Adapted from Fisher and Murray,[1] p 5)

Individual tests for each sensory modality have been presented. Reliability of these test procedures can be improved by careful adherence to consistent guidelines, administration of tests by trained individuals, and subsequent retests performed by the same examiner. Documentation of test results should address the type(s) of sensation affected, the quantity and degree of involvement, and localization of the exact boundaries of the sensory deficits. Finally, it should be emphasized that additional research related to sensory testing is warranted. The development of standardized protocols, reliability measures, and additional normative data will significantly improve the clinical applications of data obtained from sensory tests.

QUESTIONS FOR REVIEW

1. Define sensory integrity.

2. Identify six impairments or functional limitations that would warrant a sensory assessment.

3. Describe the preliminary gross screening tests used to determine mental status for each of the following areas: arousal, attention, orientation, and cognition.

4. Identify the seven types of *cutaneous* receptors, their location, and types of stimuli to which they respond.

5. Identify the four types of *muscle* receptors, their location, and types of stimuli to which they respond.

6. Identify the four types of *joint* receptors, their location, and types of stimuli to which they respond.

7. Identify the sensations mediated by the (A) anterolateral spinothalamic system and the (B) dorsal column-medial lemniscal system.

8. Describe the type of data generated from sensory testing and how it is used by the physical therapist.

9. Describe the equipment required to administer a sensory assessment.

10. Identify the information you would provide the patient prior to administration of sensory tests.

11. For each of the three groups of sensations (superficial, deep, and combined cortical) describe each sensory test, providing both the test protocol and directions for patient response.

12. Describe the method(s) you would use to record the results of sensory testing.

CASE STUDY

A 61-year-old woman presents for outpatient physical therapy. She arrives in a rented wheelchair accompanied by her son. On initial meeting, the patient greets you with a verbal "hello" and a handshake. The son speaks for his mother and recounts that she has been complaining of a burning feeling in her feet and difficulty ambulating.

The son indicates that his mother took an early retirement four years ago from her position as an elementary school teacher. This was a position she had held and enjoyed for 25 years. Her children encouraged the retirement. Their mother had frequently complained about difficulty keeping up with the teaching responsibilities and that the work had become "just too much" for her.

She has four other grown children who all live in the same suburban community. The patient lives alone in a two-bedroom apartment in a building with an elevator and level entrance to the lobby. She was widowed six years. The children recently decided that a wheelchair should be used for shopping and other outdoor travel as she had stumbled and fallen twice while walking on a level sidewalk.

You thank the son for the information and move the patient into a treatment room to begin your examination.

Guiding Questions

1. After explaining the reasons for conducting a thorough examination, you start with a brief mental status examination. Describe how you would examine: *attention, fund of knowledge,* and *memory*.

2. Your preliminary screening tests indicate that cognitive function is grossly intact and that there are no cranial nerve findings. You plan to continue your examination with the following test and measures: manual muscle test, coordination assessment, sensory tests, gait analysis, and functional assessment. Identify which test you would complete first and provide a rationale to substantiate your choice.

3. The first portion of your sensory test includes perception of pain and temperature. Describe the test protocol for each and the ascending pathway that mediate pain and temperature.

4. Your findings for pain and temperature indicate both are intact. You now progress to test proprioception and vibration. Describe the test protocol for each.

5. The test findings indicate severe loss of proprioception and vibration in the lower extremities (distal more than proximal). What receptors are responsible for these sensory modalities? Where are the receptors located? Identify the ascending pathway that mediates proprioception and vibration. What are the functional implications of the findings?

REFERENCES

1. Fisher, AG, and Murray, EA: Introduction to Sensory Integration Theory. In Fisher, et al (eds): Sensory Integration: Theory and Practice. FA Davis, Philadelphia, 1991, p 3.

2. American Physical Therapy Association: Guide to Physical Therapist Practice. Phys Ther 77, 1997.

3. Aminoff, MJ, et al: Clinical Neurology, ed 3. Appelton & Lange, Stamford, CT, 1996.

4. Jackson-Wyatt, O: Brain Function, Aging, and Dementia. In Umphred, D (ed): Neurological Rehabilitation, ed 3. Mosby, St. Louis, 1995, p 722.

5. Adams, RD, and Victor, M: Principles of Neurology, ed 5. McGraw-Hill, New York, 1993.

6. Gould, BE: Pathophysiology for the Health-Related Professions. Saunders, Philadelphia, 1997.

7. Goldman, J, and Cote, L: Aging of the Brain: Dementia of the Alzheimer's Type. In Kandel, ER, et al: Principles of

Neural Science, ed 3. Appleton & Lange, Norwalk, CT, 1991, p 974.

8. Scheibel, M, et al: Progressive dendritic changes in aging human cortex. Exp Neurol 47:392, 1975.

9. Dorfman, LJ, and Bosley, TM: Age related changes in peripheral central nerve conduction in man. Neurology 29:38, 1979.

10. Downie, AW, and Newell, DJ: Sensory nerve conduction in patients with diabetes mellitus and controls. Neurology 11:876, 1961.

11. Merchut, MP, and Toleikis, SC: Aging and quantitative sensory thresholds. Electromyogr Clin Neurophysiol 30:293, 1990.

12. Bolton, CF, et al: A quantitative study of Meissner's corpuscles in man. Neurology 16:1, 1966.

13. Craik, RL: Sensorimotor changes and adaptation in the older adult. In Guccione, AA (ed): Geriatric Physical Therapy. Mosby, Philadelphia, 1993, p 71.

14. Schmidt, RF, et al: Multiunit neural responses to strong finger pulp vibration, I. Relationship to age. Acta Physiol Scand 140:1990.

15. Mufson, EJ, and Stein, DG: Degeneration in the spinal cord of old rats. Exp Neurol 70:179, 1980.

16. Lascelles, RG, and Thomas, PK: Changes due to age in internodal length in the sural nerve of man. J Neurol Neurosurg Psychiatry 29:40, 1966.

17. Lewis, CB, and Bottomley, JM: Geriatric Physical Therapy: A Clinical Approach. Appleton & Lange, Norwalk, CT, 1994.

18. Takahsshi, J: A clinicopathologic study of the peripheral nervous system of the aged: Sciatic nerve and autonomic nervous system. J Am Geriatr Soc 21:123, 1966.

19. O'Sullivan, DJ, and Swallow, M: The fibre size and content of the radial and surae nerve. J Neurol Neurosurg Psychiatry 31:464, 1968.

20. Thornbury, JM, and Mistretta, CM: Tactile sensitivity as a function of age. J Gerontol 36:34, 1981.

21. Verrillo, RT: Age related changes in the sensitivity to vibration. J Gerontol 35:185, 1980.

22. Gellis, M, and Pool, R: Two-point discrimination distances in the normal hand and forearm. Plast Reconstr Surg 59:57, 1977.

23. Colavita, FB: Sensory Changes in Elderly. Charles C. Thomas, Springfield, MA, 1978.

24. Harkins, SW, et al: Effects of age on pain perception: Thermonociception. J Gerontol 41:58, 1986.

25. Maguire, GH: The Changing Realm of the Senses. In Lewis, CB (ed): Aging: The Health Care Challenge, ed 3. FA Davis, Philadelphia, 1996, p 126.

26. Nolan, MF: Introduction to the Neurologic Examination. FA Davis, Philadelphia, 1996.

27. Waxman, SG, and deGroot, J: Correlative Neuroanatomy, ed 22. Appleton & Lange, Norwalk, CT, 1995.

28. Gilman, S, and Newman, SW: Manter and Gatz's Essentials of Clinical Neuroanatomy and Neurophysiology, ed 9. FA Davis, Philadelphia, 1996.

29. Kiernan, JA: The Human Nervous System, ed 7. Lippincott-Raven, Philadelphia, 1998.

30. Dobkin, B: Neurologic Rehabilitation. FA Davis, Philadelphia, 1996.

31. Young, PA, and Young, PH: Basic Clinical Neuroanatomy. Williams & Wilkins, Philadelphia, 1997.

32. Fitzgerald, MJT: Neuroanatomy: Basic and Clinical, ed 2. Bailliere Tindall, Philadelphia, 1992.

33. Guyton, AC, and Hall, JE: Human Physiology and Mechanisms of Disease, ed 6. Saunders, Philadelphia, 1997.

34. Fredericks, CM: Basic Sensory Mechanism and the Somatosensory System. In Fredericks, CM, and Saladin, LK (eds): Pathophysiology of the Motor Systems: Principles and Clinical Presentations. FA Davis, Philadelphia, 1996, p 78.

35. Kandel, E, and Kupfermann, I: From Nerve Cells to Cognition. In Kandel, ER, et al (eds): Essentials of Neural Science and Behavior. Appleton & Lange, Norwalk, CT, 1995, p 321.

36. Nolan, MF: Clinical assessment of cutaneous sensory function. Clin Manage Phys Ther 4:26, 1984.

37. Werner, JL, and Omer, GE: Evaluating cutaneous pressure sensation of the hand. Am J Occup Ther 24:347, 1970.

38. Pedretti, LW: Evaluation of sensation and treatment of sensory dysfunction. In Pedretti, LW, and Zoltan, B (eds): Occupational Therapy: Practice Skills for Physical Dysfunction, ed 3. CV Mosby, St. Louis, 1990, p 177.

39. Trombly, CA, and Scott, AD: Evaluation and treatment of somatosensory sensation. In Trombly, CA (ed): Occupational Therapy for Physical Dysfunction, ed 3. Williams & Wilkins, Baltimore, 1989, p 41.

40. Kent, BE: Sensory-motor testing: The upper limb of adult patients with hemiplegia. J Am Phys Ther Assoc 45:550, 1965.

41. Nolan, MF: Limits of two-point discrimination ability in the lower limb in young adult men and women. Phys Ther 63:1424, 1983.

42. Nolan, MF: Quantitative measure of cutaneous sensation: Two-point discrimination values for the face and trunk. Phys Ther 65:181, 1985.

43. Nolan, MF: Two-point discrimination assessment in the upper limb in young adult men and women. Phys Ther 62:965, 1982.

44. Moberg, E: Evaluation of sensibility in the hand. Surg Clin North Am 40:357, 1960.

45. Moberg, E: Emergency Surgery of the Hand. E & S Livingstone, London, 1967.

46. Kandel, ER, and Jessell, TM: Touch. In Kandell, ER, et al (eds): Principles of Neural Science, ed 3. Appleton & Lange, Norwalk, CT, 1991, p 367.

47. Shumway-Cook, A, and Woollacott, M: Motor Control: Theory and Practical Applications. Williams & Wilkins, Philadelphia, 1995.

48. Ayers, JA: Tactile functions: Their relation to hyperactive and perceptual motor behavior. Am J Occup Ther 18:83, 1964.

49. Ayers, JA: Interrelations among perceptual-motor abilities in a group of normal children. Am J Occup Ther 20:288, 1966.

50. Ayers, JA: Improving academic scores through sensory integration. J Learn Disabil 5:338, 1972.

51. Ayers, JA: Sensory Integration and Learning Disabilities. Western Psychological Services, Los Angeles, 1972.

52. Ayers, JA: Cluster analysis of measures of sensory integration. Am J Occup Ther 31:362, 1977.

53. Ayers, JA: Sensory Integration and the Child. Western Psychological Services, Los Angeles, 1979.

SUPPLEMENTAL READINGS

Bennett, SE, and Karnes, JL: Neurologic Disabilities: Assessment and Treatment. Lippincott, New York, 1998.

DeMyer, WE: Technique of the Neurologic Examination: A Programmed Text, ed 4. McGraw-Hill, New York, 1994.

Hendelman, WJ: Student's Atlas of Neuroanatomy. Saunders, Philadelphia, 1994.

Jessell, TM, and Kelly, DD: Pain and analgesia. In Kandell, ER, et al (eds): Principles of Neural Science, ed 3. Appleton & Lange, Norwalk, CT, 1991, p 385.

Johansson, K, et al: Can sensory stimulation improve the functional outcome in stroke patients? Neurology 43:2189, 1993.

Kass, JH: Somatosensory system. In Paxinos, G (ed): The Human Nervous System. Academic Press, San Diego, 1990, p 813.

Magnusson, M, et al: Sensory stimulation promotes normalization of postural control after stroke. Stroke 25:1176, 1994.

Maguire, GH: The changing realm of the senses. In Bernstein Lewis, CB (ed): Aging: The Health Care Challenge, ed 3. FA Davis, Philadelphia, 1996.

Martin, JH: Coding and Processing of Sensory Information. In Kandell, ER, et al (eds): Principles of Neural Science, ed 3. Appleton & Lange, Norwalk, CT, 1991, p 329.

Martin, JH: Neuroanatomy: Text and Atlas, ed 2. Appleton & Lange, Stamford, CT, 1996.

Martin, JH, and Jessell, TM: Modality coding in the somatic sensory system. In Kandell, ER, et al (eds): Essentials of Neural Science and Behavior. Appleton & Lange, Norwalk, CT, 1995, p 341.

Martin, J, and Jessell, T: The sensory systems. In Kandell, ER, et al (eds): Essentials of Neural Science and Behavior. Appleton & Lange, Norwalk, CT, 1995, p 369.

McMahon, SB, et al: Central hyperexcitability triggered by noxious inputs. Curr Opin Neurobiol 3:602, 1993.

Nolte, J: The Human Brain: An Introduction to its Functional Anatomy, ed 3. Mosby Year Book, Philadelphia, 1993.

Schaumburg, HH, et al: Disorders of Peripheral Nerves: Contemporary Neurology Series, ed 2. FA Davis, Philadelphia, 1992.

Strub, RL, and Black, FW: The Mental Status Examination in Neurology, ed 3. FA Davis, 1993.

Vallar, G, et al: Exploring somatosensory hemineglect by vestibular stimulation. Brain 116:71, 1993.

Willard, FH, and Perl, DP: Medical Neuroanatomy: A Problem-Oriented Manual with Annotated Atlas. Lippincott, Philadelphia, 1993.

Willis, WD, and Coggeshall, RE: Sensory Mechanisms of the Spinal Cord, ed 2. Plenum, New York, 1991.

GLOSSARY

Abarognosis: Inability to recognize weight.

Acalculia: Inability to perform simple arithmetic operations; inability to calculate.

Allesthesia: Sensation experienced at a site remote from point of stimulation.

Allodynia: Pain produced by non-noxious stimulus (e.g., light touch).

Analgesia: Complete loss of pain sensibility.

Anesthesia: Loss of sensation.

Arousal: The physiological readiness of the human system for activity; alertness; the state of being prepared to act.

Astereognosis: Inability to recognize the form and shape of objects by touch (synonym, tactile agnosia).

Atopognosia: Inability to localize a sensation.

Attention: Awareness of the environment; responsiveness to a stimulus or task without being distracted by other stimuli.

Barognosis: Ability to recognize weight.

Calculation ability: Competence in foundational mathematical abilities including addition, subtraction, multiplication, and division.

Causalgia: Painful, burning sensations, usually along the distribution of a nerve.

Cognition: Process by which knowledge is acquired; includes both awareness and judgement.

Dermatome: Cutaneous areas that correspond to the spinal segments providing their innervation.

Dysesthesia: Touch sensation experienced as pain.

Dyscalculia: Impaired ability to perform simple arithmetic operations; difficulty in accomplishing calculations.

Exteroceptors: Sensory receptors that provide information from the external environment.

Fund of knowledge: Mental status screening test utilizes questions related to the patient's learning history and life experiences.

Graphesthesia (traced figure identification): Recognition of numbers, letters, or symbols traced on the skin.

Hypalgesia: Decreased sensitivity to pain.

Hyperalgesia: Increased sensitivity to pain.

Hyperesthesia: Increased sensitivity to sensory stimuli.

Hypesthesia: Decreased sensitivity to sensory stimuli.

Interoceptor: Sensory receptors that provide information about the body's internal environment (such as oxygen levels and blood pressure).

Kinesthesia (awareness of movement): Sensation and awareness of active or passive movement.

Orientation: The ability to comprehend and to adjust oneself within an unfamiliar environment with respect to awareness of time, person, and place.

Pallesthesia: Ability to perceive or to recognize vibratory stimuli.

Paresthesia: Abnormal sensation such as numbness, prickling, or tingling, without apparent cause.

Proprioception: Position sense and the awareness of the joints at rest.

Proprioceptors: Sensory receptors responsible for deep sensations; found in muscles, tendons, ligaments, joints, and fascia.

Proverb interpretation: Mental status screening that examines the patient's ability to interpret use of words outside of their usual context.

Reliability: The level of consistency of either a measuring instrument or a testing method.

Sensation: The ability to perceive stimuli through the organs of special sense (e.g., eyes, ears, nose), the peripheral cutaneous sensory system (e.g., temperature, taste, touch), or internal receptors (e.g., muscle, joint receptors).

Sensory integrity: The ability of the CNS to process and integrate incoming sensory information (from the body and environment) and use it in planning and organizing motor behavior.

Sharp/dull discrimination: Ability to discriminate between a pointed and blunt cutaneous stimuli.

Stereognosis: The ability to recognize the shape of objects by touch.

Thalamic syndrome: Vascular lesion of the thalamus resulting in sensory disturbances and partial or complete paralysis of one side of the body, associated with severe, boring-type pain. Sensory stimuli may produce an exaggerated, prolonged, and/or painful response.

Theoretical construct: A concept that helps to describe, explain, and predict unobservable events.

Thermanalgesia: Inability to perceive heat.

Thermanesthesia: Inability to perceive sensations of heat and cold.

Thermesthesia: Ability to perceive heat and cold sensations; temperature sensibility.

Thermhyperesthesia: Increased sensitivity to temperature.

Thermhypesthesia: Decreased temperature sensibility.

Thigmanesthesia: Loss of light touch sensibility.

Traced figure identification (graphesthesia): Recognition of numbers, letters, or symbols traced on the skin.

Two-point discrimination: Ability to distinguish two blunt points applied to the skin simultaneously.

Validity: The degree to which an instrument or tool measures what it is designed to measure.

APPENDIX

SUGGESTED ANSWERS TO CASE STUDY GUIDING QUESTIONS

1. After explaining the reasons for conducting a thorough examination, you start with a brief mental status examination. Describe how you would examine: *attention, fund of knowledge,* **and** *memory.*

ANSWER

Attention: Ask the patient to repeat a progressively more challenging list of items. The repetition can begin with two or three items and gradually progress to longer lists. For example, the patient could be asked to repeat a sequence of numbers (22, 57, 99, 38), a series of letters (L, R, U, A, Z,) or a series of words (desk, picture, book, clock). Another approach would be to ask the patient to spell words backward, such as card, light, food, ground, and so forth.

Fund of Knowledge: Ask the patient a series of questions related to her general knowledge base such as: Who was president of the United States the year you were born? How many cups make a quart? Where is the White House located? In what state is Detroit located?

Memory: For long-term memory, ask the patient historical information such as birth dates of her children, the date of her marriage, her mother's maiden name, and what schools she attended. For short-term memory, ask the patient to immediately repeat a series of words (radio, pen, bowl, tree, door) or a series of numbers (234, 67, 49, 34, 71), then ask her again after 5 minutes, and then again after 30 minutes.

2. Your preliminary screening tests indicate that cognitive function is grossly intact and that there are no cranial nerve findings. You plan to continue your examination with the following test and measures: manual muscle test, coordination assessment, sensory tests, gait analysis, and functional assessment. Identify which test you would complete first and provide a rationale to substantiate your choice.

ANSWER

First Examination: Sensory testing.

Rationale: Owing to the close relation between sensory input and motor output, sensory impairments will impact on motor performance. Sensory testing should occur *before* manual muscle testing, coordination assessment, gait analysis or functional assessment.

3. The first portion of your sensory test includes perception of pain and temperature. Describe the test protocol for each and the ascending pathway that mediate pain and temperature.

ANSWER

Pain: Test Protocol. The sharp end of a large-headed or safety pin, or reshaped paper clip is used. The instrument should be carefully cleaned before administering the test. The sharp point is applied to the patient's skin. All areas of the body should be tested.

Patient Response. The patient is asked to verbally indicate when a stimulus is felt.

Temperature: Test Protocol. Two test tubes with stoppers are required; one is filled with warm water and the other with crushed ice. The test tubes are randomly placed in contact with the skin area to be tested. All skin surfaces should be tested.

Patient Response. The patient is asked to indicate when a stimulus is felt and to reply "warm," "cold," or "unable to tell."

Ascending Pathway: Anterolateral Spinothalamic.

4. Your findings for pain and temperature indicate both are intact. You now progress to test proprioception and vibration. Describe the test protocol for each.

ANSWER

Proprioception: Test Protocol. The extremity or joint(s) to be assessed is moved through a range of motion and held in a static position. Small increments in range of motion are used. The words selected to identify the range of motion examined should be identified to the patient during the practice trial (e.g., initial, mid, or terminal range). Caution should be used with hand placements to avoid excessive tactile stimulation.

Patient Response: While the extremity or joint(s) under assessment is held in a static position by the therapist, the patient is asked to describe the position verbally or duplicate the position of the extremity or joint(s) with the opposite extremity.

Vibration: Test Protocol. The base of a vibrating tuning fork is placed on a bony prominence (such as the sternum, elbow, or ankle). If intact, the patient will perceive the vibration. If there is impairment, the patient will be unable to distinguish between a vibrating and nonvibrating tuning fork. Therefore, there should be a random application of vibrating and nonvibrating stimuli. Earphones may be used to reduce auditory clues from the vibrating fork.

Patient Response. The patient is asked to respond by verbally identifying the stimulus as vibrating or nonvibrating each time the base of the fork is placed in contact with a bony prominence.

5. The test findings indicate severe loss of proprioception and vibration in the lower extremities (distal more than proximal). What receptors are responsible for these sensory modalities? Where are the receptors located? Identify the ascending pathway that mediates

proprioception and vibration. What are the functional implications of the findings?

ANSWER

Receptors: Proprioceptors.

Location: Muscles, tendons, ligaments, joints, and fascia.

Ascending Pathway: Dorsal column-medial lemniscal.

Functional Implications: Impairments in balance and postural stability in standing and walking; limitations imposed on independent function; high risk for falls.

Coordination Assessment 7

Thomas J. Schmitz

LEARNING OBJECTIVES

1. Identify the general purposes of performing a coordination assessment.
2. Identify the types of data generated from a coordination assessment.
3. Describe the common coordination impairments associated with lesions of the cerebellum, basal ganglia, and dorsal columns.
4. Define the major areas of movement capabilities tested during a coordination assessment.
5. Describe the specific tests used to examine both nonequilibrium and equilibrium coordination deficits.
6. Describe the testing protocol for performing a coordination assessment.
7. Using the case study example, apply clinical decision making skills to application of coordination assessment data.

Coordination or *coordinated movement* is the ability to execute smooth, accurate, controlled motor responses. The ability to produce these motor responses is a complex process dependent on a fully intact neuromuscular system. Coordinated movements are characterized by appropriate speed, distance, direction, timing, and muscular tension. In addition, they involve appropriate synergistic influences, easy reversal between opposing muscle groups, and proximal fixation to allow distal motion or maintenance of a posture.[1] *Coordination impairments* are characterized by awkward, extraneous, uneven, or inaccurate movements.

Physical therapists are frequently involved in the examination, diagnosis, and treatment of coordination impairments, which generally represent some deficit in integration of sensory, motor, and neural processes.[2] Coordination tests assist the physical therapist in diagnosing the underlying origin of impairments. These impairments are often associated with functional limitations that are related to, and indicative of, the type, extent, and location of central nervous system (CNS) pathology.[2] Some locations of CNS involvement present very classic and stereotypical impairments, but others are much less predictable. Several examples of diagnoses that typically demonstrate coordination deficits related to CNS involvement include traumatic brain injury, parkinsonism, multiple sclerosis, Huntington's disease, cerebral palsy, Sydenham's chorea, cerebellar tumors, vestibular pathology, and some learning disabilities.

The purposes of performing a coordination assessment of motor function include the following[2]:
1. Determine muscle activity characteristics during voluntary movement.
2. Assess the ability of muscles or groups of muscles to work together to perform a task or functional activity.
3. Determine level of skill and efficiency of movement.
4. Identify the ability to initiate, control, and terminate movement.
5. Determine the timing, sequencing, and accuracy of movement patterns.
6. Assist with establishing the diagnosis of underlying impairments, functional limitations, and disability.
7. Assist with establishing *goals* to remediate impairments, formulating *outcomes* to remediate functional *limitations* and disability, and determining specific, direct *interventions*.
8. Determine the effects of therapeutic and pharmacological intervention on motor function over time.
9. Assist with determining a prognosis.

MOTOR CORTEX

The primary motor cortex (Fig. 7-1) is located in the precentral gyrus (Brodmann's area 4). It receives information from three sources: the *periphery* (receptors and muscles), the *cerebellum*, and the *basal ganglia*. Peripheral input is relayed directly to the primary motor cortex (from the thalamus) and to the primary somatosensory cortex. Peripheral input reaches the premotor areas indirectly from the sensory association areas. The cerebellum also relays information to the motor areas. This information is distributed by way of the thalamus mainly to the primary and premotor cortex. Input is also relayed through the thalamus from the basal ganglia. Note that cortical representation of different parts of the body is unequal (Fig. 7-2). Cortical representation of body segments required for fine motor skills is greater than that devoted to gross motor functions.[3,4]

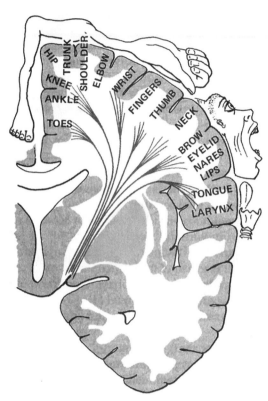

Figure 7-2. The motor homunculus indicates the somatotrophic organization of the motor cortex. The relative size of body parts reflects the proportion of the motor cortex devoted to controlling that area. (From Gilman and Winans Newman,[3] p 223 with permission; originally adapted from Penfield, W, and Rasmussen, H: The Cerebral Cortex in Man. Macmillan, New York, 1950.)

COORDINATION DEFICITS AND CENTRAL NERVOUS SYSTEM INVOLVEMENT

Figure 7-3 presents a schematic illustration of the relationship among individual components of the brain and spinal structures that use peripheral feedback to produce movement. Peripheral receptors provide information about the external environment, which is encoded and conveyed to various parts of the CNS. The information is processed based on peripheral feedback and memory, which leads to selection of a movement strategy appropriate to the task demands and environmental conditions. This motor strategy may include stored motor programs (central pattern generator). When initiated, the motor program results in activation of a preprogrammed set of instructions to produce coordinated movement. Motor programs can be called up in their entirety, modified, or reassembled in a new order. They provide the important function of freeing higher executive levels from attending to all aspects of a motor response.[3–6]

Several areas of the CNS provide input to, and act together with, the cortex in the production of coordinated movement responses. These include the cerebellum, basal ganglia, and dorsal (posterior) columns. Although it is incorrect to assign all problems of incoordination to one of these sites, lesions

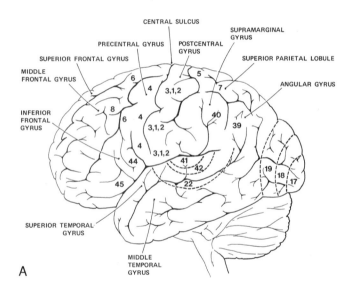

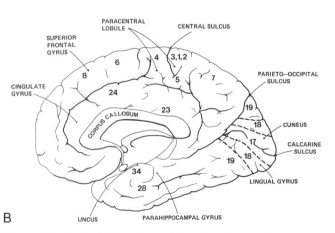

Figure 7-1. Lateral (*A*) and medial (*B*) view of the brain, indicating the numbered Brodmann's areas. (From Gilman and Winans Newman,[3] p 221, 222, with permission.)

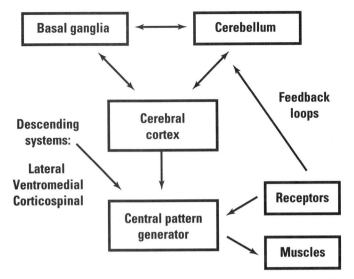

Figure 7-3. Schematic illustration of the relationship among individual components of the brain, spinal, and peripheral structures involved in production of coordinated movement. (From Newton,[4] p 83, with permission.)

in these areas are responsible for many characteristic motor deficits seen in adult populations. The following sections present an overview of the normal function of the cerebellum, basal ganglia, and posterior columns, as well as common clinical features associated with lesions in each of these areas.

Cerebellum

The primary function of the cerebellum is regulation of movement, postural control, and muscle tone. Although all of the mechanisms of cerebellar function are not clearly understood, lesions of this area have been noted to produce typical patterns of motor function deficits, impaired balance, and decreased muscle tone.

Several theories of function of the cerebellum in motor activity have been established. Among the more widely held is that the cerebellum functions as a *comparator* and *error-correcting mechanism* (Fig. 7-4).[1,7] The cerebellum compares the commands for movement transmitted from the motor cortex with the actual motor performance of the body segment. This occurs by a comparison of information received from the cortex with that obtained from peripheral feedback mechanisms. The motor cortex and brainstem motor structures provide the commands for the intended motor response.[7] Peripheral feedback during the motor response is provided by muscle spindles, Golgi tendon organs, joint and cutaneous receptors, the vestibular apparatus,[8] and the eyes and ears. This feedback provides continual input regarding posture and balance, as well as position, rate, rhythm, and force of slow movements of peripheral body segments.[8] If the input from the feedback systems does not compare appropriately (i.e., movements deviate from the intended command), the cerebellum supplies a corrective influence. This effect is achieved by corrective signals sent to the cortex, which, via motor pathways, modifies or corrects the ongoing movement (e.g., increasing or decreasing the level of activity of specific muscles).[8] The cerebellum also functions to modify cortical commands for subsequent movements.[7,9,10]

This CNS analysis of movement information, determination of level of accuracy, and provision for error correction is referred to as a **closed-loop**

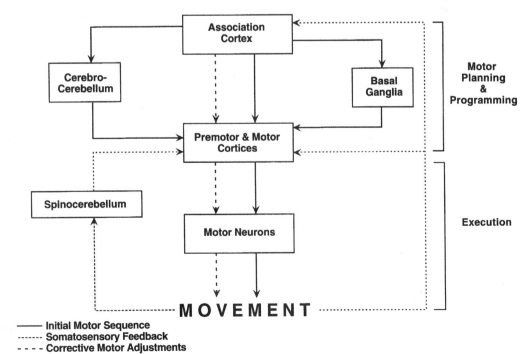

Figure 7-4. Flow chart representing the "comparator" role of the cerebellum in the planning and execution of voluntary movement. In coordinating rapid, phasic motor activity, the cerebellum (i.e., spinocerebellum) compares the movement plans formulated in the cerebral cortex and carried out through pyramidal and extrapyramidal pathways, with the actual evolution of movement. It then acts to correct any discrepancies (i.e., errors) between the *intended* and the *actual* movement. This error correction is guided by somatosensory feedback. Note that the thalamic relay of basal ganglia, cerebellar, and somatosensory input is omitted for clarity. (From Fredericks,[10] p 194, with permission.)

system.[6] It should be noted that not all movements are controlled by this system. Stereotypical movements (e.g., gait activities) and rapid, short-duration movements, which do not allow sufficient time for feedback to occur, are believed to be controlled by an **open-loop system.** In this system, control originates centrally from a **motor program,** which is a memory or preprogrammed pattern of information for coordinated movement.[6] The motor system then follows the established pattern largely independent of feedback or error-detection mechanisms.

CLINICAL FEATURES OF CEREBELLAR DYSFUNCTION

Specific clinical findings are associated with cerebellar disease. Many of these findings either directly or indirectly influence the ability to execute accurate, smooth, controlled movements. The clinical features identified emphasize the crucial influence of the cerebellum on equilibrium, posture, muscle tone, and initiation and force of movement. **Ataxia** is a general, comprehensive term used to describe the combined influence of cerebellar and sensory dysfunction (especially dysmetria and decomposition of movement)[3] on gait, posture, and patterns of movement. The following clinical signs are manifestations of cerebellar lesions:

1. **Hypotonia** is a decrease in muscle tone. It is believed to be related to the disruption of afferent input from stretch receptors and/or lack of the cerebellum's facilitory efferent influence on the fusimotor system. A diminished resistance to passive movement will be noted, and muscles may feel abnormally soft and flaccid. Diminished deep tendon reflexes also may be noted.[7]

2. **Dysmetria** is a disturbance in the ability to judge the distance or range of a movement. It may be manifested by an overestimation (**hypermetria**) or an underestimation (**hypometria**) of the required range needed to reach an object or goal.

3. **Dysdiadochokinesia** is an impaired ability to perform rapid alternating movements (RAM). This deficit is observed in movements such as rapid alternation between pronation and supination of the forearm. Movements are irregular, with a rapid loss of range and rhythm especially as speed is increased.[8]

4. **Tremor** is an involuntary oscillatory movement resulting from alternate contractions of opposing muscle groups. Two types of tremors are associated with cerebellar lesions. An **intention, or kinetic, tremor** occurs during voluntary motion of a limb and tends to increase as the limb nears its intended goal or speed is increased.[7] Intention tremors are diminished or absent at rest. **Postural (static) tremor** may be evident by back-and-forth oscillatory movements of the body while the patient maintains a standing posture. They also may be observed as up-and-down

oscillatory movements of a limb when it is held against gravity.[11,12]

5. **Movement decomposition (dyssynergia)** describes a movement performed in a sequence of component parts rather than as a single, smooth activity. For example, when asked to touch the index finger to the nose, the patient might first flex the elbow, then adjust the position of the wrist and fingers, further flex the elbow, and finally flex the shoulder. **Asynergia** is the loss of ability to associate muscles together for complex movements.

6. **Disorders of gait** involve ambulatory patterns that typically demonstrate a broad base of support. The arms may be held away from the body to improve balance (high guard position). Initiation of forward progression of a lower extremity may start slowly, and then the extremity may unexpectedly be flung rapidly and forcefully forward and audibly hit the floor.[11] Gait patterns tend to be generally unsteady, irregular, and staggering, with deviations from an intended forward line of progression.

7. **Dysarthria** is a disorder of the motor component of speech articulation. The characteristics of cerebellar dysarthria are referred to as **scanning speech.** This speech pattern is typically slow, and may be slurred, hesitant, with prolonged syllables[7] and inappropriate pauses. Word use, selection, and grammar remain intact,[7,8] but the melodic quality of speech is altered.[8]

8. **Nystagmus** is a rhythmic, oscillatory movement of the eyes. Several deficits related to eye movements are associated with cerebellar lesions. Nystagmus is the most common and causes difficulty with accurate fixation and vision. It is typically apparent as the eyes move away from a midline resting point to fix on a peripheral object. An involuntary drift back to the midline position is observed.[11,13] Nystagmus is believed to be linked to the cerebellum's influence on synergy and tone of the extraocular muscles.

9. The **rebound phenomenon** was originally described by Holmes. It is the loss of the check reflex,[11] or check factor, which functions to halt forceful active movements. Normally, when application of resistance to an isometric contraction is suddenly removed, the limb will remain in approximately the same position by action of the opposing muscle(s). With cerebellar involvement, the patient is unable to "check" the motion, and the limb will move suddenly when resistance is released. The patient may strike himself or herself or other objects when the resistance is removed.

10. **Asthenia** is generalized muscle weakness associated with cerebellar lesions.

In addition to these characteristic clinical features of cerebellar involvement, a greater length of time may also be required to initiate voluntary movements. Difficulty may be observed in stopping or changing the force, speed, or direction of movement.[14]

Basal Ganglia

The basal ganglia are a group of nuclei located at the base of the cerebral cortex. The three main nuclei of the basal ganglia include the caudate, the putamen, and the globus pallidus. These nuclei have close anatomical and functional connections with two other subcortical nuclei that are also frequently considered as part of the basal ganglia: the subthalamic nucleus and the substantia nigra.[3,15]

Although the influences of the basal ganglia on movement are not understood as clearly as those of the cerebellum, there is evidence that the basal ganglia play an important role in several complex aspects of movement and postural control.[16] These include the initiation and regulation of gross intentional movements, planning and execution of complex motor responses, facilitation of desired motor responses while selectively inhibiting others, and the ability to accomplish automatic movements and postural adjustments.[17,18] In addition, the basal ganglia play an important role in maintaining normal background muscle tone.[9] This is accomplished by the inhibitory effect of the basal ganglia on both the motor cortex and lower brainstem. The basal ganglia also are believed to influence some aspects of both perceptual and cognitive functions.[17]

The motor portion of the basal ganglia assumes a somatotopic organization. The anatomical positioning of the basal ganglia provides insight to its contribution to motor performance. The areas of the brain associated with movement (supplementary motor area, premotor cortex, motor cortex, somatosensory cortex, and the superior parietal lobe) form dense projections to the motor portion of the putamen. Output of this pathway forms the *motor circuit* of the basal ganglia, which is directed back to the supplementary motor area and the premotor cortex. These two areas and the motor cortex are all interconnected, and each has descending projections to the brainstem motor centers and spinal cord. This anatomical arrangement indicates that the influence of the basal ganglia on motor function is indirect and mediated by descending projections from the cortical motor areas (Fig. 7-5).[17-19]

Clinical observation indicates that patients with lesions of the basal ganglia typically demonstrate several characteristic motor deficits. These are (1) poverty and slowness of movement, (2) involuntary, extraneous movement, and (3) alterations in posture and muscle tone.[17-19] Common diagnostic groups that demonstrate basal ganglia involvement are parkinsonism, Wilson's disease, and Huntington's disease.

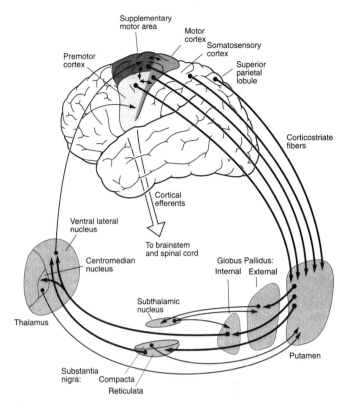

Figure 7-5. The motor circuit of the basal ganglia provides a subcortical feedback loop from the motor and somatosensory areas of the cortex, through portions of the basal ganglia and thalamus, and back to the cortical motor areas (premotor cortex, supplementary motor area, and motor cortex). (From Ghez, C, and Gordon, J: Voluntary Movement. In Kandel, ER, Schwartz, JH, and Jessell, TM (eds): Essentials of Neural Science and Behavior. Appleton & Lange, E. Norwalk, CT, 1995, p 548, with permission.)

CLINICAL FEATURES OF LESIONS OF THE BASAL GANGLIA

Disorders of the basal ganglia present a unique pattern of deficits, with characteristic involuntary movements, disturbances of muscle tone and posture, and diminished postural reactions. The following clinical signs are manifestations of basal ganglia lesions:

1. **Bradykinesia** is slowed or decreased movement. It may be demonstrated in a variety of ways, such as a decreased arm swing; slow, shuffling gait; difficulty initiating or changing direction of movement; lack of facial expression; or difficulty stopping a movement once begun; characteristic of Parkinson's disease.

2. **Rigidity** is an increase in muscle tone causing greater resistance to passive movement. Two types of rigidity may be seen: leadpipe and cogwheel. **Leadpipe rigidity** is a uniform, constant resistance felt by the examiner as the extremity is moved through a range of motion. **Cogwheel rigidity** is considered a combination of the leadpipe type with tremor. It is characterized by a series of brief relaxations or "catches'" as the extremity is passively moved.

3. **Tremor** is an involuntary, rhythmic, oscillatory

movement observed at rest (**resting tremor**). Resting tremors typically disappear or decrease with purposeful movement, but may increase with emotional stress. Tremors associated with basal ganglia lesions (e.g., parkinsonism) are frequently noted in the distal upper extremities in the form of a "pill-rolling" movement, where it looks as if a pill is being rolled between the first two fingers and the thumb. Motion of the wrist, and pronation and supination of the forearm, may be evident. Tremors also may be apparent at other body parts as well, such as the jaw; characteristic of Parkinson's disease.

4. **Akinesia** is an inability to initiate movement and is seen in the late stages of parkinsonism. This deficit is associated with assumption and maintenance of fixed postures.[17] A tremendous amount of mental concentration and effort is required to perform even the simplest motor activity.[9]

5. **Chorea** is a characteristic movement disorder associated with Huntington's disease. Features of chorea include involuntary, rapid, irregular, and jerky movements, also referred to as choreiform movements.

6. **Athetosis** is characterized by slow, involuntary, writhing, twisting, "wormlike" movements. Frequently, greater involvement in the distal upper extremities is noted; this may include fluctuations between hyperextension of the wrist and fingers and a return to a flexed position, combined with rotary movements of the extremities. Many other areas of the body may be involved, including the neck, face, tongue,[9] and trunk. The phenomena are also referred to as athetoid movements. Pure athetosis is relatively uncommon and most often presents in combination with spasticity, tonic spasms, or chorea. Athetosis can be a clinical feature of some forms of cerebral palsy.

7. **Choreoathetosis** is a term used to describe a movement disorder with features of both chorea and athetosis.

8. **Hemiballismus** is characterized by sudden, jerky, forceful, wild, flailing motions of the arm and leg of one side of the body. Primary involvement is in the axial and proximal musculature of the limb. Hemiballismus results from a lesion of the contralateral subthalamic nucleus.[3,14] Associated terms include **hyperkinesis,** which is abnormally increased muscle activity or movement; and **hypokinesis,** which is a decreased motor responses especially to a specific stimulus.

9. **Dystonia** involves twisting, sometimes bizarre, movements caused by involuntary contractions of the axial and proximal muscles of the extremities.[11] Torsion spasms also are considered a form of dystonia, with spasmotic torticollis being the most common.[11] If the contraction is prolonged at the end of the movement, it is termed a *dystonic* posture.[17]

Dorsal (Posterior) Columns

The dorsal or posterior columns (fasciculus gracilis, fasciculus cuneatus) play an important role in both coordinated movement and posture. The dorsal columns are responsible for mediating proprioceptive input from muscles and joint receptors. Proprioceptive input includes both position sense (awareness of the position of a joint at rest) and kinesthesia (awareness of movement).

CLINICAL FEATURES OF LESIONS OF THE DORSAL (POSTERIOR) COLUMNS

Coordination deficits associated with dorsal column lesions are somewhat less characteristic than those produced by other CNS lesions. However, they typically result in equilibrium and motor control disturbances related to the patient's lack of proprioceptive feedback. Because vision assists in both guiding movements and maintaining balance, visual feedback can be an effective mechanism to compensate partially for a proprioceptive loss. Thus, coordination and/or balance problems will be exaggerated in poorly lit areas or when the patient's eyes are closed (e.g., positive **Romberg sign**). In addition, some noticeable slowing of voluntary movements may be observed. This occurs because visually guided motions are generally more accurate when speed of movement is reduced.

Disturbances of gait are a common finding in dorsal column lesions. The gait pattern is usually wide-based and swaying, with uneven step lengths and excessive lateral displacement. The advancing leg may be lifted too high and then dropped abruptly with an audible impact. Watching the feet during ambulation is typical[11] and is indicative of a proprioceptive loss. Another common deficit seen with dorsal column dysfunction is dysmetria. As mentioned, this is an impaired ability to judge the required distance or range of movement and may be noted in both the upper and lower extremities. It is manifested by the inability to place an extremity accurately or to reach a target object. For example, in attempting to lock a wheelchair brake, the patient may inaccurately judge (overestimate or underestimate) the required movement needed to reach the brake handle. As with other coordination deficits associated with dorsal column lesions, visual guidance will reduce the manifestations of dysmetria.

CHANGES IN COORDINATED MOVEMENT WITH AGE

When assessing elderly persons, consideration must be given to the effects of aging on several aspects of movement abilities.[20–29] The following are typical changes associated with aging and may present either as primary or secondary components of a coordination deficit:

• *Decreased strength.* Several peripheral factors are believed to contribute to decreased muscle bulk (diminished cross-sectional area) and decreased function. These include a loss of alpha motor neurons, atrophy of type I and II myofibers (most notably type II atrophy), reduced size of muscle fibers,[30] diminished oxidative capacity of exercising muscle, and a subsequent reduction in ability to produce torque.[26]

• *Slowed reaction time.* The time interval between application of a stimulus and initiation of movement is increased.[31] This finding is also linked to degenerative changes in the motor unit. In addition, premotor time (time interval between onset of a stimulus and initiation of a response) and movement time (time interval between the initiation of movement and the completion of movement) are lengthened with normal aging.[32] Some evidence suggests that reaction times are slower in sedentary versus active elderly persons,[33] and that delayed reaction times are more often seen in fine motor versus gross motor activities.[34]

• *Loss of flexibility.* Increased tightness of joints is particularly evident toward the end range of motion and may influence the overall skill in coordinated movement. Loss of flexibility has been linked to degenerative changes in collagen fibers, dietary deficiencies, general paucity of movement, and arthritic joint changes.[25]

• *Faulty posture.* Diminished strength and flexibility are precursors to poor postural alignment. Faulty posture is further influenced by inactivity and prolonged sitting. Of particular importance is the potential loss of ability to accomplish preparatory postural adjustments prior to execution of a movement.

• *Impaired balance* (postural control). Decreased balance and increased postural sway[20–22,24,35] (the small, oscillating movements of the body over the feet during relaxed standing) both occur with advancing age. As a result, coordinated movements within the limits of stability for an elderly person will be altered (i.e., the magnitude of displacement that will disrupt stability will be decreased).

These changes may be accentuated further by alterations in sensation, perceptual skills, and visual and hearing acuity. Several recent texts[25,36,37] provide important references and further details of the physiological, neurological, and musculoskeletal changes associated with advancing age. These changes have important implications for how directions are provided to the patient during application of coordination tests. Knowledge of these anticipated age-related changes will improve the therapist's ability to establish effective communication to optimize performance during coordination tests as well as interpret the results. Sensitive and accurate communication is central to the role of the physical therapist. Because elderly clients experience changes in sensory function, communication skills that enhance the therapeutic interaction should be adopted. This involves conveying information in a language or context that is meaningful and intelligible to the patient and communicates trust, respect,

and compassion. DeMont and Peatman[38] suggest several important strategies to improve communication with elderly clients (Box 7–1).

Testing Procedures

PRELIMINARY CONSIDERATIONS

Accurate and careful observation is an important preliminary to performing a coordination assessment. Inasmuch as treatment activities will be geared toward improving functional activity levels, initial observations should focus here. Before initiation of specific testing procedures, the patient should first be observed performing a variety of functional activities: bed mobility, self-care routines (e.g., dressing, combing hair, brushing teeth), transfers, eating, writing, changing position from lying or sitting to standing, maintaining a standing position, walking, and so forth. During the initial observation, general information can be obtained that will assist in localizing specific areas of deficit. This information will include:

1. Level of skill in each activity (including amount of assistance or assistive devices required)
2. The occurrence of extraneous movements, oscillations, swaying, or unsteadiness

---

Box 7–1 STRATEGIES TO IMPROVE COMMUNICATION WITH ELDERS

1. Do not stereotype. Do not assume a level of decreased mental function or confusion. Posture, gesture, and facial expressions can be deceiving.
2. Be aware of, and adapt to, any age-related physical limitations that an elder may possess. Consider the sensory deficits in sight, hearing, speech, and reaction time, which may be barriers to communication.
3. Secure the elder's attention by eye contact or a gentle touch.
4. Identify yourself when greeting an elder.
5. Request information from each elder on how best to communicate, e.g., "Should I speak louder?" or "Would you like your glasses?"
6. Ask each individual what form of address is preferred. Do not use generic or pet names such as "Grampa" or "Mama." Each individual has a unique identity.
7. Request permission to adjust the volume of the television or radio or to change the amount or angle of light.
8. Maintain eye contact.
9. Do not pretend to understand an elder's response. Request confirmation or clarification of a message you do not understand.
10. Avoid speaking to elders as if they were children. Do not use a singsong voice, baby talk, or give orders.
11. Do not ignore individuals or talk about them in the presence of others as if they were not there.
12. Respect an elder's routines and control of his life. Schedule and keep appointments at mutually agreed-on times.

From DeMont and Peatman,[38] p 24, with permission.

3. Number of extremities involved
4. Distribution of coordination impairment: proximal and/or distal musculature
5. Situations or occurrences that alter (increase or decrease) coordination deficits
6. Amount of time required to perform an activity
7. Level of safety
8. History of any falls (frequency, precipitating events, injuries sustained)

From this initial observation, the therapist will be guided in selecting the most appropriate tests for the deficit areas noted. An initial screening of strength, sensation, and range of motion before the coordination assessment will improve validity because weakness, sensory deficits, and decreased range of motion all may influence coordinated movement. It is also important to note that coordination deficits may occur in the presence of normal muscle strength and intact sensation.

Coordination tests generally can be divided into two main categories: gross motor activities and fine motor activities. Gross motor tests involve assessment of body posture, balance, and extremity movements involving large muscle groups. Examples of gross motor activities include crawling, kneeling, standing, walking, and running. Fine motor tests involve assessment of extremity movements concerned with utilization of small muscle groups. Examples of fine motor activities include manipulating objects with the hands (such as buttoning a shirt), and finger dexterity, which involves skillful, controlled manipulation of objects (such as those required for handwriting).

Coordination tests can be subdivided into nonequilibrium and equilibrium tests. Nonequilibrium coordination tests assess both static and mobile components of movements when the body is not in an upright (standing or sitting) position. These tests involve both gross and fine motor activities. Equilibrium tests assess both static and dynamic components of posture and balance when the body is in an upright (standing or sitting) position. They involve primarily gross motor activities and require observation of the body in both static (stationary) and dynamic (body in motion) postures.

Coordination tests incorporate assessment of the four basic motor task requirements, including mobility, stability (static postural control), controlled mobility (dynamic postural control), and skill. *Mobility* refers to initial movement occurring within a functional pattern. Examples of mobility deficits include insufficient motor unit activity to initiate a contraction, problems sustaining a movement, and difficulty moving against gravity. *Stability* (static postural control) is the ability to maintain a steady position in a weight-bearing, antigravity posture. Deficits present as instability or increased postural sway in sitting or standing (inability to maintain a posture), episodes of loss of balance, and risk of falls. *Controlled mobility* (dynamic postural control) is the ability to alter a position or change positions while maintaining stability. Deficits in controlled mobility include difficulty maintaining balance dur-

ing weight shifting or rocking within a posture (e.g., sitting), and the inability to assume a posture independently (e.g., sitting up from a supine position). This latter activity requires movement against gravity through a large range of motion. Static dynamic control is a variation of controlled mobility and refers to the ability to shift weight onto one limb and free the contralateral limb for non-weight bearing dynamic activities. The inability to lift one upper or lower limb off the supporting surface from a quadruped position is an example of a static dynamic control deficit. *Skill* refers to highly coordinated movement that allows interaction with the environment. Deficits include (1) an inability to stabilize proximal segments while distal segments move, and (2) movements that are inconsistent, require increased effort, and lack appropriate direction and timing. In addition, skill deficits impose limitations on precise control of movement, maintenance of movement for extended periods, and the ability to combine several movement sequences.

Coordination tests focus on assessment of movement capabilities in five main areas: (1) *alternate or reciprocal motion*, which tests the ability to reverse movement between opposing muscle groups; (2) *movement composition*, or synergy, which involves movement control achieved by muscle groups acting together; (3) *movement accuracy*, which assesses the ability to gauge or judge distance and speed of voluntary movement; (4) *fixation or limb holding*, which tests the ability to hold the position of an individual limb or limb segment; and (5) *equilibrium (postural stability)*, which assesses the ability to maintain balance in response to alterations in center of gravity and/or base of support. The progression of difficulty of coordination tests (gradual increases in challenge to the patient) typically utilizes the following sequence: (1) unilateral tasks, (2) bilateral symmetrical tasks, (3) bilateral asymmetrical tasks, and (4) multi-limb tasks (these constitute the highest level of difficulty).

Coordination assessment of equilibrium (postural stability) identifies movement deficits in stability, balance, and function. As the postural control system is composed of multiple components, impairments identified during a coordination assessment will assist in identifying other specific tests and measures required to obtain sufficient data to complete an evaluation. The postural control system includes (1) the sensory systems required for detection of body motion, (2) CNS integrative function, and (3) the motor system responsible for execution of movement responses controlling body position. Analysis of postural stability coordination deficits will guide selection of appropriate tests and measures to elicit additional information from one or more components of the postural control system. The reader is referred to Chapter 8, Assessment of Motor Function, for a more detailed discussion of postural control and balance.

Box 7–2 presents a sample of tests appropriate for nonequilibrium coordination testing, and Box 7–3 presents suggested tests for assessing equilibrium

---

Box 7–2 NONEQUILIBRIUM COORDINATION TESTS[a]

---

1. Finger to nose	The shoulder is abducted to 90 degrees with the elbow extended. The patient is asked to bring the tip of the index finger to the tip of the nose. Alterations may be made in the initial starting position to assess performance from different planes of motion.
2. Finger to therapist's finger	The patient and therapist sit opposite each other. The therapist's index finger is held in front of the patient. The patient is asked to touch the tip of the index finger to the therapist's index finger. The position of the therapist's finger may be altered during testing to assess ability to change distance, direction, and force of movement.
3. Finger to finger	Both shoulders are abducted to 90 degrees with the elbows extended. The patient is asked to bring both hands toward the midline and approximate the index fingers from opposing hands.
4. Alternate nose to finger	The patient alternately touches the tip of the nose and the tip of the therapist's finger with the index finger. The position of the therapist's finger may be altered during testing to assess ability to change distance, direction, and force of movement.
5. Finger opposition	The patient touches the tip of the thumb to the tip of each finger in sequence. Speed may be gradually increased.
6. Mass grasp	An alternation is made between opening and closing fist (from finger flexion to full extension). Speed may be gradually increased.
7. Pronation/supination	With elbows flexed to 90 degrees and held close to body, the patient alternately turns the palms up and down. This test also may be performed with shoulders flexed to 90 degrees and elbows extended. Speed may be gradually increased. The ability to reverse movements between opposing muscle groups can be assessed at many joints. Examples include active alternation between flexion and extension of the knee, ankle, elbow, fingers, and so forth.
8. Rebound test	The patient is positioned with the elbow flexed. The therapist applies sufficient manual resistance to produce an isometric contraction of biceps. Resistance is suddenly released. Normally, the opposing muscle group (triceps) will contract and "check" movement of the limb. Many other muscle groups can be tested for this phenomenon, such as the shoulder abductors or flexors, elbow extensors, and so forth.
9. Tapping (hand)	With the elbow flexed and the forearm pronated, the patient is asked to "tap" the hand on the knee.
10. Tapping (foot)	The patient is asked to "tap" the ball of one foot on the floor without raising the knee; heel maintains contact with floor.
11. Pointing and past pointing	The patient and therapist are opposite each other, either sitting or standing. Both patient and therapist bring shoulders to a horizontal position of 90 degrees of flexion with elbows extended. Index fingers are touching or the patient's finger may rest lightly on the therapist's. The patient is asked to fully flex the shoulder (fingers will be pointing toward ceiling) and then return to the horizontal position such that index fingers will again approximate. Both arms should be tested, either separately or simultaneously. A normal response consists of an accurate return to the starting position. In an abnormal response, there is typically a "past pointing," or movement beyond the target. Several variations to this test include movements in other directions such as toward 90 degrees of shoulder abduction or toward 0 degrees of shoulder flexion (finger will point toward floor). Following each movement, the patient is asked to return to the initial horizontal starting position.
12. Alternate heel to knee; heel to toe	From a supine position, the patient is asked to touch the knee and big toe alternately with the heel of the opposite extremity.
13. Toe to examiner's finger	From a supine position, the patient is instructed to touch the great toe to the examiner's finger. The position of finger may be altered during testing to assess ability to change distance, direction, and force of movement.
14. Heel on shin	From a supine position, the heel of one foot is slid up and down the shin of the opposite lower extremity.
15. Drawing a circle	The patient draws an imaginary circle in the air with either upper or lower extremity (a table or the floor also may be used). This also may be done using a figure-eight pattern. This test may be performed in the supine position for lower extremity assessment.
16. Fixation or position holding	Upper extremity: The patient holds arms horizontally in front (sitting or standing). Lower extremity: The patient is asked to hold the knee in an extended position (sitting).

[a]Tests should be performed first with eyes open and then with eyes closed. Abnormal responses include a gradual deviation from the "holding" position and/or a diminished quality of response with vision occluded. Unless otherwise indicated, tests are performed with the patient in a sitting position.

coordination. It should be noted that a single test is often appropriate to assess several different deficit areas, and areas may be tested simultaneously to conserve time. The tests mentioned here are intended as samples and are not all-inclusive. Other activities may be developed that are equally effective in assessing a particular impairment and may be more appropriate for an individual patient. It also should be emphasized that careful observation during performance of functional activities (e.g.,

Box 7–3 EQUILIBRIUM COORDINATION TESTS

1. Standing in a normal, comfortable posture.
2. Standing, feet together (narrow base of support).
3. Standing, with one foot directly in front of the other in tandem position (toe of one foot touching heel of opposite foot).
4. Standing on one foot.
5. Arm position may be altered in each of the above postures (i.e., arms at side, over head, hands on waist, and so forth).
6. Displace balance unexpectedly (while carefully guarding patient).
7. Standing, alternate between forward trunk flexion and return to neutral.
8. Standing, laterally flex trunk to each side.
9. Standing: eyes open (EO) to eyes closed (EC); ability to maintain an upright posture without visual input is referred to as a *positive Romberg sign.*
10. Standing in tandem position eyes open (EO) to eyes closed (EC) *(Sharpened Romberg).*
11. Walking, placing the heel of one foot directly in front of the toe of the opposite foot (tandem walking).
12. Walking along a straight line drawn or taped to the floor, or place feet on floor markers while walking.
13. Walk sideways, backward, or cross-stepping.
14. March in place.
15. Alter speed of ambulatory activities; observe patient walking at normal speed, as fast as possible, and as slow as possible.
16. Stop and start abruptly while walking.
17. Walk and pivot (turn 90, 180, or 360 degrees).
18. Walk in a circle, alternate directions.
19. Walk on heels or toes.
20. Walk with horizontal and vertical head turns.
21. Step over or around obstacles.
22. Stairclimbing with and without using handrail; one step at-a-time versus step-over-step.
23. Agility activities (coordinated movement with upright balance); jumping jacks, alternate flexing and extending the knees while sitting on a Swiss ball.

self-care routines, wheelchair propulsion, transfers, etc.) often provide an effective means for assessing many coordination deficits.

The two subdivisions of coordination tests presented here (nonequilibrium and equilibrium) have traditionally been used for providing structure and organization to administration of the tests. However, it should be noted that "nonequilibrium" division is somewhat of a misnomer in that elements of posture and balance are required during these tests. Although each subdivision places particular emphasis on certain components of movement, there will clearly be overlap between assessment findings from the two subdivisions. Table 7–1 includes selected coordination deficits and suggested tests that would be appropriate to assess the given problem.

In addition to the specific tests presented in Boxes 7–2 and 7–3, gait analysis measures also add important data to the coordination assessment. A systematic gait analysis will assist with identification of (1) abnormalities in muscle tone, (2) influence of

abnormal synergistic patterns and nonintegrated reflexes, (3) control of sequential timing of muscular activity, (4) control of body movements as a whole and of body segments in relation to each other, and (5) deviations from normal posture and motion (e.g., leaning, lurching, or excessive or diminished motion at a specific joint). A variety of standardized gait

Table 7–1 SAMPLE TESTS FOR SELECTED COORDINATION IMPAIRMENTS

Impairment	Sample Test
1. Dysdiadochokinesia	Finger to nose
	Alternate nose to finger
	Pronation/supination
	Knee flexion/extension
	Walking, alter speed or direction
2. Dysmetria	Pointing and past pointing
	Drawing a circle or figure eight
	Heel on shin
	Placing feet on floor markers while walking
3. Movement decomposition (dyssynergia)	Finger to nose
	Finger to therapist's finger
	Alternate heel to knee
	Toe to examiner's finger
4. Hypotonia	Passive movement
	Deep tendon reflexes
5. Tremor (intention)	Observation during functional activities (tremor will typically increase as target is approached or movement speed increased)
	Alternate nose to finger
	Finger to finger
	Finger to therapist's finger
	Toe to examiner's finger
6. Tremor (resting)	Observation of patient at rest
	Observation during functional activities (tremor will diminish significantly or disappear with movement)
7. Tremor (postural)	Observation of steadiness of normal standing posture
8. Asthenia	Fixation or position holding (upper and lower extremity)
	Application of manual resistance to assess muscle strength
9. Rigidity	Passive movement
	Observation during functional activities
	Observation of resting posture(s)
10. Bradykinesia	Walking, observation of arm swing and trunk motions
	Walking, alter speed and direction
	Request that a movement or gait activity be stopped abruptly
	Observation of functional activities: timed tests
11. Disturbances of posture	Fixation or position holding (upper and lower extremity)
	Displace balance unexpectedly in sitting or standing
	Standing, alter base of support (e.g., one foot directly in front of the other; standing on one foot)
12. Disturbances of gait	Walk along a straight line
	Walk sideways, backward
	March in place
	Alter speed and direction of ambulatory activities
	Walk in a circle

assessments or functional measures (which include a gait component) can be used, such as The Timed Up and Go test,[39,40] The Functional Independence Measure (FIM),[41–43] The Sickness Impact Profile,[44,45] and the Physical Performance and Mobility Examination (PPME).[46] The reader is referred to Chapter 8 for additional information on examination of motor function, Chapter 10 for a more detailed discussion of gait measures and assessment instruments, and Chapter 11 for additional examples of functional assessments.

Testing Protocol

The following progression should be used in performing a coordination assessment:
A. *Gather equipment.*
   1. Coordination assessment form
   2. Pen or pencil to record data
   3. Stopwatch (for timed performance)
   4. Two chairs
   5. Mat or treatment table
   6. Method of occluding vision (if needed)
B. *Select location.* The most appropriate setting is a quiet, well-lit room, free of distractions.
C. *Test selection.* Tests should be selected (see Boxes 7–2 and 7–3) to assess the specific components of movement appropriate for the individual patient. This activity will be guided by an initial observation of functional activities completed before formal coordination testing.
D. *Patient preparation.* Preferably, testing should be conducted when the patient is well rested. The testing procedures should be fully explained to the patient. Each coordination test should be described and demonstrated by the therapist before actual testing. Because testing procedures require mental concentration and some physical activity, fatigue, apprehension or fear may adversely influence test results.
E. *Testing.* Generally, nonequilibrium tests are completed first, followed by the equilibrium tests. Attention should be given to carefully guarding the patient during testing; use of a safety belt may be warranted. During the testing activities the following questions can be used to help direct the therapist's observations. The findings should be included in the comment section of the assessment form.
   1. Are movements direct, precise, and easily reversed?
   2. Do movements occur within a reasonable or normal amount of time?
   3. Does increased speed of performance affect quality of motor activity?
   4. Can continuous and appropriate motor adjustments be made if speed and direction are changed?
   5. Can a position or posture of the body or specific extremity be maintained without swaying, oscillations, or extraneous movements?
   6. Are placing movements of both upper and lower extremities exact?
   7. Does occluding vision alter the quality of motor activity?
   8. Is there greater involvement proximally or distally? On one side of body versus the other?
   9. Does the patient fatigue rapidly? Is there a consistency of motor response over time?
F. *Documentation.* The results of each test activity should be recorded.

Recording Test Results

Protocol for assessing and recording results from coordination tests vary considerably among institutions and individual therapists. Owing to the nature of the assessment and the wide variation in types and severity of deficits, observational coordination assessments are not highly standardized. However, a number of standardized tests are available for upper extremity assessment. These tests assess specific components of manual dexterity through the use of functional or work-related tasks. Many of these tests were developed originally to assess personnel for recruitment to various employment activities. Several examples of these tests are discussed later in this chapter.

Several options are available for recording results from a coordination assessment. A coordination assessment form is frequently useful to provide a composite picture of the deficit areas noted. These forms are often developed within clinical settings. They may be general (a sample is included in Appendix A), or they may be specific to a given group of patients, such as those with head injuries.[47] Generally, these forms tend to lack reliability testing. However, they do provide a systematic method of data collection and documentation. These forms frequently include some type of rating scale in which level of performance is weighted using an arbitrary scale. An example of such a scale follows:
- 4 = Normal performance is demonstrated.
- 3 = Movement is accomplished with only slight difficulty.
- 2 = Moderate difficulty is demonstrated in accomplishing activity; movements are arrhythmic, and performance deteriorates with increased speed.
- 1 = Severe difficulty is noted: movements are very arrhythmic; significant unsteadiness, oscillations, and/or extraneous movements are noted.
- 0 = Patient is unable to accomplish activity.

A score from the rating scale would then be assigned to each component of the coordination assessment. An advantage of using rating scales is that they provide a mechanism for qualitatively describing patient performance. However, several inherent limitations exist in using such scales. Often the descriptions are not reflective of exact patient performance. Alternatively, the rating scale may not be defined adequately or detailed appropriately, thus decreasing reliability of repeated or interexaminer testing. Frequently, coordination forms include a comments section. This component of the form allows for additional narrative descriptions of patient performance. Using a combination of a rating scale and narrative comments or summary will ensure that all deficit areas are adequately documented.

The use of a series of timed tests is an important parameter or measurement for assessing coordination. Because accomplishing an activity in a reasonable amount of time is a component of performance, the length of time required to accomplish certain activities is recorded by use of a stopwatch. A few standardized measurement tools have been developed based on timed activities (e.g., timed up and go test[39]). However, specific timed performance measures may be incorporated into a more general assessment form as well.

Computer-assisted force-plates also have been used to measure one component of equilibrium coordination. This approach provides a qualitative assessment of sway (a measure of postural stability).[27,48] The force-plates are capable of monitoring fluctuations in vertical pressure exerted by the feet. They offer the important advantage of providing an objective measure of postural stability.

Finally, videotape recordings have been used effectively for periodic assessment of coordination deficits. Videotapes provide a permanent, visual record of patient performance. They are particularly useful for assessing treatment and/or drug management via preintervention and postintervention recordings.

Although several options for documenting results are available, a written record using some type of assessment form is most common. An important consideration in establishing a protocol for recording test results is that each therapist is interpreting the form and/or rating scale in the same manner. This will require developing an instrument that is well defined, with distinct rating scale categories. Training sessions for new staff members and periodic reviews for the entire staff will improve interrater reliability.

STANDARDIZED INSTRUMENTS FOR ASSESSING MANUAL DEXTERITY AND COORDINATION

Several standardized tests have been developed to assess upper extremity coordination and hand dexterity through the use of functional activities. Many of these tests include normative data to assist with interpretation of test results. Strict adherence to the prescribed method of administration is imperative when using standardized tests. Any deviations from the established protocol will affect the validity and reliability of the measures and consequently make comparisons with published norms invalid. The skill of the examiner is another important consideration. The tests should be administered by an individual

specifically trained in administration and interpretation of results. Subsequent retests should be performed by the same individual. These standardized tests are particularly useful in providing objective measures of patient progress over time. The following is a description of several of these tests.

The Jebsen-Taylor Hand Function Test[49–53] measures hand function using seven subtests of functional activities: writing; card turning; picking up small objects; simulated feeding; stacking; picking up large, lightweight objects; and picking up large, heavy objects. The test is easy to construct, administer, and score. Normative data are included relating to age, sex, maximum time, and hand dominance. It allows assessment of hand function in seven common activities of daily living.

The Minnesota Rate of Manipulation Test[53–55] was originally designed to select personnel for jobs requiring arm and hand dexterity. This test assesses ability in five operations: placing, turning, displacing, one-hand turning and placing, and two-hand turning and placing. The test requires use of a form board with wells and round disks.

The Purdue Pegboard[53,56] test assesses dexterity by placement of pins in a pegboard and assembly of pins, washers, and collars (Fig. 7-6). There are several subtests, including right-hand prehension, left-hand prehension, prehension test with both hands, and assembly. The test has been used to select personnel for industrial jobs that require manipulative skills. Normative values are available, and both unilateral and bilateral dexterity can be assessed. This test requires use of a testing board, pins, collars, and washers.

The Crawford Small Parts Dexterity Test[53,55] uses the manipulation of small tools as a component of the test. The test uses pins, collars, and screws as well as a board into which these small objects fit. Use of tweezers is required both to place the pins in holes and to place a collar over the pin. The screws must be placed with the fingers and screwed in with a screwdriver. This test has been useful in prevocational testing. Normative data are available. This test is scored by time.

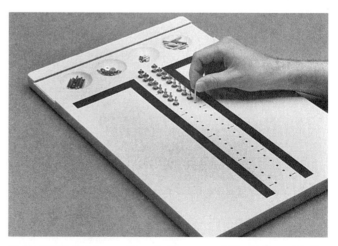

Figure 7-6. Purdue pegboard. (Courtesy of North Coast Medical, San Jose, CA.)

There are a variety of other standardized and commercially distributed tests available. Selection should be based on the individual needs of a given facility and the diagnostic groups most frequently seen. Additionally, careful assessment should be made of criteria used for standardization of the testing instrument.

SUMMARY

Coordination assessments provide the physical therapist with important information related to motor performance. They assist in identifying the source of motor deficits (although some clinical findings may not be attributable to a single area of CNS involvement). They also assist with establishing goals and outcomes, determining a treatment plan, and periodic reassessment to determine the effectiveness of treatment interventions. Because observational coordination tests are not highly standardized, there is a potential for error and misinterpretation of results. Sources of potential error can be reduced by the use of well-defined rating scales, administration of tests by skilled examiners, and subsequent retesting performed by the same therapist.

A variety of observational coordination tests have been presented. The majority of these tests can be used to assess more than one type of motor deficit. Documentation should include the type, severity, and location of the deficit as well as factors that alter the quality of performance. It is evident that multiple influences affect movement capabilities. As such, the results of coordination tests must be carefully considered with respect to data obtained from other assessments, such as sensation, muscle strength, tone, and range of motion.

QUESTIONS FOR REVIEW

1. Describe the clinical features of coordination deficits associated with lesions of the cerebellum, basal ganglia, and dorsal columns.

2. Explain the purpose of an initial observation of the patient before a formal coordination assessment. What types of activities should be observed? What information should be gathered?

3. Identify and describe the five general areas of movement capabilities assessed during a coordination assessment.

4. Differentiate between the types of activities included in equilibrium versus nonequilibrium coordination tests.

5. What questions related to patient performance should be considered during a coordination assessment to help direct the examiner's observations?

6. Define each of the following terms. Identify at least two coordination tests that would be appropriate for assessing each deficit. Explain the testing protocol you would use for each.
   A. Dysdiadochokinesia
   B. Dysmetria
   C. Movement decomposition
   D. Tremor (intention, resting, postural)
   E. Rigidity
   F. Bradykinesia

CASE STUDY

The patient is a 62 year-old man with a 5-year history of Parkinson's disease. Since the time of the diagnosis, he reports a progressive decline in functional activity level. With encouragement from his wife and children, he took an early retirement 3 years ago from his career as a commercial airline pilot. He lives with his wife of 38 years in a one-level suburban home. His four adult children all live in neighboring communities.

Initial examination reveals the following:
- Movements are decreased and slowed.
- A uniform, constant resistance is felt as the extremities are moved passively; patient reports an overall feeling of "stiffness."
- Involuntary, rhythmic, oscillatory movements of the distal upper extremities are noted at rest.
- Regular incidence of falls (2 to 3 times per week) is reported; standing balance is easily displaced with tendency to fall stiffly; difficulty changing direction of movement or stopping a movement.
- Patient has difficulty alternating distal upper extremity movements required for buttoning shirts, using eating utensils, and writing.
- Patient has difficulty making movement transitions, such as standing up from a chair or rolling from prone to supine.

The patient's medication is about to be changed from L-dopa alone to a combination of L-dopa with carbidopa (Sinemet). The physical therapy referral is for an assessment prior to the change in medication to document base-line function. Following the medication change, the assessment will be repeated and treatment initiated.

Guiding Questions

1. Identify the terms used to describe the following features of basal ganglia disorders: (1) decreased and slowed movement; (2) a uniform constant resistance to passive movement; and (3) involuntary, rhythmic, oscillatory movements of the distal upper extremities at rest.

2. What general movement deficits would be evident in the presence of bradykinesia?

3. Identify a sample of nonequilibrium coordination tests appropriate to assess the patient's difficulty alternating distal upper extremity movements.

4. Identify a sample of equilibrium coordination tests appropriate to assess this patient's altered postural reactions and balance.

5. Describe a plan for documenting findings from the examination.

REFERENCES

1. Ghez, C, and Gordon, J: Voluntary Movement. In Kandel, ER, et al (eds): Essentials of Neural Science and Behavior. Appleton & Lange, Norwalk, CT, 1995, p 529.
2. American Physical Therapy Association. Guide to physical therapist practice. Phys Ther 77, 1997.
3. Gilman, S, and Winans Newman, S: Manter and Gatz's Essential of Clinical Neuroanatomy and Neurophysiology, ed 9. FA Davis, Philadelphia, 1996.
4. Newton, RA: Contemporary Issues and Theories of Motor Control: Assessment of Movement and Balance, In Umphred, DA: Neurological Rehabilitation, ed 4. Mosby-Year Book, St. Louis, 1995, p 81.
5. Klapp, ST: Reaction Time Analysis of Central Motor Control. In Zelaznik, HN (ed): Advances in Motor Learning and Control. Human Kinetics, Champaign, IL, 1996, p 13.
6. Schmidt, RA, and Lee, TD: Motor Control and Learning: A Behavioral Emphasis. Human Kinetics, Champaign, IL 1999.
7. Ghez, C: The Cerebellum. In Kandel, ER, et al (eds): Principles of Neuroscience, ed 3. Appleton & Lange, Norwalk, CT, 1991, p 626.
8. Urbscheit, NL, and Oremland, BS: Cerebellar Dysfunction. In Umphred, DA: Neurological Rehabilitation, ed. 4. Mosby-Year Book, St. Louis, 1995, p 23.
9. Guyton, AC, and Hall, JE: Human Physiology and Mechanisms of Disease, ed 6. Saunders, Philadelphia, 1997.
10. Fredericks, CM: Cerebellar Mechanisms. In Fredericks, CM, and Saladin, LK: Pathophysiology of the Motor Systems: Principles and Clinical Presentations. FA Davis, Philadelphia, 1996, p 181.
11. Waxman, SG, and deGrot, J: Correlative Neuroanatomy, ed 22. Appleton & Lange, Norwalk, CT, 1995.
12. Aminoff, MJ, et al: Clinical Neurology, ed 3. Appleton & Lange, Stamford, CT, 1996.
13. Young, PA, and Young PH: Basic Clinical Neuroanantomy. Williams & Wilkins, Baltimore, 1997.
14. Nolte, J: The Human Brain: An Introduction to its Functional Anatomy, ed 3. Mosby-Year Book, St. Louis, 1993.
15. Martin, JH: Neuroanatomy Text and Atlas, ed 2. Appleton & Lange, Stamford, CT, 1996.
16. Shumway-Cook, A, and Woollacott, MH: Motor Control: Theory and Practical Applications. Williams & Wilkins, Baltimore, 1995.
17. Melnick, ME: Basal ganglia disorders: Metabolic, hereditary, and genetic disorders in adults. In Umphred, DA (ed): Neurological Rehabilitation, ed. 4. Mosby-Year Book, St. Louis, 1995, p 606.
18. Cote, L, and Crutcher, MD: The Basal Ganglia. In Kandel, ER, et al (eds): Principles of Neural Science and Behavior, ed 3. Appleton & Lange, Norwalk, CT, 1991, p 647.
19. Lundy-Ekman, L: Neuroscience: Fundamentals for Rehabilitation. Saunders, Philadelphia, 1998.
20. DiFabio, RP, and Emasithi, A: Aging and the mechanisms underlying head and postural control during voluntary motion. Phys Ther 77:458, 1997.
21. Woollacott, MH, and Tang, PF: Balance control during walking in the older adult: Research and its implications. Phys Ther 77:646, 1997.
22. Woollacott, MH: Changes in posture and voluntary control in the elderly: Research findings and rehabilitation. Top Geriatr Rehabil 5:1, 1990.
23. Salthouse, TA, et al: Interrelations of age, visual acuity, and cognitive functioning. J Gerontol B Psychol Soc Sci 51B:317, 1996.
24. Pyykko, I, et al: Postural control in elderly subjects. Age Ageing 19:215, 1990.
25. Lewis, CB, and Bottomley, JM: Geriatric Physical Therapy: A Clinical Approach. Appleton & Lange, East Norwalk, CT, 1994.
26. Craik, RL: Sensorimotor Changes and Adaptation in the Older Adult. In Guccione, AA (ed): Geriatric Physical Therapy. Mosby-Year Book, St. Louis, 1993, p 71.
27. Hughes, MA, et al: The relationship of postural sway to sensorimotor function, functional performance, and disability in the elderly. Arch Phys Med Rehabil 77:567, 1996.
28. Braun, BL: Knowledge and perception of fall-related risk factors and fall-reduction techniques among community-dwelling elderly individuals. Phys Ther 78:1262, 1998.
29. Chaput, S, and Proteau, L: Aging and motor control. J Gerontol B Psychol Sci Soc Sci 51B:P346, 1996.
30. Bortz, WM: Disuse and aging. JAMA 248:1203, 1982.
31. Stelmach, GE, and Worthingham, CJ: Sensory motor deficits related to postural stability. Clin Geriatr Med 1:679, 1985.
32. Welford, AT: Between bodily changes and performance: Some possible reasons for slowing with age. Exp Aging Res 10:73, 1984.
33. Spirduso, WW: Physical fitness, aging, and psychomotor speed: A review. J Gerontol 35:850, 1980.
34. Weiss, AT: Between bodily changes and performance: Some possible reasons for slowing with age. Exp Aging Res 10:73, 1984.
35. Bohannon, RW: Clinical implications of neurologic changes during the aging process. In Lewis, CB (ed): Aging: The Health Care Challenge, ed 3. FA Davis, Philadelphia, 1996, p 177.
36. Guccione, AA (ed): Geriatric Physical Therapy. Mosby-Year Book, St. Louis, 1993.
37. Lewis, CB (ed): Aging: The Health Care Challenge, ed 3. FA Davis, Philadelphia, 1996.
38. DeMont, ME, and Peatman, NL: Communication, values, and the quality of life. In Guccione, AA (ed): Geriatric Physical Therapy. Mosby-Year Book, St. Louis, 1993, p 21.
39. Podsiadlo, D, and Richardson, S: The timed "up and go": A test of basic functional mobility for frail elderly persons. J Am Geriatr Soc 39:142, 1991.
40. Mathias, S, et al: Balance in elderly patients: The "get-up and go" test. Arch Med Rehabil 67:387, 1986.
41. Granger, CV, et al: Functional assessment scales: A study of persons with multiple sclerosis. Arch Phys Med Rehabil 71:870, 1990.
42. Granger, CV, et al: Advance in functional assessment for medical rehabilitation. Top Ger Rehabil 1:59, 1986.
43. Keith, RA, et al: The functional independence measure. Advances in Clinical Rehabilitation 1:6, 1987.
44. Bergner, M, et al: The sickness impact profile: Development and final revision of a health status measure. Med Care 19:787, 1981.
45. Follick, MJ, et al: The sickness impact profile: A global measure of disability in chronic low back pain. Pain 21:67, 1985.
46. Winograd, CH, et al: Development of a physical performance and mobility examination. J Am Geriatr Soc 42:743, 1994.
47. Cruz, VW: Evaluation of coordination: A clinical model. Clinical Management in Physical Therapy 6:6, 1986.
48. Shumway-Cook, A, et al: The effects of two types of cognitive tasks on postural stabilty in older adults with and without a history of falls. J Gerontol A Biol Sci Med Sci 52(A):M232, 1997.
49. Jebson, RH, et al: An objective and standardized test of hand function. Arch Phys Med Rehabil 50:311, 1969.
50. Hackel, ME, et al: Changes in hand function in the aging adult as determined by the Jebsen test of hand function. Phys Ther 72:373, 1992.

51. Mathiowetz, V: Role of physical performance component evaluations in occupational therapy functional assessment. Am J Occup Ther 47:228, 1993.
52. Taylor, N, et al: Evaluation of hand function in children. Arch Phys Med Rehabil 54:129, 1973.
53. Asher, IE: Occupational Therapy Assessment Tools: An Annotated Index, ed 2. The American Occupational Therapy Association, Bethesda, MD, 1996.
54. Fess, EE: Documentation: Essential elements of an upper extremity assessment battery. In Hunter, JM, et al (eds): Rehabilitation of the Hand, ed 2. CV Mosby, St. Louis, 1984, p 49.
55. Smith, HD: Assessment and evaluation: An overview. In Hopkins, HL, and Smith, HD (eds): Willard and Spackman's Occupational Therapy, ed 8. Lippincott, Philadelphia, 1993, p 169.
56. Mathiowetz, V, et al, C: The purdue pegboard: Norms for 14- to 19-year-olds. Am J Occup Ther 40:174, 1986.

SUPPLEMENTAL READINGS

Adams, JH, et al (eds): Greenfield's Neuropathology, ed 5. Oxford University Press, New York, 1992.

Adams, RD, and Victor, M: Principles of Neurology, ed 5. McGraw-Hill, New York, 1993.

Bastian, AJ: Mechanisms of ataxia. Phys Ther 77:672, 1997.

Bohannon, RW, et al: Decrease in timed balance test scores with aging. Phys Ther 64:1067, 1984.

Bohannon, RW: Stopwatch for measuring thumb-movement time. Percept Mot Skills 81:211, 1995.

Chafetz, MD, et al: The cerebellum and cognitive function: Implications for rehabilitation. Arch Phys Med Rehabil 77:1303, 1996.

Chandler, JM, et al, SA: Balance performance on the postural stress test: Comparison of young adults, healthy elderly, and fallers. Phys Ther 70:410, 1990.

DeMeyer, WE: Techniques of the Neurologic Examination: A Programmed Text, ed 4. McGraw-Hill, Inc., New York, 1994.

Glick, TH: Neurologic Skills. Blackwell Scientific, Boston, 1993.

Harada, N, et al: Screening for balance and mobility impairment in elderly individuals living in residential care facilities. Phys Ther 75:462, 1995.

Kauffman, T: Impact of aging-related musculoskeletal and postural changes on falls. Top Ger Rehabil 5:34, 1990.

Kinzey, SJ, and Armstrong, CW: The reliability of the star-excursion test in assessing dynamic balance. J Orthop Sports Phys Ther 27:356, 1998.

Kurlan, R (ed): Movement Disorders. Lippincott, Philadelphia, 1995.

Lovgreen, B, et al: Muscle vibration alters the trajectories of voluntary movements in cerebellar disorders: A method of counteracting impaired movement accuracy? Clin Rehabil 7:327, 1993.

Luchies, CW, et al: Stepping responses of young and old adults to postural disturbances: Kinematics. J Am Geriatr Soc 42:506, 1994.

Mayo Clinic and Mayo Foundation: Clinical Examinations in Neurology, ed 6. Mosby Year Book, St. Louis, 1991.

Morris, ME, et al: Temporal stability of gait in Parkinson's disease. Phys Ther 76:763, 1996.

Neistadt, ME: The effects of different treatment activities on functional fine motor coordination in adults with brain injury. Am J Occup Ther 48:877, 1994.

Nolte, J: The Human Brain: An Introduction to its Functional Anatomy, ed 3. Mosby Year Book, St. Louis, 1993.

Schmahmann, JD: An emerging concept: The relationship of the cerebellum to behavior and mental processes. Arch Neurol 48:1178, 1991.

Schols, L, et al: Motor evoked potentials in the spinocerebellar ataxias type 1 and type 3. Muscle Nerve 20:226, 1997.

Shumway-Cook, A, and Woollacott, M: Motor Control: Theory and Practical Application. Williams & Wilkins, Philadelphia, 1995.

Swaine, BR, and Sullivan, J: Relation between clinical and instrumented measures of motor coordination in traumatically brain injured persons. Arch Phys Med Rehabil 73:55, 1992.

Swaine, BR, and Sullivan, SJ: Reliability of the scores for the finger-to-nose test in adults with traumatic brain injury. Phys Ther 73:71, 1993.

Willoughby, C, and Polatajko, HJ: Motor problems in children with developmental coordination disorder: Review of the literature. Am J Occup Ther 49:787, 1994.

Zupan, A: Assessment of the functional abilities of the upper limbs in patients with neuromuscular diseases. Disabil Rehabil 18:69, 1996.

GLOSSARY

Akinesia: Inability to initiate movement; seen in Parkinson's disease.

Asthenia: Generalized muscle weakness associated with cerebellar lesions.

Asynergia: Loss of ability to associate muscles together for complex movements.

Ataxia: A general term used to describe uncoordinated movement; may influence gait, posture, and patterns of movements.

Athetosis: Slow, involuntary, writhing, twisting, "wormlike" movements; clinical feature of some forms of cerebral palsy (also called *athetoid movements*).

Bradykinesia: Abnormally slow movements.

Chorea: Involuntary, rapid, irregular, jerky movements; clinical feature of Huntington's disease (also called *choreiform movements*).

Choreoathetosis: Movement disorder with features of both chorea and athetosis; seen in some forms of cerebral palsy.

Closed-loop system (servomechanism, servo): A movement control process that employs feedback against a reference for correctness for computation of error and subsequent movement correction.

Dysarthria: Disorder of the motor component of speech articulation.

Dysdiadochokinesia: Impaired ability to perform rapid alternating movements.

Dysmetria: Impaired ability to judge the distance or range of a movement.

Dyssynergia: Impaired ability to associate muscles together for complex movement; decomposition of movement.

Dystonia: Impaired or disordered tonicity; tone fluctuates in an unpredictable manner from low to high.

Hemiballismus: Sudden, jerky, forceful, wild, flailing motions of one side of the body.

Hyperkinesia: A general term used to describe abnormally increased muscle activity or movement; restlessness.

Hypermetria: Excessive distance or range of a movement; an overestimation of the required motion needed to reach a target object.

Hypokinesia: A general term used to describe decreased motor responses (especially to a specific stimulus); sluggishness, listlessness.

Hypometria: Shortened distance or range of a movement; an underestimation of the required motion needed to reach a target object.

Hypotonia (hypotonus): Reduced muscle tension below normal resting levels.

Motor program: A set of prestructured commands that when initiated results in the production of a coordinated movement sequence.

Movement decomposition: Performance of a movement in a sequence of component parts rather than as a single smooth activity.

Nystagmus: Rhythmic, oscillatory movement of the eyes.

Open-loop system: A control mechanism that uses preprogrammed instructions to regulate movement independent of a feedback and error-detection process.

Rebound phenomenon: Absence of a check reflex; when resistance to an isometric contraction is suddenly removed, the body segment moves forcibly in the direction in which effort was focused.

Rigidity: Increase in muscle tone; results in greater resistance to passive movement. Resistance is felt as constant and uniform (leadpipe rigidity), or as jerky "catches" (cogwheel rigidity).

Romberg sign: Inability to maintain standing balance when vision is occluded.

Tremor: An involuntary oscillatory movement resulting from alternate contractions of opposing muscle groups.

Tremor; types include: Intention (kinetic) tremor: Occurs during voluntary motion.

Postural (static) tremor: Back-and-forth oscillatory movements of the body while patient maintains a standing posture.

Resting tremor: Present when involved body segment is at rest; typically disappears or decreases with purposeful movement.

Scanning speech: A speech pattern that is slow, and may be slurred, hesitant, with prolonged syllables and inappropriate pauses; the melodic quality of speech is altered.

APPENDIX A

Sample Coordination Assessment Form

Name:
Examiner: _____ Date _____ .

PART I NONEQUILIBRIUM TESTS
Key to Grading
5. Normal performance.
4. Minimal impairment: able to accomplish activity with slightly less than normal speed and skill.
3. Moderate impairment: able to accomplish activity, but coordination deficits very noticeable; movements are slow, awkward and unsteady.

Grade:Left	Coordination Test	Grade:Right	Comments
	Finger to nose.		
	Finger to therapist's finger.		
	Finger to finger.		
	Alternate nose to finger.		
	Finger opposition.		
	Mass grasp.		
	Pronation/supination (RAM).		
	Rebound test of Holmes.		
	Tapping (hand).		
	Tapping (foot).		
	Pointing and past pointing.		
	Alternate heel to knee; heel to toe.		
	Toe to examiner's finger.		
	Heel on shin.		
	Drawing a circle (hand).		
	Drawing a circle (foot).		
	Fixation/position holding (upper extremity).		
	Fixation/position holding (lower extremity).		

Additional Comments:

2. Severe impairment: able only to initiate activity without completion.
1. Activity impossible.

Continued

PART II EQUILIBRIUM TESTS
Key to Grading
4. Able to accomplish activity
3. Can complete activity; minor physical contact guarding required to maintain balance.
2. Can complete activity; significant (moderate to maximal) contact guarding required to maintain balance.
1. Activity impossible.

Grade	Coordination Test	Comments
	Standing in a normal, comfortable posture.	
	Standing, feet together (narrow base of support).	
	Standing on one foot.	
	Standing, with one foot directly in front of the other in tandem position (toe of one foot touching heel of opposite foot).	
	Standing, forward trunk flexion and return to neutral.	
	Standing, laterally flex trunk to each side.	
	Standing: eyes open (EO) to eyes closed (EC); *Romberg*.	
	Standing in tandem position: eyes open (EO) to eyes closed (EC); *Sharpened Romberg*.	
	Walk at normal speed.	
	Walk as fast as possible.	
	Walk as slow as possible.	
	Walk: stop and start abruptly.	
	Walk and pivot (turn 90, 180, or 360 degrees).	
	Walking, placing the heel of one foot directly in front of the toe of the opposite foot (tandem walking).	
	Walking along a straight line drawn or taped to the floor.	
	Walking, placing feet on floor markers.	
	Walk: sideways.	
	Walk: backwards.	
	Walk: cross-stepping.	
	Walk: in a circle, alternate directions.	
	Walk: on heels.	
	Walk: on toes.	
	March in place.	
	Walk with horizontal and vertical head turns.	
	Step over or around obstacles.	
	Stairclimbing with handrail.	
	Stairclimbing without handrail.	
	Stairclimbing: one step at-a-time.	
	Stairclimbing: step-over-step.	

Additional Comments:

NOTE: Notations should be made under comments section if
1. Lack of visual input renders activity impossible or alters quality of performance.
2. Verbal cuing is required to accomplish activity.
3. Alterations in speed affect quality of performance.
4. An excessive amount of time is required to complete activity.
5. Changes in arm position influence equilibrium tests.
6. Any extraneous movements, unsteadiness, or oscillations are noted in head, neck, or trunk.
7. Fatigue alters consistency of response.

APPENDIX B

Suggested Answers to Case Study Guiding Questions

1. Identify the terms used to describe the following features of basal ganglia disorders:
(1) decreased and slowed movement.
ANSWER: Bradykinesia.

(2) a uniform constant resistance to passive movement.
ANSWER: Leadpipe rigidity.

(3) involuntary, rhythmic, oscillatory movement of the distal upper extremities at rest.
ANSWER: Resting tremor.

2. What movement deficits would be evident in the presence of bradykinesia?
ANSWER: Bradykinesia may be demonstrated in a variety of ways, such as a decreased arm swing; slow, shuffling gait; difficulty initiating or changing direction of movement; lack of facial expression; or difficulty stopping a movement once begun.

3. Identify a sample of nonequilibrium coordination tests appropriate to assess the patient's difficulty alternating distal upper extremity movements.
ANSWER: Finger to nose, finger to therapist finger, finger to finger, alternate nose to finger, finger opposition, mass grasp, pronation/supination, alternate heel to knee, heel to toe, toe to examiner's finger, and heel to shin.

4. Identify a sample of equilibrium coordination tests appropriate to assess this patient's altered postural reactions and balance.
ANSWER: Functional gait assessment—standing with feet together (narrow base of support), standing with one foot directly in front of the other (toe of one foot touching heel of opposite foot), standing on one foot, altering arm position in various upright postures, perturb balance unexpectedly, standing with alternation between forward trunk flexion and return to neutral, standing while laterally flexing trunk to each side, walking while placing the heel of one foot directly in front of the toe of the opposite foot, walking along a straight line, walking sideways and backward, marching in place, altering speed of walking, and stopping and starting abruptly.

5. Describe a plan for documenting findings from the examination.
ANSWER: Several options are available for recording results from a coordination assessment. A coordination assessment form will provide a composite picture of the deficit areas noted. These forms generally include some type of rating scale in which level of performance is weighted using an arbitrary scale (e.g., 4 = normal performance; 3 = movement accomplished with only slight difficulty; 2 = moderate difficulty is demonstrated in accomplishing activity, etc.). Because functional limitations for this patient include decreased and slowed movements, another useful option for documentation is a series of timed tests. Because accomplishing an activity in a reasonable amount of time is a component of performance, the length of time required to accomplish certain activities is recorded by the use of a stopwatch. Videotape recordings are particularly effective for periodic assessment of coordination deficits, as will be required for this patient. Videotapes will provide a permanent, visual record of patient performance before and after the change in medication.

Assessment of 8
Motor Function

Susan B. O'Sullivan

LEARNING OBJECTIVES

1. Identify the purposes and components of the examination of motor function (motor control and motor learning).
2. Describe the examination process and specific measures of motor function.
3. Describe common deficits associated with disorders of motor function.
4. Discuss factors that influence the complexity of the examination and evaluation process.
5. Discuss factors that influence determination of the physical therapy diagnosis.
6. Using the case study example, apply clinical decision making skills in evaluating motor function assessment data.

OVERVIEW OF MOTOR FUNCTION (MOTOR CONTROL AND MOTOR LEARNING)

Motor control evolves from a complex set of neurological and mechanical processes that govern posture and movement. Some movements are genetically predetermined and emerge through processes of normal growth and development. Examples of these include the reflex patterns that predominate during much of our early life. Other movements, termed **motor skills,** are learned through interaction and exploration of the environment. Practice and feedback are important variables in defining motor learning and motor skill development. Sensory information about movement is used to guide and shape the development of the motor program. A **motor program** is "an abstract representation that, when initiated, results in the production of a coordinated movement sequence."[1p416] A **motor plan** is an idea or plan for purposeful movement that is made up of several component motor programs. Motor memory involves the storage of motor programs or subprograms and includes information on how the movement felt (sense of effort), movement components, and movement outcome. Memory allows for continued access of this information for repeat performance or modification of existing patterns of movement.

Both reflex patterns and motor skills are subject to control by the central nervous system (CNS), which organizes and integrates vast amounts of sensory information. **Feedback** is response-produced information received during or after the movement and is used to monitor output for corrective actions. **Feedforward,** the sending of signals in advance of movement to ready the sensorimotor systems, allows for anticipatory adjustments in postural activity. Processing of information by the CNS is both serial and parallel, leading to the production of coordinated movement. **Coordination** refers to "the patterning of body and limb motions relative to the patterning of environmental objects and events."[2p416] **Coordinative structures** are "functionally specific units of muscles and joints that are constrained by the nervous system to act cooperatively to produce an action."[2p416]

Various different interacting systems of the CNS are engaged in cooperative actions to produce movement that accommodates to the demands of the specific task and of the environment. Hierarchical theory proposes a flexible system of command hierarchies. The highest level includes the association cortex and basal ganglia (caudate loop), which organize sensory information and elaborate the overall motor plan. The middle level includes the sensorimotor cortex, cerebellum, basal ganglia (putamen loop), and brainstem. These areas shape and define the specific motor programs and initiate commands. The lowest level is the spinal cord, which executes the commands, translating them into the final muscle actions.[3] These CNS levels do not function in a rigid top-down hierarchic manner, as once thought, but rather appear flexible. Control commands operate through numerous feedback loops and proceed in both an ascending and a descending manner. Systems theory suggests a distributed mode of motor control. A basic concept of this theory is that units of the CNS are organized around specific task demands (termed *task systems*). The entire CNS may be necessary for complex tasks, whereas only small portions may be needed for simple tasks. Command levels vary depending on the specific task executed. Thus, the highest level of command may not be required in the execution of some simple movements.[4]

Damage to the CNS interferes with motor control processes. Lesions affecting areas of the CNS can produce specific, recognizable deficits that are consistent among patients (e.g., patients with upper motor neuron syndrome). Individual differences in CNS adaptation, recovery, and functional outcomes can be expected. In conditions with widespread damage to the CNS (e.g., traumatic brain injury) the resultant problems in motor function are numerous, complex, and difficult to delineate. An accurate picture of the scope of deficits may not be readily apparent on initial examination. A process of reexamination over time will generally yield an understanding of the patient's performance capabilities and deficits. The comprehensive examination should focus on functional limitations and disabilities and on those impairments that directly impact on function. Goals, outcomes, and treatments can then be developed that directly impact on what the patient can and cannot accomplish.

EXAMINATION OF MOTOR FUNCTION

An examination of motor function is required prior to any intervention. It has three components: (1) patient history, (2) a review of relevant systems, and (3) specific tests and measures.[5]

The history includes both past and current health status. Information is commonly gathered from the patient and interested persons (family members, significant others, or caregivers). If the patient is unable to communicate accurate and meaningful information, as is frequently the case with injury to the brain, data must be gathered from other sources. A review of the medical record can be used to verify and triangulate data obtained from personal communications. Often, the medical record of a patient with pronounced deficits in motor function (e.g., the patient with traumatic brain injury) is filled with volumes of data that can be unwieldy and difficult to sort through. The therapist can benefit from the application of a framework to identify and classify problems. The model of disablement, including impairments, functional limitations, and disabilities, provides such a useful framework and is an important element of the *Guide to Physical Therapist Practice*[5] (see Chapter 1).

A systems review serves the purpose of a screening examination; that is, a brief or limited examination of the body systems. The physical therapist can then use this information to identify potential problems that will require more extensive testing. For example, screening examinations for posture and tone may reveal significant impairments and functional limitations. More detailed tests and measures are then required to delineate the exact nature of the problems uncovered. Sometimes screening examinations reveal problems in communication and/or cognition that preclude further testing. For example, the patient with stroke and severe communication and cognitive impairments will be unable to follow directions and cooperate with many individual tests of physical function. The therapist will document this in the medical record as "unable to test at the present time due to severe communication/cognitive deficits."

Specific parameters of dyscontrol should be closely examined using appropriate tests and measures. If the test accurately measures the parameter of performance being examined, it is said to have *validity*. The *reliability* of an instrument is reflected in the consistency of results obtained by a single examiner over repeat trials (intrarater reliability) or among multiple examiners (interrater reliability). Therapists should select standardized instruments with established validity and reliability whenever possible.[5]

An examination of motor function is a multifaceted process that requires a number of different specific tests and measures. Assessments can be qualitative, utilizing observations of complex aspects of performance. Insights and understanding of patterns of movement or postures are developed from inductive reasoning (formulating generalizations from specific observations). The experienced therapist or expert clinician is far more efficient in reaching decisions about qualitative performance than the novice therapist.[6] Quantitative assessment uses measurement as a way of understanding and assessing performance. Characteristics of performance are defined by measured values. Documentation constraints imposed by the health care system and third party payers increasingly emphasize objective, quantitative assessments as proof of the need for services and the effectiveness of services. However, many aspects of motor function are not easily measured. For example, motor learning is not directly measurable but rather is inferred from measures of performance, retention, generalizability, and adaptability. Thus these constructs are used to infer changes in the CNS that occur with learning. The therapist must be sensitive to the nature of the variables being assessed and identify appropriate measures that provide a meaningful analysis of patient function. It is not likely that any one measure will provide all of the data needed for the assessment of motor function.

Reexaminations are performed to determine if goals and outcomes are being met, and if the patient is benefiting from the intervention plan. Interventions can then be modified or redirected as appropriate. Successful achievement of anticipated goals and outcomes is an indication for discharge and referral for follow-up or additional services. Reexamination is also an important quality assurance measure.

The success or failure of interventions can be carefully documented through reexaminations. The following sections present individual elements of the assessment of motor function.

Consciousness and Arousal

An assessment of consciousness and arousal is important in determining the degree to which an individual is able to respond. The ascending reticular activating system (ARAS) in the brainstem acts on the cortex to maintain the conscious state, controlling different degrees of wakefulness. Low levels of activity are associated with sleep or drowsiness, whereas high levels of activity are associated with extreme excitement (high arousal). The descending reticular activating system (DRAS) functions to maintain autonomic and somatic motor systems. Sympathetic and parasympathetic outflow is modulated, establishing baseline values for a number of body functions and homeostasis. Sympathetic activity allows actions to be initiated to protect the individual under varying circumstances. Motor systems become engaged in carrying out defensive commands, producing **fight or flight responses.** Balanced interaction of the autonomic and somatic systems allows for reactive yet stable responses of an individual.[7]

Consciousness is a state of awareness and implies orientation to person, place, and time. The conscious patient is clearly awake and responds quickly and appropriately to varying stimuli. There is full awareness of self and surroundings. Different stages of consciousness have been identified. **Lethargy** refers to a general slowing of motor processes, including speech and movement. The patient appears drowsy and does not fully appreciate the environment. The patient can easily fall asleep if not continually stimulated. Attempts to communicate with the patient are difficult owing to deficits in maintaining focus or attention. **Obtunded** refers to

dulled or blunted sensitivity. The patient is difficult to arouse from sleeping and once aroused, appears confused. Attempts to interact with the patient are generally nonproductive. **Stupor** refers to a state of semiconsciousness. The patient lacks responsiveness, and can be aroused only by intense stimuli (e.g., painful stimuli such as sharp pressure over a bony prominence). The patient demonstrates little in the way of voluntary motor responses. Mass movement responses can be observed in response to painful stimuli or loud noises. The unconscious patient is said to be in a **coma** and does not perceive or respond to the environment or intense stimuli. The eyes remain closed and there are no sleep/wake cycles. The patient is ventilator dependent. Reflex reactions may or may not be seen, depending on the location of the lesion(s) within the CNS.[8]

Clinically the patient can progress from one level of consciousness to another. For example, with an intracranial bleed, the swelling and mass effect compress the brain resulting in decreasing levels of consciousness. The patient progresses from lethargy to stupor, and finally to coma. If medical interventions are successful, recovery is evidenced by a reverse progression. True coma is generally time limited. Patients emerge into a **vegetative state,** characterized by return of irregular sleep/wake cycles and normalization of the so-called vegetative functions—respiration, digestion, and blood pressure control. The patient in a vegetative state may be aroused, but remains unaware of his or her environment. There is no purposeful attention or cognitive responsiveness. Individuals in a **persistent vegetative state** remain in a vegetative state 1 year or more after brain injury. This is caused by severe brain injury or anoxic cerebral insult.

The Glasgow Coma Scale (GCS) is the gold standard used to document level of consciousness. Three areas of function are examined: eye opening, best motor response, and verbal response (see Table 24–1). Total GCS scores range from a low of 3 to a high of 15. A total score of 8 or less is indicative of severe brain injury and coma; a score between 9 and 12 is indicative of moderate brain injury, whereas a score from 13 to 15 is indicative of mild brain injury.[9]

An imbalance in the autonomic nervous system (ANS), with high levels of sympathetic activity, results in an individual with high arousal and a high level of **fight or flight responses** (alarm or stress responses). Specific responses include hyperalertness, increased heart rate (HR), increased blood pressure (BP), increased respiratory rate (RR), dilated pupils, sweating, and so forth. Whereas a certain level of arousal is necessary for optimal motor performance, high levels cause a deterioration in performance. This is referred to as the **inverted-U theory (Yerkes-Dodson law).**[10] Excess levels of arousal can also yield unexpected responses. This theory was originally proposed by Wilder as the Law of Initial Value (LIV).[11] Patients at either end of an arousal continuum (either very high or very low) may not respond at all or may respond in an unpredictable manner. Stockmeyer[12] suggests that this phenomenon may explain the reactions of patients who are labile and lack homeostatic controls for normal function. Assessment of baseline levels of central state should, therefore, precede other aspects of assessment in the patient suspected of autonomic instability (e.g., brain injury).

Critical components for baseline assessment include (1) a representative sampling of ANS responses, including HR, BP, RR, pupil dilation, and sweating; (2) a determination of patient reactivity, including the degree and rate of response to sensory stimulation; and (3) a determination of compensatory mechanisms in response to physiological stressors.[12] Careful monitoring during motor performance can also assist in defining homeostatic stability. More specific guidelines for assessment of vital functions can be found in Chapter 4.

Attention

Attention is the capacity of the brain to process information from the environment or from long-term memory. An individual with intact **selective attention** is able to screen and process relevant sensory information about both the task and the environment while screening out irrelevant information. The complexity and familiarity of the task determines the degree of attention required. If new information is presented, concentration and effort are increased. Patients who are inattentive will have difficulty concentrating. Deficits become more apparent with new or complex tasks.

Selective attention can be assessed by asking the patient to attend to a particular task. For example, the examiner may ask the patient to repeat a short list of items. The examiner can also read a list of items while the patient is asked to identify or signal each time a particular item is mentioned.[8] *Sustained attention* (or vigilance) can be assessed by determining how long the patient is able to maintain attention on a particular task. *Alternating attention* (attentional flexiblity) can be assessed by requesting the patient alternate back and forth between two different tasks, for example, add the first two pairs of numbers, then subtract the next two pairs of numbers. *Divided attention* can be assessed by requesting the patient perform two tasks simultaneously. For example, the patient talks while walking (walkie-talkie test), or walks while locating an object placed to the side (simulated grocery shopping). Documentation should include the specific component of attention assessed, any slowness or hesitation, the duration and frequency of attentional abilities, the environmental conditions that contribute to or hinder attentional abilities, and the amount of required redirection to the task.[13]

COGNITION AND COMMUNICATION

In patients with CNS lesions, mental status and communication may be affected. Cognitive deficits can range from orientation and memory deficits to poor judgment, distractibility, and difficulties in information processing, abstract reasoning, and learning, to name just a few. A detailed assessment by a neuropsychologist, occupational therapist and/or speech-language pathologist may be necessary to obtain a complete and accurate picture of these deficits. Lack of attention to cognitive problems by the physical therapist can render an assessment of motor function in a patient with brain damage invalid and unreliable.

One of the first assessments that should be conducted is an assessment of orientation. Questions are posed to ascertain the patient's awareness of self (what is your name? how old are you? where were you born?), place (where are you? what city are we in? what state are we in? what is the name of this place?), and time (what time is it? what day of the week is it? what month is it? what season is it? what is today's date?).[8] Findings are documented as oriented times 3 ($\times$ 3), times 2 ($\times$ 2), or times 1 ($\times$ 1) depending on the domains correctly identified. An additional sphere that should be examined includes an assessment of circumstance (what happened to you? what kind of a place is this? why do people come here? how long have you been here?). To answer these last questions correctly, the individual must be able to take in, store, and recall new information. This may be severely disrupted in the patient with traumatic brain injury who demonstrates post-traumatic amnesia (PTA).

The patient's ability to communicate and follow directions should be ascertained. The therapist should assess spontaneous speech during the initial examination sessions. Patients can demonstrate problems with articulation (dysarthria), evidenced by speech errors, difficulties with timing, vocal quality, pitch, volume, and breath control. Problems of fluency, word flow without pauses or breaks, should be noted. Speech that flows smoothly but contains errors, neologisms (nonsense words), paraphasias (misuse of words), and circumlocutions (word substitution) is indicative of fluent aphasia (e.g., Wernicke's aphasia). The patient typically demonstrates deficits in auditory comprehension with well-articulated speech marked by word substitutions. Speech that is slow and hesitant with limited vocabulary and impaired syntax is indicative of nonfluent aphasia (e.g., Broca's aphasia). Articulation is labored and word finding difficulties are apparent. In some settings, especially the acute hospital setting, the physical therapist may be the first to become aware of communication deficits. Referral to a speech-language pathologist for evaluation is indicated. See Chapter 30 for a thorough discussion of this topic.

To ensure the validity of the physical therapy examination, it is necessary to identify an appropriate means of communicating with the patient. Consultation with the speech-language pathologist is essential. This may include simplifying instructions, using written instructions, or using alternate forms of communication such as gestures, pantomime, or communication boards. A common error is to assume that the patient understands the task at hand when he or she really has no idea what is expected. To ensure accuracy of testing, frequent checks for comprehension should be performed throughout the assessment. For example, the use of message discrepancies (saying one thing and gesturing another) can be used to test the patient's level of understanding.

An assessment of **memory,** the mental registration, retention, and recall of past experience, knowledge, and ideas, is indicated. **Declarative memory** involves the conscious recollection of facts and events (explicit memory) while **nondeclarative memory** involves recall of skills and procedures (nonconscious or implicit memory). The length of time between recall and initial acquisition into memory distinguishes short-term and long-term memory. Short-term memory (STM) involves immediate recall (seconds to minutes) while long-term memory (LTM) involves a longer time span (days, months, years). There is a limited capacity in STM (7 ± items); LTM has unlimited capacity. Patients with **amnesia** typically demonstrate pronounced memory deficits in LTM while STM is normal. Patients may demonstrate **anterograde amnesia,** characterized by deficits in new learning of material acquired after the onset of amnesia or precipitating trauma. Deficits in **retrograde amnesia,** previous learning acquired prior to the onset of amnesia, are less common but may also occur. A simple test of STM involves presenting the patient with a short list of words of unrelated objects (e.g., pony, coin, pencil) and asking the patient to repeat those words immediately after presentation and again a short time later (e.g., 5 minutes after presentation). LTM can be assessed by having the patient recall events or persons from his or her past (where were you born? where did you go to school? where did you work?). The patient's fund of general knowledge can also be assessed (who is the president? who was president during world war II?). The questions selected should represent sensitivity to the cultural and educational background of the patient. It is important to consider that memory may be influenced by attention, motivation, rehearsal, fatigue, and other factors. Certain drugs can improve memory (e.g., CNS stimulates, cholinergic agents) while other drugs can degrade memory (e.g., benzodiazepines, anticholinergic drugs). Patients who demonstrate difficulty retreiving information will often relate that the information is on the "tip of their tongue" (known as the tip of the tongue phenomena). Various different strategies can be used to facilitate recall of information (e.g., prompting, rehearsal, and repetition, etc.). Use of any memory enhancing strategy during examination should be carefully documented. The Mini-Mental Status Examination (MMSE) provides a valid and reliable quick screen of cognitive function.[14]

If attention and memory are impaired, instructions during the examination should be kept simple and brief (one-level commands versus two- or three-level commands). The therapist should structure or choose an environment in which distractors are reduced (closed environment) to ensure maximum performance during assessment. Demonstration and positive feedback can assist the patient to understand what is expected, and can be used to motivate and improve performance. Whenever modifications and cognitive strategies are necessary, they should be documented in the patient's chart.

Sensory Integrity and Integration

Sensory information is a critical component of motor control because it provides the necessary feedback used to monitor and shape performance. This is termed a **closed-loop system** and is defined as "a control system employing feedback, a reference of correctness, computation of error, and subsequent correction in order to maintain a desired state."[1p412] A variety of feedback sources are used to monitor movement including visual, vestibular, proprioceptive, and tactile inputs. The term **somatosensation** (or somatosensory inputs) is sometimes used to refer to sensory information received from the skin and musculoskeletal systems. The CNS analyzes all available movement information, determines error, and institutes appropriate corrective actions when necessary. Thus, a thorough sensory assessment of each of these systems is an important preliminary step in a motor control assessment (see Chapter 6 for more specific guidelines).

The primary role of closed-loop systems in motor control appears to be the monitoring of constant states such as posture and balance, and the control of slow movements, or those requiring a high degree of accuracy. Feedback information is also essential for the learning of new motor tasks. Patients who have deficits in any movement-monitoring sensory system may be able to compensate with other sensory systems. For example, the patient with major proprioceptive losses can use vision as an error-correcting system to maintain a stable posture. When vision is occluded, however, postural instability becomes readily apparent (e.g., positive Romberg test). Significant sensory losses and inadequate compensatory shifts to other sensory systems may result in severely disordered movement responses. The patient with proprioceptive losses and severe visual disturbances, such as diplopia (commonly seen in the patient with multiple sclerosis), may be unable to maintain a stable posture at all. An accurate assessment, therefore, requires that the therapist not only look at each individual sensory system but also at the overall interaction and integration of these systems and the adequacy of compensatory adjustments. Postural tasks, balance, slow (ramp) movements, tracking tasks, or new motor tasks provide the ideal challenge in which to test feedback control and closed-loop processes.

Joint Integrity and Mobility

Joint range of motion (ROM) and soft tissue flexibility are important elements of functional movement. Limitations restrict the normal action of muscles as well as alter the biomechanical alignment of body segments and posture. Long-standing immobilization results in contracture, a fixed resistance resulting from fibrosis of tissues surrounding a joint. The resultant compensatory movement patterns are frequently dysfunctional, producing additional stresses and strains on the musculoskeletal system. They are also more energy costly and may limit functional mobility.

Arthrokinematic assessment is used to assess movement of the joint surfaces (slides [glides], spins, and rolls). Osteokinematic motions (movements of the shafts of bones) can be measured by goniometry. Both active range of motion (AROM) and passive range of motion (PROM) are measured. Standardized testing positions, alternative positioning, testing procedures, and average ROM values for individual motions have been well described (e.g., the American Academy of Orthopedic Surgeons[5] and Norkin and White's *Measurement of Joint Motion*[16]). The reliability of goniometric measurements can be influenced by a number of factors, including measurement procedure, difficulty palpating landmarks, complexity of the joint tested, measurement device used, passive versus active ROM, and patient characteristics.[16,17] In addition to goniometric measurements, the therapist should determine the cause of limitation (e.g., pain, spasm, adhesion, etc.) and end-feel. End-feel refers to the characteristic feel each specific joint has at the end ROM. It is assessed by the application of slight overpressure at the end of range. Determination of normal end-feels (soft, firm, and hard) and pathological end-feels (soft, firm, hard, empty) is enhanced by the use of standardized descriptions[16] and requires practice and sensitivity. Some motions are limited by the joint capsule (termed capsular patterns of ROM limitation). For example, loss of elbow flexion or shoulder lateral/external rotation are common findings with capsular involvement. Other motions may be limited by ligaments, muscle contractures, ligament shortening, muscle tension, and so forth (termed noncapsular patterns of ROM limitation). An example of a noncapsular pattern is limitation and pain in elbow extension with biceps strain.[16] Active ROM, unassisted voluntary joint motion, can be influenced by willingness to move, available muscle strength, postural stabilization, and coordination. The therapist should determine (1) the presence of pain with motion (when pain appears, severity of the pain, and the patient's reaction to the pain), (2) the pattern and quality of the movement, (3) movement of associated joints or substitutions, (4) postural stabilization, and (5) the cause of limitation.[18] As a general rule, active movements are assessed before passive movements. If a patient is able to perform full active ROM without pain or discomfort, passive ROM testing is not necessary.[19]

Painful movements should be tested last to avoid limitation of movements from overflow of painful symptoms.[18]

Documentation should indicate that ROM is normal or within normal limits (WNL) or limited. Limitations of ROM are indicated by the number of degrees of motion from start to finish (e.g., 0 to 90 degrees). Joint ROM may be less than normal (hypomobile) but still functional. For example, a range in shoulder flexion of 120 degrees is considered functional for most activities. Documentation would then state ROM is within functional limits (WFL). Joint ROM that has greater than normal ROM is termed hypermobile. A complete description of any deviations from normal is warranted.

Special tests are available to assess involved joints. Generally, these tests assist in determination of joint ligamentous integrity and/or muscle flexibility. The results of these tests, when considered with all other assessments can be used to detect specific injuries, diseases, or conditions. Magee's Orthopedic Physical Assessment[18] and Hoppenfeld's Physical Examination of the Spine and Extremities[19] are two excellent references that describe these numerous tests. See Chapter 5 for a complete discussion of musculoskeletal assessment.

Tone

Tone is defined as the resistance of muscle to passive elongation or stretch. It represents the degree of residual contraction in normally innervated, resting muscle, or steady-state contraction. Resistance is due to a number of factors including (1) physical inertia, (2) intrinsic mechanical-elastic stiffness of muscle and connective tissues, and (3) reflex muscle contraction (tonic stretch reflexes).[20] Because muscles rarely work in isolation, the term *postural tone* is preferred by some clinicians to describe a pattern of muscular tension that exists throughout the body and affects groups of muscles.[21] Tonal abnormalities are categorized as **hypertonia** (increased above normal resting levels), **hypotonia** (decreased below normal resting levels), or **dystonia** (impaired or disordered tonicity).

TONAL ABNORMALITIES

Spasticity arises from injury to corticofugal pathways (pyramidal tracts) and occurs as part of **upper motoneuron (UMN) syndrome.** Loss of inhibitory control on lower motor neurons results in disordered spinal segmental reflexes, including increased alpha motoneuron excitability, increased spindle (Ia) and flexor reflex afferent excitability, altered synaptic activity, decreased presynaptic Ia inhibition, and so forth. Additional signs and symptoms of **UMN syndrome** include brisk tendon reflexes, involuntary flexor and extensor spasms, clonus, Babinski's sign, exaggerated cutaneous reflexes, and loss of precise autonomic control. Dyssynergic movement patterns also occur, including coactivation of agonist and antagonist muscle groups, abnormal timing, paresis, loss of dexterity, and fatigability. Chronic spasticity is associated with contracture, abnormal posturing and deformity, and functional limitation.[20,22,23]

In spasticity, resistance increases with increasing amplitude and velocity of stretch. Thus the larger and quicker the stretch, the stronger the resistance of the spastic muscle. Initially stretch produces high resistance, followed by a sudden inhibition or letting go of resistance, termed the **clasp-knife response.** **Clonus** is characterized by cyclical, spasmodic alternation of muscular contraction and relaxation in response to sustained stretch of a spastic muscle. Clonus is common in the plantarflexors, but may also occur in other areas of the body such as the jaw or wrist. The **Babinski sign** is dorsiflexion of the great toe with fanning of the other toes on stimulation of the lateral sole of the foot.

Corticospinal lesions can also result in decorticate or decerebrate rigidity. **Decorticate rigidity** refers to sustained contraction and posturing of the trunk and lower limbs in extension, and the upper limbs in flexion. **Decerebrate rigidity** refers to sustained contraction and posturing of the trunk and limbs in a position of full extension. Decorticate rigidity is indicative of corticospinal tract lesion at the level of diencephalon (above the superior colliculus), and decerebrate rigidity indicates a brainstem lesion between the superior colliculus and vestibular nucleus. **Opisthotonus** is strong and sustained contraction of the extensor muscles of the neck and trunk. The patient assumes a rigid hyperextended posture. All of these conditions are exaggerated and severe forms of hypertonicity.

Rigidity originating from basal ganglia lesions is characterized by resistance to passive movement involving both agonist and antagonist muscles. Lesions of the nigrostriatal dopamine system of the basal ganglia produce the rigidity commonly seen in Parkinson's disease. Although the etiology is not well understood, it appears the rigidity is the result of excessive supraspinal drive acting on a normal spinal reflex mechanism.[24] Patients demonstrate stiffness, inflexibility, and functional limitation. **Cogwheel rigidity** is a rachetlike response to passive movement characterized by an alternate letting go and increasing resistance to movement, and is common in patients with Parkinson's disease. Bradykinesia, tremor, and loss of postural stability are associated motor deficits in patients with Parkinson's disease. **Leadpipe rigidity** is the term used to refer to constant rigidity. Rigidity is independent of the velocity of passive movement.

Hypotonia and **flaccidity** are the terms used to define decreased or absent muscular tone. Resistance to passive movement is diminished, stretch reflexes are dampened or absent, and limbs are easily moved (floppy). Hyperextensibility of joints is common. **Lower motor neuron (LMN) lesions** affecting the anterior horn cell or peripheral nerve produce decreased or absent tone along with associated symptoms of paralysis, muscle fasciculations and fibrillations with dennervation, and neurogenic

atrophy. Decreased or absent tone is also associated with UMN lesions affecting the cerebellum or pyramidal tracts. These may be temporary states, termed **spinal shock** or **cerebral shock,** depending on the location of the lesion. The duration of the CNS depression that occurs with shock is highly variable, lasting days or weeks. It is typically followed by the development of spasticity and other UNM signs.

Dystonia is a hyperkinetic movement disorder characterized by impaired or disordered tone, accompanied by repetitive involuntary movements. Movements are usually twisting or writhing motions. Tone fluctuates in an unpredictable manner from low to high. **Dystonic posturing** refers to sustained abnormal postures caused by co-contraction of agonist and antagonist muscles that may last for several minutes or permanently. Dystonia results from a CNS lesion (commonly the basal ganglia) and can be inherited (primary idiopathic dystonia), associated with other neurodegenerative disorders (Wilson's disease, Parkinson's disease), or metabolic disorders (amino acid or lipid disorders). Dystonia is also seen in dystonia musculorum deformans or spasmodic torticollis (wry neck).[25]

TONAL ASSESSMENT

Tone can be influenced by a number of factors including (1) volitional effort and movement, (2) stress and anxiety, (3) position and interaction of tonic reflexes, (4) medications, (5) general health, (6) environmental temperature, and (7) state of CNS arousal or alertness. In addition, urinary bladder status (full or empty), fever and infection, and metabolic and/or electrolyte imbalance can also influence tone. Variability of tone is common. For example, patients with spasticity can vary in their presentation from morning to afternoon, day to day, or even hour to hour depending on the presence of these factors. The therapist should therefore consider the impact of each of these factors in arriving at a determination of tone. Tonal assessment requires repeat examinations and a consistent approach to examination to improve the reliability of test results.

Initial observation of the patient can reveal abnormal posturing of the limbs or body. Careful assessment should be made regarding the position of the limbs, trunk, and head. Posturing in fixed, antigravity positions is common; for example, the upper extremity is held fixed against the body in flexion, adduction, and supination with elbow and wrist/finger flexion. In the supine position a lower extremity held in extension, adduction with plantarflexion, and inversion may also indicate spasticity. Limbs that appear floppy and lifeless (e.g., a lower extremity rolled out to the side in external rotation) may indicate hypotonicity. Palpation of the muscle belly may yield additional information about the resting state of muscle. Consistency, firmness, and turgor should all be examined. Hypotonic muscles will feel soft and flabby, whereas hypertonic muscles will feel taut and harder than normal.

Assessment of passive motion reveals subjective

information about the responsiveness of muscles to stretch. Because these responses should be examined in the absence of voluntary control, the patient is instructed to relax, letting the therapist support and move the limb. During a passive motion test, the therapist should maintain firm and constant manual contact, moving the limb in all motions. When tone is normal, the limb moves easily and the therapist is able to alter direction and speed without feeling abnormal resistance. The limb is responsive and feels light. Hypertonic limbs generally feel stiff and resistant to movement, while flaccid limbs feel heavy and unresponsive. Older adults may find it difficult to relax; their stiffness should not be mistaken for spasticity. Varying the speed of movement is an important aspect of the assessment of spasticity. Faster movements will intensify the resistance to passive motion. Clonus, a phasic stretch response, is assessed using a quick stretch stimulus that is then maintained. For example, ankle clonus is tested by sudden dorsiflexion of the foot and maintaining the foot in dorsiflexion. The presence of a clasp-knife response should also be noted. All limbs and body segments are assessed, with particular attention given to those identified as problematic in the initial observation. Comparisons should be made between upper and lower limbs and right and left extremities. Documentation should include a determination of whether the tonal abnormalities are symmetrical or asymmetrical. Asymmetrical tonal abnormalities are always indicative of neurological dysfunction.[8] Comparison to the unaffected side in the patients with hemiplegia is common. These comparisons may not be valid, however, because abnormal findings have been reported on these supposedly normal extremities.[26] It is also important to remember that measurement of tone in one position does not ensure that measurement will be the same in other positions or during functional activities. A change in position such as sitting up or standing up substantially alters the requirements for postural support (postural tone).

A qualitative determination of the degree of tone should be made. Therapists need to be familiar with the wide range of normal and abnormal tonal responses to develop an appropriate frame of reference to assess tone. A common clinical rating scale used to assess tone is:

0   No response (flaccidity)
1+ Decreased response (hypotonia)
2+ Normal response
3+ Exaggerated response (mild to moderate hypertonia)
4+ Sustained response (severe hypertonia)

Spastic hypertonia can be assessed using the Ashworth Scale, a 5-point ordinal scale[27] or the modified Ashworth Scale.[28] This latter scale was developed to reduce the clustering effect around the middle grades of the original Ashworth Scale. It provides an additional intermediate grade and has been shown to have high interrater reliability (Table 8–1).

A pendulum test can also be used to assess

Table 8–1 MODIFIED ASHWORTH SCALE FOR GRADING SPASTICITY

Grade	Description
0	No increase in muscle tone.
1	Slight increase in muscle tone, manifested by a catch and release or by minimal resistance at the end of the ROM when the affected part(s) is moved in flexion or extension.
1+	Slight increase in muscle tone, manifested by a catch, followed by minimal resistance throughout the remainder (less than half) of the ROM.
2	More marked increase in muscle tone through most of the ROM, but affected part(s) easily moved.
3	Considerable increase in muscle tone, passive movement difficult.
3	Affected part(s) rigid in flexion or extension.

From Bohannon and Smith,[28] p 207, with permission from the APTA.

spasticity. With the patient seated or lying with knees flexed over the end of a table, the patient's knee is fully extended and allowed to drop and swing like a pendulum. A normal and hypotonic limb will swing freely for several oscillations. Hypertonic limbs are resistant to the swinging motion and will quickly return to the initial dependent starting position. Movements can be quantified using an electrogoniometer (ROM oscillations) and an electromyograph (EMG) (motor unit activity).[29] The pendulum test has also been performed using an isokinetic dynamometer with high test-retest reliability.[30]

Reflex Integrity

DEEP TENDON REFLEXES

Muscle stretch reflexes, termed deep tendon reflexes (DTRs), are assessed by tapping over the muscle tendon with a standard reflex hammer or with the tips of the therapist's fingers. To ensure adequate response, the muscle is positioned in midrange and the patient is instructed to relax. Stimulation can result in visable movement of the joint (brisk or strong responses). Weak responses may only be evident with palpation (slight or sluggish responses with little or no joint movement). The quality and magnitude of responses should be carefully documented.[8] A 6-point grading scale for muscle stretch reflexes is presented in Table 8–2. Reflexes commonly examined include the jaw, biceps, triceps, hamstrings, patellar, and ankle reflexes, and are presented in Table 8–3. Use of standardized testing allows the therapist to accurately isolate and examine radicular integrity of muscles.

If DTRs are difficult to elicit, responses can be enhanced by specific reinforcement maneuvers. In the *Jendrassik maneuver*, the patient hooks together the fingers of the hands and attempts to pull them apart. While this pressure is maintained, lower extremity reflexes can be tested. Maneuvers that can be used to reinforce responses in the upper extremi-

Table 8–2 GRADING SCALE FOR MUSCLE STRETCH REFLEXES

Grade	Evaluation	Response Characteristics
0	Absent	No visible or palpable muscle contraction with reinforcement.
1+	Hyporeflexia	Slight or sluggish muscle contraction with little or no joint movement. Reinforcement may be required to elicit a reflex response.
2+	Normal	Slight muscle contraction with slight joint movement.
3+	Hyperreflexia	Clearly visible, brisk muscle contraction with moderate joint movement.
4+	Abnormal	Strong muscle contraction with one to three beats of clonus. Reflex spread to contralateral side may be noted.
5+	Abnormal	Strong muscle contraction with sustained clonus. Reflex spread to contralateral side may be noted.

ties include squeezing the knees together, clenching the teeth, or making a fist with the contralateral extremity. The use of any reinforcing maneuvers to elicit responses in patients with hyporeflexia should be carefully documented.

SUPERFICIAL CUTANEOUS REFLEXES

Superficial cutaneous reflexes are elicited with a noxious stimulus, usually a light scratch, applied to the skin. The expected response is brief contraction of muscles innervated by the same spinal segments receiving the afferent inputs from the cutaneous receptors. A stimulus that is too strong may produce irradiation of cutaneous signals with activation of protective withdrawal reflexes. Several reflexes commonly tested are the plantar reflex, confirming toe signs (Chaddock), and superficial abdominal reflexes. The *plantar reflex* is tested by applying a noxious stroking stimulus on the sole of the foot along the lateral border and up across the ball of the foot. A normal response consists of flexion of the big toe; sometimes the other toes will demonstrate a downgoing response, or no response at all. An abnormal response **(positive Babinski sign)** consists of dorsiflexion (upgoing) of the big toe, with fanning of the lateral four toes. In adults, it is always indicative of corticospinal dysfunction. The **Chaddock sign** is elicited by stroking around the lateral ankle and up the lateral dorsal aspect of the foot. It also produces dorsiflexion of the big toe and is considered a confirmatory toe sign. The *abdominal reflex* is elicited with quick, light strokes over the skin of the abdominal muscles. A localized contraction under the stimulus is produced, with a resultant deviation of the umbilicus toward the area stimulated. Each quadrant should be tested in a diagonal direction. Umbilical deviation in a superior/lateral direction indicates integrity of spinal segments T6 to T9. Umbilical deviation in an inferior/lateral direction indicates integrity of spinal segments T11 to L1. Loss of response is abnormal, indicative of corticospinal pathology. Asymmetry from side to side is highly significant with respect to neurological disease.[8] Examples of superficial cutaneous reflex tests are summarized in Table 8–4.

DEVELOPMENTAL REFLEXES AND REACTIONS

Information about the function and integration of the developmental reflexes and reactions is obtained through a systematic examination. Assessment begins with the *primitive* and *tonic reflexes*. These reflexes are normally present during gestation or infancy and become integrated by the CNS at an early age. Once integrated, these reflexes are not generally recognizable in their pure form. They do continue, however, as adaptive fragments of behavior, underlying normal motor control and aiding volitional movement.[31] In adults, they may become apparent under some conditions of fatigue or effort[32,33] or following damage to the CNS.[34,35] Adult patients with brain injury who present with stereotypical reflexive behaviors demonstrate limitations in voluntary movement control and abnormal postures. Reflexes in this category include (1) spinal level or elemental reflexes (flexor withdrawal, extensor thrust, crossed extension) and (2) brainstem level or tuning reflexes (tonic neck, tonic labyrinthine, and associated reactions). Spinal level reflex responses are generally the simplest to observe and

Table 8–3 REFLEX ASSESSMENT—MYOTATIC REFLEXES

Myotatic Reflexes (Stretch)	Stimulus	Response
Jaw (trigeminal n)	Patient is sitting, with jaw relaxed and slightly open. Place finger on top of chin; tap downward on top of finger in a direction which causes the jaw to open.	Jaw rebounds.
Biceps (C5, C6)	Patient is sitting with arm flexed and supported. Place thumb over the biceps tendon in the cubital fossa, stretching it slightly. Tap thumb or directly on tendon.	Slight contraction of muscle normally occurs (elbow flexes).
Triceps (C7, C8)	Patient is sitting with arm supported in abduction, elbow flexed. Palpate triceps tendon just above olecranon. Tap directly on tendon.	Slight contraction of muscle normally occurs (elbow extends).
Hamstrings (L5, S1, S2)	Patient is prone with knee semiflexed and supported. Palpate tendon at the knee. Tap on finger or directly on tendon.	Slight contraction of muscle normally occurs (knee flexes).
Patellar (L2, L3, L4)	Patient is sitting with knee flexed, foot unsupported. Tap tendon of quadriceps muscle between the patella and tibial tuberosity.	Contraction of muscle normally occurs (knee extends).
Ankle (S1, S2)	Patient is prone with foot over the end of the plinth or sitting with knee flexed and foot held in slight dorsiflexion. Tap tendon just above its insertion on the calcaneus. Maintaining slight tension on the gastrocnemius-soleus group improves the response.	Slight contraction of muscle normally occurs (foot plantarflexes).

Table 8–4 REFLEX ASSESSMENT—SUPERFICIAL REFLEXES

Superficial Reflexes (Cutaneous)	Stimulus	Response
Plantar (S1, S2)	With a large pin or fingertip, stroke up the lateral side of the foot, moving from the heel to the base of the little toe and then across the ball of the foot.	Normal response is slow flexion (plantarflexion) of the great toe, and sometimes the other toes. Abnormal response, termed a positive Babinski, is extension (dorsiflexion) of the great toe with fanning of the four other toes (typically seen in upper motor neuron (corticospinal) lesions).
Chaddock	Stroke around lateral ankle and up lateral aspect of foot to the base of the little toe.	Same as for plantar.
Abdominal (T7–12)	Position patient in supine position, relaxed. Make quick, light stroke with a large pin or fingertip over the skin of the abdominals from the periphery to the umbilicus (test each abdominal quadrant separately).	Localized contraction under the stimulus, causing the umbilicus to move toward the quadrant stimulated.

are typically judged by their appearance as part of an overt movement response. Brainstem reflexes on the other hand serve to bias the musculature and may not be visible through overt movement responses. In fact, movement is rarely produced but rather posture is more typically influenced through tonal adjustments. Thus the term "tuning reflexes" is an appropriate description of their function.

To obtain an accurate assessment, the therapist must be concerned with several factors. The patient must be positioned appropriately to allow for the expected movement response. An adequate test stimulus is essential, including both an adequate magnitude and duration of stimulation. Keen observation skills are needed to detect what may be subtle movement changes and abnormal responses. Obligatory and sustained responses that dominate motor behavior are always considered pathological in the adult patient. Palpation skills can assist in identifying tonal changes not readily apparent to the eye.

Objective scoring of responses is essential. A reflex scoring key suggested by Capute et al.[36,37] is as follows:

0+ Absent
1+ Tone change: slight, transient with no movement of the extremities
2+ Visable movement of extremity
3+ Exaggerated, full movement of extremities
4+ Obligatory and sustained movement, lasting for more than 30 seconds

Higher level reactions (righting, equilibrium, protective) are controlled by centers in the midbrain and cortex and are important components of normal postural control and movement. The term **reaction** is commonly used to refer to those reflexes that appear during infancy or early childhood and remain throughout life. *Righting reactions* (RR) serve to maintain the head in its normal upright posture (face vertical, mouth horizontal) or to maintain the normal alignment of the head and trunk. Assessment procedures focus on positioning or manipulating the body and observing the automatic adjustments necessary to restore normal alignment and head position. *Equilibrium reactions* (ER) serve to maintain balance in response to alterations in the body's center of gravity (COG) and/or base of

support (BOS). They can be tested by using a movable surface that alters the patient's base of support with respect to the body's center of gravity (termed tilting reactions). Equilibrium boards are commonly used to assess tilting reactions. Equilibrium reactions can also be tested by altering the patient's position through voluntary movements or by perturbation (manual displacement). *Protective reactions* (PR, protective extension reactions) serve to stabilize and support the body in response to a displacing stimulus when the COG exceeds the BOS. Thus, the arms or legs extend in an effort to support the body weight when the BOS is exceeded. Reflex testing procedures have been effectively described by a number of authors.[36,38–40] Table 8–5 presents an overview of the assessment of developmental reflexes.

Cranial Nerve Integrity

There are 12 pairs of cranial nerves, all distributed to the head and neck with the exception of CN X (vagus), which is distributed to the thorax and abdomen. Cranial nerves I, II, and VIII are purely sensory and carry the special senses of smell, vision, hearing, and equilibrium. Cranial nerves III, IV, and VI are purely motor and control pupillary constriction and eye movements. Cranial nerves XI and XII are also purely motor, innervating the sternocleidomastoid, trapezius, and tongue muscles. Cranial nerves V, VII, IX, and X are mixed, containing both motor and sensory fibers. Motor functions include chewing (V), facial expression (VII), swallowing (IX, X), and vocal sounds (X). Sensations are carried from the face and head (V, VII, IX), alimentary tract, heart, vessels, and lungs (IX, X), and tongue, mouth, and palate (VII, IX, X). Parasympathetic secretomotor fibers (ANS) are carried in cranial nerve III for control of smooth muscles in the eyeball, VII for control of salivary and lacrimal glands, IX to the parotid salivary gland, and X to the heart, lungs, and most of the digestive system.

An examination of cranial nerve function should be performed with suspected lesions of the brain, brainstem, and cervical spine. Deficits in olfactory

Table 8–5 REFLEX ASSESSMENT—DEVELOPMENTAL REFLEXES

Primitive/Spinal Reflexes	Stimulus	Response
Flexor withdrawal	Noxious stimulus (pinprick) to sole of foot. Tested in supine or sitting position.	Toes extend, foot dorsiflexes, entire leg flexes uncontrollably. Onset: 28 weeks gestation. Integrated: 1–2 months.
Crossed extension	Noxious stimulus to ball of foot of extremity fixed in extension; tested in supine position.	Opposite lower extremity flexes, then adducts and extends. Onset: 28 weeks gestation. Integrated: 1–2 months.
Traction	Grasp forearm and pull up from supine into sitting position.	Grasp and total flexion of the upper extremity. Onset: 28 weeks gestation. Integrated: 2–5 months.
Moro	Sudden change in position of head in relation to trunk; drop patient backward from sitting position.	Extension, abduction of upper extremities, hand opening, and crying followed by flexion, adduction of arms across chest. Onset: 28 weeks gestation. Integrated: 5–6 months.
Startle	Sudden loud or harsh noise.	Sudden extension or abduction of arms, crying. Onset: birth. Integrated: persists.
Grasp	Maintained pressure to palm of hand (palmar grasp) or to ball of foot under toes (plantar grasp).	Maintained flexion of fingers or toes. Onset: palmar, birth; plantar, 28 weeks gestation. Integrated: palmer, 4–6 months; plantar, 9 months.

Tonic/Brainstem Reflexes	Stimulus	Response
Asymmetrical tonic neck (ATNR)	Rotation of the head to one side.	Flexion of skull limbs, extension of the jaw limbs, "bow and arrow" or "fencing" posture. Onset: birth. Integrated: 4–6 months.
Symmetrical tonic neck (STNR)	Flexion or extension of the head.	With head flexion: flexion of arms, extension of legs; with head extension: extension of arms, flexion of legs. Onset: 4–6 months. Integrated: 8–12 months.
Symmetrical tonic labyrinthine (TLR or STLR)	Prone or supine position.	With prone position: increased flexor tone/flexion of all limbs; with supine: increased tone/extension of all limbs. Onset: birth. Integrated: 6 months.
Positive supporting	Contact to the ball of the foot in upright standing position.	Rigid extension (co-contraction) of the lower extremities. Onset: birth. Integrated: 6 months.
Associated reactions	Resisted voluntary movement in any part of the body.	Involuntary movement in a resting extremity. Onset: birth–3 months. Integrated: 8–9 years.

Midbrain/Cortical Reflexes	Stimulus	Response
Neck righting action on the body (NOB)	Passively turn head to one side; tested in supine.	Body rotates as a whole (log rolls) to align the body with the head. Onset: 4–6 months. Integrated: 5 years.
Body righting acting on the body (BOB)	Passively rotate upper or lower trunk segment; tested in supine.	Body segment not rotated follows to align the body segments. Onset: 4–6 months. Integrated: 5 years.
Labyrinthine head righting (LR)	Occlude vision; alter body position by tipping body in all directions.	Head orients to vertical position with mouth horizontal. Onset: birth–2 months. Integrated: persists.
Optical righting (OR)	Alter body position by tipping body in all directions.	Head orients to vertical position with mouth horizontal. Onset: birth–2 months. Integrated: persists.
Body righting acting on head (BOH)	Place in prone or supine position.	Head orients to vertical position with mouth horizontal. Onset: birth–2 months. Integrated: 5 years.
Protective extension (PE)	Displace center of gravity outside the base of support.	Arms or legs extend and abduct to support and to protect the body against falling. Onset: arms, 4–6 months; legs, 6–9 months. Integrated: persists.
Equilibrium reactions—tilting (ER)	Displace the center of gravity by tilting or moving the support surface (e.g., with a movable object such as an equilibrium board or ball).	Curvature of the trunk toward the upward side along with extension and abduction of the extremities on that side; protective extension on the opposite (downward) side. Onset: prone 6 months; supine 7–8 months; sitting 7–8 months; quadruped 9–12 months; standing 12–21 months. Integrated: persists.
Equilibrium reactions—postural fixation	Apply a displacing force to the body, altering the center of gravity in its relation to the base of support; can also be observed during voluntary activity.	Curvature of the trunk toward the external force with extension and abduction of the extremities on the side to which the force was applied. Onset: prone 6 months; supine 7–8 months; sitting 7–8 months; quadruped 9–12 months; standing 12–21 months. Integrated: persists.

function should be suspected with lesions of the nasal cavity, and anterior/inferior cerebrum. Lesions of the optic pathways (optic nerve, optic chiasma, optic tract, lateral geniculate body, superior colliculus) and visual cortex may produce visual deficits. Midbrain (mesencephalic) lesions may result in deficits of cranial nerves III and IV. Pontine lesions may involve several cranial nerves, including V (ophthalmic, maxillary, and mandibular branches) and VI. Nuclei of cranial nerves VII and VIII (vestibular and cochlear branches) are located at the junction of the pons and medulla. Lesions affecting the medulla may involve IX, X, XI, and XII. The spinal root of XI is found in the upper five cervical segments. Clinical examination of the cranial nerves is presented in Table 8–6.

Muscle Performance

STRENGTH AND POWER

Muscle performance is "the capacity of a muscle to do work (force × distance)."[5p2–14] **Muscle strength** is "the measurable force exerted by a muscle or group of muscles to overcome a resistance in one maximal effort."[5p2–14] The resultant force can be used in the production of movement. Isotonic contractions involve active shortening of muscles, and eccentric contractions involve active lengthening of muscles. Isometric contractions produce high levels of tension without movement. **Muscle power** is "work produced per unit of time or the product of strength and speed."[5p2–14] **Muscle endurance** is "the ability to contract the muscle repeatedly over a period of time."[5p2–14] Muscle performance depends on a number of interrelated factors including length-tension characteristics, velocity, metabolic adequacy (fuel storage and delivery) as well as integrated actions of the CNS. The number of motor units recruited, firing rate, timing, sequencing, and postural stabilization are all important factors in defining muscle performance.

Analysis of muscle strength, power, and endurance can be performed using manual muscle testing (MMT). Standardized methods and protocols have been developed to address issues of validity and reliability.[41,42] MMT grades are presented in Table 5–6. Both hand-held and isokinetic dynamometers have also been shown to provide objective, reliable, and sensitive measurements of muscle performance. Analysis of muscle timing including amplitude, duration, waveform, and frequency can be performed using EMG. Analysis of functional performance can also yield important data about muscle strength, power, and endurance. Timed performance (e.g., timed self-care tasks; time to walk a particular distance; 5-minute walk test) provides objective and reproducible measures of endurance. These topics are discussed in Chapters 5, 9, and 11.

Patients with neurological dysfunction pose unique challenges for the assessment of muscle performance. Weakness is a common finding of UMN syndrome along with spasticity, hyperactive reflexes, and so forth. Weakness with decreased tone is evident with lower motor injury or peripheral nerve disease. Strength testing measures (MMT) were originally developed for the assessment of diseases involving lower motor neurons (e.g., polio). Their usefulness in assessment of patients with UMN disorders has been questioned.[43,44] Bobath[21] suggested that weakness of muscles in patients with stroke may not be actual muscle weakness but may be the result of opposition by spastic antagonists, the presence of mass patterns of movements, sensory deficit, and/or lack of synergistic fixation. Literature suggests that activity of the agonist muscle seems more related to interference of force production.[43–47] Altered recruitment and decreased motor unit firing rate have been identified.[48,49] Patients with stroke show up to a 50 percent decrease in motor units of affected extremities within two months after insult.[50] Changes in muscle viscoelasticity and the presence of denervated muscle fibers are also evident in weakness.[51] Neurogenic atrophy, primary muscle atrophy, is the direct result of denervation and occurs in LMN lesions. Patients with UMN lesions may develop disuse atrophy as a result of the loss of functional mobility.

Clinical measurement of strength in patients with CNS lesions is a necessary part of the examination. Patients with CNS lesions are a diverse group with varying levels of impairments and functional limitations. Strength testing using standardized protocols may be appropriate for some patients, but not for others. Appropriate criteria are therefore critical in determining whether the standards of validity and reliability are met. First and foremost, the therapist must consider the patient's movement capabilities. Individual joint movements, mandated by standardized MMT procedures and isokinetic protocols, may not be possible in the presence of stereotypic movement patterns, abnormal co-activation, spasticity, and abnormal posturing. The mandated test positions may also be precluded by the presence of abnormal reflex activity (e.g., supine testing influenced by presence of the tonic labyrinthine reflex). Muscle and soft tissue changes in viscoelasticity offer a form of passive restraint and may also preclude the use of standardized testing. In these instances, an estimation of strength can be made from observations of active movements during functional tasks. Movements can be graded using the following ordinal scale[52]:

  0 = no movement
  1 = palpable contraction or flicker
  2 = movement with gravity eliminated
  3 = movement against gravity
  4 = movement against some resistance
  5 = normal strength

If standardized MMT is to be used, therapists must utilize correct positioning. If a modified position is required (e.g., the patient lacks full ROM or adequate stabilization), it should be carefully documented. Substitutions (muscle actions that compensate for specific muscle weakness) should be identified, eliminated whenever possible, and carefully

Table 8–6 CRANIAL NERVE ASSESSMENT

Nerve	Function	Assessment	Signs and Symptoms of Damage
I Olfactory	Smell	Assess sense of smell common odorants	Anosmia—inability to detect smells
II Optic	Vision	Assess visual acuity: Central: Snellen eye chart	Blindness, impaired vision
		Peripheral vision, visual fields	Visual field defects
	Pupillary reflexes	Test corneal light reflex Assess pupillary size/shape	Absence of light reflexes on shining light in eye
III Oculomotor	Elevates eyelid	Assess position of eyelid	Ptosis (drooping)
	Turns eye up, down, in	Test pursuit eye movements	Eye deviates down and out Diplopia with attempted lateral gaze to contralateral side
	Constricts pupil	Test pupillary light reflex	Loss of light and accommodation reflexes (ipsilateral eye)
	Accommodates lens	Test accommodation reflex	
IV Trochlear	Turns adducted eye down	Test pursuit eye movement	Diplopia with attempted downward/adducted gaze
	Intorsion of eye		Adductor paralysis (ipsilateral eye)
V Trigeminal	Somatosensation: Face Cornea Anterior tongue	Test sensation: forehead, cheeks, chin Test corneal reflex	Loss of facial sensations, numbness Loss of corneal reflex ipsilaterally (blinking in response to corneal touch)
	Mastication	Have patient clench jaws, hold against resistance	Weakness, wasting muscles of mastication Deviation of jaw when opened to ipsilateral side
VI Abducent	Turns eye out	Test pursuit eye movement	Diplopia with attempted lateral gaze to ipsilateral side Convergent strabismus Abductor paralysis—ipsilateral eye
VII Facial	Facial expression	Assess motor function: Raise eyebrows Show teeth, smile Close eyes tightly Puff cheeks	Paralysis ipsilateral facial muscles Inability to close eye Drooping corner of mouth Difficulty with speech articulation
	Tearing: lacrimal gland Salivary secretion: submandibular and sublingual glands		Loss of lacrimation, pain with blinking Decreased salivation—dry mouth
	Taste from anterior tongue	Test taste—sweet, salty, sour, bitter	Loss of taste (ageusia) anterior two-thirds of tongue
	Somatosensation		
VIII Vestibulocochlear	Equilibrium	Assess balance Eye-head coordination (VOR) Assess for nystagmus	Vertigo, dysequilibrium, nystagmus Gage instability with head rotations
	Hearing	Assess auditory acuity Weber test: conduction Rinne test: sensorineural	Deafness, impaired hearing, tinnitus
IX Glossopharyngeal	Elevates pharynx Salivary secretion: parotid gland		Dysphagia Dry mouth
	Taste: posterior third of tongue	Assess taste: sweet, salty, sour, bitter	Loss of taste posterior third of tongue Anesthesia of pharynx and larynx Dysphonia
	Somatosensations: posterior tongue oropharynx		
	Reflexes	Test gag reflex	
X Vagus	Deglutition, phonation	Assess phonation, articulation Observe movements soft palate Swallowing	Dysphagia Dypsphonia, hoarseness Palatal paralysis
	Cardiac depressor		Cardiac dysryhythmia, respiratory disturbances (bilateral vagal dysfunction)
	Bronchoconstrictor GI tract peristalsis, secretion Taste Visceral sensations and reflexes		
	Reflexes	Test gag reflex	Loss of gag reflex
	Somatosensations	Test pharyngeal sensation	
XI Accessory Cranial: part	Deglutition and phonation		
Spinal: part	Head movements: sternocleidomastoid trapezius	Assess muscle strength, size, tone	Muscle weakness: inability to shrug ipsilateral shoulder turn head to opposite side
XII Hypoglossal	Tongue movements	Assess strength of tongue movements, tongue protrusion	Wasting of tongue Deviation to ipsilateral side on protrusion Difficulty with lingual sounds "la, la" Dysphagia

documented. Reliability of manual muscle testing in the clinical setting has been low. In one study, the investigators found the percentage of therapists, obtaining the same muscle grade, only ranged from 50 to 60 percent. Factors that influence the reproducibility of the results include difficulty with determining the magnitude of resistive force (subjectivity of good and normal grades), differences in testing method, differences in force application (point, line of force, speed), duration of the contraction, patient factors (cooperation, fatigue), therapist factors (experience, instructions, volume of commands, interactions with patient), and environment (distracting influences).[53] It is important to note that generalizability of strength measurements taken in one position to performance of functional tasks in other positions is problematic.[44]

Hand-held dynamometers are small portable devices that measure mechanical force; they have been incorporated clinically into manual muscle testing procedures. The therapist reads the exact amount of force applied to the muscle during tests for good and normal grades instead of estimating the amount of resistance. High intra- and intertester reliability scores have been reported.[54–56] Limitations in their use include difficulty in stabilizing both the limb and device, controlling the rate of muscle tension development, and applying sufficient force for a break test. These may be factors in reports that indicate the portable dynamometer is less reliable for testing lower extremity muscle groups.[57,58]

The use of an isokinetic dynamometer allows the therapist to monitor many important parameters of motor control, including peak torque at varying speeds and ROM or arc of excursion as a function of time. Rate of tension development (time to peak torque) and shape of the torque curve can also be determined. Reciprocal contractions (agonist/antagonist relationships) can be analyzed. Corrections for weight of the limb (gravity effects) are necessary to arrive at an accurate relationship. However, comparison to reciprocal actions of muscles in more functional patterns of movement may not be valid as these two modes of action are very dissimilar.[59] An assessment of muscle performance varying types of contractions is important for an understanding of functional performance. Isokinetic equipment allows for testing of concentric as well as isometric and eccentric torques. To ensure the validity of the measurements, calibration of the equipment is necessary and should be performed each day testing is done. Proper alignment of the joint axis and machine axis is required. Isokinetic testing has been shown to have high reliability for testing maximum torque production.[60–65] At least one practice session is recommended to acquaint the patient with the equipment and testing protocol. Repeat test sessions should utilize the identical protocol.

Patients with neurological insult demonstrate a variety of deficits on testing with an isokinetic dynamometer, including decreased torque development, decreased limb excursion, extended times to peak torque development and the time peak torque is held, increased time intervals between reciprocal contractions, and/or problems in torque development at higher speeds.[26,66] For example, many patients with hemiplegia are unable to develop tension above 70 to 80 degrees per second. When this value is compared to the speed needed for normal walking (100 degrees per second), reasons for gait difficulties become readily apparent. Normative data, when available, can provide an appropriate reference for evaluating and interpreting patient data.[67–70] Watkins et al.[26] studied a group of patients with hemiplegia and found, in addition to many of the above changes, diminished torque values on the supposedly normal extremities. These findings cast doubt as to the validity of using the uninvolved side as a reference for normal control in patients with hemiplegia.

ENDURANCE

An assessment of muscle endurance is important in determining functional capacity. **Fatigue** has been defined as "the failure to generate the required or expected force during sustained or repeated contractions."[71p463] Although fatigue is protective and serves a useful function in guarding against overwork and injury, it is a serious problem for some individuals. For example, patients with postpolio syndrome or chronic fatigue syndrome may experience significant restrictions in their functional activities and work due to debilitating fatigue. Other groups of individuals who may also experience limitations due to fatigue include those with multiple sclerosis, amyotrophic lateral sclerosis, Duchenne muscular dystrophy, and Guillain-Barré syndrome.[72–76]

The assessment of fatigue should be included during routine initial interview and functional assessment. The patient can be asked questions pertaining to the frequency and severity of fatigue episodes, and the circumstances surrounding the onset and cessation of fatigue. Precipating activities should be established within the context of habitual daily activity. It is important to document **threshold for fatigue,** defined as "that level of exercise that cannot be sustained indefinitely."[77p691] In most cases, the onset of fatigue is gradual, not abrupt, and dependent upon the intensity and duration of the activity attempted. Additional factors that can influence fatigue include health status, environmental context (e.g., stressful environment), and temperature (e.g., heat stress in the patient with multiple sclerosis). The therapist should carefully document the patient's level of performance, including complete independence, modified independence, or level of assistance required (minimal, moderate, or maximal). Perceived level of fatigue can be recorded using a visual analog scale or the Borg Scale for Ratings of Perceived Exertion.[78]

Exhaustion is defined as the limit of endurance, beyond which no further performance is possible. Most patients can report with great accuracy the point at which exhaustion is reached. Of concern with some patients is **overwork weakness (injury),** defined as "a prolonged decrease in absolute strength and endurance due to excessive activity of partially denervated muscle."[79p22] For example, patients with postpolio syndrome may experience weakness following strenuous activity that is not recovered with ordinary rest. They report having to spend the entire next day or two in bed following an exhaustive exercise session. It is therefore important to document the type, length, and effectiveness of rest attempts. Delayed onset muscle soreness is common in patients with overwork weakness, peaking between 1 and 5 days post-activity.[75,76] The Fatigue Impact Scale (FIS) is a useful instrument to assess quality-of-life problems related to fatigue. It includes questions on the cognitive and social domains, as well as physical performance.[80]

Clinical assessment of muscle fatigue can also include both volitional and electrically elicited fatigue tests using an isokinetic dynamometer. This equipment permits quantification of torque outputs. Patients are asked to perform repetitive, submaximal isokinetic contractions. A drop-off of peak torque by 50 percent can be used as an index of fatigue. Electrically induced fatigue tests can also be used to assess muscle performance and may provide a more reliable measure in individuals with low motivation or who have a disorder of central drive (e.g., stroke). The muscle is stimulated with groups of electrical pulses (pulse trains) and percentage of decline in force production is measured.[81–83]

Voluntary Movement Patterns

Coordinative structures are defined as functionally specific units of muscles and joints **(synergies)** that are constrained by the CNS to act cooperatively to produce an action.[84] The CNS is able to reduce the **degrees of freedom,** defined as the number of separate independent dimensions of movement that must be controlled,[1] by engaging cooperative units of action. These units are defined by precise spatial and temporal organization. Coordination involves control of speed, distance, direction, rhythm, and levels of muscle tension. Both discrete skills (skills that have definite beginning and end points) and continuous skills (skills that have no recognizable beginning or end) can be executed with ease. Patterns of upper and lower limb coordination interlimb coordination including bilateral (bimanual) tasks and symmetrical, asymmetrical, or reciprocal patterns are important elements of control. Coordination of limb movements with needed proximal stabilization and postural support and with events in the environment (evidenced by coincident timing) is also necessary. Coordination assessment is discussed fully in Chapter 7.

ABNORMAL SYNERGISTIC PATTERNS

Synergistic organization of movement may be disturbed in cases of UMN syndrome. **Abnormal synergies** are defined as obligatory, highly stereo-typed mass patterns of movement. Selective movement control (isolated joint movements) becomes severely disordered or disappears completely. For example, patients with hemiplegia typically demonstrate obligatory flexion synergies (characterized by flexion, abduction, external rotation) and extension synergies (characterized by extension, adduction, internal rotation). Abnormal synergies are highly predictable and characteristic of middle stages of recovery of stroke.[21,34]

Assessment of synergies is both qualitative and quantitative. The therapist observes whether movement can be initiated, completed, and how the movement is carried out. If movement is stereotypical, what muscle groups are linked together? How strong are the linkages between muscle groups? Are the movements influenced by other components of UMN syndrome, primitive reflexes? spasticity? paresis? by position? For example, do elbow, wrist, and finger flexion always occur when shoulder flexion is initiated? Is head turning used to initiate or reinforce upper extremity flexion? Therapists also need to identify when these patterns occur, under what circumstances, and what variations are possible. As CNS recovery progresses, synergies become more variable and may only reemerge under certain conditions such as stress or fatigue. Lessening of synergy dominance and emergence of selective movement control are used to document sequential recovery in patients with stroke. The Fugl-Meyer Post-Stroke Assessment of Physical Performance[85] provides an objective and quantifiable assessment of motor function after stroke (see Chapter 17, Appendix A).

Postural Control and Balance

Postural orientation involves the control of relative positions of body parts by skeletal muscles, with respect to gravity and each other. **Postural stability (equilibrium)** is defined as the condition in which all the forces acting on the body are balanced such that the center of mass (COM) is within the stability limits, boundaries of the BOS.[84] The overall goals of the balance control system are stability and function, achieved through integrated CNS systems of control. **Reactive control** occurs in response to external forces (threats, perturbations) displacing the COM or movement of the BOS (moveable platform). **Proactive (anticipatory) control** occurs in anticipation of internally generated, destabilizing forces imposed on the body's own movements.[86] An individual's prior experiences allow the various elements of the postural control system to be pretuned or readied for upcoming movements. Postural requirements vary depending on the characteristics of the task and the environment. **Adaptive postural control** allows the individual to appropriately "modify sensory and motor systems in response to changing task and environmental demands."[84p121] Components of the postural control system include (1) sensory systems responsible for the detection of body motion, (2) CNS integration processes, and (3) motor systems responsible for the execution of motor responses for controlling body position. Assessment of balance should focus on each of these components.

POSTURAL ALIGNMENT AND WEIGHT DISTRIBUTION

Normal postural alignment in standing can be assessed by observation in the sagittal plane using a plumbline or line with a weight. More sophisticated analysis can be achieved using radiography, photography, and electromyography. The vertical line of gravity (LOG) falls close to most joint axes: slightly anterior to the ankle and knee joints, at or slightly posterior to the hip joint, through midline trunk, just anterior to the shoulder joint, and through the external auditory meatus.[87] Natural spinal curves are present but flattened in upright stance depending on the level of postural tone, lumbar and cervical lordosis, and thoracic or dorsal kyphosis. The pelvis is in neutral position, with no anterior or posterior tilt. There is symmetry and equal weight distribution between feet. Normal alignment minimizes the need for active muscle contraction during erect stance. Muscles that are active during quiet stance include: tibialis anterior and gastronemius-soleus, gluteus medius and tensor fascia latae, iliopsoas, and abdominals and erector spinae.[88] In sitting, the head and trunk are vertical with a midline orientation and symmetrical weight bearing on the lower extremities (buttocks, thighs, and feet). Natural spinal curves are present with the pelvis maintained in neutral.

Limits of stability (LOS) is defined as "the maximum angle from vertical that can be tolerated without loss of balance."[89p5] Thus the individual is able to shift forward and backward or side to side without losing balance or taking a step. In normal individuals, the anteroposterior (AP) LOS in standing is approximately 12 degrees while the medial-lateral (ML) LOS is approximately 16 degrees from side to side (normal stance width, 4 inches). LOS is influenced by individual characteristics such as height and foot length for AP LOS and distance between the feet and height for ML LOS.[89] During standing, an individual normally exhibits small range postural shifts (postural sway) and cycles intermittently from side to side and from heel to toe. During walking, there are minimal COM movements up and down and side to side, resulting in a smooth sinusoidal curve.[87] In sitting, the BOS is larger and COM lower (just above the support base), resulting in greater LOS.[89] The midpoint of LOS is termed the **COM alignment.** Steadiness refers to the ability to maintain a given posture with minimum movement (sway).[90]

Postural sway can be measured simply by visual inspection with the patient standing against a postural grid.[91] More sophisticated instrumentation, static posturography, utilizes forceplates to measure ground reaction forces, either center of force (COF) measures or center of pressure (COP)

measures. COF is calculated using only vertical forces, and COP is calculated using both vertical and horizontal shear forces. The weight of each foot is determined, forces calculated, and converted into a visual image (see Figure 8-1). Audio signals are available on some devices. Software allows analysis of data and typically includes protocols that can be used for training. Measures of the initial stance position (center of alignment), mean sway path, total excursion (LOS), and the zone of stability can be obtained and are valid and reliable measures of postural control.[92,93] Using this information, the therapist can objectively determine the patient's postural symmetry, which is a reflection of the amount of weight placed on each foot. Patients with asymmetry present with the COP positioned away from midline; for example, the patient with stroke typically stands with most of the weight on the sound limb. Steadiness can be determined by using postural sway measures. The larger the sway path the greater the postural unsteadiness.[90] For example, the patient with ataxia typically demonstrates hypermetric responses, with large sway paths and little postural steadiness. The patient with Parkinson's disease presents with the opposite problem—hypometric responses, with little sway excursion and excessive stabilization.[86] Dynamic stability can be determined by using LOS information. Patients with deficits in motor function (e.g., the patient with stroke) typically have reduced LOS.[90,94,95] LOS and COM alignment are also typically altered in other pathological states (e.g., muscle weakness, skeletal

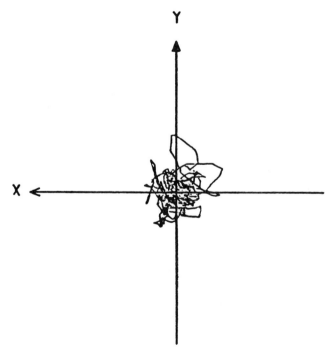

Figure 8-1. Postural sway. Recording of the movement of the center of pressure for 60 seconds in a subject standing on a balance platform. Values: mean amplitude of sway path in inches = .13 × .15 Y; length of path = 32.2; velocity = .45 in/s. (From Smith, L, et al: Brunnstrom's Clinical Kinesiology, ed 5. FA Davis, Philadelphia, 1996, p 406, with permission.)

deformity, and tonal abnormalities). Reexamination following training using force platform biofeedback has been used to demonstrate the effectiveness of training using such devices.[94,96,97]

SENSORY ORGANIZATION

Information from the sensory systems is received and integrated by the CNS. A determination of postural orientation and stability is made and necessary postural strategies to maintain or restore balance are initiated. Peripheral inputs are received from the visual, somatosensory, and vestibular systems.

The visual system detects the relative orientation of the body parts and the orientation of the body with reference to the environment (termed **visual proprioception**). It also relays information about the organization of the external environment. Motor functions include righting reactions of the head, trunk, and limbs (optical righting reactions), and visually guided movement. Visual acuity (focal vision) should be assessed using a Snellen eye chart. A distance acuity poorer than $^{20}/_{50}$ will have a significant effect on postural stability.[99] Ambient vision, or sensorimotor vision, plays a major role in localizing features in the environment and movement control. Whereas focal vision is detected by the central retina only, ambient vision is detected by the entire visual field (central and peripheral).[1] Patients with loss of peripheral vision (e.g., the patient with glaucoma or the patient with brain injury and optic ataxia) may demonstrate deficits in visual proprioception. Patients with visual field defects (e.g., the patient with stroke and hemianopsia) also typically demonstrate impairments in visual proprioception, visual neglect, and functional performance. Peripheral vision can be assessed using the confrontation method. The patient sits in front of the therapist and is instructed to focus gaze on the therapist's nose. The therapist then slowly brings a target (finger or pencil) slowly into the patient's field of view from the right or left side. The patient is instructed to indicate (point or declare) when and where the target is detected.

Somatosensory inputs include the cutaneous and pressure sensations from the body segments in contact with the support surface (e.g., the feet in standing or buttocks, thighs, and feet in sitting) and muscle and joint proprioceptors. They detect the relative orientation and movement of body parts, and orientation of the support surface. Motor functions include the stretch reflexes (myotatic and inverse myotatic reflexes), flexor withdrawal and crossed extensor reflexes, and automatic postural reactions. Assessment should include a sensory examination of the extremities and trunk. Cutaneous function (touch and pressure) and proprioceptive responses of the foot and ankle are particularly important in ascertaining information about standing position and movement. Sensory assessment techniques are discussed fully in Chapter 6.

The vestibular system detects angular acceleration and deceleration forces acting on the head (semicircular canals [SCC]). The otolith organs detect linear acceleration and orientation of the head with reference to gravity. The SCC are sensitive to fast (phasic) movements of the head, and the otoliths respond to slow head movements and position. The primary motor functions of the vestibular system include the stabilization of gaze during head movements (vestibulo-ocular reflex [VOR]), righting reactions of the head, trunk, and limbs (labyrinthine righting reactions), and regulation of muscle tone and postural muscle activation. Tests for vestibular function can include positional and movement testing, use of a rotary chair (Barany test) and **caloric testing.** These tests stimulate the SCC, either through movement or temperature changes. The patient is observed for symptoms of vestibular dysfunction (e.g., dizziness, vertigo, nystagmus).[100] See Chapter 25 for a complete discussion of this topic.

CNS INTEGRATION

Sensory organization by the CNS is flexible; although all inputs are important, the CNS weights the various inputs as needed. During quiet stance, defined as a stable support surface and surroundings, all inputs contribute to the maintenance of posture. For intact adults under normal conditions, greater weighting is placed by the CNS on somatosensory inputs.[84] Somatosensory inputs assume a major role when platform perturbations are introduced. If sensory conflict is introduced (e.g., standing on dense foam) or if somatosensory inputs are impaired (e.g., the patient with peripheral neuropathy), vision assumes a greater role. The role of vision can be assessed by having the patient stand first eyes open, then eyes closed **(Romberg test).** If both somatosensory and visual inputs become impaired or distorted, vestibular inputs, which are referenced to gravity, become dominant and resolve sensory conflict.[89] Balance responses are therefore task and context dependent and are triggered by availability and accuracy of specific sensory inputs. Because these inputs are redundant, stable balance can be maintained in the absence of vision, on unstable surfaces, or in sensory conflict situations. If more than one sensory system is deficient, however, lack of balance control will be evident.[101]

The Clinical Test for Sensory Interaction in Balance (CTSIB) is a simple, inexpensive test that can be used to assess sensory organization.[102,103] This test, also known as the foam and dome test, assesses standing balance under six different sensory conditions (Fig. 8-2). The support surface varies from normal to standing on dense foam, which distorts orientational information. Visual inputs vary from eyes open to eyes closed (similiar to a Romberg test), to wearing a dome that provides visually incorrect information by moving in phase with the patient's head movement. Condition 1 provides the baseline reference, and each of the other five conditions systematically varies the sensory inputs, increasing the level of sensory conflict. Conditions 2 (eyes closed) and 3 (visual surround moving with body sway) vary the availability and accuracy of visual information. Conditions 4 through 6 repeat the eye conditions in 1 through 3 with altered support surface (standing on dense foam). Conditions 5 and 6 (altered visual and somatosensory inputs) provide the greatest challenges; maintenance of posture depends on availability and accuracy of vestibular inputs. Thus, patients with vestibular dysfunction will demonstrate maximum instability in conditions 5 and 6. Each condition is maintained for 30 seconds. The CTSIB is scored by observing changes in the amount and direction of postural sway. A numerical scoring system (1 = minimal sway, 2 = mild sway, 3 = moderate sway, 4 = fall) can be used. Alternatively, the time in balance can be scored using a stopwatch, or the amount of sway can be estimated using a plumb line and postural grid. Subjective complaints of the patient (e.g., nausea, dizziness) and changes in movement strategy should be documented during each of the test conditions.

Dynamic posturography measures dynamic standing balance under conditions of changing sensory conditions of movement. A moving platform introduces mechanical perturbations (sliding or tilting movements). A moving visual surround can be sway referenced, introducing visual conflict. Both the surround and force-plate are referenced to the patient by means of hydraulic mechanisms. *The Sensory Organization Test (SOT)* uses the same six sensory conditions as the CTSIB (Fig. 8-2). A printed bar graph indicates how well the patient performed during each of the six conditions in terms of postural sway. Ratios comparing one condition to another can provide information regarding reliance on one sensory system over another. Additional analyses concerning available motor coordination can also be performed.[103–105]

MOTOR STRATEGIES

Postural responses during perturbed stance vary from the simple monosynaptic stretch reflex to the activation of motor strategies. Postural strategies function in either a feedback mode (as a reaction to a specific stimulus) or in a feedforward mode (in

preparation for voluntary movement). As the LOS are reached with a COM disturbance, the magnitude of the postural response increases. Specific motor strategies have been described by Nashner and others.[103,106–108] The specific patterns are achieved through synergistic activation of muscles. The *ankle strategy* involves shifting the COM forward and back by rotating the body as a relatively fixed pendulum about the ankle joints. Muscles are activated in a distal-to-proximal sequence. With forward sway, gastrocnemius is activated first, followed by hamstrings, then paraspinal muscles. With backward sway, the anterior tiabialis is activated first, followed by quadriceps, then abdominals. The ankle strategy is the most commonly used strategy when disturbances are small, well within the LOS. The *hip strategy* involves shifts in the COM by flexing or extending at the hips. It has a proximal pattern of muscle activation. With forward sway abdominals are activated first, followed by quadriceps. With backward sway, paraspinal muscles are activated first, followed by hamstrings. With lateral destabilization, hip abductors provide primary control. The hip strategy is recruited with larger and faster disturbances of the COM. Both of these strategies are termed *fixed-support strategies*, in that the COM is controlled over a fixed BOS.

Change-in-support strategies are defined as movements of the lower or upper limbs to make a new contact with the support surface.[109] The *stepping strategy* realigns the BOS under the COM by using rapid steps or hops in the direction of the displacing force, for example, forward or backward steps. In instances of lateral destabilization, the individual takes a side step or a cross step to bring the BOS back under the COM. The stepping strategies are recruited in response to fast, large postural perturbations (Fig. 8-3). Change-in-support movements of the upper limb can assist in stabilizing the COM over the BOS, and serve a protective function in absorbing impact and protecting the head in a fall event. Grasping movements assist in extending the BOS and stabilizing posture. Maki and McIlroy found that these reactions are very prevalent in

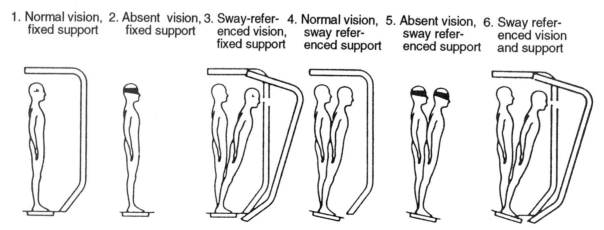

1. Normal vision, fixed support 2. Absent vision, fixed support 3. Sway-referenced vision, fixed support 4. Normal vision, sway referenced support 5. Absent vision, sway referenced support 6. Sway referenced vision and support

Figure 8-2. The sensory organization test.

destabilization situations, occurring in over 85 percent of trials. Stepping strategies were also frequent, leading these researchers to suggest that change-in-support strategies should not be viewed as strategies of last resort. They are often initiated well before the COM nears or exceeds the LOS, contrary to the traditional view.[109]

In sitting, postural strategies to regain balance include movement of the trunk about the hips. Backward sway elicits responses in hip flexors, quadriceps, abdominals, and neck flexors. In forward sway, extensor muscles of the neck, trunk, and hips are activated along with ankle plantarflexors if the feet are in contact with the support surface. Somatosensory inputs from backward rotation of the pelvis may have an important role in triggering the postural strategies in sitting.[110]

The examination of motor strategies should first begin with an assessment of musculoskeletal elements (ROM, postural tone, and strength). Weakness and limited ROM in the ankles will affect successful use of an ankle strategy, whereas weakness and limited ROM about the hips will influence the hip strategy. Limitations of neck ROM can be expected in patients with primary vestibular disorders. Available motor strategies in response to destabilizations (anteroposterior, medial-lateral) should be determined.

Dynamic posturography provides the ideal way to study motor strategies. The *Movement Coordination Test (MCT)* developed by Nashner and co-workers[108] provides information about postural responses to control the COM when the platform moves, including symmetry of weight bearing and forces generated, latency of postural responses, amplitude of response in relation to the stimulus size, and strategy utilized (ankle or hip). Optional EMG monitoring can reveal specific muscle activation patterns and latencies. The main disadvantage is that the equipment is very expensive and not portable. Correlation with functional performance is also lacking.

The therapist needs to determine if the strategies are (1) present and normal, (2) present but limited or delayed, (3) present but inappropriate for the particular context or situation, (4) abnormal, or (5) absent.[91] Differences in responses can be seen by systematically varying sensory inputs and the size and type of perturbations. Anticipatory postural control should also be examined. For example, the patient can be asked to raise the arms overhead or lift a weighted ball.[91] The destabilizing effects of voluntary movement and strategies used to maintain position should be documented. Finally, the ability to adapt postural strategies should be examined. For example, the patient can be asked to stand first with normal stance width, then with a narrowed BOS. The ability to improve performance with repeat trials should be documented.

FUNCTIONAL BALANCE TESTS

Traditional tests of balance have focused on the maintenance of posture (static balance), balance during weight shifting or movement (dynamic balance), and responses to manual perturbations. Items for static control typically include double limb stance, single limb stance, tandem stance (heel-toe position), Romberg test (eyes open to eyes closed [EO > EC]), and sharpened Romberg test (tandem foot position, EO > EC). Dynamic test items include standing up, walking, turning, stopping, and starting. Subjective grading scales are typically used and can range from a simple 3-point ordinal ranking (absent, impaired, present) to a scale with grades of normal, good, fair, poor, and absent. Reliability measures are lacking for most subjective grading scales.[91,92] Comparison of responses to other patients or to a normal population is difficult owing to the subjectivity of grades. A more definitive scale of functional balance includes descriptors that define performance (see Table 8–7). Objectivity can be increased by using timed performance to document postural stability. For example, a stopwatch can be used to time a 30-second trial of a static balance task (e.g., single limb stance).[112]

Standardized tests and measures of balance are available that emphasize functional performance. It is important to consider measures with established reliability, validity, and responsiveness. Responsiveness is the ability to detect meaningful change in the patient's status.[113] Tests particularly deserving of attention include the Functional Reach, the Berg Balance Scale, the Tinetti

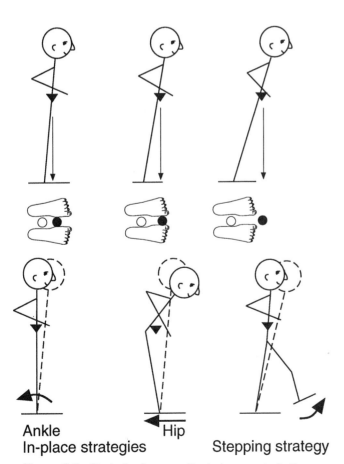

Ankle   **Hip**
In-place strategies   **Stepping strategy**

Figure 8-3. Strategies for correcting balance perturbations.

Table 8–7 FUNCTIONAL BALANCE GRADES

Normal	Patient is able to maintain steady balance without support (static).
	Accepts maximal challenge and can shift weight in all directions (dynamic).
Good	Patient is able to maintain balance without support (static).
	Accepts moderate challenge; able to maintain balance while picking object off floor (dynamic).
Fair	Patient is able to maintain balance with handhold (static).
	Accepts minimal challenge; able to maintain balance while turning head/trunk (dynamic).
Poor	Patient requires handhold and assistance (static).
	Unable to accept challenge or move without loss of balance (dynamic).

Performance-Oriented Mobility Assessment, and the Get Up and Go Test.

The *Functional Reach Test (FR)* developed by Duncan et al.[114] is a test of dynamic standing balance. Functional reach is defined as the maximal distance one can reach forward beyond arm's length while maintaining a fixed BOS in the standing position. It uses a leveled yardstick mounted on the wall and positioned at the patient's shoulder height (acromion). The patient stands next to the wall (without touching) with the shoulder flexed to 90° and elbow extended. The hand is fisted. An initial measurement is made of the position of the 3rd metacarpal along the yardstick. The patient is then instructed to lean as far forward as possible without losing balance or taking a step. A repeat measurement is made in the forward reach position. This measurement is then subtracted from the initial measurement. Three trials of FR are performed and the average of all three trials recorded. The FR test has a reported test-retest reliability of 0.92 and an interrater reliability of 0.98.[113] Age-related norms for FR have been determined. These include:

20 to 40 years old: 14 to 17 inches
41 to 69 years old: 13 to 16 inches
70 to 87 years old: 10 to 13 inches

The FR was originally developed for use with an elderly population. Scores of less than 7 are indicative of a frail individual who is limited in mobility and ADL skills and demonstrates increased fall risk.[115–117]

The Balance Scale developed by Berg et al.[118,119] is an objective measure of static and dynamic balance abilities. The scale consists of 14 functional tasks commonly performed in everyday life. The items range from sitting or standing unsupported, to movement transitions (sitting to standing, standing to sitting), variations in standing position (eyes closed, feet together, reaching forward, retrieving an object from the floor, turning, standing on one foot) to placing the foot on a stool. Scoring uses a 5-point ordinal scale, with scores ranging from 0 to 4. Descriptive criteria are provided for scoring each level: a score of 4 is used to indicate that the patient *performs independently and meets time and distance criteria,* and a score of 0 is used for *unable to perform*

(see Appendix A). A maximum of 56 points is possible. Both intrarater and interrater reliability scores are reported to be high (0.95), while the range of scores for individual items is between 0.71 and 0.99. The Balance Scale was originally developed for use with elderly patients with stroke and has been shown to be a sensitive measure of recovery. Balance scale scores were also shown to be useful in predicting falls in the elderly[120] and evaluating changes in patients undergoing physical therapy.[122]

The *Performance-Oriented Mobility Assessment (POMA)* developed by Tinetti[123,124] provides a simple, brief, and reliable assessment of position changes, response to perturbations, and gait movements during daily activity (see Appendix B). It includes both static and dynamic balance items organized into two subtests of balance and gait. Balance tests include sitting balance, rising from and sitting down in a chair, standing balance (eyes open to eyes closed, withstanding a perturbation, single limb stance, tandem stance, reaching, bending over) and turning 360 degrees. Gait tests include an assessment of initiation of gait, path deviation, stepping, turning, and walking time. Some items are scored on a 0 to 2 scale, and some items are timed. The original POMA I scale has a total possible score of 28. It was developed for use with the frail elderly, especially nursing home residents with a propensity to fall.[125] Interrater reliability, as scored by a physician and nurse, is high with a reported 85 percent agreement. A revised form, the POMA IA, expanded the items for use as a predictor of falls among community dwelling elderly (total possible score of 40). The POMA II was developed as an outcome measure in a frailty and injury prevention trial (the Yale FICSIT trial).[126,127] This expanded version has a total possible score of 54.

The *Get Up and Go (GUG) Test* developed by Mathias et al.[128] is a quick measure of basic mobility and balance. The patient is seated comfortably in a firm chair with arms and back resting against the chair. The patient is then instructed to rise, stand still momentarily, and then walk 3 meters toward a wall at normal walking speed, turn without touching the wall, return to the chair, turn and sit down. Tape is used to mark the walking distance and turning point. The original GUG test was scored using a 5-point ordinal scale with scores of 1 normal (no risk of falls), 2 very slightly abnormal, 3 mildly abnormal, 4 moderately abnormal, and 5 severely abnormal (high risk of falls). If an assistive device is required, the type is recorded. Reliability was reported to be high for a group of physical therapists (0.85) while only moderate (0.69) for a group of physicians examining videotaped performance. Efforts by Podsiadlo and Richardson[129] to improve the objectivity and reliability resulted in the *Timed Up and Go test.* Timing with a stopwatch begins when the patient is instructed with "go" and ends when the patient returns to the start position in the chair. Both test-retest and interrater reliability of the timed Timed Up and Go Test are reported to be very high

(0.98). Research indicates that most adults can complete the test in 10 seconds. Scores of 11 to 20 seconds are considered within normal limits for frail elderly or individuals with a disability; scores over 20 seconds are indicative of impaired functional mobility. The Timed Up and Go Test provides a reliable quick screening measure; abnormal scores warrant additional comprehensive assessment.[113]

An investigation of postural control during gait should include an assessment of level walking. Gait speed has been shown to be a sensitive measure of functional performance. There is a wide range of normal gait speeds reported, ranging from 1.2 to 1.5 m/s in healthy young adults. Gait speeds decrease in older adults (0.9 to 1.3 m/s), in individuals with a disability and those requiring assistive devices.[87,130] Gait speed was used to distinguish between household and community ambulators in an elderly population.[130] A timed 8-foot walk test was used as a predictor of subsequent disability in individuals over the age of 70.[131] The *Three Minute Walk Test* can be used to document functional performance. The total distance achieved in 3 minutes of walking at a self-selected speed, number of times of loss of balance (LOB), pulse rate, and symptoms of exertional intolerance (chest pain, shortness of breath) are recorded.[84]

Examination of postural control also includes *observational gait analysis.* A complete description of normal gait parameters and gait analysis can be found in Chapter 10. The therapist should determine the BOS, step width, stride length, cadence, and position and movements of the extremities. Gait abnormalities should be carefully documented. Inconsistency and arrhythmicity of stepping and arm movements, guardedness, weaving, waddling, staggering, widely spaced steps, and arms held out to the side (guard position) are all indicative of decreased balance control.[132] The *Gait Assessment Rating Scale (GARS)* developed by Wolfson et al.[133] has been used to document gait abnormalities in the elderly and to identify those at risk for falls.

The ability to modify gait **(adaptive control)** can be assessed by changing task demands. The *Dynamic Gait Index* developed by Shumway-Cook[134] includes variations in speed (slow, fast), head turning (looking right, left, up, and down), turning (pivot turn, 360-degree turn), stepping over an obstacle, stepping around obstacles, stairclimbing, picking an object up from the floor, and alternate step-ups on a stool. The Index appears sensitive in predicting likelihood for falls with older adults. Attentional demands should also be assessed. In the *Walky-Talky Test,* the therapist walks alongside the patient on indoor walk. A conversation is begun. The test is positive if the patient has difficulty walking and talking or has to stop walking in order to talk. The introduction of secondary task interference reveals important information about the level of conscious awareness required for response programming of the first task.[135]

Functional Mobility Skills

Analysis of function focuses on the measurement and classification of functional abilities and the identification of functional limitations and disabilities. Testing can focus on any of four dimensions of function: physical, mental, or affective/social. Performance-based measures of physical function yield important information about motor control. Numerous instruments are available with objective scoring systems. The selection of an appropriate tool will depend on specific patient characteristics and treatment focus and may vary with practice setting. This topic is discussed fully in Chapter 11.

Progression through a sequence of functional mobility skills typically includes:
- rolling from side-to-side
- moving from supine to sitting and sitting to supine
- maintaining sitting posture
- transfers
- moving from sitting to standing and standing to sitting
- maintaining standing posture
- walking

Control can also be assessed in other postures including prone on elbows, quadruped (hands and knees), kneeling, half-kneeling, and standing up from the floor. It is important to note that there is considerable variability in motor performance of functional tasks across the lifespan.[136–140] Changes are influenced by such factors as changing body dimensions, age, health, level of physical activity, and so forth. Thus, the activities of rolling over and sitting up may vary considerably between two adults of different size, age, or health.

Qualitative assessment of functional patterns should be performed. Patterns may be normal, abnormal but compensatory (task is accomplished), abnormal/non-compensatory, or absent. The presence of impairments may alter the way movements are performed and should be carefully documented. For example, the patient with hemiplegia will attempt to sit up from supine using the sound side. The affected extremities may lag behind, not well integrated into the movement pattern. Differing environments can also alter the way the task is performed.

Assessment and documentation should consider four basic task requirements: (1) mobility, (2) stability, (3) controlled mobility, and (4) skill. **Mobility** is a term used to describe initial movement in a functional pattern. In assessing mobility, adequate range of motion must be available for the movement to occur as well as sufficient muscle activity. Patients with deficits in initial mobility demonstrate movements that are not sustained or well coordinated. Antigravity control is generally lacking. Thus, patients may be able to roll but are unable to move from supine to sitting against gravity.

Stability is a term used to describe the ability to maintain a steady position in a weight bearing, antigravity posture (also referred to as *static postural control*). For example, the patient demonstrates stability in sitting or standing posture if he or she is able to maintain the posture with minimum sway or instability. Episodes of LOB and fall safety risk should be documented in each posture.

Controlled mobility (CM) describes the ability to alter a position or move into a new position while maintaining stability (also termed *dynamic postural control*). Thus an individual is able to shift weight or rock in a posture (e.g., sitting). Full ROM and balanced control in all directions is expected. Independent assumption of a posture is also an example of controlled mobility. This is a more difficult activity, because it requires the patient to move through a greater range of movement and against the effects of gravity. The patient who is unable to sit up from supine without assistance demonstrates a deficiency in controlled mobility function. If assistance is required, the type and amount is recorded. **Static-dynamic control,** a variation of controlled mobility, is defined as the ability to shift weight onto one side and free up a limb for non-weight bearing, dynamic activities. Unilateral weight bearing places increased demands for dynamic stability because the support limb assumes the full weight bearing load while the dynamic limb challenges control. For example, a patient in quadruped who is unable to lift either an upper or lower limb, or lift the opposite upper and lower limbs together, demonstrates a deficit in static-dynamic control.

Skill is highly coordinated movement that allows for investigation and interaction with the physical and social environment. Proximal segments stabilize while distal segments are free for function (e.g., manipulation and transport). Movements are consistent, with an economy of effort, and regulated with precise timing and direction (coordination). Skilled movements can be discrete, continuous, or serial. Kicking a ball is an example of a discrete skill, with a recognizable beginning and end. Walking is a continuous skill (no recognizable beginning and end), and playing a piano represents a serial skill (a series of discrete actions put together). Movements are shaped to the specific environments in which they occur: movement in a stable, nonchanging environment is called a **closed skill,** while movement in a variable, changing environment is called an **open skill.** A skilled individual is able to perform single or simultaneous movement tasks. Thus the skilled individual is able to move with precise control (e.g., feeding or dressing), maintain movement sequences for extended periods (e.g., walking or running), perform equally well in different types of environments (e.g., in the clinic or at home), and combine different movement sequences (e.g., walking while reaching for an object).[141]

The qualitative analysis of functional skills can be enhanced by the use of video equipment. Patient responses recorded on videotape provide a permanent record of motor performance and allow the therapist the opportunity to compare responses over time. Recordings made at 3 or 6 weeks of recovery can be compared easily without reliance on the therapist's memory or written notes. Accuracy of observations can be improved. A therapist who is closely involved in assisting or guarding during performance may not be attentive enough to observe all movement parameters (e.g., when assisting the patient with traumatic brain injury with severe ataxia). Depending on equipment capabilities, videotapes can be viewed repeatedly at different speeds to determine control during different tasks and at different body segments. For example, a patient's performance in a task such as sitting up from supine can be observed first at regular speeds, then at slow motion speeds. Stop-action or freezing a frame can be used to isolate a problematic point in the movement sequence. This may be helpful, particularly for the inexperienced therapist, in improving both the quality and reliability of observations. Repeat trials on a functional performance test may needlessly tire the patient while yielding a decrease in performance. Sequential video recordings over the course of rehabilitation provide visual documentation of patient progress and can be important motivational and learning tools in therapy. This equipment can also be a valuable tool in educating family members and staff.[142,143]

Reliability of taping for intersession comparisons can be improved by the following measures. Placement of equipment should be planned in advance to achieve the best location and should be consistently placed over subsequent sessions. Use of a tripod can improve the stability of the recording. During the session, repeat trials of the same task (e.g., at least three trials) will provide information about the consistency of performance. Verbal descriptions of the performance during each trial can be edited directly onto the tape or documented in a written summary.[144]

Motor Learning

Motor learning has been defined as "a set of internal processes associated with practice or experience leading to relatively permanent changes in the capability for skilled behavior."[1p416] Learning is a complex process that requires spatial, temporal, and hierarchical organization within the CNS. Changes in the CNS are not directly observable, but rather are inferred from improvement in performance as a result of practice or experience.

Individual differences in learning are expected and influence both the rate and degree of learning possible. Motor abilities among individuals vary across three main foundational categories of abilities: cognitive abilities, perceptual speed ability, and psychomotor ability.[145] Differences occur as a result of both genetics and experience. The therapist should be sensitive to such factors as alertness, anxiety, memory, speed of processing information, speed and accuracy of movements, uniqueness of the setting, and so forth.[2] In addition, patients may vary in their learning potential according to the pathology present, the number and type of impairments, and general health status and co-morbidities. Although most skills can be learned through practice or experience, the therapist should be sensitive to the patient's underlying capabilities (abilities) that support certain skills. For example, some patients with spinal cord injury are never able to learn to manage curbs or "wheelies" because of the difficulty of the task, their residual abilities, and general health status.

PRACTICE OBSERVATIONS

Motor learning is typically assessed by documenting improvements in performance that result from practice or experience. Performance criteria are established and used for comparison when assessing learning outcomes. The therapist must then select an appropriate motor skill performance measure (see Table 8–8 for sample measures). For example, an individual is able to demonstrate functional independence in transfers after a series of training sessions. Improvement in functional scores (e.g., FIM scores) documents changes in the level of assistance needed. The number of practice trials or practice time required to achieve skill mastery can be documented. Qualitative changes in performance are determined by comparing changes in the spatial and temporal organization of movements with the criterion skill (e.g., how the transfer should be performed). Error measures can be used to docu-

ment accuracy of movement. Thus, therapists can report the number and type of errors (constant, variable) that occur within a given practice session and across practice sessions. A decrease in the frequency of errors is consistent with improvements in learning. One common measurement problem in skill learning is the speed-accuracy trade-off. Typically initial practice sessions are characterized by slowed performance in order to improve movement accuracy. As learning progresses, performance speed can be increased once accuracy demands are satisfied. Thus number of errors should be considered along with speed of performance. Magill[2] suggests that for tasks that require speed, the number of errors and time to complete the task can be added and then divided by two to achieve a speed-accuracy score.[2] Reduced effort and concentration are indicative of learning and should be documented. Whereas a high degree of cognitive monitoring is necessary in early learning (cognitive stage), performance in the associative and autonomous stages of learning is characterized by reduced cognitive monitoring and increasingly more automaticity.[146] As learning progresses, performance is increasingly characterized by persistence and consistency. Thus the acquired skills are observed for more than one performance trial and trial-to-trial variability decreases.

Practice observations can be misleading in that performance is not always an accurate reflection of

Table 8–8 TWO CATEGORIES OF MOTOR SKILL PERFORMANCE MEASURES

Category	Examples of Measures	Performance Examples
1. Response outcome measures	Time to complete a response e.g., sec, min, hr	Amount of time to run a mile, type a word
	Reaction time	Time between starter's gun and beginning of movement
	Amount of error in performing criterion movement e.g., AE, CE, VE	Number of cm away from the target in reproducing a criterion limb position
	Number or percentage of errors	Number of free throws missed
	Number of successful attempts	Number of times the beanbag hit the target
	Time on/off target	Number of seconds stylus in contact with target on pursuit rotor
	Time on/off balance	Number of seconds stood in stork stance
	Distance	Height of vertical jump
	Trials to completion	Number of trials it took until all responses correct
2. Response production measures	Displacement	Distance limb traveled to produce response
	Velocity	Speed limb moved while performing response
	Acceleration	Acceleration/deceleration pattern while moving
	Joint angle	Angle of each joint of arm at impact in hitting ball
	Electromyography (EMG)	Time at which the biceps initially fired during a rapid flexion response
	Electroencephalogram (EEG)	Characteristic of the P300 for a choice RT response

The events and time intervals related to typical measurement of reaction time (RT) and movement time (MT).
Absolute error (AE), constant error (CE), variable error (VE).
From Magill, R: Motor Learning Concepts and Applications, ed 4. WCP Brown & Benchmark, Madison, 1993, p 17, with permission.

learning. It is possible to practice enough to temporarily improve performance but not retain the learning. Conversely, factors such as fatigue, anxiety, poor motivation, boredom, or drugs can cause performance to deteriorate while learning may still occur. Thus the patient who is fatigued or stressed performs very poorly during scheduled treatment but returns after the weekend rested and calm, and is able to perform the task with ease. Performance plateaus, defined as a leveling off of performance after a period of steady improvement, characterize normal practice and can be expected to occur.[2] During plateaus, learning may still be going on. Typically these are temporary steady states and performance will begin to show improvement again. Plateaus can also be the result of ceiling effects (a high level of performance in which further improvement cannot be detected by the performance measure) or floor effects (when decreasing scores demonstrate improved performance). More reliable inferences about learning can be made through the use of retention tests and transfer tests.

RETENTION TESTS

A **retention test,** defined as "a performance test administered after a retention interval for the purposes of assessing learning,"[1p418] provides an important measure of learning. The learner is asked to demonstrate the skill after a period of no practice **(retention interval).** Retention intervals can be of varying lengths. For example, the patient who is seen only once a week in an outpatient clinic is asked to demonstrate a skill practiced the previous week. Performance after the retention interval is compared to performance on the initial practice session. Performance may show a slight initial decrease (termed warm-up decrement) but should return to original performance levels within relatively few practice trials if learning has occurred. It is important not to provide any verbal cueing or knowledge of results during the retention trial. This same patient may have been given a home exercise program (HEP) that includes daily practice of the desired skill. If upon return to the clinic some weeks later, performance of the desired skill has not been maintained or has deteriorated, the therapist might reasonably conclude that the patient has not been diligent with the HEP and learning has not been retained.

TRANSFER TESTS

Learning can be assessed by determining if the skill acquired can be generalized. **Generalizability** is defined as the "extent to which practice on one task contributes to the performance of other, related skills.[1p280] Thus the individual is able to apply a learned skill to the learning of other similar tasks. Individuals who learn to transfer from wheelchair to platform mat can apply that learning to other variations of transfers (e.g., wheelchair to car, wheelchair to tub). The number of practice trials, time, and effort required to perform these new types of transfers should be reduced from that required to perform the initial skill.

Learning can be assessed by determining the **resistance to contextual change.** This is the adaptability required to perform a motor task in altered environmental situations. Thus an individual who has learned a skill (e.g., walking with a cane) should be able to apply that learning to new and variable situations (e.g., walking at home, walking outdoors, walking downtown on a busy street). The therapist documents how successful the individual is in performing the skill in the new situations. The patient who is only able to perform the skill in one type of environment, for example, the patient with traumatic brain injury who is only able to function within a tightly controlled, closed environment, demonstrates limited and largely nonfunctional learning. This patient is not likely to return home independent in the community environment, and will likely require placement in an assisted living (structured) setting.

The patient who is able to engage in active introspection and self-evaluation of performance and reach decisions independently about how to improve performance demonstrates an important element of learning. Often physical therapists overemphasize guided movements and errorless practice. Although this may be important for safety reasons, lack of exposure to performance errors may preclude the patient from developing capabilities for self-assessment. In an era of fiscal responsibility and limitations on the amount of physical therapy sessions allowed, many patients are able to learn only the very basic skills while in active rehabilitation. Much of the necessary learning of functional skills occurs after discharge and during outpatient episodes of care. The therapist cannot possibly structure practice sessions to meet all of the functional challenges the patient may face. The acquisition of independent problem solving/decision making skills ensures that the final goal of rehabilitation—independent function—can be achieved.

Learning Styles

Individuals vary in their learning style, defined as their characteristic mode of gaining, processing, and storing information. Learning styles differ according to a number of factors, including personality characteristics, reasoning styles (inductive versus deductive), initiative (active versus passive), and so forth. Some individuals utilize an analytical/objective learning style. They process information in a step-by-step order and learn best with factual information and structure. Other individuals are more intuitive/global learners. They tend to process information all at once, and learn best when information is personalized and presented in the context of practical, real-life examples. They may have difficulty in ordering steps and comprehending details. Some individuals rely heavily on visual processing and demonstration to learn a task.

Others depend more on auditory processing, talking themselves through a task. These characteristics are best determined by talking with the patient and family, and using careful listening and observation skills. The medical record may also provide information concerning relevant premorbid history (occupation, interests). A thorough understanding of each of these factors allows the therapist to appropriately structure the learning environment and therapist-patient interactions.

EVALUATION

Evaluation refers to the clinical judgments therapists make based on the data gathered from the examination.[5] Numerous factors influence the judgments therapists make when working with patients with neurological dysfunction, including complexity and understanding of the nervous system, clinical findings, extent of loss of function, social considerations, and overall physical function and health. Therapists evaluate data in terms of severity of problems, level of chronicity, and possibility for multisystem failure and disability. Potential discharge placement and resources can also influence evaluation of the data and development of the plan of care. There is a clear need for the therapist to focus on those problems that directly impact on function and can be remediated. The therapist must also consider the consequences of failure to intervene appropriately when the patient is at risk for additional impairments, functional limitations, and disabilities.

DIAGNOSIS

The physical therapy diagnosis is determined from evaluation of the findings and is based on a cluster of signs, symptoms, or categories. The *Guide to Physical Therapist Practice*,[5] a consensus document developed by expert physical therapy clinicians, identifies diagnostic categories and preferred practice patterns that delineate appropriate interventions. For example, Impaired Motor Function and Sensory Integrity Associated with Acquired Nonprogressive Disorders of the Central Nervous System includes patients with traumatic brain injury, cerebrovascular accident, tumor, and so forth.[5pB-1] The reader is referred to this document for comparison and refinement of his or her own practice. Novice therapists can gain understanding and insights into the complex practice issues facing therapists who work with patients with deficits in motor function.

SUMMARY

Assessment of motor function is a difficult, multifaceted process, critically related to the therapist's ability to accurately examine and categorize behaviors. An understanding of normal motor control and motor learning mechanisms is essential to this process. Determining the causative factors responsible for abnormal movement patterns must be based upon comparison of expected or normal responses (norm-referenced behaviors) with the patient's abnormal ones. This can best be achieved by a systematic and thorough approach to assessment with emphasis on the use of valid, reliable, and responsive measurement tools. A number of different factors are analyzed, ranging from consciousness and arousal, attention, cognition and communication, sensory integrity, joint integrity, tone and reflex integrity, cranial nerve integrity, muscle performance, voluntary movement patterns, postural control and balance, and functional mobility skills. Traditional clinical testing of individual systems can yield valuable information about the integrity of individual components. However, normal motor control and motor learning is achieved through the integrated action of CNS systems. Evaluation must therefore also focus on integrated function. Our theoretical understanding of the CNS, motor control, and motor learning processes is both incomplete and imperfect. Therapists must, therefore, be constantly aware of the changing knowledge base in neuroscience and in neurological rehabilitation to incorporate new ideas into their therapeutic approach to assessment and treatment.

QUESTIONS FOR REVIEW

1. What are the components of the examination of motor function? How can the components be structured (ordered) to improve validity and reliability of results?

2. Describe the examination of consciousness and arousal, and cognition, and communication. How can deficits in each of these areas influence the assessment of motor function?

3. What tests can be used for a screening examination of motor function of the cranial nerves? sensory function?

4. The presence of abnormal tone, reflexes, or synergy may impair normal movement. How can each be assessed? What interaction effects between them are likely to influence the examination?

5. Describe the reasons, both pro and con, for using strength testing (MMT) in patients with neurological dysfunction.

6. Lesions of the dorsal columns/lemniscal system can result in decreased or absent discriminative touch and proprioception. In the lower extremities how can these losses contribute to deficits in balance, coordination, and gait? What are the expected deficits, and how can each be examined?

7. Describe balance testing measures that can be used to assess static balance control? dynamic

balance control? reactive versus anticipatory control?

8. Following neurological injury, functional mobility skills are typically impaired. How can task requirements be assessed for stability, controlled mobility, and skill in sitting? How can the examination be structured to obtain information about adaptability of skills?

9. Differentiate between practice observations, retention tests, and transfer tests in the assessment of motor learning. What is the relative importance of each in determining learning?

10. Discuss factors that can influence the evaluation of data and determination of the physical therapy diagnosis for patients with deficits of motor function.

CASE STUDY

The patient is a 17-year-old female who is 10 months post motor vehicle accident (MVA). At the time of admission to the hospital, she was comatose and decerebrate. CT scan revealed intracranial bleeding into the right occipital horn. She received a tracheostomy and a gastrostomy. Two months post MVA, she was transferred to a long-term care facility specializing in traumatic brain injury.

On initial admission she was able to open her eyes to verbal and tactile stimuli but was unable to visually track. She withdrew her upper and lower extremities in response to stimulation but was not able to move them on command. She was alert but confused, and was unable to carry on a conversation. ROM was within normal limits (WNL) except for right elbow flexion (20 to 100 degrees) and right knee flexion (10 to 110 degrees). She demonstrated increased tone on Modified Ashworth Scale: 3 in her left upper extremity (LUE), 4 in her right upper extremity (RUE), and 4 in both lower extremities (BLEs). She exhibited 4+ bilateral ankle clonus. She was unable to sit unsupported. In the wheelchair her head and trunk control was poor, with persistent posturing to the left side. She has received daily physical and occupational therapy consisting of PROM, upright positioning, and sensory/cognitive stimulation. She is currently being assessed for transfer to active rehabilitation status.

PHYSICAL THERAPY EXAMINATION FINDINGS

° **Consciousness/Arousal**

Fully awake; responds appropriately to varying stimuli.

Oriented to person; some confusion with orientation to place and time.

Can become agitated with minimal stimulation, especially when tired.

° **Cognition/Behavior**

Demonstrates difficulty with concentration and attention.

Able to follow simple instructions (one- or two-level commands) but occasionally forgets what is asked of her.

Reaction time is slowed as the number of choices is increased.

Easily forgets what she is doing.

° **Sensory Integrity**

Aware of sensory input (pinprick, vibration, light touch) to all extremities.

Unable to discern common objects placed in either hand for stereognosis discrimination.

° **Joint Integrity and Mobility**

Decreased PROM:

RLE: plantar flexion contracture (-40 degrees to neutral), hip and knee flexion contractures (-10 degrees to full knee and hip extension).

RUE: right elbow has a flexor contracture (-10 degrees to full extension).

Full PROM in the LUE and LLE.

° **Tone**

Increased bilaterally (R > L).

On Modified Ashworth Scale: RUE and RLE 3; LUE and LLE 2.

° **Reflex Integrity**

Hyperactive, 3+ DTRs RUE, RLE.

3+ bilateral ankle clonus.

° **Cranial Nerve Integrity**

Dysphagia and dysphonia are present.

° **Muscle Performance**

Strength is decreased in the RUE, RLE, and trunk (unable to test with MMT). She is unable to sustain R knee extension during standing.

° **Voluntary Movement Patterns**

RUE moves in partial range, obligatory flexor synergy pattern only.

RLE moves in flexor and extensor synergy patterns with no variation.

LUE and LLE demonstrate full voluntary control with isolated joint movements. Coordination is decreased. Unable to reach directly to an object that is held out to her and demonstrates foot placement problems with the LLE in sitting or in standing.

Demonstrates problems with coordinating limb and trunk movements.

° **Postural Control and Balance**

Demonstrates good head control in all positions.

Sitting: can sit independently for up to 5 minutes. Demonstrates difficulty in maintaining weight equally on both buttocks. Tends to list to the right side while placing weight primarily on her left buttock. Able to reach to the left and forward; demonstrates loss of balance (LOB) with minimal reaching to right.

Standing: able to stand in parallel bars with min assistance × 1 for up to 2 minutes. Has to be reminded to place weight on her RLE. Tends to lose her balance easily if she moves quickly; associated with brief episodes of dizziness and vertigo.

° **Functional Mobility Skills**

Rolling: requires supervision and occasional minimal assistance with rolling to the right; she requires maximal assist when rolling to the left.

Supine-to-sit: able to come to sitting by rolling to the L side and pushing up with her LUE; requires minimal assistance.

Transfers: able to perform stand pivot transfers with minimal assistance × 1.

Gait: does not initiate ambulation on her own. Can ambulate the length of the parallel bars (6 feet) with maximal assistance × 2. Requires posterior splint to stabilize R knee.

Propels wheelchair by using the LUE and both feet for pushing; requires supervision for safety.

° **Motor Learning**

Demonstrates profound deficits in short-term memory; unable to remember new information presented during therapy. Her memory for events and learning prior to the MVA is good.

Guiding Questions

Based on your evaluation of the data presented in the case history and the physical therapy examination, answer the following questions:

1. Categorize her level of consciousness upon admission to the long-term care facility using the Glasgow Coma Scale.

2. Establish a clinical problem list. Categorize the problems in terms of direct impairments, indirect impairments, composite impairments, and functional limitations (see Chapter 1 for definitions of these terms).

3. Prioritize the problems in terms of possible functional goals and outcomes.

4. Determine the physical therapy diagnosis using the preferred practice pattern identified by the *Guide to Physical Therapist Practice*.[5]

REFERENCES

1. Schmidt, R, and Lee, T: Motor Control and Learning, ed 3. Human Kinetics, Champaign, IL, 1999.
2. Magill, R: Motor Learning Concepts and Applications, ed 4. WCB Brown & Benchmark, Madison, WI, 1993.
3. Brooks, V: The Neural Basis of Motor Control. Oxford University Press, New York, 1986.
4. Bernstein, N: The Coordination and Regulation of Movements. Pergamon Press, New York, 1967.
5. American Physical Therapy Association. Guide to Physical Therapist Practice. APTA, Alexandria, VA, 1998.
6. Riolo, L: Skill differences in novice and expert clinicians in neurologic physical therapy. Neurology Report 20:60, 1996.
7. Dell, P: Reticular homeostasis and critical reactivity. In Moruzzi, B, et al (eds): Progress in Brain Research, vol 1, Brain Mechanisms. Elsevier, New York, 1963, p 82.
8. Nolan, M: Introduction to the Neurological Examination. FA Davis, Philadelphia, 1996.
9. Jennett, B, and Bond, M: Assessment of outcome after severe head injury: A practical scale. Lancet 1:480, 1975.
10. Yerkes, R, and Dodson J: The relation of strength of stimulus to rapidity of habit-formation. J Comp Neurol Psychol 18:459, 1908.
11. Wilder, J: Basimetric approach (law of initial value) to biological rhythms. Ann N Y Acad Sci 98:1211, 1961.
12. Stockmeyer, S: Clinical decision making based on homeostatic concepts. In Wolf, S (ed): Clinical Decision Making in Physical Therapy. FA Davis, Philadelphia, 1985, p 79.
13. Zoltan, B: Vision, Perception, and Cognition. A Manual for the Evaluation and Treatment of the Neurologically Impaired Adult, ed 3. Slack, Thorofare, NJ, 1986.
14. Folstein, M: Mini-mental state: A practical method for grading the cognitive state of patients for the clinician. J Psychiatr Res 12:189, 1975.
15. American Academy of Orthopaedic Surgeons: Joint Motion: Method of Measuring and Recording. American Academy of Orthopaedic Surgeons, Chicago, 1965.
16. Norkin, C, and White, D: Measurement of Joint Motion: A Guide to Goniometry, ed 2. FA Davis, Philadelphia, 1995.
17. Gajdosik, R, and Bohannon R: Clinical measurement of range of motion: Review of goniometry emphasizing reliability and validity. Phys Ther 67:1867, 1987.
18. Magee, D: Orthopedic Physical Assessment, ed 3. Saunders, Philadelphia, 1997.
19. Hoppenfeld, S: Physical Examination of the Spine and Extremities. Appleton-Century-Crofts, Norwalk, CT, 1976.
20. Katz, R, and Rymer, Z: Spastic hypertonia: Mechanisms and measurement. Arch Phys Med Rehabil 70:144, 1989.
21. Bobath, B: Adult Hemiplegia: Evaluation and Treatment, ed 2. Heinemann, London, 1978.
22. Burke, D: Spasticity as an adaptation to pyramidal tract injury. In Waxman, S (ed): Advances in Neurology, 47: Functional Recovery in Neurological Disease. Raven, New York, 1988.
23. Dobkin, B: Neurologic Rehabilitation. FA Davis, Philadelphia, 1996.
24. Jankovic, J: Pathophysiology and clinical assessment of motor symptoms in Parkinson's disease. In Koller, W (ed): Handbook of Parkinson's Disease. Marcel Dekker, New York, 1987, p 99.
25. Jankovic, J, and Fahn, S: Dystonic syndromes. In Jankovic, J, and Tolosa, E (eds): Parkinson's Disease and Movement Disorders. Urban & Schwarzenburg, Baltimore, 1988, p 283.
26. Watkins, M, et al: Isokinetic testing in patients with hemiparesis. Phys Ther 64:184, 1984.
27. Ashworth, B: Preliminary trial of carisoprodol in multiple sclerosis. Practitioner 192:540, 1964.
28. Bohannon, R, and Smith, M: Interrater reliability of a modified Ashworth scale of muscle spasticity. Phys Ther 67:206, 1987.
29. Bajd, T, and Vodovnik, L: Pendulum testing of spasticity. J Biomech Eng 6:9, 1984.
30. Bohannon, R: Variability and reliability of the pendulum test for spasticity using a Cybex II Isokinetic Dynamometer. Phys Ther 67:659, 1987.
31. Easton, T: On the normal use of reflexes. Am Sci 60:591, 1972.
32. Hellebrandt, F, et al: Methods of evoking the tonic neck reflexes in normal human subjects. Am J Phys Med 35:144, 1956.
33. Hellebrandt, F, and Waterland, J: Expansion of motor patterning under exercise stress. Am J Phys Med 41:56, 1962.
34. Brunnstrom, S: Movement Therapy in Hemiplegia. Harper & Row, New York, 1970.
35. Bobath, B: Abnormal Postural Reflex Activity Caused by Brain Lesions. Heinemann, London, 1965.
36. Capute, A, et al: Primitive Reflex Profile. University Park Press, Baltimore, 1978.
37. Capute, A, et al: Primitive Reflex Profile: A Pilot Study. Phys Ther 58:1061, 1978.
38. McGraw, M: From reflex to muscular control in the assumption of an erect posture and ambulation in the human infant. Child Dev 3:291, 1932.
39. Barnes, M, et al: The Neurophysiological Basis of Patient Treatment, vol II, Reflexes in Motor Development. Stokesville Publishing, Atlanta, 1978.
40. Fiorentino, M: Reflex Testing Methods for Evaluating C.N.S. Development, ed 2. Charles C Thomas, Springfield, IL, 1973.
41. Kendall, F, and McCreary E: Muscle Testing and Function, ed 4. Williams & Wilkins, Baltimore, 1993.

42. Hislop, H, and Montgomery, J: Muscle Testing: Techniques of Manual Examination, ed 6. Saunders, Philadelphia, 1995.

43. Rothstein, J, et al: Commentary. Is the measurement of muscle strength appropriate in patients with brain lesions? Phys Ther 69:230, 1989.

44. Bohannon, R: Is the measurement of muscle strength appropriate in patients with brain lesions? Phys Ther 69:225, 1989.

45. Sahrmann, S, and Norton, B: The relationship of voluntary movement to spasticity in the upper motor neuron syndrome. Ann Neurol 2:460, 1977.

46. Knuttsson, E, and Martensson, A: Dynamic motor capacity in spastic paresis and its relation to prime mover dysfunction, spastic reflexes and antagonist co-activation. Scand J Rehabil Med 12:93, 1980.

47. Rosenfalck, A, and Andreassen, S: Impaired regulation of force and firing pattern of single motor units in patients with spasticity. J Neurol Neurosurg Psychiatry 43:907, 1980.

48. Gowland, C, et al: Agonist and antagonist activity during voluntary upper-limb movement in patients with stroke. Phys Ther 72:624, 1992.

49. Bourbonnais, D, et al: Abnormal spatial patterns of elbow muscle activation in hemiparetic human subjects. Brain 112:85, 1989.

50. Bourbonnais, D, and Vanden Noven, S: Weakness in patients with hemiparesis. Am J Occup Ther 43:313, 1989.

51. Craik, R: Abnormalities of motor behavior. In Contemporary Management of Motor Control Problems. Proceedings of the II Step Conference. Foundation for Physical Therapy, Alexandria, VA, 1991.

52. Post-Stroke Rehabilitation Guideline Panel: Post-Stroke Rehabilitation Clinical Practice Guideline. Aspen, Gaithersburg, MD, 1996. (Formerly published as AHCPR Publication No. 95-0662, May 1995.)

53. Frese, E, et al: Clinical reliability of manual muscle testing: Middle trapezius and gluteus medius muscles. Phys Ther 67:1072, 1987.

54. Riddle, D, et al: Intrasession and intersession reliability of hand-held dynamometer measurements taken on brain-damaged patients. Phys Ther 69:182, 1989.

55. Bohannon, R: Test-retest reliability of hand-held dynamometry during a single session of strength assessment. Phys Ther 66:206, 1986.

56. Bohannon, R, and Andrews, A: Interrater reliability of handheld dynamometry. Phys Ther 67:931, 1987.

57. Kloos, A: Measurement of muscle tone and strength. Neurology Report 16:9, 1992.

58. Agre, J, et al: Strength testing with a portable dynamometer: reliability for upper and lower extremities. Arch Phys Med Rehabil 68:454, 1987.

59. Rothstein, J, et al: Clinical uses of isokinetic measurements. Phys Ther 67:1840, 1987.

60. Mawdsley, R, and Knapik, J: Comparison of isokinetic measurements with test repetitions. Phys Ther 62:169, 1982.

61. Moffroid, M, et al: A study of isokinetic exercise. Phys Ther 49:735, 1969.

62. Farrell, M, and Richards, J: Analysis of the reliability and validity of the isokinetic communicator exercise device. Med Sci Sports Exer 18:44, 1986.

63. Johnson, J, and Siegal, D: Reliability of an isokinetic movement of the knee extensors. Research Quarterly 49:88, 1978.

64. Tredinnick, T, and Duncan, P: Reliability of measurements of concentric and eccentric isokinetic loading. Phys Ther 68:656, 1988.

65. McCrory, M, et al: Reliability of concentric and eccentric measurements on the Lido Active Isokinetic Rehabilitation System. Med Sci Sports Exer 21(suppl):52, 1989.

66. Armstrong, L, et al: Using isokinetic dynamometry to test ambulatory patients with multiple sclerosis. Phys Ther 63:1274, 1983.

67. Goslin, B, and Charteris, J: Isokinetic dynamometry: Normative data for clinical use in lower extremity (knee) cases. Scand J Rehabil Med 11:105, 1979.

68. Murray, M, et al: Strength of isometric and isokinetic contractions: Knee muscles of men aged 20 to 86. Phys Ther 60:412, 1980.

69. Griffin, J, et al: Sequential isokinetic and manual muscle testing in patients with neuromuscular disease: A pilot study. Phys Ther 66:32, 1986.

70. Kozlowski, B: Reliability of isokinetic torque generation in chronic hemiplegic subjects. Phys Ther 64:714, 1984.

71. Edwards, R: Physiological analysis of skeletal muscle weakness and fatigue. Clin Sci Mol Med. 54:463, 1978.

72. Curtis, C, and Weir, J: Overview of exercise responses in healthy and impaired states. Neurology Report 20:13, 1996.

73. Wade, C, and Forstch, J: Exercise and Duchenne muscular dystrophy. Neurology Report 20:20, 1996.

74. Costello, E, et al: Exercise prescription for individuals with multiple sclerosis. Neurology Report 24:13, 1996.

75. Bassile, D: Guillain-Barre syndrome and exercise guidelines. Neuro Report 24:31, 1996.

76. McDonald, M: Exercise and postpolio syndrome. Neurology Report 24:37, 1996.

77. Bigland-Richie, B, and Woods, J: Changes in muscle contractile properties and neural control during human muscular fatigue. Muscle Nerve 7:691, 1984.

78. Borg, G: Psychophysical bases of perceived exertion. Med Sci Sports Exer 14:377, 1982.

79. Bennett, R, and Knowlton, G: Overwork weakness in partially denervated skeletal muscle. Clin Orthop 12:22, 1958.

80. Fisk, J, et al: The impact of fatigue on patients with multiple sclerosis. Le Journal Canadien Des Sciences Neurologiques 21:9, 1994.

81. Barnes, S: Isokinetic fatigue curves at different contractile velocities. Arch Phys Med Rehabil 62:66, 1981.

82. Binder-Macleod, S, and Synder-Mackler, L: Muscle fatigue: Clinical implications for fatigue assessment and neuromuscular electrical stimulation. Phys Ther 73:902, 1993.

83. McDonnell, M, et al: Electrically elicited fatigue test of the quadriceps femoris muscle. Phys Ther 67:941, 1987.

84. Shumway-Cook, A, and Woollacott, M: Motor Control Theory and Practical Application. Williams & Wilkins, Baltimore, 1995.

85. Fugl-Meyer, A: The post-stroke hemiplegic patient, I. A method for evaluation of physical performance. Scand J Rehabil Med 7:13, 1975.

86. Horak, F, et al: Postural perturbations: New insights for Treatment of Balance Disorders. Phys Ther 77:517, 1997.

87. Norkin, C, and Levangie, P: Joint Structure & Function, ed 2. FA Davis, Philadelphia, 1992.

88. Smith, L, et al: Brunnstrom's Clinical Kinesiology, ed 5. FA Davis, Philadelphia, 1996.

89. Nashner, L: Sensory, neuromuscular, and biomechanical contributions to human balance. In Duncan, P (ed): Balance. American Physical Therapy Association, Alexandria, VA, 1990, p 5.

90. Nichols, D: Balance retraining after stroke using force platform biofeedback. Phys Ther 77:553, 1997.

91. Horak, F: Clinical measurement of postural control in adults. Phys Ther 67:1881, 1987.

92. Goldie, P, et al: Force platform measures for evaluating postural control: Reliability and validity. Arch Phys Med Rehabil 70:510, 1989.

93. Liston, R, and Brouwer, B: Reliability and validity of measures obtained from stroke patients using the Balance Master. Arch Phys Med Rehabil 77:425, 1996.

94. Dettman, M, et al: Relationships among walking performance, postural stability, and functional assessments of the hemiplegic patient. Am J Phys Med 66:77, 1987.

95. Dickstein, R, et al: Foot-ground pressure pattern of standing hemiplegic patients: Major characteristics and patterns of movement. Phys Ther 64:19, 1984.

96. Shumway-Cook, A, et al: Postural sway biofeedback: Its effect on reestablishing stance stability in hemiplegic patients. Arch Phys Med Rehabil 69:395, 1988.

97. Moore, S, and Woollacott, M: The use of biofeedback devices to improve postural stability. Physical Therapy Practice 2:1, 1993.

98. Winstein, C, et al: Standing balance training effect on

balance and locomotion in hemiparetic adults. Arch Phys Med Rehabil 70:755, 1989.

99. Brandt, T, et al: Visual acuity, visual field and visual scene characteristics affect postural balance. In Igarash, M, and Black, F (eds): Vestibular and Visual Control on Posture and Locomotor Equilibrium. Karger, Basel, 1985.
100. Herdman, S: Vestibular Rehabilitation. FA Davis, Philadelphia, 1994.
101. Horak, F, et al: Postural strategies associated with somatosensory and vestibular loss. Exp Brain Res 82:167, 1990.
102. Shumway-Cook, A, and Horak, F: Assessing the influence of sensory interaction on balance: Suggestion from the field. Phys Ther 66:1548, 1986.
103. Cohen, H, et al: A study of CTSIB. Phys Ther 73:346, 1993.
104. Nashner, L: Adaptive reflexes controlling human posture. Exp Brain Res 26:59, 1976.
105. Nashner, L: A Systems Approach to Understanding and Assessing Orientation and Balance. NeuroCom International, Clackamas, OR, 1987.
106. Nashner, L, and McCollum, G: The organization of human postural movements: A formal basis and experimental synthesis. Behavioral and Brain Sciences 8:135, 1985.
107. Horak, F, and Nashner, L: Central programming of postural movements: Adaptation to altered support-surface configuration. J Neurophysiol 55:1369, 1986.
108. Nashner, L: Fixed patterns of rapid postural responses among leg muscles during stance. Exp Brain Res 30:13, 1977.
109. Maki, B, and McIlron, W: The role of limb movements in maintaining upright stance: The "change-in-support" strategy. Phys Ther 77:488, 1977.
110. Forssberg, H, and Hirschfeld, H: Postural adjustments in sitting humans following external perturbations: Muscle activity and kinematics. Exp Brain Res 97:515, 1994.
111. Lee, W, et al: Quantitative and clinical measures of static standing balance in hemiparetic and normal subjects. Phys Ther 68:970, 1988.
112. Bohannon, R, et al: Decrease in timed balance test scores with aging. Phys Ther 64:1967, 1984.
113. Berg, K, and Norman, K: Functional assessment of balance and gait. Clinics Geriatr Med 12:705, 1996.
114. Duncan, P, et al: Functional reach: A new clinical measure of balance. J Gerontol 85:529, 1990.
115. Weiner, D, et al: Functional reach: A marker of physical frailty. J Am Geriatr Soc 40:203, 1992.
116. Weiner, D, et al: Does functional reach improve with rehabilitation? Arch Phys Med Rehabil 74:796, 1991.
117. Duncan, P, et al: Functional reach: Predictive validity in a sample of elderly male veterans. J Gerontol 47:M93, 1992.
118. Berg, K, et al: Measuring balance in the elderly: Preliminary development of an instrument. Physiotherapy Canada 41:304, 1989.
119. Berg, K, et al: A comparison of clinical and laboratory measures of postural balance in an elderly population. Arch Phys Med Rehabil 73:1073, 1992.
120. Berg, K, et al: Measuring balance in the elderly: Validation of an instrument. Can J Public Health 83(suppl 2):S7, 1992.
121. Berg, K, et al: The Balance Scale: Reliability assessment for elderly residents and patients with an acute stroke. Scand J Rehabil Med 27:27, 1995.
122. Harada, N, et al: Physical therapy to improve functioning of older people in residential care facilities. Phys Ther 75:830, 1995.

123. Tinetti, M: Performance-oriented assessment of mobility problems in elderly patients. J Am Geriatr Soc 34:119, 1986.
124. Tinetti, M, et al: A fall risk index for elderly patients based on number of chronic disabilities. Am J Med 80:429, 1986.
125. Tinetti, M: Factors associated with serious injury during falls by ambulatory nursing home residents. J Am Geriatr Soc 35:644, 1987.
126. Tinetti, M, et al: Risk factors for falls among elderly persons living in the community. N Engl J Med 319:1701, 1988.
127. Tinetti, M, et al: Yale FISCIT: Risk factor abatement strategy for fall prevention. J Am Geriatr Soc 41:315, 1993.
128. Mathias, S, et al: Balance in elderly patients: The "Get-up and go" test. Arch Phys Med Rehabil 67:387, 1986.
129. Podsiadlo, D, and Richardson, S: The timed "Up and Go": A test of basic mobility for frail elderly persons. J Am Geriatr Soc 39:142, 1991.
130. Murray, M, et al: Comparison of free and fast speed walking patterns of normal men. Am J Phys Med 45:8, 1966.
131. Imms, F, and Edholm, O: Studies of gait and mobility in the elderly. Age Ageing 10:147, 1981.
132. Guralnick, J, et al: Lower-extremity function over the age of 70 years as a predictor of subsequent disability. N Engl J Med 332:556, 1995.
133. Wolfson, L, et al: Gait assessment in the elderly: A gait abnormality rating scale and its relation to falls. J Gerontol 45:M12, 1990.
134. Shumway-Cook, A: Reducing the risk for falls in the elderly. Boston, APTA Combined Sections Meeting, 1998.
135. Abernethy, B: Dual-task methodology and motor skills research: Some applications and methodological constraints. J of Human Movement Studies 14:101, 1988.
136. VanSant, A: Life span development in functional tasks. Phys Ther 70:788, 1990.
137. Shenkman, M, et al: Whole-body movements during rising to standing from sitting. Phys Ther 70:638, 1990.
138. VanSant, A: Rising from a supine position to erect stance: Description of adult movement and a developmental hypothesis. Phys Ther 68:185, 1988.
139. Green, L, and Williams, K: Differences in developmental movement patterns used by active vs sedentary middle-aged adults coming from a supine position to erect stance. Phys Ther 72:560, 1992.
140. Richter, R, et al: Description of adult rolling movements and hypothesis of developmental sequences. Phys Ther 69:63, 1989.
141. Gentile, A: Skill acquisition: Action, movement and neuromotor processes. In Carr, J, et al (eds): Movement Science: Foundations for Physical Therapy in Rehabilitation. Aspen, Rockville, MD, 1987, p. 93.
142. Pink, M: High speed video applications in physical therapy. Clinical Management 5:14, 1985.
143. Turnbull, G, and Wall, J: The development of a system for the clinical assessment of gait following stroke. Physiotherapy 71:294, 1985.
144. Lewis, A: Documentation of movement patterns used in the performance of functional tasks. Neurology Report 16:13, 1992.
145. Ackerman, P: Individual differences in skill learning: An integration of psychometric and information processing perspectives. Psychological Bulletin 102:3, 1988.
146. Fitts, P, and Posner, M: Human Performance. Brooks/Cole, Belmont, CA, 1969.

SUPPLEMENTAL READINGS

American Physical Therapy Association. Guide to Physical Therapist Practice. APTA, Alexandria, VA, 1997.
Gilman, S (ed): Clinical Examination of the Nervous System. McGraw-Hill, New York, 2000.
Magill, R: Motor Learning Concepts and Applications, ed 4. WCB Brown & Benchmark, Madison, 1993.
Nolan, M: Introduction to the Neurological Examination. FA Davis, Philadelphia, 1996.

Schmidt, R, and Lee, T: Motor Control and Learning, ed 3. Human Kinetics, Champaign, IL, 1999.
Shumway-Cook, A, and Woollacott, M: Motor Control Theory and Practical Application. Williams & Wilkins, Baltimore, 1995.
Strub, R, and Black, F: The Mental Status Examination in Neurology, ed 3. FA Davis, Philadelphia, 1993.

GLOSSARY

Amnesia: Loss of memory.

    Anterograde amnesia: Amnesia for events that occurred after a precipitating trauma.

    Retrograde amnesia: Amnesia for events that occurred before the precipitating trauma.

Arousal: Internal state of alertness or excitement.

Attention: Capacity of the brain to process information from the environment or from long-term memory.

    Selective attention: Ability to screen and process relevant sensory information about both the task and the environment while screening out irrelevant information.

Babinski sign: Dorsiflexion of the great toe with fanning of the other toes on stimulation of the lateral sole of the foot.

Caloric testing: A procedure used to assess vestibular function. With the patient supine, each ear is irrigated with warm (44°C) water for 30 sec., followed by irrigation with cold (30°C) water. Warm water elicits rotatory nystagmus to the side being irrigated; cold water produces the opposite reaction.

Cerebral shock: Transient hypotonia following injury to the brain.

Chaddock sign: Dorsiflexion of the big toe elicited by stroking around the lateral ankle and up the lateral aspect of the foot.

Clasp-knife response: A sudden relaxation or letting go of a spastic muscle in response to a stretch stimulus.

Clonus: Cyclical, spasmodic alteration of muscular contraction and relaxation in response to a sustained stretch of a spastic muscle.

Closed-loop system: A control system employing feedback as a reference for correctness, commutation of error, and subsequent correction in order to maintain a desired state.

Coma: A state of unconsciousness or abnormal deep stupor, occurring as a result of illness or injury; the patient cannot be aroused by external stimuli.

Consciousness: A state of awareness; implies orientation to person, place, and time.

Controlled mobility (dynamic postural control): The ability to maintain postural control during weight shifting and movement.

Coordination: The patterning of body and limb motions relative to the patterning of environmental objects and events.

Coordinative structures: Functionally specific units of muscles and joints that are constrained by the nervous system to act cooperatively to produce an action.

Decerebrate rigidity: Sustained contraction and posturing of the trunk and limbs in a position of full extension; results from a lesion in the brainstem between the superior colliculi and vestibular nucleus.

Decorticate rigidity: Sustained contraction and posturing of the trunk and lower limbs in extension, and the upper limbs in flexion; results from a lesion at the level of the diencephalon (above the superior colliculus).

Degrees of freedom: The number of separate independent dimensions of movement that must be controlled.

Dystonia: A hyperkinetic movement disorder characterized by impaired or disordered tone, accompanied by repetitive involuntary movements; typically twisting or writhing motions.

Dystonic posturing: Sustained abnormal postures caused by cocontraction of agonist and antagonist muscles; may last for several minutes or permanently.

Exhaustion: The limit of endurance, beyond which no further performance is possible.

Fatigue: The failure to generate the required or expected force during sustained or repeated contractions.

    Fatigue threshold: That level of exercise that cannot be sustained indefinitely.

Feedback: Response-produced information received during or after the movement used to monitor output for corrective actions.

Feedforward: The sending of signals in advance of movement to ready the sensorimotor systems and allow for anticipatory adjustments in postural activity.

Fight or flight response (alarm or stress response): Defensive responses initiated by discharge by large portions of the sympathetic nervous system (mass discharge) to protect the individual under varying circumstances.

Flaccidity: Absence of muscle tone.

Generalizability: The extent to which practice on one task contributes to the performance of other, related skills.

Hypertonia: State of increased tone above normal resting levels.

Hypotonia: State of decreased tone below normal resting levels.

Inverted-U theory (Yerkes-Dodson law): There is an optimal level of arousal for performance; too much or too little arousal can cause marked deterioration in performance.

Lethargy: A state of general slowing of motor responses, including speech and movement.

Limits of stability (LOS): The maximum angle from vertical that can be tolerated without a loss of balance.

    COM alignment: The midpoint of LOS.

Lower motor neuron (LMN) lesions: Lesions affecting the anterior horn cell or peripheral nerve produce decreased or absent tone along with associated symptoms of paralysis, muscle fasciculations and fibrillations with denervation, and neurogenic atrophy.

Memory: The mental registration, retention, and recall of past experience, knowledge, and ideas.

Declarative memory: The conscious recollection of facts and events (explicit memory).

Nondeclarative memory (motor memory): The recall of skills and procedures (nonconscious or implicit memory).

Mobility: Initial movement in a functional pattern; range of motion is available for movement to occur and there is sufficient motor unit activity to initiate muscle contraction.

Motor learning: a set of internal processes associated with practice or experience leading to relatively permanent changes in the capability for skilled behavior.

Motor program: A set of commands that, when initiated, results in the production of a coordinated movement sequence.

Motor plan: An idea or plan for purposeful movement that is made up of several component motor programs.

Muscle performance: The capacity of a muscle to do work (force × distance).

Muscle power: Work produced per unit of time or the product of strength and speed.

Muscle endurance: The ability to contract the muscle repeatedly over a period of time.

Obtunded: Dulled or blunted sensitivity.

Opisthotonus: Strong and sustained contraction of the extensor muscles of the neck and trunk.

Overwork weakness (injury): A prolonged decrease in absolute strength and endurance due to excessive activity of partially denervated muscle.

Postural orientation: The control of relative positions of body parts by skeletal muscles, with respect to gravity and to each other.

Postural stability (equilibrium): The condition in which all the forces acting on the body are balanced such that the center of mass (COM) is within stability limits, the boundaries of the base of support (BOS).

Adaptive control: Control that allows the individual to appropriately modify the sensorimotor systems in response to changing task and environmental demands.

Proactive (anticipatory) control: Control that occurs in anticipation of internally generated, destabilizing forces imposed on the body's own movements.

Reactive control: Control that occurs in response to external forces displacing the COM or movement of the BOS.

Reaction: An involuntary movement response to a stimulus.

Resistance to contextual change: The adaptability required to perform a motor task in altered environmental situations.

Retention test: A performance test administered after a period of no practice (retention interval) for the purposes of assessing learning.

Rigidity: Stiffness; inability to bend or be bent.

Cogwheel rigidity: A rachetlike response to passive movement characterized by an alternate giving and increased resistance to movement; seen in disorders of the basal ganglia.

Leadpipe rigidity: A constant resistance to movement; seen in disorders of the basal ganglia.

Romberg test: An assessment of the role of vision in balance control; standing balance is assessed first with eyes open, then eyes closed.

Skill: Highly coordinated movement that allows for investigation and interaction with the physical and social environment.

Closed skill: Motor skill performed in a stable, nonchanging environment.

Open skill: Motor skill performed in a variable, changing environment.

Somatosensation: Sensory information received from the skin and musculoskeletal systems.

Spasticity: Increased tone or resistance of muscle causing stiff awkward movements; the result of an upper motor neuron lesion.

Spinal shock: Transient hypotonia following injury to the spinal cord.

Stability (static postural control): The ability to maintain a steady position in a weight bearing, antigravity posture.

Static-dynamic control: The ability to shift weight onto support segments, freeing up a limb for dynamic activities.

Stupor: A state of semiconsciousness.

Synergy: Normal association of functionally linked muscles to produce coordinated movement.

Abnormal synergy: An obligatory, highly stereotyped mass pattern of movement.

Tone (muscle): The resistance of muscles to passive elongation or stretch.

Upper motor neuron (UMN) syndrome: Motor dysfunction observed in patients with lesions of the corticospinal or pyramidal tract in the brain or spinal cord. Characterized by spasticity, abnormal reflex behaviors, loss of precise autonomic control, impaired muscle activation, paresis, decreased dexterity, and fatigability.

Vegetative state: A continuing and unremitting condition of complete unawareness of self and the environment, accompanied by sleep-wake cycles with preservation of hypothalamic and brainstem autonomic functions.

Persistent vegetative state: A vegetative state with a duration of 1 year or more, the result of severe brain injury or diffuse cerebral hypoxia.

Visual proprioception: Detection of the relative orientation of the body parts and orientation of the body with reference to the environment by the visual system; provides a basis for movement control.

APPENDIX A

Berg Balance Scale

1. Sitting to standing

INSTRUCTIONS: *Please stand up, try not to* use *your* hands *for support.*

( ) 4 able to stand without using hands and stabilizes independently
( ) 3 able to stand independently using hands
( ) 2 able to stand using hands after several tries
( ) 1 needs minimal aid to stand or stabilize
( ) 0 needs moderate or maximal assist to stand

2. Standing unsupported

INSTRUCTIONS: *Please stand for 2 minutes without holding.*

( ) 4 able to stand safely 2 minutes
( ) 3 able to stand 2 minutes with supervision
( ) 2 able to stand 30 seconds unsupported
( ) 1 needs several tries to stand unsupported 30 seconds
( ) 0 unable to stand 30 seconds without support

3. Sitting with back unsupported but feet supported on floor or on a stool

INSTRUCTIONS: *Please sit with arms folded for 2 minutes.*

( ) 4 able to sit safely and securely 2 minutes
( ) 3 able to sit 2 minutes with supervision
( ) 2 able to sit 30 seconds
( ) 1 able to sit 10 seconds
( ) 0 unable to sit without support 10 seconds

4. Standing to sit

INSTRUCTIONS: *Please sit down.*

( ) 4 sits safely with minimal use of hands
( ) 3 controls descent by using hands
( ) 2 uses back of legs against chair to control descent
( ) 1 sits independently, but has uncontrolled descent
( ) 0 needs assistance to sit

5. Transfers

INSTRUCTIONS: *Arrange chairs for a pivot transfer. Ask the patient to transfer one way toward a seat without armrests and one way toward a seat with arms. You may use two chairs or a bed/mat and a chair.*

( ) 4 able to transfer safely with minor use of hands
( ) 3 able to transfer safely with definite need of hands
( ) 2 able to transfer with verbal cuing and/or supervision
( ) 1 needs one person to assist
( ) 0 needs two people to assist or supervise to be safe

6. Standing unsupported with eyes closed

INSTRUCTIONS: *Please close your eyes and stand still for 10 seconds.*

( ) 4 able to stand 10 seconds safely
( ) 3 able to stand 10 seconds with supervision
( ) 2 able to stand 3 seconds
( ) 1 unable to keep eyes closed for 3 seconds but stands safely
( ) 0 needs help to keep from falling

7. Standing unsupported with feet together

INSTRUCTIONS: *Place your feet together and stand without holding.*

( ) 4 able to place feet together independently and stand safely 1 minute
( ) 3 able to place feet together independently and stand with supervision for 1 minute
( ) 2 able to place feet together independently but unable to hold for 30 seconds
( ) 1 needs help to assume the position but can stand for 15 seconds, feet together
( ) 0 needs help to assume the position and unable to stand for 15 seconds

8. Reaching forward with outstretched arm while standing

INSTRUCTIONS: *Lift arm to 90°. Stretch out your fingers and reach forward as far as you can. (Clinician places a ruler at the tips of the outstretched fingers—subject should not touch the ruler when reaching.) Distance recorded is from the fingertips with the subject in the most forward position. The subject should use both hands when possible to avoid trunk rotation.*

( ) 4 can reach forward confidently 20–30 cm (10 inches)
( ) 3 can reach forward safely 12 cm (5 inches)
( ) 2 can reach forward safely 5 cm (2 inches)
( ) 1 reaches forward but needs supervision
( ) 0 loses balance when trying, requires external support

9. Pick up object from the floor from a standing position

INSTRUCTIONS: *Pick up the shoe slipper which is placed in front of your feet.*

( ) 4 able to pick up the slipper safely and easily
( ) 3 able to pick up the slipper but needs supervision
( ) 2 unable to pick up the slipper, but reaches 2–5 cm (1–2 inches) from the slipper and keeps balance independently
( ) 1 unable to pick up and needs supervision while trying
( ) 0 unable to try/needs assistance to keep from losing balance/falling

Continued

10. Turning to look behind over your left and right shoulders while standing

INSTRUCTIONS: *Turn and look directly behind you over toward the left shoulder. Repeat to the right. Examiner may pick an object to look at directly behind the subject to encourage a better twist.*

( ) 4 looks behind from both sides and weight shifts well

( ) 3 looks behind one side only, other side shows less weight shift

( ) 2 turns sideways only but maintains balance

( ) 1 needs close supervision or verbal cuing

( ) 0 needs assistance while turning

11. Turn 360 degrees

INSTRUCTIONS: *Turn completely around in a full circle, pause, then turn a full circle in the other direction.*

( ) 4 able to turn 360 degrees safely in 4 seconds or less

( ) 3 able to turn 360 degrees safely, one side only, 4 seconds or less

( ) 2 able to turn 360 degrees safely, but slowly

( ) 1 needs close supervision or verbal cuing

( ) 0 needs assistance while turning

12. Place alternate foot on step or stool while standing unsupported

INSTRUCTIONS: *Place each foot alternately on the step stool. Continue until each foot has touched the step stool 4 times.*

( ) 4 able to stand independently and safely and complete 8 steps in 20 seconds

( ) 3 able to stand independently and complete 8 steps >20 seconds

( ) 2 able to complete 4 steps without aid with supervision

( ) 1 able to complete >2 steps needs minimal assistance

( ) 0 needs assistance to keep from falling/unable to try

13. Standing unsupported one foot in front

INSTRUCTIONS: *(Demonstrate to subject). Place one foot directly in front of the other. If you feel that you cannot place your foot directly in front, try and step far enough ahead that the heel of your forward foot is ahead of the toes of your other foot. (To score three points, the length of the step should exceed the length of the other foot and the width of the stance should approximate the subject's normal stance width.)*

( ) 4 able to place foot tandem independently and hold 30 seconds

( ) 3 able to place foot ahead of the other independently and hold 30 seconds

( ) 2 able to take a small step independently and hold 30 seconds

( ) 1 needs help to step but can hold 15 seconds

( ) 0 loses balance while stepping or standing

14. Standing on one leg

INSTRUCTIONS: *Stand on one leg as long as you can without holding*

( ) 4 able to lift leg independently and hold >10 seconds

( ) 3 able to lift leg independently and hold 5–10 seconds

( ) 2 able to lift leg independently and hold = or >2 seconds

( ) 1 tries to lift leg unable to hold 3 seconds but remains standing independently

( ) 0 unable to try or needs assistance to prevent fall

_____ TOTAL SCORE (Maximum = 56)

APPENDIX B

Performance-Oriented Assessment of Mobility I—POMA I (Tinetti)

Balance

INSTRUCTIONS: Subject is seated in hard armless chair. The following maneuvers are tested.

1. Sitting balance
0 = leans or slides in chair
1 = leans in chair slightly or slight increased distance from buttocks to back of chair
2 = steady, safe, upright

2. Arising
0 = unable without help or loses balance
1 = *able* but uses arm to help or requires more than two attempts *or* excessive forward flexion
2 = *able* without use of arms in one attempt

3. Immediate standing balance (first five seconds)
0 = unsteady marked staggering, moves feet, marked trunk sway or grabs object for support
1 = steady but uses walker or cane *or* mild staggering but catches self without grabbing object
2 = steady without walker or cane or other support

4. Side-by-side standing balance
0 = unsteady
1 = unsteady, but wide stance (medial heels more than 4 inches apart) or uses cane, walker or other support
2 = narrow stance without support

5. Pull test (subject at maximum position as above, examiner stands behind and exerts mild pull back at wrist)
0 = begins to fall
1 = staggers, grabs, but catches self
2 = steady

6. Turn 360°
0 = unsteady (grabs, staggers)
1 = steady but steps discontinuous
2 = steady and steps continuous

7. Able to stand on one leg for 5 seconds (pick one leg)
0 = unable or holds onto any object
1 = some staggering, swaying or moves foot slightly
2 = able

8. Tandem stand
0 = unable to stand with one foot in front of other or begins to fall

1 = some staggering, swaying, moves arms, or moves foot slightly
2 = able to tandem stand × five seconds

9. Reaching up—Examiner holds 5-pound weight at height of subject's fully extended reach
0 = unable or holds onto any object
1 = some staggering, swaying or moves foot slightly
2 = able

10. Bending over (place 5-pound weight on floor and ask subject to pick it up)
0 = unable or is unsteady
1 = able and is steady

10a. Time required _____ seconds

11. Sit down
0 = unsafe (misjudged distance; falls into chair)
1 = uses arms or not a smooth motion
2 = safe, smooth motion

11a. Timed rising
Time required to rise from chair three times _____ seconds

Gait

INSTRUCTIONS: Subject stands with examiner. Walks down 15 foot walkway (measured). Ask subject to walk down walkway, turn and walk back. Subject should use customary walking aid.

1. Initiation of gait (immediately after told to "go")
0 = any hesitancy or multiple attempts to start
1 = no hesitancy

2. Path (estimated in relation to line on floor or rug). Observe excursion of one foot over middle 10 feet of course.
0 = marked deviation
1 = mild/moderate deviation *or* uses walking aid
2 = straight without walking aid

3. Missed step (trip or loss of balance)
0 = yes and inappropriate attempt to recover balance
1 = yes, but appropriate attempt to recover
2 = no

4. Turning (while walking)
0 = staggers, unsteady
1 = discontinuous, but no staggering, or uses walker or cane
2 = steady, continuous without walking aid

Continued

5. Timed walk performed after 1–7 complete (measure out 15 foot walkway)
   a) Ask subject to walk at normal pace _____ seconds
   b) Ask subject to walk as "fast as feels safe" _____ seconds

6. Step over obstacle (to be assessed in a separate walk with a block placed on course)
   0 = begins to fall or unable
   1 = able but uses walking aid or some staggering but catches self
   2 = able and steady

APPENDIX C

Suggested Answers to Case Study Guiding Questions

Based on your evaluation of the data presented in the case history and the physical therapy examination, answer the following questions.

1. Categorize her level of consciousness upon admission to the long-term care facility using the Glasgow Coma Scale.

ANSWER: The eye opening response is a 3; the best motor response is a 4; the verbal response is a 4. The total score on the Glasgow Coma Scale is 11, indicating this patient is out of coma and exhibits moderate head injury.

2. Categorize the problems in terms of:

Direct impairments
ANSWER: Impaired cognition:
   pronounced deficits in attention, concentration
   short-term/anterograde memory deficits
   confusion
   pronounced learning deficits
autonomic instability (agitation when tired)
impaired sensory discrimination (stereognosis)
increased tone:
   RUE and RLE (Modified Ashworth grade 3)
   LUE and LLE (Modified Ashworth grade 2)
   hyperactive DTRs, bilateral ankle clonus
   abnormal synergistic movements RUE and RLE
   abnormal posturing sitting and standing

Indirect impairments
ANSWER: decreased PROM RUE and RLE

Composite impairments
ANSWER: decreased muscle strength
decreased dynamic balance in sitting
decreased static and dynamic balance control in standing

Functional limitations
ANSWER: Impaired functional mobility skills:

rolling: supervision/min assist to R; max assist to L
supine-to-sit transitions: min assist
stand-pivot transfers: min assist
gait: max assist × 2
wheelchair propulsion: supervision

3. Prioritize the problems in terms of possible functional goals and outcomes.

ANSWER: Highly prioritized problems include the limitations in functional mobility skills, including bed mobility (rolling, supine-to-sit), transfers, and wheelchair management. Physical impairments that are directly linked to these functional limitations include deficits in ROM, strength, postural alignment, and balance. Based on her current status (4 months post injury), it is not likely that she will become an independent ambulator. However, assisted ambulation can be promoted for physiological and motivational reasons. Cognitive deficits will directly impact on overall rehabilitation outcomes and on the amount of learning possible. Frequent reexaminations of cognitive and physical function will be needed to document recovery, treatment effectiveness, and the presence of expanding multisystem involvement (emerging indirect impairments). Frequent reexaminations will also be necessary to determine prognosis and final discharge placement. A review of the findings in this case indicates referral to occupational therapy and speech-language pathology is indicated.

4. Determine the physical therapy diagnosis using the preferred practice pattern identified by the Guide to Physical Therapist Practice.

ANSWER: Patients/clients with traumatic brain injury fall under the category Impaired Motor Function and Sensory Integrity Associated with Acquired Nonprogressive Disorders of the Central Nervous System. Clinical indications, anticipated goals, and specific direct interventions are outlined.[5]

Electromyography and Nerve Conduction Velocity Tests

9

Leslie G. Portney
Serge H. Roy

LEARNING OBJECTIVES

1. Describe the instrumentation system used to record EMG signal data for clinical and kinesiologic uses.
2. Describe the general methodology used to perform an EMG and nerve conduction velocity (NCV) examination.
3. Describe the characteristics of normal and abnormal EMG potentials.
4. Describe the EMG signal and NCV findings typically seen with neuromuscular disorders.
5. Discuss the implications of clinical EMG signal findings for goal setting and treatment planning in rehabilitation.
6. Discuss the relationship between the EMG signal EMG and force with different types of contractions.
7. Discuss procedural, technical, and physiological considerations for interpreting clinical and kinesiologic EMG data.
8. Describe the uses of kinesiologic EMG for evaluation of movement.
9. Using the case study example, apply clinical decision making skills in evaluating EMG assessment data.

Luigi Galvani presented the first report on electrical properties of muscles and nerves in 1791.[1] He demonstrated that muscle activity followed stimulation of neurons and recorded potentials from muscle fibers in states of voluntary contraction in frogs. This information was disregarded for close to a century because conflicting theories were accepted and did not become part of medical technology until the early part of this century, when instrumentation was developed to make recording such activity reliable and valid. Today, the electromyographic signal, or electromyogram (EMG), is used to evaluate the scope of neuromuscular disease or trauma, and as a kinesiologic tool to study muscle function.

As an assessment procedure, clinical **electromyography** involves the detection and recording of electrical potentials from skeletal muscle fibers. **Nerve conduction velocity (NCV)** tests determine the speed with which a peripheral motor or sensory nerve conducts an impulse. Together with other clinical assessments, these two electrodiagnostic procedures can provide information about the extent of nerve injury or muscle disease, and the prognosis for surgical intervention and rehabilitation. These data can be valuable for diagnosis and determination of rehabilitation goals for patients with musculoskeletal and neuromuscular disorders.

Kinesiologic EMG is used to study muscle activity and establish the role of various muscles in specific activities. Although the concepts are the same, the focus of kinesiologic EMG is quite different from that of clinical EMG in terms of instrumentation requirements and data analysis techniques. Basmajian and De Luca[2] have provided a thorough review of literature in this area. Selective topics in the use of surface EMG in the occupational setting are available in the literature as well.[3]

CONCEPTS OF ELECTROMYOGRAPHY

Electromyography is, in essence, the study of motor unit activity. Motor units are composed of one anterior horn cell, one axon, its neuromuscular junctions, and all the muscle fibers innervated by that axon (Fig. 9-1). The single axon conducts an impulse to all its muscle fibers, causing them to depolarize at relatively the same time. This depolarization produces electrical activity that is manifested as a **motor unit action potential** (MUAP) and recorded graphically as the EMG. Recording the EMG requires a three-phase system: an input phase that includes electrodes to pick up electrical potentials from contracting muscle; a processor phase, during which the small electrical signal is amplified; and an output phase, in which the electrical signal is converted to visual and/or audible signals so that the data can be displayed and analyzed (Fig. 9-2).

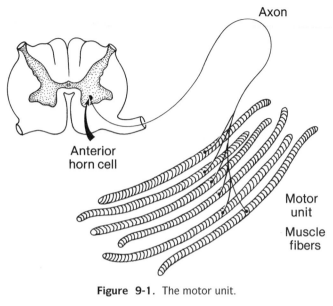

Figure 9-1. The motor unit.

Instrumentation

DETECTING THE EMG SIGNAL: ELECTRODES

An **electrode** is a transducer, a device for converting one form of energy into another. Several types of electrodes can be used to monitor the myoelectric signal. **Surface electrodes** are used to test NCV and in kinesiologic investigations. They are generally considered adequate for monitoring large superficial muscles or muscle groups. They are not considered selective enough to record activity accurately from an individual **motor unit** or from specific small or deep muscles, unless special recording procedures using multielectrode arrays and spatial filtering techniques are utilized.[4,5] **Fine-wire indwelling electrodes** can be used for kinesiologic study of small and deep muscles. Needle electrodes are necessary to record single motor unit potentials for clinical EMG.

In addition to a **recording electrode** (either surface or needle), a **ground electrode** must be applied to provide a mechanism for canceling out the interference effect of external electrical noise such as that caused by fluorescent lights, broadcasting facilities, elevators, and other electrical apparatus. The ground electrode is a surface electrode that is attached to the skin near the recording electrodes, but usually not over muscle.

Surface electrodes are applied to the skin overlying the appropriate muscle (Fig. 9-3). The sensor is configured either as a small metal disc, commonly made of silver/silver chloride, or as a bipolar **active electrode** of fixed interelectrode geometry with preamplifiers at the detection site (Fig. 9-4). Silver/silver chloride electrodes are typically 3 to 5 millimeters (mm) in diameter (effective surface area), and are often contained within a casing that can be affixed to the surface of the skin with adhesive collars or tape. In a bipolar arrangement, two electrodes are placed over one muscle, usually over

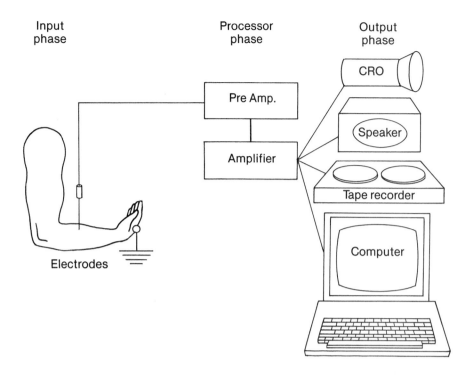

Figure 9-2. The EMG recording system.

the belly, in a longitudinal direction parallel to the muscle fibers. Electrode gel is applied beneath surface electrodes to facilitate the conduction of electrical potentials. Often, some skin preparation is necessary to reduce **skin resistance,** which can interfere with the quality of recording. This may include washing, rubbing with alcohol, and abrading the superficial skin layer to remove dead, dry skin cells. Active electrodes, developed in response to this inconvenience, do not require skin preparation.[6]

Fine-wire indwelling electrodes were introduced in the early 1960s for kinesiologic study of small and deep muscles.[7] The electrodes are made with two strands of small-diameter wire (approximately 100 µm). These are coated with a polyurethane or nylon insulation and threaded through a hypodermic needle. The tips of the wires are bared for 1 to 2 mm and bent back against the needle shaft (Fig. 9-5). The needle is inserted into the muscle belly and immediately withdrawn, leaving the wires embedded in the muscle. Because of the small diameter of these wires, which are as thin as a hair, subjects cannot feel the presence of the wires in the muscle. The wires form a bipolar electrode configuration that can record from a localized area and are capable of picking up single motor unit potentials. Fine-wire electrodes are necessary for monitoring

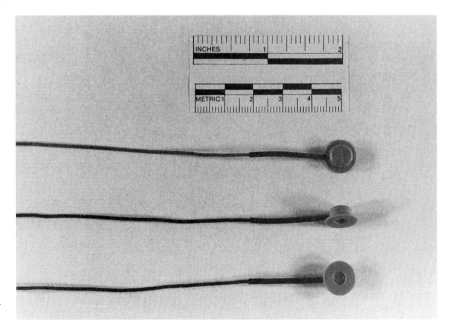

Figure 9-3. Silver-silver chloride surface electrodes.

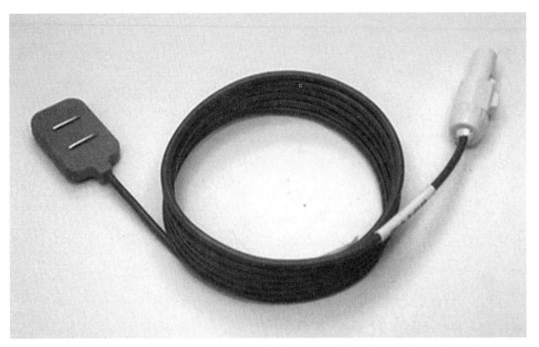

Figure 9-4. Active electrode, composed of two parallel bars, each 1.0 cm long, 1.0 mm wide, and spaced 1.0 cm apart. The housing contains a preamplifier at the detection site, reducing cable noise and eliminating the need for skin preparation. (Courtesy of DelSys, Inc.)

activity from deep muscles, such as the soleus, or small or narrow muscles, such as the finger flexors. They may not be as useful for larger muscles because they sample motor unit activity from such a small area of the muscle.

A needle electrode is required for clinical EMG, so that single motor unit potentials can be recorded from different parts of a muscle. The first studies of motor unit activity were done in 1929 by Adrian and Bronk,[8] who used a **concentric (coaxial) needle electrode.** This type of electrode consists of a stainless steel cannula, similar to a hypodermic needle, through which a single wire of platinum or silver is threaded (Fig. 9-6A). The cannula shaft and wire are insulated from each other, and only their tips are exposed. The wire and the needle cannula act as electrodes, and the difference in potential between them is recorded. A *bipolar concentric needle electrode* can also be used, with two wires threaded through the cannula (Fig. 9-6B). The bared tips of both wires act as the two electrodes, and the needle serves as the ground.

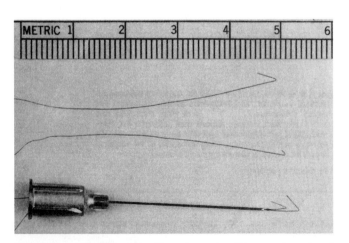

Figure 9-5. Fine-wire indwelling electrode: 27-gauge hypodermic needle through which two strands of polyurethane-coated wire are threaded. Insulation is removed from the tips of the wires, and hooks are created to keep the wires imbedded while the needle is removed from the muscle. (From Soderberg, GL, and Cook, TM: Electromyography in biomechanics. Phys Ther 64:1814, 1984, with permission.)

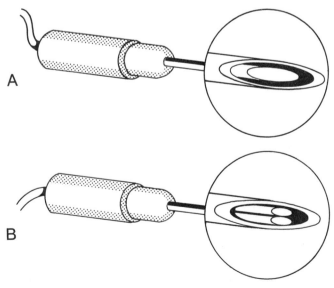

Figure 9-6. Concentric needle electrodes, showing single (A) and bipolar (B) wire configurations.

Another commonly used approach for clinical EMG involves the use of a **monopolar needle electrode,** which is composed of a single fine needle, insulated except at the tip. A second surface electrode placed on the skin near the site of insertion serves as the **reference electrode.** These electrodes are less painful than concentric electrodes because they are much smaller in diameter. Because monopolar configurations record much larger potentials than bipolar, the type of electrode must be specified to avoid misinterpretation of data relative to the size of potentials and the area of pickup. Clinical EMG can also be used to record from single muscle fibers. *Single-fiber needle electrodes* are concentric, but have wires 25 micrometers (µm) in diameter (as compared to 0.1 mm for standard concentric electrode wires).

Needle electrodes are not useful for kinesiologic study because of the discomfort caused by the needle remaining in the muscle during contraction. Fine-wire electrodes are inappropriate for use in clinical EMG because the examiner has neither good control over placement of the electrode, nor the ability to move the electrode within the muscle once it is placed. Ultrasound imaging has recently been used with great success in helping to guide the placement of fine-wire electrodes in deeply situated muscles, such as the iliopsoas.[9] Guidelines for insertion of electrodes have been published[10,11] and anatomical references should always be consulted to assure accurate and safe placement when using needles. Because they pierce the skin, all needle and fine-wire electrodes must be sterilized.

THE MYOELECTRIC SIGNAL

EMG electrodes convert the bioelectric signal resulting from muscle or nerve depolarization into an electrical potential capable of being processed by an **amplifier.** It is the difference in electrical potential between the two recording electrodes that is processed.

The unit of measurement for difference of potential is the **volt** (V). The **amplitude,** or height, of potentials is usually measured in microvolts (1 µV = 10^{-6} V). The greater the difference in potential seen by the electrodes, the greater the amplitude, or voltage, of the electrical potential. The amplitude of a MUAP is usually measured from peak to peak (i.e., from the highest to the lowest point). The **duration** of the potential is a measure of time from onset to cessation of the electrical potential. Typical peak-to-peak ranges for MUAP amplitude are 5 microvolts to 5 µV; their duration varies from 2 to 14 milliseconds.[2]

The Motor Unit Action Potential (MUAP)

It is of interest to analyze the process by which a MUAP is transmitted to an amplifier in order to understand how such potentials can be interpreted. Because of the dispersion of the fibers in a single motor unit, the muscle fibers from several motor units may be interspersed with one another (Fig. 9-7). Therefore, when one motor unit contracts, the

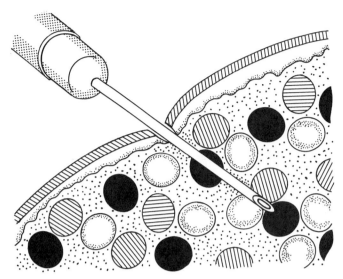

Figure 9-7. Cross-sectional view of muscle belly with needle electrode inserted. Differently shaded fibers represent different motor units.

depolarizing fibers are not necessarily close together. Consequently, a needle or surface electrode cannot be situated precisely within or over any one motor unit.

All the fibers of a single motor unit contract almost synchronously, and the electrical potentials arising from them travel through body fluids as a result of the excellent conducting properties of the electrolytes surrounding the fibers. This process is called **volume conduction.** The electrical activity will flow through the conducting medium, the *volume conductor,* in all directions, not just in the direction of the inserted needle electrode or the surface electrodes on the skin. Fibrous tissue, fat, and blood vessels act as insulation against the flow. Therefore, the actual pattern of the flow of electrical activity within the volume conductor is not predictable. The signals that do reach the electrode are transmitted to the amplifier. All others are simply not recorded, although they are present. The activities produced by all the individual fibers contracting at any one time are summated since they reach the electrode almost simultaneously. Electrodes only record potentials they pick up, without differentiating their origin. Therefore, if two motor units contract at the same time, from the same or adjacent muscles, the activity from fibers of both units will be summated and recorded as one large potential.

Myoelectric signals recorded from a multi-electrode array as a function of time (Fig. 9-8) demonstrate that the EMG signal is generated from the point of innervation of the muscle and propagates in opposing directions until it dies at the tendonous zones of the muscle fibers. Although still in an early state of development, Fig. 9-8 demonstrates how this technique can be used clinically as a means of estimating muscle fiber conduction velocity, locating the innervation and tendonous zones, and noninvasively identifying individual MUAPs.[4,5,12,13]

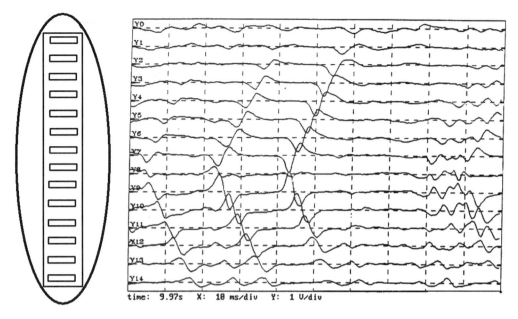

Figure 9-8. Illustration of recording from a multi-electrode array demonstrating the propagation of the motor unit action potential during a voluntary isometric contraction of the biceps brachii sustained at constant force. The drawing on the left illustrates how the array was positioned on the surface over the muscle. Each EMG channel (numbered Y0 to Y14) is a differential recording from two consecutive parallel detection "bars" or electrodes. The EMG data indicate the presence of an innervation zone at channel Y8 and tendonous zones at approximately Y1 (proximal) and Y13 (distal). The time delay between successive EMG waveforms represents the conduction velocity of the EMG signal.

Variables That Affect the MUAP

What variables, then, influence how much electrical activity is seen by the electrodes, and consequently, the amplitude and shape of the recorded potential? First, the proximity of the electrodes to the fibers that are firing will affect the amplitude and duration of the recorded potential. Fibers that are further away will contribute less to the recorded potential. Second, the number and size of the fibers in the motor unit will influence the potential's size. A larger motor unit will produce more activity. Third, the distance between the fibers will affect the output, because if the fibers are very spread out, less of their total activity is likely to reach the electrodes. The size of the electrodes may also be a consideration. If the recording surface is larger, the electrodes will pick up from a larger area, making the size of the recorded signal greater. Therefore, to record from smaller muscles, a smaller electrode should be used.

The distance between the electrodes is another major factor affecting the size of the recorded potential. Greater electrode spacing will increase the surface, width, and depth of the recording area. Because voltage is dependent on the difference in potential between the electrodes, the greater the distance, the greater the voltage, or amplitude. There is, of course, a critical limit to this distance above which the electrodes will not be able to record a valid signal. Lynn et al.[14] have theoretically shown that any active fiber at a depth of approximately half of the interelectrode spacing will dominate the surface EMG signal. Furthermore, the recording from fibers at a depth of more than 1.5 times the interelectrode spacing will be obliterated by inadequate signal to noise. Some surface electrode assemblies have been developed where the two electrodes are fixed within a casing, so that interelectrode distance is standardized. Needle electrodes have a fixed distance between the wires and the needle shaft; this distance never changes, even when the electrode is moved. Fine-wire indwelling electrodes are the least reliable in this aspect, because there is little control over the interwire distance within the muscle. The wires are often prone to change position within the muscle after repeated contractions, a situation that compromises the validity of the signals.

The shape, size, and duration of the recorded motor unit potential is actually a graphic representation of the electrical activity being picked up by the electrodes, relative to the structure of the motor unit and the electrode placement (Fig. 9-9). Therefore, with a given electrode placement, each motor unit potential will look distinctly different. The implications of this process for repeated EMG testing should be evident. It is impossible to recognize a motor unit potential as the same one if electrodes have been reinserted or moved, because the spatial and temporal relationships between the electrodes and the muscle fibers cannot be validly duplicated. This holds true for surface electrodes as well, although reapplication of surface electrodes has been shown to be more reliable than reinsertion of wire electrodes.[15]

Cross-talk

Another important consideration is the ability of electrodes to record activity selectively from a single muscle. Because of volume conduction, electrical activity from nearby contracting muscles, other than the muscle of interest, may reach the electrodes and be processed simultaneously. There is no way to distinguish this activity by looking at the output signal. Careful electrode placement and spacing, and choice of size and type of electrode will help control such **cross-talk** or electrical overflow.[2] Empirical evidence from the research literature has identified cross-talk between lower leg muscles as high as nearly 20 percent.[16]

Recent innovations using a three-bar electrode can eliminate the presence of cross-talk through a

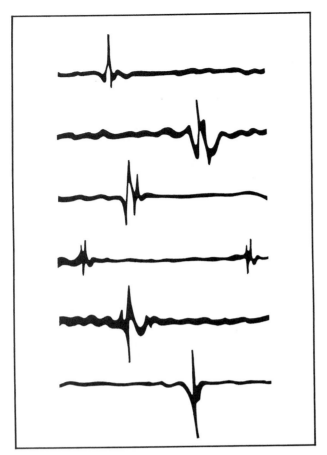

Figure 9-9. Single motor unit potentials as seen on an oscilloscope.

limiting factor is the directionality of the transmitting antenna. Multiple antennas or omnidirectional antennas are used to alleviate this problem.

The decision to invest in telemetered EMG systems must be made by considering the significant added expense versus the advantage of greater freedom of movement of the subject. A recent alternative, still under development, is *portable data loggers*. These are small battery-operated devices worn on the person that provide on-board storage of multichannel EMG data (via magnetic or digital tape or a digital signal processing card). The stored data can then be downloaded after acquisition to a mainframe system for analysis.

ARTIFACTS

The EMG signal should be a true representation of motor unit activity occurring in the muscle of interest. Unfortunately, many excess signals, or **artifacts** can be recorded and processed simultaneously with the EMG. These artifacts can be of sufficient voltage to distort the output signal markedly. Electromyographers will usually observe the output signal on an oscilloscope to monitor artifacts. Some newer commercial devices have built-in artifact suppression circuitry, or produce an audible signal and/or LED display to indicate the presence of

process referred to as *double-differentiation* (DD).[17] As shown in Fig. 9-10*A*, the EMG is recorded in two ways: first, using the bipolar signal from bars 1 and 3 (single differentiation [SD]), and second, by subtracting the SD signal from electrode bars 1 and 2 from the SD signal from electrode bars 2 and 3. Figure 9-10*B* shows that there is a difference between the SD and DD signals when recording from wrist flexors during wrist extension. The fact that the DD signal is near baseline indicates that the SD recording is cross-talk from wrist extensors. During wrist flexion, shown in Fig. 9-10*C*, no cross-talk is present, as the SD and DD signals are similar in magnitude.

TELEMETRY

When EMG recordings are considered for environments in which it is not practical to have the subject tethered, **telemetry** of the EMG signal via radio frequency transmitter and receiver is an option. Typically, a small battery-powered transmitter combines the EMG signal with an FM radio signal. This combined signal is then broadcast at the FM carrier frequency to the receiver. The receiver, in turn, demodulates the FM signal to recover the EMG information. The power output of the transmitter and the **sensitivity** of the receiver determine the range of the telemetry link. Although transmitter range is more than adequate for most indoor applications (30 m or more), a far more serious

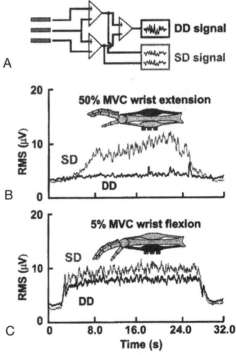

Figure 9-10. Illustration of the double differential technique to eliminate the presence of cross-talk. (*A*) Surface EMG is recorded from flexor carpi ulnaris muscle using both single-differentiated (between electrode bars 1 and 3) and double-differentiated signals (the difference between 1–2 and 2–3). The activity is recorded during wrist extension (*B*), showing cross-talk with single-differentiated signal, and during wrist flexion (*C*), showing no cross-talk, as single- and double-differentiated signals are of nearly equal magnitude. (Adapted from DeLuca, CJ: The use of surface electromyography in biomechanics. J Appl Biomech 13:135, 1997, with permission.)

an artifact such as 60-cycle interference in near real-time.

Movement Artifact

All electrodes are composed of a metallic detecting surface that is in contact with an electrolyte. This electrolyte may be the conductive electrode gel placed between a surface electrode and the skin, or it may be the tissue fluids surrounding an inserted needle or fine-wire electrode. An ion exchange occurs at the interface between the electrode and electrolyte, and this is recorded as a bioelectric event when a difference of potential exists between the two electrodes. If no muscle activity is present, therefore, and the ionization that exists at each electrode-electrolyte interface is stable, then no difference of potential exists, resulting in **electrical silence.**

If, however, some disturbance occurs at one or both electrode-electrolyte interfaces, so as to produce a difference of potential, a low-frequency signal will be recorded that does not represent EMG activity. This signal is called **movement artifact.** It may result from movement of the skin beneath a surface electrode, pressure on or movement of the electrodes, or movement of a needle or fine-wire electrode within a contracting muscle. For example, if hamstring muscle activity is being monitored during an activity in the sitting position, pressure on the electrodes on the posterior aspect of the thigh may cause movement artifact. Some form of padding under the thigh, placed proximal and distal to the electrodes, can help alleviate this pressure. Most movement artifact occurs at signal **frequencies** below 10 to 20 hertz (Hz), causing minimal interference with the amplitude of the signal, but creating a wavy baseline. These artifacts can usually be eliminated with firm fixation of the electrodes and proper high-pass filtering of the signal to attenuate frequencies below a specified frequency, such as 20 Hz (see discussion of frequency response in the next section).

Movement of electrode cables can also cause a high-voltage, high-frequency artifact as a result of disturbance in the electromagnetic field that surrounds the conducting lead wires. These artifacts produce wide, large-amplitude spikes, and are not easily filtered. Active electrodes eliminate this problem by placing the preamplification stage as close as possible to the detection surface. This signal is then fed to the EMG amplifier on a low impedance section of the circuit. For nonactive electrode use during activities requiring broad movements, cables should be taped down as much as possible, either to a table or chair, or along the limb itself, to avoid artifacts caused by cable movement.

Power Line Interference

The human body acts as an antenna, attracting electromagnetic energy from the surrounding environment. This energy is most commonly drawn from power lines and electrical equipment operating under an alternating current at 60 cycles per second (60 Hz). An artifact caused by this interference current resembles a sine wave and can cause a constant hum in the recorded signal if it is not eliminated through appropriate amplification techniques. A 60 Hz signal can occur if electrode attachments become loose, or if electrodes are broken or frayed. Electrode wires often break beneath the protective tubing that connects the electrode itself to the lead wire. If raw data are not monitored, this condition may not be noticed. Other equipment in the area also may be the source of electrical interference. Diathermy equipment, electrical stimulators, and vibrators are examples of devices that generate electrical noise. Sometimes, using isolated power lines will help with this situation. A *notch filter* can be used to remove 60 Hz signals, although this will also eliminate some of the EMG signal within that frequency range.

Electrocardiogram

A third type of artifact, from the electrocardiogram, can occur when electrodes are placed on the trunk, upper arm, or upper thigh. Correct application of the ground electrode and use of an amplifier with appropriate characteristics should help reduce these potentials, but may not be able to eliminate them. Their amplitude will vary depending on placement of electrodes. Electrocardiogram artifacts are generally regular, however, and their effect may be successfully cancelled out. If the EMG is being analyzed for frequency characteristics, this signal will provide significant interference.

Amplifying the EMG Signal

DIFFERENTIAL AMPLIFIER

Before the motor unit potential can be visualized, it is necessary to amplify the small myoelectric signal. An amplifier converts the electrical potential seen by electrodes to a voltage signal large enough to be displayed. This electrical potential is composed of the EMG signal from muscle contraction and unwanted **noise** from static electricity in the air and power lines. To control for the unwanted part of the signals, the recording electrodes each transmit electrical potentials to two sides of a **differential amplifier,** each electrode supplying input to one side. The difference in potential between each input and ground is processed in opposite directions. The difference between these signals is amplified and recorded, hence the name of the amplifier. If the two electrodes receive equal signals, no activity is recorded. Noise is transmitted to both ends of the amplifier as a *common mode signal*. The noise, being equal at both ends of the amplifier, is cancelled out when the difference of potential between the two sides is recorded.

COMMON MODE REJECTION RATIO

In reality, however, the noise is not eliminated completely in a differential amplifier. Some of the recorded voltage will include noise. The **common** mode rejection ratio (CMRR) is a measure of how much the desired signal voltage is amplified relative to the unwanted signal. A CMRR of 1000:1 indicates that the wanted signal is amplified 1000 times more than the noise. The CMRR may also be expressed in decibels (dB) (1000:1 = 60 dB). The higher this value, the better. A good differential amplifier should have a CMRR exceeding 100,000:1.

SIGNAL-TO-NOISE RATIO

Noise also can be internally generated by the electronic components of an amplifier, including resistors, transistors, and integrated circuits. This noise is often manifested as a hissing sound on an oscilloscope. The factor that reflects the ability of the amplifier to limit this noise relative to the amplified signal is the **signal-to-noise ratio,** or the ratio of the wanted signal to the unwanted signal.

GAIN

This characteristic refers to the amplifier's ability to amplify signals. The gain refers to the ratio of the output signal level to the input level. A higher gain will make a smaller signal appear larger on the display. The gain is often larger for clinical EMG where individual motor units must be distinctly visible and their amplitude measured.

INPUT IMPEDANCE

Impedance is a resistive property, opposing current flow, that occurs in alternating current circuits (such as an amplifier). It is analogous to resistance, which is exhibited by direct circuits. Electrodes provide one source of impedance and are affected by such variables as electrode material, electrode size, length of the leads, and the electrolyte. If the electrode impedance is too great, the signal will be attenuated. Electrode impedance can be reduced by using larger electrodes of good conductivity with shorter leads. Fine-wire and needle electrodes generally have much greater impedance than surface electrodes because of their much smaller surface area.

Body tissues, including adipose tissue, blood, and skin, also provide a source of resistance to the electrical field. Resistance and impedance are measured in units called ohms (Ω). Skin impedance can be measured with an ohmmeter and its value reduced by proper preparation. Most researchers have reported acceptable skin impedance under 20,000 Ω, although with proper preparation and good electrodes, resistance can usually be reduced to between 1000 and 5000 Ω. Some skin areas, such as those with darker pigments or those that are more exposed, generally have higher impedance. Skin impedance obviously is only a concern with surface electrodes.

Impedance is also present at the input of an amplifier. The muscle action potential is effectively divided into voltage changes at the electrode and amplifier input terminals. Because of the direct relationship between voltage and impedance (based on Ohm's law), if the impedance at the amplifier is greater than the impedance at the electrode, the voltage drop will be greater at the amplifier (the recorded potential) and more accurately represent the true signal voltage. If the electrode impedance is too great, the voltage will drop at the source of the signal and less of the electrical energy will be transmitted to the amplifier. Therefore, the amplifier input impedance should be substantially greater (at least 1000 times) than the impedance recorded at the electrodes. An input impedance of 1 megaohm (1 MΩ = $10^6\Omega$) is acceptable for surface electrodes, but should be greater with fine-wire and needle electrodes. Active electrodes use amplifiers with high **input impedance** (>100 MΩ) to compensate for the unwanted noise and signal attenuation that is produced by the high resistance of the skin. Because skin resistance contributes to the impedance measured at the electrodes, greater input impedance decreases the need for skin preparation with surface electrodes.

FREQUENCY BANDWIDTH

The EMG waveforms processed by an amplifier are actually the summation of signals of varying frequencies, measured in **hertz** (1 Hz = 1 cycle per second). A MUAP can be likened to a piano chord, which is composed of many notes, each at a different frequency (sound). If we vary the notes, the chord will sound different. Similarly, the shape and amplitude of an action potential are, in part, a function of the frequencies that compose the waveform. Amplifiers usually have variable filters that can be adjusted to limit the range of frequencies they will process. The main reason for using filters is to reduce noise.

The **frequency bandwidth** delineates the highest and lowest frequency components that will be processed, or the upper and lower cutoff frequencies. If the full range of frequencies that make up the major portion of a waveform are not processed, the potential will be distorted. Amplifiers should be able to respond to signals between 10 and 10,000 Hz to accurately record nerve and muscle potentials for clinical EMG.[18]

For kinesiologic purposes, however, where specific waveform characteristics are not of major interest, lower bandwidths are used. The frequency content of an EMG signal is inversely proportional to the interelectrode separation distance. Consequently, the frequency spectrum extends from 10 to 500 Hz for most surface electrodes, and from 10 to 1000 Hz for fine-wire electrodes. Limiting signals to these frequency ranges by a filter is helpful for reducing the effects of low- and high-frequency artifacts.

Displaying the EMG Signal

The amplified signal must be displayed in a useful fashion. The form of output used is dependent on the type of information desired and instrumentation available.

Computers sample and store EMG data for display and analysis. Data may be stored in *analog* form (i.e., as a continuous varying signal) or in *digital* form (i.e., the continuous signal is converted into a series of numbers, each of which represents the amplitude of the signal at a particular instant in time). The conversion process is referred to as analog-to-digital (A-to-D) conversion, and the device that performs this task is called an A-to-D converter. The process involves sampling the signal at a frequency of at least 1 KH_2, and converting it into numerical form with a 10- or 12-bit A-to-D converter, or higher. When working with A-to-D converters, it is necessary to specify the sampling rate for EMG data acquisition. An important rule, referred to as the *Nyquist sampling rate*, is to select a sampling rate that is at least twice the highest frequency component of the signal. Because surface EMG signals may have frequency components as high as 300 to 500 Hz, a sampling rate of at least 1000 Hz should be selected. If the sampling rate is specified lower than the Nyquist rate, the signal will be distorted.

The electrical signal can be displayed visually on a cathode ray oscilloscope or computer monitor for analysis. The motor unit potential can also be converted into sound in the same way that a radio signal is processed. For the same reason that every motor unit potential will look different, it will also sound different. Normal and abnormal potentials have distinctive sounds that are helpful in distinguishing them. These will be described in the next section.

Several types of recorders have been used in kinesiologic study. Graphic recorders, such as pen or chart recorders, provide a permanent written record of the output. These recorders rarely have a full-scale bandwidth greater than 60 Hz, but are more useful for integrated or averaged waveforms. An oscilloscope is often used in conjunction with a pen recorder to allow visual inspection of raw signals for artifacts. With the advent of computer workstations and digital processors, pen and chart recorders are not commonly used today.

Unlike graphic recorders, machine-interpretable recorders, such as FM magnetic tape recorders or digital recorders, store information in a form that cannot be read or analyzed without a machine interface. The advantage of the FM tape recorder is that it can store the EMG signal in its original analog form. When using FM recorders, it is important to be aware that the bandwidth of the tape recorder is directly proportional to the tape speed. Therefore, a recording speed must be selected that provides a bandwidth adequate for the signal being recorded. Second, FM recorders have an input dynamic range (typically ± 1 V) that cannot be exceeded; otherwise that portion of the waveform that exceeds the input dynamic range will be clipped. This means that the investigator must adjust the gain of the amplifier appropriately. Too large a gain will result in distortion of the signal due to clipping. Inadequate gain will result in poor signal-to-noise ratio.[6]

Digital recorders can store data on digital magnetic tape or disc following A-to-D conversion of the signal. Their primary advantages are that they avert the noise and distortion problems of FM recorders and they provide data in a digital format that can be directly input to a computer for analysis and display. The fidelity of the digitally recorded data is dependent primarily on the performance of the A-to-D converter.

CLINICAL ELECTROMYOGRAPHY

The Electromyographic Examination

An EMG examination assesses the integrity of the neuromuscular system, including upper and lower motor neurons, the neuromuscular junction, and muscle fibers. The test usually involves observation of muscle action potentials from several muscles in different stages of muscle contraction. The EMG is only part of a complete examination, however, which will include assessment of muscle strength and atrophy, pain, reflexes and sensory deficits, as well as functional abilities in extremity and trunk musculature. These screens will suggest which muscles or neurons should be tested.

INSERTION ACTIVITY

Initially, the patient is asked to relax the muscle to be examined during insertion of the needle electrode. Insertion into a contracting muscle is uncomfortable, but bearable. At this time, the electromyographer will observe a spontaneous burst of potentials, which is possibly caused by the needle breaking through muscle fiber membranes. This is called **insertion activity** and normally lasts less than 300 ms.[19] This activity is also seen during examination as the needle is repositioned in the muscle. It usually stops when the needle stops moving. Insertion activity can be described as normal, reduced, or increased, in part depending on the magnitude and speed of movement of the needle in the muscle. It is considered a measure of muscle excitability and may be markedly reduced in fibrotic muscles or exaggerated when denervation or inflammation is present (Fig. 9-11).

THE MUSCLE AT REST

Following cessation of insertion activity, a normal relaxed muscle will exhibit electrical silence, which is the absence of electrical potentials. Observation of silence in the relaxed state is an important part of the EMG examination. Potentials arising spontaneously during this period are significant abnormal findings. It is often difficult for a patient to relax sufficiently to observe complete electrical silence. However, the potentials seen will be distinct motor unit potentials, whereas **spontaneous potentials** can be differentiated by their low amplitude, shape, and sound.

One exception to finding no activity in normal resting muscle occurs when the needle is in the

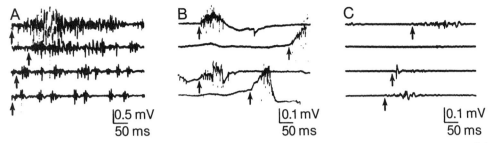

Figure 9-11. Increased (*A*), normal (*B*), and decreased (*C*) insertion activity induced by movements of the needle electrode (*arrows*). The tracings were obtained from the first dorsal interosseus in a patient with tardy ulnar palsy (*A*), tibialis anterior in a control subject (*B*), and fibrotic deltoid of a patient with severe dermatomyositis (*C*). (From Kimura, J: Electrodiagnosis of Diseases of Nerve and Muscle: Principles and Practice, ed 2, FA Davis, Philadelphia, 1989, p 231, with permission.)

end-plate region. Such activity may be reflected as a constant low-amplitude noise or high-amplitude intermittent spikes. It usually disappears by repositioning the needle slightly. End-plate potentials may be excessive in denervated muscle.[19]

NORMAL MOTOR UNIT ACTION POTENTIALS

After observing the muscle at rest, the patient is asked to contract the muscle minimally (Fig. 9-12). This weak voluntary effort should cause individual motor units to fire. These motor unit potentials are assessed with respect to amplitude, duration, shape, sound, and frequency (Fig. 9-13). These five parameters are the essential characteristics that will distinguish normal and abnormal potentials. Finally, the patient is asked to increase levels of contraction progressively to a strong effort, allowing assessment of recruitment patterns.

A motor unit potential is actually the summation of electrical potentials from all the fibers of that unit close enough to the electrodes to be recorded. The voltage amplitude is affected by the number of fibers involved. The duration and shape are functions of the distance of the fibers from the electrodes, the more distant fibers contributing to terminal phases of the potential.

In normal muscle, the peak-to-peak amplitude of a single MUAP, recorded with a concentric needle,

may range from 300 μV to 5 mV. The amplitude is primarily determined by a limited number of fibers located close to the electrode tip. Therefore, motor units must be sampled from different sites to determine their amplitude accurately.

The total duration, measured from initial baseline deflection to return to baseline, will normally range from 3 to 16 ms. Duration is a function of the synchrony with which individual muscle fibers fire within a motor unit. This is affected by the length and conduction velocity of the axon terminals and muscle fibers. Duration can be affected significantly by electrical activity originating in fibers distant to the electrode. The *rise time* of the potential, measured from the initial positive peak to the following negative peak, provides an indication of the distance between the electrode and the contracting motor unit. A normal unit close to the electrode should have a rise time between 100 and 200 μs. Distant discharges will have a longer rise time, and will not be useful for assessing motor unit properties.

The typical shape of an MUAP is diphasic or triphasic, with a **phase** representing a section of a potential above or below the baseline. It is not abnormal to observe small numbers of **polyphasic potentials,** having four or more phases, in normal muscle. However, when polyphasic potentials repre-

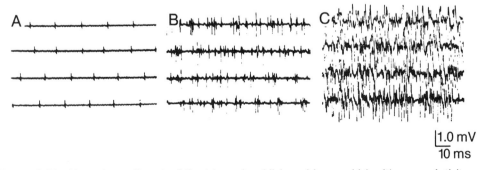

Figure 9-12. Normal recruitment of the triceps brachii in a 44 year-old healthy man. Activity was recorded during minimal contraction (*A*) where single motor unit activity is evident, during moderate contraction (*B*) when motor units are recruited, and during maximal contraction (*C*) when an interference pattern is visible. (From Kimura, J: Electrodiagnosis of Diseases of Nerve and Muscle: Principles and Practice, ed 2, FA Davis, Philadelphia, 1989, p 241, with permission.)

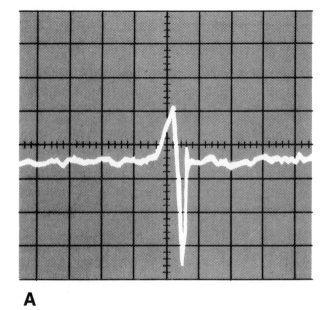

A

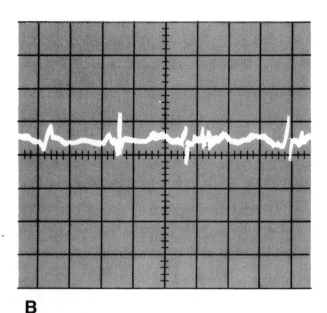

B

Figure 9-13. Single motor unit action potentials. The characteristics of amplitude, duration, and shape are examined by the electromyographer. (*A*) Normal biphasic potential, (*B*) Normal triphasic potentials. (From Yanof, HM: Biomedical Electronics, ed 2, FA Davis, Philadelphia, 1972, p 438, with permission.)

sent more than 10 percent of a muscle's output, it may be an abnormal finding.

The normal motor unit will fire up to 15 times per second with strong contraction. The identifying sound is a clear, distinct thump. Gradually increasing the force of contraction will allow the electromyographer to observe the pattern of recruitment in the muscle. With greater effort, increasing numbers of motor units fire at higher frequencies, until the individual potentials are summated and can no longer be recognized, and an **interference pattern** is seen (see Fig. 9-12). This is the normal finding

with a strong contraction. Highest amplitudes for interference patterns typically vary between 2 and 5 mV.

One of the disadvantages of conventional assessment methods is that the examination of single motor unit potentials can be made only during weak voluntary effort, essentially restricting the analysis to low-threshold type I motor units. An interesting alternative involves the use of *automatic quantitative assessment*, which further analyzes the interference pattern by assessing the number of directional changes of the waveform that do not necessarily cross the baseline.[20,21] These data are processed by a computer to display the number of reversals and the intervals between reversals within a given time period. Such ratios can vary between normal and pathological conditions, allowing for greater diagnostic precision in the differentiation of primary muscle disease and neurogenic lesions.[22,23] This approach allows the electromyographer to observe the behavior of motor units even during maximal effort, when individual potentials cannot be delineated.

An electromyographer, therefore, examines insertion activity, as well as activity with the muscle at rest and in states of minimal, moderate, and maximal contraction. The needle electrode is moved to different areas and depths of each muscle to sample different muscle fibers and motor units. This is necessary because of the small area from which a needle electrode will pick up electrical activity, and because the effects of pathology may vary within a single muscle. Up to 25 different points within a muscle may be examined by moving and reinserting the needle electrode.

ABNORMAL POTENTIALS

Spontaneous Activity

Because a normal muscle at rest exhibits electrical silence, any activity seen during the relaxed state can be considered abnormal. Such activity is termed spontaneous because it is not produced by voluntary muscle contraction. Four types of spontaneous potentials have been identified: **fibrillation potentials, positive sharp waves, fasciculation potentials,** and **repetitive discharges.**

Fibrillation Potentials. Fibrillation potentials are believed to arise from spontaneous depolarization of a single muscle fiber. This theory is supported by the small amplitude and duration of the potentials. They are not visible through the skin. Fibrillation potentials are classically indicative of lower motor neuron disorders, such as peripheral nerve lesions, anterior horn cell disease, radiculopathies, and polyneuropathies with axonal degeneration. They are also found to a lesser extent in myopathic diseases such as muscular dystrophy, dermatomyositis, polymyositis, and myasthenia gravis.

Fibrillation potentials may have up to three phases, and their spikes may vary in amplitude from 20 to 300 μV, with an average duration of 2 ms

(Fig. 9-14). Their sound is a high-pitched click, which has been likened to rain falling on a roof or wrinkling tissue paper. Fibrillation potentials have been recorded at frequencies of up to 30 per second.

Positive Sharp Waves. Positive sharp waves have been observed in denervated muscle at rest, usually accompanied by fibrillation potentials. However, they are also reported in primary muscle disease, especially muscular dystrophy and polymyositis. The waves are typically diphasic, with a sharp initial positive deflection (below baseline) followed by a slow negative phase (see Fig. 9-14). The negative phase is of much lower amplitude than the positive phase, and of much longer duration, sometimes up to 100 ms. The peak-to-peak amplitude may be variable, with voltages approaching 1 mV. The discharge frequency may range from 2 to 100 per second. The sound has been described as a dull thud. Positive sharp waves are recorded when the tip of the recording electrode is in contact with the depolarized muscle membrane.[24]

Evidence indicates that fibrillation potentials and positive sharp waves may also be present with upper motor neuron lesions, creating a need for alternative explanations for their occurrence.[25] Researchers have observed both types of potentials in patients with spinal cord lesions and attributed their occurrence to the lack of some trophic factor from higher centers to the anterior horn cell. The occurrence of the denervation activity with central involvement supports the assumption of a trans-synaptic degeneration of alpha-motoneurons. Berman suggests that spinal cord trauma can cause loss of motor axons in regions several segments caudal to the site of injury.[26] This interpretation may have implications for the design of rehabilitation strategies. Speilholz[27] postulated that these findings may also explain the observation of fibrillations and positive sharp waves with myopathies, and that the presence of these potentials indicates that muscle disease also affects the neuron. A similar hypothesis was formulated to explain the finding of spontaneous potentials in patients who had sustained a cerebral vascular accident.[28,29]

Investigators have also demonstrated spontaneous potentials in normal muscles of healthy subjects, primarily in muscles of the feet.[30] They have suggested that pathological changes involving axonal loss, segmental demyelination, and collateral sprouting may be associated with aging or mechanical trauma to the feet. Their findings have important clinical implications in that interpretation of the pattern of EMG and other assessments is necessary for accurate evaluation of pathology.

Fasciculations. Fasciculations are spontaneous potentials seen with irritation or degeneration of the anterior horn cell, nerve root compression, and muscle spasms or cramps. They are believed to represent the involuntary asynchronous contraction of a bundle of muscle fibers or a whole motor unit. Although their origin is not clearly known, there is evidence that the spontaneous discharge originates in the spinal cord or anywhere along the path of the peripheral nerve, causing contraction of the muscle fibers.[31]

Fasciculations are often visible through the skin, seen as a small twitch. They are not by themselves a definitive abnormal finding, however, because they are also seen in normal individuals,[32] particularly in calf muscle, eyes, hands, and feet.[33] When seen with other abnormal factors, such as fibrillations and positive sharp waves, fasciculations do contribute information indicating pathology. The amplitude and duration of these potentials may be similar to a motor unit potential (Fig. 9-15). They may be diphasic, triphasic, or polyphasic. Their firing rate is usually irregular, up to 50 per second. Their sound has been described as a low-pitched thump.

Repetitive Discharges. Repetitive discharges, also called bizarre high-frequency discharges, are seen with lesions of the anterior horn cell and peripheral nerves, and with myopathies. The discharge is characterized by an extended train of potentials of various form (Fig. 9-16). The feature that distinguishes these discharges from other spontaneous potentials is their frequency, which usually ranges from 5 to 100 impulses per second. The amplitude can vary from 50 µV to 1 mV, and duration may be up to 100 ms. Repetitive discharges that increase and decrease in amplitude in a waxing and waning fashion are typical of myotonias, and sound like a "dive-bomber." High-frequency discharges are probably triggered by movement of the needle electrode within unstable muscle fibers, or by volitional activity.

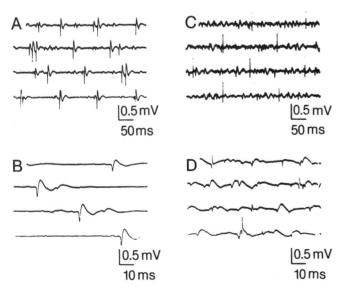

Figure 9-14. Spontaneous activity of the anterior tibialis in a 68 year-old woman with amyotrophic lateral sclerosis. Positive sharp waves (A,B) have a consistent configuration with a sharp positive deflection followed by a long-duration, low-amplitude negative deflection (B). Fibrillation potentials (C, D) are low-amplitude biphasic spikes. (From Kimura, J: Electrodiagnosis of Diseases of Nerve and Muscle: Principles and Practice, ed 2, FA Davis, Philadelphia, 1989, p 256, with permission.)

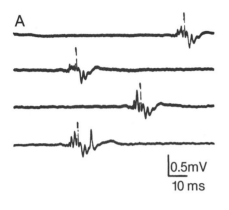

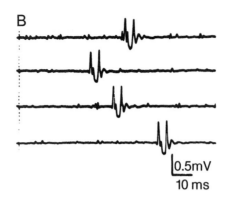

Figure 9-15. Fasciculation potentials in two patients with polyneuropathy. Recordings were obtained from the tibialis anterior in both patients, showing a very polyphasic potential of long duration (A) and a double-peaked, complex discharge (B). Fasciculation potentials are not always abnormal in waveform, as shown here, and are usually indistinguishable in shape from voluntarily activated motor unit potentials. (From Kimura, J: Electrodiagnosis of Diseases of Nerve and Muscle: Principles and Practice, ed 2, FA Davis, Philadelphia, 1989, p 260, with permission.)

Abnormal Voluntary Potentials

Polyphasic potentials are generally considered abnormal, but they are elicited on voluntary contraction, not at rest. They are typical of myopathies and peripheral nerve involvement. In primary muscle disease, these potentials are generally of smaller amplitude than normal motor units, and of shorter duration. These multiphasic changes occur because of the decrease in the number of active muscle fibers within the individual motor units due to pathology. Although the entire unit will fire during voluntary contraction, fewer fibers are available in each unit to contribute to the total voltage and the duration of the potential. The polyphasic configuration is a result of the slight asynchrony of muscle fibers within a motor unit. This phenomenon is probably due to the difference in the length of the terminal branches of the axon extending to each individual fiber. The effects of this are normally not seen because the time differences are so slight. When some fibers are no longer contracting, however, these differences become more apparent, resulting in a fragmentation of the motor unit potential (Fig. 9-17).

Polyphasic potentials may also be seen after regeneration of a peripheral nerve. As some muscle fibers become reinnervated, they will generate action potentials with voluntary contraction. However,

there are significantly fewer fibers acting than were present in the original unit, and these fibers will clearly reflect asynchronous depolarization. These polyphasic potentials are also much smaller in amplitude and duration than normal units, and they have been termed *nascent motor units*. Although polyphasic potentials are generally considered an abnormal finding, they are a positive finding in patients with peripheral nerve lesions because they indicate reinnervation.

Some forms of neuropathic involvement, such as anterior horn cell disease, will result in hypertrophy of an intact motor unit by collateral sprouting of axons to fibers of denervated motor units, forming **giant motor units.** Because these sprouts are of small diameter and have slow conduction velocities, there is a dispersion in the recorded potential, which increases the amplitude and duration and results in

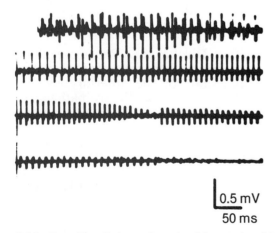

Figure 9-16. Repetitive discharge from the right anterior tibialis in a 39 year-old man with myotonic dystrophy. The waxing and waning quality of these discharges is evident. (From Kimura, J: Electrodiagnosis of Diseases of Nerve and Muscle: Principles and Practice, ed 2, FA Davis, Philadelphia, 1989, p 254, with permission.)

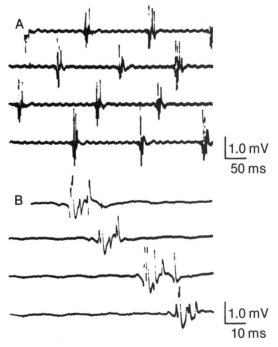

Figure 9-17. Polyphasic motor unit potentials from the anterior tibialis in a 52 year-old man with amyotrophic lateral sclerosis, recorded at fast (A) and slow (B) sweep speeds. (From Kimura, J: Electrodiagnosis of Diseases of Nerve and Muscle: Principles and Practice, ed 2, FA Davis, Philadelphia, 1989, p 265, with permission.)

a polyphasic shape. These potentials are often seen in post-polio syndrome.[34–36] If this situation is sufficiently prevalent, the interference pattern may be increased in amplitude.

Single Fiber Electromyography

Some properties of muscle can be examined using extracellular recordings from individual muscle fibers within the same motor unit using a technique called *single fiber electromyography (SFEMG)*. This procedure was developed to study neuromuscular transmission in the end-plate region in patients with myasthenia gravis, but has become a routine adjunct to the EMG examination in patients with myopathies, myasthenic syndromes, and motor neuron disease.[37]

SFEMG requires the use of a small electrode (25 μm in diameter), which is inserted via a steel canula. During a slight voluntary contraction, recordings are taken from a single site. Because consecutive discharges from a single fiber have reproducible properties, timed measurements are able to accurately record the potentials. To assess neuromuscular transmission, the electrode is positioned to record from two fibers in the motor unit. A trigger is used to control the tracings of these potentials, allowing the measurement of latency between the two discharges. This latency, called *jitter*, represents the variable conduction time across the neuromuscular junction. For normal muscle contraction, mean values for jitter fall between 5 and 60 μs. In a patient with myasthenia gravis, normal and increased values for jitter have been recorded. Impulse blocking can occur as well, with intermittent failure of some axons.[37]

SFEMG has also been used to assess changes in muscle morphology as a function of *fiber density*, by counting the number of spikes in a single muscle fiber potential. With conditions causing changes in the organization of motor units, such as myopathies or reinnervation, fiber density will appear higher than normal.

MACRO EMG

Another technique, called *macro EMG*, is used to assess the overall status of the motor unit. Using a modification of the SFEMG electrode, recordings are made from as many fibers from one motor unit as possible. Two channels of EMG are recorded, one from the needle canula, and the other as a difference of potential between the needle tip and the canula. Using timed recordings and averaging techniques, the peak-to-peak amplitude and area of the macro EMG signal will reflect the number and size of the muscle fibers within the entire motor unit.

With normal muscle, the macro EMG motor unit potentials will differ in shape from one motor unit to another.[38] With myopathy, the macro EMG potential is decreased. Studies of patients with post-polio syndrome have identified dramatic increases in motor unit size, often more than 20 times normal.[35,39]

NERVE CONDUCTION TESTS

Hodes et al.[40] first developed the technique for calculating the conduction velocity of the ulnar nerve in 1948. Dawson and Scott[41] further refined the procedure a year later, recording nerve potentials from the ulnar and median nerves through the skin at the wrist. This EMG technique has since become a valuable tool for assessing abnormalities and lesions of peripheral nerves, as well as localizing the site of involvement.

NCV tests involve direct stimulation to initiate an impulse in motor or sensory nerves. The **conduction time** is measured by recording the **evoked potential** either from the muscle innervated by the motor nerve or from the sensory nerve itself. NCV can be tested on any peripheral nerve that is superficial enough to be stimulated through the skin at two different points. Most commonly it is performed on the ulnar, median, peroneal, and posterior tibial nerves; and less commonly on the radial, femoral, and sciatic nerves. Complete guidelines for performing NCV tests are available in comprehensive references.[42,43]

Instrumentation

Whereas EMG records the spontaneous or volitional potentials of motor units, nerve conduction measurements involve evoked potentials, produced by direct electrical stimulation of peripheral nerves. The instrumentation, therefore, includes a stimulator in addition to all the components of the electromyograph already described (Fig. 9-18).

The **stimulating electrode** is typically a two-pronged bipolar electrode with the cathode (−) and the anode (+) extending from a plastic casing (Fig. 9-19). A single cathodal stimulating electrode can also be used in conjunction with an inactive electrode. A needle electrode can be used to stimulate the nerve. The stimulus is provided by a square-wave generator, with pulses typically delivered at a duration of 0.1 ms and a frequency of 1 pulse per second (up to 20 pulses per second). The intensity needed will vary with the nerve and the individual patient, usually between 100 and 300 V, or 5 and 40 mA.[19] Diseased nerves with decreased excitability may require as much as 500 volts or 75 mA. These intensities are considered safe for most patients. With a cardiac pacemaker, however, grounding should be checked and stimulation should be a sufficient distance from the pacemaker.[44] With indwelling cardiac catheters or central venous pressure lines, nerve conduction studies are contraindicated, because the electrical current may directly reach the cardiac tissue.

A trigger mechanism is incorporated into the recording system, so that the oscilloscope sweep is

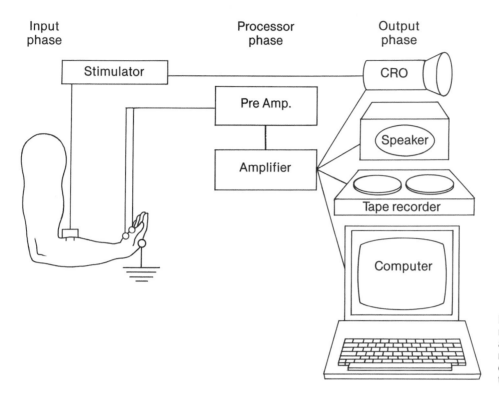

Figure 9-18. Recording system for nerve conduction velocity test, showing addition of the stimulator. Note the connection between the stimulator and the cathode ray oscilloscope, which is the triggering mechanism.

triggered by the stimulator. This means that the sweep begins when the stimulus is delivered, producing a stimulus artifact on the screen with each successive stimulus. This allows the measurement of time from stimulus onset to response. The sweep makes one complete excursion across the screen for each pulse put out by the stimulator.

Motor Nerve Conduction Velocity

STIMULATION AND RECORDING

Recording potentials directly from a peripheral nerve makes monitoring of purely sensory or motor

fibers impossible. Therefore, to isolate the potentials conducted by motor axons of a mixed nerve, the evoked potential is recorded from a distal muscle innervated by the nerve. Although the stimulation of the nerve will evoke sensory and motor impulses, only the motor fibers will contribute to the contraction of the muscle. For the ulnar nerve, the test muscle is the abductor digiti minimi; for the median nerve, the abductor pollicis brevis; for the peroneal nerve, the extensor digitorum brevis; and for the posterior tibial nerve, the abductor hallicus or abductor digiti minimi.

Small surface electrodes are usually used to record the evoked potential from the test muscle,

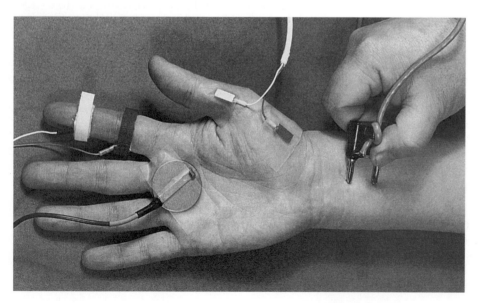

Figure 9-19. Set up for motor and sensory conduction velocity tests of the median nerve. Recording electrodes are placed over the muscle belly of the abductor pollicis brevis for motor conduction, and ring electrodes are placed over the proximal and distal interphalangeal joints of the second digit for sensory conduction. The ground electrode is located between the stimulating and recording electrodes on the hand. The nerve is stimulated at the wrist (shown) and at the elbow to obtain motor latencies. Only stimulation at the wrist is necessary for sensory latency. (From Kimura, J: Electrodiagnosis of Diseases of Nerve and Muscle: Principles and Practice, ed 2, FA Davis, Philadelphia, 1989, p 106, with permission.)

although needle electrodes may be used when responses are very weak. The *recording electrode* (sometimes called the pickup electrode) is placed over the belly of the test muscle. Accurate location of this electrode is important to the accuracy of the test, and the belly of the muscle should be carefully palpated, preferably against slight resistance. A second electrode, the *reference electrode,* is taped over the tendon of the muscle, distal to the active electrode. The skin should be cleaned with alcohol to reduce skin resistance before applying electrodes. A ground electrode is placed over a neutral area between the electrodes and the stimulation sites, usually over the dorsum of the hand or foot, or over the wrist or ankle.

For the purposes of illustration, the test procedure for the motor NCV of the median nerve will be described. The technique is basically the same for all nerves, except for the sites of stimulation and placement of the electrodes. The recording electrode is taped over the belly of the test muscle, the abductor pollicis brevis, and the reference electrode is taped over the tendon just distal to the metacarpophalangeal joint. The stimulating electrode is placed over the median nerve at the wrist, just proximal to the distal crease on the volar surface, with the cathode directed toward the recording electrodes (see Fig. 9-19). The **cathode** is the stimulating electrode (usually black) and the **anode** is the inactive electrode (usually red). It is important that the cathode be directed toward the recording electrodes to stimulate depolarization toward the muscle (orthodromic conduction).

At the moment the stimulus is produced, the **stimulus artifact** is seen at the left of the screen. The trigger mechanism controls this and it will, therefore, always appear in the same spot on the screen, facilitating consistent measurements. This spike is purely mechanical and does not represent any muscle activity (Fig. 9-20).

The stimulus intensity starts out low and is slowly increased until the evoked potential is clearly observed. When the stimulating electrode is properly placed over the nerve, all muscles innervated distal to that point will contract, and the patient will see and feel his hand "jump." The intensity is then increased until the evoked response no longer increases in size. At that time, the intensity is increased further by about 25 percent to be sure that the stimulus is *supramaximal*. Because the intensity must be sufficient to reach the threshold of all motor fibers in the nerve, a supramaximal stimulus is required. It is also essential that the cathode be properly placed over the nerve trunk so that the stimulus reaches all the motor axons.

As in the EMG, the potentials seen on the **oscilloscope** represent the electrical activity picked up by the recording electrode. The signal will represent the difference in electrical potential between the recording and reference electrodes. When the supramaximal stimulus is applied to the median nerve at the wrist, all the axons in the nerve will

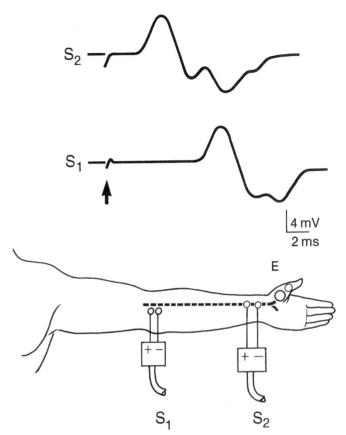

Figure 9-20. Illustration of the recording of median nerve motor conduction velocity, with recording electrodes (E) over the thenar muscles. The M wave is recorded after stimulation at the wrist (S2) and elbow (S1). Nerve conduction time from the elbow to the wrist is determined as the difference between the latencies recorded from the distal (S2) and proximal (S1) stipulations. Latency is measured from the stimulus artifact (*arrow*) to the onset of the M wave. The motor nerve conduction velocity is then calculated by dividing the surface distance between the two points by the conduction time.

depolarize and begin conducting an impulse, transmitting the signal across the motor end plate, initiating depolarization of the muscle fibers. During these events, the two recording electrodes do not record a difference in potential because no activity is taking place beneath the electrodes. When the muscle fibers begin to depolarize, the electrical potentials are transmitted to the electrodes through the volume conductor, and a deflection is seen on the oscilloscope. This is the evoked potential, which is called the **M wave** (Fig. 9-20). The M wave represents the summated activity of all motor units in the muscle that responds to stimulation of the nerve trunk. The amplitude of this potential is, therefore, a function of the total voltage produced by the contracting motor units. The initial deflection of the M wave is the negative portion of the wave, above the baseline.

Motor NCV tests can be performed on more proximal segments of the nerve trunk by stimulating at more proximal points, such as Erb's point and the axilla (see Fig. 9-20), but these areas are tested less frequently.

CALCULATION OF MOTOR NERVE CONDUCTION VELOCITY

The point at which the M wave leaves the baseline indicates the time elapsed from the initial propagation of the nerve impulse to the depolarization of the muscle fibers beneath the electrodes. This is called the response **latency.** The latency is measured in milliseconds from the stimulus artifact to the onset of the M wave. This time alone is not a valid measurement of nerve conduction because it incorporates other events besides pure nerve conduction—namely, transmission across the myoneural junction and generation of the muscle action potential. There is also evidence that the distal segments and terminal branches of nerves conduct at much slower rates than the main axon.[45] Therefore, these extraneous factors must be eliminated from the calculation of the motor NCV, so that the measurement reflects only the speed of conduction within the nerve trunk.

To account for these distal variables, the nerve is stimulated at a second, more proximal point. This will produce a response similar to that seen with distal stimulation (see Fig. 9–20). The stimulus artifact will appear in the same spot on the screen, but the M wave will originate in a different place because the time for the impulses to reach the muscle would, obviously, be longer. Subtraction of the **distal latency** from the **proximal latency** will determine the conduction time for the nerve trunk segment between the two points of stimulation. **Conduction velocity (CV)** is determined by dividing the distance between the two points of cathodal stimulation (measured along the surface) by the difference between the two latencies (velocity = distance/time).

$$CV = \frac{\text{Conduction distance}}{\text{Proximal latency} - \text{distal latency}}$$

Conduction velocity is always expressed in meters per second (m/s), although distance is usually measured in centimeters and latencies in milliseconds. These units must be converted during calculation.

To compute the motor NCV for the test illustrated in Fig. 9–20, the proximal and distal latencies are determined by measuring the time from the stimulus artifact to the initial M wave deflection, according to the calibration scale, or sweep speed. The conduction time is calculated by taking the difference between these latencies. **Conduction distance** is then determined by measuring the length of the nerve between the two points of stimulation. For example:

- Proximal latency: 7 msec
- Distal latency: 2 msec
- Conduction distance: 30 cm

$$CV = \frac{30 \text{ cm}}{7 \text{ msec} - 2 \text{ msec}} = \frac{30 \text{ cm}}{5 \text{ msec}} = 60 \text{ m/sec}$$

Interpretation of the motor NCV is made in relation to normal values, which are usually expressed as mean values, standard deviations, and ranges. Norms have been determined by many investigators in different laboratories. Even so, average values seem to be fairly consistent. The motor NCV for the upper extremity has a fairly wide range, with values reported from 45 to 70 ms. The average normal value is about 60 m/s. For the lower extremity, the average value is about 50 ms. Distal latencies and average normal amplitudes of M waves are also found in such tables, but these must be viewed with caution, because technique, electrode setup, instrumentation, and patient size can affect these values. The reader is referred to more comprehensive discussions for complete tables of normal values.[42,43]

It is important to note that the value calculated as the conduction velocity is actually a reflection of the speed of the fastest axons in the nerve. Although all axons are stimulated at the same point in time, and supposedly fire at the same time, their conduction rates vary with their size. Not all motor units will contract at the same time; some receive their nerve impulse later than others. Therefore, the initial M wave deflection represents the contraction of the motor unit, or units, with the fastest conduction velocity. The curved shape of the M wave is reflective of the progressively slower axons reaching their motor units at a later time.

The M wave can also provide useful information about the integrity of the nerve or muscle. Three parameters should be examined: amplitude, shape, and duration. Any change occurring in these characteristics is called **temporal dispersion.** These parameters reflect the summated voltage over time produced by all the contracting motor units within the test muscle. Therefore, if the muscle is partially denervated, fewer motor units will contract after nerve stimulation. This will cause the M wave amplitude to decrease. Duration may change depending on the conduction velocity of the intact units. Similar changes may also be evident in myopathic conditions, in which all motor units are intact, but fewer fibers are available in each motor unit.

The shape of the M wave can also be variable. Deviation from a smooth curve need not be abnormal, and it is often useful to compare the proximal and distal M waves with each other as well as with the contralateral side. They should be similar. In abnormal conditions, changes in shape may be the result of a significant slowing of conduction in some axons, repetitive firing, or asynchronous firing of axons after a single stimulus.

Sensory Nerve Conduction Velocity

Sensory neurons demonstrate the same physiological properties as motor neurons, and NCV can be measured in a similar way. However, some differences in technique are necessary to differentiate between sensory and motor axons. Although sensory fibers can be tested using **orthodromic conduction** (physiological direction) or **antidromic conduction** (opposite to normal conduction), orthodromic measurements appear to be more common. For the same reason that motor axons are examined by recording over muscle, sensory axons are either stimulated or recorded from digital sensory nerves. This eliminates the activity of the motor axons from the recorded potentials.

STIMULATION AND RECORDING

The stimulating electrode used for motor NCV tests can be used for sensory NCV tests, or the stimulus may be provided by ring electrodes placed around the base of the middle of the digit innervated by the nerve (see Fig. 9-19). The recording electrodes can be surface or needle electrodes. Surface electrodes are placed over the nerve trunk, where it is superficial to the skin. The active electrode is placed distally, and a ground electrode is usually set between the stimulating and recording electrodes.

The electrode positions can be reversed, measuring antidromic conduction. If electrode sites are consistent, the latencies should be essentially equivalent in both directions. Orthodromic stimulation of fingertips appears to be more uncomfortable than stimulation of the nerve trunk.

Sensory potentials for the median and ulnar nerves can be recorded at the wrist and elbow. The ulnar nerve can also be monitored at the axilla, although it is rather unreliable and difficult to differentiate between median and ulnar nerves. In lower extremities, the toes can be stimulated and sensory potentials recorded at various sites along the tibial and sciatic nerves. The path of the main nerve trunk can often be determined by electrical stimulation and observation of motor responses.

CALCULATION OF SENSORY NERVE CONDUCTION VELOCITY

Latencies are usually measured from the stimulus artifact to the peak of the evoked potential, rather than to the initial deflection, because of the uneven baseline seen with sensory tests (Fig. 9-21). The baseline is more uneven because sensory tests require much greater amplifier sensitivity than do motor tests, and this allows more noise to interfere with recording. Although sensory NCV can be determined in the same way as motor NCV (dividing distance by difference between latencies), often latencies are sufficient measurements, because terminal branching does not seem to be a significant limitation. Therefore, the latency essentially represents sensory nerve conduction activity only.

Normal sensory NCV ranges between 45 and 75 ms. Amplitude, measured with surface electrodes, may be 10 to 60 µV, and duration should be short, less than 2 ms. Sensory evoked potentials are usually sharp, not rounded like the M wave. Sensory NCVs have been found to be slightly faster than motor NCVs because of the larger diameter of sensory nerves.[46]

H Reflex

The **H reflex** (named for Hoffmann[47]) is a useful diagnostic measure for radiculopathy and peripheral neuropathy. Its most common application is in testing the integrity of the sensory and motor monosynaptic pathways of S1 nerve roots, and to a lesser extent at C6 and C7.[48] A submaximal stimulus is applied to the tibial nerve at the popliteal fossa, and a motor response is recorded from the medial portion of the soleus muscle. The action potentials travel along the IA afferent neurons toward the spinal cord, synapsing onto alpha-motoneurons within the anterior horn. The consequent activation of the motor neuron leads to an impuse traveling peripherally to the response muscle, resulting in a muscle contraction. Because the stimulus causes impulses to travel both distally and proximally within a mixed motor and sensory neuron, the

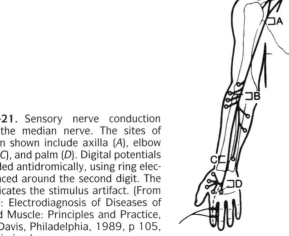
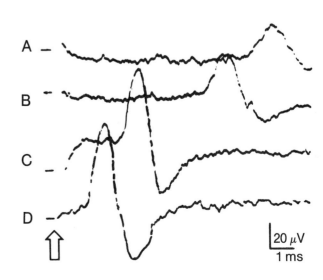

Figure 9-21. Sensory nerve conduction study of the median nerve. The sites of stimulation shown include axilla (*A*), elbow (*B*), wrist (*C*), and palm (*D*). Digital potentials are recorded antidromically, using ring electrodes placed around the second digit. The arrow indicates the stimulus artifact. (From Kimura, J: Electrodiagnosis of Diseases of Nerve and Muscle: Principles and Practice, ed 2, FA Davis, Philadelphia, 1989, p 105, with permission.)

latency of this response is a measure of the integrity of both sensory and motor fibers.

Because the initial phase of the H reflex is the afferent arc along IA fibers, its response is linked to the presence of muscle spindles. Muscles with slow-twitch fibers contain an abundance of muscle spindles and are able to demonstrate the H reflex most consistently. Therefore, the soleus muscle, composed predominantly of slow-twitch fibers, is most often used. Sabbahi and Khalil[49] have also demonstrated the H reflex in the flexor carpi radialis muscle to test the median nerve.

The H-reflex response latency is a function of age and leg length, according to the equation:

$$\text{H-reflex latency} = 0.46\,(\text{leg length [cm]}) + 9.14 + 0.1\,(\text{Age [yr]})$$

A normal response falls within ± 5.5 ms of this calculated latency. An average response is 29.8 ms (± 2.74 ms).[50] A slowed latency is indicative of abnormal dorsal root function, often from a herniated disc or impingement syndrome. Because of this central involvement, the peripheral motor and sensory NCV would not be affected. This latency would also identify nerve root compression sooner than EMG denervation potentials would be obvious. The H-reflex latency is elicited using fixed stimulus parameters, resulting in a stable response from trial to trial. Latency can be affected by facilitory and inhibitory techniques, reflecting the excitability of the motor neuron pool; however, the response will be more variable.[51]

The F Wave

The **F wave** was first described by Magladary and McDougal in 1950.[52] It is elicited by the supramaximal stimulus of a peripheral nerve at a distal site, leading to both orthodromic and antidromic impulses. While the orthodromic impulse travels to the distal muscle, the antidromic response travels to the anterior horn cell. This impulse is thought to reverberate; that is, the axon hillock is depolarized, leading to depolarization of dendrites, which in turn depolarizes the axon hillock once again, generating an orthodromic volley back to the muscle. No synapse is involved, so the F wave is not considered a reflex, but only a measure of motor neuron conduction.

The F wave is a useful supplement to nerve conduction and EMG measures, and is most helpful in the diagnosis of conditions where the most proximal portion of the axon is involved, including Guillain-Barré syndrome, thoracic outlet syndrome, brachial plexus injuries, and radiculopathies with more than one nerve root involved.[42] The F response has also been used in pharmacological studies of spasticity, as a measure of alpha motor neuron excitability.[53,54]

The latency of the F wave is normally approximately 30 seconds in the upper limb and less than 60 seconds in the lower limb. This total time includes the M wave elicited as part of the motor NCV. Only a small percent of motor neurons actually participate in the F response.[55] Because it is an inconsistent response, it must be calculated on the basis of at least 10 successive trials.

Effects of Age and Temperature

Age and temperature are the two most influential factors that can cause variations in conduction velocity. Nerve conduction is slowed considerably in infants, young children, and elderly individuals. At birth, the motor NCV is approximately one half of normal adult values, gradually increasing until reaching adult rates at 5 years of age.[56] Motor and sensory conduction velocities have been shown to decrease slightly after age 35, with larger, significant differences noted after age 70.[57,58]

Lower temperature can also decrease motor and sensory conduction velocities significantly.[59] Drops of 1.8°F (1°C) in intramuscular temperature have been correlated with changes of 2 to 2.4 ms in conduction velocity. It is advisable to warm a cool limb before examination to stabilize the limb's temperature.

REPORTING THE RESULTS OF THE CLINICAL ELECTROMYOGRAPHY EXAMINATION

The performance of reliable and valid EMG examinations requires extensive experience and expertise with biomedical instrumentation, as well as neuromuscular anatomy and pathology. The material presented here, however brief, is intended to provide sufficient background for the reader to intelligently utilize information from an EMG report and to apply these data to other aspects of patient care specifically related to prognosis, goal setting, and treatment planning. With this in mind, it seems appropriate to review how such reports are presented.

The EMG report is typically found in a patient's chart or medical record. The essential data include (1) the specific muscle or muscles tested, including side of the body and the innervation of these muscles; (2) the response seen during electrode insertion; (3) the response at rest (spontaneous activity, specifying type of potentials or electrical silence); and (4) responses with voluntary contraction (motor unit potentials and recruitment) (Fig. 9-22). The data provided should relate to the five parameters of electrical potentials previously described: amplitude, duration, shape, sound, and frequency.

Reports of nerve conduction measurements should include (1) location of recording and stimulating electrodes, (2) the calculated velocity in meters per second, (3) the distal latency and distance between recording and stimulating electrodes, and (4) the amplitude and duration of the M wave or

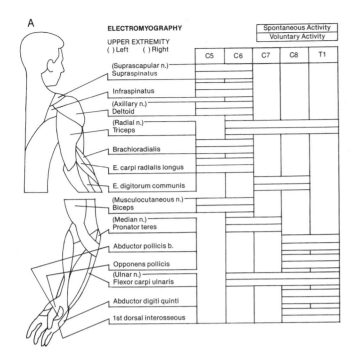

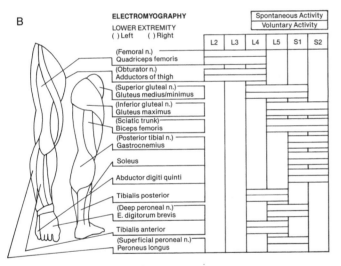

Figure 9-22. Sample report form for EMG. This pictorial form demonstrates the relative position and peripheral nerve and root innervation of the commonly tested upper extremity and lower extremity muscles. Information about spontaneous and voluntary activity can be recorded for each muscle. (From Brumback, RA, et al: Pictorial report form for needle electromyography. Phys Ther 63:224, 1983, with permission.)

evoked sensory potential (Fig. 9-23). Comments should follow the data, stating the impression or implications of findings.

It is extremely important to stress here that diagnoses are not made solely on the basis of EMG data. All other appropriate assessment procedures performed on the patient are used to provide a complete picture of the patient's disorder. These include a history and laboratory tests, as well as physical therapy examinations, such as the manual muscle test,

sensory tests, a range of motion test, pain assessment, and so forth. Electrodiagnostic findings will often provide objective evidence to support clinical observations.

CLINICAL IMPLICATIONS OF ELECTROMYOGRAPHY TESTS

Typical findings with neurogenic or myogenic disorders can be described. The following discussion will focus on selected disorders that typify EMG and NCV results, and their implications for evaluation and treatment planning.

Disorders of the Peripheral Nerve

Electrophysiological findings usually correlate with clinical signs in patients with neuropathic involvement. Some differences exist between types of neuropathies in terms of relative onset of sensory and motor symptoms and nerve conduction changes. EMG findings are usually significant only if axonal damage is a factor. Often electrophysiological changes are seen before clinical manifestations, with sensory nerves being affected before motor; this makes the EMG unremarkable. The sensory NCV test may then provide the most helpful information. Clinicians will find such information useful in following progression or remission of the existing condition.

PERIPHERAL NERVE LESIONS

Lesions of the peripheral nerve fall into three categories: neurapraxia, axonotmesis, and neurotmesis. They may be due to traumatic injury or entrapment. Such disorders typically cause weakness and atrophy of all muscles innervated distal to the lesion. Sensory findings often occur first, but may not be as definitive as motor deficits in localizing the site of the lesion. EMG data can assist in the identification and prognosis of such cases.

Neurapraxia

A neurapraxia involves some form of local blockage, which stops or slows conduction across that point in the nerve. Conduction above and below the blockage is usually normal. Compression disorders (e.g., Bell's palsy [facial nerve], Saturday night palsy [radial nerve compression in spiral groove], pressure over the peroneal nerve at the fibula head, carpal tunnel syndrome [median nerve entrapment]) are the most common causes of neurapraxic lesions. NCV tests can detect evidence of demyelinization prior to axonal degeneration, which may occur with long-standing compression. Nerve conduction measurements will usually reveal increased latencies across the compressed area, but normal conduction velocity above and below. In acute conditions with no denervation, the EMG will be

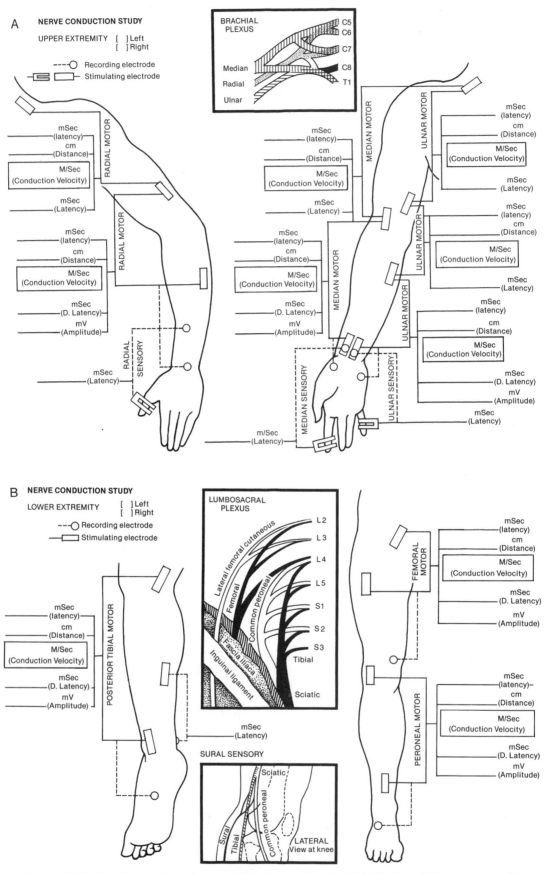

Figure 9-23. Sample report form for nerve conduction studies, containing listings of latencies, electrode distances, potential amplitudes, and calculated conduction velocities, followed by interpretation. Forms for upper and lower extremity show relationship of anatomy to nerve conduction velocity data. (From Brumback, RA, et al: Pictorial report form for nerve conduction studies. Phys Ther 61:1457, 1981, with permission.)

normal at rest. This should be considered a positive prognostic sign. The interference pattern may be decreased or absent if there is severe blockage.

Axonotmesis

With axonotmesis the neural tube is intact, but axonal damage has occurred, with wallerian degeneration distal to the lesion. This may be a progressive condition as a result of long-standing neurapraxia, or it may occur from a traumatic lesion. The deficit in NCV will depend partly on the number of axons affected. If the larger diameter fibers remain intact, the conduction velocity may be normal. However, M-wave amplitude will be decreased because fewer motor units are contracting. Fibrillation potentials and positive sharp waves are typically seen on EMG 2 to 3 weeks after denervation, depending on the distance of the axon from the cell body.

Neurotmesis

Neurotmesis involves total loss of axonal function, with disruption of the neural tube. Conduction ceases below the lesion. A conduction velocity test cannot be performed because no evoked response can be elicited. Recovery is dependent on proper orientation of axons as they regenerate. Spontaneous potentials will appear with the muscle at rest, and no activity is produced with attempted voluntary contraction.

Regeneration of peripheral nerves will be signaled by the presence of small polyphasic potentials (nascent units) with voluntary contraction. These may be seen before clinical recovery is evident through the results of clinical assessments, such as the manual muscle test. After clinical recovery is established, polyphasic potentials may persist, often as giant potentials, due to collateral sprouting. Rehabilitation goals for patients with peripheral nerve injuries can be influenced by results of serial EMG findings. Evidence of regeneration will suggest that motor function is improving and treatment plans should address minimal exercise for the weak and easily fatigued muscles. Positive signs of regeneration will also help in setting realistic outcomes for functional recovery.

POLYNEUROPATHIES

Polyneuropathies typically result in sensory changes, distal weakness, and hyporeflexia. Neuropathies can be related to general medical conditions, such as diabetes, alcoholism, renal disease, or malignancies; they may result from infections, such as leprosy or Guillain-Barré syndrome; and they may be associated with metabolic abnormalities, such as malnutrition or the toxic effects of drugs or chemicals.

Neuropathic conditions may be manifested as axonal damage or demyelination of axons. With axonal lesions, recruitment will be severely affected. A partial interference pattern may be observed with maximal effort, or single motor unit potentials may still be identifiable (Fig. 9-24). The motor unit duration and amplitude may be decreased. Fibrillation potentials, positive sharp waves, and fasciculations are typical (see Fig. 9-14).

With demyelinization, nerve conduction measurements will often provide the most useful data. Sensory fibers are often affected before motor fibers, and significant slowing of sensory conduction velocity may be seen. The evoked potential will typically be reduced in amplitude.

Motor Neuron Disorders

Motor neuron disorders most commonly involve degenerative diseases of the anterior horn cells. These include poliomyelitis, syringomyelia, and some diseases that are characterized by degeneration of both upper and lower motor neurons, such as amyotrophic lateral sclerosis, progressive muscular atrophy, and progressive bulbar palsy. Spinal muscular atrophies are another classification of motor neuron disease. The reader is referred to comprehensive texts to review clinical features of these diseases.

Diseases of the anterior horn cell are classically indicated by fibrillation potentials and positive sharp waves at rest (see Fig. 9-14), and by reduced recruitment with voluntary contraction, due to loss of motor neurons. Newer techniques for estimation of the number of motor units in a muscle have allowed electromyographers to examine the progressive nature of many motor neuron diseases.[60-62]

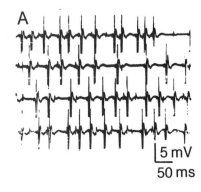

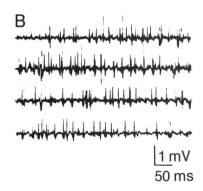

Figure 9-24. Large amplitude, long duration motor unit potentials from the first dorsal interosseus (*A*) compared with relatively normal motor unit potentials from orbicularis oculi (*B*) in a patient with polyneuropathy. Note discrete single unit interference pattern during maximal voluntary contraction. (From Kimura,[19] p 267, with permission.)

Single MUAPs that can still be seen with maximal effort are called a **single motor unit pattern.** Motor NCV may be slowed, depending on the distribution of degeneration among motor fibers, but sensory evoked potentials are unaffected.

Polyphasic motor unit potentials of increased amplitude and duration are often seen later in the course of motor neuron disease (see Fig. 9-15), due to reinnervation and collateral sprouting. This is a typical finding in post-polio syndrome and amyotrophic lateral sclerosis, where enlarged motor units are found in partially denervated muscle.[63,64] Macro EMG has shown signs of reinnervation in these groups,[35,39] although denervation often continues and has been found in affected and supposedly unaffected limbs.[65] Individuals with post-polio syndrome often exhibit functional decline many years after their acute episode. These individuals experience new muscle weakness and atrophy in extremities, bulbar and respiratory muscles, and excessive fatigue. This syndrome appears to manifest when the reinnervation process crosses a critical threshold, whereby remaining neurons cannot support all their muscle fibers.[65]

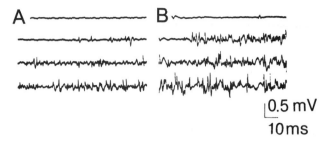

Figure 9-25. Low-amplitude, short-duration motor unit potentials recorded during minimal voluntary contraction from the biceps brachii (*A*) and tibialis anterior (*B*) in a 7-year-old boy with Duchenne's dystrophy. A high number of discharging motor units during minimal contraction reflects early recruitment. (From Kimura, J: Electrodiagnosis of Diseases of Nerve and Muscle: Principles and Practice, ed 2, FA Davis, Philadelphia, 1989, p 268, with permission.)

in documenting the extent of deterioration over time. Electromyography will help delineate the distribution of the involvement, assisting the therapist in focusing treatment and planning adaptations for functional activities.

Myopathies

In primary muscle diseases, such as the dystrophies or polymyositis, the motor unit remains intact, but degeneration of muscle fibers is evident. Therefore, the number of fibers innervated by one axon is diminished. Motor nerve conduction is typically normal, although the amplitude of the M wave will be decreased because fewer fibers are responding to stimulation. Sensory nerve potentials and neuromuscular transmission are normal. In the early stages, the EMG examination shows prolonged insertion activity, perhaps due to the instability of muscle fibers or of the muscle membrane itself. Fibrillations and positive sharp waves are also seen, sometimes with repetitive discharges. Voluntary contraction typically elicits short-duration, low-amplitude polyphasic potentials, reflecting random loss of muscle fibers. Less than maximal effort will require early recruitment, and an interference pattern is evoked because more motor units are needed to create the necessary tension within the muscle (Fig. 9-25). The total amplitude of the interference pattern, however, will be diminished. Use of single-fiber EMG, macro EMG, and motor unit estimation are often used to assess the course of myopathic disease.[21]

In advanced stages of polymyositis and muscular dystrophy, when contractile tissue is replaced by fibrous and other tissues, no electrical potentials may be seen at all. On insertion, the needle will meet some resistance as it enters the fibrotic tissue. Motor nerve conduction measurements will also be impossible under such conditions because no evoked potential can be elicited.

Because most myopathies are progressive, clinicians will find EMG and motor NCV findings helpful

Myotonia

Myotonia is a disorder characterized by delayed relaxation of previously contracted muscle. It results in a pathological muscle stiffness. Myotonia dystrophica exhibits EMG changes typical of myopathy as well. Myotonic disorders do not have a known etiology, although research suggests that a defect in the sarcolemmal membrane causes after-depolarization following activation of the muscle membrane.[66]

As a part of the generalized membrane abnormality, myotonia may result in mildly slowed motor NCV, and a marked reduction in motor unit activity and strength.[67,68] The typical EMG response in myotonia, however, is the persistence of high-frequency repetitive discharges with alternately increasing and decreasing amplitude (see Fig. 9-16). This "waxing and waning" is a distinctive feature, producing the classic "dive-bomber" sound. These trains of potentials can discharge at frequencies up to 150 pulses per second. The **myotonic discharge** follows voluntary contraction or may be provoked by needle insertion or movement. Myotonic symptoms can be abolished or lessened pharmacologically.

Myasthenia Gravis

Myasthenia gravis and myasthenic syndrome are disorders of neuromuscular transmission characterized by weakness following repetitive contractions, and recovery following rest or administration of an anticholinesterase. Myasthenia gravis is thought to be an autoimmune disorder, often associated with other immunological diseases.[19] It is characterized by weakness and excessive fatigability, often confined to ocular muscles, or palatal and pharyngeal muscles.

Myasthenic syndrome often is associated with small cell carcinoma of the bronchus, and is more prevalent in males. Weakness and fatigability primarily affect the lower extremities, particularly the pelvic girdle and thigh muscles.[19]

Myasthenic disorders demonstrate a normal EMG at rest, although fibrillation potentials and positive sharp waves may be present in severely affected muscles, indicating loss of innervation. Motor unit potentials will appear normal at first and then progressively decrease in amplitude with continued effort. Repetitive stimulation during a motor nerve conduction test will cause progressive decreases in the amplitude of the M wave (Fig. 9-26). Pharmacological intervention often will normalize the response.

Radiculopathy

Nerve root involvement, or radiculopathy, is not an uncommon condition at all spinal levels. Electromyography can often assist in identifying this condition, determining the etiology for radiating pain, persistent weakness, hyporeflexia, and fasciculations. Sensory symptoms accompany motor signs, and may range from mild paresthesias to complete loss of sensation.

The fundamental feature in the determination of motor nerve root involvement is the delineation of the distribution of abnormal findings within muscles receiving their peripheral innervation from the same myotome. For example, abnormal potentials seen in the extensor muscles of the hand may suggest involvement of the radial nerve. However, if the biceps brachii is examined (musculocutaneous nerve), as well as the opponens pollicis (median nerve), and these muscles also exhibit some abnormal EMG potentials, the common feature could be considered the C6 nerve root. These findings would have significant implications for treatment planning in terms of addressing the cause of muscle weakness or fatigue.

EMG abnormalities are those typical of neuropathic involvement. Compression of a nerve root can result in irritation or degeneration of nerve fibers. If the lesion is of sufficient severity and duration, the EMG will show increased insertion activity, fibrillation potentials, and positive sharp waves at rest, as well as low-amplitude polyphasic potentials. In later stages, high-amplitude polyphasic potentials may appear, reflecting reinnervation. Polyphasic potentials have been documented within 1 to 3 weeks of the onset of radicular symptoms,[69] perhaps resulting from inflammation, causing activation of two to three motor units that appear as a single potential. Electrodiagnostic examination has shown that patients with cervical or lumbosacral radiculopathy will often have abnormalities in paraspinal muscles as well.[70]

Electromyography is especially valuable in differentiating between disorders of the peripheral nerve trunk and more proximal involvement. It may be more useful than NCV studies, which may not show any remarkable changes at distal segments of these peripheral nerves unless diffuse degeneration has occurred. The F wave and the H reflex have been shown to be clinically useful in the assessment of radiculopathy, independent of clinical EMG.[71] For

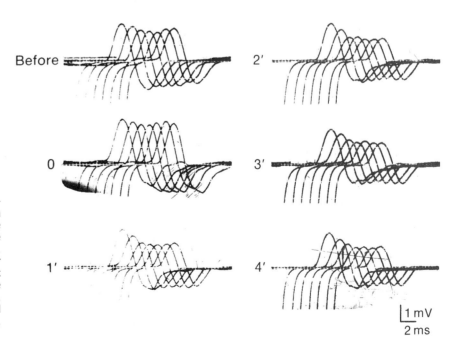

Figure 9-26. Decremental evoked motor responses before and after voluntary exercise in a patient with generalized myasthenia gravis. The median nerve was stimulated at the rate of three shocks per second for seven shocks in each train. The M wave was recorded from the thenar muscles. Comparing the amplitude of the last response with the amplitude of the first, the decrement was 25 percent at rest. (From Kimura, J: Electrodiagnosis of Diseases of Nerve and Muscle: Principles and Practice, ed 2, FA Davis, Philadelphia, 1989, p 191, with permission.)

1 mV

2 ms

example, even with normal distal EMG, if the H reflex is diminished and the F wave is normal, that would be evidence of dorsal root involvement.

KINESIOLOGIC ELECTROMYOGRAPHY

In addition to being a standard method for neuromuscular assessment, surface electromyography can also be used as a kinesiologic tool to examine muscle function during specific, purposeful tasks or therapeutic regimens. For this purpose, the therapist looks at patterns of muscle response, onset, and cessation of activity, muscle fatigue, and the level of muscle response in relation to effort, type of muscle contraction, and position. With the growing need for evidence-based practice, kinesiologic EMG presents an objective means for documenting the effect of treatment on muscle impairments. The therapist should have a basic understanding of kinesiologic EMG to critically assess methods and data analysis procedures in published studies. Many professional journals and societies exist for clinicians and researchers with a common interest centered on the use of EMG for kinesiologic studies.*

While the principles of recording and instrumentation are the same for clinical and kinesiologic EMG, several additional factors must be considered to interpret kinesiologic EMG data.

Surface and Fine-Wire Recording

As described, surface and fine-wire indwelling electrodes are used in kinesiologic study, although surface electrodes are used more. Once a muscle is selected for study, its size and location must be considered in choosing and applying or inserting electrodes. Based on previous discussions of volume conduction and the factors affecting the motor unit potential, the following determinations must be made: (1) electrode size, (2) interelectrode distance, (3) location of electrode sites (including the ground), and (4) skin preparation (for some surface electrodes). There is currently no agreement on the preferred configuration and dimensions of a surface EMG electrode, although researchers have attempted to promote standardization.[17,72,73]

Smaller muscles obviously require the use of smaller electrodes, with a small interelectrode distance. If electrodes are too far apart, even on larger muscles, activity from nearby muscles may be recorded. This cross-talk would confound interpretation of the output by making activity look greater than it actually was. The ground electrode should be located reasonably close to the recording electrodes, preferably on the same side of the body. Skin should be prepared to reduce impedance, although newer amplifiers may have sufficient input impedance to make this unnecessary.

Locating Electrode Sites

Criteria for location of electrode sites are not universally accepted. Fine-wire electrodes should be inserted into the muscle belly using guidelines similar to those used for clinical EMG. For surface electrodes, Basmajian and DeLuca[2] and DeLuca[17] recommend placing the electrodes in the region halfway between the center of the innervation zone and the furthest tendon. Many investigators and clinicians have found it efficient to use palpation for locating surface electrode sites over the muscle belly, if the subject can voluntarily contract the muscle to facilitate this process. However, if repeated measurements are attempted, requiring reapplication of surface electrodes, this method may be unreliable. When electrodes are not oriented to the muscle in the same way with repeated testing, the output will look different, even with identical levels of contraction.

Some investigators have used electrical stimulation of motor points to locate optimal electrode sites. Some have marked the skin with indelible solutions to be able to relocate electrodes. Still others have used body landmarks and measured specific distances to standardize application sites (Fig. 9-27). Basmajian and Blumenstein[74] provide guidelines for placement of surface electrodes for use with biofeedback that can be useful for kinesiologic study as well, but do not adjust locations for variation in body parameters and muscle bulk. Verification of surface electrode placement is usually attempted using manual muscle testing procedures to see if the EMG responds when appropriate resistance is applied. The technique is only partially effective, however, because muscles cannot effectively be isolated.

The distance between electrodes must also be standardized so that repeated EMG analysis is valid. The best way to achieve this is to use electrodes that have their bipolar detection surfaces fixed as a single unit. If interelectrode separation is altered from session to session, the same level of contraction may produce higher or lower amplitude readings, or a different frequency content. DeLuca[17] recommended that the surface EMG electrode be standardized such that electrode centers are separated by 10 mm and detection surfaces are arranged as two parallel "bars" 1 cm long and 1 to 2 mm wide (see Fig. 9-4).

When using surface electrodes, the therapist must also consider problems related to the displacement of skin overlying muscle during movement. The spatial relationship between the electrodes and the muscle can change greatly as a muscle contracts through its range. This will, of course, affect the

---

*The International Society for Electrophysiological Kinesiology maintains a website at <http://shogun.bu.edu/isek/>.

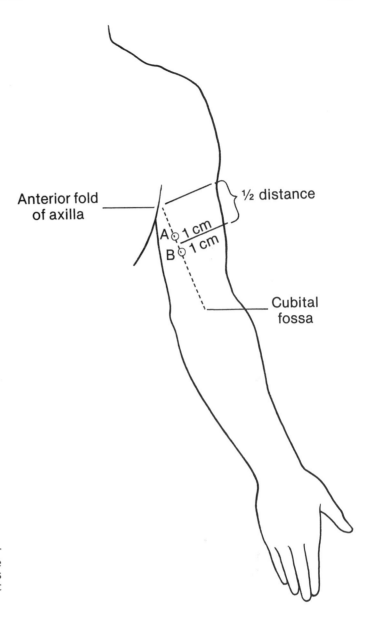

Anterior fold
of axilla

½ distance

A 1 cm
B 1 cm

Cubital
fossa

Figure 9-27. Example of standardized electrode placement for the biceps brachii. A line is drawn from the anterior axillary fold to the center of the cubital fossa, and a point marked at the center of this line. Electrodes are then placed 1 cm above and below this point along this line.

EMG signal. The electrode sites should be determined with this in mind. Such problems are often seen when monitoring the biceps brachii, sternocleidomastoid, or scapula muscles, for instance. Electrodes should be applied to the skin with the limb or body part positioned as it will be during the procedure.

When placement criteria are specified, researchers have shown fairly good test-retest reliability for surface electrodes,[15,75] although submaximal contractions have demonstrated better reproducibility than maximal contractions.[76] Reapplication of indwelling electrodes is less reliable than that of surface electrodes because of the difficulty in consistently placing a needle within muscle tissue on reinsertion.[15,77] Reapplication of surface EMG electrodes on different days or test sessions is also less reliable than when reliability is assessed without removing the electrodes.[78]

Signal Processing

Technology has advanced sufficiently today that microcomputers are now readily applied to the processing of conditioned signals, including integration and display. Personal computers can be easily adapted to interface with EMGs of all types. The EMG signal can be stored, averaged, and sampled in a variety of ways to permit detailed and complete analysis. Digital techniques are becoming more common than analog techniques but they require A-to-D conversion. All analog processing schemes can be replaced by a digital equivalent.

QUANTIFICATION

For clinical EMG, the raw signal is displayed to allow visual examination of the size and shape of individual muscle and nerve potentials. For kinesiologic EMG, however, the therapist is generally interested in looking at overall muscle activity during specific activities, and quantification of the signal is often desired to describe and compare changes in the magnitude and pattern of muscle response.

Rectification and Linear Envelope

The EMG signal can be manipulated electronically in several ways to facilitate quantification, and to eliminate problems of processing raw data (Fig. 9-28). Through a process called **rectification,** both the negative and positive portions of the raw signal appear above the baseline; the signal is then full-wave rectified. The rectified signal can be "smoothed" through low-pass filtering to produce a *linear envelope*, which describes a curve outlining the peaks of the full-wave rectified signal.[18] With the correct type of filter and cut-off frequency, the linear envelope profile closely follows muscle tension.[79] Many authors and electronic equipment companies call this an "integrated" signal, but that is a misnomer, because the linear envelope is a moving average of the EMG output over time.

Integration

Another type of signal conditioning is produced through mathematical **integration** of the EMG signal over the time of the contraction. Its units (mV*s) represent the area under the full-wave-rectified signal.[18] The integrated EMG (IEMG) signal is produced either through digital signal processing or through the accumulation of electrical energy on a capacitor, or condensor. IEMG can be processed in several ways (see Fig. 9-28). The simplest method is integration throughout the period of muscular activity. The total accumulated activity can be determined for a series of contractions or a single contraction. The slope of the curve, or ramp, is a direct function of the amount of electrical energy being processed.

Alternatively, the condenser can be set to discharge at predetermined intervals based on time or voltage amplitude. Time intervals can be set so that the capacitor resets to zero on a regular basis, within periods as small as 200 milliseconds or as long as 10 seconds. The height of each peak, or ramp, then represents the accumulated activity over that time interval. Integration can also be based on a preset voltage level. When the condenser reaches this voltage, it resets to zero, without regard to time. If the EMG signal is very weak, the condenser may continue to collect electrical energy for indefinite periods until its discharge threshold is finally reached. The frequency with which the condenser resets is an indication of the level of EMG activity. Each ramp can also be depicted as a pulse, and the frequency of pulses can be counted to determine the level of activity (see Fig. 9-28).

Average EMG

Closely related to the IEMG is the average EMG, which is the time integral of the full-wave-rectified signal divided by the integration period. This parameter provides a single number with which to report the general level of activity of any given muscle over a predetermined time, such as a period of movement. For example, Kellis[80] studied the effect of fatigue on agonist and antagonist EMG patterns at

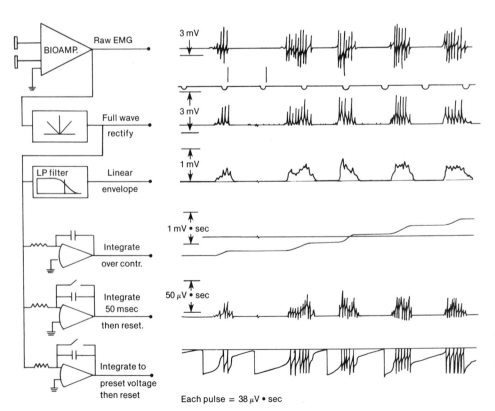

Figure 9-28. Illustration of the raw EMG and several methods of signal processing. The raw EMG was full-wave rectified and expressed as a linear envelope and integrated data. (From Winter, DA: Biomechanics of Human Movement. John Wiley & Sons, New York, 1979, p 140, with permission.)

the knee during 90 degrees of dynamic knee extension. He averaged the EMG within arcs of 10 to 35 degrees, 36 to 55 degrees, and 56 to 80 degrees to characterize differences in EMG at shortened, middle, and lengthened ranges.

Cycle-to-cycle averages of EMG profiles, such as during walking, running, or cycling, can be obtained through ensemble averaging. The full-wave-rectified and linear envelope EMGs are averaged for each cycle, where each cycle is normalized to 100 percent. To illustrate this, MacIntyre and Robinson[81] studied patterns of the quadriceps muscles in female runners diagnosed with patellofemoral pain syndrome. Linear envelope EMGs from vastus medialis, vastus lateralis, and rectus femoris were recorded as each subject ran on a treadmill at 80 percent of their normal running pace. Each stride period was normalized to 100 percent, then the linear envelopes for 10 trials were ensemble averaged to achieve a mean ensemble for each muscle from each subject.

Root-Mean-Square

The root-mean-square (RMS), an electronic average, represents the square root of the average of the squares of the current or voltage over the whole cycle. The RMS provides a nearly instantaneous output of the power of the EMG signal.[18] This EMG parameter is considered by some researchers to be the preferred estimate of muscle tension.[2]

Frequency Parameters

A method of signal processing commonly used to interpret changes in the EMG signal resulting from fatigue or abnormalities in the neuromuscular system is to analyze the *frequency spectrum* of the signal by Fourier analysis. Because any continuous signal can be represented as a summation of sine and cosine waveforms of different frequencies, an interference pattern can be decomposed into its different frequency components. With localized fatigue (i.e., fatigue from within the muscle, rather than central), there is a reduction in the high-frequency components of the spectrum, and an increase in the low-frequency components (Fig. 9-29). This frequency shift may be monitored by tracking a statistical parameter, such as the median frequency. The median frequency is defined as the frequency that divides the frequency spectrum into two parts of equal area, as illustrated in Fig. 9-29. The *muscle fatigue index* is represented by the decay in the median frequency during a sustained contraction.

Timing of Muscle Activity

A number of different computer-based analysis procedures have been described for quantifying latencies and amplitude of EMG signals during purposeful activities. The timing of a muscle's response is often of interest to determine the latency of responses between different muscles, or relative to some other parameter (e.g., the command to

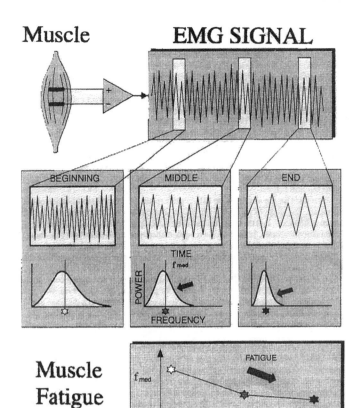

Figure 9-29. Diagrammatic explanation of the change to the EMG signal and its frequency spectrum that occurs as a result of localized fatigue. The upper panel represents the EMG signal sampled at the beginning, middle, and end of a sustained contraction. Each sample "window" of data is analyzed to calculate the frequency spectrum, as illustrated by the POWER vs. FREQUENCY plot in the center panel. The median frequency, or midpoint of the spectrum, is indicated as a vertical line and star in each of the three figures. These three median frequency data points are plotted as a function of contraction time in the lower panel. The Muscle Fatigue Index is represented by the decay in EMG median frequency. (From DeLuca, CJ: The use of surface electromyography in biomechanics. J Appl Biomech 13:135, 1997, with permission).

move) or specific task components. Measurement of EMG onset to assess muscle activation time requires knowledge of the amount of noise present. An epoch of noise must be recorded before the EMG signal is activated to estimate the noise level. Figure 9-30 provides an example of EMG signal activation for a slowly increasing isometric contraction.[17] The top trace represents the raw EMG signal and the bottom trace the RMS value. The amplitude of the noise has been represented by the shaded area in the lower RMS time plot. This area was calculated as ±2 standard deviations of the mean value, thus capturing approximately 95 percent of the amplitude of the noise signal. The raw signal is not sufficient to mark a clear differentiation between noise and EMG. Using the RMS value, however, the specific time at which the EMG signal exceeds this noise level for a minimally defined amount of time (e.g., at least 20 ms) can be determined. This can be considered the "on" time of the muscle, indicated as t_0 in Fig. 9-30.[17]

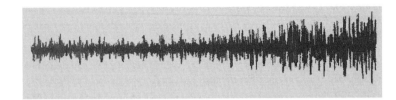

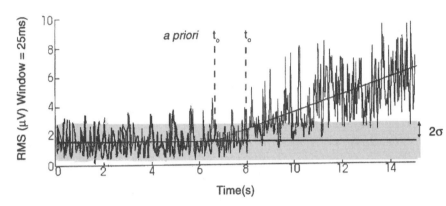

Figure 9-30. Example of background noise before initiation of EMG signal activation (t_0) from the erector spinae muscles during slowly increasing isometric extension of the trunk. The raw EMG signal is presented in the upper trace. The shaded area in the lower trace represents ±2 standard deviations from the average RMS before initiation at t_0. Muscle initiation is identified as the time when the RMS signal exceeds a threshold of 2 standard deviations of the background signal. (Adapted from DeLuca, CJ: The use of surface electromyography in biomechanics. J Appl Biomech 13:135, 1997, with permission.)

This differentiation is essential to an accurate appraisal of EMG activity.

Normalization

For many studies, the quantified EMG signal is used to compare activity between sessions, muscles, or subjects. Because of the variability inherent in the EMG signal, and interindividual differences in anatomy and movement, however, it is not reasonable to compare the EMG activity of one muscle to another, or from one person to another. Therefore, some form of **normalization** is necessary to validate these comparisons. This is usually done by first recording the EMG of a muscle during a maximal voluntary isometric contraction (MVIC), or some known submaximal level of contraction, and then expressing all other EMG values as a percentage of this contraction. This *control value* serves as a standard against which all comparisons can be made, even if test values exceed the control. In this way subjects and muscles can be compared, and activity on different days can be correlated by repeating the control contraction at each test session. This helps eliminate some of the problems related to reapplication of electrodes as well.

Other methods of normalization have included using a series of submaximal contractions,[82] contractions during defined reference tasks,[83] or one of the tasks being tested.[84] Although no standard method has been developed for this normalization, most investigators use MMT positions, resisting isometric contractions either manually or against some fixed resistance. In a comparison of various normalization methods, Knutson et al.[85] found that an MVIC provided the greatest reproducibility.

When using dynamic movements, this issue becomes cloudier. Because the changing muscle length through a movement alters the length-tension rela-

tionships and consequently the EMG activity, a static contraction may not be a reasonable "control" condition when assessing movement. Researchers have shown that measurements of dynamic EMG will vary with different normalization procedures, suggesting that it is more appropriate to normalize EMG activity over specific arcs of movement.[86] For example, investigators have looked at maximal activity through a range of motion, and quantified the EMG within arcs of 10 or 30 degrees. This maximal EMG within each arc is then used as the control value, and EMG measured during the test activity is normalized as a percentage of this value at the same angle.

The Relationship Between Electromyography and Force

The relationship between EMG and muscle tension has been studied since 1952.[87,88] It is generally accepted that a direct relationship exists between EMG and muscular effort, but this relationship must be discussed in terms of muscle length and type of contraction.

Isometric Contractions

Several early studies have demonstrated that when muscles contract while maintaining a constant length, EMG signal amplitude varies directly with muscle tension. Many investigators have documented a linear relationship between muscle tension and IEMG.[88–90] Others have reported curvilinear relationships.[90–92] The linear slope or the degree of nonlinearity seems to vary with the muscle tested, the joint position or muscle length, the electrode placements, and the method of measurement of force.[90,91,93] DeLuca[17] adds that when the detection volume of the electrode is much smaller than the cross-sectional area of the active muscle (e.g., in large muscles), newly recruited motor units located close to the muscle will contribute proportionally greater increases to the EMG signal than to the muscle force. This effect will therefore result in a curvilinear relationship between EMG amplitude and force. Conversely, when the detection area of the electrode is closer to the active cross-sectional area of the muscle, an approximate one-to-one relationship between the EMG amplitude and force will result, thereby producing a linear relationship.

Although methods vary among studies, they all support the general conclusion that an increase in EMG output is observed with increasing muscle tension, as long as the muscle length does not change (i.e., during an isometric contraction). When muscle length is varied, however, this relationship between EMG amplitude and tension does not hold. Generally, less EMG amplitude is seen with greater tension as a muscle is lengthened and, conversely, greater EMG amplitude is seen with decreased tension as a muscle is shortened (Fig. 9-31).[88] Theoretically, therefore, we can assume that fewer motor units are needed to produce the same level of tension in the lengthened position.

If it is impossible for the investigator to constrain the test contractions to isometric conditions, EMG signal processing for estimation of muscle force should be limited to portions of the activity that are near isometric. Furthermore, if the anisometric activity is cyclical, such as during gait or cycling, then a fixed epoch in the period of the contraction should be chosen for analysis, and all comparisons should be made for this epoch.[17]

ISOTONIC CONTRACTIONS

The relationship between EMG and force is further confounded during isotonic contractions, which are defined as contractions producing average constant force or torque.[18] When muscle length continually changes during movement, several factors must be considered. The force-length relationship of the muscle varies throughout the contraction, thereby constantly altering the motor unit activity in proportion to tension. The axis of rotation of the joint changes as the limb moves through its range, so as to change the moment arm and resulting force components. The movement of the skin over the muscle and the variation in shape of the muscle as it contracts will also affect the spatial relationship between the electrodes and muscle fibers, and change the amount of electrical activity actually recorded at different muscle lengths. It is difficult, therefore, to validly quantify muscle activity when movement is occurring.

The EMG-force relationship has also been examined in terms of eccentric and concentric contractions. Eccentric, or lengthening, contractions utilize elastic elements and metabolic processes more efficiently than concentric contractions. Therefore, for the same amount of muscle tension, an eccentric

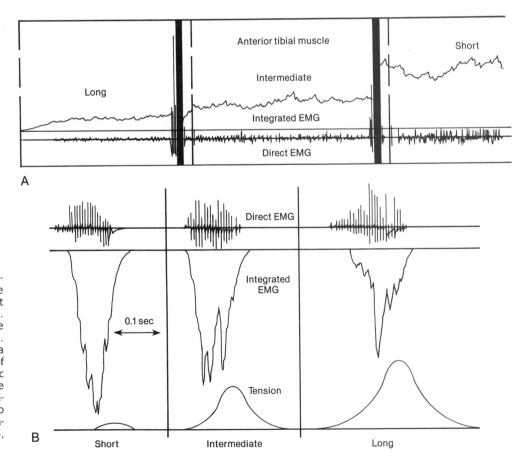

Figure 9-31. (*A*) Maximal voluntary isometric contraction of the anterior tibialis of a normal subject with the muscle at different lengths. Note the rise in EMG activity as the muscle is progressively shortened. The integrated EMG is really a linear envelope. (*B*) EMG activity of the triceps brachii of a cineplastic amputation, illustrating the same effect. (From Inman, VT, et al: Relation of human electromyogram to muscular tension. Electroencephalogr Clin Neurophysiol 4:193, 1952, with permission.)

contraction will require fewer motor units (i.e., less overall EMG activity) than a concentric contraction.

The rate of muscle shortening is another consideration. During eccentric contractions, the level of EMG activity remains constant for a given load, independent of the velocity of the contraction.[94] Concentric EMG activity, on the other hand, is greater for a given force as velocity is increased, and probably reflects a need for greater recruitment to accommodate for a faster contraction time. However, only when velocity is kept constant is the EMG proportional to tension.[94] Therefore, with isotonic movement at uncontrolled velocity, the EMG signal will not be a direct reflection of muscle tension. This is an important point when we consider clinical applications of EMG signals.

MUSCLE FATIGUE

When a muscle exhibits localized fatigue after a sustained contraction, one might expect to see a decrease in overall EMG output. The opposite is generally observed, however. Typically, an increase in EMG amplitude is seen as a muscle fatigues. In an attempt to maintain the level of active tension in the muscle, additional motor units are recruited, and active motor units fire at increasing rates to compensate for the decreased force of contraction of the fatigued fibers. After maximal contraction, when the entire motor unit pool is supposedly recruited, force declines and EMG amplitude stays constant and eventually declines. The presence of constant EMG amplitude suggests that the maximal number of motor units is still contracting. Eventually, however, as the contraction continues, the contractile elements within the muscle will fail and EMG activity will simultaneously start to decrease. EMG indications of fatigue can occur very quickly, within the first several seconds of both submaximal and maximal contractions.

Researchers have observed both linear[89,91] and nonlinear[90,95] EMG-force relationships during fatiguing contractions. The slope of this relationship varies with the degree of fatigue. Studies have also demonstrated a relationship between predominance of fiber type within a muscle and its EMG fatigue characteristics.[90] Muscles composed of primarily type I (slow-twitch) fibers fatigue at a slower rate and demonstrate only small increases in EMG signal amplitude.

FREQUENCY ANALYSIS

EMG evidence of local muscle fatigue may also be quantified by frequency analysis of the EMG signal during constant-force isometric contractions. It has been proposed that spectral indices of fatigue are a more direct representation of localized fatigue than amplitude parameters.[2,96] The spectral modification to the signal appears as compression toward lower frequencies is accompanied by a skewing of the power density spectrum. Essentially, the high-frequency components of the signal are diminished and there is a gradual increase in the low-frequency components of the spectrum.[96]

Using shifts in EMG median frequency to determine whether a muscle is exhibiting local fatigue has at least two advantages over mechanical indices of fatigue: (1) it provides a noninvasive, muscle-specific measure of fatigue; and (2) spectral EMG indices of fatigue change continuously from the initiation of a sustained contraction and do not require the subject to expend considerable effort for long periods of time.

Researchers have been able to document muscle fatigue during specific tasks using this technique.[97–101] By measuring frequency shifts in the electrical potentials of an impaired muscle during treatment, a therapist can determine whether the muscle is being sufficiently exercised.[2,96,102] If the frequency spectrum does not change over time, then synergists may be responsible for the force being generated, rather than the involved muscle. If a decrease in the frequency is seen at first, and the frequency then abruptly levels off without a decrease in output force, the involved muscle may have stopped participating, and other muscles may have taken over to generate the force. Such a technique could be helpful in discriminating which muscles are truly contributing the force output that is measured over a joint. Of course, appropriate instrumentation for recording and analysis must be available. These types of data will not be analyzed with conventional EMG units or biofeedback devices. More and more commercially available EMG systems, however, include spectral analysis as a component of their analysis software.

ELECTROMYOGRAPHY AND STRENGTH

The above factors are of great significance for interpreting EMG amplitude during activities that require muscles to operate at different lengths or speeds, or that utilize different types of contractions. Those who use EMG signals to study muscle function during activities are often tempted to make statements regarding the muscle's "strength." Although this term is used clinically, it must be used with caution. Strength is a construct that must be defined as torque or force produced under a specific set of conditions. Clinicians must be very careful, therefore, about concluding that a muscle is "working harder" or that a muscle is "stronger" just because the EMG activity is greater. Within a single session, when electrode positions remain constant, the position of the limb, the type of contraction, and the speed of movement will affect the level of EMG activity recorded.

The significance of these factors becomes apparent when comparisons are made between isometric exercises performed at different joint angles. The recorded EMG activity from a single muscle positioned at different points in the range may have varied amplitudes, but may in fact represent contractions of similar tension levels. Therefore, the EMG, which records motor unit activity, must be distinguished from muscle tension, which is a function of contractile processes. Therapists often use the term "optimal" to describe a biomechanically advantageous position for a muscle; however, EMG could be lower at this optimal position because fewer motor units are required to create a given level of force. Greater EMG activity may actually indicate that a muscle's efficiency is decreased.

Therapists should also be cognizant of the fact that EMG can record activity of individual muscles, whereas the force or torque measured across a joint may represent the resultant interaction of agonists, antagonists, and synergists. Adjacent muscles make differential contributions to the strength, stability, and coordination of a contraction. The EMG signals from the agonists may not necessarily be a valid representation of activity around a joint. Therefore, EMG data cannot be expected to provide direct information about an individual muscle's "strength."

MUSCLE TONE

Therapists must also resist the temptation to make inferences about muscle tone based on EMG activity. Normal muscle "tonus" refers to resting tension within a muscle due to the elastic and viscoelastic properties of muscle fibers. Tone also reflects the level of gamma input to the muscle spindle, or readiness of a muscle to contract. Essential to a definition of tone is the fact that even though a relaxed muscle shows no electrical activity on EMG, it still maintains a passive state of tone. Therefore, tone is not a function of motor unit activity, and cannot be measured with EMG. This means that when the term spasticity is used to indicate a state of hypertonia, it actually refers to the potential for an overactive muscle response to a stimulus, and not motor unit activity per se. Just as in a normal muscle at rest, a "relaxed" spastic muscle will exhibit electrical silence. This is true of the rigid muscles of patients with parkinsonism as well.[103]

MOVEMENT PATTERNS

Kinesiologic electromyography helps us interpret the role of muscles in various movements, specifically related to amplitude, timing, and changes in the power spectrum. When used in combination with biomechanical measures (e.g., force or torque instrumentation, three-dimensional motion analysis systems, foot switches, electrogoniometers, video), these studies provide a rich understanding of muscle function. With an appreciation for the concepts of recording and of the limitations of interpretation previously discussed, the therapist will find EMG a valuable clinical tool to help validate intervention.

It is impossible to provide a comprehensive review of these applications; however, it is useful to consider some examples to illustrate the utility and limitations of EMG methodology.

EMG and Exercise

MOTOR LEARNING

EMG has been used to assess changes in motor unit recruitment patterns with skill acquisition and coordination. Studies in motor learning have looked at EMG activity over time to determine how muscle activity changes as skill improves. Researchers have shown changes in premovement electrical activity, in sequential firing of various muscles, and other myotemporal variations with motor learning.[104,105] Bernardi et al.[106] examined the median frequency power spectrum recorded from biceps and triceps as subjects learned to control levels of force during elbow flexion. They found that repeated functional use of the muscle resulted in slower, prolonged recruitment of motor units in the agonist muscle, allowing a more precise and accurate control of force increments. The authors suggested that these findings have significant implications for rehabilitation, reinforcing the concepts of plasticity of motor unit control according to the functional demands imposed on the muscle.[107]

PRINCIPLES OF EXERCISE

Many exercise principles are based on anatomical and biomechanical considerations, providing the foundation for assumptions that guide our choices of interventions. EMG data allow us to determine whether these assumptions should be supported. For example, the concepts of co-contraction and joint stability are often applied to specific exercises. Santello and McDonagh[108] documented co-contraction of ankle musculature during jumps from different heights, suggesting that this pattern was responsible for increasing ankle joint stiffness as fall height was increased. Hefzy et al.[109] saw co-contraction with hamstrings and quadriceps muscles during a maximal lunge activity.

Therapeutic concepts such as co-contraction must be operationally defined, however. For example, Isear et al.[110] looked at quadriceps and hamstring muscles during an unloaded squat in healthy individuals, measuring EMG during 30-degree arcs through the range. They found minimal hamstring activity (4–12% MVIC) as compared to quadriceps activity (22–68% MVIC). They suggested that the low hamstring activity reflected low demand placed on the hamstrings to counteract anterior shear forces acting on the proximal tibia. So is this co-contraction? How much activity must be present in a group of muscles around a joint for "co-contraction" to be present? Must all the muscles be equally active? Other important considerations for this question include the difficulty in interpreting EMG when the force of the antagonist is not measurable, velocity of movement is variable, position changes, and cross-talk may be evident.[111]

Consideration of concepts of muscle function must include a discussion about the roles of agonist and antagonist. Is a muscle an antagonist by virtue of being attached on the opposite side of a joint, or is it defined by its action? Can a muscle normally considered an antagonist be a synergist? These questions cause us to consider aspects of motor control that are not clearly understood. For instance, in a study of triceps brachii activation during elbow flexion and extension, Garland et al.[112] showed that the same motor units were activated whether the muscle was functioning as an agonist or antagonist, controlling both acceleration and deceleration of the movement.

The closed-chain exercise is another concept that has been used to reinforce the application of increased weight bearing and facilitation of co-contraction around a joint. In 1993, Lutz et al.[113] demonstrated that a closed kinetic chain exercise produced significantly greater compression forces at the knee with muscle co-contraction, compared to open-chain activities at similar angles, which produced maximal shear forces and minimal co-contraction. These benefits have been supported in other investigations as well. For example, in a comparison of the squat, leg press, and open knee extension, Escamilla et al.[114] found that the squat generated approximately twice as much hamstring activity as the leg press and knee extensions. Quadriceps muscle activity was greatest in the closed-chain activity when the knee was near full flexion, and in the open-chain activity when the knee was near full extension. The open-chain movement produced more rectus femoris activity, whereas the closed chain produced more vasti muscle activity. The authors suggest that an understanding of these results can help in choosing appropriate exercises for rehabilitation and training.

In a study of patients with patellofemoral dysfunction, improvements in peak torque were observed in patients who had performed either open- or closed-chain exercises, but only the closed-chain group showed significant improvement in functional status.[115] An important contrast to these findings was demonstrated in a study of upper extremity tasks, where no difference in EMG was found between open- and closed-chain activities, suggesting that load was more of an issue in determining muscle activity than the boundary of the task.[116] This type of conflict illustrates the need to consider specific measurement methods and activities before generalizations are drawn.

Proximal stability is also an issue that lends itself readily to EMG investigation. For instance, researchers have looked at synergistic shoulder activity elicited during maximal hand grip. Sporrong et al.[117] examined four shoulder muscles—the supraspinatus, infraspinatus, the middle portion of the deltoid, and the descending part of the trapezius—with EMG in adducted and flexed arm positions in healthy subjects. They demonstrated that shoulder activity was greatest with the arm elevated during grip, suggesting that the stabilizing function of the shoulder was an important consideration during manual tasks. In another example, Krebs et al.[118] examined EMG activity during gait with and without a cane in an 85 year-old man with a left-instrumented femoral head prosthesis. They found highest acetabular contact pressures at the postero-superior acetabulum, just prior to peak EMG, during late stance phase. Their data identified a small area of high acetabular and femoral head stress during gait, and suggested that muscle activity, rather than solely body weight, drives hip loading. Therefore, therapeutic goals to limit hip loads should include reduction in both hip muscle contraction and weight-bearing in late stance.

Neuromuscular Dysfunction

EMG has also been a useful adjunct for investigating elements of motor control in patients who have experienced neuromuscular dysfunction. For example, many researchers have compared motor activity in patients with hemiplegia and control subjects, with varying results. Levin and Hui-Chan[119] studied the co-contraction ratio between plantar and dorsiflexors, and found an inverse correlation with force in paretic dorsiflexors. They also established that the EMG output was reproducible over time, suggesting that this type of assessment could be useful for tracking change with treatment.

Gowland et al.[120] looked at upper extremity tasks in patients with hemiplegia, and found that the inability to perform these tasks was due to inadequate recruitment of the agonist muscle, not increased activity of the antagonist. A similar outcome was obtained in a study of knee EMG during isometric and isokinetic exercises, where co-contraction was low or absent, and was similar for patients and control subjects.[121] These findings support aiming treatment at improving recruitment of the agonist, rather than concentrating on inhibition of the antagonist. A contradictory finding was obtained in a study of isometric wrist extension and flexion, where researchers found increased antagonist activity with decreased agonist activity in the paretic arm, concluding that intervention should address decreasing antagonist activity. Once again, we must be cautious in drawing any generalizations. Perhaps the most important message these findings provide is the need to attend to potential methodological and physiological differences that might account for conflicting results. As with any other research method, the consumer must consider the samples studied, the instrumentation used, the muscles selected, and the operational definitions of the activities, to determine whether direct comparisons are warranted.

Pain-Related Muscle Impairments

Clinical research has demonstrated the usefulness of incorporating EMG parameters, such as activation time, amplitude, and median frequency, into a classification scheme for musculoskeletal pain disorders. By understanding the interaction between pain and motor performance, clinicians can directly address motor impairments that will impact function. For example, Madeliene et al.[122] examined mechanisms leading to chronic neck and shoulder pain during upper extremity activities. They found shifts in patterns of muscle synergy and higher EMG frequency components, suggesting altered motor unit recruitment with painful conditions. Wadsworth and Bullock-Saxton[123] studied competitive swimmers, comparing those with unilateral shoulder injuries and noninjured athletes, to determine differences in shoulder EMG patterns with pathology. They demonstrated significant variation or delays in muscle activation with injury, indicating that temporal recruitment patterns are related to injury of the scapular rotators, interfering with consistency of movement. They were also able to identify muscle function deficits on the unaffected side. These outcomes suggest intervention strategies that focus on functional tasks, and the need to examine the effect of injury on other joints as part of these tasks.

Patellofemoral pain has also been a major topic of interest for EMG researchers. Questions regarding the most effective exercises, or the role of various knee muscles during functional activities, lend themselves to EMG study. Many clinical approaches to this problem have focused on the ratio of activity between the vastus medialis oblique and vastus lateralis. Interestingly, in studies of isometric exercises (even with hip adduction),[124] sitting and standing,[125] weight-bearing and non-weight-bearing activities,[126] and running,[81] several researchers have found no difference between symptomatic and nonsymptomatic subjects. Clinicians have also tried to document the effect of specific interventions for improving knee strength. For instance, Werner et al.[127] studied the effects of taping on patients with patellar hypermobility, and found significant increases in knee extensor torque after taping. In terms of general exercise positions, studies have shown us that the vastus medialis is more active during a quadriceps setting exercise than during a straight leg raise in subjects with healthy and painful knees.[128,129] These data provide a useful guide for making intervention choices.

EMG research has been used extensively to study paraspinal muscle impairment in patients with low back pain.[99,102] Declines in mean and median frequency have been identified in those with chronic low back pain, indicative of increased fatigability.[130–132] These same parameters have been used to establish the success of exercise programs as well.[133] Functional assessments, such as gait, have also demonstrated differences in those with low back pain, including greater lumbar muscle activity during swing, as compared to normals, in whom these muscles are relatively silent.[134] Researchers have suggested that EMG changes during gait may be interpreted as a functional adaptation to muscle pain, although the consequences of these altered muscle patterns are not known.

SUMMARY

Electromyography provides a powerful tool for documenting the role of muscle in physical activity, and for assessing the integrity of the neuromuscular system. Despite its common use in movement research, however, therapists must use EMG wisely, recognizing its limitations as a measurement tool. Interpretation of EMG must account for the effect of velocity and acceleration, type of muscle contraction, instrumentation, and a host of anatomical, physiological, and neurogenic factors that can influence the output signal.[6] Electromyography can show that a muscle is working, but not why it is working, and it can only be interpreted as a measure of motor unit activity. Electromyography cannot determine that a treatment is "effective" in the sense of achieving predicted functional outcomes. Electromyography by itself cannot provide information as to whether a muscle has gotten stronger or weaker, or if it is hypertonic or hypotonic. Under most circumstances, with repeated testing over short time periods, small changes will be hard to assess. These must be determined through clinical assessment. But the EMG can provide information that may increase efficacy during treatment or assessment. It is a form of feedback for the therapist that can be invaluable in situations where overt movement or muscle contraction is not observable.

Kinesiologic literature abounds with studies concerning the use of EMG to examine muscle function under different conditions.[2] Therapists should be familiar with this body of literature in order to interpret and utilize EMG data. These studies can also be used as guides for setting up EMG as part of treatment plans. One must be critical of EMG studies, however, because many of them demonstrate methodological faults that can invalidate findings. In addition, the results of EMG studies may not always be generalized to a specific patient, and should not be considered the "correct" responses in all cases. Obviously, the therapist's clinical judgment must prevail when observing responses of individual patients.

The clinician is encouraged to explore the uses of EMG in any situation where response of superficial muscles is of interest. As long as the limitations of interpretation of EMG are kept in mind, this tool can be a major adjunct to therapeutic intervention and assessment.

QUESTIONS FOR REVIEW

1. What are the basic components of a recording system for EMG and NCV tests?

2. What are the stages in a clinical EMG examination?

3. Describe how motor and sensory nerve conduction velocities are calculated.

4. What are the typical EMG and NCV findings with peripheral nerve lesions, myopathy, and motor neuron disease?

5. What are the possible causes of movement artifact? How can these effects be reduced or eliminated?

6. Describe four types of signal processing for EMG.

7. What is the effect of changing muscle length on the relationship between EMG and force?

8. What types of changes are seen in the EMG signal when a muscle fatigues?

9. Assume you are including EMG to monitor muscle response as a component of a treatment program. What considerations are important for setting up your procedure in terms of:
    A. Choice and placement of electrodes?
    B. Type of contractions?
    C. Patient position?
    D. Timing of activities?
    E. How the EMG will be interpreted?

CASE STUDY

It is widely recognized that muscle dysfunction can result from direct neuromuscular injury, pain, or disuse. Some muscles may compensate for this deficit, resulting in a relative alteration in their EMG activity during sustained tasks that cause localized fatigue. A case report is described to provide an example of how surface EMG signal measurements were used to assess paraspinal muscle impairment in a patient with low back pain (LBP).

PATIENT DESCRIPTION: The patient, a 36 year-old male with subacute, nonspecific lower back pain (LBP), was initially examined by his general practitioner and was treated with rest for several days, a home program of stretching exercise, cold packs as needed, and a prescription for a nonsteroidal anti-inflammatory drug (NSAID). The patient was in otherwise good health with no history of neurological disorders or serious musculoskeletal injuries. The onset of his back pain symptoms occurred 6 weeks before the EMG assessment. The patient did not associate this episode of LBP with a specific triggering event, but described that he has had LBP off and on for more than 8 years. Previous examinations using radiographic imaging procedures have been unremarkable. At the time of his EMG assessment, which was conducted as part of a clinical research study, the patient reported pain symptoms bilaterally in the lower lumbar region and upper buttock area which was most severe on arising in the morning or while standing. At the time of the EMG assessment, the patient completed a self-report of pain intensity (6/10 using the Visual Analog Scale) and pain-related function (38% using the Oswestry Disability Scale[135]).

MEASUREMENT PROCEDURE: A surface EMG-based dynamometer, referred to as the Back Analysis System (BAS), was used to acquire and process the surface EMG signals. The technique is described in detail in previous reports,[136] and is based on monitoring the change in fatigue indices from EMG signals acquired simultaneously from a lumbar electrode array during a sustained isometric extension of the trunk. The efficacy of the technique has been described in recent review articles[99,102] and in specific research publications in which the BAS was used to monitor treatment progression in patients with subacute and chronic LBP undergoing work-hardening rehabilitation,[100] in patients with chronic LBP while in remission,[132] and in competitive rowers with subacute and chronic LBP.[137]

The BAS device, depicted in Fig. 9-32, includes the following key components: (1) an adjustable test frame to maintain static posture and isolate the paraspinal muscles; (2) a torque feedback system to maintain constant muscle force; and (3) an EMG acquisition and processing system designed for near-real-time display of EMG median frequency and RMS. With the patient positioned in the device

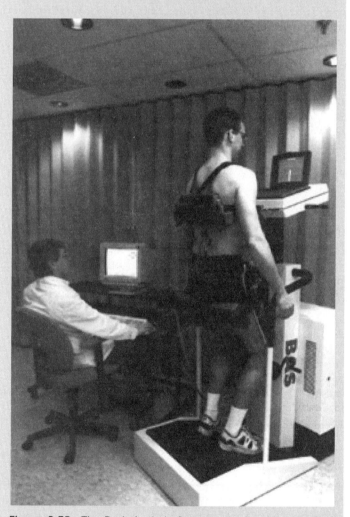

Figure 9-32. The Back Analysis System used for acquiring EMG signals and force during sustained isometric extension of the trunk. A subject is shown positioned in the postural restraint apparatus with six surface EMG electrodes positioned bilaterally on the lower back. The subject's task is to produce a trunk extension torque against the scapular pad according to a target force set on the visual feedback display facing him. The EMG signals are automatically sampled and analyzed from a computer workstation shown in front of the operator. The test results are compared to a database for classification of back muscle impairment. (Courtesy of Neuromuscular Research Center, Boston University, Boston, MA.)

as illustrated in the figure, six active surface EMG electrodes (see Fig. 9-4) were placed at anatomical locations corresponding to contralateral longissimus thoracis (L1 spinal level), iliocostalis lumborum (L2 spinal level), and multifidus (L5 spinal level) muscles. A padded strap, connected at each end to a noncompliant force transducer, was placed across the scapular region for the subject to push against during the test contractions. A monitor was positioned in front of the subject to provide force feedback and a target force level, which was set according to the test protocol.

The test protocol began with a set of warm-up and training exercises in the BAS device. The patient practiced the task of exerting isometric trunk extension at targeted force levels using the feedback display to guide them. After these preliminary trials were successfully completed, the patient was instructed to exert several attempts at producing a maximal voluntary contraction in trunk extension. After a brief rest period, the subject was instructed to follow a "staircase" protocol in which he had to exert a series of sustained isometric trunk extensions in the device at force levels set at 20, 50, 70, and 90 percent of his ideal body weight, respectively. Ideal body was calculated from a weight table established for men and women according to frame size.[138] The use of ideal body weight to standardize the protocol task was adopted to eliminate the confounding effects of subject motivation when previous test contractions were based on the maximal voluntary contraction. Each contraction was sustained for 30 seconds. A rest period of 15 seconds was provided between each contraction.

RESULTS: Using the "staircase" protocol described, results showed altered neuromuscular control of paraspinal muscles for the patient (Fig. 9-33A) as compared to a control subject (Fig. 9-33B) matched for age, sex, ideal body weight, and strength. The results are displayed for the force (lower plot), the EMG median frequency (MF), and the EMG and root mean square (RMS). EMG data from the six electrode sites are plotted separately.

The example demonstrates that despite the ability of the two subjects to produce similar forces,

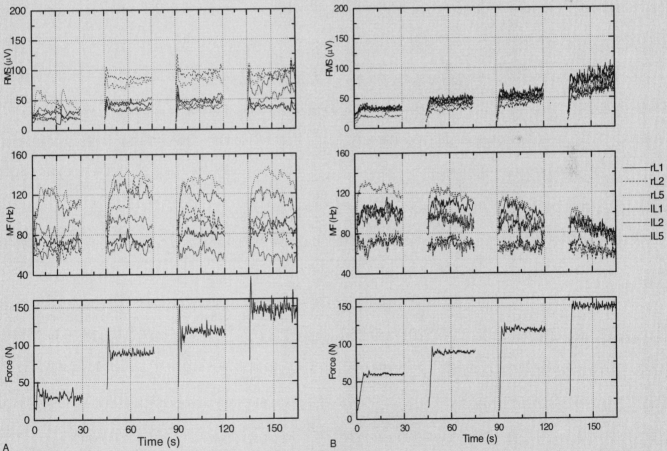

Figure 9-33. Examples of RMS, median frequency (MF) and force data recorded during a "staircase" protocol in the Back Analysis System in (A) a patient with subacute LBP and (B) a control subject without LBP. The staircase protocol requires the subject to sustain a constant-force isometric contraction for progressively higher target force levels. In this instance, the subjects were tested at 20, 50, 70, and 90 percent of their ideal body weight. Each contraction was held for 30 seconds. (From Roy, SH, and Oddsson, LI: Classification of paraspinal muscle impairments by surface electromyography. Phys Ther 78:838, 1998, with permission.)

Continued

there are obvious differences in neuromuscular control and/or muscle fatigability. A consistent pattern of increasing RMS with increasing force was seen in the control subject, whereas in the patient with LBP, the changes in RMS with force were highly variable and asymmetric. Similar results were apparent for the median frequency curves. For the control subject, the MF decreased more rapidly as the force increased, and the pattern was highly symmetric and well ordered in contralateral muscle groups. In contrast, in the patient with LBP, the MF appeared to stay more or less constant for most muscles, decreasing slightly near the end of the contraction at the higher force levels.

SIGNIFICANCE: In this instance, the lack of a gradual, orderly fatigue response in the patient with LBP may represent a characteristic loss of the ability of paraspinal muscles to produce greater forces as needed when external loads or torque is increased. Based on large-scale clinical trials, it has been proposed that these differences in EMG measurements reflect a characteristic signature of pain-related impairments that is likely the result of muscle inhibition and avoidance behavior. The hypothesis for this model of impairment is that in the presence of pain, muscles respond by reducing their level of activity and thereby accommodate a lesser share of the mechanical loads displaced across the joints they support. As a result, normal patterns of muscle activity among synergistic muscles become recognizably altered, the so-called favoring of muscle use.

The assessment and treatment of LBP-related impairments have always assumed a common role among physical therapists. Treatment approaches to LBP disorders are based for the most part on reversing and preventing recurrence of the musculoskeletal components to LBP, with the expectation that such change will lead to improved function and reduced disability. Back pain specialists have traditionally relied on a variety of qualitative and quantitative methods to characterize the musculoskeletal integrity of the spinal complex and identify related impairments. Paraspinal muscle impairments have been quantitatively assessed by the use of dynamometers in an attempt to supplement standard clinical assessment procedures and provide greater objectivity. The measurements are based entirely on mechanical output, such as torque, velocity, or displacement of the trunk. Consequently, they share a common flaw: The kinematic and force variables can be cognitively perceived by the subject and purposefully altered in a manner that compromise validity. Therefore maximal physical performance capability cannot be completely isolated from factors related to motivation and secondary gain.

The developers of the BAS propose that muscle performance objectivity is enhanced by specifying that the test be limited to the performance of submaximal, constant-force, isometric contractions in which the duration of the contraction is predetermined.[132] Furthermore, the useful information from the EMG signals is not derived from a single muscle group or a single parameter, but rather is the result of the concurrent behavior or mapping of many coactive muscle groups. It is assumed that the subject is likely to be unaware of, and cannot volitionally control, parameters derived from such a measurement scheme.

Guiding Questions

1. What do you consider to be the minimal requirements for an assessment procedure to be meaningful?

2. How well does the EMG procedure described in the case satisfy these requirements?

3. Specifically, how would the information derived from the results of the EMG assessment be used to guide therapeutic intervention?

4. How else might this EMG assessment technique be used to describe other kinds of muscle impairments associated with LBP?

REFERENCES

1. Green, RM: Commentary on the Effect of Electricity on Muscular Motion. Elizabeth Licht, Cambridge, 1953.
2. Basmajian, JV, and DeLuca, CJ: Muscles Alive, ed 2. Williams & Wilkins, Baltimore, 1985.
3. Soderberg, GL: Selected Topics in Surface Electromyography for Use in the Occupational Setting. U.S. Department of Health and Human Services, Public Health Service, Centers for Disease Control, Washington, DC, NIOSH, Publication No. 91-100, 1992.
4. Reucher, H, et al: Spatial filtering of noninvasive multi-electrode EMG: Part I—Introduction to measuring technique and applications. IEEE Trans Biomed Eng 34:98, 1987.
5. Reucher, H, et al: Spatial filtering of noninvasive multielectrode EMG: Part II—Filter performance in theory and modeling. IEEE Trans Biomed Eng 34:106, 1987.
6. Gerleman, DG, and Cook, TM: Instrumentation. In Soderberg, GL (ed): Selected Topics in Surface Electromyography for Use in the Occupational Setting: Expert Perspectives. U.S. Department of Health and Human Services, Public Health Service, Centers for Disease Control, Washington, DC, NIOSH, Publication No. 91-100, 1992, p 44.
7. Basmajian, JV, and Stecko, G: A new bipolar electrode for electromyography. J Appl Physiol 17:849, 1962.
8. Adrian, ED, and Bronk, DW: The discharge of impulses in motor nerve fibers. J Physiol (Lond) 67:119, 1929.
9. Andersson, E, et al: EMG activities of the quadratus lumborum and erector spinae muscles during flexion-relaxation and other motor tasks. Clin Biomech 11:392, 1996.
10. Goodgold, J: Anatomical Correlates of Clinical Electromyography. Williams & Wilkins, Baltimore, 1974.
11. Geiringer, SR: Anatomic Localization for Needle Electromyography. Mosby-Year Book, St. Louis, 1999.
12. Merletti, RM, and Roy, SH: Myoelectric and mechanical manifestations of muscle fatigue in voluntary contractions. J Ortho Sports Phys Ther 24:342, 1996.
13. Merletti, R, et al: Modeling of surface myoelectric signals. Part II: Model based interpretation of EMG signals. IEEE Trans Biomed Engineer 46:7:821, 1999.

14. Lynn, PA, et al: Influences of electrode geometry on bipolar recordings of the surface electromyogram. Med Biol Eng Comput 16:651, 1978.

15. Komi, PV, and Buskirk, ER: Reproducibility of electromyographic measurements with inserted wire electrodes and surface electrodes. Electromyography 10:357, 1970.

16. DeLuca, CJ, and Merletti, R: Surface myoelectric signal cross-talk among muscles of the leg. Electroencephalogr Clin Neurophysiol 69:568, 1988.

17. DeLuca, CJ: The use of surface electromyography in biomechanics. J Appl Biomech 13:135, 1997.

18. Ad Hoc Committee of the International Society of Electrophysiological Kinesiology: Units, Terms and Standards in the Reporting of EMG Research. Department of Medical Research, Rehabilitation Institute of Montreal, Montreal, 1980.

19. Kimura, J: Electrodiagnosis of Diseases of Nerve and Muscle: Principles and Practice, ed 2. FA Davis, Philadelphia, 1989.

20. McGill, KC, and Dorfman, LJ: Automatic decomposition electromyography (ADEMG): Validation and normative data in brachial biceps. Electroencephalogr Clin Neurophysiol 61:453, 1985.

21. Liguori, R, et al: Electromyography in myopathy. Neurophysiol Clin 27:200, 1997.

22. Fuglsang-Frederiksen, A, et al: Electrical muscle activity during a gradual increase in force in patients with neuromuscular diseases. Electroencephalogr Clin Neurophysiol 57:320, 1984.

23. Hausmanowa-Petrusewicz, I, and Kopec, J: EMG parameters changes in the effort pattern at various load in dystrophic muscle. Electromyogr Clin Neurophysiol 24:121, 1984.

24. Terebuh, BM, and Johnson, EW: Electrodiagnosis (EDX) consultation including EMG examination. In Johnson, EW, and Pease, WS (eds): Practical Electromyography. Williams & Wilkins, Baltimore, 1997, p 1.

25. Cruz Martinez, A: Electrophysiological study in hemiparetic patients. Electromyography, motor conduction velocity, and response to repetitive nerve stimulation. Electromyogr Clin Neurophysiol 23:139, 1983.

26. Berman, SA, et al: Injury zone denervation in traumatic quadriplegia in humans. Muscle Nerve 19:701, 1996.

27. Spielholz, NI, et al: Electrophysiological studies in patients with spinal cord lesions. Arch Phys Med Rehabil 53:558, 1972.

28. Brown, WF, and Snow, R: Denervation in hemiplegic muscles. Stroke 21:1700, 1990.

29. Johnson, EW, et al: Sequence of electromyographic abnormalities in stroke syndrome. Arch Phys Med Rehabil 56:468, 1975.

30. Falck, B, and Alaranta, H: Fibrillation potentials, positive sharp waves and fasciculation in the intrinsic muscles of the foot in healthy subjects. J Neurol Neurosurg Psychiatry 46:681, 1983.

31. Wettstein, A: The origin of fasciculations in motoneuron disease. Ann Neurol 5:295, 1979.

32. Wenzel, S, et al: Surface EMG and myosonography in the detection of fasciculations: A comparative study. J Neuroimaging 8:148, 1998.

33. Van der Heijden, A, et al: Fasciculation potentials in foot and leg muscles of healthy young adults. Electroencephalogr Clin Neurophysiol 93:163, 1994.

34. Rodriquez, AA, et al: Electromyographic and neuromuscular variables in post-polio subjects. Arch Phys Med Rehabil 76:989, 1995.

35. Stalberg, E, and Grimby, G: Dynamic electromyography and muscle biopsy changes in a 4-year follow-up: Study of patients with a history of polio. Muscle Nerve 18:699, 1995.

36. Roeleveld, K, et al: Motor unit size estimation of enlarged motor units with surface electromyography. Muscle Nerve 21:878, 1998.

37. Stalberg, E: Needle electromyography. In Johnson, EW, and Pease, WS (eds): Practical Electromyography. Williams & Wilkins, Baltimore, 1997, p 89.

38. Stalberg, E, and Fawcett, PRW: Macro EMG changes in healthy subjects of different ages. J Neurol Neurosurg Psychiatry 45:870, 1982.

39. Luciano, CA, et al: Electrophysiologic and histologic studies in clinically unaffected muscles of patients with prior paralytic poliomyelitis. Muscle Nerve 19:1413, 1996.

40. Hodes, R, et al: The human electromyogram in response to nerve stimulation and the conduction velocity of motor axons. Arch Neurol Psychiatry 60:340, 1948.

41. Dawson, GD, and Scott, JW: The recording of nerve action potentials through the skin in man. J Neurosurg Psychiatry 12:259, 1949.

42. Echternach, JL: Introduction to Electromyography and Nerve Conduction Testing: A Laboratory Manual. SLACK, Thorofare, N.J., 1994.

43. Johnson, EW, and Pease, WS: Practical Electromyography, ed 3. Williams & Wilkins, Baltimore, 1997.

44. AEEE: Guidelines in Electrodiagnostic Medicine. Professional Standard Committee, American Association of Electromyography and Electrodiagnosis, Rochester, MN, 1984.

45. Trojaborg, W: Motor nerve conduction velocities in normal subjects with particular reference to the conduction in proximal and distal segments of median and ulnar nerves. Electroencephalogr Clin Neurophysiol 17:314, 1964.

46. Dawson, GD: The relative excitability and conduction velocity of sensory and motor nerve fibers in man. J Physiol (Lond) 131:436, 1956.

47. Hoffman, P: Uber die beziehungen der sehnen reflexe zur wilkurlichen bewegung und zum tonus. Z Biol 68:351, 1918.

48. Sabbahi, MA, and Khalil, M: Segmental H-reflex studies in upper and lower limbs of patients with radiculopathy. Arch Phys Med Rehabil 71:223, 1990.

49. Sabbahi, MA, and Khalil, M: Segmental H-reflex studies in upper and lower limbs of healthy subjects. Arch Phys Med Rehabil 71:216, 1990.

50. Braddom, RL, and Johnson, EW: Standardization of H-reflex and diagnostic use in S1 radiculopathy. Arch Phys Med Rehabil 55:161, 1974.

51. Abbruzese, M, et al: Changes in central delay of soleus H-reflex after facilitory or inhibitory conditioning in humans. J Neurophysiol 65:1598, 1991.

52. Magladery, JW, and McDougal, JB: Electrophysiological studies of nerve and reflex activity in normal man. I. Identification of certain reflexes in the electromyogram and the conduction velocity of peripheral nerve fibers. Bull Johns Hopkins Hosp 86:265, 1950.

53. Milanov, I, and Georgiev, D: Mechanisms of trizanidine action on spasticity. Acta Neurol Scand 89:274, 1994.

54. Nance, PW: A comparison of clonidine, cyproheptadine and baclofen in spastic spinal cord injured patients. J Am Paraplegic Soc 17:150, 1994.

55. Dumitru, D: Electrodiagnostic Medicine. Hanly Belfus, Philadelphia, 1995, p 191.

56. Gamstorp, I: Normal conduction velocity of ulnar, median and peroneal nerves in infancy, childhood and adolescence. Acta Paediatrica 146(suppl):68, 1963.

57. Buchthal, F, and Rosenfalck, A: Evoked action potentials and conduction velocity in human sensory nerves. Brain Res 3:1, 1966.

58. Norris, AH, et al: Age changes in the maximum conduction velocity of motor fibers of human ulnar nerves. J Appl Physiol 5:589, 1953.

59. Halar, EM, et al: Nerve conduction studies in upper extremities: Skin temperature corrections. Arch Phys Med Rehabil 64:412, 1983.

60. McComas, AJ: Motor-unit estimation: The beginning. J Clin Neurophysiol 12:560, 1995.

61. Daube, JR: Estimating the number of motor units in a muscle. J Clin Neurophysiol 12:585, 1995.

62. Doherty, T, et al: Methods for estimating the numbers of motor units in human muscles. J Clin Neurophysiol 12:565, 1995.

63. McComas, AJ, et al: Early and late losses of motor units after poliomyelitis. Brain 120:1415, 1997.

64. Bromberg, MB, et al: Motor unit number estimation, isometric strength, and electromyographic measures in amyotrophic lateral sclerosis. Muscle Nerve 16:1213, 1993.
65. Dulakas, MC: Pathogenetic mechanisms of post-polio syndrome: morphological, electrophysiological, virological and immunological correlations. Ann NY Acad Sci 753:167, 1995.
66. Rowland, LP: Pathogenesis of muscular dystrophies. Arch Neurol 33:315, 1976.
67. Chisari, C, et al: Sarcolemmal excitability in myotonic dystrophy: Assessment through surface EMG. Muscle Nerve 21:543, 1998.
68. Orizio, C, et al: Muscle surface mechanical and electrical activities in myotonic dystrophy. Electromyogr Clin Neurophysiol 37:231, 1997.
69. Colachis, SC, et al: Polyphasic motor unit action potentials in early radiculopathy: Their presence and ephaptic transmission as an hypothesis. Electromyogr Clin Neurophysiol 32:27, 1992.
70. Czyrny, JJ, and Lawrence, J: The importance of paraspinal muscle EMG in cervical and lumbosacral radiculopathy: Review of 100 cases. Electromyogr Clin Neurophysiol 36:503, 1996.
71. Toyokura, M, et al: Follow-up study on F-wave in patients with lumbosacral radiculopathy. Comparison between before and after surgery. Electromyogr Clin Neurophysiol 36:207, 1996.
72. Hermens, HJ, et al: Applications of Surface ElectroMyography. In Second General SENIAM Workshop, Stockholm, 1997.
73. Hermens, HJ, et al: European Activities on Surface ElectroMyography. In First General SENIAM Workshop, Torino, Italy, 1996.
74. Basmajian, JV, and Blumenstein, R: Electrode Placement for EMG Biofeedback. Williams & Wilkins, Baltimore, 1980.
75. Graham, GP: Reliability of electromyographic measurements after surface electrode removal and replacement. Percept Mot Skills 49:215, 1979.
76. Yang, JF, and Winter, DA: Electromyography reliability in maximal and submaximal isometric contractions. Arch Phys Med Rehabil 64:417, 1983.
77. Kadaba, MP, et al: Repeatability of phasic muscle activity: Performance of surface and intramuscular wire electrodes in gait analysis. J Orthop Res 3:350, 1985.
78. Viitasalo, JH, and Komi, PV: Signal characteristics of EMG with special reference to reproducibility of measurements. Acta Physiol Scand 93:531, 1975.
79. Winter, DA: The Biomechanics and Motor Control of Walking, ed 2. University of Waterloo Press, Waterloo, Canada, 1991.
80. Kellis, E: The effects of fatigue on the resultant joint moment, agonist and antagonist electromyographic activity at different angles during dynamic knee extension efforts. J Electromyogr Kinesiol 9:191, 1999.
81. MacIntyre, DL, and Robertson, DG: Quadriceps muscle activity in women runners with and without patellofemoral pain syndrome. Arch Phys Med Rehabil 73:10, 1992.
82. Perry, J, and Bekey, GA: EMG-force relationships in skeletal muscle. Crit Rev Biomed Eng 7:22, 1981.
83. Winkel, J, and Bendix, T: Muscular performance during seated work evaluated by two different EMG methods. Eur J Appl Physiol 55:167, 1986.
84. Janda, DH, et al: Objective evaluation of grip strength. J Occup Med 29:569, 1987.
85. Knutson, LM, et al: A study of various normalization procedures for within day electromyographic data. J Electromyography Kinesiol 4:47, 1994.
86. Kellis, E, and Baltzopoulos, V: The effects of normalization method on antagonistic activity patterns during eccentric and concentric isokinetic knee extension and flexion. J Electromyogr Kinesiol 6:235, 1996.
87. Lippold, OCJ: The relation between integrated action potentials in a human muscle and its isometric tension. J Physiol (Lond) 117:492, 1952.
88. Inman, VT, et al: Relation of human electromyogram to muscular tension. Electroencephalogr Clin Neurophysiol 4:187, 1952.

89. Edwards, RG, and Lippold, OCJ: The relation between force and integrated electrical activity in fatigued muscle. J Physiol (Lond) 132:677, 1956.
90. Woods, JJ, and Bigland-Ritchie, B: Linear and non-linear surface EMG/force relationships in human muscles. Am J Phys Med Rehabil 62:287, 1983.
91. Vredenbregt, J, and Rau, G: Surface electromyography in relation to force, muscle length and endurance. In Desmedt, JE (ed): New Developments in Electromyography and Clinical Neurophysiology, Vol 1. Karger, BaSEL, 1973, p 606.
92. Zuniga, EN, and Simons, DG: Nonlinear relationship between averaged electromyogram potential and muscle tension in normal subjects. Arch Phys Med Rehabil 50:613, 1983.
93. Lawrence, JH, and DeLuca, CJ: Myoelectric signal vs. force relationship in different human muscles. J Appl Physiol 54:1653, 1983.
94. Bigland, B, and Lippold, OCJ: The relation between force, velocity and integrated electrical activity in human muscles. J Physiol (Lond) 123:214, 1954.
95. Petrofsky, JS, et al: Evaluation of the amplitude and frequency components of the surface EMG as an index of muscle fatigue. Ergonomics 25:213, 1982.
96. DeLuca, CJ: Myoelectrical manifestations of localized muscular fatigue in humans. Crit Rev Biomed Eng 11:251, 1985.
97. Kuorinka, I: Restitution of EMG spectrum after muscular fatigue. Eur J Appl Physiol 57:311, 1988.
98. Huijing, PA, et al: Triceps source EMG spectrum changes during sustained submaximal isometric contractions at different muscle lengths. Electromyogr Clin Neurophysiol 26:181, 1986.
99. Roy, SH, et al: Classification of back muscle impairment based on the surface electromyographic signal. J Rehabil Res Dev 34:405, 1997.
100. Roy, SH, et al: Spectral electromyographic assessment of back muscles in patients with low back pain undergoing rehabilitation. Spine 20:38, 1995.
101. Oddsson, LI, et al: Development of new protocols and analysis procedures for the assessment of LBP by surface EMG techniques. J Rehabil Res Dev 34:415, 1997.
102. Roy, SH, and Oddsson, LI: Classification of paraspinal muscle impairments by surface electromyography. Phys Ther 78:838, 1998.
103. Shimazu, H, et al: Rigidity and spasticity in man: Electromyographic analysis with reference to the role of the globus pallidus. Arch Neurol 6:10, 1962.
104. Vorro, J, and Hobart, D: Kinematic and myoelectric analysis of skill acquisition: I. 90cm subject group. Arch Phys Med Rehabil 62:575, 1981.
105. Hobart, DJ, et al: Modifications occurring during acquisition of a novel throwing task. Am J Phys Med 54:1, 1975.
106. Bernardi, M, et al: Force generation performance and motor unit recruitment strategy in muscles of contralateral limbs. J Electromyogr Kinesiol 9:121, 1999.
107. Bernardi, M, et al: Motor unit recruitment strategy changes with skill acquisition. Eur J Appl Physiol 74:52, 1996.
108. Santello, M, and McDonagh, MJ: The control of timing and amplitude of EMG activity in landing movements in humans. Exp Physiol 83:857, 1998.
109. Hefzy, MS, et al: Co-activation of the hamstrings and quadriceps during the lunge exercise. Biomed Sci Instrum 33:360, 1997.
110. Isear, JA, Jr, et al: EMG analysis of lower extremity muscle recruitment patterns during an unloaded squat. Med Sci Sports Exerc 29:532, 1997.
111. Kellis, E: Quantification of quadriceps and hamstring antagonist activity. Sports Med 25:37, 1998.
112. Garland, SJ, et al: Motor unit activity during human single joint movements. J Neurophysiol 76:1982, 1996.
113. Lutz, GE, et al: Comparison of tibiofemoral joint forces during open-kinetic-chain and closed-kinetic-chain exercises. J Bone Joint Surg Am 75:732, 1993.
114. Escamilla, RF, et al: Biomechanics of the knee during closed kinetic chain and open kinetic chain exercises. Med Sci Sports Exerc 30:556, 1998.

115. Stiene, HA, et al: A comparison of closed kinetic chain and isokinetic joint isolation exercise in patients with patellofemoral dysfunction. J Orthop Sports Phys Ther 24:136, 1996.
116. Blackard, DO, et al: Use of EMG analysis in challenging kinetic chain terminology. Med Sci Sports Exerc 31:443, 1999.
117. Sporrong, H, et al: Hand grip increases shoulder muscle activity: An EMG analysis with static hand contractions in 9 subjects. Acta Orthop Scand 67:485, 1996.
118. Krebs, DE, et al: Hip biomechanics during gait. J Orthop Sports Phys Ther 28:51, 1998.
119. Levin, MF, and Hui-Chan, C: Ankle spasticity is inversely correlated with antagonist voluntary contraction in hemiparetic subjects. Electromyogr Clin Neurophysiol 34:415, 1994.
120. Gowland, C, et al: Agonist and antagonist activity during voluntary upper-limb movement in patients with stroke. Phys Ther 72:624, 1992.
121. Davies, JM, et al: Electrical and mechanical output of the knee muscles during isometric and isokinetic activity in stroke and healthy adults. Disabil Rehabil 18:83, 1996.
122. Madeleine, P, et al: Shoulder muscle co-ordination during chronic and acute experimental neck-shoulder pain. An occupational pain study. Eur J Appl Physiol 79:127, 1999.
123. Wadsworth, DJ, and Bullock-Saxton, JE: Recruitment patterns of the scapular rotator muscles in freestyle swimmers with subacromial impingement. Int J Sports Med 18:618, 1997.
124. Laprade, J, et al: Comparison of five isometric exercises in the recruitment of the vastus medialis oblique in persons with and without patellofemoral pain syndrome. J Orthop Sports Phys Ther 27:197, 1998.
125. Thomee, R, et al: Quadriceps muscle performance in sitting and standing in young women with patellofemoral pain syndrome and young healthy women. Scand J Med Sci Sports 6:233, 1996.
126. Karst, GM, and Willett, GM: Onset timing of electromyographic activity in the vastus medialis oblique and vastus lateralis muscles in subjects with and without patellofemoral pain syndrome. Phys Ther 75:813, 1995.
127. Werner, S, et al: Effect of taping the patella on concentric and eccentric torque and EMG of knee extensor and flexor muscles in patients with patellofemoral pain syndrome. Knee Surg Sports Traumatol Arthrosc 1:169, 1993.
128. Soderberg, GL, and Cook, TM: An electromyographic analysis of quadriceps femoris muscle setting and straight leg raising. Phys Ther 63:1434, 1983.
129. Soderberg, GL, et al: Electromyographic analysis of knee exercises in healthy subjects and in patients with knee pathologies. Phys Ther 67:1691, 1987.
130. Kankaanpaa, M, et al: Back and hip extensor fatigability in chronic low back pain patients and controls. Arch Phys Med Rehabil 79:412, 1998.
131. Mannion, AF, et al: The use of surface EMG power spectral analysis in the evaluation of back muscle function. J Rehabil Res Dev 34:427, 1997.
132. Roy, SH, et al: Lumbar muscle fatigue and chronic lower back pain. Spine 14:992, 1989.
133. Mooney, V, et al: Relationships between myoelectric activity, strength, and MRI of lumbar extensor muscles in back pain patients and normal subjects. J Spinal Disord 10:348, 1997.
134. Arendt-Nielsen, L, et al: The influence of low back pain on muscle activity and coordination during gait: A clinical and experimental study. Pain 64:231, 1996.
135. Fairbank, JC, et al: The Oswestry low back pain disability questionnaire. Physiotherapy 66:271, 1980.
136. DeLuca, CJ: Use of the surface EMG signal for performance evaluation of back muscles. Muscle Nerve 16:210, 1993.
137. Roy, SH, et al: Fatigue, recovery, and low back pain in varsity rowers. Med Sci Sports Exerc 22:463, 1990.
138. Society of Actuaries and Association of Life Insurance Medical Directors of America: Build Study, 1979. New York: Metropolitan Life Insurance Company, 1983.
139. Rothstein, JM, and Echternach, JL: Primer on Measurement: An Introductory Guide to Measurement Issues. American Physical Therapy Association, Washington, DC, 1993, p. 66.
140. Rainville, J, et al: Altering beliefs about pain and impairment in a functionally oriented treatment program for chronic low back pain. Clin J Pain 9:196, 1993.
141. Soderberg, GL, and Cook, TM: Electromyography in biomechanics. Phys Ther 64:1813, 1984.

GLOSSARY

Amplifier: A device used to process an electrical signal, converting it to a voltage output that can be displayed.

  Differential amplifier: An amplifier that processes the voltage difference between two input terminals, effectively rejecting common mode voltages that appear between each input terminal and the common ground.

Amplitude: Of an action potential, the maximum voltage difference between two points, usually measured baseline to peak, or peak to peak; expresses the level of the signal activity.

Anode: The positive terminal of a source of electrical current.

Antidromic conduction: Propagation of an action potential in a direction opposite the normal (orthodromic) direction for that fiber (i.e., conduction along motor fibers toward the spinal cord, and conduction along sensory fibers away from the spinal cord).

Artifacts: Voltage signals generated by a source other than the one of interest.

  Movement artifact: An electrical signal resulting from the movement of the recording electrodes or their cables.

  Stimulus artifact: A potential recorded at the time the stimulus is applied.

Cathode: The negative terminal of a source of electrical current.

Common mode rejection ratio (CMRR): A ratio expressing an amplifier's ability to reject unwanted noise while amplifying the wanted signal, for example, a ratio of 1000:1 indicates the wanted signal will be amplified 1000 times more than noise, can also be expressed in decibels (1000:1 equals 60 dB).

Conduction distance: Distance measured (in centimeters) between two points of stimulation along a nerve in a nerve conduction velocity test.

Conduction time: Time difference (in milliseconds) between the distal and proximal latencies in a nerve conduction velocity test (i.e., the time it takes for an impulse to travel between the two points of stimulation along a nerve trunk).

Conduction velocity (CV): Speed of propagation of an action potential along a nerve or muscle fiber. Calculated in meters per second by dividing the conduction distance by the conduction time. The calculated velocity represents the conduction velocity of the fastest axons in the nerve.

Cross-talk: Activity seen at one electrode site that is generated by a muscle other than the one being monitored.

Duration: The duration of an action potential is measured as the interval from the first deflection from the baseline to its final return to the baseline.

Electrical silence: The absence of measurable EMG activity, typically recorded at rest in normal muscles.

Electrode: A device capable of recording electrical potentials or conducting electricity to provide a stimulus.

Active electrode: A bipolar electrode configuration with fixed interelectrode geometry and preamplifiers at the detection site.

Concentric (coaxial) needle electrode: Recording electrode consisting of a steel cannula through which is threaded a single platinum wire that is insulated from the needle shaft. The wire and shaft are bared at the tip, and the potential difference between them is recorded in the presence of electrical activity. The electrode can also be configured with two wires (bipolar) threaded through the cannula, recording the difference of potential between these wires.

Fine-wire indwelling electrodes: Small-diameter insulated wires inserted into the muscle belly by means of a hypodermic needle.

Ground electrode: An electrode connected to a common source, used to reduce the effect of electrical noise in a recording system; an arbitrary zero potential reference point.

Monopolar needle electrode: A solid wire, usually of stainless steel, coated, except at its tip, with insulating material. Voltage is measured between the tip of the needle and some other electrode, usually placed on the skin (reference electrode).

Recording electrode: Needle or surface electrode used to record electrical activity from nerve and muscle.

Reference electrode: In motor nerve conduction velocity test, the electrode placed over the tendon of the test muscle. In monopolar recording of EMG, the inactive electrode placed over a neutral area.

Stimulating electrode: Device used to apply electrical current to stimulate propagation of a nerve impulse or muscle contraction; requires positive (anode) and negative (cathode) terminals.

Surface electrodes: Small metal disks applied to the skin overlying the appropriate muscle and used to monitor EMG signals from large, superficial muscles.

Electromyography: The recording and study of the electrical activity of muscle. It is commonly used to refer to nerve conduction studies as well. The electromyograph is the instrument used to record and display the EMG.

Evoked potential: Waveform elicited by a stimulus.

Fasciculation potentials: Electrical activity characterized by random, spontaneous twitching of a group of muscle fibers which may be visible through the skin. The amplitude, configuration, duration, and frequency are variable.

Fibrillation potentials: Electrical activity associated with fibrillating muscle and reflecting the activity of a single muscle fiber; associated with denervation and myopathy. Classically, these potentials are biphasic spikes of short duration (<5 milliseconds), with a peak-to-peak amplitude less than 1 millivolt, a firing rate ranging from 1 to 50 hertz, and a high-pitched regular sound likened to "rain on the roof."

Frequency: Number of complete cycles of a repetitive waveform in 1 second. Measured in hertz (Hz).

Frequency bandwidth: Frequency response of an amplifier, referring to the limits on the range of signal frequencies processed; for example, 10 to 1000 hertz.

Giant motor units: Motor unit potentials with a peak-to-peak amplitude and duration much greater than normal ranges. Often seen after collateral sprouting with regeneration of peripheral nerves.

Hertz: Unit of frequency representing number of cycles per second.

Input impedance: A form of resistance to current flow in an alternating current circuit. Skin, electrodes, and amplifier input terminals provide sources of impedance to EMG potentials.

Insertion activity: Electrical activity caused by insertion or movement of a needle electrode in a muscle. Can be described as normal, reduced, increased, or prolonged.

Integration: Mathematical processing of a rectified EMG signal that allows quantification. Integration can be performed over set time intervals or within preset voltage threshold levels.

Interference pattern: Electrical activity, recorded from a muscle during maximal voluntary effort, in which identification of each of the contributing motor unit potentials is not possible.

Latency: In nerve conduction velocity tests, the interval between onset of a stimulus and the onset of a response, measured from the stimulus artifact to the onset of the M wave.

Distal latency: The time (in milliseconds) for an action potential to travel from the distal point of stimulation along a nerve to the recording electrode; used in calculating nerve conduction velocity.

Proximal latency: The time (in milliseconds) for an action potential to travel from the proximal point of stimulation along a nerve to the recording electrode; used in calculating nerve conduction velocity.

Motor unit: The anatomical unit of an anterior horn cell, its axon, the neuromuscular junctions, and all the muscle fibers innervated by that axon.

Motor unit action potential: Action potential reflecting the electrical activity of a single motor unit capable of being recorded by an electrode. Characterized by its amplitude, configuration, duration, frequency, and sound.

M wave: A compound action potential evoked from muscle by a single electrical stimulus to its motor nerve.

Myotonic discharge: A high-frequency discharge, characterized by repetitive firing (2080 Hz) of biphasic or monophasic potentials recorded after needle insertion or after voluntary muscle contraction, with a waxing and waning amplitude and frequency and a sound likened to a "dive-bomber."

Nerve conduction velocity (NCV): The speed with which a peripheral motor or sensory nerve conducts an impulse.

Noise: An unwanted electrical signal that is detected along with the desired signal.

Normalization: Use of a reference value for kinesiological EMG to allow for comparison of EMG activity across subjects or muscles.

Orthodromic conduction: Propagation of an action potential in the same direction as physiological conduction (i.e., motor nerve conduction away from the spinal cord and sensory nerve conduction toward the spinal cord).

Oscilloscope: A device for displaying electronic signals on a screen, composed of a cathode ray tube within which horizontal and vertical beams strike a phosphorescent surface, allowing visualization of the signal. Control of the values for vertical and horizontal divisions permits quantification of the amplitude and duration of signals.

Phase: That portion of a wave between the departure from and the return to the baseline.

Polyphasic potentials: Action potentials having five or more phases.

Positive sharp waves: Electrical potentials associated with fibrillating muscle fibers, recorded as a biphasic, positive-negative action potential initiated by needle movement and recurring in uniform patterns. The initial positive phase is of short duration (< 5 ms) and large amplitude (up to 1 mV); the second negative phase is of long duration (10,100 ms) and low amplitude.

Rectification: A process whereby the negative portion of an EMG wave is inverted and superimposed on the positive portion, so that the signal is seen only above the baseline. This allows further processing and integration.

Repetitive discharges: An extended train of potentials, generally 5 to 100 impulses per second, commonly seen in lesions of the anterior horn cell and peripheral nerves, and with some myopathies. Also called bizarre high-frequency discharges.

Sensitivity: Characteristic of a system, expressing its ability to record and display signals of different sizes, usually expressed as a range, for example, 20 microvolts to 30 millivolts.

Signal-to-noise ratio: The relationship (proportion) between the signal power and the power of the noise.

Single motor unit pattern: An interference pattern, recorded at maximal effort, when single motor unit potentials can still be identified.

Skin resistance: The opposition to electrical conduction offered by skin cells and other substances on the skin, usually necessitating some form of skin preparation before application of surface electrodes.

Spontaneous potentials: Action potentials recorded from muscle or nerve at rest after insertional activity has subsided and when there is no voluntary contraction or external stimulus.

Telemetry: Transmission of the EMG signal via radio frequency transmitter and receiver.

Temporal dispersion: Distortion of duration, amplitude, or shape of the M wave potential in a motor nerve conduction velocity test.

Volt: The difference of potential between two points; the unit of measurement for EMG amplitude.

Volume conduction: Spread of current from a potential source through a conducting medium, such as body tissues.

APPENDIX A

Suggested Answers to Case Study Guiding Questions

1. What do you consider to be the minimal requirements for an assessment procedure to be meaningful?

ANSWER: Muscle impairment classification systems should provide a consistent method of identifying the presence of abnormal muscle functioning in a manner that will suggest a form of treatment. Classification systems are typically based on models or procedures that converge toward a particular impairment type based on a single measurement or a group of measurements. The system should, at the very least, provide a reliable method to identify whether a deviation from normality is present on the basis of the measurements considered. It is preferable, however, if the system can also characterize the type of abnormality present as well as provide a measure of confidence for the classification.

For impairment classifications to be meaningful to clinicians, they should describe categories or types of conditions that provide a basis for treatment.[139] Simply assigning measurements to groups "A, B, C, D, . . . n" is of little clinical value, even if these assignments are without error. For instance, it would be of little value to a physical therapist to know only that the EMG spectral parameters from a test of their patients' back muscles was not assignable to a "normal" classification; it would be more helpful if a specific classification of impairment were made, such as muscle inhibition consistent with a pain-related behavior. This example of impairment classification would suggest a specific method of treatment.

2. How well does the EMG procedure described in the case satisfy these requirements?

ANSWER: As described in the results of the case, it can be argued that the EMG signals can be analyzed in a manner that describes a specific kind of muscle impairment. More importantly, the type of impairment is suggestive of a treatment approach that would, for instance, take into consider-ation that the patient must overcome his or her inhibition or avoidance of back muscle use. Therapeutic exercise should therefore incorporate methods to relearn the proper coordinated use of muscles when performing tasks involving sustained extension of the trunk. Comprehensive functionally oriented treatment programs for chronic low back pain have been proposed that include altering beliefs about pain and impairment.[140] The results as presented did not include a procedure for quantifying the degree of impairment or probability of misclassification. Statistical methods have been derived to realize this capability on the basis of discriminant analysis procedures.[102]

3. Specifically, how would the information derived from the results of the EMG assessment be used to guide therapeutic intervention?

ANSWER: The possible relevance of this impairment to LBP injury, treatment, and prevention are two-fold: (a) pain-related behaviors characterized by unreasonable fear and avoidance of activity is considered to be a significant source of disability among some patients with LBP; and (b) alterations in muscle activation during tasks which significantly load the spine may lead to overuse injuries due to inadequate stabilization of the spine by muscles which normally function in this capacity.

4. How else might this EMG assessment technique be used to describe other kinds of muscle impairments associated with LBP?

ANSWER: Other distinct impairment categories have been proposed based on surface EMG analysis.[102] For instance, since the median frequency parameter can be used as a fatigue index, patients with muscle atrophy and other detrimental effects of deconditioning typically present with much higher fatigue indices as measured by the rate of decay in the EMG median frequency than healthy control subjects.[132] Patients and controls were tested in BAS device using a protocol similar to the one described in the case.

Gait Analysis 10

Cynthia C. Norkin

LEARNING OBJECTIVES

1. Define the terms used to describe normal gait.
2. Define reliability, validity, sensitivity, and specificity in relation to gait analysis.
3. Describe the variables that are assessed in each of the following types of gait analyses: kinematic qualitative analysis, kinematic quantitative analysis, and kinetic analysis.
4. Describe and give examples of some of the most commonly used types of gait profiles.
5. Compare and contrast the advantages and disadvantages of kinematic qualitative and kinematic quantitative gait analyses.
6. Using the case study example, apply clinical decision making skills in evaluating gait analysis data.

INTRODUCTION

One of the major purposes of the rehabilitative process is to help patients achieve as high a level of functional independence as possible within the limits of their particular impairments. Human ambulation or gait is one of the basic components of independent functioning that is commonly affected by either disease processes or injury. Consequently, one of the desired outcomes of many physical therapy intervention strategies is either to restore or to improve a patient's ambulatory status.

CONTENT OF GAIT ANALYSIS

To establish realistic outcome measures and to develop and implement a treatment plan directed toward improving or restoring a patient's gait, the physical therapist must be able to assess ambula-

tory status. A comprehensive analysis should include:

1. An accurate description of gait pattern and gait variables.
2. An identification and description of all gait deviations.
3. An analysis of the deviations and identification of the mechanisms responsible for producing abnormalities in gait.
4. Assessment of balance, endurance, energy expenditure, and safety.
5. Determination of the functional ambulation capabilities of the patient in relation to functional ambulation demands of the patient's home, community, and work environments.

The analysis should provide objective and valid data that can be used as a basis for describing a patient's present status, assessing a patient's progress over time, and in some instances for predicting a patient's future status.

SELECTION OF A GAIT ANALYSIS

Gait is a complex activity, and many articles regarding methods of gait analysis are contained in the physical therapy literature.[1–35] The type of gait analysis the clinician selects depends on the purpose of the analysis, the type of equipment available, and the experience, knowledge, and skills of the clinician. General as well as specific clinical indications for conducting a gait analysis may be found in the *Guide to Physical Therapist Practice*.[36]

The purpose of a gait analysis may include, but is not limited to, the following:

1. Description of the differences between a patient's performance and the parameters of normal gait.
2. Identification of the mechanisms causing dysfunction.
3. Classification of the severity of disability.
4. Prediction of a patient's future status.
5. Determination of the need for adaptive, assistive, orthotic, prosthetic, protective, or supportive devices or equipment.
6. Assessment of the effectiveness and fit of the devices or equipment selected (to provide joint protection and support, to correct deviations and dysfunctions, to reduce energy expenditure, and to promote safe locomotor functioning).
7. Assessment of the effects of interventions such as therapeutic exercise aerobic endurance activities, developmental activities, strengthening or stretching, electrostimulation, balance training, surgical procedures, and medication.
8. Enhancement of performance.

Many examples of these purposes are found in the literature; descriptions of the differences between a patient's performance and the parameters of normal gait,[37–40] identification of the mechanisms causing dysfunction,[40–44] assessment of the fit of a lower extremity prosthesis,[1] comparison of the effects of different types of assistive devices,[2] determination of either the need for or the effectiveness of an orthotic device,[45–48] assessment of the effects of treatment interventions,[49–55] assessment of energy expenditure,[56–63] and prediction of future status.[23,64] To determine the need for either a prosthetic or an orthotic adjustment, the therapist may need to assess the forces acting during gait. To determine if a patient should increase ambulating endurance, the therapist needs to assess time and distance variables as well as physiological parameters such as energy expenditure.

The type of equipment necessary for performing a gait analysis depends on the purpose of the analysis, equipment availability, and the amount of time the therapist can expend. Equipment used in a gait analysis may be either as simple as a pencil, paper,[3] and stopwatch[65] or as complex as an electronic imaging system with force plates embedded in the floor.[4,5,37,66] Therefore, the therapist must be aware of the types of analyses that are available and should determine which methods are reliable and valid so that the appropriate method may be selected.

Reliability

Reliability as applied to gait analysis refers to the level of consistency of either a measuring instrument (footswitches, force plates, motion analysis systems, electrogoniometers) or a method of analysis (observational gait analysis checklists, ambulation profiles, and formulas for measuring stride length). To determine if a measuring instrument is reliable, the measurements obtained from successive and repeated use of the instrument must be consistent. For example, if an electrogoniometric measurement of a known angle of 60 degrees consistently measures 60 degrees on every Monday morning for 2 months, the instrument is said to be reliable. If, however, the measurement obtained on the first Monday is 60 degrees, 30 degrees on the second Monday morning, and 40 degrees on the third Monday morning, the instrument would have very low reliability.

To make a definitive determination of the reliability of an instrument, one must make certain to rule out factors other than the instrument that could influence the measurement, (e.g., that a subject has not injured his or her knee between successive measurements or that the placement of the instrument had not changed).

To determine whether an assessment method is reliable, two different forms of reliability need to be determined: *intratester* and *intertester reliability*. The intratester reliability of an assessment method can be determined by examining the consistency of the results obtained when one individual uses a particular method repeatedly. For example, Sue Jones, PT, uses a particular method to assess a student physical therapist's gait. Sue repeats her assessment at 2-week intervals for 2 weeks and obtains the same results during each analysis. In this instance the method would be considered as having high intratester reliability because the results obtained by the same person are consistent over time. (The preceding example is a hypothetical one because factors other than the therapist's skill such as fatigue, time of day, and other variables may affect performance and must be controlled in any analysis.)

Intertester reliability is determined by examining the consistency of the data obtained from repeated analyses performed by a number of different persons. If the results obtained by the numerous examiners are in agreement, and no significant differences in the results exist among testers, the method has high intertester reliability.

Sensitivity and Specificity

Two other terms, sensitivity and specificity, are important to consider when selecting a method of analysis. *Sensitivity* as it relates to gait analysis refers to the proportion of times that a method of analysis correctly identifies a gait abnormality or condition when that abnormality or condition is actually present. *Specificity* refers to the proportion of times that a method of analysis correctly identifies the abnormality as being absent when it is absent.[67]

Validity

The other aspect of gait analysis that must be considered is validity. Generally, **validity** refers to the degree that a measurement reflects what it is supposed to measure. There are several types of validity—construct validity, content validity, and criterion-based validity (concurrent, predictive, and prescriptive). *Construct validity* is determined through logical argumentation based on theoretical research evidence (the ability of an instrument to measure an abstract concept or construct). *Content validity* is determined by providing evidence that the measuring instrument contains all relevant elements of a construct and no extraneous elements. In this instance, the test developer might justify the test by demonstrating that all items in the test were correlated with each other. *Criterion-based validity* is a type of validity whereby validity is established by comparisons of either one instrument with another or with data obtained from other forms of testing. *Concurrent validity* is a form of criterion-based validity in which the inference is justified by comparisons between the results of a specific test (gait analysis) and another test (functional test) taken at approximately the same time. *Predictive validity* is a form of criterion-based validity in which one must justify the capability of the instrument to predict future events, such as falls.[68]

The therapist should determine if the reliability and validity of an instrument or method of analysis has been established by either looking in the literature or by contacting other investigators who are using the particular method or instrument. If the instrument or method has not been tested, therapists may wish to perform their own tests for reliability and validity.

GAIT TERMINOLOGY

To assess gait, a therapist must be familiar with the terminology used to describe gait. The largest unit used to describe gait is called a *gait cycle*, which has both distance (spatial) and temporal parameters. In normal walking a gait cycle commences when the heel of the reference extremity contacts the supporting surface. The gait cycle ends when the heel of the same extremity contacts the ground again. In some abnormal gaits, the heel may not be the first part of the foot to contact the ground. Therefore, the gait cycle may be considered to begin when some portion of the reference extremity contacts the ground. The cycle ends when that same

portion of the extremity contacts the ground again. The gait cycle is divided into two phases, stance and swing, and two periods of double support. In normal gait the **stance phase,** which constitutes 60 percent of the gait cycle, is defined as the interval in which the foot of the reference extremity is in contact with the ground. For example, if the right lower extremity is the reference extremity, the left lower extremity will be in the swing phase when the right lower extremity is in its stance phase. Therefore, a single gait cycle contains right and left stance phases. The **swing phase,** which constitutes 40 percent of the gait cycle, is that portion in which the reference extremity does not contact the ground. For example, if the right lower extremity is the reference extremity, the left lower extremity will be in the stance phase when the right lower extremity is in its swing phase. Therefore, a single gait cycle includes both right and left swing phases. The term **double support time** refers to the two intervals in a gait cycle in which body weight is transferred from one foot to the other and both right and left feet are in contact with the ground at the same time (Fig. 10-1). Each of these variables may be measured in time; for example, stance time (right and left) **swing time** (right and left), double support time, and cycle time.

Two steps, a right step and a left step, comprise a **stride,** and a stride is equal to a gait cycle. **Step** and stride may be defined in two dimensions: distance and time. **Step length** is the distance from the point of heel strike of one extremity to the point of heel strike of the opposite extremity, whereas **stride length** is the distance from the point of heel strike of one extremity to the point of heel strike of the same extremity. **Stride time** and **step time** refer to the length of time required to complete a step and a stride, respectively (Fig. 10-2).

Traditionally, each phase of gait (stance and swing) has been divided into the following units: stance (heel strike, footflat, midstance, heel off, and toe off) and swing (acceleration, midswing, and deceleration). The Los Amigos Research and Education Institute, Inc. of Rancho Los Amigos Medical Center has developed a different terminology in which the subdivisions have been redefined and named as follows: stance (initial contact, loading response, midstance, terminal stance, and preswing) and swing (initial swing, midswing, and terminal swing).[20,24] The similarities and differ-

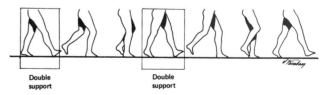

Figure 10-1. Double support is defined as the period in which some portion of the feet of both extremities are in contact with the supporting surface at the same time. Two periods of double support occur within a single gait cycle. One period occurs early in the stance phase of the reference extremity and the other occurs late in the stance phase of the reference extremity. (From Norkin, and Levangie,[75] p 452, with permission.)

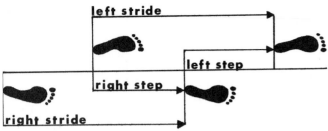

Figure 10-2. A right stride and a left stride. Right stride length is the distance between the point of contact of the right heel (at the lower left corner of the diagram) and the next contact of the right heel. Left stride length is the distance between the point of contact of the left heel (at the top left of the diagram) to the point of contact of the next left heel. Each stride contains two steps, but only both steps in the left stride are labeled. The left stride contains a right step and a left step. The right step length (shown in the middle of the diagram) is the distance between left heel contact to the point of right heel contact. Left step length is the distance between right heel contact and the next left heel contact. Step and stride times refer to the amount of time required to complete a step and to complete stride, respectively.

ences between the two terminologies are presented in Table 10–1.

Angular rotations at the joints in each portion of both swing and stance phases as well as muscle activity and function are presented in Tables 10–2 to

10–6. The clinician should be familiar with ranges and patterns of motion associated with normal gait to identify deviations from published standards. The clinician also should be familiar with the muscle activity and function associated with normal gait in order to perform an analysis of the causes of the deviations.

TYPES OF ANALYSES

The types of gait analyses in use today can be classified under two broad categories: **kinematic** and **kinetic.** Kinematic gait analyses are used to describe movement patterns without regard for the forces involved in producing the movement.[3] A kinematic gait analysis consists of a description of movement of the body as a whole and/or body segments in relation to each other during gait. Kinematic gait analyses can be either qualitative or quantitative. Kinetic gait analyses are used to determine the forces involved in gait.[69] In some instances, kinematic and kinetic gait variables may be assessed in one analysis. In addition to assessing kinematic and kinetic variables, physiological variables such as heart rate, and oxygen consumption should be considered in any comprehensive analysis.

Table 10–1 GAIT TERMINOLOGY

Traditional	Rancho Los Amigos	Traditional	Rancho Los Amigos
Stance Phase		*Swing Phase*	
Heel strike: The beginning of the stance phase when the heel contacts the ground. The same as initial contact.	Initial contact: The beginning of the stance phase when the heel or another part of the foot contacts the ground.	Acceleration: The portion of beginning swing from the moment the toe of the reference extremity leaves the ground to the point when the reference extremity is directly under the body.	Initial swing: The portion of swing from the point when the reference extremity leaves the ground to maximum knee flexion of the same extremity.
Foot flat: Occurs immediately following heel strike, when the sole of the foot contacts the floor. This event occurs during loading response.	Loading response: The portion of the first double support period of the stance phase from initial contact until the contralateral extremity leaves the ground.	Midswing: Portion of the swing phase when the reference extremity passes directly below the body. Midswing extends from the end of acceleration to the beginning of deceleration.	Midswing: Portion of the swing phase from maximum knee flexion of the reference extremity to a vertical tibial position.
Midstance: The point at which the body passes directly over the reference extremity.	Midstance: The portion of the single limb support stance phase that begins when the contralateral extremity leaves the ground and ends when the body is directly over the supporting limb.	Deceleration: The swing portion of the swing phase when the reference extremity is decelerating in preparation for heel strike.	Terminal swing: The portion of the swing phase from a vertical position of the tibia of the reference extremity to just prior to initial contact.
Heel off: The point following midstance at which time the heel of the reference extremity leaves the ground. Heel off occurs prior to terminal stance.	Terminal stance: The last portion of the single limb support stance phase that begins with heel rise and continues until contralateral extremity contacts the ground.		
Toe off: The point following heel off when only the toe of the reference extremity is in contact with the ground.	Preswing: The portion of stance that begins the second double support period from the initial contact of the contralateral extremity to lift off of the reference extremity.		

Table 10–2 ANKLE AND FOOT: STANCE PHASE, SAGITTAL PLANE ANALYSIS

Portion of Phase	Normal Motion[24]	Normal Moment	Normal Muscle Activity	Result of Weakness	Possible Compensation
Heel strike to foot flat	0–15 degrees plantarflexion	Plantarflexion	Pretibial group acts eccentrically to oppose plantarflexion moment and thereby to prevent foot slap by controlling plantarflexion.	Lack of ability to oppose the plantarflexion moment causes the foot to slap the floor.	To avoid foot slap and to eliminate the plantarflexion moment, the foot may be placed flat on the floor or placed with the toes first at initial contact.
Foot flat through midstance	15 degrees plantarflexion to 10 degrees dorsiflexion	Plantarflexion to dorsiflexion	Gastrocnemius and soleus act eccentrically to oppose the dorsiflexion moment and to control tibial advance.	Excessive dorsiflexion and uncontrolled tibial advance.	To avoid excessive dorsiflexion, the ankle may be maintained in plantarflexion.
Midstance to heel off	10–15 degrees dorsiflexion	Dorsiflexion	Gastrocnemius and soleus contract eccentrically to oppose the dorsiflexion moment and control tibial advance.	Excessive dorsiflexion and uncontrolled forward motion of tibia.	The ankle may be maintained in plantarflexion. If the foot is flat on the floor, the dorsiflexion moment is eliminated and a step-to gait is produced.
Heel off to toe off	15 degrees dorsiflexion to 20 degrees plantarflexion	Dorsiflexion	Gastrocnemius, soleus, peroneus brevis, peroneus longus, flexor hallicus longus contract to plantarflex the foot.	No roll off. Decreased contralateral step.	Whole foot is lifted off the ground.

Table 10–3 ANKLE AND FOOT: SWING PHASE, SAGITTAL PLANE ANALYSIS

Portion of Phase	Normal Motion	Normal Moment	Normal Muscle Action	Result of Weakness	Possible Compensation
Acceleration to midswing	Dorsiflexion to neutral	None	Dorsiflexors contract to bring the ankle into neutral and to prevent the toes from dragging on the floor.	Foot drop and/or toe dragging.	Hip and knee flexion may be increased to prevent toe drag, or the hip may be hiked or circumducted. Sometimes vaulting on the contralateral limb may occur.
Midswing to deceleration	Neutral	None	Dorsiflexion	Foot drop and/or toe dragging.	Hip and knee flexion may be increased to prevent toe drag. The swing leg may be circumducted, or vaulting may occur on the contralateral side.

Table 10–4 KNEE: STANCE PHASE, SAGITTAL PLANE ANALYSIS

Portion of Phase	Normal Motion	Normal Moment	Normal Muscle Action	Result of Weakness	Possible Compensation
Heel strike to foot flat	Flexion 0–15 degrees	Flexion	Quadriceps contracts initially to hold the knee in extension and then eccentrically to oppose the flexion moment and control the amount of flexion.	Excessive knee flexion because the quadriceps cannot oppose the flexion moment.	Plantarflexion at ankle so that foot flat instead of heel strike occurs. Plantarflexion eliminates the flexion moment. Trunk lean forward eliminates the flexion moment at knee and therefore may be used to compensate for quadriceps weakness.
Foot flat through midstance	Extension 15–5 degrees	Flexion to extension	Quadriceps contracts in early part, and then no activity is required.	Excessive knee flexion initially.	Same as above in early part of midstance. No compensation required in later part of phase.
Midstance to heel off	5 degrees of flexion to 0 degrees (neutral)	Flexion to extension	No activity required.		None required.
Heel off to toe off	0–40 degrees flexion	Extension to flexion	Quadriceps required to control amount of knee flexion.		

Table 10–5 KNEE: SWING PHASE, SAGITTAL PLANE ANALYSIS

Portion of Phase	Normal Motion	Normal Moment	Normal Muscle Action	Result of Weakness	Possible Compensation
Accleration to mid-swing	40–60 degrees flexion	None	Little or no activity in quadriceps. Biceps femoris (short head), gracilis, and sartorius contract concentrically.	Inadequate knee flexion.	Increased hip flexion, circumduction, or hiking.
Midswing	60–30 degrees extension	None			
Deceleration	30–0 degrees extension	None	Quadriceps contracts concentrically to stabilize knee in extension, in preparation for heel strike.	Inadequate knee extension.	

Table 10–6 HIP: STANCE PHASE, SAGITTAL PLANE ANALYSIS

Portion of Phase	Normal Motion	Normal Moment	Normal Muscle Action	Result of Weakness	Possible Compensation
Heel strike to foot flat	30 degrees flexion	Flexion	Erector spinae, gluteus maximus, hamstrings.	Excessive hip flexion and anterior pelvis tilt owing to inability to counteract flexion moment.	Trunk leans backward to prevent excessive hip flexion and to eliminate the hip flexion moment.

Continued

Table 10–6 HIP: STANCE PHASE, SAGITTAL PLANE ANALYSIS *Continued*

Portion of Phase	Normal Motion	Normal Moment	Normal Muscle Action	Result of Weakness	Possible Compensation
Foot flat through midstance	30 degrees flexion to 5 degrees (neutral)	Flexion to extension	Gluteus maximus at beginning of period to oppose flexion moment, then activity ceases as moment changes from flexion to extension.	At the beginning of the period, excessive hip flexion and anterior pelvic tilt owing to inability to counteract flexion moment.	At beginning of the period, subject may lean trunk backward to prevent excessive hip flexion; however, once the flexion moment changes to an extension moment, the subject no longer needs to incline the trunk backward.
Midstance to heel off		Extension	No activity.	None.	None required.
Heel off to toe off	10 degrees of hyperextension to neutral	Extension	Illiopsoas, adductor, magnus, and adductor longus.	Undetermined.	Undetermined.

KINEMATIC QUALITATIVE GAIT ANALYSIS

The most common method used in the clinic is a **qualitative gait analysis.** This method usually requires only a small amount of equipment and a minimal amount of time. The primary variable that is assessed in a qualitative kinematic analysis is **displacement,** which includes a description of patterns of movement, deviations from normal body postures, and joint angles at specific points in the gait cycle.

Observational Gait Analysis

The most commonly used clinical method of performing a kinematic qualitative analysis is through observation. Some of the most well-known observational gait analysis (OGA) schemes that have been used in the past were developed by Brunnstrom,[25] and at New York University's Post-Graduate Medical School Prosthetics and Orthotics,[26] at Temple University,[27] and at Rancho Los Amigos Medical Center.[20,24] Recently an OGA system was developed for use by podiatrists.[28] The Brunnstrom and Rancho Los Amigos OGA systems are still being used today. However, the Rancho Los Amigos OGA system is probably the most commonly used OGA method used by physical therapists. The Rancho Los Amigos OGA method involves a systematic assessment of the movement patterns of the following body segments at each point in the gait cycle: ankle, foot, knee, hip, pelvis, and trunk. The Rancho Los Amigos form consists of 48 descriptors of common gait deviations such as toe drag, excessive plantarflexion and dorsiflexion, excessive varus or valgus at the knee or foot, hip hiking, and trunk flexion. The observing therapist must decide whether or not a deviation is present and note the occurrence and timing of the deviation on the form.[24]

Considerable training and constant practice are necessary to develop the observational skills that are needed for performing any OGA. Therapists who wish to learn the Rancho method either may elect to attend a workshop or the therapist can learn independently by studying the Rancho Los Amigos Observational Gait Analysis Handbook.[24] Forms for recording an assessment are included in the handbook and a sample form is included in this chapter (Fig. 10-3). Practice gait film strips useful for learning how to use the recording forms may be obtained by writing to Rancho Los Amigos.[24]

The biomechanical gait assessment form described by Southerland is presented in Figure 10-4. This form is used in conjunction with a static quantitative analysis which includes measurements of the range of motion (ROM) of all joints from the hip to the toes, as well as measurements of limb length. Detailed information is also collected on both the dorsal and plantar surfaces of the feet such as callus formation and corns. The examiner is expected to document abnormalities such as hallux valgus and hammer toes. The dynamic qualitative component of the assessment uses a shorthand system for recording the details of the OGA. The acronym GHORT (gait, homunculus, observed, relational, and tabular) is used to assist the rater in recording information gathered from the observational analysis (Fig. 10-5). An example of the recording method is shown in Figure 10-6. Following completion of the dynamic portion, the rater's qualitative impressions of the patient's gait are compared with the results of the static assessment to verify the accuracy of the findings and analysis of the causes of abnormal function. The author states

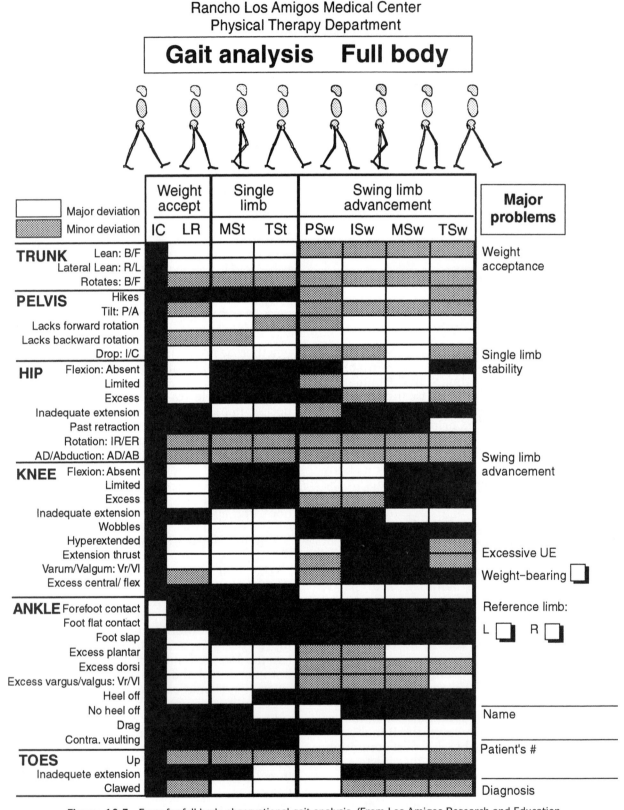

Figure 10-3. Form for full body observational gait analysis. (From Los Amigos Research and Education Institute of Rancho Los Amigos Medical Center,[24] p 55, with permission.)

that after the first five analyses, a new rater's results are the same or similar to other raters; however, the author did not reference any reliability and/or validity studies.[28]

In general, these protocols provide the therapist with a systematic approach to observational gait analysis by directing the therapist's attention to a specific joint or body segment during a given point

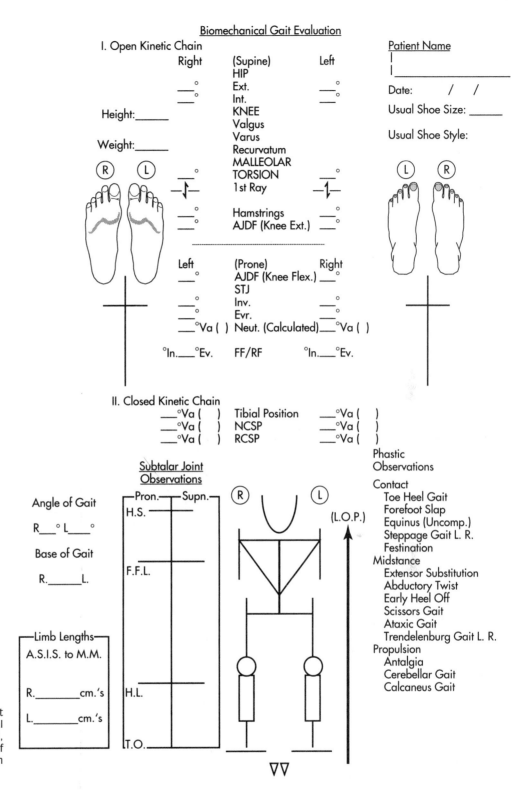

Figure 10-4. Biomechanical Gait Evaluation Form for Observational Gait Analysis (From Sutherland, Chapter 7 in Clinical Biomechanics of the Lower Extremities,[28] p 155, with permission.)

in the gait cycle. Most of the methods use checklists or profiles in which the examiner notes the presence or absence of a particular deviation or critical event at a particular point in the patient's gait cycle.

ADVANTAGES AND DISADVANTAGES

The advantages of OGAs are that they require little or no instrumentation, are inexpensive to use, and can yield general descriptions of gait variables.

The disadvantages are that the technique, being dependent on both the therapist's training and observational skills, is subjective, has only low to moderate reliability, and validity has not been demonstrated.[70] Difficulties involved in observing and making accurate judgements about the motions occurring simultaneously at numerous body segments, the lack of a standardized form, and inadequate training in OGA methods are thought to

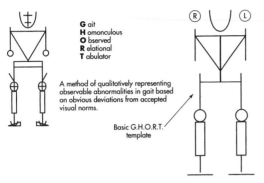

Figure 10-5. GHORT (From Sutherland, Chapter 7 in Clinical Biomechanics of the Lower Extremities,[28] p 159, with permission.)

contribute to the low reliability. Also, therapists differ in their observational skills. Only moderate reliability between therapists (intertester reliability) was found when a modification of the New York University (NYU) orthotic gait analysis method was used to assess the gait of 10 patients with hemiplegia. The authors suggested that training of therapists in gait analysis was necessary to improve reliability.[71] In another study, only moderate interrater and intrarater reliability was found when three physical therapists with at least 5 years' experience used an observational gait form created from the NYU, Temple, and Rancho forms to examine the gaits of 15 children with disabilities with knee-ankle-foot orthoses.[72] The reliability of the Rancho Los Amigos OGA technique has not been published. Gronley and Perry[4] reported that differences among raters were resolved through discussion and consensus.

If therapists decide to use an OGA method, they should seriously consider videography. The camcorder should have the capability of slowing or stopping motion. A visual record is especially important when using the Rancho format because of the time involved in assessing a large number of vari-

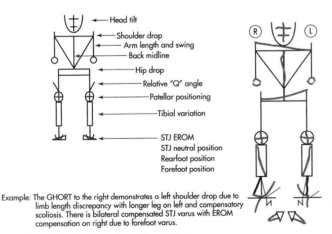

Recorded Points of Evaluation on GHORT

Example: The GHORT to the right demonstrates a left shoulder drop due to limb length discrepancy with longer leg on left and compensatory scoliosis. There is bilateral compensated STJ varus with EROM compensation on right due to forefoot varus.

Top-to-bottom, front-to-rear sequence on GHORT.

Figure 10-6. Recording Points of Evaluation on GHORT (From Sutherland, Chapter 7 in Clinical Biomechanics of the Lower Extremities,[28] p 164, with permission.)

ables at six different body parts. Most patients cannot walk continuously for the length of time required to complete a detailed, full-body observational analysis. Furthermore, the observers cannot either rate or score a large number of variables while a subject is walking. Videotape records of a patient's initial assessment that can be replayed in slow motion, allow therapists the time needed to make judgments about gait events.

Although the use of videotape may provide an opportunity for the observers to assess the reliability of their scoring, unless therapists are knowledgeable about normal gait parameters and variables and are adequately trained to use the measuring instrument, reliability will probably remain in the low to moderate range. Russell et al.[73] found that when observers were trained in the scoring of a Gross Motor Function Measure (GMFM) a significant improvement occurred following training compared with the observers' pretraining scoring of the videotape. On the other hand, Eastlack et al.[18] found only low to moderate interrater reliability among 54 practicing physical therapists who rated 10 gait variables while observing the videotaped gait of three patients. These therapists reported that they were comfortable performing observational gait analyses. However, more than half of the therapists were unfamiliar with any of the following three commonly used observational gait analysis formats: (1) New York University's Child Prosthetic-Orthotic Studies Observational Analysis Form, (2) Temple University's The Visual Examination of Pathologic Gait, and (3) Rancho Los Amigos' Observational Gait Analysis Handbook. Thirteen of the 22 therapists who were familiar with one of the three observational gait analysis methods indicated exposure to the Rancho Los Amigos format.[18] The lack of agreement among raters found in this study as well as the rater's lack of knowledge of normal gait parameters and terminology have serious implications for patient treatments based on the results of observational gait analyses. Krebs[74] argues that OGA performed clinically is impossible.

If OGA is used it should be used in conjunction with quantitative measures. Videotape or film can provide a permanent record of the patient's gait. Also videography or cinematography may be used to assess joint range of motion at the hip, knee, and ankle by taking goniometric measurements directly from the screen. Stuberg et al.[15] found no significant differences between goniometric measurements taken from videotaped gait and measurements taken from film for 10 children with cerebral palsy and 9 normal children. Examples of the process involved in an OGA will be presented in the following section.

Kinematic Gait Analysis and Assessment of Variables

The purpose of this section is to introduce the process involved in an OGA. The first step in the process involves the identification and accurate description of the patient's gait pattern and any deviations. The second step involves a determination of the causes. To identify and describe a patient's gait, the therapist must have a good knowledge of gait terminology and an accurate mental picture of normal gait postures and normal displacements of the body segments in each portion of the two phases of gait and in each plane of analysis (saggital, coronal, and transverse). To determine the causes of a patient's gait pattern and specific deviations, the therapist must understand the normal roles and functions of muscles during gait and the normal forces involved.[20,21,75] A patient's deviations from normal occur because of an inability to perform the tasks of walking in a normal fashion. For example, a patient with paralysis of the dorsiflexors (which causes a foot drop) cannot use the dorsiflexors to attain the normal neutral position of the ankle necessary to complete the task of clearing the floor during the swing phase. Therefore, the patient must find some other method of clearing the floor. The patient could compensate for the inability to dorsiflex the ankle by some method such as increasing the amount of hip and knee flexion above the normal amount, by **circumduction** of the entire limb, or by hiking the hip. The type of compensation that a particular individual selects depends on the specific disability. Increased hip and knee flexion may be used if the patient has an isolated problem in the ankle and adequate muscle strength and range of motion in the extremity. Circumduction or hip hiking may be used if the patient has either a stiff knee or extensor thrust, which prevents use of increased knee flexion to raise the plantarflexed foot above the floor.[42] The therapist needs to be aware that patients may use a variety of methods to compensate for joint or muscle deficits.

Tables 10–2 to 10–7 provide a review of the normal sagittal plane joint displacements, moments of force, and muscle activity and function as well as the results of isolated muscle weaknesses and possible compensations. Tables 10–8 to 10–14 present a few of the common deviations observed in a sagittal plane analysis and probable causes for the devia-

tions. Tables 10–15 and 10–16 provide sample gait analysis recording forms. If the reader decides to use the gait analysis recording forms presented in this text, reliability tests should be conducted because these forms are presented only as guides and have not been evaluated.

In Tables 10–2 to 10–7, the phase of gait, the normal joint displacements, moments of force, and muscle activity are presented in the first four columns, and the effects of muscle weakness and possible compensations are presented in the last two columns. (The reader should be aware that only the effects of isolated muscle weaknesses and associated compensations are presented.) The intent of the tables is to identify factors of normal gait that must be considered when observing gait and an example of how to proceed with an analysis of the causes of an atypical gait pattern or particular deviation.

Tables 10–8 to 10–14 present some of the common gait deviations, as well as possible causes and analyses. Notice that the sample recording form presented in Table 10–16 is formatted in the same manner as Tables 10–8 to 10–14. Therefore, the clinician can use the sample analyses presented in the tables as guides.

Observational Gait Analysis Procedure

Directions for performing an OGA for the sagittal and coronal planes are enumerated below.

1. Select the area in which the patient will walk, and measure the distance that you want the patient to cover.
2. Position yourself to allow an unobstructed view of the subject. If filming, the cameras should be positioned to view the patient's lower extremities and feet as well as the head and trunk from both the sagittal and coronal perspectives.
3. Select the joint or segment to be assessed first (e.g., ankle and foot), and mentally review the normal displacement patterns and muscle functions.

Text continued on page 271

Table 10–7 HIP: SWING PHASE, SAGITTAL PLANE ANALYSIS

Portion of Phase	Normal Motion	Normal Moment	Normal Muscle Activity	Result of Weakness	Possible Compensation
Acceleration to midswing	20–30 degrees flexion	None	Hip flexor activity to initiate swing illiopsoas, rectus, femoris, gracilis, sartorius, tensor fascia lata.	Diminished hip flexion causing an inability to initiate the normal forward movement of the extremity and to raise the foot off the floor.	Circumduction and/or hip hiking may be used to bring the leg forward and to raise the foot high enough to clear the floor.
Midswing to deceleration	30 degrees flexion to neutral	None	Hamstrings.	A lack of control of the swinging leg. Inability to place limb in position for heel strike.	

Table 10–8 COMMON DEVIATIONS, ANKLE AND FOOT: STANCE PHASE, SAGITTAL PLANE ANALYSIS

Portion of Phase	Deviation	Description	Possible Causes	Analysis
Initial contact	Foot slap	At heel strike, forefoot slaps the ground.	Flaccid or weak dorsiflexors or reciprocal inhibition of dorsiflexors; atrophy of dorsiflexors.	Look for low muscle tone at ankle. Look for steppage gait (excessive hip and knee flexion) in swing phase.
	Toes first	Toes contact ground instead of heel. The tip-toe posture may be maintained throughout the phase, or the heel may contact the ground.	Leg length discrepancy; contracted heel cord; plantarflexion contraction; spasticity of plantarflexors; flaccidity of dorsiflexors; painful heel.	Compare leg lengths and look for hip and/or knee flexion contractures. Analyze muscle tone and timing of activity in plantarflexors. Check for pain in heel.
	Foot flat	Entire foot contacts the ground at heel strike.	Excessive fixed dorsiflexion; flaccid or weak dorsiflexors; neonatal/proprioceptive walking.	Check range of motion at ankle. Check for hyperextension at the knee and persistence of immature gait pattern.
Midstance	Excessive positional plantarflexion	Tibia does not advance to neutral from 10 degrees plantarflexion.	No eccentric contraction of plantarflexors; could be due to flaccidity/weakness in plantarflexors; surgical overrelease, rupture, or contracture of Achilles tendon.	Check for spastic or weak quadriceps; hyperextension at the knee; hip hyperextension; backward- or forward-leaning trunk. Check for weakness in plantarflexors or rupture of Achilles tendon.
	Heel lift in midstance	Heel does not contact ground in midstance.	Spasticity of plantarflexors.	Check for spasticity in plantarflexors, quadriceps, hip flexors, and adductors.
	Excessive positional dorsiflexion	Tibia advances too rapidly over the foot, creating a greater than normal amount of dorsiflexion.	Inability of plantarflexors to control tibial advance. Knee flexion or hip flexion contractures.	Look at ankle muscles, knee and hip flexors, range of motion, and position of trunk.
	Toe clawing	Toes flex and "grab" floor.	Could be due to a plantar grasp reflex that is only partially integrated; could be due to positive supporting reflex; spastic toe flexors.	Check plantar grasp reflex, positive supporting reflexes, and range of motion of toes.
Push-off (heel off to toe off)	No roll off	Insufficient transfer of weight from lateral heel to medial forefoot.	Mechanical fixation of ankle and foot. Flaccidity or inhibition of plantarflexors, inverters, and toe flexors. Rigidity/cocontraction of plantarflexors and dorsiflexors. Pain in forefoot.	Check range of motion at ankle and foot. Check muscle function and tone at ankle. Look at dissociation between posterior foot and forefoot.

Table 10–9 COMMON DEVIATIONS, ANKLE AND FOOT: SWING PHASE, SAGITTAL PLANE ANALYSIS

Portion of Phase	Deviation	Description	Possible Causes	Analysis
Swing	Toe drag	Insufficient dorsiflexion (and toe extension) so that forefoot and toes do not clear floor.	Flaccidity or weakness of dorsiflexors and toe extensors. Spasticity of plantarflexors. Inadequate knee or hip flexion.	Check for ankle, hip, and knee range of motion. Check for strength and muscle tone at hip, knee, and ankle.
	Varus	The foot is excessively inverted.	Spasticity of the invertors. Flaccidity or weakness of dorsiflexors and evertors. Extensor pattern.	Check for muscle tone of invertors and plantarflexors. Check strength of dorsiflexors and evertors. Check for extensor pattern of the lower extremity.

Table 10–10 COMMON DEVIATIONS, KNEE: STANCE PHASE, SAGITTAL PLANE ANALYSIS

Portion of Phase	Deviation	Description	Possible Causes	Analysis
Initial contact (heel strike)	Excessive knee flexion	Knee flexes or "buckles" rather than extends as foot contacts ground.	Painful knee; spasticity of knee flexors or weak or flaccid quadriceps. Short leg on contralateral side.	Check for pain at knee; tone of knee flexors; strength of knee extensors; leg lengths; anterior pelvic tilt.
Foot flat	Knee hyperextension (genu recurvatum)	A greater than normal extension at the knee.	Flaccid/weak quadriceps and soleus compensated for by pull of gluteus maximus. Spasticity of quadriceps. Accommodation to a fixed ankle plantarflexion deformity.	Check for strength and muscle tone of knee and ankle flexors, and range of motion at ankle.
Midstance	Knee hyperextension (genu recurvatum)	During single limb support, tibia remains in back of ankle mortice as body weight moves over foot. Ankle is plantarflexed.	Same as above.	Same as above.
Push-off (heel off to toe off)	Excessive knee flexion	Knee flexes to more than 40 degrees during push-off.	Center of gravity is unusually far forward of pelvis. Could be due to rigid trunk, knee/hip flexion contractures; flexion-withdrawal reflex; dominance of flexion synergy in middle recovery from CVA.	Look at trunk posture, knee and hip range of motion, and flexor synergy.
	Limited knee flexion	The normal amount of knee flexion (40 degrees) does not occur.	Spastic/overactive quadriceps and/or plantarflexors.	Look at tone in hip, knee, and ankle muscles.

CVA = cerebrovascular accident.

Table 10–11 COMMON DEVIATIONS, KNEE: SWING PHASE, SAGITTAL PLANE ANALYSIS

Portion of Phase	Deviation	Description	Possible Causes	Analysis
Acceleration to midswing	Excessive knee flexion	Knee flexes more than 65 degrees	Diminished preswing knee flexion, flexor-withdrawal reflex, dysmetria.	Look at muscle tone in hip, knee, and ankle. Test for reflexes and dysmetria.
	Limited knee flexion	Knee does not flex to 65 degrees	Pain in knee, diminished range of knee motion, extensor spasticity. Circumduction at the hip.	Assess for pain in knee and knee range of motion. Test muscle tone at knee and hip.

Table 10–12 COMMON DEVIATIONS, HIP: STANCE PHASE, SAGITTAL PLANE ANALYSIS

Portion of Phase	Deviation	Description	Possible Causes	Analysis
Heel strike to foot flat	Excessive flexion	Flexion exceeding 30 degrees.	Hip and/or knee flexion contractures. Knee flexion caused by weak soleus and quadriceps. Hypertonicity of hip flexors.	Check hip and knee range of motion and strength of soleus and quadriceps. Check tone of hip flexors.
Heel strike to foot flat	Limited hip flexion	Hip flexion does not attain 30 degrees.	Weakness of hip flexors. Limited range of hip flexion. Gluteus maximus weakness.	Check strength of hip flexors and extensors. Analyze range of hip motion.

Continued

Table 10–12 COMMON DEVIATIONS, HIP: STANCE PHASE, SAGITTAL PLANE ANALYSIS *Continued*

Portion of Phase	Deviation	Description	Possible Causes	Analysis
Foot flat to midstance	Limited hip extension	The hip does not attain a neutral position.	Hip flexion contracture, spasticity in hip flexors.	Check hip range of motion and tone of hip muscles.
	Internal rotation	An internally rotated position of the extremity.	Spasticity of internal rotators. Weakness of external rotators. Excessive forward rotation of opposite pelvis.	Check tone of internal rotators and strength of external rotators. Measure range of motion at both hip joints.
	External rotation	An externally rotated position of the extremity.	Excessive backward rotation of opposite pelvis.	Assess range of motion at both hip joints.
	Abduction	An abducted position of the extremity.	Contracture of the gluteus medius. Trunk lateral lean over the ipsilateral hip.	Check for abduction pattern.
	Adduction	An adducted position of the lower extremity.	Spasticity of hip flexors and adductors such as seen in spastic diplegia. Pelvic drop to contralateral side.	Assess tone of hip flexors and adductors. Test muscle strength of hip abductors.

Table 10–13 COMMON DEVIATIONS, HIP: SWING PHASE, SAGITTAL PLANE ANALYSIS

Portion of Phase	Deviation	Description	Possible Causes	Analysis
Swing	Circumduction	A lateral circular movement of the entire lower extremity consisting of abduction, external rotation, adduction, and internal rotation.	A compensation for weak hip flexors or a compensation for the inability to shorten the leg so that it can clear the floor.	Check strength of hip flexors, knee flexors, and ankle dorsiflexors. Check range of motion in hip flexion, knee flexion, and ankle dorsiflexion. Check for extensor pattern.
	Hip hiking	Shortening of the swing leg by action of the quadratus lumborum.	A compensation for lack of knee flexion and/or ankle dorsiflexion. Also may be a compensation for extensor spasticity of swing leg.	Check strength and range of motion at knee, hip, and ankle. Also check muscle tone at knee and ankle.
	Excessive hip flexion	Flexion greater than 20–30 degrees.	Attempt to shorten extremity in presence of foot drop. Flexor pattern.	Check strength and range of motion at ankle and foot. Check for flexor pattern.

Table 10–14 COMMON DEVIATIONS, TRUNK: STANCE, SAGITTAL PLANE ANALYSIS

Portion of Phase	Deviation	Description	Possible Causes	Analysis
Stance	Lateral trunk lean	A lean of the trunk over the stance extremity (gluteus medius gait/ Trendelenberg gait).	A weak or paralyzed gluteus medius on the stance side cannot prevent a drop of pelvis on the swing side, so a trunk lean over the stance leg helps compensate for the weak muscle. A lateral trunk lean over the affected hip also may be used to reduce force on hip if a patient has a painful hip.	Check strength of gluteus medius and assess for pain in the hip.
	Backward trunk lean	A backward leaning of the trunk, resulting in hyperextension at the hip (gluteus maximus gait).	Weakness or paralysis of the gluteus maximus on the stance leg. Anteriorly rotated pelvis.	Check for strength of hip extensors. Check pelvic position.

Continued

Table 10–14 COMMON DEVIATIONS, TRUNK: STANCE, SAGITTAL PLANE ANALYSIS *Continued*

Portion of Phase	Deviation	Description	Possible Causes	Analysis
	Forward trunk lean	A forward leaning of the trunk, resulting in hip flexion.	Compensation for quadriceps weakness. The forward lean eliminates the flexion moment at the knee. Hip and knee flexion contractures.	Check for strength of quadriceps.
		A forward flexion of the upper trunk.	Posteriorly rotated pelvis.	Check pelvic position.

4. Select either a sagittal plane observation (view from the side) or a coronal plane observation (view from the front and/or back).
5. Observe the selected segment during the initial part of the stance phase and make a decision about the position of the segment. Note any deviations from the normal pattern.
6. Observe either the same segment during the next part of the stance phase or another segment at the initial part of the stance phase. Progress through the same process as in number five.

7. Repeat the process described in number six until you have completed an assessment of all segments in the sagittal and coronal planes. Remember to concentrate on one segment at a time in one part of the gait cycle. Do not jump from one segment to another or from one phase to another.
8. Always perform observations on both sides (right and left). Although only one side may be involved, the other side of the body may be affected.

Table 10–15 GAIT ANALYSIS RECORDING FORM

Fixed Postures Observed During Gait			
Patient's Name		Age	Sex
Head	Tilt	To the right _____	To the left _____
		Forward _____	Backward _____
Trunk	Lean	To the right _____	To the left _____
		Forward _____	Backward _____
Pelvis	Tilt	To the right _____	To the left _____
		Anterior _____	Posterior _____
Hip	Flexion	On the right _____	On the left _____
		Bilateral _____	
	Extension	On the right _____	
		Bilateral _____	
	Abduction	On the right _____	On the left _____
		Bilateral _____	
	Adduction	On the right _____	On the left _____
		Bilateral _____	
	External rotation	On the right _____	
		Bilateral _____	
	Internal rotation	On the right _____	On the left _____
		Bilateral _____	
Knee	Flexion	On the right _____	On the left _____
		Bilateral _____	
	Extension	On the right _____	On the left _____
		Bilateral _____	
	Hyperextension	On the right _____	On the left _____
		Bilateral _____	
	Valgum	On the right _____	On the left _____
		Bilateral _____	
	Varum	On the right _____	On the left _____
		Bilateral _____	
Ankle/foot	Dorsiflexion	On the right _____	On the left _____
		Bilateral _____	
	Plantarflexion	On the right _____	On the left _____
		Bilateral _____	
	Varus	On the right _____	On the left _____
		Bilateral _____	
	Valgus	On the right _____	On the left _____
		Bilateral _____	
	Pes planus	On the right _____	On the left _____
		Bilateral _____	
	Pes cavus	On the right _____	On the left _____
		Bilateral _____	

Table 10–16 RECORDING FORM FOR OBSERVATIONAL GAIT ANALYSIS

Patient's name _____ Age _____ Sex _____ Height _____ Weight _____
Diagnosis _____
Footwear _____ Assistive devices _____
Date _____ Therapist _____
DIRECTIONS: Place a check in the space opposite the deviation if the deviation is observed.

Body Segment	Deviation	Stance HS R	HS L	FF R	FF L	MST R	MST L	HO R	HO L	TO R	TO L	Swing ACC R	ACC L	MSW R	MSW L	DEC R	DEC L	Possible Cause	Analysis
Ankle and foot	None																		
Observations	Foot flat																		
In the sagittal plane	Foot slap																		
	Heel off																		
	No heel off																		
	Excessive plantarflexion																		
	Excessive dorsiflexion																		
	Toe drag																		
	Toe clawing																		
	Contralateral vaulting																		
Observations in the frontal plane	Varus																		
	Valgus																		
Knee	None																		
Observations in the sagittal plane	Excessive flexion																		
	Limited flexion																		
	No flexion																		
	Hyperextension																		
	Genu recurvatum																		
	Diminished extension																		
Observations in the frontal plane	Varum																		
	Valgum																		
Hip	None																		
Observations in the sagittal plane	Excessive flexion																		
	Limited flexion																		
	No flexion																		
	Diminished extension																		
Observations in the frontal plane	Abduction																		
	Adduction																		
	External rotation																		
	Internal rotation																		
	Circumduction																		
	Hiking																		

Continued

Table 10–16 RECORDING FORM FOR OBSERVATIONAL GAIT ANALYSIS *Continued*

Body Segment	Deviation	Stance HS	FF	MST	HO	Swing TO	ACC	MSW	DEC	Possible Cause	Analysis
Pelvis	None										
Observations in sagittal plane	Anterior tilt										
	Posterior tilt										
	Increased backward rotation										
	Increased forward rotation										
	Limited backward rotation										
	Limited forward rotation										
	Drops on contralateral side										
Trunk	None										
Observations in frontal plane	Backward rotation										
	Lateral lean										
	Forward rotation										
	Backward lean										
	Forward lean										

ACC, acceleration; DEC, deceleration; FF, foot flat; HO, heel off; HS, heel strike; MST, midstance; MSW, midswing; TO, toe off.

Observational Gait Analysis in Neuromuscular Disorders

The gait patterns of individuals with neuromuscular deficits are influenced primarily by abnormalities in muscle tone and synergistic organization, influences of nonintegrated early reflexes, diminished influence of righting and balance reactions, diminished dissociation among body parts, and diminished coordination. If proximal stability (cocontraction of the postural muscles of the trunk) is threatened by atypically low or high muscle tone, or muscle tone that fluctuates, controlled mobility is lost. In gait, a loss of control over the sequential timing of muscular activity may result in asymmetrical step and stride lengths. In addition, deviations from normal posture and motion may occur such as forward or backward trunk leaning, excessive flexion or extension at the hip and knee in the stance phase, and diminished dorsiflexion or excessive plantarflexion.

In the presence of multiple muscle involvement or neurological deficits that affect balance, coordination, and muscle tone, the deviations observed and the analysis of these deviations will be more complex than indicated in the tables. Examples of gait patterns observed in association with spasticity and with hypotonus follow.

An individual with hypertonia (e.g., an individual with diplegic cerebral palsy) may have a posteriorly tilted pelvis, forward flexion of the upper trunk, protracted scapulae, and somewhat excessive neck extension. Excessive hip flexion, with adduction and internal rotation (scissoring) may be observed during stance and may be accompanied by either excessive knee flexion or hyperextension. If excessive knee flexion occurs during stance, dorsiflexion at the ankle may be exaggerated during late stance/preswing to advance the tibia over the ankle and clear the toes and forefoot from the ground after push-off (heel off to toe off).

In other individuals with hypertonia, hyperextension at the knee occurs in stance and may be accompanied by plantarflexion and inversion at the ankle and foot. Electromyographic recordings may show prolonged activity in the quadriceps and in the gastroc-soleus muscle groups. The hamstrings and gluteal and dorsiflexor muscle groups may be reciprocally inhibited.

In individuals with low muscle tone (hypotonia) in the trunk, proximal stability (tonic extension and cocontraction of axial muscles) is diminished. The pelvis may be anteriorly tilted so that the upper trunk is slightly extended. The scapulae may be retracted and the head may be forward. The hip may be flexed during stance and the knee may be hyperextended accompanied by plantarflexion at the ankle. The foot may be pronated with the majority of the body weight borne on the medial border. Frequently, these individuals show diminished longitudinal trunk rotation and sluggish balance reactions in the trunk. They tend to rely on protective extension reactions of the limbs to maintain balance. The staggering or stepping reactions of the lower extremities may be pronounced. Stride length and step length may be uneven. Gait may be wide based and unsteady.

Although the gait patterns in neurological gait may be complex and an analysis of the causes may be difficult, a detailed OGA can provide valuable data. Generally, to analyze gait patterns in persons who have sustained neurological damage, the following preliminary questions need to be asked:

1. How does the position of the head influence muscle tone and position in the trunk and the limbs?
2. How does weight-bearing influence muscle tone and position in the upper and lower extremities and in the pelvis and trunk?
3. What is the influence of abnormal (obligatory) synergistic activity on position and movement?
4. What is the influence of weakness (paresis) on position and movement?
5. What is the influence of impaired balance reactions on position and movement?

Ambulation Profiles and/or Scales

Profiles and rating scales constitute gait analyses that often include both qualitative (observational) and quantitative (time and distance) measures. Profiles and scales are used for a variety of reasons; for example, assessment of ambulation skills,[30] determination of the patient's need for assistance, identification of a change in a patient's status, screening for identification of the patient's need for physical therapy,[76] and identification of elderly individuals who are at risk for falling.[64] Gait analyses of one type or another may be either the sole focus of a profile or the gait analysis may constitute only a small portion of a broad assessment profile that includes balance skills as well as other functional activities. One particular advantage of some of these profiles is that subordinate gait skills such as standing balance may be assessed in individuals who may not be able to walk unassisted. Because many of these profiles were developed for use with specific populations, comparative data may also be available to the therapist.

The following profiles have been selected for review in this chapter because they are in current use and have been assessed for reliability and/or validity: the Functional Ambulation Profile (FAP),[30] the Iowa Level of Assistance Score,[77] the Functional Independence Measure (FIM),[78] the Functional Independence Measure for Children (WEEFIM),[79] the Gait Abnormality Rating Scale (GARS),[80] and the Modified GARS (GARS-M),[23]

the Dynamic Gait Index, Berg Balance Scale,[64] and the Fast Evaluation of Mobility, Balance and Fear (FEMBAF).[81]

The **Functional Ambulation Profile (FAP)** developed by Nelson is designed to assess gait skills on a continuum from standing balance in the parallel bars to independent ambulation. A stopwatch is used to measure the amount of time required either to maintain a position or perform a task. The test consists of three phases. In the first phase the patient is asked to perform the following three tasks in the parallel bars: bilateral stance, uninvolved leg stance, and involved leg stance. In the second phase, the patient is asked to transfer weight from one extremity to another as rapidly as possible. In the third phase the patient is asked to walk 20 feet (6 m) in the parallel bars, walk 20 feet (6 m) with an assistive device, and if possible to walk a distance of 20 feet (6 m) independently. The interrater and intrarater reliability of the FAP was found to be high when tested on 31 patients with neurological deficits.[30]

The *Iowa Level of Assistance Scale* is an instrument in which gait is included as one of the following four functional tasks: getting out of bed, standing from bed, ambulating 15 feet (4.57 m), and walking up and down three steps. The patient's performance on the tasks is rated according to the following seven levels: not tested for safety reasons, activity attempted but not completed, maximum assistance (therapist applies three or more points of control), moderate assistance (therapist applies two points of contact), minimal assistance (therapist provides one point of contact), standby assistance (no therapist contact but therapist not comfortable leaving patient), and independence (therapist comfortable leaving room). The scale was found to be highly reliable, valid, and responsive when used with patients following total hip or knee replacements.[77]

The *Functional Independence Measure (FIM)* is the result of a project funded by The National Institute of Handicapped Research to develop a uniform data system for medical rehabilitation[78] (see Chap. 11: Functional Assessment for a complete description of the FIM). The FIM Locomotion: Walk/Wheelchair Guide is that portion of the FIM that is related to gait (see Box 10–1 for scoring information).

The *Functional Independence Measure for Children (WEEFIM)* is designed to measure functional independence in children. It consists of 18 items involving the following 6 subscales: self-care, sphincter control, transfers, locomotion, communication, and social cognition. Agreement and stability of the **WEEFIM** was found to be excellent across trained raters and time when tested on 205 children (11 to 87 months of age) diagnosed with cerebral palsy, developmental disabilities, mental retardation, Down's Syndrome, and other cognitive impairments. The validity and sensitivity of the WEEFIM were not examined by these authors.[79]

The **Gait Abnormality Rating Scale (GARS)** was designed to identify patients at risk for falling in a nursing home population where time, space, and

---

Box 10–1 GUIDE FOR UNIFORM DATA SET FOR MEDICAL REHABILITATION VERSION 5.0

Locomotion: Walk/wheelchair
Includes walking, once in a standing position, or if using a wheelchair, once in a seated position, on a level surface. Performs safely. Indicate the most frequent mode of locomotion (Walk or Wheelchair). If both are used about equally, code Both.

No helper

7   Complete Independence—Subject *walks* a minimum of *150* feet (50 meters) without assistive devices. Does not use a wheelchair. Performs safely.

6   Modified Independence—Subject *walks* a minimum of *150* feet (50 meters) but uses a brace (orthosis) or prosthesis on leg, special adaptive shoes, cane, crutches, or walkerette; takes more than reasonable time or there are safety considerations.
    If not walking, subject operates manual or motorized wheelchair independently for a minimum of *150* feet (50 meters); turns around; maneuvers the chair to a table, bed, toilet; negotiates at least a 3 percent grade; maneuvers on rugs and over door sills.

5   Exception (Household Ambulation)—Subject walks only short distances (a minimum of *50* feet or 17 meters) *independently* with or without a device. Takes more than reasonable time, or there are safety considerations, or operates a manual or motorized wheelchair independently only short distances (a minimum of *50* feet or 17 meters).

Helper

5   Supervision
    If walking, subject requires standby supervision, cueing, or coaxing to go a minimum of *150* feet (50 meters).
    If not walking, requires standby supervision, cueing, or coaxing to go a minimum of *150* feet (50 meters) in wheelchair.

4   Minimal Contact Assistance—Subject performs 75% or more of locomotion effort to go a minimum of *150* feet (50 meters).

3   Moderate Assistance—Subject performs 50% to 74% of locomotion effort to go a minimum of *150* feet (50 meters).

2   Maximal Assistance—Subject performs 25% to 49% of locomotion effort to go a minimum of *50* feet (17 meters). Requires assistance of one person only.

1   Total Assistance—Subject performs less than 25% of effort, or requires assistance of two people, or does not walk or wheel a minimum of *50* feet (17 meters).

Comment: If the subject requires an assistive device for locomotion: wheelchair, prosthesis, walker, cane, AFO, adapted shoe, etc., the Walk/Wheelchair score can never be higher than level 6. The mode of locomotion (Walk or Wheelchair) must be the same on admission and discharge. If the subject changes mode of locomotion from admission to discharge (usually wheelchair to walking), record the admission mode and scores based on the *more frequent mode of locomotion at discharge.*

From: Guide for the Uniform Data Set for Medical Rehabilitation (including the FIM™ instrument), version 5.0. Buffalo, NY 14214: State University of New York at Buffalo; 1997, with permission.

resources are often very limited. The expenses include purchase of a camcorder and videotapes, and the therapist's time to film, review, and rate the videotapes. The test developers selected the following 16 features of the gait pattern as being associated with the risk of falling:

1. Variability of stepping and arm movements
2. Guardedness (lack of propulsion or commitment to stepping)
3. Weaving
4. Waddling
5. Staggering
6. Percentage of time in the stance phase
7. Foot contact
8. Hip range of motion
9. Knee range of motion
10. Elbow extension
11. Shoulder extension
12. Shoulder abduction
13. Arm-heel strike synchrony
14. Head held forward
15. Shoulder held elevated
16. Upper trunk flexed forward

These features are scored on a 0 to 3 rating scale where 0 = normal, 1 = mildly impaired, 2 = moderately impaired, and 3 = severely impaired. All except

three of the variables (head forward, shoulder elevation, and upper trunk forward) showed high interrater reliability. Furthermore, because the GARS scores correlated well with walking speed, stride length and with history of falling, the instrument appears to have validity for predicting the history of falling when used with nursing home residents. Arm-swing amplitude, upper and lower extremity synchrony, and guardedness best distinguished between older fallers and other subjects. However, as Woolacott et al.[80] have observed, the GARS does not provide information regarding the type of falls (trips, slips, losing balance) sustained by this population. Therefore it is not helpful in determining the cause of the falls.

The **Modified GARS (GARS-M),** which is a modified 7-item version of the GARS, contains the following 7 variables: variability, guardedness, staggering, foot contact, hip range of motion, shoulder extension, and arm-heelstrike synchrony. These variables were selected for inclusion because they had been found to be the most reliable in the original GARS. The scoring is the same as used in the original profile with the total score representing a rank ordering for risk of falling. A higher score is associated with a more abnormal gait. Van Swearingen et al.[23]

used the GARS-M with 52 community-dwelling elderly residents to determine its reliability, and concurrent and construct validity. Interrater and intrarater reliability were determined for GARS-M scores by three physical therapist raters. Concurrent validity was determined by quantitative measures of speed and stride length, and construct validity was obtained by the ability of the GARS-M scores to distinguish between subjects with a history of falls and those without a history of falls. The authors concluded that the GARS-M was reliable and valid and could be used to predict persons at risk for falls.[23]

Shumway-Cook et al.[64] examined the following four assessments in an attempt to develop a model for predicting the likelihood of falls among community-dwelling elderly (aged 65 and over): (1) **Balance Self Perceptions Test,** (2) Berg Balance Scale, (3) mobility (timed walking at self-paced preferred speed and at fast speed for 50 feet [15.2 m]), and (4) the Dynamic Gait Index. The Balance Self Perceptions Test is a self-rating assessment of the degree to which balance and perceived risk for falls interfere with daily activities. The **Berg Balance Scale** is a performance based assessment of balance and mobility in which subjects are rated on a 0 to 4 scale (0, cannot perform to 4, normal performance) on 14 different tasks such as ability to sit, stand, reach, turn, look over each shoulder, and turn a complete circle (gait assessment is not included). The total possible score on the Berg Balance Scale is 56 indicating excellent balance. The 50-foot walk test for mobility was timed and mean speed was calculated for both self-paced and fastest speed. The **Dynamic Gait Index** is designed to assess the ability to adapt gait to changes in task demands. Performance is rated on a 0 to 3 scale with 0 = poor to 3 = excellent. Individuals are rated on eight different tasks including gait on even surfaces, gait while changing speeds, gait and head turns in a vertical or horizontal direction, stepping over obstacles, and gait with pivot turns and steps. Although the Dynamic Gait Index was included as one of the factors that predicted a risk of falling, the final model included only the Berg Balance Scale and history of falling, with the Berg Balance Scale being the best single predictor of fall status. The Berg Balance Scale and history of falling had a sensitivity of 91 percent (20 of the 22 fallers correctly classified) and a specificity of 82 percent (18 of the nonfallers correctly classified). Patients who have high scores on the Berg Balance Scale have a relatively low fall risk. Patients with a score of 40 or less have a high risk for falls and would appear to be candidates for physical therapy.[64]

Fast Evaluation of Mobility Balance and Fear (FEMBAF) is another instrument designed to identify risk factors, functional performance, and factors that hinder mobility. It consists of a 22-item risk factor questionnaire and an 18-item performance component, which includes among other measures stair climbing and descending, stepping over an obstacle, and one-legged standing. According to DiFabio and Seay,[81] the FEMBAF provides a valid and reliable measurement of risk factors, functional performance, and factors that hinder mobility. However, further testing is required to validate its predictive capacity.

KINEMATIC QUANTITATIVE GAIT ANALYSIS

Kinematic **quantitative gait analyses** are used to obtain information on time and distance gait variables as well as motion patterns. The data obtained through these analyses are quantifiable and therefore provide the therapist with baseline data that can be used to plan treatment programs and assess progress toward goals or goal attainment. The fact that the data are quantifiable is important because third-party payers are demanding that therapists use measurable parameters when assessing patient function, establishing treatment strategies, and documenting the outcomes of a treatment program. However, data derived from qualitative observations may be necessary to classify degrees of motor impairment and to check the validity of the quantitative variables measured. Therefore, both qualitative and quantitative kinematic gait analyses should be performed to provide a more comprehensive picture of an individual's gait.

Distance and Time Variables

The variables measured in a quantitative gait analysis are listed and described in Table 10–17. Because distance and time variables are affected by a number of factors such as age,[82–89] gender,[90,91] height, weight,[29,92,93] level of physical activity,[94,95] and level of maturation,[96] attempts have been made to take some of these factors into account. Ratios such as stride-length divided by functional lower extremity length are used to normalize for differences in patients' leg lengths. Step length divided by the subject's height is used in an attempt to normalize differences among patients' heights. In an attempt to control for both height and weight, body weight is divided by standing height to yield the **body mass index (BMI).** Other ratios are used to assess symmetry; for example, right swing time divided by left swing time and swing time divided by stance time. Sutherland et al.[96] list the ratio of pelvic span to ankle spread as one of the determinants of mature gait in children.

Methods Used for Measuring Variables

The physical therapy literature contains a number of studies describing techniques for measuring distance (spatial) and temporal gait variables.[8–13,22,38,44,48,50,54,66,76,87,97–100] as well as studies investigating the uses and reliability of different

Table 10-17 GAIT VARIABLES: QUANTITATIVE GAIT ANALYSIS

Variable	Description
Speed	A scalar quantity that has magnitude but not direction.
Free speed	A person's normal walking speed.
Slow speed	A speed slower than a person's normal speed.
Fast speed	A rate faster than normal.
Cadence	The number of steps taken by a patient per unit of time. Cadence may be measured in centimeters as the number of steps per second $$Cadence = \frac{number\ of\ steps}{time}$$ A simple method of measuring cadence is by counting the number of steps taken by the patient in a given amount of time. The only equipment necessary is a stopwatch, paper, and pencil.
Velocity	A measure of a body's motion in a given direction.
Linear velocity	The rate at which a body moves in a straight line.
Angular velocity	The rate of motion in rotation of a body segment around an axis.
Walking velocity	The rate of linear forward motion of the body. This is measured in either centimeters per second or meters per minute. To obtain a person's **walking velocity,** divide the distance traversed by the time required to complete the distance. $$Walking\ velocity = \frac{distance}{time}$$ Walking velocity may be affected by age, level of maturation, height, sex, type of footwear, and weight. Also, velocity may affect cadence, step, stride length, and foot angle as well as other gait variables.
Acceleration	The rate of change of velocity with respect to time. Body acceleration has been defined by Smidt and Mommens[2] as the rate of change of velocity of a point posterior to the sacrum. Acceleration is usually measured in meters per second per second (m/s^2).
Angular acceleration	The rate of change of the angular velocity of a body with respect to time. Angular acceleration is usually measured in radians per second per second $(radians/s^2)$.
Stride time	The amount of time that elapses during one stride: that is, from one foot contact (heel strike if possible) until the next contact of the same foot (heel strike). Both stride times should be measured. Measurement is usually in seconds.
Step time	The amount of time that elapses between consecutive right and left foot contacts (heel strikes). Both right and left step times should be measured. Measurement is in seconds.
Stride length	The linear distance between two successive points of contact of the same foot. It is measured in centimeters or meters. The average stride length for normal adult males is 1.46 meters. The average stride length for adult females is 1.28 meters.
Swing time	The amount of time during the gait cycle that one foot is off the ground. Swing time should be measured separately for right and left extremities. Measurement is in seconds.
Double support time	The amount of time spent in the gait cycle when both lower extremities are in contact with the supporting surface. Measured in seconds.
Cycle time (stride time)	The amount of time required to complete a gait cycle. Measured in seconds.
Step length	The linear distance between two successive points of contact of the right and left lower extremities. Usually a measurement is taken from the point of heel contact at heel strike of one extremity to the point of heel contact of the opposite extremity. If a patient does not have a heel strike on one or both sides, the measurement can be taken from the heads of the first metatarsals. Measured in centimeters or meters.
Width of walking base (step width)	The width of the walking base (base of support) is the linear distance between one foot and the opposite foot. Measured in centimeters or meters.[7]
Foot angle (degree of toe out or toe in)	The angle of foot placement with respect to the line of progression. Measured in degrees.[7]
Bilateral stance time (for the FAP)	The length of time up to 30 seconds that a person can stand upright in the parallel bars bearing weight on both lower extremities.
Uninvolved stance time (for the FAP)	The length of time up to 30 seconds that an individual can stand in the parallel bars while bearing weight on the uninvolved lower extremity (involved extremity is raised off the supporting surface).
Involved stance time (for the FAP)	The length of time up to 30 seconds that an individual can stand in the parallel bars on the involved lower extremity (uninvolved lower extremity is raised off the supporting surface).
Dynamic weight transfer rate (for the FAP)	The rate at which an individual standing in the parallel bars can transfer weight from one extremity to another. Measured in seconds from the first lift-off to the last lift-off.
Parallel bar ambulation (for the FAP)	Length of time required for an individual to walk the length of the parallel bars as rapidly as possible. Two trials are averaged to obtain this measurement. Measurement is in seconds.

FAP = Functional Ambulation Profile.

methods of measurement.[34,65,101,102] Two types of variables (distance and temporal) are frequently included in a kinematic quantitative gait analysis and are necessary for the interpretation of kinetic and electromyographic (EMG) data. The techniques and equipment required for measurement of these variables range from simple to complex. The time requirements also vary, and the therapist must be familiar with different methods of assessing these variables in order to select the method most appropriate to each situation. Prior to selecting a method of measurement, the therapist should understand the variable in question and how that variable is related to the patient's gait.

DISTANCE VARIABLES

Measurement of the distance completed within a set time frame is one of the simplest methods that can be used to assess distance variables. Schenkman et al. used the distance covered in a 6-minute walk at a comfortable pace *(Six-Minute Walk Test)* to assess the physical performance of patients with Parkinson's disease.[65] These authors found that test-retest reliability was high and suggested that this simple test, used in combination with other physical performance and impairment measures (i.e., ROM and muscle force) could be used to either monitor decline, or assess improvement due to treatment interventions. For individuals with limited endurance, a *Three-Minute Walk Test* has been used.[103]

Measurement of variables such as degree of foot angle, width of base of support, step length, and stride length also can be assessed simply and inexpensively in the clinic by recording the patient's footprints during gait. Many different methods for recording footprints (footfall) have been described in the literature, for example, walkway marking methods include the absorbent paper method[7]; commercially available carbon paper system[3]; painting,[6] inking,[34,99] or chalking of the feet; and felt-tipped markers attached to the shoes.[12,23]

Walkways for recording footprints may be created either by the application of various materials to the floor or by using an uncarpeted floor or hallway. A few of the materials used to create walkways include absorbent paper,[7] commercially produced carbon paper,[3] and aluminum.[13] In the absorbent paper method, three layers of material are placed over a carpeted floor to form a walkway. The first layer is brown paper, the second layer is moistened paper or terry cloth, and the third layer is absorbent paper such as a paper tablecloth. When the subject walks along the walkway, the pressure of the body weight causes the water from the second layer to be absorbed by the dry top layer. The therapist outlines the footprints with a felt-tipped pen immediately following the walking trail. The resulting record permits measurement of step and stride lengths, stride width, and foot angle. The commercially made carbon paper and aluminum paper provide a similar type of footprint record.

Other simple methods of recording footprints require the application of paints, ink, or chalk to the bottom of the patient's foot or shoe or the attachment of inked pads or other markers. For example, the bottoms of a patient's feet may be covered with Tempera paint[6] prior to walking along a paper-covered walkway, or a felt-tipped marker may be taped to the back of a patient's shoe.[12,23] In both methods, measurements of step length, stride length, step width, and foot angle may be obtained.

Another way of obtaining step length and stride length data is by placing a grid pattern on the floor.[9] A strip of masking tape about 1 foot (30 centimeters) wide and 32 feet (10 m) long is laid down in a straight line. The tape is marked off in 1-inch (3 cm) increments for its entire length, and the segments are numbered consecutively so that the patient's heel strikes can be identified. The therapist calls out the heel strike locations from the numbers on the grid pattern and the numbers are recorded by a tape recorder.

TEMPORAL VARIABLES

In most of the listed methods of assessing stride and step lengths, temporal variables such as cadence, velocity, and stride times may be calculated if the elapsed time it takes the subject to walk a measured distance *(d)* is obtained using a stopwatch. **Cadence** *(c)* can be determined by dividing the number of steps *(n)* taken during the walking trial by the elapsed time *(tn)* between the first and last heel strikes using the following formula $c = n/tn$. **Velocity** *(v)* can be calculated by taking the total distance *(d)* between the first and last heel strikes and dividing it by the elapsed time *(td)* for the distance *(v = d/td)*. To obtain a normal walking speed, the patient should be allowed to take a few steps prior to the beginning of any measurements.

Todd et al.,[89] who tested 84 normal children (41 girls and 43 boys) ages 13 months to 12 years, and analyzed data from over 200 other children ages 11 months to 16 years, developed a two-dimensional gait graph that provides a visual record of a child's walking performance. The gait graph is similar in appearance to graphs used for height and weight, however, the gait graph shows norms for gait dimensions of cadence and stride length adjusted by height (Fig. 10-7).

Instrumented Systems

Instrumented systems for measuring spatial and temporal variables include: two types of walkways and three types of footswitch systems. The first type of walkway has an electrically conductive surface. This type of walkway is used in conjunction with conductive strips on the patient's feet. Foot contact and foot-off are measured through starting and stopping of the electrical current. The information obtained is transmitted via a cable to a strip chart recorder that records and analyzes the data. The variables measured are swing time, stance time, cycle time, single support time, and double support time. The advantages of this type of system is that it is inexpensive and easy to use. The disadvantages are that it measures only temporal parameters and requires the patient to be attached to a cable. The drag of the cable may modify a patient's gait.

The second type of walkway is embedded with pressure-sensitive switches that open and close in response to contact with the patient's feet. The time of openings and closures of the switches are recorded by a computer thus providing information on step length, step time, and average walking speed. **GAITMAT** (produced by EQ., Inc., Plymouth Meeting, PA) is an example of a commercially available walkway with embedded switches. A new version of the GAITMAT, the GAITMAT II has .5-inch (15 mm) square pressure sensitive switches ar-

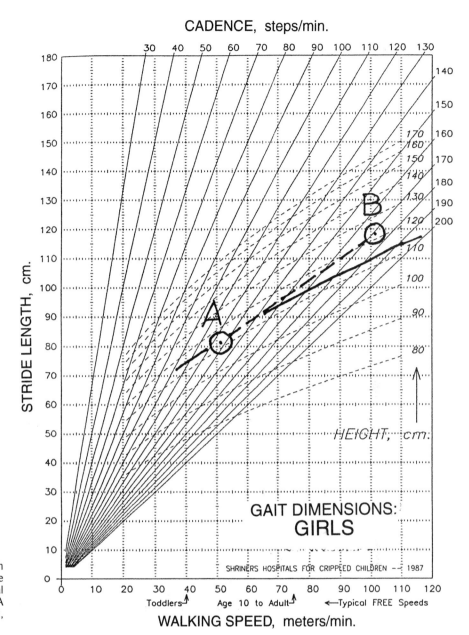

Figure 10-7. The *solid line* on the gait graph represents normal parameters for height. The *dashed line* represents data plotted for a normal 6 year-old girl whose height was 114 cm. A similar chart is available for boys. (From Todd, et al.,[89] p 201, with permission.)

ranged in a matrix of 256 transverse rows with 40 switches to a row. The display produced from the GAITMAT II system shows recognizable footprints, identifies individual footprints, distinguishes left from right, and provides information on step length, stride length, base of support, step time, swing time, stance time, single support time, and double support time for each extremity. The advantages of this system are that it measures both spatial and temporal gait parameters, and the patient is unencumbered by equipment attached to either the feet or body. The main disadvantage is cost.

Foot switches are pressure-sensitive switches that are placed either on the inside or outside of a patient's shoes or feet. The switches do not require a walkway, but the patient usually has to carry a data collection device. Foot switches consist of transducers and a semiconductor and are used to signal such

events as heel strike. One type of foot switch device that has been used to assess both temporal and loading variables is the Krusen Limb Load Monitor.[8] Originally this device was designed to monitor the amount of weight a patient placed on an affected extremity. When the weight exceeded a predetermined magnitude, the instrument emitted a warning signal. Later, the device was modified and used to obtain data on temporal and loading gait variables. This device consists of a pressure-sensitive force plate that can be worn within a patient's shoe. It can be connected to a strip chart recorder to yield a permanent record of temporal and distance gait variables.[8]

The Timer-Logger Communicator (TLC) Gait Monitor is another commercially available foot switch system. It consists of digital foot switches from MIE Electronics (Biokinetics, Bethesda, MD) that are connected to the TLC (a battery-operated portable microcomputer). The TLC weighs less than 2.20 pounds (1 kg) and is carried on a belt fastened around the subject's waist. This system was used by Roth et al.[44] to investigate the relationship between velocity and 18 temporal gait variables in 25 patients with a first hemispheric stroke resulting in hemiplegia. These authors concluded that although velocity is a critical component of hemiplegic gait assessment, and significantly correlated with 12 of the 18 variables measured (cadence, mean cycle duration, mean cycle length, hemiplegic limb stance phase duration, non-hemiplegic limb stance phase duration and percent, non-hemiplegic limb swing phase percent, double support phase duration and percent, hemiplegic limb swing/stance phase ratio, non-hemiplegic limb swing/stance phase ratio, and swing phase symmetry ratio) velocity should not be used as the only indicator of a patient's gait status. Characterization of the degree of asymmetry, and descriptions of individual phase durations and proportions of subject's hemiplegic stance and swing percentages in addition to velocity should be included in a gait analysis of patients with hemiplegia.

The **Stride Analyzer** is a footswitch system available from B and L Engineering (Santa Fe Springs, CA). This system uses special insoles that contain four pressure sensitive switches placed under the heel, at the heads of the first and fifth metatarsals, and at the great toe. The parameters measured by this system include stride length, velocity, cadence, cycle time, single limb support time, swing time, double support time, and stance time. These measurements are recorded automatically and the information is transmitted to a computer, which analyzes the data. Times are presented in seconds, and as a percent of the gait cycle. The computer analysis also includes a percentage of normal using a built-in data base (Box 10–2).

The advantages of the Stride Analyzer system are that measurements from both feet are available, the system is easy to move from place to place, and, because it has been used by a large number of physical therapists with different populations, data comparisons may be possible.[38,48,50,54,76,97,98] A few of the recent studies in which the Stride Analyzer was used are included in Table 10–18. The sample studies appear to indicate that the Stride Analyzer apparently is suitable for use with various age groups as well as for patients with either neurologic or orthopedic problems.

Joint displacement can be measured relatively simply by using an electrogoniometer. The electrogoniometer is composed of two rigid links connected by a potentiometer that converts movement into an electrical signal that is proportional to the degree of movement. The rigid links or arms of the electrogoniometer are attached to the proximal and distal limb segments. Data obtained from the electrogoniometer can be displayed either as angle/angle diagrams or on a strip chart recorder. **Angle/angle diagrams** are produced by plotting the angular sagittal plane displacements of adjacent joints against each other. Strip chart recorders provide a record of the displacement patterns of gait. According to Perry,[20] electrogoniometers, which cost approximately $3000, are the "most convenient and least expensive" means of measuring knee and ankle motion during walking.

Imaging based systems are the most sophisticated method of assessing joint displacement and patterns of motion. In these computerized motion analysis systems, markers placed on body segments such as the knee, ankle, and hip are tracked by automated multicamera systems. Two types of motion analysis systems are available: **optoelectric** and **video-based.** Optoelectric systems use active markers while video-based systems use passive markers. Active markers are generally **light emitting diodes (LEDs)** that flash at given frequencies. Passive markers require an external source of illumination.

An imaging system using LEDs for assessing sagittal plane motion has been used at the University of Iowa.[10] The following two optoelectronic systems are commercially available: the Waterloo Spatial Motion Analysis and Recording Technique **(WATSMART)** system may be obtained from Northern Digital, Inc. (Waterloo, Ontario, Canada) and the **Vicon Motion Analysis System** is available from Oxford Metrics Ltd. (Botleg, Oxford, England).

The Peak Motus used with the 3-D Gait Analysis Module produced by Peak Performance Technologies, Inc., is an example of a video-based imaging system. It provides information on displacement for right and left hip, knee and ankle joint centers of rotation as well as joint angles for hip, knee, ankle, and pelvic motions. In addition, this system is able to measure kinetic variables in addition to temporal and spatial variables. Figure 10-8 provides an example of passive marker placement on a subject as well as a graph of linear velocities of the shoulder, hip, and knee, and angular velocities of the shoulder, elbow, and knee. In Figure 10-9 the degrees of motion for the ankle and knee are plotted against time. In Figure 10-10, stick figures are shown with accompanying knee angles. The **Expert Vision System** (Motion Analysis Corporation, Santa Rosa, CA) and the **Ariel Performance Analysis System** are other commercially available video-based systems.

A sample of recent studies using various motion analysis systems for gait analysis is presented in Table 10–19. The table includes the variables measured as well as the methods used to measure each variable. In the majority of studies, motion analysis systems were used in conjunction with other methods of measurement, such as dynamometers to measure muscle force, footswitches to measure temporal and/or distance gait parameters, and scales to measure pain.

EMG is used to analyze the timing and peak activity of muscle activity during gait.[32,35,104] Usually, EMG is used in combination with other instrumentation such as the Stride Analyzer and/or an imaging system to identify the particular portion of the gait cycle in which the muscle activity occurs.[48]

Box 10–2 SIMPLE TABULATED OUTPUT FROM THE STRIDE ANALYZER SYSTEM

YOUR DEPARTMENT'S NAME
YOUR INSTITUTION'S NAME
STRIDE ANALYZER REPORT—WALKING

NAME:	JOHN SMITH	RUN:	JS01
I.D. NUMBER:	1234	STRIDES:	4
DATE:	05/13/93	DISTANCE (M):	6.00
AGE:	29	TEST CONDITIONS:	
SEX:	M	WALK	
DIAGNOSIS:	Sprained Right Ankle		

STRIDE CHARACTERISTICS	ACTUAL	%NORMAL
VELOCITY (M/MIN):	60.3	74.0
CADENCE (STEP/MIN):	100.4	92.7
STRIDE LENGTH (M):	1.201	79.8
GAIT CYCLE (SEC):	1.20	106.8

	-R-	-L-
SINGLE LIMB SUPPORT		
(SEC):	0.429	0.418
(%NORMAL):	86.4	84.2
(%GC):	35.9	35.0
SWING (%GC):	33.5	34.5
STANCE (%GC):	66.5	65.5
DOUBLE SUPPORT		
INITIAL (%GC):	15.2	15.4
TERMINAL (%GC):	15.4	15.2
TOTAL (%GC):	30.6	30.6

LEFT FOOT (stance = 65.5% GC)
  HEEL   -- Normal contact at 0.0% GC (0.0% Stance)
                     Delayed cessation at 50.6% GC (77.2% Stance)
  5TH METATARSAL -- Premature contact at 3.8% GC (5.7% Stance)
                     Delayed cessation at 63.3% GC (96.6% Stance)
  1ST METATARSAL -- Normal contact at 22.4% GC (34.2% Stance)
                     Delayed cessation at 63.9% GC (97.5% Stance)
  TOE   -- Normal contact at 33.7% GC (51.4% Stance)
                     Delayed cessation at 65.5% GC (100.0% Stance)

RIGHT FOOT (stance = 66.5% GC)
  HEEL   -- Normal contact at 0.0% GC (0.0% Stance)
                     Delayed cessation at 50.8% GC (76.4% Stance)
  5TH METATARSAL -- Premature contact at 4.0% GC (6.0% Stance)
                     Delayed cessation at 64.8% GC (97.5% Stance)
  1ST METATARSAL -- Normal contact at 19.6% GC (29.4% Stance)
                     Delayed cessation at 63.8% GC (96.0% Stance)
  TOE   -- Normal contact at 38.1% GC (57.3% Stance)
                     Delayed cessation at 65.2% GC (98.1% Stance)

Source: From Craik and Oatis,[21] p 133, with permission.

An example of how EMG is used in combination with a motion analysis system (Vicon) is presented in Figure 10-11. The figure shows the EMG output and ROM on the graph while the computer generated figures provide a visual image. The differences in muscle activity among the three types of walking patterns are easily seen in the graphs. The deviations from normal ROM at the knee are also easy to identify. A careful observation of the figures in the extension thrust pattern show an extension thrust of the knee immediately after initial contact and excessive plantarflexion at the ankle both at heel strike and throughout the gait cycle. Refer to Chapter 9 for a detailed presentation on EMG.

RELIABILITY AND VALIDITY

Reliability of the absorbent paper and felt-tipped pen methods has not been reported. In a study of 61 patients with neurological impairments, Holden et al.[34] used ink footprints on a paper-covered walkway. High interrater and test-retest reliability was reported using the inked footprint method to determine the following variables: velocity, cadence, step length, and stride length. These investigators also

Table 10–18 STUDIES USING THE STRIDE ANALYZER

Authors	Purpose	Method	Variables	Subjects	Results
Evans, Goldie, and Hill[102]	To obtain intersession estimates of error for time and distance parameters of gait.	Stride Analyzer	Velocity, cadence, stride length, gait cycle duration, single limb support time, and double limb support time	Thirty-one patients with stroke who were four months post-stroke and involved in inpatient rehabilitation	Patients would have to increase gait velocity by more than 6.8 m/min. or decrease velocity more than 6.8 m/min. before it could be assumed with 95% confidence that genuine change beyond limits of error had occurred. Alternative strategies such as serial measurements may be required for measuring changes in velocity.
Harada, et al.[70]	To identify persons for referral for physical therapy evaluation.	Stride Analyzer, Berg Balance Scale, Tinetti Performance Oriented Mobility Assessment and the Tinetti Fall Efficiency Scale	Velocity	Fifty-three patients with stroke living in two residential facilities	A combination of the Berg Balance Scale results and gait velocity yielded the highest sensitivity level of 91% and therefore might be the best combination for screening. The sensitivity of gait velocity was 80% and the specificity was 89%.
Morris, et al.[54]	To determine how a patient's medication cycle affects gait.	Stride Analyzer	Velocity, cadence, stride length, gait cycle duration, single limb support time, and double limb support time	Thirty-one patients with stroke who were 4 months post-stroke and involved in inpatient rehabilitation	Patients would have to increase gait velocity by more than 6.8 m/min. or decrease velocity more than 6.8 m/min. before it could be assumed with 95% confidence that genuine change beyond limits of error had occurred. Alternative strategies such as serial measurements may be required for measuring changes in velocity.
Powers, et al.[50]	To establish the relationship between isometric muscle force and temporal/spatial gait characteristics for individuals with below knee amputations.	Stride Analyzer	Velocity, cadence, and stride length	Fifteen males and seven females with below knee amputations	Mean walking speed was limited to 59% of normal. Hip extensor torque of the residual limb was the only predictor for both free speed and fast gait. Cadence was equal to 83% of normal. Hip abductor torque of the sound limb was the only predictor of cadence for free and fast speed. Stride length was 69% of normal.
Powers, et al.[98]	To compare stride characteristics and joint motion in subjects with patellofemoral pain with and without patellar taping.	Stride Analyzer Vicon Motion Analysis System	Velocity, stride length and cadence Sagittal plane joint motion of the pelvis, hip, knee and ankle	Fifteen female subjects with the diagnosis of patellofemoral pain	No significant differences were found in gait velocity or cadence between the taped and untaped trials. Patellar taping resulted in a small but significant increase in knee flexion loading response. The increase in knee flexion could help with shock absorption at heel strike.

Author	Purpose	Instrumentation	Measurements	Subjects	Results
Powers, et al.[100]	To determine the influence of pain and muscle weakness on gait variables in subjects with patellofemoral pain.	Stride Analyzer; Vicon Motion Analysis System; Lido Dynamometer; Visual Analog Pain Scale; Functional Assessment Questionnaire	Velocity, stride length and cadence; Sagittal plane joint motion of the hip, knee and ankle; Isometric knee extensor torque; Knee pain; Patellofemoral joint symptoms	Nineteen female subjects with a diagnosis of patellofemoral pain and 19 female subjects without patellofemoral pain	The primary compensation in the patellofemoral pain group was a decrease in walking speed which was a function of decreased stride length and cadence. Knee extensor torque was the only predictor of gait function with increased torque correlating with improved stride characteristics.
Radtka, et al.[48]	To compare the effects of dynamic AFO's with a plantar flexion stop, solid AFO's and no AFO's.	Stride Analyzer; 3-D Motion Analysis	Velocity, cadence, and stride length; Joint motion at ankle, knee, hip and pelvis; Muscle timing	Ten children (four boys and six girls) with spastic cerebral palsy who had a dynamic equinus gait pattern with excessive plantarflexion during stance	Both orthoses increased stride length, decreased cadence and reduced ankle plantarflexion when compared to the no AFO condition. No differences were found between the two orthoses.
Von Schroeder, et al.[38]	To compare gait parameters and patterns in patients with stroke and controls.	Surface EMG; Stride Analyzer	Velocity, cadence, stride length, gait cycle time, double support time, single limb support and swing phase time	Forty-nine ambulatory patients with stroke and 24 age-matched controls	Patients walked significantly slower than control subjects. The patients had decreased cadence, increased cycle time, and increased double support time. The unaffected limb had significantly more time spent in stance and single limb support.

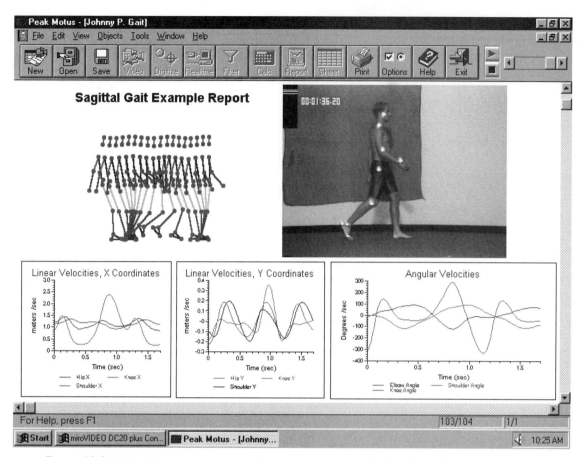

Figure 10-8. A typical computer screen from an automated video-based motion-analysis system. Marker placement on the individual whose gait is being analyzed can be seen in the video image at the right upper side of the screen. Computer-generated stick figure representations of the person's gait are shown in the left upper side of the screen. The bottom half of the screen provides linear and angular velocities. (Courtesy of Peak Performance Technologies, Englewood, CO.)

found a strong linear relationship between the variables tested and a Functional Ambulation Classification test protocol that was developed at Massachusetts General Hospital. The grid pattern method of gait analysis is reported to be a feasible clinical research tool as well as a good method for quantitative analysis of temporal and distance measures.[9] Soderberg and Gabel[10] report that the LED system has high interrater and intrarater reliability for temporal and distance measures. Stuberg et al.[15] found no significant differences in measurements of stride length and walking velocity using cinematography and measurements using moleskin foot markers on a paper walkway and a stopwatch. Subjects in the study were 10 children with cerebral palsy and 9 normal children.

Wilson et al.[105] investigated the accuracy of reconstructed angular estimates of the Ariel Performance Analysis System and found that the mean errors of the reconstructed angles were consistently within the range of plus or minus 1 degree regardless of angular velocity. The authors believe this was within an acceptable range of measurement error for imaging systems, but cautioned that the users of these systems need to establish strict guidelines for quality control. Potential errors can be introduced by obstruction of markers by body segments, skin/soft tissue motion, marker vibration, and improper placement of markers in relation to the joint center of motion. Owing to the use of passive markers, these video-based systems are especially susceptible to errors due to marker obstruction when markers are in close proximity to one another.

ADVANTAGES AND DISADVANTAGES

The primary advantages of assessing time and distance are that these measures can be assessed simply and inexpensively in the clinic and that they yield an objective and reliable baseline upon which to formulate goals and outcomes and to assess progress or lack of progress toward outcomes (goals). For example, gait patterns displayed by patients with arthritis often are characterized by a reduced rate and range of knee motion compared with those of normal subjects, and they have a slower than normal gait velocity. Brinkmann and Perry[106] found that following joint replacement the rate and range of knee motion and gait velocity increased above preoperative levels but did not reach normal levels. Usually increases in measures such as cadence and velocity indicate improvement in a patient's gait. However, comparisons with

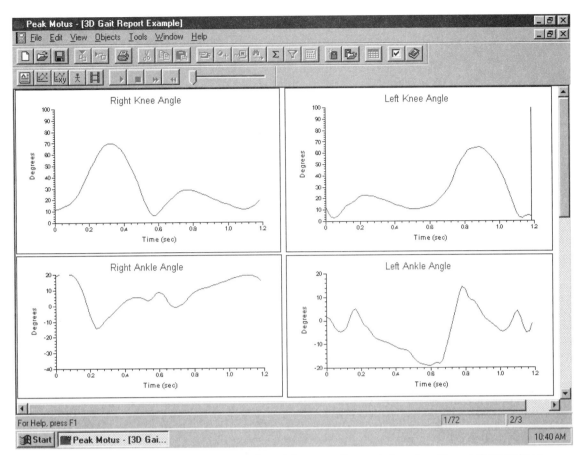

Figure 10-9. A typical computer-generated graph from a motion-analysis system. The graph shows knee and ankle range-of-motion patterns, which are plotted against time for both lower extremities. (Courtesy of Peak Performance Technologies, Englewood, CO.)

normal standards are appropriate only if the goal of treatment is to restore a normal gait pattern (e.g., for a patient recovering from a meniscectomy). Comparison with normative standards may not be appropriate for a patient who has had a cerebral vascular accident. The appropriate norms for assessing the gait of a patient with hemiplegia may be either a population of patients with hemiplegia who are of similar age, gender, and involvement, or the patient's pretreatment gait.

Therapists need to be extremely cautious when selecting a norm or standard by which to measure patient progress. Significant age-, gender-, weight-, and activity-level-related differences have been found in both temporal and distance measures.[82–85] Hinman et al.[83] examined the gait of 289 males and females ages 19 to 102 years and found that the oldest group (63 years and older) had a significantly slower self-selected walking speed and smaller step length in comparison to the younger group. Age was a significant determinant of walking speed after age 62, but height was a significant determinant prior to age 62. In a study of 15 healthy elderly individuals, ages 62 to 78 (10 males, 5 females), the authors found that step length was significantly shorter and the double support stance period significantly increased in this sample compared to a database of young adults.[85] Leiper and Craik[94] compared the effects of physical activity level on gait variables in 81 women (64.0 to 94.5 years of age) and found that the normal walking speeds of all the women tested were slower than values reported for younger women. In addition, the women with the highest activity level were able to walk at a significantly slower pace than women with lower levels of activity. Bohannon et al.[87] found that gender, body weight, and nondominant hip flexor strength were the best predictors of both comfortable and maximum gait speed for a group of 77 healthy men and 79 healthy women ages 50 to 79 years. However, these variables only accounted for a small percentage of the variance in gait speed: 13 percent for comfortable walking and 21 percent for maximum speed walking. Furthermore, muscle strength correlated more highly with maximal gait speed than with comfortable speed. Age was not correlated with gait speed in this group of subjects.[87] In a study of 152 community-dwelling adults ranging in age from 65 to 85 years, Buchner et al.[93] found that changes in gait speed were related to changes in depressive symptoms and physical health status, but not to changes in strength and aerobic capacity.

Therefore, one way to determine if the normative standard is appropriate for use with an individual patient is to compare the characteristics of the population used to establish the norm with the

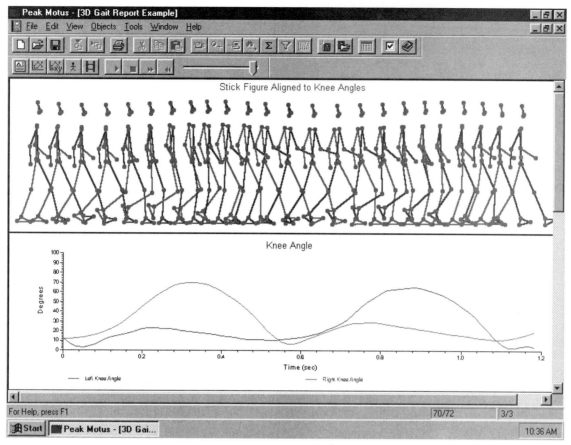

Figure 10-10. Another format for presentation of the data from a motion-analysis system is computer-generated stick figure representations of one complete gait cycle. In this particular case, the pattern of knee motion is graphically presented below the stick figures. (Courtesy of Peak Performance Technologies, Englewood, CO.)

patient's characteristics. For example, is the age of the patient in the same range as the sample population? Is the patient's gender the same as that of the sample population? Holden et al.[34] have recommended that gait performance goals and outcomes for patients with neurological problems should not only be based on norms derived from patients with the same diagnosis, but also should consider etiological factors, type of ambulation aid, and functional category.[34]

The interpretation of motion patterns obtained through motion analysis systems usually involves comparisons of an individual's data with a mean curve for normal subjects using one standard deviation (SD) for boundaries. Sutherland et al.[107] believe motion patterns cannot be fully analyzed without consideration of all points along the curve. Therefore, they propose the use of prediction regions (multiples of the SD above and below the mean curve of data for each point in the gait cycle) (Fig. 10-12). Within a prediction region, if any point along the curve of joint motion falls outside of the defined region, the patient's gait is considered to be abnormal. Testing of the prediction region model with 38 children (31 with cerebral palsy, 7 with various other disorders) demonstrated that the sensitivity was satisfactory. The regions predicted a high per-

centage of abnormal motion curves (true positives).

Temporal and distance measures may be critical factors in determinations of a patient's independence in ambulation. For example, a patient may need to attain a certain velocity of gait to cross a local street within the limit of the time allotted by a crossing light. A patient may need to walk a certain distance to shop in the local supermarket. Changes in velocity may affect step length, cadence, and other gait variables. Therapists need to survey the community to determine the distances and time requirements for accessing stores and public buildings prior to making a judgement about a patient's functional ambulation status.[108] Robinett and Von Dran[107] found that target goals on a sample of gait assessment forms were low compared to distance and velocity requirements found in a community survey. For example, the fastest walking velocity found on the forms was 18.2 m/min whereas the minimum safe street crossing velocity that the investigators found in a survey of rural and urban communities was 30 m/min with a range of 30 to 82.5 m/min.[108] Walsh et al.,[110] in a study of 29 individuals at 1 year post total knee arthroplasty, found that these individuals achieved over 80 percent of the normal walking speeds of their age- and gender-matched counterparts. However, for 62 percent of

Table 10–19 STUDIES USING MOTION ANALYSIS SYSTEMS

Authors	Purpose	Method	Variables	Subjects	Results
Damiano, et al.[52]	To determine the effects of a quadriceps strengthening program on producing improvements in gait performance by reducing the degree of knee crouch during gait.	Hand-held dynamometer	Quadriceps and hamstrings isometric muscle force	Fourteen children with spastic diplegia ranging in age from 6 to 14	Mean force gains of fifty percent over initial values were produced in the quadriceps without a concurrent force gain in the hamstrings. Knee extension was increased at initial floor contact at self-selected gait speeds for ten of the fourteen children. Also stride length increased at both free and fast speeds.
Eng and Pierrynowski[47]	To examine the effects of foot orthotics on the ROM of the talocrural, subtalar and knee joints during walking and running.	Expert Vision Motion Analysis System WATSMART Motion Analysis System	Joint motion at the pelvis, hips, knees and ankles in the coronal, transverse and sagittal planes Cadence, velocity and stride length ROM at the knee, talocrural and subtalar joints in the sagittal, coronal and transverse planes	Ten females mean age 14.4 years who had been prescribed orthotics for patellofemoral pain	Foot orthotics had no significant effect on the ROM, but the orthotic reduced the talocrural and subtalar joint motion in the coronal plane during walking and running. The orthotic reduced knee joint motion in the coronal plane during walking but increased knee joint motion during running.
Mueller, et al.[37]	To compare gait characteristics, plantar-flexor peak torques and ankle ROM of subjects with diabetes mellitus and age matched controls.	Lido Active Isokinetic Table Foot switches Expert Vision Motion Analysis System Calculations using a two-dimensional link segment model	Plantarflexion peak torque Initial floor contact and toe off Kinematics of the trunk and lower extremities and the ground reaction force Moments and power at the ankle, knee, and hip	Ten patients with diabetes and peripheral neuropathy whose mean age was 57.7 years and 10 subjects with no history of diabetes whose mean age was 56.8 years	The subjects with diabetes showed less ankle mobility, moment, and power than nondiabetic subjects. Also patients with diabetes had slower velocity and shorter stride length than nondiabetic subjects. The subjects with diabetes appeared to use a hip strategy rather than an ankle strategy. The hip strategy may be a safer method for ambulation for these patients because it provides more stability and reduces pressure on the plantar surface of the foot.

Continued

Table 10–19 STUDIES USING MOTION ANALYSIS SYSTEMS *Continued*

Authors	Purpose	Method	Variables	Subjects	Results
Mueller, et al.[41]	To determine the relationship of plantarflexor peak torque and dorsiflexion ROM to peak ankle moments and power during the late phase of walking	Plastic goniometer	Dorsiflexion ROM	Six subjects with diabetes and peripheral neuropathies whose mean age was 57.9 years and 10 subjects with no history of diabetes whose mean age was 56.8 years	Plantarflexor peak torque made the greatest contribution to the variance of the plantarflexor peak moment and power during the late stage of walking. A strong correlation existed between plantarflexor peak torque and dorsiflexor ROM and ankle power. The mean plantarflexor peak torque in patients was three standard deviations lower than in the non-diabetic subjects.
		Lido Isokinetic Table	Plantarflexion peak torque		
		Foot switches	Initial contact and toe off		
		Expert Vision Motion Analysis System and force plate	Ankle motion and plantarflexor moment during walking		
Powers, et al.[98]	To examine the effects of patellar taping on stride characteristics and joint motion in subjects with patellofemoral pain	Vican Motion Analysis System	Sagittal plane motion of the pelvis, hip, knee and ankle	Fifteen female subjects between the ages of 14 and 41 years with a diagnosis of patellofemoral pain	Pain decreased with taping but taping was not effective in increasing gait velocity or any other gait variables. However, taping compared to nontaping, resulted in a significant increase in knee flexion during loading. The increase in knee flexion should serve to assist in shock absorption during loading.
		Stride Analyzer	Velocity, cadence and stride length		
		Visual Analog Pain Scale	Knee pain		

Slow gait velocity

Extension Thrust Pattern

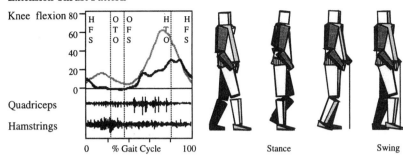

Stiff-Knee Pattern

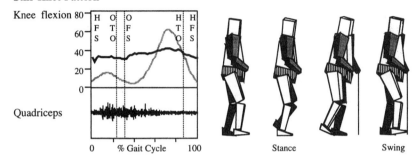

Buckling-Knee Pattern

Figure 10-11. Graphs and electromyographic data for motion of the knee in the sagittal plane for one gait cycle of three patients. Each patient represents only one of the three motion patterns (extension thrust, stiff knee, and buckling knee) associated with a slow gait velocity. The solid black line indicates the motion pattern and the gray line represents the normal. HFS, foot strike (initial contact) on the hemiplegic side; OTO, toe off on the contralateral (unaffected) side; OFS, foot strike (initial contact) on the contralateral (unaffected) side; HTO, toe off on the hemiplegic side. (From De Quervain, et al.,[42] with permission.)

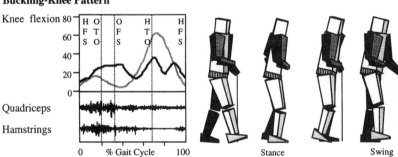

the females and 25 percent of the males, the normal walking speed attained would not be sufficient to cross a street intersection safely.

Few disadvantages exist regarding kinematic quantitative gait analysis except for the expense involved in instrumentation and the fact that a certain amount of uncertainty exists about how to normalize for leg length, height, age, sex, weight, level of maturation, and disability. Temporal and distance assessments should be used as an integral part of or in conjunction with both observational and kinetic assessments to provide a complete picture of gait. A sample recording form for time and distance variables is presented in Table 10–20.

KINETIC GAIT ANALYSIS

Kinetic gait analyses are directed toward assessment and analysis of the forces involved in gait, i.e., ground reaction forces, joint torques, center of pressure (COP), center of mass (COM), mechanical

energy, moments of force, power, support moments, work, **joint reaction forces** and intrinsic foot pressure (Table 10–21). Although in the past, kinetic gait analyses have been used primarily for research purposes, at the present time they are being used clinically as well.

The instrumentation required to assess kinetic variables is complex and expensive. Force plates are the most commonly used devices for force measurement in gait analysis. These plates contain load transducers that measure ground reaction forces and the **center of pressure (COP)** and **center of mass (COM)** during gait. Typically the force plates are based on either strain gage or piezoelectric technology. The **ground (floor) reaction force (GRF)** is defined as the net vertical and shear or horizontal forces acting between the foot and the supporting surface. The force is three-dimensional and can be resolved into three components: vertical, anterior-posterior, and medial-lateral. Each component varies throughout the gait cycle and is affected by velocity, cadence, and body mass. The averaged

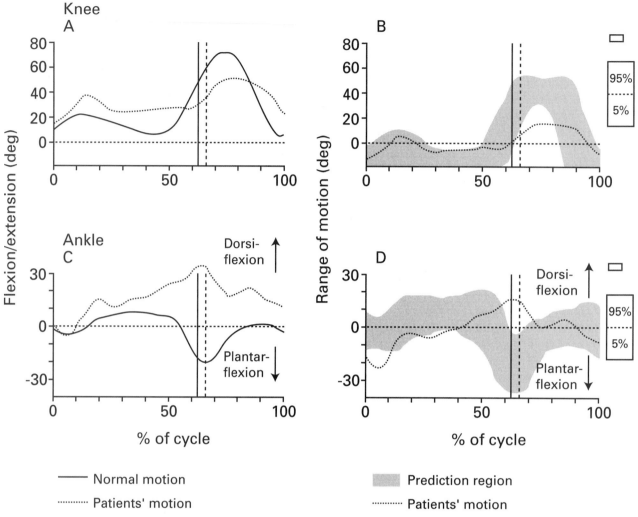

Figure 10-12. Prediction regions (from Sutherland, et al.,[107] with permission.)

wave forms of the vertical and anterior-posterior force components presented as a percentage of body weight show consistent patterns across normal subjects for loading rate, peak force, average force, and unloading rate. The anterior-posterior force has a characteristic negative phase followed by a positive phase. The negative phase represents deceleration, and the positive phase represents deceleration of the body mass. The vertical force waveform shows a characteristic double hump (Fig. 10-13). The medial-lateral force waveforms are variable even in normal individuals. **Force plate** technology such as that produced by Kistler Instrument Corporation (Amherst, NY) is capable of measuring the GRF as well as calculating the COM, acceleration, velocity, displacement, power, and work. A graphics display is also possible showing the waveforms of the GRF. Kistler also markets a treadmill called the Gaitway, which has piezoelectric force plates and charge amplifiers built into the unit. The treadmill is capable of measuring the GRF and COP during both walking and running. In addition to graphical presentation and statistics functions, the treadmill system can calculate temporal and spatial

parameters. Another corporation that produces force-plates is Genisco Technology Corporation (Northridge, CA).

Cook et al.[55] used a force plate to investigate the effect of angle of knee flexion restriction (using a brace) and walking speed on the GRF. These authors found that the loading rate, peak force, unloading rate, and average values of the GRF were significantly affected by walking speed. Faster walking increased both the loading rate and the GRF in both limbs. The authors concluded that the application of a brace to restrict knee flexion for the purpose of protection after injury or while surgically repaired structures were healing may actually increase the stress on both the braced and unbraced limbs.

Hesse et al.,[40] in a study that compared the trajectories of the COP and the COM in 10 healthy and 14 subjects with hemiparesis, found that the healthy subjects showed no differences in the behavior of the COP, COM, temporal parameters, and step length when initiating gait with either the right or left extremity. In comparison, patients with hemiparesis showed pronounced asymmetric behavior depending on which limb was the starting limb

Table 10–20 GAIT ANALYSIS RECORDING FORM: TEMPORAL AND DISTANCE MEASURES

Patient's name _____ Age _____ Sex _____

Height _____ Weight _____

Diagnosis: _____

Ambulatory aids: Yes _____ No _____

Type: Crutch(es) _____ Cane(s): R _____ Walker: _____

L _____

Other: _____

Date																	
Therapist's initials																	
Distance walked (distance from first to last heel strike)																	
Elapsed time (time from first to last heel strike)																	
Walking velocity (distance walked divided by elapsed time)																	
Left stride length (distance between two consecutive left heel strikes)																	
Right stride length (distance between two consecutive right heel strikes)																	
Left step length (distance between a right heel strike and the next consecutive left heel strike)																	
Right step length (distance between a left heel strike and the next consecutive right heel strike)																	
Step length difference (difference between right and left step lengths)																	
Cadence (total number of steps taken divided by the elapsed time)																	
Width of walking base (perpendicular distance between right and left heel strike)																	
Left foot angle (angle formed between a line bisecting the left foot and the line of progression)																	
Right foot angle (angle formed between a line bisecting the right foot and the line of progression)																	
Right stride length to right lower extremity length (right stride length divided by right lower extremity length)																	
Left stride length to left lower extremity length (left stride length divided by left lower extremity length)																	

The therapist may obtain averages for stride and step lengths, width of walking base, and foot angles.

(affected vs. nonaffected). When patients started with the affected limb the resulting trajectory of the COM in the medial-lateral plane was similar to healthy subjects. However, when the patients started gait with the nonaffected limb, the movements of the COP were inconsistent and incapable of producing directional movement of the body's COM. Anterior-posterior displacement of the COM was delayed. The authors concluded that for patients with hemiparesis starting gait with the unaffected leg is characterized by a higher degree of uncertainty owing to weakness of the supporting affected limb. Therefore, therapists should be cautioned about promoting this type of gait initiation. Rossi et al.[43] investigated the COM, COP, and GRF in a study of gait initiation in patients with transtibial amputations. These authors found that the patients consistently loaded the intact limb more than the prosthetic limb regardless of which limb initiated gait.[43]

Force plates are usually used either as part of, or in combination with, motion analysis systems and may be used with temporal-distance analysis systems as well as in conjunction with electromyography and electrogoniometry for a comprehensive analysis of kinematic and kinetic gait variables.

Pressure measurement systems may also be used with force plates. Pressure is equal to force divided by area and is measured by pressure sensors. There-

Table 10–21 GAIT VARIABLES: KINETIC GAIT ANALYSIS

Ground reaction forces	Vertical, anterior-posterior, and medial-lateral forces created as a result of foot contact with the supporting surface. These forces are equal in magnitude and opposite in direction to the force applied by the foot to the ground. Ground reaction forces are measured with force platforms in newtons (N) or pound force.
Pressure	Pressure = force per unit area. In gait analysis the pressure parameter that is usually measured is the pressure distribution under the foot.
Center of Pressure (COP)	The point of application of the resultant force. Movement of the COP as a function of time is used as a measure of stability of a subject who is either standing or walking on a force plate.
Torque (moment of force)	The turning or rotational effect produced by the application of a force. The greater the perpendicular distance from the point of application of a force from the axis of rotation, the greater the turning effect, or torque, produced. Torque is calculated by multiplying the force by the perpendicular distance from the point of application of the force and the axis of rotation. Torque = force × perpendicular distance or moment arm

fore pressure is equal to the force on the sensor divided by the area of the sensor. The most common uses of pressure measurements in gait are the pressure distribution under the foot (foot to ground contact), foot to shoe contact, and shoe to ground contact. Pressure measurement may be used for such purposes as determining orthotic efficacy and ulceration risk, and for regulating weight-bearing following surgery. Many different types of measurement techniques have been developed for measuring contact pressures. Tekscan, Incorporated (South Boston, MA) has a system called the **F-Scan In-Shoe Pressure Measurement System** that measures bipedal plantar pressures using paper thin disposable pressure sensors placed in patient's shoes. The sensor is ultrathin, flexible, and trimmable with 960 sensing locations distributed across the entire plantar surface. An example of the type of information that is provided from the F-Scan system is presented in Figure 10-14. Another system produced by Tekscan is called **Mat-Scan,** which is a pressure-sensing floor mat that allows the clinician to identify barefoot pressures. Mueller et al.[111] used the In-Shoe Pressure Measurement System in the management of patients with neuropathic ulcers or metatarsalgia. Armstrong et al.[112] investigated the influence of peak pressures on the healing time of diabetic ulcers treated with total contact casts.

Patients found to have high plantar pressures and wounds greater than 3.12 inches (8 cm) took significantly longer to heal than other patients. Wertsch et al.[113] described a portable insole plantar pressure measurement system which also could be used to study cane cadence and stump pressures of below-knee prosthesis.

Simple hand-held dynamometers and isokinetic systems can be used to obtain static and dynamic peak torques prior to a gait analysis of temporal and distance measures. Connelly et al.[95] found that decreases in isometric and dynamic quadriceps strength led to significant decreases in fast-paced and self-selected speed walking in a group of 10 female nursing home residents whose mean age was 82.8 years.

ENERGY COST DURING AMBULATION

Generally, conditions that affect either the motor control of gait and posture and/or conditions that affect joint and muscle structure and function will increase the energy cost of gait.[56–63] The type of footwear,[114] use of assistive devices, and speed of gait also affect energy expenditure.[64] Thus, energy expenditure is an important consideration in any gait analysis. The two parameters usually measured to determine energy expenditure are oxygen cost and oxygen rate.[22] The **oxygen cost** or energy expenditure per unit of distance walked (in mL/kg/m) defines the physiological work involved in the task.[59] The **oxygen rate** or energy expenditure per unit of time (in mL/kg/min) defines the power requirement.[59,60] The preferred method of measuring oxygen uptake is called open spirometry. The Douglas Bag Technique, in which expired air is collected during walking and subsequently analyzed, has been the classic method of analysis.[22,62] Modifications of this technique including metabolic carts are in use today.[22,64]

Davies and Dalsky[62] found no gender differences in submaximal oxygen uptake between sedentary men and women when gait speed was controlled. However, the same authors found that older individuals compared to younger individuals had higher energy costs to walk 1 mile.

The relative energy cost of gait can be estimated by monitoring heart rate during ambulation. Heart rate is directly and linearly related to oxygen consumption during exercise,[59] and can provide information as to how the patient's cardiovascular system is adapting to the stress of ambulation. Relative energy consumption has been found to be highly correlated with heart rate and absolute level of energy consumption has been found to be highly correlated with heart rate and maximum walking speed. Simple measures of heart rate and maximum ambulatory velocity allowed accurate prediction ($R = 0.89$) of energy consumption in 35 children with myelomeningocele.[60] However, Herbert et al.[61] found no difference in heart rate between children with transtibial amputations and those with intact

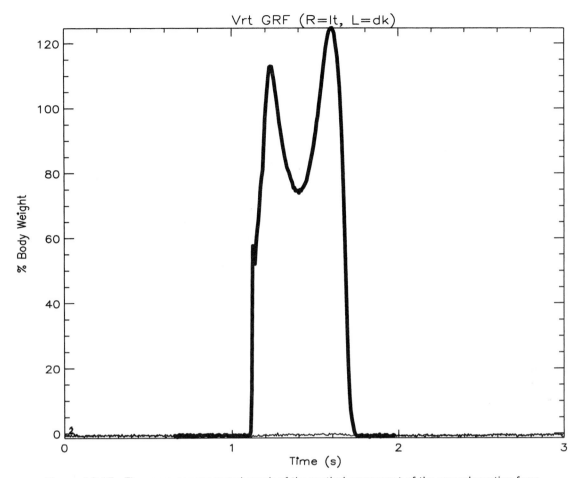

Figure 10-13. The computer-generated graph of the vertical component of the ground-reaction force was obtained using a force plate. (Courtesy of Dr. David Krebs, Motion Analysis Laboratory, MGH Institute of Health Professions, Boston, MA.)

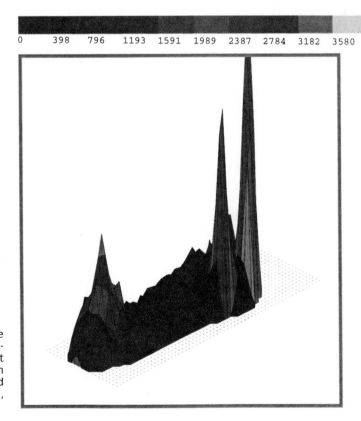

Figure 10-14. This figure shows the magnitude and location of peak pressure during one complete left foot strike. The highest pressures are shown on the heel, first metatarsal head and great toe. (Courtesy of Tekscan, Inc., South Boston, MA.)

lower extremities even though energy consumption was 15 percent higher in children with amputations compared to children without amputations. Waters et al.[57] found that in patients with hip arthrodesis oxygen consumption was 32 percent greater than normal and that heart rate also was significantly greater than normal.[57]

The most accurate way to assess heart rate is to use a telemetry system that produces beat-by-beat information as well as electrocardiographic activity. The intensive care or cardiac care units in many hospitals have telemetry systems that could be utilized for monitoring a patient during gait. If the therapist does not have access to telemetry monitoring, heart rate responses to ambulation can be assessed by palpation of the radial or carotid arteries. A pulse measurement should be taken at rest, just prior to ambulation, immediately post ambulation, and at various intervals after ambulation (e.g., 1, 3, and 5 min of recovery). The palpation method allows the therapist to determine how hard the heart had to work to accomplish a given gait activity and how long the heart takes to return to resting level.

SUMMARY

An overview of some methods for kinematic and kinetic gait analyses have been presented in this chapter. Many of the common variables assessed in gait analyses have been described and examples of studies using gait analyses have been presented. Observational gait analysis and time and distance variables have been emphasized because they appear to be the most common types of analyses used in the clinical setting. A brief overview of some of the motion analysis systems has been provided but readers are encouraged to consult references such as Perry[20] and Craik and Oatis[21] for more information. The ability to perform a gait analysis that accurately describes a patient's gait will provide important quantifiable information necessary for adequate treatment planning.

QUESTIONS FOR REVIEW

1. Describe each of the three different types of gait analyses (kinematic qualitative, kinematic quantitative, and kinetic).

   a. List the variables assessed in each of the three types of gait analyses.

   b. Select one variable from each type of analysis and describe a method of assessment for each variable selected.

2. Explain the difference between intratester and intertester reliability and give examples of how a test might be set up for each form of reliability.

3. Compare the advantages and disadvantages of a kinematic qualitative gait analysis with the advantages and disadvantages of a kinematic quantitative analysis.

4. Using the model presented in Tables 10–1 to 10–11, perform an OGA that includes both identification of observed deviations and an analysis to determine the causes of the deviations.

5. Which type of gait analysis would be appropriate for assessing: velocity and cadence? stride length? peak plantar pressures? ground reaction forces? Describe the analysis system you selected and justify your reason for selecting that particular system or method of analysis.

6. What distances must people in the community walk to get into stores, banks, and post offices?

7. How quickly must one walk to cross a street before the light changes?

8. Explain validity and how it relates to gait analysis. Give an example of each of the different types of validity.

9. How could a gait analysis of temporal parameters be used to demonstrate a patient's progress or lack of progress?

CASE STUDY
HISTORY

This 65 year-old woman is 5 days post right total hip arthroplasty. The surgery was performed following a femoral neck fracture incurred during a fall on the ice in front of her home. She has had daily bedside physical therapy for the past 3 days and now is independent in transfers. However, she needs to be independent in walking before she goes home.

She has a past history of diabetes mellitus (onset age 50), which is controlled with daily insulin injections. She denies any history of "heart problems." She does not participate in any regular exercise program and spends a great deal of time sitting during her work as a seamstress. She is alert and oriented to time and place and has a pleasant demeanor. She is 5 feet 3 inches tall, and weighs 160 pounds.

EXAMINATION RESULTS

PASSIVE RANGE OF MOTION ASSESSMENT

Goniometric Assessment (ROM): Lower Extremities			
Range of Motion (Degrees)		Left	Right
Hip	Flexion	WFL	0–40
	Extension	WFL	0–10
	Abduction	WFL	0–20
	Adduction	WFL	0–10
	Medial Rotation	WFL	Not tested
	Lateral Rotation	WFL	0–20
Knee	Flexion	WFL	0–120
Ankle	Dorsiflexion	WFL	0–15
	Plantarflexion	WFL	0–45
	Inversion	WFL	0–5
	Eversion	WFL	0–20

WFL, within functional limits; upper extremities: All ROM measurements are WFL.

STRENGTH ASSESSMENT

Manual Muscle Test (MMT): Lower Extremities			
		Left	Right
Hip	Flexion	G	F
	Extension	G–	P
	Abduction	G–	P
	Adduction	G	F+
	Lateral Rotation	G	G–
	Medial Rotation	G	G–
Knee	Flexion	G	G–
	Extension	G–	G–
Ankle	Dorsiflexion	G	P
	Plantarflexion	G–	G–
	Inversion	G–	F
	Eversion	G	F+
Toes	Flexion	G–	G–
	Extension	G	P

MMT Upper Extremities: All muscle grades are within the G to G– range.

SENSATION

RIGHT LOWER EXTREMITY: Deficits noted primarily along the medial aspect of right foot and two medial toes. Numeric values refer to the Sensation Scale below.

SENSORY ASSESSMENT

	Medial Aspect R Foot	Two Medial Toes
Sharp/dull:	5	5
Light touch	5	5
Temperature	5	5
Proprioceptive sensations	4	4

Sensation Scale:
1. Intact: normal, accurate
2. Decreased: delayed response
3. Exaggerated: increased sensitivity
4. Inaccurate: inappropriate perception of stimuli
5. Absent: no response
6. *Inconsistent or ambiguous*

INSPECTION

Patient has an ulcer on the medial aspect of the right plantar surface which is 0.7 × 6.0 centimeters in diameter and 1.5 millimeters deep.

FUNCTIONAL ASSESSMENT

Transfers
  FIM level = 7
Activities of daily living
  Eating: FIM = 7
  Bathing: FIM = 7
  Dressing: FIM = 7

GUIDING QUESTIONS

1. Develop a physical therapy problem list.
2. Complete the sample OGA form based on the information presented (see Appendix A).
3. Present your recommendations for physical therapy intervention.

REFERENCES

1. Ogg, LH: Gait analysis for lower-extremity child amputees. Phys Ther 45:940, 1965.
2. Smidt, GL, and Mommens, MA: System of reporting and comparing influence of ambulatory aids on gait. Phys Ther 60:551, 1980.
3. Craik, RL, and Otis, CA: Gait assessment in the clinic: Issues and approaches. In Rothstein, JM (ed): Measurement in Physical Therapy. Churchill Livingstone, London, 1985, p 169.
4. Gronley, JK, and Perry, J: Gait analysis techniques. Rancho Los Amigos Hospital Gait Laboratory. Phys Ther 64:1831, 1984.
5. Laughman, RK, et al: Objective clinical evaluation of function. Phys Ther 64:35, 1984.
6. Shores, M: Footprint analysis in gait documentation: An instructional sheet format. Phys Ther 60:1163, 1980.
7. Clarkson, BH: Absorbent paper method for recording foot placement during gait. Phys Ther 63:345, 1983.
8. Wolf, SL, and Binder-Macleod, SA: Use of the krusen limb load monitor to quantify temporal and loading measurements of gait. Phys Ther 62:976, 1982.
9. Robinson, JL, and Smidt, GL: Quantitative gait evaluation in the clinic. Phys Ther 61:351, 1981.

10. Soderberg, GL, and Gabel, RH: A light emitting diode system for the analysis of gait: A method and selected clinical examples. Phys Ther 58:426, 1978.
11. Little, H: Gait analyses for physiotherapy departments: A review of current methods. Physiotherapy 67:334, 1981.
12. Cerny, K: A clinical method of quantitative gait analysis. Phys Ther 63:1125, 1983.
13. Chodera, JD: Analysis of gait from footprints. Physiotherapy 60:179, 1974.
14. Harris, GF, and Wertsch, JJ: Procedures for gait analysis. Arch Phys Med Rehabil 75:216, 1994.
15. Stuberg, WA, et al: Comparison of a clinical gait analysis method using videography and temporal-distance measures with 16-mm cinematography. Phys Ther 68:1221, 1988.
16. Gunderson, LA, et al: Bilateral analysis of the knee and ankle during gait: An examination of the relationship between lateral dominance and symmetry. Phys Ther 69:640, 1989.
17. Stanerson, B, et al: Reliability of a system to measure gait variables in children with cerebral palsy. Abstract Phys Ther 17(suppl): 1990.
18. Eastlack, ME, et al: Interrator reliability of videotaped observational gait-analysis assessments. Phys Ther 71:465, 1991.
19. Rose, SSA, et al: Strategies for the assessment of pediatric gait in the clinical setting. Phys Ther 71:961, 1991.
20. Perry, J: Gait Analysis: Normal and Pathological Function. Slack Inc., Thorofare, NJ, 1992.
21. Craik, RL, and Oatis, CA: Gait Analysis: Theory and Application. Mosby, St. Louis, 1995.
22. Wall, JC, and Scarbrough, J: Use of a multimemory stopwatch to measure temporal gait parameters. J Orthop Sports Phys Ther 25:277, 1997.
23. Van Swearingen, JM, et al: The Modified Gait Abnormality Rating Scale for recognizing the risk of recurrent falls in community-dwelling elderly adults. Phys Ther 76:994, 1996.
24. Pathokinesiology Service and Physical Therapy Department: Observational Gait Analysis Handbook. Professional Staff Association of Rancho Los Amigos Medical Center, Downey, CA, 1981.
25. Brunnstrom, S: Movement Therapy in Adult Hemiplegia. Harper & Row, New York, 1970.
26. Lower Limb Prosthetics. New York University Medical strengthening on crouch gait in children with spastic diplegia. Phys Ther 75:658, 1995.
27. Bampton, S: A Guide to the Visual Examination of Pathological Gait. Temple University Rehabilitation Research and Training Center #8, Moss Rehabilitation Hospital, Philadelphia, 1979.
28. Sutherland, CC: Gait Evaluation. In Valmassy, RL (ed): Clinical Biomechanics of the Lower Extremities. Mosby-Yearbook, St. Louis, 1996.
29. Spyropoulos, P, et al: Biomechanical gait analysis in obese men. Arch Phys Med Rehabil 72:1065, 1991.
30. Nelson, AJ: Functional ambulation profile. Phys Ther 54:1059, 1974.
31. Grieve, DW, et al: The analysis of normal stepping movements as a possible basis for locomotor assessment of the lower limbs. J Anat 127:515, 1978.
32. Peat, M, et al: Electromyographic temporal analysis of gait: Hemiplegic locomotion. Arch Phys Med Rehabil 57:421, 1976.
33. Yack, HJ: Techniques for clinical assessment of human movement. Phys Ther 64:17, 1984.
34. Holden, MK, et al: Clinical gait assessment in the neurologically impaired, reliability and meaningfulness. Phys Ther 64:35, 1984.
35. Waters, RL, et al: Electromyographic gait analysis before and after operative treatment for hemiplegic equinus and equinovarus deformity. J Bone Joint Surg 64A:284, 1982.
36. Guide to Physical Therapist Practice. Phys Ther 77:1163, 1997.
37. Mueller, MJ, et al: Differences in gait characteristics of patients with diabetes and peripheral neuropathy compared with age-matched controls. Phys Ther 74:299, 1994.
38. Von Schroeder, HP: Gait parameters following stroke: A practical assessment. J Rehabil Res Dev 32:25, 1995.
39. Walker, SC, et al: Gait Pattern alteration by junctional sensory substitution in healthy and in diabetic subjects with peripheral neuropathy. Arch Phys Med Rehabil 78: 853, 1997.
40. Hesse, S, et al: Asymmetry of gait initiation in hemiparetic stroke subjects. Arch Phys Med Rehabil 78:719, 1997.
41. Mueller, MJ, et al: Relationship of plantar flexor peak torque and dorsiflexion range of motion to kinetic variables during walking. Phys Ther 75:684, 1995.
42. De Quervain, IAK, et al: Gait pattern in the early recovery period after stroke. J Bone Joint Surg 78A:10:1506, 1996.
43. Rossi, SA, et al: Gait initiation of persons with below-knee amputations: The characterization and comparison of force profiles. J Rehabil Res 32:120, 1995.
44. Roth, EJ, et al: Hemiplegic gait: Relationships between walking speed and other temporal parameters. Am J Phys Med Rehabil 76:128, 1997.
45. Zachazewski, JE, et al: Effects of tone inhibiting casts and orthoses on gait. Phys Ther 62:453, 1982.
46. McCulloch, M, et al: The effect of foot orthotics and gait velocity on lower limb kinematics and temporal events. J Orthop Sports Phys Ther 17:2, 1993.
47. Eng, JJ, and Pierrynowski, MR: The effect of soft foot orthotics on three-dimensional lower limb kinematics and kinetics during walking and running. Phys Ther 74:836, 1994.
48. Radka, SA, et al: A comparison of gait with solid, dynamic and no ankle-foot orthoses in children with spastic cerebral palsy. Phys Ther 77:395, 1997.
49. Bogataj, U, et al: Restoration of gait during two to three weeks of therapy with multichannel electrical stimulation. Phys Ther 69:319, 1989.
50. Powers, CM, et al: The influence of lower-extremity muscle force on gait characteristics in individuals with below-knee amputations secondary to vascular disease. Phys Ther 76:369, 1996.
51. Selby-Silverstein, L, et al: Gait analysis and bivalved serial casting of an athlete with shortened gastrocnemius muscles: A single case design. J Orthop Sports Phys Ther 25:282, 1997.
52. Damiano, DL, et al: Effects of quadriceps muscle strengthening on crouch gait in children with spastic diplegia. Phys Ther 75:658, 1995.
53. Malezic, M, et al: Application of a programmable dual-channel adaptive electrical stimulation system for the control and analysis of gait. J Rehabil Res Devel 29:4, 1992.
54. Morris, ME, et al: Temporal stability of gait in Parkinson's disease. Phys Ther 76:7, 1996.
55. Cook, TM, et al: Effects on restricted knee flexion and walking speed on the vertical ground reaction force during gait. Phys Ther 25:236, 1997.
56. Findley, TW, and Agre, JC: Ambulation in the adolescent with spina bifida II: Oxygen cost of mobility. Arch Phys Med Rehabil 69:855, 1988.
57. Waters, RL, et al: Comparable energy expenditure after arthrodesis of the hip and ankle. J Bone Joint Surg 70A:1032, 1988.
58. Gussoni, M, et al: Energy cost of walking with hip joint impairment. Phys Ther 70:295, 1990.
59. Olgiati, R, et al: Increased energy cost of walking in multiple sclerosis: Effect of spasticity, ataxia, and weakness. Arch Phys Med Rehabil 69:846, 1988.
60. Marsolais, MD, and Edwards, BG: Energy costs of walking and standing with functional neuromuscular stimulation and long leg braces. Arch Phys Med Rehabil 69:243, 1988.
61. Herbert, LM, et al: A comparison of oxygen consumption during walking between children with and without below-knee amputations. Phys Ther 74:943, 1994.
62. Davies, MJ, and Dalsky, GP: Economy of mobility in older adults. J Ortho Sports Phys Ther 26:69, 1997.
63. Torburn, L, et al: Energy expenditure during ambulation in dysvascular and traumatic below-knee amputees: A comparison of five prosthetic feet. J Rehabil Res Develop 32:111, 1995.
64. Shumway-Cook, A, et al: Predicting the probability for falls in community-dwelling older adults. Phys Ther 77:812, 1997.

65. Schenkman, M, et al: Reliability of impairment and physical performance measures for persons with parkinson's disease. Phys Ther 77:19, 1997.

66. Olney, SJ, et al: Temporal kinematic and kinetic variables related to gait speed in subjects with hemiplegia. Phys Ther 74:872, 1994.

67. Strube, MJ, and DeLitto, A: Reliability and Measurement Theory. In Craik, R, and Oatis, C (eds): Gait Analysis: Theory and Application. Mosby Yearbook, St. Louis, 1995, p 88.

68. Rothstein, JM, Roy, SH, and Wolf, SL: The Rehabilitation Specialist's Handbook (ed 2). FA Davis, Philadelphia, 1998.

69. Rodgers, MM, and Cavanough, PR: Glossary of biomechanical terms: Concepts and units. Phys Ther 64:182, 1984.

70. Bernhardt, J, et al: Accuracy of observational kinematic assessment of upper-limb movements. Phys Ther 78:3, 1998.

71. Goodkin, R, and Diller, L: Reliability among physical therapists in diagnosis and treatment of gait deviations in hemiplegics. Percept Mot Skills 37:727, 1973.

72. Krebs, D, et al: Observational gait analysis reliability in disabled children. Phys Ther (Abstract) 64:741, 1984.

73. Russell, DJ, et al: Training users in the gross motor function measure: Methodological and practical issues. Phys Ther 74:630, 1994.

74. Krebs, DE: Interpretation standards in locomotor studies. In Craik, R, and Oatis, C (eds): Gait Analysis: Theory and Application. Mosby Yearbook, St. Louis, 1995, p 334.

75. Norkin, C, and Levangie, P: Joint Structure and Function: A Comprehensive Analysis, ed 2. FA Davis, Philadelphia, 1992.

76. Harada, N, et al: Screening for balance and mobility impairment in elderly individuals living in residential care facilities. Phys Ther 75:462, 1995.

77. Shields, RK, et al: Reliability, validity and responsiveness of functional tests in patients with total joint replacement. Phys Ther 75:169, 1995.

78. Morton, T: Uniform data system for rehab begins: First tool measures dependence level. Progress Report, American Physical Therapy Association, Alexandria, VA, 1986.

79. Ottenbacher, KJ, et al: Interrater agreement and stability of the functional independence measure for children (WeeFIM): Use in children with developmental disabilities. Arch Phys Med Rehabil 78:1309, 1997.

80. Woolacott, MA, and Tang, PF: Balance control during walking in the older adult: Research and its implications. Phys Ther 77:646, 1997.

81. Di Fabio, RP, and Seay, R: Use of the **"Fast Evaluation of Mobility, Balance and Fear"** in elderly community dwellers: Validity and reliability. Phys Ther 77:904, 1997.

82. Finley, FR, et al: Locomotive patterns in elderly women. Arch Phys Med Rehabil 50:140, 1969.

83. Hinmann, JE, et al: Age-related changes in speed of walking. Med Sci Sports Exercise 20:161, 1988.

84. Hageman, PA, and Blanke, DJ: Comparison of gait of young women and elderly women. Phys Ther 66:1382, 1986.

85. Winter, DA, et al: Biomechanical walking pattern changes in the fit and healthy elderly. Phys Ther 70:340, 1990.

86. Blanke, DJ, and Hageman, PA: Comparison of gait of young men and elderly men. Phys Ther 69:144, 1989.

87. Bohannon, RW, et al: Walking speed: Reference values and correlates for older adults. J Orthop Sports Phys Ther 77:86, 1996.

88. Ostrosky, JM, et al: A comparison of gait characteristics in young and old subjects. Phys Ther 74:637, 1994.

89. Todd, FN, et al: Variations in the gait of normal children: A graph applicable to the documentation of abnormalities. J Bone Joint Surgery 71A:196, 1989.

90. Murray, M, et al: Walking patterns in normal men. J Bone Joint Surg 46A:335, 1964.

91. Murray, M, et al: Walking patterns of normal women. Arch Phys Med Rehabil 51:637, 1970.

92. Hills, AP, and Parker, AW: Gait characteristics of obese children. Arch Phys Med Rehabil 72:403, 1991.

93. Buchner, DM, et al: Factors associated with changes in gait speed in older adults. J Geron Med Sci 51A:M297, 1966.

94. Leiper, CI, and Craik, RL: Relationship between physical activity and temporal-distance characteristics of walking in elderly women. Phys Ther 71:791, 1991.

95. Connelly, DM, and Vandervoort, AA: Effects of detraining on knee extensor strength and functional mobility in a group of elderly women. J Orthop Sports Phys Ther 26:340, 1997.

96. Sutherland, DH, et al: The development of mature gait. J Bone Joint Surg 61A:336, 1980.

97. Titianova, AEB, and Tarka, IM: Asymmetry in walking performance and postural sway in patients with chronic unilateral cerebral infarction. J Rehabil Res 32:236, 1995.

98. Powers, CM, et al: The effect of patellar taping on stride characteristics and joint motion in subjects with patellofemoral pain. J Orthop Sports Phys Ther 26:286, 1997.

99. Sekiya, N, et al: Optimal walking in terms of variability of step length. J Orthop Sports Phys Ther 26:266, 1997.

100. Powers, CM, et al: Are patellofemoral pain and quadriceps femoris muscle torque associated with locomotor function? Phys Ther 77:1063, 1997.

101. Fransen, M, et al: Reliability of gait measurements in people with osteoarthritis of the knee. Phys Ther 77:944, 1997.

102. Evans, MD, et al: Systematic and random error in repeated measurements of temporal and distance parameters of gait after stroke. Arch Phys Med Rehabil 78:725, 1997.

103. Shumway-Cook, A, and Woollacott, WJ: Motor Control Theory and Practical Applications. William & Wilkins, Baltimore, 1995.

104. Lyons, K, et al: Timing and relative intensity of hip extensor and abductor muscle action during level and stair ambulation. Phys Ther 64:1597, 1983.

105. Wilson, DJ, et al: Accuracy of reconstructed angular estimates obtained with the Ariel Performance Analysis System. Phys Ther 77:1741, 1997.

106. Brinkmann, JR, and Perry, J: Rate and range of knee motion during ambulation in healthy and arthritic subjects. Phys Ther 65:7, 1985.

107. Sutherland, DH, et al: Clinical use of prediction regions for motion analysis. Develop Med Child Neurol 38:773, 1996.

108. Lerner-Frankiel, MB, et al: Functional community ambulation: What are your criteria? Clinical Management 6:12, 1986.

109. Robinett, CS, and VonDran, MA: Functional ambulation velocity and distance requirements in rural and urban communities: A clinical report. Phys Ther 63:1371, 1988.

110. Walsh, M, et al: Physical impairments and functional limitations: A comparison of individuals 1 year after total knee arthroplasty with control subjects. Phys Ther 78:248, 1998.

111. Mueller, MJ: Use of an in-shoe pressure measurement system in the management of patients with neuropathic ulcers or metatarsalgia. J Orthop Sports Phys Ther 21:328, 1995.

112. Armstrong, DG, et al: Peak foot pressures influence the healing time of diabetic foot ulcers treated with total contact casts. J Rehab Res Develop 35:1, 1998.

113. Wertsch, JJ, et al: A portable insole plantar measurement system. J Rehab Res Dev 29:13, 1992.

114. Ebbling, CJ, et al: Lower extremity mechanics and energy cost of walking in high-heeled shoes. J Orthop Sports Phys Ther 19:190, 1994.

GLOSSARY

Acceleration: The rate of change of velocity with respect to time. Body acceleration has been defined by Smidt and Mommens[2] as the rate of change of velocity of a point posterior to the sacrum. Acceleration is usually measured in meters per second per second (m/s^2).

Accelerometer: A device used to measure the vertical, anterior-posterior, and medial-lateral accelerations of body.

Angle/angle diagrams: Diagrams in which angular displacements of adjacent joints in the sagittal plane are plotted against each other.

Angular acceleration: The rate of change of the angular velocity of a body segment with respect to time. Angular acceleration is usually measured in radians per second per second (radians/s^2).

Angular velocity: The rate of motion in rotation of a body segment around an axis.

Ariel Performance Analysis System: A video-based system used for assessing joint displacements and patterns of motion during gait.

Balance Self Perceptions test: A self-rating assessment of the degree to which balance and perceived risk for falls interfere with daily activities.

Berg Balance scale: A performance based assessment of balance and mobility.

Bilateral stance time: The length of time (up to 30 s) that a subject can stand upright in the parallel bars bearing weight on both lower extremities.

Body mass index: This index, which is used to control for both height and weight, is determined by dividing body weight by standing height.

Cadence: Number of steps per unit of time; may be measured in centimeters as the number of steps per second (cadence = number of steps/time). A simple method of measuring cadence is by counting the number of steps taken by the patient in a given amount of time. The only equipment necessary is a stopwatch, paper, and pencil.

Center of mass (COM): The center of mass or center of gravity where the weight of the body is said to be concentrated. In the erect standing posture the center of mass of the entire body is said to be located at the level of the second sacral segment.

Center of pressure (COP): The point of application of the ground reaction force vector which is located between the feet in bilateral stance.

Circumduction: A circular motion of the swinging lower extremity that includes the hip motions of abduction, external rotation, adduction, and internal rotation. This gait deviation may be used to compensate for inadequate hip or knee flexion and/or insufficient dorsiflexion.

Cycle time (stride time): The amount of time required to complete a gait cycle; measured in seconds.

Displacement: The change in position of the body as a whole (linear, or translational, displacement) or its segments (rotational displacement). Linear, or translational, displacement is measured in meters, whereas rotational displacement is measured in degrees.

Double support time: The period of the gait cycle when both lower extremities are in contact with the supporting surface (double support); measured in seconds.

Dynamic weight transfer rate: The speed at which an individual standing in the parallel bars can transfer weight from one extremity to another; measured in seconds from the first lift off to the eighth lift off.

Dynamic Gait Index: An instrument designed to examine a person's ability to adapt his or her gait to changes in task demands.

Expert Vision System: A video-based motion analysis system produced by Motion Analysis Corporation, Santa Rosa, CA.

Fast Evaluation of Mobility Balance and Fear: An instrument designed to identify risk factors, functional performance and factors that hinder mobility.

Foot angle: Degree of toe out or toe in; the angle of foot placement with respect to the line of progression; measured in degrees.

Force plates: Load transducers that are capable of measuring ground reaction forces and the center of pressure. Force plates are manufactured by Kistler Instrument Corporation, Amherst, New York and by Genisco Technology Corporation in Northridge, CA, among others.

Free speed: An individual's normal walking speed.

F-Scan In-Shoe Pressure Measurement System: A system produced by Tecksan, Inc., South Boston, MA, that uses pressure sensors in a person's shoes to measure plantar pressures during gait.

Functional Ambulation Profile: A profile that is designed to assess ambulation skills on a continuum from standing balance in the parallel bars to independent ambulation.

Gait Abnormality Rating Scale (GARS): A profile designed to identify residents in nursing homes who are at risk for falling.

GAITMAT: An instrumented walkway that has pressure sensitive switches embedded for measuring spatial and temporal gait variables. The walkway is produced by EQ, Inc., Plymouth Meeting, PA.

Ground (floor) reaction force: Vertical, anterior-posterior, and medial-lateral forces created as a result of foot contact with the supporting surface. These forces are equal in magnitude and opposite in direction to the force applied by the foot to the ground. Ground reaction forces are measured with force platforms in newtons (N) or pound force.

Involved stance time: The length of time (up to 30 seconds) that an individual can stand in the parallel bars on the involved lower extremity (uninvolved lower extremity is raised off the supporting surface).

Joint reaction forces: The forces between articular surfaces that are created by muscle, gravity, and inertial forces; measured in Newtons.

Kinematics: A description of the type, amount, and direction of motion; does not include the forces producing the motion.

Kinetics: The study of the forces that cause motion.

Light-emitting diode (LED): System for assessing sagittal-plane motion and temporal and distance variables. The system consists of LEDs, foot switches, and a 35-mm single-frame color-slide photographic technique.

Linear velocity: The rate at which a body moves in a straight line.

Mat-Scan: A pressure sensing floor mat produced by Tekscan, Incorporated, South Boston, MA.

Modified GARS (GARS-M): A modification of the GARS that is appropriate for use for persons in the community.

Optoelectric (or optoelectronic) Motion Analysis System: A type of motion analysis system that uses active markers on body segments.

Oxygen cost: The energy expenditure per unit of distance walked (milliliters per kilogram of body weight per meter [mL/kg/m]).

Oxygen rate: The energy expenditure per unit of time (millimeters per kilogram of body weight per minute [mL/kg/min]).

Parallel bar ambulation: Length of time required for an individual to walk the length of the parallel bars as rapidly as possible. Two trials are averaged to obtain this measurement; measured in seconds.

Qualitative gait analysis: The identification and description of gait patterns.

Quantitative gait analysis: The measurement in distance and time of gait variables.

Reliability: The degree of consistency between successive measurements of the same variable (e.g., the position of the knee at heel strike), in the same individual, and under the same conditions.

Speed: A scalar quantity; has magnitude but not direction. Slow speed is a speed slower than an individual's normal speed; fast speed is a rate faster than normal.

Stance phase: The portion of gait in which one extremity is in contact with the ground. The phase is divided into the following segments: heel strike, foot flat, midstance, heel off, and toe off. The Rancho Los Amigos divisions are initial contact, loading response, midstance, terminal stance, and preswing.

Step: Consists of two dimensions; a distance (step length) and time (step time); two steps comprise a stride.

Step length: The linear distance between two successive points of contact of the right and left lower extremities. Usually a measurement is taken from the point of heel contact at heel strike on one extremity to the point of heel contact of the opposite extremity. If a patient does not have a heel strike on one or both sides, the measurement can be taken from the heads of the first metatarsals; measured in centimeters or meters. Both right and left step lengths should be obtained. When the right foot is leading, it is a right step. When the left foot is leading, it is a left step.

Step time: The number of seconds between consecutive right and left foot contacts; both right and left step times should be measured.

Stride: Consists of two dimensions; a distance (stride length) and a time (stride time).

Stride Analyzer: A footswitch system for analyzing temporal gait variables that is produced by B and L Engineering, Santa Fe Springs, CA.

Stride length: The linear distance between two consecutive foot contacts of the same lower extremity. Usually a measurement is taken from the point of one heel contact at heel strike and the next heel contact of the same extremity. However, stride length may be measured by using other events such as two consecutive toe offs; measured in centimeters or meters. Both right and left stride lengths should be measured.

Stride time: The number of seconds that elapses during one stride (from one foot contact until the next contact of the same foot). Stride time is synonymous with cycle time. Both right and left stride times should be measured.

Swing phase: The phase of gait during which the reference limb is not in contact with the supporting surface.

Swing time: The number of seconds during the gait cycle that one foot is off the ground. Swing time should be measured separately for right and left extremities.

Timer-logger Communicator Gait Monitor: A system consisting of foot switches which are connected to a battery operated portable microcomputer. The system is produced by Biokinetics, Bethesda, Maryland and is able to monitor temporal gait variables.

Torque (moment of force): The turning or rotational effect produced by the application of a force. The greater the perpendicular distance of the point of application of a force from an axis of rotation, the greater the turning effect or torque produced. Torque is calculated by multiplying the force by the perpendicular distance from the point of application of the force and the axis of rotation.

$$\text{Torque} = f \times \text{perpendicular distance} \\ \text{or moment arm}$$

Measurement is in newton meters.

Uninvolved stance time: The length of time (up to 30 seconds) that an individual can stand in the parallel bars while bearing weight on the uninvolved lower extremity (involved extremity is raised off the supporting surface).

Validity: The degree that a measurement reflects what it is supposed to measure.

Velocity: A measure of a body's motion in a given direction.

Vicon Motion Analysis System: A optoelectronic imaging system for assessing sagittal plane motion. This system is available from Oxford Metrics Ltd., Oxford, England.

Video-based Motion Analysis System: A type of motion analysis system that uses passive markers placed on body segments.

Walking velocity: The rate of linear forward motion of the body; measured in either centimeters per second or meters per minute.

$$\text{Walking velocity} = \text{distance/time}$$

Walking velocity may be affected by age, level of maturation, height, gender, type of footwear, and weight. Also, velocity may affect cadence, step, stride length, and foot angle as well as other gait variables.

WATSMART: An optoelectric imaging system for motion analysis produced by Northern Digital, Inc., Waterloo, Ontario, Canada.

WeeFIM: A profile designed to measure functional independence in children.

Width of walking base (step width; base of support): The linear distance between one foot and the opposite foot; measured in centimeters or meters.

Work: The application of a force through a distance; accomplished whenever a force moves an object through a distance.

$$\text{Work} = \text{force} \times \text{distance}$$

APPENDIX A

BLANK SAMPLE RECORDING FORM FOR OBSERVATIONAL GAIT ANALYSIS

Patient's name _____ Age _____ Sex _____ Height _____ Weight _____

Diagnosis _____

Footwear _____ Assistive devices _____

Date _____ Therapist _____

DIRECTIONS: Place a check in the space opposite the deviation if the deviation is observed.

Body Segment	Deviation	Stance HS R	HS L	FF R	FF L	MST R	MST L	HO R	HO L	TO R	TO L	ACC R	ACC L	Swing MSW R	MSW L	DEC R	DEC L	Possible Cause	Analysis
Ankle and foot	None																		
Observations in the sagital plane	Foot flat																		
	Foot slap																		
	Heel off																		
	No heel off																		
	Excessive plantarflexion																		
	Excessive dorsiflexion																		
	Toe drag																		
	Toe clawing																		
	Contralateral vaulting																		
Observations in the frontal plane	Varus																		
	Valgus																		
Knee	None																		

Continued

BLANK SAMPLE RECORDING FORM FOR OBSERVATIONAL GAIT ANALYSIS *Continued*

Body Segment	Deviation	Stance HS R	L	FF R	L	MST R	L	HO R	L	TO R	L	Swing ACC R	L	MSW R	L	DEC R	L	Possible Cause	Analysis
Observations in the sagittal plane	Excessive flexion																		
	Limited flexion																		
	No flexion																		
	Hyperextension																		
	Genu recurvatum																		
	Diminished extension																		
Observations in the frontal plane	Varum																		
	Valgum																		
Hip	None																		
Observations in the sagittal plane	Excessive flexion																		
	Limited flexion																		
	No flexion																		
	Diminished extension																		
Observations in the frontal plane	Abduction																		
	Adduction																		
	External rotation																		
	Internal rotation																		
	Circumduction																		
	Hiking																		
Pelvis	None																		

BLANK SAMPLE RECORDING FORM FOR OBSERVATIONAL GAIT ANALYSIS *Continued*

Body Segment	Deviation	Stance						Swing			Possible Cause	Analysis
		HS	FF	MST	HO	TO	ACC	MSW	DEC		
Observations in the sagittal plane	Anterior tilt										
	Posterior tilt										
	Increased backward rotation										
	Increased forward rotation										
	Limited backward rotation										
	Limited forward rotation										
	Drops on contralateral side										
Trunk	None										
Observations in the frontal plane	Backward rotation										
	Lateral lean										
	Forward rotation										
	Backward lean										
	Forward lean										

303

COMPLETED SAMPLE RECORDING FORM FOR OBSERVATIONAL GAIT ANALYSIS

Patient's name _Edna Smith_
Diagnosis _Post total Hip Arthroplasty – Peripheral Neuropathy – Diabetes_ Age _65_ Sex _F_ Height _5'3"_ Weight _160 lbs._
Footwear _Shoes_   Assistive devices _None_
Date _5/6/98_   Therapist _North_
DIRECTIONS: Place a check in the space opposite the deviation if the deviation is observed.

Body Segment	Deviation	HS (R)	HS (L)	FF (R)	FF (L)	MST (R)	MST (L)	HO (R)	HO (L)	TO (R)	TO (L)	ACC (R)	ACC (L)	MSW (R)	MSW (L)	DEC (R)	DEC (L)	Possible Cause	Analysis
		Stance										**Swing**							
Ankle and foot	None																		
Observations in the sagittal plane	Foot flat	✓																weakness dorsiflexors	
	Foot slap																		
	Heel off																		
	No heel off																		
	Excessive plantarflexion			✓		✓						✓		✓		✓		weakness dorsiflexors	
	Excessive dorsiflexion																		
	Toe drag											✓		✓				weakness dorsiflexors	
	Toe clawing																		
	Contralateral vaulting																		
Observations in the frontal plane	Varus																		
	Valgus																		
Knee	None																		

COMPLETED SAMPLE RECORDING FORM FOR OBSERVATIONAL GAIT ANALYSIS *Continued*

Body Segment	Deviation	Stance HS R	HS L	FF R	FF L	MST R	MST L	HO R	HO L	TO R	TO L	Swing ACC R	ACC L	MSW R	MSW L	DEC R	DEC L	Possible Cause	Analysis
Observations in the sagittal plane	Excessive flexion																		
	Limited flexion																		
	No flexion																		
	Hyperextension																		
	Genu recurvatum																		
	Diminished extension																		
Observations in the frontal plane	Varum																		
	Valgum																		
Hip	None																		
Observations in the sagittal plane	Excessive flexion																		
	Limited flexion																		
	No flexion																		
	Diminished extension																		
Observations in the frontal plane	Abduction																		
	Adduction					✓												Drop of pelvis	
	External rotation																		
	Internal rotation																		
	Circumduction																		
	Hiking																		
Pelvis	None																		

Continued

COMPLETED SAMPLE RECORDING FORM FOR OBSERVATIONAL GAIT ANALYSIS *Continued*

Body Segment	Deviation	Stance					Swing			Possible Cause	Analysis
		HS	FF	MST	HO	TO	ACC	MSW	DEC		
Observations in the sagittal plane	Anterior tilt										
	Posterior tilt										
	Increased backward rotation										
	Increased forward rotation										
	Limited backward rotation										
	Limited forward rotation										
	Drops on contralateral side		TO THE	LEFT ✓	✓					Weakness Right hip abductors	
Trunk	None										
	Backward rotation										
Observations in the frontal plane	Lateral lean										
	Forward rotation			✓						weakness	compensation to counteract
	Backward lean	✓	✓							hip extensors	flexion moment
	Forward lean										

APPENDIX C

Suggested Answers to Guiding Questions

1. Develop a physical therapy problem list.
ANSWER: Limited ROM right ankle/and hip.
Decreased muscle strength right hip abductors, flexors and extensors, ankle dorsiflexors, and invertors and toe extensors.
Diminished sensation right foot and toes.
Ulcer right foot.
Obesity.
Pronation on right.

2. Complete the sample OGA form based on the information present.
ANSWER: The findings of an OGA were consistent with the muscle weakness found in the physical examination (see Fig. 1 in Appendix B). The excessive plantar flexion observed (on the right) through most of the stance phase, and the toe drag observed from acceleration to midswing reflect the weakness found in the patient's right dorsiflexors. At heel strike the excessive plantarflexion resulted in a toes first floor contact. The slight backward lean of the trunk at right heel strike represents an attempt to compensate for weakness of the right hip extensors. The contralateral drop of the pelvis during right stance is due to the weakness of the right hip abductors.

An analysis of temporal and distance measures showed prolonged stance time on the left, shortened stance on the right, decreased velocity as well as left/right asymmetry. A measurement of plantar pressures during walking showed peak pressures under the first metatarsal head on the right foot.

3. Present your recommendations for physical therapy intervention.
ANSWER: The patient will probably require intervention to reduce and/or redistribute plantar pressures and allow for healing of the ulcer. She may also require custom-made shoes, and an orthosis to reduce foot drop. An exercise program to strengthen her hip, ankle, and toe musculature should be implemented; however, the damage to her dorsiflexors and toe extensors may be irreversible. The patient should be encouraged to implement a daily exercise program and to consult her physician regarding a weight control program. Once she has her orthotic devices she should have repeated gait analyses to determine if the plantar pressures have been relieved and if the ankle foot orthosis and muscle strengthening have improved her gait (her temporal and distance gait parameters as well as her excessive plantarflexion, backward trunk lean, pelvic drop, and pronation). Optimally, she should have a comprehensive gait analysis using motion analysis to verify the OGA findings as well as kinetic, plantar pressure gait analysis, EMG, and energy cost assessment.

Functional Assessment *11*

Andrew A. Guccione

LEARNING OBJECTIVES

1. Discuss the concepts of health status, impairment, functional limitation, and disability.
2. Define functional activity, and discuss the purposes and components of a functional assessment.
3. Select activities and roles appropriate to an individual's particular characteristics and condition to guide a functional assessment.
4. Compare and contrast characteristics of various formal tests of function, including physical function tests and multidimensional functional assessment instruments.
5. Identify factors to be considered in the selection of formal instruments for testing function.
6. Compare and contrast various scoring methods used in functional assessment.
7. Discuss the issues of reliability and validity as they relate to functional assessment.
8. Using the case study example, apply clinical decision making skills in evaluating functional assessment data.

INTRODUCTION

The ultimate objective of any rehabilitation program is to return the individual to a lifestyle that is as close to the premorbid level of function as possible or, alternatively, to maximize the current potential for function and maintain it. For an otherwise healthy patient with a fractured arm, this may be a reasonably simple process: improving range of motion and strength will reestablish skills in dressing and feeding. However, considering the patient with a stroke as an example, the task is much more complex because the problems are much more extensive, complicated, and interwoven. The two cases, however, are broadly similar. In both instances, the therapist begins by describing the patient's problem in functional terms obtained from the patient history, performing a systems review and detailed examination using selected tests and measures, evaluating the data, establishing a diagnosis and prognosis, implementing interventions to reduce or to eliminate the problems identified, and documenting the progress of the patient toward the desired functional outcome.[1]

Every individual values the ability to live independently. Functional activities encompass all those tasks, activities and roles that identify a person as an independent adult or as a child progressing toward adult independence. These activities require the integration of both cognitive and affective abilities with motor skills. Functional activity is a patient-referenced concept and is dependent on what the individual self-identifies as essential to support physical and psychological well-being as well as to create a personal sense of meaningful living. Function is not totally individualistic, however; there are certain categories of activities that are common to everyone. Eating, sleeping, elimination, and hygiene are major components of survival and protection common to all animals. Particular to humans are the evolutionary advancements of bipedal locomotion and complex hand activities, which permit independence in the personal environment. Work and recreation are functional activities in a social context.

This chapter presents a conceptual framework for assessing functional status and introduces the reader to terminology used in the field. It presents an overview of the purposes of functional assessment and the range and rigor of formal test instruments currently available to clinicians and researchers. Considerations in test selection and principles of administration are also presented.

A CONCEPTUAL FRAMEWORK

Chronically ill and disabled persons represent a large segment of the population in this country. Approximately 35 million individuals suffer from physical or mental impairments that limit their capacity to perform some daily functional activity.[2] Traditionally, these individuals have been categorized or classified according to their medical diseases or conditions. Medical assessment procedures such as physical examination and laboratory tests are the primary tools to delineate the problems created by disease. Strict focus on a biomedical model, with its emphasis on the characteristics of **disease** (etiology, pathology, and clinical manifestations), may contribute to reducing patients to the medical labeling of these individuals; for example, referring to people as amputees, paraplegics, arthritics, or CVAs rather than as individuals with these conditions. This model virtually ignores the equally important psychological, social, and behavioral dimensions of the **illness,** which accompanies the disease. Illness refers to the personal behaviors that emerge when the reality of having a disease is internalized and experienced by an individual.[3] Factors related to illness often play a key role in determining the success or failure of rehabilitation efforts well beyond the nature of the medical condition that prompted a patient's referral to physical therapy. In helping the individual with a disease, physical therapists come to understand each person's illness as well.

A broad conceptual framework is necessary to fully understand the concept of health and its relationship to functional disability. Terms such as well-being, health-related quality of life, and functional status are often used interchangeably to describe health status. The most global definition of **health** has been provided by the World Health Organization (WHO). This organization defined health as "a state of complete physical, mental, and social well-being, and not merely the absence of diseases and infirmity."[4] Although such global definitions are useful as philosophical statements, they lack the precision necessary for a clinician or researcher. Factors that are often used to define health in more measurable terms include (1) physical signs, (2) symptoms, and (3) functional disability.[5] Full consensus on the meaning of these terms, however, has not been reached. The WHO adopted an International Classification of Impairments, Disability, and Handicaps (ICIDH)[6] with the goal of promoting the use of consistent terminology and to

provide a framework for discourse among health professionals by standardizing four key terms: disease, impairment, disability, and handicap. Although quite often found as a framework in the research and clinical literature in other parts of the world, this classification system has not been generally adopted by rehabilitation specialists in the United States.[7] Nagi has been particularly influential in developing a model found throughout the American literature that explicates health status and the relationship among the various terms used to describe health status (Fig. 11-1).[8–10]

Nagi's conceptual model, used in this chapter to capture the concept of health status, begins with the pathology or disease process that mobilizes the body's defenses and response mechanisms. Physical signs and symptoms set the individual's clinical presentation apart as abnormal and indicate the body's attempts to cope with this attack on its normal functioning. **Physical signs** are the directly observable or measurable changes in an individual's organs or systems. **Symptoms** are the more subjective reactions to the changes experienced by the individual. Thus the individual demonstrates an elevated blood pressure (a physical sign) and reports feeling dizzy (a symptom). Many medical conditions are, in fact, not labels for a single pathologic entity, but clusters of signs and symptoms that designate a syndrome. Two common examples of "diseases" that are really syndromes are congestive heart failure (CHF) and acquired immune deficiency syndrome (AIDS). Although the definition of disease presented above implies an active condition, many of the physical signs and symptoms that are important to physical therapy assessment and treatment are not associated with active or ongoing medical conditions. For example, a resolved myocardial infarction is a fixed lesion with great importance for physical therapists, but is not an active disease process in itself.

Impairments, as described within Nagi's model, evolve as the natural consequence of pathology or disease and are defined as any alteration or deviation from normal in anatomical, physiological, or psychological structures or functions.[8–10] The partial or complete loss of a limb or an organ, or any disturbance in body part, organ, or system function are examples of impairments. Physical therapists are primarily concerned with impairments of the musculoskeletal, neuromuscular, cardiopulmonary, and integumentary systems; for example, loss of range of motion, strength, endurance, or scar formation. Impairments may be temporary or permanent

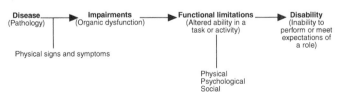

Figure 11-1. Schematic representation of Nagi's model of the process of disablement.

and represent an overt manifestation of the disease or pathological state. Some impairments are themselves sequelae of other impairments. For example, the patient with a swollen and stiff joint may eventually develop weakness in the muscles surrounding the joint. Therefore, impaired muscle strength would be the result of impaired joint mobility, rather than a specific disease or pathological process.[11,12]

A **functional limitation** is the inability of an individual to perform an action or activity in the way it is done by most people, usually as the result of an impairment.[8–10] Accurate judgement about the relationship between impairments and functional limitations is at the heart of all physical therapist examination, evaluation, and intervention.[1,7] Three main categories of function have been delineated: physical function, psychological function, and social function. **Physical function** refers to those sensory-motor skills necessary for the performance of usual daily activities. Getting out of bed, walking, and climbing stairs are examples of physical functional activities. Physical therapists are traditionally most involved with this category of functional assessment and intervention. These sensory-motor skills underlie the tasks of daily self-care such as feeding, dressing, hygiene, and physical mobility that are known as **basic activities of daily living (BADL).** Advanced skills that are considered vital to an individual's independent living in the community are termed **instrumental activities of daily living (IADL).** These include a wide range of high-level tasks and activities such as managing personal affairs, cooking and shopping, home chores, and driving.

Psychological function has two components: mental and affective. **Mental function** refers to the intellectual or cognitive abilities of an individual. Factors such as initiative, attention, concentration, memory, problem solving, or judgement are important components of normal mental function. **Affective function** refers to the affective skills and coping strategies needed to deal with the everyday "hassles" as well as the more traumatic and stressful events each person encounters over the course of a lifetime. Factors such as self-esteem, attitude toward body image, anxiety, depression, and the ability to cope with change are examples of affective functions. Finally, **social function** refers to an individual's performance of social roles and obligations. Categories of roles and activities relevant to assessing an individual's social function include social activity, including participation in recreational activities and clubs; social interaction, such as telephoning or visiting relatives or friends; and social roles created and sustained through interpersonal relationships specific to one's personal life and occupation.

When an individual is limited in a number of functional activities and unable to engage in critical social roles (e.g., worker, student, spouse), this person may be regarded as disabled as conceptualized within the Nagi model.[8–10] **Disability** is characterized by a discordance between the actual performance of an individual in a particular role and the expectations of the community regarding what is "normal" for an adult. Thus, disability is a term that takes its meaning from the community in which the individual lives and the criteria for "normal" within that social group. Many factors can influence the connections among disease, impairment and function, not the least of which will be the individual's personal response. Patients with the same disease and the same impairments may not always have the same functional limitations. Furthermore, although an individual may perform functional activities differently than is "normal," this person may successfully accomplish expected social roles and escape the label of being "disabled." Physical therapists most often think of "normal" adulthood in terms of independence in self-care activities, competence and autonomy in decision making, and productivity. In some cultural subgroups, social expectations may be quite different, particularly if the individual has certain impairments or functional limitations. Physical therapists should account for the effects of culture and social expectations in determining what is "normal" function for an individual, especially when the therapist and the patient do not share the same social or cultural backgrounds. Nagi's model has no term to cover the concept of **handicap,** which is the social disadvantage of disability and a function of a society's response to needs of people with different abilities which label an individual as handicapped.[13] In some instances, even a person who is functioning independently may still be handicapped by the social stigma of using an assistive device such as a wheelchair. Physical therapists can help to change social attitudes and environmental restrictions like architectural barriers that stigmatize individuals as "handicapped."

The ICIDH is currently under its most extensive revision to date. Draft revisions of the ICIDH that were circulated for review internationally in 1998 continue using the term "impairment," but abandon the terms "disability" and "handicap" in favor of the terms "activity limitation" and "participation restriction," respectively.[14] These proposed changes in ICIDH terminology, if adopted, would be closer, respectively, to the notions of "functional limitation" and "disability" used in the Nagi model and greatly reduce the overall differences between the two sets of concepts.

Although deficits in behavioral or motor skills or limitations in function may typically exist in certain disease categories, the exact empirical relationship between a particular set of impairments and a specific functional disability is not yet known. The "cause-and-effect" relationship between an impairment and a functional limitation is most often inferred in the clinic from empirical evidence. For example, physical therapists may assume that the reason a patient cannot transfer independently is causally linked to the fact that the individual has lost enough lower extremity range of motion at the hip (e.g., hip flexion contractures) to prevent balancing in a fully upright posture. The return of function following remediation of the impairment of joint mobility is then considered clinical evidence of a causal relationship between the impairment and the functional limitation. For data to be clinically useful, functional assessment must be linked to the other tests and measures which are used by a physical therapist to examine a patient.

ASSESSMENT OF FUNCTION

Purpose of Functional Assessment

Analysis of function focuses on the identification of pertinent **functional activities** and measurement of an individual's ability to successfully engage in them. In essence, functional assessment measures how a person does certain tasks or fulfills certain roles in the various dimensions of living described above. Functional assessment is accomplished through the application of selected tests and measures that yield data that can be used as (1) baseline information for setting function-oriented goals and outcomes of intervention, (2) indicators of a patient's initial abilities and progression toward more complex functional levels, (3) criteria for placement decisions, for example, the need for inpatient rehabilitation, extended care, or community services, (4) manifestations of an individual's level of safety in performing a particular task and the risk of injury with continued performance, and (5) evidence of the effectiveness of a specific intervention (medical, surgical, or rehabilitative) on function.

General Considerations

Physical therapists possess a unique body of knowledge related to the identification, remediation, and prevention of movement dysfunction. Thus, they have traditionally been involved in the assessment of physical function. Other members of the rehabilitation team, including the occupational therapist, nurse, rehabilitation counselor, and recreational therapist, are also typically involved in administering and interpreting functional assessments. Some formal instruments for functional assessment are designed to be completed collectively by the team. Other tests are compiled in separate sections by specific health professionals and housed together in the patient's chart. Where teams exist, physical therapists are typically responsible for the assessment of **functional mobility skills,** that is, bed mobility, transfers, and locomotion (wheelchair mobility, ambulation, and negotiation of stairs and graded elevations). Overlap among team members exists, however. For example, the assessment of toilet transfers may be done by the physical therapist, occupational therapist, or the nurse as a component of care for a patient with incontinence. In these instances, testing should be coordinated to reduce duplication and unnecessary patient stress. In noninstitutional settings or where there is no team, the physical therapist is often responsible for assessing all aspects of physical function.

Assessment Perspectives

The assessment of function can utilize two highly divergent perspectives on what is to be tested or measured by the physical therapist. It is extremely important that the therapist determine in advance whether data are needed to describe the habitual level of a patient's ability to do certain tasks and activities, or to identify the patient's capacity to perform certain tasks and activities, whether the patient habitually performs up to that level or not, or even performs them at all.

These divergent viewpoints directly affect what types of tests and measures should be chosen and what parameters of measurement are appropriate to yield data useful to making clinical judgements. Most importantly, physical therapists must consider the differences between capacity for function and habitual function in determining the prognosis for rehabilitation and estimating the likelihood of the success of an intervention. Patients only accept a therapist's recommendations regarding the goals of treatment if there is the perceived need and motivation to function habitually at the highest level of ability. Understanding the difference between what a person actually does or would be willing to do, and what that person potentially could do, is an essential component of designing realistic, and achievable, functional goals. For example, even though a person might have the capacity to climb stairs, there may not be any willingness to do so. Ultimately, physical therapists must abide by each patient's own decision regarding which tasks and activities will be incorporated into a daily routine and what is a meaningful level of function, regardless of the therapist's professional opinion.

Irrespective of the particular instrument used, there are several basic considerations to be kept in mind. The setting chosen must be conducive to the type of testing and free of distractions. Instructions should be precise and unambiguous. Assessments may be biased by fatigue. If a patient performs best in the morning but tires by afternoon, an accurate assessment of functional ability must consider the variation in the patient's performance. Therapists should be aware of patients whose energy fluctuates during the day, and interpret the data accordingly. In general, functional assessments should always be interpreted in the context provided by other data generated during the initial examination (e.g., tests and measures of joint integrity and mobility, motor function, muscle performance and sensory integrity). Retesting should occur at regular intervals during treatment to document progress and at discharge from the episode of care.

Types of Instruments

PERFORMANCE-BASED ASSESSMENTS

A **performance-based assessment** may be administered by a therapist who observes the patient during the performance of an activity. Generally speaking, the therapist who chooses a performance-based assessment is searching for an indication of what a patient can do under a specific set of circumstances, which may or may not be similar to the natural environment in which the patient functions. If performance-based assessment is chosen with the intention of making inferences about how the patient will perform at home, then the conditions and setting should be as similar as possible to the actual environment in which the patient usually performs the tasks and activities. A performance-based approach may be used either to describe the patient's current level of function or to identify the maximum level of function possible.

During the administration of the test, each task is presented and the patient is asked to perform it. For example, to assess current level of function in wheelchair mobility, a patient would receive this instruction, "Push your wheelchair over to that red chair and stop." To determine the patient's maximum level of function in this activity, the instruction might specify a particular manner of performance: "Push your wheelchair over to that red chair *as quickly as you can* and stop." Understanding the difference between these two commands, even though both are observation-based assessments of wheelchair mobility, is essential to sound clinical decision making. Data from the first example identifies only what the patient can do under specific circumstances, but does not support the inference that the patient will be able to wheel across a busy intersection in the short time-span allotted to a typical pedestrian walkway. The form of the instruction determines whether an inference can be made about the patient's maximal level of function in formulating the goals for intervention and the treatment plan.

In either case, a patient is given no additional instructions or assistance unless he or she is unable or unsure of how to perform. Then only as much direction or assistance as is needed is given. Appropriate safety precautions should be taken during the session so that the patient does not attempt tasks that are potentially dangerous.

There are a number of tests of impairments which are sometimes also referred to as performance measures, including the Six Minute Walk Test,[15] the Physical Performance and Mobility Examination,[16] the Functional Reach Test,[17,18] the Get Up and Go Test,[19] the Timed Up and Go Test,[20] and the Physical Performance Battery.[21] A performance measure of this sort is a quantification of the complex integration of systems that permits an individual to maintain a posture, transition to other postures, or sustain safe and efficient movement. The data from such a test, gathered under controlled conditions, characterize a person's performance limitations as a result of impairments, and are purported to predict the success or failure of an individual in performing goal-directed activities under natural conditions, using a score that summates the combined impacts of impairments throughout and across systems on movement dysfunction. Each of these tests can contribute to an understanding of a person's function, but they do not assess a functional limitation in a particular BADL or IADL. Although these tests employ the method of direct observation of performance, they most often do not measure the task or activity as it might be accomplished in the "real" world of the patient, which is also influenced by motivation and habit.

SELF-ASSESSMENTS

In contrast to the method of direct observation used in performance-based measures of function, useful data on how a person functions may also be gathered by self-assessment, where the patient is asked directly either by the therapist or a trained interviewer (**interviewer assessment**) or through the use of a **self-administered assessment** instrument. The critical issue in the ability of a self-assessment to capture function correctly and completely lies in providing clearly worded questions without language bias, concise directions on completing the questions, and a format that encourages accurate reporting of answers to all questions. Self-assessment is a valid method of assessing function, and may be preferable to performance-based methods in some circumstances.[22] Self-assessments should be designed so that questions are asked in a standard format and answers are recorded as specified by the predetermined choices. Long paper-and-pencil tests may be difficult for those with upper extremity disability.

Clinical personnel who will act as interviewers must be trained to administer a questionnaire and should practice until they have reached a high degree of agreement with expert assessors of the same cases. Periodic retraining may be necessary if interviewers do not have frequent practice administering the instrument. The interview should be scheduled with the patient in advance and conducted in an environment conducive to complete concentration. Interviews may be conducted by phone or in person, but the mode of administration should be kept consistent if comparisons of the data are to be made. Ad lib prompting by the interviewer or caregivers for answers is discouraged because these intrusions into the patient's *self*-assessment tend to bias results. If the patient has had help in filling out a form or responding to questions, this should be noted. Similarly, if the data have been provided by a spouse, family member, or caregiver, this should be documented as well.

The distinction in perspectives on function that was discussed regarding performance-based measures of function also holds for self-assessments. It is extremely important to distinguish between questions that indicate a person's habitual performance (e.g., "*Do* you cook your own meals?") and those that identify a person's perceived capacity to perform a task (e.g., "If you had to, *could* you cook your own meals?").

The time frame reference of self-assessment is also a relevant consideration. A therapist should decide in advance if the relevant "window" on a person's functional level is the past 24 hours, last week, last month, or the previous year. One can easily imagine how the same person might respond differently regarding the same functional activity depending on frame of reference. Instruments that assess only short-term objectives may not relate well to the long-term objectives of a rehabilitation program.

Instrument Parameters and Formats

Performance-based and self-assessment instruments grade performance on a number of different criteria in a variety of formats. There is no one parameter or format that is perfect for every type of clinical encounter or research need. It is particularly important that documentation of a patient's progress not be blunted by "floor" or "ceiling" effects of various descriptors. For example, if a therapist wishes to measure changes in function among generally well elderly patients and the most advanced functional activity on an instrument measures "independent ambulation on level surfaces," there would be no room to demonstrate either progression or decline except around ambulation on level surfaces. Similarly, a patient who was severely debilitated might improve in transfers from needing the maximum assistance of two persons to maximum assistance of one. If the instrument only measures change from "maximum assistance" to "moderate assistance," this patient's real improvement will not be recorded.

DESCRIPTIVE PARAMETERS

Therapists should use descriptive terms that are well-defined and unambiguous. Meanings of descriptive terms should be clear to all others using the medical record. Table 11–1 provides a sample set of acceptable terms and definitions. Additional terms used to qualify function include **dependence** and **difficulty.** Most often, the term *independent* refers to the complete absence of a need for human or mechanical assistance to accomplish a task, but some scoring systems consider reliance on devices and aids as a modified form of independence when used without the help of another person. The use of equipment during the performance of a functional task should be explicitly noted; for example, independent in ambulation with axillary crutches or independent in dressing with adapted clothing and a long-handled shoe-horn.

"Difficulty" is a hybrid term that suggests an activity poses an extra burden for the patient, regardless of dependence level. It is unclear whether it is a measure of overall perceptual-motor skill,

Table 11–1 FUNCTIONAL ASSESSMENT AND IMPAIRMENT TERMINOLOGY

DEFINITIONS
1. **Independent:** patient is able consistently to perform skill safety with no one present.
2. **Supervision:** patient requires someone within arm's reach as a precaution; low probability of patient having a problem requiring assistance.
3. **Close guarding:** person assisting is positioned as if to assist, with hands raised but not touching patient; full attention on patient; fair probability of patient requiring assistance.
4. **Contact guarding:** therapist is positioned as with close guarding, with hands on patient but not giving any assistance; high probability of patient requiring assistance.
5. **Minimum assistance:** patient is able to complete majority of the activity without assistance.
6. **Moderate assistance:** patient is able to complete part of the activity without assistance.
7. **Maximum assistance:** patient is unable to assist in any part of the activity.

DESCRIPTIVE TERMINOLOGY
A. Bed mobility
  1. Independent—no cuing[a] is given
  2. Supervision
  3. Minimum assistance   } may require cues
  4. Moderate assistance
  5. Maximum assistance
B. Transfers: ambulation
  1. Independent—no cuing is given
  2. Supervision
  3. Close guarding
  4. Contact guarding   } may require cues
  5. Minimum assistance
  6. Moderate assistance
  7. Maximum assistance
C. Functional Balance Grades

1. Normal	Patient is able to maintain steady balance without support (static).	
	Accepts maximal challenge and can shift weight in all directions (dynamic).	
2. Good	Patient is able to maintain balance without support (static).	
	Accepts moderate challenge; able to maintain balance while picking object off floor (dynamic).	
3. Fair	Patient is able to maintain balance with handhold (static).	
	Accepts minimal challenge; able to maintain balance while turning head/trunk (dynamic).	
4. Poor	Patient requires handhold and assistance (static).	
	Unable to accept challenge or move without loss of balance (dynamic).	
5. No balance		

[a]Types of cues: verbal, visual, or tactile. In some instances (e.g., a person with a memory deficit, short attention, learning disability, visual loss), a decrease in the number of cues may represent treatment progress, even though the level of dependence remains the same. Interim progress notes can denote these changes by citing frequencies (e.g., 2 out of 3 tries) or an arbitrarily defined rank order scale (e.g., always/occasionally/rarely).

coordination, endurance, efficiency, or a combination of measures. Difficulty can be measured in two ways. One approach assumes that difficulty is likely to be present and quantifies the degree of difficulty that the individual experiences while performing the activity (e.g., "How much difficulty do you have while doing household chores? None, some, or a great deal?"). The other approach quantifies the frequency that the difficulty is encountered (e.g., "How often do you have difficulty putting on your shoes? Never, sometimes, very often, or always?").

Often it is helpful to qualify a person's performance by linking observations with nonspecific indicators of impairments such as the energy consumption required to complete the functional task and the degree to which patients must exert themselves to engage in the activity. Simple measurements of a patient's physiological response to activity generally include heart rate, respiratory rate, and blood pressure, both at rest (baseline measurements) and during the most stressful elements of the functional task. For example, "heart rate increased to 100 beats per minute with independent ambulation on stairs; no increase in respiratory rate." In addition, the patient's fatigue, perception of exertion, and overt signs of physiological stress, such as shortness of breath, also should be noted. These notations may assist the therapist in a quick identification of some obvious impairments that limit function, which should be followed by more specific tests and measures of impairment.

Additional descriptors that are frequently used to qualify functional performance further include (1) pain, (2) fluctuations according to the time of day, (3) medication level, and (4) environmental influences. Any factors that modify a patient's function should be carefully noted and considered by the physical therapist evaluating examination data.

QUANTITATIVE PARAMETERS

The time it takes to complete a series of functional activities is often used to enhance a therapist's quantification of function when a given speed of performance is required or an improvement in performance speed is expected. A common example of timed assessments is found in pre- and post-medication assessments of individuals with Parkinson's disease who are placed on L-dopa therapy. Examples of activities that may be timed include (1) walking a set distance, (2) writing one's signature, (3) donning an article of clothing, and (4) crossing a street during the time of a "Walk" light. Scores of timed tests should not be taken as absolute, but rather as one dimension of performance. Although the ability to complete a particular activity in a specified period of time does provide one kind of important data on a patient's overall ability, it may not always be correct to conclude that what is being measured as "quicker" can be interpreted as "better." For example, the patient may get dressed quickly (within seconds), but do so with poorly coordinated movements and a haphazard outcome. When the task is slowed down, the movements may become more coordinated, with a more satisfactory functional outcome, even though the time taken to do the task increases. Similarly, certain medical conditions that affect energy expenditure may require that the patient properly pace a functional activity to complete it successfully. Thus, time scores alone do not always yield the complete

functional picture. When interpreted in light of other aspects of the patient's clinical presentation, they do provide an added dimension to the evaluation of data collected during a functional assessment.

RESPONSE FORMATS

Nominal Measures

One of the simplest formats in functional assessment uses a **nominal** level of measurement by presenting a **checklist** of various functional tasks on which the patient is simply scored as able to do/not able to do, independent/dependent, completed/incomplete, or the like. The results are not particularly descriptive of the exact nature of an individual's limitations and usually require further examination prior to interpretation.

Ordinal Measures

A few tests use descriptive scales that describe a range of performance or the degree to which a person can perform the task. Most commonly, the scales are **ordinal or rank-order scales** (e.g., "no difficulty," "some difficulty," or "unable to do"; or "always," "sometimes," "rarely," or "never"). Scales may be graded in ascending or descending order. The primary drawback in using such a system to score function is that these grades do not define categories that are separated by equal intervals. For example, it is not possible to tell whether the patient who went from maximal assistance to moderate assistance changed as much as a patient who also went one level between moderate assistance and minimal assistance.

SUMMARY OR ADDITIVE MEASURES

Summary or **additive** measures grade a specific series of skills, award points for part or full performance, and sum the subscores as a proportion of the total possible points, such as 60/100 or 6/24 and so forth. One example, which is well-known to physical therapists, is the Barthel Index (Table 11–2).[23] Some formal, standardized instruments for assessing function summarize detailed information about a complex area of function into an overall index score. Use of these instruments facilitates the interpretation of complex data and enables the clinician to perform cross-disease, cross-program, and cross-population comparisons of function. Caution must be exercised in considering only summated scores, however, because potentially important individual differences in functional ability can be masked.[24] A patient who is limited in only a few of the many tasks covered on a functional assessment will most likely score well, despite what could be substantial limitations in discrete functional activities, which

Table 11–2 BARTHEL INDEX[a]

Date _____
Initial _____

FEEDING
10 = Independent. Able to apply any
necessary device. Feeds in reasonable time.
5 = Needs help (e.g., for cutting).   _____

BATHING
5 = Independent   _____

PERSONAL TOILET
5 = Independently washes face,
combs hair, brushes teeth,
shaves (manages plug if elec-
tric).   _____

DRESSING
10 = Independent. Ties shoes, fastens
fasteners, applies braces.
5 = Needs help, but does at least
half of work in reasonable time.   _____

BOWELS
10 = No accidents. Able to use enema or suppository, if needed.
5 = Occasional accidents or needs
help with enema or suppository.   _____

BLADDER
10 = No accidents. Able to care for
collecting device if used.   _____
5 = Occasional accidents or needs
help with device.   _____

TOILET TRANSFERS
10 = Independent with toilet or bedpan. Handles clothes, wipes,
flushes, or cleans pan.
5 = Needs help for balance, han-
dling clothes or toilet paper.   _____

TRANSFERS—CHAIR AND BED
15 = Independent, including locking
of wheelchair, lifting footrests.
10 = Minimum assistance or supervision.
5 = Able to sit, but needs maximum
assistance to transfer.   _____

AMBULATION
15 = Independent for 50 yards. May
use assistive devices, except for
rolling walker.
10 = With help, 50 yards.
5 = Independent with wheelchair
for 50 yards if unable to walk.   _____

STAIR CLIMBING
10 = Independent. May use assistive
devices.   _____
5 = Needs help or supervision.   _____

Totals _____

[a]A score of zero (0) is given in any category in which the patient
does not achieve the stated criterion. (From Mahoney and Barthel,[23]
pp 62–65, with permission.)

are pertinent to the physical therapist's anticipated goals of treatment. Similarly, two patients with the same numeric score might be quite different in their functional deficits, having gained (or lost) their points on different activities. Although these measures yield a "hard number," which is regarded statistically as an interval level of measurement, the degree to which "points" are truly equal intervals apart should be carefully scrutinized.

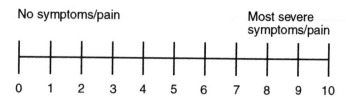

Figure 11-2. A visual analog scale for measuring pain or other symptoms. The patient is instructed to mark the line at the point that corresponds to the degree of pain or severity of symptoms that are experienced.

VISUAL ANALOG SCALES

Visual or linear analog scales attempt to represent measurement quantities in terms of a straight line placed horizontally or vertically on paper (Fig. 11-2). The endpoints of the line are labeled with descriptive or numeric terms to anchor the extremes of the scale and provide a frame of reference for any point in the continuum between them. Some scales will also use descriptors or numeric intervals between the endpoints to assist the individual in grading responses. Commonly the entire visual analog line is 10 centimeters long, but distances of 15 and 20 cm are also used. The patient is asked to bisect the line at a point representing self-assessed position on the scale. The patient's score is then obtained by measuring from the zero mark to the mark bisecting the scale.

VIDEO RECORDINGS

With ever-increasing application of technology to clinical data collection, new tools are available to clinicians and researchers for recording changes in function. Although more costly than traditional methods, videotaping or filming can be a valuable adjunct to functional assessment. Visual recordings are appropriate methods for assessing and validating the effectiveness of new interventions or treatment approaches. They are also useful to patients in displaying the quality of their movement patterns and in depicting the true extent of their disability. Video recordings are valuable tools for training staff to score tasks reliably by reaching agreement on observed performance.

INTERPRETING TEST RESULTS

Clearly, the single most important consideration in functional assessment is using the test results correctly to establish and revise the goals and outcomes of intervention and the plan of care. The therapist should carefully delineate the contributing factors that result in the functional deficit. When diminished ability is evident, the therapist must attempt to ascertain the cause of the problem. Some important questions to ask include:

1. What are the normal movements necessary to perform the task?

2. Which impairments inhibit performance or completion of the task? For example, do factors such as poor motor planning and execution, decreased strength, decreased range of motion, or altered joint integrity impede function? Does fatigue hamper functional ability?
3. Are the patient's functional deficits the result of impaired communication, perception, vision, hearing, or cognition?

Examples of the kinds of questions a therapist must pose to assess function and integrate findings into a comprehensive treatment program are found in the case vignettes that follow:

Case A	Case B
36 year-old male construction worker	72 year-old female homemaker
dx: traumatic right transtibial amputation; post fracture left femur	dx: CVA with right hemiplegia with global aphasia
Partial Examination Findings	
Motor Control and Muscle Performance:	
decreased all extremities following prolonged immobilization	flaccid paralysis right extremities
Functional limitations: unable to transfer from bed to wheelchair	unable to transfer from bed to wheelchair

Although the functional disability in each case is in fact identical, the contributing factors, goals and outcomes, and the interventions would be markedly different. In case A, the patient's inability to transfer can reasonably be attributed to decreased strength. When ameliorated, it is likely that the patient will go on to achieve an outcome of independent ambulation with a prosthesis. The patient in case B has factors that cannot be addressed solely through physical therapy. In addition, it may be difficult to determine whether it is the paralysis or the aphasia that compromises efforts to assess and improve function. Although a similar goal of independence in wheelchair mobility and transfers may be proposed, reexamination throughout the episode of care may demonstrate that functional deficits persist, despite improvement in motor function. In that case, the impairments in comprehension and language function may be the more important factors contributing to functional limitation. Thus, the design of rehabilitation programs is based on the impairments that presumably underlie the functional deficits. If remediation of the impairment does not solve the functional problem, the therapist needs to reexamine the initial clinical impression by looking for other potentially causative factors.

Some functional tasks may need to be analyzed more precisely. Activities can be broken down into subordinate parts, or subroutines. A **subordinate part** is defined as an element of movement without which the task cannot proceed safely or efficiently. For example, bed mobility includes the following subordinate parts: (1) scooting in bed (changing position for comfort or skin care and getting to the edge), (2) rolling onto the side, (3) lowering the legs, (4) sitting up, and (5) balancing at the edge of the bed. A functional loss of independent bed mobility may result from an inability to perform any or all of these subroutines. These are not only checkpoints for examining patients, but they also later represent the anticipated goals of various interventions. The more involved the patient, the slower the learner, or complex the task, the more the functional task may need to be broken down into subordinate parts.

Assessing the Quality of Instruments

Within the rehabilitation setting, many tools have been developed primarily for in-house use and may have spread from facility to facility as staff have moved. In most instances, the instruments underwent many modifications and the original sources have been lost. Other tests have been designed more rigidly and tested in clinical trials, assessing the instrument's psychometric properties and providing documentation of its **reliability** and **validity** in the literature. If the reliability and validity of an instrument are not established, little faith can be put in the results obtained or in the conclusions drawn from the results.[25] A poorly constructed instrument can produce data that are questionable, if not worthless. In light of the fact that the viability of physical therapy as a reimbursable service rests on the demonstration of functional outcomes, the importance of these concepts to functional assessment becomes clear. Some of the more recently developed instruments have undergone extensive testing of their measurement properties. In accordance with the American Physical Therapy Association's Standards of Measurement, physical therapists should use only those instruments whose reliability and validity are known.[26] Although no instrument will have perfect reliability or validity, therapists must be able to gauge the certainty of their data and the appropriate scope of inferences drawn from the data.

RELIABILITY

A reliable instrument measures a phenomenon dependably, time after time, accurately, predictably, and without variation. If a functional assessment or any test is not reliable, the patient's initial baseline status or the true effect of treatment can be concealed. An instrument with acceptable *test-retest reliability* is stable and will not indicate change when none has occurred. Assessments performed by the same therapist of the same performance should be highly correlated (*intrarater reliability*). Instruments should also have strong *interrater reliability*, or agreement among multiple observers of the same event. If a particular patient is examined by several therapists in the course of treatment, or reexamined over time to determine long-term change, the reliability of the functional assessment tool must be known.

A flaw in the clinical use of most types of standardized tests and measures is the tendency to disregard interrater reliability. To use functional assessments with maximum accuracy, (1) scoring criteria must be defined clearly and must be mutually exclusive, (2) criteria must be strictly applied to each clinical situation, and (3) all therapists in a facility must be retrained periodically in the use of the instrument to ensure similarity.

VALIDITY

Validity is a multifaceted concept and established in many different ways. Questions regarding an instrument's validity attempt to determine (1) whether an instrument designed to measure function truly does just that, (2) what the appropriate applications of the instrument are, and (3) how the data should be interpreted. First, the valid instrument should, on the face of it, appear to measures what it purports to measure (*face validity*).[25] Another critical dimension is whether the assessment instrument measures all the important or specified dimensions of function (*content validity*). Through the use of various statistical procedures, it is also possible to demonstrate the degree to which items on the instrument group together to measure concepts which can be labeled as physical mobility or social interaction (*construct validity*). If there were a **gold standard** (an unimpeachable measure of a phenomenon, such as a laboratory test with normative values), then a new instrument could be tested against the results of this standard. Such a gold standard does not exist for functional assessment instruments. New functional assessment tools can, however, be compared to existing ones that are accepted measures of the same functional activities. The degree to which the two instruments agree helps to establish *concurrent validity*. Concurrent validity can also be demonstrated by showing that an instrument corresponds appropriately to measures of other phenomena. This method is particularly relevant for self-assessment instruments. The concurrent validity of some self-assessment instruments has been determined by comparison with clinician ratings and other clinical findings; for example, a person's level of function as indicated by an instrument correlates directly with clinician's ratings of improvement and inversely with the patient's reports of pain. Finally, there is the *predictive validity* of a test or measure, which indicates the likelihood of a subsequent phenomenon or event (e.g., return to work) on the basis of a prior phenomenon (e.g., a baseline measure of function).

OTHER FACTORS

In addition to reliability and validity, a measure of functional status should be (1) sufficiently sensitive to reflect meaningful changes in patient status, and (2) concise enough to be clinically useful.

Considerations in Selection of Instruments

A large number of instruments have been developed to assess and to classify functional ability.

Given the plethora of instruments that currently exist, it is quite reasonable to ask how these instruments compare with one another. It is important to remember that no instrument is perfect for all patients or all situations. No instrument can assess all the items potentially relevant to a particular individual and provide the perfect composite picture. For example, one instrument may provide an extensive assessment of **activities of daily living (ADL),** but not deal with psychological or social dimensions of function. Another instrument may investigate social functioning while omitting some ADL tasks. Many items overlap from instrument to instrument. For example, a question on the ability to ambulate is a common item found in most physical function instruments. Although instruments may cover the same kind of activity, the questions posed about the performance of the same activity may be quite different. For example, one instrument may investigate the degree of difficulty and of human assistance required to "dress yourself, including handling of closures, buttons, zippers, snaps." Another may ask, "How much help do you need in getting dressed?" As discussed, differences also may exist in the time frames sampled in the various instruments.

Critical questions to ask, therefore, in selecting an instrument include:

1. What are the domains or categories that the assessment instrument focuses on?
2. How adequately does the instrument measure the domain or domains being sampled?
3. What areas of physical function are included? Does the instrument measure ADL? IADL? Functional mobility skills?
4. What aspect of function is being measured? Is the level of dependence-independence considered? What is the length of time required to complete the functional task? Degree of difficulty? Influence of pain?
5. What is the time frame sampled in the assessment?
6. What is the mode of administration?
7. What type of scoring system is used?
8. Are multiple instruments necessary to provide a more complete assessment?

Extrapolating items from a variety of instruments may provide the kind of data desired but should be considered with extreme caution inasmuch as this process changes reliability or validity of the assessment. Factors such as the theoretic orientation of the user, the purpose for using the instrument, and the relevance of particular functional items to certain patient populations all enter into the decision making process. In the final analysis, the choice of instrument may be dictated by practical considerations. For example, self-report instruments, which rely on information from the patient, are limited in use to mentally competent individuals. Time and resources for administration also may influence test selection. In any case, there are many suitable instruments available for assessing functional status, some of which are quite commonly used by clinicians as well as researchers.

Selected Instruments
Assessing Physical Function

BARTHEL INDEX

The Barthel Index was developed by a physical therapist over 30 years ago.[23] Although not as commonly used today as some other instruments, this assessment tool represents one of the earliest contributions to the functional status literature and identifies physical therapists' long-standing inclusion of functional mobility and ADL measurement within their scope of practice. The Barthel Index specifically measures the degree of assistance required by an individual on 10 items of mobility and self-care ADL (see Table 11-2). Levels of measurement are limited to either complete independence or needing assistance. Each performance item is assessed on an ordinal scale with a specified number of points assigned to each level or ranking. Variable weightings were established by the developers of the Barthel Index for each item based on clinical judgment or other implicit criteria. An individual who uses human assistance in eating, for example, would receive 5 points; independence in eating would receive a score of 10 points. A single global score, ranging from 0 to 100, is calculated from the sum of all weighted individual item scores, so that a 0 equals complete dependence for all 10 activities, and 100 equals complete independence in all 10 activities. The Barthel Index has been used widely to monitor functional changes in individuals receiving in-patient rehabilitation, particularly in predicting the functional outcomes associated with stroke.[27,28] Although its psychometric properties have never been fully assessed, the Barthel Index has demonstrated strong interrater reliability (0.95) and test-retest reliability (0.89) as well as high correlations (0.74 to 0.80) with other measures of physical disability.[29]

KATZ INDEX OF ACTIVITIES OF DAILY LIVING

The Katz Index of ADL focuses on patient performance and the degree of assistance required in six categories of basic ADL: bathing, dressing, toileting, transferring, continence, and feeding[30,31] (Table 11-3). Using both direct observation and patient self-report over a 2-week period, the examiner scores 1 point for each activity that is performed without human help. A score of 0 is given if the activity is performed with human assistance or is not performed. Activity scores are combined to form a cumulative scale in letter grades (A through G) in order of increasing dependency. An individual's global letter score indicates an exact pattern of responses to the list of items. A score of B in the Katz Index, for example, means that the individual is independent in performing all but one of the six basic ADL categories. On the other hand, a score of D means that the individual is independent in all but bathing, dressing, and one additional function. The combination of categoric deficits in the Katz Index reflects a particular theoretical orientation. The developers of the Katz Index assumed a developmental and hierarchical organization of function in constructing their instrument. This organizational model is based on the empirically noted integration of neurological and locomotor responses seen in children. One version of the scale demonstrated agreement ratios of 0.68 and 0.98 between different professional raters. Test-retest reliability of respondent self-reports produced intraclass correlation coefficients ranging from 0.61 to 0.78.[32]

The Katz Index, originally developed for use with institutionalized patients, has been adapted for use in community-based populations.[33] A major disadvantage of using the Katz Index in rehabilitation settings is its failure to include an item on ambulation. The predictive validity of the instrument for long-term survival also has been reported.[31]

SUMMARY OF PHYSICAL FUNCTION TESTS

Neither of the single physical functional assessment instruments presented above covers all areas of physical function (Table 11–4). Even items that appear to assess the same function may, depending on how the item is worded, be concerned with a different aspect of performance.[34] Therefore, one of these instruments may be chosen to match the specific needs of the clinician for a brief, unidimensional functional assessment, but only if the likely functional limitations of the clinical population served are described by the items on the instrument.

Multidimensional Functional Assessment Instruments

The previous discussion of functional assessment instruments that describe only one dimension of health status highlights a clinician's need to understand a patient's health status in all its domains. Further instrument development in the last 20 years has resulted in the emergence of multidimensional health status instruments to measure the spectrum of health status domains more comprehensively. Most concentrate on two or three dimensions of a patient's function, and record little about a person's disease or impairments. Therefore, to some small degree the term *health status* frequently used to describe these instruments is a misnomer, inasmuch as these instruments actually measure multiple dimensions of function as they contribute to a person's health and not "health" in, and of, itself. Similarly, these instruments are also sometimes referred to as measuring health-related quality of life. Without bringing in the patient's perspective on personal meaningfulness to the individual, the gold standard quality of life, such terminology may overstate the value of these instruments. However, used in conjunction with traditional clinical methods of assessing signs and symptoms, multidimensional functional status instruments can add an important comprehensive view of a patient's function to the overall health assessment process. In this

Table 11–3 THE KATZ INDEX OF ADL

Name _____ Day of evaluation _____

For each area of functioning listed below, check description that applies. (The word "assistance" means supervision, direction, or personal assistance.)

Bathing—either sponge bath, tub bath, or shower.

☐	☐	☐
Receives no assistance (gets in and out of tub by self if tub is usual means of bathing).	Receives assistance in bathing only one part of the body (such as back or a leg).	Receives assistance in bathing more than one part of the body (or not bathed).

Dressing—gets clothes from closets and drawers—including underclothes, outer garments and using fasteners (including braces if worn).

☐	☐	☐
Gets clothes and gets completely dressed without assistance.	Gets clothes and gets dressed without assistance except for assistance in tying shoes.	Receives assistance in getting clothes or in getting dressed, or stays partly or completely undressed.

Toileting—going to the "toilet room" for bowel and urine elimination, cleaning self after elimination, and arranging clothes.

☐	☐	☐
Goes to "toilet room," cleans self, and arranges clothes without assistance (may use object for support such as cane, walker, or wheelchair and may manage night bedpan or commode, emptying same in morning).	Receives assistance in going to "toilet room" or in cleansing self or in arranging clothes after elimination or in use of night bedpan or commode.	Doesn't go to room termed "toilet" for the elimination process.

Transfer

☐	☐	☐
Moves in and out of bed as well as in and out of chair without assistance (may be using object for support such as cane or walker).	Moves in and out of bed or chair with assistance.	Doesn't get out of bed.

Continence

☐	☐	☐
Controls urination and bowel movement completely by self.	Has occasional "accidents."	Supervision helps keep urine or bowel control; catheter is used, or is incontinent.

Feeding

☐	☐	☐
Feeds self without assistance.	Feeds self except for getting assistance in cutting meat or buttering bread.	Receives assistance in feeding or is fed partly or completely by using tubes or intravenous fluids.

The Index of Independence in Activities of Daily Living is based on an evaluation of the functional independence or dependence of patients in bathing, dressing, going to toilet, transferring, continence, and feeding. Specific definitions of functional independence and dependence appear below the index.

A—Independent in feeding, continence, transferring, going to toilet, dressing, and bathing.
B—Independent in all but one of these functions.
C—Independent in all but bathing and one additional function.
D—Independent in all but bathing, dressing, and one additional function.
E—Independent in all but bathing, dressing, going to toilet, and one additional function.
F—Independent in all but bathing, dressing, going to toilet, transferring, and one additional function.
G—Dependent in all six functions.
Other—Dependent in at least two functions, but not classifiable as C, D, E, or F.

Independence means without supervision, direction, or active personal assistance, except as specifically noted below. This is based on actual status and not on ability. A patient who refuses to perform a function is considered as not performing the function, even though he is deemed able.

Bathing (sponge, shower, or tub)
Independent: assistance only in bathing a single part (as back or disabled extremity) or bathes self completely
Dependent: assistance in bathing more than one part of body; assistance in getting in or out of tub or does not bathe self

Dressing
Independent: gets clothes from closets and drawers; puts on clothes, outer garments, braces; manages fasteners; act of tying shoes is excluded
Dependent: does not dress self or remains partly undressed

Going to toilet
Independent: gets to toilet; gets on and off toilet; arranges clothes; cleans organs of excretion (may manage own bedpan used at night only and may or may not be using mechanical supports)
Dependent: uses bedpan or commode or receives assistance in getting to and using toilet

Transfer
Independent: moves in and out of bed independently and moves in and out of chair independently (may or may not be using mechanical supports)
Dependent: assistance in moving in or out of bed and/or chair; does not perform one or more transfers

Continence
Independent: urination and defecation entirely self-controlled
Dependent: partial or total incontinence in urination or defecation; partial or total control by enemas, catheters, or regulated use of urinals and/or bedpans

Feeding
Independent: gets food from plate or its equivalent, into mouth (precutting of meat and preparation of food, as buttering bread, are excluded from evaluation)
Dependent: assistance in act of feeding (see above); does not eat at all or parenteral feeding

From Katz, S, et al.[31] p 20, with permission.

Table 11–4 ITEMS COVERED IN SELECTED PHYSICAL FUNCTION INSTRUMENTS

	Barthel	Katz
Mobility		
Transfers	+	+
Ambulation	+	−
Inclines/stairs	+	−
ADL		
Bathing	+	+
Grooming	+	−
Dressing	+	+
Feeding	+	+
Toileting	+	+

respect they add a crucial, and previously missing, component in evaluating the health of individuals. A few of these instruments representative of the current "state of the art" are discussed below.

THE FUNCTIONAL INDEPENDENCE MEASURE

The Functional Independence Measure (FIM)[35,36] is an 18-item measure of physical, psychological, and social function which is part of the Uniform Data System for Medical Rehabilitation (UDS$_{MR}$).[37] The UDS$_{MR}$ collects data from participating rehabilitation facilities and issues summary reports of the records that have been entered into the UDS$_{MR}$ database. The FIM uses the level of assistance an individual needs to grade functional status from total independence to total assistance (Fig. 11-3). A person may be regarded as independent if a device is used, but this is recorded separately from "complete" independence. The instrument lists six self-care activities: feeding, grooming, bathing, upper body dressing, lower body dressing, and toileting. Bowel and bladder control, aspects of which some may consider as impairments rather than function, are categorized separately. Functional mobility is tested through three items on transfers. Under the category of locomotion, walking and using a wheelchair are listed equivalently, while stairs are considered separately. The FIM also includes two items on communication and three on social cognition.

The FIM measures what the individual does, not what that person could do under certain circumstances. The interrater reliability of the FIM has been established at an acceptable level of psychometric performance (intraclass correlation coefficients ranging from 0.86 to 0.88). The face and content validity of the FIM as well as its ability to capture change in a patient's level of function have also been determined. Any clinical worker can administer the FIM after appropriate training in using the response set for each item.

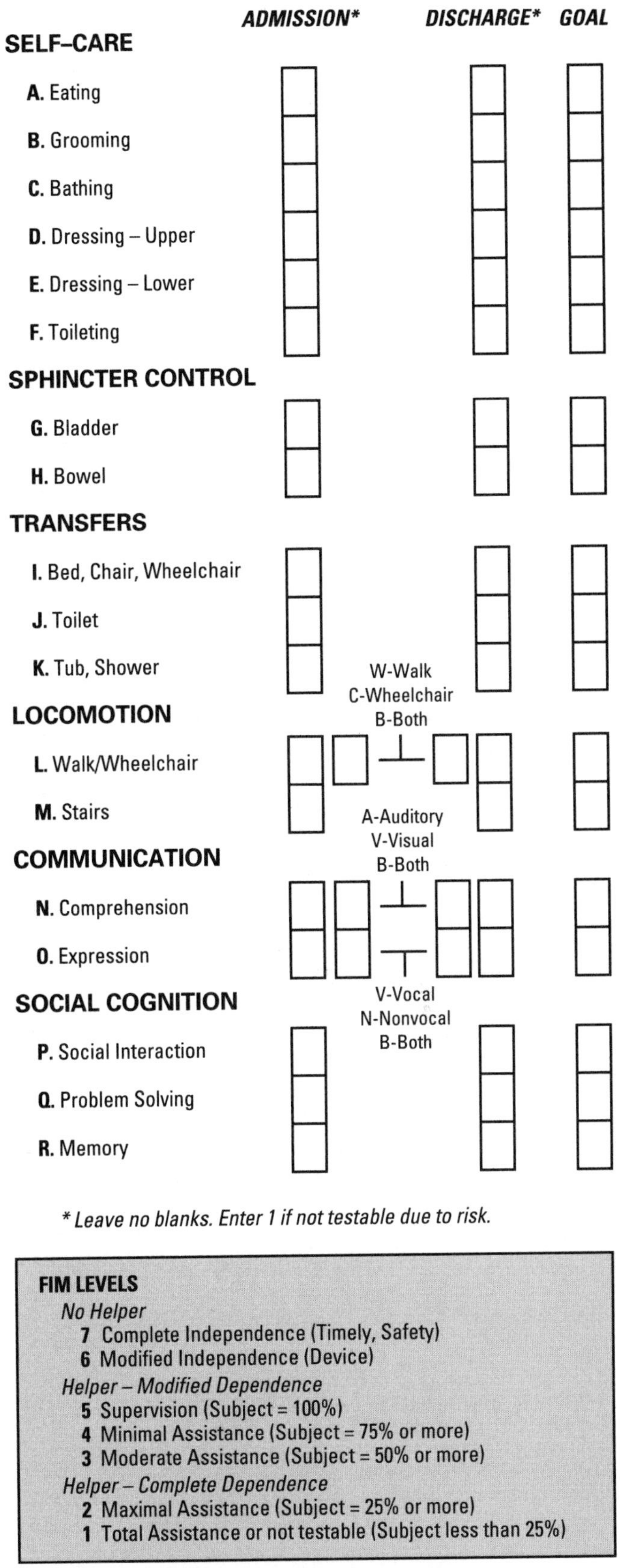

THE SICKNESS IMPACT PROFILE

The Sickness Impact Profile (SIP) was developed to address the need for an instrument that was precise enough to detect meaningful changes in perceived function.[36–43] Intended for use across types and severities of illness, it is designed to detect

Figure 11-3. The Functional Independence Measure (FIM™) instrument scores function using a seven-point scale based on percentage(s) of active participation from patient. (From the Uniform Data System for Medical Rehabilitation, a division of UB Foundation Activities, Inc. [UDS$_{MR}$™]. Guide for the Uniform Data Set for Medical Rehabilitation [including the FIM™ instrument], Version 5.1. Buffalo, NY 14214: State University of New York at Buffalo; 1997, with permission.)

Table 11–5 SICKNESS IMPACT PROFILE (SIP): AFFECTIVE FUNCTION

Please respond to (check) *only* those statements that you are *sure* describe you today and are related to your state of health.

1. I say how bad or useless I am; for example, that I am a burden on others. _____
2. I laugh or cry suddenly. _____
3. I often moan and groan in pain or discomfort. _____
4. I have attempted suicide. _____
5. I act nervous or restless. _____
6. I keep rubbing or holding areas of my body that hurt or are uncomfortable. _____
7. I act irritable and impatient with myself; for example, talk badly about myself, swear at myself, blame myself for things that happen. _____
8. I talk about the future in a hopeless way. _____
9. I get sudden frights. _____

CHECK HERE WHEN YOU HAVE READ ALL STATEMENTS ON THIS PAGE ☐

Reprinted by permission of Marilyn Bergner, PhD.[42]

small impacts of illness. The SIP contains 136 items in 12 categories of activities. These include sleep and rest, eating, work, home management, recreation, ambulatory mobility, body care and movement, social interaction, alertness, emotional behavior, and communication. A sample SIP measure of affective functioning specific to emotional behavior is found in Table 11–5. The entire test can be either self-administered or administered by an interview in 20 to 30 minutes. SIP scores are percentage ratings based on the ratio of the summed scale scores to the summed values of all SIP items. Higher scores indicate greater dysfunction.

The SIP test-retest reliability coefficients range from 0.75 to 0.92 for the overall score and from 0.45 to 0.60 for items checked.[40] Validity has been determined using subjective self-assessment, clinician assessment, and subjects' scores on other instruments. Correlations relevant to establishing multiple forms of validity range from a low of 0.35 to a high of 0.84.[39] The SIP has been used to describe

the physical and psychosocial functions of individuals in an outpatient setting in relation to the duration of disease[44] and the efficacy of using transcutaneous electrical nerve stimulation (TENS) with low back pain patients.[45] There are, however, some concerns regarding its use and suitability in certain kinds of studies. In assessing disability, SIP focuses only on ability versus inability to perform an activity; for example, "I am not going into town." It neglects the range of performance in between, with some potential loss of precision. The SIP also combines many functional activities into a single item, which may also reduce its discriminatory ability, such as "I have difficulty doing handwork; for example, turning faucets, using kitchen gadgets, sewing, carpentry." A few investigators have noted that the SIP may be more sensitive to detecting deterioration of status than to improvement, which may diminish its suitability as an instrument for monitoring individuals over time.[46]

THE SF-36

The SF-36 contains 36 items based on questions used in the RAND Health Insurance Study. These 36 items were culled from the 113 questions used by RAND in the Medical Outcomes Study (MOS) to explore the relationship between physician practice styles and patient outcomes.[47] Thus, it was named the SF-36, because it was a short form of the MOS instrument with only 36 questions. The MOS provided important data on the functional status of adults with specific chronic conditions[48] and the well-being of patients experiencing depression compared to subjects with a chronic medical condition.[49] The SF-36 demonstrated high reliability and validity (correlation coefficients ranging from 0.81 to 0.88).[50–53] Normative data for these self-report items have been collected.[54] The development of the SF-36 stands as the premier example of a complete and published exploration of the psychometric properties of an instrument as an essential part of its development, and a testament to the

Table 11–6 THE SF-36: PHYSICAL AND ROLE FUNCTION

The following questions are about activities you might do during a typical day. Does *your health* limit you in these activities? If so, how much? (Mark one box on each line.)	Yes, limited a lot	Yes limited a little	No, not limited at all
a. *Vigorous activities,* such as running, lifting heavy objects, participating in strenuous sports	1☐	2☐	3☐
b. *Moderate activities,* such as moving a table, pushing a vacuum cleaner, bowling, or playing golf	1☐	2☐	3☐
c. Lifting or carrying groceries	1☐	2☐	3☐
d. Climbing *several* flights of stairs	1☐	2☐	3☐
e. Climbing *one* flight of stairs	1☐	2☐	3☐
f. Bending, kneeling, or stooping	1☐	2☐	3☐
g. Walking *more than a mile*	1☐	2☐	3☐
h. Walking *several blocks*	1☐	2☐	3☐
i. Walking *one block*	1☐	2☐	3☐
j. Bathing or dressing yourself	1☐	2☐	3☐

During the *past 4 weeks,* have you had any of the following problems with your work or other regular daily activities *as a result of your physical health?* (Mark one box on each line.)	Yes	No
a. Cut down the *amount of time* you spent on work or other activities	1☐	2☐
b. *Accomplished less* than you would like	1☐	2☐
c. Were limited in the *kind* of work or other activities	1☐	2☐
d. Had *difficulty* performing the work or other activities (for example, it took extra effort)	1☐	2☐

With permission.

Table 11–7 OUTCOME AND ASSESSMENT INFORMATION SET (OASIS): ADL/IADLs

(M0640) Grooming: Ability to tend to personal hygiene needs (i.e., washing face and hands, hair care, shaving or make up, teeth or denture care, fingernail care).

Prior	Current	
☐	☐	0—Able to groom self unaided, with or without the use of assistive devices or adapted methods.
☐	☐	1—Grooming utensils must be placed within reach before able to complete grooming activities.
☐	☐	2—Someone must assist the patient to groom self.
☐	☐	3—Patient depends entirely upon someone else for grooming needs.
☐		UK—Unknown

(M0650) Ability to Dress *Upper* Body (with or without dressing aids) including undergarments, pullovers, front-opening shirts and blouses, managing zippers, buttons, and snaps:

Prior	Current	
☐	☐	0—Able to get clothes out of closets and drawers, put them on and remove them from the upper body without assistance.
☐	☐	1—Able to dress upper body without assistance if clothing is laid out or handed to the patient.
☐	☐	2—Someone must help the patient put on upper body clothing.
☐	☐	3—Patient depends entirely upon another person to dress the upper body.
☐		UK—Unknown

(M0660) Ability to Dress *Lower* Body (with or without dressing aids) including undergarments, slacks, socks or nylons, shoes:

Prior	Current	
☐	☐	0—Able to obtain, put on, and remove clothing and shoes without assistance.
☐	☐	1—Able to dress lower body without assistance if clothing and shoes are laid out or handed to the patient.
☐	☐	2—Someone must help the patient put on undergarments, slacks, socks or nylons, and shoes.
☐	☐	3—Patient depends entirely upon another person to dress lower body.
☐		UK—Unknown

(M0670) Bathing: Ability to wash entire body. ***Excludes*** **grooming (washing face and hands only).**

Prior	Current	
☐	☐	0—Able to bathe self in *shower or tub* independently.
☐	☐	1—With the use of devices, is able to bathe self in shower or tub independently.
☐	☐	2—Able to bathe in shower or tub with the assistance of another person: (a) for intermittent supervision or encouragement or reminders, *OR* (b) to get in and out of the shower or tub, *OR* (c) for washing difficult to reach areas.
☐	☐	3—Participates in bathing self in shower or tub, *but* requires presence of another person throughout the bath for assistance or supervision.
☐	☐	4—*Unable* to use the shower or tub and is bathed in *bed or bedside chair*.
☐	☐	5—Unable to effectively participate in bathing and is totally bathed by another person.
☐		UK—Unknown

(M0680) Toileting: Ability to get to and from the toilet or bedside commode.

Prior	Current	
☐	☐	0—Able to get to and from the toilet independently with or without a device.
☐	☐	1—When reminded, assisted, or supervised by another person, able to get to and from the toilet.
☐	☐	2—*Unable* to get to and from the toilet but is able to use a bedside commode (with or without assistance).
☐	☐	3—*Unable* to get to and from the toilet or bedside commode but is able to use a bedpan/urinal independently.
☐	☐	4—Is totally dependent in toileting.
☐		UK—Unknown

(M0690) Transferring: Ability to move from bed to chair, on and off toilet or commode, into and out of tub or shower, and ability to turn and position self in bed if patient is bedfast.

Prior	Current	
☐	☐	0—Able to independently transfer.
☐	☐	1—Transfers with minimal human assistance or with use of an assistive device.
☐	☐	2—*Unable* to transfer self but is able to bear weight and pivot during the transfer process.
☐	☐	3—Unable to transfer self and is *unable* to bear weight or pivot when transferred by another person.
☐	☐	4—Bedfast, unable to transfer but is able to turn and position self in bed.
☐	☐	5—Bedfast, unable to transfer and is *unable* to turn and position self.
☐		UK—Unknown

(M0700) Ambulation/Locomotion: Ability to *SAFELY* walk, once in a standing position, or use a wheelchair, once in a seated position, on a variety of surfaces.

Prior	Current	
☐	☐	0—Able to independently walk on even and uneven surfaces and climb stairs with or without railings (i.e., needs no human assistance or assistive device).
☐	☐	1—Requires use of a device (e.g., cane, walker) to walk alone *or* requires human supervision or assistance to negotiate stairs or steps or uneven surfaces.
☐	☐	2—Able to walk only with the supervision or assistance of another person at all times.
☐	☐	3—Chairfast, *unable* to ambulate but is able to wheel self independently.
☐	☐	4—Chairfast, unable to ambulate and is *unable* to wheel self.
☐	☐	5—Bedfast, unable to ambulate or be up in a chair.
☐		UK—Unknown

Continued

Table 11–7 OUTCOME AND ASSESSMENT INFORMATION SET (OASIS): ADL/IADLs *Continued*

(M0710) Feeding or Eating: Ability to feed self meals and snacks. **Note: This refers only to the process of** *eating, chewing,* **and** *swallowing, not preparing* **the food to be eaten.**

Prior	*Current*	
□	□	0—Able to independently feed self.
□	□	1—Able to feed self independently but requires:
		(a) meal set-up; *OR*
		(b) intermittent assistance or supervision from another person; *OR*
		(c) a liquid, pureed or ground meat diet.
□	□	2—*Unable* to feed self and must be assisted or supervised throughout the meal/snack.
□	□	3—Able to take in nutrients orally *and* receives supplemental nutrients through a nasogastric tube or gastrostomy.
□	□	4—*Unable* to take in nutrients orally and is fed nutrients through a nasogastric tube or gastrostomy.
□	□	5—Unable to take in nutrients orally or by tube feeding.
□		UK—Unknown

(M0720) Planning and Preparing Light Meals (e.g., cereal, sandwich) or reheat delivered meals:

Prior	*Current*	
□	□	0—(a) Able to independently plan and prepare all light meals for self or reheat delivered meals; *OR*
		(b) Is physically, cognitively, and mentally able to prepare light meals on a regular basis but has not routinely performed light meal preparation in the past (i.e., prior to this home care admission).
□	□	1—*Unable* to prepare light meals on a regular basis due to physical, cognitive, or mental limitations.
□	□	2—Unable to prepare any light meals or reheat any delivered meals.
□		UK—Unknown

(M0730) Transportation: Physical and mental ability to *safely* use a car, taxi, or public transportation (bus, train, subway).

Prior	*Current*	
□	□	0—Able to independently drive a regular or adapted car; *OR* uses a regular or handicap-accessible public bus.
□	□	1—Able to ride in a car only when driven by another person; *OR* able to use a bus or handicap van only when assisted or accompanied by another person.
□	□	2—*Unable* to ride in a car, taxi, bus, or van, and requires transportation by ambulance.
□		UK—Unknown

(M0740) Laundry: Ability to do own laundry—to carry laundry to and from washing machine, to use washer and dryer, to wash small items by hand.

Prior	*Current*	
□	□	0—(a) Able to independently take care of all laundry tasks; *OR*
		(b) Physically, cognitively, and mentally able to do laundry and access facilities, *but* has not routinely performed laundry tasks in the past (i.e., prior to this home care admission).
□	□	1—Able to do only light laundry, such as minor hand wash or light washer loads. Due to physical, cognitive, or mental limitations, needs assistance with heavy laundry such as carrying large loads of laundry.
□	□	2—*Unable* to do any laundry due to physical limitation or needs continual supervision and assistance due to cognitive or mental limitation.
□		UK—Unknown

(M0750) Housekeeping: Ability to safely and effectively perform light housekeeping and heavier cleaning tasks.

Prior	*Current*	
□	□	0—(a) Able to independently perform all housekeeping tasks; *OR*
		(b) Physically, cognitively, and mentally able to perform *all* housekeeping tasks but has not routinely participated in housekeeping tasks in the past (i.e., prior to this home care admission).
□	□	1—Able to perform only *light* housekeeping (e.g., dusting, wiping kitchen counters) tasks independently.
□	□	2—Able to perform housekeeping tasks with intermittent assistance or supervision from another person.
□	□	3—*Unable* to consistently perform any housekeeping tasks unless assisted by another person throughout the process.
□	□	4—Unable to effectively participate in any housekeeping tasks.
□		UK—Unknown

(M0760) Shopping: Ability to plan for, select, and purchase items in a store and to carry them home or arrange delivery.

Prior	*Current*	
□	□	0—(a) Able to plan for shopping needs and independently perform shopping tasks, including carrying packages; *OR*
		(b) Physically, cognitively, and mentally able to take care of shopping, but has not done shopping in the past (i.e., prior to this home care admission).
□	□	1—Able to go shopping, but needs some assistance:
		(a) By self is able to do only light shopping and carry small packages, but needs someone to do occasional major shopping; *OR*
		(b) *Unable* to go shopping alone, but can go with someone to assist.
□	□	2—*Unable* to go shopping, but is able to identify items needed, place orders, and arrange home delivery.
□	□	3—Needs someone to do all shopping and errands.
□		UK—Unknown

Table 11–7 OUTCOME AND ASSESSMENT INFORMATION SET (OASIS): ADL/IADLs *Continued*

(M0770) Ability to Use Telephone: Ability to answer the phone, dial numbers, and *effectively* use the telephone to communicate.

Prior	Current	
☐	☐	0—Able to dial numbers and answer calls appropriately and as desired.
☐	☐	1—Able to use a specially adapted telephone (i.e., large numbers on the dial, teletype phone for the deaf) and call essential numbers.
☐	☐	2—Able to answer the telephone and carry on a normal conversation but has difficulty with placing calls.
☐	☐	3—Able to answer the telephone only some of the time or is able to carry on only a limited conversation.
☐	☐	4—*Unable* to answer the telephone at all but can listen if assisted with equipment.
☐	☐	5—Totally unable to use the telephone.
☐	☐	NA—Patient does not have a telephone.
☐		UK—Unknown

Source: OASIS-B, Center for Health Services and Policy Research, Denver, CO, 1997. With permission.

responsibility of its creators in verifying the quality of the SF-36 as a scientific tool.

All but one of the 36 questions of the SF-36 are used to form eight different scales: physical function, social function, role function, mental health, energy/fatigue, pain, and general health perceptions. The last question considers self-perceived change in health during the past year. Items are scored on nominal (yes/no) or ordinal scales. Each possible response to an item on a scale is assigned a number of points. The total points for all items within a scale are then added and transformed mathematically to yield a percentage score, with 100 percent representing optimal health. Sample items on physical function and role function are presented in Table 11–6 on page 322. The SF-36 has been used in a number of studies that describe the health status and physical functioning of patients with a variety of impairments receiving physical therapy services.[55–60]

THE OUTCOME AND ASSESSMENT INFORMATION SET

The Outcome and Assessment Information Set (OASIS) was designed to assure the collection of pertinent data on the adult patient in the home care setting that would allow home health agencies to assess the quality of care by measuring the outcomes of care.[61,62] During the years of its initial development, use of the OASIS by home health agencies had been voluntary. However, beginning on January 1, 1999, home health agencies were mandated to use the OASIS as a Condition of Participation in the Medicare program by the Health Care Financing Administration. Developed over a 10-year period, the current version of OASIS, known as OASIS-B, contains 79 core items covering sociodemographic characteristics, environmental factors, social support, health status, and functional status. Future revisions of OASIS will be labeled OASIS-C, OASIS-D, and so on. OASIS is not designed to be a comprehensive assessment of a patient, or an "add-on" assessment. OASIS items are meant to be integrated into the clinical record to highlight various aspects of a patient's status that identify particular needs for care upon admission to the home health service, at follow-up every 60 days, and at discharge. The OASIS was intended to be a discipline-neutral record, administered by any health professional including physical therapists. Created as part of a research program to develop outcomes measures applicable to home health, the OASIS has been field-tested through demonstration projects and refined by a panel of experts. Reliability testing is ongoing.

Ease of administration increases with familiarity with the instrument. Unlike most other instruments, the response sets that accompany each item are specifically matched to the item. Some response sets have only two possible descriptions of behavior, whereas others have as many as nine possible descriptions of behavior. Therefore, the user must be familiar with the possible response set to each item, and anticipate that comfort level in using this instrument will increase over a learning curve. The ADL/IADL section is composed of 14 different items (Table 11–7, pages 323–325) including grooming, dressing the upper body, dressing the lower body, bathing, toileting, transfers, ambulation/locomotion, feeding, meal preparation, transportation, laundry, housekeeping, shopping, and the ability to use the telephone. The format of the instrument in this section allows recording of both prior and current functional status on each of the items.

SUMMARY OF MULTIDIMENSIONAL FUNCTIONAL ASSESSMENT INSTRUMENTS

For the purposes of illustration, four multidimensional instruments have been presented. Choice of a multidimensional instrument carries the same caveats mentioned for instruments assessing physical function.[63] No instrument assesses all potentially relevant items. Table 11–8 presents a comparison of items covered. In the physical function area, questions on the ability to ambulate are the only items these instruments have in common. Aspects of physical function not covered in any of these instruments include bed mobility and dexterity. The FIM and the OASIS include more BADL items than either the SIP or the SF-36. The SIP and the SF-36 investigate work performance, whereas the FIM and the OASIS do not. This is not surprising, given that the FIM was originally developed as a tool for the in-patient rehabilitation setting and the OASIS was expressly designed for home health agencies, both

Table 11–8 ITEMS COVERED IN SELECTED MULTIDIMENSIONAL FUNCTIONAL ASSESSMENT INSTRUMENTS

	FIM	SIP	SF-36	OASIS
Symptoms	−	+	+	+
Physical function				
Transfers	+	−	−	+
Ambulation	+	+	+	+
ADL				
Bathing	+	+	+	+
Grooming	+	−	−	+
Dressing	+	−	+	+
Feeding	+	−	−	+
Toileting	+	−	−	+
IADL				
Indoor home chores	−	+	+	+
Outdoor home chores/shopping	−	+	+	+
Community travel/drive car	−	+	+	+
Work/school	−	+	+	−
Affective function				
Communication	+	+	−	+
Cognition	+	+	−	+
Anxiety	−	+	+	+
Depression	−	+	+	+
Social function				
Interaction	+	+	+	−
Activity/leisure	−	+	+	−
General health perceptions	−	−	+	−

generally serving older patients. In contrast, the development of the SIP and SF-36 was focused on younger adult populations in ambulatory care.

Anxiety and depression are addressed as areas of psychological function in the SIP, the SF-36, and the OASIS, but not in the FIM. The OASIS does not explore social function, while the other three instruments do. Finally, only the SF-36 records general health perceptions.

SUMMARY

This chapter has presented a conceptual framework for understanding health status and functional assessment. The traditional medical model with its narrow focus on disease and its symptoms fails to consider the broader social, psychological, and behavioral dimensions of illness. All these factors have an impact on an individual's function. Functional assessment, therefore, must be viewed as a broad, multidimensional process. Three main categories of function have been delineated—physical, psychological, and social. Instrumentation has been presented that addresses the physical dimension of function, the area of examination that physical therapists are traditionally most involved with, as well as other dimensions. Finally, specific aspects of functional assessment have been discussed, including purpose, selection of instruments, aspects of test administration, interpretation of test results, and assessment of instrument quality.

QUESTIONS FOR REVIEW

1. How do functional status and functional assessment relate to health status?

2. Your rehabilitation facility uses the FIM. How can reliability be ensured so that the results can be used with confidence in both treatment planning and research?

3. What criteria can be used in the selection of a functional instrument?

4. Discuss the uses, advantages, and disadvantages of performance-based assessments, interviewer assessments, and self-administered assessments.

5. Explain how environment, fatigue, and other related issues affect a functional assessment. Suggest ways to control these factors in the clinic.

6. Identify the major types of scoring systems used in functional assessments. What are some common errors in interpretation of testing results?

7. Review Tables 11–2 through 11–8. Hypothesize a caseload in a particular setting and indicate how and when you could use each of these instruments with the proposed population. Describe the advantages and disadvantages of each. Imagine that you are looking to follow the progress of these same patients to another setting. Which instruments would you choose?

8. Using one of the instruments, develop a set of results and use them to identify treatment goals and outcomes and to formulate a plan for intervention.

9. For each of the following, identify particular physical tasks relevant to that individual's functional status.

    a. a 22 year-old female file clerk

    b. a 31 year-old male physical therapist assistant

    c. a 39 year-old female homemaker with children

    d. a 45 year-old male construction worker

    e. a 56 year-old female school teacher

    f. a 65 year-old male journalist

10. Discuss the relationship among disease, impairment, functional limitations, and disability.

CASE STUDY

A 78 year-old woman with a diagnosis of osteoarthritis was admitted for a right total hip replacement. The patient reported a long-standing history of discomfort. She described the hip pain as radiating posteriorly to the buttock and low back and exacerbated by weight-bearing and stair climbing. Over the past 12 months she has experienced a very marked increase in pain and stiffness. Radiographic findings demonstrated degenerative changes of both the acetabulum and femoral head consistent with osteoarthritis. The surgical intervention replaced the right femoral head and neck with a metallic prosthesis and the acetabulum was resurfaced with a plastic cup. Past medical history is unremarkable.

Social History: The patient is a retired manager of a small accounting firm that she and her husband established. Her husband is deceased. She has three grown children who all live in neighboring communities. Prior to the functional limitations imposed by the hip pain, the patient had been independent in all ADL and IADL. She also volunteered her accounting services 1 day per week to a local charity that provides meals to homebound individuals. She was a regular participant in family outings, enjoyed going to the theater, concerts, and special museum events, and was an active member of the community historical preservation society. Recently, these activities had to be curtailed owing to the increased hip discomfort. She essentially had no activities outside the home for 3 months prior to admission and used a walker to minimize weight bearing and reduce pain. She also required the assistance of a home care aide 4 hours a day two times per week (primarily for shopping, errands, and some household management tasks). She expressed considerable distress at being unable to take a bath and having to rely on the assistance of another person for some basic care activities. She had been using aspirin for its analgesic and anti-inflammatory effects. However, the pain experienced in recent months was not alleviated by the aspirin and other conservative measures. She has been instructed to use local applications of heat, periodic rest intervals, and gentle range of motion exercises. The patient has extensive medical insurance coverage and is without financial concerns.

Post-surgical Right Hip Precautions

No hip flexion beyond 90 degrees.

Avoid crossing one leg or ankle over the other.

Avoid internal rotation of right lower extremity.

Review of Systems

Communication, Affect, Cognition, Learning Style: Fully communicative and oriented × 3. Cooperative and motivated. Hearing intact. Wears corrective lens; experiences "night blindness," which she describes as seeing poorly in dim light and her eyes take several seconds longer than normal to adjust from brightness to dimness.

Cardiopulmonary: HR = 84; BP = 130/78; RR = 16; No appreciable increases with activity.

Integumentary: Surgical wound healing well; staples removed.

Musculoskeletal: Upper extremity gross ROM is WNL. Gross strength generally good to normal, except hands. Heberden's nodes noted at the DIP and PIP joints of the left index finger. Left hip, knee, and ankle at least good on break test. Partial weight-bearing on right lower extremity.

Functional Status: Impaired bed mobility (modified independence device), sit-to-stand, transfers (min assist).

Tests and Measures:

Joint Integrity and Mobility: Patient reports some sporadic episodes of wrist and finger stiffness upon awakening in the morning and after periods of immobility. Crepitus noted in right knee.

Range of Motion: Right knee and ankle within functional limits; right hip not tested).

Muscle Performance: Grip strength is reduced bilaterally (G-).

Pain: Patient denies pain in wrist or fingers, or right hip.

Gait, Locomotion and Balance: The patient is ambulating on level surfaces with supervision using bilateral standard aluminum axillary crutches with partial weight bearing on the right lower extremity. Stair climbing also requires minimal assistance. It is anticipated the patient will be independent with ambulation on level surfaces at time of discharge from the hospital.

Patient Goals: The patient is extremely motivated to once again be an independent manager of her personal care and household management needs. The prosthetic replacement has successfully relieved much of the pain experienced in the hip prior to surgery (most of her current discomfort is described as minor and associated with the surgical incision). She would also like to return to her family, volunteer, social, and leisure activities. She is very determined to discontinue the home care assistance as soon as possible.

Home Environment: The patient lives alone in a fifth-floor apartment in a building with an elevator. The living space is a one-bedroom apartment on a single level.

Guiding Questions

1. Based on the findings of the initial examination, discuss the links between the patient's impairments, functional limitations, and disability as presented in the Nagi model of the process of disablement.

2. Identify the specific ADL and IADL skills that would need to be assessed to return this patient to the highest level of function and achieve the patient's goals for rehabilitation. Discuss the appropriateness of the instruments presented in this chapter for assessing her function and documenting the outcomes of patient management.

REFERENCES

1. The Guide to Physical Therapist Practice. Phys Ther 77:1163, 1997.
2. Pope, AM, and Tarlov, AR (eds): Disability in America: Toward a National Agenda for Prevention. National Academy Press, Washington DC, 1991.
3. Duckworth, D: The need for a standard terminology and

classification of disablement. In Granger, C, and Gresham, G (eds): Functional Assessment in Rehabilitation Medicine. Williams & Wilkins, Baltimore, 1984, p 1.

4. World Health Organization (WHO): The First Ten Years of the World Health Organization. World Health Organization, Geneva, 1958.

5. Jette, A: Concepts of health and methodological issues in functional assessment. In Granger, C, and Gresham G (eds): Functional Assessment in Rehabilitation Medicine. Williams & Wilkins, Baltimore, 1984, p 46.

6. World Health Organization (WHO): International Classification of Impairments, Disabilities, and Handicaps. World Health Organization, Geneva, 1980.

7. Guccione, AA: Physical therapy diagnosis and the relationship between impairments and function. Phys Ther 71:499, 1991.

8. Nagi, S: Disability concepts revisited. In Pope, AM, and Tarlov, AR (eds): Disability in America: Toward a National Agenda for Prevention. National Academy Press, Washington DC, 1991, p 309.

9. Nagi, S: Disability and Rehabilitation. Ohio State Univ. Pr., Columbus, 1969.

10. Nagi, S: Some conceptual issues in disability and rehabilitation. In Sussman, M: Sociology and Rehabilitation, Ohio State Univ. Pr., Columbus, 1965, p 100.

11. Schenkman, M, and Butler, RB: A model for multisystem evaluation, interpretation, and treatment of individuals with neurologic dysfunction. Phys Ther 69:538, 1989.

12. Schenkman, M, and Butler, RB: A model for multisystem evaluation and treatment of individual's with Parkinson's disease. Phys Ther 69:932, 1989.

13. Granger, C: A conceptual model for functional assessment. In Granger, C, and Gresham, G (eds): Functional Assessment in Rehabilitation Medicine. Williams & Wilkins, Baltimore, 1984, p 14.

14. ICIDH-2: International Classification of Impairments, Activities and Participation. A Manual of Dimensions of Disablement and Functioning. Beta-1 draft for field trials. World Health Organization, Geneva, 1997.

15. Cahalin, LP, et al: The six-minute walk test predicts peak oxygen uptake and survival in patients with advanced heart failure. Chest 110:325, 1996.

16. Winograd, CH, et al: Development of a physical performance and mobility examination. J Am Geriatr Soc 42:743, 1994.

17. Duncan, PW, et al: Functional reach: A new clinical measure of balance. J Gerontol 45:192, 1990.

18. Duncan, PW, et al: Functional reach: Predictive validity in a sample of elderly male veterans. J Gerontol 47:93, 1992.

19. Mathias, S, et al: Balance in elderly patients: The "Get Up and Go" test. Arch Phys Med Rehabil 67:387, 1986.

20. Podsiadlo, D, and Richardson, S: The timed "Up and Go": A test of basic functional mobility for frail elderly persons. J Am Geriatr Soc 39:142, 1991.

21. Guralnik, JM, et al: A short physical performance battery assessing lower extremity function: Association with self-reported disability and prediction of mortality and nursing home admission. J Gerontol 49:85, 1994.

22. Tager, IB, et al: Reliability of physical performance and self-reported functional measures in an older population. J Gerontol 53:295, 1998.

23. Mahoney, F, and Barthel, D: Functional evaluation: The Barthel Index. Md Med J 14:61, 1965.

24. Guccione, AA, et al: Defining arthritis and measuring functional status in elders: Methodological issues in the study of disease and disability. Am J Public Health 80:949, 1990.

25. Rothstein, JM: Measurement and clinical practice: Theory and application. In Rothstein, JM (ed): Measurement in Physical Therapy. New York, Churchill Livingstone, 1985, p 1.

26. Standards for Tests and Measurements in Physical Therapy Practice. Phys Ther 71:589, 1991.

27. Granger, CV, et al: The Stroke Rehabilitation Outcome Study—Part I: General Description. Arch Phys Med Rehabil 69:506, 1988.

28. Granger, CV, et al: The Stroke Rehabilitation Outcome Study: Part II. Relative merits of the total Barthel Index score and a four-item subscore in predicting patient outcomes. Arch Phys Med Rehabil 70:100, 1989.

29. Granger, C, et al: Outcome of Comprehensive Medical Rehabilitation: Measurement by Pulses Profile and the Barthel Index. Arch Phys Med Rehabil 60:145, 1979.

30. Katz, S, et al: Studies of illness in the aged. The Index of ADL: A standardized measure of biological and psychosocial function. JAMA 185:914, 1963.

31. Katz, S, et al: Progress in the development of the Index of ADL. Gerontologist 10:20, 1970.

32. Liang, M, and Jette, A: Measuring functional ability in chronic arthritis. Arthritis Rheum 24:80, 1981.

33. Branch, L, et al: A prospective study of functional status among community elders. Am J Public Health 74:266, 1984.

34. Guccione, AA, and Jette, AM: Assessing limitations in physical function in patients with arthritis. Arthritis Care Research 1:170, 1988.

35. Granger, CV, et al: Advances in functional assessment for medical rehabilitation. Topics in Geriatric Rehabilitation 1:59, 1986.

36. Granger, CV, et al: Functional assessment scales: A study of persons with multiple sclerosis. Arch Phys Med Rehabil 71:870, 1990.

37. Guide for the Uniform Data Set for Medical Rehabilitation (Adult FIM), Version 4.0. Buffalo, Uniform Data System for Medical Rehabilitation, UB Foundation Activities, Inc., 1993.

38. Gilson, B, et al: The Sickness Impact Profile: Development of an outcome measure of health care. Am J Public Health 65:1304, 1975.

39. Bergner, M, et al: The Sickness Impact Profile: Validation of a health status measure. Med Care 14:57, 1976.

40. Pollard, W, et al: The Sickness Profile: Reliability of a health status measure. Med Care 14:146, 1976.

41. Carter, W, et al: Validation of an interval scaling: The Sickness Impact Profile. Health Serv Res 11:516, 1976.

42. Bergner, M, et al: The Sickness Impact Profile: Development and final revision of a health status measure. Med Care 19:787, 1981.

43. Deyo, R, et al: Measuring functional outcomes in a chronic disease: A comparison of traditional scales and a self-administered health status questionnaire in patients with rheumatoid arthritis. Med Care 21:180, 1983.

44. Deyo, R, et al: Physical and psychosocial function in rheumatoid arthritis. Clinical use of a self-administered health status instrument. Arch Intern Med 142:870, 1982.

45. Deyo, R, et al: A controlled trial of transcutaneous electrical stimulation (TENS) and exercise for chronic low back pain. New Engl J Med 322:1627, 1990.

46. MacKenzie, C, et al: Can the Sickness Impact Profile measure change: An example of scale assessment. Journal of Chronic Diseases 39:429, 1986.

47. Tarlov, AR, et al: The Medical Outcomes Study: An application of methods for monitoring the results of medical care. JAMA 262:925, 1989.

48. Stewart, AL, et al: Functional status and well-being of patients with chronic conditions: Results from the Medical Outcomes Study. JAMA 262:907, 1989.

49. Wells, KB, et al: The functioning and well-being of depressed patients: Results from the Medical Outcomes Study. JAMA 262:914, 1989.

50. Stewart, AL, et al: The MOS short general health survey: Reliability and validity in a patient population. Med Care 26:724, 1988.

51. Ware, JE, and Sherbourne, CD: The MOS 36-item short form health survey (SF-36): I. Conceptual framework and item selection. Med Care 30:473, 1992.

52. McHorney, CA, et al: The MOS 36-item short form health survey (SF-36): II. Psychometric and clinical tests of validity in measuring physical and mental health constructs. Med Care 31:247, 1993.

53. McHorney, CA, et al: The MOS 36-item short form health survey (SF-36): III. Tests of data quality, scaling assumptions, and reliability across diverse patient groups. Med Care 32:40, 1994.

54. Ware, JE, et al: SF-36 Health Survey: Manual and Intepretation Guide. Boston, The Health Institute, New England Medical Center, 1993.

55. Mossberg, KA, and McFarland, C: Initial health status of patients at outpatient physical therapy clinics. Phys Ther 75:1043, 1995.

56. Jette, DU, and Downing, J: Health status of individuals entering a cardiac rehabilitation program as measured by the Medical Outcomes Study 36-item short form survey (SF-36). Phys Ther 74:521, 1994.

57. Jette, DU, and Downing, J: The relationship of cardiovascular and psychological impairments to the health status of patients enrolled in cardiac rehabilitation programs. Phys Ther 76: 130–139, 1996.

58. Jette, DU, and Jette, AM: Physical therapy and health outcomes in patients with spinal impairments. Phys Ther 76:930, 1996.

59. Jette, DU, and Jette, AM: Physical therapy and health outcomes in patients with knee impairments. Phys Ther 76:1178, 1996.

60. Jette, DU, et al: The disablement process in patients with pulmonary disease. Phys Ther 77:385, 1997.

61. Krisler, KS, et al: OASIS Basics: Beginning to Use the Outcome and Assessment Information Set. Center for Health Services and Policy Research, Denver, 1997.

62. Shaughnessy, PW, and Crisler, KS: Outcome-based Quality Improvement. A Manual for Home Care Agencies on How to Use Outcomes. National Association for Home Care, Washington, DC, 1995.

63. Guccione, AA, and Jette, AM: Multidimensional assessment of functional limitations in patients with arthritis. Arthritis Care Research 3:44, 1990.

SUPPLEMENTAL READINGS

Dittmar, S, and Bresham, G: Functional Assessment and Outcome Measures for the Rehabilitation Health Professional. Aspen Publishers, Inc., Gaithersburg, MD, 1997.

GLOSSARY

Activities of daily living (ADL): Activities necessary for daily self-care, personal maintenance, and independent community living, such as feeding, dressing, hygiene, and physical mobility. Sometimes also referred to as basic activities of daily living (BADL).

Affective function: Mental and emotional skills and coping strategies needed to manage everyday tasks and stresses as well as the more traumatic events each person encounters over the course of a lifetime; includes such factors as self-esteem, body image, anxiety, depression, and the ability to cope with change.

Checklist: Assessment tool format in which a description of various tasks is simply scored with a nominal measure (e.g., present/absent; completed or not completed).

Dependence: Requiring some level of human assistance.

Difficulty: Hybrid term that suggests that an activity poses an extra burden for an individual, regardless of dependence level.

Disability: Inability to perform social roles typical of independent adults relative to age, gender, social and cultural factors.

Disease: Pathological condition of the body that presents a group of characteristic signs and symptoms that sets the condition apart as abnormal.

Functional activities: Activities identified by an individual as essential to support physical and psychological well-being as well as to create a personal sense of meaningful living.

Functional limitation: Deviation from normal in the way an individual performs an activity, usually as the result of impairment.

Functional mobility skills (FMS): Skills required for daily function, such as bed mobility (rolling, turning supine to prone and prone to supine, supine to sit, sit to supine), sitting, standing, transferring, locomotion, and walking.

Gold standard: Accepted, accurate measure of a particular phenomenon that can serve as the normative standard for other measures.

Handicap: Social disadvantage for a given individual of an impairment, functional limitation, or disability.

Health: State of complete physical, mental, and social well-being, and not merely the absence of disease and infirmity.

Illness: Forms of personal behavior that emerge as the reality of having a disease is internalized and experienced by an individual.

Impairments: Any loss or abnormality of anatomical, physiological, or psychological structure or function; the natural consequence of pathology or disease.

Instrumental activities of daily living (IADL): Advanced skills considered vital to an individual's independent living in the community, including managing personal affairs, cooking and shopping, and home chores.

Interviewer assessment: Process in which the assessor interviews or questions a subject and records answers.

Mental function: Intellectual or cognitive abilities of an individual, including initiative, attention, concentration, memory, problem solving, and judgment.

Nominal measures: Classification scheme based on categories without order or rank, the simplest of which are dichotomous response sets such as "present/absent" and "yes/no" but may also have more than two categories, for example, marital status (never married, married, separated, widowed, divorced).

Ordinal (or rank order) measures: Classification scheme that rates observations in terms of the relationship between items (e.g., less than, equal to, or greater than).

Performance-based assessment: Assessment of a

particular skill based on observation of an actual attempt, as compared to acceptance of a self-report of skill level.

Physical function: Sensory-motor skills necessary for the performance of usual daily activities.

Physical signs: Directly observable or measurable changes in an individual's organs or systems as a result of pathology or disease.

Psychological function: Ability to use mental and affective resources effectively relative to the requirements of a particular situation.

Reliability: Degree to which an instrument can consistently measure the same parameter under specific conditions.

Self-administered assessment: Survey or series of questions constructed to be answered directly by the respondent without additional input or direction.

Social function: Ability to interact successfully with others in the performance of social roles and obligations; includes social interactions, roles, and networks.

Subordinate part (subroutine): Element of movement without which the task cannot proceed safely or efficiently.

Summary (or additive) measure: Approach to grading a specific series of skills by awarding points for each task or activity; totals the score as a percentage of 100 or as a fraction.

Symptoms: Subjective reactions to the changes experienced by an individual as a result of pathology or disease.

Validity: The degree to which data or results of a study are correct or true.

Visual (or linear) analog scale: Linear rating designed to capture a subject's judgment of his or her position on a continuum. A line is presented horizontally or vertically on paper, with the end points anchored with descriptive words representing the extremes of the parameter of interest.

APPENDIX A

Suggested Answers to Case Study Guiding Questions

1. Based on the findings of the initial examination, discuss the links between the patient's impairments, functional limitations, and disability as presented in the Nagi model of the process of disablement.

ANSWER: The patient's problems stem from a particular pathological condition that has predictable effects on the musculoskeletal and neuromuscular systems, resulting in characteristic impairments of joint integrity and mobility, range of motion, and muscle performance (strength). Difficulty in all weight-bearing activities, presenting as deficits in gait, locomotion, and balance, is also typical in these patients due to the degenerative changes in the joint itself, as well as the composite effects of impairments of joint integrity and mobility and strength. Although this particular patient does not have evidence of secondary impairments of the cardiopulmonary system, it would not be surprising if long-term curtailment of function led to impaired aerobic capacity and endurance.

This patient exhibits limitations in all basic functional mobility skills including bed mobility, transfers, and walking that are essential to independent performance of most self-care ADL and IADL required to function independently in the community. In addition to the physical functional deficits, this patient exhibits some evidence of social functional limitations that have reduced her social activities and opportunities for social interaction. She appears to be experiencing substantial role disability as a mother to a family as well as a community volunteer.

2. Identify the specific ADL and IADL skills that would need to be assessed to return this patient to the highest level of function and achieve the patient's goals for rehabilitation. Discuss the appropriateness of the instruments presented in this chapter for assessing her function and documenting the outcomes of patient management.

ANSWER: This patient will need to have regained independence in the full array of ADL and IADL required to live alone in the community. Specifically, she will need to be able to get out of bed, walk across her apartment, and engage in all her personal hygiene, grooming, and dressing activities. To maintain her status as an independent adult, she will also need to be able to negotiate stairs, curbs, and ramps as she goes into the community to perform errands and shop. At some point, it would be appropriate to examine her ability to travel through her community either by driving a car or using public transportation.

Although each of the instruments reviewed in this chapter have some relevance to assessing the outcomes of care, none of the instruments capture the full array of activities, tasks, and roles that capture the specific details of this particular individual's independent function in the community. Therefore, if a therapist wished to use a particular instrument to capture the same data on all patients by using a standardized instrument, the data collection on initial examination would also have to gather supplemental information in order to identify the particular problems of this patient, design an individualized plan of care, and identify the anticipated goals and expected outcomes of intervention.

Environmental *12* Assessment

Thomas J. Schmitz

LEARNING OBJECTIVES

1. Understand the importance of environmental accessibility in optimizing patient function.
2. Identify common environmental barriers that impact patient function.
3. Describe the tests and measures used to identify environmental barriers.
4. Identify strategies to improve patient function through environmental modifications.
5. Recognize the importance of an environmental assessment in overall rehabilitation planning.

The **physical environment** in which an individual functions consists of a complex variety of both built and natural objects. Built objects refer to buildings and structures created by humans; natural objects include other humans as well as geographical objects such as vegetation, mountains, rivers, uneven terrain, and so forth.[1] The environment encompasses a substantial range of components that impact human function and includes the individual's home, neighborhood, community, and method(s) of transportation, in addition to the individual's education, workplace, entertainment, commercial, and natural settings.[2]

Environmental barriers are defined as physical impediments that prevent individuals from functioning optimally in their surroundings, and include safety hazards, access problems, and home or workplace design difficulties.[3] **Accessibility** is the degree to which an environment affords use of its resources with respect to an individual's level of function. **Accessible design** typically refers to structures that meet prescribed standards for accessibility. In the United States, these standards are available from the American National Standards Institute (Accessible and Usable Buildings and Facilities, ICC/ANSI A117.1-1998), the Fair Housing Amendments Act of

1988, and the Uniform Federal Accessibility Standards (UFAS). Requirements for public and commercial buildings are regulated by the accessibility guidelines of the Americans with Disabilities Act (ADA). The term **universal design** (also called *life-span* design and *inclusive* design) designates structures and dwellings that meet the requirements of all people including those with a disability. Universal design features provide environmental access to a wide range of individuals of different ages, stature, sizes, and abilities and take into consideration the changing needs of human beings across the life span.

Reflective of the importance of **environmental accessibility,** an internationally recognized symbol identifies buildings accessible to individuals with a disability (Fig. 12-1A). Other international symbols identify the availability of assistive listening devices (Fig. 12-1B) such as telephones with interactive text capabilities (TTY), which allow the user to communicate using a keyboard and visual display (Fig. 12-1C), and volume-controlled telephones (Fig. 12-1D).

A primary outcome of rehabilitation intervention is for the patient to be fully functional in a former environment and life-style. To achieve this outcome, continuity of accessibility must exist within the

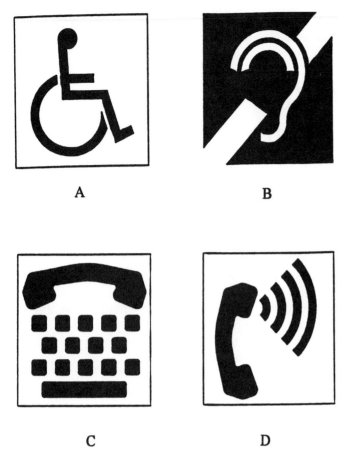

Figure 12-1. (*A*) International Symbol of Accessibility. (*B*) International Symbol of Access for Hearing Loss. (*C*) International TTY Symbol. (*D*) Volume-Controlled Telephone.

individual's environmental context. With full accessibility as a goal, environmental assessments must address the individual needs of each patient. The purposes of an environmental assessment are multiple and serve to:

1. Assess the degree of safety and level of function of the patient in the physical environment.
2. Make realistic recommendations regarding environmental accessibility to the patient, support network (family, friends, caregivers, significant others, co-workers, professional colleagues, neighbors), employer, and/or government agencies, and third party payers.
3. Assess the patient's need for additional **adaptive equipment.**
4. Assist in preparing the patient and support network for the patient's return to a former environment and to help determine whether further services may be required (i.e., outpatient treatment, home health services, etc.).

ASSESSMENT STRATEGIES

Physical therapists can use several specific tests and measures to assess the environment and subsequently suggest potential modifications. These tests

and measures together with the data generated are presented in Box 12–1.

Depending on the nature of the patient's disability, data collection during the environmental assessment may be gathered through one or more of the following strategies: (1) *interview,* (2) *self-assessment and performance-based tests,* (3) *visual depictions and dimensions of physical space,* and (4) *on-site visits.* Depending on patient need, a combination of two or more of these strategies may be warranted to generate all needed data. The current era of cost containment has placed restrictions on time and travel allocations for on-site visits. In such situations, several data collection alternatives (e.g., interview, self-assessment, and performance-based tests, and use of visual depictions and physical dimensions) can be implemented to achieve the goals of the environmental assessment.

Interview

Environmental assessments are typically initiated by interviewing the patient and support network members. If the patient's functional limitations impact only isolated tasks or activities or if accessibility issues involve limited environmental barriers, an interview may be all that is needed to assess the physical impediments and provide suggestions and guidelines for improving performance and resolving access problems. In the presence of more formidable functional limitations, the interview may be the first of several strategies used to collect data about the patient's environment. The interview can be used to establish the general characteristics of the environ-

---

Box 12–1 TESTS AND MEASURES USED AND DATA GENERATED DURING ENVIRONMENTAL ASSESSMENT

Tests and measures may include:
Analysis of physical space using photography or videotape
Assessment of current and potential barriers
Measurement of physical space
Physical inspection of the environment
Questionnaires completed by and interviews conducted with patient and others as appropriate

Data generated may include:
Adaptations, additions, or modifications that would enhance safety
Level of compliance with standards set forth in federal and state laws and regulations
Recommendations for eliminating environmental barriers
Space limitations and other barriers including their dimensions, that limit ability to perform specific movement tasks during home, work, (job/school/play), and leisure activities

From American Physical Therapy Association,[3] p 2–8, with permission.

ment to be assessed (number of levels, stairs, railings, and so forth), identify any special environmental problems previously encountered by the patient, alert the therapist to potential safety hazards, and identify the need for additional assessment and treatment strategies. The interview process also provides the therapist an opportunity to gain knowledge of support network characteristics including: (1) attitude toward the patient, (2) the extent of their desire to have the patient return to his or her environment, (3) their caregiving goals and capabilities,[1] and (4) attitude toward rehabilitation team members, which may influence receptivity to suggested environmental modifications.

Self-assessment and Performance-based Tests

Self-assessments involve asking the patient to provide information about his or her ability to perform certain tasks and activities in various environments. Administration can be either in a paper-and-pencil format or by way of an interview conducted by the therapist. An inherent shortcoming of self-assessment instruments is that an individual may overestimate performance capabilities or underestimate the impact of environmental barriers. Accuracy of reporting can be improved by (1) requesting the patient focus the performance assessment on a recent time interval (e.g., *within* the previous week); and (2) by distinguishing between actual performance of an activity (e.g., *daily* use of shower for bathing) versus perceived ability in the absence of consistent execution of the task.

Performance-based assessments are administered by the therapist who observes patient performance of the activity (examples include the Functional Reach Test,[4] the Get Up and Go test,[5] and the Physical Performance Battery[6]). The assessments address the impact of impairments on function and help predict patient performance within his or her natural environment. The reader is referred to Chapter 11: Functional Assessment for additional information on both self-assessments and performance-based assessments.

Visual Depictions and Dimensions of Physical Space

The therapist may request support network members provide visual depictions (e.g., photographs, videotapes, diagrams) and physical dimensions (obtained with a tape measure) of the environment in which the patient is expected to function. If photography equipment is unavailable, an inexpensive disposable camera works well for this purpose. Suggestions for modifications can be made from the visual depictions and measured dimensions of the patient's environment. Such environmental information will allow the therapist to simulate aspects of the patient's surroundings for practicing tasks while directing attention to maximizing safety and func-

tion. This will also allow the therapist to assess the need for adaptive equipment.

On-site Visit

The on-site visit is the preferable assessment strategy for many patients because it allows observation of performance in the actual environment in which the activities must be accomplished. On-site visits are often useful in reducing patient, support network, and employer apprehension concerning the patient's ability to function within the environment. The on-site visit also provides an excellent opportunity for the therapist to identify safety hazards and make recommendations regarding altering, coping with, or adapting specific environmental barriers.

Whichever assessment strategy or combination of strategies are applied, the scope and breadth of the assessment will be enhanced by involvement of members of the patient's support network. Because it is usually not feasible for the therapist to assess all aspects of the patient's total environment, involvement of other individuals can be instrumental in assuring that the goal of maximum accessibility is met. This is particularly important for assessment of general community access. The therapist can direct and encourage an investigation of access to community recreational, educational, and commercial facilities as well as availability of public transportation. The therapist can also provide guidance in the essential role of exploring funding sources for needed environmental modifications (potential funding sources will be addressed later in this chapter).

OVERVIEW OF INTERVENTION STRATEGIES FOR ENVIRONMENTAL MODIFICATIONS

Data from an environmental assessment are used to evaluate the need for specific interventions. Corcoran and Gitlin[1] identify five major areas of intervention strategies to modify the environment. These include (1) *assistive devices* or *adaptive equipment* such as **grab bars,** reachers, adapted eating utensils (e.g., rocker knife), canes, or walkers; (2) *safety devices* such as lighting, smoke detectors, or sensing devices; (3) *structural alterations*, which include widening doors, installing railings or ramps, or removing a doorway threshold; (4) *modification* or *altered location of environmental objects* such as disabling a stove, placing locks on doors, use of extension levers on door handles, removing throw rugs, or moving furniture; and (5) *task modification* such as use of visual, auditory, or other sensory cuing, and energy conservation techniques.

On-site Assessments

The following two sections offer suggestions for home and workplace assessments. The information presented is neither exhaustive nor inclusive of the needs of every patient. The environmental considerations are intended to direct attention to some of the most common concerns encountered during on-site visits.

HOME ASSESSMENT

Prior to the on-site visit, occupational and physical therapy treatment sessions should be scheduled that will include participation from support group members. These visits serve several functions. They provide an opportunity to become familiar with the patient's capabilities and limitations. They give the support network members time to learn safe methods of assisting with ambulation, transfers, exercise, and functional activities. During these visits the therapist will have an opportunity to provide instruction in the use of assistive devices and adaptive equipment. The time spent in support network education will facilitate the patient's transition from the inpatient facility to the home and community. When realistic, weekend passes for the patient should be encouraged prior to the on-site assessment. During these visits problems not previously anticipated by the therapist or support network may be uncovered. Emphasis can then be placed on solving these problems prior to actual return to the environment.

Preceding the on-site assessment, information should be gathered about several important areas that will influence both the preparation for and the types of suggestions made during the visit. This information should include:

1. Knowledge of the patient's performance needs and goals.[1]
2. Detailed information about present level of function as judged by the patient and all involved disciplines (occupational therapist, physical therapist, speech-language pathologist, etc.).
3. Characteristics and dimensions of assistive devices or adaptive equipment.
4. Knowledge of the projected prognosis for the patient's disability (e.g., whether the disability is static or progressive, and what long-term functional capabilities are expected).
5. Information about the patient's insurance coverage and financial resources (in terms of capacity to modify environment).
6. Knowledge of the patient's future plans (household management, family care, employment outside the home, school, vocational training, and so forth).

This information can be gathered from interviews with the patient, conferences with members of the patient's support network, medical records, social service interviews, and specific assessment procedures (e.g., functional assessments). Once this information is gathered, decisions can be made concerning the assistive devices or adaptive equipment required for the on-site visit and the appropriate team members to accompany the patient on the visit.

Ideally, the physical and occupational therapist accompany the patient on the home visit. They assume shared responsibility for assessing the physical structure and the patient's functional level at home. Depending on the specific needs of the patient and/or support network members, a speech-language pathologist, social worker, or nurse also may be included on the home visit. The visit should be broken into two components. The first portion should deal with accessibility of the dwelling's *exterior*, and the second half should be concerned with an assessment of the home's *interior*. A tape measure and home assessment form are valuable tools during the visit. Many rehabilitation departments develop their own home assessment forms to meet the particular needs of their patient population. The forms help to organize the visit and are useful in directing attention to all necessary details. A variety of home assessment forms and checklists are available. A sample is provided in Appendix A. This form can be expanded or modified, depending on the specific needs of the individual or patient population. Some caution must be used in interpreting data from home assessment forms because they generally lack reliability and standardization.

Upon arrival at the home for the on-site visit, the patient may need to rest for a short while before beginning the assessment. This is an important consideration, because many patients become very excited or emotional when returning home after a lengthy absence. This may be true even if previous passes were issued for weekend home visits.

One method of accomplishing the interior assessment is to begin with the patient in bed as though it were morning. Simulation of all daily activities, including dressing, grooming, bathroom activities, and preparation of meals can ensue. The patient should attempt to perform all transfer, exercise, ambulation, self-care, and homemaking activities as independently as possible to facilitate the assessment. This will provide an additional opportunity to teach the support network members how and when to assist the patient.

EXTERIOR ACCESSIBILITY: GENERAL CONSIDERATIONS

1. It is important to note whether the house or apartment is owned or rented. The type and ownership of the home may preclude any modifications the patient may require.
2. The relative permanence of the dwelling should be considered. If the patient plans to move in the near future, it will influence the type of modifications recommended (e.g., installing permanent ramps versus removable ones, or paving a gravel driveway).

EXTERIOR ACCESSIBILITY: SPECIFIC CONSIDERATIONS

Route of Entry

1. If there is more than one entry to the dwelling, the most accessible should be selected (closest

to driveway, most level walking surface, fewest stairs, available handrails, etc.).

2. Ideally, the driveway should be a smooth, level surface with easy access to the home. Walking surfaces to the entrance should be carefully assessed. Cracked and uneven surfaces should be repaired or an alternate route selected.

3. The entrance should be well lighted and provide adequate cover from adverse weather conditions.

4. The height, number, and condition of stairs should be noted. Ideally, steps should not be greater than 7 inches (180 mm) high with a minimum depth of 11 inches (280 mm).[7] **Nosings,** also referred to as "lips," are the ½ inch (13 mm) curved overhangs on the front edge of stairs. These overhangs are often problematic because they can cause a patient's toe to "catch" and prevent smooth transition to the next step. Nosings should be removed or reduced, if possible. Nosing can be minimized by installing small wood bevels under the overhangs that taper down toward the lower step and provide a smoother contour (Fig. 12-2A). The steps also should have a nonslip surface to improve traction. This can be accomplished by adding abrasive strips to improve traction (Fig. 12-2B).

5. Handrails should be installed, if needed. In general, the handrails should measure between a minimum of 34 inches (865 mm) and a maximum of 38 inches (965 mm) high. This range in handrail height allows for modifications to accommodate needs of particularly tall or short individuals. At least one handrail should extend a minimum of 12 inches (305 mm) beyond the foot and top of the stairs. Outside cross-sectional diameter of circular handrails should be between a minimum of 1.25 inches (32 mm) and a maximum of 2 inches (51 mm). If mounted adjacent to a wall, clearance between the handrail and wall should be a minimum of 1.50 inches (38 mm).[7]

6. If a ramp is to be installed, there should be adequate space. Large ramps are typically constructed of wood or concrete; smaller ramps can be made from aluminum or fiberglass. The minimum **grade** (incline or slope) for wheelchair ramps is that for every inch of threshold height there is a corresponding 12 inches of ramp length (a running slope of 1:12).[7] Outdoor ramps exposed to inclement weather such as snow or ice formation require a more gradual running slope of approximately 1:20. Ramps should be a minimum of 36 inches (915 mm) wide, with a nonslip surface. The overall rise of any ramp should be no greater than 30 inches (760 mm). Handrails also should be included on the ramp with a minimum height of 34 inches (865 mm) and a maximum height of 38 inches (965 mm) and extend 12 inches (305 mm) beyond the top and

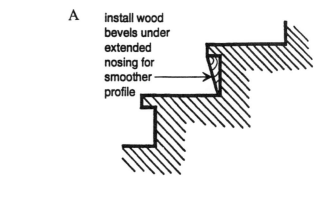

A install wood bevels under extended nosing for smoother profile

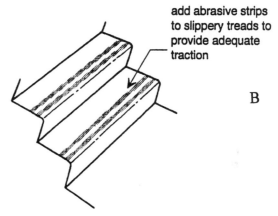

add abrasive strips to slippery treads to provide adequate traction

B

Figure 12-2. (A) Wood bevels under nosings minimize the danger of "toe-catching" during transition to the next higher step. (B) Abrasive strips improve traction. (From U.S. Department of Housing and Urban Development [HUD], Office of Policy Development and Research [PD&R]: Residential Remodeling and Universal Design: Making Homes More Comfortable and Accessible, 1996, p 79, with permission.)

bottom of the ramp (Fig. 12-3).[7] Small commercially available ramps can be used for traversing curbs and small step heights.

7. *Vertical platform lifts* and *stairway inclined lifts* are commercially available and may be a consideration when inadequate space is available for a ramp. Vertical platform lifts travel approximately 8 feet straight up and down. Both open and enclosed models are available. Platform lifts are often installed adjacent to stairs with an upper landing. The lift (approximately 30 × 40 inches) brings the patient from the ground level to the landing level to access the entrance to the home (these lifts can be used indoors as well). Stairway inclined lifts are installed directly onto existing stairways and are typically used indoors. The stairway lifts are mounted on runners that traverse the length of the stairs and slightly beyond. Many models allow the platform to fold up against an adjacent wall to allow free stair access for other members of the home. Residential elevators are another more costly option; they require construction of an enclosed shaft.

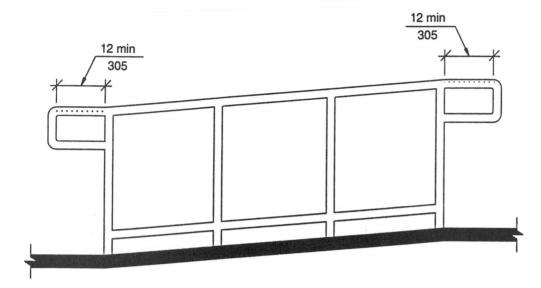

Figure 12-3. Handrail extensions run a minimum of 12 inches (305 mm) beyond the top and bottom edge of ramp. (From American National Standards Institute, Inc.,[7] p 37, with permission.)

ENTRANCE

1. For individuals using a wheelchair, the entrance should have a platform large enough to allow the patient to rest and to prepare for entry. This platform area is particularly important when a ramp is in use. It provides for safe transit from the inclined surface to the level surface. If an individual using a wheelchair is required to open a door that swings out, this area should be at least 5 × 5 feet (153 × 153 cm). If the door swings away from the patient, a space at least 3 feet (91.5 cm) deep and 5 feet (153 cm) wide is required.
2. The door locks should be accessible to the patient. The height of the locks should be assessed as well as the amount of force required to turn the key. Alternative lock systems (e.g., voice- or card-activated, remote control locks, keypad electronic security systems, and push-button padlocks) may be an important consideration for some patients.
3. The door handle should be turned easily by the patient. Rubber doorknob covers (which stretch over doorknob and provide a textured grip) or lever-type handles (Fig. 12-4) are often easier to use for patients with limited grip strength (screw fastened, slip-on lever-type handles are also available).
4. The door should open and close in a direction that is functional for the patient. A cane may be hung outside the door to help an individual using a wheelchair to close the door when leaving.
5. If there is a raised **threshold** in the doorway, it should be removed. If removal is not possible, the threshold should be lowered to no greater than ½ inch (13 mm) in height, with **beveled** edges.[7] If needed, weatherstripping the door will help prevent drafts.
6. The doorway width should be measured. Generally, 32 to 34 inches (815 to 865 mm) is an acceptable doorway width to accommodate most wheelchairs.
7. If the door is weighted to aid in closing, the pressure should not exceed 8 pounds to be functional for the patient.
8. **Kick plates** may be added to doors frequently entered by individuals using a wheelchair or ambulatory assistive devices. The kick plate should measure 12 inches (305 mm) in height from the bottom of the door.

INTERIOR ACCESSIBILITY: GENERAL CONSIDERATIONS

Furniture Arrangement

1. Sufficient room should be made available for maneuvering a wheelchair or ambulating with an assistive device.

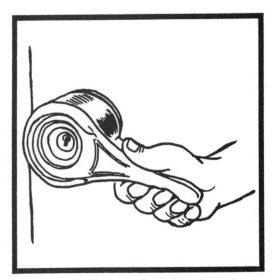

Figure 12-4. Door knob lever. Screw-fastened, slip-on models are also available. (From Krantz, GC, et al: Assistive Products: An Illustrated Guide to Terminology. The American Occupational Therapy Association, Inc., Bethesda, MD, 1998, p 25, with permission.)

2. Clear passage must be allowed from one room to the next.
3. Unrestricted access should be provided to telephones, wall switches, and electrical outlets. Power strip receptacles can be used to increase the number of outlets as well as improve access. Outlets may need to be raised and wall switches lowered. For individuals using a wheelchair, use of pull cord extensions may allow control of some high electrical switches.

Floors

1. All floor coverings should be glued or tacked to the floor. This will prevent bunching or rippling under wheelchair use. When carpeting is used, a dense, low pile generally provides for easiest movement of a wheelchair or ambulatory assistive device.
2. Scatter rugs should be removed.
3. Use of nonskid waxes should be encouraged.

Doors

1. Raised thresholds should be removed to provide a flush, level surface.
2. Doorways may need to be widened (if less than 32 inches [815 mm] wide) to allow clearance for a wheelchair or assistive device. In instances in which this is not possible, wheelchair users may benefit from a narrowing device attached directly to the chair. This allows the width of the chair to be temporarily reduced by turning a crank handle.
3. Doors may have to be removed, reversed (e.g., to open outward for easier exit, especially in the case of an emergency), or replaced with folding doors, or a door of lighter weight. Several other options are available to increase door clearance. These options include (a) installation of pocket doors, which slide into the adjacent wall when not in use; (b) use of offset hinges, which swing the open door clear of the frame and provide approximately 2 additional inches (51 mm) of clearance; and (c) removal of the door with installation of a curtain (inexpensive spring-loaded curtain rods and a fabric or plastic shower curtain can be used).
4. As mentioned in regard to exterior doors, handles inside the home should also be assessed. Rubber doorknob covers or lever-type handles may be important considerations. **Knurled surface** (roughened) door handles are used on interiors of buildings and dwellings when frequented by persons with visual impairments. These abrasive, knurled surfaces indicate that the door leads to a hazardous area and alerts the individual to danger.

Stairs

1. All indoor stairwells should have handrails and should be well lighted. Battery-operated wall lamps are a practical supplement to electrical light sources. Inexpensive track lighting provides multiple adjustable lamps and requires only a single electrical source. Lighting should be bright with glare and reflection minimized. Motion detection lights that automatically turn on when the patient approaches the stairs (or other area of the home) can also be an important safety consideration.
2. For patients with decreased visual acuity or age-related visual changes, tactile warnings provided by contrasting textures on the surface of the top and bottom stair(s) will alert them that the end of the stairwell is near (they can also be used on each step to identify its edge). Circular bands of tape also can be placed at the top and bottom of the handrail for the same purpose. Tactile warning strips placed on the floor can also be used to signal a change in level of the walking surface or entrance to another area or room of the dwelling.
3. Many patients with visual impairment will benefit also from bright, contrasting color tape on the border of each stair. Warm colors (reds, oranges, and yellows) are generally easier to see than cool colors (blues, greens, and violets).

Heating Units

1. All radiators, heating vents, and hot water pipes should be appropriately screened off or insulated with pipe covers to prevent burns, especially for patients who have sensory impairments.
2. Adaptations may be required to allow patient access to heat controls (e.g., use of reachers or enlarged, extended, or adapted handles on heat control valves).

INTERIOR ACCESSIBILITY: SPECIFIC CONSIDERATIONS

Bedroom Area

1. The bed should be stationary and positioned to provide ample space for transfers. Stability may be improved by placing the bed against a wall or in the corner of the room (except when the patient plans to make the bed). Additional stability may be achieved by placing rubber suction cups under each leg.
2. The height of the sleeping surface must be considered to facilitate transfer activities. The height of the bed may be raised by use of wooden blocks with routed depressions to hold each leg. The use of another mattress or box springs also will provide additional height to the bed. Blocks may be used to raise the height of chairs, as well.
3. The mattress should be carefully assessed. It should provide a firm, comfortable surface. If the mattress is in relatively good condition, a bed board inserted between the mattress and box springs may suffice to improve the sleeping surface adequately. If the mattress is badly worn, a new one should be suggested.

4. A bedside table or cabinet should be available; it can be used to hold a lamp, telephone (preferably cordless with a memory dial for frequently used numbers or emergency phone numbers), necessary medications, and call bell if assistance is needed from a caregiver.

5. The closet clothes bar may require lowering to provide wheelchair accessibility. The bar should be lowered to 52 inches (132 cm) from the floor. Wall hooks also may be a useful addition to the closet area and should be placed between 40 inches (101.6 cm) and 56 inches (142.2 cm) from the floor. Shelves also can be installed at various levels in the closet (Fig. 12-5). The highest shelf should not exceed 45 inches (115.5 cm). Clothing and grooming articles frequently used by the patient should be placed in the most easily accessible bureau drawer. Free-standing modular storage units are also commercially available in a variety of dimensions. These units typically provide clothes bar, shelves, and drawers that can be adjusted to meet the needs of the user.

6. A portable commode, urinal, or bedpan also may be an appropriate consideration.

Figure 12-6 illustrates the basic components and dimensions of a wheelchair-accessible bedroom.

Bathroom Area

1. If the doorframe prohibits passage of a wheelchair, the patient may transfer at the door to a chair with **casters** attached. As mentioned under general considerations for door modifications, several other solutions are available to address the problem of narrow door frames, including a wheelchair adaptor that allows the

width of the chair to be narrowed, pocket doors, offset hinges, and removal of doors (with a curtain hung in door frame).

2. An elevated toilet seat will facilitate transfer activities.

3. Grab bars (securely fastened to a reinforced wall) will assist in both toilet and tub transfers. Grab bars should have a circular cross section diameter of 1.25 inches (32 mm) minimum and 2 inches (51 mm) maximum and be knurled. For use in toilet transfers, the bars should be mounted horizontally 33 to 36 inches (840 to 915 mm) from the floor. The length of the grab bars should be between 42 and 54 inches (1065 and 1370 mm) on the side wall and between 24 and 36 inches (610 and 915 mm) on the back wall (Fig. 12-7). Ideally, two grab bars are secured horizontally to the back wall for use in tub transfers. One is placed 33 to 36 inches (840 to 915 mm) from the floor of the tub and the second 9 inches (230 mm) above the rim of the bathtub. Grab bars may also be mounted horizontally at the foot-end wall of the bathtub (recommended length is 24 inches [610 mm] with placement at the front edge of the bathtub) and at the head-end wall of the bathtub (recommended length is 12 inches [305 mm] with placement at the front edge of the bathtub).

4. A tub transfer bench (tub seat) may be recommended for bathing. Many types of commercially produced benches are available. In selecting a tub transfer bench (tub seat), function and safety are primary considerations. The bench should provide a wide base of support (some are designed with suction feet; and some provide height adjustment), a back rest, and an appropriate seating surface to facilitate transfers in and out of the tub (Fig. 12-8A and B). Tub transfer benches with relatively long seating surfaces are typically positioned with two legs in the tub and two legs on the floor adjacent to the tub. Smaller benches are available that require all four legs be placed inside the bathtub.

5. A bathmat or nonskid adhesive strips may be placed on the floor of the tub (these are easily attainable at most hardware stores).

6. Additional bathroom considerations may include a handspray attachment to the bathtub faucet (Fig. 12-9), anti-scald valves to prevent water temperature from rising above a preset limit (also referred to as *high temperature stops*), enlarged faucet handles on the tub or sink (single-lever system faucets are optimal owing to their ease of use), and a towel rack and small shelf, which places toilet articles within easy reach of the patient.

7. An enlarged mirror over the sink also may be useful. A wall mirror with an adjustment hinge to tilt the top away from the wall facilitates use from a sitting position. Hinged-wall, goose-

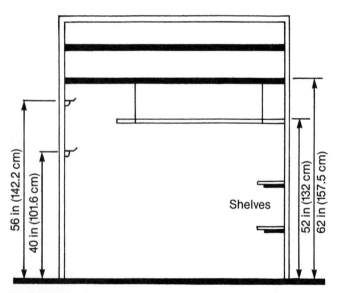

Figure 12-5. Closet modifications to provide accessibility for an individual using a wheelchair. Values denoted in inches and centimeters. (From Cotler, SR, and DeGraff, AH: Architectural Accessibility for the Disabled of College Campuses. New York State University Construction Fund, Albany, 1976, p 57, with permission.)

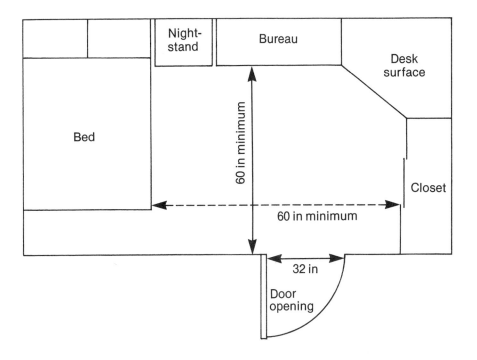

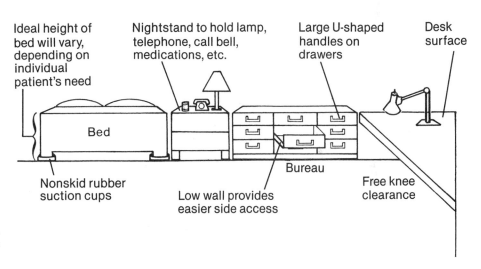

Figure 12-6. Sample dimensions and features of a bedroom area providing access to an individual using a wheelchair.

neck, or accordion fold-up mirrors (with one side magnified) are also helpful for close work.

8. Any exposed hot water pipes under the sink should be insulated to avoid burns.

Figure 12-10 illustrates the basic components and minimum space requirements of a wheelchair accessible bathroom.

Kitchen

1. The height of countertops (work space) should be appropriate for the individual using a wheelchair; the armrests should be able to fit under the working surface. The ideal height of counter surfaces should be no greater than 31 inches (794 mm) from the floor with a knee clearance of 27.5 to 30 inches (705 to 769 mm). Counter space should provide a depth of at least 24 inches (615 mm). All

surfaces should be smooth to facilitate sliding of heavy items from one area to another. Slide-out counter spaces are useful in providing an over-the-lap working surface. For patients who are ambulatory, stools (preferably with back and footrests) may be placed strategically at the main work area(s).

2. A small cart with casters may be suggested to improve ease of movement of articles from refrigerator to counter and other such activities.

3. The height of tables also should be checked and the tables may have to be raised or lowered.

4. Equipment and food storage areas should be selected with optimum energy conservation in mind. All frequently used articles should be within easy reach, and unnecessary items

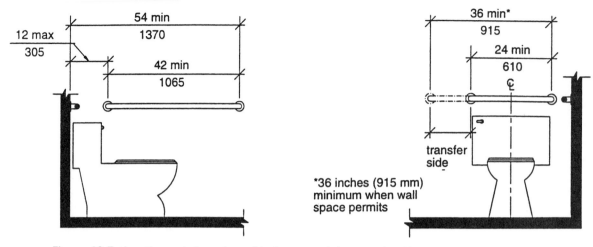

Figure 12-7. Location and dimensions of bathroom grab bars on the side wall (*A*) and rear wall (*B*). Values denoted in inches and millimeters. The bars should be mounted horizontally 33 inches (840 mm) to 36 inches (915 mm) from the floor. (From American National Standards Institute, Inc.,[7] p 41, with permission.)

should be eliminated. Additional storage space may be achieved by installation of open shelving or use of pegboards for pots and pans. If shelving is added, adjustable shelves are preferable and should be placed 16 inches (410 mm)[8] above the countertop. Electronically powered storage cabinets are also available which automatically lower for countertop access.

5. Electric stoves are generally preferable to open-flame gas burners. Controls may require adaptation and should be located on the front or side border of the stove (to eliminate the need for reaching across the burners). Burners that are placed beside each other provide a safer arrangement than those placed one behind the other. A burn-proof counter surface adjacent to the burners will facilitate movement of hot items once cooking is completed. Smooth, ceramic cooktop surfaces also reduce the amount of lifting required while cooking. If cooktops provide knee clearance beneath, exposed or potential contact surfaces must be insulated. Electromagnetic stoves are also available that heat food without flames or heating elements.[9]

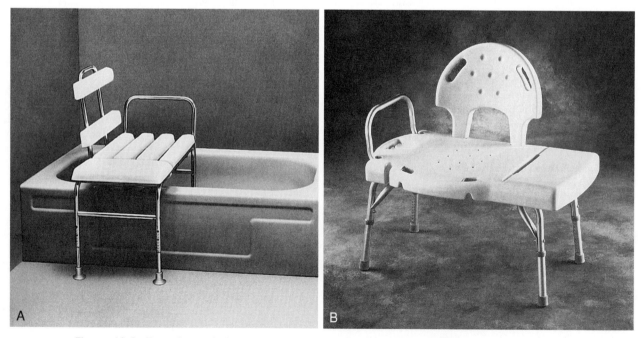

Figure 12-8. Two tub transfer bench designs each providing a wide base of support, a secure back rest, and a long seating surface to facilitate transfers. (Courtesy of Lumex, Bay Shore, NY.)

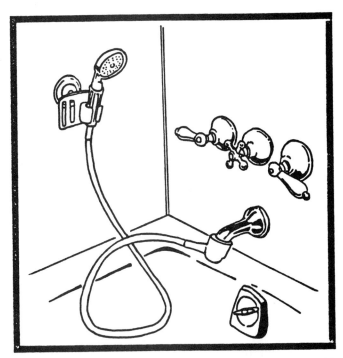

Figure 12-9. Handspray attachment to the bathtub faucet with shower hose and head. (From Krantz, GC, et al: Assistive Products: An Illustrated Guide to Terminology. The American Occupational Therapy Association, Inc., Bethesda, MD, 1998, p 72, with permission.)

6. For patients with visual impairments, large-print label-making devices and large-print stencil overlays can be used to enlarge appliance control indicators and dials (e.g., on/off or temperature indicators on thermostats, microwaves, stoves, and ovens). Timers, wall clocks, and telephones with large-print numbers are also available.[9]

7. A split-level cooking unit is generally more easily accessible than a single, low-level combined oven and burner unit. Oven units should be self-cleaning.

8. A countertop microwave oven also may be an important consideration for some patients.

9. Improved function and safety may be provided by a sink equipped with large blade-type handles, a spray-hose fixture, anti-scald valves, or electronic sensors that automatically turn water off and on. Shallow sinks 5 to 6 inches (128 to 153 mm)[8] deep will improve knee clearance below. Providing sink access to an individual using a wheelchair may require removal of under-sink cabinets. As in the bathroom, hot water pipes under the kitchen sink should be insulated to prevent burns. Motorized adjustable sinks are also commercially available. These adjustable sinks are designed to be mounted against a wall between two stationary cabinets with free space beneath. By activating the control switch, the sink height can be adjusted for the individual user whether seated in a wheelchair or standing.

10. Dishwashers should be front loading, with pull-out shelves and front-mounted controls.

11. Clothes washers and dryers should also be front loading with front-mounted controls.

12. Access to the refrigerator will be enhanced by use of a side-by-side (refrigerator-freezer) model.

13. A smoke detector and one or more easily accessible, portable fire extinguishers should be available. For patients with hearing impairments, the smoke detector can be at-

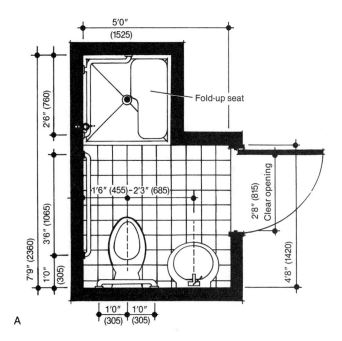

A

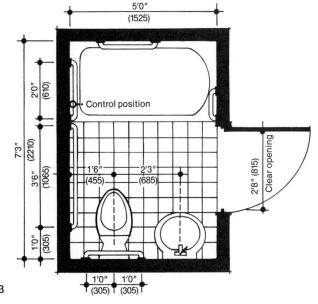

B

Figure 12-10. Sample features and minimum space requirements of a residential bathroom with (A) a shower stall and (B) a bathtub. The dotted line indicates lengths of wall that require reinforcement to receive grab bars or supports. (From Nixon, V: Spinal Cord Injury: A Guide to Functional Outcomes in Physical Therapy Management. Aspen Systems Corporation, Rockville, MD, p 186, with permission.)

tached to a signaling system that activates both an audible and strobe light response to visually warn of danger (these signaling systems also can be used to activate flashing lights in response to a doorbell, knock on the door, telephone ring, or burglar alarm).

Figure 12–11 presents sample features of a kitchen designed for an individual using a wheelchair.

Adaptive Equipment

A large variety of **adaptive equipment** is commercially available to increase independence, speed, skill, and efficiency in performing activities of daily living (ADL). Adaptive equipment is available to assist performance in such areas as bathing, personal care, dressing, meal preparation, and general household tasks. Typically, adaptive equipment is a component of a *compensatory training approach* that focuses on achieving the highest level of function possible by using remaining abilities. This approach involves considering alternate ways to accomplish a task, use of intact segments to compensate for those lost, use of energy conservation techniques, and adapting the patient's environment to optimize performance.[10]

Table 12–1 presents suggestions for adaptive equipment to improve function in several areas of ADL. The table is organized around adaptive equipment recommendations and compensatory strategies for four impairments including (1) one upper extremity or body side involvement; (2) reduced upper extremity range of motion and strength; (3) incoordination of upper extremities; and (4) mobility limitations without upper extremity involvement. The table also identifies common diagnoses associated with each impairment together with the rationale for the suggested compensatory strategies.[11]

REMOTE CONTROLS AND ENVIRONMENTAL CONTROL UNITS

Inexpensive remote control units can be used in any room of the home to control lights or small appliances. They are readily available from hardware or electrical supply stores and provide user control by a portable hand-held keypad or button. The simplest designs of these remote control units send signals through existing wires (receiver modules are plugged into existing outlets and appliances are plugged into the receiver and controlled by a hand-held remote) or are wireless and utilize radio signals. Others require additional wiring (receiver modules are wired directly into the electrical system of the dwelling).[12]

An **environmental control unit (ECU)** is an electronic interface that allows the user to control a variety of appliances and devices (e.g., telephones, bed controls, various components of an entertainment unit, room temperature and lighting, open and close curtains, open doors, full computer access). These devices combine operation of all appliances into a central control panel providing increased independence for individuals with severe disability.[13]

The three main components of an ECU (Fig. 12–12) include (1) the input device, (2) the control unit, and (3) the appliance. The *input device* controls the ECU using whatever voluntary movement the individual has available (e.g., joystick, control panel, keypad, keyboard [ECU computer software programs are available], a series of switches, touch pads and screens, light pen, optical pointers, and voice, mouthstick, and eye control). The *control unit* is the central processor that translates the input signal to an output signal to regulate the target appliance. The *appliance* can be virtually any device that can be controlled electronically.[13]

Workplace Assessment

An investigation of the workplace is an important component of the environmental assessment. It is used to determine if the individual can return to his or her former workplace. The most effective means of assessing the patient's work environment is an on-site visit. However, a variety of standardized work capacity instruments are commercially available that can be used to gather preliminary data prior to an on-site assessment. These tools are used to measure performance in specific components of work-related tasks. The specificity of the individual's job will dictate the types of functional activities needed to perform the required tasks. Work capacity instruments are selected based on these requirements. They assess the group of skills that comprise an employment task (e.g., eye-hand coordination needed for clerical tasks; reach, grasp, and manipulation capability for assembly work). Integrated with information from other assessments (e.g., manual muscle testing, range of motion, functional assessments, cardiopulmonary assessment), data from these test batteries help predict the individual's work capacity and parameters of the physical environment needed to optimize function. Examples of physical work capacity assessments include the *Valpar Component Work Sample Series and Dexterity Modules* (Valpar Corporation, 3801 East 34th Street, Tucson, AZ, 85713), the *BTE Work Simulator* (Baltimore Therapeutic Equipment Co., 7455-L New Ridge Rd., Hanover, Maryland, 21076-3105) and the *Physical Work Performance Evaluation* (Ergo Science Inc., 4131 Cliff Road, Birmingham, Alabama, 35222).

As with the home assessment, the work assessment should begin with an interview. The purpose of the interview is to gather preliminary data about the functional requirements of the job and the physical space in which the individual is required to work. Interview questions are developed based on the type of employment and task requirements. A sample of suggested interview questions appropriate for a clerical position are presented in Box 12–2.

When assessing level of function in the work environment, the principles of energy conservation,

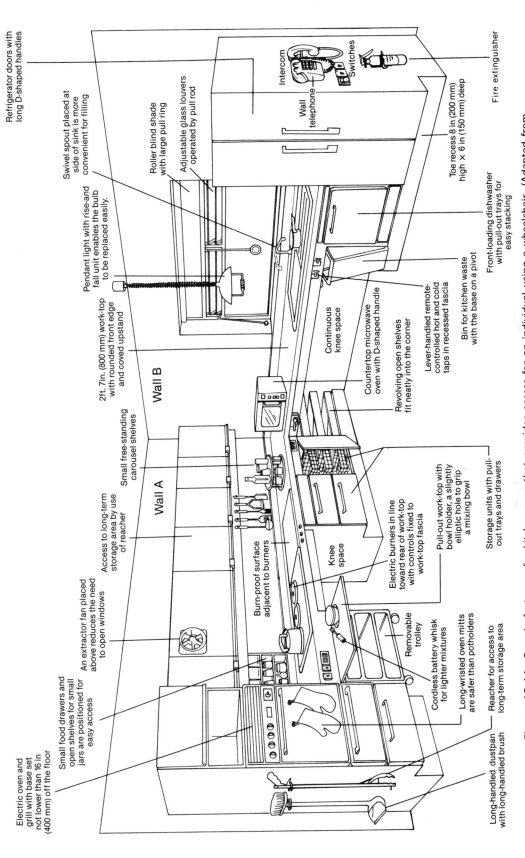

Refrigerator doors with long D-shaped handles

Swivel spout placed at side of sink is more convenient for filling

Pendant light with rise-and fall unit enables the bulb to be replaced easily.

Roller blind shade with large pull ring

Adjustable glass louvers operated by pull rod

Intercom

Wall telephone

Switches

Toe recess 8 in (200 mm) high × 6 in (150 mm) deep

Fire extinguisher

Front-loading dishwasher with pull-out trays for easy stacking

Bin for kitchen waste with the base on a pivot

Lever-handled remote-controlled hot and cold taps in recessed fascia

Revolving open shelves fit neatly into the corner

Countertop microwave oven with D-shaped handle

Continuous knee space

2ft. 7in. (800 mm) work-top with rounded front edge and coved upstand

Wall B

Wall A

Small free-standing carousel shelves

Access to long-term storage area by use of reacher

An extractor fan placed above reduces the need to open windows

Small food drawers and open shelves for small jars are positioned for easy access

Electric oven and grill with base set not lower than 16 in (400 mm) off the floor

Burn-proof surface adjacent to burners

Knee space

Electric burners in line toward rear of work-top with controls fixed to work-top fascia

Pull-out work-top with bowl holder, a slightly elliptic hole to grip a mixing bowl

Storage units with pull-out trays and drawers

Removable trolley

Cordless battery whisk for lighter mixtures

Long-wristed oven mitts are safer than potholders

Reacher for access to long-term storage area

Long-handled dustpan with long-handled brush

Figure 12-11. Sample features of a kitchen area that provides access for an individual using a wheelchair. (Adapted from Conran, T: The Kitchen Book, Mitchell Beazley, London, 1977, pp 118–119.)

345

Table 12–1 ADAPTIVE EQUIPMENT AND COMPENSATORY STRATEGIES FOR SELECTED AREAS OF ADL

Impairment
One upper extremity or body side involvement.

Common Diagnoses Associated with Impairment
Hemiplegia (cerebrovascular accident [CVA] or head injury), unilateral trauma or amputation, temporary conditions such as burns and peripheral neuropathy.

Rationale for Using Compensatory Strategies
To allow for safe, one-handed performance; to stabilize objects for task completion; with hemiplegia, to compensate for loss of balance and mobility

ADL Area	Adaptive Equipment	Adaptive Techniques
Meal preparation and cleanup	To stabilize objects, consider use of: • Adapted cutting board with stainless steel or aluminum nails for cutting or peeling. Raised corners on the board can stabilize bread to spread ingredients or make a sandwich. • Sponge dishes, Dycem™ or suction devices to stabilize bowls or dishes during food preparation. • Pot stabilizer. To allow for safe, one-handed performance: • Adapted jar openers. • Electric appliances such as food processor and hand mixer save time and energy. *Note:* patient safety and judgement need to be considered when electrical appliances are considered. • Rocker knife. • Whisk to mix food. To compensate for decreased standing tolerance and mobility, consider use of: • Utility cart to transport objects. • If cooking is done at wheelchair level or seated, use angled mirror over the stove to watch food on the stove. For cleanup, consider use of: • Hand-held spray for rinsing dishes. • Rubber mat at bottom of sink to reduce breakage. • Suction-type brush to clean glassware. • Laundry can be transported to and from washer and dryer using a wheeled cart.	If balance is affected, it is recommended that the task be done in a seated position. • Objects can be stabilized by using the knees. • Pots and pans can be slid across counters, rather than lifted. • To open a jar, place it in a drawer, then lean against it to stabilize it before opening. • Scissors can be used to open plastic bags. • Milk cartons can be opened by using a fork. • An egg can be cracked by holding it in the palm of the hand, hitting the egg against the edge of the bowl, and separating the egg shell with the index and middle fingers. For clean-up: • Soak and air-dry dishes for easier clean-up.
Clothing management (laundry, ironing, clothing repair) Housecleaning	• Long-reach duster. • Long-handled dustpan and brush. • Self-wringing mop.	• Incorporate energy conservation by making bed completely at each corner before progressing to the next corner. • No-wax floors are easier to care for. • If balance and ambulation problems are present, some floor care can be managed from a seated position.

Table 12–1 ADAPTIVE EQUIPMENT AND COMPENSATORY STRATEGIES
FOR SELECTED AREAS OF ADL *Continued*

Impairment
Reduced upper-extremity range of motion and strength.

Common Diagnoses Associated with Impairment
Quadriplegia, burns, arthritis, upper-extremity amputation, multiple sclerosis, amyotrophic lateral sclerosis, orthopedic and other traumatic injuries.

Rationale for Using Compensatory Strategies
To compensate for lack of reach or hand grip; to compensate for lack of strength or tolerance for prolonged activity; to allow gravity to assist; to compensate for decreased balance.

ADL Area	Adaptive Equipment	Adaptive Techniques
Meal preparation and cleanup	Consider the use of: • Adapted jar opener. • Foam or built-up handles on utensils. • Universal cuff to hold utensils to compensate for reduced grip. • Long-handled reacher to obtain lightweight objects from overhead or low places. • Wheeled cart to transport objects. • Adapted cutting board. • Loop handles can be added to utensils to substitute for reduced grasp. • If using a walker, a walker basket can help transport objects. For marketing: • Marketing by phone, mail or computer is recommended because many objects may be out of reach in store.	• Joint protective measures for rheumatoid arthritis. • Position electrical appliances within easy reach. This helps to conserve energy. • To conserve energy, work at a seated position. • Use teeth to open containers. • Purchase convenience foods to eliminate food preparation. • Tenodesis action (wrist extension and finger flexion; wrist flexion and finger extension) can be used to pick up lightweight objects. • Use a fork to open milk cartons. • Use lightweight pots, pans, and utensils.
Housecleaning	• Long-handled reacher allows objects to be picked up from the floor. • Long-handled sponge to clean bath tub. • Self-wringing mop. • Use lightweight tools such as sponge mops and brooms for floor care.	• Use aerosol cleaners to dissolve dirt before cleaning surfaces. • When making the bed, do not tuck sheets in.
Laundry	• If patient is ambulatory, the preference is for a top-loading washer to avoid the need to bend. • Push-button controls on the washer and dryer are easier to use than knobs. If knobs are present, they may need to be adapted. • If patient chooses to iron, set iron at a low temperature setting. An asbestos pad can be placed at the end of the ironing board to eliminate the need to stand iron up after each ironing stroke.	• Use premeasured packages of soap or bleach to avoid handling large containers. It may be more economical to buy larger containers and have someone else measure soap or bleach into single packets. Use energy conservation: • Place hangers near dryer to hang permanent press items as they come out of the dryer. Remain seated to do ironing.

Continued

**Table 12–1 ADAPTIVE EQUIPMENT AND COMPENSATORY STRATEGIES
FOR SELECTED AREAS OF ADL** *Continued*

Impairment
Incoordination of upper extremities.

Common Diagnoses Associated with Impairment
Head injury, cerebral palsy, CVA, multiple sclerosis, tumors, other neurological conditions.

Rationale for Using Compensatory Strategies
To stabilize proximal portion of limbs; to reduce movements distally by using weight; to stabilize objects for task completion; to provide an
    environment in which patient is safe and proficient; to avoid breakage or accidents with sharp utensils or hot food or equipment.

ADL Area	Adaptive Equipment	Adaptive Techniques
Meal preparation and cleanup	• Use heavy cookware, ironstone dishes to aid with distal stabilization. • Use pots and casseroles with double handles to provide greater stability. • Weighted wrist cuffs may reduce tremors. • Use nonslip materials such as Dycem™ to provide stability. • Use adapted cutting board to stabilize food while cutting. • A serrated knife is less likely to slip than a straight-edged knife. • Using a frying basket to cook foods, such as vegetables, makes for safe removal and reduces the chance of burns. • Free-standing appliances, electric skillet, and countertop mixer are safer than transferring objects out of oven or using handheld mixer. • Use a milk carton holder with handles to pour milk. • A stove with front controls is preferred so the client does not need to reach over hot pots to the back of the stove. • A wheeled cart that is weighted is one alternative for transporting food. • Place a rubber mat or sponge cloth at the bottom of the sink to cushion fall of dishes.	• During food preparation such as cutting and peeling, stabilize arms proximally to reduce tremors. • Start the stove after the food has been placed on the burner. • Sliding food and dishes over a counter is preferable to lifting to transport food item. • To avoid breakage, soak dishes, rinse with hand sprayer and drip dry; eliminate dish handling.
Housecleaning	• Heavier work tools are useful. A dust mitt is easier to handle than gripping a duster. • Fitted sheets on a bed are recommended.	• Eliminate or store excess household decorations to reduce dusting.

Table 12–1 ADAPTIVE EQUIPMENT AND COMPENSATORY STRATEGIES FOR SELECTED AREAS OF ADL *Continued*

Impairment
Mobility limitations without upper extremity involvement.

Common Diagnoses Associated with Impairment
Paraplegia, osteoarthritis, lower-extremity amputation, burns, leg and knee fractures and replacement.

Rationale for Using Compensatory Strategies
Mobility may be provided by a wheelchair. Wheelchair accessibility includes consideration of work heights, maneuverability, and access to storage, equipment, and supplies.
Other types of mobility devices (walker, crutches) may require increased endurance.

ADL Area	Adaptive Equipment	Adaptive Techniques
Meal preparation and cleanup	• Transport items using a wheelchair lap-tray. The laptray can be used as a work surface to protect lap from hot pans. • Stove controls should be in the front of the stove. • Use an angled mirror to see the contents of pots.	• Remove cabinet doors to eliminate need to maneuver around them. • Place frequently used items on easy-to-reach shelves, above and below counter-top level. Increase height of wheelchair to allow use of standard height countertops.
Laundry Housekeeping	• Use front-loading washer and dryer. • Use self-propelled lightweight vacuums.	

Adapted from Culler,[11] p 371, with permission.

ergonomics, and anthropometrics are of prime importance in prevention of injury and maximizing the worker's efficiency and comfort. Capabilities should be weighed against the physical demands of the work environment, and the therapist, using knowledge of adaptive equipment and applied biomechanics, may suggest changes appropriate to the situation.

Intervention in the workplace is an expanding area of interest within physical therapy.[14–21] The on-site assessment of the workplace typically includes (1) a **job analysis** to identify the specific components of the work task and features of the environment in which they must be accomplished, and (2) an **ergonomic assessment** to identify the immediate or predicted risks of musculoskeletal injury for an individual worker. Data from the on-site assessment will allow the therapist to establish a *plan for risk reduction* that provides recommendations to eliminate the potential for injury, and a *plan to optimize function* that includes suggestions for adaptive equipment and recommendations for improving performance within the work environment.[14,15]

Many of the assessments and adaptive strategies employed in the home will be used in the work environment as well. Several considerations specific to the work setting are described below.

EXTERNAL ACCESSIBILITY

1. A parking space should be available within a short distance of the building if the patient plans to drive to and from work. Parking spaces should be a minimum of 96 inches (2440 mm) wide, with an adjacent access aisle 60 inches (1525 mm) wide (Fig. 12-13).[7] The location should be clearly marked as a reserved parking area.
2. External accessibility of the building should be addressed using guidelines similar to those presented for home exteriors.

INTERNAL ACCESSIBILITY

1. Initially, the component requirements of the work task must be identified. The complexity of some tasks or the needed interface with the work environment may render the analysis of such tasks prior to the on-site visit inappropriate. This will include determination of mobility requirements (movement within and outside the primary work area), as well as determination of demands or skill required in each of the

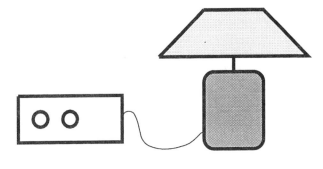

Figure 12-12. The three main components of an environmental control unit. (From Angelo and Lane,[13] p 178, with permission.)

Input Device   Control Unit   Appliance

Box 12–2 SUGGESTED INTERVIEW QUESTIONS APPROPRIATE FOR A CLERICAL POSITION. INTERVIEW QUESTIONS ARE USED TO GATHER GENERAL DATA ABOUT FUNCTIONAL REQUIREMENTS OF THE JOB AND THE PHYSICAL SPACE IN WHICH THE INDIVIDUAL IS REQUIRED TO WORK.

1. Y N Do you frequently lift more than 35 pounds?
2. Y N Are you required to lift objects from below knee level or above shoulder level on an occasional or frequent basis?
3. Y N When you lift, do you reach across other objects or at arms' length in order to accomplish the lift?
4. Y N Do you frequently reach for objects above shoulder level during the day?
5. Y N Do you sit for more than 4 hours per day?
6. Y N Does your job require you to maintain one position or posture for 30 to 60 minutes or longer at one time? If yes, what posture is it? _____

7. Y N Are repetitive exertions required on a regular basis (e.g., typing, 10-key)?
8. Y N Does your job require frequent motions of the fingers, wrists, elbows, or shoulders? (If yes, circle all that apply.)
9. Y N Do you feel that your desk height is at a comfortable level?
10. Y N a) Is your chair comfortable for you?
    Y N b) Do you feel that it fits you properly?
    Y N c) Do you know how to adjust your chair?
11. Y N Is there ample space for you to perform your job?
12. Y N Does your job involve frequent bending, twisting, or jerking movements?

Source: From Hunter,[16] p 68, with permission.

---

following areas: strength (trunk, upper versus lower extremities), posture, endurance, manual dexterity, eye-hand coordination, vision, hearing, and communication.

2. The immediate work area should be carefully examined. This will include lighting, temperature, seating surface (if other than a wheelchair), the height and size of the work counter (some patients may benefit from a variable height or tilting work surface), and exposure to noise, vibration, or fumes. Access to supplies, materials, or equipment should be considered with respect to the patient's vertical and horizontal reaching capabilities. From an upright wheelchair sitting position, the unobstructed high forward reach is a maximum of 48 inches (1220 mm) from the floor and the low forward reach is a minimum of 15 inches (380 mm) from the floor (Fig. 12-14). When the high forward reach is over a work surface of not greater than 20 inches (510 mm), the maximum reach distance is 48 inches (1220 mm) from the floor (Fig. 12-15A). Progressively deeper work surfaces will alter the forward reach accordingly. For example, a work surface depth between 20 and 25 inches allows a maximum forward reach of not greater than 44 inches (1120 mm) from the floor (Fig. 12-15B).[7] For individuals with

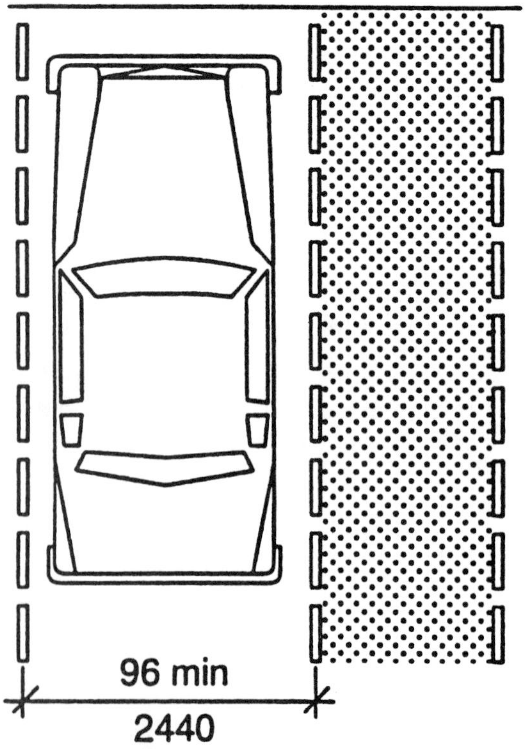

Figure 12-13. Vehicle parking spaces should be a minimum of 96 inches (2440 mm) wide, with an adjacent access aisle 60 inches (1525 mm) wide. Values denoted in inches and millimeters. (From American National Standards Institute, Inc.,[7] p 33, with permission.)

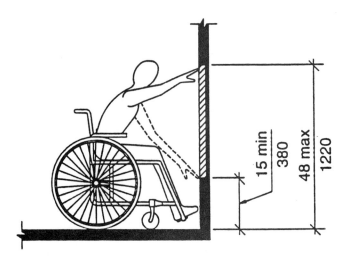

Figure 12-14. Unobstructed high forward reach is a maximum of 48 inches (1220 mm) from the floor and the low forward reach is a minimum of 15 inches (380 mm) from the floor. Values denoted in inches and millimeters. (From American National Standards Institute, Inc.,[7] p 11, with permission.)

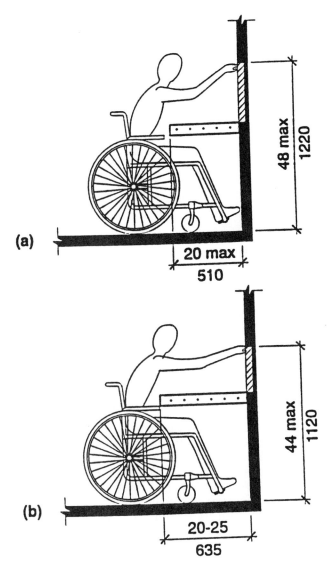

Figure 12-15. (*A*) High forward reach over a 20-inch (510 mm) deep work surface is a maximum of 48 inches (1220 mm) from the floor. (*B*) A work surface depth of 20 to 25 inches (510–635 mm) allows a maximum forward reach of not greater than 44 inches (1120 mm) from the floor. Values denoted in inches and millimeters. (From American National Standards Institute, Inc.,[7] p 11, with permission.)

good trunk control, reaching capacity will be increased.

3. Access to public telephones, drinking fountains, and bathrooms should be addressed.

Alpert[14] suggests four potential approaches to facilitating optimum function in the work environment. These include (1) modification in the work space design or tools and equipment; (2) administrative changes such as rotation of job assignments, staggered breaks, lower production rates, and limited overtime; (3) education on effective work habits (e.g., correct posture, altered size of handled tools, and frequent equipment maintenance); and (4) use of protective or adaptive equipment.

A variety of building survey forms have been developed to facilitate the on-site assessment of the workplace. These forms assist with attending to all

necessary details during the visit. A sample of such a form is provided in Appendix B.

Community Assessment

To attain the goal of full accessibility for the patient, the availability of community resources, services, and facilities must be investigated. As mentioned, when a direct involvement by the therapist is not possible, this may best be accomplished by providing the support network members with guidelines for exploring access to local facilities.

Another important consideration is to refer the patient and/or the support network members to community organizations such as the Arthritis Foundation, National Easter Seal Society, Multiple Sclerosis Society, Chamber of Commerce, or the Veterans Administration. These groups can provide information on services available to individuals with a disability who reside in the community. Individuals who are returning to school should be encouraged to contact the campus student services office, which addresses the needs of students with disabilities. Information will be offered on housing, special services, and general campus resources.

TRANSPORTATION

Currently the availability of accessible public transportation varies considerably among geographic areas. As such, careful exploration by the patient and support network will be needed to determine what resources are obtainable in specific locales. Some communities provide part-time service of partially or completely accessible buses. These include the so-called kneeling buses equipped with a hydraulic unit that lowers the entrance to curb level for easier boarding. Some buses, although fewer in number, are designed with hydraulic lifts to allow direct entry by an individual using a wheelchair. In communities where these buses are available, they typically operate on specific time schedules and are frequently limited to highly trafficked routes. Careful planning is usually necessary to benefit from such service.

Unfortunately, the majority of public transportation systems in the United States do not allow use by individuals who are nonambulatory or by those with limited ambulatory capacity. Most urban transit systems are virtually inaccessible to individuals with mobility impairments. As an alternative, many areas provide door-to-door van transportation to residents of the community with disabilities. Again, availability of such services may be scarce in some locations.

Some patients will want to master driving an adapted automobile or van. This, of course, will improve opportunities for community travel significantly. Motor vehicle adaptations are selected based on the physical capabilities of the individual. Common adaptive equipment includes hand controls to operate the brakes and the accelerator; steering wheel attachments, such as knobs or universal cuffs, for individuals with limited grip strength; lifting units to assist with placement of the wheelchair into the vehicle; and, for patients with quadriplegia or high-level paraplegia, self-contained lifting platforms for entry to a van while remaining seated in a wheelchair.

For patients whose capacity for long-distance ambulation is limited and/or whose endurance is low, commercially available city-going electric carts (Fig. 12-16) may be a practical alternative for travel within a reasonable proximity of the home.

ACCESS TO COMMUNITY FACILITIES

A few elements considered for workplace assessment warrant attention for general community access, as well. Briefly, these area facilities should be assessed for the availability of appropriate parking areas, beveled curbs, external and internal structural accessibility of buildings, and availability of accessible public telephones, drinking fountains, bathrooms, and restaurants. Theaters, auditoriums, and lecture halls must be considered with respect to accessible seating areas. Many such public presentation spaces are now designed with an accessible isle leading to open floor space interspersed within a row of standard seats to accommodate a wheelchair. This allows the individual using a wheelchair the option of sitting next to a person who is ambulatory or someone using a wheelchair. Locations of emergency exits should also be noted for all facilities. In addition to these general considerations, stores and shopping areas should also be inspected for access to merchandise (especially for individuals using a wheelchair), appropriate aisle widths, and adequate space at checkout counters.

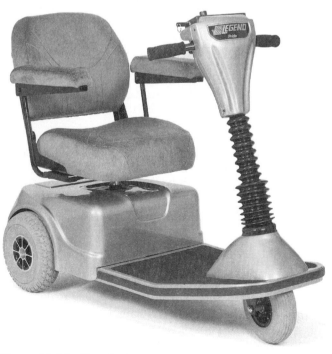

Figure 12-16. Motorized scooter suitable for outdoor travel. (Courtesy of Pride Health Care, Exeter, PA.)

Another useful source of information on community access is the guidebook offered by many larger cities (funded as a community service by local businesses). These books provide information on accessibility of local cultural, civic, and religious institutions, government offices, theaters, hotels, restaurants, shopping areas, transportation, and social and recreational facilities. These publications usually can be obtained from the city's chamber of commerce, the mayor's office, or the office of tourism. Combined use of such guides and phoning ahead for details of accessibility will facilitate travel both within and outside the local community.

DOCUMENTATION

Upon completion of the environmental assessment, a final collaborative report is prepared and includes data from each team member who participated in the on-site visit. This report consists of information obtained from the home and, if applicable, the workplace assessment. Information should be included about the measures taken to explore general community accessibility.

Documentation of the on-site visit should incorporate a completed home assessment or building survey form. Additional information that should be provided includes (1) a description of the methods used to assist the patient in ambulation or functional activities, (2) a description of the type and quantity of adaptive equipment required (including source and cost), and (3) suggested environmental modifications with precise specifications.

Documentation related to community access entails a verification that the patient is aware of available community resources. The sources of this information, as well as whether the therapist was directly or indirectly involved in assessment, should be documented.

The completed report should then be included as part of the patient's medical record. Copies of the report should be submitted to the patient's support network, the physician, third party payer(s), and any community-based health care or social service agencies that will be providing care.

FUNDING FOR ENVIRONMENTAL MODIFICATIONS

The patient and support network may require assistance in locating appropriate financial resources to achieve environmental accessibility. Typically, the social service department within the patient care facility will provide direction in this area. Information on resource organizations can also be obtained from the National Council on Disabilities. Potential sources of funding include private medical insurance companies, home equity or other types of bank loans, Veterans Administration Housing Grants, the Division of Vocational Rehabilitation (DVR), the Worker's Compensation Commission, and local chapters of national civic groups such as Kiwanis International, Veteran's of

Foreign Wars, Masons/Shriners Lodges, and Lions International.

An important consideration is that not all patients will have current housing that is amenable to modification (e.g., an individual who previously lived in a third-floor walk-up apartment and now uses a wheelchair). In such instances, the local Housing and Urban Development (HUD) Office will be an important resource. This office can provide a listing of accessible housing within the community. Because there are often waiting lists for such dwellings, early application is warranted.

Finally, some "creative funding" for specific items (such as specialized adaptive equipment not covered by other resources) may be available through private organizations or foundations. Considerable time, research, and perseverance may be required in locating a receptive organization. General suggestions the patient and support network might consider in seeking assistance include contacting local businesses or corporate giving offices, civic or service clubs, churches or synagogues, labor unions, Jaycees, and the Knights of Columbus.

LEGISLATIVE ACTION RELATED TO ENVIRONMENTAL ACCESS

Much attention has been focused on the importance of environmental accessibility. Through legislation and a variety of private organizations, significant strides have been made in this area. In 1990 the *Americans with Disabilities Act* (ADA) was signed into law. This legislation is among the most comprehensive of the civil rights laws enacted for individuals with disabilities. It guarantees civil rights protection and equal opportunity in the areas of government services, employment, public transportation, privately owned transportation available to the public, telephone service, and public accommodations.[22] This law requires that all "public places of accommodation" be made accessible to people with a disability unless it imposes "undue hardship" to the establishment. This law includes compliance by restaurants, movie theaters, hotels, professional offices, and retail stores.

With respect to an individual, disability is defined in the ADA as "a physical or mental impairment that substantially limits one or more major life activities of such an individual; a record of such impairment; or being regarded as having such impairment."[22] p 4 Undue hardship includes excessive direct cost of adapting the environment, limited resources of the establishment, or situations where these changes would fundamentally alter the nature or daily operation of a business. Connolly[23] suggests that the cost of changes cannot be used as a defense during litigation unless the financial burden would threaten the very existence of the business. The ADA also provides a federal tax credit incentive for measures taken by businesses to comply with this law.

The Fair Housing Act, as amended in 1988, prohibits discrimination in housing on the basis of race, color, religion, gender, disability, familial status, and national origin. It requires landlords to allow individuals with disabilities to make reasonable, access-related modifications to their living space, as well as common areas of the building. However, the landlord is not required to pay for these modifications. The Fair Housing Act also provides accessible construction standards for multifamily housing units built for first occupancy after March, 1991.

The Rehabilitation Act of 1973 provided that access must be established in all federally funded buildings and transportation facilities constructed after 1968. The law requires nondiscrimination in federal employment, accessibility within federal buildings, and established the Architectural Transportation Barriers and Compliance Board. Because many federally funded institutions provided low compliance with the 1973 Rehabilitation Act, an amendment was passed in 1978. The Comprehensive Rehabilitation Services Amendments (P.L. 95-602) of 1978 strengthened the enforcement of the original 1973 Rehabilitation Act. The Architectural and Transportation Barriers Compliance Board is the governing body responsible for enforcing this legislation.[14]

The Architectural Barrier Act of 1968 (P.L. 90-480) provided that certain buildings that were financed by federal funds be designed and constructed "to insure that physically handicapped persons will have ready access to, and use of, such buildings."[24] p 719 Another important item of legislation related to environmental accessibility is the Public Buildings Act of 1983, which functioned to establish public building policies for the federal government. This act (section 307) provided several amendments to the Architectural Barrier Act of 1968 to further strengthen and delineate the importance of accessibility. The term *fully accessible* in this act was defined as "the absence or elimination of physical and communications barriers to the ingress, egress, movement within, and use of a building by handicapped persons and the incorporation of such equipment as is necessary to provide such ingress, egress, movement, and use and, in a building of historic, architectural, or cultural significance, the elimination of such barriers and the incorporation of such equipment in such a manner as to be compatible with the significant architectural features of the building to the maximum extent possible."[25] p 373

Despite the recent gains made in architectural accessibility, many barriers continue to exist. Inasmuch as most public transportation systems were built before 1968, accessibility is not required by law.[14] However, the ADA indicates that all concerns that offer public transit along a fixed route must also provide buses that are accessible to individuals with disabilities, including access by wheelchairs. Other areas that continue to be problematic include revolving doors, the design of many supermarkets and shopping areas (barriers imposed by checkout areas and items displayed on high shelves), lack of available parking spaces, multiple levels of stairs at the entrance to some buildings, and the design of many theaters and auditoriums that do not have specifically designated areas for individuals using a wheelchair.

In response to recent legislation related to accessibility, several important publications have been developed to assist in planning new construction, provide guidelines for modification of existing facilities, and answer frequently asked questions about federal accessibility requirements.[26–31] The US Department of Justice also established an ADA information line (800.514.0301), which provides technical assistance on accessibility standards and a 24-hour automated service for ordering ADA material. Additional ADA information can be obtained from the sources provided in Appendix C.

Although increasing numbers of buildings are being designed to provide accessibility, this area warrants further involvement from therapists. Both physical and occupational therapists are equipped to provide leadership in compliance with existing and new laws. They have important knowledge and skills to enable them to provide valuable input into the modification and/or initial planning of barrier-free designs.

SUMMARY

Information obtained from an environmental assessment is an important factor in facilitating the patient's transition from the rehabilitation setting to the home and community. Such assessments assist in determining the level of patient access, safety, and function within specific components of the environment. They also assist in determining the need for additional treatment interventions, environmental modifications, outpatient services, and adaptive equipment. Additionally, they assist in preparing the patient, support network members, and/or colleagues for the individual's return to a given setting.

This chapter has presented a sample approach to environmental assessment. Common environmental features that typically warrant consideration have been highlighted. Inasmuch as a return to a former environment is often a primary goal of rehabilitation, early consideration of these issues is warranted. Collaboration among team members, the patient, and support network members will ensure an optimum and highly individualized approach to community reintegration.

QUESTIONS FOR REVIEW

1. Define each of the following terms: environmental barrier, accessibility, environmental accessibility, accessible design, and universal design.
2. Identify the purposes of an environmental assessment.
3. Identify the tests and measures used and the types of data generated during an environmental assessment.
4. In addition to an on-site visit, what other assessment strategies can be used to gather data about the environment?
5. Identify and provide examples of the five major areas of intervention strategies used to modify the environment.
6. What information should be obtained prior to an on-site visit?
7. Who should be involved in the on-site visit?
8. What specific aspects of the *exterior* of a patient's home should be assessed during an on-site visit? Your response should address the route to the entrance and actual entrance to the home.
9. What specific aspects of the *interior* of a patient's home should be assessed during an on-site visit? Your response should address furniture arrangement, floor surfaces, doors, stairs, and considerations specific to the bedroom, bathroom, and kitchen areas of the dwelling.
10. Explain the importance of an environmental assessment in overall rehabilitation planning.
11. Describe the information that should be included in documentation of an on-site environmental assessment.
12. What civil rights of individuals with disabilities are protected by the 1990 Americans with Disabilities Act?

CASE STUDY

A 78 year-old woman with a diagnosis of osteoarthritis was admitted for a right total hip replacement. The patient reported a long-standing history of discomfort. She described the hip pain as radiating posteriorly to the buttock and low back and was exacerbated by weight-bearing and stair climbing. Over the past 12 months she has experienced a very marked increase in pain and stiffness. Radiographic findings demonstrated degenerative changes of both the acetabulum and femoral head consistent with osteoarthritis. The surgical intervention replaced the right femoral head and neck with a metallic prosthesis and the acetabulum was resurfaced with a plastic cup. Past medical history is unremarkable.

Social History: The patient is a retired manager of a small accounting firm that she and her husband established. Her husband is deceased. She has three grown children who all live in neighboring communities. Prior to the functional limitations imposed by the hip pain, the patient had been independent in all BADL and IADL. She also volunteered her accounting services one day per week to a local charity which provides meals to homebound individuals, she was a regular participant in family outings, enjoyed going to the theater, concerts, and special museum events, and was an active member of the community historical preservation society. Recently, these activities had to be curtailed owing to the increased hip discomfort. She essentially had no activities outside the home for three months prior to admission and used a walker to minimize weightbearing and reduce pain. She also required the assistance of a home care aide four hours a day two times per week (primarily for shopping, errands, and some household management tasks). She expressed considerable distress at being unable to take a bath and having to rely on the assistance of another person for some basic care activities. She had been using aspirin for its analgesic and anti-inflammatory effects. However, the pain experienced in recent months was not alleviated by the aspirin and other conservative measures she has been instructed to use (e.g., local applications of heat, periodic rest intervals, and gentle range of motion exercises). The patient has medical insurance coverage and is without financial concerns.

REVIEW OF SYSTEMS

Cognitive Function: Intact.

Vision: Wears corrective lens; experiences "night blindness," which she describes as seeing poorly in dim light and her eyes take several seconds longer than normal to adjust from brightness to dimness.

Hearing: Intact.

Strength

1. Upper Extremities: Generally within functional limits; patient reports some sporadic episodes of wrist and finger stiffness upon awakening in the morning and after periods of immobility. Grip strength is reduced bilaterally (MMT of finger flexors = G-). Heberden's nodes noted at the DIP and PIP joints of the left index finger. Patient denies pain in wrist or fingers.
2. Lower Extremities:
    1. Left: within functional limits.
    2. Right: within functional limits (hip motions not tested owing to surgical intervention); crepitus noted in right knee.

Range of Motion

Within functional limits (with the exception of the right hip, which was not tested)

Post-surgical Right Hip Precautions

No hip flexion beyond 90 degrees.
Avoid crossing one leg or ankle over the other.
Avoid internal rotation of right lower extremity
Coordination: Within normal limits.
Sensation: Intact.
Weight-bearing status
on right lower extremity: Partial weight-bearing

Gait

The patient is ambulating on level surfaces with supervision using bilateral standard aluminum axillary crutches with partial weight-bearing on the right lower extremity. Stair climbing also requires minimal assistance. It is anticipated the patient will be independent with ambulation on level surfaces at time of discharge from the hospital.

Patient Goals: The patient is extremely motivated to once again be an independent manager of her personal care and household management needs. The prosthetic replacement has successfully relieved much of the pain experienced in the hip prior to surgery (most of her current discomfort is described as "minor" and associated with the surgical incision). She would also like to return to her family, volunteer, social, and leisure activities. She is very determined to discontinue the home care assistance as soon as possible.

Home Environment: The patient lives alone in a fifth-floor apartment in a building with an elevator. The living space is a one-bedroom apartment on a single level. At your request, one of the patient's children has provided dimensions of door frames and height of sleeping and seating surfaces together with several photographs of each room of the patient's home. The physical dimensions and photographs indicate the following:

1. Bedroom: two small area rugs, a nightstand with an alarm clock, a bureau, a wooden platform bed with a sleeping surface 1½ feet from the floor, and a ceiling lamp fixture controlled by a switch adjacent to the door.
2. Bathroom: an area rug, standard toilet and sink, bathtub does not include a shower, a doorway entrance 30 inches wide.
3. Kitchen: polished linoleum floors, adequate counter space, and a dining table in the center of the room.
4. Livingroom: overstuffed upholstered furniture with low seating surfaces, a large carpet that appears to ripple in several areas, a centered coffee table, a telephone with an extra-long extension wire placed on the coffee table, a manual control television, two end-tables and a bookcase.
5. Hallway (between rooms): poorly lit with a long, narrow area rug.

Guiding Questions

With general knowledge of the patient's living space, what environmental modifications, adaptive equipment, or additional instruction would you suggest or provide to optimize safety and function in each of the following areas of the home?

1. Bedroom
2. Bathroom
3. Kitchen
4. Livingroom
5. Hallway

REFERENCES

1. Corcoran, M, and Gitlin, L: The role of the physical environment in occupational performance. In Christiansen, CH, and Baum, CM (eds): Occupational Therapy Enabling Function and Well-Being, ed 2. Slack, Thorofare, NJ, 1997, p 336.
2. Lawton, MP, et al: Assessing environments for older people with chronic illness. Journal of Mental Health and Aging 3:83, 1997.
3. American Physical Therapy Association: Guide to Physical Therapist Practice. APTA, Alexandria, VA, 1999.
4. Duncan, PW, et al: Functional reach: Predictive validity in a sample of elderly male veterans. J Gerontol 47:M93, 1992.
5. Mathias, S, et al: Balance in elderly patients: The "Get Up and Go" test. Arch Phys Med Rehabil 67:387, 1986.
6. Guralnik, JM, et al: A short physical performance battery assessing lower extremity function: Association with self-reported disability and prediction of mortality and nursing home admission. J Gerontol 49(2):M85-94, 1994.
7. American National Standards Institute, Inc: American National Standard: Accessible and Usable Buildings and Facilities (ICC/ANSI A117.1-1998). International Code Council, Inc., Falls Church, VA, 1998.
8. Building Design. Requirements for the Physically Handicapped, rev ed. Eastern Paralyzed Veterans Association, New York, undated.
9. Beaver, KA, and Mann, WC: Overview of technology for low vision. Am J Occup Ther 49:913, 1995.
10. O'Sullivan, SB, and Schmitz, TJ: Physical Rehabilitation Laboratory Manual: Focus on Functional Training. FA Davis, Philadelphia, 1999.
11. Culler, KH: Treatment for Work and Productive Activities: Home and Family Management. In Neistadt, ME, and Crepeau, EB (eds): Willard & Spackman's Occupational Therapy, ed 9. Lippincott-Raven, Philadelphia, 1998, p 369.
12. NAHB Research Center, Inc. (Upper Marlboro, MD) and Barrier Free Designs (Raleigh, NC): Residential Remodeling and Universal Design: Making Homes More Comfortable and Accessible. US Department of Housing and Urban Development, Office of Policy Development and Research, 451 Seventh Street, S.W., Washington, DC, 1996.
13. Angelo, J, and Lane, S (eds): Assistive Technology for Rehabilitation Therapists. FA Davis, Philadelphia, 1997.
14. Alpert, J: The physical therapist's role in job analysis and on-site education. Orthop Phys Ther Pract 5:8, 1993.
15. Owens, TR, et al: An ergonomic perspective on accomodation in accessibility for people with disability. Disabil Rehabil 18:402, 1996.
16. Hunter, S: Using CQI to improve worker's health. PT Magazine 3:64, 1995.
17. Helm-Williams, P: Industrial rehabilitation: Developing guidelines. PT Magazine 1:65, 1993.
18. Wynn, KE: A continuum of care to treat the injured worker. PT Magazine 2:52, 1994.
19. Hebert, LA: OSHA ergonomics guidelines and the PT consultant. PT Magazine 3:54, 1995.
20. Wynn, KE: Setting corporate trends with on-site PT. PT Magazine 4:66, 1996.
21. Lawrence, LP: Practicing where industry lives. PT Magazine 6:28, 1998.
22. The Americans with Disabilities Act of 1990 (As Amended): Public Law 101-336.
23. Connolly, JB: Understanding the ADA. Clinical Management 12:40, 1992.
24. Architectural Barriers Act, Public Law 90-480, 1968.
25. Public Buildings Act, 98th Congress, 1st session, 1983.
26. The Americans with Disabilities Act: Title II Technical Assistance Manual Covering State and Local Government Programs and Services. US Department of Justice, Civil Rights Division (PO Box 66738, Washington, DC, 20035-68738), 1993.
27. The Americans with Disabilities Act: Title III Technical Assistance Manual 1994 Supplement. US Department of Justice, Civil Rights Division (PO Box 66738, Washington, DC, 20035-68738), 1994.
28. Common ADA Errors and Omissions in New Construction and Alterations. US Department of Justice, Civil Rights Division (PO Box 66738, Washington, DC, 20035-68738), 1997.
29. Americans with Disabilities Act: ADA Guide for Small Businesses. US Department of Justice, Civil Rights Division (PO Box 66738, Washington, DC, 20035-68738), 1997.
30. Americans with Disabilities Act: Questions and Answers. US Equal Employment Opportunity Commission (1801 L Street, NW, Washington, DC, 20507) and US Department of Justice, Civil Rights Division (PO Box 66738, Washington, DC 20035-68738), 1997.
31. Enforcing the ADA: A Status Report from the Department of Justice. US Department of Justice, Civil Rights Division (PO Box 66738, Washington, DC, 20035-68738), 1998.

SUPPLEMENTAL READINGS

Clemson, L, et al: Types of hazards in the homes of elderly people. Occupational Journal of Research 17:200, 1997.

Durham, DP: Occupational and physical therapist's perspective of the perceived benefits of a therapeutic home visit program. Physical & Occupational Therapy in Geriatrics 10:15, 1992.

El-Faizy, M, and Reinsch, S: Home safety intervention for the prevention of falls. Physical & Occupational Therapy in Geriatrics 12:33, 1994.

Hendricks, S, et al: Implementation of the Americans with Disabilities Act into physical therapy programs. Journal of Physical Therapy Education 12:9, 1998.

Iwarsson, S, and Isacsson, A: Housing standards, environmental barriers in the home and subjective general apprehension of housing situation among the rural elderly. Scandinavian Journal of Occupational Therapy 3:52, 1996.

Johnson, KL, et al: Assistive technology in rehabilitation. Phys Med Rehabil Clin N Am 8:389, 1997.

Keleher, KC: Primary care for women: Environmental assessment of the home, community, and workplace. J Nursemidwifery 40:88, 1995.

Lach, HW: Alzheimer's disease: Assessing safety problems in the home. Geriatric Nursing 16:160, 1995.

Lawton, MP, et al: Assessing environments for older people with chronic illness. Journal of Mental Health and Aging 3:83, 1997.

Lubinski, P, and Higginbotham, DJ: Communications Technologies for the Elderly: Vision, Hearing and Speech. Singular Publishing Group, San Diego, CA, 1997.

Mann, WC, et al: The relationship of functional independence to assistive device use of elderly persons living at home. Journal of Applied Gerontology 14:225, 1995.

Mann, WC, et al: The use of phones by elders with disabilities: Problems, interventions, costs. Assist Technol 8:23, 1996.

Mann, WC, et al: Assistive devices used by home-based elderly persons with arthritis. Am J Occup Ther 49:810, 1995.

Mann, WC, et al: Environmental problems in homes of elders with disabilities. The Occupational Therapy Journal of Research 14:191, 1994.

Mital, A, and Shrey, DE: Cardiac rehabilitation: Potential for ergonomic interventions with special reference to return to work and the Americans with Disabilities Act. Disabil Rehabil 18:149, 1996.

Monga, TN, et al: Driving: A clinical perspective on rehabilitation technology. Physical Medicine and Rehabilitation 11:69, 1997.

Narayan, MC, and Tennant, J: Environment assessment. Home Health Nurse 15:799, 1997.

Ottenbacher, KJ, and Christiansen, C: Occupational Performance Assessment. In Christiansen, CH, and Baum, CM (eds): Occupational Therapy Enabling Function and Well-Being, ed 2. Slack, Thorofare, NJ, 1997, p 104.

Painter, J: Home environment considerations for people with Alzheimer's disease. Occupational Therapy in Health Care 10:45, 1996.

Rogers, JC, and Holm, MB: Evaluation of Occupational Performance Areas. In Neistadt, ME, and Crepeau, EB (eds): Willard & Spackman's Occupational Therapy, ed 9. Lippincott-Raven, Philadelphia, 1998, p 185.

Shrey, DE: Disability management in industry: The new paradigm in injured worker rehabilitation. Disabil Rehabil 18:408, 1996.

Trefler, E, and Hobson, D: Assistive Technology. In Christiansen, CH, and Baum, CM (eds): Occupational Therapy Enabling Function and Well-Being, ed 2. Slack, Thorofare, NJ, 1997, p 482.

Turner-Stokes, L, et al: Secondary safety of car adaptations for disabled motorists. Disabil Rehabil 18:317, 1996.

Ward RS, et al: Accommodations for students with disabilities in physical therapy and physical therapist assistant programs: A pilot study. Journal of Physical Therapy Education 12:16, 1998.

Wieland, K, et al: The integration of employees with disabilities in Germany and the importance of workplace design. Disabil Rehabil 18:429, 1996.

GLOSSARY

Accessibility: The degree to which an environment affords use of its resources with respect to an individual's level of function.

Accessible design: The structural plan of buildings or dwellings that meet prescribed standards for accessibility such as those recommended by the American National Standards Institute, the Fair Housing Amendments Act of 1988, and the Uniform Federal Accessibility Standards (UFAS).

Adaptive equipment: Devices or equipment designed and fabricated to improve performance in activities of daily living.

Beveled: Smooth, slanted angle between two surfaces; for example, a slant or inclination between two uneven surfaces to allow easier passage of a wheelchair.

Casters: Small revolving wheels on the legs of a chair; such a chair may allow mobility in an area that is unable to accommodate a wheelchair; term also refers to the small front wheels of a wheelchair.

Environmental accessibility: Absence or removal of physical barriers from the entrance and within a building or dwelling to allow use by individuals with disabilities.

Environmental barrier: Physical impediments that prevent individuals from functioning optimally in their surroundings and include safety hazards, access problems, and home or workplace design difficulties (e.g., revolving doors, stairways, narrow doorways).

Environmental control unit (ECU): An electrical interface that allows the user to control a variety of electrical appliances and devices; operation is accomplished by use of a central control panel.

Ergonomic assessment: Data collection concerned with fitting a job to a person's anatomical and physiological characteristics in a way that enhances human efficiency and performance; identifies potential risks of injury for an individual worker.

Grab bars: Wall supports used to assist a person in both toilet and tub transfers; can be mounted vertically, horizontally, or diagonally.

Grade, gradient: Degree of inclination or slope of a ramp. (1:12 or 1 inch of threshold height for every 12 inches of ramp length).

Job analysis: An assessment that identifies the specific components of work tasks and features of the environment in which they must be accomplished.

Kick plate: Metal guard plate attached to the bottom of a door.

Knurled surface: Roughened area, often in a criss-crossed pattern; used on either doorknobs or grab bars. On doorknobs it is used to provide tactile clues to visually impaired persons to indicate that passage leads to an area of danger. On grab bars it is used to improve grasp and to prevent slipping.

Nosing: Edge or brim of a step that projects out over the lower stair surface.

Physical environment: The surroundings in which an individual functions; consists of both built (e.g., buildings and structures created by humans) and natural (e.g., vegetation, mountains, rivers, uneven terrain) objects.

Threshold: Elevated surface on floor of doorway; a doorsill.

Universal design (*life-span* design, *inclusive* design): A structural plan for buildings and dwellings which meet the requirements of all people including those with functional limitations; takes into consideration the needs of a wide range of individuals as well as the changing needs of human beings across the life-span.

APPENDIX A

Home Assessment Form

TYPE OF HOME

_____ Apartment
              Is elevator available? _____
              What floor does patient live on? _____
_____ One floor home.
_____ Two or more floors.
_____ Does patient live on first floor, second floor, or use
              all floors of home?
_____ Basement. Does patient have or use basement area?

ENTRANCES TO BUILDING OR HOME

Location   Front   Back   Side   (Circle one)
    Which entrance is used most frequently or easily? _____
    Can patient get to entrance? _____
Stairs
    Does patient manage outside stairs? _____
    Width of stairway _____
    Number of steps _____ Height of steps _____
    Railing present as you go up? R _____ L _____
    Both _____
    Is ramp available for wheelchair? _____
Door
    Can patient unlock, open, close, lock door? (Circle for yes)
    If doorsill is present, give height _____ and
        material _____
    Width of doorway _____
    Can patient enter _____ leave _____ via door?
Hallway
    Width of hallway _____
    Are any objects obstructing the way? _____

APPROACH TO APARTMENT OR LIVING AREA

    (Omit if not applicable)
Hallway
    Width _____
    Obstructions? _____
Steps
    Width of stairway _____
    Number of steps _____ Height of steps _____
    Railing present as you go up? R _____ L _____
    Both _____
    Is ramp available? _____
Door
    Can patient unlock, open, close, lock door? (Circle one)
    Doorsill? Give height _____ material _____
    Width of doorway _____
    Can patient enter _____ leave _____ via door?
Elevator
    Is elevator present? _____ Does it land flush with
        door? _____
    Width of door opening _____
    Height of control buttons _____
    Can patient use elevator alone? _____

INSIDE HOME

Note width of hallways and of door entrances.
Note presence of doorsills and height.
Note if patient must climb stairs to reach room.
Can patient move from one part of the house to another?
    Hallways _____
    Bedroom _____
    Bathroom _____
    Kitchen _____
    Livingroom _____
    Others _____

Can patient move safely?
    Loose rugs _____
    Electrical cords _____
    Faulty floors _____
    Highly waxed floors _____
    Sharp-edged furniture _____
Note areas of particular danger for patient.
    Hot water pipes _____
    Radiators _____

BEDROOM

    Is light switch accessible? _____
    Can patient open and close windows? _____
Bed
    Height _____ Width _____
    Both sides of bed accessible? _____ Headboard
        present? _____ footboard? _____
    Is bed on wheels? _____ Is it stable? _____
    Can patient transfer from wheelchair to bed? _____ and
        bed to wheelchair? _____
    Is night table within patient's reach from bed _____ Is tele-
        phone on it? _____
Clothing
    Is patient's clothing located in bedroom? _____
    Can patient get clothes from dresser? _____
        closet? _____ elsewhere? _____

BATHROOM

Does patient use wheelchair _____ walker _____ in
    bathroom?
Does wheelchair _____ walker _____ fit into bathroom?
Light switch accessible? _____ Can patient open and close
    window? _____
What material are bathroom walls made of? _____
    If tile, how many inches does it extend from the floor beside the
        toilet? _____
How many inches from the top of the rim of the bathtub? _____
Does patient use toilet? _____
    Can patient transfer independently to and from toilet? _____
    Does wheelchair wheel directly to toilet for transfers? _____
    What is height of toilet seat from floor? _____
    Are there bars or sturdy supports near toilet? _____
    Is there room for grab bars? _____
Can patient use sink? _____ What is height of sink? _____
    Is patient able to reach and turn off faucets? _____
    Is there knee space beneath sink? _____
    Is patient able to reach necessary articles? _____
        mirror? _____ electrical outlet? _____
Bathing
    Does patient take tub bath? _____ shower? _____ sponge
        bath? _____
    If using tub, can patient safely transfer without
        assistance? _____
    Bars or sturdy supports present beside tub? _____
    Is equipment necessary? (tub seat, handspray attachment,
        tub rail, no-skid strips, grab rails, other _____)
    Can patient manage faucets and drain plug? _____
    Height of tub from floor to rim _____
    Is tub built-in _____ or on legs? _____
    Width of tub from the inside _____
    If uses separate shower stall, can patient transfer independently
        and manage faucets? _____
    If patient takes sponge bath, describe method. _____
    _____
    _____

LIVING ROOM AREA

Light switch accessible? _____ Can patient open and close window? _____

Can furniture be rearranged to allow manipulation of wheelchair? _____

Can patient transfer from wheelchair to and from sturdy chair? _____
Height of chair _____

Can patient transfer from wheelchair to and from sofa? _____
Height of sofa _____

Can ambulatory patient transfer to and from chair? _____ sofa? _____

Can patient manage television and radio? _____

DINING ROOM

Light switch accessible? _____

Is patient able to use table? _____ Height of table _____

KITCHEN

What is the table height? _____ Can wheelchair fit under? _____

Can patient open refrigerator door and take food? _____

Can patient open freezer door and take food? _____

Sink
   Can patient be seated at sink? _____
   Can patient reach faucets? _____ Turn them on and off? _____
   Can patient reach bottom of basin? _____

Shelves and cabinets
   Can patient open and close? _____
   Can patient reach dishes, pots, silver, and food? _____
   Comments:

Transport
   Can patient carry utensils from one part of kitchen to another? _____
Stove
   Can patient reach and manipulate controls? _____
   Light pilot on oven? _____
   Manage oven door? _____
   Place food in oven and remove? _____
   Manage broiler door? _____
   Put food in and remove? _____
Other Appliances
   Can patient reach and turn on appliances? _____
   Can patient use outlets? _____
Counter space: Is there enough for storage and work area? _____
Diagram (include stove, refrigerator, sink, table, counters, others if applicable)

LAUNDRY

If patient has no facilities, how will laundry be managed?

Location of facilities in home or apartment and description of facilities present:

Can patient reach laundry area? _____

Can patient use washing machine and dryer? _____
   Load and empty? _____
   Manage doors and controls? _____

Can patient use sink? _____
   What is height of sink? _____
   Able to reach and turn on faucets? _____
   Knee space beneath sink? _____
   Able to reach necessary articles? _____

Is laundry cart available? _____

Can patient hang clothing on line? _____

Ironing board _____
   Location: _____
      Is it kept open? _____
      If not kept open, can patient set up and take down ironing board? _____
   Can patient reach outlet? _____

CLEANING

Can patient remove mop, broom, vacuum, pail from storage? _____

Use equipment? (mop, broom, vacuum and so forth) _____

EMERGENCY

Location of telephone in house:

Could patient use fire escape or back door in a hurry if alone? _____

Does patient have numbers for neighbors, police, fire and physician? _____

OTHER

Will patient be responsible for child care? _____
   If so, give number of children _____ and ages: _____
Will patient do own shopping? _____
   Is family member or friend available? _____
   Is delivery service available? _____
Does family have automobile? _____
Is family member or friend available to help with lawn care, changing high light bulbs, and so forth? _____

APPENDIX B

Building Survey Form

Name of building: _____ Date of survey: _____

Location: _____ Surveyor: _____

	Yes	No

PARKING AREA

1. Are accessible parking spaces with adjacent access aisle to accommodate a wheelchair available? _____ _____
2. Are curb cutouts available and appropriately labeled? _____ _____
3. Are parking spaces easily accessible to walkway without requiring negotiating behind parked cars? _____ _____
4. Indicate number of accessible parking spaces available. _____ _____

ENTRANCES TO BUILDING

1. Is at least one major entrance available for use by an individual using a wheelchair? _____ _____
2. Does the entrance provide access to a level where elevators are available? _____ _____

ELEVATORS

1. Is a passenger elevator available? _____ _____
2. Does the elevator reach all levels of the building? _____ _____
3. Are control buttons (both inside and outside of the elevator) no more than 48 in (122 cm) from the floor? _____ _____
4. Are control buttons raised and easy to push? _____ _____
5. Is an emergency telephone accessible? _____ _____

PUBLIC TELEPHONES

1. Are an appropriate number of phones available and accessible to individuals using a wheelchair? _____ _____
2. Are they dial or pushbutton? _____ _____
3. Is the height of the dial mechanism no more than 44 in (112 cm) from the floor? _____ _____
4. Is a receiver volume control available? _____ _____

FLOOR SURFACES

1. Are surfaces nonslip? _____ _____
2. If carpeting is present, is it tightly woven and securely glued to floor (to prevent rippling under wheelchair)? _____ _____

REST ROOMS

1. Is there an adequate number of accessible rest rooms available? _____ _____
2. Is there at least 48 in (122 cm) between inside wall and partitions enclosing toilet? _____ _____
3. Is entrance to cubicle at least 48 in (122 cm) wide? _____ _____
4. Are grab bars present and securely mounted? _____ _____
5. Is height of seat not more than 17.5 in (44.5 cm)? _____ _____
6. Is toilet paper holder within easy reach? _____ _____
7. Is adequate turning space (6 ft × 6 ft [183 cm × 183 cm]) available in main area of rest room? _____ _____
8. Is there adequate space for clearance of knees under sink? _____ _____
9. Are drain and hot-water pipes covered or shielded to avoid burns? _____ _____
10. Are faucet handles large (blade-type) and accessible? _____ _____

WATER FOUNTAINS

1. Is the fountain height appropriate for use by someone in a wheelchair? _____ _____
2. Are controls pushbutton or blade-type? _____ _____
3. Is a foot control available? _____ _____
4. Is adequate space (at least 3 ft [92 cm]) provided near fountain to permit wheelchair mobility? _____ _____

From Cotler, SR, and DeGraff, AH: Architectural Accessibility for the Disabled of College Campuses. New York State Univ. Construction Fund, Albany, 1976.

APPENDIX C: Americans with Disabilities Act (ADA) Information Resources

US DEPARTMENT OF JUSTICE

Civil Rights Division
Disability Rights Section
PO Box 66738
Washington, DC 20035-6738
Documents and Information:
800.514.0301 (Voice)
800.514.0383 (TDD)
Electronic Bulletin Board:
202.514.6193
Internet:
http://www.usdoj.gov/crt/ada/adahom1.htm

US EQUAL EMPLOYMENT OPPORTUNITY COMMISSION (EEOC)

1801 L Street, NW
Washington, DC 20507
Documents:
800.669.3362 (Voice)
800.800.3302 (TDD)
Questions and Information:
800.669.4000 (Voice)
800.669.6820 (TDD)
Internet:
http://www.eeoc.gov/

US DEPARTMENT OF TRANSPORTATION

Federal Transit Administration
400 Seventh Street, SW
Washington, DC 20590
Documents and Information:
202.366.1656 (Voice)
202.366.4567 (TDD)
Electronic Bulletin Board:
202.366.3764
Internet:
http://www.fta.dot.gov

US ARCHITECTURAL AND TRANSPORTATION BARRIERS COMPLIANCE BOARD

1331 F Street, NW (Suite 1000)
Washington, DC 20004-1111
Documents and Information:
800.872.2253 (Voice)
800.993.2822 (TDD)
Electronic Bulletin Board:
202.272.5448
Internet:
http://www.access-board.gov/
e-mail:
news@access-board.gov

PRESIDENT'S COMMITTEE ON EMPLOYMENT OF PEOPLE WITH DISABILITIES

Job Accommodation Network (JAN)
West Virginia University
PO Box 6080
Morgantown, West Virginia 26506-6080
Accommodation Information:
800.526.7234 (Voice and TDD)
ADA Information:
800.232.9675 (Voice and TDD)
Internet:
http://janweb.icdi.wvu.edu/english/homeus.htm
e-mail:
jan@jan.icdi.wvu.edu

FEDERAL COMMUNICATIONS COMMISSION

1919 M Street, NW, Room 254
Washington, DC 20554
Information:
202.418.0200 (Voice)
202.418.2555 (TDD)
Internet:
http://www.fcc.gov
e-mail:
psd@fcc.gov

APPENDIX D

Suggested Answers to Case Study Guiding Questions

With general knowledge of the patient's living space, what environmental modifications, adaptive equipment, or additional instruction would you suggest or provide to optimize safety and function in each of the following areas of the home?

1. Bedroom
ANSWER:
- Remove two small area rugs (recommend use of nonskid waxes).
- Recommend the addition of a cordless phone to the nightstand.
- A lamp should be placed on the nightstand (with an on/off control switch easily accessed by the patient).
- The height of the sleeping surface should be raised sufficiently to maintain the hip at no greater than a 90 degree angle when seated at bedside.

2. Bathroom
ANSWER:
- Remove area rug.
- Recommend a raised toilet seat and side grab bar.
- Recommend a tub transfer bench and hand-spray attachment to the bathtub faucet.
- Instruct the patient in techniques to cross a narrow doorway threshold using crutches.

3. Kitchen
ANSWER:
- Recommend use of nonskid waxes.

- Move centrally located dining table next to wall to provide more clear floor space.
- Suggest use of a small rolling cart to transport items from one area or surface to another.
- Provide patient instruction in task modification using energy conservation techniques.
- Recommend use of appropriate adaptive equipment such as reachers (to retrieve items both from the floor and high shelves), electric can openers, jar openers, and so forth.

4. Livingroom
ANSWER:
- Raise the seating surface of the patient's favorite chair; all seating surfaces should be firm (i.e., use of dense foam).
- Move centrally located coffee table next to wall to provide more clear floor space.
- Place telephone adjacent to the patient's chair and eliminate extra-long extension wire.
- Either remove large carpet or tack it to the floor to avoid rippling.
- Recommend a universal remote control unit for the television.

5. Hallway
ANSWER:
- Remove narrow area rug.
- Address the dim lighting by installation of track lighting, battery operated lighting units, or some other mechanism to fully illuminate the dim area.

Strategies to Improve Motor Control and Motor Learning

Susan B. O'Sullivan

LEARNING OBJECTIVES

1. Describe models for clinical decision making that incorporate components of normal motor control and motor learning.
2. Identify factors critical to motor control and describe intervention strategies designed to optimize the acquisition of motor control.
3. Identify factors critical to motor learning and describe intervention strategies designed to optimize learning.
4. Differentiate between the following approaches to intervention: compensatory training, remediation/facilitation, and functional/task-oriented training.
5. Analyze and interpret patient data, formulate realistic goals and outcomes, and develop a plan of care that presents an integrated approach to treatment when presented with a clinical case study.

Developing strategies to improve motor control and motor learning requires a thorough understanding of the neural processes involved in producing movement and learning, and the pathologies that may affect the central nervous system (CNS). In addition, knowledge of recovery processes following CNS insult is essential. Treatment models based on theories of motor control and learning allow the therapist to organize thinking and approach clinical decision making in a coherent manner. Patients with disorders of motor function frequently demonstrate a wide variety of impairments, functional limitations, and disabilities. Careful assessment of motor and learning behaviors and the environmental contexts in which they occur provides an appropriate base for planning. Many of these assessments are discussed in preceding chapters. A number of different treatment approaches and techniques have been developed by physical therapists to address disorders of motor function. An optimal plan of care must address the individual needs of the patient, maintain a focus on functional limitations and physical disabilities, and enhance overall quality of life.

OVERVIEW OF MOTOR CONTROL

Motor control has been defined as "an area of study dealing with the understanding of the neural, physical, and behavioral aspects of movement."[1] p 416 Information processing of human motor behavior occurs in stages (Fig. 13-1). The initial stage is termed the *stimulus identification*. Relevant stimuli concerning current body state and environmental context are selected and identified. Meaning is attached based on past sensorimotor experiences. Perceptual and cognitive processes including memory contact, attention, motivation, and emotional control all play an integral role in ensuring the ease and accuracy of information processing during this stage. Selection of relevant sensory input is sensitive to the clarity and intensity of the stimuli received. Thus, stronger and crisper stimuli result in enhanced attentional mechanisms and information processing. Processing is also influenced by stimulus pattern complexity. Complicated, novel patterns of stimuli prolong stimulus identification. An intrinsic knowledge of movement (e.g., position of limb, length of limb, distance to goal, etc.) is a critical characteristic of motor behavior. In the *response selection stage* the plan for movement is developed.

A **motor plan** is defined as an idea or plan for purposeful movement that is made up of component motor programs. A general rather than detailed response is selected; that is, a prototype of the final

movement. Decision making during this stage is sensitive to the number of different movement alternatives possible and the overall compatibility between the stimulus and response. The more natural the association between stimulus and response, the easier the decision making. For example, in a well-learned movement like crossing at a street light, an individual easily responds to the green light by moving forward. If a crossing guard signals the individual to move forward even though the light is red, the individual is likely to be more hesitant in responding.

The final stage is termed *response programming*. Neural control centers translate and change the idea for movement into muscular actions. The structuring of motor programs includes attention to specific parameters such as synergistic component parts, force, direction, timing, duration, and extent of movement. Parametric specification is based on the constraints of the individual, the task, and the environment. Information processing during this stage is sensitive to the complexity of the desired movement and duration. Thus, complex and lengthier movement sequences increase the duration of processing during this stage. Programming can also be affected by response-response compatibility. This is the compatibility for dual movement tasks that either occur simultaneously (e.g., bouncing a ball while walking) or when choices are required (e.g., one paired movement response must occur before another). During response execution (movement output), muscles are selected against an appropriate background of postural control. **Feedforward,** the sending of signals in advance of movement to ready the system, allows for anticipatory adjustments in postural activity. **Feedback,** response-produced information received during or after the movement, is used to monitor output for corrective actions. Although this simplified model gives the appearance that the information flow is linear, actual processing by the CNS is both serial and parallel. Thus, both single and multiple pathways are engaged to process information.[1] Figure 13-2 provides a schematic description of the major directions of information flow within the CNS during voluntary movement.

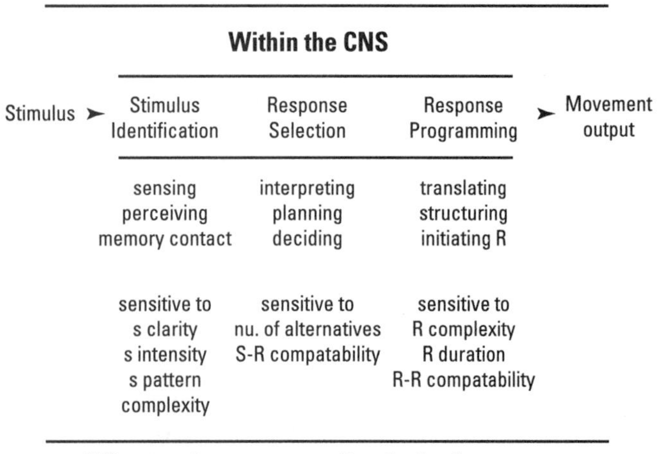

Theories of Motor Control

A theory is the orderly explanation of observations. Different theories of motor control have been developed over time, and reflect current understanding and interpretation of nervous system function. Because theories provide an important framework for clinical practice, a brief overview is warranted. The reader is also referred to the excellent works of Schmidt[1] and Shumway-Cook and Woollacott[2] for further review and study.

An early theory of motor control, *reflex theory,* was established by Sherrington.[3] His research on sensory receptors led to the view that movement was the result of a stimulus-response sequence of events or **reflex** based. Complex movements were nothing

---

Within the CNS

Stimulus ➤	Stimulus Identification	Response Selection	Response Programming	➤ Movement output
	sensing perceiving memory contact	interpreting planning deciding	translating structuring initiating R	
	sensitive to s clarity s intensity s pattern complexity	sensitive to nu. of alternatives S-R compatability	sensitive to R complexity R duration R-R compatability	

CNS = central nervous system, S = stimulus, R = response

Figure 13-1. Model of information-processing stages of movement control.

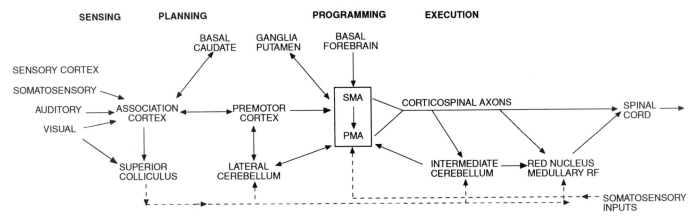

Figure 13-2. Major directions of information flow during a voluntary movement to and from the primary motor areas (PMA) and supplementary motor areas (SMA), only some of the connections of the superior colliculus are shown. (RF = reticular formation.) From Brooks,[5] p 199, with permission.

more than the coupling or chaining together of a number of reflexes to produce the final outcome. Thus, sensation assumed a primary role in the initiation and production of movement. Limitations in reflex theory abound. It fails to consider that voluntary movements can be activated in the absence of a sensory stimulus. It also fails to consider that some movements occur so fast as to not allow use of available feedback. Finally, it fails to consider the infinite variability that allows for different movements in response to the same stimulus.[2]

Hierarchical theory dates back to the work of Hughlings Jackson.[4] This theory is based on the assumption that the CNS is organized into three primary levels of control: high, middle, and low centers. Control was viewed as proceeding in a descending direction from higher to lower centers, a "top-down" progression. Reflex theory integrated with hierarchical theory presents the view that reflexes are components of the lower centers that became integrated during normal maturation and development as higher centers assumed control. Conversely reflexes reemerge in control of movement when higher centers become damaged. A more current interpretation of this model proposes a theory of *flexible hierarchies*.[5] Within this theory, the command hierarchies have been more fully described. The association cortex operates as the highest level (elaborating perceptions and planning strategies), while the sensorimotor cortex in association with portions of the basal ganglia, brainstem, and cerebellum function as the middle level (converting strategies into motor programs and commands). The spinal cord functions as the lowest level, translating commands into muscle actions resulting in the execution of movement (see Fig. 13-2). Modern hierarchical theory proposes that the three levels do not operate in a rigid, top-down order but rather as a flexible system in which each level can exert control on the others. Shifts in control are dependent on the demands and complexity of the task with the higher centers assuming control whenever the task requires.

Systems theory, proposed by Bernstein,[6] is based on the view that motor control is the result of the cooperative actions of many interacting systems, working to accommodate the demands of the specific task. Both internal factors (joint stiffness, inertia, movement-dependent forces) and external factors (gravity) must be taken into consideration in the planning of movements. It assumes a shifting locus of neural control, referred to as a *distributed model of control*. Thus, large areas of the CNS may be engaged for complex motor tasks while relatively few centers are engaged for more discrete movements. This type of multilevel control allows for the control of a number of separate independent dimensions of movement, termed **degrees of freedom.** The executive level is freed from the responsibility of control for simple movements or the demands of having to control many degrees of freedom at one time. **Coordinative structures** are used to simplify control, and to initiate coordinate patterns or synergies to produce movements. The use of synergies for the control of locomotion (central pattern generators) and posture (postural synergies) is well documented.[7]

Motor Programming

A **motor program** is defined as "an abstract representation that, when initiated, results in the production of a coordinated movement sequence."[1] p 225 Motor programs allow for movements to occur in the absence of sensation (deafferentation) or in situations where limitations in speed of processing feedback negates control (rapid movements). Motor programs also free up the nervous system from conscious decisions about movement, reducing the problem of multiple degrees of freedom. Motor programs can be run off virtually without the influence of peripheral feedback or error detection processes, termed an **open-loop control system** (Fig. 13-3). This is in contrast to a **closed-loop control system** (Fig. 13-4), which employs feedback and a reference for correctness to compute error and initiate subsequent corrections. Feedback and closed-loop pro-

MOTOR FUNCTION

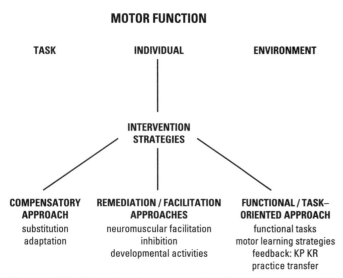

Figure 13-3. Motor function emerges from interaction among the task, the individual, and the environment. Intervention strategies to improve motor function consist of compensatory, remediation/facilitation, and functional/task-oriented strategies. KP = knowledge of performance, KR = knowledge of results.

cesses play a critical role in the learning of new motor skills (response selection) and in the shaping and correction of ongoing movements (response execution). Feedback is also essential for the ongoing maintenance of body posture and balance.[1]

The complexity of human movement negates any simplistic model of movement control. An **intermittent control hypothesis** described by Schmidt[1] proposes a blending of both open-loop and closed-loop processes, in which both operate in concert as part of the larger system. Motor programs provide the generalized code for motor events **(schema)**, while feedback is used to refine and perfect movements. Either may assume a dominant role, depending on the task at hand. Both may operate within a given movement but at different times and with different functions.

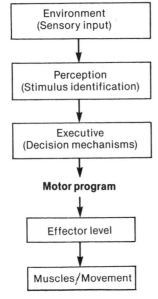

Figure 13-4. Open-loop control system.

Generalized motor programs include both invariant characteristics and parameters. **Invariant characteristics** are the unique features of the stored code: relative force, relative timing, and order of components. **Parameters** are the changeable features that ensure flexibility of motor programs and variations in movements from one performance to the next. These include overall force and overall duration of the movement. For example, walking performance can be changed by speeding up or slowing down (changes in overall duration) while the basic order of stepping cycle and relative timing of the components (invariant characteristics) are maintained.[8] Patients with deficits in motor function may demonstrate impairments in voluntary movements (impaired motor planning or programming) or the corrective actions (feedback adjustments) needed to initially learn and coordinate movements.

OVERVIEW OF MOTOR LEARNING

Motor learning has been defined as "a set of internal processes associated with practice or experience leading to relatively permanent changes in the capability for skilled behavior."[1] p 375 Learning a motor skill is a complex process that requires spatial, temporal, and hierarchical organization of the CNS. Changes in the CNS are not directly observable but rather are inferred from changes in motor behavior. Improvements in **performance** result from practice or experience and are a frequently used measure of learning. For example, with practice an individual is able to develop appropriate sequencing of movement components with improved timing and reduced effort and concentration. Performance, however, is not always an accurate reflection of learning. It is possible to practice enough to temporarily improve performance but not retain the learning. Conversely, factors such as fatigue, anxiety, poor motivation, or medications may cause performance to deteriorate while learning may still occur. Because performance can be affected by a number of factors, it can be reasonably defined as a "temporary change in motor behavior seen during practice sessions."[2] p 24 **Retention** provides a better measure of learning. The learner is able to demonstrate the skill over time and after a period of no practice (a **retention interval**). Performance after a retention interval may decrease slightly, but should return to original performance levels within relatively few practice trials. For example, riding a bike is a well-learned skill that is generally retained even though an individual may not have ridden a bike for years. The ability to apply a learned skill to the learning of other similar tasks, termed **generalizability,** is another important measure of learning. Individuals who learn to transfer from wheelchair to platform mat can apply that learning to other types of transfers (e.g., wheelchair to car, wheelchair to tub). The time and effort required to organize and learn these new types of transfers is reduced. Finally, learning can be measured by **resistance to contextual change.** This is the adaptability required to perform a motor task in altered environmental situations. Thus, an individual who has learned a skill (e.g., walking with a cane) should be able to apply that learning to new and variable situations (e.g., walking outdoors, walking on a busy sidewalk). Motor learning is the direct result of practice and is highly dependent on sensory information and feedback processes. The relative importance of the different types of sensory information varies according to task and to the phase of learning. Individual differences exist and may influence both the rate and degree of learning possible. Impairments in learning are common for the patient with CNS dysfunction.

Theories of Motor Learning

Adams[9] developed a theory of motor learning based on closed-loop control (closed-loop theory). He postulated that sensory feedback from ongoing movement is compared with stored memory of the intended movement (perceptual trace) to provide the CNS with a reference of correctness and error detection. Memory traces are then used to produce an appropriate action and to evaluate outcomes. The stronger the perceptual trace developed through practice, the greater the capability of the learner to use closed-loop processes and acquire movements. Adams concentrated on examining slow, linear-positioning responses. This theory does not adequately explain learning under conditions of rapid movements (open-loop control processes). It also does not explain learning that can occur in the absence of sensory feedback (deafferentation studies).

Schema theory is based on the concepts that slow movements are feedback-based while rapid movements are program-based. Schmidt[10] proposed using the term schema rather than detailed motor programs for storage into memory. He defined schema as "a rule, concept, or relationship formed on the basis of experience."[1] p 418 Schema include such things as initial conditions (body position, weight of objects, etc.), relationships between parameters of movement, environmental outcomes, and sensory consequences of movement. Recall (motor) schema are used to select and define the initial movement conditions while recognition schema are used to evaluate movement responses based on expected sensory consequences. Clinically, this theory supports the concept that practicing a variety of movement outcomes would improve learning through the development of expanded rules or schema.[1] It also provides a plausible explanation for the learning of novel and open skills performed in a variable and changing environment.

Stages of Motor Learning

The process of motor learning has been described by Fitts and Posner[11] as occurring in relatively distinct stages, termed cognitive, associated, and autonomous. These stages provide a useful framework for describing the learning process and for organizing strategies. Table 13–1 provides a summary of this model of information.

COGNITIVE STAGE

During the initial **cognitive stage** of learning, the major task at hand is to develop an overall understanding of the skill, termed the *cognitive map* or cognitive plan. This decision making phase of "what to do" requires a high level of cognitive processing as the learner performs successive approximations of the task, discarding strategies that are not successful and retaining those that are. The resulting trial-and-error practice initially yields uneven performance. Processing of sensory cues and perceptual-motor organization eventually leads to the selection of a motor program that proves reasonably successful. Because the learner progresses from an initially disorganized and often clumsy pattern to more organized movements, improvements in performance can be readily observed during this acquisition phase. The learner relies primarily on vision to guide learning and movement. A stable environment free from distractors optimizes learning during this initial stage.

ASSOCIATIVE STAGE

During the middle or **associative stage** of learning, refinement of the motor program is achieved through practice. Spatial and temporal aspects become organized as the movement develops into a coordinated pattern. Performance improves, with greater consistency and fewer errors and extraneous movements. The learner is now concentrating on "how to do" the movement rather than on what movement to do. Proprioceptive cues become increasingly important, while dependence on visual cues decreases. The learning process takes varying lengths of time depending on a number of factors. The nature of the task, prior experience and motivation of the learner, available feedback, and organization of practice can all influence acquisition of learning.

AUTONOMOUS STAGE

The final or **autonomous stage** of learning is characterized by motor performance that after considerable practice is largely automatic. There is only a minimal level of cognitive monitoring of movement, with motor programs so refined they can almost "run themselves." The spatial and temporal components of movement are becoming highly organized, and the learner is capable of coordinated motor patterns. The learner is now free to concentrate on other aspects, such as "how to succeed" at a competitive sport. Movements are largely error-free with little interference from environmental distractions. Thus the learner can perform equally well in an unchanging, predictable environment (termed **closed skills**) or in a changing, unpredictable environment (termed **open skills**).

Table 13–1 STAGES OF MOTOR LEARNING AND TRAINING STRATEGIES

Cognitive Stage Characteristics	Training Strategies
The learner develops an understanding of task; **cognitive mapping** assesses abilities, task demands; identifies stimuli, contacts memory; selects response; performs initial approximations of task; structures motor program; modifies initial responses *"What to do"* decision	Highlight purpose of task in functionally relevant terms. Demonstrate ideal performance of task to establish a **reference of correctness.** Have patient verbalize task components and requirements. Point out similarities to other learned tasks. Direct attention to critical task elements. Select appropriate feedback. • Emphasize intact sensory systems, intrinsic feedback systems. • Carefully pair extrinsic feedback with intrinsic feedback. • High dependence on vision: have patient watch movement. • **Knowledge of Performance** (KP): focus on errors as they become consistent; do not cue on large number of random errors. • **Knowledge of Results** (KR): focus on success of movement outcome. Ask learner to evaluate performance, outcomes; identify problems, solutions. Use reinforcements (praise) for correct performance, continuing motivation. Organize feedback schedule. • Feedback after every trial improves performance during early learning. • Variable feedback (summed, fading, bandwidth designs) increases depth of cognitive processing, improves retention; may decrease performance initially. Organize initial practice. • Stress controlled movement to minimize errors. • Provide adequate rest periods (distributed practice) if task is complex, long, or energy costly or if learner fatigues easily, has short attention, or poor concentration. • Use manual guidance to assist as appropriate. • Break complex tasks down into component parts, teach both parts and integrated whole. • Utilize bilateral transfer as appropriate. • Use blocked (repeated) practice of same task to improve performance. • Use variable practice (serial or random practice order) of related skills to increase depth of cognitive processing and retention; may decrease performance initially. • Use mental practice to improve performance and learning, reduce anxiety. Assess, modify arousal levels as appropriate. • High or low arousal impairs performance and learning. • Avoid stressors, mental fatigue. Structure environment. • Reduce extraneous environmental stimuli, distractors to ensure attention, concentration. • Emphasize closed skills initially gradually progressing to open skills.
Associated Stage Characteristics	**Training Strategies**
The learner practices movements, refines motor program: spatial and temporal organization; decreases errors, extraneous movements Dependence on visual feedback decreases, increases for use of proprioceptive feedback; cognitive monitoring decreases *"How to do"* decision	Select appropriate feedback. • Continue to provide KP; intervene when errors become consistent. • Emphasize proprioceptive feedback, "feel of movement" to assist in establishing an internal reference of correctness. • Continue to provide KR; stress relevance of functional outcomes. • Assist learner to improve self-evaluation, decision making skills. • Facilitation techniques, guided movements may be counterproductive during this stage of learning. Organize feedback schedule. • Continue to provide feedback for continuing motivation; encourage patient to self-assess achievements. • Avoid excessive augmented feedback. • Focus on use of variable feedback (summed, fading, bandwidth) designs to improve retention. Organize practice. • Encourage consistency of performance. • Focus on variable practice order (serial or random) of related skills to improve retention. Structure environment. • Progress toward open, changing environment. • Prepare the learner for home, community, work environments.
Autonomous Stage Characteristics	**Training Strategies**
The learner practices movements, continues to refine motor responses, spatial and temporal highly organized, movements are largely error-free, minimal level of cognitive monitoring *"How to succeed"* decision	Assess need for conscious attention, automaticity of movements. Select appropriate feedback. • Learner demonstrates appropriate self-evaluation, decision making skills. • Provide occasional feedback (KP, KR) when errors evident. Organize practice. • Stress consistency of performance in variable environments, variations of tasks (open skills). • High levels of practice (massed practice) are appropriate. Structure environment. • Vary environments to challenge learner. • Ready the learner for home, community, work environments. Focus on competitive aspects of skills as appropriate, e.g., wheelchair sports.

DEVELOPMENTAL PERSPECTIVE

Control of posture and movement is a continuously evolving process that proceeds throughout the life-span. Fundamentals of movement skills are learned as a child with the emergence of specific markers of developmental maturation.[12–15] In the adult, age-related factors result in modification and adaptation of motor behaviors.[16–19] Skills are modified when changes in body dimensions occur (e.g., changes in body weight and height). All stages of information processing are affected by aging.[20] Sensory losses (decline in receptor sensitivity, recognition, and sensory encoding) affect stimulus identification. Response selection and programming are also affected by CNS changes. An age-related slowing of movements is well documented with increases noted in both reaction and movement times.[21] Coordination changes result from changes in motor unit size with deficits particularly noticeable in fine motor control. Older adults are also more sensitive to complexity of movement.[22] Decreasing levels of cardiovascular fitness and strength commonly associated with a sedentary life-style can also affect the performance of motor skills.[22–25] Finally, older adults often experience multiple disease pathologies and insults that may affect their ability to move and learn.[26] For example, an older adult may alter the method used to roll over and sit up secondary to an increase in body weight, a decrease in overall strength and fitness, or an emerging pathology.

Developmental theory focuses on the orderly acquisition of motor skills. As children develop, practice and experience of a number of different skills is required. These postures and activities are often termed **developmental activities or skills** although they remain important functional skills throughout life. Rolling, rising from supine to sitting, prone-on-elbows, quadruped, sitting, kneeling, half-kneeling, plantigrade, sitting to standing, standing, and walking are examples of these activities. Progression through a sequence of activities can be used to address the degrees of freedom problem in the acquisition of motor control and in treatment. For example, the prone-on-elbows posture focuses on development of shoulder, upper trunk, and head control while eliminating all demands for movement control in the lower body. Because the center of gravity is low and the base of support wide in many of the early developmental activities, they are inherently safe and reduce the likelihood of injury from falls when control is lacking. It is clear that considerable variability exists in the development of children and that there is no rigid developmental sequence of events for all children. It is also true that although these activities provide an important base for functional training in older adults, a specific sequence of activities cannot be applied. Because motor programs, subroutines, and postural sets already exist in the adult patient, the major issues in relearning a motor skill following brain injury include accessing, reorganizing, and utilizing this information. This is a very different situation from that of the child who has not yet developed motor skills.

RECOVERY OF FUNCTION

Recovery of function is the "re-acquisition of movement skills lost through injury."[2] p 23 In its strictest definition, the performance of the reacquired skills is identical in every way to pre-injury performance. In a less strict interpretation of recovery, performance is achieved through variations in the original premorbid movement patterns. *Compensation* is defined as "behavioral substitution, that is, alternative behavioral strategies are adopted to complete a task."[2] p 38 For example, the patient recovering from stroke may learn to dress independently using the non-affected upper extremity.

Brain injury was for a long time thought to be permanent with little potential for brain repair and recovery. This is now viewed as incorrect and can represent a dangerous self-fulfilling prophecy when applied to the individual who suffers from such injuries. **Neural plasticity** has been defined as "the ability of the brain to change and repair itself."[27] p 134 Several explanations have been offered to account for plasticity. Different and underutilized areas of the brain can take over the functions of damaged tissue, a process called **vicariance.** Another view holds that the CNS has back-up or fail-safe systems that become operational when the primary system breaks down, called **redundancy.** The unmasking of new (redundant) neuron pathways permits function to be maintained. Areas of the brain are also capable of becoming reprogrammed, a process termed **functional substitution.** An example of functional substitution is the increased sensitivity of the hands as a sensory information system for the person who becomes blind. The adoption of compensatory strategies leads to structural reorganization within the brain and enhanced function. The term **diaschisis** is used to refer to the recovery of brain activity after the resolution of temporary blocking factors (i.e., shock, edema, decreased blood flow, decreased glucose utilization). Evidence from positive emission tomography (PET scan) studies suggest that recovery is a complex process, and may involve all of the above processes. Following injury, changes in the brain are widespread. Blood flow changes suggestive of neural activity have been found to exist on both sides of the brain and in both cortical and subcortical structures, areas that are remote from the injured site. Nerve growth and repair of brain tissue have been demonstrated following brain injury. These responses may be adaptive (functional) or maladaptive (nonfunctional). The presence of trophic molecules (nerve growth factors) has been shown to play a key role in the development of growth and repair processes and is a topic of ongoing research. For an excellent review of brain repair processes the reader is referred to the work of Stein et al.[27]

Factors Contributing to Recovery of Function

Recovery of function is influenced by multiple factors. Age is an important determinant of recovery. A general belief exists that the younger the age, the greater the plasticity of the nervous system. However, regional variability in brain maturation may influence the results of injury-induced recovery. Once maturation is complete and specialized function of brain tissue is present, plasticity is reduced.

An injury that occurs slowly over time is likely to produce an improved recovery outcome when compared to an injury that is rapid. For example, slow-growing lesions like tumors are linked to better conservation of function and improved recovery outcomes in comparison to rapid lesions such as stroke. In this example, the brain is able to functionally adapt over time. Smaller lesions and lesions serially induced (with time intervals in between) also result in improved functional outcomes when compared to a single large lesion.

Beneficial effects have been demonstrated in animal studies by placement in enriched environments. The sensory experiences from exposure to an enriched environment provide a level of brain stimulation that appears to assist in brain development, maintenance of function, and brain repair after injury. Animals exposed to impoverished or standard cage environments demonstrated less recovery than those placed in enriched settings. Active participation is critical in obtaining positive benefits from an enriched environment. Animals that were restrained and passively moved in the enriched environments demonstrated less recovery than animals allowed to actively interact with the enriched environments. Use of specific training activities as opposed to nonspecific environmental exposure has also been shown to assist recovery. Animals exposed to training tasks (e.g., general activity on a training wheel) demonstrated improved recovery, although not as great as those exposed to environmental and sensory enrichment. Thus, both environment and activity assist in inducing functional reorganization of the cerebral cortex. This has been expressed as "changing behavior also changes physiology."[27] p 131 For an excellent discussion of this topic as it applies to the field of rehabilitation the reader is referred to the work of Held.[28]

FRAMEWORK FOR INTERVENTION

Various different therapeutic approaches have been developed for the rehabilitation of patients with disorders of motor function (Fig. 13-5). Historically many practical treatment ideas have resulted from empirical-clinical knowledge. Theory has been applied to explain the success of these interventions and to organize them into a coherent treatment philosophy. Differences result from the interpretation of theory and on the assumptions made regarding function of the CNS.

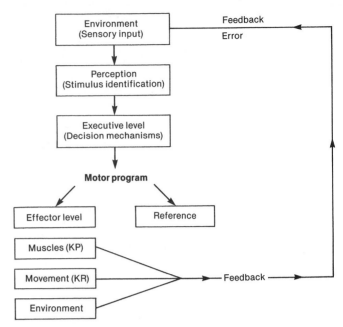

Figure 13-5. Closed-loop control system. KP = knowledge of performance, KR = knowledge of results.

Compensatory Training Approach

The focus of a **compensatory training approach** is on the early resumption of functional independence using the uninvolved or less involved segments for function. For example, the patient with left hemiplegia is taught to dress using the right upper extremity; the patient with paraplegia regains functional mobility and wheelchair independence using the upper extremities. Central to this approach is the concept of substitution. The patient is first made aware of movement deficiencies (cognitive awareness is developed). Changes are then made in the patient's overall approach to functional tasks. Alternate ways to accomplish the task are suggested, simplified, and adopted. The patient practices and relearns the task using the new pattern. The patient then practices the new pattern in the environment in which the function is expected to occur. Energy conservation techniques are incorporated to ensure the patient can successfully complete all daily tasks.

A second central tenet of this approach is modification of the environment **(adaptation)** to facilitate relearning of skills, ease of movement, and optimal performance. For example, the patient with unilateral neglect is assisted in dressing by color coding of the shoes (red tape on the left shoe, yellow tape on the right shoe). The wheelchair brake toggle is extended and color coded to allow the patient easy identification.

One of the major criticisms of this approach is the focus on uninvolved segments may suppress recovery and contribute to **learned nonuse** of impaired segments.[29] For example, the patient with stroke fails to learn to use the involved extremities. Focus on task-specific learning may also lead to development of **splinter skills,** which are skills that cannot be easily generalized to other environments or to variations of the same task.

A compensatory training approach may be the only realistic approach possible when the patient presents with severe impairments and functional losses with very little expectation for additional recovery. Patients with severe sensorimotor deficits and extensive co-morbidities (e.g., severe cardiac and respiratory compromise or memory deficits associated with Alzeimer's disease) may be limited in their ability to actively participate in rehabilitation and to relearn motor skills.

Remediation/Facilitation Approaches

Traditional remediation/facilitation approaches, also termed "neurotherapeutic approaches" or "neurophysiological approaches," have as their primary focus the use of therapeutic exercises and neuromuscular facilitation techniques to reduce sensorimotor deficits and promote motor recovery and improved function. The affected body segments are targeted to prevent learned nonuse[29] and overcompensation by intact segments. Thus, training using these approaches requires some degree of voluntary movement control of affected segments. Manual techniques are used to enhance control in the primary functional or developmental skills (e.g., rolling over, sitting up, standing, etc.). Training focuses on the remediation of specific impairments and the promotion of "normal" patterns of movement. These approaches include: neurodevelopmental treatment (NDT), movement therapy in hemiplegia, and proprioceptive neuromuscular facilitation (PNF) and the sensory stimulation techniques.

Neurodevelopmental treatment (NDT), a treatment approach initially developed by Drs. Karl and Berta Bobath,[30,31] identified the essential problems of the patient with neurological dysfunction (cerebral palsy and stroke) as abnormal tone and coordination. The primary cause of disordered control was thought to be the release of abnormal postural reflexes (primitive spinal cord and brainstem reflexes) with loss of higher level postural reactions (righting, equilibrium, protective extension), a concept that has been called into question.[32–34] In NDT, the patient learns to control movement through the use of the developmental sequence using activities that promote "normal" selective movements. Automatic higher level postural reactions are facilitated through the use of postural *handling* and *key points of control* (e.g., shoulders, pelvis, hands, and feet). Excessive tone is inhibited through the use of *dynamic reflex inhibiting patterns* (patterns opposite of the expected reflex influence). Sensory stimulation, specifically kinesthetic, proprioceptive, tactile, and vestibular feedback, is used to facilitate normal movement experiences. Activities are varied in terms of difficulty and environmental context. Compensatory training strategies (use of the less involved segments) are avoided for fear that development or recovery and use of the involved segments will be suppressed. Carryover is promoted through a strong emphasis on patient, family, and caregiver education.[35,36]

Movement therapy in hemiplegia, developed by Brunnstrom,[37] was designed to promote recovery in patients with stroke. Patients relearn movement control through structured activities that promote normal function. Brunnstrom was one of the first to describe the recovery stages and the stereotypical patterns of abnormal synergistic control in patients with stroke (knowledge that is applied by almost all therapists today). Many practical training activities are suggested to stimulate out-of-synergy combinations. Initially, Brunnstrom suggested that patients with low-level function should be first encouraged to gain control of the basic limb synergies and then progressed to out-of-synergy combinations simulating normal recovery. Because the repeated use of synergies made isolated joint control more difficult to obtain, this concept is now viewed as inappropriate. Sensory stimulation techniques (stretch, tapping, stroking, pressure) are used to initiate and enhance desired movement responses. Concepts of motor learning such as positive reinforcement and repetition are stressed.[38]

Coordinated movement can also be promoted using proprioceptive neuromuscular facilitation (PNF), an approach initially developed by Dr. Herman Kabat and Maggie Knott and later expanded on by Dorothy Voss.[39] PNF incorporates functional patterns of movement that are spiral and diagonal, based on normal movements. A battery of techniques, largely proprioceptive, were developed to facilitate movement (e.g., stretch, maximal resistance). Precise manual contacts are used to enhance the function of underlying muscles and completion of the desired patterns. A developmental emphasis was added later to include practice in the various different patterns of the developmental sequence (e.g., rolling, prone-on-elbows, quadruped, etc.). Individual patterns of motion and combinations of patterns are practiced to develop and reinforce needed control. PNF also incorporates a number of motor learning strategies (e.g., practice, repetition, visual guidance of movement, etc.).[40]

The incorporation of sensory stimulation techniques into the remediation/facilitation approaches is based largely on the work of Margaret Rood.[41,42] Stimuli were organized into phasic or tonic categories and applied during treatment based on the stage of control the patient exhibited. Rood utilized the terminology mobility, stability, mobility superimposed on stability, and skill to categorize stages of motor control development. This terminology has widespread application in physical therapy today. Tonic stimuli like approximation or steady resistance were used to assist the development of control in stability activities like holding in a sitting position. Phasic stimuli like quick ice and quick stretch were used to facilitate mobilizing actions of muscles, such as rolling over. Either facilitatory or inhibitory stimuli could be applied to achieve the desired movement responses.

Gordon[32] points out the dominant treatment philosophy at the time these approaches were developed was one of muscular reeducation (e.g., Kenny method), which could not be easily adapted to patients with CNS disorders. As therapists sought to develop more appropriate approaches for this group of patients, the facilitation approaches evolved. A common base was the view that the motor behavior of patients with brain damage was largely unchecked with the reflex and automatic behaviors predominating. Recovery was viewed as a process of reintegration of the CNS (progressive encephalization) to allow the higher centers to resume control. The primacy of the neurophysiological explanation for all motor phenomena following brain damage resulted in inattention to other systems and to important parameters of movement, such as biomechanical factors, strength, and so forth. Interventions were often impairment focused (e.g., tone, **posture**, etc.) rather than on function. Responding to these criticisms, current emphasis in the clinical application of NDT and PNF is more functionally based. Educational strategies for patients and caregivers are emphasized to promote carry-over of function into real life environments.

It is important to recognize that many of these treatment techniques are appropriate to use within a functional framework for patients with low function. These patients require a more "hands-on" approach to assist in their early movement attempts. This can include the use of techniques for manual assistance (guided movements) or facilitated movement. The reader is referred to Appendices A and B for more detailed description of techniques. Patients with high function capable of independent movement would not benefit from a hands-on approach. Quite the opposite, functional recovery may be impaired through the inappropriate use of assisted or facilitated movement with these patients. The prolonged nature of treatment using remediation/facilitation approaches applied to patients with low function is a frequently voiced criticism, especially in today's cost-conscious health care environment.

Functional/Task-Oriented Training Approach

A more contemporary approach is functional/task-oriented training, sometimes referred to as a **motor control/motor learning approach.** This approach integrates systems theory with motor learning theory. Its central tenet is the idea that the interacting systems within the CNS are organized around essential functional tasks and the environment in which the task is performed. Thus an understanding of tasks, the essential elements within each task, and the environment is key to understanding and promoting motor control.[43] This approach is also based on the theory that action systems within the CNS are organized to control function.[44] Advocates of this approach utilize a

training program that focuses on specific functional tasks to engage the systems (musculoskeletal, neuromuscular, etc.). Patients are instructed to practice those tasks that present difficulties for them, and to practice them in varying environments. Different strategies may be used by different individuals and should be allowed if they achieve the desired functional outcome.[45] For example, the patient with brain injury practices the functional mobility task of rising from supine-to-sitting or from sitting-to-standing. A variety of cognitive, perceptual, motor learning, and biomechanical strategies are used to enhance function. This approach represents a shift away from a focus on impairments. A hands-on approach is taken to facilitate movement and active participation of patients in learning task-specific functional skills. The patient is encouraged to be an active participant in the learning process, using perceptual-cognitive information processing to decide on the best approach to movement. Patients with severe neurological damage and cognitive impairments would not benefit from this approach.

The *motor relearning programme* (MRP) for stroke developed by Janet Carr and Roberta Shephard[46] is a good example of this approach. These authors selected several basic functional tasks including sitting up, balanced sitting, standing up and sitting down, balanced standing, and walking. The reader will recognize from previous descriptions these activities as developmental tasks. In addition they included upper limb activities (reach and grasp, etc.) and oromotor activities (jaw and lip closure, swallowing, etc.). Task performance is analyzed and activities selected for practice. The environment is modified to create an appropriate setting to promote learning and goal-directed behaviors. Complex movements are broken down into discrete parts and then practiced as a whole. Use of motor learning training strategies is an important component of this approach. Visual guidance of movement and verbal feedback (corrections) are stressed. Manual guidance of movement is limited to only those absolutely essential assists to movement. Consistency of practice, appropriate feedback and positive reinforcement, and mental stimulation are key to promoting independent function (see Table 17–10).

Integrated Approach

An understanding of how the brain regulates movement is essential to making sound clinical decisions in selecting from the diversity of approaches and interventions. Therapists must be cautious not to develop a "disciple-like" adherence to one approach. Therapists who become certified in, and a proponent of, a particular approach must be particularly cautious about over-reliance on a single group of treatment interventions. The diversity of problems experienced by patients with disordered motor function negates the idea that any one approach would be equally successful for all patients.

Although it is important to acknowledge the contributions of early theorists, contemporary management must be based on an accurate understanding of motor control and information processing. A model that emphasizes the importance of integrated functioning of the CNS where sensory, perceptual, cognitive, and motor systems cannot be separated is critical. As Mulder[47] points out, therapists need to look at an *integrated, theory-based model* for restoration of motor function. Interventions must be function based and environmentally realistic for the patient. The choice of interventions must consider those that have the greatest chance of promoting successful motor function. The choice of interventions must also take into consideration other factors, including ease of delivering care, cost-effectiveness in terms of length of stay and number of alloted physical therapy visits, age of the patient and number of co-morbidities, and potential discharge placement. The remainder of this chapter will focus on specific interventions within the framework of an integrated model.

INTERVENTION STRATEGIES TO IMPROVE MOTOR CONTROL

Arousal and Attention

The consciousness system of the body governs arousal, sleep, and attention. The reticular formation and its ascending reticular activating system (RAS) integrates sensory and cortical inputs and maintains the consciousness system. **Arousal** refers to the overall level of alertness or excitement of the cerebral cortex. Low arousal is associated with sleep or drowsiness, whereas high arousal is associated with extreme excitement or stress. **Attention** is the capacity of the brain to process information from the environment or from long-term memory. An individual with intact **selective attention** is able to screen and process relevant sensory information about both the task and the environment while screening out irrelevant information. If new information is presented, concentration and effort is increased. The autonomic nervous system (ANS) functions to establish baseline values for a number of body functions, to maintain equilibrium (homeostasis), and to initiate actions designed to adapt and protect the individual under varying conditions **(fight-or-flight response).** Overt physiological manifestations of a fight-or-flight response indicative of high arousal include elevated heart rate, increased sweating, and dilated pupils, to name but a few.

A number of factors can influence arousal including emotions, medications, time of day, or fatigue. Stimulus-specific arousal responses are activated by cortical activity (thinking) and by novel, unexpected, or threatening stimuli. A certain level of arousal is necessary for optimal motor performance. High states of arousal cause a deterioration in performance, whereas low states fail to yield the necessary responsiveness needed for effective performance. This is referred to as the **inverted U hypothesis (Yerkes-Dodson law).**[48] Different motor tasks may require different levels of arousal. For example, high arousal may improve performance on rapid, power activities. However, the same level of arousal would decrease performance on precision or fine motor tasks. Tasks that require a high degree of steadiness or decision processing are also impaired by high arousal levels. Examples of these include postural holding responses and complex motor skills. Open skills are more impaired by high arousal levels than are closed skills. Optimal arousal levels also vary according to the stage of learning, with higher arousal being more disruptive during early cognitive learning.[1]

Patients with brain damage may show decreased alertness and arousal levels (vegetative or low-level functioning states). Poor attention, selection, and identification of sensory information are characteristic. These patients may benefit from a stimulation program designed to improve generalized response levels, sometimes called a **coma stimulation program** or **early recovery management program.** Two different types of stimulation are used: environmental stimulation and structured sensory stimulation. *Environmental stimulation* involves structuring the patient's environment to provide ongoing, pleasant (nonadversive) stimuli such as music, soft lights, familiar pictures of loved ones, and so forth. **Structured sensory stimulation** involves the presentation of stimuli to the patient in an organized manner. Tactile, visual, vestibular, auditory, olfactory, and gustatory stimuli may be used[49] (see Table 13–2 and Appendix B). The therapist must examine the patient's ability to respond to a particular stimulus and carefully grade the response in terms of the behaviors produced. Decisions must be reached concerning the type of stimulation that evokes the best response in the patient, the optimal time of the day for treatment, and general length of the session. Premorbid interests often provide an important source of information in determining which stimuli are most meaningful to the patient. Stimuli should be carefully presented, one at a time, and extraneous environmental stimuli minimized. Verbal explanations should focus the patient's attention on the specific stimulus and should be kept brief and to the point. Once responsiveness (cognitive awareness) increases, the therapist should have the patient begin to discriminate particular types of stimuli and respond to stimuli with specific motor responses. Thus, touching two different textured objects, discriminating between them, and then holding the one selected requires the patient to make choices and initiate actions. Response times are frequently delayed after stimulus presentation, so extra time should be allowed for the patient to respond.[49] Overstimulation should be avoided because stimulation can also yield unexpected or paradoxical responses. For example, a patient with a brain injury does not respond to a stimulus. Re-

Table 13–2 SENSORY STIMULI USED IN MODIFYING AROUSAL LEVELS

Low Arousal State: Sensory Stimuli Are High Intensity, High Frequency Intermittent, Phasic	Response Is One of Generalized Arousal; Brief, Phasic

Auditory
  Verbal commands
  Brisk music
  Different sounds
	Orientation to sound

Visual
  Stationary targets
  Tracking targets (horizontal and vertical)
  Bright colors
	Orientation to objects

Cutaneous
  Light, moving touch
  Different textured, shaped materials
	Activation of total withdrawal patterns

Kinesthetic
  Upright positioning (wheelchair, tilt table)
  ROM, ADL tasks
	Orientation to environment and body

Vestibular
  Fast movements: angular or transient linear acceleration
  Mobile surfaces (large ball, bolster, equilibrium board)
	Increased tone
	Increased postural reactions

Olfactory/gustatory
  Different scents, tastes
  Noxious odors
	Orientation to stimuli

High Arousal State: Sensory Stimuli Are Low Intensity, Low Frequency Maintained, Tonic	**Response Is One of Generalized Calming; Maintained, Tonic**

Auditory
  Soft, soothing voice
  Soft music
  Quiet environment
	Decreased tone, decreased activity

Visual Soft, low lights	

Cutaneous
  Maintained touch
  Neutral warmth
  Slow stroking down back	

Kinesthetic Highly structured activity	Organized response

ADL, activities of daily living; ROM, range of motion.

peated stimulation may result in decreased responsiveness or a shutting down of the system. Thus, the central state of the CNS can affect the reaction of somatic systems to external stimuli.[50,51] The effectiveness of stimulation programs in influencing recovery from brain injury is inconclusive. Available research has produced variable results. Studies are flawed with methodological problems[52] and more definitive research is needed.

Agitated patients with brain injury who demonstrate excess levels of arousal and poor attention may also benefit from intervention. Frequently, sources of stimulation from the environment precipitate bouts of agitation and disorganization. The patient is generally unable to effectively process stimuli and is similarly unable to control his or her responses, which are often bizarre and combative.

Careful assessment of the environment can distinguish the offending stimuli and those that have a calming influence. The environment should be modified to eliminate or reduce irritative stimuli. For example, the patient with brain injury is often treated in a *quiet room* rather than in a busy, noisy, cluttered physical therapy gym. Because unexpected events often precipitate outbursts, consistency in total management is very important. It is important to establish a daily routine and provide overall structure. Each new activity should be carefully explained before the activity is attempted. During treatment, verbal reassurances should be provided and each successful effort should be rewarded with positive reinforcement. When agitated outbursts occur, the therapist should calmly redirect the patient's attention away from the cause of irritation. Selection of a task over which the patient has some control often helps the patient's composure. The therapist should at all times model calm, controlled behavior.[53] Therapeutic stimuli can be selected that attempt to restore homeostatic balance by promoting generalized relaxation. These include maintained touch, slow stroking, neutral warmth, or slow vestibular stimulation (see Table 13–2; Appendix B). In general, these stimuli are applied in a slow, maintained manner and are thought to produce a calming effect by influencing brainstem activity and parasympathetic outflow.

Patients with attention deficits following brain damage are unable to attend to important stimuli and process information. They often appear erratic in thought and action and are unable to concentrate on the task at hand. Impairments in cognitive function and general mental slowing are common. Deficits may be present in **focused attention** (the ability to respond to different kinds of stimulation), **sustained attention** or **vigilance** (the ability to maintain attention for a long time), selective attention (the ability to discriminate sensory information), or **divided attention** (the ability to do several tasks at one time).[54] Effective remediation of attention deficits requires careful assessment. The occupational therapist is particularly important during the assessment and planning of intervention strategies. General strategies include carefully structuring of the environment to eliminate distractors (a closed environment) and limiting information presented to the patient. Concise verbal commands with adequate volume and inflection should be used. Instructions should be short and simple. Combining instructions with demonstration is frequently a more effective strategy to engage the patient's attention than instructions alone. Eye contact with the patient should be maintained to indicate the therapist's full interest and attention. Controlled sensory cues should be provided to ensure that the important parts of the skill are attended to. Focus should be on key task elements and previous knowledge to help the patient organize new information. The patient should verbalize skills step-by-step to assist in concentration. Therapy sessions should be planned that work within the limitations of the patient's attention span. Thus, shorter periods of treatment and simple activities are more beneficial than longer treatment times and more complex tasks. Familiar activities and activities of special interest to the patient are generally more successful than novel tasks. It is important to establish a consistent daily routine, and promptly reward desired behaviors. For example, provide rewards when the patient is able to reach a predetermined time on a task.[54]

Patients who **perseverate** appear to get stuck on a thought or action and persist in repeating themselves over and over again. For example, the patient recovering from stroke persists in locking the brake on a wheelchair over and over again. These patients should be gently guided into a new activity. Use interesting activities to help refocus attention and well-defined sequences of activities to limit perservation episodes. Successful completion of a task or sequence of movements should be positively rewarded.

Cognition

Response selection follows stimulus identification and is the result of decision processing in the CNS. During this cognitive phase, an individual must determine the idea of the movement (motor plan). Components of the motor plan (motor programs) are assembled, modified, or reassembled in different order, to form the new motor pattern. General strategies to improve the cognitive phase of learning are discussed later in this chapter in the section on motor learning, the cognitive stage.

Patients who experience memory impairments demonstrate significant deficits in learning. They are unable to retrieve from memory stored perceptions of movements or previous interactions with the environment. They are also typically unable to automatically rehearse and encode new information. For example, the patient with brain damage returns to therapy the next day as if each day were totally new, with the previous daily session forgotten. Memory function may be affected by attention deficits, emotional state, or level of motivation. Thus, the use of attentional training strategies typically results in improved memory function for many patients. Organization of the task and the environment is important because patients with memory impairments typically cannot organize for themselves. The therapist should select simple, familiar tasks (e.g., activities of daily living [ADL] skills) as opposed to complex or novel tasks. Similarly, it is important to ensure a calm emotional state and employ motivational strategies to assist memory training. The major emphasis should be on assisting the patient in regaining rehearsal skills for active encoding. Strategies can be used to assist the patient to form associations (e.g., rhyming mnemonics). Adaptive strategies that focus on the use of external aids to assist memory are an important part of any intervention program. These devices can include storage devices (e.g., notebooks, diaries, lists, audiotapes, computers), cueing devices (e.g., alarm clocks, timers, watch alarms), and structured environments (e.g., labels in the patient's room on drawers or cabinets, posted therapy schedule).[54] Strategies to improve memory function are discussed more fully in Chapter 29.

Sensory Integrity and Integration

Several general concepts are important to an understanding of the role of sensation in movement. Sensation allows one to interact with the environment, guides the selection of movements, and prevents or minimizes injury. Sensory inputs are also used to modify movements and shape motor programs through corrective actions. Variability and adaptability of movements to environmental change are made possible by the information processing of sensory inputs. Interaction of sensory and motor systems occurs throughout the CNS. The term *somatosensation* (or somatosensory inputs) refers to the sensory information received from the skin and musculoskeletal systems. Much of the somatosensory information received is not consciously perceived. Spinal-level interactions are largely reflexive in nature, whereas supraspinal centers modulate more complex levels of sensorimotor behavior. Conscious perception and interpretation of sensory information occurs at the highest level, the cortex.

Sensory stimulation of movement is an important element of the early remediation/facilitation approaches.[30,37,39,41] Movements are elicited and modified through the use of specific stimuli (e.g., stretching, tapping). Because these movements rely on augmented inputs, their greatest use is as a temporary bridge for the patient with absent or severely disordered voluntary control. Once a desired motor response is obtained, active movements that utilize naturally occurring intrinsic sensory information will serve to reinforce and strengthen the response. Active movements also allow for sensation to be used for feedforward movement adjustments, rather than for strictly feedback adjustments. Thus, sensory stimulation may be effective to assist early attempts at movement but should be withdrawn as soon as possible. Repeated use of sensory stimulation long after it is necessary can result in movements that become stimulus dependent, and can further limit the patient's ability to regain voluntary control.

The various types of sensory receptors demonstrate differential sensitivity. Each receptor is highly sensitive to a preferential stimulus while being relatively insensitive to other stimuli at normal intensities. Use of appropriate intensities of sensory stimulation is important to ensure that the desired receptors are stimulated. Excess stimulation can activate unwanted sensory receptors and produce undesired responses, including generalized arousal and sympathetic fight-or-flight reactions. Another special characteristic of sensory receptors is their adaptation to stimuli over time. Generally, they can be divided into two categories, slow- or fast-adapting receptors. In treatment, fast-adapting, phasic receptors such as touch receptors are generally more effective in initiating movement sequences, whereas slow-adapting, tonic receptors such as joint receptors, Golgi tendon organs, and muscle spindles are used more in monitoring and regulating movement responses (e.g., postural corrections). Velocity of movement is also a consideration. At slow velocities, afferent stimuli can contribute to movement responses, while at high velocities there is insufficient time to allow for afferent information to effect motor control (open skills). Certain body segments such as the face, palms of the hands, and soles of the feet demonstrate both high concentrations of tactile receptors and increased representation in the sensory cortex. These areas are highly responsive to stimulation and are closely linked to both protective and exploratory functions.

Damage to the CNS can produce deficits in sensory function. Alterations in tactile, proprioceptive, visual, or vestibular systems can affect a patient's ability to move and learn new activities. Deafferentiation in animals and in humans is associated with nonuse of a limb, although gross movements are possible under forced situations. Learning of new movements through corrective actions is impaired. The therapist must focus on forced training of sensory-deficient limbs even though the patient may have little interest in moving the limb. The movements obtained should not be expected to be normal, however, because significant deficits have been noted in fine motor control in deafferentiated limbs.

FACILITATION TECHNIQUES

Physical therapists have a number of therapeutic techniques that can be used to facilitate, activate, or inhibit muscle contraction. These have been collectively called facilitation techniques, although this term is a misnomer, because they also include techniques used for inhibition. The term **facilitation** refers to the enhanced capacity to initiate a movement response through increased neuronal activity and altered synaptic potential. An applied stimulus may lower the synaptic threshold of the alpha motor neuron but may not be sufficient to produce an observable movement response. **Activation** on the other hand refers to the actual production of a movement response and implies reaching a critical threshold level for neuronal firing. **Inhibition** refers to the decreased capacity to initiate a movement response through altered synaptic potential. The synaptic threshold is raised, making it more difficult for the neuron to fire and produce movement. The combination of spinal inputs and supraspinal inputs acting on the alpha motor neuron (final common pathway) will determine whether a muscle response is facilitated, activated, or inhibited.

Several general guidelines are important. First, facilitative techniques can be additive. That is, several inputs applied simultaneously, such as quick stretch, resistance, and verbal commands that are commonly combined in PNF patterns, may produce

the desired motor response, whereas use of a single stimulus may not. This demonstrates the property of spatial summation within the CNS. Repeated application of the same stimulus (e.g., repeated quick stretches) may also produce the desired motor response due to the property of temporal summation within the CNS, whereas a single stimulus does not. Thus, stretch is used repeatedly to ensure that the patient is able to move from the lengthened to the shortened range. The application of a given facilitation technique does not always produce the predicted response. The response to stimulation or inhibition is unique to each patient and dependent on a number of different factors, including level of intactness of the CNS, arousal, and the specific level of activity of the motoneurons in question. For example, a patient who is depressed and hypoactive may require large amounts of stimulation to achieve the desired response, whereas a patient with hyperactivity may require very little stimulation, if any, to generate a movement response. The intensity, duration, and frequency of simulation need to be adjusted to meet the individual needs of the patient. Unpredicted responses can also be the result of inappropriate techniques. For example, stretch applied to a spastic muscle may increase spasticity and fail to increase voluntary movement.

Very little controlled research is available to guide the therapist in the application of facilitation techniques. Therefore, it is critical that keen observation skills and good judgement be applied to each clinical situation. Initial selection of stimuli should be based on a careful assessment of the patient and the environment. Careful observation during stimulus application can be compared with the therapist's knowledge of expected responses. If the responses are not as expected, adjustments in either stimulus intensity, duration, or frequency may be necessary to improve the response. If no response is obtained or an inappropriate opposite occurs, continued stimulation is contraindicated. Sensory stimulation is also contraindicated in patients who demonstrate adequate voluntary control.

Facilitation techniques can be grouped according to the sensory system and receptors that are preferentially activated during application of the stimuli. Thus, techniques are classified as exteroceptive, proprioceptive, and vestibular (see Appendix B for a complete description of these techniques). The special senses of vision, hearing, or smell can also be stimulated (see Table 13–2).

Joint Integrity and Mobility

Joint **range of motion (ROM)** and muscle flexibility must be adequate to allow for functional excursions of muscle and normal biomechanical alignment. Deficiencies can lead to changes in muscle and postural alignment (e.g., muscle tightness, atrophy, fibrosis, contracture, joint ankylosis, postural deformity). Both static and dynamic flexibility are required for normal motor function. Early therapeutic intervention is critical in maintaining full and pain-free ROM, joint integrity, muscle flexibility, and function. Additional benefits include increased circulation to the limbs and temporary relief of pain and spasticity.

Techniques to improve joint mobility and flexibility include ROM exercises, passive stretching, and peripheral joint mobilization.[55,56] The use of a preliminary therapeutic heat modality (e.g., hot pack or ultrasound) increases muscle temperature and elasticity, and collagen extensibility.[57,58] A warm-up period of exercise can also be used. For example, calisthenics or low-resistance cycling will gradually increase tissue temperatures and elasticity, thereby enhancing the safety of stretching. Cold modalities can be used to cool muscles and decrease muscle spasm and physiologic splinting.[59] Patients with spasticity may benefit from preliminary prolonged icing and relaxation techniques (e.g., rhythmic rotation, cognitive relaxation). Icing can also be added following stretching, if necessary, to reduce tissue inflammation.

ROM exercises should be performed with the limb well supported to prevent joint trauma. The exercises should be slow, smooth, and applied within the available range. The therapist may choose to use passive, active-assistive, or active ROM. Active ROM techniques are an important part of the home exercise program (HEP). ROM movements can be taught using anatomic planes of motion or in patterns of motion (PNF patterns). The latter is more efficient in that ROM can be administered throughout a limb, combining motions at more than one joint. Because PNF patterns focus on motion in multiple planes of motion and model functional patterns of movement, they may also be more effective for improving function.

Passive stretching involves applying a mechanical force at the physiological end of range, elongating the resting length of tissues. The term *static stretching* is used to refer to a low-load maintained stretch applied for an extended period of time (i.e., at least 15 to 30 seconds or longer depending upon the patient's tolerance[55]). Therapists can use manual stretching applied for several repetitions. Long duration mechanical stretching can be applied for 30 minutes up to several hours using mechanical pulleys and weights, or a tilt table with wedges and straps. Inhibitory casting or splinting is another form of static stretching used to increase range and decrease tone. The benefits of static stretching using low loads include less danger of tearing the tissues, less muscle soreness, and decreased energy requirements.[60–64] **Ballistic stretching,** the use of a high-load, short-duration bouncing stretch, can increase range but is generally contraindicated because it is associated with high rates of microtrauma and injury. It is particularly hazardous for the elderly and the chronically ill who present with prolonged immobilization.

Facilitated stretching refers to the use of active inhibition in conjunction with passive stretching. Facilitated stretching techniques were originally developed within the PNF approach[39] and now are widely applied across clinical specialities. Maximal contraction of the tight agonist muscle in the range-limiting pattern is followed by voluntary relaxation. Muscle inhibition is the result of autogenic inhibition from golgi tendon organ (GTO) receptors and conscious relaxation. The limb is then passively moved into the antagonist pattern (elongated position). Hold-relax utilizes isometric contraction of agonist muscles, while contract-relax utilizes isotonic contraction of the rotators accompanied by isometric contraction of all other muscles in the agonist pattern. A variation is hold-relax-active contraction (HRAC) or contract-relax-active contraction (CRAC). In this technique active movement into the antagonist pattern follows the relaxation phase. This produces the additional reciprocal inhibition effects (i.e., antagonist contraction further inhibits the tight agonist). Although these techniques were originally meant to be applied as the patient moved in functional (PNF) patterns, clinically they have also been applied during ROM exercises in anatomical planes of motion. Investigators have demonstrated the effectiveness and superiority of facilitated stretching techniques over static and ballistic stretching techniques.[65–67] An additional benefit is that patients frequently report less discomfort with the application of facilitated stretching techniques as compared to other stretching techniques. Because the inhibitory mechanisms affect primarily muscle and depend on voluntary contraction, these techniques are not effective in very weak or paralyzed muscles, in spastic muscles, or for tightness primarily associated with connective tissue changes.

Flexibility exercises should be performed daily to achieve optimal benefits. Flexibility exercises should always be followed by active functional movements that maximize the mobility gained in the newly gained range. This serves to further maintain the range through reciprocal inhibition effects. Patients and/or their families should be taught flexibility exercises as part of the HEP to maintain carryover outside of the clinic setting.

Tone and Reflex Integrity

Tone is the resistance of muscle to passive elongation or stretch. The term **muscle tone** is used to refer to the level of tension in muscle while the term **postural tone** is used to refer to the overall level of tension in the body musculature necessary to maintain body posture against gravity. Changes in tone are common in neurological conditions and can vary from higher than normal tone (hypertonia, i.e., spasticity, hyperreflexia, rigidity) to lower than normal tone (i.e., hypotonia, flaccidity, hyporeflexia). Fluctuating tone (dystonia) can also occur, for example, in some patients with extrapyramidal lesions. Tonal changes affect movement control and function. For example, the patient with significant spasticity will present with a stiff limb held or fixed in an antigravity posture. The upper extremity typically assumes a flexor posture while the lower extremity typically assumes an extensor posture. There is very little spontaneous movement of the limb. Spasms, clonus, a positive Babinski sign, hyperactive stretch reflexes, and exaggerated cutaneous and autonomic reflexes also occur with spasticity in varying combinations. The antagonist muscles are typically weak and the patient demonstrates poor volitional control (dyssynergic patterns of activation, excessive cocontraction of agonist/antagonist muscles), and limited functional use of the limb. If left untreated, abnormal tone can lead to the development of secondary impairments such as contracture, postural asymmetries, and deformity. The patient with hypotonia typically demonstrates weak or paralyzed muscles with associated joint instability and deformity. Following neurological insult, tone may vary relative to recovery stage. For example, the patient with a new or recent spinal cord injury will present with flaccidity during the stage of spinal shock while the same patient in the post-acute stage will demonstrate spasticity. Patients may present with asymmetries of tone between limbs, between the two sides of the body, or between limbs and the trunk. Asymmetries may also occur within a limb from muscle to muscle. For example, the proximal muscles are spastic while the distal hand muscles are flaccid. Careful assessment of tone is warranted.

A number of techniques have been developed within the remediation/facilitation approaches to address problems of tone, some with a neurophysiological basis and some empirically. Traditional techniques to decrease tone for patients with spasticity include prolonged icing, prolonged stretch, inhibitory pressure, neutral warmth, or slow vestibular stimulation (see Appendix B for a complete description of these techniques). Rhythmic rotation is also a highly effective technique in reducing hypertonicity. The application of these techniques precedes ROM and active exercises. Precise handling is important. The therapist should use constant, firm manual contacts on nonspastic areas whenever possible to avoid stimulating spastic muscles. Movements are directed out of the spastic pattern. Johnstone[68] advocates the use of inflatable pressure splints to decrease hypertonicity and maintain limbs in optimal tone-reducing positions during functional training. At best, inhibitory techniques produce a temporary reduction in tone, with results that can last 20 to 30 minutes or up to a few hours. They do not result in a permanent alteration in tone or permanent changes within the CNS. Thus, these techniques must be viewed as preparatory for ROM and movement reeducation, not a primary focus of treatment. For example, ROM exercise for the patient with severe lower extremity spasticity resulting from multiple sclerosis will likely be ineffective without first applying a tone-reducing technique. Relaxation can be obtained through rhythmic rotation with both lower extremities positioned on a ball and gently rocked side-to-side. Once relaxation

occurs, the therapist can effectively range the limbs to ensure adequate length of muscle and joint position. Resting splints can then be applied to maintain the muscles in an elongated state with positioning of the feet in a neutral position.

Strengthening of antagonist muscles is necessary to maintain tone inhibition and promote movement reeducation. The following guidelines can be used:

- First, all unnecessary muscle activity should be eliminated. Primary focus should be on contraction of antagonist muscles (muscles opposite the spastic muscles).
- Movements should be slow and well controlled, and should emphasize increasing control over newly gained range and direction.
- Assistance (active assistive or guided movements) can be used initially as needed but should be withdrawn as soon as the patient is able to move on his or her own.
- Once active movement in the antagonist pattern is possible, reciprocal actions can then be attempted. Agonist (spastic muscle) contractions are initiated in small ranges, with emphasis on reversing the movement and moving back into the antagonist pattern. Smooth, reciprocal movements are practiced while relaxation is maintained.
- Highly stressful activities and intense effort are contraindicated; they may reinforce abnormal tone.
- Functional muscle synergies should be enhanced to promote attainment of specific functional skills. For example, the patient practices slow and controlled reciprocal hand to mouth movements.

Patients and their family or caregivers should be educated about the need to maintain length of spastic muscles. Daily slow passive ROM exercises should be stressed as well as effective use of positioning and splinting techniques. Triggers (noxious stimuli that initiate spasms and increased tone) should be identified and eliminated whenever possible. These can include extrinsic factors (e.g., tight, restrictive clothing, a blocked catheter) or intrinsic factors (e.g., bladder infection, bowel impaction, pressure sores, pain).

Additional interventions to manage spasticity include static stretching with splints and serial casts, electric stimulation, and biofeedback. Static splints are typically used to maintain a functional position, for example, of the hand and wrist or foot. They are applied after inhibitory and ROM techniques. Casting is used when traditional techniques fail and the patient is at risk for development of contractures and deformity, or demonstrates ineffective movement patterns or severe limitations in hygiene and skin care. Inhibitory techniques are first used to move the limb into its fully lengthened range. Casting is then applied while the limb is held at the end of available range. The sustained position produces relaxation of the spastic muscles, thought to be the result of GTO autogenic inhibition and adaptation of stretch receptors.[69–71] Neutral warmth and continuous even pressure may also be contributing factors. Inhibitory casting has also been found to promote changes in muscle or tendon length and sarcomere distribution.[72,73] The casts are typically changed every 7 to 10 days (serial application) to gradually increase available range.[74,75] Serial casts have been utilized for either upper or lower limb spasticity and have been shown effective in reducing tone and improving ROM in patients with traumatic brain injury, quadriplegia, and stroke.[69,71,72,76–77] Poor casting techniques include loose-fitting casts, insufficient padding, or poor patient positioning. They may result in lack of treatment results or even increased tone, skin breakdown especially on bony prominences, or nerve compression. An overly restrictive cast may result in decreased circulation and peripheral edema. Highly agitated patients may potentially injure themselves and demonstrate increased risk of skin breakdown and cast breakage. Patients with cognitive or communication impairments should be monitored closely because they will be unable to indicate pain or discomfort and potential skin breakdown. Casting is contraindicated in patients with severe heterotropic ossification; skeletal muscle rigidity; skin conditions such as open wounds, blisters, or abrasions; impaired circulation and edema; uncontrolled hypertension; unstable intracranial pressure; pathological inflammatory conditions such as arthritis or gout; or in individuals at risk for compartment syndrome or nerve impingement.[78] Application to individuals with long-standing contractures (longer than 6 to 12 months) is also contraindicated.

Neuromuscular electrical stimulation (NMES) has also been used to reduce spasticity.[79] Applications to the tibialis anterior muscle or to the common peroneal nerve have been shown to reduce spasticity in the plantarflexor muscles and ankle clonus.[80,81] Electrical stimulation of forearm muscles can reduce flexor tone and posturing of the hand. Spinal cord stimulators have also been utilized to reduce severe flexor and extensor spasms, with variable results.[79] Dobkin[82] suggests that intrathecal baclofen administration is a more effective treatment for this problem. Pharmacological approaches to spasticity are the mainstay of medical management (e.g., dantrolene, baclofen, benzodiazepines, etc.). Chemical blocks (e.g., phenol, botulinum toxin) injected into a nerve, motor point, or muscle can also reduce spasticity, clonus, and dystonic postures. The effects of blocking agents are temporary, generally lasting for 6 to 12 months for phenol agents and up to 3 months for Botox. Biofeedback has also been used to train voluntary inhibition of spastic muscles.[83,84] Its greatest benefit is achieved when used in combination with a balanced neuromuscular reeducation program to restore movement control. See Chapter 33 for a more complete discussion of this topic.

Intervention techniques to increase tone for patients with hypotonia (flaccidity) can include quick stretch, tapping, resistance, approximation, and positioning (see Appendix B). Patients typically also demonstrate weakness and at times it is difficult to differentiate between the two states. Strengthening exercises that do not overload the weak, hypotonic muscles are indicated. Postural instability is a common problem. Interventions should be designed to improve postural stability in functional positions (see the section on stability). Initial assistance into weight-bearing postures may be needed to ensure satisfactory postural alignment. Supportive and protective devices may be necessary to prevent injury to limbs and postural asymmetries (e.g., a Swedish knee cage can be used to prevent hyperextension). Patients with hypotonia may also present with severe sensory deficits and inattention to affected limbs and body segments. Sensory stimulation techniques and early and continued movement experiences can be used to optimize available sensory inputs and promote movement. NMES can also be used to activate hypotonic muscles, improve strength, and generate movement in paralyzed limbs while preventing disuse atrophy.[85–87] It is important to focus the patient's attention on the desired movement and verbally cue the patient to attempt volitional contraction. Without such cueing, functional carryover is not possible. Electrical stimulation should ideally be coupled with functional training activities to optimize outcomes. For example, a weak triceps can be stimulated in sitting with weight-bearing on an extended upper extremity.

Muscle Performance: Strength, Power, and Endurance

Muscle performance is defined as the capacity of a muscle to do work (force × distance).[88] Strength is the ability of muscle to produce force necessary to overcome a resistance in one maximal effort.[88] **Muscle power** is the work produced per unit of time (strength × speed), and **muscle endurance** is the ability to contract the muscle repeatedly over time.[88] Muscle performance is regulated by a number of factors, including motor unit recruitment, motoneuron firing patterns, muscle length and tension, muscle fiber composition, fuel storage and delivery, speed and type of contraction, and movement arm.[89] Techniques that optimize these factors will yield maximum functional outcomes.

Strength training methods for patients with weakness have been well described and documented.[55] These include isometric, isotonic, and isokinetic training sequences. Exercise training produces a number of neuromuscular changes. There is an increase in the production of maximal force due to changes in neural drive (recruitment of additional motor units and/or firing rate) and changes in muscle (hypertrophy of individual muscle fibers, improved metabolic/enzymatic adaptations). The effectiveness of a strengthening program is dependent upon achieving an adequate training stimulus. The loads placed on muscle must be greater than those normally incurred (**overload principle**). Free weights, pulley systems, elastic resistance bands, mechanical resistance machines, isokinetic dynamometers, and manual resistance all provide sources of external load on muscle. The physiological responses to training are specific to the particular muscles and type of exercise used (**specificity principle**). Thus, a training program that uses an aerobic protocol will not improve anaerobic performance. Nor will exercise training of the upper extremities transfer to improved lower extremity performance. For strength and power training, an exercise prescription should include the following elements: the type of strengthening exercise, the required force quantified in terms of a percentage of maximal voluntary contraction, and the frequency (number of repetitions, number of sets).

Selection of a particular training sequence must be based on the specific needs of the patient and the potential benefits of a particular method. For example, isometric training will result in gains in static strength without added joint motion. This may be important during early rehabilitation when pain is a factor or protection of an injured part is necessary. For patients with significant weakness and an inability to initiate or sustain a contraction, early training should focus on isometric and eccentric contractions because muscle tension is better maintained than with concentric contractions. This is primarily due to the improved peripheral reflex support of contraction as opposed to the spindle unloading, which occurs as the muscle moves into the shortened range of a concentric contraction. The patient is asked to actively hold at midrange where the greatest tension can be generated. The therapist may need to assist initial efforts through stabilization of proximal segments and/or direct muscle stimulation. Progression is to isometric holding at various different angle positions because isometric strength adaptations are joint-angle specific. The patient is then asked to slowly lower the limb (an eccentric contraction) and hold (an isometric contraction). Once control is achieved in both of these types of contractions, concentric contractions can be attempted. Prestretching the muscle by starting contraction in the lengthened range optimizes tension development through increased use of viscoelastic forces (length-tension relationship) and peripheral reflex support. Concentric movements should therefore be progressed from the lengthened range to midrange and then to movement through the range into the fully shortened range. Movements can be initially assisted, progressing to lightly resisted (*tracking resistance*), to finally active control. Control of velocity is also important to ensure efficiency of initial movement attempts. In concentric contractions total tension decreases as velocity increases. Thus, patients may be able to generate a contraction at slow speeds but not at high speeds. The patient should be instructed to begin with slow movements that can be controlled. As movements become more efficient, they can be progressed to faster speeds.

Gains in strength can be obtained through progressive resistive exercises (PRE) using free weights or fixed mechanical resistance machines. A major disadvantage of this type of training is that the weight selected is determined by the amount that can be lifted by the muscle at the weakest point of the range. Isokinetic training devices offer the advantage of providing accommodating resistance throughout the range. Muscle performance is therefore not limited to the weakest part of the range. The amount of force generated is recorded, providing an important objective measure of performance. Different protocols using isometric, concentric, and eccentric contractions have been developed. The speed of movement can be set by using predetermined movement speeds. This can be an important consideration for training the patient who demonstrates neuromuscular impairments in timing and velocity control. For example, the patient recovering from stroke may be unable to generate the acceleration and deceleration forces needed during the different phases of gait. This results in delayed sequencing of muscle components and a general slowing of **gait.** Isokinetic training that focuses on the timing of these various components is important. Carryover to improved functional performance with any of these resistance training methods is not assured. Additional functional training is necessary to ensure effective transference of strength and timing parameters to improved functional performance (specificity principle).

Resistance exercises using patterns of movement (PNF patterns) offer the advantage of functionally based movements. Patterns of motion are spiral and diagonal in nature as opposed to straight planes of motion. The therapist can accommodate to the patient's specific level of weakness by providing variable manual resistance throughout the range and by adding additional facilitation as needed to improve or maintain performance. Effective verbal commands have been shown to improve the magnitude of muscle contraction.[90] Stretch is applied in the lengthened range to assist in the initiation of contraction and throughout the range to sustain contraction. Approximation is applied to assist extensor patterns while traction is applied to assist flexor patterns. Specific PNF techniques (e.g., slow reversal, repeated contractions, etc.) are described in Appendix A. Elastic resistance bands can also be used to provide resistance in functional patterns of movement.

Strength gains can be achieved through a functional training program that uses task-oriented activities and postures.[91] Resistance is provided by gravity, body weight, manual resistance of the therapist, or elastic resistance bands. Activities are selected that focus on specific body segments and progressed to involve larger and larger body segments. Increased demands are placed on postural control and balance as the base of support (BOS) is narrowed and the center of mass (COM) elevated. Functional training helps the patient develop control of muscle groups in multiple axes and planes of movements. Different types and combinations of muscle contractions (concentric, eccentric, isometric, etc.) are used to impose demands that simulate normal movement. There are several advantages of this type of program. The movements selected are complex movements in which the primary focus is on coordinated action of synergistic muscles, not isolated muscle or joint control. This is a very different focus from the straight planes of motion and isolated movements commonly employed in PRE and isokinetic machines. There is increased sensory input from the body (somatosensory, vestibular, visual) to assist in movement control. The practice of functional patterns maximizes carry-over into real-life skills. The promotion of functional independence becomes the central focus of treatment. See following section outlining the use of functional training strategies to improve movement control.

Muscle endurance can be improved with low-resistance submaximal contractions repeated over longer periods of time. Any of the resistance training sequences discussed above can be used to improve muscle endurance. Aerobic endurance activities using treadmills, ergometers, steps, or pools can also be used to induce a training effect. For endurance exercise, an exercise prescription should include the following inter-dependent elements: frequency, intensity, time or duration, and type or exercise mode (the FITT equation).

Patients who demonstrate poor exercise capacity and fatigue can benefit from endurance training. *Fatigue* is defined as the inability to contract muscle repeatedly over time. Thus exercise cannot be sustained. The onset of fatigue is variable from patient to patient. Although many different factors may play a role, among the most important are the type and intensity of exercise. With the onset of fatigue, patients will demonstrate a decrement in force production progressing to total exhaustion (a ceiling effect). Fatigue can arise from neuromuscular disease affecting three primary sites: (1) the CNS (central fatigue), (2) the peripheral nerves or neuromuscular junction, or (3) the muscle itself.[92] Examples of conditions that can produce debilitating fatigue include Guillain-Barré syndrome, chronic fatigue syndrome, and post-polio syndrome. Patients typically present with a number of other variable symptoms including muscle weakness and are therefore difficult to assess. The real danger of exercise training with these patients is **overwork weakness,** defined as a prolonged decrease in absolute strength and endurance as a result of excessive activity.[93] For example, following an exercise session a patient with post-polio syndrome may demonstrate prolonged weakness and fatigue that does not recover with rest. If exercise is exhaustive, the patient may be unable to get out of bed the next day or perform normal ADLs. In general, low to moderate intensities of exercises are safe, whereas high levels are contraindicated for patients with chronic fatigue.[94–96] Close attention to activity pacing is necessary to carefully balance activity with rest. Energy conservation, stress management, and life-style modification are also essential components of any rehabilitation program. Even a simple conditioning program should be carefully monitored and progressed slowly to avoid overexertion and injury.

Functional Training to Improve Movement Control

The adult patient with deficits in motor function is likely to present with a unique and often variable pattern of functional limitations and disabilities. A careful and accurate functional assessment is therefore essential for planning (see Chapter 11). Underlying impairments must be linked to functional performance. Functional limitations may vary by task, environment, or the individual. Thus, performance may be affected by the degree of involvement, stage of recovery, type of environment, and so forth. A conceptual framework for intervention allows various different postures, activities, and techniques to be classified according to function. The terms mobility, stability, controlled mobility, and skill will be used to organize task-oriented activities and interventions. Progression is through increasingly more difficult postures and activities (Table 13–3). The use of techniques to assist or facilitate movement should decrease as active control emerges.

STRATEGIES AND TECHNIQUES TO IMPROVE MOBILITY

Initial **mobility** is characterized by the ability to move into stable postures. Patients with problems in initial mobility demonstrate poorly controlled movements that deteriorate as the demands for antigravity control and synergistic control of multiple body segments increase. Thus, a patient may be able to complete bed mobility activities with assistance in gravity-minimized planes but be unable to sit up or stand up. Postures and activities that minimize the demands for postural control (wide BOS and low center of mass [COM]) should be attempted first. For example, the patient can practice partial range (sidelying) or full range (supine-to-prone) rolling. Scooting in bed and moving from supine-to-sit or supine-to-sidelying on elbow are also important early mobility activities. For patients unable to stand, lower trunk/lower extremity control can be developed first using hooklying and bridging activities. Once control is obtained in these early activities, progression can be to higher level postures and controlled mobility activities. For example, sit-to-stand and transfers are important functional activities that may present significant challenges for the patient and require increasing amounts of assistance from the therapist. Interim postures like kneeling, half-kneeling, and plantigrade can be used to bridge the gap between sitting and standing by limiting the degrees of freedom (in this example, the number of body segments that must be controlled).

Patients who demonstrate problems with mobility control may be too stiff to move, the result of

Table 13–3 DEVELOPMENTAL SEQUENCE POSTURES AND TREATMENT BENEFITS

Posture	Treatment Benefits
1. Prone on elbows	• Improve upper trunk, UE, and neck/head control • Facilitate flexor tone • Increase ROM at hip extensors • Improve shoulder stabilizers strength • Wide BOS, low COG
2. Quadruped	• Improve upper trunk, lower trunk, LE, UE, and neck/head control • Weight bearing through hips • Increase hip stabilizers strength • Decrease extensor tone at knees by weight-bearing • Increase shoulder stabilizers strength • Weight-bearing through shoulders, elbows, and wrists • Increase extensor ROM at wrists and fingers • Wide BOS, low COG
3. Bridging	• Improve lower trunk and LE control • Increase hip stabilizers strength • Weight-bearing through feet and ankles • Lead up activity for bed mobility • Wide BOS, low COG
4. Sitting	• Improve upper trunk, lower trunk, LE, and head/neck control • Weight-bearing through UE • Functional posture • Improve balance reactions • Medium BOS, medium COG
5. Kneeling and half-kneeling	• Improve head/neck, upper trunk, lower trunk, and LE control • Weight-bearing through hips • Inhibit extensor tone at knees • Increase hip stabilizers strength • Improve balance reactions • Weight-bearing through ankle in half-kneeling • Narrow BOS, high COG (kneeling) • Wide BOS, high COG (half-kneeling)
6. Modified plantigrade	• Improve head/neck, upper trunk, lower trunk, and UE and LE control • Weight-bearing through UE and LE • Improve balance reactions • Functional posture • Increase extensor ROM at wrists and fingers • Wide BOS, high COG
7. Standing	• Improve head/neck, upper trunk, lower trunk, and LE control • Weight-bearing through LE • Improve balance reactions • Functional posture • Narrow BOS, high COG

BOS, base of support; COG, center of gravity; LE, lower extremity; ROM, range of motion; UE, upper extremity.

hypertonia (spasticity, rigidity). Patients may also exhibit impairments in flexibility (contractures) or pain (painful spasm) that result in decreased mobility and desire to move. These patients may benefit from techniques designed to decrease tone or painful spasm and increase active movements and ROM. Decreased mobility function may also result from another set of problems arising from decreased tone (hypotonia), weakness, motor programming deficits (dyspraxia), or decreased responsiveness to sensory stimulation (low-level cognitive functioning in patients with traumatic brain injury or hyposensitivity

following stroke). These patients may benefit from techniques designed to improve mobility control by increasing sensory responsiveness, tone, strength, and initiation of movement.

The therapist may choose to use any of a number of facilitation techniques that enhance initial muscle contraction through motor unit recruitment and/or peripheral reflex support. These include quick stretch, tapping, resistance, approximation, manual contacts, light touch, or dynamic verbal commands (see Appendix B). Electrical stimulation and biofeedback can also be used to enhance initial contractions. These techniques should be viewed as a temporary bridge to voluntary control, withdrawn as soon as active control emerges. Continued practice of task-directed movements and appropriate feedback will serve to strengthen neuromuscular associations and enhance motor learning.

The patient's initial movement attempts can be assisted using active assistive movement (AAM). The therapist first explains the task goal and then manually guides the patient through the desired movement to ensure that the patient has the correct idea of the task. Assistance allows the patient to preview the sensations of movement (e.g., tactile and kinesthetic inputs) without fear of failure. The patient is then asked to actively participate in the movement, an essential requirement for learning. The key to success is knowing when to provide assistance and how much. Generally, the greatest assistance is needed at the point in the range where maximum effects of gravity are acting on the body. Equally important is knowing when to remove assistance and let the patient move on his or her own. For example, in supine-to-sit transfers, the therapist will need to provide maximum support and assistance to the upper trunk in the first half of the movement while decreasing assistance as the patient approaches the upright position. It is important to remember that initial movement attempts may be quite stressful for the patient who may feel "out of control." The therapist needs to model confidence and ensure the patient that the movements will be safe and controlled. Close observation and heightened kinesthetic awareness from appropriate manual contacts will allow the therapist to adjust movements as needed. A videotape record of performance is an effective tool to further instruct the patient and modify performance.

Therapeutic guiding is an expansion of AAM developed and described by Affolter.[97,98] This technique has been applied in the treatment of brain-damaged individuals to promote interaction with the environment and initial mobility. A key element is engaging the patient's hands for active exploration. The therapist guides the patient's hands to contact the support surface and engage him or her fully in the task (e.g., feeding, dressing). This promotes increased tactile and kinesthetic inputs and awareness of the task and the environment. The therapist provides manual assistance to ensure body support and stability during movement attempts. Real-life functional tasks are practiced and the patient is engaged in active problem solving. Davies[99] offers numerous examples of how therapeutic guiding can be implemented during recovery from brain injury, including examples of guiding the patient while still in the intensive care unit.

The PNF techniques of rhythmic initiation, repeated contractions, and hold-relax active motion[39] can also be used to assist initial mobility (see Appendix A). Rhythmic initiation (RI) is a PNF technique that involves voluntary relaxation followed by passive, active-assistive, and finally mildly resisted movements of the agonist pattern. Transition into the next stage is dependent on the patient's ability to (1) relax completely and be moved passively before attempting active assisted movement, and (2) participate in the movement actively before attempting mildly resisted movement. RI was developed for use with hypertonia, for example, the patient with rigidity from Parkinson's disease. It is an effective technique for the initial stages of motor learning to guide and stimulate correct motor patterns. Thus, the patient with dyspraxia or receptive aphasia can benefit from use of RI. *Repeated contraction* (RC) is a PNF technique that involves repeated isotonic contractions of the agonist pattern. The movements are resisted, and repeated stretch is added to reinforce voluntary contraction during the weak parts of the range. Hold-relax active motion (HRA) involves first obtaining an isometric contraction in the shortened range, followed by active relaxation, and passive movement into the lengthened range. The patient is instructed to move isotonically back through the range against resistance. Repeated stretch is added as needed. The technique of HRA is effective in enhancing stretch sensitivity and contraction of a weak or hypotonic agonist.

STRATEGIES AND TECHNIQUES TO IMPROVE STABILITY

Stability (static postural control) is characterized by the ability to maintain a stable posture. Muscles co-contract to stabilize joints to ensure maintenance of upright posture against gravity. Stability control is developed in weight-bearing postures. The prone-on-elbows posture facilitates the development of head, upper trunk, and proximal joint (shoulder) control; the quadruped (all fours) posture adds the components of lower trunk, hip, and elbow control; sitting focuses on upper trunk control; kneeling adds lower trunk and hip control. A plantigrade position (weight-bearing in standing with extended arm and lower extremity support) and full standing add the components of knee and foot-ankle stability control. Hooklying and bridging can be used to develop control in hip and foot-ankle stability while limiting the actions of other body segments.

Patients who demonstrate problems with stability control may be unable to hold steady for a number of reasons, including tonal imbalances (hypotonia, spasticity), decreased strength, impaired voluntary control and hypermobility (ataxia, athetosis), sensory hypersensitivity (tactile-avoidance reactions), or increased arousal (high sympathetic state).

The therapist may chose to use any of a number of facilitation techniques that enhance muscle co-contraction and stability. These include quick stretch, tapping, resistance, approximation, manual contacts, or dynamic verbal commands (see Appendix B). For the patient with poor extensor muscle control, the therapist may need to initially start with isometric contractions of postural extensors starting in midrange and progressing to the shortened range (termed shortened held resisted contraction). The sidelying modified pivot prone position can be used for the patient unable to support body weight in any upright position (e.g., the patient with severe instability following traumatic brain injury). The therapist can then progress training through postures that demand co-contraction and increasing amounts of upright (antigravity) postural control.

Specific exercise techniques used to enhance stability control include (1) alternating isometrics and rhythmic stabilization (PNF), (2) slow reversal hold through decrements of ROM (PNF), and (3) placing and holding or hold-after-positioning (NDT) (see Appendix A). Alternating isometrics (AI) consist of alternate isometric contractions of first the agonist and then the antagonist muscles. The patient is instructed to hold and the therapist resists the hold first in one direction, then in the other. The holding can be challenged in all directions; that is, anterior-posterior, medial-lateral, or diagonal directions. Rhythmic stabilization (RS) similarly employs isometric contractions of antagonist patterns but differs from AI in that resistance is applied simultaneously to alternate muscle groups. For example, in standing, resistance can be applied simultaneously to the upper trunk flexors/rotators and to the lower trunk extensors/rotators. The therapist's hands are then switched to the opposite surfaces and resistance is applied. This occurs without any distinct relaxation phase between opposing contractions. Slow reversal hold (SRH) is a technique that involves alternate isotonic and isometric contractions of both agonists and antagonists. The patient is instructed to hold (agonist contraction) followed by stretch and resisted movement in the opposite direction ending with a corresponding contraction of the antagonists. When SRH is used as a stability technique, the isometric contractions are stressed and the range of movement becomes progressively more limited. SRH applied through a decreasing range (decrements of range) is effective in helping patients with hyperkinetic disorders (ataxia, athetosis) progress toward steady holding (stability). In placing and holding, the patient is assisted into position and asked to hold the position against the resistance of gravity. Tapping can be used to help the patient maintain the position.

Additional strategies to improve stability include the use of elastic resistance bands or weights to provide proprioceptive loading and enhance contraction of stabilizing muscles. For example, in the prone-on-elbows position, bands can be placed around the forearms. The patient is instructed to push out against the band and maintain the forearms apart. This selectively loads and facilitates contraction of the shoulder stabilizers (abductors and rotator cuff muscles). In bridging, kneeling, or standing, elastic resistance bands can be placed around the thighs. The patient is instructed to maintain the thighs apart against the resistance of the bands. This selectively loads and facilitates contraction of the hip stabilizers (abductors, extensors), improving stability control at the hips. Stability control can also be enhanced by having the patient sit on a Swiss ball and gently bouncing. This provides gentle joint approximation through the vertebral joints, facilitating extensors and an upright posture. Pool therapy can also be used to enhance postural antigravity support. The water provides a degree of unweighting and resistance to movement. This is a form of proprioceptive loading that can be quite effective in reducing hyperkinetic movements and enhancing postural stability. For example, the patient recovering from traumatic brain injury who demonstrates significant ataxia may be able to sit or stand in the pool with minimal assistance while these same activities are not possible on land.

STRATEGIES AND TECHNIQUES TO IMPROVE CONTROLLED MOBILITY

The ability to move while maintaining a stable upright posture is referred to as **controlled mobility (dynamic stability).** It represents the combined function of both mobilizing and stabilizing muscles and is characterized by smooth coordinated movements with appropriate synergistic stabilization. Movements can be easily reversed, demonstrating good interplay between antagonist muscles. Examples of activities in which controlled mobility function is utilized include rocking, weight shifting, or movement transitions (i.e., shifting from one posture to another). In sitting, for example, the patient weight shifts slowly from side-to-side or forward-backward. Diagonal shifts are more advanced because they represent a combination of both flexion-extension and abduction-adduction elements. Thus, in a quadruped position the patient can rock forward and diagonally over one shoulder and backward and diagonally over the opposite leg. Examples of movement transitions include assuming a quadruped position from the side-sitting position or a standing position from sitting. A variation of controlled mobility is termed **static-dynamic control.** While maintaining a static posture, one limb is freed to move through space (e.g., reaching or stepping). The patient in a quadruped position lifts one arm or lifts one arm and the opposite leg off of the support surface. This increases the demand for dynamic stability because the overall BOS is reduced and the COG is shifted over the remaining support limbs. Additional movement challenges, such as PNF extremity patterns, can be added to the dynamic limb to increase the level of difficulty (*dual-task training*). For example,

in sitting the patient moves the dynamic limbs in a chop/reverse chop pattern while maintaining a stable posture. Swiss ball activities can also be used to develop controlled mobility function and balance reactions. For example, the patient sits on a Swiss ball and gently moves the ball side-to-side or forward and back. Or the patient sits on the ball and bounces while moving the arms in a reciprocal overhead pattern.

Patients who demonstrate problems with controlled mobility are unable to maintain their posture while moving the body or the limbs. A number of factors can produce deficits in controlled mobility, including tonal imbalances (spasticity, rigidity, hypotonia), ROM restrictions, impaired voluntary control and hypermobility (ataxia, athetosis), impaired reciprocal actions of the antagonists (cerebellar dysfunction), or impaired proximal stabilization.

During controlled mobility activity training, the therapist emphasizes movements with smooth directional changes that engage antagonist actions. The movement is gradually expanded through an increasing range (increments of range). Movements can be facilitated using light tracking resistance, stretch, or with the resistance of gravity. Although active movement is desired, assistance may be indicated during initial instruction of the movement pattern. During training of movement transitions, the patient can be initially assisted into the posture. Focus should then be on achieving active eccentric control first (moving out of a posture) before concentric control (moving into a posture). Specific task-oriented training (e.g., standing and reaching to an overhead cabinet) will prove more motivating, especially if the task is desirable to the patient.

Specific PNF exercise techniques can be used to assist patients in gaining controlled mobility through the use of resistance and proprioceptive loading and include slow reversals, slow reversal-hold, repeated contractions, and agonist reversals (see Appendix A). Slow reversals (SR) consists of applying light resistance to alternating isotonic contractions of first agonist, then antagonist patterns. The movements are reversed without any relaxation phase. The patient is directed toward gaining full range of motion. The addition of a hold (SRH) can be used to promote stability at end ranges. RC are appropriate to improve controlled mobility when muscle imbalances exist and the movements are stronger in one direction than the other. Agonist reversals (AR) is a technique that incorporates resistance to both concentric and eccentric contractions of agonists; for example, in bridging, assuming the posture involves concentric contraction of the hip extensor muscles, while movement from the bridged position back down to the starting position involves a controlled eccentric contraction. AR provides resistance to both types of contractions. Functional activities that require eccentric control include bridging, sitting from standing, descending stairs, and moving from kneeling to heel-sitting.

STRATEGIES AND TECHNIQUES TO IMPROVE SKILL

Skill level function enables the individual to produce highly coordinated movement, characterized by precise timing and direction. Movements are highly consistent and efficient, allowing goal attainment with an economy of effort. Activities considered skilled include investigatory behaviors that allow exploration of the environment. For example, an individual learns about the environment through eye and head movements, grasp and manipulation, and oromotor exploration. Skilled behaviors also allow for adaptive functions and interaction with the environment through body orientation, position, and movement. For example, locomotion (reciprocal creeping, walking with a heel-toe gait pattern, and a reciprocal arm swing) are considered skilled movements. Oromotor activities of speech and feeding are also skilled movements. Progression to skill level activities normally occurs after control in stability and controlled-mobility activities have been achieved.

Skill movements can be defined by various different parameters. Movements that have a clearly defined beginning and end point defined by the task itself are termed *discrete motor skills*. For example, the individual locks the brakes on a wheelchair. Discrete skills put together into a sequence are termed *serial motor skills*. A transfer is an example of several component skills put together (i.e., locking the brake, standing up, pivoting, and sitting down). Motor skills that have an arbitrary beginning and end point defined by the performer or some external person are termed *continuous motor skills*. For example, an individual runs or walks an arbitrary distance. Skilled function can include single tasks or simultaneous tasks (dual task control). An individual walking and bouncing a ball is an example of dual task control. Motor skills can be self-paced or externally paced (e.g., by a metronome, escalator). Closed skills are movements performed in a fixed environment in which the regulatory conditions are stable and unchanging. Open skills are movements performed in a changing or variable environment.

There are many reasons why patients fail to develop motor skills. Potential for performance may be seriously or irreversibly limited with significant cognitive impairments. For example, the individual with traumatic brain injury may present with serious learning-based difficulties. Noncognitive reasons may include any of the problems previously mentioned. In addition, individuals may demonstrate impaired balance (postural synergies and reactions), impaired motor planning (apraxia, dyspraxia), or impaired coordination.

In general, a hands-on approach using remediation/facilitation techniques should have a limited role during skill training. Active practice of specific task-oriented activities progressing to task variations and variable environments is needed to promote successful learning and develop problem solving skills (see discussion on Strategies to Improve Motor Learning). In planning interventions, the therapist can include, as appropriate,

1. Coordination tasks, stressing synergistic control with sequential and temporal organization of movements (e.g., upper extremity reciprocal tasks, manual dexterity).
2. Multilimb tasks, stressing simultaneous control of multiple body segments (e.g., dual task training, walking while moving the head right or left, walking while talking).
3. Tasks that focus on postural control mechanisms, balance, and gait (e.g., Swiss ball activities, balance activities on computerized platforms, equilibrium or wobble boards, etc.).
4. Agility tasks that combine both coordination and balance (e.g., jumping jacks); many Swiss ball activities appropriately challenge agility while providing novelty and diversity.[100,101]
5. Tasks that focus on overall timing can be used to develop velocity control by varying speed of movements (e.g., a stationery bike, isokinetic device, or treadmill).
6. PNF patterns can be used to improve overall timing and coordination of movements and skill level function. Carefully graded resistance promotes balanced contributions of agonists and antagonists during the spiral, diagonal, and patterns of movement. PNF patterns are functionally based and more easily transferred into real-life skills as compared to the movements permitted on most exercise machines. For example, the D1 extension pattern of the upper extremity (extension, abduction, internal rotation) can be used as an appropriate lead-up activity to weight-bearing on an extended arm for crutch use. Specific deficits can be addressed using techniques of SR, SRH, RC with timing for emphasis, and resisted progression. Timing for emphasis (TE) promotes normal timing of pattern components by reinforcing or resisting the stronger components to augment the weaker ones. Completion of a diagonal pattern of motion emphasizes all components with normal distal to proximal timing. When an imbalance exists, the stronger components are maximally resisted to create overflow and enhance contractions of the weaker segments. The stronger components can also be isometrically "locked in" at a point in the range where they are the strongest, while repeated contractions are then applied simultaneously to improve contraction of the weaker components. Resisted progression (RP) involves the use of stretch and resistance to enhance gait. The therapist's manual contacts are positioned to resist both forward progression and pelvic rotation. Gait patterns can be resisted in any direction, that is, forward-backward, sideways, or diagonally. Crossed-step walking and *braiding* (a PNF activity that combines side-stepping with alternate cross-stepping in front and be-

hind) are appropriate skill level training activities.

CONTROL OF ABNORMAL MOVEMENT PATTERNS

Stereotypical movement synergies are characterized by muscles firmly linked together in obligatory and primitive synergistic patterns. There is a loss of selective movement and individual joint control. They are common in patients with neurological dysfunction (e.g., stroke, traumatic head injury). Alterations in synergistic control can arise from deficits in central programming, altered peripheral inputs, or both. Reduced firing rates, muscle fiber atrophy (predominately type II), and abnormal firing patterns may also contribute to the problem. In addition, the deficits may be influenced by alterations in biomechanical properties (e.g., increased muscle and joint stiffness).

The primary goal of intervention is to break up stereotypical synergies by altering and reorganizing movement components. Strong linkages are identified and modified first. For example, elbow flexion is typically strongly associated with shoulder flexion and abduction (flexion synergy). An early treatment activity would be practicing elbow extension with shoulder flexion or abduction (e.g., weight-bearing on an extended upper extremity in sitting). Training begins in a supported position with control of small ranges, and progresses to full range control and more challenging movement combinations. Once strong elements are broken up, focus can be shifted to weaker elements. Gradually more and more varieties of movements are introduced.[31,35,36,38,68] The main goal of rehabilitation is to rebuild functional patterns of movement. Practice must therefore be specific to the movement combinations needed for functional skills. For example, knee flexion with hip extension is needed for toe-off during gait and is not typically seen in stereotypical synergies in the patient with stroke. Bridging activities are important lead-up skills that can be used to promote knee flexion with hip extension and functional toe-off.

Postural Control and Balance

An intervention program to improve **balance** must be based on an accurate assessment of deficits (see Chapter 8). Balance training activities can be used to:

1. Improve trunk stability, biomechanical alignment, and symmetrical weight distribution.
2. Improve awareness and control of COM and limits of stability (LOS).
3. Improve musculoskeletal responses necessary for balance including functional ROM, strength, and synergistic patterns.
4. Promote use of functional balance strategies during static and dynamic activities and in varying environmental conditions.
5. Improve utilization of sensory systems (somatosensory, visual, vestibular inputs) and CNS sensory integration mechanisms for balance.
6. Improve safety awareness and compensatory strategies for effective fall prevention.

POSTURAL ALIGNMENT AND WEIGHT DISTRIBUTION

Musculoskeletal impairments can affect postural control and balance. Physical therapy interventions should focus first on improving ROM, muscle strength, endurance, and stabilization control. For example, active exercises to improve standing balance can include standing heel-cord stretches, heel-rises, toe-offs, partial wall squats, chair rises, side kicks, back kicks, and marching in place.[91] Faulty postures such as forward head posture, kyphosis, swayback (increased lordosis), scoliosis, or pelvic asymetries can result in pain and altered kinesthetic awareness of position. Although mild deficits may not affect balance control,[102] deficits that significantly alter the COM position can impair balance.[2] Patients are typically unable to self-correct faulty postures. Postural reeducation requires practice and repetition. Patient awareness of position and normal alignment can be facilitated through appropriate use of feedback (verbal and visual cues). Mirrors can be effective aids to assist the patient in achieving a correct position providing visuospatial perceptual deficits are not present. Tactile and proprioceptive inputs can also be used to help reinforce appropriate muscle activity. Teaching strategies should address control of essential postural elements, that is, axial extension, shoulder and pelvic position, and normal spine alignment. Application of correct postures to real-life functional situations is important to ensure carryover and lasting change.[55]

The therapist should focus on obtaining symmetrical weight-bearing and static balance control. Patients may present with specific directional instabilities, such as weight-bearing more on one side than the other. For example, after a stroke the patient typically keeps weight centered toward the sound side. Practice should include redirecting the patient into a centered position by moving toward the affected side. **Limits of stability (LOS)** should be explored. For example, in sitting or standing, the patient is instructed to slowly sway forward and back and side-to-side. The outer point at which the COM is still maintained within the BOS is termed the LOS. Loss of balance occurs when the LOS have been exceeded, for example, when the COM extends beyond the BOS. Practice of volitional body sway is important to assist the patient in developing accurate perceptual awareness of stability limits, an important component of an overall CNS internal model of postural control. Because the LOS change with different tasks, a variety of functional activities should be practiced in different environmental settings.

Force-platform devices can be used to provide center of pressure (COP) biofeedback.[103–107] The weight on each foot is computed and converted into visual feedback regarding the locus and movement of the patient's COP. Some units provide auditory feedback. A computer analyzes the data and provides relevant biofeedback data (sway path and COP position) on a visual monitor. Postural sway movements can be shaped and modified to enhance symmetry, steadiness, and expand stability limits. The patient can be instructed to increase or decrease sway movements or move the COP cursor on the computer screen to achieve a designated range or to match a designated target. Force-platform biofeedback is an effective training device for patients who demonstrate problems in force generation. For example, the patient with decreased force generation (hypometria) as typically demonstrated by individuals with Parkinson's disease is directed toward achieving larger and faster sway movements during force-platform training. The patient with too much force (hypermetria), as typically demonstrated by the individual with cerebellar ataxia, is directed toward decreasing sway movements progressing to holding a stable, centered posture.[105–107] It is important to remember that balance retraining using force-platform biofeedback does not automatically transfer to functional skills like gait. Winstein[108,109] found that a reduction in standing balance asymmetry did not result in a concomitant reduction in asymmetrical limb movement patterns associated with hemiparetic locomotion. Given the specificity of training principle, this is not a surprising finding. Alternate and less expensive strategies can also be used to provide weight information and achieve symmetrical weight-bearing by using a set of bathroom scales or limb load monitors.[110,111]

FUNCTIONAL BALANCE STRATEGIES

Retraining functional balance strategies is an important goal of treatment. Muscle synergy patterns used for the maintenance of balance are specific to the demands of the task. Nashner[112,113] first described synergy patterns for standing balance in response to anterior/posterior platform perturbations. Small shifts in the COM alignment and/or slow body sway motions are normally achieved by an ankle strategy. This is characterized by early activation of ankle dorsiflexors or plantarflexors followed by activation of more proximal limb and trunk muscles in ascending order. Lateral perturbations involve early activation of hip abductors rather than ankle muscles. Larger shifts in the COM, which approach the LOS, and/or faster body sway motions, recruit a hip strategy, characterized by early activation of proximal hip and trunk muscles.[112–114] Stepping strategies are described as occurring when the COM exceeds the LOS, a strategy of last resort. The unweighting and stepping movements are accompanied by early activation of hip abductors and ankle co-contraction for medial-lateral stability during single limb support.[115] Maki and McIlroy[116] investigated the role of limb movements in maintaining upright stance, specifically compensatory stepping and grasping movements of the upper

limbs, which they termed change-in-support strategies (as opposed to the fixed-support strategies at the ankle and hip). These investigators found that both stepping and arm movements were very common reactions to loss of balance. Moreover they were initiated well before the COM reached the LOS, contradicting the traditional view that they are strategies of last resort. They also found that stepping may actually be a preferred strategy to using a hip strategy. The direction and magnitude of change-in-support strategies were found to vary according to the magnitude and direction of the perturbation. For example, stepping may occur forward or backward in response to anterior or posterior displacements. Lateral displacements typically resulted in cross-stepping pattern (seen in 87 percent of lateral stepping responses) as opposed to straight side-steps. Lateral destabilization with its increased demands for lateral weight transfer is particularly problematic for a large portion of older adults who experience falls. Arm reactions in response to whole-body instability were also found to be prevalent with activation of shoulder muscles occurring in 85 percent of destabilizing trials. Increased understanding of the range and variability of postural strategies for balance negates any simplistic view based on a developmental perspective of reflex control of balance (i.e., righting and equilibrium reactions). Overall, the organization of balance strategies must be viewed as flexible, not rigid, involving multiple body segments. In that context observable patterns will vary according to a number of different factors including initial conditions, perturbation characteristics, learning, and intention.[117] A continuation of strategies may also be present, for example, the patient first responds with an ankle strategy but quickly progresses to a hip or stepping strategy.

Patients may demonstrate a variety of deficits. Delays in activating postural responses may accompany such conditions as peripheral neuropathy, multiple sclerosis, brain injury, or aging. Patients may also show deficits in spatiotemporal coordination. For example, the patient with stroke, brain injury, or cerebellar lesion may demonstrate disordered synergistic patterns. The patient with Parkinson's disease will demonstrate decreased amplitude (hypometric) responses secondary to rigidity, whereas the patient with cerebellar dysfunction typically demonstrates ataxic (hypermetric) responses. The postural strategies of patients with neurological impairments are typically characterized by overcompensation. Thus, the patient with a balance deficiency will increase the magnitude of the overt response, demonstrating large-scale or abrupt movements. Patients can also compensate by relying on more anticipatory control to regulate strategies. Thus, unexpected events are likely to produce greater impairments in balance responses.[117–119]

Therapists historically have used two main training strategies to promote balance responses: (1) manual perturbation, a force that displaces the COM, and (2) a moveable surface that displaces the

BOS (e.g., Swiss ball, equilibrium board, standing tilt or wobble board). It is important to select challenges (displacements) appropriate for the patient's range and speed of control. For example, the patient is sitting on a Swiss ball and instructed to move the ball side-to-side or in a circle starting with small range shifts and progressing to large range shifts. These movements require automatic postural readjustments to maintain a stable position on the ball. Repeated practice can result in more organized and efficient responses. Feedback should be provided to assist the patient in recruiting the correct synergies. For example, to recruit ankle strategies in standing, the patient should be encouraged to practice small-range, slow-velocity shifts. Attention should be directed to the action of ankle muscles to move the body (COM) over the fixed feet (BOS). The patient should practice hip motions (flexion and extension) during balance tasks that normally recruit a hip strategy (e.g., in sitting, anterior/posterior perturbations).

A number of different functional training activities should be utilized, because most demands for balance come with normal everyday activities. Considerations in selection of training activities include (1) patient safety and level of control, and (2) variety in terms of real-life functional tasks and environments. It is important to remember that some activities may cause the patient distress initially. The patient will feel threatened when placed in situations where he or she is in jeopardy of losing balance. The therapist should ensure patient confidence by providing a clear explanation of what is going to happen, and what is expected of the patient in terms that are easy to understand. Support may be given initially to reduce fear if using a new posture, but should be withdrawn as soon as possible to allow focus on active control (e.g., light touch-down support of both hands progressing to one hand and finally no support). Feedback should be directed toward achieving appropriate functional responses and eliminating those strategies that are ineffective. Activities can be organized as beginning-level, intermediate-level, and advanced-level activities.[91] The therapist can vary the level of activities, selecting activities that both provide success as well as appropriately challenge the patient. Postures should be selected based on the patient's level of control and the need to limit degrees of freedom. For example, sitting balance training typically preceeds standing balance training. The complexity of the task can be altered to increase difficulty (e.g., weight shifting in sitting to picking up objects off the floor). The patient's attention can be redirected during the balance task (e.g., ball throwing and/or catching while standing). Anticipatory postural adjustments should also be practiced, because predictive control must be operational for functional balance. The patient is provided with advance information about the upcoming demands of the movement. For example, "I want you to catch this 5-pound weighted ball while maintaining your sitting position." The prior knowledge serves as an important source of information in initiating correct postural patterns. Practice should occur in a variety of environments. For example, training can progress from a closed or fixed environment to a more variable environment such as the physical therapy gym. Balance training must ultimately be context specific to real-life settings of home or community to ensure functional carryover.

SENSORY ORGANIZATION

An important focus of a balance training program is the utilization and integration of appropriate sensory systems. Normally three sources of inputs are utilized to maintain balance: somatosensory inputs (proprioceptive and tactile inputs from the feet and ankles), visual inputs, and vestibular inputs.[120] Careful assessment can identify the patient's use of inputs to maintain balance (e.g., Clinical Test for Sensory Interaction and Balance [CTSIB]).[121] Treatment can then be directed to using varying sensory conditions to challenge the patient. For example, patients who demonstrate a high degree of dependence on vision can practice balance tasks with eyes open and eyes closed, in reduced lighting, or in situations of inaccurate vision (petroleum-coated lenses or prism glasses). Altering the visual inputs allows the patient to shift focus and reliance to other sensory inputs, in this case to intact somatosensory and vestibular inputs. Patients can practice varying somatosensory inputs by standing and walking on varying surfaces, from flat surfaces (floor) to compliant surfaces (low to high carpet pile), to dense foam. Closing the eyes eliminates use of visual cues. A patient who is barefoot or wearing thin-soled shoes is better able to attend to sensation from the feet than if wearing thick-soled shoes. Challenges to the vestibular system can be introduced by reducing both visual and somatosensory inputs through sensory conflict situations. The patient can practice standing or walking on varying heights of dense foam. The thicker the foam, the less the reliance on somatosensory inputs, the greater the challenge to the vestibular system. The patient can also be directed to stand or walk on foam with eyes closed, a condition that requires maximum use of vestibular inputs. Patients should also practice walking outside, progressing from relatively smooth terrain (sidewalks) to uneven terrain. Stepping onto moving surfaces (escalator, elevator) can also be practiced. Repetition and practice are important factors in assisting in CNS adaptation.

Patients with significant loss of sensory information will require assistance in shifting toward the intact systems to monitor and adjust balance (a compensatory training strategy). For example, the patient with proprioceptive losses will need to learn to shift focus onto the visual system to monitor balance. Thus, the patient with bilateral amputations learns to rely heavily on visual inputs to maintain standing balance. The patient must then be cautioned to maintain adequate lighting while walking. If deficits exist in more than one of the major sensory systems, compensatory shifts are generally inadequate and balance deficits will be more pronounced.[2] Thus, the patient with diabetic neuropathy and retinopathy will be at high risk for loss of balance and falls. Compensatory training with an assistive device is indicated. Other patients must be encouraged to ignore distorted information (e.g., impaired proprioception accompanying stroke) in favor of more accurate sensory information (e.g., vision). Augmented feedback can be used to provide additional sensory information for balance (e.g., verbal commands, light-touch finger contact, a biofeedback cane with auditory signals, or visual monitors).

SAFETY AND FALL PREVENTION

Prevention of falls for the patient with balance deficiency is an important goal of therapy. Life-style counseling is important to help recognize potentially dangerous situations and reduce the likelihood of falls. For example, high-risk activities likely to result in falls include turning, sit-to-stand transfers, reaching and bending over, and stair climbing. Patients should also be discouraged from clearly hazardous activities such as climbing on step stools, ladders, and chairs, or walking on slippery or icy surfaces. The education plan should stress the harmful effects of a sedentary life-style. Patients should be encouraged to maintain an active life-style, including a program of regular exercise and walking. Medications should be reviewed and those medications linked to increased risk of falls (e.g., medications that result in postural hypotension) should be addressed. A consult with the physician for medication review may be indicated.

Compensatory training strategies should be utilized. The patient should be instructed in how to maintain an adequate BOS at all times. For example, the patient should widen BOS when turning or sitting down. If a force is expected, the patient should be instructed to widen the BOS in the direction of the expected force (e.g., leaning into the wind). If greater stability is needed, instruction should be provided in how to lower the COM (e.g., crouching down to reduce the likelihood of a fall). Greater stability can also be achieved if friction is increased between the body and the support surface. The patient should therefore be instructed to wear shoes with low heels and rubber-soles for better gripping (e.g., athletic shoes). Assistive devices should be used to assist balance when necessary. Consideration should always be given to using the least restrictive device while at the same time ensuring safety. Light touch-down support using a vertical or slant cane (similar to that used by individuals who are blind) has been shown to improve balance.[122]

A fall prevention program must also address environmental factors that contribute to falls. The following recommendations are of major importance in reducing falls in the home environment.

1. Ample light should be provided. Both low light and glare can be hazardous, particularly for the elderly. Glare can be reduced with translucent shades or curtains.
2. Inaccessible light switches should be repositioned at the entrance to a room. Timers can ensure that lights come on routinely at dusk. Clapper devices can be used to enable the patient to turn on lights from across the room. Nightlights typically used in bathrooms or hallways do not provide enough light to ensure adequate balance.
3. Carpets with loose edges should be tacked down. Scatter or throw rugs should be removed.
4. Furniture that obstructs walkways should be removed or repositioned.
5. Chairs should be of adequate height and firmness to assist in sit-to-stand transfers. Chairs with armrests and elevated seat heights may be required. Motorized chairs that elevate the patient into standing may be hazardous for some patients who are unable to initiate active balance responses in a timely manner during initial standing.
6. Stairs are the site of many falls. Adequate lighting is essential. Contrast tape using bright warm colors (red, orange, or yellow) can be used to highlight steps. Handrails are important for safety on stairs and, if not present, may need to be installed.
7. Grab bars or rails reduce the incidence of falls in the bathroom. Nonskid mats or strips in the bathtub along with a tub or shower seat can also improve safety. Toilet seats can be elevated to facilitate independent use.

Gait and Locomotion

Substantial rehabilitation efforts are directed toward improving gait to restore or improve a patient's functional mobility and independence. Walking is frequently the number one goal of patients who "want to walk" above all other considerations. Ability to ambulate independently is often a significant factor in determining discharge placements (e.g., return to home or extended care facility). To establish a realistic intervention plan and outcome measures, the physical therapist must accurately analyze gait. Comprehensive gait analysis including gait variables and common gait deviations is discussed in Chapter 10. The functional demands of the patient's home, community, or work environment must be considered in planning successful interventions and in predicting a patient's future status.

Gait is a complex skill that requires the functioning of many interacting systems. Multiple muscle groups are active in alternating synergistic patterns. Stabilizing muscles contribute to stability of the stance limb and trunk during weight acceptance and single limb support. Other muscles contribute to limb advancement of the dynamic limb during the swing phase. The pattern is then reversed as the gait cycle progresses. As the speed of walking increases, the requirements for timing and control increase. Interventions must first be directed at improving function of individual components. For example, attention is directed first at improving strength of weak muscles such as hip abductors or knee extensors, or ankle joint range. Emphasis can then shift to improving synergistic control of gait through functional training activities.[91]

Important functional lead-up activities that improve strength, range, and control necessary for gait include bridging; sit-to-stand transfers; stabilizing and weight shifting in kneeling, half-kneeling, modified plantigrade, and standing; and stepping in modified plantigrade and standing (see Chapter 14). Walking is typically practiced first under supportive conditions using parallel bars or assistive devices (e.g., walker, cane, crutches). The goal is early mobilization of the patient out of bed or out of chair to prevent further indirect impairments (e.g., weakness, decreased endurance, loss of mobility, etc.). Gait is typically slow and deliberate with a great deal of conscious effort. Therapists often assist required gait elements, including the weight shift, stabilization of the stance limb, or advancement of the dynamic limb. These compensatory strategies are effective in promoting early ambulation but do little to promote the balance and the dynamic control needed for independent gait. The patient must be gradually progressed out of the parallel bars to the least restrictive assistive device, and finally to no device at all.

Active walking should be practiced in both forward and backward directions. Side-stepping or crossed-stepping can be practiced first holding on to the outside of the parallel bars or to an oval bar progressing to no support. The PNF[39] activity of braiding is a skill-level gait activity that involves alternating side-steps with cross-steps. One limb steps out to the side while the other limb alternates between stepping up and across in front of the other leg (in a D1 flexion pattern) or back and around the other leg (in a D2 extension pattern). The alternating patterns result in improved pelvic/lower trunk rotation. **Locomotion** can also be resisted using the PNF technique of RP. Manual contacts placed on the pelvis first lightly stretch and then resist motion. Improved timing and control of pelvic rotation is the goal. Resistance can also be provided using elastic resistance bands either wrapped around the pelvis or held in the patient's hands. The therapist walks behind and holds the other end of the resistance bands. Gait can be resisted in any direction, that is, forward, backward, or sideways.

Walking should be practiced on varying surfaces, from smooth surfaces to uneven terrain outside. Additional challenges to balance can be achieved by having the patient walk on a thick rug or floor mat. Walking can be challenged by varying the BOS from wide to narrow to tandem walking. Visual inputs can be varied by having the patient walk with eyes open progressing to eyes closed. Vestibular inputs can be varied by having the patient walk while moving the head right and left or up and down. Turns should also be practiced, progressing from wide turns to more narrow turns and partial turns (90-degree turns) to full turns (180-degree turns). Attention can be varied by having the patient practice walking with full attention to walking while performing a second task (dual-task training). For example, the patient walks and carries an object or bounces a ball. Attention can also be diverted by talking to the patient while walking. Walking through an obstacle course around and over objects can also be used to challenge control. Although close stand-by guarding may be necessary, a hands-off, task-oriented training approach is definitely recommended at this point. Initially, the patient may need to use light touch-down (fingertip) support of the hands to maintain balance. For example, the patient can walk in a corridor next to a wall while lightly touching the wall. Progression is then to walking away from the wall. The therapist verbally cues the patient to maintain the pace and symmetry of gait. Treadmill walking is an effective strategy to achieve velocity control. The patient begins by walking at self-selected comfortable speeds and is gradually progressed to faster and more functional speeds of walking.

Climbing stairs is an important functional skill. For many patients, it may mean the difference between going home or going to an alternate living environment. Important lead-up activities for stair climbing include sit-to-stand transfers, and standing weight shifting and stepping activities. Initially upper extremity support on handrails may be used to compensate for any instability the patient may experience. However, pulling forward with the hand during ascent or pushing during descent masks active control of trunk and lower extremity muscles. As soon as possible stair climbing should be practiced without upper extremity support. Initial practice can begin with step-ups or lateral step-ups using a low aerobic step or platform. The height of the step can be raised to increase the challenge of the activity. Practice can begin in the parallel bars or next to a treatment table or wall for light touch-down support. Progression can then be to no upper extremity support, practicing ascent and descent using a limited number of steps, to finally practicing the number of steps required in the patient's home environment. It is important to stress the patient maintain a wide BOS throughout stair-climbing practice. Practice on ramps may also be necessary for some patients. For patients with knee extension instability, ramps pose an increased challenge during descent while knee stabilization is enhanced during ascent.

INTERVENTION STRATEGIES TO IMPROVE MOTOR LEARNING

Motor learning involves a significant amount of practice and feedback, and a high level of information processing related to control, error detection, and correction.[123] Motor learning can be facilitated through the use of effective training strategies (summarized in Table 13–2).

Strategy Development

The overall goal during the early cognitive stage of learning is to facilitate task understanding and organize early practice. The patient's knowledge of the skill and any existing problems must be ascertained. The therapist should highlight the purpose of the action in a functionally relevant context. The task should seem important, desirable, and realistic to learn. The therapist should demonstrate the task exactly as it should be done (i.e., smoothly, completely, and at ideal performance speeds). This helps the patient develop an internal cognitive map or *reference of correctness*. Attention should be directed to the desired outcome and critical task elements. The therapist should point out similarities to other learned tasks so that subroutines that are part of other motor programs can be retrieved from memory. Features of the environment critical to performance should also be highlighted.

During initial practice, the therapist should give clear and simple verbal instructions and not overload the patient with excessive or wordy commands. It is important to reinforce correct performance and intervene when movement errors become consistent or when safety is an issue. The therapist should attempt to correct all the numerous errors that characterize this stage. Feedback, particularly visual feedback, is important during early learning. The patient should be directed to watch the movements closely. Augmented visual feedback can be provided through the use of mirrors and videotaped demonstration providing the patient does not demonstrate visuospatial impairments. The patient's initial performance trials can be recorded for later review, or audiovisual materials such as videotapes or films of other patients can be used for demonstration. Highly skilled patients (e.g., rehabilitation graduates) called upon for demonstration can provide meaningful motivation to patients just starting the rehabilitation process. Demonstration has also been shown to be effective in producing learning even with unskilled patient models. In this situation the learner/patient benefits from the cognitive processing and problem solving he or she uses while watching the unskilled model attempt to correct errors and arrive at the desired movement.[124]

Initial performance may be improved by manually guiding the patient's movements. Guidance allows the patient to preview the stimuli inherent in the movement pattern, that is, to learn the "sensations of movement" as described by Bobath.[31] The supportive use of hands can also allay patient fears and instill confidence. The therapist's hands can effectively substitute for the missing elements and guide the patient toward correct performance. The key to success in using manually guided movements is to provide only as much assistance as needed and remove the assistance as soon as possible. Active movements promote learning, whereas passive movements (e.g., dragging the patient through the motions) does little to ensure learning and may actually increase dependence on the therapist. For some patients, excessive or overuse of **guided movement** prevents development of independent movement. Clinically, the patient cannot move unless assisted by "my therapist" and performance is markedly reduced when assistance is removed. Guided movement is most effective for slow postural responses (positioning tasks) and least effective for rapid or ballistic tasks.

As initial practice progresses, the patient is asked to assess performance and identify problems—specifically, what difficulties exist, what can be done to correct the difficulties, and how can the movements be modified to achieve a successful outcome? If a complex task is practiced, the patient is asked to identify if the correct components were performed, how the individual components fit together, and if they were appropriately sequenced. The therapist should confirm the accuracy of the patient's assessment if the patient is able to accurately identify problems and the strategies needed to correct the problems. If the patient is unable to provide an accurate assessment of problems, the therapist can prompt the patient in decision making by utilizing key questions. Facilitation techniques (tapping, stretch, etc.) can be used to activate and focus attention on missing movement components. For example, if the patient consistently falls to the right while standing, questions can be directed (in what direction did you fall? what do you need to do to correct this problem?). If additional assistance is required, the therapist can use manual tapping or light resistance to provide directional cues to assist the patient in correcting postural responses. The patient is actively involved in self-monitoring and self-correction of movements. The development of these decision making skills is critical in ensuring adaptability of movements and generalizability of learning to other environments.

During the associated and autonomous phases of learning, the patient continues with high levels of practice. Random errors decrease. As consistent errors are identified, solutions are generated. The focus is on refinement of skills and movement consistency in a variety of environmental contexts. This will ensure an overall range of movement patterns that are adaptable and fit the changing circumstances of the environment. It is appropriate to focus the patient's attention on proprioceptive feedback, the "feel of the movement." Thus, the patient is directed to attend to the sensations intrinsic to the movement itself and to associate those sensations with the motor actions. Facilitation techniques may be counterproductive at this stage, because they maintain dependence on initiation and control of movement by the therapist and preclude the learning of intrinsic sensations of active movement. Guided movement may also be counterproductive, because it alters the normal feel of active movement. During late-stage learning, the use of distracters such as ongoing conversation or dual task training (e.g., ball skills during standing and walking) can yield important evidence of an autonomous level of control. Finally, it is important to remember that many patients undergoing active rehabilitation do not reach this final stage of learning. For example, in patients with traumatic brain injury, performance may reach consistent levels within structured environments, while performance in more open environments is not possible.

Feedback

The vast body of motor learning and therapeutic literature stresses the importance of feedback in promoting motor learning. Feedback can be either **intrinsic,** occurring as a natural result of the movement, or **augmented,** by extrinsic sensory cues not typically received in the task. Proprioceptive, visual, vestibular, and cutaneous signals are examples of types of intrinsic feedback, while verbal or tactile cuing, videotaped replays, and biofeedback are forms of augmented feedback. During therapy, both intrinsic and augmented feedback can be manipulated to enhance motor learning. *Concurrent feedback* is given during task performance, and *terminal feedback* is given at the end of task performance. Augmented feedback about the nature or quality of the movement pattern produced is termed **knowledge of performance (KP).** Augmented feedback about the end result or overall outcome of the movement is termed **knowledge of results (KR)**[1], p 415. The importance of KP and KR varies according to the skill being learned and the availability of feedback from intrinsic sources.[125–128] The learner should be assisted in perceiving and classifying movement cues that highlight final movement outcomes (KR). Performance cues (KP) should focus on key task elements that lead to a successful final outcome. Clinical decisions about feedback focus on (1) what type of sensory feedback to employ, (2) how much feedback to use (intensity), and (3) when to give the feedback (scheduling).

SELECTION

Choices here involve the selection of which intrinsic sensory systems to highlight, what type of augmented feedback to use, and how to pair augmented feedback to intrinsic feedback. The selection of sensory systems depends on specific examination findings and on the stage of learning. The sensory systems selected must provide accurate information. If intrinsic systems are impaired and provide distorted or incomplete information, then alternate sensory systems and/or augmented feedback should be utilized. Decisions should also be based on stage of learning. Early in learning, visual feedback is easily brought to conscious attention and therefore is important. Less consciously accessible sensory information such as proprioception is more useful during the middle and end stages of learning.

FREQUENCY AND SCHEDULING

Decisions about frequency and scheduling of feedback (when and how much) must be reached. Frequent feedback (e.g., given after every performance trial) quickly guides the learner to the correct performance. Too little feedback will delay learning, and too much feedback is also detrimental; it fosters feedback dependence. In this last situation, the patient may be able to perform a movement task but only when augmented feedback is present (e.g., the therapist's verbal or manual cuing). Independent function is obviously restricted. Slower postural (closed-loop) tasks may benefit from concurrent feedback whereas fast, ballistic (open-loop) tasks require terminal feedback. Research also suggests that practice with concurrent performance feedback may result in improved performance (e.g., learning a partial weight-bearing skill) while post-response feedback was detrimental for immediate performance but more beneficial for longer-lasting learning as measured by 2-day retention tests.[129]

Varied feedback schedules should be considered. These include (1) *summed feedback,* feedback given after a set number of trials (e.g., after every other trial or every third trial); (2) *faded feedback,* feedback given at first after every trial and then less frequently (e.g., after every second trial, progressing to every fifth trial); and (3) *bandwidth feedback,* feedback given only when performance is outside a given error range. Research demonstrates that varied feedback schedules slow the acquisition of a skill but result in improved learning as measured by retention tests.[1,130–134] This is most likely due to the increased depth of cognitive processing that accompanies the variable presentation of feedback. *Delayed feedback,* feedback given after a short time delay (e.g., a 3-second delay) can also be beneficial in allowing the learner a brief time for introspection and self-assessment.[135] In contrast, the therapist who bombards the patient immediately after task completion with verbal feedback stressing movement accuracy precludes active information processing by the learner. The patient's own decision making skills are minimized, while the therapist's skills predominate. Winstein[136] points out that this may well explain why many studies on the effectiveness of therapeutic approaches cite minimal carryover and limited retention of newly acquired motor skills. The delay interval should not be filled with practice of other movements; the resulting interference may decrease learning.

Practice

In general, increased **practice** leads to increased learning. The therapist needs to ensure that the patient practices desired movements. Practice of incorrect movement patterns can lead to a negative learning situation in which "faulty habits and postures" must be unlearned before the correct movements can be mastered. The organization of practice will depend upon several factors, including the patient's motivation, attention span, concentration, endurance, and the type of task. Additional factors may include the frequency of allowable therapy sessions; the latter is often dependent upon hospital scheduling and availability of services and payment. For outpatients, practice at home is highly dependent on motivation, family support, and suitable environment. Clinical decisions about practice focus on (1) what type, (2) how much, (3) when (practice order of tasks), and (4) environmental context.

PHYSICAL VERSUS MENTAL PRACTICE

Physical practice allows the patient to gain direct experience and is important for shaping elements of the motor program. **Mental practice** is the cognitive rehearsal of a motor task without any overt movement. The patient is instructed to visualize the movement and imagine how it will occur. The formation of a kinesthetic image (what the movement will feel like) is an important element that is confirmed once physical practice occurs. Mental practice has consistently been found to facilitate the acquisition of new motor skills.[137–141] Patients who fatigue easily and are unable to repeat physical practice can benefit from mental practice to aid learning. Mental practice is also effective in alleviating anxiety associated with initial practice by previewing the upcoming movement experience. Mental practice when combined with physical practice has been shown to increase the accuracy and efficiency of movements at significantly faster rates than subjects who used physical practice alone.[141] When using mental practice, it is important to make sure the patient is actively rehearsing the correct movement steps. This can be assured by having the patient verbalize aloud the steps he or she is rehearsing.

CONSTANT VERSUS VARIABLE PRACTICE

Constant practice refers to practice organized around one task performed repeatedly, and **variable practice** refers to the practice of several variations of the same task or within the same category of movements. Although both allow for motor skill acquisition, variable practice has superior long-term effects in retention and generalizability of skills. For example, a variety of different transfers (e.g., bed to wheelchair, wheelchair to toilet, wheelchair to tub transfer seat) can be practiced all within the same training session. Although skilled performance may be initially delayed, improved retention of skills can be expected. The constant challenge of varying the task demands increases the depth of cognitive processing through retrieval of variations of the motor program from memory stores.[142–144] The acquired skills can then be applied more easily to other novel variations or environments that have not yet been attempted, resulting in improved generalizability. Constant practice of only one type of transfer will improve initial performance but does not achieve the same results in terms of retention and generalizability.[1]

MASSED VERSUS DISTRIBUTED PRACTICE

Massed practice consists of a sequence of practice and rest times in which the rest time is much less than the practice time[1], p 416. Fatigue, decreased performance, and risk of injury are factors that must be considered when using massed practice. **Distributed practice** consists of spaced practice intervals in which the rest time equals or exceeds the practice time[1], p 413. Although learning is possible with both, distributed practice is preferable for many patients undergoing active rehabilitation who demonstrate limited performance capabilities and endurance. With adequate rest periods, performance can be improved without the interfering effects of fatigue. Distributed practice is also of benefit if motivation is low or if the learner has a short attention span, poor concentration, or motor planning deficits (dyspraxia). Distributed practice should also be considered if the task itself is complex, long, or has a high energy cost. Massed practice can be considered when motivation or skill level are high and when the patient has adequate attention and concentration. For example, the patient with spinal cord injury in the final stages of rehabilitation will spend long practice sessions acquiring the wheelchair skills needed for community access.

PRACTICE ORDER

The third area for clinical decision making involves practice order, the sequence in which tasks are practiced. *Blocked order* refers to the repeated practice of a task or group of tasks in a predictable order (three trials of task 1, three trials of task 2, three trials of task 3: 111222333). *Serial order* refers to a predictable but nonrepeating order (practice of multiple tasks in the following order: 123123123). *Random order* refers to a nonrepeating and nonpredictable order (123321312). Although skill acquisition can be achieved with all three, differences have been found. Blocked order produces improved early acquisition of skills while serial and random order produce better retention and generalizability of skills. This is due to contextual interference and increased depth of cognitive processing. The key element here is the degree to which the learner is actively involved in problem solving. For example, a treatment session can be organized to include several variations of the same skill (e.g., pelvic rotation) practiced in different postures (bridging, kneeling, plantigrade, and standing). Random ordering of the tasks may initially delay acquisition of the desired movements (performance) but over the long term will enhance retention and generalizability.[8,145,146]

TRANSFER TRAINING

Transfer of learning refers to the gain (or loss) of task performance as a result of practice or experience on some other task[1], p 389. This can be a useful strategy to promote learning. The most frequently used application of this principle is practicing component parts of a motor activity in order to learn the whole activity, what is known as **parts-to-whole transfer.** The success of this strategy is dependent on the nature of the task and the learner. If the task is complex, with highly independent parts that can be naturally divided into units (e.g., a transfer), or if the learner has a limited memory or attention span, then learning can be enhanced through this method of practice. If the task has highly integrated, dependent parts (e.g., gait) or is relatively simple, then practice of the integrated whole will be more successful. If the parts-to-whole method is used, it is important to alternately practice both the parts and then the whole to ensure adequate transfer. Thus, within the same session the patient should practice the component parts, then the integrated whole. Delaying practice of the integrated whole for days or weeks can interfere with transfer effects and learning.[1]

The integration of motor programs is made easier by practice that includes appropriate timing. In tasks that require speed and accuracy, both should be emphasized. Stressing accuracy first and delaying practice of speeded performance may result in inadequate transfer of learning, because accuracy tasks involve feedback processing while speed tasks involve feedforward processing.[1] For example, when gait movements are practiced at very slow speeds stressing accuracy, the timing needed for normal or fast walking may then be difficult to achieve.

Learning can be achieved through **bilateral-transfer.** The patient practices the movements first using unaffected body segments progressing to practice of involved body segments. For example, the patient with stroke first practices the desired movement pattern using the more normal (unaffected) extremity. This initial practice enhances formation of the necessary motor program, which can then be applied to the opposite, involved extremity. This method cannot, however, substitute for lack of movement potential of the affected extremities (e.g., a flaccid limb on the hemiplegic side). Transfer effects are greatest with similar parts (arm-to-arm), similar tasks (identical stimuli and responses), and similar environments. For example, optimal transfer can be expected with practice of an elbow flexion pattern first on one side, then with an identical pattern on the other side. Transfer effects can be improved by ensuring a sufficient number of practice trials of the contralateral extremity and selecting a practice environment that closely resembles the actual environment.[8]

ENVIRONMENTAL CONTEXT

Altering the environmental context is an important consideration in structuring practice sessions. Because learning is task specific within specific environments, tasks must be practiced in the environments in which they naturally occur. Practicing walking only within the physical therapy clinic might lead to successful performance in that setting but does little to prepare the patient for ambulation at home or in the community. The therapist should begin to gradually modify the environment as soon as performance becomes consistent.

Motivation

Motivation is the internal state that tends to direct or energize the system toward a goal[1], p 416. The patient must fully understand the purpose of the task at hand and want to acquire the skill. Planning that involves the patient and family in mutual goal setting can greatly enhance the desire to achieve goals. Continued motivation can also be enhanced by the effective use of feedback during treatment. Treatment successes are important and can be highlighted through the use of carefully planned positive reinforcements. Balancing more difficult tasks with easier ones allows the patient to experience feelings of success interspersed with frustrations. The therapist should plan to end each therapy session on a positive, successful note. This will promote a sense of time well spent for the patient despite the inherent frustrations. In addition, this approach typically contributes to a sense of accomplishment for the patient and a feeling that future goals are achievable.

SUMMARY

This chapter outlined a conceptual framework based on normal processes of motor control and motor learning. Clinical decision making for patients with motor control and motor learning deficits must be based upon a comparison of normal and abnormal function. The therapist must be able to examine patients accurately in terms of impairments, functional limitations, and disability. Basic elements of motor control that must be addressed include CNS readiness (arousal and attention), cognition, sensory integrity and integration, joint integrity and mobility, tone and reflex integrity, muscle performance, and motor patterns. The unique problems of each patient require that the therapist also recognize a number of interrelated factors, including individual needs, motivation, goals, concerns, and potential for independent function. Physical therapists have the knowledge and clinical skills to reduce or eliminate functional limitation and disability while improving overall quality of life. Given the tremendous variability of patients with motor control dysfunction, it is unrealistic to expect that any particular set of interventions will be successful with all patients. Interventions must be carefully chosen to address impairments that directly impact on overall function and disability. Interventions are also chosen to prevent complications, and minimize injury, future impairments, functional loss, or disability. The effective use of motor learning strategies can dramatically improve treatment outcomes. The role of the therapist using a motor learning approach is primarily one of facilitator. Carefully planned and structured education empowers the patient. Patient skills in self-evaluation and decision making are promoted whenever possible to foster independence. If patient independence is not possible because of the complexity of motor control and motor learning deficits, education of family, friends, and caregivers assumes paramount importance.

QUESTIONS FOR REVIEW

1. Differentiate between the terms motor control and motor learning. How can deficits in motor control be distinguished from those of motor learning?

2. Describe how information is processed within the CNS to arrive at an appropriate plan for movement.

3. Compare and contrast hierarchical and systems theories of motor control.

4. What is schema theory? How does it explain motor learning?

5. Differentiate between the three stages of motor learning. How should training strategies differ during each stage?

6. What is recovery of function? What are the different theories proposed to explain recovery? What factors are important in promoting recovery of function?

7. Define compensatory training. Identify three interventions that can be considered compensatory training strategies.

8. Define the remediation/facilitation approaches. Identify three interventions that are utilized in remediation/facilitation approaches.

9. Define functional/task-oriented training. Give three examples of interventions based on this approach.

10. What factors must be considered when working with patients with impaired attention and arousal? What interventions can be used to improve attention? Modify arousal levels?

11. Clinically, how would you determine if sensory stimulation is indicated? What parameters would you use to decide on application, continued use of a technique?

12. Identify three therapeutic techniques (interventions) that can be used for patients with deficits in (a) mobility, (b) stability, (c) controlled mobility, and (d) skill stages of motor control.

13. Discuss motor learning training strategies designed to improve retention and generalizability. How do they differ from strategies that optimize performance?

14. What is meant by transfer of training? Give two examples of appropriate transfer training strategies.

CASE STUDY

HISTORY: The patient is a 36 year-old man who sustained a traumatic brain injury following a motorcycle accident. On admission to a local hospital, the patient was found to have left frontal laceration with an underlying linear skull fracture. CT scan revealed edema, a right basal ganglia contusion, and a left frontal contusion. The patient was comatose on admission. His acute hospital course was complicated by increased intracranial pressure and severe spasticity which required casts and splints. A gastric tube was inserted.

The patient's neurological status did not substantially improve at the acute hospital. He was transferred to a rehabilitation hospital 4 weeks post injury for intensive rehabilitation. He had a brief readmission to the acute hospital during his sixth week post injury for stabilization of acute hypothermia and hypothyroidism. He was then returned to the rehabilitation facility for continued intensive rehabilitation. His medications consisted of Tegretol (200 mg po QID), multivitamins, and Colace.

Cognition. The patient is now semicomatose and unresponsive. He inconsistently responds to a command to "look at me" with eye opening and to "lift up your leg" with movement of the right leg only. Otherwise there is no response to auditory or visual stimulation.

Language-Communication. Unable to assess.

Social. Married with no children. Wife is a registered nurse and very supportive of her husband.

PHYSICAL THERAPY EXAMINATION—INITIAL ADMISSION:

Vital signs: Heart rate 60 bpm, blood pressure 122/70 mmHg, respiratory rate of 14 breaths per minute.

Sensation. Unable to assess; unresponsive.

Tone (modified Ashworth Scale grades)
- Severe flexor tone and spasms of the trunk that result in the patient moving in bed from a supine to a left sidelying, curled-up (fetal) position: 4
- Right upper extremity (RUE) extensor tone: 3
- Right lower extremity (RLE) extensor tone: 3
- LUE flexor tone: 3
- LLE extensor tone: 2

Range of Motion
- RUE and LUE are within normal limits.
- Both lower extremities (BLEs) are within normal limits except for ankle dorsiflexion 0–10 degrees.

Control of active movement
- The patient is agitated with restless movements and is frequently diaphoretic.
- No head or trunk control, dependent sitting balance.

- Movement of the RUE is spontaneous, purposeful at times, and out of synergy.
- Movement of the RLE is spontaneous, nonpurposeful, and out of synergy.
- LUE no active movement is noted.
- LLE movement is spontaneous, nonpurposeful, and in synergy.

Coordination. Unable to assess; unresponsive.

Posture. At times the patient displays decorticate posturing with mass patterning. The lower extremities scissor at times, especially when upper body flexor tone increases.

Reflexes. Exhibits frequent asymmetrical tonic neck reflex posturing with head rotated to the right, flexor withdrawal reflexes bilaterally in response to pain (delayed on the left with decreased intensity of response), and a positive support reflex on the left. Deep tendon reflexes are increased throughout.

Skin. Multiple healed lacerations on the knees and calves and pressure sores bilaterally on the lateral malleolus and calcaneous from bivalve positioning splints.

Bladder and bowel. Incontinent of bowel and bladder, and has a Texas catheter.

Part I (Questions 1–3)

1. Identify and prioritize the clinical problems presented in this case in terms of direct, indirect, and composite impairments, and functional limitations.

2. Identify the goals and outcomes of physical therapy intervention for this patient at this point in his recovery (initial admission).

3. Identify treatment interventions appropriate for this patient at this point in his recovery (initial admission).

REEXAMINATION: 6 MONTHS POST INJURY

Cognition: The patient is alert, oriented ×3. He is functioning at Rancho Level VI Confused-Appropriate (Rancho Levels of Cognitive Functioning). He shows some limited goal-directed behavior but is dependent on external supervision. He follows simple directions consistently and shows some carryover for new learning but at a significantly decreased rate. Memory is impaired; past memories show more depth and detail than short-term memory. Attention span is reduced; he requires repetition and structure to complete activities. He demonstrates little insight into disability or safety awareness.

Language-communication. The patient is dysarthric; speech is usually intelligible but difficult to understand and delayed in onset. Auditory comprehension is good.

PHYSICAL THERAPY ASSESSMENT

Vital signs, vision, and hearing are within normal limits.

Skin lacerations are healed.

Sensation

Absent sensation in the LUE and impaired sensation in the LLE with decreased proprioception. Sensation is intact in the RUE and RLE.

Tone (modified Ashworth Scale grades)
- Tone in the trunk is within normal limits except for occasional flexor spasms
- RUE and RLE extensor tone: 1+
- LUE flexor tone: 2
- LLE extensor tone: 1+

Range of motion: Within normal limits except for ankle dorsiflexion bilaterally of 0–15 degrees

Control of Active Movement
- Demonstrates purposeful, full, isolated motions through available ranges against gravity in the RUE and RLE. Strength is grossly F+ in the RUE and F– in the RLE.
- No active movement is present in the LUE.
- Movement in the LLE is purposeful and in synergy.
- Movement in the head and trunk is functional and strength is grossly fair.

Coordination
- Exhibits moderate to severe ataxia in the trunk and extremities.
- Demonstrates moderate impairment in finger-to-nose and toe-taping test.

Reflexes
- Exhibits strong associated reactions in the LUE and increased flexor posturing with stressful activities.

Balance
- In sitting requires contact guarding for safety; sacral sits with a posterior tilt of the pelvis.
- In standing requires moderate assist ×1 in the parallel bars.
- Impaired postural adjustments in sitting and standing, with impaired protective reactions in the RUE and absent protective reactions in the LUE.

Functional Activities
- Bed mobility: rolls to right and left with S
- Supine to sit: with S
- Transfers: Mod A in stand-pivot transfers
- Gait: walks in parallel bars 1 to 2 lengths with Mod A ×2 for balance
- Wheelchair: maneuvers power wheelchair with close S for safety

Key: Mod A, moderate assistance; S, supervision.

Part II (Questions 4–6)

4. Identify and prioritize this patient's problems in terms of direct, indirect, and composite impairments, and functional limitations (6 months post injury).

5. Identify the goals and outcomes of physical therapy intervention for this patient at this point in his recovery (6 months post injury).

6. Identify treatment interventions appropriate for this patient at this point in his recovery (6 months post injury).

REFERENCES

1. Schmidt, R: Motor Control and Learning, 3rd ed. Human Kinetics Pub., 1999.
2. Shumway-Cook, A, and Woollacott, M: Motor Control Theory and Practical Applications. Williams & Wilkins, Baltimore, 1995.
3. Sherrington, C. The Integrative Action of the Nervous System, ed 2. Yale Univ. Pr., New Haven, CT, 1947.
4. Taylor, J (ed): Selected Writings of John Hughlings Jackson. Basic Books, New York, 1958.
5. Brooks, V: The Neural Basis of Motor Control. Oxford Univ. Pr., New York, 1986.
6. Bernstein, N: The Coordination and Regulation of Movements. Pergamon Press, Oxford, 1967.
7. Kelso, JA: Dynamic Patterns: The Self-Organization of Brain and Behavior. MIT Press, Cambridge, MA, 1995.
8. Mcgill, R: Motor Learning Concepts and Applications, ed 4. Brown & Benchmark, Madison, WI, 1993.
9. Adams, J: A closed-loop theory of motor learning. J Motor Behav 3:111, 1971.
10. Schmidt, R: A schema theory of discrete motor skill learning. Psychol Rev 82:225, 1975.
11. Fitts, P, and Posner, M: Human Performance. Brooks/Cole, Belmont, CA, 1967.
12. Bayley, N: The development of motor abilities during the first three years. Monographs of the Society for Research in Child Development 1 (1, serial no 1), 1935.
13. Gesell, A, and Amatruda, C: Developmental Diagnosis. Harper, New York, 1941.
14. McGraw, M: The Neuromuscular Maturation of the Human Infant. Hafner, New York, 1945.
15. Keogh, J, and Sugden, D: Movement Skill Development. Macmillan, New York, 1985.
16. VanSant, A: Life span development in functional tasks. Phys Ther 70:788, 1990.
17. VanSant, A: Rising from a supine position to erect stance: Description of adult movement and a developmental hypothesis. Phys Ther 69:185, 1988.
18. Woollacott, M, and Shumway-Cook, A: Changes in posture control across the life span: A systems approach. Phys Ther 70:799, 1990.
19. Woollacott, M, and Shumway-Cook, A (eds): Development of Posture and Gait Across the Life span. Univ. of South Carolina Pr., Columbia, 1989.
20. Light, K: Information processing for motor performance in aging adults. Phys Ther 70:821, 1990.
21. Salthouse, T, and Somberg, B: Isolating the age deficit in speeded performance. J Gerontol 37:59, 1982.
22. Light, K, and Spirduso W: Effects of adult aging on the movement complexity factor of response programming. J Gerontol 45:107, 1990.
23. Spirduso, W: Physical fitness, aging, and psychomotor speed: A review. J Gerontol 35:850, 1980.
24. Schlendorf, S: Effects of aging and exercise on the adult central nervous system: A literature review. Neurology Report 15:24, 1991.
25. Shephard, R: Physical Activity and Aging, ed 2. Aspen, Rockville, MD, 1987.
26. Morris, J, and McManus, D. The neurology of aging: Normal versus pathologic change. Geriatrics 46:47, 1991.
27. Stein, D, et al: Brain Repair. Oxford Univ. Pr., New York, 1995.
28. Held, J: Recovery of function after brain damage: Theoretical implications for therapeutic intervention. In Carr, J, et al (eds): Movement Sciences: Foundations for Physical Therapy in rehabilitation. Aspen, Rockville, MD, 1987, p 155.
29. Taub, E: Movement in nonhuman primates deprived of somatosensory feedback. Exercise and Sports Science Reviews 4:335, 1976.
30. Bobath, B: The treatment of neuromuscular disorders by improving patterns of coordination. Physiotherapy 55:1, 1969.
31. Bobath, B: Adult Hemiplegia: Evaluation and Treatment, ed 2. Heinemann, London, 1978.
32. Gordon, J: Assumptions underlying physical therapy intervention: Theoretical and historical perspectives. In Carr, J, et al (eds): Movement Science Foundations for Physical Therapy Rehabilitation. Aspen, Rockville, MD, 1987, p 1.
33. Kesner, E: Controlling stability of a complex movement system. Phys Ther 70:844, 1990.
34. Sahrmann, S, and Norton, B: The relationship of voluntary movement to spasticity in the upper motoneuron syndrome. Ann Neurol 2:460, 1977.
35. Davies, P: Steps to Follow: A Guide to the Treatment of Adult Hemiplegia. Springer-Verlag, New York, 1985.
36. Davies, P: Right in the Middle: Selective Trunk Activity in the Treatment of Adult Hemiplegia. Springer-Verlag, New York, 1990.
37. Brunnstom, S: Movement Therapy in Hemiplegia. Harper & Row, New York, 1970.
38. Sawner, K, and LaVigne, J: Brunnstrom's Movement Therapy in Hemiplegia, ed 2. Lippincott, New York, 1992.
39. Voss, D, et al: Proprioceptive Neuromuscular Facilitation, ed 3. Harper & Row, Philadelphia, 1985.
40. Adler, S, et al: PNF in Practice. Springer-Verlag, New York, 1993.
41. Rood, M: The use of sensory receptors to activate, facilitate, and inhibit motor response, autonomic and somatic, in developmental sequence. In Satterly, C (ed): Approaches to the Treatment of Patients with Neuromuscular Dysfunction. Wm C Brown, Dubuque, IA, 1962.
42. Stockmeyer, S: An interpretation of the approach of Rood to the treatment of neuromuscular dysfunction. Am J Phys Med 46:950, 1967.
43. Green, P: Problems of organization of motor systems. In Rosen, R, and Snell, F (eds): Progress in Theoretical Biology. Academic Press, San Diego, 1972, p 304.
44. Reed E: An outline of a theory of action systems. J Motor Behavior 14:98, 1982.
45. Horak, F: Assumptions underlying motor control for neurologic rehabilitation. In: Contemporary Management of Motor Control Problems. Proceedings of the II Step Conference. APTA, Alexandria, VA, 1992.
46. Carr, J, and Shepherd, R: A Motor Relearning Programme for Stroke, ed 2. Aspen, Rockville, MD, 1987.
47. Mulder, T: A process-oriented model of human motor behavior: Toward a theory-based rehabilitation approach. Phys Ther 71:157, 1991.
48. Yerkes, R, and Dodson, J: The relationship of strength of stimulus to rapidity of habit-formation. J Comp Neurol Psychol 18:459, 1908.
49. Malkmus, D: Integrating cognitive strategies into the physical therapy setting. Phys Ther 63:1952, 1983.
50. Wilder, J: Stimulus and Response: The Law of Initial Value. John Wright & Sons, Bristol, UK, 1967.
51. Stockmeyer, S: Clinical decision making based on homeostatic concepts. In Wolf, S (ed): Clinical Decision Making in Physical Therapy. FA Davis, Philadelphia, 1985, p 79.
52. Zasler, N, et al: Coma stimulation and coma recovery. Neurorehabilitation 1:33, 1991.
53. Howard, M, and Bleiberg, J: A Manual of Behavior Management Strategies for Traumatically Brain-Injured Adults. Rehabilitation Institute of Chicago, Chicago, 1983.
54. Zoltan, B: Vision, Perception, and Cognition, ed 3. Slack Inc., Thorofare, NJ, 1996.
55. Kisner, C, and Colby, L: Therapeutic Exercise Foundations and Techniques, ed 3. FA Davis, Philadelphia, 1996.
56. Kaltenborn, F: Mobilization of the Extremity Joints: Basic Examination and Treatment Techniques, ed 4. Olaf Norlis Bokhandel, Universitetsgaten, Oslo, 1989.
57. Wessling, K, et al: Effects of static stretch versus static stretch and ultrasound combined on triceps surae muscle extensibility in healthy women. Phys Ther 67:674, 1987.
58. Lentell, G, et al: The use of thermal agents to influence the effectiveness of a low-load prolonged stretch. J Orthop Sports Phys Ther 16:200, 1992.
59. Cornelius, W, and Jackson, A: The effects of cryotherapy and PNF techniques on hip extensor flexibility. Athletic Training 19:183, 1984.

60. Kottke, F, et al: The rationale for prolonged stretching of shortened connective tissue. Arch Phys Med Rehabil 47: 345, 1982.

61. Bandy, W, and Irion, J: The effects of time on static stretch on the flexibility of the hamstring muscles. Phys Ther 74:845, 1994.

62. Bohannon, R, and Larkin, P: Passive ankle dorsiflexion increases in patients after a regimen of tilt table: Wedge board standing. Phys Ther 65:1676, 1985.

63. Gajdosik, R: Effects of static stretching on the maximal length and resistance to passive stretch of short hamstring muscles. J Orthop Sports Phys Ther 13:126, 1991.

64. Light, K, et al: Low-load prolonged stretch vs. high-load brief stretch in treating knee contractures. Phys Ther 64:330, 1984.

65. Sady, S, et al: Flexibility training: Ballistic, static or proprioceptive neuromuscular facilitation. Arch Phys Med Rehabil 63:261, 1982.

66. Markos, P: Ipsilateral and contralateral effects of proprioceptive neuromuscular facilitation techniques on hip motion and electromyographic activity. Phys Ther 59:1366, 1979.

67. Etnyre, B, and Abraham, L: Gains in range of ankle dorsiflexion using three popular stretching techniques. Am J Phys Med 65:189, 1986.

68. Johnstone, M: Restoration of Normal Movement after Stroke. Churchill Livingstone, New York, 1995.

69. Barnard, P, et al: Reduction of hypertonicity by early casting in a comatose head-injured individual: A case report. Phys Ther 64:1540, 1984.

70. Booth, BJ, et al: Serial casting for the management of spasticity in the head-injured adult. Phys Ther 63:1960, 1983.

71. Lehmkuhl, L, et al: Multimodality treatment of joint contractures in patients with severe brain injury: Cost, effectiveness, and integration of therapies in the application of serial/inhibitive cases. J Head Trauma Rehabil 5:23, 1990.

72. Hill, J: The effects of casting on upper extremity motor disorders after brain injury. Am J Occup Ther 48:219, 1994.

73. Tabary, J, et al: Physiological and structural changes in the cat's soleus muscle due to immobilization at different lengths by plaster casts. J Physiol 224:231, 1972.

74. Feldman P: Upper extremity casting and splinting. In Glenn, M, and Whyte, J (eds): The Practical Management of Spasticity in Children and Adults. Lea & Febiger, Philadelphia, 1990.

75. Giorgetti, M: Serial and inhibitory casting: Implications for acute care physical therapy management. Neurology Report 17:18, 1993.

76. Bronski, B: Serial casting for the neurological patient. Physical Disabilities Special Interest Section Newsletter 18:4, 1995.

77. Zablotny, C, et al: Serial casting: Clinical applications for the adult head-injured patient. J Head Trauma Rehabil 2:46, 1987.

78. Kent, H, et al: Case control study of lower extremity serial casting in adult patients with head injury. Physiotherapy Canada 42:189, 1990.

79. Stefanovska, A, et al: Effects of electrical stimulation on spasticity. Crit Rev Phys Rehabil Med 3:59, 1991.

80. Sieb, T, et al: The quantitative measurement of spasticity: Effect of cutaneous electrical stimulation. Arch Phys Med Rehabil 75:746, 1994.

81. Levin, M, and Hui-Chan, C: Relief of hemiparetic spasticity by TENS is associated with improvement in reflex and voluntary motor functions. Electroencephalogr Clin Neurophysiol 85:131–142, 1992.

82. Dobkin, B: Neurologic Rehabilitation. FA Davis, Philadelphia, 1996.

83. Tries, J: EMG feedback for the treatment of upper extremity dysfunction: Can it be effective? Biofeedback Self-Regulation 14:21, 1989.

84. Middaugh, S: On clinical efficacy: Why biofeedback does— and does not—work. Biofeedback Self-Regulation 15:204, 1990.

85. Delitto, A, and Robinson, A: Neuromuscular electrical stimulation for muscle strengthening. In Snyder-Mackler, L, and Robinson, A (eds): Clinical Electrophysiology: Electrotherapy and Electrophysiologic Testing. Williams & Wilkins, Baltimore, 1989, p 95.

86. Delitto, A, and Synder-Mackler, L: Two theories of muscle strength augmentation using percutaneous electrical stimulation. Phys Ther 70:158, 1990.

87. Gordon, T, and Mao, J. Muscle atrophy and procedures for training after spinal cord injury. Phys Ther 74:50, 1994.

88. American Physical Therapy Association: Guide to Physical Therapist Practice. Phys Ther 77:1163, 1997.

89. Smidt, G, and Rogers, M: Factors contributing to the regulation and clinical assessment of muscular strength. Phys Ther 62:1283, 1982.

90. Johansson, C, et al: Relationship between verbal command volume and magnitude of muscle contraction. Phys Ther 63:1260, 1983.

91. O'Sullivan, S, and Schmitz, T: Physical Rehabilitation Laboratory Manual: Focus on Functional Training. FA Davis, Philadelphia, 1999.

92. Curtis, C, and Weir, J: Overview of exercise responses in healthy and impaired states. Neurology Report 20:13, 1996.

93. Bennett, R, and Knowlton, G: Overwork weakness in partially denervated skeletal muscle. Clin Orthop 12:22, 1958.

94. Dean, E: Effect of modified aerobic training on movement energetics in polio survivors. Orthopedics 14:1253, 1991.

95. Fillyaw, M, et al: The effects of long-term non-fatiguing resistance exercise in subjects with post-polio syndrome. Orthopedics 14:1252, 1991.

96. Aitkens, S, et al: Moderate resistance exercise program: Its effects in slowly progressive neuromuscular disease. Arch Phys Med Rehabil 74:711, 1993.

97. Affolter, F: Perceptual processes as prerequisites for complex human behavior. Int Rehabil Med 3:3, 1981.

98. Affolter, F: Perception, Interaction and Language. Springer-Verlag, New York, 1991.

99. Davies, P: Starting Again. Springer-Verlag, New York, 1994.

100. Creager, C: Therapeutic Exercises using the Swiss Ball. Executive Physical Therapy, Boulder, CO, 1994.

101. Posner-Mayer, J: Swiss Ball Applications for Orthopedic and Sports Medicine. Ball Dynamics Int., Denver, CO, 1995.

102. Damis, C, et al: Relationship between standing posture and stability. Phys Ther 78:502, 1998.

103. Hocherman, S, et al: Platform training and postural stability in hemiplegia. Arch Phys Med Rehabil 65:588, 1984.

104. Shumway-Cook, A, et al: Postural sway biofeedback: Its effect on reestablishing stance stability in hemiplegic patients. Arch Phys Med Rehabil 69:395, 1988.

105. Wannstedt, F, and Herman, R: Use of augmented sensory feedback to achieve symmetrical standing. Phys Ther 58:553, 1978.

106. Moore, S, and Woollacott, M: The use of biofeedback devices to improve postural stability. Phys Ther Practice 2:1, 1993.

107. Nichols, D: Balance retraining after stroke using force platform biofeedback. Phys Ther 77:553, 1997.

108. Winstein, C, et al: Standing balance training: Effect on balance and locomotion in hemiparetic adults. Arch Phys Med Rehabil 70:755, 1989.

109. Winstein, C: Balance retraining: Does it transfer? In Duncan, P (ed): Balance. American Physical Therapy Association, Alexandria, VA, 1990, p 95.

110. Gapsis, J, et al: Limb load monitor: Evaluation of a sensory feedback device for controlling weight-bearing. Arch Phys Med Rehabil 63:38, 1982.

111. Gauthier-Gagnon, C, et al: Augmented sensory feedback in the early training of standing balance of below-knee amputees. Physiotherapy Canada 38:137, 1986.

112. Nashner, L: Fixed patterns of rapid postural responses among leg muscles during stance. Exp Brain Res 30:13, 1977.

113. Nashner, L: Adapting reflexes controlling the human posture. Exp Brain Res 26:59, 1976.

114. Horak, F, and Nashner, L: Central programming of postural movements: Adaptation to altered support surface configurations. J Neurophysiol 55:1369, 1986.
115. McIlroy, W, and Maki, B: Adaptive changes to compensatory stepping responses. Gait and Posture 3:43, 1995.
116. Maki, B, and McIlroy, W: The role of limb movements in maintaining upright stance: The "change-in-support" strategy. Phys Ther 77:488, 1997.
117. Horak, F, et al: Postural perturbations: New insight for treatment of balance disorders. Phys Ther 77:517, 1997.
118. Badke, M, and DeFabio, R: Balance deficits in patients with hemiplegia: Considerations for assessment and treatment. In Duncan, P (ed): Balance. Proceedings of the APTA Forum. American Physical Therapy Association, Alexandria, VA, 1990, p 73.
119. Herdman, S: Assessment and treatment of balance disorders in the vestibular-deficient patient. In Duncan, P (ed): Balance. American Physical Therapy Association, Alexandria, VA, 1990, p 87.
120. Nashner, L: Sensory, neuromuscular, and biomechanical contributions to human balance. In Duncan, P (ed): Balance. American Physical Therapy Association, Alexandria, VA, 1990, p 5.
121. Shumway-Cook, A, and Horak, F: Assessing the influence of sensory interaction on balance. Phys Ther 66:1548, 1986.
122. Jeka, J: Light touch contact as a balance aid. Phys Ther 77:476, 1997.
123. Winstein, C, and Sullivan, K: Some distinctions on the motor learning/motor control distinction. Neurology Report 21:42, 1997.
124. Lee, T, and Swanson, L: What is repeated in a repetition? Effects of practice conditions on motor skill acquisition. Phys Ther 71:150, 1991.
125. Salmoni, A, et al: Knowledge of results and motor learning: A review and critical appraisal. Psychol Bull 95:355, 1984.
126. Lee, T, et al: On the role of knowledge of results in motor learning: Exploring the guidance hypothesis. J Mot Behav 22:191, 1990.
127. Bilodeau, EA, et al: Some effects of introducing and withdrawing knowledge of results early and late in practice. J Exper Psych 58:142, 1959.
128. Winstein, C: Knowledge of results and motor learning: Implications for physical therapy. Phys Ther 71:140, 1991.
129. Winstein, C, et al: Learning a partial-weight-bearing skill: Effectiveness of two forms of feedback. Phys Ther 76:985, 1996.
130. Bilodeau, E, and Bilodeau, I: Variable frequency knowledge of results and the learning of a simple skill. J Exp Psychol 55:379, 1958.
131. Ho, L, and Shea, J: Effects of relative frequency of knowledge of results on retention of a motor skill. Percept Mot Skills 46:859, 1978.
132. Sherwood, D: Effect of bandwidth knowledge of results on movement consistency. Percept Mot Skills 66:535, 1988.
133. Winstein, C, and Schmidt, R: Reduced frequency of knowledge of results enhances motor skill learning. J Exp Psychol (Learn Mem Cogn) 16:677, 1990.
134. Lavery, J: Retention of simple motor skills as a function of type of knowledge of results. Can J Psych 16:300, 1962.
135. Swinnen, S, et al: Information feedback for skill acquisition: Instantaneous knowledge of results degrades learning. J Exp Psychol 16:706, 1990.
136. Winstein, C: Knowledge of results and motor learning: Implications for physical therapy. Phys Ther 71:140, 1991.
137. Feltz, D, and Landers, D: The effects of mental practice on motor skill learning and performance: A meta-analysis. J Sports Psychol 5:25, 1983.
138. Richardson, A: Mental practice: A review and discussion (Part 1). Research Quarterly 38:95, 1967.
139. Richardson, A: Mental practice: A review and discussion (Part 2). Research Quarterly 38:263, 1967.
140. Warner, L, and McNeill, M: Mental imagery and its potential for physical therapy. Phys Ther 68:516, 1988.
141. Maring, J: Effects of mental practice on rate of skill acquisition. Phys Ther 70:165, 1990.
142. Shea, J, and Morgan, R: Contextual interference effects on the acquisition, retention, and transfer of a motor skill. J Exp Psychol [Hum Learn] 5:179, 1979.
143. Wulf, G, and Schmidt, R: Variability in practice facilitation in retention and transfer through schema formation or context effects? J Mot Behav 20:133, 1988.
144. Wulf, G, and Schmidt, R: Variability of practice and implicit motor learning. J Exp Psychol: Learning, Memory, and Cognition 23:987, 1997.
145. Battig, W: The flexibility of human memory. In Cermak, L, and Craik, F (eds): Levels of Processing in Human Memory. Lawrence Erlbaum Associates, Hillsdale, NJ, 1979, p 23.
146. Lee, T, and Magill, R: The locus of contextual interference in motor skill acquisition. J Exp Psychol: Learning, Memory, and Cognition 9:730, 1983.

SUPPLEMENTAL READINGS

Carr, J, and Shephard, R: Neurological Rehabilitation Optimizing Motor Performance. Butterworth-Heinemann, Woburn, MA, 1998.
Fredericks, CM, and Saladin, LK: Pathophysiology of the Motor Systems. FA Davis, Philadelphia, 1996.
Lundy-Ekman, L: Neuroscience Fundamentals for Rehabilitation. Philadelphia, Saunders, 1998.
Magill, R: Motor Learning Concepts and Applications, ed 4. WCB Brown & Benchmark, Madison, WI, 1993.
Schmidt, R: Motor Control and Learning, ed 3. Human Kinetics Pub., Champaign, IL, 1998.
Shumway-Cook, A, and Woollacott, M: Motor Control Theory and Practical Application. Williams & Wilkins, Baltimore, 1995.

GLOSSARY

Activation: An internal state characterized by potential for action; the attainment of a critical threshold level of neuronal firing for movement.

Adaptation: The modification of the environment to facilitate relearning of skills; a component of the compensatory training approach.

Arousal: An internal state of alertness or excitement.

Associative stage (motor learning): The second or middle stage of learning in which the skill strategy has been selected; refinement of the skill is achieved through continued practice.

Attention: The capacity of the brain to process information from the environment or from long-term memory.

    Divided attention: The ability to do several tasks at one time.

    Focused attention: The ability to respond to different kinds of stimulation.

    Selective attention: The ability to screen and process relevant sensory information about both the task and the environment while screening out irrelevant information.

    Sustained attention (vigilance): The ability to maintain prolonged attention.

Automatic postural synergies: Discrete patterns of leg and trunk muscle contractions characterized by consistency in muscle combinations, timing, and intensity (e.g., to preserve standing balance).

Autonomous stage (motor learning): The third stage of learning in which the spatial and temporal aspects of movement become highly organized through practice; there is automaticity of the skill with a low degree of attention required for performance.

Balance (postural stability): The condition in which all the forces acting on the body are balanced such that the center of mass (COM) is within the stability limits, the boundaries of the base of support (BOS).

Closed-loop control system: A control system employing feedback as a reference of correctness, a computation of error, and subsequent correction in order to maintain a desired state; sometimes called a servomechanism or servo.[1] p 97

Closed skills: Motor skills performed in an unchanging, predictable environment (closed environment).[1] p 412

Cognition: The act or process of knowing, including both awareness and judgment.

Cognitive stage (motor learning): The initial stage of learning in which the cognitive plan for the skill is developed; the learner develops an understanding of the task, develops strategies, and determines how the task should be evaluated.

Coma stimulation (early recovery management) program: An organized program of sensory and environmental stimulation designed to improve the overall level of alertness and arousal of patients with brain injury who are emerging from coma and vegetative states.

Compensatory training approach: A therapeutic approach to retraining the patient with movement disorders, based on use of behavioral substitution. Alternative behavioral strategies are adopted to complete a task; involves use of uninvolved or less involved segments for function.[2] p 38

Controlled mobility (dynamic stability): The ability to move while maintaining a stable upright posture (e.g., weight shifting or rocking).

Coordinative structures (synergy): The coordination of muscle groups to act within functionally coherent units; synergistic organization of muscles by the CNS.

Degrees of freedom: The number of separate independent dimensions of movement that must be controlled.

Developmental activities or skills: Functional skills acquired during early motor development used as landmarks of progressions of change.

Diaschisis: The recovery of brain activity after the resolution of temporary blocking factors (e.g., shock, edema, decreased blood flow, decreased glucose utilization).

Facilitation: Increased capacity to initiate a movement response through increased neuronal activity and altered synaptic potential.

Feedback: Response-produced information received during or after movement used to monitor output for corrective actions. Two general types exist:

    Augmented feedback (extrinsic feedback): Feedback that supplements intrinsic feedback normally received during a movement task.

    Intrinsic feedback: The feedback normally received during the execution of movement from the various sensory systems (e.g., visual, somatosensory).

Feedforward: The sending of signals in advance of movement to ready the systems (e.g., anticipatory adjustments in postural activity).

Fight-or-flight response: Defensive responses initiated by discharge of large portions of the sympathetic nervous system (mass discharge) to protect the individual under varying circumstances.

Functional substitution: Recovery of function through reprogramming of brain areas.

Functional/task-oriented approach: A therapeutic approach to retraining the patient with movement disorders, based on theories of motor control (systems theory) and motor learning.[2] p 461

Gait: The manner in which a person walks, characterized by rhythm, cadence, step, stride, and speed.

Generalizability: The ability to apply a learned skill to the learning of other similar tasks.

Guided movement (guidance; active assisted movement): A series of techniques in which the behavior of the learner is limited or controlled by various means to prevent errors.[1] p 414

Inhibition: Decreased capacity to initiate a movement response through decreased neuronal activity and altered synaptic potential.

Intermittent control hypothesis: A theory of motor control that specifies the interaction between closed-loop and open-loop processes in controlling movement.

Inverted U hypothesis (Yerkes-Dodson law): Increasing arousal level improves performance up to a point. Further increases in the intensity of arousal result in a decrease in performance.

Knowledge of performance (KP): Augmented feedback related to the nature of the movement pattern produced.[1] p 415

Knowledge of results (KR): Augmented feedback related to the nature of the result produced in terms of the environmental goal.[1] p 415

Learned nonuse: A learned pattern of disuse that follows sensory or motor loss affecting one side of the body; accompanied by overcompensation by intact segments.

Limits of stability (LOS): The maximum angle from vertical that can be tolerated without a loss of balance or changing the base of support.

Locomotion: The ability to move from one place to another.

Mental practice: A practice method in which performance on the task is imagined or visualized without overt physical practice.[1] p 416

Mobility: Initial movement in a functional pattern; range of motion is available for movement to occur and there is sufficient motor unit activity to initiate muscle contraction (e.g., rolling over and sitting up).

Motor function (motor control and motor learning): The ability to learn or demonstrate the skillful and efficient assumption, maintenance, modification, and control of voluntary postures and movement patterns.

Motor control: An area of study dealing with the understanding of the neural, physical, and behavioral aspects of movement.[1] p 416

Motor learning: A set of internal processes associated with practice or experience and leading to relatively permanent changes in the capability for skilled behavior.[1] p 416

Motor plan (complex motor programs): An idea or plan for purposeful movement that is made up of component motor programs.

Motor program: An abstract code or set of prestructured commands that, when initiated, results in the production of a coordinated movement sequence.[1] p 416

  Invariant characteristics: The unique features of the stored code; includes relative force, relative timing, and order of components.

  Parameters: The changeable features of the stored code; includes overall force and overall duration of movement.

Motivation: The internal state that tends to direct or energize the system toward a goal.[1] p 416

Muscle endurance: The ability to contract the muscle repeatedly over a period of time.

Muscle performance: The capacity of muscle to do work (force × distance).

Muscle power: Work produced per unit of time or the product of strength and speed.

Muscle strength: The measurable force exerted by a muscle or group of muscles to overcome a resistance in one maximal effort.

Muscle tone: The resistance of muscle to passive elongation or stretch.

Neural plasticity: The ability of the brain to change and repair itself.[27] p 134

Neuromotor development: The acquisition and evolution of movement skills throughout the life span.

Open-loop control system: A control system that uses preprogrammed instructions and does not use feedback information and error-detection processes.[1] p 416

Open skills: Motor skills performed in a changing, unpredictable environment (open environment).

Overload principle: In order to strengthen muscle, the loads must be greater than normally incurred.

Overwork weakness: A prolonged decrease in absolute strength and endurance as a result of excessive activity.

Performance: A change in motor behavior, the result of practice or experience; may not be reflective of learning (i.e., in the presence of fatigue, anxiety, poor motivation, or drugs).

Perseverate: Continued repetition of a word or act not related to successive instructions or commands.

Posture: The alignment and positioning of the body in relation to gravity, center of mass, and base of support.

Postural tone: Increased level of activity in antigravity muscles that helps maintain the body vertically against the force of gravity.[2] p 460

Practice: Repeated performance trials.

  Constant practice: Practice organized around one task performed repeatedly.

  Distributed practice: An alternating sequence of practice and rest periods in which practice time is less than rest time.[1] p 422

  Massed practice: A prolonged period of practice sequence of practice and rest periods in which the rest time is much less than the practice time.[1] p 416

  Variable practice: Practice of several variations of the same task or within the same category or class of movements.[1] p 420

Range of motion (ROM; including muscle length): The space, distance, or angle through which movement occurs at a joint or series of joints. Muscle length is measured at various joint angles through the range. Muscle length, in conjunction with joint integrity and soft tissue extensibility, determines flexibility.

Recovery of function: The re-acquisition of movement skills lost through injury.[2] p 23

Redundancy: The recovery of function through use of available back-up or fail-safe systems (pathways) within the CNS.

Reflex: A stereotypic, involuntary reaction to any of a variety of sensory stimuli.

Remediation/facilitation approaches: Neurotherapeutic approaches that have as their primary focus the use of therapeutic exercises and neuromuscular facilitation techniques to reduce sensorimotor deficits and promote motor recovery and improved function (e.g., neurodevelopmental treatment [NDT], proprioceptive neuromuscular facilitation [PNF]).

Resistance to contextural change: A measure of adaptability of performance in which a task can be performed equally well in altered environmental contexts.

Retention: The ability to demonstrate a skill over time and after a period of no practice.

  Retention interval: A period of no practice.

Schema: A rule, concept, or relationship formed on the basis of experience.[1] p 418

Sensory integration: The ability to integrate information from the environment to produce movement.

Sensory integrity: Includes peripheral sensory processing (e.g., sensitivity to touch) and cortical sensory processing (e.g., two-point and sharp/dull discrimination).

Sensory strategies: An organized application of sensory information from visual, somatosensory, and vestibular systems for postural and movement control.[2p460]

Structured sensory stimulation: The presentation of stimuli to the patient in an organized manner; part of coma stimulation program.

Skill: The ability to produce highly coordinated movement, characterized by precise timing and direction; movements are highly consistent and efficient (e.g., feeding, writing, walking).

Specificity principle: The physiological responses to training are specific to the particular type of exercise used (e.g., isometric, isotonic, isokinetic), the specific body segments utilized, and the particular environment in which training occurs.

Splinter skills: Skills that cannot be easily generalized to other environments or to variations of the same task.

Stability (static postural control): The ability to maintain a stable posture (e.g., holding a posture).

Static-dynamic control: The ability to move one limb or more than one limb while maintaining a stable posture (e.g., reaching or stepping).

Stretching: Any therapeutic maneuver designed to lengthen (elongate) pathologically shortened soft tissue structures and thereby to increase range of motion.

Ballistic stretching: The application of quick stretches (high-intensity, very short duration) of muscles and tissues; bobbing or bouncing movements may rupture weakened tissues and cause reflex contraction of muscle being stretched.

Facilitated stretching: The application of techniques that promote reflex relaxation of the muscle to be elongated prior to or during the stretching maneuver (e.g., contract-relax, hold-relax).

Passive stretching: The application of a maintained external force (manual, mechanical or low-load) to stretch soft tissues beyond the free range of motion.

Selective stretching: The application of stretching techniques selectively to improve overall function; some muscles and joints are stretched while some limitation of motion is allowed to develop in other muscles or joints (e.g., for tenodesis grasp).

Stereotypical movement synergies (obligatory synergies): Muscles activated in an abnormal synergistic unit and firmly linked together; movement variations and isolated joint movements are not possible; commonly seen in patients with hemiplegia.

Transfer of learning: The gain (or loss) of task performance as a result of practice or experience on some other task.[1] p 389

Bilateral-transfer: The ability to learn a skill after the skill has been practiced with the opposite hand or foot.[8] p 148

Parts-to-whole transfer: Practice of separate component parts before practice of the integrated whole.

Vicariance: The recovery of function through the utilization of different and underutilized areas of the brain.

APPENDIX A

Therapeutic Exercise Techniques

1. **Approximation** (joint compression): Compression force applied to joints; typically applied through gravity acting on body weight; can be applied through manual contacts or weight belts.
   Indications: Instability of extensor muscles in weight-bearing and holding, poor static postural control, and/or weakness.

2. **Agonist reversals (AR):** A slow isotonic, shortening contraction through the range followed by an eccentric, lengthening contraction using the same muscle groups; performed through increments of range; typically used in bridging, sit-to-stand transitions, and stepping-up and down a step.
   Indications: Weak postural muscles, inability to eccentrically control body weight during movement transitions, poor dynamic postural control.

3. **Alternating isometrics (AI):** Isometric holding is facilitated first on one side of the joint, followed by alternate holding of the antagonist muscle groups. May be applied in any direction (anterior-posterior, medial-lateral, diagonal).
   Indications: Instability in weight-bearing and holding, poor static postural control, and/or weakness.

4. **Contract-relax (CR):** A relaxation technique usually performed at a point of limited ROM in the agonist pattern; isotonic movement in rotation is performed followed by an isometric hold of the range-limiting muscles in the antagonist pattern against slowly increasing resistance followed by voluntary relaxation, and passive movement into the new range of the agonist pattern.
   Contract-relax-active-contraction (CRAC): Similar to CR, except movement into the newly gained range of the agonist pattern is active not passive. Active contraction serves to maintain the inhibitory effects through reciprocal inhibition.
   Indications: Limitations in ROM caused by muscle tightness, spasticity.

5. **Facilitation techniques:** A group of techniques used to facilitate or inhibit muscle contraction (see Appendix B).

6. **Guided movement (active assisted movement; AAM):** Active movements are guided or assisted in some way. For example, the therapist manually assists the patient through the movement. Guidance reduces errors, promotes early learning during the acquisition phase of motor skill learning, and reduces frustration and movement anxiety.

Manual assists may be maximal, moderate, or minimal. The therapist removes support when the patient is able to take over the movement, and resumes guiding as needed. Verbal assists cue the patient through a movement.
Active movement control is the overall goal. Effective problem solving is promoted as the key to independent function.
Indications: Inability to move; impaired tactile and kinesthetic inputs that normally guide movements; perceptual dysfunction.

7. **Handling:** Physical handling techniques are used to inhibit abnormal movements, tone, or reflexes and facilitate normal tone and patterns of movement.
   Key points of control: Parts of the body the therapist chooses as optimal to control tone and movement. Proximal key points (trunk, head, shoulders and pelvis) are used to ensure control of trunk and proximal segments before facilitating active limb movements. Proximal key points are also generally effective in influencing tone throughout the entire limb. Distal key points (hands and feet) may also be used.
   Tone is normalized before active movements are attempted. Examples of key points of control to decrease tone include:
   a. Head and trunk flexion decreases shoulder retraction, trunk and limb extension (key points of control: head and trunk).
   b. Humeral external rotation and flexion to 90 degrees decreases flexion tone of the upper extremity (key point of control: humerus).
   c. Thumb abduction and extension with forearm supination decreases flexion tone of the wrist and fingers (key point of control: the thumb).
   d. Femoral external rotation and abduction decreases extensor adductor tone of the lower extremity (key point of control: hip).
   Indications: Inability to move due to spasticity, abnormal reflex activity.

8. **Hold-relax active motion (HRAM):** An isometric contraction performed in the middle to shortened range followed by voluntary relaxation and passive movement into the lengthened range; tracking resistance is applied to an isotonic contraction as movement occurs from the lengthened to the shortened range.
   Indications: An inability to initiate movement, hypotonia (poor spindle stretch sensitivity), weakness, marked imbalances between opposing muscle groups.

Continued

9. **Hold-relax (HR):** Relaxation technique usually performed at the point of limited ROM in the agonist pattern; an isometric contraction of the range-limiting antagonist pattern is performed against slowly increasing resistance, followed by voluntary relaxation, and passive movement into the newly gained range of the agonist pattern.
Hold-relax-active contraction (HRAC): Active contraction into the newly gained range of the agonist pattern can also be performed and serves to maintain the inhibitory effects through reciprocal inhibition.
Indications: Limitations in ROM caused by muscle tightness, muscle spasm, and pain.

10. **Repeated contractions (RC):** Repeated isotonic contractions induced by quick stretches and enhanced by resistance performed through the range or part of range at a point of weakness; RC is a unidirectional technique; an isometric hold can be added at a point of weakness.
Indications: Weakness, incoordination, muscle imbalances, and/or diminished muscular endurance.

11. **Resisted progression (RP):** Stretch and tracking resistance is applied to facilitate progression in walking, creeping, kneel-walking, or movement transitions.
Indications: Impaired timing and control of lower trunk/pelvic segments (pelvic rotation), and endurance.

12. **Rhythmic initiation (RI):** Voluntary relaxation followed by passive movements through increments in range, followed by active-assisted movements progressing to resisted movements using tracking resistance (light, facilitatory resistance) to isotonic contractions; RI may be unidirectional or in both directions.
Indications: Inability to relax, hypertonicity (spasticity, rigidity), inability to initiate movement (apraxia), motor learning deficits, communication deficits (aphasia).

13. **Rhythmic rotation (RRo):** Voluntary relaxation combined with slow, passive, rhythmic rotation of the body or body part around a longitudinal axis, followed by passive movement into the antagonist range (opposite to the spastic pattern). Rotation may be combined with active movements to promote relaxation and gain new range or hold in the new range.
Indications: Hypertonia with limitations in function or ROM.

14. **Rhythmic stabilization (RS):** Isometric contraction of the agonist pattern followed by the antagonist pattern; performed without relaxation using careful grading of resistance; results in cocontraction of opposing muscle groups; RS emphasizes rotational stability control.
Indications: Instability in weight-bearing and holding, poor static postural control, weakness; also limitations in ROM caused by muscle tightness, and painful muscle splinting.

15. **Shortened held resisted contraction (SHRC):** Resistance applied to an isometric contraction of muscle(s) holding in the shortened range; typically applied to extensor muscles in modified pivot prone positions (sidelying or supported sitting).
Indications: Instability in weight-bearing and holding, poor static postural control, and weakness.

16. **Slow reversals (SR):** Slow isotonic contractions of first agonist, then antagonist patterns using careful grading of resistance and optimal facilitation; reversal of antagonists; progression through increments of range.
Slow reversal hold (SRH): An isometric hold is added at the end of the range or at a point of weakness (the hold may be added in both directions or only in one direction).
Indications: Inability to reverse directions, muscle imbalances, weakness, incoordination, and lack of endurance.

17. **Tapping:** Stimulation via quick stretch to the muscle spindle; stimulus is applied directly over muscle belly.
Sweep tapping: Widespread activation of the muscle being tapped.
Indications: Weakness and/or hypotonia.

18. **Timing for emphasis (TE):** Use of maximum resistance to elicit a sequence of contractions of major muscle components of a pattern of motion; allows overflow to occur from strong to weak components; can be performed within a limb (one muscle group to another) or using overflow from limb to limb or trunk to limb. Typically combined with repeated contractions to strengthen the weaker components, TE/RC.
Indications: Weakness and/or incoordination.

19. **Traction:** A distraction force applied to joints; force is typically applied through manual contacts.
Indications: Inability of flexor muscles to function in mobilizing patterns, weakness.

APPENDIX B

Neuromuscular Facilitation Techniques

A group of techniques used to facilitate or inhibit muscle contraction or responses.

Proprioceptive Facilitation Techniques

1. Quick Stretch

STIMULUS

Quick stretch applied to a muscle.

ACTIVATES

Muscle spindles (facilitates Ia endings); sensitive to velocity and length changes. Muscle spindle provides input to higher centers.

RESPONSE

Phasic, facilitates or enhances muscle contraction due to largely peripheral reflex effects (facilitates agonist, inhibits antagonists, facilitates synergists, reciprocal innervation effects).

TECHNIQUES

Quick stretch (more effective applied in the lengthened range)

Tapping over muscle belly or tendon

COMMENTS

A low threshold response, relatively short-lived; can add resistance to maintain contraction.

Apply resistance in the lengthened range to initiate contraction.

ADVERSE EFFECTS

May increase spasticity

2. Prolonged Stretch

STIMULUS

Slowly applied maintained stretch especially in lengthened ranges

ACTIVATES

Muscle spindles (Ia and II endings), golgi tendon organs (Ib endings); sensitive to length changes

Muscle spindle provides input to higher centers

RESPONSE

Inhibits or dampens muscle contraction and tone due largely to peripheral reflex effects.

TECHNIQUES

Manual contacts

Inhibitory splinting, casting

Reflex-inhibiting patterns

Mechanical low-load weights

COMMENTS

Higher threshold response.

May be more effective in extensor muscles than flexors due to the added effects of II inhibition.

To maintain inhibitory effects, activate antagonist muscles.

3. Resistance

STIMULUS

A force exerted to muscle

ACTIVATES

Muscle spindles (Ia and II endings) and golgi tendon organs (Ib endings); sensitive to velocity and length changes.

Muscle spindle provides input to higher centers.

RESPONSE

Facilitates or enhances muscle contraction due to peripheral reflex effects (facilitates agonist, inhibits antagonists, facilitates synergists, reciprocal innervation effects).

Suprasegmental effects: recruits both alpha and gamma motoneurons, additional motor units.

Hypertrophies extrafusal muscle fibers.

Enhances kinesthetic awareness.

TECHNIQUES

Manual resistance

Use of body weight and gravity

Mechanical weights

COMMENTS

Light (tracking) resistance is used to facilitate very weak muscles.

With weak hypotonic muscles, eccentric and isometric contractions are used before concentric (enhances muscle spindle support of contraction with less spindle unloading).

Maximal resistance may produce overflow to other muscles.

ADVERSE EFFECTS

Too much resistance can easily overpower weak, hypotonic muscles and prevent voluntary movement, encourage substitution.

May increase spasticity.

4. Joint Approximation

STIMULUS

Compression of joint surfaces

ACTIVATES

Joint receptors (static, type I receptors)

RESPONSE

Facilitates postural extensors and stabilizers

Enhances joint awareness

TECHNIQUES

Joint compression, either manual or mechanical using weight cuffs or belts

Bouncing while sitting on a Swiss ball

COMMENTS

Applied in extensor patterns, weight-bearing positions, in middle to shortened ranges of extensors

ADVERSE EFFECTS

Contraindicated in inflamed joints.

Continued

5. Joint Traction

STIMULUS
Distraction of joint surfaces

ACTIVATES
Joint receptors (possibly phasic, type II)

RESPONSE
Facilitates agonists, enhances contraction
Enhances joint awareness

TECHNIQUES
Manual distraction

COMMENTS
Used as a facilitatory stimulus in flexor patterns, pulling actions.
Slow, sustained traction to joints can be used to improve mobility, relieve muscle spasm, and reduce pain with techniques of joint mobilization.

6. Inhibitory Pressure

STIMULUS
Prolonged pressure to long tendons

ACTIVATES
Muscle receptors (muscle spindles, golgi tendon organs) and tactile receptors

RESPONSE
Inhibition, dampens muscle tone

TECHNIQUES
Firm pressure can be applied manually or with body weight; positioning at end ranges
Mechanical: firm objects (cones) in hand inhibitory splints, casts

COMMENTS
Weight-bearing postures are used to provide inhibitory pressure, for example:
• Quadruped or kneeling postures can be used to promote inhibition of quadriceps and long finger flexors.
• Sitting, with hand open, elbow extended, and upper extremity supporting body weight can be used to promote inhibition of long finger flexors.

ADVERSE EFFECTS
Sustained positioning may dampen muscle contraction and affect functional performance.

EXTEREOCEPTIVE STIMULATION TECHNIQUES

7. Light Touch

STIMULUS
Brief, light contact to skin

ACTIVATES
Fast adapting tactile receptors, autonomic nervous system, sympathetic division

RESPONSE
Phasic withdrawal responses, flexion and adduction of the extremities withdrawing away from the stimulus; increased arousal

TECHNIQUES
Brief, light stroke of the fingertips
Brief swipe with ice cube
Light pinch or squeezing

Applied to areas of high tactile receptor density (hands, feet, lips) that are more sensitive to stimulation

COMMENTS
Low threshold response, accommodates rapidly
Effective in initially mobilizing patients with low response levels, for example, the patient with traumatic brain injury during early recovery
Application of resistance to maintain contraction

ADVERSE EFFECTS
Increased sympathetic arousal, may produce fight or flight responses.
Contraindicated in patients with generalized arousal or autonomic instability, for example, the patient with traumatic brain injury who is agitated and combative.

8. Maintained Touch

STIMULUS
Maintained contact or pressure

ACTIVATES
Tactile receptors, autonomic nervous system, parasympathetics

RESPONSE
Calming effect, generalized inhibition
Desensitizes skin

TECHNIQUES
Firm manual contacts
Firm pressure to midline abdomen, back, lips, palms, and/or soles of feet
Firm rubbing

COMMENTS
Useful for patients with high arousal, patients with a hypersensitivity to sensory stimulation.
Can be applied to hypersensitive areas to normalize responses; for example, the patient with peripheral nerve injury and paresthesias.
Brief touch stimuli should be avoided.
Can be used in combination with other maintained stimuli.

9. Slow Stroking

STIMULUS
Slow stroking, applied to paravertebral spinal region (over posterior primary rami)

ACTIVATES
Tactile receptors, autonomic nervous system, parasympathetics

RESPONSE
Calming effect, generalized inhibition

TECHNIQUES
The patient is placed in a supported position such as prone, or sitting head and arms supported and resting forward on a table top. A flat hand is used to apply firm, alternate strokes downward to paravertebral region for approximately 3 to 5 minutes.

COMMENTS

Useful with patients who demonstrate high arousal, increased sympathetic (fight-or-flight) responses.

10. Manual Contacts

STIMULUS

Firm, deep pressure of the hands in contact with the body

ACTIVATES

Tactile receptors, muscle proprioceptors

RESPONSE

Facilitate contraction in muscle directly under the hands

Provide sensory awareness, directional cues to movement

Provide security and support to unstable body segments

COMMENTS

Can be used with or without resistance. *Contraindicated* over spastic muscles, and open wounds.

11. Prolonged Icing

STIMULUS

Cold applications

ACTIVATES

Thermoreceptors

RESPONSE

Decreases neural, muscle spindle firing

Provides inhibition of muscle tone and painful muscle spasm

Decreases metabolic rate of tissues

TECHNIQUES

Immersion in cold water, ice chips

Ice towel wraps

Ice packs

Ice massage

COMMENTS

Monitor effects carefully

ADVERSE EFFECTS

Sympathetic nervous system arousal, protective withdrawal responses, fight or flight responses.

Contraindicated in patients with sensory deficits, generalized arousal, autonomic instability, vascular problems.

12. Neutral Warmth

STIMULUS

Retention of body heat

ACTIVATES

Thermoreceptors

Autonomic nervous system, primarily parasympathetics

RESPONSE

Generalized inhibition of tone; produces a calming effect, relaxation, decreases pain

TECHNIQUES

Wrapping body or body parts: ace wraps, towel wraps

Application of snug fitting clothing (gloves, socks, tights) or air splints

Tepid baths

Applied for approximately 10 to 20 minutes

COMMENTS

Useful for patients with high arousal, or increased sympathetic activity; spasticity.

ADVERSE EFFECTS

Overheating should be avoided, may produce rebound effects (increased arousal or tone).

VESTIBULAR STIMULATION TECHNIQUES

13. Slow Maintained Vestibular Stimulation

STIMULUS

Low-intensity vestibular stimulation, for example, slow rocking

ACTIVATES

Facilitates primarily otolith organs (tonic receptors); less effects on semicircular canals (phasic receptors)

RESPONSE

Generalized inhibition of tone

Decreased arousal, calming effect

TECHNIQUES

Slow, repetitive rocking movements; assisted rocking in a weight-bearing position, for example, rocking with equipment:

rocking chair, Swiss ball, equilibrium board, hammock

Slow rolling movements

COMMENTS

Useful with patients who are hypertonic, hyperactive, or who demonstrate high arousal, or tactile defensiveness.

Combine with cognitive relaxation techniques.

14. Fast Vestibular Stimulation

STIMULUS

High-intensity vestibular stimulation, for example, fast spinning, irregular movements with acceleration and deceleration component

ACTIVATES

Facilitates semicircular canals (phasic receptors), less effects on otoliths (tonic receptors)

RESPONSE

Generalized facilitation of tone

Improves motor coordination

Improves retinal image stability, decreases post-rotatory nystagmus

TECHNIQUES

Fast spinning, for example, spinning in a chair, mesh net or hammock

Fast acceleration/deceleration movements, for example, prone on a scooter board

Fast rolling movements

COMMENTS

Useful with:

Hypotonic patients (for example, the individual with Down's syndrome)

Continued

Patients with sensory integrative dysfunction

Patients with coordination problems (e.g., stroke, cerebral palsy)

Helpful in overcoming the effects of akinesia or bradykinesia in patients with Parkinson's disease

ADVERSE EFFECTS

Behavioral changes, seizures, sleep disturbances may occur.

Contraindicated for patients with recurrent seizures or who are intolerant to sensory stimulation.

APPENDIX C

Suggested Answers to Case Study Guiding Questions
Part I (Questions 1–3)

1. Identify and prioritize the clinical problems presented in this case in terms of direct, indirect, and composite impairments, and functional limitations—initial admission.

1. Increased tone throughout (direct).
2. Decreased ROM both ankles (indirect).
3. Decreased active, purposeful movement (direct).
4. Decreased head control (direct).
5. Decreased trunk control (direct).
6. Decreased bed mobility (functional limitation).
7. Abnormal posturing (direct).
8. Decreased response to sensory and environmental stimulation (direct).

2. Identify the goals and outcomes of physical therapy intervention for this patient at this point in his recovery—initial admission.

1. Patient is assisted in early recovery.
2. Patient's baseline data on alertness is determined.
3. Communication system is established.
4. Caregiver support is provided to assist in coping adjustment and understanding of the recovery process.
5. Patient is positioned as needed to avoid contractures, skin breakdown, heterotrophic ossification, and to reduce tone.
6. Patient's lung fields remain clear.
7. Patient increases passive range of motion (PROM) ankle dorsiflexion in both lower extremities by 5 degrees.
8. Patient's need for splints and/or serial casting is determined.
9. Patient is fitted with appropriate wheelchair (w/c) with supportive devices.
10. Patient tolerates w/c sitting for up to 2 hours.
11. Patient tolerates standing program on tilt table for up to 30 minutes.
12. Patient tolerates sitting on edge of mat for up to 15 minutes at a time with min. assistance.
13. Patient is able to localize and display purposeful responses at least 25 percent of the time in response to sensory stimulation.
14. Written and verbal instruction is given to caregiver on various aspects of early recovery rehabilitation program.

3. Identify treatment interventions appropriate for this patient at this point in his recovery—initial admission.

The patient will be seen 1½ to 2 hours daily for the following:

1. Bed positioning to control for abnormal tone, maintain ROM and skin integrity.
2. Passive range of motion (PROM) to active (AROM) AEs as tolerated.
3. Upright positioning in tilt-in-space wheelchair with adaptations to stabilize head and trunk.
4. Upright positioning on tilt table with adaptations to stabilize trunk and LEs.
5. Relaxation of tone using rhythmic rotation techniques during PROM; slow rocking on a vestibular board can be tried.
6. Activities to increase head and trunk control in supported sitting: active-assisted (AA) holding of head with therapist supporting the trunk in sitting.
7. AA bed mobility activities: rolling, supine to sit.
8. AA transfer activities.
9. Inhibitive casting when indicated (complete wound healing).
10. Caregiver education on ROM, positioning, and skin care.

Commentary

The patient is only 7 weeks post traumatic head injury. Significant spontaneous recovery may occur, and benefits are expected from intensive rehabilitation programming. The patient will be reexamined weekly with modification of goals and the plan of care as indicated by progress or lack thereof. The expected functional outcomes of rehabilitation will continue to be formulated as the patient's recovery progresses. Treatment activities were selected to (1) relax tone and promote *mobility* control and (2) begin *stability* control in sitting. The patient is in the *precognitive phase* of learning and demonstrates significant cognitive deficits. He will benefit from a highly structured, closed environment. Sensory stimulation techniques (normally part of an early recovery management program) will be of use to stimulate movement and awareness. Positioning tasks will benefit from guided movement to control extraneous movements and reduce the degrees of freedom problem. Careful structuring and consistency of sensory cues (augmented feedback) is necessary. True learning and carryover from one treatment session to the next cannot be expected at this stage of recovery.

Part II (Questions 4–6)

4. Identify and prioritize the clinical problems presented in this case in terms of direct, indirect, and composite impairments, and functional limitations (6 months post injury).

1. Increased tone: trunk, left extremities greater than right (direct).
2. Ataxia: trunk, extremities (direct).

Continued

3. Impaired active control: left greater than right (direct).
4. Impaired postural reactions (composite).
5. Abnormal LUE posturing (direct).
6. Decreased PROM ankle dorsiflexion in both lower extremities (indirect).
7. Impaired functional ability: sitting, transfers, gait, safety during wheelchair mobility.

5. Identify the goals and outcomes of physical therapy intervention for this patient at this point in his recovery (6 months post injury).
1. The patient will be able to live in an assisted living environment with the assistance of a personal care attendant for the performance of:
   a. all BADLs with appropriate assistive devices with Min A or S
   b. transfers, stand-pivot with S only
2. Patient is independent in wheelchair mobility (electric).
3. Patient tolerates physical therapy while sitting for up to 60 minutes.
4. Patient is able to perform sit-to-stand transfers with S only.
5. Patient is able to perform w/c transfers stand-pivot to bed or mat with S only.
6. Patient is able to maintain sitting balance without back support for up to 10 minutes with close S.
7. Patient is able to maintain standing balance in parallel bars with UE support for up to 5 minutes with close S.
8. Patient is able to perform w/c mobility using electric hand controls for RUE for a minimum of 100 feet with S.
9. Patient is able to maintain position of LUE and LLE out of mass patterning for a minimum of 10 minutes.
10. Patient is able to maintain static stability in quadruped and high kneeling positions for a minimum of 2 minutes with Min A.
11. Patient increases PROM ankle dorsiflexion in BLEs by 5 degrees.
12. Patient is compliant 50 percent of the time with behavior management plan.
13. Patient is able to participate in all therapies off hospital unit.
14. Patient is able to attend to task for 5 minutes out of a 30-minute treatment session.
15. Patient recalls daily tasks and names of therapists with up to 25 percent accuracy.
16. Patient demonstrates appropriate safety with mobility activities with Min S.
17. Caregiver is able to identify patient's schedule and rehabilitation services, and expected treatment outcome.

6. Identify treatment interventions appropriate for this patient at this point in his recovery (6 months post injury).
1. Inhibitory handling techniques for reduction of tone: rhythmic rotation (RRO).
2. Sitting balance activities: holding, reaching for objects; use of techniques to improve stability control/reduce ataxia: alternating isometrics (AI), rhythmic stabilization (RS).
3. Postural exercises: correction of posterior pelvic tilt, forward head in sitting.
4. Standing balance activities in parallel bars: holding, weight shifting with bilateral arm support; use of techniques to improve stability control.
5. Trunk activities: holding in quadruped, high-kneeling; independent assumption of postures.
6. Wheelchair mobility training.
7. PROM with contract-relax technique to improve range in ankle dorsiflexion.
8. Consistency, structure, and repetition: scheduling, choice of treatment techniques, closed environment.
9. Use of memory training devices: printed daily schedule, memory log.

Commentary
The patient is now 6 months post-injury. Consultation and close communication with other members of the rehabilitation team is essential for coordinated care and optimal treatment outcomes. Treatment activities are focused on (1) relaxation of tone and maintenance of functional *mobility;* (2) improving *stability* control in sitting, standing, quadruped, and high kneeling; (3) promoting *controlled mobility* function in those same postures with weight-shifting activities and independent assumption; and (4) promoting balance, a *skill-level* function, in sitting and standing. The patient's increasing cognitive abilities allow the implementation of additional motor learning strategies for the *cognitive/associative phases* to help the patient develop movement strategies and begin to utilize his own sensory cues, detect errors, and generate solutions to movement problems. A primary focus of training is on functional tasks and safety. The patient performs reasonably well in a closed environment, with increasing difficulty noted in more open environments. A goal of treatment is to maintain environmental structure during practice until such time as cognitive recovery and learning allow for environmental modification. Additional benefits of an intensive rehabilitation program are expected.

Preambulation and **14** Gait Training

Thomas J. Schmitz

LEARNING OBJECTIVES

1. Identify the major elements of physical therapy intervention for patients with gait impairments.
2. Identify the goals of a preambulation exercise program.
3. Describe the characteristic features of each posture included in the preambulation exercise program.
4. Explain the sequence of activities included in the parallel bar progression.
5. Describe the guidelines for selection and measurement of canes, crutches, and walkers.
6. Describe the common gait patterns and guarding technique used with each assistive device.
7. Using the case study example, apply clinical decision making skills to gait training activities.

Ambulation is a primary functional goal for many patients. The physical therapy gait analysis presented in Chapter 10 includes identification of problems that limit or prevent ambulation as well as determination of their causes. Evaluation of gait analysis data allows the therapist to develop an appropriate plan of therapeutic intervention. This intervention typically includes preambulation exercises and gait training. The purpose of preambulation exercises and gait training activities is to provide the patient with a method of ambulation that allows maximum functional independence and safety at a reasonable energy cost.

Interventions to address problems that limit or prevent ambulation are applicable to physical therapy management of a broad spectrum of diagnostic groups. The preferred practice patterns contained in the *Guide to Physical Therapist Practice*[1] is replete with examples of gait training as a suggested intervention for multiple diagnostic groups. Gait training is included as an element of patient management for impairments and disabilities of the musculoskeletal, neuromuscular, cardiopulmonary, and integumentary systems.

This chapter presents a general discussion of preambulation exercises and gait training with assistive devices that can be modified to meet the needs of an individual patient. Several factors will be of major influence in determining the extent and type of gait training activities required to achieve desired outcomes. These factors include information obtained from the gait analysis and subsequent evaluation of these data, diagnosis, prognosis, weight-bearing status, as well as the patient's goals for ambulation. For example, the progression of gait training activities indicated for an otherwise healthy individual with a non-weight-bearing tibial fracture would be very different from those developed for a patient with paraplegia.

The major elements of physical therapy intervention for gait impairments are outlined in Box 14–1. It should be noted that the entire sequence of intervention will not be indicated for each patient. Depending on individual patient need, multiple segments may be accomplished concurrently (i.e., a more rapid progression may be indicated), or portions may be completely omitted.

PREAMBULATION MAT PROGRAM: PREPARATION FOR STANDING

Preambulation exercises prepare the patient for assuming the upright position and typically involve a large component of mat work. Many of these mat activities are based on a developmental framework and progress from initial activities with a large base of support (BOS) and a low center of gravity (COG) through later activities which have a smaller BOS and high COG. The techniques utilized within each posture of the mat program are sequenced according to the four stages of motor control and progress from (1) *mobility*, which incorporates initiation of movement techniques, including *assist to position* in which the therapist manually assists the patient to achieve a given posture; to (2) *stability*, characterized by the ability to maintain a posture against gravity; to (3) *controlled mobility*, which is the ability to maintain postural control during weight shifting and movement; and finally to (4) *skill*, which is the highest level, characterized by discrete motor control superimposed on proximal stability. The techniques used within each posture typically progress from assisted or guided movement to active movement to resisted movement.

These mat or lead-up activities (the term *lead-up* implies that the activities are preparatory for or "lead up" to ambulation) have important functional carryover to other daily activities as well, such as relieving pressure, dressing, and bed mobility. The development of successful mat programs will require the therapist to draw on several different exercise approaches. The work of Voss et al.,[2] Sullivan and Markos,[3] and O'Sullivan and Schmitz,[4] is particularly helpful in this regard. Additionally, many other forms of exercise provide important components of an overall program of preambulation exercises (e.g., progressive resistive exercises, endurance and cardiovascular training, and mobility, flexibility, coordination, and breathing exercises).

Depending on the level of patient involvement, the goals of a preambulation exercise program will be to:

1. Improve strength, power, and endurance.
2. Increase or maintain range of motion.
3. Improve motor function (motor control and motor learning).
4. Enhance sensory integration.
5. Instruct the patient in handling and moving the affected extremity or extremities.

Box 14–1 MAJOR ELEMENTS OF PHYSICAL THERAPY INTERVENTION FOR GAIT IMPAIRMENTS

A. PREAMBULATION MAT PROGRAM
Activities and techniques to:
Improve strength, coordination, and range of motion.
Enhance sensory integration.
Improve flexibility and endurance.
Develop postural stability.
Develop controlled mobility in movement transitions.
Develop static-dynamic control.
Develop dynamic balance control and skill.

B. PARALLEL BAR PROGRESSION
Instruction and training in:
Moving from sitting to standing and reverse.
Standing balance and weight shifting activities.
Use of appropriate gait pattern, forward progression, and turning.
Moving from sitting to standing, and reverse, with assistive device.[a]
Standing balance and weight-shifting activities with assistive device.[a]
Use of assistive device (with appropriate gait pattern) for forward progression and turning.[a]

C. ADVANCED PARALLEL BAR ACTIVITIES
Walking forward and backward.
Side-stepping and crossed-stepping.
Braiding.
Resisted progression.

D. INDOOR PROGRESSION
Instruction and training in:
Use of assistive device for ambulation on level surfaces.
Elevation activities, including climbing stairs and, if available indoors, negotiating ramps and curbs.
Opening doors and passing through doorways (including elevators) and over thresholds.
Falling techniques (generally included for individuals who are active ambulators; particularly important for individuals who require long-term use of an assistive device).

E. OUTDOOR PROGRESSION
Instruction and training in:
Opening doors and passing through thresholds that lead outdoors.
Use of assistive device on outdoor terrain and uneven surfaces.
Elevation activities including stair climbing and negotiating curbs.
Crossing a street within the time allocated by a traffic light.
Entering an automobile and/or public transportation.

---

[a]Because of limited space, use of the parallel bars may not be possible. However, when adjustable-width bars are available, they provide added security for preliminary use of the assistive device. An alternative approach would be to begin use of the device outside and next to standard parallel bars or oval-shaped parallel bars.

6. Develop postural stability in sitting and standing.
7. Develop controlled mobility function as evidenced by the ability to move within postures.

8. Develop controlled mobility function in movement transitions such as rolling and moving from a supine position to a sitting position.
9. Improve trunk and pelvic control.
10. Develop static and dynamic balance control.

A general outline of suggested preambulation mat exercises follows. The activities should be ordered from easiest to most difficult and should reflect the spiral nature of the development of motor control; that is, total mastery of one activity is not necessary before moving to the next higher level. Sequences may be planned in such a way that multiple postures may be overlapped and used in a mat program concurrently. Although the activities are described here in a general order of easiest to more difficult, it is not uncommon for the order to be changed, or for several activities to be worked on simultaneously. With adult patients it is common to work on several levels of activities concurrently. The specific activities and techniques selected, as well as the sequence, will be determined by goals established for the individual patient. Chapter 13 should be consulted for descriptions of the individual techniques and additional treatment suggestions. The mat sequence that follows uses a number of activities and postures, including rolling, prone-on-elbows (and prone-on-hands), hooklying and bridging, quadruped, sitting, kneeling and half-kneeling, modified plantigrade, and, finally, standing.

Rolling

Rolling may be the initial starting point for a preambulation mat program for some patients with significant impairment. This activity provides a large BOS and low COG without bearing weight through the joints. Mat work may begin in a sidelying position at first, particularly if initiation of rolling is difficult. Resisted isometric contractions in shortened ranges (termed *shortened held resisted contraction*) are a useful early technique in sidelying. This technique uses sustained isometric contractions of the postural extensors. Manual contacts are posteriorly on the shoulder and pelvis. The patient is asked to "hold" maximally against the resistance of the therapist through increments of range. Additionally, the proprioceptive neuromuscular facilitation (PNF) techniques of hold-relax-active movement and rhythmic stabilization also may be used in sidelying to facilitate contraction and proximal stability.

Rolling activities may include a progression from *log rolling* to *segmental rolling*. **Log rolling** produces movement of the entire trunk as a unit around the longitudinal axis of the body. **Segmental rolling** is an alternative form of rolling during which either the upper or the lower segment of the trunk moves independently while the other segment is stabilized. As the progression continues, **counterrotation** will develop. *Counterrotation* involves si-

multaneous movement of the upper and lower segments of the trunk in opposite directions. Several suggested activities follow that can be used and/or combined to facilitate rolling.

1. Flexion of the head and neck with rotation may be used to assist movement from supine to prone positions.
2. Extension of the head and neck with rotation may be used to assist movement from prone to supine positions.
3. Bilateral upper extremity activities that cross the midline will produce a pendular motion and can be used to rock the body from a supine position toward a prone position. To create this momentum, both elbows are extended and the shoulders are flexed to approximately 110 degrees with the hands clasped together. The upper extremities are then swung from side-to-side.
4. Crossing the ankles will also facilitate rolling. The ankles are crossed so that the upper leg is toward the direction of the roll (e.g., the right ankle would be crossed over the left when rolling toward the left).
5. Several PNF patterns are useful during early rolling activities. The upper extremity PNF patterns of D1 flexion, D2 extension, reverse chop, and lift will facilitate rolling. The lower extremity pattern of D1 flexion will also facilitate rolling.

Prone-on-elbows Position

In the prone-on-elbows position there continues to be a large BOS and low COG. This position is very stable and provides weight-bearing on the elbows and forearms. The posture is useful to facilitate proximal stability of the glenohumeral and scapular musculature; this is an important prerequisite for using the upper extremities in weight-bearing. Although head and neck control is required to assume a prone-on-elbows position, it can be further improved in this posture. The prone-on-elbows position must be used cautiously because some patients will find it difficult to tolerate (e.g., in the presence of spasticity following a stroke). Alternate positioning includes (1) using a wedge cushion to reduce loading and (2) sidelying on one elbow. Additionally, this position may be problematic for patients with shoulder or elbow pathology, cardiac or respiratory impairment, hip flexor tightness, or low back discomfort (which may be exacerbated by the increased **lordotic** curve required of the prone-on-elbows position).

To assist in initial assumption of the prone-on-elbows position, the patient should be in the following starting position: prone, both lower extremities extended, the shoulders abducted, elbows flexed, forearms pronated, palms flat on supporting surface, and the head in a neutral position (or turned to one side for comfort). The therapist is positioned to the side of the patient or, if the supporting surface permits, straddling the patient's trunk with one foot on either side of the patient's body. The therapist's hips and knees should be flexed and manual contacts placed over the pectoral muscles with fingers pointing toward the sternum. The therapist then assists the patient to assume the position by lifting and supporting the upper trunk as the patient adducts the shoulders to allow weight-bearing on the elbows (Fig. 14-1). Several suggested activities that can be used as a progression within this posture follow.

1. Initial activities should include assisted assumption and maintenance of the posture.
2. Manually applied approximation force can be used to facilitate holding of proximal musculature. Rhythmic stabilization or alternating isometrics may be used to increase stability of head, neck, and scapula.
3. A progression can be made to independent maintenance of the posture while altering head position and depressing the scapula.
4. Weight shifting in this position will improve dynamic stability through increased joint approximation (Fig. 14-2). Weight shifting is usually easiest in a lateral direction but may also be accomplished in an anterior or posterior direction. Light tracking resistance using slow reversals can be applied to the upper

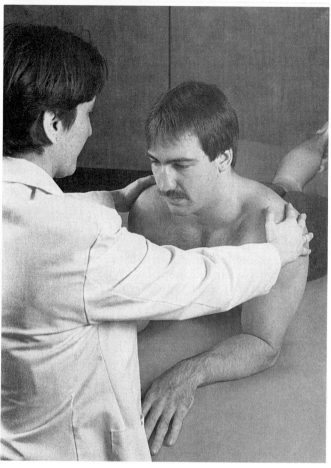

Figure 14-2. Prone-on-elbow position. Lateral weight shifting will improve dynamic stability secondary to increased joint approximation.

trunk during weight shifting to assist proprioceptive loading.

5. Activities that require resisted grasp in this position such as squeezing a ball or a cone will reinforce co-contraction at the shoulder.
6. Theraband® tubing can be positioned around the patient's forearms. The patient is instructed to hold against the tubing keeping the forearms apart. This will increase proprioceptive loading of the shoulder stabilizers.
7. Controlled mobility activities of the scapula can be used to promote proximal dynamic stability (e.g., prone-on-elbows push-ups).
8. Static-dynamic activities should be included in the prone-on-elbows position. This involves unilateral weight-bearing on the static limb while the dynamic limb is freed. This will further facilitate co-contraction in the weight-bearing limb.
9. Movement within this posture (*"commando walking"*) can be achieved by an on-elbows side-to-side (lateral) progression. These lateral semicircular movements have several important functional implications. For example, an individual with a spinal cord in-

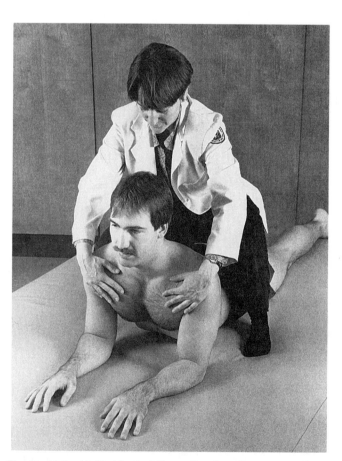

Figure 14-1. Method for assisting patient into the prone-on-elbows position.

jury may use these movements to assist with bed mobility, dressing activities, and movement transitions. Movement within this posture can be practiced in a forward-and-backward direction as well.

10. Movement into and out of the posture should be a final component of the prone-on-elbows sequence.

Prone-on-hands Position

This position is considered an intermediate step between the prone-on-elbows and quadruped positions. In the prone-on-hands position a smaller BOS and higher COG is achieved. Weight is now borne through the elbows to the hands and wrists. As with the prone-on-elbows position, this position also will be inappropriate for some patients owing to the excessive lordosis required to assume and to maintain the position. However, this position has several important functional implications. The functional carryover of the prone-on-hands position includes development of the initial hyperextension of the hips and low back for patients requiring this type of postural alignment during ambulation (e.g., patients with paraplegia), and standing from a wheelchair or rising from the floor with crutches and bilateral knee-ankle-foot orthoses (KAFOs).

To assist to the prone-on-hands position, the patient should first assume the prone-on-elbows position. The therapist's position and manual contacts are the same as for assisting to prone-on-elbows. Initially, work in this position often requires starting with the patient's supporting hand placement further away from the body (i.e., with greater than 90 degrees of shoulder flexion) until the patient becomes accustomed to the position. This type of early positioning may require contact guarding from the therapist to allow maintenance of the position. Several suggestions follow for activities that may be completed while the patient is in the prone-on-hands position.

1. Initial activities should include assisted assumption and assisted maintenance of the posture.
2. Additional approximation force can be applied through manual contacts to further facilitate tonic holding of proximal musculature.
3. Independent maintenance of the posture should be practiced; a progression can be made to maintaining the posture with alterations in head position and during scapular depression.
4. Lateral weight shifting with weight transfer between hands will increase joint approximation.
5. Resisted scapular depression and prone-on-hands push-ups may be used as strengthening exercises in this position.
6. A progression can be made to movement within this posture in both forward and lateral

directions. This activity has useful functional implications for patients with paraplegia. An important example is floor-to-stand transitions. The prone-on-hands position provides the functional skills to allow the patient to reposition the body and the crutches to prepare for standing.

Hooklying

In this posture, the patient is supine with hips and knees flexed and feet flat on the mat. This position involves lower trunk, hip, and knee control and provides a large BOS with a low COG. Lower trunk rotation can be facilitated by movement of the lower extremities across the midline. It is useful in activating both the lower abdominals, low back extensors, and hip abductors/adductors as well as increasing range of motion in the low back and hips. Activities within this posture are initiated with assisted or guided movement. A progression is then made to application of resistance applied in each direction away from the midline. Manual contacts at the knees must be altered from the medial to lateral surfaces as the direction of movement is changed. Several suggestions that may be used and/or combined in the hooklying position follow.

1. Tonic holding activities within a shortened range will improve stability (shortened held resisted contraction).
2. Rhythmic stabilization may be used with manual contacts at the knees to facilitate co-contraction and stability.
3. Active assisted, guided, or resisted movement in each direction away from the midline may be used to increase range of motion (Fig. 14-3).
4. Hip abduction and adduction can be facilitated by use of alternating isometrics with manual contacts at the knees.
5. The level of difficulty of this activity may be increased by decreasing the amount of hip and

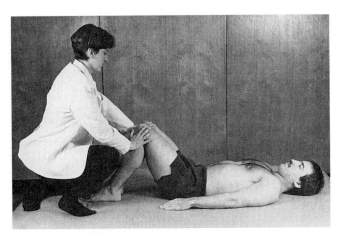

Figure 14-3. Hooklying. In this position lower trunk rotation and range of motion is facilitated by movement of the lower extremities in each direction from the midline.

knee flexion and moving manual contacts for application of resistance to the ankles.

Bridging, Pelvic Elevation

This activity is a progression from hooklying. It allows weight-bearing through the feet and is an important precursor to assuming the kneeling position and in developing sit-to-stand control. For this activity the patient is in a hooklying position and elevates the pelvis off the mat (Fig. 14-4). The BOS is thus reduced and the COG is raised. This activity is particularly useful for facilitating pelvic motions and strengthening the low back and hip extensors in preparation for the stance phase of gait. In addition, bridging has several important functional implications, including bed mobility, use of a bedpan, pressure relief, lower extremity dressing, and movement from a sitting to a standing position. Specific pelvic motions (e.g., pelvic forward motion, rotation, and lateral shift) required during gait also can be initiated and facilitated in this position. Several suggestions that can be used as a progression within this posture follow.

1. Initial activities will involve assisted assumption and assisted maintenance of the position. Manual contacts to assist to position are at the pelvis. Assistance during early bridging activities also can be provided by having the patient abduct the arms on the mat to provide a larger BOS.
2. The ability to maintain, or to hold, the posture can be facilitated by use of isometric contractions. The techniques of alternating isometrics and rhythmic stabilization can be used to promote stability.
3. Independent maintenance of the posture should be practiced with a progressive decrease in the BOS provided by the upper extremities (i.e., moving arms closer to body).
4. The techniques of slow reversal and slow

reversal-hold can be used to facilitate pelvic rotation and lateral shifting.

5. Strengthening can be accomplished during bridging by application of resistance with manual contacts at the anterior superior iliac spines. Resistance also can be applied diagonally (greater emphasis of resistance to one side) to facilitate pelvic rotation and/or to increase range of motion selectively on one side.
6. Bridging also can be used to facilitate hip abduction and adduction. This can be accomplished either symmetrically (resistance applied against the same motion in each extremity) or asymmetrically (resistance applied against opposing motions) by use of alternating isometrics with manual contacts at the knees. Theraband® tubing can be placed around the patient's distal thighs to increase contraction of the hip abductor muscles (gluteus medius) and to increase proprioceptive loading.
7. Unassisted or resisted (e.g., using agonist reversal) movement into and out of the posture should be practiced.
8. Several modifications to bridging can be made to make the activity more demanding by altering the BOS. These modifications include (a) performing the activity with support from only one lower extremity in preparation for weight acceptance during the stance phase of gait, and (b) decreasing the angle of hip and knee flexion (i.e., moving the feet distally).

Quadruped Position

This on-all-fours (hands and knees) position further decreases the BOS and raises the COG with weight-bearing through multiple joints. The **quadruped** position is the first position in the mat progression that allows weight-bearing through the hips. This posture is particularly useful for facilitating initial control of the musculature of the lower trunk and hips.

Assumption of the quadruped position can be achieved from two positions. If the patient is able to sit, the patient may be guided into sidesitting by rotating the trunk to allow weight-bearing on the hands with the elbows extended. The therapist then guides the lower trunk into the quadruped position, with manual contacts on the pelvis to assist movement of the pelvis over the knees.

The quadruped position also may be assumed from a prone-on-elbows position. Using this approach the therapist straddles the patient's lower extremities with one foot placed parallel to each thigh. With the therapist's hips and knees bent, he or she then lifts and guides the pelvis over the knees as the patient "walks" backward on elbows. Once the pelvis is positioned over the knees, the patient assumes or is assisted into weight-bearing on hands with full elbow extension. Several suggested tech-

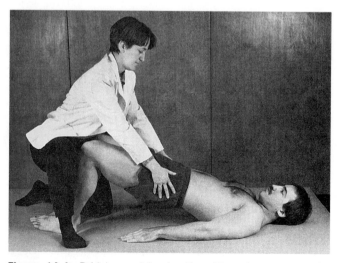

Figure 14-4. Bridging, pelvis elevation. Manual contacts at the pelvis can be used to assist or to resist pelvic elevation.

niques and activities that can be incorporated into the quadruped position follow.

1. Initial activities involve assisted assumption and assisted maintenance of the position. If these activities are difficult, a gymnastic ball can first be used to support the patient's trunk during the movement transition from sidesitting to the quadruped position and then during maintenance of the position. The ball can be placed centrally under the trunk or moved toward the upper or lower extremities, depending on the area of greatest weakness.

2. Rhythmic stabilization or alternating isometrics will facilitate co-contraction of shoulder, hip, and trunk musculature.

3. Weight shifting can be used in a forward, backward, and side-to-side direction to increase weight-bearing over two extremities simultaneously to improve dynamic stability.

4. Manual application of approximation force can be used to facilitate co-contraction through both upper and lower extremities.

5. For patients with spasticity, this position can be used to provide inhibitory pressure to the quadriceps and long finger flexors (using an open-hand position) to diminish tone.

6. Rocking through increments of range (forward, backward, side-to-side, and diagonally) will facilitate balance and proprioceptive responses as well as increase range of motion at the proximal weight-bearing joints.

7. Static-dynamic activities, such as freeing one or more extremities from a weight-bearing position, may be used in the quadruped position. A progression is frequently made from unweighting one upper extremity to unweighting one lower extremity to unweighting opposite upper and lower extremities simultaneously. This activity will provide greater joint approximation forces on the supporting extremities and increase dynamic holding of postural muscles (Fig. 14-5).

8. Unassisted movement into and out of the quadruped posture can be practiced.

9. Movement within the quadruped position

(creeping) has several important implications for ambulation. It is typically the first activity that requires trunk counterrotation, an important prerequisite for ambulation. Creeping can also be used to improve strength (resisted progression), facilitate dynamic balance reactions, and improve coordination and timing. Movement within the quadruped position is also an important precursor to assuming a standing position from the floor (e.g., after a fall a patient can "creep" to a chair or sofa prior to again assuming an upright posture).

Sitting

A program of mat activities typically includes work in the sitting position. Sitting can be used effectively to develop balance, trunk control, and weight bearing on the upper extremities. In addition, improved stability of the head and neck can be achieved in this position. Two types of sitting are often incorporated into a preambulation mat program:

1. **Short sitting.** In this position the patient's hips and knees are flexed with the feet flat on the floor.

2. **Long sitting.** In this position the hips are flexed and the knees are extended on the supporting surface. The sitting position provides a small BOS and high COG. However, it should be noted that the BOS for the two types of sitting is different and may influence selection for an individual patient. For example, the long sitting position provides a relatively large BOS as compared with the short sitting position. This larger BOS in long sitting is provided by placement of the lower extremities in contact with the supporting surface.

Another factor that warrants consideration in selection of a sitting posture is the range of motion required to assume the position. The long sitting position will be difficult for some patients owing to limited range of motion in the low back and/or hamstrings. Hamstring tightness in the long sitting position will also result in alterations in pelvic position, causing the patient to "sit back" on the ischia (this is referred to as *sacral sitting*).

The BOS in sitting may be altered by changing the position of upper extremity support. Upper extremity support may be placed posterior to the pelvis (large BOS), lateral to the pelvis (small BOS), or anterior to the pelvis (intermediate BOS). Several suggestions that can be incorporated into a progression of activities used in the sitting positions follow.

1. Initial activities will focus on assisted assumption and assisted maintenance of the position. For patients with proprioceptive loss and intact vision, use of a mirror during sitting activities may provide important visual feedback.

2. Manual application of approximation force

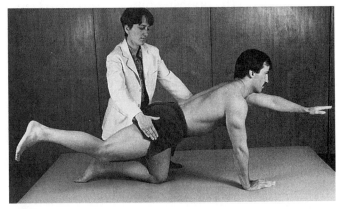

Figure 14-5. Quadruped. Static-dynamic activities facilitate dynamic holding of postural muscles by increasing weight-bearing demands on the static limbs.

may be used at the shoulders to promote co-contraction.

3. A variety of PNF techniques may be used. Specifically, alternating isometrics and rhythmic stabilization are important in promoting early stability in this posture.

4. For patients with spasticity, sitting with extended arm support and with the hand open and flat will provide inhibitory input to the long finger flexors to dampen tone.

5. The position of upper extremity support may be altered with subsequent transfer of weight in each position (e.g., posteriorly, anteriorly, and laterally). This activity also will promote co-contraction as well as alter the BOS.

6. Unassisted maintenance of the posture should be included with a gradual reduction and then elimination of upper extremity support.

7. Balancing activities may be practiced in the sitting position without upper extremity support. The position of the upper extremities may be altered by having the patient move into shoulder flexion, abduction, and so forth while maintaining trunk balance. A progression may be made to movement of the trunk (forward, backward, and side-to-side) without upper extremity support. As a component of these activities, the patient's balance may be manually challenged at the trunk or by passive movement of the lower extremities. Balance also may be challenged by asking the patient to practice throwing and catching a ball to and from various directions, or by completing functional activities such as putting on a pair of socks, tying shoes, and so forth.

8. Unassisted movement into and out of the sitting position should be practiced.

9. When indicated, the sitting position is often used for partial instruction in self-range-of-motion exercises. Both long sitting and *tailor sitting* (Indian style sitting, which places the hips in flexion, abduction and external rotation, with the knees flexed and the ankles crossed) can be used for this purpose. Forward flexion of the trunk with the knees extended in long sitting will maintain length of the low back and hamstring muscles. The tailor sitting position facilitates range of motion in hip external rotation, abduction, and knee flexion, and allows easier access to the ankle and foot.

10. Sitting push-ups are an important preliminary activity for transfers and ambulation with assistive devices as well as for improving ability in positional changes. This activity is accomplished by placing arms at sides, extending the elbows, and depressing the shoulders to lift the buttock from the mat. The activity can be accomplished initially with bearing weight on the base of the hands placed directly on the mat, with weight-bearing on sand bags, or progressed to the use of push-up blocks with graded increments in height (for patients with a disproportionately long trunk and/or short arms, sitting push-ups with hands placed directly on the mat will be difficult and sandbags or push-up blocks will be needed). A modification of the sitting push-up is placement of both hands on one side of the body in a long sitting position (sidesitting). The patient then pushes down on both upper extremities to lift the buttocks off the mat. This facilitates lower trunk rotation in preparation for gait. The functional implications of this activity are also related to movement transitions from sitting to quadruped positions. In addition, it is an important preliminary activity prior to sit-to-stand activities for patients with paraplegia (initial trunk rotation is often required before standing).

11. Movement within this posture has direct functional carryover to transfers, ambulation, and positional changes. However, these activities require good bilateral upper extremity strength (e.g., patients with paraplegia). Many of these activities are included in a mat program for patients with spinal cord injury and may incorporate the use of mat crutches. For patients with spinal cord injury, movement within sitting can be accomplished by using a seated push-up in combination with movement from the head and upper body. Momentum is created by throwing the head and shoulders forcefully in the direction opposite to the desired direction of motion. For example, while performing a push-up on the mat from the long sitting position, simultaneous rapid and forceful extension of the head and shoulders will move the lower extremities forward; movement in a posterior direction can be achieved by use of a sitting push-up with simultaneous rapid and forceful flexion of the head and trunk. This same progression of movement is used with the **swing-to** and **swing-through gait** patterns. Movement in the sitting position also may be accomplished by hiking one hip and shifting weight forward or backward and then repeating with the opposite hip.

12. A number of additional exercises may be included in the sitting position. With manual contacts at the shoulder, resistance may be applied to active trunk extension, flexion, and rotation. Combining PNF patterns of the head, trunk, and extremities in sitting (e.g., chopping or lifting activities) can be used to improve controlled mobility function, as well as to assist the patient in achieving functional goals related to this posture.

Kneeling

The kneeling position further decreases the BOS and raises the COG. It provides weight-bearing at the hips and knees simulating the requirements of normal upright standing alignment. This position is particularly useful for establishing lower trunk and pelvic control and further promoting upright balance control. The position also facilitates the lower extremity pattern (initiated during bridging) of combined hip extension with knee flexion necessary for gait activities.

It is usually easiest to assist the patient into a kneeling position from a quadruped position. From the quadruped position, the patient moves or "walks" the hands backward until the knees further flex and the pelvis drops toward the heels. The patient will be "sitting" on the heels. From this position the patient may be assisted to kneeling by using the upper extremities to climb stall bars (wall ladder) while the therapist guides the pelvis. Another method is for the therapist to assume a heel-sitting position directly in front of the patient. The patient's upper extremities are supported on the therapist's shoulders while the therapist manually guides the pelvis. Several suggested techniques and activities that can be utilized during kneeling follow.

1. Initial activities concentrate on assisted assumption and assisted maintenance of the position.
2. Approximation force may be used at the hips to facilitate co-contraction.
3. The PNF technique of slow reversal or slow reversal-hold is effective in facilitating pelvic forward motion, lateral shifting, and rotation.
4. Eccentric hip control can be facilitated by agonist reversals. This technique uses a smooth reversal between concentric and eccentric contractions. With manual contacts at the pelvis, the hips are moved into increments of flexion with a return to extension. The excursion of movement is gradually increased. This technique also improves ability to move from heel-sitting to the kneeling position.
5. Transfer of weight from one knee to the other will facilitate co-contraction on the supporting limb.
6. Balancing activities may be practiced, progressing from support with one upper extremity to balancing without upper extremity support. The patient's balance may be challenged in this position. Throwing and catching a ball from various directions also can be used as a component of these balance activities.
7. Unassisted assumption of the posture can be facilitated by use of reverse chop or lift trunk patterns.
8. Hip hiking and forward progression, or "kneel walking," while the upper extremities are supported on the therapist's shoulders can be included in this position. A resisted progression can be used to facilitate forward movement. A progression is then made to a resisted progression with the upper extremities freed.
9. A variety of mat crutch activities can be used in the kneeling position (most commonly used with individuals who have sus-

tained spinal cord injuries). Examples include weight shifting anteriorly, posteriorly, and laterally with emphasis on lower trunk and pelvic control, by placing the crutches forward, backward, and to the side with weight shifts in each direction; alternately raising one crutch at a time and returning it to the mat; hip hiking; instruction in selected gait patterns; and forward progression using crutches.

10. Kneeling can be used to provide inhibition to the quadriceps muscle and thus to dampen tone in patients with spasticity. Reduction of extensor tone may be an important preparatory activity to standing and walking for some patients.

Half-kneeling

In half-kneeling (Fig. 14-6) the COG is the same as in kneeling; however, the BOS is widened. Greater demands are now placed on the posterior weight-bearing limb in preparation for weight acceptance during the stance phase of gait. Weight on the forward limb is now borne through the ankle. This position allows facilitation of hip extension, lateral pelvic control, and ankle movements, and it increases proprioceptive input through the foot. The following techniques and activities are appropriate for use in the half-kneeling position.

1. Initial activities will include assisted assumption and assisted maintenance of the posture.
2. Rhythmic stabilization or alternating isometrics may be used in this position to improve stability. Several combinations of manual contacts may be used: shoulder and pelvis, shoulder and anterior knee, and pelvis and anterior knee.
3. Anterior-posterior diagonal weight shifting in this position will facilitate range of motion

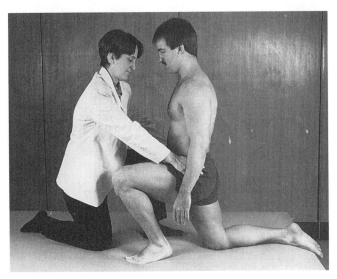

Figure 14-6. Half-kneeling. Anterior weight shifting onto forward limb.

of the hip, knee, and especially the ankle (see Fig. 14-6).

4. Resistance may be introduced with manual contacts at the pelvis during weight shifting (e.g., slow reversal or slow reversal-hold).
5. Practice in assuming the posture (moving from kneeling to half-kneeling) is an important prerequisite to accomplishing movement transitions from the floor to upright standing (e.g., after a fall).

Modified Plantigrade

Modified plantigrade (Fig. 14-7) is an early weight-bearing posture that can be used in preparation for erect standing and walking. In this position there is a relatively small BOS and high COG. This posture inherently promotes stability because weight-bearing demands are placed on all four extremities. Modified plantigrade posture is an important precursor to walking inasmuch as it superimposes close to full weight-bearing on an advanced lower extremity pattern. This pattern, required during gait, combines hip flexion with knee extension and ankle dorsiflexion.

Initial assist-to-position activities are usually easiest from a sitting position, using a chair with

arms. The chair is positioned directly in front of a treatment table or other stable surface of appropriate height. A guarding belt is warranted during early transitions from sitting to plantigrade positions. The patient is asked or assisted to move forward in the chair. The feet should be flat on the floor and the hands placed on the armrests of the chair. The patient then pushes down on the armrests and moves toward the modified plantigrade posture (placing one hand at a time onto the supporting surface). The therapist provides the needed level of assistance by use of the guarding belt and/or manual contacts. Several suggested activities and techniques that can be used in this posture follow.

1. Initial activities involve assisted assumption and assisted maintenance of the posture.
2. Stability can be enhanced by use of manual approximation force at both the shoulders and the pelvis. Rhythmic stabilization and alternating isometrics also can be used to promote stability in this position. Manual contacts are at the pelvis, shoulders, or both shoulders and pelvis.
3. Range of motion can be increased and dynamic stability further enhanced by controlled mobility techniques such as rocking through increments of range. Rocking can be used in multiple directions (e.g., forward, backward, diagonally) and is effective in increasing weight-bearing over one or more extremities. Guided weight shifting is effectively accomplished by the therapist standing behind the patient with manual contacts at the pelvis.
4. A progression can be made to static-dynamic activities. Freeing one lower extremity (e.g., side-stepping) will place increased demands on the three remaining weight-bearing limbs. In addition to side-stepping, lower extremity positions can also be altered by stepping with the dynamic limb in both forward and backward directions. Body weight is then shifted over the dynamic limb while the static limb remains stationary. This will facilitate pelvic motion and lateral shifting. Rotation of the lower trunk also can be emphasized during static-dynamic lower extremity activities.

Standing

In erect standing the BOS is small with a high COG, requiring maximum balance control. Standing activities are most often initiated in the parallel bars (described in the next section). However, for many patients these activities can be initiated next to a treatment table or other supporting surface. Some patients may demonstrate sufficient stability to maintain a standing posture prior to being able to assume the position independently.

It should be noted that achieving a specific level of motor control within an individual posture of the exercise sequence *does not guarantee translation of gains to standing.* Subcomponents (e.g., hip stability

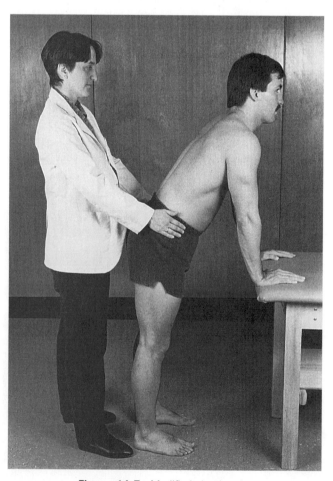

Figure 14-7. Modified plantigrade.

in quadruped) do not translate into ambulatory function without practice within a specific context. Motor learning relies on sensory information and feedback provided by practice and experience to shape specific functions. Components of the lead-up activities must be incorporated in upright standing to ensure transfer of subcomponents into a functional whole. The amount of practice required and the rate of learning vary among patients. The following activities and techniques can be used in the standing position.

1. Initial activities involve assisted assumption (described under parallel bar progression) and assisted maintenance of the position.
2. The ability to maintain the posture can be promoted by stability techniques such as rhythmic stabilization and alternating isometrics with manual contacts at the pelvis, scapula, or both scapula and pelvis. With the lower extremities in a symmetrical stance position, Theraband® tubing can be placed around the thighs to increase proprioceptive loading and pelvic stabilization by the hip abductors.
3. Guided weight shifting onto alternate lower extremities with manual contacts on the pelvis also will improve stability. Additional support may be provided by placement of the patient's hands on the therapist's shoulders. As stability improves, upper extremity support should be reduced or eliminated.
4. Controlled-mobility activities of the trunk can be practiced in standing with the feet symmetrical or in stride. Anterior-posterior, lateral, and rotational movements of the trunk can be emphasized.
5. Static-dynamic activities (e.g., stepping) will promote weight acceptance by advancing the dynamic limb forward and moving body weight over the advanced limb. This activity also will promote forward rotation and lateral shift of the pelvis (Fig. 14-8). Upper extremity movements can also be superimposed on these activities (e.g., reciprocal arm swing).

Walking

Walking represents the final and highest level of motor control (skill). Manual contacts can be placed at the pelvis to guide and to assist with control of pelvic movement. Upper extremity support should be gradually decreased and then eliminated. The sequence of activities in standing typically includes resisted progression; walking backward, sidestep, cross-step; and braiding. These activities are described in the following section.

This section presented a sample of mat activities to improve control. The incremental emphasis of control from proximal to distal body segments is summarized in Table 14–1. It should be noted that this basic sequence will require adaptation and modification depending on the unique needs of each individual patient. In addition to the preambulation

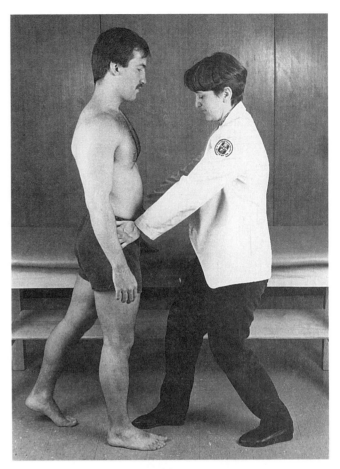

Figure 14-8. Standing. Static-dynamic activities will promote weight acceptance on the dynamic limb, forward pelvic rotation, and lateral shift.

mat activities outlined, a program of strengthening and coordination exercises are important concurrent activities during preparation for ambulation. Transfer training and wheelchair management also can be initiated in conjunction with mat activities once the patient has begun work on movement within the sitting position. Box 14–2 presents an overview of the preambulation exercise program. For a more detailed description of therapeutic exercise interventions for gait impairments the reader is referred to *Physical Rehabilitation Laboratory Manual: Focus on Functional Training.*[4]

PARALLEL BAR PROGRESSION

Upright activities in the parallel bars can be initiated as soon as adequate motor control is achieved. All mat activities may not be warranted or feasible before initiating upright activities. Prior to standing, two important preliminary activities include fitting the patient with a guarding belt and adjusting the parallel bars. The initial adjustment of the parallel bars is an estimate based on the patient's height. Ideally the bars should be adjusted to allow 20 to 30 degrees of elbow flexion and come to about the level of the greater trochanter. Considering individual variations in body proportions and arm

Table 14–1 FOCUS OF CONTROL WITHIN EACH POSTURE OF THE PREAMBULATION MAT PROGRESSION

Posture	Focus of Control
Rolling	Trunk
	Segmental rotation
	Counterrotation
Prone-on-elbows	Head
	Neck
	Upper trunk
	Scapula
	Shoulders
Prone-on-hands	Elbows (intermediate control of upper extremities)
Hooklying	Lower trunk
	Proximal lower extremities
Bridging	Lower trunk
	Hips/pelvis
	Lower extremities
Quadruped	Trunk
	Proximal and intermediate upper extremities
	Proximal lower extremities
Sitting	Trunk
	Proximal and intermediate upper extremities
Kneeling	Trunk
	Pelvis
	Proximal lower extremities
Half-kneeling	Trunk
	Pelvis
	Proximal and distal lower extremities (knee and ankle)
	Reciprocal control of lower extremities
Plantigrade	Trunk
	Proximal and intermediate control of lower extremities
Standing	Trunk
	Lower extremities

length, the elbow measurement is usually most accurate. Once the patient is standing, the height of the bars can be checked. If adjustments are required, the patient should be returned to a sitting position. Prior to beginning work in the parallel bars, two important preparatory activities include *wheelchair positioning* and *placement of the guarding belt*.

The patient's wheelchair should be positioned at the end of the parallel bars. The brakes should be locked, the footrests placed in an upright position, and the patient's feet should be flat on the floor. The guarding belt should be fastened securely around the patient's waist. Guarding belts provide several critical functions. They increase the therapist's effectiveness in controlling or preventing potential loss of

balance; they improve patient safety; they facilitate the therapist's use of proper body mechanics in untoward circumstances; and finally, they are an important consideration regarding issues of liability. The safety implications of the guarding belt should be explained to the patient carefully. A sequence of activities for use in the parallel bars follows.

1. *Initial instruction/demonstration.* In initiating instruction in parallel bar activities, the entire progression should be presented before breaking it into component parts. This will include instruction and demonstration in how to assume a standing position in the parallel bars, guarding techniques to be used by the therapist, the components of initial standing balance activities, the gait pattern to be used, how to turn in the parallel bars, and how to return to a sitting position. Demonstrating these activities by assuming the role of the patient during verbal explanations will facilitate learning. Each component of the parallel bar progression should then be reviewed prior to the patient's actual performance of the activity.

2. *Assuming the standing position.* To prepare for standing, the patient should be instructed to move forward in the chair. The therapist is positioned directly in front of the patient. A method of guarding should be selected that does not interfere with the patient's use of the upper extremities while moving to standing. One useful approach is to grasp the guarding belt anteriorly (an "underhand" grasp will provide the most security). With unilateral involvement, the therapist's opposite wrist should be placed on the lateral trunk near the axillary region on the patient's stronger or unaffected side with the hand at the lateral border of the scapula. Care should be taken not to exert any upward pressure into the axilla. Although the correct position for guarding is typically on the patient's weaker side, the therapist may stand closer to the unaffected side to brace or to guard the patient's sound lower extremity and to ensure one strong supporting limb. For example, this approach would be indicated in situations in which one lower extremity requires a non-weight-bearing status. If bilateral involvement exists, the therapist should be positioned more centrally to

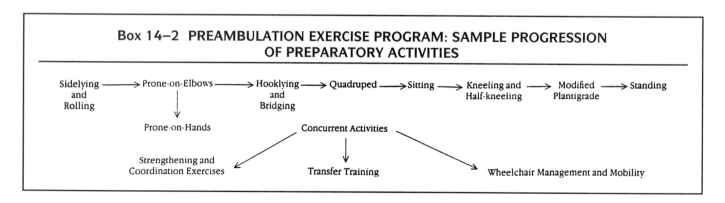

Box 14–2 PREAMBULATION EXERCISE PROGRAM: SAMPLE PROGRESSION OF PREPARATORY ACTIVITIES

Sidelying and Rolling → Prone-on-Elbows → Hooklying and Bridging → Quadruped → Sitting → Kneeling and Half-kneeling → Modified Plantigrade → Standing

Prone-on-Hands

Concurrent Activities

Strengthening and Coordination Exercises

Transfer Training

Wheelchair Management and Mobility

brace both of the patient's knees. If necessary, the patient's feet may be braced (by the therapist's feet) to prevent sliding. An alternate hand placement particularly useful with bilateral involvement is one hand at the posterior hip, the opposite hand on the lateral aspect of the guarding belt or lateral trunk below the axilla. Having moved forward in the chair with the supporting foot or feet flat on the floor, the patient should be instructed to come to a standing position by leaning forward and pushing down on the armrests of the wheelchair. The patient should not be allowed to stand by pulling up on the parallel bars. As the patient nears an erect posture, the hands should be released from the armrests one at a time and placed on the parallel bars. The patient's COG should be guided over the BOS to promote a stable standing posture.

3. *Initial parallel bar activities*. During parallel bar activities, the therapist usually stands inside the bars facing the patient or outside the bars on the patient's weaker side. In guarding the patient from inside the bars, one hand should grasp the guarding belt anteriorly, and the opposite hand should be in front of, but not touching, the patient's shoulder. From outside the bars one hand should grasp the belt posteriorly with the opposite hand in front of, but not touching, the patient's shoulder. This method of guarding provides effective hand placement for an immediate response should the patient lose his or her balance. It also eliminates the patient's feeling of being "held back" or "pushed forward," which may occur with manual contacts at the shoulders. The following initial balancing activities in the parallel bars can be modified relative to the patient's weight-bearing status and the specific requirements of a treatment (e.g., use of a prosthesis or orthosis). Guarding techniques are maintained by the therapist during these activities.
   a. *Standing balance*. Initially, the patient should be allowed time to become acclimated to the upright posture. During initial standing activities, the therapist should be alert to complaints of nausea or lightheadedness, which may indicate an onset of **orthostatic (postural) hypotension** caused by a drop in blood pressure. These symptoms typically disappear as tolerance to the upright posture improves. However, if the patient has been confined to bed and/or a wheelchair for a prolonged period, these symptoms may be severe. In these situations a gradual progression of tilt-table activities and careful monitoring of vital signs may be warranted prior to standing. Use of compressive stockings or wraps and an abdominal support or binder will further minimize these effects.
   b. *Limits of stability (LOS)*. Exploration of LOS involves determining how far the patient's COG can be displaced while balance is maintained. Early exploration is accomplished by use of *anterior-posterior* and *lateral weight shifts*, and *alteration in hand placement* on the parallel bars.
      1. *Lateral weight shift*. The patient shifts weight from side-to-side without altering the BOS; hand placement on the parallel bars is not altered.
      2. *Anterior-posterior weight shift*. The patient shifts weight forward and backward without altering the BOS; hand placement on the parallel bars is not altered.
      3. *Anterior-posterior hand placement and weight shift*. The patient moves the hands forward on the bars and shifts weight anteriorly. This is alternated with a posterior hand placement, and weight is shifted backward.
      4. *Single-hand support*. The patient balances with support from only one hand on the parallel bars; hands are alternated. A progression of this activity involves gradual changes in position of the freed hand and upper extremity. For example, begin the activity by moving the freed hand several inches above the bar and gradually progress to alternate positions such as shoulder flexion, abduction, crossing the midline, and so forth. A progression can be made to balancing with both hands freed from the bars.
   c. *Hip hiking*. The patient maintains the BOS and alternately hikes one hip at a time; hand placement on the parallel bars is maintained. Resistance can be applied by manual contacts at the pelvis.
   d. *Standing push-ups*. The patient's hands are placed just anterior to the thighs on the parallel bars. Body weight is lifted by simultaneous elbow extension and shoulder depression. Additional height may be gained by forward flexion of the head. Return to the starting position is made by a controlled lowering of the body. This activity requires significant upper extremity strength and builds on the controlled mobility developed in preambulation activities. It is usually reserved for younger patient groups, such as those with paraplegia, and selected patients with lower extremity amputation.
   e. *Stepping forward and backward*. The patient steps forward with one leg, shifts weight anteriorly, and returns to the starting position (normal BOS). This is alternated with stepping backward with one leg, shifting the weight posteriorly, and returning to the starting position. Resistance can be applied with manual contacts at the pelvis.
   f. *Forward progression*. The patient begins ambulation in the parallel bars using the se-

lected gait pattern and appropriate weight-bearing on the affected lower extremity. The patient should be instructed to push down rather than to pull on the parallel bars while ambulating, inasmuch as this is the motion that eventually will be required with an assistive device. This will be easier if the patient is instructed to use a loose or open grip on the bars rather than a tight grip; the loose or open grip facilitates correct use of the parallel bars and, ultimately, the assistive device.

g. *Turning*. Once the desired distance in the parallel bars has been reached, the patient should be instructed to turn toward the stronger side. For example, with a non-weight-bearing left lower extremity, the turn should be toward the right. The patient should be instructed to turn by stepping in a small circle and not to pivot on a single extremity. This technique will carry over to ambulation outside the bars, when pivoting will always be discouraged because of the potential loss of balance by movement on a small BOS. Guarding while turning in the parallel bars can be accomplished two ways. The therapist can remain in front of the patient, maintain the same hand positions, and turn with the patient. This will keep the therapist positioned in front of the patient. A second method is not to turn with the patient but, rather, to guard from behind on the return trip. In this method hand placements will change during the turn. Hand placement is changed gradually by first placing both hands on the guarding belt as the patient initiates the turn. One hand then remains on the posterior aspect of the belt and the freed hand is placed anterior to, but not touching, the shoulder on the patient's weaker side for the return trip toward the chair. Although both techniques are acceptable, the latter is probably more practical, considering the limited space available in the parallel bars.

As mentioned, guarding also may be accomplished from outside the parallel bars. This positioning of the therapist is particularly useful during later stages of gait training. However, it presents several inherent problems for early training. If unilateral involvement exists, it is frequently difficult to remain close to the patient's weaker side (especially if the patient is not able to ambulate the full length of the parallel bars). In addition, the distance between the therapist and patient imposed by the intervening bar renders the therapist less effective in guarding and in using appropriate, safe body mechanics to help support the patient during periods of unsteadiness or loss of balance.

h. *Returning to the seated position*. When reaching the chair the patient should again turn as described earlier. Once completely turned, patients are typically instructed to continue backing up until they feel the seat of the chair on the back of their legs (this will require substitution with visual or auditory clues for patients with impaired sensation). At this point the patient releases the stronger hand from the parallel bar and reaches back for the wheelchair armrest. Once this hand has securely grasped the armrest, the patient should be instructed to bend forward slightly, release the opposite hand from the parallel bar and place it on the other armrest. Keeping the head and trunk forward, the patient gently returns to a seated position.

4. *Advanced parallel bar activities*. Although not appropriate for every patient, several more advanced activities also can be incorporated into gait training in the parallel bars. These include the following.

a. *Resisted forward progression*. Resistance can be applied through manual contacts at the pelvis and/or shoulder as the patient walks forward.

b. *Walking backward*. Walking backward can be initiated actively and can progress to application of resistance through manual contacts at the pelvis. This activity also combines hip extension with knee flexion and is particularly useful for patients with hemiplegia with synergy influence in the lower extremities.

c. *Side-stepping*. Initially, this activity is performed actively. A progression can then be made to application of resistance with manual contacts at the pelvis and thigh. Side-step (sidewards) walking facilitates active abduction of the moving limb, combined with controlled mobility and weight-bearing of the opposite supporting extremity.

d. *Braiding*. This activity requires a crossed and side-step progression with one limb advancing alternately anteriorly and posteriorly across the other while the second limb sidesteps. It incorporates lower trunk rotation as well as crossing the midline. For braiding activities, the patient can be either inside or outside standard parallel bars with both hands placed on a single bar or by placing both hands on an oval bar.

5. *Stepping up*. An aerobic step is placed directly in front of the patient inside the parallel bars. The patient weight shifts laterally toward the support limb and places the dynamic limb on the step. The limb is then returned to the original stance position. Stepping up is an important lead-up activity for stair climbing. The height of the step can be varied to increase or decrease the difficulty of the activity. For example, a 4 inch (10 cm) step can be used initially with a gradual progression to a standard 7 inch (17.5 cm) step.

ASSISTIVE DEVICES AND GAIT PATTERNS

Before continuing with the progression of gait training activities outside the parallel bars, consideration will be given to (1) selection and measurement of assistive devices, and (2) selection and description of gait patterns used with each ambulatory device.

Selection, Measurement, and Gait Patterns for Use of Ambulatory Assistive Devices

There are three major categories of ambulatory assistive devices: canes, crutches, and walkers. Each has several modifications to the basic design, many of which were developed to meet the needs of a specific patient problem or diagnostic group. Assistive devices are prescribed for a variety of reasons, including problems of balance, pain, fatigue, weakness, joint instability, excessive skeletal loading, and cosmesis. Another primary function of assistive devices is to eliminate weight-bearing fully or partially from an extremity. This unloading occurs by transmission of force from the upper extremities to the floor by downward pressure on the assistive device.

CANES

Most canes used in current clinical practice are constructed of lightweight aluminum. The function of a cane is to *widen the BOS* and *improve balance*.[5] Canes are not intended for use with restricted weight-bearing gaits (such as non- or **partial-weight-bearing**). Patients are typically instructed to hold a cane in the hand *opposite the affected extremity*. This positioning of the cane most closely approximates a normal reciprocal gait pattern with the opposite arm and leg moving together. It also widens the BOS with less lateral shifting of the COG than when the cane is held on the ipsilateral side.

Contralateral positioning of the cane is particularly important in reducing forces created by the abductor muscles acting at the hip.[6] During normal gait, the hip abductors of the stance extremity contract to counteract the gravitational moment at the pelvis on the contralateral side during swing. This prevents tilting of the pelvis on the contralateral side but results in a compressive force acting at the stance hip. Use of a cane in the upper extremity opposite the affected hip will reduce these forces. The floor (ground) reaction force created by the downward pressure of body weight on the cane counterbalances the gravitational movement at the affected hip.[7] Thus, the need for tension in the abductor muscles is reduced, with a subsequent decrease in joint compressive forces.

Several components of floor reaction forces that create joint compression at the hip can be reduced by use of a cane. In a study by Ely and Smidt,[8] contralateral use of a cane was found to decrease the vertical and posterior components of the floor reaction force produced by the affected foot. They noted that the reductions in vertical floor reac-

tion peaks were probably due to a shifting of body weight toward the cane, which was a contributing factor in reducing contact force at the affected hip. Neumann[6] found that contralateral use of a cane reduced the average hip abductor muscle EMG activity to 31 percent below that generated when not using a cane.

Research suggests that use of a cane is an effective method of reducing forces acting at the hip.[6,8] This concept is particularly important for activities such as stair climbing, when the forces generated at the hip are significantly increased.[7] Clearly, use of a cane has important implications for hip involvement such as joint replacements or degenerative joint disease.

In addition to altering the forces on the affected extremity, canes are selected on the basis of their ability to improve gait by providing increased dynamic stability and improving balance. This is achieved by the increased BOS provided by the additional points of floor contact. The level of stability provided by canes is on a continuum. The greatest stability is provided by the broad-based canes and the least by a standard cane. The following section presents several of the more common types of canes in clinical use and identifies their advantages and disadvantages.

Standard Cane

This assistive device also is referred to as a regular or conventional cane (Fig. 14-9A). It is made of aluminum, wood or plastic and has a half circle ("crook") handle. The distal rubber tip is at least 1 inch in diameter or larger.

Advantages. This cane is inexpensive and fits easily on stairs or other surfaces where space is limited.

Disadvantages. The standard cane is not adjustable and must be cut to fit the patient. Its point of support is anterior to the hand, not directly beneath it.

Standard Adjustable Aluminum Cane

This assistive device (Fig. 14-9B) has the same basic design as the regular or standard cane. It is made of aluminum tubing and has a half-circle handle with a molded plastic covering. The telescoping design of this cane enables the height to be adjusted by placing the locking-pin mechanism into the proper notch. Variations in available height range differ slightly with manufacturers. However, they are generally adjustable within the range of approximately 27 to 38.5 inches (68 to 98 cm). The distal rubber tip is at least 1 inch in diameter or larger. (*Note:* Most adjustable aluminum assistive devices use a push-button pin or notch mechanism to alter height; some include a reinforcing cuff that is tightened by a thumbscrew or a rotation sleeve.)

Advantages. This cane is quickly adjustable, facilitating ease of determining appropriate height. It is particularly useful for measurement prior to altering the length of a standard cane. It is lightweight and fits easily on stairs.

Disadvantages. The point of support is anterior to the hand, not directly beneath it. This cane is more costly than a standard cane.

Adjustable Aluminum Offset Cane

The proximal component of the body (shaft) of this cane is offset anteriorly creating a *straight* (or *offset*) handle. It is made of aluminum tubing with a plastic or rubber molded grip-shaped handle (Fig. 14-9C). The telescoping design allows the height to be adjusted from approximately 27 to 38.5 inches (68 to 98 cm) by a pin or notch mechanism. The diameter of the distal rubber tip is at least 1 inch.

Advantages. The design of this cane allows pressure to be borne over the center of the cane for greater stability. This cane also is quickly adjusted, lightweight, and fits easily on stairs.

Disadvantages. This cane is more costly than standard or adjustable aluminum canes.

Quad (Quadruped) Cane

This assistive device is constructed of aluminum and aluminum tubing and is available in a variety of designs depending on the manufacturer. Both large-

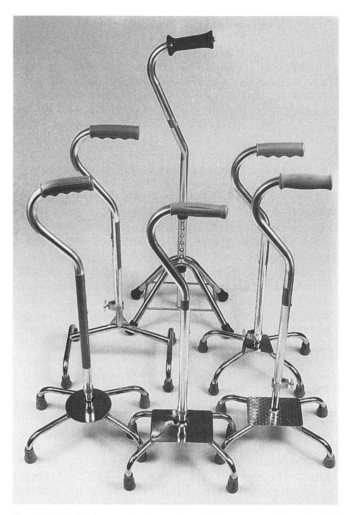

Figure 14-10. Shown here are a variety of large-based quadruped canes.

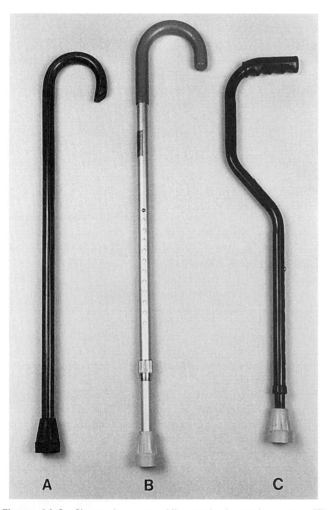

Figure 14-9. Shown here are (A) standard wooden cane, (B) standard adjustable aluminum cane, and (C) adjustable offset cane.

based quad canes (LBQC) and small-based quad canes (SBQC) are commercially available (Figs. 14-10 and 14-11). The characteristic feature of these canes is that they provide a broad base with four points of floor contact. Each point (leg) is covered with a rubber tip. The legs closest to the patient's body are generally shorter and may be angled to allow foot clearance. On many designs the proximal portion of the cane is offset anteriorly. The handpiece is usually one of a variety of contoured plastic grips. A telescoping design allows for height adjustments. Quad canes are generally adjustable from approximately 28 to 38 inches (71 to 91 cm).

Advantages. This cane provides a broad-based support. Bases are available in several different sizes. This cane is also easily adjustable.

Disadvantages. Depending on the specific design of the cane, the pressure exerted by the patient's hand may not be centered over the cane and may result in patient complaints of instability. As a result of the broad BOS, some quad canes may not be practical for use on stairs. Another disadvantage of broad-based canes is that they warrant use of a slower gait pattern. If a faster forward progression is

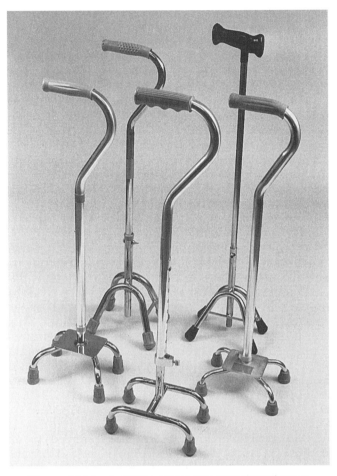

Figure 14-11. A variety of small-based quadruped canes.

Hand Grips

A general consideration relevant to all canes is the nature of the handgrip. There are a variety of styles and sizes available. The type of handgrip should be judged and selected primarily on the basis of patient comfort and on the grip's ability to provide adequate surface area to allow effective transfer of weight from the upper extremity to the floor. The more common types of handgrips are (1) the *crook* handle, (2) the *straight* (or *offset*) handle, (3) the *shovel* handle, and (4) the *pistol* handle, which conforms to the patient's hand. It is useful to have several handgrip styles available for assessment with individual patients.

Measuring Canes

In measuring cane height, the cane (or center of a broad-based cane) is placed approximately 6 inches from the lateral border of the toes. Two landmarks typically are used during measurement: the *greater trochanter* and the *angle at the elbow*. The top of the cane should come to approximately the level of the greater trochanter, and the elbow should be flexed to about 20 to 30 degrees. Because of individual variations in body proportion and arm

used, the cane often "rocks" from rear legs to front legs, which decreases effectiveness of the cane. Patients should be instructed to place all four legs of the cane on the floor simultaneously to obtain maximum stability.

Walk Cane

The walk cane (sometimes referred to as a *hemi-walker*) also is constructed of aluminum and aluminum tubing (Fig. 14-12). It provides a very broad base with four points of floor contact. Each point (leg) is covered with a rubber tip. The legs farther from the patient's body are angled to maintain floor contact and to improve stability. The handgrip is molded plastic around the uppermost segment of aluminum tubing. Walk canes fold flat and are adjustable in height from approximately 29 to 37 inches (73 to 94 cm).

Advantages. Walk canes provide very broad-based support and are more stable than a quad cane. These canes also fold flat for travel or storage.

Disadvantages. As with the quad canes, the specific design of a walk cane or handgrip placement may not allow pressure to be centered over the cane. Walk canes cannot be used on most stairs. They require use of a slow forward progression and are generally more costly than quad canes.

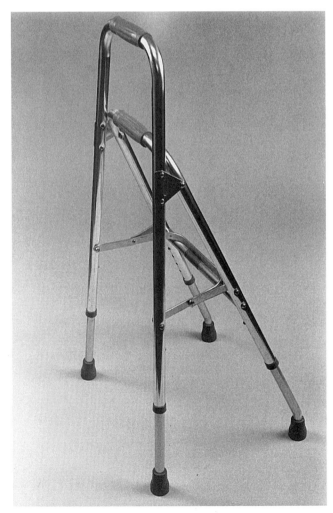

Figure 14-12. Walk cane.

lengths, the degree of flexion at the elbow is the more important indicator of correct cane height. This elbow flexion serves two important functions. It allows the arm to shorten or to lengthen during different phases of gait, and it provides a shock-absorption mechanism. Finally, as with all assistive devices, the height of the cane should be assessed with regard to patient comfort and the cane's effectiveness in accomplishing its intended purpose.

Gait Pattern for Use of Canes

As discussed, the cane should be held in the upper extremity opposite the affected limb. For ambulation on level surfaces, the cane and the involved extremity are advanced simultaneously (Fig. 14-13). The cane should remain relatively close to the body and should not be placed ahead of the toe of the involved extremity. These are important considerations, because placing the cane too far forward or to the side will cause lateral and/or forward bending, with a resultant decrease in dynamic stability.

When bilateral involvement exists, a decision must be made as to which side of the body the cane will be held. This question is most effectively resolved by a problem-solving approach with input from both the patient and therapist. Questions to be considered include:

1. On which side is the cane most comfortable?

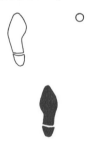

(4) Cycle is repeated.

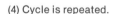

(3) The uninvolved extremity is advanced.

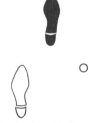

(2) The cane and involved extremity are moved forward simultaneously.

(1) Starting position. In this example, the left lower extremity is the involved limb.

Figure 14-13. Gait pattern for use of cane.

2. Is one placement superior in terms of improving balance and/or ambulatory endurance?
3. If gait deviations exist, is one position more effective in improving the overall gait pattern?
4. Is safety influenced by cane placement (e.g., during transfers, stair climbing, or ambulation on outdoor surfaces)?
5. Is there a difference in grip strength between hands?
6. Are two canes needed for stability?

Consideration of these questions will generally provide sufficient information to determine the most effective cane placement and use when bilateral involvement exists.

CRUTCHES

Crutches are used most frequently to improve balance and to either relieve weight-bearing fully or partially on a lower extremity. They are typically used bilaterally, and function to increase the BOS, to improve lateral stability, and to allow the upper extremities to transfer body weight to the floor. This transfer of weight through the upper extremities permits functional ambulation while maintaining a restricted weight-bearing status. There are two basic designs of crutches in frequent clinical use: axillary and forearm crutches.

Axillary Crutches

These assistive devices also are referred to as regular or standard crutches (Fig. 14-14A). They are made of lightweight wood or aluminum. Their design includes an axillary bar, a handpiece, and double uprights joined distally by a single leg covered with a rubber suction tip (which should have a diameter of 1.5 to 3 inches). The single leg allows for height variations. Height adjustments for wooden and some aluminum crutches are accomplished by altering the placement of screws and wing bolts in predrilled holes. The design of most aluminum crutches incorporates a push-button pin or notch mechanism for height adjustments similar to those found on aluminum canes. Some aluminum crutches also have patient height markers adjacent to the notches to assist in adjustment. The height of the handgrips for wooden and some aluminum crutches is adjusted by placement of screws and wing bolts in predrilled holes. The handgrip height on some aluminum crutches is adjusted using a push-button mechanism with a reinforcing clip-lock (Fig. 14-15). Both the overall height of the crutch as well as the height of the handgrip typically adjust in 1-inch increments. Axillary crutches are generally adjustable in adult sizes from approximately 48 to 60 inches (122 to 153 cm), with children's and extra-long sizes available.

A modification to this basic design is the ortho crutch (Fig. 14-14B). This type of axillary crutch is made of aluminum. Its design includes a single upright, an axillary bar covered with sponge-rubber padding, and a handgrip covered with molded plastic. The crutch adjusts both proximally (to alter elbow angle) and distally (to alter height of crutch).

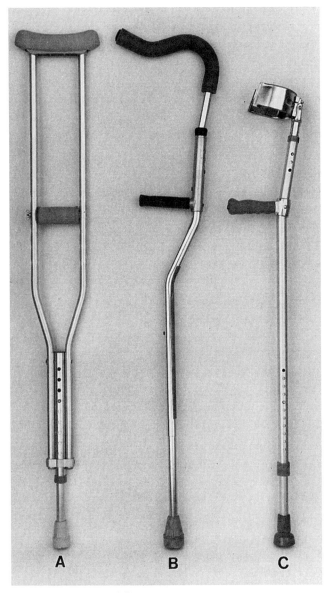

Figure 14-14. (A) Axillary crutch, (B) ortho crutch, and a (C) forearm crutch.

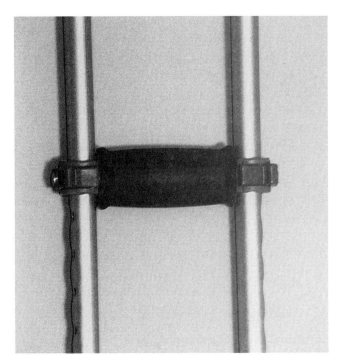

Figure 14-15. Push-button handgrip adjustment with reinforcing clip-lock.

Platform Attachments

These attachments (Fig. 14-16) are also referred to as forearm rests or troughs. Although they are described here, they also are used with walkers. Their function is to allow transfer of body weight through the forearm to the assistive device. A platform attachment is used when weight-bearing is contraindicated through the wrist and hand (e.g., some patients with arthritis). The forearm piece is usually padded, has a dowel or handgrip, and has Velcro straps to maintain the position of the forearm. Trough crutches are also commercially available.

Forearm Crutches

These assistive devices are also known as Lofstrand and Canadian crutches (Fig. 14-14C). They are constructed of aluminum. Their design includes a single upright, a forearm cuff, and a handgrip. This crutch adjusts both proximally to alter position of the forearm cuff and distally to alter the height of the crutch. Adjustments are made using a pin or notch mechanism. The available heights of forearm crutches are indicated from handgrip to floor and are generally adjustable in adult sizes from 29 to 35 inches (74 to 89 cm), with children's and extra-long sizes available. The distal end of the crutch is covered with a rubber suction tip. The forearm cuffs are available with either a medial or anterior opening. The cuffs are made of metal and can be obtained with a plastic coating.

Advantages. The forearm cuff allows use of hands without the crutches becoming disengaged. They are easily adjusted and allow functional stair-climbing activities. Many patients feel they are more

Adjustments are made using a push-button pin or notch mechanism. The distal end of the crutch is covered with a rubber suction tip.

Advantages. Axillary crutches improve balance and lateral stability, and provide for functional ambulation with restricted weight-bearing. They are easily adjusted, inexpensive when made of wood, and can be used for stair climbing.

Disadvantages. Because of the tripod stance required to use crutches and the resultant large BOS, crutches are awkward in small areas. For the same reason, the safety of the user may be compromised when ambulating in crowded areas. Another disadvantage is the tendency of some patients to lean on the axillary bar. This causes pressure at the radial groove (spiral groove) of the humerus, creating a situation of potential damage to the radial nerve as well as to adjacent vascular structures in the axilla.

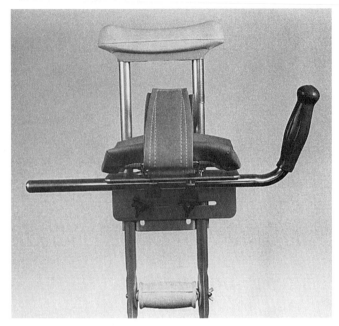

Figure 14-16. Platform attachment to axillary crutch.

cosmetic and they fit more easily into an automobile owing to the overall decreased height. They are also the most functional type of crutch for stair-climbing activities for individuals wearing bilateral KAFOs.

Disadvantages. Forearm crutches provide less lateral support owing to the absence of an axillary bar. The cuffs may be difficult to remove.

Measuring Crutches

Axillary Crutches. Several methods are available for measuring axillary crutches. The most common use a standing or a supine position. Measurement from standing is most accurate and is the preferred approach.

Standing. From the standing position in the parallel bars, crutches should be measured from a point approximately 2 inches below the axilla. The width of two fingers is often used to approximate this distance. During measurement, the distal end of the crutch should be resting at a point 2 inches lateral and 6 inches anterior to the foot. A general estimate of crutch height can be obtained prior to standing by subtracting 16 inches from the patient's height. With the shoulders relaxed, the handpiece should be adjusted to provide 20 to 30 degrees of elbow flexion.

Supine. From this position the measurement is taken from the anterior axillary fold to a surface point (mat or treatment table) 6 to 8 inches (5 to 7.5 cm) from the lateral border of the heel.

Forearm Crutches. Standing is the position of choice for measuring forearm crutches. From a standing position in the parallel bars, the distal end of the crutch should be positioned at a point 2 inches lateral and 6 inches anterior to the foot. With the shoulders relaxed the height should then be adjusted to provide 20 to 30 degrees of elbow flexion. The forearm cuff is adjusted separately. Cuff placement

should be on the proximal third of the forearm, approximately 1 to 1.5 inches below the elbow.

Gait Patterns for Use of Crutches

Gait patterns are selected on the basis of the patient's balance, coordination, muscle function, and weight-bearing status. The gait patterns differ significantly in their energy requirements, BOS, and the speed with which they can be executed.

Prior to initiating instruction in gait patterns, several important points should be emphasized to the patient:

1. During axillary crutch use, body weight should always be borne on the hands and not on the axillary bar. This will prevent pressure on both the vascular and nervous structures located in the axillary region.
2. Balance will be optimal by always maintaining a wide (tripod) BOS. Even when in a resting stance, the patient should be instructed to keep the crutches at least 4 inches (10 cm) to the front and to the side of each foot. The foot should not be allowed to achieve parallel alignment with the crutches. This will jeopardize anterior-posterior stability by decreasing the BOS.
3. When using standard crutches, the axillary bars should be held close to the chest wall to provide improved lateral stability.
4. The patient should also be cautioned about the importance of holding the head up and maintaining good postural alignment during ambulation.
5. Turning should be accomplished by stepping in a small circle rather than pivoting.

Three-point Gait. In this type of gait three points of support contact the floor. It is used when a non-weight-bearing status is required on one lower extremity. Body weight is borne on the crutches instead of on the affected lower extremity. The sequence of this gait pattern is illustrated in Figure 14-17.

Partial Weight-Bearing Gait. This gait is a modification of the three-point pattern. During forward progression of the involved extremity, weight is borne partially on both crutches and on the affected extremity (Fig. 14-18). During instruction in the partial weight-bearing gait, emphasis should be placed on use of a normal heel-toe progression on the affected extremity. Often the term *partial weight-bearing* is interpreted by the patient as meaning that only the toes or ball of the foot should contact the floor. Use of this positioning over a period of days or weeks will lead to heel cord tightness. Limb load monitors are often a useful adjunct to partial weight-bearing gait training and are described later in this chapter. These devices provide auditory feedback to the patient regarding the amount of weight borne on an extremity.

Four-point Gait. This pattern provides a slow, stable gait as three points of floor contact are maintained. Weight is borne on both lower extremities and typically is used with bilateral involvement due to poor balance, incoordination, or muscle weak-

(5) Cycle is repeated.

(4) Both crutches are advanced.

(3) Weight is shifted through the upper extremities onto the crutches, and the uninvolved limb advances beyond the crutches. If this presents difficulty, the unaffected limb may initially be brought to the crutches and later progress beyond.

(2) Weight is shifted onto the uninvolved right lower extremity, and the crutches are advanced.

(1) Starting position. In this example, the left lower extremity is non-weight-bearing.

Figure 14-17. Three-point gait pattern.

(4) Cycle is repeated.

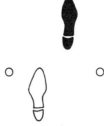

(3) Weight is shifted onto the crutches and partially to the affected extremity, and the unaffected limb advances.

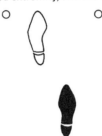

(2) Weight is shifted onto the uninvolved limb. The crutches and the affected extremity are advanced simultaneously as shown or can be broken into two components: (a) advance crutches, (b) advance affected extremity.

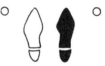

(1) Starting position. In this example, the left lower extremity is partial-weight-bearing.

Figure 14-18. Partial weight-bearing gait; modification of the three-point gait pattern.

ness. In this gait pattern one crutch is advanced and then the opposite lower extremity is advanced. For example, the left crutch is moved forward, then the right lower extremity, followed by the right crutch and then the left lower extremity (Fig. 14-19).

Two-point Gait. This gait pattern is similar to the four-point gait. However, it is less stable because only two points of floor contact are maintained. Thus, use of this gait requires better balance. The two-point pattern more closely simulates normal gait, inasmuch as the opposite lower and upper extremity move together (Fig. 14-20).

Two additional, less commonly used crutch gaits are the *swing-to* and *swing-through* patterns. These gaits are often used when there is bilateral lower extremity involvement, such as in spinal cord injuries. The swing-to gait involves forward movement of both crutches simultaneously, and the lower extremities "swing to" the crutches. In the swing-through gait, the crutches are moved forward together, but the lower extremities are swung beyond the crutches. Both these crutch patterns are discussed in greater detail in Chapter 27.

WALKERS

Walkers are used to improve balance and relieve weight-bearing either fully or partially on a lower extremity. Of the three categories of ambulatory assistive devices, walkers afford the greatest stability. They provide a wide BOS, improve anterior and lateral stability, and allow the upper extremities to transfer body weight to the floor.

Walkers are typically made of tubular aluminum with molded vinyl handgrips and rubber tips. They are adjustable in adult sizes from approximately 32 to 37 inches (81 to 92 cm), with children's, youth, and tall sizes available. Several modifications to the standard design are available and are described below.

1. A folding mechanism. Folding walkers are particularly useful for patients who travel. These walkers can be easily collapsed to fit in an automobile or other storage space.

(6) Cycle is repeated.

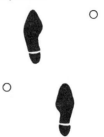

(5) The left lower extremity is advanced.

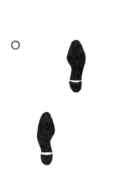

(4) The right crutch is advanced.

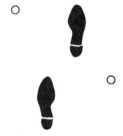

(3) The right lower extremity is advanced.

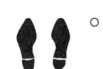

(2) The left crutch is advanced.

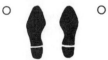

(1) Starting position. Weight is borne on both lower extremities and both crutches.

Figure 14-19. Four-point gait pattern.

2. Handgrips. Enlarged and molded handgrips are available, and may be useful for some patients with arthritis.
3. Platform attachments. This adaptation is used when weight-bearing is contraindicated through

(4) Cycle is repeated.

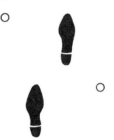

(3) The right crutch and left lower extremity are advanced together.

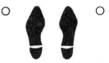

(2) The left crutch and right lower extremity are advanced together.

(1) Starting position. Weight is borne on both lower extremities and both crutches.

Figure 14-20. Two-point gait pattern.

the wrist and hand (described in crutch section).
4. Reciprocal walkers. These walkers are designed to allow unilateral forward progression of one side of the walker. A disadvantage of this design is that some inherent stability of the walker is lost. However, they are useful for patients incapable of lifting the walker with both hands and moving it forward.
5. Wheel attachments. This adaptation to walkers (sometimes called a *rolling* walker), should be used judiciously because the stability of the walker will be reduced. However, the addition of wheels (either to the two front wheels only or to all four wheels) may allow functional ambulation for patients who are unable to lift and to move a conventional walker (e.g., frail elderly). *Swivel wheels* turn freely in a complete circle. *Fixed wheels* rotate around a central axis and turn in a single direction (Fig. 14-21). Wheels are generally available in 3- and 5-inch diameters. Pressure brakes should be considered with wheels placed on two walker legs and should *always* be used with wheels placed on all four walker legs.
6. Stair-climbing walkers. Walkers designed for use on stairs are commercially available. Regardless of design, walkers tend to be extremely unsafe on stairs and should be avoided.

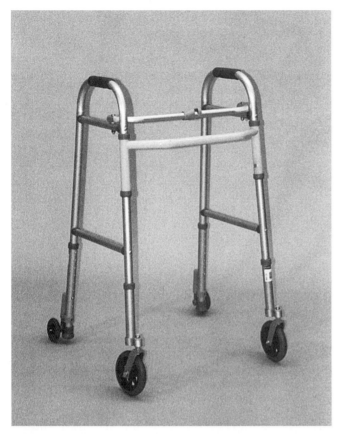

Figure 14-21. Walker with wheel attachments. The front legs have *swivel wheels*, which turn freely in a complete circle. The back legs have *fixed wheels*, which turn in a single direction. Note that the back legs are equipped with pressure brakes.

7. Baskets. Baskets can be attached to the anterior portion of the walker to provide storage for frequently needed personal items. This walker modification may be an important consider-ation for individuals ambulating outside the home. Vinyl or nylon storage bags and pouches secured to the walker by Velcro straps are also available (Fig. 14-22).

8. Seating surface. A variety of seat designs are available that attach to walkers. These seats generally fold to the side or front of the walker when not in use (Fig. 14-23). Seats may be an important consideration for individuals with limited endurance (i.e., post-polio syndrome). Walker seats should be carefully assessed for stability and safety with respect to individual patient needs.

9. Glides. Glides are small, plastic attachments placed on the bottom of walker legs. For patients unable to lift and to move a walker forward, they allow the walker to more easily "slide" across a smooth floor surface. Glides are made of high-density plastic and replace the rubber tips on the walker legs to provide a smoother floor surface contact. The two most common designs are (1) a 1-inch diameter "disk" with a central stem that slides into the tubular leg and is tightened into place with a screwdriver; and (2) a fitted cap that is placed directly onto the walker leg (in the same manner the rubber tip is attached).

Advantages. Walkers provide four points of floor contact with a wide BOS. They provide a high level of stability. They also provide a sense of security for patients fearful of ambulation. They are relatively lightweight and easily adjusted.

Disadvantages. Walkers tend to be cumbersome, are awkward in confined areas, and are difficult to maneuver through doorways and into cars. They eliminate normal arm swing and cannot be used safely on stairs.

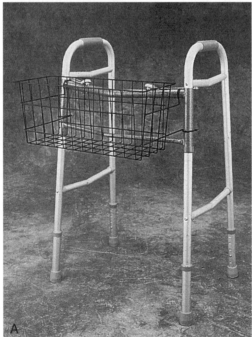
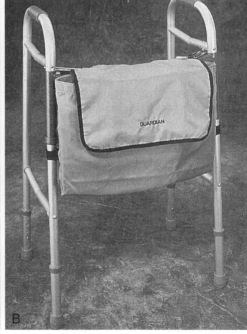

Figure 14-22. Walker basket (*left*) and walker pouch (*right*). (Courtesy of Sunrise Medical, Longmont, CO.)

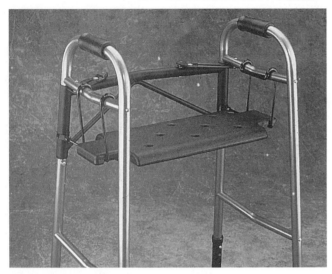

Figure 14-23. Walker seat. The seat folds to the side when not in use. (Courtesy of Sunrise Medical, Longmont, CO.)

Measuring Walkers

The height of a walker is measured in the same way as that of a cane. The walker should come to approximately the greater trochanter and allow for 20 to 30 degrees of elbow flexion.

Gait Patterns for Use of Walkers

Prior to initiating instruction in gait patterns, several points related to use of the walker should be emphasized with the patient:

1. The walker should be picked up and placed down on all four legs simultaneously to achieve maximum stability. Rocking from the back to front legs should be avoided because it decreases the effectiveness and safety of the assistive device.
2. The patient should be encouraged to hold the head up and to maintain good postural alignment.
3. The patient should be cautioned not to step too close to the front crossbar. This will decrease the overall BOS and may result in a fall.

There are three types of gait patterns used with walkers. These are the full, partial, and non-weight-bearing gaits. The sequence for each pattern follows.

Full Weight-Bearing Gait
1. The walker is picked up and moved forward about an arm's length.
2. The first lower extremity is moved forward.
3. The second lower extremity is moved forward past the first.
4. The cycle is repeated.

Partial Weight-Bearing Gait
1. The walker is picked up and moved forward about an arm's length.
2. The involved lower extremity is moved forward, and body weight is transferred partially onto this limb and partially through the upper extremities to the walker.

3. The uninvolved lower extremity is moved forward past the involved limb.
4. The cycle is repeated.

Non-Weight-Bearing Gait
1. The walker is picked up and moved forward about an arm's length.
2. Weight is then transferred through the upper extremities to the walker. The involved limb is held anterior to the patient's body but does not make contact with the floor.
3. The uninvolved limb is moved forward.
4. The cycle is repeated.

Use of Assistive Devices on Level Surfaces and Stairs

LEVEL SURFACES

Gait training activities on indoor surfaces are begun once the patient has achieved appropriate skill and balance in parallel bar activities (including moving to and from standing and sitting positions, turning, and use of the selected gait pattern). Use of the parallel bars often continues concurrently with initial gait training on indoor surfaces. At this point in the progression, continued use of the parallel bars typically emphasizes advanced activities and/or work on specific deviations.

Several important preparatory activities should precede ambulation on level surfaces with the assistive device. These activities may be completed in the parallel bars for added security. However, if the width of the bars is not adjustable, the BOS of the assistive device may make movement within the bars difficult and unsafe. An alternative is to move the patient outside but next to the parallel bars (or oval bar) or near a treatment table or wall. These preparatory activities include:

1. Instruction in assuming the standing and seated positions with use of the assistive device. These techniques are outlined in Box 14–3 for each category of assistive device.
2. Standing balance activities with the assistive device (similar to those using the parallel bars, described earlier).
3. Instruction in use of assistive device (with selected gait pattern) for forward progression and turning.

As mentioned, demonstrating these activities by assuming the role of the patient during verbal explanations is an effective teaching approach. Following the demonstration, verbal cuing and explanations can be used again to guide performance of the activity. **Mental practice** (mental rehearsal of a task) is another important strategy to assist in the learning and performance of motor tasks.[9–15] The literature suggests that mental practice facilitates acquisition of a motor skill as well as improves retention. The physiological basis for mental practice remains in question. However, it has been suggested that mental rehearsal may be functionally similar to motor preparation.[9] Kohl and Roenker[10] suggest that imagined movements and actual performance are closely re-

---

**Box 14–3 BASIC TECHNIQUES FOR ASSUMING STANDING AND SEATED
POSITIONS WITH ASSISTIVE DEVICES**

I. CANE
  A. *Coming to standing*
    1. Patient moves forward in chair.
    2. Cane is positioned on uninvolved side (broad-based cane) or leaned against armrest (standard cane).
    3. Patient leans forward and pushes down with both hands on armrests, comes to a standing position, and then grasps cane. With use of a standard cane, the cane may be grasped loosely with fingers prior to standing and the base of the hand used for pushing down on armrests.
  B. *Return to sitting*
    1. As the patient approaches the chair, the patient turns in a small circle toward the uninvolved side.
    2. The patient backs up until the chair can be felt against the patient's legs.
    3. The patient then reaches for the armrest with the free hand, releases the cane (broad-based), and reaches for the opposite armrest. A standard cane is leaned against the chair as the patient grasps the armrest.
II. CRUTCHES
  A. *Coming to standing*
    1. The patient moves forward in the chair.
    2. Crutches are placed together in a vertical position on the *affected* side.
    3. One hand is placed on the handpieces of the crutches; one on the armrest of the chair.
    4. The patient leans forward and pushes to a standing position.
    5. Once balance is gained, one crutch is cautiously placed under the axilla on the unaffected side.
    6. The second crutch is then carefully placed under the axilla on the affected side.
    7. A tripod stance is assumed.
  B. *Return to sitting*
    1. As the patient approaches the chair, the patient turns in a small circle toward the uninvolved side.
    2. The patient backs up until the chair can be felt against the patient's legs.
    3. Both crutches are placed in a vertical position (out from under axilla) on the *affected* side.
    4. One hand is placed on the handpieces of the crutches; one on the armrest of the chair.
    5. The patient lowers to the chair in a controlled manner.
      [*Note:* See Chapter 27 for alternative methods using bilateral knee ankle orthoses.]
III. WALKER
  A. *Coming to standing*
    1. The patient moves forward in the chair.
    2. The walker is positioned directly in front of the chair.
    3. The patient leans forward and pushes down on armrests to come to standing.
    4. Once in a standing position, the patient reaches for the walker, one hand at a time.
  B. *Return to sitting*
    1. As the patient approaches the chair, the patient turns in a small circle toward the stronger side.
    2. The patient backs up until the chair can be felt against the patient's legs.
    3. The patient then reaches for one armrest at a time.
    4. The patient lowers to the chair in a controlled manner.

---

lated and may partially share a common physiological substrate. Mental practice is generally considered most effective when combined with physical practice.

Following these preliminary instructions, gait training using the assistive device can be begun on level surfaces. The following guarding technique (Fig. 14-24) should be used.

1. The therapist stands posterior and lateral to the patient's weaker side.
2. A wide BOS should be maintained with the therapist's leading lower extremity following the assistive device. The therapist's opposite lower extremity should be externally rotated and follow the patient's weaker lower extremity.
3. One of the therapist's hands is placed posteriorly on the guarding belt and the other anterior to, but *not touching*, the patient's shoulder on the weaker side.

Should the patient's balance be lost during gait training, the hand guarding at the shoulder should make contact. Frequently, the support provided by the therapist's hands at the shoulder and on the guarding belt will be enough to allow the patient to regain balance. If the balance loss is severe, the therapist should move in toward the patient so that the body and guarding hands can be used to provide stabilization. The patient should be allowed to regain balance while "leaning" against the therapist. If balance is not recovered and it is apparent the patient is going to fall, further attempts should not be made to hold the patient up because this is likely to result in injury to the patient and/or the therapist. In this situation, the therapist should continue to brace the patient against the body to break the fall and to protect the head and move with the patient to a sitting position on the floor. It is also important to talk to the patient ("Help me lower you to the floor") so that the patient does not continue to struggle to regain balance.

Gait training activities on level surfaces should include instruction and practice in passage through doorways, elevators, and over thresholds. When

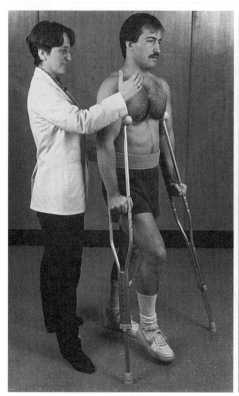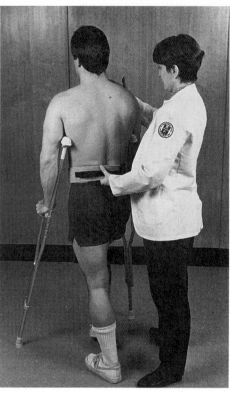

Figure 14-24. Anterior (*left*) and posterior (*right*) views of guarding technique for level surfaces, demonstrated with use of crutches. The same positioning is used with canes and walkers.

using crutches, doorways are most easily approached from a diagonal. A hand must be freed to open the door and one crutch must be placed in a position to hold it open. The patient then gradually proceeds through the doorway, using the crutch to open the door wider if necessary.

Because many patients using a walker or cane may have balance problems, careful assessment will determine the safest methods for passage through doorways. A patient using a walker with sufficient balance may be able to use a technique similar to that described above.

STAIR CLIMBING

The next activity in the gait training progression is stair climbing (as mentioned earlier, *step-ups* inside the parallel bars may be a beneficial lead-up activity to stair climbing for some patients). Ideally, firsthand information from a home visit will provide information about the type and number of stairs the patient will be required to use. However, careful questioning of the patient and/or family members generally will provide sufficient information on which to plan. The information obtained should include the height and number of stairs, presence and stability of railings, and condition and type of floor covering or pavement leading to and on the stairs.

Several general guidelines should be relayed to the patient during instruction in stair climbing. First, if a railing is available it should always be used. This is true even if it requires placing an assistive device in the hand in which it is not normally used. For stair climbing with axillary

crutches using a railing, both crutches are placed together under one arm. Second, the patient should be cautioned that the stronger lower extremity always leads going up the stairs, and the weaker or involved limb always leads coming down ("up with the good and down with the bad").

The progressions of stair-climbing techniques are presented in Box 14–4. The following guarding technique should be used by the therapist during stair climbing.

Ascending Stairs (Fig. 14-25)
1. The therapist is positioned posterior and lateral on the affected side behind the patient.
2. A wide **BOS** should be maintained with each foot on a different stair.
3. A step should be taken only when the patient is not moving.
4. One hand is placed posteriorly on the guarding belt and one is anterior to, but not touching, the shoulder on the weaker side.

Descending Stairs (Fig. 14-26)
1. The therapist is positioned anterior and lateral on the affected side in front of the patient.
2. A wide **BOS** should be maintained with each foot on a different stair.
3. A step should be taken only when the patient is not moving.
4. One hand is placed anteriorly on the guarding belt and one is anterior to, but not touching, the shoulder on the weaker side.

Should the patient's balance be lost during stair climbing, the following procedure should be fol-

---

Box 14–4 STAIR-CLIMBING TECHNIQUES[a]

I. CANE
   A. *Ascending*
      1. The unaffected lower extremity leads up.
      2. The cane and affected lower extremity follow.
   B. *Descending*
      1. The affected lower extremity and cane lead down.
      2. The unaffected lower extremity follows.
II. CRUTCHES: THREE-POINT GAIT (non-weight-bearing gait)
   A. *Ascending*
      1. The patient is positioned close to the foot of the stairs. The involved lower extremity is held back to prevent "catching" on the lip of the stairs.
      2. The patient pushes down firmly on both handpieces of the crutches and leads up with the unaffected lower extremity.
      3. The crutches are brought up to the stair that the unaffected lower extremity is now on.
   B. *Descending*
      1. The patient stands close to the edge of the stair so that the toes protrude slightly over the top. The involved lower extremity is held forward over the lower stair.
      2. Both crutches are moved down *together* to the *front* half of the next step.
      3. The patient pushes down firmly on both handpieces and lowers the unaffected lower extremity to the step that the crutches are now on.
III. CRUTCHES: PARTIAL WEIGHT-BEARING GAIT
   A. *Ascending*
      1. The patient is positioned close to the foot of the stairs.
      2. The patient pushes down on both handpieces of the crutches and distributes weight partially on the crutches and partially on the affected lower extremity while the unaffected lower extremity leads up.
      3. The involved lower extremity and crutches are then brought up together.
   B. *Descending*
      1. The patient stands close to the edge of the stair so that the toes protrude slightly over top of the stair.
      2. Both crutches are moved down *together* to the *front* half of the next step. The affected lower extremity is then lowered (depending on patient skill, these may be combined). *Note:* When crutches are not in floor contact, greater weight must be shifted to the uninvolved lower extremity to maintain a partial weight-bearing status.
      3. The uninvolved lower extremity is lowered to the step the crutches are now on.
IV. CRUTCHES: TWO- AND FOUR-POINT GAIT
   A. *Ascending*
      1. The patient is positioned close to the foot of the stairs.
      2. The right lower extremity is moved up and then the left lower extremity.
      3. The right crutch is moved up and then the left crutch is moved up (patients with adequate balance may find it easier to move the crutches up together).
   B. *Descending*
      1. The patient stands close to the edge of the stair.
      2. The right crutch is moved down and then the left (may be combined).
      3. The right lower extremity is moved down and then the left.

[a]The sequences presented here describe stair-climbing techniques without the use of a railing. When a secure railing is available, the patient should be instructed to use it always.

---

lowed. First, contact should be made with the hand guarding at the shoulder. Next, the therapist should move toward the patient to help brace the patient (the patient should never be pulled toward the therapist on stairs) or leaned toward the wall of the stairwell (if available). Finally, if needed, the therapist can move with the patient to sit the patient down on the stairs. Remember to inform the patient of your intentions ("I'm going to sit you down").

CURBS AND RAMPS

The technique for climbing curbs is essentially the same as that of climbing a single stair (see Box 14–4). A useful lead-up activity to curb climbing is provided by a series of small, freestanding, wooden platforms (approximately 3 × 3 ft) with nonslip coverings. These can be fabricated easily in increments of height. For additional security they can be placed next to or within the parallel bars, and a progression can be made from a 3- or 4-inch (7.62-cm or 10.16-cm) increment to a 7-inch (17.78-cm) curb height.

Ramps can be negotiated in several ways. If the incline is very gradual, it may be sufficient simply to instruct the patient to use smaller steps. However, for steeper inclines the patient should be instructed to use smaller steps and to traverse the ramp (use a diagonal, zigzag pattern) for both ascending and descending.

OUTDOOR SURFACES

Activities on outdoor surfaces are among the final components of a gait training progression. They must be specifically assessed to determine their appropriateness for an individual patient. Basic outdoor activities include:

1. Exit and entrance through outside doors and thresholds.
2. Gait training on outdoor, uneven surfaces (e.g., sidewalks, grassy surfaces, parking lots, etc.).

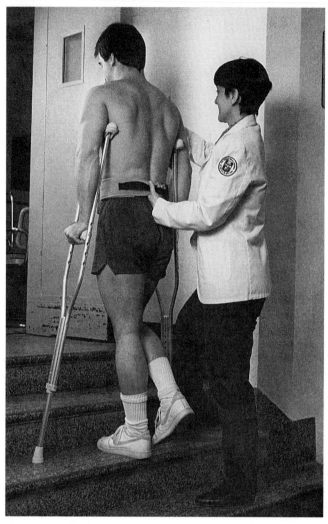

Figure 14-25. Guarding technique for ascending stairs.

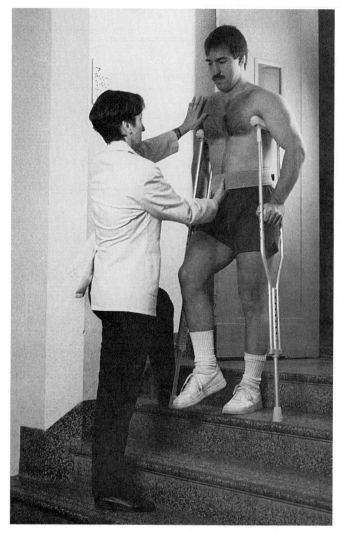

Figure 14-26. Guarding technique for descending stairs.

3. Curbs, ramps, and stair climbing.
4. Crossing the street in the time allotted by a traffic light.
5. Entering and exiting public or private transportation.

ADJUNCT TRAINING DEVICES

Limb Load Monitors

A limb load monitor is a form of biofeedback used clinically as an adjunct intervention during gait training. The limb load monitor incorporates a strain gauge attached to the sole or heel of the shoe. When a force or pressure is applied, the strain gauge is deformed and an auditory signal provides feedback to the wearer. As pressure increases, the signal becomes louder or more rapid. This feedback provides information about the amount of weight-bearing on a limb. Limb load monitors can also be used to reinforce the correctness or timing of a movement. For example, an audible noise or buzzer

sounding when the heel makes contact with the floor can provide immediate feedback on foot placement. Similar devices can also be attached to a cane (often referred to as a *biofeedback cane*). The principle of operation is the same and incorporates a strain gauge. Auditory signals provide the patient with information on placement as well as pressure applied to the cane. Biofeedback is discussed in detail in Chapter 33.

ORTHOTICS

A wide variety of orthotic devices are incorporated within gait training programs to improve efficiency and safety, diminish or eliminate gait deviations, and decrease energy expenditure. These devices span a wide spectrum of functions from a relatively simple Swedish knee cage designed to control recurvatum to the more specialized reciprocating gait orthosis. This later device provides important advantages during early gait training for patients with bilateral lower extremity involvement. As the patient shifts weight onto one leg, the opposite leg is advanced forward via cable attachments. During this early training, the parallel bars or a walker is typically used. The reader is referred to Chapter 31 for a thorough discussion of orthotic applications.

SUMMARY

This chapter presented a general framework of preambulation exercises and gait training activities. Each component should be considered during treatment planning. Through a process of careful assessment, the appropriate elements of the mat progression, specific treatment techniques, and segments of the upright progression can be selected for an individual patient. Additional factors that will influence treatment planning include the patient's diagnosis, prognosis, weight-bearing status, and input from the patient regarding ambulatory goals.

QUESTIONS FOR REVIEW

1. What factors influence the extent and type of gait training activities required to achieve desired outcomes for an individual patient?

2. What are the major elements of physical therapy intervention for patients with gait impairments?

3. What are the goals of a preambulation exercise program?

4. Outline a general parallel bar progression that would be appropriate for a patient preparing to use a partial weight-bearing crutch gait.

5. Contrast and compare the advantages and disadvantages of each category of ambulatory assistive device: canes, crutches, and walkers.

6. Explain the guidelines used for measuring a cane, crutches, and a walker.

7. Describe the sequence for instructing a patient to rise from and return to a sitting position with a cane, crutches, and a walker.

8. Describe therapist positioning and hand placement for guarding the patient on level surfaces and stairs.

9. Describe the sequence for the following crutch gaits: four-point, two-point, three-point, and partial weight-bearing.

CASE STUDY

The patient is a 26 year-old male who was involved in a motorcycle accident 3 days ago. He sustained closed transverse fractures of the left tibia and fibula secondary to angulatory forces acting on the limb during the accident. Disruption of the periosteum and surrounding soft tissue was evident. The mid-shaft fractures were reduced and a long leg cast applied with the knee flexed to 30 degrees (to help control rotation at the fracture site). The cast is to remain in place for 4 weeks with progression to a below-knee patellar tendon weight-bearing cast.

A Colles fracture of the right wrist was also sustained as the patient attempted to break his fall landing on an open hand with the forearm pronated. The main transverse fracture line is at the flared-out distal metaphysis of the radius with avulsion of the ulnar styloid. The fracture was reduced and a cast applied to the wrist and forearm. The thumb and fingers were left free. A series of repeat radiographs are planned at 2 week intervals to ensure satisfactory alignment is maintained. The plan is to progress to functional fracture bracing of the right wrist within 4 weeks.

Past Medical History: Unremarkable.

Social History: The patient lives with his mother, stepfather, and two younger siblings. He has a bachelor's degree in engineering, is employed by a large automotive manufacturer, and is working part-time toward a master's degree. He plans to be married in 6 months. The patient is an avid sportsman with particular interests in sailing, archery, and skiing.

Review of Systems:			
Vision:	Intact	*Respiration:*	14/minute
Hearing:	Intact	*Coordination:*	Intact
Blood *Pressure:*	124/80	*Sensation:*	Intact
Pulse:	60/minute	*Cognition:*	Intact

Weight-bearing Status: Non-weight-bearing left lower extremity; no weight is to be borne on the right wrist.

Range of Motion Assessment: The left lower extremity and right wrist and fingers not tested owing to fractures. Range of motion for all other joints is within normal limits (WNL).

Manual Muscle Testing: The left lower extremity and right wrist and fingers not tested owing to fractures. All other strength values are within normal limits (WNL).

Plan: The patient is to remain hospitalized for another 48 to 72 hours for observation and physical therapy intervention. He will then be followed as an out-patient through the orthopedic clinic. The patient has been referred for gait training activities. Assume you have selected axillary crutches as the assistive device for this patient.

Guiding Questions

1. What advantages would selection of the axillary crutches have for this patient?

2. Would you recommend any special attachments to the axillary crutches? If yes, give the rationale for your selection.

3. What type of gait pattern would you select for this patient? Provide a rationale for your selection.

4. As you plan the parallel bar progression for this patient, you decide to provide a verbal description of the gait pattern while you concurrently demonstrate proper use of the crutches. Identify how you would *verbally describe* the sequencing of crutches and foot placement for the gait pattern selected.

5. Prior to initiating instruction in use of the axillary crutches, what general guidelines for their use would you emphasize with the patient?

6. Are there any special considerations or modifications you would need to make to the parallel bar progression for this patient? Describe an appropriate sequence and progression of parallel bar activities.

7. Describe the appropriate therapist positioning and hand placements for guarding the patient during gait training on level surfaces.

8. Describe the sequence of crutch and foot placement for ascending and descending stairs using both crutches (for this response, assume a railing is unavailable).

9. Describe the appropriate therapist positioning and hand placements for guarding the patient while ascending and descending stairs.

10. What basic outdoor activities would you include during gait training for this patient?

REFERENCES

1. American Physical Therapy Association: Guide to physical therapist practice. APTA, Alexandria, VA 1999.
2. Voss, DE, et al: Proprioceptive Neuromuscular Facilitation: Patterns and Techniques, ed 3. Harper & Row, Philadelphia, 1985.
3. Sullivan, PE, and Markos, PD: Clinical Decision Making in Therapeutic Exercise. Appleton & Lange, Norwalk, CN, 1995.
4. O'Sullivan, SB, and Schmitz, TJ: Physical Rehabilitation Laboratory Manual: Focus on Functional Training. FA Davis, Philadelphia, 1999.
5. Milczarek, JJ, et al: Standard and four-point canes: Their effect on the standing balance of patients with hemiparesis. Arch Phys Med Rehabil 74:281, 1993.
6. Neumann, DA: Hip abductor muscle activity as subjects with hip prostheses walk with different methods of using a cane. Phys Ther 78:490, 1998.
7. Norkin, CC, and Levangie, PK: Joint Structure and Function: A Comprehensive Analysis, ed 2. FA Davis, Philadelphia, 1992.
8. Ely, DD, and Smidt, GL: Effect of cane on variables of gait for patients with hip disorders. Phys Ther 57:507, 1977.
9. Stephan, KM, et al: Functional anatomy of the mental representation of upper extremity movements in healthy subjects. J Neurophysiol 73:373, 1995.
10. Kohl, RM, and Roenker, DL: Behavioral evidence for shared mechanisms between actual and imaged motor responses. J Hum Mov Stud 17:173, 1989.
11. Decety, J, et al: Central activation of autonomic effectors during mental simulation of motor actions in man. J Physiol 461:549, 1993.
12. Yaguez, L, et al: A mental route to motor learning: Improving trajectorial kinematics through imagery training. Behav Brain Res 90:95, 1998.
13. Maring, J: Effects of mental practice on rate of skill acquisition. Phys Ther 70:165, 1990.
14. Decety, J, et al: The cerebellum participates in mental activity: Tomographic measurements of regional cerebral blood flow. Brain Res 535:313, 1990.
15. Wulf, G, et al: Does mental practice work like physical practice without information feedback? Res Q Exerc Sport 66:262, 1995.

SUPPLEMENTAL READINGS

Basmajian, JV: Crutch and care exercise and use. In Basmajian, JV, and Wolf, SL (eds): Therapeutic Exercise, ed 5. Williams & Wilkins, Baltimore, 1990, p 125.

Chung, CY, et al: Comparisons of cane handle designs for use by elders with arthritic hands. Technology and Disability 7:183, 1997.

Dean, E, and Ross, J: Relationships among cane fitting, function, and falls. Phys Ther 73:494, 1993.

Foley, MD, et al: Effects of assistive devices on cardiorespiratory demands in older adults. Phys Ther 76:1313, 1996.

Gussoni, M, et al: Energy cost of walking with hip impairment. Phys Ther 70:295, 1990.

Minor, MAD, and Minor, SD: Patient Care Skills, ed 3. Appleton & Lange, Norwalk, CN, 1995.

Finch, L, et al: Influence of body weight support on normal human gait: Development of a gait retraining strategy. Phys Ther 71, 1991.

Forbes, WF, et al: Factors associated with self-reported use and non-use of assistive devices among impaired elderly residing in the community. Canadian Journal of Public Health 84:53, 1993.

Jeka, JJ: Light touch contact as a balance aid. Phys Ther 77:476, 1997.

Kisner, C, and Colby, LA: Therapeutic Exercise Foundations and Techniques, ed 3. FA Davis, Philadelphia, 1996.

Kumar, R, et al: Methods for estimating the proper length of a cane. Arch Phys Med Rehabil 76:1173, 1995.

Mann, WC, et al: An analysis of problems with walkers encountered by elderly persons. Physical & Occupational Therapy in Geriatrics 13:1, 1995.

Palmer, ML and Toms, JE: Manual for Functional Training, ed 3. FA Davis, Philadelphia, 1992.

Soderberg, GL: Gait and gait retraining. In Basmajian, JV, and Wolf, SL (eds): Therapeutic Exercise, ed 5. Williams & Wilkins, Baltimore, 1990, p 139.

Sullivan, PE, and Markos, PD: Clinical Procedures in Therapeutic Exercise, ed 2. Appleton & Lange, Norwalk, CN, 1996.

Vargo, MM, et al: Contralateral vs ipsilateral cane use: Effects on muscle crossing the knee joint. Am J Phys Med Rehabil 71:170, 1992.

Winter, DA, et al: Biomechanical walking pattern changes in the fit and healthy elderly. Phys Ther 70:340, 1990.

Winter, DA, et al: A technique to analyze the kinetics and energetics of cane-assisted gait. Clin Biomech 8:37, 1993.
Woollacott, MH, and Tang, PF: Balance control during walking in the older adult: Research and its implications. Phys Ther 77(6), 1997.

GLOSSARY

Counterrotation (in rolling): Simultaneous movement of the upper and lower segments of the trunk in opposite directions.

Developmental sequence: An established pattern of developmental activities by which a child acquires the control needed for functional movement.

Elevation activities: A general term used in gait training to describe an ambulatory activity requiring movement from one level surface to another (e.g., negotiating curbs, climbing stairs or ramps).

Four-point gait: One crutch is moved forward, the opposite lower extremity is advanced, the other crutch is moved forward and opposite lower extremity advanced; slow, stable gait pattern.

Log rolling: Rolling in which movement of the entire trunk rotates as a unit around the longitudinal axis of the body.

Long sitting: Sitting with knees extended on a supporting surface.

Lordosis (lordotic): Abnormally increased anterior curvature of the lumbar spine.

Mental practice: Cognitive rehearsal of a physical task; an adjunctive method for learning a motor skill.

Orthostatic (postural) hypotension: A lower than normal drop in blood pressure as a result of movement to a standing position; may be severe after prolonged bed rest or confinement to a sitting position.

Partial weight-bearing (PWB) gait: A modification of the three-point gait pattern; during stance phase on the affected extremity, weight is borne partially on the affected extremity and partially on the crutches; the crutches and affected lower extremity are advanced together, the uninvolved lower extremity steps past the crutches; a partial weight-bearing gait may also be achieved with a walker.

Quadruped: All-fours position; weight-bearing on hands and knees.

Segmental rolling: Rolling in which the upper or lower segment of the trunk moves independently while the opposite segment is stable.

Short sitting: Sitting with knees flexed over a supporting surface such as a mat or bed.

Swing-through gait: Both crutches are moved forward together, both lower extremities then swing beyond the crutches; typically used with severe involvement or paralysis of both lower extremities.

Swing-to gait: Both crutches are moved forward together, both lower extremities then swing to the crutches; typically used with severe involvement or paralysis of both lower extremities.

Three-point gait: A non-weight-bearing (NWB) gait; weight is borne on the crutches instead of on the affected lower extremity; both crutches are advanced and the unaffected lower extremity steps past the crutches.

Two-point gait: One lower extremity and the opposite crutch are advanced together; this is repeated with the other crutch and lower extremity.

APPENDIX

Suggested Answers to Case Study Guiding Questions

1. What advantages would selection of the axillary crutches have for this patient?

ANSWER

Axillary crutches improve balance and lateral stability and provide for functional ambulation with restricted weight-bearing. They are easily adjusted and can be used for stair climbing.

2. Would you recommend any special attachments to the axillary crutches? If yes, identify the rationale for your selection.

ANSWER

Platform attachment (forearm rest or trough) placed on right axillary crutch. *Rationale:* The platform attachment will allow transfer of body weight through the forearm to the assistive device and will eliminate weight-bearing directly through the right wrist.

3. What type of gait pattern would you select for this patient? Provide a rationale for your selection.

ANSWER

Three-point gait pattern.

Rationale: In this type of gait three points of support contact the floor. The three-point gait pattern will allow maintenance of the non-weight-bearing status required for the left lower extremity. Body weight will be borne on the crutches instead of the affected left lower extremity.

4. As you plan the parallel bar progression for this patient, you decide to provide a verbal description of the gait pattern while you concurrently demonstrate proper use of the crutches. Identify how you would *verbally describe* the sequencing of crutches and foot placement for the gait pattern selected.

ANSWER

- Starting position is a tripod stance with the left lower extremity non-weight bearing.
- Weight is shifted onto the uninvolved right lower extremity, and the crutches are advanced.
- Weight is then shifted through the upper extremities onto the crutches, and the uninvolved right limb advances beyond the crutches.
- Both crutches are advanced.
- The cycle is repeated.

5. Prior to initiating instruction in use of the axillary crutches, what general guidelines for their use would you emphasize with the patient?

ANSWER

- Body weight should always be borne on the left handpiece and right platform attachment and not on the axillary bar. This will prevent pressure on both the vascular and nervous structures located in the axillary region.
- To optimize balance, a wide (tripod) BOS should always be maintained. When in a resting stance, the crutches should be kept at least 4 inches (10 cm) to the front and to the side of each foot. The foot should not be allowed to achieve parallel alignment with the crutches. This will jeopardize anterior-posterior stability by decreasing the BOS.
- The axillary bars should be held close to the chest wall to provide lateral stability.
- The head should be held upright and good postural alignment maintained during ambulation.
- Turning should be accomplished by stepping in a small circle (toward the right unaffected lower extremity) rather than pivoting.

6. Are there any special considerations or modifications you would need to make to the parallel bar progression for this patient? Describe an appropriate sequence and progression of parallel bar activities.

ANSWER

Special considerations or modifications:

Owing to the right Colles fracture, limitations will be experienced in grasping the parallel bar. In this situation, a logical approach would be to incorporate use of the right crutch (with platform attachment) into the parallel bar progression (the patient would grasp the parallel bar with the left hand in the usual fashion and the right upper extremity would be supported by the platform attachment to the right axillary crutch).

Sequence and progression of parallel bar activities:

- Initial instruction and demonstration in how to assume a standing position, guarding techniques to be used by the therapist, the components of initial standing balance activities, the gait pattern to be used, how to turn in the parallel bars, and how to return to a sitting position.
- Practice in assuming the standing position (initially, assistance may be required).
- Standing balance activities, exploration of limits of stability (LOS) including lateral weight shift, anterior-posterior weight shift, anterior-posterior hand (and right crutch) placement and weight shift, single-hand support (alternating between support provided by parallel bar on left and the axillary crutch on the right).
- Stepping forward and backward with right lower extremity.
- Forward progression using the selected gait pattern maintaining a non-weight-bearing status on the left lower extremity.
- Turning toward the stronger right side.

7. Describe the appropriate therapist positioning and hand placements for guarding the patient during gait training on level surfaces.

ANSWER
- The therapist stands posterior and lateral to the patient's left (non-weight-bearing) side.
- A wide BOS is maintained with the therapist's leading lower extremity following the left crutch. The therapist's opposite lower extremity should be externally rotated and follow the patient's left (non-weight-bearing) lower extremity.
- One of the therapist's hands is placed posteriorly on the guarding belt and the other anterior to, but *not touching*, the patient's shoulder on the weaker side.

8. Describe the sequence of crutch and foot placement for ascending and descending stairs using both crutches (for this response, assume a railing is unavailable).

ANSWER
Ascending:
- The patient is positioned close to the foot of the stairs (the left non-weight-bearing lower extremity is held back slightly to prevent "catching" on the lip of the stairs).
- The patient pushes down on the right platform attachment and the left crutch handpiece and leads up with the right (unaffected) lower extremity.
- The crutches are brought up to the stair that the right (unaffected) lower extremity is now on.

Descending:
- The patient stands close to the edge of the stair with the left (non-weight-bearing) lower extremity held forward over the next lower stair.
- Both crutches are moved down together to the front half of the next lower step.
- The patient pushes down on the right platform attachment and the left crutch handpiece and lowers the right (unaffected) lower extremity to the step that the crutches are now on.

9. Describe the appropriate therapist positioning and hand placements for guarding the patient while ascending and descending stairs.

ANSWER
Ascending:
- The therapist is positioned posterior and lateral on the left (non-weight-bearing) side behind the patient.
- A wide BOS is maintained by the therapist with each foot on a different stair.
- The therapist takes a step only when the patient is not moving.
- One of the therapist's hands is placed posteriorly on the guarding belt and one is anterior to, but *not touching*, the shoulder on the left (non-weight-bearing) side.

Descending:
- The therapist is positioned anterior and lateral on the left (non-weight-bearing) side in front of the patient.
- A wide BOS is maintained by the therapist with each foot on a different stair.
- The therapist takes a step only when the patient is not moving.
- One of the therapist's hands is placed anteriorly on the guarding belt and one is anterior to, but *not touching*, the shoulder on the left (non-weight-bearing) side.

10. What basic outdoor activities would you include during gait training for this patient?

ANSWER
- Exit and entrance through outside doors and thresholds.
- Gait training on outdoor, uneven surfaces (e.g., sidewalks, grassy surfaces, parking lots, and so forth).
- Curbs, ramps, and stair climbing.
- Crossing the street in the time allotted by a traffic light.

Chronic Pulmonary Dysfunction

Julie Ann Starr

LEARNING OBJECTIVES

1. Define the disease processes (including definition, etiology, pathophysiology, clinical presentation, and clinical course) of chronic obstructive pulmonary disease, asthma, cystic fibrosis, and restrictive lung disease.
2. Describe assessment procedures (including patient interview, vital signs, observation, inspection, palpation, auscultation, and laboratory tests) for a patient with pulmonary disease.
3. Identify the potential goals and outcomes of pulmonary rehabilitation.
4. Describe the rehabilitative management of a patient with chronic pulmonary dysfunction.
5. Value the therapist's role in the management of a patient with chronic pulmonary dysfunction.
6. Analyze and interpret patient data, formulate realistic goals and outcomes, and develop a plan of care when presented with a clinical case study.

Pulmonary rehabilitation is a multidimensional continuum of services directed toward persons with pulmonary disease and their families, usually by an interdisciplinary team of specialists, with the goal of achieving and maintaining the individual's maximum level of independence and functioning in the community.[1]

Years ago, patients with chronic pulmonary disease were given a standard prescription for rest and avoidance of exercise.[2] Well into the 1960s, the stress imposed by exercise was considered deleterious to people with pulmonary disorders.[3] They were treated as invalids, sometimes being referred to as "respiratory cripples."[4] A 1964 study by Pierce et al.[3] provided the impetus to change direction in the treatment of pulmonary dysfunction. The authors documented exercise training effects in their subjects with chronic obstructive pulmonary disease (COPD). These training effects included decreases in exercising heart rate, respiratory rate, minute ventilation, oxygen consumption, and carbon dioxide production at a given workload.[3] Increased exercise tolerance has also been documented.[3,5–11] Reconditioning of patients with pulmonary disease was found to be possible. Rehabilitation for patients with chronic lung disease is now a well-established and widely accepted means of optimizing function.[12–14]

COPD and asthma are the most common chronic lung diseases for which pulmonary rehabilitation is rendered. Patients with restrictive lung disease have also demonstrated improvement in functional abilities following pulmonary rehabilitation.[15] Advances in medical management of cystic fibrosis have resulted in a longer survival rate, albeit with an increased pulmonary dysfunction. Some of these patients are candidates for pulmonary rehabilitation.[16] Pulmonary rehabilitation is currently part of preparation for, and recovery from, surgical interventions such as lung transplantation and lung volume reduction surgery.[17]

In this chapter, chronic pulmonary diseases (COPD, asthma, cystic fibrosis, and restrictive lung disease) will be discussed, as well as the physical therapy assessment and treatment of patients with chronic pulmonary disease. A brief review of ventilation and respiration are warranted for a better understanding of the disease pathologies, and for understanding the rationale of the physical therapy assessment procedures. The supplemental readings list at the end of this chapter contains references for a more in-depth and thorough review of respiratory physiology.

RESPIRATORY PHYSIOLOGY

Ventilation

Air is inspired through the nose or mouth, through all of the conducting airways until it reaches the distal respiratory unit, which contains the respiratory bronchiole, alveolar ducts, alveolar sacs, and the alveoli (Fig. 15-1).

LUNG VOLUMES AND CAPACITIES

At full inspiration, the lungs contain their maximum amount of gas. This volume of air is called **total lung capacity (TLC),** which can be divided into four separate volumes of air: (1) tidal volume, (2) inspiratory reserve volume, (3) expiratory reserve

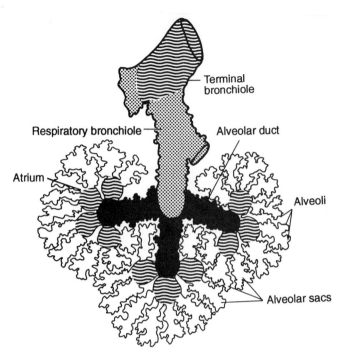

Figure 15-1. The anatomy of the distal conducting airway, the terminal bronchiole and the respiratory unit, the respiratory bronchiole, alveolar ducts aveolar sacs, and alveoli. (From Brannon, FJ, et al. Cardiopulmonary Rehabilitation: Basic Theory and Application, ed 2. FA Davis, Philadelphia, 1993, p 43, with permission.)

volume, and (4) residual volume. Combinations of two or more of these lung volumes are termed capacities. Figure 15-2 illustrates the relationship of lung volumes and capacities.

Tidal Volume

The amount of air inspired and expired during normal resting ventilation is termed **tidal volume (TV).** As this tidal volume of air enters the respiratory system, it travels through the conducting airways to reach the respiratory units. Tidal volume is about 500 mL/breath for a young, healthy, white male. The amount of inspired air that actually reaches the distal respiratory unit and takes part in gas exchange is about 350 mL of the 500 mL total. The remaining 150 mL of the inhaled tidal breath remains in the conducting airways and does not take part in gas exchange.

Inspiratory Reserve Volume

When only a tidal breath occupies the lungs, there is "room" for additional air that can be further inhaled. This volume in excess of that used in tidal breathing is the **inspiratory reserve volume (IRV).** Aptly named, it is the volume of air that can be inspired when needed, but is usually kept in reserve.

Expiratory Reserve Volume

There is a quantity of air that can potentially be exhaled beyond the end of a tidal exhalation. Although it is kept in reserve, the volume of air that

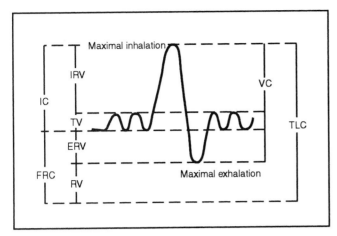

Figure 15-2. Lung volumes and capacities; IRV, inspiratory reserve volume; TV, tidal volume; ERV, expiratory reserve volume; RV, residual volume; IC, inspiratory capacity; FRC, functional residual capacity; VC, vital capacity; TLC, total lung capacity.

can be exhaled in excess of tidal breathing is called the **expiratory reserve volume (ERV).**

Residual Volume

The lungs are not completely emptied of air even after maximally exhaling the expiratory reserve volume. The volume of air remaining within the lungs when ERV has been exhaled is called the **residual volume (RV).**

Inspiratory Capacity

The sum of the tidal volume plus the inspiratory reserve volume is known as the **inspiratory capacity (IC).** This refers to the volume of air that can be inspired beginning from a tidal exhalation.

Functional Residual Capacity

The combination of residual volume and expiratory reserve volume is the **functional residual capacity (FRC).** Functional residual capacity is the volume of air that remains in the lungs at the end of a tidal exhalation.

Vital Capacity

The sum of inspiratory reserve volume, tidal volume, and expiratory reserve volume is called the **vital capacity (VC).** It is the total volume of air within the lungs that is under volitional control. The common method of measuring VC is to achieve maximal inspiration, then forcibly exhale all of the air into a measuring device as hard and as fast as possible until ERV has been exhausted. Because this is a forced expiratory maneuver, it is termed the forced vital capacity (FVC).

FLOW RATES AND MECHANICS

Flow rate measures the volume of gas moved in a period of time. Expiratory flow rates, therefore, are measurements of exhaled gas volume divided by the amount of time required for the volume to be exhaled. Flow rates reflect the ease with which the lungs can be ventilated and are related to the elasticity of the lung parenchyma.[18] An important airflow measurement is the volume of air that can be forcefully exhaled during the first second of a forced vital capacity maneuver. This is called the **forced expiratory volume** in one second **(FEV$_1$).** This flow rate is thought to reflect the status of the larger airways of the lungs. In healthy individuals, FEV$_1$ is 80 percent of the total FVC (FEV$_1$/FVC = 80%).[18]

Forced expiratory flow from 25 to 75 percent of FVC (FEF$_{25-75\%}$) is the flow rate found in the middle of the forced expiratory flow volume curve. This flow rate is thought to reflect the status of the smaller, more fragile airways of the lung.

Inspiratory flow rates can also be determined by measuring the amount of air inspired and the amount of time necessary for the inhalation. **Maximum inspiratory pressure (PI$_{max}$)** reflects the greatest inspiratory effort that can be generated from residual volume. It is measured as a pressure in millimeters of mercury or cubic centimeters of water.

Lung volumes, capacities, flow rates, and mechanics depend on the size and configuration of the thorax. Therefore, height, gender, and race influence static and dynamic lung measurements. Any alteration in the properties of the lungs or chest wall due to the aging process or a disease process will change the lung volumes, capacities, flow rates, or mechanics.

RESPIRATION

Respiration is a term used to describe the gas exchange within the body. This should not be confused with ventilation, which describes only the movement of air. External respiration is the exchange of gas that occurs at the alveolar capillary membrane between atmospheric air and the pulmonary capillaries. Internal respiration takes place at the tissue capillary level between the tissues and the surrounding capillaries. The following discussion traces the course of gas exchange, specifically that of oxygen and carbon dioxide, during both external and internal respiration.

For external respiration to take place, there must first be an inhalation of air from the environment, through the conducting airways, and into the alveoli. Oxygen diffuses through the alveolar wall, through the interstitial space, and through the pulmonary capillary wall. Most of the oxygen (98.5%) then travels through the blood plasma into red blood cells where it occupies one of the gas-carrying sites of hemoglobin. A small portion of dissolved oxygen (1.5%) is carried in the plasma.

The oxygenated blood returns to the left side of the heart via the pulmonary veins; from there it travels through the aorta, and then through a network of connecting arteries, arterioles, and capillaries, until its destination, the tissue, is reached. Internal respiration begins when the arterial blood reaches the tissue level. Oxygen diffuses from the gas-carrying sites of hemoglobin, out of the red blood cell, out of the capillary, through the cell membranes, and into the mitochondria of the working cells. Again, this process occurs through diffusion.

Carbon dioxide (CO_2), which is produced at the tissue level as a by-product of metabolism, diffuses out of the working cells and into the capillaries. Carbon dioxide is transported through the venous system into the right side of the heart. Once the carbon dioxide makes its way to the pulmonary capillary, it diffuses out through the capillary membrane, through the interstitial space, and into the alveoli, where it is finally exhaled into the atmosphere.

When the cycle of external and internal respiration has occurred, oxygen has been provided to the body tissues and carbon dioxide has been removed. Of course, this system is dependent upon an intact cardiovascular system to pump the blood through the lungs, deliver it to the working cells, and then return it back to the lungs, all in a timely fashion.

CHRONIC LUNG DISEASES

Chronic Obstructive Pulmonary Disease

Chronic obstructive pulmonary disease (COPD) is the most common chronic pulmonary disorder, afflicting 10 to 15 percent of adults over the age of 55, and its prevalence is increasing.[12] COPD is a disorder characterized by the presence of airflow obstruction that is generally progressive, may be accompanied by airway hyperreactivity, and may be partially reversible.[20] The pulmonary components that comprise COPD are chronic bronchitis and emphysema.

According to the American Thoracic Society, **chronic bronchitis** is defined as chronic cough and expectoration, when other specific causes of cough can be excluded, which persists for at least a 3-month period for at least 2 consecutive years.[21] **Emphysema** is defined as abnormal enlargement of the distal respiratory unit accompanied by destructive changes of the alveolar walls without obvious fibrosis.[20,21] Overdistension of the air spaces without destruction of the alveolar walls, as normally seen in aging, is not included in the definition of emphysema. Because chronic bronchitis and emphysema can coexist, and their clinical signs and symptoms overlap, the term COPD is useful in the clinical setting to describe the combination of these disorders.

ETIOLOGY

Chronic inflammation caused by the irritation of inhaled cigarette smoke is the major causal agent in the development of COPD.[22] There is a direct relationship between the amount and duration of cigarette smoking and the severity of the lung disease, although significant individual variation does exist.[20] The etiological role of other factors, such as agents inhaled from occupational exposure without the effects of smoking, appears to be relatively insignificant.[20,22]

PATHOPHYSIOLOGY

The pathophysiology of COPD is characterized by a number of impairments that contribute to the overall disease process. Chronic inflammation from inhaling pollutants causes glands and goblet cells within the bronchial walls to hypertrophy. Excessive secretions are then produced, which either partially or completely obstruct the airway. As air enters the lungs, the airways are pulled open, increasing the diameter of the lumen. As the air exits, airways decrease in size. When excessive secretions are present in an airway, air can be inspired around the secretions. During exhalation, however, only some of the air escapes before the airway closes down around the secretions, trapping air distal to the obstruction. Partial obstruction of an airway by mucus, that is, obstruction only during exhalation, accounts for the **hyperinflation** (an abnormal increase in the amount of air within the lung tissue) seen in these patients. Complete obstruction of the airways will result in absorption **atelectasis.**

Decreases in ciliary function and alterations in physiochemical characteristics of bronchial secretions also impair airway clearance and contribute to airway obstruction.[23] Stagnant bronchial secretions predispose the patient to recurrent respiratory tract infections. Damaged and inflamed mucosa shows an increased sensitivity of the irritant receptors within the bronchial walls, which in turn cause bronchial **hyperreactivity.** Destruction of pulmonary tissue results in loss of the normal elastic recoil properties of the lungs. During expiration, some airways collapse from a lack of support by the surrounding elastic parenchyma.[23] Premature airway collapse causes hyperinflation or air trapping and reduced expiratory flow rates.

In advanced stages of the disease, destruction of the alveolar capillary membrane may be present. Ventilation of the alveoli and **perfusion** of the capillary membrane are no longer matched. This results in **hypoxemia,** a condition in which a decreased amount of oxygen is carried by the blood to the tissues. As the disease progresses and more areas of the lung become involved, hypoxemia will worsen and **hypercapnea,** a condition in which there is an increased amount of carbon dioxide within the arterial blood, will develop. Increased pulmonary vascular resistance secondary to capillary destruction and reflex vasoconstriction in the presence of hypoxemia and hypercapnea results in right ventricular hypertrophy, or **cor pulmonale.** *Polycythemia,* an increase in the amount of circulating red blood cells, is another complication of advanced COPD.[24]

CLINICAL PRESENTATION

Patients with COPD will present with symptoms of chronic cough, expectoration, and exertional dyspnea. The intensity of each symptom varies according to the patient's unique combination of individual diseases (e.g., chronic bronchitis and/or emphysema) that contribute to the clinical diagnosis of COPD.

Cough and expectoration appear slowly and insidiously. Dyspnea is first evidenced during exertion. As the disease progresses, symptoms worsen. Respiratory infections are common. Dyspnea occurs at progressively lower activity levels. Severely involved patients may appear dyspneic even at rest.

On physical examination, the thorax appears enlarged owing to loss of lung elastic recoil. The anterior-posterior diameter of the chest increases and a dorsal kyphosis is noted. These anatomical changes give the patient a "barrel-chest" appearance. As a result of lung hyperinflation, breath sounds and heart sounds are usually distant and somewhat difficult to hear. Increased secretions that partially obstruct the bronchi may result in expiratory **wheezing. Crackles** may also be present. Hypertrophy of accessory muscles of ventilation, pursed-lip breathing, **cyanosis,** and **digital clubbing** may all be present in the advanced stages of COPD. (See the section on pulmonary assessment for clarification of terms.)

A significant and progressive increase in airway obstruction is reflected in decreases in expiratory flow rates, especially FEV_1. Pulmonary function studies reveal that these changes do not show a major reversibility in response to pharmacological agents. Inspiratory flow rates may also be reduced as a result of increased secretions in the airways. There is an increase in residual volume, which may be several times the normal value due to air trapping.[25] As a result, functional residual capacity is also increased. Figure 15-3 shows the changes in lung volumes and capacities that occur in obstructive pulmonary disease.

Arterial blood gas analyses may reflect hypoxemia in the early stages of COPD. Hypercapnea appears as the disease progresses. With disease progression, chest radiographs show several characteristic findings. These include depressed and flattened hemidiaphragms; alteration in pulmonary vascular markings; hyperinflation of the thorax, evidenced by an increased anterior-posterior diameter of the chest; and an increased retrosternal airspace, **hyperlucency,** elongation of the heart, and right ventricular hypertrophy.

COURSE AND PROGNOSIS

The clinical course of COPD can run for 30 years or more.[23,24] Several researchers suggest that changes in flow rates of the small peripheral airways, the $FEF_{25-75\%}$, may actually be a precursor to the development of COPD.[21,26,27] Early detection of abnormalities in the peripheral airway may allow

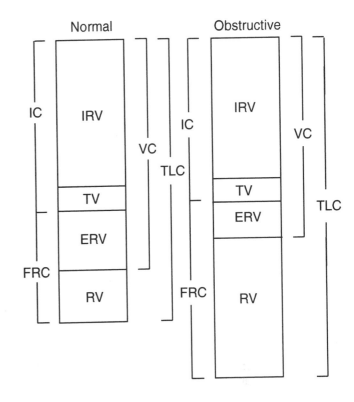

ERV: Expiratory reserve volume
FRC: Functional residual capacity
IC: Inspiratory capacity
IRV: Inspiratory reserve volume
RV: Residual volume
TLC: Total lung capacity
TV: Tidal volume

Figure 15-3. Lung volumes of a healthy pulmonary system compared with the lung volumes found in obstructive disease. (From Rothstein, J, et al: The Rehabilitation Specialist's Handbook. FA Davis, Philadelphia, 1991, p 604, with permission.)

for a timely alteration in the patient's personal life-style and environment. Such intervention may prevent development of COPD.[28]

Without intervention, some, but not all, patients with abnormalities in their peripheral airways will show progression of lung dysfunction. Patients may develop the symptoms of chronic bronchitis, chronic cough, and expectoration. Some patients may demonstrate these findings for many years before developing signs or symptoms of emphysema. The progression to emphysema is evidenced by an increase in the severity of airway obstruction, deterioration of pulmonary function test values, and more frequent respiratory tract infections.[29]

Expiratory flow rates measured during stable periods are good indicators of the progression of COPD. There is also a good correlation between the severity of airway obstruction, as judged by FEV_1, and mortality rates. The rate of decrease in FEV_1, was found to be approximately 54 mL/year in a cross-sectional study.[30] Smoking cessation has been shown to delay this decline in function.[31,32] With an FEV_1 below 750 mL/sec, few patients survive 5 years.[23]

Asthma

Asthma is a clinical syndrome characterized by increased reactivity of the tracheobronchial tree in the presence of various stimuli.[21] The most remarkable feature of asthma is the episodic attacks of wheezing and dyspnea. These attacks improve either spontaneously or with medical intervention and are interspersed with intervals that are symptom free.

ETIOLOGY

Asthma is a common respiratory disease, affecting 14 to 15 million people in the United States.[33] Symptoms may begin at any age. Although the exact mechanism of airway hyperreactivity is unknown, genetic predisposition,[34] environmental contributions (house dust, animal and mite proteins, molds, cigarette smoke, pollens and perhaps chemical and particulate air pollutants),[33] autonomic nervous system imbalance, and mucosal epithelial damage[23] have been implicated in the development of asthma. The airways of patients with asthma are hypersensitive to a variety of factors including allergens, respiratory tract infections, respiratory irritants, cold, emotional stresses, exercise, and chemical substances. Any or all of these may precipitate or aggravate the symptoms of asthma.

PATHOPHYSIOLOGY

The major physiological manifestation of asthma is widespread narrowing of the airways. The airway narrowing occurs as a result of **bronchospasm,** inflammation of the bronchial mucosa, and increased bronchial secretions. The narrowed airways increase the resistance to airflow and cause air trapping, leading to hyperinflation. These narrowed airways provide an abnormal distribution of ventilation to the alveoli.

CLINICAL PRESENTATION

The clinical symptom of asthma is airway narrowing with varying degrees of dyspnea and wheezing. During an acute exacerbation, the chest is usually held in an expanded position, indicating that hyperinflation of the lungs has occurred. Accessory muscles of ventilation are used for breathing and expiratory wheezes can be heard over the entire chest. Sometimes crackles can be heard as well. With severe airway obstruction, breath sounds may markedly decrease due to poor air movement; wheezing may occur on inspiration as well as expiration; and intercostal, supraclavicular, and substernal **retractions** may be present on inspiration. Chest radiographs taken during an asthmatic exacerbation usually indicate hyperinflation, as evidenced by an increase in the anterior-posterior diameter of the chest and hyperlucency of the lung fields. Less commonly, chest radiographs may reveal

areas of atelectasis from the bronchial obstruction or infiltrates. Normal chest radiographs can be seen between asthmatic exacerbations.

The most consistent change during an exacerbation of asthma is decreased expiratory flow rates (FEV_1). Residual volume and functional residual capacity are increased because of air trapping at the expense of vital capacity and inspiratory reserve volume, which are reduced. The reversibility of these pulmonary function test abnormalities is characteristic of asthma. During remission, the patient with asthma may have normal or near-normal values.

The most common arterial blood gas finding during an asthmatic exacerbation is mild to moderate hypoxemia. Usually some degree of **hypocapnea** is present secondary to hyperventilation. With severe attacks, hypoxemia may be more pronounced and with further clinical deterioration, hypercapnea occurs, indicating the patient is exhausted and respiratory failure may follow.[23,35,36]

CLINICAL COURSE AND PROGNOSIS

By the time adulthood is reached, 33 percent of children with asthma do not have symptoms of the disease.[23] When the onset of symptoms begins later in life, the clinical course is usually more progressive, showing changes in pulmonary function tests even during periods of remission. Although the morbidity and mortality of asthma are on the rise, it is still a relatively infrequent cause of death.[37]

Cystic Fibrosis

Cystic fibrosis (CF) is a disease characterized by an exocrine gland dysfunction that results in abnormally viscid secretions. CF affects many organ systems. Viscous secretions obstruct the airways and pancreatic ducts; obstruction of the former causes chronic pulmonary disease, and of the latter results in malabsorption of food and nutritional compromise.

ETIOLOGY

CF is a hereditary disease transmitted as an autosomal recessive (Mendelian) trait. The incidence of disease in white children is approximately 1 in 2000 live births, with a carrier rate of 1 in 20 persons. CF is less common in the African-American population (1 in 17,000 live births) and is rare in the Asian population.[38] The CF gene has been identified on the long arm of chromosome 7 making prenatal testing, testing for the presence of disease, and testing to determine carriers of the gene possible.

PATHOPHYSIOLOGY

Chronic pulmonary disease in CF is related to the abnormally viscous mucus secreted by the tracheobronchial tree. The function of the mucociliary transport is impaired by the altered secretions and results in airway obstruction, recurrent infection, and hyperinflation. Partial or complete obstruction of the airways reduces ventilation to the alveolar units. Ventilation and perfusion within the lungs are uneven. Fibrotic changes are also found in the lung parenchyma.

CLINICAL PRESENTATION

The diagnosis of CF may be suspected in patients who present with a positive family history of the disease, with recurrent respiratory infections from *Staphylococcus aureus* and *Pseudomonas aeruginosa*, or with a diagnosis of malnutrition and/or failure to thrive. A chloride concentration of 60 mEq/L found in the sweat of children is a positive test for the diagnosis of CF.

Pulmonary function studies show obstructive impairments: decreased FEV_1, decreased FVC, increased residual volume, and increased FRC. The abnormal ventilation-perfusion relationship within the lungs results in hypoxemia and hypercapnea, as shown by arterial blood gas analysis. As the disease progresses, destruction of the alveolar capillary network causes pulmonary hypertension and cor pulmonale. In advanced disease, chest radiographs show diffuse hyperinflation, increased lung marking, and atelectasis.

COURSE AND PROGNOSIS

Respiratory failure is the most frequent cause of death in patients with CF. Although some patients still die in infancy and early childhood, the majority of patients currently survive into adulthood. Life expectancy continues to increase owing to advances in early diagnosis and improved medical management. The mean survival age of patients with CF in 1995 was 30.1 years.[39] Treatment of the pulmonary dysfunction administered by CF centers includes removal of the abnormal secretions and prompt treatment of pulmonary infections. Gastrointestinal dysfunction from CF can be aided by proper diet, vitamin supplements, and replacement of pancreatic enzymes.

Restrictive Lung Disease

Restrictive lung disease is actually a group of diseases with differing etiologies. What these disorders have in common is a difficulty in expanding the lungs and a reduction in lung volume. This restriction can come from diseases of the alveolar parenchyma and/or the pleura that result in fibrosis of the alveoli, interstitial lung parenchyma, and pleura. The restriction can also be caused by changes in the chest wall or in the neuromuscular apparatus.[18] For the purpose of this discussion, those diseases most likely to be encountered in a rehabilitation setting—restrictive diseases of the lung parenchyma and pleura—will be presented.

ETIOLOGY

This group of disorders has a variety of causes. Numerous agents, such as radiation therapy, inorganic dust, inhalation of noxious gases, oxygen toxicity, asbestos exposure, and tuberculosis can cause damage to the pulmonary parenchyma and pleura and result in restrictive pulmonary disease. The most common restrictive lung disease is idiopathic pulmonary fibrosis (IPF). The etiology of IPF is not known; however, there is an immunological reaction in some cases.[18]

PATHOPHYSIOLOGY

The particular changes occurring within the lungs depends on the etiological factors of restrictive disease. Parenchymal changes often begin with chronic inflammation and a thickening of the alveoli and interstitium. As the disease progresses, distal air spaces become fibrosed making them more resistant to expansion (i.e., less distensible). Consequently, lung volumes are reduced. A reduced pulmonary vascular bed eventually leads to hypoxemia and cor pulmonale.

In pleural diseases, thickened plaques of collagen fibers cause fibrosis, which may be found in various locations. In asbestos exposure, for example, the plaques are found on the parietal pleura. The mechanism responsible for plaque development is not completely clear. There may also be parenchymal alterations that accompany pleural diseases. These changes may be due to injury or inflammatory reactions that lead to fibrosis.

CLINICAL PRESENTATION

Dyspnea is the classic symptom of restrictive lung diseases. A nonproductive cough is often encountered; weakness and early fatigue are also common. Signs of restrictive lung disease include rapid, shallow breathing; limited chest expansion; crackles, especially over the lower lung fields; digital clubbing; and cyanosis.[40]

In the early stages of parenchymal restrictive disease, the chest radiograph reveals fine interstitial markings that look like ground glass. In longstanding fibrosis there is radiographic evidence of diffuse infiltrates, and the appearance of the lung has been likened to that of a honeycomb. Reduction in lung volumes can be seen serially on chest radiographs. Radiographic evidence of pleural thickening can also be seen, especially on oblique films.

Pulmonary function tests reveal a reduction in VC, FRC, and TLC. Residual volume may be normal or near normal, and expiratory flow rates remain normal. Figure 15-4 shows the changes in lung volumes and capacities that occur in restrictive pulmonary disease.

Arterial blood studies show varying degrees of hypoxemia and hypocapnea. Hypoxemia at rest is usually exacerbated by exercise. Exercise may significantly lower oxygenation, even for patients with normal oxygenation at rest.

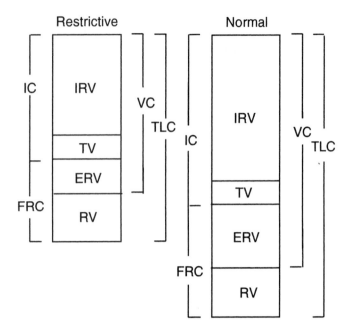

ERV: Expiratory reserve volume
FRC: Functional residual capacity
IC: Inspiratory capacity
IRV: Inspiratory reserve volume
RV: Residual volume
TLC: Total lung capacity
TV: Tidal volume

Figure 15-4. Lung volumes of a healthy pulmonary system compared with the lung volumes found in restrictive disease. (From Rothstein, J, et al: The Rehabilitation Specialist's Handbook. FA Davis, Philadelphia, 1991, p 604, with permission.)

COURSE AND PROGNOSIS

Restrictive pulmonary disease may have a slow onset but is chronic and progressive in nature. Survival depends on the type of restrictive disease, the etiological factor, and the treatment. Almost 50 percent of patients with IPF die within 5 years of diagnosis.[40] Chest radiographs are insensitive indicators of the extent of the disease. Hypercapnea is an ominous sign, indicating the terminal stage of pulmonary fibrosis.

MEDICAL MANAGEMENT OF PULMONARY DISEASE

Pharmacological Management

Pharmacological agents provide the foundation for the medical management of pulmonary disease. These drugs can affect exercise performance, heart rate, and blood pressure, both at rest and with exercise. It is important to know the medications used in pulmonary care and their effects on the pulmonary system.

Broad classifications of drugs often used in the care of patients with pulmonary disease are found in Table 15–1. It is not unusual for patients to be on a combination of drugs for the management of their pulmonary disease.

Bronchodilators, classified as anticholinergics, beta 2 agonists, and theophylline are commonly prescribed drugs for patients with pulmonary disease. Bronchodilators are used to reduce airway obstruction and resistance to airflow by increasing the size of the airway lumen.

Inhaled anticholinergics are a commonly prescribed first-line drug for patients with COPD.[41] Their action is to decrease airway smooth muscle contractions and reduce the secretion of mucus, thus promoting bronchodilation. Anticholinergics have a slower onset of these actions but maintain the effects longer than beta 2 agonists. Therefore, they should be taken on a regular schedule, 2 to 4 puffs, 3 to 4 times per day for a consistent level of bronchodilation.[20]

Inhaled short-acting beta 2 agonists are used for a more immediate relief of symptomatic bronchospasm and bronchial edema.[42] They are sometimes referred to as "rescue" drugs. Salmeterol is an inhaled longer acting beta 2 agonist that is used to decrease the frequent use of other beta 2 agonists and should be taken on a more scheduled basis. Oral beta 2 agonists, such as metaproterenol sulfate (Alupent) and montelukast (Singulair), are also available for a longer acting bronchodilation, with perhaps more systemic effects. Patients should be advised to use their prescribed inhaled short acting beta 2 agonist prior to the onset of activity to enhance exercise performance. [43]

Theophylline is a weak bronchodilator that also promotes collateral ventilation, mucociliary clearance, and may have anti-inflammatory effects.[42] It is generally used as an addition to a regimen of inhaled agents owing to the fine line between therapeutic and toxic effects. Patients who take a theophylline preparation should have their blood levels monitored regularly to avoid toxicity.[18]

Although the mechanism of each bronchodilator is different, there may be an increase in resting heart rate with their use. Employing the Karvonen formula for exercise intensity, the elevated resting heart rate is acknowledged and a more appropriate target heart rate is calculated. The use of the rate of perceived shortness of breath may also be used as a reliable indicator of exercise intensity.

Anti-inflammatory drugs, such as cromolyn sodium and corticosteroids, are often used in the treatment of asthma. Cromolyn sodium (Intal) has the ability to block inflammation of the airways in some patients.[18] Because of its action, cromolyn sodium is a prophylactic drug, not one to be used in an acute situation. Its preventative capacity makes it useful in maintenance therapy. In chronic pulmonary disease, corticosteroids may be prescribed for an acute exacerbation with high doses for a short duration, possibly 5 to 7 days.[42] For some patients, low-dose administration of corticosteroids is used for long-term management of symptoms. Side ef-

Table 15–1 PULMONARY DRUGS[a]

Use	Side Effects	Drug Names	Routes of Administration
I. Beta 2 agonist			
Smooth muscle relaxation	Tachycardia	Isoproterenol	Inhaled
Bronchodilation	Palpitations	Epinephrine (Ephedrine)	PO
	GI distress	Isoetharine (Bronkosol)	IM
	Nervousness	Metaproterenol (Alupent)	IV
	Tremor	Terbutaline (Brethine)	
	Headache	Albuterol (Proventil, Ventolin)	
	Dizziness	Salmeterol (Serevent)	
		Montelukast sodium (Singulair)	
II. Theophyllin			
Smooth muscle relaxation	Tachycardia	Aminophylline (Aminodur)	Inhaled
Bronchodilation	Arrhythmias	Theophylline (Elixophyllin)	PO
	GI distress	(Slo-phyllin, Theodur)	IV
	Nervousness	(Fleet Theophyllin)	PR
	Headache	Oxtriphyllin (Choladril)	
	Dizziness		
III. Anticholinergic			
Blocks smooth muscle	Tachycardia	Ipratropium bromide (Atrovent)	Inhaled
constriction	Palpitations	Atropine sulfate	IM
bronchodilation	Drying of tracheal secretions		IV
	Throat irritation		Subcutaneous
	Photophobia		
	Urinary retention		
	Constipation		
IV. Anti-inflammatory agents			
Corticosteroids	Increased BP	Prednisone	Inhaled
Reduces mucosal edema	Sodium retention (edema)	Hydrocortisone (Cortisol)	PO
Reduces inflammation	Muscle wasting	Triamcinolone acetonide (Azmacort)	IM
Reduces immune response	Osteoporosis	Beclomethasone (Vanceril, Beclovent)	IV
	GI irritation		
	Atherosclerosis		
	Hypercholesteremia		
	Increased susceptibility to infections		
Cromolyn Sodium	Throat irritation	Intal	Inhaled
Reduces inflammation	Cough	Fivent	
	Bronchospasm		

[a]Generic drugs are known by other proprietary names in addition to those given above.
GI, gastrointestinal; IM, intramuscular; IV, intravenous; PO, oral; PR, parenteral.

fects of systemic steroids, including osteoporosis, myopathies, and muscle wasting, may require modifications to an exercise program such as muscle strengthening and low-impact exercise.[43]

Pulmonary infections can be devastating to the patient and cause major setbacks in pulmonary rehabilitation efforts. The early signs of an infection are often noted by some change in the patient's baseline (i.e., a change in exercise ability, change in dyspnea, change in the color or amount of sputum). Fever, chest roentgenograms, or sputum cultures are not necessary to begin treatment with antibiotics. Antibiotics may be divided into five basic categories: penicillins, cephalosporins, aminoglycosides, tetracyclines, and erythromycins. The action of these drugs is either bacteriostatic or bactericidal. Organisms can be sensitive to some antibiotics but resistant to others.

Supplemental oxygen is used to prevent tissue hypoxia. An absolute indication for use of long-term oxygen therapy is an arterial partial pressure of oxygen (Pao_2) of 55 mmHg or less, which correlates with an Sao_2 of 88 percent or less.[42] The normal value for Pao_2 is 95 to 100 mmHg, which corresponds to an Sao_2 of between 98 and 100 percent. If a patient is found to have an Sao_2 of 90 percent or greater at rest but desaturates with exercise, then supplemental oxygen should be used during the exercise session because it has been shown to decrease dyspnea and improve exercise tolerance.[45] The amount of oxygen used should be titrated individually to maintain an Sao_2 of at least 90 percent if possible.[20] There are various delivery methods available: continuous flow, pulsed flow, and reservoir are among the most common.

Surgical Management

There are few surgical options for the patient with pulmonary disease. Surgical resection of giant bullae is a well-accepted surgical technique designed to remove abnormally dilated, nonfunctional lung tissue to decompress the adjacent functional lung tissue.[46] Inclusion criteria for this surgical procedure recommend that the bullae occupy at least one third to one half of a hemithorax.[47] Although this surgical procedure can provide impressive results, it is an option for only a small number of patients with lung disease.

Lung volume reduction surgery (LVRS), also called pneumonectomy, is a surgical technique introduced in the 1950s, but was not widely performed until quite recently. Patients with heterogeneous emphysema have the relatively nonfunctional aspects of each lung, approximately 20 to 30 percent, removed to reestablish more normal chest wall and lung mechanics.[46] Postoperative results show improved FEV_1, decreased TLC and RV, a decrease in symptoms of dyspnea, and an increase in exercise tolerance.[17,20] A 6-week preoperative pulmonary rehabilitation program is advocated to reduce complications postoperatively.[17,46]

Lung transplantation for end-stage pulmonary disease remains the definitive "cure."[20,48] The goals of lung transplantation are to restore normal lung function, restore normal exercise capacity, and prolong life.[49] The largest population of people awaiting a lung transplant are patients with emphysema but, owing to the strict inclusion criteria and the small number of organs available for transplantation, this option becomes a reality for only a small number of individuals.[49]

REHABILITATION FOR THE PATIENT WITH PULMONARY DISEASE

Chronic pulmonary disease and its associated dysfunction have a slow onset and a progressive course. The person with pulmonary dysfunction avoids activities that result in the uncomfortable sensation of dyspnea. A slow but steady decrease in these patients' activities follows. It is not uncommon for someone with pulmonary disease to have lost many functional abilities before ever seeking medical help. The intended outcome of pulmonary rehabilitation is to interrupt this downward spiraling of physical ability.[50]

Goals and Outcomes

The *Guide for Physical Therapist Practice* provides a complete list of anticipated goals and outcomes of physical therapy intervention for patients with impaired ventilation and respiration, and aerobic capacity and endurance.[51] The following is a concise list of goals and outcomes for physical therapy intervention for the patient with pulmonary disease.

1. Increased understanding of patient and family of disease process, expectations, goals, and outcomes.
2. Increased cardiovascular endurance.
3. Increased strength, power, and endurance of peripheral muscles.
4. Improved performance of physical tasks, both basic activities of daily living and instrumental activities of daily living.
5. Increased strength, power, and endurance of ventilatory muscles.
6. Improved independence in airway clearance.
7. Decreased work of breathing.

8. Improved decision making ability regarding the use of health care resources.
9. Enhanced self-management of symptoms and self-management of pulmonary disease.

PULMONARY ASSESSMENT

The assessment of a patient's pulmonary status has several purposes: (1) to evaluate the appropriateness of the patient's participation in a pulmonary rehabilitation program; (2) to determine the therapeutic measures most appropriate for the participant's treatment program; (3) to monitor the participant's physiological response to exercise; and (4) to appropriately progress the participant's treatment program over time.

Patient Interview

A patient interview should begin with the "chief complaint," the patient's perception of why pulmonary rehabilitation is being sought. Commonly, the chief complaint is often shortness of breath and/or loss of function. Quantifying dyspnea at the beginning and the end of a rehabilitation program and during periods of exacerbation can be accomplished through a visual analog scale[52] (Fig. 15-5) or the Baseline Dyspnea Index[53] (Table 15–2). A medical history contains pertinent pulmonary symptoms specific to that patient: cough, sputum production, wheezing, and shortness of breath. Occupational, social, medication, and family histories should also be recorded.

Figure 15-5. The visual analogue scale is an empty vertical line with end caps labeled Greatest Breathlessness and No Breathlessness. The patient is asked to mark the point on the line that reflects his level of breathlessness. (From Mahler, D, et al: The impact of dyspnea and physiologic function in general health status in patients with chronic obstructive pulmonary disease. Chest 102:215, 1992, with permission.)

Table 15–2 BASELINE DYSPNEA INDEX

Functional Impairment

_____ Grade 4: *No Impairment.* Able to carry out usual activities and occupation without shortness of breath.

_____ Grade 3: *Slight Impairment.* Distinct impairment in at least one activity but no activities completely abandoned. Reduction in activity at work *or* in usual activities that seems slight or not clearly caused by shortness of breath.

_____ Grade 2: *Moderate Impairment.* Patient has changed jobs *and/or* has abandoned at least one usual activity due to shortness of breath.

_____ Grade 1: *Severe Impairment.* Patient unable to work *or* has given up most or all customary activities due to shortness of breath.

_____ Grade 0: *Very Severe Impairment.* Unable to work *and* has given up most or all customary activities due to shortness of breath.

_____ W: *Amount Uncertain.* Patient is impaired owing to shortness of breath, but amount cannot be specified. Details are not sufficient to allow impairment to be categorized.

_____ X: *Unknown.* Information unavailable regarding impairment.

_____ Y: *Impaired for Reasons Other than Shortness of Breath.* For example, musculoskeletal problem or chest pain.

Magnitude of Task

_____ Grade 4: *Extraordinary.* Becomes short of breath only with extraordinary activity, such as carrying very heavy loads on the level, lighter loads uphill, or running. No shortness of breath with ordinary tasks.

_____ Grade 3: *Major.* Becomes short of breath only with such major activities as walking up a steep hill, climbing more than three flights of stairs, or carrying a moderate load on the level.

_____ Grade 2: *Moderate.* Becomes short of breath with moderate or average tasks, such as walking up a gradual hill, climbing less than three flights of stairs, or carrying a light load on the level.

_____ Grade 1: *Light.* Becomes short of breath with light activities, such as walking on the level, washing, standing, or shopping.

_____ Grade 0: *No Task.* Becomes short of breath at rest, while sitting, or lying down.

_____ W: *Amount Uncertain.* Patient has limited exertional capacity due to shortness of breath, but amount cannot be specified. Details are not sufficient to allow impairment to be categorized.

_____ X: *Unknown.* Information unavailable regarding limitation of magnitude of task.

_____ Y: *Impaired for Reasons Other than Shortness of Breath.* For example, musculoskeletal problem or chest pain.

Magnitude of Effort

_____ Grade 4: *Extraordinary.* Becomes short of breath only with the greatest imaginable effort. No shortness of breath with ordinary effort.

_____ Grade 3: *Major.* Becomes short of breath with effort distinctly submaximal, but of major proportion. Tasks performed without pause unless the task requires extraordinary effort that may be performed with pauses.

_____ Grade 2: *Moderate.* Becomes short of breath with moderate effort. Tasks performed with occasional pauses and requiring longer to complete than the average person.

_____ Grade 1: *Light.* Becomes short of breath with little effort. Tasks performed with little effort or more difficult tasks with frequent pauses and requiring 50–100% longer to complete than the average person might require.

_____ Grade 0: *No Effort.* Becomes short of breath at rest, while sitting, or lying down.

_____ W: *Amount Uncertain.* Patient has limited exertional capacity due to shortness of breath, but amount cannot be specified. Details are not sufficient to allow impairment to be categorized.

_____ X: *Unknown.* Information unavailable regarding limitation of effort.

_____ Y: *Impaired for Reasons Other than Shortness of Breath.* For example, musculoskeletal problem or chest pain.

From Mahler, D, et al.[52] p 399.

Physical Examination

VITAL SIGNS

Temperature and resting blood pressure, heart rate, and respiratory rate should be determined and recorded (see Chapter 4). An individual's height should be measured because there is a direct relationship between height and lung volume.

Weight should be measured on a standard balance scale and each assessment of weight should be performed on the same scale.

OBSERVATION, INSPECTION, AND PALPATION

By observing the neck and shoulders of a patient with pulmonary disease, the use of accessory muscles of ventilation can be observed. A normal configuration of the thorax reveals a ratio of anterior-posterior (AP) to lateral diameter of 2:1. Emphysema causes destruction of the lung parenchyma, which results in an increase in the AP diameter and a reduction of this ratio (up to 1:1). During inhalation and exhalation both sides of the thorax should move symmetrically.

Cyanosis is a bluish discoloration of the skin that can be observed periorally, periorbitally, and in nail beds; it indicates hypoxemia. In digital clubbing of the fingers and toes, an indicator of chronic hypoxemia, there is an increase in the angle created by the distal pharynx and the point where the nail exits from the digit. The tip of the distal pharynx becomes bulbous.

AUSCULTATION OF THE LUNGS

Auscultation involves listening over the chest wall to the airways as gas enters and exits the lungs. To perform auscultation of the lungs, a stethoscope is placed firmly on the patient's thorax over the lung tissue. The patient is asked to inspire fully through an open mouth, then to exhale quietly. Inhalation and the beginning of exhalation normally produce a soft rustling sound. The end of exhalation is silent. This characteristic of a normal breath sound is termed **vesicular.** When a louder, more hollow and echoing sound occupies a larger portion of the ventilatory cycle, the breath sounds are referred to as **bronchial.** When the breath sounds are very quiet and barely audible, they are termed **decreased.** These three terms—vesicular, bronchial, and decreased—allow the listener to describe the intensity of the breath sound.[54]

In addition to the normal and abnormal intensity of the breath sound, there may be additional sounds and vibrations heard during auscultation. These are called **adventitious breath sounds.** These sounds are superimposed on the already-described intensity of the breath sound. According to the American College of Chest Physicians and the American Thoracic Society, there are two types of adventitious sounds: crackles and wheezes.[55] **Crackles,** historically termed rales, sound like the rustling of cellophane and are thought to occur when previously closed small airways and alveoli are rapidly reopened.[56] **Wheezes** are more musical in nature. A decrease in the size of the lumen of the airway will create a wheezing sound, much as stretching the neck of an inflated balloon narrows the passageway through which air must escape and produces a whistling sound.

MEASUREMENT OF STRENGTH

Patients with pulmonary disease may show peripheral and/or ventilatory muscle weakness due to inactivity or long-term steroid use. Peripheral and ventilatory muscle weakness can contribute to exercise limitations and an inability to perform activities of daily living.[57-59] Therefore, manual muscle testing and measurement of maximal inspiratory pressure will assess the need for strength training during the rehabilitation sessions.

LABORATORY TESTS

Various laboratory studies may be performed to examine patients with pulmonary disease. These include chest radiographs, pulmonary function tests (PFTs), graded exercise tests (GXT), arterial blood gas (ABG) analysis, oxygen saturation measurements (Sao_2), and electrocardiograms.

Exercise Testing in Patients with Pulmonary Disease

A determination of functional capacity is part of the assessment of a patient with pulmonary disease. A **graded exercise test** (exercise tolerance test) can provide the objective information to (1) document a patient's symptomatology and physical impairment, (2) prescribe safe exercise, (3) document changes in oxygenation during exercise and determine the need for supplemental oxygen, and (4) identify any changes in pulmonary function during exercise intervention.

EXERCISE TESTING PROTOCOLS

There are a number of testing methods available to assess the maximal oxygen consumption and functional abilities of patients with pulmonary disease. The 12- or 6-minute walk has been shown to be a good predictor of functional abilities.[60,61] The patient is asked to cover as much distance as possible in the time frame given, either 12 or 6 minutes. The ease of application and availability of the required equipment has made it a common pre- and post-program assessment technique.

A GXT gradually increases intensity stressing the patient with pulmonary dysfunction to the point of limitation, while vital signs are monitored to ensure safety. ABGs measured during exercise provides the best method for determining arterial oxygenation and the adequacy of alveolar ventilation. The ECG, continuously recorded during exercise, records the exercise heart rate and electrical activity of the cardiac conduction system. Blood pressure measurements, recorded at 1- to 3-minute intervals during exercise and during recovery from the test provide information on the hemodynamic status of the patient. These protocols are outlined in Table 15–3.[62-68]

Procedures and equipment requirements for measuring functional ability range from the very simple 6- or 12-minute walk test to more sophisticated treadmill and cycle protocols. (Refer to the section on exercise testing protocols in Chapter 16 for more information on exercise protocols.)

TEST TERMINATION

The symptom-limited GXT requires the patient to continue the exercise protocol until symptoms dictate cessation. Criteria for stopping a pulmonary exercise test are listed in Box 15–1.[69,70]

Table 15–3 PROTOCOLS USED FOR EXERCISE TESTING THE PATIENT WITH PULMONARY DISEASE

Mode	Author	Protocol
Walk test	Cooper[62]	Ambulate as far as possible in 12 min
	Guyatt, et al.[63]	Ambulate as far as possible in 6 min
Cycle test	Jones[64]	Begin with 100 kpm (17 W), increase 100 kpm
	Jones and Campbell	Begin with 25 W, increase 15 W/min
	Berman and Sutton[66]	Begin with 100 kpm, increase 100 kpm every min or 50 kg/min every min when FEV_1 less than 1 L/sec
	Massachusetts Respiratory Hospital	Begin at 25 W, 10 W every 20 sec or 5 W every 20 sec when FEV_1 less than 1 L/sec
Treadmill tests	Naughton[67]	2 mph constant 0 grade
		3.5% grade every 3 min
	Balke[68]	3.3 mph constant 0 grade
		3.5% grade every 2 min
	Massachusetts Respiratory Hospital	1.5 mph constant 0 grade
		4% grade every 2 min
		2% grade every 2 min if FEV_1 is less than 1 L/sec

From Brannon, F, et al: Cardiac Rehabilitation: Basic Theory and Application. FA Davis, Philadelphia, 1998, p 299, with permission.

INTERPRETATION OF GRADED EXERCISE TEST RESULTS

Functional capacity assessed by an exercise test allows for appropriate vocational counseling assessment and provides the documentation necessary for addressing disability.[71] The need for supplemental oxygen is indicated if a patient becomes hypoxemic during the exercise test session. A decrease in the Pao_2 of less than 55 mmHg, corresponding to an Sao_2 of 88 percent or less, are indications of a need for oxygen supplementation during exercise.[20]

PFTs performed prior to and following an exercise test document the effects of exercise on lung function. A reduction of 10 percent in FEV_1 is an indication to provide bronchodilator therapy.[72] Finally, a prescription for exercise that will safely promote cardiopulmonary fitness can be developed based on the GXT. This is the topic of the next section.

Box 15–1 GRADED EXERCISE TEST TERMINATION CRITERIA

1. Maximal shortness of breath
2. A fall in Pao_2 of greater than 20 mmHg or a Pao_2 less than 55 mmHg
3. A rise in $Paco_2$ of greater than 10 mmHg or greater than 65 mmHg
4. Cardiac ischemia or arrhythmias
5. Symptoms of fatigue
6. Increase in diastolic blood pressure readings of 20 mmHg, systolic hypertension greater than 250 mmHg, decrease in blood pressure with increasing workloads
7. Leg pain
8. Total fatigue
9. Signs of insufficient cardiac output
10. Reaching a ventilatory maximum

From Brannon, F, et al: Cardiopulmonary Rehabilitation: Basic Theory and Application. FA Davis, Philadelphia, 1998, p 300, with permission.

EXERCISE PRESCRIPTION

Exercise prescription incorporates four variables that together provide an individually tailored exercise formula designed to produce an increase in functional capacity. These variables are mode, intensity, duration, and frequency.

Mode

Any type of sustained **aerobic exercise** is recommended for pulmonary rehabilitation. Lower extremity (LE) activities, including walking, jogging, rowing, cycling, and swimming, are recommended to improve exercise tolerance.[20] Upper extremity (UE) aerobic exercise, arm ergometry, or free weights should also be included to improve arm exercise performance.[20] The combination of UE and LE training in a rehabilitation program resulted in improved functional status compared to either exercise alone.[12,73,74] Many programs utilize a circuit approach to train different muscle groups and maintain the participant's interest.

Intensity

Three techniques used to prescribe and monitor exercise intensity are *target heart rate range (THRR)*, percent of maximum oxygen consumption (Vo_2), and a rating of perceived exertion/shortness of breath (RPE).[70,75–84]

HEART RATE

The THRR defines safety guidelines for exercise intensity during the treatment session. The **target heart rate (THR)** for a specific patient defines the most appropriate heart rate within the prescribed target heart rate range to ensure endurance training.

The most commonly used method to determine the THRR and the THR is the **heart rate reserve method** (Karvonen formula).[76] The heart rate reserve is the difference between the resting heart rate (HR_{rest}) in the seated position and the maximal heart rate (HR_{max}) achieved on a GXT. To calculate the THRR, percentages of the heart rate reserve are added to the resting heart rate. The equation for determining the THRR is:[70]

$$THRR = [(HR_{max} - HR_{rest}) \times 0.40 \text{ and } 0.85] + HR_{rest}$$

For example, on a GXT a patient achieved a maximal heart rate of 165 beats per minute. Resting heart rate was 85 beats per minute. The heart rate reserve is calculated to be 165 − 85 = 80 beats per minute; 40 percent of 80 + resting heart rate = 117 beats per minute; 85 percent of 80 + resting heart rate = 153 beats per minute. Thus, for this patient, a THRR of 117 to 153 beats per minute has been calculated.

Determining the appropriate THR (i.e., where in this wide range of 117 to 153 beats per minute to exercise) requires careful consideration of individual abilities and disabilities. For patients with mild to moderate pulmonary disease, the THR should be calculated using a minimum of 50 percent and a maximum of 60 to 70 percent of the heart rate reserve.[81] Because mild to moderate disease does not provide a pulmonary limitation to exercise, a maximal cardiovascular exercise test is likely to have been performed. Exercise intensity can be in the mid-range of THRR (in the example 120 to 136 beats/min) to ensure cardiovascular training. Patients with moderate to severe pulmonary impairment will reach their ventilatory maximum before their cardiovascular maximum is approached; that is, their maximal exercise heart rate is lower than their cardiovascular heart rate maximum would be. For these patients, exercise intensities that approach their maximum ventilatory limits or the upper end of the THRR, 70 to 85 percent of heart rate reserve, can be used.[11,82] In the example, this would be a THR of 136 to 148 beats per minute. It should be emphasized that exercise intensity should be prescribed with an upper and lower heart rate limit, not a single number because a patient can demonstrate HR fluctuations of up to 10 percent during a single exercise session.

EXERCISE AS A PERCENT OF Vo_{2MAX}

A GXT reports functional capacity in terms of Vo_2, or maximum **metabolic equivalents** (**METs**), attained during exercise. Exercise intensity can be prescribed using a percent of the maximum Vo_2 achieved on a GXT. Owing to the pulmonary limitations of patients with COPD, research has shown that some patients can exercise up to 95 percent of their Vo_{2max}.[83]

There are some difficulties using METs to prescribe exercise intensity for patients with pulmonary disease. Often, a normative table is used to categorize an activity according to the **oxygen consumption,** or the number of METs, required to perform that activity (one MET equals 3.5 mL of oxygen used per kilogram of body weight). Patients with pulmonary dysfunction may not respond to exercise in a normative fashion. The participant has an individual oxygen consumption for each activity, and this may vary considerably from the normative chart. Day-to-day variations in environmental conditions, patient abilities, and stress level may change the metabolic cost of an activity. The difference between the actual oxygen expenditure and predicted norms makes prescribing exercise intensity by METs somewhat imprecise.

RATING OF PERCEIVED SHORTNESS OF BREATH

Patients with pulmonary disease can use a scale for rating perceived shortness of breath, a variation of the Borg scale for rating of perceived exertion (RPE), to prescribe exercise intensity (Table 15–4). Because patients with pulmonary disease may have poor ventilatory reserves but adequate heart rate reserves, the use of a scale of perceived shortness of breath becomes a useful tool for monitoring exercise intensity by subjective means.[84] Ratings between 3 (moderately short of breath) and 6 (between severely and very severely short of breath) define the range within which patients with pulmonary dysfunction generally exercise. A rating of 3 corresponds approximately to 50 percent of Vo_{2max}. A rating of 6 corresponds approximately to 85 percent of Vo_{2max}[70] (see also Chapter 16 for more information about the Borg scale of perceived exertion).

The prescription for exercise intensity should incorporate symptoms of shortness of breath and fatigue rather than being based strictly on THR, fixed work levels, or METs.[82,83] Clinicians often prefer to prescribe exercise by utilizing a combination of prescription by heart rate and the rating of perceived exertion or perceived shortness of breath.

Duration

Exercising within the target heart rate for at least 20 minutes is recommended. The duration of the training session varies according to patient tolerance, with some participants not being able to

Table 15–4 THE BORG SCALE FOR RATING PERCEIVED SHORTNESS OF BREATH

0	Nothing at all
0.5	Very, very slight (just noticeable)
1	Very slight
2	Slight
3	Moderate
4	Somewhat severe
5	Severe
6	
7	Very severe
8	
9	Very, very severe (almost maximal)
10	Maximal

Reprinted with permission from Borg, G.[80]

maintain the exercise intensity prescribed for the full 20 minutes. Frequent rest periods can be interspersed with exercise to accomplish a total of 20 minutes of exercise.

Frequency

The frequency of exercise refers to the number of sessions performed on a weekly basis during the exercise training period. The frequency of exercise is often dependent on the intensity that can be achieved and the duration that can be maintained. If 20 minutes of aerobic exercise can be accomplished within the THR, then three to five evenly spaced workouts per week are recommended. More frequent exercise sessions are recommended for patients with lower functional abilities. One to two daily sessions are advisable for patients with very low functional work capacities.

PULMONARY REHABILITATION SESSION

Aerobic Training

The aerobic training portion of a pulmonary rehabilitation session includes the following components: check-in, warm-up, aerobic exercise, and cool-down periods. The check-in period is a time to take vital signs, including resting heart rate, respiratory rate, blood pressure, auscultation of the lungs, and weight. It is also the time to discuss with patients their medication schedule, any problems they have encountered, and any changes that need to be noted and addressed by a member of the pulmonary rehabilitation team. If the patient was found to have a decrease in FEV_1 of 10 percent or more on the GXT, a prescribed inhaler should be used at this time. If a patient was found to have a decrease in oxygenation with exercise, the supplemental oxygen should be readied at this time.

Prior to the aerobic period of exercise, the participant performs stretching exercises to help prevent musculoskeletal injuries. Stretching exercises should be performed during exhalation to prevent a valsalva maneuver, which would worsen a participant's pulmonary capabilities. Patients often use accessory muscles of ventilation during the exercise program; therefore, the neck and upper extremities should be incorporated into the stretching program. The warm-up component is a time to slowly increase the HR and BP to ready the cardiovascular system for aerobic exercise. This is usually accomplished by performing the same mode of exercise that will be used in the aerobic portion of the program but at a lower intensity, with an emphasis on controlled breathing. For example, cycling with no resistance could be used as a warm-up activity for a patient with a biking program. The warm-up portion of the program lasts between 5 and 15 minutes.

The aerobic portion of the rehabilitation session consists of a mode or modes of aerobic exercise at the appropriate intensity to maintain the THR of the exercise prescription for the advised duration. This portion of the program lasts from at least 20 minutes up to 60 minutes. The participant can be monitored by using a rating of perceived shortness of breath, heart rate values, respiratory rate, and oximetry to measure Sao_2. The aerobic training period should be followed immediately by a cool-down period. This consists of 5 to 15 minutes of low-level aerobic activities that slowly return the cardiovascular system to near pre-exercise levels. Again, there is an emphasis on controlled breathing. Finally, stretching exercises are repeated to maintain joint and muscle integrity and to help prevent injury.

Strength Training

Strength of both upper and lower extremities will increase with appropriate training. Strength training can use similar modes of exercise as the endurance training with a change to higher resistance and lower repetitions (i.e., increase the grade of treadmill, increase resistance on stationary cycle or arm ergometer), or weight training of the involved muscle groups can be prescribed. Patients with COPD who desaturated during graded exercise testing have shown stable Sao_2 values during weight training.[85] Participants should be encouraged to refrain from using the valsalva maneuver during training as this may impair ventilatory exchange and effect exercise performance.

Exercise Progression

Modifications in the duration and intensity of the exercise session should be made as an individual physiologically adapts to exercise. Exercise progression is appropriate when the individual perceives the intensity of the exercise session to be easier or when the same exercise intensity is performed with a lesser degree of shortness of breath and lower heart rate.

The duration of exercise should be increased by extending the amount of time spent in continuous aerobic activity and decreasing the amount of time spent in rest periods. The goal of duration progression would be a continuous 20 minutes of aerobic activity without the need for a rest. When at least 20 minutes of activity can be accomplished, then an increase in exercise intensity can be proposed. Frequency should be adjusted as necessary, based on duration and intensity.

A patient's age, functional ability, symptoms, and severity of disease must be considered prior to any change in the exercise prescription. It is advisable, when considerable change in a participant's ability has occurred, to perform a new GXT. The new exercise prescription will allow for a safe and comfortable progression of exercise under controlled guidance.

Program Duration

Improved exercise tolerance can occur during an inpatient hospital admission, as an outpatient, or with a program of home-based care. Because of the limited length of stays in many hospital admissions, most increases in functional capacity occur during an outpatient or home program. Generally, conditioning exercises are conducted three times per week over a course of 6 to 8 weeks. At the end of the rehabilitation program, patients are reevaluated. A second exercise test may be performed to assess the exercise prescription for continuation of care. Although GXTs may provide a wealth of information, a 6- or 12-minute walk test, with its ease of administration, makes it a valuable pre- and post-pulmonary rehabilitation program outcome measure.

Home Exercise Programs

A home exercise program (HEP) usually begins while the participant is still enrolled in an outpatient pulmonary rehabilitation program. When the staff deems it feasible (based on exercise and laboratory data), the participant can be assigned exercise activities to be done at home. The patient returns to the outpatient clinic with an exercise log containing the heart rate, RPEs, exercise parameters, and any problems that may have occurred during the home program. The staff analyzes this data and adjusts the home program if necessary. Progression of the patient to a home program and to independent exercise is an important goal of the rehabilitation program.

An unfortunate reality is that patients with pulmonary dysfunction often have respiratory setbacks from exacerbations of their disease. Continued contact and encouragement in the form of periodic evaluation are essential to maintain the new level of physical activity. However, reimbursement for such care can be difficult to obtain. Patients are encouraged to join community-based groups that facilitate compliance with their medical and exercise regimens (e.g., the Better Breathing Club, sponsored by the American Lung Association).

Multispecialty Team

A diversity of health professionals is essential to meet the medical, physical, social, and psychological needs of the patient with pulmonary disease. The team may include nurses, physicians, physical therapists, occupational therapists, nutritionists, respiratory care practitioners, exercise physiologists, psychiatrists, psychologists, social workers, recreational therapists, clergy, and most importantly, the patient and the patient's family.

Although aerobic exercise training is integral to pulmonary rehabilitation, patients may require additional services and information to optimize their exercise capability and to improve quality of life.

The following section addresses other elements of a pulmonary rehabilitation program: patient education, secretion removal techniques, ventilatory muscle training and breathing re-education, pacing, and smoking cessation.

Patient Education

The concept of self-management is promoted in the educational sessions of a pulmonary rehabilitation program. By using both individual and group sessions for education, the benefits of both types of interaction can be attained. Participants are given individual, one-on-one time to identify their own needs and address issues that are particular to themselves. Benefits from group discussions include support from peers regarding the patient's feelings or needs, learning from others' experiences and questions, and the socialization only a group can provide. Key components of an education program can be found in Box 15–2.

Education makes it possible for a patient to assume responsibility for his or her own wellness. An individual will carry out the required activities to produce the desired outcome only if he or she knows what to do, how to do it, and also wants to do it.[86] This theory of self-efficacy for the patient with pulmonary disease begins with a daily routine that includes self-assessment, adherence to a medication schedule, and performing airway clearance, activities of daily living with pacing, and an exercise session.

Self-assessment is used to recognize the first sign of an exacerbation of the disease (increased dyspnea, decreased exercise tolerance, change in sputum color or consistency, pedal edema, or any other significant change from baseline).[42] An exacerbation protocol is devised for each patient that includes a set of standard instructions consistent with the participant's disease and abilities. Depending on the

---

Box 15–2 EDUCATION SESSION TOPICS

Anatomy and physiology of respiratory disease
Airway clearance techniques
Nutritional guidelines
Energy-saving techniques
Stress management and relaxation
Benefits of being smoke free
Environmental factors
Pharmacology/use of MDIs
Oxygen delivery systems
Psychosocial aspects of COPD
Diagnostic techniques
Management of COPD
Community resources
Exercise: Effects, contraindications, compliance

COPD, chronic obstructive pulmonary disease; MDIs, metered dose inhalers.

skill of the participant, these behaviors may include a call to the primary care physician or nurse practitioner, as well as the initiation of certain medications (bronchodilators, antibiotics, corticosteroids) that the participant should have on hand at all times.

Patients should understand the action of each prescribed medication, as well as how it is to be taken. The specific medication schedule must be set up to realistically bridge the sometimes opposing issues of optimal timing of the drug and patient compliance. A different type of patient education is required for medications that are taken on an "as needed" (PRN) basis.

Patients should perform independent airway clearance techniques on a regular basis. Dependent airway clearance provided by a family member or therapist should be scheduled on a regular basis. Independent home exercise sessions should be performed on a regular basis as well as those scheduled at a rehabilitation program. Activities of daily living should be practiced at all times using pacing techniques (described later in this chapter) when indicated.

Individuals can be taught to manage their lung disease with a well-designed educational program.[87] Compared to education alone, education as part of a comprehensive pulmonary rehabilitation program produced significantly improved exercise abilities, decreased dyspnea, and greater self-efficacy.[88]

Secretion Removal Techniques

Secretion retention can interfere with ventilation and the diffusion of oxygen and carbon dioxide. An assessment of the pulmonary system will identify the areas of secretion retention. An individualized program of secretion removal techniques directed to the areas of involvement can optimize ventilation and therefore gas exchange capabilities. Patients with secretion retention may improve their performance on an exercise regimen if the proper secretion removal techniques are provided prior to the exercise session.

POSTURAL DRAINAGE

Positioning a patient so that the bronchus of the involved lung segment is perpendicular to the ground is the basis for **postural drainage.** Using gravity, these positions assist the mucociliary transport system in removing excessive secretions from the tracheobronchial tree. Standard postural drainage positions are presented in Figure 15-6. Although these postural drainage positions are optimal for gravity drainage of specific lung segments, they may not be realistic for some patients. The standard position for postural drainage could make a patient's respiratory status, or a concomitant problem, worse. Modification of these standard positions may prevent any untoward effects and still enhance secretion removal. Box 15–3 lists precautions that should be considered prior to instituting postural drainage

with patients enrolled in an outpatient pulmonary rehabilitation program. These are not absolute contraindications, but relative precautions. The list is not meant to be inclusive; however, it does provide the reader with a range of dysfunction that should be considered prior to instituting postural drainage.

PERCUSSION

Percussion is a force rhythmically applied with the therapist's cupped hands to the patient's chest wall. The percussion technique is applied to a specific area on the thorax that corresponds to an underlying involved lung segment. The technique is typically administered for 3 to 5 minutes over each involved lung segment. Percussion is thought to release the pulmonary secretions from the wall of the airways and into the lumen of the airway.[89] Unfortunately, this process seems to be nondirectional. That is, the secretions may be moved closer to the glottis or deeper into the pulmonary parenchyma. By coupling percussion with the appropriate postural drainage position for a specific lung segment, the probability of secretion removal is enhanced.[90–92] Because percussion is a force directed to the thorax, there are precautions that need to be considered prior to its use. These precautions are outlined in Box 15–4. The list is again by no means inclusive. It does provide some general guidelines that deserve consideration when percussion is part of the therapeutic regimen. It should be noted also that some modification of this technique can be made to enhance patient tolerance.

SHAKING

Following a deep inhalation, a bouncing maneuver is applied to the rib cage throughout the expiratory phase of breathing. This **shaking** is applied to a specific area on the thorax that corresponds to the underlying involved lung segment. Five to seven trials of shaking are appropriate to hasten the removal of secretions via the mucociliary transport system and prevent possible hyperventilation. Shaking is commonly used following percussion in the appropriate postural drainage position. Because this technique consists of a force applied to the thorax, the same considerations are needed as in the application of percussion.

AIRWAY CLEARANCE

Once the secretions have been mobilized with postural drainage, percussion, and shaking or vibration, the task of removing the secretions from the airways is undertaken. *Coughing* is the most common and easiest means of clearing the airway. *Huffing* is another method of airway clearance that is useful for patients with COPD. High intrathoracic pressures, such as those generated during coughing, can force the closing of small airways in some patients. By trapping air behind the closed airway, the forced expulsion of air during a cough becomes ineffective in clearing secretions. A huff uses many of the same steps of coughing, without creating the

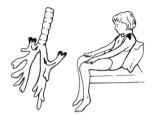

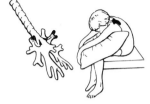

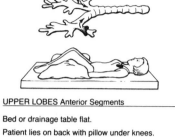

UPPER LOBES Apical Segments

Bed or drainage table flat.

Patient leans back on pillow at 30° angle against therapist.

Therapist claps with markedly cupped hand over area between clavicle and top of scapula on each side.

UPPER LOBES Posterior Segments

Bed or drainage table flat.

Patient leans over folded pillow at 30° angle.

Therapist stands behind and claps over upper back on both sides.

UPPER LOBES Anterior Segments

Bed or drainage table flat.

Patient lies on back with pillow under knees.

Therapist claps between clavicle and nipple on each side.

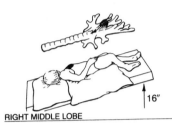

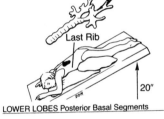

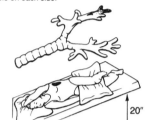

RIGHT MIDDLE LOBE

Foot of table or bed elevated 16 inches.

Patient lies head down on left side and rotates ¼ turn backward. Pillow may be placed behind from shoulder to hip. Knees should be flexed.

Therapist claps over right nipple area. In females with breast development or tenderness, use cupped hand with heel of hand under armpit and fingers extending forward beneath the breast.

LEFT UPPER LOBE Lingular Segments

Foot of table or bed elevated 16 inches.

Patient lies head down on right side and rotates ¼ turn backward. Pillow may be placed behind from shoulder to hip. Knees should be flexed.

Therapist claps with moderately cupped hand over left nipple area. In females with breast development or tenderness, use cupped hand with heel of hand under armpit and fingers extending forward beneath the breast.

LOWER LOBES Anterior Basal Segments

Foot of table or bed elevated 20 inches.

Patient lies on side, head down, pillow under knees.

Therapist claps with slightly cupped hand over lower ribs. (Position shown is for drainage of left anterior basal segment. To drain the right anterior basal segment, patient should lie on the left side in same posture.)

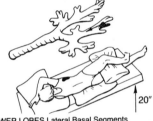

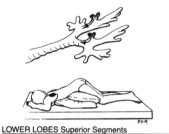

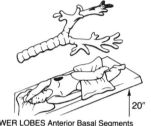

LOWER LOBES Lateral Basal Segments

Foot of table or bed elevated 20 inches.

Patient lies on abdomen, head down, then rotates ¼ turn upward. Upper leg is flexed over a pillow for support.

Therapist claps over uppermost portion of lower ribs. (Position shown is for drainage of right lateral basal segment. To drain the left lateral basal segment, patient should lie on his right side in the same posture.)

LOWER LOBES Posterior Basal Segments

Foot of table or bed elevated 20 inches.

Patient lies on abdomen, head down, with pillow under hips. Therapist claps over lower ribs close to spine on each side.

LOWER LOBES Superior Segments

Bed or table flat.

Patient lies on abdomen with two pillows under hips.

Therapist claps over middle of back at tip of scapula on either side of spine.

Figure 15–6. Positions used for postural drainage. (From Rothstein, J, et al: The Rehabilitation Specialist's Handbook. FA Davis, Philadelphia, 1991, pp 624–625, with permission.)

Box 15–3 PRECAUTIONS FOR POSTURAL DRAINAGE

Precautions for the use of the *Trendelenberg* position
  Circulatory: pulmonary edema, congestive heart failure, hypertension
  Abdominal: obesity, abdominal distention, hiatal hernia, nausea, recent food consumption
  Shortness of breath made worse with the Trendelenberg position
Precautions for the use of the side-lying position
  Vascular: axillofemoral bypass graft
  Musculoskeletal: arthritis, recent rib fracture, shoulder bursitis, or tendonitis, any conditioning that would make appropriate postural drainage positioning uncomfortable

---

high intrathoracic pressures. The patient is asked to take a deep breath and rapidly contract the abdominal muscles and forcefully saying "HA HA HA." This allows a forced expiration through a stabilized open airway and makes secretion removal more effective.[93]

Ventilatory Muscle Training and Breathing Re-Education

The inability to sufficiently increase ventilation and a sense of breathlessness are often limiting factors in functional activities and exercise tolerance of patients with pulmonary dysfunction. Optimizing ventilatory function can decrease the work of breathing, decrease the severity of breathlessness, and improve the ability to perform work.[94–96] Ventilatory muscle training has been utilized to improve the strength and endurance of the muscles of ventilation, thus increasing the efficiency of breathing.

There are specific devices, *ventilatory muscle trainers (VMTs)*, that provide inspiratory resistance via graded aperture openings. The patient breathes in through this narrowed opening, which loads the inspiratory muscles and thereby trains the muscles of ventilation.[96] By changing the size of the aperture opening, training programs for both strength and endurance of the inspiratory muscles can be formulated. Although VMT is not seen as an essential component of pulmonary rehabilitation, it may be used in some patients who show decreased strength of the ventilatory muscles or constraints on exercise owing to breathlessness.[12]

Although not a physiological training technique, breathing re-education teaches a more efficient pattern of breathing and can decrease the work of breathing. Breathing pattern training, enhanced with visual feedback, has been shown to increase the FEV_1 and FVC in patients with COPD.[97] Encouraging the use of the diaphragm, the principle and most efficient muscle of inspiration, can decrease the oxygen cost of breathing. Decreasing the use of accessory muscles also decreases the work of breathing. Biofeedback can be used to discourage accessory muscle firing during the ventilatory cycle, thus emphasizing the proper use of the diaphragm.

Pursed-lip breathing, when used by patients with COPD, has been shown to decrease respiratory rate and increase tidal volume.[98] Pursed-lip breathing may delay or prevent airway collapse, allowing for better gas exchange.[99]

PACING

Pacing refers to the performance of an activity within the limits or boundaries of that patient's breathing capacity. Often, this means that the activity needs to be broken down into component parts such that each component can be performed at a rate that does not exceed breathing abilities. By breaking activities down into component parts, interspersing rest periods between each component, the total activity can be safely completed without dyspnea and fatigue. Pacing can and should be part of every activity that would otherwise cause dyspnea. Pacing refers to daily tasks such as activities of daily living, ambulation, stair climbing, and so forth.

Pacing is not a technique to be used during the aerobic portion of a pulmonary rehabilitation program. During exercise, some shortness of breath should and will occur.

Smoking Cessation

Smoking is the leading cause of the development of COPD, as well as a contributing cause to many other disease processes. Therefore, a special focus on the effects of smoking and smoking cessation should be included in pulmonary rehabilitation programs.

There are many types of smoking cessation programs, such as behavior modification, "cold turkey," diversion therapy, aversion therapy, nicotine gum, or nicotine patch.[100–106] No single method of smoking cessation can claim a higher success rate over another in the long run. A comprehensive treatment approach incorporating many different smoking cessation strategies has a higher abstention rate than any single specific technique.[104–106] It is the role of the clinician to guide the patient in his or her efforts to quit smoking, not necessarily to provide this service. The regional offices of the American Lung Association and the American Cancer Society are good resources for local smoking cessation programs.

SUMMARY

Pulmonary rehabilitation programs have become well established in recent years. Components of these programs typically include exercise training, respiratory care instruction, education, and psychosocial support. The slow and steady decreases in a person's activity secondary to increases in pulmonary discomfort can be interrupted by pulmonary rehabilitation. Increases in exercise tolerance have been documented and maintained in follow-up studies.[59,107–109] Pulmonary rehabilitation resulted in an improvement in symptoms, specifically dyspnea, during exercise and activities of daily living.[110–113] Increases in functional abilities can make the difference between a life-style of independence and one of dependence. Haas and Cardon[114] reported that, for patients who did not receive pulmonary rehabilitation, the percentage who were admitted to nursing homes and were not able to provide their own self-care was greater than for patients who did receive pulmonary rehabilitation. A reduction in the number of hospitalizations or hospital days by patients following pulmonary rehabilitation has been reported.[20,114–118] Increases in the quality of life for patients who have participated in pulmonary rehabilitation programs have also been reported.[10,61,119,120] Physical therapists have the important role of assessing patients, determining their potential, and through exercise prescription and exercise programs, ensuring that rehabilitation goals are realized.

QUESTIONS FOR REVIEW

1. How does the clinical presentation of obstructive disease differ from the clinical presentation of restrictive disease?

2. Explain how increased secretions within the tracheobronchial tree in chronic bronchitis lead to emphysema.

3. What would be the expected breath sounds of a patient with emphysema? With asthma during an exacerbation? (Remember to describe intensity as well as adventitious sounds.)

4. Identify the tests and measures required to determine the extent of pulmonary disease.

5. What are the pulmonary end points to a symptom-limited graded exercise test?

6. How does exercise prescription differ for a patient with mild pulmonary disease and the patient with severe pulmonary disease?

7. How do you know when to progress a patient's exercise program? What is the nature of that progression? When is another exercise test warranted?

8. How would you explain stair climbing that utilizes the principles of pacing to a patient with pulmonary disease? How would you combat the patient's assumption that it would take longer to climb stairs with pacing than without?

9. Design a secretion removal treatment plan for a patient with CF that can be carried out by his or her family prior to coming to pulmonary rehabilitation.

10. What evidence is presented in the current literature regarding the benefits of pulmonary rehabilitation?

CASE STUDY: PATIENT WITH COPD

A 67 year-old white female was admitted to the hospital with a diagnosis of acute bacterial pneumonia. She was treated with mechanical ventilation for 5 days, steroids, antibiotics, and bronchodilators. After the acute care hospital stay of 7 days, the patient was transferred to a rehabilitation facility for 5 days. She is now referred to outpatient physical therapy.

PAST MEDICAL HISTORY: COPD, pneumonia × 4 over the past 2 years, s/p lumpectomy of right breast 8 years ago, smoking history of 45 pack/years, quit on day of admission to hospital for acute bacterial pneumonia.

MEDICATIONS: 2 L/min of pulsed oxygen, atrovent 4 puffs QID, ventilin PRN, prednisone 5 mg/d.

OCCUPATION: Secretary, works 32 hours/week. Presently on medical leave.

SOCIAL: Lives with husband in own home. Ramp to front door, 6 stairs within the home.

OBJECTIVE FINDINGS

INTERVIEW: Mental Status: awake, alert, talks in 3 to 4 word sentences. Adequate historian. Chief complaint: shortness of breath limiting function. Patient is able to walk short distances before needing to rest to catch her breath. No complaints of increased secretions. Baseline dyspnea index: functional impairment, grade 1; magnitude of task, grade 1; magnitude of effort, grade 1. Patient's desired functional outcome is to be oxygen free and able to care for grandchildren without shortness of breath.

VITAL SIGNS: HR 72, BP 96/74, Sao$_2$ 98% on 2 L/min pulsed O$_2$ on 1 pulse/breath, RR 34, Temp 98.5°F.

OBSERVATION, INSPECTION, PALPATION: Thin, frail-looking female wearing nasal cannula. Kyphosis noted. Patient uses posture of forward sitting with arms supported to enhance ventilatory accessory muscle use. Increased AP diameter, increased accessory muscle use. Labored, symmetrical breathing pattern. No venous distention, no edema, no cyanosis, clubbing evident.

AUSCULTATION: Decreased breath sounds throughout both lung fields, especially at bases. End expiratory wheezes at left lateral base.

STRENGTH: Lower extremity manual muscle testing grossly 4/5 (good) except bilateral quadriceps strength 3/5 (fair). Upper extremity grossly 4/5 (good). Maximal inspiratory effort: 52 mmHg.

FUNCTIONAL INDEPENDENCE MEASUREMENTS (FIM SCORES): Ambulation: 6 (modified independence—slow gait with pacing necessary). Stairs: 6 (modified independence: requires pacing and railing). Patient is dependent in shopping, house cleaning, and laundry.

EXERCISE TEST DATA: Patient performed a 7-minute, staged (3 min/stage) exercise test using a modified protocol. Miles per hour was held constant at 2 mph, grade increased from 0 to 2 to 3 percent. ECG was within normal limits. RHR was 84 beats per minute, HR$_{MAX}$ 121 beats per minute. Sao$_2$ resting 98 percent on 2 liters pulsed 1:1. Sao$_2$ decreased to 93 percent at max exercise and decreased to 90 percent during the first minute of cool down on 2 liters pulsed oxygen. Rate of perceived shortness of breath at max exercise was 7. Exercise was terminated due to patient request.

LABORATORY TEST DATA: None available.

Guiding Questions

1. Generate a physical therapy problem list.
2. Identify anticipated treatment goals.
3. Identify functional outcomes of physical therapy.
4. Formulate a physical therapy plan of care for week 1. Patient will be seen 3 times/week for this first week of therapy.

REFERENCES

1. Fishman, AP: Pulmonary rehabilitation research. Am J Respir Crit Care Med 149:825, 1994.
2. Hughes, R, and Davison, R: Limitation of exercise reconditioning in COLD. Chest 83:241, 1983.
3. Pierce, A, et al: Responses to exercise training in patients with emphysema. Arch Intern Med 114:28, 1964.
4. Hale, T, et al: The effects of physical training in chronic obstructive pulmonary disease. Bull Eur Physiopath Resp 14:593, 1978.
5. Reis, A, et al: Effects of pulmonary rehabilitation on physiologic and psychosocial outcomes in patients with Chronic Obstructive Pulmonary Disease. Ann Intern Med 122:823, 1995.
6. Wijkstra, P, et al: Effects of home rehabilitation on physical performance in patients with Chronic Obstructive Pulmonary Disease (COPD). Eur Respir J 9:104, 1996.
7. Bass, H, et al: Exercise training: Therapy for patients with chronic obstructive pulmonary disease. Chest 57:116, 1970.
8. Vyas, M, et al: Response to exercise in patients with chronic airway obstruction, I. Effects of exercise training. Am Rev Respir Dis 103:390, 1971.
9. O'Donnell, D, et al: The impact of exercise reconditioning on breathlessness in severe chronic airflow limitation. Am J Respir Crit Care Med 152:2005, 1995.
10. Bebout, D, et al: Clinical and physiological outcomes of a university hospital pulmonary rehabilitation program. Respiratory Care 28:1468, 1983.
11. Carter, R, et al: Exercise conditioning in the rehabilitation of patients with chronic obstructive pulmonary disease. Arch Phys Med Rehabil 69:118, 1988.
12. Pulmonary rehabilitation: Joint ACCP/AACVPR evidence-based guidelines. Chest 112:1363, 1997.
13. Ries, A: Position paper of the American Association of Cardiovascular and Pulmonary Rehabilitation: Scientific basis of pulmonary rehabilitation. J Cardiopulmonary Rehabil 10:418, 1990.
14. Casaburi, R, and Petty, T: Principles and Practice of Pulmonary Rehabilitation. WB Saunders, Philadelphia, 1993.
15. Foster, S, and Thomas, H: Pulmonary rehabilitation in lung disease other than chronic obstructive pulmonary disease. Am Rev Respir Dis 141:601, 1990.
16. Orenstein, D, and Noyes, B: Cystic Fibrosis. In Casaburi, R, and Petty, T (eds): Principles and Practice of Pulmonary Rehabilitation. WB Saunders, Philadelphia, 1993, p 439.
17. Gaissert, H, et al: Comparison of early functional results after volume reduction or lung transplantation for chronic obstructive pulmonary disease. J Thorac Cardiovasc Surg 111:293, 1996.
18. West, J: Pulmonary Pathophysiology: The essentials, ed 5. Williams & Wilkins, Baltimore, 1995.
19. Martin, D, and Youtsey, J: Respiratory Anatomy and Physiology. Mosby, St. Louis, 1988.
20. American Thoracic Society: Standards for the diagnosis and care of patients with chronic obstructive pulmonary disease (COPD) and asthma. Am J Respir Crit Care Med 152:S77, 1995.
21. American Thoracic Society: Standards for the diagnosis and care of patients with chronic obstructive pulmonary disease (COPD) and asthma. Am Rev Respir Dis 136:225, 1987.
22. Hammon, W, and Hasson S: Cardiopulmonary Pathophysiology. In Frownfelter, D, and Dean, E: Principles and Practice of Cardiopulmonary Physical Therapy, ed 3. Mosby-Year Book, St. Louis, 1996, p 71.
23. Farzan, S: A Concise Handbook of Respiratory Diseases, ed 2. Reston, Reston, VA, 1985.
24. Sheldon, J: Boyd's Introduction to the Study of Disease, ed 10. Lea & Febiger, Philadelphia, 1988.
25. Morris, J (Chairman): Chronic obstructive pulmonary disease. American Lung Association Publication, New York, 1981.
26. Thurlbeck, Z: Chronic airflow obstruction in lung disease, Vol 5, Major Problems in Pathology. WB Saunders, Philadelphia, 1976, p 378.
27. Wright, J, et al: The detection of small airways disease. Am Rev Respir Dis 129:989, 1984.
28. Cosio, M, et al: The relationship between structural changes in small airways and pulmonary function tests. N Engl J Med 298:1277, 1977.
29. Bates, D: The fate of the chronic bronchitic: A report of the 10-year follow-up in the Canadian department of veteran's affairs coordinated study of chronic bronchitis. Am Rev Respir Dis 108:1043, 1973.
30. Travers, G, et al: Predictors of mortality in chronic obstructive pulmonary disease. Am Rev Respir Dis 119:902, 1979.
31. Nemeny, B, et al: Changes in lung function after smoking cessation: An assessment from a cross sectional survey. Am Rev Respir Dis 125:122, 1982.
32. Anthonisen, N, et al: Effects of smoking intervention and the use of an inhaled anticholinergic bronchodilator on the rate of decline of FEV_1: The Lung Health Study. JAMA 272:1497, 1994.
33. Ziment, I: Editorial review, asthma. Curr Opin Pulm Med 3:1, 1997.
34. Sibbaid, B, et al: Genetic factors in childhood asthma. Thorax 35:671, 1980.
35. Berte, J: Critical Care, the Lungs, ed 2. Appleton-Century-Crofts, Norwalk, CT, 1986.
36. Burki, N: Pulmonary Diseases. Medical Examination, Garden City, NY, 1982.
37. Mezac, D, and Gershwin, E: Why is asthma becoming more of a problem? Curr Opin Pulm Med 3:6, 1997.
38. Tecklin, J: Pediatric Physical Therapy, ed 2. JB Lippincott, Philadelphia, 1994, p 275.
39. Aitken, M: Editorial overview: Cystic fibrosis. Curr Opin Pulm Med 2:435, 1996.
40. Sharma, O: Editorial review: Ideopathic pulmonary fibrosis. Curr Opin Pulm Med 2:343, 1996.
41. Chapman, K: An international perspective on anticholinergic therapy. Am J Med 100:2S, 1996.
42. Tiep, B: Disease management of COPD with pulmonary rehabilitation. Chest 112:1630, 1997.
43. Belman, M, et al: Inhaled bronchodilators reduce dynamic hyperinflation during exercise in patients with chronic obstructive pulmonary disease. Am J Respir Crit Care Med 153:967, 1996.
44. Kotarski, M, et al: Bone density site comparison in a pulmonary rehabilitation program and the implications for therapy. Abstract. J Cardiopulmonary Rehabil 16:326, 1996.
45. Rooyachers, P, et al: Training with supplemental oxygen in patients with COPD and hypoxemia at peak exercise. Eur Respir J 10:1278, 1997.
46. Bendett, J, and Albert, R: Surgical options for patients with advanced emphysema. Clin Chest Med 18:577, 1997.
47. Connolly, J: Results of bullectomy. Chest Surgery Clinics of North America 5:765, 1995.
48. American Thoracic Society Statement: Lung transplantation. Am Rev Respir Dis 147:772, 1993.
49. Kesten, S: Pulmonary rehabilitation and surgery for end stage lung disease: Clin Chest Med 18:173, 1997.
50. Ludwick, S: Exercise testing and training: Primary cardiopulmonary dysfunction. In Frownfelter, D, and Dean, E (eds): Principles and Practice of Cardiopulmonary Physical Therapy, ed 3. Mosby-Year Book, St. Louis, 1996, p 417.
51. American Physical Therapy Association: Guide to Physical Therapist Practice. APTA, Alexandria, VA, 1999, 6F1.
52. Mahler D, et al: The impact of dyspnea and physiologic function in general health status in patients with chronic obstructive pulmonary disease. Chest 102:395, 1992.
53. Mahler D: Dyspnea: Diagnosis and management. Clin Chest Med 8:215, 1987.
54. Murphy, R: Auscultation of the lung: Past lessons, future possibilities. Thorax 36:99, 1981.
55. ACCP-ATS joint committee on pulmonary nomenclature: Pulmonary terms and symbols: A report of the ACCP-ATS joint committee on pulmonary nomenclature. Chest 67:583, 1975.

56. Forgacs, P: Crackles and wheezes. Lancet 2:203, 1967.
57. Gosslink, R, et al: Peripheral muscle weakness contributes to exercise limitation in COPD. Am J Respir Crit Care Med 153:976, 1996.
58. Killian, J, et al: Exercise capacity and ventilatory, circulatory and symptom limitation in patient with chronic airflow limitation. Am Rev Respir Dis 146:935, 1992.
59. Simpson, K, et al: Randomized controlled trial of weight lifting exercise in patients with chronic airflow limitation. Thorax 47:70, 1992.
60. Cahalin, L, et al: The relationship of the 6 min walk test to maximum oxygen consumption in transplant candidates with end stage lung disease. Chest 108:452, 1995.
61. Steele, B: Timed walking test of exercise capacity in chronic cardiopulmonary illness. J Cardiopulmonary Rehabil 16:25, 1996.
62. Cooper, K: A means of assessing maximal oxygen intake: Correlation between held and treadmill walking. JAMA 203:201, 1968.
63. Guyatt, G, et al: Long-term outcome after respiratory rehabilitation. Can Med Assoc J 137:1089, 1987.
64. Jones, N: Exercise testing in pulmonary evaluation: Rationale, methods and the normal respiratory response to exercise. N Engl J Med 293:541, 1975.
65. Carter, R, et al: Exercise gas exchange in patients with moderate severe to severe chronic obstructive pulmonary disease. J Cardiopulmonary Rehabil 9:243, 1989.
66. Berman, L, and Sutton, J: Exercise for the pulmonary patient. J Cardiopulmonary Rehabil 6:55, 1986.
67. Naughton, J, et al: Modified work capacity studies in individuals with and without coronary artery disease. J Sports Med 4:208, 1964.
68. Balke, B, and Ware, R: An experimental study of physical fitness of air force personnel. US Armed Forces Med J 10:675, 1959.
69. American Thoracic Society: Evaluation of impairment secondary to respiratory disease. Am Rev Respir Dis 126:945, 1982.
70. American College of Sports Medicine: Guidelines for Exercise Testing and Prescription, ed 5. Lea & Febiger, Philadelphia, 1995.
71. Hodgkins, J, et al: Pulmonary rehabilitation: Guidelines to success. Butterworth, Boston, 1984.
72. Wilson, P, et al: Rehabilitation of the Heart and Lungs. Beckman Instruments, Fullerton, CA, 1980.
73. Lake, F, et al: Upper limb and lower limb exercise training in patients with chronic airflow obstruction. Chest 97:1077, 1990.
74. Reis, A, et al: Upper extremity exercise training in chronic obstructive pulmonary disease. Chest 93:688, 1988.
75. Fletcherr, G, et al: American Heart Association Medical Scientific Statement: Special report-exercise standards: A statement for health professionals. The American Heart Association. Circulation 82:2286, 1990.
76. American College of Sports Medicine 1990: Position stand: The recommended quantity and quality of exercise for developing and maintaining cardiorespiratory and muscular fitness in healthy adults. Med Sci Sports Exerc 22:265, 1990.
77. Faryniarz, K, and Mahler D: Writing an exercise prescription for patients with COPD. J Respir Dis 11:638, 1990.
78. Horowitz, M, and Mahler, D: The validity of using dyspnea ratings for exercise prescription in patients with COPD. Am Rev Respir Dis 147(Suppl)A:744, 1993.
79. Hodgkins, J, and Litzau, K: Exercise training target heart rates in chronic obstructive pulmonary disease. Chest 94:305, 1988.
80. Borg, G: Psychophysical basis of perceived exertion. Med Sci Sports Exerc 14:377, 1982.
81. Hodgkins, J: Prognosis in chronic obstructive pulmonary disease. Clin Chest Med 11:555, 1990.
82. Reis, A: Endurance exercise training at maximal targets in patients with chronic obstructive pulmonary disease. J Cardiopulmonary Rehabil 7:594, 1987.
83. Punzal, P, et al: Maximum intensity exercise training in patients with chronic obstructive pulmonary disease. Chest 100:618, 1991.
84. Noble, B: Clinical applications of perceived exertion. Med Sci Sports Exerc 14:406, 1982.
85. Manetz, C, et al: Effects of weight training exercises on cutaneous arterial oxygen saturation in patients with chronic obstructive pulmonary disease (Abstract). J of Cardiopulmonary Rehabil 16:323, 1996.
86. Bandura, A: Self-efficacy mechanisms in human agency. American Psychology 37:122, 1982.
87. Zimmerman, B, et al: A self-management program for chronic obstructive pulmonary disease: Relationship to dyspnea and self-efficacy. Rehabilitation Nursing 21:253, 1996.
88. Ries, A, et al: Effects of pulmonary rehabilitation of physiologic and psychosocial outcomes in patients with chronic obstructive pulmonary disease. Ann Intern Med 122:823, 1995.
89. Kigin, C: Advances in chest physical therapy. In O'Donohue, W: Current Advances in Respiratory Care, American College of Chest Physicians, Parkridge, IL, 1983, p 44.
90. Chopra, S, et al: Effects of hydration and physical therapy on tracheal transport velocity. Am Rev Resp Dis 115:1009, 1977.
91. Denton, R: Bronchial secretions in cystic fibrosis. Am Rev Resp Dis 86:41, 1962.
92. Mazzocco, M, et al: Physiologic effects of chest percussion and postural drainage in patients with bronchiectasis. Chest 88:360, 1985.
93. Hietpas, B, et al: Huff coughing and airway patency. Resp Care 24:710, 1979.
94. Harver, A, et al: Targeted inspiratory muscle training improves respiratory function and reduces dyspnea in patient with Chronic Obstructive Pulmonary Disease. Ann Intern Med 111:117, 1989.
95. Pardy, R, et al: Inspiratory muscle training compared to physiotherapy in patients with chronic airflow limitation. Am Rev Respir Dis 123:421, 1981.
96. Smith, K, et al: Respiratory muscle training in chronic airflow limitation: A meta-analysis. Am Rev Respir Dis 145:533, 1992.
97. Esteve, F, et al: The effects of breathing pattern training on ventilatory function in patients with COPD. Biofeedback and Self Regulation 21:311, 1996.
98. Thoman, R, et al: The efficacy of pursed-lips breathing in patients with chronic obstructive pulmonary disease. Am Rev Respir Dis 93:100, 1966.
99. Kigin, C: Breathing exercises for the medical patient: The art and the science. Phys Ther 70:700, 1990.
100. Harris, M, and Rothberg, C: A self-control approach to reducing smoking. Psychol Rep 31:165, 1972.
101. Horn, D, and Waingrow, S: Some dimensions of a model for smoking behavior change. Am J Public Health 56 (Suppl 12):21, 1966.
102. Relinger, J, et al: Utilization of adverse rapid smoking in groups: Efficacy of treatment and maintenance procedures. J Consult Clin Psychol 45:245, 1977.
103. Russell, M, et al: Clinical use of nicotine chewing gum. BMJ 280:1599, 1980.
104. Guilford, J: Group treatment versus individual initiative in the cessation of smoking. J Appl Psychol 56:162, 1972.
105. Peters, J, and Lim, V: Smoking cessation techniques. In Hodgkins, J, et al (eds): Pulmonary Rehabilitation: Guidelines to Success. Butterworth, Boston, 1984, p 91.
106. Lando, J: Successful treatment of smokers with a broad spectrum behavior approach. J Consult Clin Psychol 45:361, 1977.
107. Eakin, E, et al: Clinical trial of rehabilitation in chronic obstructive pulmonary disease: Compliance as a mediator of change in exercise endurance. J Cardiopulmonary Rehabil 12:105, 1992.
108. Swerts, M, et al: Exercise training as a mediator of increased exercise performance in patients with chronic obstructive pulmonary disease. J Cardiopulmonary Rehabil 12:188, 1992.
109. Tydeman, D, et al: An investigation into the effects of exercise tolerance training on patients with chronic airway obstruction. Physiotherapy 70:261, 1984.

110. Martinez, F, et al: Supported arm exercise vs unsupported arm exercise in the rehabilitation of patients with severe chronic airflow obstruction. Chest 103:1397, 1993.

111. Readron, J, et al: The effect of comprehensive outpatient pulmonary rehabilitation on dyspnea. Chest 105:1046, 1994.

112. Lareau, C, et al: Development and testing of the pulmonary functional status and dyspnea questionaire (PFSDQ). Heart Lung 23:242, 1994.

113. Lacassey, Y, et al: Meta analysis of respiratory rehabilitation in chronic obstructive pulmonary disease. Lancet 348:1115, 1996.

114. Haas, A, and Cardon, H: Rehabilitation in chronic obstructive pulmonary disease: A 5-year study of 252 male patients. Med Clin North Am 53:593, 1969.

115. Burns, M, et al: Hospitalization rates of patients before and after a program of pulmonary rehabilitation (Abstract). Am J Respir Crit Care Med 153:A127, 1996.

116. Sneider, R, et al: Trends in pulmonary rehabilitation at Eisenhower Medical Center: An 11-year experience 1976–1987. J Cardiopulmonary Rehabil 8:453, 1988.

117. Lertzman, M, and Cherniack, R: Rehabilitation of patients with chronic obstructive pulmonary disease. Am Rev Respir Dis 114:1145, 1976.

118. Hudson, L, et al: Hospitalization needs during an outpatient rehabilitation program for severe chronic airway obstruction. Chest 70:606, 1976.

119. Jensen, P: Risk, protective factors, and supportive interventions in chronic airway obstruction. Arch Gen Psychiatry 40:1203, 1983.

120. Mall, R, and Medeiros, M: Objective evaluation of results of a pulmonary rehabilitation program in a community hospital. Chest 94:1156, 1988.

SUPPLEMENTAL READINGS

American College of Chest Physicians/American Association of Cardiovascular and Pulmonary Rehabilitation: Evidence Based Guidelines. Chest 112:1363, 1997.

American College of Sports Medicine. Guidelines for Exercise Testing and Prescription, ed 5. Lea & Febiger, Philadelphia, 1995.

American Thoracic Society: Standards for the diagnosis and care of patients with chronic obstructive pulmonary disease (COPD) and asthma. Am J Respir Crit Care Med. 152:S77, 1995.

Brannon, F, et al: Cardiopulmonary Rehabilitation: Basic Theory and Application. FA Davis, Philadelphia, 1998.

Casaburi, R, and Petty, T: Principles and Practice of Pulmonary Rehabilitation. WB Saunders, Philadelphia, 1993.

Ciccone, C: Pharmacology in Rehabilitation, ed 2. FA Davis, Philadelphia, 1996.

Frownfelter, D, and Dean, E: Principles and Practice of Cardiopulmonary Physical Therapy, ed 3. Mosby-Yearbook, St. Louis, 1996.

Goodman, C, and Boissonnault, W: Pathology: Implications for the Physical Therapist. WB Saunders, Philadelphia, 1998.

Tiep, B: Disease management of COPD with pulmonary rehabilitation. Chest 112:1630, 1997.

GLOSSARY

Adventitious breath sounds: Crackles or wheezes; heard during auscultation, in addition to the overall quality of the breath sound.

Aerobic exercise: Any sustained exercise where the required energy is supplied by the available oxygen within the system.

Asthma: A clinical syndrome characterized by increased reactivity of the tracheobronchial tree to various stimuli.

Atelectasis: Alveolar collapse involving part or all of the lung due to the complete absorption of gas or the inability of the alveoli to expand.

Auscultation: Listening through the chest wall to air movement by means of a stethoscope.

Bronchial breath sounds: A hollow or echoing breath sound that occupies more of the ventilatory cycle than normal.

Bronchospasm: Contraction of the smooth muscle within the walls of the airways to cause narrowing of the lumen.

Chronic bronchitis: A clinical syndrome characterized by persistent cough and expectoration for at least a 3-month period for at least 2 consecutive years.

Chronic obstructive pulmonary disease (COPD): A disease process that decreases the ability of the lungs to perform ventilation. Diseases that cause this condition are chronic bronchitis and pulmonary emphysema.

Cor pulmonale: Right ventricular enlargement from a primary pulmonary cause.

Crackles: An adventitious sound heard during lung auscultation and related to the opening of previously closed small airways and alveoli.

Cyanosis: A bluish coloration of the skin in response to hypoxemia.

Cystic fibrosis: A genetic disorder characterized by an exocrine gland dysfunction that results in abnormally viscid secretions.

Decreased breath sounds: Diminished or distant sounds heard during lung auscultation.

Digital clubbing: A sign of hypoxemia in which the tip of the distal pharynx (finger or toe) becomes bulbous and the nail of that digit exits at an increased angle.

Emphysema: An abnormal enlargement of the distal respiratory unit that is accompanied by destructive changes of the alveolar walls without obvious fibrosis.

Exercise prescription: An individualized exercise program specifying mode, intensity, frequency, and duration.

Expiratory reserve volume (ERV): The volume of air that can be exhaled following a normal resting exhalation.

Flail chest: Two or more ribs broken in two or more places.

Forced expiratory flow rate from 25 to 75 percent ($FEF_{25-75\%}$): The volume of air forcibly exhaled during the middle portion of expiration; 25 to 75 percent of the forced vital capacity maneuver.

Forced expiratory volume (FEV_1): The volume of air forcibly exhaled during the first second of a forced vital capacity maneuver.

Functional residual capacity (FRC): The amount of air remaining in the lung after a normal resting exhalation. Expiratory reserve volume plus the residual volume equals functional residual capacity.

Graded exercise test (GXT, exercise tolerance test): The observation and recording of an individual's cardiopulmonary responses during gradually increasing exercise challenges to determine the body's capacity to adapt to physical work. Tests may be maximal or submaximal.

Heart rate reserve method (Karvonen formula): Resting heart rate (HR_{rest}) is subtracted from maximal heart rate (HR_{max}) to obtain the heart rate reserve. The conditioning intensity, 40 percent and 85 percent of heart rate reserve, is calculated. These values are added to HR_{rest} to obtain the target heart rate range (THRR).

Hemoptysis: The presence of blood in the sputum.

Hypercapnia: An increase in the amount of carbon dioxide within the arterial blood.

Hyperinflation: An abnormal increase in the amount of air within the lung tissue.

Hyperlucency: An increase in the penetration of x-rays seen on a good-quality chest radiograph; it indicates hyperinflation of the chest.

Hyperreactivity: An increase in the sensitivity of the airway walls to stimuli.

Hypocapnea: A decrease in the amount of carbon dioxide within the arterial blood.

Hypoventilation: An increase in the amount of carbon dioxide within the arterial blood due to a decrease in alveolar ventilation.

Hypoxemia: A decrease in the amount of oxygen within the arterial blood.

Inspiratory capacity: The total amount of air that can be inspired after a tidal exhalation. Inspiratory reserve volume plus residual volume equals inspiratory capacity.

Inspiratory reserve volume (IRV): The amount of air that can be inspired after a tidal inspiration.

Maximum inspiratory pressure (PI_{max}): The greatest amount of inspiratory pressure that can be generated by a person who is beginning the breath from residual volume.

Metabolic equivalent (MET): A rating of energy expenditure for a given activity based on oxygen consumption. One MET equals 3.5 milliliters of oxygen used per kilogram of body weight per minute.

Oxygen consumption (Vo_2): The volume of oxygen that is used by the tissues in 1 minute.

Pacing: The breaking down of an activity of daily living into manageable components, with rest periods interspersed between each component such that the activity can be completed without any occurrence of dyspnea.

Percussion: A force rhythmically applied with the therapist's cupped hands to the patient's thorax and thought to release secretions from the wall of the airways.

Perfusion (pulmonary): Blood flow through the pulmonary vascular bed.

Peripheral airways disease: Inflammation, fibrosis, and narrowing of the terminal and respiratory bronchioles.

Postural drainage: Positioning a patient such that the bronchus is perpendicular to the ground and the mucociliary transport of secretions is facilitated.

Rate of perceived shortness of breath: A subjective assessment of shortness of breath as it relates to exercise intensity.

Residual volume (RV): The amount of air that remains in the lungs at the end of a full exhalation.

Respiration: The exchange of gas within the body. *External respiration* is the exchange of gas between the alveoli and the pulmonary capillaries. *Internal respiration* is the exchange of gas between the capillary and the tissue.

Restrictive lung disease: A group of pulmonary disorders characterized by difficulty in expanding the lungs and a reduction in total lung volume.

Retractions: The inward movement of the intercostal spaces during inspiration, usually during respiratory distress.

Shaking: A bouncing maneuver applied to the rib cage throughout the expiratory phase of breathing by the hands of the therapist. It is thought to assist the mucociliary transport system.

Target heart rate (THR): For a specific patient, the most appropriate heart rate within the prescribed heart rate range to ensure endurance training.

Tidal volume (TV): The amount of air that is inspired or expired during normal resting ventilation.

Total lung capacity (TLC): The volume of air that is within the lungs at full inspiration.

Trendelenberg position: An inclined bed position such that the head of the bed is lower than the foot.

Ventilation: The act of moving air in and out of the lungs.

Vesicular breath sounds: The normal intensity of a breath sound heard during auscultation of the lungs.

Vital capacity (VC): The greatest volume of air that can be exhaled from a full inspiration, or the greatest volume of air that can be inhaled from a full exhalation.

Wheeze: A musical adventitious sound heard during lung auscultation when expired air is forced through a narrowed airway.

APPENDIX A

Suggested Answers to Case Study Guiding Questions

1. Generate a physical therapy problem list.
ANSWER
- Decreased strength of ventilatory muscles
- Decreased strength of upper and lower extremities, especially quadriceps
- Dyspnea on exertion
- Decreased endurance
- Decreased function
- (6/7 on functional independent measures [FIM])
- Sao_2 less than 88 percent on room air

2. Identify anticipated treatment goals.
ANSWER
- Patient will demonstrate a 20% increase in PI_{max} within 4 weeks.
- Patient will increase the strength of quadriceps muscles bilaterally to 3+/5 in 2 weeks.
- Patient will report decreased dyspnea at similar workloads on exercise test within 4 weeks.
- Patient will be able to ambulate 15 minutes at 2 mph with an RPE of 5 within 4 weeks.
- Patient will be able to maintain an Sao_2 greater than 88 percent on 2 liters/min pulsed oxygen at 4:1 ratio within 4 weeks.

3. Identify functional outcomes of physical therapy.
ANSWER
- Patient will be able to verbally describe an exacerbation protocol within 1 week.
- Patient will be able to carry out exacerbation protocol when necessary within 6 weeks.
- Patient will be able to climb one flight of stairs with pacing without railing within 4 weeks.
- Patient will remain smoke free.
- Patient will be able to return to work.

4. Formulate a physical therapy plan of care for week 1. Patient will be seen 3 times/week for this first week of therapy.
ANSWER
1. Ventilatory muscle training, beginning with 30 percent or PI_{max} for 10 to 15 minutes, as tolerated.

2. Therapeutic exercises for UE and LE strength training with Theraband for home, PRE during treatment session. Emphasis on muscle contraction during exhalation phase of ventilatory cycle.

3. Endurance training will use a target heart rate range of 110 to 116 beats per minute. Because this patient did not achieve a cardiovascular end point to her exercise test (age adjusted max heart rate would be 153), she did not plateau at any point in the exercise session, and her reason for stopping the test was patient request with RPE of 7 (very severely short of breath), her THRR was calculated using 70 to 85 percent of heart rate reserve. On her exercise test, the reported RPE scale at a heart rate of 114 beats per minute was 5 (severely short of breath), which is an appropriate RPE guideline for exercise intensity. Circuit training includes UE and LE endurance training at work loads that will achieve a heart rate of between 110 and 116, and an RPE of 5. These workloads were established to be as follows: treadmill 2 mph, 0 percent grade; cycle ergometer 50 watts; and arm ergometer 20 watts. Patient was instructed to perform 10 minutes of treadmill walking, 10 minutes of cycling, and 2 minutes forward and 2 minutes of backward cycling on the arm ergometer. Rest periods of 2 to 3 minutes were offered whenever needed to accomplish the prescribed amount of time in exercise.

4. An exacerbation protocol that included antibiotics and bronchodilators as well as a call to the primary care physician was written and approved by the primary care physician and implemented.

5. A home exercise program (HEP) will be written to include Theraband exercises for general strengthening, inspiratory muscle training, and a walking program.

Kate Grimes

LEARNING OBJECTIVES

1. Describe the etiology, pathophysiology, symptomatology, and sequelae of heart disease.
2. Identify and describe the examination procedures used to evaluate patients with heart disease to establish a diagnosis, prognosis, and plan of care.
3. Describe the role of the physical therapist in assisting the patient in recovery from heart disease in terms of interventions, patient-related instruction, coordination, communication, and documentation.
4. Identify and describe strategies of intervention during various phases of cardiac rehabilitation.
5. Analyze and interpret patient data, formulate realistic goals and outcomes, and develop a plan of care when presented with a clinical case study.

Cardiovascular disease is the leading cause of death in the United States today. It accounts for nearly 1 million deaths each year (approximately 43% of all deaths). An estimated 70 million Americans have one or more forms of heart or blood vessel disease.[1] Heart disease is the leading cause of death for whites, blacks, Asians, American Indians, and Hispanics.[2] The term *heart disease* includes a variety of clinical diagnoses including myocardial infarction (MI; heart attack), angina, heart failure, arrhythmias, sudden death, and valvular dysfunction.[3] The most prevalent type of heart disease is disease of the coronary arteries, also known as **coronary heart disease (CHD), coronary artery disease (CAD),** or ischemic heart disease. The World Health Organization identifies coronary heart disease as either an acute or chronic cardiac disability resulting from a reduction (or arrest) of blood supply to the myocardium with associated coronary arterial disease.[4, p 2] In the United States, an estimated 13.7 million people have CHD; half of these individuals present with a MI and half with angina.[2] In 1996, the US Department of Health and Human Services reported that CHD caused 800,000 new heart attacks per year and 450,000 recurrent attacks.[5]

The pathophysiological conditions that underlie cardiovascular disease are atherosclerosis, valvular dysfunction, arrhythmias, altered myocardial muscle mechanics, and hypertension. Hypertension is "the most prevalent cardiovascular disease in the United States and one of the most powerful contributors to cardiovascular morbidity and mortality."[6, p 8] Besides its contribution to coronary artery disease, atherosclerosis is also a primary contributor to cerebrovascular disease (stroke) and peripheral arterial disease.

The clinical presentations of cardiovascular disease are diverse; perhaps the most common cardiac diagnoses that are referred for direct physical therapy intervention are CAD and heart failure. Physical therapists may also be involved with patients with risk factors for CAD such as hypertension, hyperlipidemia, or diabetes either as part of a **primary prevention** program or as a comorbidity with other physical therapy diagnoses. Heart failure is commonly referred to as **congestive heart failure (CHF)**; heart failure may be due to either inadequate ventricular contractility (i.e., systolic dysfunction) or inadequate ventricular compliance (i.e., diastolic dysfunction).

Common signs and symptoms associated with heart disease are chest pain, dyspnea, fatigue, syncope, presyncope, and palpitations. Although strongly associated with heart disease, these clinical manifestations are not exclusive to heart disease; therefore, taking a thorough patient history and performing appropriate assessments are crucial to establishing the physical therapy diagnoses.

The functional limitations associated with CAD and heart failure may vary widely and depend on the amount of intact, perfused left ventricle (LV) function. A patient with heart failure may have difficulty performing activities of daily living (ADLs), whereas a patient with a MI with well-preserved LV function may actively participate in recreational activities including endurance events such as marathons and cross-country biking.

NORMAL CARDIAC ANATOMY AND PHYSIOLOGY

The heart functions as a pump, the goal of which is to provide the energy necessary for tissue metabolism by delivering adequate oxygenated blood to the body, as well as to the heart itself. The working of this pump is dependent on several interrelated physiological responses: (1) the oxygen supply to the heart, (2) the contractility of the ventricles, and (3) the electrical conduction of an impulse from the sinus node to the ventricles.

Myocardial Oxygen Supply/Demand

An increase in systemic oxygen demand (e.g., exercise) requires an increase in myocardial oxygen demand. Unlike skeletal muscle, which has the capability of both aerobic and anaerobic metabolism, the heart muscle (the myocardium) is essentially dependent on aerobic metabolism and has very limited anaerobic capacity. Myocardial oxygen supply is dependent upon the delivery of oxygenated blood through the coronary arteries, the oxygen carrying capacity of arterial blood, and the ability of the myocardial cells to extract oxygen from the arterial blood. The myocardium is routinely very efficient at extracting oxygen from its blood supply; therefore, during times of increased energy demand very little further increase in extraction can occur. The primary mechanism for increasing myocardial oxygen supply during times of increased demand is by an increase in **coronary blood flow (CBF).**[7] In general, there is a linear relationship between CBF and myocardial oxygen demand. During exercise, CBF may increase 5 times above resting level in response to the increased demand.[8]

Myocardial oxygen demand **(MVo_2),** the energy cost to the myocardium, is dependent on many factors.[9] Clinically, however, MVo_2 may be assessed by the product of heart rate (HR) and systolic blood pressure (SBP) known as the **rate pressure product (RPP),** sometimes this is also referred to as the double product.[8] Any activity that increases heart rate and/or blood pressure (BP) will increase myocardial oxygen demand. Understanding this relationship is important in prescribing exercise programs for patients with impaired myocardial oxygenation. Physical therapy exercise prescriptions, which increase myocardial oxygen demand, must not exceed the patient's available myocardial oxygen supply. When a patient's oxygen demand exceeds the available supply, a condition known as **ischemia** occurs (Fig. 16-1).

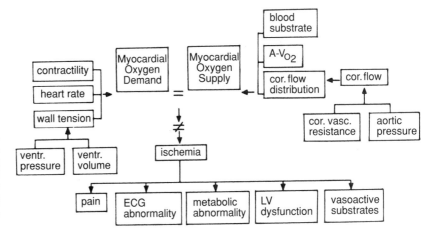

Figure 16-1. Myocardial oxygen supply and demand (MVo₂) relationship. Myocardial oxygen supply and demand are influenced by many factors; demand is strongly influenced by contractility, heart rate and wall tension; supply is primarily influenced by coronary blood flow. (Adapted from Ellestad M: Stress Testing Principles and Practice, ed 2. FA Davis, Philadelphia, 1980, p 24, with permission.)

Contractility

From a clinical perspective, the property of contractility is essentially a function of the ventricles. Throughout the cardiac cycle, diastole and systole place different demands on the ventricles. During diastole, the ventricles must be compliant, being able to stretch to accommodate the blood entering the ventricles (the preload). During systole, the ventricles must be able to contract adequately to eject the appropriate stroke volume. The principles of Starling's length-tension relationship is applicable to the myocardium. **Starling's length-tension relationship** combines the properties of diastole and systole. As muscle length increases (i.e., the ventricular chamber size increases) during diastole the ability of the myocardium to generate contractile force during systole is increased, up to a point. Beyond that point the muscle becomes actively insufficient with a resultant decrease in contractile force owing to the inadequate coupling of the actin and myosin. If the ventricle is impaired in its diastolic properties, myocardial function will be diminished; too little compliancy, such as with pericarditis or diabetes will tend to stiffen the LV, too much compliancy such as with cardiomyopathies will tend to overstretch and dilate the LV.

During systole, the energy cost to the myocardium is increased due to the active, forceful contraction of the ventricles. The work of the LV in overcoming the resistance of aortic pressure to eject the stroke volume into the aorta is significantly greater than that of the RV, which must overcome the resistance of the lower pressure of the pulmonary artery (PA). Clinically, impaired contractility, (i.e., systolic dysfunction) more commonly presents as LV failure than right ventricle (RV) failure.

The amount of blood that leaves the ventricles per minute is known as the **cardiac output** (CO; expressed in L/min). It is influenced by heart rate (expressed as beats per minute [bpm]) and stroke volume (expressed as mL/min). **Stroke volume** is the amount of blood that is ejected with each myocardial contraction and is influenced by three factors: **preload,** the amount of blood in the ventricle during diastole; **contractility,** the ability of the ventricle to contract; and **afterload,** the force the LV must generate during systole to overcome aortic pressure and open the aortic valve. Afterload may also be described as the "load . . . against which the LV contracts during left ventricular ejection."[10, p 378] In general, stroke volume will increase with an increase in preload or contractility and will decrease with an increase in afterload. Clinically, especially in critical care settings, the concept of **cardiac index (CI)** is often preferred to CO. Cardiac index is the relationship of CO to body surface area (BSA; CO ÷ BSA), and provides a more complete assessment of a specific individual's perfusion capability, For example, in comparing a 6-foot tall individual and a 5-foot tall individual each with a CO of 3 L/min, the 5-foot tall person will have better tissue perfusion because the CI is higher.

Electrical Conduction

Contraction depends on an intact electrical conduction system that results in depolarization of the myocardium and timely repolarization. In **normal sinus rhythm (NSR)** the impulse begins in the sinus node, travels through the atria, the A-V node, bundle of His, Purkinjie fibers, septum, and ventricles.

Electrical conduction can be viewed via the electrocardiogram (ECG) complex. Each component of the complex reflects a certain phase of conduction: P wave, atrial depolarization; PR segment, conduction through AV node; QRS complex, ventricular depolarization; ST segment, ventricular repolarization, absolute refractory period; and T wave, ventricular repolarization, relative refractory period (Fig. 16-2).

Clinically, the ECG is most useful in identifying impulse initiation abnormalities such as arrhythmias (e.g., atrial fibrillation) and ectopy (e.g., premature ventricular contractions); conduction abnormalities such as conduction delays (e.g., A-V blocks); and perfusion abnormalities such as ischemia (e.g.,

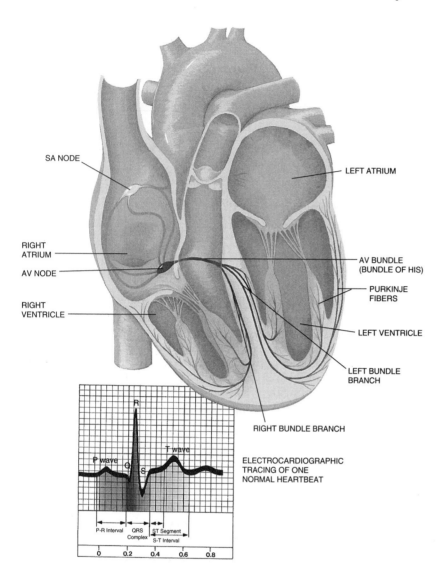

SA NODE

RIGHT ATRIUM

AV NODE

RIGHT VENTRICLE

LEFT ATRIUM

AV BUNDLE (BUNDLE OF HIS)

PURKINJE FIBERS

LEFT VENTRICLE

LEFT BUNDLE BRANCH

RIGHT BUNDLE BRANCH

R

P wave

Q

S

T wave

ELECTROCARDIOGRAPHIC TRACING OF ONE NORMAL HEARTBEAT

P-R Interval   QRS Complex   ST Segment   S-T Interval

0   0.2   0.4   0.6   0.8

Figure 16-2. Schematic representation of the heart and normal cardiac electrical activity. The ECG is the body surface manifestation of the depolarization and repolarization waves of the heart. The P wave is generated by atrial depolarization, the QRS by ventricular muscle depolarization, and the T wave by ventricular repolarization. The PR interval is a measure of conduction time from atrium to ventricle, and the QRS duration indicates the time required for all of the ventricular cells to be activated. The QT interval reflects the duration of the ventricular action potential. (From Tabor's Cyclopedic Medical Dictionary, 18th ed, FA Davis Co., Philadelphia, PA, 1997, p 852, with permission.)

depressed ST segment or inverted T wave), or MIs (e.g., abnormal Q wave and elevated ST segment).

Blood Flow through the Heart

Blood enters the heart via the superior and inferior vena cava. Forward flow is the movement of blood from the right atrium (RA), to right ventricle, pulmonary artery, pulmonary veins, left atrium (LA), left ventricle, and finally out through the aorta. **Retrograde flow,** the movement of blood from a chamber or vessel to the chamber or vessel preceding it, may occur with valvular disease (e.g., regurgitant valves) or LV dysfunction (e.g., CHF). An example of retrograde flow is the movement of blood from the LV to the LA that occurs with mitral regurgitation or LV failure.

Blood volume in any chamber or vessel generates a pressure; the normal pressure recordings for the cardiovascular system are presented in Table 16–1. Because of the known correlation of blood volumes and pressures, assessment of blood vol-umes within the heart may therefore be done by invasive monitoring of the intravascular or chamber pressures. In invasive monitoring, a catheter with pressure-sensitive recording ability is placed within the chamber or vessel. Common sites for invasive monitoring in a clinical setting are the RA, PA, and pulmonary capillaries **(pulmonary capillary wedge pressure [PCWP])** to assess filling pressures via a **right heart catheterization** and the radial or femoral artery to assess systemic arterial blood pressure via an **arterial line.** Invasive monitoring of the filling pressures of the heart is commonly assessed via the internal jugular or subclavian veins into the right side of the heart (RA to PCWP). An advantage of a right heart catheterization is the ability to monitor filling pressures not only on the right side but also, by estimation, of left heart pressures without the need for the more difficult and risky LV catheterization. The most sensitive measure of LV function is the left ventricular end diastolic volume (LVEDV), which can be indirectly assessed by the PCWP taken from the right heart catheterization.

Table 16–1 HEMODYNAMIC VARIABLES

Right Heart Catheterization	Normal Ranges
Central Venous Pressure (CVP)	0–8 mmHg
Right Atrial (mean)	0–8 mmHg
Pulmonary Artery (PA)	Systolic 20–25 mmHg
	Diastolic 6–12 mmHg
	Mean 9–19 mmHg
Pulmonary Capillary Wedge Pressure (PCWP)	6–12 mmHg
Left Heart Catheterization	
Left ventricular end diastolic pressure	5–12 mmHg
Left ventricular peak systolic pressure	90–140 mmHg
Systemic Arterial Pressure	Systolic 110–120 mmHg
	Diastolic 70–80 mmHg
	Mean 82–102 mmHg
Cardiac Output (CO)	4–5 L/min
Cardiac Index (CO ÷ Body surface area)	2.5–3.5 L/min
Stroke Volume	55–100 ml/beat
Systemic Vascular Resistance	800–1200 dynes/sec/cm^{-5}

Adapted from Braunwald, E (ed): Heart Disease: A Textbook of Cardiovascular Medicine. Saunders, Philadelphia 1997, p 188; and Parrillo, JE: Current Therapy in Critical Care Medicine. BC Decker Inc, 1987, p 36.

Neurohumoral Influences

The autonomic nervous system (ANS) influences the heart and blood vessels through direct neural and indirect neurohumoral mechanisms. The heart has dual direct innervation from the sympathetic and parasympathetic nervous systems.[11] The sympathetic receptors for the heart are primarily beta-adrenergic receptors.[12] Stimulation of the beta receptors by the sympathetic neurotransmitter norepinephrine (noradrenaline) increases the overall activity of the heart by increasing the rate (chronotropy) and force of contraction (inotropy), and also results in coronary artery dilatation.[13] Sympathetic stimulation to the alpha-adrenergic receptors of peripheral blood vessels will result in vasoconstriction and therefore an increase in peripheral vascular resistance (PVR). The status of the peripheral vascular system strongly influences the cardiovascular system. Systemic arterial blood pressure is a factor of CO and peripheral vascular resistance (CO × PVR); therefore, an increase in PVR will contribute to an increase in systemic blood pressure.

The sympathetic nervous system may also stimulate the adrenal cortex to secrete the catecholamine epinephrine. This blood-borne hormone will have sympathetic effects that at times may even be more long lasting and potent than direct sympathetic fiber activation. Epinephrine is released as part of the normal exercise response, especially when exercise is continued beyond a few minutes. The role of the catecholamine epinephrine in myocardial functioning, especially during the exercise response, is especially crucial for the patient who has undergone a heart transplant. In this surgical procedure the direct sympathetic fibers to the heart are excised, and sympathetic influence on the denervated heart is therefore solely dependent on catecholamine stimulation of the beta-adrenergic myocardial receptors.

The normal parasympathetic influence via the vagus nerve has a primary impact on the resting heart, influencing resting heart rate substantially more than the sympathetic nervous system. During exercise, the effects of the sympathetic nervous system and catecholamine release significantly override any effect from the parasympathetic system. Parasympathetic stimulation results in a depression of heart rate, decreased force of atrial contraction, and decreased conduction speed through the A-V node. Vagal fiber innervation of ventricular myocardium is relatively small, and therefore the effect on LV function is minimal.[14] The impact of direct parasympathetic influence on peripheral blood vessels is limited to a vasodilatory effect on the bowel, bladder, and genitals.

A more influential factor for the regulation of coronary artery vasomotor tone than either the neurotransmitters or hormones released by the sympathetic system is autoregulation. Active hyperemia, a type of autoregulation, results in arteriolar vasodilation in response to a decrease in local oxygen concentration or an increase in carbon dioxide and hydrogen ions. Another form of autoregulation is pressure autoregulation, in which a local decrease in arterial blood flow results in arteriolar dilation. Coronary artery disease as well as peripheral atherosclerotic blood vessel disease results in a decrease in local arterial blood flow owing to a decrease in lumen size. Autoregulation provides a mechanism to maintain adequate capillary bed filling of the diseased arteries by influencing local arteriolar vasodilation. It is important to remember that autoregulation is a local not systemic effect; it influences the arterioles of the diseased vessels only. Autoregulation provides a mechanism for a quick and direct response to a change in local metabolism or blood flow alterations and can thereby be more specific and faster responding than sympathetic neurotransmission or blood-borne catecholamines.

Systemic arterial blood pressure is a product of CO and peripheral vascular resistance; the influences on blood pressure, however, are multifactorial.[15] The central nervous system (CNS) regulatory site for blood pressure control is the vasomotor center primarily located within the medulla. The vasomotor center mediates sympathetic and vagal inputs and is influenced by neural impulses arising in the baroreceptors, chemoreceptors, hypothalamus, cerebral cortex, and skin, and can be altered by changes in the blood concentrations of oxygen and carbon dioxide.[16] The baroreceptor reflex is activated by either pressure or stretch receptors located within the internal carotids (carotid sinus) and aortic arch. They are more responsive to constantly changing pressure than to sustained constant pressure; therefore, they play a key role in the short-term adjustment of blood pressure, which was altered abruptly and not in long-term blood pressure control.[13] These receptors respond to an increase in arterial pressure by facilitating a compensatory decrease in CO and PVR. Activation of the baroreceptor reflex results in a decrease in sympathetic activation of the heart, arterioles, and veins, and an increase in parasympathetic activation. A decrease in arterial pressure results in a decrease in firing of the arterial baroreceptors resulting in an increase in sympathetic activation of the heart, veins, and arterioles, and a decrease in parasympathetic activity of the heart, facilitating a compensatory increase in PVR and CO and therefore an increase in systemic blood pressure. **Chemoreceptors** located in the internal carotids (carotid bodies), aortic arch, and PA monitor the carbon dioxide and oxygen concentration of the blood; this information is processed in the respiratory and cardiovascular centers in the medulla. In response to a decrease in arterial oxygen content, the depth and rate of ventilation increases and usually results in an increase in heart rate as well. Stimulation of the carotid chemoreceptors by hypercapnia, hypoxemia, or acidosis may also result in coronary artery vasodilation.[14] Blood pressure may also increase as a result of a decrease in arterial oxygen concentration or an increase in arterial carbon dioxide concentration.[17] Stimulation of the motor cortex, hypothalamus, or other higher nerve centers in response to exertion, emotions, or an alarm pattern may also influence the vasomotor center resulting in either its excitation or inhibition.

Many cardiovascular drugs either enhance or suppress sympathetic functioning. Those that mimic the action of the sympathetic nervous system are known as **sympathomimetics,** those that suppress sympathetic functioning are known as **sympatholytics.** Frequently used sympathomimetics are dopamine, epinephrine, and atropine, which are common in critical care settings. Dopamine and epinephrine increase CO; atropine increases heart rate in the presence of critical **bradycardia.** Frequently used sympatholytics are the category of drugs known as beta blockers (beta-adrenergic antagonists), which suppress beta-adrenergic activity; they are commonly used as part of an anti-ischemic drug regime and for the medical management of hypertension.

Coronary Arteries

During systole, blood flows from the left ventricle, through the open aortic valve into the aorta. During diastole, the aortic valve is closed, exposing the coronary ostium located behind the aortic leaflets in the wall of the aorta. The right and left ostium are the openings for the right and left coronary arteries respectively. The coronary arteries receive the majority of their blood flow during diastole; thus, diastolic pressure and duration are important determinants of CBF. Tachycardia, which decreases diastolic filling time, may predispose patients with CAD to myocardial ischemia, not only because of the increase in myocardial oxygen demand but also because of the reduced coronary filling time.[18]

The left coronary artery begins as the left main (LM) and then branches into the left anterior descending (LAD) and the circumflex (CX). The LAD may have further divisions known as diagonal branches that come off of the primary LAD. The LAD and its diagonal branches primarily supply the anterior and superior surfaces of the LV as well as portions of the interventricular septum. The circumflex may also have branches; they are known as marginal branches. The circumflex and its marginal branches supply the lateral and part of the inferior surfaces of the left ventricle and portions of the left atrium. The posterior wall may be supplied by either the circumflex or the posterior descending branch of the right coronary.

The right coronary artery (RCA), beginning in the right ostium, supplies the RA, most of the right ventricle, part of the inferior wall of the left ventricle, portions of the interventricular septum, and the conduction system. The posterior descending artery (PDA) is most commonly a branch of the RCA and perfuses the posterior heart. If the RCA does not perfuse the posterior heart, the circumflex will supply this area. When the PDA comes from the RCA, the anatomy is referred to as being right dominant (Fig. 16-3).

The inner diameter of the arteries through which the blood flows is the *lumen*. The size of the lumen is critical for adequate blood flow; a narrowing of the lumen, such as occurs with a fixed atherosclerotic lesion of CAD, will decrease the available blood supply to the myocardium. Lumen size may also be altered by the action of the smooth muscles in the wall of the arteries; vasodilation will increase lumen diameter, and vasoconstriction will decrease diameter. The responsiveness of arterial smooth muscle is also influenced by the integrity of the endothelium, the lining of the coronary artery that is in direct contact with the lumen. The etiology of the clinical condition known as **coronary spasm,** in which

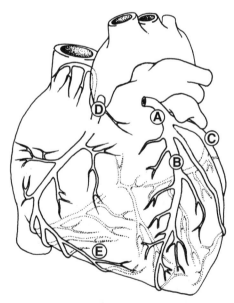

Figure 16-3. Coronary circulation. (*A*) Left main (LM); (*B*) left anterior descending (LAD); (*C*) left circumflex (Circ) (*D*) right coronary (RCA); (*E*) posterior descending (PDA). The branches of the LAD are known as diagonals; the branches of the Circ are known as marginals.

smooth muscle contraction results in occlusion of the coronary artery, is not clearly understood but may in part be due to a disruption of the endothelial surface. During the past 20 years, awareness of the importance of the endothelium to the integrity of the arterial wall has heightened: "the endothelium plays the central role in controlling the biology of the vessel wall."[19, p 1264] The endothelium has a number of normal functions to stabilize the arterial wall: anti-inflammatory actions, growth inhibition, anti-thrombotic activity, as well as vasodilation.

Atherosclerosis is a progressive inflammatory disease of primarily large- and medium-sized arteries, whose lesions will become more complex if the inflammatory process is not abated. The earliest stage of the lesion, the fatty streak, consists of macrophages and specific T lymphocytes; the advanced, complicated lesion consists of lipids, macrophages, lymphocytes, smooth muscle, and necrotic tissue covered by a fibrous cap (Fig. 16-4). The etiology of atherosclerosis is hypothesized to occur in response to endothelial dysfunction or even perhaps denudation.[20] The causes of endothelial dysfunction are varied and again not clearly understood. Proposed possible causes include elevated and modified low-density lipoprotein (LDL) levels, elevated plasma homocysteine, the presence of free radicals in response to hypertension, cigarette smoking, diabetes mellitus, genetic abnormalities, and infectious microorganisms such as herpes viruses or *Chlamydia pneumonia*.[20] Passive exposure to cigarette smoking is also associated with loss of endothelium-dependent vasodilation. As compared to premenopausal women, postmenopausal women exhibit impaired endothelial motor function.[21] The presence of atherosclerosis itself appears to result in a dysfunction of the endothelium resulting in, among other things, decreased vasodilation capacity. The cause of this is not completely understood, but may be attributed to the production of oxygen-free radicals; Alexander and Griendling noted that "excessive production of oxygen radicals may be a general metabolic feature of atherosclerotic arteries that may explain, in part, the abnormal vasomotor control and tendency toward vasospasm."[19, p 1265] A potent endothelial vasodilator is **endothelium-derived relaxing factor (EDRF),** a form of which is nitric oxide (NO). NO facilitates vascular smooth muscle relaxation; atherosclerosis, however, may interfere with the availability of NO and therefore result in a decreased vasodilatory capacity of the coronary arteries.

Surface Anatomy

The heart is in the left thoracic cavity, the base of the heart is cephalic, and the apex is caudal. The heart is rotated (in the sagittal plane) so that the right ventricle is positioned anteriorly to the left ventricle, a fact that will be important when viewing a chest x-ray (CxR) and recognizing that most of what is seen in the posterior-anterior (PA) view is the

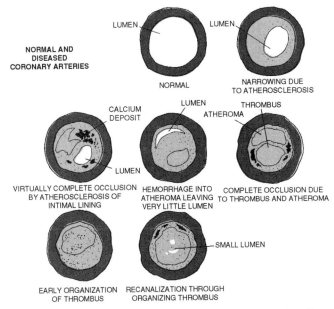

Figure 16-4. Normal and atherosclerotic coronary arteries. (From Tabor's Cyclopedic Medical Dictionary, 18th ed, FA Davis, Philadelphia, PA, 1997, p 446, with permission.)

RV. The RA is generally located in the area of the second rib, intercostal space, and the **angle of Louis.** When palpating the sternum, the angle of Louis is the "bump" that demarcates the manubrium from the body of the sternum. The RA is the clinical reference point for the filling pressures of the heart; for example, the amount of distention of the jugular vein (an indication of increased filling pressure) is measured from the angle of Louis. The second intercostal spaces are lateral and slightly below the angle of Louis. The second intercostal space is an important auscultatory landmark. The second right intercostal is known as the aortic area, the second left as the pulmonic area. The auscultatory intensity of the normal **heart sounds** S_1 and S_2 varies and depends in part on the location of the stethoscope on the chest. Although both sounds can be heard in all areas of the chest, there are designated areas in which one sound will be relatively louder than another.[22] The areas for auscultation of heart sounds are not directly over the valves themselves. The second heart sound (S_2), resulting from the closure of the aortic and pulmonic valves, is usually loudest in the second right intercostal and second left intercostal areas. S_2 marks the end of systole and the beginning of diastole. The first heart sound (S_1) results from closure of the mitral and tricuspid valves and marks the beginning of systole. The tricuspid area is found in the fourth and fifth intercostal areas adjacent to the left sternal border. The mitral area is located in the left fifth intercostal space medial to the midclavicular line but clinical auscultation often uses the cardiac apex as the mitral area.[23] S_1 is therefore loudest in the mitral, tricuspid, and apical areas. The apex of the normal heart is in the fifth intercostal space at the mid-clavicular line. In a healthy heart this area is where the contraction of the LV is most pronounced; it is also known as the **point of maximal impulse (PMI).**

Anatomical classifications for MIs may be somewhat confusing. An anterior MI involves the anterior surface of the LV, an inferior MI involves the inferior surface of the LV (the diaphragmatic region), a lateral MI may be referred to as involving the free wall of the LV (i.e., the myocardial wall not adjacent to another structure), a septal MI involves the septum, and a posterior MI involves the LV posterior wall.

Connective Tissue Structures

The cardiovascular system is composed of muscle, blood vessels, nerves, and connective tissue structures. The most prominent connective tissue structures are the endocardium, epicardium, pericardium, and valves. The endocardium serves as a lining for the chambers of the heart and formation of the valves, the valves are composed not only of endocardium but dense connective tissue as well. The epicardium lines the outer surface of the heart and forms the visceral layer of the pericardial sac. The pericardium surrounds and cushions the heart; its two layers are the outer parietal layer and the inner visceral layer (the epicardium). Between these two layers is pericardial fluid, which serves as a lubricant allowing the two surfaces to slide past one another. The status of the pericardium primarily influences the diastolic behavior of the heart, specifically compliance. A decrease in compliance of the pericardium may limit ventricular filling. Connective tissue is also found within the walls of blood vessels, in particular, surrounding arterial smooth muscle cells. It is important to note that any disease that affects the connective tissue of the body may also affect any of the connective tissue structures within the cardiovascular system.

CLINICAL TESTS AND MEASUREMENTS

A number of clinical tests and measures are used to assess myocardial function. A few of the more commonly used are described below.

Electrocardiogram

The ECG is used to assess heart rate, rhythm, conduction delays, and coronary perfusion. Two of the most common types of ECG are the single lead and the 12-lead (Fig. 16-5). In the single lead, only one area of the heart (e.g., anterior, lateral, inferior, etc.) may be viewed at a time; this area may be changed, however, by altering the location of the electrodes. In the 12-lead, 12 areas may be viewed almost simultaneously. The single lead is sensitive to rate and rhythm changes and is commonly used for monitoring patients during ambulation and activity. Monitoring is accomplished either via *telemetry*

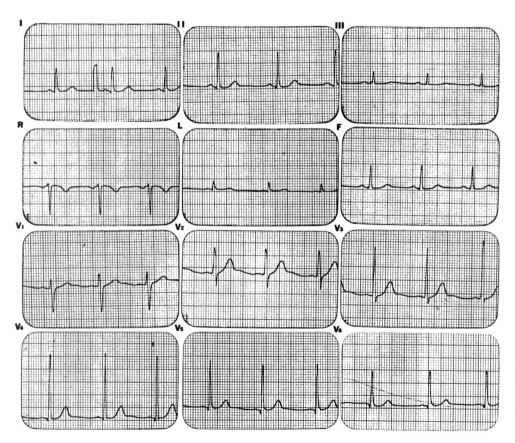

Figure 16-5. Normal 12-lead ECG. Counting from the fourth complex to the fifth complex (300,150,100,75, 60, 50), the fifth complex falls between (60–50 bpm) the HR would be approximately 53. (From Brannon, F et al: Cardiopulmonary Rehabilitation: Basic Theory and Application, 3rd ed, FA Davis, Philadelphia, PA, p 192, with permission.)

Table 16–2 ELECTROCARDIOGRAPHIC CHANGES FOLLOWING MYOCARDIAL INFARCTION

A. Sequential phases in infarction	
1. Acute	ST elevation (earliest change)
	Tall, hyperacute T waves
	New Q or QS wave
2. Evolving	Deep T wave inversions may persist; usually returns to normal (months)
	ST elevation returns to baseline (days)
	Q or QS waves may decrease in size, rarely disappear
B. Infarction type	
1. Subendocardial intramural	ST-T changes: ST depression or T wave inversion
	Without QRS changes
2. Transmural	Abnormal Q or QS waves in leads overlying the infarct
	ST-T changes
C. Infarction site*	
1. Anterior infarction:	Q or QS in V1 to V4
2. Lateral infarction:	Q or QS in lead I, aV1
3. Inferior infarction:	Q or QS in leads II, III, aVf
4. Posterior infarction:	Large R waves in V1–V3
	ST depression V1, V2, or V3

Adapted from Goldberger and Goldberger,[16] and Conover.[17]

*Standard 12-lead electrocardiogram: leads I to III, aVr, aV1, and aVf are limb leads; V1 to V6 are chest leads.

(radio transmission) allowing the patient freedom to move around when wearing this portable device, or by hardwire, where the patient is attached to the monitor by a cable approximately 15 feet long, and mobility is therefore limited. A variation of the single lead is the 3-lead, which is usually hardwire and is used for monitoring in an inpatient setting; it can be worn continuously throughout an entire treatment session or throughout the entire hospitalization.

The 12-lead ECG is sensitive to changes in perfusion as well as rate, rhythm, and conduction. Each coronary artery is represented by a cluster of leads, which, although not absolutely correlated with each individual's anatomy, gives a general schema for myocardial perfusion. For example, changes in the perfusion of the right coronary artery affects the inferior part of the heart and are generally displayed in leads II, III, AVF; left coronary perfusion of the anterior, anterior-lateral, and anterior-septal parts of the heart are displayed by various combinations of the other leads (Table 16–2). Unlike the single-lead system, the 12-lead does not provide continuous monitoring (except during an **exercise tolerance test [ETT]**). Two common uses for the 12-lead are the resting ECG taken with the patient quietly supine and the ETT. Twelve-lead ECGs are invaluable in identifying perfusion impairments in the coronary arteries and in assisting with arrhythmia detection. During the ETT, the ECG is continuously monitored to assess the presence of ischemia or arrhythmias with each increase in workload.

ECG interpretation is an important component of the evaluation process. For a more thorough understanding of ECGs and for guided practice there are several excellent texts available on ECG interpreta-

tion.[24–26] The following section presents a summary of the basic concepts of ECG interpretation.

RATE

The ECG graph paper consists of a series of small boxes (represented by light black lines) and large boxes (represented by heavy black lines). Each large box is made up of five small boxes. The horizontal axis represents time; when the ECG paper is moving at the usual speed of 25 mm/sec, five large boxes constitutes one second. Knowing that time is on the x axis there are therefore many ways to calculate a heart rate from the ECG graph paper. The ECG paper has markings every 3 seconds. An easy way to calculate a minute rate is to count the number of complexes in 6 seconds and multiply by 10. An alternative approach is to identify an R wave from one ECG complex that is close to or on a heavy black line (i.e., a large box) and then assign each of the following heavy black lines (large boxes) a number: 300, 150, 100, 75, 60, 50, 40. The heavy line closest to the next R wave will provide an approximation of heart rate. Finally, dividing 300 by the number of large boxes between two R waves will also indicate the heart rate (see Fig. 16-6).

A heart rate that is greater than 100 bpm is known as **tachycardia;** a heart rate less than 60 bpm is known as **bradycardia.** Exercise commonly results in a tachycardia as part of the normal response to the increased systemic oxygen demand (Vo_2). Volume loss such as with surgery or dehydration may

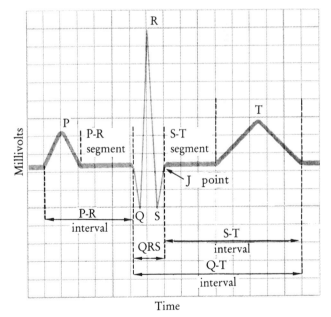

Figure 16-6. Normal ECG complex. The horizontal axis represents time, one large box denotes 0.2 seconds; the vertical axis denotes voltage, one small box denotes l mm. Characteristics of normal sinus rhythm are as follows: PR interval (0.12 to 0.20 seconds); QRS durations (0.04 to 0.1 seconds); QT interval depends on HR. At heart rates between 60 and 100 bmp, QT interval would be between 0.43 and 0.27 seconds. The ST segment is on the isoelectric (i.e., baseline) line; it measures the time from the end of ventricular depolarization to the beginning of ventricular repolarization.

result in a **compensatory tachycardia** to maintain cardiac output in the presence of a reduced stroke volume. Bradycardia at rest is commonly seen in people with good aerobic capacities as a result of regular endurance exercise; with exercise, however, the heart rate response will appropriately increase with an increased systemic oxygen demand (Vo_2). Patients may have bradycardia because of impaired conduction, a sick sinus node, or medications. If the heart rate does not increase appropriately when systemic oxygen demand is increased, CO will decrease. Altered mental status, peripheral vasoconstriction, lightheadedness, angina, and decreased blood pressure are some indicators of inadequate CO. An inadequate heart rate response in the presence of increased oxygen demand is known as **chronotropic incompetence.**

RHYTHM

A rhythm is either regular or irregular. A regular rhythm indicates a consistent relationship between each QRS complex as measured by the R to R interval between ECG complexes; an irregular rhythm indicates an inconsistent relationship between each QRS complex. There are many different arrhythmias and conduction delays. The most common types are the atrial arrhythmias of atrial fibrillation (a-fib), paroxysmal atrial tachycardia (PAT), and supraventricular tachycardia (SVT) and the ventricular arrhythmias of bigeminy, trigeminy, ventricular tachycardia (v-tach), and ventricular fibrillation (v-fib). The severity of any arrhythmia is assessed by its impact on CO. Because the ventricular arrhythmias are more likely to cause a decrease in CO, particularly if prolonged, they usually have a more detrimental effect on cardiac functioning than atrial arrhythmias.

Ectopic Beats

A beat that originates from a site other than the sinus node is known as an ectopic beat. The common ectopic beats are atrial **(premature atrial contractions [PACs])** and ventricular **(premature ventricular contractions [PVCs]).** PVCs may occur either by themselves, or in groups such as couplets or triplets, or alternating with sinus beats such as bigeminy or trigeminy. There may also be a premature junctional beat from the A-V node, but at times this is difficult to differentiate from the atrial beat so they are commonly referred to as ectopic **supraventricular beats** (occurring above the ventricles in either the atria or A-V node). The presence of ectopic beats results in an irregular rhythm. Usually ectopic beats are transient, and their severity depends on their impact on CO. It is certainly common to have a few PVCs even in a normal heart. Many people may have ectopic beats during times of stress or with stimulants such as nicotine and caffeine. Even though this may be a common response, it is important to educate patients who may have ectopic beats or irregular rhythms as a result of their myocardial impairments to avoid these aggravators. An increase

in ectopy is undesired. It is unwise for any patient with cardiac disease to engage in exercise following recent cigarette smoking. Although the specific time frame that a patient may be at risk for increased ectopy is not clearly known, a good rule of thumb may be abstinence of smoking for 2 hours either before or after exercise.

CONDUCTION

Changes in the length of the PR interval, the width of the QRS complex, and the length of the QT interval are some of the measurements indicative of conduction abnormalities. Conduction delays through the A-V node are classified as first-, second-, or third-degree A-V block and display a prolonged PR interval (first degree), dropped beats (second degree), and a mismatch of atrial and ventricular conduction (third degree). Patients with third-degree A-V block are candidates for pacemakers. Patients should not exercise when third-degree A-V block is present; patients may exercise when first-degree block is present. Whether or not exercise is permitted with second-degree A-V block depends on the etiology and subsequent hemodynamic response; this patient population should be cleared by the attending physician before beginning exercise. Examples of ectopy and arrhythmias are shown in Figure 16-7.

Atrial Fibrillation (see Fig. 16-7A)

A-fib is the classic irregular rhythm, characterized by a varied number of non-sinus originating P waves (known as flutter waves) for each QRS complex. Patients may exhibit this rhythm continuously as their baseline rhythm. Physical therapy intervention may be appropriate for patients in a-fib who have a good ventricular response at rest, with appropriate hemodynamic and heart rate increase with exercise. A good rule of thumb is to avoid physical therapy interventions if the patient's heart rate is greater than 115 bpm, if the patient appears uncomfortable, or if there is an inadequate hemodynamic response. Because this rhythm is irregular, it is important to monitor the heart rate for a full minute.

Premature Atrial Contraction (see Fig. 16-7B)

A PAC is an ectopic beat that originates in the atria and may present as an irregular rhythm; usually PACs will not compromise CO and therefore physical therapy intervention may be appropriate if accompanied by adequate hemodynamics and an appropriate ventricular response. A run of PACs occurring at a fast rate (100–200 bpm) is known as **paroxysmal atrial tachycardia (PAT).** A common cause of PAT is digoxin toxicity. It may be difficult to distinguish a PAC from a premature junctional contraction (PJC), an ectopic beat that originates in the A-V node. A run of either PACs or PJCs at a rate of 150 to 250 bpm is known as **supraventricular tachycardia (SVT)** (see Fig. 16-7c). In some cases it may be difficult to distinguish PAT from SVT; SVT usually responds to a carotid massage whereas PAT

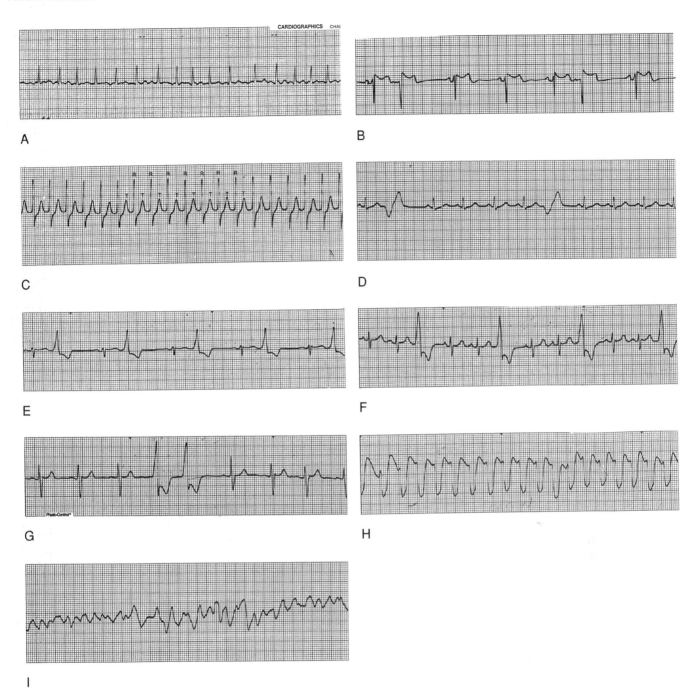

Figure 16-7. Examples of ectopy and arrhythmias. (*A*) Atrial fibrillation. (*B*) Atrial premature beat, also known as premature atrial contraction (PAC) (note third complex). (*C*) Supraventricular tachycardia (SVT). (*D*) Premature ventricular contraction (PVC) (note third complex). (*E*) Bigeminy (note second, fourth, and sixth complexes are PVCs). (*F*) Trigeminy (note second, fifth, and eighth complexes are PVCs). (*G*) Couplets (note fourth and fifth complexes are PVCs). (*H*) Ventricular tachycardia (v-tach). (*I*) Ventribular fibrillation (v-fib) (v-tach deteriorates into v-fib). (From Brown, K and Jacobson, S: Mastering Dysrhythmias: A Problem-Solving Guide, FA Davis, Philadelphia, 1988, pp 30–127, with permission.)

does not. No physical therapist should ever initially instruct a patient in the use of a carotid massage; due to the adverse rhythm changes that may occur with its use, a physician must first carefully screen patients with ECG monitoring. No physical therapy intervention should occur during an episode of SVT or PAT; these rhythms usually last for a short time (minutes, not hours) and activity may usually be resumed after the patient has been examined and the etiology determined and corrected if possible.

Premature Ventricular Contraction (see Fig. 16-7D)

A PVC is an ectopic beat that originates in the ventricle and may present as an irregular rhythm. Usually single PVCs will not compromise CO if less than 7 per minute. Therefore physical therapy intervention may be appropriate if accompanied by adequate hemodynamics. If PVCs increase with activity, the activity should be stopped and the patient assessed for possible myocardial ischemia. PVCs that come from different ectopic sites within the ventricle are known as multifocal PVCs. They are more serious than unifocal PVCs and therefore the patient should be medically cleared before beginning an activity.

Ventricular Bigeminy (see Fig. 16-7E)
Ventricular Trigeminy (see Fig. 16-7F)

In ventricular bigeminy, every other beat is a PVC (bigeminy); in trigeminy, every third beat is a PVC. These rhythms occur transiently or episodically, and many patients have frequent bursts of these rhythms. Altered LV function and ischemia are two of the more common causes; therefore, medical management is directed toward improved LV function and perfusion whenever possible as well as arrhythmia control. Physical therapy intervention is conservative at best and depends on the hemodynamic stability of the patient. If ectopy increases with activity, then activity should be immediately stopped.

Ventricular Couplets (Figure 16-7G) and
Ventricular Triplets

When two PVCs occur together, it is known as a couplet; when three PVCs occur together, it is known as a triplet. Couplets and triplets are worrisome in that they suggest a higher level of ventricular irritability than bigeminy or trigeminy. In general activity should be stopped for anyone who has a couplet or triplet and the patient should be examined for myocardial ischemia. Activity should not continue until the patient has received medical clearance.

Ventricular Tachycardia (see Fig. 16-7H)

A run of four or more PVCs in a row is known as v-tach. V-tach may be either sustained or nonsustained. **Sustained v-tach** by definition occurs at a heart rate of at least 100 bpm and lasts for at least 30 seconds.[27] The patient may or may not have a palpable pulse and, if present, it will be very weak. Because of the severe decrease in CO associated with this rhythm and the rapid hemodynamic deterioration of the patient in this rhythm, the presence of sustained v-tach is considered an emergency situation. Medical intervention must be initiated as soon as possible. No physical therapy intervention is appropriate except to assist in stabilizing the patient if possible, initiating CPR when indicated, and activating the advanced cardiac life support (ACLS) system.

Nonsustained V-Tach occurs either in groups of three to five PVCs known as salvos, or a run of six or more PVCs lasting for up to 30 seconds.[28] Nonsustained v-tach is considered a high-risk indicator for potentially lethal arrhythmias. Because the rhythm is nonsustained the decrease in CO may not be

sufficient to cause symptoms. However, until the etiology of the arrhythmia is identified and the rhythm controlled, physical therapy intervention is generally inappropriate.

Ventricular Fibrillation (see Fig. 16-7I)

When the ventricles do not contract, but instead fibrillate, there is no effective CO. The patient will expire if this rhythm is not altered immediately; the treatment of choice is activation of ACLS including electrical defibrillation and medication.

ST Segment

The clinical usefulness of the ST segment is to identify the presence of impaired coronary perfusion, either ischemia or injury. The J point, the point where the S wave turns into the ST segment, is the point of reference for interpreting the ST segment. On the ECG paper, if the ST segment is depressed (1–2 small boxes) at 2 small boxes beyond the J point, then ischemia is likely present. Ischemia is transient and when myocardial supply and demand are rebalanced, the ST segment will return to baseline. Unlike the ST depression of ischemia, a transmural myocardial injury (i.e., infarction) presents as ST segment elevation (Fig. 16-8). A non-transmural myocardial injury, however, presents as ST depression and is usually accompanied by laboratory values (e.g., CPK MB, troponin) that indicate infarction has occurred.

Left Heart Catheterization/
Coronary Angiogram

Left heart cardiac catheterization or **cath,** as it is commonly referred to, involves insertion of a catheter into a major artery (often the femoral or radial artery) and advancing it retrograde through the aorta until it reaches the LV. The catheter may then proceed into the LV and is used to measure hemodynamic pressures during systole and diastole and to assess LV function. The **ejection fraction (EF)** is a clinically useful measure of LV function. The EF is the relationship between the stroke

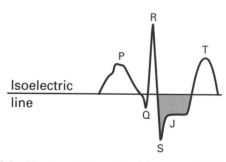

Figure 16-8. ST segment depression. The amount of ST depression is determined by measuring the amount of deflection at the J point from the isoelectric line (baseline). The J point is the point where the S wave and ST segment meet. This diagram illustrates horizontal ST depression of about 2 millimeters.

volume and the left ventricular end diastolic volume (LVEDV – LVESV; i.e., the preload); therefore EF = SV/LVEDV. Normal EF is 55 to 75 percent, meaning that with each contraction 55 to 75 percent of the volume of blood that was in the left ventricle at the end of diastole has been ejected into the aorta during systole. In systolic dysfunction a general rule of thumb is that the lower the EF the more impaired the LV function. The **angiogram** component involves injecting a radiopaque dye into the ostium of each coronary artery and then videorecording blood flow through each of the arteries to determine the presence of lesions or blood flow obstructions. Depending on the information desired and the patient's status, a cardiac cath procedure may last from 1 to 3 hours.

Echocardiogram

With ultrasound technology, the echocardiogram is used to assess wall motion integrity, valvular status, wall thickness, chamber size, and LV function. The EF may also be calculated using the data obtained from the echocardiogram. An echocardiogram may accompany a stress test and is known as a **stress echo.** The purpose of a stress echo is to compare LV function and wall motion between rest and exercise when an increased systemic oxygen demand (Vo_2) results in an increased myocardial oxygen demand. A positive stress echo indicates a worsening of LV function as activity increases; a negative stress echo indicates that the LV has adequately adapted to the increase in energy demand.

Invasive Monitors

When is it not feasible to perform a left heart catheterization to assess LV function, or if continuous monitoring of myocardial function is desired, a catheter may be inserted through the vessels entering the right side of the heart to record the following pressures: central venous pressure (CVP), pulmonary artery (PA) pressure, and pulmonary capillary wedge pressures (PCWP). This catheter is referred to as a central line. A common type of central line for hemodynamic monitoring is the Swan-Ganz catheter. Because the cardiovascular system is a closed loop and the LV depends on the integrity of the RV to function appropriately, recording right-sided pressures gives an indirect indication of the status of the LV. By comparing the actual readings from the patient to the expected norm, a failing LV may be identified by elevated pressures; a volume-depleted LV may be identified by lowered pressures. Patients in intensive care settings are frequently invasively monitored to assess minute-to-minute hemodynamic changes over extended periods of time. If the patient is relatively hemodynamically stable, physical therapy intervention may be appropriate; activity is limited, however, to bed or possibly chair activity.

Exercise Tolerance Test

To assess the ability of the cardiovascular system to accommodate to increasing systemic oxygen demands, an exercise tolerance test (**ETT;** stress test or graded exercise test) is useful. The patient exercises through stages of increasing workloads, expressed in units of oxygen. Oxygen cost may be expressed in L/min, mL/kg/min, kcal, or metabolic equivalents (METs); a **MET** represents the basic systemic oxygen requirement at rest, roughly 3.5 mL O_2/kg/min. The clinical usefulness of METs is that an activity can be expressed in comparison to resting energy cost; for example, the first stage of the Bruce protocol requires roughly 5 METs of energy (i.e., it requires five times the energy expended at rest). The most common modalities used in exercise testing of patients with cardiac impairments are the treadmill, bicycle, and arm ergometer (Fig. 16-9). In the earlier years of exercise testing for assessment of CAD, the step test was routinely used; however, it has for the most part been replaced by the other modalities. The step test is useful for fitness screening in the relatively healthy population and in exercise training for both the cardiac and non-cardiac populations.

Knowledge of systemic energy requirements is important in prescribing exercise and activity guidelines, as well as in exercising testing, for patients with cardiac impairments. Many charts are available that express systemic energy requirements using a variety of oxygen equivalents (Table 16–3).

The two major goals of exercising testing are to detect the presence of ischemia and to determine the functional aerobic capacity of the individual. The patient is monitored with a 12-lead ECG throughout the test and recovery; information regarding perfusion, rhythm, or conduction changes is therefore immediately available. In addition to the ECG, other diagnostic tools may be used, most commonly the echocardiogram and nuclear imaging. The stress echo assesses wall motion abnormalities that may or may not be present at rest but may become more pronounced with increasing workloads. Nuclear imaging (e.g., thallium sestamibi) compares coronary perfusion between rest and exercise; if there is no decrease in perfusion with increasing workloads, the test is negative; if there is a decrease in coronary perfusion with increasing workloads, the test is considered positive.

Stress tests are interpreted as either positive (+) or negative (–). A **positive ETT** indicates that there is a point at which the myocardial oxygen supply is inadequate to meet the myocardial oxygen demand, and the test is therefore positive for ischemia. A **negative ETT** indicates that at every tested physiological workload there is a balanced oxygen supply and demand. Patients are often confused regarding this grading system; it is helpful to reassure them that in this case, a negative test is in fact good. Stress tests are not unlike other diagnostic tools, however; they are not 100 percent specific and sensitive in identifying the presence of ischemia. A **false negative ETT** is one that is interpreted as negative but

Figure 16-9. Estimated oxygen requirements for step, bicycle, and treadmill. The standard Bruce protocol begins at 1.7 mph and 10 percent grade (roughly 5 METs). Oxygen requirements increase with progressive increases in workload for all modalities. (Adapted from American Heart Association: Circulation 91:580, 1985; *Circulation*, 91:580, 1995; American Heart Association: The Exercise Standards Book, 1979, p 11; and Braunwald, E (ed): Heart Disease: A Textbook of Cardiovascular Medicine. Saunders, Philadelphia, 1997, p 156.)

FUNCTIONAL CLASS	CLINICAL STATUS	O2 COST ml/kg/min	METS	STEP TEST Nagle Balke Naughton (Height cm)	BICYCLE ERGOMETER (KPDS)	Bruce (MPH / %GR)	Cornell (MPH / %GR)	Balke-Ware (% grad at 3.3 mph)	ACIP (MPH / %GR)	mACIP (MPH / %GR)	Naughton (%GR at 2 / 3 / 3.4 MPH)	Ware (MPH / %GR)
Normal and I	Healthy dependent on age, activity	56.0	16				5.0 / 18	26		3.4 / 24			
		52.5	15			5.5 / 20	4.6 / 17	25	3.1 / 24	3.1 / 24		
		49.0	14				24				
		45.5	13			5.0 / 18	4.2 / 16	23	3 / 21	2.7 / 24		
		42.0	12	40	1500		22				
		38.5	11	36	1350	4.2 / 16	3.8 / 15	21	3 / 17.5	2.3 / 24		
		35.0	10	32	1200		20				
	Sedentary healthy	31.5	9	28	1050	3.4 / 14	19	3 / 14	2 / 24			
								18			
		28.0	8	24	900	3.0 / 13	17				
								16			
		24.5	7	20	750	2.5 / 12	2.5 / 12	15	3 / 10.5	2 / 18.9	17.5 / 32.5 / 26	3.4 / 14.0
II		21.0	6	16	600	2.1 / 11	14			14 / 30 / 24	3.0 / 15.0
								13			10.5 / 27.5 / 22	3.0 / 12.5
		17.5	5	12	450	1.7 / 10	1.7 / 10	12	3.0 / 7.0	2 / 13.5	7 / 25 / 20	3.0 / 10.0
III								11			3.5 / 22.5 / 18	3.0 / 7.5
	Limited	14.0	4	8	300	1.7 / 5	1.7 / 5	10	3.0 / 3.0	2 / 7	0 / 20 / 16	2.0 / 10.5
								9			/ 17.5 / 14	2.0 / 7.0
		10.5	3	4	150	1.7 / 0	1.7 / 0	8	2.5 / 2.0	2 / 3.5	/ 15 / 12	2.0 / 3.5
								7			/ 12.5 / 10	
	Symptomatic	7.0	2					6	2.0 / 0	2 / 0	/ 10 / 8	1.5 / 0
								5			/ 7.5 / 6	
IV								4			/ 5 / 4	1.0 / 0
								3			/ 2.5 / 2	
		3.5	1					2			/ 0	
								1				

Treadmill protocol stage durations: Bruce = 3-min stages; Cornell = 2-min stages; Balke-Ware = 1-min stages; ACIP = 2-min stages (first 2 stages 1 min); Naughton = 2-min stages; Ware = 2-min stages. Bicycle ergometer: 1 watt = 6 kpds; KPDS for 70 kg body weight. Step test: 2-min stages, 30 steps/min; step height increased 4 cm q 2 min.

Table 16–3 METABOLIC EQUIVALENT (MET) CHART

Intensity (70-kg Person)	Endurance Promoting	Occupational	Recreational
1½–2 METs 4–7 mL/kg/min 2–2½ kcal/min	Too low in energy level	Desk work, driving auto, electric calculating machine operation, light housework, polishing furniture, washing clothes	Standing, strolling (1 mph), flying, motorcycling, playing cards, sewing, knitting
2–3 METs 7–11 mL/kg/min 2½–4 kcal/min	Too low in energy level unless capacity is very low	Auto repair, radio and television repair, janitorial work, bartending, riding lawn mower, light woodworking	Level walking (2 mph), level bicycling (5 mph), billiards, bowling, skeet shooting, shuffleboard, powerboat driving, golfing with power cart, canoeing, horseback riding at a walk
3–4 METs 11–14 mL/kg/min 4–5 kcal/min	Yes, if continuous and if target heart rate is reached	Brick laying, plastering, wheelbarrow (100-lb load), machine assembly, welding (moderate load), cleaning windows, mopping floors, vacuuming, pushing light power mower	Walking (3 mph), bicycling (6 mph), horseshoe pitching, volleyball (6-person, noncompetitive), golfing (pulling bag cart), archery, sailing (handling small boat), fly fishing (standing in waders), horseback riding (trotting), badminton (social doubles)
4–5 METs 14–18 mL/kg/min	Recreational activities promote endurance; occupational activities must be continuous, lasting longer than 2 minutes	Painting, masonry, paperhanging, light carpentry, scrubbing floors, raking leaves, hoeing	Walking (3½ mph), bicycling (8 mph), table tennis, golfing (carrying clubs), dancing (foxtrot), badminton (singles), tennis (doubles), many calisthenics, ballet
5–6 METs 18–21 mL/kg/min	Yes	Digging garden, shoveling light earth	Walking (4 mph), bicycling (10 mph), canoeing (4 mph), horseback riding (posting to trotting), stream fishing (walking in light current in waders), ice or roller skating (9 mph)
6–7 METs 21–25 mL/kg/min 7–8 kcal/min	Yes	Shoveling 10 times/min (4½ kg or 10 lb), splitting wood, snow shoveling, hand lawn mowing	Walking (5 mph), bicycling (11 mph), competitive badminton, tennis (singles), folk and square dancing, light downhill skiing, ski touring (2½ mph), water skiing, swimming (20 yards/min)
7–8 METs 25–28 mL/kg/min 8–10 kcal/min	Yes	Digging ditches, carrying 36 kg or 80 lb, sawing hardwood	Jogging (5 mph), bicycling (12 mph), horseback riding (gallop), vigorous downhill skiing, basketball, mountain climbing, ice hockey, canoeing (5 mph), touch football, paddleball
8–9 METs 28–32 mL/kg/min 10–11 kcal/min	Yes	Shoveling 10 times/min (5½ kg or 14 lb)	Running (5½ mph), bicycling (13 mph), ski touring (4 mph), squash (social), handball (social), fencing, basketball (vigorous), swimming (30 yards/min), rope skipping
10+ METs 32+ mL/kg/min 11+ kcal/min	Yes	Shoveling 10 times/min (7½ kg or 16 lb)	Running (6 mph = 10 METs, 7 mph = 11½ METs, 8 mph = 13½ METs, 9 mph = 15 METs, 10 mph = 17 METs), ski touring (5+ mph), handball (competitive), squash (competitive), swimming (greater than 40 yards/min)

From Fox, SM, et al: Physical activity and cardiovascular health: 3. The exercise prescription: Frequency and type of activity. Mod Con Cardiovasc Dis 41:26, 1972, with permission.

the patient in fact has ischemia; conversely, a **false positive ETT** is one that is interpreted as positive but the patient does not have ischemia. Although relatively safe for a vast majority of patients, there are certain contraindications to exercise testing that should be noted (Box 16–1).

When a patient is unable to perform an exercise test because of limitations such as musculoskeletal or neurological impairments, a pharmacological stress test such as a **persantine thallium** test is often recommended. Persantine when given intravenously decreases coronary vascular resistance by causing arterioles to vasodilate, and therefore increases the blood flow through the capillary beds. If an artery is atherosclerotic, its arteriole may have

gradually dilated over time in an attempt to increase capillary blood flow by means of pressure autoregulation. Therefore, when persantine is given, the diseased arteries may have a limitation in the amount of further arteriolar dilation that can occur. In comparison to the nondiseased arteries there will be a relative decrease in blood flow through the capillary beds of the diseased arteries. Imaging studies will thus detect a relative decrease in blood flow to the area of the myocardium that is perfused by the diseased artery compared to the nondiseased. Adenosine, which is a coronary and peripheral vasodilator (as well as an antiarrhythmic), has similar effects as persantine and may be used instead.[29]

Box 16–1 CONTRAINDICATIONS TO EXERCISE TESTING

Absolute contraindications
1. A recent significant change in the resting ECG suggesting infarction or other acute cardiac event
2. Recent complicated myocardial infarction (unless patient is stable and pain free)
3. Unstable angina
4. Uncontrolled ventricular arrhythmia
5. Uncontrolled atrial arrhythmia that compromises cardiac function
6. Third-degree AV heart block without pacemaker
7. Acute congestive heart failure
8. Severe aortic stenosis
9. Suspected or known dissecting aneurysm
10. Active or suspected myocarditis or pericarditis
11. Thrombophlebitis or intracardiac thrombi
12. Recent systemic or pulmonary embolus
13. Acute infections
14. Significant emotional distress (psychosis)

Relative contraindications
1. Resting diastolic blood pressure >115 mmHg or resting systolic blood pressure >200 mmHg
2. Moderate valvular heart disease
3. Known electrolyte abnormalities (hypokalemia, hypomagnesemia)
4. Fixed-rate pacemaker (rarely used)
5. Frequent or complex ventricular ectopy
6. Ventricular aneurysm
7. Uncontrolled metabolic disease (e.g., diabetes, thyrotoxicosis, or myxedema)
8. Chronic infectious disease (e.g., mononucleosis, hepatitis, AIDS)
9. Neuromuscular, musculoskeletal, or rheumatoid disorders that are exacerbated by exercise
10. Advanced or complicated pregnancy

From the American College of Sports Medicine, Guidelines for Exercise Testing and Prescription, ed 5. Williams & Wilkins, Baltimore, 1995, p 42, with permission.

CARDIOVASCULAR ASSESSMENT

History and Present Status

Review of the medical record is helpful in understanding the patient's status and in planning physical therapy interventions. Depending on the type of setting (inpatient, outpatient, acute, rehabilitation, etc.), the specific contents of the medical record may vary; the acute inpatient record is generally the most thorough regarding medical/surgical interventions. Items important to note include the following:

1. Medical problems, past medical history, physician's examination
2. Medications including type, dosage, and schedule
3. Laboratory tests
   A. Blood tests for specific cardiac enzymes that may indicate an MI has occurred such as a positive CPK MB or troponin level.
   B. Electrolytes, especially potassium (K) if ventricular arrhythmias are present and albumin if CHF is present.
   C. Complete blood count (CBC), which may indicate the presence of anemia via the hemoglobin and hematocrit values and also the status of kidney and liver function.
   D. Presence of CAD risk factors such as elevated lipid values (cholesterol, triglycerides, LDLs, high-density lipoproteins (HDL), and elevated blood sugars (glucose).
4. Diagnostic studies
   A. CxR
   B. ECGs
   C. ETT results
   D. Cardiac catheterization
   E. Surgical reports
   F. Hemodynamic monitors (central line, etc.)
   G. Arterial blood gases (ABGs)
5. Nursing and other health care provider notes

The medical record contains information regarding what has happened to the patient as well as the status of the patient within the last 24 hours, or since the last health care provider intervention. It often is not up to date enough to give the immediate status. The use of flow charts, which record vital signs, temperature, oxygenation requirements, and volume status, provide more up-to-date patient data and may therefore provide invaluable information for the physical therapist, especially when working with the more medically challenged patient.

Patient Interview

Although a review of the medical record is generally regarded as the first step in the patient assessment, it can be helpful to spend a few minutes with the patient prior to the review. The purpose of this is to introduce yourself and observe to actually see the patient before becoming potentially biased by the medical record. It also serves as an opportunity to ask the patient how he or she is feeling and what the activity level has been. After a few minutes, it is reasonable to excuse yourself to review the medical record and to let the patient know when you are planning to return. The medical record of a patient with cardiovascular impairments may at times be so overwhelming and time-consuming that to have a picture of the person and a quick assessment of their cognition and activity level prior to the review is very helpful in sorting out the information. Without this insight, it is very possible to assume either a lower or higher functioning status of the patient based on the medical record alone.

The formal patient interview should follow the medical record review. An assessment of overall cognition (orientation, memory, learning needs, comprehension, etc.) should be made. Information regarding the patient's life-style, previous level of functioning, recreational interests, work requirements, and goals is important in establishing the intervention. Data should also be obtained about the patient's response to health and illness, coping status, support systems, and knowledge of heart disease. It is important to note that not all the information from the interview needs to be obtained on the first session. During subsequent sessions the patient may begin to feel better and less anxious, and may therefore be able to communicate more easily. Patient education can often be woven into the interview process, either subtly or overtly.

The patient should describe in his or her own words the quality and location of the symptom for which they sought medical attention. It is common for physical therapists to ask a patient about his or her pain; in those patients with cardiac disease, one should be cautious about assuming that the patient's symptom is pain. Many patients will not use pain as their qualifier but instead describe their symptoms as pressure, heaviness, shortness of breath (dyspnea), aching, heartburn, or general malaise, to identify a few. Knowing the symptom presentation for each individual will make patient education and activity progression easier. It is also important to identify any consistent precipitating factors and alleviators as well as duration and frequency of symptoms.

The interview also helps to establish rapport and trust between therapist and patient, creating an environment for mutual goal setting and facilitating easier compliance with the overall rehabilitation program. The total cardiac rehabilitation program should be outlined and explained so that the patient may have a clearer perspective of time frames for healing and convalescence when necessary. Education for family members and significant others is also crucial for patient compliance and understanding.

Physical Examination

The cardiac physical examination is generally completed by the physician and includes observation, inspection of precordium, neck vessels, and periphery, palpation of pulses, peripheral vascular status and auscultation of heart sounds. Specific details of the examination may be found in many medical or nursing texts for physical assessments such as those by Bates[30] and Mosby.[31] The physical therapist will take and monitor vital signs at rest and with activity, auscultate the heart (and lungs), as well as perform a general inspection of the patient. An overview of the pertinent components of the physical examination and the impact on the physical therapy intervention will be presented.

VITAL SIGNS

Chapter 4 provides a discussion of vital signs and how they are assessed.

HEART RATE AND RHYTHM

In taking an initial heart rate either by palpation or auscultation, it is important to count for a full minute. When assessing the patient's response to an activity and no arrhythmia is present, an immediate post-exercise heart rate can be taken for 10 seconds. Always note if the rhythm is regular or irregular and report it as such; unless there is ECG monitoring, it is impossible to identify a specific rhythm by palpation or auscultation alone. Note that there is a normal respiratory variation in heart rate; inspiration results in an increase in heart rate, exhalation in a slowing down of heart rate. Obviously the patient is going to be both inhaling and exhaling throughout the counting; therefore, do not identify the rhythm as irregular.

Exercise Response

There is a direct, almost linear relationship between heart rate and workload (Fig. 16-10); therefore, if the physical therapy intervention requires an increase in systemic oxygen consumption (i.e., an increase in MET levels, kcal, mL O_2/kg/min, etc.) then heart rate should also increase. Although some cardiac medications, particularly the **beta blockers,** which suppress the sympathetic nervous systems' effect on the heart, will limit the actual amount of increase, the heart rate should rise nonetheless. Failure of the heart rate to increase with increasing workloads (chronotropic incompetence) should be of concern for the physical therapist. And other physiological parameters should be quickly assessed, such as blood pressure, respiratory rate, skin color and temperature, patient's level of cognition, and patient's level of perceived exertion. An adverse response in any of these parameters is an indication of the patient's inability to hemodynamically respond to the given amount of work.

RESPIRATORY RATE, RHYTHM, AND SHORTNESS OF BREATH

As with the heart, both rate and rhythm of respirations should be noted. Patients with cardiac impairments frequently complain of shortness of breath **(dyspnea)** and report that it is anxiety provoking. The patient needs to seek immediate medical care if dyspnea occurs at rest. Frequently dyspnea is associated with activity and is known as **dyspnea on exertion (DOE);** it is important for the physical therapist to document and understand the amount and types of activity that provoke DOE. Patients may also describe a type of dyspnea that awakens them from sleep but is relieved when they assume an upright posture; this is known as **paroxysmal nocturnal dyspnea (PND)** and is associated with LV failure. It is also important to ask the number of pillows that a patient needs to sleep with to feel comfortable breathing. Patients with LV failure frequently use more than one pillow to sleep; by elevating the trunk, venous return is slightly delayed and the work of the LV is temporarily decreased. This is recorded as **"two pillow orthopnea"** (or whatever number of pillows are needed). **Orthopnea** refers to the dyspnea that is influenced by gravity's effect on increased venous return (e.g., occurs in the supine but not in the upright position).

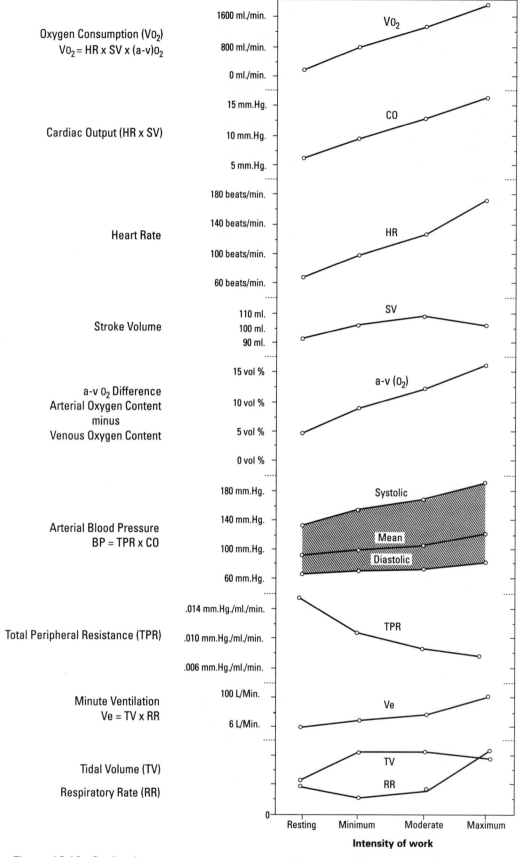

Figure 16-10. Cardiopulmonary response to acute aerobic exercise. (Adapted from Berne, RM and Levy, MN: Cardiovascular Physiology, 5th ed. CV Mosby, St. Louis, 1986, p 237; Zadai, CC: Clinics in Physical Therapy, Pulmonary Management in Physical Therapy, Churchill Livingstone, New York, 1992, p 27; and McArdle WD et al: Essentials of Exercise Physiology, Lea & Febiger, Philadelphia, 1994, p 230.

In heart failure, orthopnea may be exacerbated by the shift of blood volume from the periphery to the pulmonary circulation.[32] Some patients may experience dyspnea as their anginal equivalent; that is, they do not have the typical chest discomfort often associated with ischemia but instead experience shortness of breath. Treatment should be immediate and follow the guidelines for ischemia.

RESPIRATORY EXERCISE RESPONSE

As systemic oxygen requirements increase, the depth of respirations will normally increase from rest (i.e., tidal volume) as well as the rate (Fig. 16-10).

BLOOD PRESSURE

Arterial **blood pressure** is a product of CO and peripheral vascular resistance (BP = CO × PVR). An increase in either of these factors will increase blood pressure and a decrease in either may decrease blood pressure. Blood pressure is normally slightly higher in supine than in either sitting or standing because of the increase in venous return in the gravity-minimized position. This increase in venous return contributes to an increase in CO. In the upright position, gravity will delay venous return and there will be a transient, brief, asymptomatic decrease in blood pressure until peripheral muscle contractions and sympathetic venoconstriction are able to increase venous return and sympathetic arteriolar vasoconstriction increases PVR. Although difficult to substantiate, clinical observation indicates that blood pressure usually normalizes within seconds to a minute of standing.

Orthostatic or Postural Hypotension

This is the sudden prolonged drop in blood pressure that accompanies a position change from lying to either sitting or standing. Common symptoms of **postural hypotension** include lightheadedness, dizziness, and loss of balance.[33] A drop of systolic blood pressure of more than 20 mmHg between measurements (lying vs. sitting vs. standing) is unacceptable; a standing blood pressure less than 100 mmHg systolic may be abnormal; both situations require further clinical assessment and intervention.[33] If the patient has any of the above symptoms with position change, she or he should be managed as if there was an orthostatic response, even if blood pressure is only minimally decreased. Patients at risk for orthostatic changes are those who have been on prolonged bed rest, who may be volume depleted, who may have peripheral vascular disease or muscle atrophy, or who may be taking vasodilators or antihypertensive medications. Management of postural hypotension involves a gradual, step-wise progression from supine to sit, gradually elevating the head of the bed to allow a slow physiological adaptation to occur. When sitting on the side of the bed, the feet should be supported and the patient encouraged to take deep breaths and perform ankle pumps, all of which facilitate venous return. Use of support stockings or ace wraps to increase venous return may also be indicated for some patients.

Exercise Response

Blood pressure should be taken before and immediately after exercise with the patient in the same position (i.e., supine, sitting, standing) and in the same arm each time. Ideally blood pressure should be taken during exercise to assess the actual hemodynamic response to the increased workload. However, depending on the type of exercise modality, this is often technically difficult. If heart rate and blood pressure are both to be taken following exercise, heart rate should be taken first. Whenever possible it is a more accurate assessment of blood pressure and heart rate response to exercise if these measurements can be taken during exercise. As with heart rate, a linear increase in systolic pressure is expected with increasing levels of work (Fig. 16-10). Hellerstein[34] reported that for each 10 percent increment of maximal heart rate, systolic blood pressure increased 12 to 15 mmHg. Naughton[35] interpreted an increase in systolic blood pressure in excess of 12 mmHg/MET as a hypertensive exercise response and an increase below 5 mmHg as a hypotensive exercise response. Diastolic pressures exhibit limited changes with exercise; they may increase or decrease by 10 mmHg or stay the same.

The American College of Sports Medicine[36] defines abnormal blood pressure responses to exercise as an indication to stop activity. These abnormal responses include: (1) failure of the systolic pressure to rise as exercise continues, (2) a hypertensive blood pressure response including a systolic pressure of greater than 200 mmHg and/or a diastolic pressure greater than 110 mmHg, or (3) a progressive fall in systolic pressure of 10 to 15 mmHg. In addition to the criteria identified in Box 16–2 for terminating an exercise session, a significant change in cardiac rhythm detected either by palpation or by ECG monitoring warrants termination of an exercise session.

OBSERVATION, INSPECTION, AND PALPATION

The patient's skin color should be inspected. **Cyanosis,** a bluish color of the skin, nailbeds, and possibly lips and tongue, may be present when arterial oxygen saturation is 85 percent or less.[37] **Pallor,** the absence of a pink, rosy color may indicate a decrease in CO. **Diaphoresis** (excess sweating) or cool clammy skin should also be noted because they may indicate excessive effort or inadequate cardiovascular response. Cold fingertips may be due to compensatory vasoconstriction in response to a decreased CO or from the suppressed beta sympathetic response of some beta blockers.

Pulses, especially the femoral, dorsalis pedis, and posterior tibialis, should be compared bilaterally and documented as normal, weak, or strong. A diminished pulse may be due to a decrease in CO or a local arterial occlusion. The strength of the carotid pulse is palpated by the physician as well as auscultated. Auscultation is done to determine the

---

Box 16–2 CRITERIA FOR TERMINATION OF AN INPATIENT EXERCISE SESSION

1. Fatigue
2. Failure of monitoring equipment
3. Light-headedness, confusion, ataxia, pallor, cyanosis, dyspnea, nausea, or any peripheral circulatory insufficiency
4. Onset of angina with exercise
5. Symptomatic supraventricular tachycardia
6. ST displacement (3 mm) horizontal or downsloping from rest
7. Ventricular tachycardia (3 or more consecutive PVCs)
8. Exercise-induced left bundle branch block
9. Onset of second-degree and/or third-degree A-V block
10. R on T PVCs (one)
11. Frequent multifocal PVCs (30% of the complexes)
12. Exercise hypotension (>20 mmHg drop in systolic blood pressure during exercise)
13. Excessive blood pressure rise: systolic ≥220 mmHg or diastolic ≥110 mmHg
14. Inappropriate bradycardia (drop in heart rate greater than 10 bpm) with increase or no change in work load
15. Significant change in cardiac rhythm

Adapted from American College of Sports Medicine: Guidelines for Exercise Testing and Training, ed 4. Lea & Febiger, Philadelphia, 1991, p 127, with permission.

presence of an abnormal sound known as a **bruit,** which is associated with a narrowing within the carotid artery commonly owing to atherosclerosis.

The heart borders are palpated to assess its size. This is commonly done by the physician. The location of the apex and PMI is noted; if the LV has increased in size as frequently occurs with patients in LV failure, the PMI will be displaced laterally toward the axilla. The extremities are inspected for the presence of edema; patients with LV failure may have an increase in peripheral edema owing to the increase in hydrostatic intravascular pressure associated with increased pressure from the LV transmitted back through the heart and venous system. Edema is assessed for its level of **pitting** (indentation) when moderate pressure is applied. Bilateral peripheral edema may be a result of congestive heart failure; edema of one leg, however, is usually associated with local factors within the same leg such as varicose veins, lymphedema, or thrombophlebitis.[37] The patient with chronic CHF who has a weight gain owing to sodium and water retention may notice edema of the ankles and lower legs during the day (due to an increase in hydrostatic pressure) that diminishes during the night.

AUSCULTATION

Invaluable information as to the status of the heart is obtained from **auscultation** of the heart (listening to) the heart. Normal heart sounds are identified as S_1 (**"lub"**), which occurs at the time of the closure of the mitral (and tricuspid) valve and marks the beginning of systole and S_2 (**"dub"**),

which occurs at the time of aortic (and pulmonic) valve closure and marks the end of systole.

Abnormal Heart Sounds

S_1 and S_2 are usually heard as separate and distinct sounds; a systolic murmur will present as audible turbulence between S_1 and S_2, and a diastolic murmur as turbulence between S_2 and S_1. Murmurs are commonly the result of a valve that is either too tight (**stenotic**) or too loose (**regurgitant**) with resulting changes in blood flow around and through the altered valve.

Other abnormal sounds are S_3 and S_4. S_3, which is also known as a **ventricular gallop,** occurs after S_2 and is clinically associated with LV failure. S_4, which is also known as an **atrial gallop,** occurs before S_1 and is clinically associated with an MI or chronic hypertension. The abnormal heart sounds are therefore positioned on either side of the normal heart sounds such that they would be ordered as (S_4, S_1, S_2, S_3).

Another type of auscultatory finding is the **pericardial friction rub.** These friction sounds are high pitched with a leathery and scratchy quality although they may vary in intensity from hour to hour or day to day, or may even transiently disappear.[38] The pericardial rub has been described as "like the squeak of leather on a new saddle under a rider or grating in the knee joint on moving the patella over the femoral condyles."[39, p 5] This rub results from an inflammation of the pericardial sac, either with or without excessive fluid. Pericardial disease may result from many causes such as trauma, infections, tumors, collagen diseases, anticoagulants, and MI. Post-MI pericarditis is known as **Dressler's syndrome.**[40] An example of documentation for heart sounds would be: *Cor: RRR ∅ m, r, g,* which would be interpreted as *Heart: regular rate and rhythm without murmurs, rubs, or gallops.*

Auscultating the lungs is an important component of the cardiac physical examination. Patients who have LV failure often have the adventitious sounds of **crackles (rales).** A patient with decreased breath sounds or consolidations may have a decrease in the oxygen content of his or her blood; a decrease in oxygenation may result in an increase in myocardial work and aggravate a preexisting cardiac impairment.

As mentioned, if there is a blockage in a major peripheral artery a distinctive sound may be heard through the stethoscope; this sound is called a **bruit.** It is heard most commonly in the carotid and femoral arteries and indicates the probable presence of atherosclerotic disease.

PATHOPHYSIOLOGY

The pathophysiology of the heart, for the most part, can be viewed as a failure of any of the three interrelated factors: (1) the oxygen supply to the heart, (2) the contractility of the ventricles, or (3) impulse initiation or conduction. Clinically, an inadequate myocardial oxygen supply to meet the myocardial demand is the hallmark of CAD. Inadequate compliancy or contractility is the primary myocardial impairment in heart failure. Altered impulse initiation or conduction is the basis for many arrhythmias. Because the work of the LV is really the powerhouse of the entire heart, most clinical problems are a result of some type of LV pathology, whether it be inadequate perfusion through the coronary arteries, or inadequate contractility of the myocardium. Impaired RV functioning can also occur, either in combination with the LV as in **biventricular failure,** or separately as seen in either **cor pulmonale,** which is right-sided failure owing to pulmonary abnormalities, or right-sided valvular disorders (tricuspid, pulmonic). Clinically, however, LV failure is more common than RV failure.

CORONARY ARTERY DISEASE

The primary impairment in CAD is an imbalance of myocardial oxygen supply to meet the myocardial oxygen demand. The decrease in supply is due to a narrowing of the **lumen** of the coronary artery usually due to a fixed atherosclerotic lesion attached to the endothelial surface of the coronary artery. This lesion is composed of platelets, lipids, monocytes, plaque, and other debris. One hypothesis as to the etiology of atherosclerosis is that it is an inflammatory reaction in response to an injury.[41] The lesion therefore contains elements of the inflammatory response such as macrophages, monocytes, and platelets as well as fibroproliferative response cells such as fibroblasts, connective tissue, calcium, and lipids. The cause of this initial injury is not well understood, but risk factors have been identified that are associated with an increased risk for the formation of an **atherosclerotic lesion.** The earliest identified risk factors by epidemiological studies such as The Framingham Heart Study included smoking, high cholesterol, hypertension, diabetes, emotional stress, and family history. In recent years, obesity, sedentary life-style, and elevated blood homocysteine and fibrinogen levels have also been identified as possible contributors.

Premenopausal women appear to have added protection from atherosclerosis. Initial clinical manifestation of coronary disease is delayed an average of 10 years for woman compared to men; the incidence of MIs presents as much as two decades later.[42] The use of estrogen replacement therapy (ERT) in postmenopausal women is a topic of much discussion without clear answers. Hennekens[43] reviewed 31 observational studies and estimated that there was a 44 percent reduction in coronary heart disease among postmenopausal women receiving ERT. Although hormone replacement therapy appears beneficial for coronary disease, there may be an increased risk of certain gynecological cancers. The risk of CAD increases with age for both men and women. Beyond age 65, females are nearly as vulnerable to cardiovascular mortality as men.

Clinical Manifestations of Coronary Artery Disease

Patients may have occlusions within their coronary arteries and not have symptoms; in general, symptoms are not experienced until the lumen is at least 70 percent occluded. There are, therefore, many patients who are unaware of their subacute occlusions. It is imperative that an individual's risk factors are known and interventions and monitoring adjusted accordingly.

The clinical conditions resulting from CAD are due to inadequate myocardial oxygen supply to meet the myocardial oxygen demand. The most common clinical presentations of CAD are ischemia, infarction, or arrhythmias. It has been estimated, however, that as many as 25 percent of patients with CAD present with **sudden death** (cardiac arrest) as their first symptom. The majority of sudden deaths are believed to be precipitated by an arrhythmia, specifically, ventricular fibrillation.[44]

ISCHEMIA

Ischemia is a result of insufficient oxygenated blood flow to tissues. Ischemia is a temporary condition; when the balance of myocardial oxygen supply and demand is reestablished, ischemia will cease. Recall that the factors that influence myocardial demand are heart rate and systolic blood pressure (the RPP). When ischemia is present, reducing the RPP by stopping the aggravating activity and decreasing the systemic oxygen demand may correct the myocardial oxygen imbalance. A blockage of 70 percent or more of the coronary artery reduces blood flow enough to cause ischemia. This blockage is most commonly due to the presence of an atherosclerotic lesion. A less common cause of coronary narrowing is spasm of the smooth muscle in the walls of the vessels. As a result of myocardial ischemia, the patient will feel the symptom of **angina.** The classical presentation of angina is substernal chest pressure accompanied by the **Levine sign** (the patient clenching his or her fist over the sternum). The Levine sign has a high diagnostic accuracy for ischemia.[45] For some patients, angina does not present in the classic way but rather may present as a pain or heaviness in the shoulder, jaw, arm, elbow, or upper back between scapulae. Angina may radiate from the chest to the arm or up to the throat; it may present as indigestion or even shortness of breath (Fig. 16-11). The patient is often asked to rank his or her discomfort on a scale of 1 to 10, with 10 being the most pain/discomfort that they have ever had. The term **stable angina** is used when the angina occurs at a predictable RPP and is alleviated by decreasing RPP, commonly by stopping the activity and resting and the possible use of nitroglycerin (NTG). **Unstable angina,** sometimes referred to as preinfarction angina, does not occur at a predictable RPP; it typically occurs at rest without any obvious precipitating factors or with minimal exertion; it does not necessarily respond to a decrease in RPP and is therefore more difficult to manage medically. Unstable angina usually warrants immediate medical intervention, because the patient may be at risk for further complications such as a MI or a lethal arrhythmia (v-tach, v-fib).

Ischemic myocardium demonstrates both systolic and diastolic dysfunctions. During the time of ischemia, there is a marked depression in contractility and an increase in myocardial stiffness (decreased compliance) in the affected area. Reversal of these myocardial dysfunctions will occur if the myocardial oxygen supply is reestablished after a short interruption. The longer the ischemic period, the longer it will take for normal contractility and relaxation to occur.[46]

INFARCTION

Individual myocardial cells may differ in their tolerance for ischemia; however, irreversible changes with resultant cell death occurs in most myocardial cells when ischemia lasts from 20 min-

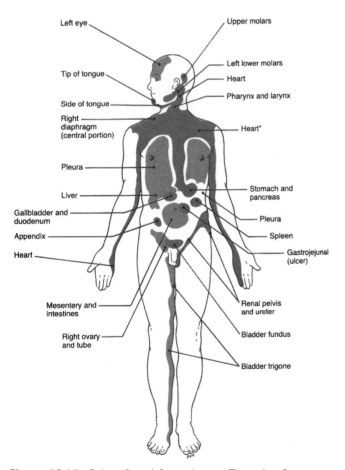

PAIN REFERRED FROM VISCERA
Anterior View

Left eye
Upper molars
Tip of tongue
Left lower molars
Heart
Side of tongue
Pharynx and larynx
Right diaphragm (central portion)
Heart*
Pleura
Liver
Stomach and pancreas
Gallbladder and duodenum
Pleura
Appendix
Spleen
Heart
Gastrojejunal (ulcer)
Mesentery and intestines
Renal pelvis and ureter
Right ovary and tube
Bladder fundus
Bladder trigone

Figure 16-11. Pain referred from viscera. The pain of coronary insufficiency can involve any aspect of the anterior chest: interscapular, retrosternal, shoulders, arms, and epigastric area. Another site for myocardial ischemia is jaw discomfort. Also note the varieties of differential diagnosis that may present in the same locations as myocardial ischemic pain. (From Rothstein, J et al: The Rehabilitation Specialist's Handbook, 2nd ed, F.A. Davis, Philadelphia, PA, 1998, p 484, with permission.)

utes to 2 hours.[9] The actual process of an infarction evolves over a period of hours. Angina commonly precedes an MI, but the intensity of the symptoms are dramatically increased. Patients frequently describe their discomfort as a 10 out of 10 on the pain scale. Infarction is irreversible. Whereas ischemia is due to a partial blockage of the coronary artery, an infarction results from complete occlusion of the vessel. This occlusion may result from a variety of factors such as a fixed atherosclerotic lesion, a fixed atherosclerotic lesion with a superimposed **thrombus** (blood clot), plaque rupture with thrombus formation, or coronary spasm. The cause of plaque rupture is not clearly understood. As a result of the rupture, however, thrombosis occurs. There may be several mechanisms for thrombosis formation such as mechanical obstruction of the lumen, release of tissue thromboplastin and the initiation of the clotting cascade, and platelet plug formation from the contact of platelets and exposed collagen.[47] Often pictured as three concentric circles (although not absolutely histologically correct), the area of infarction would be at the center of the circle surrounded first by an area of injury and then an outside area of ischemia (Fig. 16-12). The effects on the ventricle as a result of the infarction often extend beyond the acute infarction period; these long-term effects occur primarily in ventricles that have sustained a moderate to large MI. As the ventricle heals a process of **remodeling** occurs as a result of the presence of the infarcted tissue and subsequent dilation. Over time this reengineering process produces an alteration in ventricular size, shape, and function; thus, the resultant ventricle often operates at an increased myocardial energy cost owing to its inefficient mechanics.

MIs are identified as either **transmural** (full thickness of the myocardium) or **non-transmural** (involving the subendocardial area); their location (anterior, inferior, lateral, etc.), and the resulting EF. An EF of less than 35 percent is considered a large MI with significant systolic dysfunction and with the potential for LV failure. Although initially most MIs heal without incident, the major complications following an MI are ongoing ischemia, LV failure, and ventricular arrhythmias. The ultimate complication would be **cardiogenic shock** with inadequate CO and arterial blood pressure to perfuse the major organs as a result of severe LV failure. This may necessitate extraordinary medical interventions such as the **intra-aortic balloon pump (IABP)**.[48] The IABP facilitates CO and decreases MVo_2 by decreasing afterload via deflation of the intra-aortic balloon in early systole; the IABP increases coronary artery perfusion via inflation of the intra-aortic balloon during diastole. The IABP may be used in other conditions besides post-MI cardiogenic instability, for example, patients with hemodynamic decompensation who are awaiting heart transplantation; patients with unstable angina and malignant arrhythmias (such as v-tach and v-fib); or post-cardiac surgical patients with severe hemodynamic instability.[8]

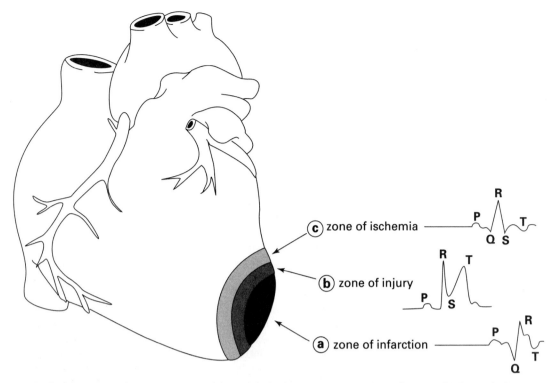

Figure 16-12. ECG following an MI. *(A)* Zone of infarction: causes a large Q wave. *(B)* Zone of injury: causes ST elevation. *(C)* Zone of ischemia: causes T wave inversion.

Once an MI has occurred, the wound healing process begins. In general, the stability of the wound is established within the first 4 to 6 weeks. During this time the patient may engage in low-level activity but aerobic training activity should generally be avoided. After 4 to 6 weeks, it is common for the patient to undergo a symptom-limited maximal ETT. Most patients will have a **negative ETT** at this time meaning that there is no apparent ischemic myocardium at the workload achieved. If ischemia is present, the physician may suggest altering the patient's medications or suggest a cardiac catheterization to assess the feasibility of a revascularization procedure such as **coronary artery bypass grafting (CABG)** or angioplasty (see next section). After the ETT, patients may undergo an aerobic and strength training program for the next 2 to 4 months followed by a maintenance program. Cardiac rehabilitation and maintenance programs include not just exercise but education and support for the suggested behavioral changes and the patient's individual pharmacological management.

Medical Management, Revascularization, and Diagnostic Tests

The classic tool for assessing a patient's complaint of suspected angina is the 12-lead ECG. If ischemia is present, the ST segment will be depressed, and the T wave may be inverted (flipped) in those leads corresponding to the coronary perfusion pattern of the involved artery. If a transmural MI is present, a series of changes will occur; the ST will initially elevate indicating an area of injury (more serious than ischemia, less serious than an infarction), and a pathological Q wave will emerge within 6 to 36 hours of the MI (see Fig. 16-12). A **nontransmural (non-Q wave) MI** will not have a Q wave and the ECG will exhibit ST depression in the leads corresponding to the artery with decreased perfusion.

If the patient presents to the emergency room with the symptom of angina supported by ECG (ST depression) the goal is to decrease myocardial oxygen demand and/or increase myocardial oxygen supply. The patient is given supplemental oxygen by nasal cannula and administered NTG, a potent vasodilator that will (a) decrease myocardial work (i.e., energy requirements) of the heart by decreasing blood pressure (afterload) and venous return (preload) and (b) increase coronary blood supply by dilating coronary arteries. Patients not responsive to these and other interventions are at risk for an MI; they may therefore be candidates for an emergent cardiac catheterization to locate and identify the critical lesion. Having done so, the patient may be a candidate for one of several types of revascularization procedures to decrease the atherosclerotic lesion such as **percutaneous transluminal coronary angioplasty (PTCA), rotational atherectomy** of the lesion, or laser surgery. Bypass surgery may also be an option **(CABG),** in which a donor vessel is used to bypass the involved lesion and establish an alternate blood supply. The donor vessel may be either the patient's completely detached saphenous vein or radial artery, or the internal mammary artery, which maintains its proximal attachment while its distal segment is unattached from its insertion and rerouted to bypass the involved segment of the coronary artery. Bypass surgery techniques are constantly changing; traditionally, the full sternum was cut and retracted, but newer mildly invasive techniques have emerged that involve less sternal cutting and some techniques involve no sternal cutting at all but access the heart via the intercostal space. Most CABG procedures involve placing the patient on the artificial heart-lung machine (bypass pump), which maintains the oxygenation and circulation of the blood while the heart is stopped for the surgical procedure. As a result of the bypass pump, patients may have additional fluid weight gain following surgery, may feel fatigued, and some patients may have transient atrial fibrillation.

If the patient's ECG is consistent with a pattern of injury without evidence of infarction, a **thrombolytic agent** such as streptokinase or tissue plasminogen activase (TPA) may be given. The effect of the thrombolytics is to lyse the new active thrombus being formed within the coronary artery; this reduction in thrombus size will help to restore at least partial blood flow to the myocardium and either avert an MI or reduce its potential size.

Two of the most common methods for determining whether a patient has had an MI are ECG findings and blood work; specific to the latter is the presence of elevated levels of **CPK MB,** an enzyme released with intracellular myocardial damage. Unlike an MI, there are no blood tests that indicate the presence of ischemia or injury. Other markers that may be used to diagnosis an acute MI are **troponin I, troponin T,** and myoglobin. In reporting on the results of the Diagnostic Marker Cooperative Study (DMCS) Alexander et al.[49] note that total CPK-MB, troponin I, and troponin T have a high sensitivity for the diagnosis of an MI 12 to 16 hours from the onset of symptoms. In patients with concomitant skeletal muscle and myocardial injury, troponin I may be a more specific marker for MI than CPK MB.[49]

Once the diagnosis of an MI has been reached (i.e., the patient has "ruled in" for an MI), the goal of medical management is to keep the patient hemodynamically stable and optimize the wound healing of the myocardium. Usually after an uneventful 24 hours of bed rest, the patient may gradually begin to increase his or her activity, ideally under the supervision of a physical therapist.

Pharmacological Management of Coronary Artery Disease

Cardiovascular pharmacological agents are critical in the medical management of patients with CAD. There are a variety of drugs designed to reestablish the balance of myocardial supply and demand, with new drugs being added all the time. The major anti-ischemic categories are beta blockers, calcium channel blockers, and nitrates. **Beta blockers** decrease beta sympathetic activity on the heart resulting in a decrease in heart rate and contractility and therefore energy demand (MVo_2). **Calcium channel blockers** reduce blood pressure and therefore decrease the work of the heart. Calcium channel blockers are also somewhat unique in preventing coronary smooth muscle spasm and thereby may increase myocardial blood supply. **Nitrates,** one of the oldest categories of drugs, are potent vasodilators that decrease preload and afterload, and therefore myocardial work, as well as dilating coronary arteries. **Afterload reducers,** particularly angiotensin converting enzyme, **ACE inhibitors,** are frequently used to counteract the adverse effects of ventricular remodeling that occurs following MIs.

For further study of pharmacological management, the reader is referred to excellent texts by Ciccone,[50] Malone,[51] Kupersmith,[52] or Hillegass and Sadowsky.[53] Therapists working with patients who have CAD must be familiar with these medications and their side effects, especially their effect on exercise response. The effect of some of the more widely used cardiac drugs on heart rate, blood pressure, ECG findings, and exercise are effectively discussed in *Guidelines for Exercise Testing and Prescription* by the American College of Sports Medicine (Table 16–4).[36]

Physical Therapist Intervention

GOALS AND OUTCOMES

According to the APTA *Guide to Physical Therapist Practice,* the preferred practice pattern for management of patients with cardiovascular disease depends on whether the impairment of the cardiovascular pump results in pump dysfunction (Pattern 6-D) or pump failure (Pattern 6-E).[54] The status of the LV and the adequacy of the CO are the key factors for this determination. The medical diagnosis of CAD may therefore be included in either pattern, depending on the resultant functioning of the LV. The following is an adapted list from the *Guide* of goals that are appropriate for patients with CAD.

1. Aerobic capacity is increased.
2. Ability to perform physical tasks related to self-care, home management, community and work integration or reintegration and leisure activities is increased.
3. Physiological response to increased oxygen demand is improved.
4. Strength, power, and endurance are increased.
5. Symptoms associated with increased oxygen demand are decreased.
6. Ability to recognize a recurrence is increased and intervention is sought in a timely manner.
7. Risk of recurrence is reduced.
8. Behaviors that foster healthy habits, wellness, and prevention are acquired.
9. Decision making is enhanced regarding health of patient and the use of health care resources

Table 16–4 EFFECTS OF MEDICATIONS ON HEART RATE, BLOOD PRESSURE, ECG, AND EXERCISE CAPACITY

Medications	Heart Rate	Blood Pressure	ECG	Exercise Capacity
I. Beta blockers (including labetalol)	↓* (R and E)	↓ (R and E)	↓ HR* (R) ↓ ischemia† (E)	↑ in patients with angina; ↓ or ←→ in patients without angina
II. Nitrates	↑ (R) ↑ or ←→ (E)	↓ (R) ↓ or ←→ (E)	↑ HR (R) ↑ or ←→ HR (E) ↓ ischemia† (E)	↑ in patients with angina; ←→ in patients without angina; ↑ or ←→ in patients with congestive heart failure (CHF)
III. Calcium channel blockers Felodipine Isradipine Nicardipine Nifedipine	↑ or ←→ (R and E)	↓ (R and E)	↑ or ←→ HR (R and E) ↓ ischemia† (E) ↓ HR (R and E) ↓ ischemia† (E)	↑ in patients with angina; ←→ in patients without angina
Bepridil Diltiazem Verapamil	↓ (R and E)			
IV. Digitalis	↓ in patients w/atrial fibrillation and possibly CHF Not significantly altered in patients w/sinus rhythm	←→	May produce nonspecific ST-T wave changes (R) May produce ST segment depression (E)	Improved only in patients with atrial fibrillation or in patients with CHF
V. Diuretics	←→	←→ or ↓ (R and E)	←→ (R) May cause PVCs and "false positive" test results if hypokalemia occurs. May cause PVCs if hypomagnesemia occurs (E)	←→ except possibly in patients with CHF
VI. Vasodilators, non-adrenergic	↑ or ←→ (R and E)	↓ (R and E)	↑ or ←→ HR (R and E)	←→ except ↑ or ←→ in patients with CHF
ACE inhibitors	←→	↓ (R and E)	←→	←→ except ↑ or ←→ in patients with CHF
Alpha-adrenergic blockers	←→	↓ (R and E)	←→	←→
VII. Nicotine	↑ or ←→ (R and E)	↑ (R and E)	↑ or ←→ HR May provoke ischemia, arrhythmias (R and E)	←→ except ↓ or ←→ in patients with angina

Adapted from American College of Sports Medicine: Guidelines for Exercise Testing and Prescription, ed 5. Williams & Wilkins, Baltimore, 1995, pp 246, 247, 251, with permission.

Key: ↑ = increase; ←→ = no effect; ↓ = decrease.

*Beta-blockers with ISA lower resting HR only slightly.

†May prevent or delay myocardial ischemia.

R = rest; E = exercise.

by patient/client, family, significant others, and caregivers.

Physical therapists not only treat patients who have a primary diagnosis of heart disease but also, and perhaps more commonly, patients with multiple medical diagnoses, only one of which is cardiac. Physical therapy intervention may be the traditional cardiac rehabilitation: following the patient while an inpatient recovering from his or her cardiac event such as an MI and then providing discharge guidelines and follow up as an outpatient. However, patients with cardiac histories commonly have physical therapy needs at other points throughout their lives other than at the time of their acute cardiac diagnosis. For example, the patient with a previous MI might require ambulation training as a result of a fractured hip, an outpatient knee rehabilitation program following a skiing injury, tennis elbow intervention, prosthetic ambulation training, or intervention following a cerebrovascular accident (CVA). If the physical therapist understands the pathophysiology of the cardiac condition and the energy de- mands that are being placed on the patient then the therapist will be able to adjust the plan of care accordingly.

Patients with Coronary Artery Disease

It is important to remember that a patient with known CAD may not have symptomatic ischemia. The goal of anti-ischemic medications is to keep the patient's physiological response to activity below his or her ischemic threshold; therefore, the patient will ideally remain asymptomatic with activity. Following a noncomplicated MI, ischemia should not occur because infarcted tissue cannot become ischemic; however, if there are other diseased vessels then ischemia can occur in any noninfarcted tissue that has a compromised blood supply. A physical therapist working with patients with CAD must be aware that their basic cardiac impairment is an imbalance of myocardial oxygen supply and demand for the given systemic energy demand and that any increase in systemic oxygen consumption will increase myocardial oxygen consumption. Patients should there-

---

Box 16–3 CONTRAINDICATIONS FOR ENTRY INTO INPATIENT AND OUTPATIENT EXERCISE PROGRAMS

1. Unstable angina
2. Resting systolic blood pressure >200 mmHg or resting diastolic blood pressure >100 mmHg
3. Orthostatic blood pressure drop of ≥20 mmHg
4. Moderate to severe aortic stenosis
5. Acute systemic illness or fever
6. Uncontrolled atrial or ventricular dysrhythmias
7. Uncontrolled sinus tachycardia (>120 beats/min^{-1})
8. Uncontrolled congestive heart failure
9. Third-degree A-V heart block
10. Active pericarditis or myocarditis
11. Recent embolism
12. Thrombophlebitis
13. Resting ST displacement (>3 mm)
14. Uncontrolled diabetes
15. Orthopedic problems that would prohibit exercise

From American College of Sports Medicine: Guidelines for Exercise Testing and Training, ed 4. Lea & Febiger, Philadelphia, 1991, p 126, with permission.

---

fore be progressed gradually, in a logical step-wise fashion of increasing energy costs (METS, kcalories, etc.) with appropriate HR and SBP monitoring. Refer to Box 16–3 for contraindications for either an inpatient or outpatient exercise program. Risk stratification for cardiac patients was published by the American Association of Cardiovascular and Pulmonary Rehabilitation (AACVPR) and the American College of Physicians and is presented in Table 16–5.

Patients with Symptoms during Physical Therapy

If a patient becomes symptomatic with angina during a physical therapy intervention, the immediate goal is to decrease myocardial oxygen demand; therefore, the activity should be immediately stopped. The patient should sit or, if possible, lie down on a bed or plinth; the physical therapist should take the patient's heart rate and blood pressure as soon as possible to assess the ischemic threshold. If the patient is in an inpatient facility, help should be sought immediately to ensure that facility guidelines may be initiated; such guidelines may include supplemental oxygen, a 12-lead ECG, administration of NTG, and other anti-ischemic medications. If the patient is an outpatient and has his or her own NTG (which patients should be carrying at all times), he or she should take it themselves and follow the guidelines given to him or her by the physician. NTG should produce a tingling or burning sensation if it is effective, failure of the NTG to produce these may indicate that the NTG is outdated. Patients are generally instructed to take one NTG sublingually (under the tongue), although some patients use an NTG spray, wait 5 minutes and repeat if the symptoms are not completely gone. A third NTG may also be taken after waiting another 5 minutes. Patients are frequently told that if the

Table 16–5 RISK STRATIFICATION CRITERIA FOR CARDIAC PATIENTS BY THE AMERICAN COLLEGE OF PHYSICIANS (ACP), AND AMERICAN ASSOCIATION OF CARDIOVASCULAR AND PULMONARY REHABILITATION (AACVPR)

ACP	AACVPR
Low Risk	
Uncomplicated MI or CABG	Uncomplicated MI, CABG, angioplasty, or atherectomy
Functional capacity ≥8 METs 3 weeks after clinical event	Functional capacity ≥6 METs 3 or more weeks after clinical event
No ischemia, left ventricular dysfunction or complex arrhythmias	No resting or exercise-induced myocardial ischemia manifested as angina and/or ST segment displacement
	No resting or exercise-induced complex arrhythmias
Asymptomatic at rest with exercise capacity adequate for most vocational and recreational activities	No significant left ventricular dysfunction (EF ≥50%)
Intermediate (Moderate) Risk	
Functional capacity <8 METs 3 weeks after clinical event	Functional capacity <5–6 METs 3 or more weeks after clinical event
Shock or CHF during recent MI (<6 months)	Mild to moderately depressed left ventricular function (EF 31–49%)
Failure to comply with exercise prescription	Failure to comply with exercise prescription
Inability to self-monitor heart rate	
Exercise-induced ST-segment depression <2 mm	Exercise-induced ST-segment depression of 1–2 mm or reversible ischemic defects (echocardiography or nuclear radiography)
High Risk	
Severely depressed LV function (EF <30%)	Severely depressed LV function (EF ≤30%)
Resting complex ventricular arrhythmias (low grade IV or V)	Complex ventricular arrythmias at rest or appearing or increasing with exercise
PVCs appearing or increasing with exercise	
Exertional hypotension (≥15 mmHg decrease in systolic pressure during exercise)	Decrease in systolic blood pressure of >15 mmHg during exercise or failure to rise consistent with exercise workloads
Recent MI (<6 months) complicated by serious ventricular arrhythmias	MI complicated by CHF, cardiogenic shock, and/or complex ventricular arrhythmias
Exercise-induced ST-segment depression >2 mm	Patients with severe CAD and marked (>2 mm) exercise-induced ST-segment depression
Survivor of cardiac arrest	Survivor of cardiac arrest

From American College Sports Medicine: Guidelines For Exercise Testing, ed 5. Williams & Wilkins, Baltimore, 1995, pp 20, 21, with permission.

Abbreviations: CABG, coronary artery bypass graft: MET, metabolic equivalent; EF, ejection fraction; CHF, congestive heart failure; LV, left ventricular; PVC, premature ventricular contraction.

symptoms have not resolved completely after three doses of NTG they should come to the emergency room for further management. If the patient does not have his or her own NTG, is in an outpatient setting, and has symptoms that do not resolve after a few minutes of rest, then quickly follow the facility guidelines to activate advanced care for the patient. If the patient's symptoms escalate, even after the first NTG, emergency care needs to be initiated immediately. If the patient is climbing stairs, the patient should stop, take a few easy deep breaths, and then descend when the symptoms have abated and walk slowly to the first available support. However, if the patient's symptoms are quickly accelerating despite stopping the activity and taking deep breaths then the patient should be assisted to a position of comfort and further medical assistance sought immediately. The therapist should present a calm demeanor, reassuring the patient that this situation can be handled efficiently and easily (which it can).

Physical therapists must be sensitized to the fact that not all chest pain is necessarily cardiac in origin (Fig. 16-11). They must therefore be able to differentiate musculoskeletal from cardiac pain, which at times may be difficult. Listening to the patient's subjective report of his or her symptoms, identifying pertinent risk factors, and performing screening tests to clear the musculoskeletal system are good assessment procedures to utilize. Generally, cardiac pain is associated with an increase in myocardial demand, that is, an increase in heart rate and blood pressure, and therefore is often associated with activity. When the intensity of the activity decreases, the symptoms should resolve or decrease. Breathing patterns, body positions, or range of motion generally do not effect the pain of cardiac origin. The absolute measure of ischemia is the ECG; the ST segment will depress with ischemia and stay depressed as long as ischemia is occurring or the T wave will invert.

INAPPROPRIATE EXERCISE RESPONSE

The American College of Sports Medicine has identified signs and symptoms of excessive effort (Box 16-4). Obviously if a patient experiences any of these symptoms, the activity should be stopped and the patient stabilized. It is also important to inform patients that some responses may be delayed for as long as several hours after exercise. Observation of the patient throughout the physical therapy intervention provides a mechanism for on-going assessment. By paying attention to any subtle changes in the patient's facial expression, tone of voice, or thought processing that may indicate activity intolerance, the physical therapist may quickly respond and modify the intervention.

Myocardial Infarction Rehabilitation

Although it is common today to take cardiac rehabilitation for granted, it really was not that long ago that treatment for patients with MIs included weeks of prolonged bed rest. In the pivotal 1952 study by Levine and Lown,[55] chair rest and low-level activity was found to be more beneficial than the traditional 8 weeks of bed rest. Today, the patient

---

Box 16–4 SIGNS AND SYMPTOMS OF EXCESSIVE EFFORT

- Persistent dyspnea
- Dizziness or confusion
- Pain
- Severe leg claudication
- Excessive fatigue
- Pallor, cold sweat
- Ataxia
- Pulmonary rales

Responses that may be delayed for as long as several hours include:
- Prolonged fatigue
- Insomnia
- Sudden weight gain owing to fluid retention

From American Colleges of Sports Medicine: Guidelines for Exercise Testing and Training, ed 4. Lea & Febiger, Philadelphia, 1991, with permission.

---

with a noncomplicated MI may be hospitalized for as few as 5 days.

Cardiac rehabilitation (cardiac rehab) is multidisciplinary and may include the physician, nurse, physical and occupational therapists, exercise physiologist, nutritionist, and social service case worker. Cardiac rehab begins in the hospital and extends indefinitely into the maintenance phase. The inpatient component is typically referred to as **phase 1.** There are three outpatient phases: **phase II** (immediately post-discharge) lasts around 12 weeks; **phase III** (intermediate) lasts 4 to 6 months; and **phase IV** (maintenance) lasting indefinitely as the patient maintains heart healthy life-style and dietary habits. The American Association of Cardiovascular and Pulmonary Rehabilitation[56] makes the following distinction between phases II and III: phase II occurs immediately after discharge, requires intensive monitoring and supervision including monitoring of ECGs, and intensive risk factor interventions. In phase III, the patient has stabilized and requires ECG monitoring only if signs and symptoms necessitate; endurance training and risk factor modification continue. Ideally phase II is initiated within 2 weeks of hospital discharge. It is important to note that these phases are not absolutes and the timelines and activities of these phases may change according to managed care models, contracts with payers, and treatment protocol designs. Because of insurance coverage, some patients do not enter into a formal cardiac rehab program until after their symptom-limited maximum ETT at 4 to 6 weeks post MI.

INPATIENT/PHASE 1

The length of hospital stay for a patient with an MI has changed dramatically in the last decade and today is commonly under a week for an **uncomplicated MI** (no post MI angina, malignant arrhythmias, or heart failure) compared to at least twice that time in the early 1980s. Inpatient cardiac rehab uses a team approach based on activity progression, patient education, hemodynamic and ECG monitoring, and medical and pharmacological management. The role of the physical therapist is to monitor activity tolerance, prepare for discharge, educate the patient to recognize adverse symptoms with activity, support risk factor modification techniques, provide emotional support, and collaborate with other team members.

Vital sign monitoring occurs before and after activity and, if possible, during as well. The intensity of the activity is considered to be low level, perceived exertion for the patient should be comparable to the "fairly light range" of the **Borg Rate of Perceived Exertion (RPE) Scale.**[57] A heart rate increase of 10 to 20 bpm above resting is typical, depending on medications. If a beta blocker is used, the increase is generally 10 bpm or less. Following the physical therapy intervention, an assessment statement regarding the patient's tolerance of activity and hemodynamic stability should be documented. Inappropriate exercise responses are listed in Table 16–6.

There are a variety of inpatient cardiac rehab programs, frequently based on levels of increasing energy costs. Each facility will establish their own levels and criteria for activity progression and education; an example of an inpatient program is shown in Table 16–7. Following are some general comments and recommendations about the various levels.

Level 1

The patient is in the intensive care unit (ICU) and is stable; generally the physical therapy intervention does not begin until after the first 24 hours from admission or until the patient has been stable for 24 hours. Prior to this, the patient is on bed rest, but may use the bedside commode as needed, depending on hemodynamic stability. Physical therapy intervention should begin after the blood work

has indicated the MI is completed. CPK levels are monitored. Commonly, three sets of CPK levels, collected 8 hours apart, are drawn. Because CPK is released very quickly into the bloodstream with cellular damage, it is typical for the first and second CPK levels to show a progressive increase and the third set to be less than the second; that is, the **CPK peak** has occurred and the values are now trending downward. Because CPK may be released with cellular damage other than to the myocardium, specific myocardial isoenzymes known as CPK MB are monitored. The surgical patient or the patient that has fallen will have elevated CPK levels but should have normal CPK MB levels indicating that no myocardial damage has occurred. If the surgical patient or the patient who has fallen does in fact have elevated CPK MB in conjunction with elevated CPK levels, then it is probable that an MI has occurred. Appropriate activity for the patient in the ICU is to move comfortably within the bed, perform ankle pumps, deep breathing exercises, and limited personal care.

Level 2

Signs of **orthostatic hypotension** should be assessed when the patient changes position from supine to sitting on the side of the bed. The patient's feet should be supported on a stool to assist venous return if they are not able to touch the floor. The patient sits in an upright chair for up to 30 minutes a few times a day. There is a real temptation by many health care providers to have the patient "do" something while seated, such as washing, eating, or visiting with family. It is probably wise to just let the patient sit for the first time, without being encumbered with other tasks. The therapist is thus better able to evaluate the patient's response to being upright. If the patient has had a large MI or requires a slow progression to upright posture, then the use of a reclining chair is a gradual way to assume the upright position. The patient performs LE exercises such as ankle pumps, knee extensions, or marching in place. Vital signs are assessed for hemodynamic stability and appropriate activity response. The importance of healing time, pacing activities, and creating a healthful environment are components of patient education.

Level 3

Patients are gradually increasing their ambulation. One approach is to document ambulation in terms of time instead of duration. Time is a more reproducible measurement; distance may be difficult to judge (e.g., "I want you to walk for 2 minutes" vs. "I want you to walk 200 feet"). It also allows for an easier transition to the home exercise program, which is commonly based on length of time. Information regarding CAD risk factors allows patients to begin to take responsibility for their choices in regard to activity and life-style. Use of the Borg RPE scale or any other measure of perceived exertion empowers the patient in assessment of activity intensity.

Table 16–6 BORG'S ORIGINAL RATE OF PERCEIVED EXERTION SCALE AND REVISED SCALE

	Rate of Perceived Exertion	Scale	Revised Rating Scale
6		0	Nothing at all
7	Very, very light	0.5	Very, very weak
8		1	Very weak
9	Very light	2	Weak
10		3	Moderate
11	Fairly light	4	Somewhat strong
12		5	Strong
13	Somewhat hard	6	
14		7	Very strong
15	Hard	8	
16		9	
17	Very hard	10	Very, very strong
18			Maximal
19	Very, very hard		

From Borg, GV: Psychophysical bases of perceived exertion. Med Sci Sports Exerc 14:377, 1982, with permission.

Table 16–7 INPATIENT CARDIAC REHABILITATION PROGRAM

CCU—Essentially Bedrest

Level 1
1–1.5 METs
  Evaluation and patient education
  Arms supported for meals and ADLs
  Bed exercises and dangle with feet supported (if CPKs have peaked and patient has no complications)
Education
  Introduction to inpatient cardiac rehab and role of physical therapy
    Education
    Monitored progression of activity
    Home exercise/activity guidelines/outpatient cardiac rehab

Sitting—Limited Room Ambulation

Level 2
1.5–2 METs
  Sitting 15–30 min, 2–4 times/day
  Leg exercises
  Commode privileges
  Reclining upright chair
  Limited ADL
  Electric razor
  Limited supervised room ambulation for small uncomplicated MI
Education
  Identification of CAD risk factors
  Concept of "healing interval" and need to pace activities

Room—Limited Hall Ambulation

Level 3
2–2.5 METs
  Room or hall ambulation up to 5 min as tolerated 3–4 times/day
  Standing leg exercises optional[a]
  Sit on side of bed or in bathroom to wash (per discretion nurse/P.T.)
  Manual shave
  Bathroom privileges
  Independent or assisted ambulation in room or hall as advised by P.T.
Education
  Size of infarct and how it relates to the need for gradual resumption of activities
  Impact of exercise on reducing the patient's risk factors
  Teach use of Borg's Scale for Rating of Perceived Exertion and appropriate parameters with activity

Progressive Hall Ambulation

Level 4
2.5–3 METs
  Hall ambulation 5–7 min as tolerated 3–4 times/day
  Standing trunk exercises optional[a]
  Independent or assisted ambulation in hall as advised by P.T.
Education
  Teach pulse taking and appropriate parameters with activity
  Reinforce benefits of outpatient cardiac rehabilitation

Progressive Hall Ambulation

Level 5
3–4 METs
  Hall ambulation 8–10 min as tolerated
  Arm exercises optional[a]
  Standing shower
  Independent hall ambulation as advised by P.T.
Education
  Written home exercise/activity guidelines reviewed
  Patient given written information on outpatient cardiac rehab

Stair Climbing

Level 6
4–5 METs
  Progressive hall ambulation as tolerated
  Full flight of stairs (or as required at home) up and down one step at a time[b]
Education
  Answer patient's questions
  Check for understanding of activity guidelines

Continued

Table 16–7 INPATIENT CARDIAC REHABILITATION PROGRAM *(Continued)*

Patient Outcome—No Evidence of Hemodynamic Compromise with Activity Progression (All Levels)
No systolic drop in BP >10 mmHg or increase >30 mmHg
No HR increase >12 if beta blocked, or no HR increase >20 if not beta blocked
No complaints of dizziness, lightheadedness, or angina
Perceived exertion <13/20

Hemodynamic Monitoring
Level 1
HR and BP before and after supine bed exercises
Orthostatic signs supine and dangling at bedside
Level 2
Orthostatic signs (supine, sit, and stand) before exercises and transfer
HR and BP after leg exercises/transfer to chair
HR and BP after return to bed
Levels 3–6
HR and BP in sitting and standing prior to activity
HR and BP immediately following activity
HR and BP 5 min after activity

From Rehabilitation Services Department, Newton Wellesley Hospital, Newton, MA, with permission.

[a]Optional exercises are at the discretion of the physical therapist (PT) and may be used to establish the patient's CV response in the room, prior to moving on to more challenging hallway ambulation; or in those patients who require general strengthening exercises.

[b]Stair climbing activities should take place after the ETT if the scheduling of the ETT permits. Otherwise patients may, at the discretion and supervision of the P.T., climb stairs on the day prior to the ETT.

Levels 4 through 6

Patients gradually increase the frequency and time of their walks at a comfortable and leisurely pace. Stairs may be climbed foot over foot with a planned rest half way or so, or one foot at a time depending on the status of the patient. Patients are often hesitant to move, especially in stretching their arms overhead; therefore performing a variety of trunk, arm, and standing leg exercises for a few repetitions each often allays the fear and helps the patient feel more comfortable moving.

The patient needs to be made aware of the fatigue that often accompanies seemingly innocuous activities (e.g., showering) and plan their rests accordingly. Visitors are often a hidden energy cost. Patients are often very excited and reassured to have visitors but the fatigue that follows is sometimes very disconcerting to the patient. Helping the patient understand the concept of energy and the cost of not just physical but emotional and mental activities is invaluable. Comparing energy costs to money may help the patient to pace activity. Patients are told that they have a dollar's worth of energy and everything they do is going to cost them some part of that dollar; however they can never spend more than 50 or 60 cents at one time. Every time they rest, it is like going to the ATM for a quick refill. In this way, patients become knowledgeable about the expendability of energy and yet are given the responsibility to spend (and save) as they choose.

Home Exercise Program

Perhaps two of the more important concepts for a patient to understand at the time of discharge are symptom recognition and appropriate activity guidelines. It is crucial that the patient be aware of and recognize cardiac symptoms and understand the action to take if they occur.

Physical therapists establish activity guidelines for the first 4 to 6 weeks post MI while the myocardium is healing. During this healing phase physical activity involves a gradual increase in ambulation time with a goal of 20 to 30 minutes of ambulation 1 to 2 times per day at 4 to 6 weeks post MI. Patients are encouraged to walk comfortably, dress appropriately, and to try to exercise in ambient temperature at indoor malls if weather is not appropriate (i.e., below 40°F, including wind chill factor, over 80°F, or excessive humidity and poor air quality). Some patients are very sensitive to environmental factors and should exercise in ambient conditions or indoors only.

The patient's days will be a combination of rest and low-level activity including ambulation and LE and UE mobility. The patient should be encouraged to try and change positions or activity every 1 to 2 hours or so. For example, it is generally not a good idea for the patient to be up all morning and then rest all afternoon. It is invaluable to have the patients verbally outline what their days will include once they are discharged. This affords an opportunity to better understand the interests of the patient and to make specific suggestions, as well as provide an opportunity to assess the patient's understanding of activity guidelines.

Aerobic Exercise Prescription for Patients with Coronary Artery Disease (Phases 2 through 4)

The Clinical Practice Guidelines for Cardiac Rehabilitation were established after extensive and critical review of published scientific literature.[58] These guidelines support the beneficial effect of exercise training on exercise tolerance for patients with heart disease. The most consistent benefit appeared to occur with exercise training at least three times per week for 12 or more weeks' duration. The duration of aerobic exercise training sessions varied from 20 to 40 minutes, at an intensity approximating 70 to 85 percent of the baseline maximal exercise test heart rate. Exercise prescriptions are based on intensity, duration, and frequency.

INTENSITY

Intensity may be prescribed by either heart rate or RPE. One of the more commonly used scales of exertion was created by Borg.[57] Subjective ratings of intensity of exertion have been used to quantify effort during exercise. The original **Rate of Perceived Exertion scale (RPE)** developed by Borg has been used extensively (Table 16–6). It consists of numbers ranging from 6 to 20, which patients use to rate their perceptions of how hard they are working. Descriptive words accompany the numbers, such as hard or very hard. Commonly, patients are asked to limit their exertion to between fairly light and somewhat hard. A more recent version, also developed by Borg, is the 10-point scale. Both local symptoms such as muscle aches, cramps, pain, or fatigue and central symptoms such as feelings of fatigue or breathlessness contribute to the overall feelings of work performance. High correlation of RPE ratings with HR and aerobic power have been found in normal individuals and in patients with cardiac disease.

A common aerobic exercise prescription based on heart rate is (70 to 85%) of heart rate max (HRmax). However the more deconditioned patient may be aerobically trained at as low as 50 to 60 percent of HRmax. Any patient who has documented CAD should have a medically supervised ETT before beginning an aerobic exercise program. Without an ETT it is impossible to assume what the maximum heart rate would be for a patient with cardiac disease. The ECG monitoring during the ETT is useful in the detection of exercise-induced ischemia. If there are no ETT data available, it is unwise to prescribe an exercise based on heart rates. Cautious progression of activity is warranted, along with use of RPE and knowledge of adverse signs and symptoms for exercise intolerance. Symptom-limited maximal ETTs are commonly done at 4 to 6 weeks post MI. If a patient is enrolled in an early phase II program, then continuation of the HEP, including low-level activity at a RPE of "fairly light" intensity is appropriate. Close monitoring of blood pressure and heart rhythm as well as rate is important. Generally heart rate increase is limited to 10 to 20 bpm above resting if the patient is otherwise hemodynamically stable. An easy tool for self-monitoring is for the patient to be able to talk without becoming breathless while exercising. This provides a fair indication that the patient is appropriately exercising below his or her maximal oxygen capacity.

FREQUENCY

Exercise is commonly prescribed 3 to 5 times per week. The patient should not experience increased fatigue as a result of exercise. If fatigue does exist, then the frequency and/or intensity of exercise should be decreased.

DURATION

The goal of 30 to 40 minutes of aerobic exercise with an additional 5 to 10 minutes of warm-up and an adequate cool-down is appropriate. If this amount of activity is uncomfortable for the patient, then whatever amount he or she can do comfortably without adverse symptoms is appropriate. Patients who are deconditioned may require brief rests every 5 minutes during their early training. Adequate warm-up is crucial for all patients with heart disease, especially CHD. By gradually increasing the myocardial oxygen demand and allowing the coronary arteries time to adequately vasodilate, a balanced myocardial supply and demand may be possible with subsequent activity.

Modality

Exercise equipment has literally exploded in the last 20 years of the twentieth century. The good news is that the patient has the opportunity to experience a variety of equipment including treadmills, stair climbers, bicycles, rowers, cross country ski simulators, reclining bicycles and steppers, arm ergometers, and others. Patients frequently ask which is the best equipment. The one that they enjoy and the one that they will use is by far the best for them.

STRENGTH TRAINING

The inclusion of strength training in a cardiac rehab program is a relatively recent development to the traditional cardiac rehabilitation program.[59] Initial concern was that resistance work would inordinately increase myocardial oxygen demands and ventricular arrhythmias and therefore be detrimental. A publication by Beniamini and Rubenstein[60] gives excellent insight into this area. The AACVPR's thorough review of the literature on this topic concluded that "resistance exercise has been shown to be a safe and effective method for improving strength and cardiovascular endurance, modifying risk factors and enhancing self efficacy in low-risk cardiac patients."[56] Some guidelines for resistance training are identified in Box 16–5. The American Heart Association, American College of Sports Medicine, and the AACVPR advocate the importance of muscular fitness for the patient with cardiac impairment and support the inclusion of resistance training into the patient's exercise program.[56,61–63]

PATIENT WITH A POSITIVE EXERCISE TOLERANCE TEST

If a patient has had a **positive ETT** the exercise prescription becomes relatively simple: keep the myocardial oxygen demand represented by the

---

Box 16–5 INDICATIONS FOR RESISTANCE EXERCISE TRAINING FOR OUTPATIENTS

1. Four to six weeks after myocardial infarction or CABG
2. One to two weeks following PTCA or other revascularization procedure, except for CABG, without myocardial infarction
3. Four to six weeks in supervised aerobic program or completion of phase II
4. Diastolic blood pressure <105 mmHg
5. Peak exercise capacity of >5 METs
6. Not compromised by CHF, unstable symptoms, or arrhythmias

From American College of Sports Medicine: Guidelines for Exercise Testing and Prescription, ed 5. Williams & Wilkins, Baltimore, 1995, p 190, with permission.

RPP below the patient's ischemic RPP (HR × SBP). A good rule of thumb is to not exceed 90 percent of the ischemic RPP. The remainder of the exercise prescription may follow the common guidelines for aerobic training in regards to frequency, intensity, and duration for patients with cardiac involvement.

REVASCULARIZATION

There are presently no strict guidelines for when a patient may resume aerobic training exercise following an angioplasty (PTCA). Conventional wisdom, however, favors waiting approximately 2 weeks to allow the inflammatory process time to subside. The new exercise prescription should be based on the results of the post-revascularization ETT, not the pre-angioplasty ETT, which was more than likely positive. Certainly patients may continue to ambulate at a low intensity and comfortable pace during their recovery time, avoiding the moderate to high intensities associated with aerobic training.

For patients who have had bypass surgery (CABG) recovery is somewhat slower than that for PTCA owing to the complexity of the surgical procedure and the incisional healing. The number and location of incisions depends on the surgeon's technique (i.e., either a full sternal cut, partial sternal cut, or intercostal approach). The donor graph site may require additional incisions: a leg incision if saphenous vein is used, a nondominant arm incision if radial artery is used, or no additional incision if grafted with the internal mammary artery. Physical therapy intervention should address any soft tissue impairments that may be affected by the incision to maintain appropriate flexibility and postures. If a sternal wound is present, appropriate posture, scapula retraction, and functional shoulder movements should be encouraged. Use of Proprioceptive Neuromuscular Facilitation (PNF) upper extremity diagonal patterns often works well. Patients should be reminded that a few repetitions at a time throughout the day are better tolerated than 5 to 10 reps 1 to 2

times per day; the latter regime often results in incisional soreness. Patients will also appreciate information regarding energy conservation and rest periods. Even though the functioning of their heart is perhaps the best it has been in quite some time, the effects of major surgery on energy level and mobility must be emphasized. The impact of fatigue on sense of well-being may be profound and it is important that patients understand the need for rest periods as well as ambulation periods. To avoid sternal discomfort, patients will benefit from splinting the incision with a hand or pillow when laughing, coughing, or sneezing. Patients will be instructed to avoid lifting, pushing, and pulling objects until 4 to 6 weeks post surgery when their sternum is well healed. Early ambulation and mobility beginning the first day post surgery will assist in the patient's physical and emotional recovery.

Home Exercise Program (HEP)

FIRST 6 WEEKS POST SURGERY

The early in-hospital limitations following cardiac surgery have perhaps more to do with the surgical procedure and less to do with the heart itself, which is theoretically healthier than it was before the surgery. Postoperative fatigue may be due to a combination of factors including anesthesia, blood loss, initial weight gain due to cardiopulmonary bypass machine, common arrhythmias such as atrial fibrillation, and the energy cost of healing. As with the post MI recovery period, when the surgical patient returns home it is a good idea to break the day into many subunits including rest, leisure activity, and perhaps visiting with friends by phone as well as in person. Developing a schedule but keeping it flexible helps the patient exert some control over the day and his or her energy level.

The patient is encouraged to gradually increase walking with a goal of 30 minutes of ambulation 1 to 2 times per day at 6 weeks post surgery. If the patient is walking in his or her neighborhood, suggest that the initial walks be back and forth in front of the house rather than around the block. In this way if the patient overestimated his or her energy level, the close proximity of home will provide a welcomed rest and prevent overexertion. Many patients ambitiously begin their walk only to find themselves suddenly fatigued and further from home than they would like. Continuing their exercises for posture, UE and trunk mobility, and sternal protection are also important components of the HEP.

CARDIAC REHABILITATION AFTER 6 WEEKS

Once a patient's incisions have healed, and his or her blood counts including hematocrit and hemoglobin are in acceptable ranges, then a patient may have a maximal ETT and begin aerobic and strength training according to the general guidelines.

HEART FAILURE

With the marked improvement in anti-ischemic medications, increased knowledge and management of CAD risk factors, availability of sophisticated monitoring, and revascularization techniques, more patients are living longer with coronary disease than similar patients 20 or 30 years ago. New technology and medications continually improve the understanding and management of CAD; however, an undesired effect of long-term CAD may be the increased prevalence of heart failure also known as congestive heart failure (CHF). Coronary disease may well be the most common etiology of CHF.[64] More than 2 million Americans are effected by heart failure and about 400,000 new cases are diagnosed each year. Five-year mortality rates are in the range of 50 percent. Heart failure has surpassed MI as the leading cause of cardiac deaths in the United States; heart failure is also the most frequent cardiac diagnosis for hospital admissions and readmissions. Although the term heart failure most commonly refers to LV failure, heart failure may also include both right and left ventricles or be limited to the right ventricle alone. As a result of LV failure, increased pressure gradients may occur not only in the LV but may continue in a retrograde fashion to include the RV as well. When left and right heart failure coexist, **biventricular** failure is present. Right heart failure may occur independently of left heart failure with pulmonary disease such as chronic obstructive pulmonary disease (COPD) in which chronically elevated PA pressures result in RV failure; this is referred to as cor pulmonale.

Left ventricles that have had significant myocardial scarring as a result of a large MI or multiple MIs undergo a process of **ventricular remodeling** in which the ventricle gradually dilates and myocytes hypertrophy. Over time ventricular dilation leads to a worsening of LV function owing to the altered ventricular length-tension relationship and an increased myocardial oxygen cost. The dilated, inefficient LV presents as a cardiomyopathy with a decreased contractile force (i.e., systolic dysfunction). Besides the dilated ischemic cardiomyopathy of coronary artery disease, there are other categories of **cardiomyopathies.** The three common classifications are dilated, hypertrophic, and restrictive.[65] Dilated cardiomyopathies due to reasons other than CAD also present as systolic dysfunction, and are characterized by an enlarged, inefficient LV. Alcohol abuse is a common cause of a dilated cardiomyopathy.

Hypertrophic cardiomyopathy presents as diastolic dysfunction with an increased ventricular mass, frequently a decrease in LV chamber size, but often with preserved LV systolic function; restrictive cardiomyopathy also results in diastolic dysfunction as a result of excessively rigid ventricular walls.[65,66] The EF of patients with ischemic or dilated cardiomyopathies (systolic dysfunction) are decreased from normal, usually less than 30 percent; patients with hypertrophic or restrictive cardiomyopathies (diastolic dysfunctions) may have a normal or even above normal EF. Because of the decreased LVEDV, diastolic dysfunction may present with a normal EF (EF = SV ÷ LVEDV); in this case, however, it is important to remember that an EF in the normal range of 55 to –70 percent does not mean a normal LV. Patients may also present with a combination of these classifications (i.e., systolic and diastolic dysfunction may coexist).[66] Besides coronary disease, cardiomyopathy may result from alcohol, viral or bacterial infections, chronic hypertension, or an unknown (idiopathic) cause. Cardiomyopathies are not exclusive to the older population.

A common classification system for heart failure is the 4-class scale established by the New York Heart Association (Table 16–8). Patients in Class 4 are potential candidates for heart transplantation, whereas patients in Class 1 may be working full time and enjoying light recreational activities. Once signs of overt failure appear, approximately 50 percent of patients will die within 5 years, despite medical management.[67]

Pathophysiology of Congestive Heart Failure

In response to the decrease in LV function, a series of compensatory events occur in an attempt to maintain adequate CO: ventricular dilation and hypertrophy, sympathetic nervous system stimulation, and activation of the renin-angiotensin system. As a result of decreased contractility, the LVEDV increases and over time results in a dilated LV. The increased work of the myocardium as a result of the ineffective contractility contributes to myocardial hypertrophy. The increase in LVEDV also contributes to a rise in LV pressure; the increased pressure is transmitted retrograde toward the left atrium and then the pulmonary veins. This increase in hydrostatic pressure in the pulmonary veins causes fluid to move out of the veins and into the interstitial space of the lung resulting in **pulmonary edema.** This increased pressure may in fact continue from the pulmonary veins, capillaries and into the pulmonary artery, right heart and the peripheral venous system; the increase in the hydrostatic pressure in the peripheral veins will result in peripheral edema.

Sympathetic nervous system activation in heart failure results in tachycardia and blood flow redistribution. As a result of decreased contractility, stroke volume decreases and, in an attempt to maintain CO, there is a compensatory increase in heart rate. A resting tachycardia, therefore, may not be an unusual finding for patients in Class 3 or 4 heart failure. Blood flow redistribution occurs in response to a depressed CO. In an effort to maintain perfusion to the central circulation and major organs, peripheral vasoconstriction occurs, redistributing blood to the central circulation and resulting in a decreased peripheral blood flow.

Table 16–8 FUNCTIONAL AND THERAPEUTIC CLASSIFICATIONS OF PATIENTS WITH DISEASES OF THE HEART

Functional	Continuous-Intermittent Permissible Work Loads	Maximal
Class I	4.0–6.0 cal/min Patients with cardiac disease but without resulting limitations of physical activity. Ordinary physical activity does not cause undue fatigue, palpitation, dyspnea, or anginal pain.	6.5 METs
Class II	3.0–4.0 cal/min Patients with cardiac disease resulting in slight limitation of physical activity. They are comfortable at rest. Ordinary physical activity results in fatigue, palpitation, dyspnea, or anginal pain.	4.5 METs
Class III	2.0–3.0 cal/min Patients with cardiac disease resulting in marked limitation of physical activity. They are comfortable at rest. Less than ordinary physical activity causes fatigue, palpitation, dyspnea, or anginal pain.	3.0 METs
Class IV	1.0–2.0 cal/min Patients with cardiac disease resulting in inability to carry on any physical activity without discomfort. Symptoms of cardiac insufficiency or of the anginal syndrome may be present even at rest. If any physical activity is undertaken, discomfort is increased.	1.5 METs
Therapeutic		
Class A	Patients with cardiac disease whose physical activity need not be restricted in any way.	
Class B	Patients with cardiac disease whose ordinary physical activity need not be restricted but who should be advised against severe or competitive efforts.	
Class C	Patients with cardiac disease whose ordinary physical activity should be moderately restricted, and whose more strenuous efforts should be discontinued.	
Class D	Patients with cardiac disease whose ordinary physical activity should be markedly restricted.	
Class E	Patients with cardiac disease who should be at complete rest or confined to bed or chair.	

Reprinted by permission of the American Heart Association, New York.

The renin-angiotensin-aldosterone system is activated by a decrease in renal artery perfusion as a result of the decrease in CO. This decrease in kidney function as a result of heart failure is known as **pre-renal failure,** meaning the mechanism for renal failure occurred in the organ preceding the kidneys (i.e., the heart). In response to the perceived inadequate volume, the renin-angiotensin system stimulation and activation of aldosterone results in retention of salt and water. In reality, however, there is not too little blood volume but rather an inappropriate allocation of volume (within the heart or venous system) resulting in a decrease in arterial blood flow. Activation of the renin-angiotensin, especially owing to the contribution of angiotensin, also causes peripheral vasoconstriction. Vasoconstriction redistributes blood to the central circulation and by the increased peripheral vascular resistance may contribute to an increase in blood pressure and therefore peripheral perfusion pressure.

CHF is really a systemic disease. Although the precipitating cause is LV dysfunction, the sequelae of the disease process involves far more than the LV, including the kidneys, peripheral vascular system, skeletal muscle, and neurohormonal influences.

Clinical Presentation of Congestive Heart Failure

The clinical presentation of the patient with CHF depends not only on the amount of LV failure but also on the status of compensatory mechanisms and drug therapy (Table 16–9). Common signs and symptoms include fatigue, dyspnea, edema (pulmonary and peripheral), fluid weight gain, presence of an S_3 heart sound, and renal dysfunction. In patients with mild failure (Class 1) the compensatory mechanisms may actually facilitate cardiac functioning and result in improved organ perfusion and arterial blood pressure, and provide an adequate CO for moderate exercise without symptoms. However, many of the associated symptoms and signs of moderate to severe heart failure (Class 3 or 4) may result from these very compensatory mechanisms. For example, increased sympathetic activity may present as tachycardia, and activation of the renin-angiotensin-aldosterone system results in sodium and water retention, which contributes to the formation of pulmonary edema (and its associated shortness of breath), and peripheral edema.[68] However, although the terminology may be somewhat confusing, it is important to appreciate that when a patient is referred to as being in **compensated heart failure,** this means that the patient's congestive symptoms are relieved by medical therapy.[69] Common medical therapy includes a combination of drugs such as diuretics, a positive inotropic agent such as digoxin, ACE inhibitors, vasodilators or anti-ischemic medications if high blood pressure or ischemia require management, and an alpha/beta blocker such as Carvedilol. A patient who is noncompensated is showing signs and symptoms of congestion and requires medical readjustment.

The usual abnormal heart sound associated with CHF is the presence of an S_3 probably resulting from altered LV compliance. Heart murmurs, especially that of mitral regurgitation, may also be present owing to the effect of the enlarged LV pulling on the mitral valve. Pulmonary edema may be assessed by the presence of rales on auscultation and via CxR. Dyspnea, either positional (orthopnea, paroxysmal nocturnal) or exertional, is frequently associated with pulmonary edema. Dyspnea may also result

Table 16–9 COMPARISON OF SIGNS AND SYMPTOMS BETWEEN CLASS I, II, III, IV HEART FAILURE

	Class I: No Limitations	Class II: Slight Limitations	Class III: Marked Limitations	Class IV: Complete Limitations
Neck veins	Flat at 45° angle			Distended at 45°
Respirations	10–20 at rest	20–30 at rest	20–30 at rest	Over 30 at rest
Rales	Absent			Present
Position	Able to lie flat without distress			Unable to lie flat without distress
Edema	No dependent edema	1+ pitting edema	2+ pitting edema	3+ pitting edema
Ventricular rate	60–80 at rest	80–100 at rest	80–100 at rest	Over 100 at rest
Blood pressure	WNL for patient			+/– 10 mmHg of normal for patient
Ventricular ectopic beats	None	Occasional	—	Frequent
Cyanosis	None			Present with exertion
Pedal pulses	Easily palpable			Minimal (non palpable)
Affect	Tranquil			Restless
Weight	Stable or decreasing			Increasing

from the increased energy cost of activity as a result of decreased peripheral endurance and peripheral muscle changes. Weight gain and peripheral edema are among the signs of systemic volume overload. Increased arteriolar and arterial resistance results in an increase in afterload and therefore in myocardial oxygen demand. The increased resistance may result from a combination of factors, including increased sympathetic adrenergic stimulation; decreased vasodilation of vascular smooth muscle as a result of a decrease in the availability of the endothelium-derived relaxant factor nitric oxide; an increase in the endothelial-derived smooth muscle vasoconstrictor, endothelin-1; an increase in vascular stiffness as a result of salt and water retention; and the presence of the powerful peripheral vasoconstrictors angiotensin II and vasopressin.[68] One of the common complaints of patients with CHF that affects their activity tolerance is easy muscle fatigue. The cause of their muscle fatigue may be multifactorial, including a decrease in peripheral blood flow, changes within the peripheral vascular beds, peripheral vasoconstriction, atrophy of muscle fibers, or increased utilization of anaerobic metabolism.[70,71] Most recently, the contributions to muscle fatigue of intracellular mechanisms such as an alteration in the control of calcium release and reuptake have been studied.[72] Besides peripheral muscle functioning in patients with heart failure, exercise studies have also investigated various other factors including oxygen uptake kinetics, neurohumoral parameters, and endothelial function that may influence the exercise response.[73–75]

Pharmacological Management of CHF

The principles of drug management with CHF are quite simple—increase contractility and relieve congestion. Drugs that increase contractility are known as **positive inotropes;** the common oral drug in this category is digoxin. Diuretics decrease preload, thereby decreasing LVEDV; patients are often on a sliding scale dosage of diuretics depending on their amount of fluid weight gain. Afterload reducers, particularly those that block the effects of the renin-angiotensin system (angiotensin converting enzyme inhibitors, ACE inhibitors) are often a critical component of drug management in this population by decreasing preload (blocking salt and water retention), as well as afterload (peripheral vasoconstriction). The increase in sympathetic activity that accompanies heart failure causes (1) an increase in myocardial oxygen demand (from beta receptor stimulation) and (2) peripheral vasoconstriction and resultant reduction in peripheral blood flow (from alpha receptor stimulation). To diminish these undesired effects a new drug is being assessed for management of heart failure, a combined beta blocker and alpha blocker (Carvedilol). Beta-adrenergic receptor blockade will result in a decrease in myocardial oxygen demand; alpha-adrenergic receptor blockade will result in peripheral vascular vasodilation.

Physical Therapist Intervention

GOALS AND OUTCOMES

According to the APTA *Guide to Physical Therapist Practice*, the management of CHF would be included under the category of Impaired Aerobic Capacity and Endurance Associated with Cardiovascular Pump Failure (Pattern 6-E).[54] The following is an adapted list from the *Guide* of goals that are appropriate for patients with CHF.

1. Physiological response to increased oxygen demand is improved.
2. Self-management of symptoms is improved.
3. Ability to perform physical tasks is increased.
4. Behaviors that foster healthy habits, wellness, and prevention are acquired.
5. Disability associated with acute or chronic illness is reduced.
6. Risk of secondary impairments is reduced.
7. Awareness and use of community resources is improved.
8. Performance of and independence in ADLs and instrumental ADLs is increased.

Exercise Prescription

Exercise programs for patients with CHF are relatively recent. Studies have shown that patients with heart failure can exercise safely and regular exercise may improve functional status and decrease symptoms.[76–81] With the advent of new medications in the management of CHF such as combined alpha and beta blockers, ACE inhibitors, and vasodilators, the symptoms of volume overload are more effectively managed.[82–83] Patients whose cardiac status was once thought to be too fragile to participate in organized exercise are now cautiously participating. Using a multidisciplinary approach that includes a thorough physical assessment before each exercise session with a review of symptoms and medications, low-level exercise may be begun if the patient is hemodynamically stable. Components of the exercise program may include systemic conditioning, peripheral endurance training, low-level resistance training, and respiratory muscle training.[84–87] Monitoring oxygen saturation via pulse oximetry is a valuable tool in assessing the system's ability to provide adequate tissue oxygenation. Patients may desaturate if their CO is inadequate, if pulmonary gas exchange is decreased owing to pulmonary congestion, or if peripheral vasoconstriction occurs to redistribute blood flow toward the central core and away from the periphery. Regardless of the reason, it is prudent to stop and reassess the intensity of the activity as well as determine the need for supplemental oxygen if the patient desaturates more than 2 percent from resting levels. Some patients with CHF eventually require not just supplemental oxygen with activity but home oxygen for sleeping as well. Patient assessment should include vital sign monitoring, auscultation, observation, and recording of RPE.

A recommendation for an exercise prescription would be to keep intensity low and duration gradually increasing as the patient tolerates. Heart rate may be limited to resting heart rate plus 10 to 20 bpm. RPE is a valuable assessment tool in this population and should be kept to a rating of fairly light. Because of the decrease in diastolic filling time and the potential alteration in cardiac function at higher heart rates, keeping the exercise heart rate below 115 bpm is prudent. In the normal heart, an increase in heart rate is accompanied by an increase in inotropy. In the failing heart, an increase in heart rate may actually result in a decrease in force; this is known as the negative treppe effect.[88] Duration of exercise depends on the physiological response of the patient. A compensated Class 3 patient may be able to complete 20 continuous minutes of low-level sustained activity such as treadmill walking or recumbent biking. Another patient may require an intermittent schedule with planned rests after every minute of exercise. Light calisthenics in the sitting position are often a good initial exercise for the most compromised of patients. A prolonged warm-up and cool-down period are recommended.[89] Besides systemic conditioning exercises, inclusion of light resistance work has been recommended for inclusion in the conditioning program for the patient with CHF.[90] Modalities for resistance training may include Theraband or elastic bands for mild upper and lower extremity resistance work or light weights. A patient's hemodynamic status may change quickly with activity; therefore, it is prudent to be prepared for signs/symptoms of exertional hypotension, chronotropic incompetence, and significant dysrhythmias.[89]

Functional assessment of this population may be done with the **6 minute walk test (6MWT)**.[84,89,91] One study reported that in patients with heart failure, the oxygen consumption (Vo_2) measured at the end of a standardized 6MWT was on average only 15 percent less than the peak Vo_2 attained on an ETT.[92] Patients are asked to walk as far as they can in 6 minutes, taking as many rests as needed during this time. Quality of life questionnaires such as the Minnesota Living with Heart Failure Questionnaire are valuable for tracking patients' responses over time, although anecdotally, functional improvements do not always translate into improved quality of life scores. Relative contraindications to exercise training in this patient population are identified in Box 16–6.

Box 16–6 RELATIVE CONTRAINDICATIONS TO EXERCISE TRAINING FOR PATIENTS WITH CARDIAC MUSCLE DYSFUNCTION

Resting HR >130 bpm, <40 bpm
Resting SBP >180 mmHg
  DBP >100 mmHg
Any recent ECG change
Electrolyte abnormalities (e.g., hypokalemia or hyperkalemia)
Easily provoked angina or nocturnal angina
Extreme dyspnea (resting respiratory rate >35 breaths/min)
Profound fatigue
Mental confusion
Hemoglobin <8 gm/100 mL, hematocrit <26%
Frequent arrhythmias (premature ventricular contractions, rapid atrial fibrillation)
Acute ventricular aneurysm
Moderate to severe valvular heart disease (e.g., aortic stenosis and/or insufficiency, and mitral stenosis and/or insufficiency)
Acute systemic illness or fever >100°F
Profound and debilitating musculoskeletal, neuromuscular, or rheumatoid disorders
Pulmonary artery pressure >35 mmHg

HR, heart rate; SBP, systolic blood pressure; DBP, diastolic blood pressure; ECG, electrocardiogram; bpm, beats per minute.
From Cahalin L: In Hillegass, E, and Sadowsky, S (eds): *Essentials of Cardiopulmonary Physical Therapy.* Saunders, Philadelphia, 1994, p 166, with permission.

EXERCISE CONSIDERATIONS FOR SPECIAL CARDIAC POPULATIONS

For a brief overview of areas for consideration when designing an exercise prescription for patients following a CABG, valvular surgery, PTCA, pacemaker, automatic implantable defibrillator (AICD), or heart transplant[93] and for those patients with a diagnosis of silent ischemia or severe LV dysfunction, refer to Table 16–10.[94] Patients who have undergone a heart transplant may present with the following:

(1) calf cramps (occurring in approximately 15 percent of patients) owing to the immunosuppressive drug cyclosporine, (2) decreased lower extremity strength, (3) obesity owing to long-term corticosteroid use, (4) increased risk of fracture owing to osteoporosis associated with long-term, high-dose corticosteroids, and (5) an increased probability of developing atherosclerosis in the coronary arteries of the donor heart after the first year post surgery.[95] Because the heart is denervated, heart rate alone is an inappropriate measure of exercise intensity; therefore, blood pressure and perceived exertion should be included in the routine data collection.

Automatic implantable cardioverter defibrillators (also referred to as AICD or ICD) are placed in patients who have life-threatening ventricular tachycardia; the AICD is programmed to deliver an electric shock if it detects a heart rate higher than its programmed heart rate limit. Therefore, it is important for the physical therapist to know this limit and to avoid an exercise intensity that may inadvertently activate the device.[96] Besides knowing the heart rate settings for the patient with a pacemaker, other considerations include the following: (1) ST segment changes on the ECG may be common and are not specific for ischemia and therefore other diagnostic studies must be done, and (2) UE aerobic or strengthening exercises should be avoided initially after placement of the pacer to avoid inadvertently dislodging the device or the lead wires.[96] Checking with the physician when these exercises may be included is prudent. There may be a danger for patients with AICDs or pacemakers from electromagnetic signals such as anti-theft devices either causing the AICD to fire or causing pacers to slow down or speed up. It may be no problem for patients to walk through these devices but lingering within a few feet could be dangerous.[97]

PATIENT EDUCATION FOR PATIENTS WITH HEART DISEASE

For patients with cardiac disease, patient and family education develops along a continuum depending on the patient's baseline status and readiness to attend to the information. The physical therapist, along with other members of the health care team, needs to assess the patient's and family's ability

Table 16–10 SPECIAL CONSIDERATIONS FOR EARLY REHABILITATION

Classification	Key Factors	Exercise Prescription
CABG or valvular surgery	• Incisional discomfort • Infectious processes • Anemia	• RPE of 11–14 • Range of motion for trunk and upper extremities • Muscular strength and endurance for upper extremities
PTCA (or similar procedure), MI, or angina	• Intravascular inflammation post procedure • Signs or symptoms of continued ischemia • Anxiety • Symptom denial • New ischemia (signs or symptoms) • Resting (unstable) angina	• HR criteria if below ECG signs of ischemia • Limited by symptoms • RPE
Silent ischemia	• Associated signs (e.g., shortness-of-breath, nausea, general malaise) • Sudden decrease in exercise capacity • Sudden changes in overall condition or "sense of well-being" (prodromal symptoms)	• RPE preferred for monitoring
Severe LV dysfunction and CHF	• Significant weight gain (>4 lb) over short duration (1–2 days) • Decreased (or failure to increase) SBP during exercise • Resting or abnormal exercise shortness-of-breath	• RPE • SBP response to exertion • Symptoms
Pacemakers or AICDs	• Pacemaker type and method of function • Symptoms similar to pacemaker insertion • AICD threshold discharge rate • Ectopy or ventricular tachycardia	• RPE • HR (if available from post-insertion GXT) • HR and intensity threshold for exercise-induced ventricular tachycardia • Ventricular ectopy pattern(s)
Heart transplant	• Delayed and attenuated exercise HR response • Elevated resting HR • Signs of rejection • Infection • Medication side effects	• RPE • Signs and symptoms

Adapted from American College of Sports Medicine: Guidelines for Exercise Testing and Training, ed 5, Williams & Wilkins, Baltimore, 1995, pp 191–192, with permission.

to understand the information and, when needed, to bring in home care personnel for supervision and safety. Appropriate discharge or ongoing outpatient topics to be addressed include the following:

1. **Activity guidelines.** Patients (and family) need to be able to understand specific activity guidelines, which include planned exercise sessions as well as leisure time and rests.

2. **Self-monitoring.** Patients may monitor the intensity of their activity in a variety of ways; two of the more common ways are palpating a pulse and RPE. Because many older patients have decreased sensitivity in their palpation skills, the use of RPE may be easier and more reliable. Those patients that are able to take a pulse or choose to invest in a heart rate monitor may prefer to do so. Self-monitoring not only involves heart rate or RPE but awareness of other symptoms/signs that may suggest exercise intolerance such as lightheadedness, mental confusion, dyspnea, and inability to carry on a brief conversation while performing an activity. Patients with CHF commonly use the dyspnea scale or the Borg RPE scale.

3. **Symptom recognition and response.** Being able to recognize their specific cardiac symptoms and to know how to respond is a key component in patient education. Patients should have written information regarding the action they should take when symptoms occur, when to call their physician, or go to the hospital. Angina is the most common symptom associated with coronary heart disease, while weight gain (2 pounds over 1 to 2 days), dyspnea, lower extremity edema, and increased pillows for sleep are common signs/symptoms for CHF.

4. **Nutrition.** Patients commonly meet with a nutritionist to assess their usual dietary habits and to make recommendations when needed for a more heart-healthy diet. Most commonly, patients with coronary heart disease are instructed to reduce their fat intake; patients with CHF are instructed to monitor their salt and fluid intake.

5. **Medications.** Patients should receive written information regarding the desired action of their medications, potential side effects, dosage, and timing of medications. Patients should also know which nonprescription drugs such as cold, sinus, allergy, or anti-inflammatory medications they should avoid because of possible interactions with their prescription drugs.

6. **Life-style issues.** Many factors influence whether a patient will return to work after a cardiac event. Many patients with CAD return to work if they were employed before their event; patients with CHF are, in general, an older population when compared to patients with CAD and therefore may have already retired.

   Resumption of sexual activity may be an uncomfortable discussion for some patients. There may be many issues of concern for the patient (e.g., fear, anxiety, performance concerns, lack of libido). Patients and their partners are encouraged to verbalize their concerns to each other and to seek appropriate information from their health care team. Some medications (e.g., beta blockers) may blunt the sexual response and it is important that patients communicate this with their physician. Often, another medication or category of medication may be better tolerated. When patients feel ready for sex, when their energy level throughout the day is satisfying for them and they are able to walk outdoors and climb stairs comfortably, they are probably ready. It may be helpful for patients to remember that sexual activity is not unlike other physical activity in regards to energy cost and therefore planning, pacing, and warm-up are powerful contributors for a more comfortable outcome.

7. **Psychological/social issues.** Cardiac disease may not only create new emotional issues but also enhance some that might have existed before the cardiac event. Reassure patients that many of these issues are normal sequelae of their event. Encourage them to seek guidance and counseling in whatever arena they feel appropriate (health care, counseling, religion, etc.).

As listed in Box 16–7, the US Department of Health & Human Services Clinical Practice Guidelines for Patients with CHF[56] suggest additional topics for patient and family education for patients with LV dysfunction.

PRIMARY PREVENTION OF CORONARY ARTERY DISEASE

Patients who do not have documented CAD but who have identifiable risk factors should be encouraged to adopt life-style behaviors that can modify their risk factors. Health education and primary prevention programs through individualized education and exercise guidelines attempt to modify an individual's risk factors and thereby prevent CAD.

Patients are instructed in appropriate dietary guidelines including low fat, adequate fiber, minerals and vitamins, and decreased salt, particularly if the patient has high blood pressure. Besides lowering total dietary fat, patients are often instructed to decrease their percentage of saturated fats and to avoid trans fatty acids. Although the data regarding the benefits of their use is not definitive, many patients are encouraged to include anti-oxidants such as the vitamins E, C, co-enzyme Q10, and mixed carotenes (controversial), as well as folic acid into their diet. Elevated levels of the amino acid homocysteine appear to increase the risk of arterial endothelial disease; one of the B vitamins, folic acid, lowers homocysteine levels. If weight loss is needed, patients are encouraged to see a nutritionist to design a sensible eating plan. Patients are encouraged to begin increasing their endurance activity such as walking 30 to 40 minutes (not including warm-up and cool-down) 4 times a week. The American Col-

Box 16–7 SUGGESTED TOPICS FOR PATIENT, FAMILY, AND CAREGIVER EDUCATION AND COUNSELING

General counseling
Explanation of heart failure and the reason for symptoms
Cause or probable cause of heart failure
Expected symptoms
Symptoms of worsening heart failure
What to do if symptoms worsen
Self-monitoring with daily weights
Explanation of treatment/care plan
Clarification of patient's responsibilities
Importance of cessation of tobacco use
Role of family members or other caregivers in the treatment/care plan
Availability and value of qualified local support group
Importance of obtaining vaccinations against influenza and pneumococcal disease

Prognosis
Life expectancy
Advance directives
Advice for family members in the event of sudden death

Activity recommendations
Recreation, leisure, and work activity
Exercise
Sex, sexual difficulties, and coping strategies

Dietary recommendations
Sodium restriction
Avoidance of excessive fluid intake
Fluid restriction (if required)
Alcohol restriction

Medications
Effects of medications on quality of life and survival
Dosing
Likely side effects and what to do if they occur
Coping mechanisms for complicated medical regimens
Availability of lower cost medications or financial assistance

Importance of compliance with the treatment care plan

From Clinical Practice Guidelines, Number 11, Heart Failure: Evaluation and Care of Patients With Left-Ventricular Systolic Dysfunction, AHCPR Publication No. 94-0612, p 42.

lege of Sports Medicine and the American Heart Association recommend that anyone over the age of 40 with two or more risk factors should have an ETT before beginning an aerobic or strengthening exercise program. The purpose of the ETT is to identify the presence of any latent ischemia.

If no ischemia is present, a typical aerobic exercise prescription might be: intensity (70 to 85%) of heart rate max as the aerobic training zone; duration of 30 to 40 minutes in the aerobic training zone; appropriate warm-up of 5 to 10 minutes, and cool-down, at a frequency of 3 to 4 times per week. Maximum heart rate may be estimated by subtracting the person's age from

220; this cannot be done, however, if the person is on any cardiac medications, such as beta blockers, that may decrease the maximum heart rate. Supplemental resistance work is also encouraged at moderate intensities, with initial monitoring of heart rate and blood pressure.

Modification of the other CAD risk factors is also key to the success of any primary prevention intervention. Patients are encouraged to identify their risk factors and to seek resources to assist in modifying them. There are many community-based smoking cessation programs or medically supervised programs that a patient might want to explore. Stress management programs are also varied and can be adapted to the individual's needs. Proper and consistent use of any medications that might be used in controlling risk factors such as antihypertensives, anti-hypercholesterolemias, blood glucose lowering agents (hypoglycemics), and anti-anxiety or antidepressants is crucial to the success of any program.

Hypertension, as the most prevalent cardiovascular disease in the United States, is one of the most powerful contributors to cardiovascular morbidity and mortality.[6] The Joint National Committee on Detection, Evaluation and Treatment of High Blood Pressure recommends a multifactorial approach and suggests that "lifestyle modifications such as weight reduction, physical activity and moderation of dietary sodium are recommended as definitive or adjunctive therapy for hypertension."[98]

SUMMARY

Physical activity is important for all individuals and is especially beneficial for those individuals who are at risk for the development of CAD.[99] When a person has heart disease it does not necessarily mean that they cannot participate in physical activity either recreationally or as a prescribed exercise. Rather it means that the person needs to understand

Box 16–8 DECONDITIONING EFFECTS OF PROLONGED BEDREST

A decrease in physical work capacity
An increase in the heart rate response to effort
A decrease in adaptability to change in posture, which is manifested primarily as orthostatic hypotension
A decrease in the circulation blood volume (with plasma volume decreasing to a greater extent than red cell mass)
A decrease in lung volume and vital capacity
A decrease in serum protein concentration
A negative nitrogen and calcium balance
A decrease in the contractile strength of the body musculature

From Wenger, N: Coronary Care: Rehabilitation after Myocardial Infarction. American Heart Association, New York, 1973, with permission.

the parameters in which he or she may participate in activity. The person with heart disease should understand that a consistent exercise program is part of the management for their disease and is as necessary as their medications. The role of the physical therapist is to provide a safe exercise prescription for all patients.

During the time of illness, the effects of decreased activity can be devastating (Box 16–8). A paradox exists, however, in that the less activity that is done, the less activity that can be done as a result of a decreased work capacity. Deconditioning results in a decrease in functional aerobic capacity. Therefore, the relative energy cost of all activities increases and the heart actually works harder for any given task. Not encouraging the patient to assume an activity level when he or she is medically stable, is a disservice. As physical therapists, our role is clear: to understand the pathophysiology of the disease process, to obtain an accurate assessment of the patient, and to establish a safe exercise program. The ultimate goal is to improve the patient's physiological response to increased oxygen demand and in doing so decrease the work of the cardiovascular system, particularly the myocardial oxygen cost.

QUESTIONS FOR REVIEW

1. Discuss the role of the endothelium in atherosclerosis.

2. Describe the evolutionary process of an MI, addressing plaque formation, plaque rupture, thrombus formation, and the role of TPA.

3. Compare all the pertinent findings in the medical record: ECG, physical examination, heart sounds, lung sounds, peripheral pulses, blood work, presenting clinical symptoms, and so forth between ischemia, infarction, and CHF.

4. Discuss the physical therapy management if your patient has angina during a treatment session.

5. Design a HEP for a patient who has a positive ETT.

6. Design a HEP for a patient with Class 3 CHF.

7. Identify the various potential presentations of angina. Discuss how you would instruct your patient in symptom recognition.

8. What is the usual clinical course following a non-complicated MI? What is a complicated MI?

9. Discuss the HEP for a patient being discharged from the hospital 5 days post CABG.

10. Identify and discuss the components of cardiac output. (a) How does a patient respond to an increase in systemic oxygen demand? (b) What symptoms/signs may your patient present when there is a decrease in cardiac output?

11. Discuss factors regulating blood pressure. Discuss what actions you may take and why if your patient becomes hypotensive.

CASE STUDY

A 58 year-old male presents to the local emergency room with chief complaint of SOB and difficulty sleeping last night; patient had to sit up all night to make symptoms even a little better. Patient came to ER because he was unable to get ready for work owing to increased SOB. Patient reports that he has felt SOB off and on for a couple of months, usually associated with physical activity; symptoms, however, usually resolved with rest. Today's episode was the first related to sleeping.

PAST MEDICAL HISTORY
- Coronary artery disease: Anterior MI 4 years ago
- Hypercholesterolemia
- Peripheral vascular disease

MEDICATIONS: Digoxin, captopril, furosemide (Lasix), diltiazem, simvastatin (Zocor)

FAMILY/SOCIAL
- Patient is adopted; works full-time as an engineer; travels 3 to 4 days per month.
- Married, lives with his wife in a two story home on a 2-acre lot; three college-aged children.
- Patient is an avid golfer; enjoys gardening and landscaping.

PRESENT ILLNESS
Physical Exam

Heart Sounds:	S_1, S_2 normal; S_3 present, no S_4; 2/6 systolic murmur
Lung sounds:	Crackles 1/3 way
Rhythm/rate:	Irregular, irregular 140
Blood pressure:	100/60
Respiratory rate:	26 breaths/minute
Spo_2	90%
JVD	5 cm

Echocardiogram: akinetic apex, akinetic distal septum and anterior wall; dilated atria and LV,
Chest X-ray: unavailable.
Laboratory Data: enzyme pending; CBC WNL except BUN and creatinine slightly elevated.

Patient remained in the hospital for 2 days while medications were adjusted. During this time patient underwent further testing, including an ETT.

Results of ETT: Bruce protocol: 4 minutes; estimated Vo_2 max; 20 ml O_2/kg/min (~6 METs)
Max VS: 130 HR; 120/60 BP
ECG: (−) negative for ischemia, chest pain
Reason for stopping: absolute exhaustion.

Exam immediately post ETT: (+) S_3

Physical and occupational therapy were requested to assist with exercise guidelines and discharge planning.

PATIENT'S GOALS
- Return to work.
- Resume hiking.
- Begin to prepare his garden for spring planting within the next 5 weeks.

PHYSICAL THERAPY INTERVENTION: Exercise tolerance via low level exercises sitting and standing, as well as 5-minute walk.

VS	HR	BP
Rest	90	110/60
Sitting exercises	108	110/60
Standing (rest)	110	108/60
Standing exercise	116	110/60
5-minute walk	120	116/60

HOME INSTRUCTIONS: Meetings planned with patient and his family to discuss discharge guidelines over the next 4 to 8 weeks.

FOLLOW UP: Patient returns to his PCP 3 months after discharge. Echocardiogram is unchanged with EF 30 percent. Patient states that he has been following discharge guidelines.

VS HR 100; BP 116/70/ (resting).

Patient states that he feels great and just wants to get on with his life.

Guiding Questions

1. What is a reasonable presenting diagnosis? Identify each piece of information (and how you interpreted it) that you used to make this diagnosis.

2. Explain the pathophysiology of the patient's presenting symptoms.

3. If the patient's symptoms and signs worsened and he was admitted to the CCU,
   a) What do you think his Swan-Ganz reading could reasonably look like?
   b) What would you expect these signs/symptoms would be that would bring the patient to the CCU?
   c) What might be a reasonable cause of his signs/symptoms worsening?
   d) What other drugs/interventions might be given in the CCU?

4. What rhythm do you think the patient is in and why? What do you think might be a reason that he is in this rhythm?

5. What do you think the CxR would look like and why?

6. What is your assessment of the patient's vital sign response to PT intervention? What is your plan for your next session?

7. What exercise prescription would you recommend for the patient at home (modality, intensity, duration, frequency)?

REFERENCES

1. American Heart Association: Fact Sheet on Heart Attack, Stroke, and Risk Factors. American Heart Association, Dallas, 1993.
2. American Heart Association: Heart and Stroke Facts. 1995 Statistic Supplement. American Heart Association, Dallas, 1995.
3. Adams, PF, and Marano, MA: Current Estimates from the National Health Survey, United States 1994. Vital and Health Statistics. Vol. DHHS pub no (PHS) 96-1521: US Government Printing Office, Washington, DC, 1995.
4. WHO: MONICA Manual revised edition, Cardiovascular Diseases Unit. WHO MONICA Project. Geneva, 1990.
5. National Heart Lung and Blood Institute: Mortality and Morbidity in Cardiovascular, Lung and Blood Diseases: US Department of Health and Human Services, Washington, DC, 1996.
6. Thom, TJ, et al: Incidence, Prevalence and Mortality of Cardiovascular Disease in the United States. In Alexander, RW, Schlant, RC (eds): Hurst's The Heart, 9th ed. McGraw-Hill, New York, 1998, p 8.
7. Schlant, RC, et al: Normal Physiology of the Cardiovascular System. In Alexander, RW, et al (eds): Hurst's The Heart. McGraw-Hill, New York, 1998, p 108.
8. Fletcher, GF, and Schlant, RC: The Exercise Test. In Schlant, RC, and Alexander, RW (eds): Hurst's The Heart, 8th ed. McGraw-Hill, New York, 1994, p 424.
9. Alpert, JS: Physiology of the Cardiovascular System. Boston. Little, Brown and Co, Boston, 1984, p 20.
10. Opie, L: Mechanisms of cardiac contraction and relaxation. In Braunwald, E (ed): Heart Disease: A Textbook of Cardiovascular Medicine. Saunders, Philadelphia, 1997, p 378.
11. Noback, CR: The Human Nervous System. McGraw-Hill, New York, 1967, p 112.
12. Schlant, RC, and Sonnenblick, EH: Normal Physiology of the Cardiovascular System. In Schlant, RC, and Alexander, RW (eds): Hurst's The Heart, 8th ed. McGraw-Hill, New York, 1994, p 127.
13. Berne, RM, and Levy, MN: Cardiovascular Physiology, ed 4. Mosby, St. Louis, 1981, p 140.
14. Schlant, RC, and Sonnenblick, EH: Normal physiology of the cardiovascular system. In Schlant, RC, and Alexander, RW (eds): Hurst's The Heart, 8th ed. McGraw-Hill, New York, 1994, p 137.
15. Berne, RM, and Levy, MN: Cardiovascular Physiology, ed 4. Mosby, St. Louis, 1981 p 98.
16. Berne, RM, and Levy, MN: Cardiovascular Physiology. Mosby, St. Louis, 1981 p 136.
17. Vander, AJ, et al: Human Physiology. McGraw-Hill, New York, 1990, p 407.
18. Schlant, RC, and Sonnenblick, EH: Normal physiology of the cardiovascular system. In Schlant, RC, and Alexander, RW, (eds): Hurst's The Heart, 8th ed: McGraw-Hill, New York, 1994, p 135.
19. Alexander, RW. Coronary Ischemic Syndromes: Relationship to the Biology of Atherosclerosis. In Alexander, RW, et al (eds): Hurst's The Heart, 9th ed. McGraw-Hill, New York, 1998, p 1265.
20. Ross, R: Atherosclerosis: An inflammatory disease. N Engl J Med 340:115, 1998.
21. Charo, S, et al: Endothelial dysfunction and coronary risk reduction. J Cardiopulm Rehabil 18:60, 1998.
22. Guyton, AC: Heart sounds: Dynamics of valvular and congenital heart defects. Textbook of Medical Physiology. Saunders, Philadelphia, 1991, p 256.
23. Shaver, JA, and Salerni, R: Auscultation of the heart. In Schlant, RC, and Alexander, RW (eds): Hurst's The Heart, 8th ed. McGraw-Hill, New York, 1994, p 254.
24. Thaler, MS: The Only EKG Book You'll Ever Need. Lippincott, Philadelphia, 1998.

25. Golderberger, A, and Golderberger, E: Clinical Electrocardiography: A Simplified Approach. Mosby, St. Louis, 1981.
26. Dubin, D: Rapid Interpretation of EKGs. Cover, Tampa, 1974.
27. Myerburg, RJ, et al: Recognition, clinical assessment, and management of arrhythmias and conduction disturbances. In Schlant, RC, and Alexander, RW (eds): Hurst's The Heart, 8th ed. McGraw-Hill, New York, 1994, p 737.
28. Myerburg, RJ, et al: Recognition, clinical assessment, and management of arrhythmias and conduction disturbances. In Schlant, RC, and Alexander, RW (eds): Hurst's The Heart, 8th ed. McGraw-Hill, New York, 1994, p 736.
29. Kupersmith, J: Antiarrhythmic Drugs. The Pharmacologic Management of Heart Disease: Williams & Wilkins, Baltimore, 1997, p 449.
30. Bates, B: A Guide To Physical Examination and History Taking. Lippincott, Philadelphia, 1995.
31. Seidel, HM, et al: Mosby's Guide to Physical Examination. Mosby, St. Louis, 1995.
32. Alexander, RW: Dyspnea and Fatigue. In Schlant, RC, and Alexander, RW (eds): Hurst's The Heart, 8th ed. McGraw-Hill, New York, 1994, p 473.
33. Perry, AG, and Potter, PA: Vital Signs and Clinical Assessment. Clinical Nursing Skills and Techniques. Mosby, St. Louis, 1998, p 269.
34. Hellerstein, HK, et al: Principles of exercise prescription. In Naughton, JP (ed): Exercise Testing and Exercise Training in Coronary Heart Disease. Academic, New York, 1973, p 153.
35. Naughton, J, and Haider, R: Methods of exercise testing. In Naughton, JP, and Hellerstein, HK (eds): Exercise Testing and Exercise Training in Coronary Heart Disease. Academic, New York, 1973, p 82.
36. American College of Sports Medicine: Guidelines for Exercise Testing and Prescription. Lea & Febiger, Philadelphia, 1991.
37. Hurst, JW, and Morris, DC: The history: Symptoms and past events related to cardiovascular disease. In Schlant, RC, and Alexander, RW (eds): Hurst's The Heart, 8th ed. McGraw-Hill, New York, 1994, pp 212–213.
38. Shaver, JA, and Salerni, R: Auscultation of the heart. In Schlant, RC, and Alexander, RW (eds): Hurst's The Heart. McGraw-Hill, New York, 1994, p 284.
39. Collin, V: Contribution to diseases of the heart and pericardium: I. Historical Introduction. Bull NY Med Coll 18:1, 1955.
40. Shabetai, R: Diseases of the pericardium. In Alexander, RW, et al (eds): Hurst's The Heart, 9th ed. McGraw-Hill, New York, 1998, p 2171.
41. Ross, R: The pathogenesis of atherosclerosis: A perspective for the 1990's. Nature 362:801, 1993.
42. Wenger, NK: Coronary heart disease in women: Evolving knowledge is dramatically changing clinical care. In Julian, DG, and Wenger, NK (eds): Women and Heart Disease. Mosby, St. Louis, 1997, p 22.
43. Hennekens, CH: Coronary disease: Risk intervention. In Julian, DG, and Wenger, NK (eds): Women and Heart Disease. Mosby, St. Louis, 1997, p 45.
44. Cobb, LA: The mechanisms, predictors and prevention of sudden cardiac death. In Schlant, RC, and Alexander, RW (eds): Hurst's The Heart, 8th ed. New York: McGraw-Hill, 1994, p 947.
45. Schlant, RC, and Alexander, RW: Diagnosis and management of patients with chronic ischemic heart disease. In Alexander, RW, et al (eds): Hurst's The Heart, 9th ed. McGraw-Hill, New York, 1998, p 1277.
46. Alpert, JS: Physiology of the Cardiovascular System. Little, Brown and Co, Boston, 1984, p 36.
47. Factor, SM, and Bache, RJ: Pathophysiology of Myocardial Ischemia. In Alexander, RW, et al (eds): Hurst's The Heart, 9th ed. McGraw-Hill, New York, 1998, p 1252.
48. Richenbacher, WE, and Pierce, WS: Assisted circulation and the mechanical heart. In Braunwald, E (ed): Heart Disease: A Textbook of Cardiovascular Medicine, ed 5. Saunders, Philadelphia, 1997, p 535.
49. Alexander, RW, et al: Diagnosis and management of patients with acute myocardial infarction. In Alexander, RW, et al (eds): Hurst's The Heart, 9th ed. McGraw-Hill, New York, 1998, p 1356.
50. Ciccone, C: Pharmacology in Rehabilitation. FA Davis, Philadelphia, 1990.
51. Malone, T: Physical and Occupational Therapy: Drug Implications for Practice. Lippincott, Philadelphia, 1989.
52. Kupersmith, J: Antiarrhythmic Drugs. The Pharmacologic Management of Heart Disease. Williams & Wilkins, Baltimore, 1997.
53. Grimes, K, and Cohen, M: Cardiac pharmacology. In Hillegass, E (ed): Essentials of Cardiopulmonary Physical Therapy. Saunders, Philadelphia, 1995.
54. American Physical Therapy Association: Guide to Physical Therapist Practice APTA, Alexandria, VA, 1999.
55. Levine, SA, and Lown, B: Armchair treatment of acute coronary thrombosis. JAMA 1948:1356, 1952.
56. American Association of Cardiovascular and Pulmonary Rehabilitation: Guidelines for Cardiac Rehabilitation Programs: Human Kinetics, Champaign, IL, 1995, p 49.
57. Borg, GV: Psychophysical basis of perceived exertion. Med Sci Sports Exer 14:377, 1982.
58. US Department of Health and Human Services: Effects of Cardiac Rehabilitation Exercise Training. Clinical Practice Guidelines, Cardiac Rehabilitation, AHCPR No. 17 publication No. 96-0672, October 1995.
59. McCartney, N: Role of resistance training in heart disease. Med Sci Sports Exerc S396, 1998.
60. Beniamini, Y, et al: Effects of high intensity strength training on quality of life parameters in cardiac rehabilitation patients. Am J Cardiol 841, 1997.
61. American Association of Cardiovascular and Pulmonary Rehabilitation: Guidelines for Cardiac Rehabilitation Programs. Human Kinetics Publishers, Champaign, IL, 1991, pp 27–56.
62. American College of Sports Medicine: ACSM's Resource Manual for Guidelines for Exercise Testing and Prescriptions. Williams & Wilkins, Baltimore, 1998, p 448.
63. Fletcher, GF, et al: Exercise standards: A statement for healthcare professionals from the American Heart Association. Circulation 91:580, 1995.
64. Kannel, WB: Epidemiological aspects of heart failure. Cardiol Clin 7:1, 1989.
65. Cahalin, LP: Cardiac muscle dysfunction. In Hillegass, E (ed): Essentials of Cardiopulmonary Physical Therapy. Saunders, Philadelphia, 1995, p 126.
66. Wynne, J, and Braunwald, E: The cardiomyopathies and myocarditides. In E B (ed): Heart Disease: A Textbook of Cardiovascular Medicine, vol 2. Saunders, Philadelphia, 1997, p 1404.
67. Thom, TJ, et al: Incidence, prevalence and mortality of cardiovascular disease in the United States. In Alexander, RW, et al (eds): Hurst's The Heart, 9th ed. McGraw-Hill, New York, 1998, pp 12–13.
68. Schlant, RC, and Sonnenblick, EH: Pathophysiology of heart failure. In Schlant, RC, and Alexander, RW (eds): Hurst's The Heart, 8th ed. McGraw-Hill, New York, 1994, p 522.
69. Schlant, RC, and Sonnenblick, EH: Pathophysiology of heart failure. In Schlant, RC, and Alexander, RW (eds): Hurst's The Heart, 8th ed. McGraw-Hill, New York, 1994, p 519.
70. Atsumi, H, et al: Cardiac sympathetic nervous disintegrity is related to exercise intolerance in patients with chronic heart failure. Nucl Med Commun 19:451, 1998.
71. Linjiing, X, et al: Effect of heart failure on muscle capillary geometry: Implications for O_2 exchange. Med Sci Sports Exerc 30:1230, 1998.
72. Lunde, PK, et al: Skeletal muscle fatigue in normal subjects and heart failure patients. Is there a common mechanism? Acta Physiol Scand 162:215, 1998.
73. Rocca, HPBL, et al: Oxygen uptake kinetics during low level exercise in patients with heart failure: Relation to neurohormones, peak oxygen consumption, and clinical findings. Heart 81:121, 1999.
74. Bank, AJ: Effects of short-term forearm exercise training on resistance vessel endothelial function in normal subjects and patients with heart failure. J Card Fail 4:193, 1998.
75. Genth-Zotz, S, et al: Changes of neurohumoral parameters and endothelin-1 in response to exercise in patients with

mild to moderate congestive heart failure. Int J Cardiol 30:137, 1998.

76. Coats, A, et al: Controlled trial of physical training in chronic heart failure: Exercise performance, hemodynamics, ventilation and autonomic function. Circulation 85: 2119, 1992.

77. Rossi, P: Physical training in patients with CHF. Chest 101:350s, 1992.

78. Cahalin, LP. Exercise training in chronic heart failure, the European experience. AACN Clin Issues 9:225, 1998.

79. Kavanagh, T: Exercise training in chronic heart failure: The European experience. Eur Heart J 19:363, 1998.

80. Tyni-Lenne, R, et al: Improved quality of life in chronic heart failure patients following local endurance training with leg muscles. J Card Fail 2:111, 1996.

81. Afzal, A, et al: Exercise training in heart failure. Prog Cardiovasc Dis 41:175, 1998.

82. Avezum, A, et al: Beta-blocker therapy for congestive heart failure: A systemic overview and critical appraisal of the published trials. Can J Cardiol 14:1045, 1998.

83. Cleland, JG, et al: Beta-blockers for chronic heart failure: From prejudice to enlightenment. J Cardiovasc Pharmacol 32:S36, 1998.

84. Cahalin, LP: Heart failure. Phys Ther 76:516, 1996.

85. Cahalin, L: The six-minute walk test predicts peak oxygen uptake and survival in patients with advanced heart failure. Chest 110:325, 1996.

86. Johnson, PH, et al: A randomized controlled trial of inspiratory muscle training in stable chronic heart failure. Eur Heart J 19:1249, 1998.

87. Balady, GJ: Exercise training in the treatment of heart failure: What is achieved and how? Ann Med 30(suppl 1):61, 1998.

88. Schlant, RC, and Sonnenblick, EH: Pathophysiology of heart failure. In Schlant, RC, and Alexander, RW (eds): Hurst's The Heart, 8th ed. New York: McGraw-Hill, 1994, p 530.

89. American College of Sports Medicine: ACSM's Exercise Management for Persons with Chronic Diseases and Disabilities. Human Kinetics, Champaign, IL, 1997, p 50.

90. McKelvie, RS, et al: Comparison of hemodynamic responses to cycling and resistance exercises in congestive heart failure secondary to ischemic cardiomyopathy. Am J Cardiol 76:977, 1995.

91. Schaufelberger, SM, and Swedberg, K: Is six-minute walk test of value in congestive heart failure? Am Heart J 136:371, 1998.

92. Faggiano, P, et al: Assessment of oxygen uptake during the six-minute walking test in patients with heart failure: Preliminary experience with a portable device. Am Heart J 134:203, 1997.

93. Braith, RW: Exercise training in patients with CHF and heart transplant recipients. Med Sci Sports Exerc 30(suppl 10), 1998.

94. American College of Sports Medicine: ACSM's Guide For Exercise Testing and Prescription. Williams & Wilkins, Baltimore, 1995, pp 191–192.

95. American College of Sports Medicine: ACSM's Exercise Management for Persons with Chronic Diseases and Disabilities. Human Kinetics, Champaign, IL, 1997, p 55.

96. American College of Sports Medicine: ACSM's Exercise Management for Persons with Chronic Diseases and Disabilities. Human Kinetics, Champaign, IL, 1997, p 38.

97. Harvard Heart Letter: Hazards for patients with cardiac pacemakers and defibrillators. Harvard Heart Letter 9:6, 1999.

98. National High Blood Pressure Education Program: The Fifth Report of The Joint National Committee on Detection, Evaluation and Treatment of High Blood Pressure, NHLBI Obesity Education Initiative, US Government Printing Office, Washington, D.C., 1993.

99. Miller, T, et al: Exercise and its role in the prevention and rehabilitation of cardiovascular disease. Ann Behav Med 19:220, 1997.

SUPPLEMENTAL READINGS

Alexander, RW, et al (eds): Hurst's The Heart, 9th ed. McGraw-Hill, New York, 1998.

American Association of Cardiovascular and Pulmonary Rehabilitation: Guidelines for Cardiac Rehabilitation Programs. Human Kinetics, Champaign, IL, 1991.

American College of Sports Medicine: ACSM's Exercise Management for Persons with Chronic Diseases and Disabilities. Human Kinetics, Champaign, IL, 1997.

American College of Sports Medicine: ACSM's Guidelines for Exercise Testing and Prescription, ed 5. Williams & Wilkins, Baltimore, 1995.

Braunwald, E: Heart Disease: A Textbook of Cardiovascular Medicine, ed 5. Saunders, Philadelphia, 1997.

Frownfelter, D, and Dean, E: Principles and Practice of Cardiopulmonary Physical Therapy. Mosby-Year Book, St. Louis, 1996.

Hillegass, EA, and Sadowsky, HS: Essentials of Cardiopulmonary Physical Therapy. Saunders, Philadelphia, 1994.

Kupersmith, J, and Deedwania, PC: Pharmacologic Management of Heart Disease. Williams & Wilkins, Baltimore, 1997.

Robergs, RA, and Roberts, SO: Exercise Physiology, Mosby, St. Louis, 1997.

US Department of Health and Human Services: Clinical Practice Guideline, Number 17, Cardiac Rehabilitation, AHCPR Publication No. 96-0672, October, 1995.

US Department of Health and Human Services: Clinical Practice Guideline, Number 11, Heart Failure: Management of Patients with Left Ventricular Systolic Dysfunction, AHCPR Publication No. 94-0613, June, 1994.

Watchie, J: Cardiopulmonary Physical Therapy: A Clinical Manual. Saunders, Philadelphia, 1995.

GLOSSARY

ACE inhibitors: A category of drug that inhihibits the renin-angiotensin system.

Active hyperemia: Autoregulation in response to metabolic changes.

Afterload: The resistance against which the ventricle contracts; blood pressure is a measure of afterload.

Afterload reducers: A category of medications that decrease afterload.

Angina: Caused by deficiency of oxygen supply to heart muscle; typically presents as substernal chest pressure (SSCP) or pain, but there are also varied atypical presentations.

Stable angina: Angina that is a result of an imbalance of myocardial oxygen supply and myocardial oxygen demand; when the myocardial demand is decreased, the angina will abate.

Unstable angina: Angina that is unable to be controlled by decreasing myocardial oxygen demand; may occur at rest; may indicate a preinfarction state.

Angiogram: A component of a left heart catheterization in which a dye is injected into the coronary arteries to assess blood flow and the presence of occlusions.

Angle of Louis: Anatomical landmark on the chest wall for the RA; the bony demarcation of the manubrium from the body of the sternum.

Arterial line: Invasive monitoring of arterial blood pressure via insertion of a catheter into an artery.

Atherosclerotic lesion: The site of an arterial endothelial injury undergoes an inflammatory process and creates a lesion consisting of lipids, macrophages, necrotic tissue, and calcium.

Auscultation: The process of listening to the heart, lungs, blood vessels, and so forth, with a stethoscope.

Autoregulation: A type of vascular regulation that occurs at the local level.

Baroreceptor reflex: A stretch-sensitive reflex that is activated by an increase in arterial pressure.

Beta blockers: A category of anti-ischemic medications that block the sympathetic beta receptors and decrease myocardial work.

Blood pressure: The amount of pressure within the arteries throughout the cardiac cycle; a product of CO and peripheral vascular resistance.

Bradycardia: A heart rate below 60 bpm.

Bruit: An abnormal auscultatory finding that is associated with a blockage within an artery; most commonly found within the carotid or femoral arteries.

Coronary artery bypass graft (CABG): Surgical revascularization procedure to restore coronary blood flow through new grafts.

Calcium channel blockers: A category of drug that prevents coronary spasm and decreases blood pressure.

Cardiac index (CI): CO expressed in relation to body surface area.

Cardiac output (CO): The volume of blood that leaves the LV per minute; it is a product of heart rate and stroke volume; expressed in L/min.

Cardiogenic shock: Life-threatening event; inadequate CO and arterial blood pressure to perfuse the major organs.

Cardiomyopathies: Cardiac muscle dysfunction; three basic categories are dilated cardiomyopathy, hypertrophic cardiomyopathy, and restrictive cardiomyopathy.

Catecholamine: Formed from the amino acid tyrosine, they contain a catechol ring (six-sided carbon ring with two hydroxyl groups); the three catecholamines are dopamine, norepinephrine, and epinephrine. Norepineprhine and epinephrine are hormones secreted from the adrenal medulla.

Catheterization

   Left heart catheterization: Insertion of a thin tube (catheter) into an artery, usually femoral or radial, and advancing it retrograde either to the LV to assess LV function or to the coronary ostium to assess coronary blood flow and the presence of coronary atherosclerotic lesions.

   Right heart catheterization: Insertion of a catheter into the right side of the heart via the internal jugular or subclavian vein for the purpose of hemodynamic monitoring.

Chemoreceptors: Monitors the concentrations of oxygen, carbon dioxide, and H^+ ions.

Chronotropic incompetence: Inability to increase heart rate appropriately in response to an increase in oxygen demand.

Chronotropy: Heart rate.

Compensated heart failure: LV dysfunction in which the compensatory mechanisms have provided an adequate CO and blood pressure response and in which there are no systemic signs of congestion.

Compensatory tachycardia: A condition in which the heart rate increases in response to a decrease in stroke volume to maintain CO.

Congestive heart failure (CHF): The presence of pulmonary or peripheral congestion due to heart failure, most commonly LV dysfunction.

Contractility: The ability of the LV to contract; a factor of stroke volume.

Cor pulmonale: Right heart failure owing to a primary pulmonary cause such as pulmonary hypertension.

Coronary artery disease (CAD): Heart disease owing to a narrowing of the coronary arteries sufficient to prevent adequate blood supply to the heart.

Coronary blood flow (CBF): The amount of blood flow through the coronary arteries; a critical factor in increasing myocardial oxygen supply.

Coronary heart disease (CHD, ischemic h.d.): A lack of oxygen supply to the heart, with consequent altered cardiac function; the most common cause is atherosclerosis of the coronary arteries.

Coronary spasm: Transient occlusion of a coronary artery due to spasm of the arterial smooth muscle.

CPK MB: An intracellular enzyme that is released with tissue damage, specifically myocardial tissue. CPK levels usually peak within the first 12 to 24 hours of an MI.

Crackles (rales): An abnormal auscultatory finding within the lungs commonly associated with the pulmonary congestion of CHF although its presence may also indicate a pulmonary dysfunction.

Cyanosis: A bluish color of the skin, nailbeds and lips associated with a decrease in arterial oxygenation.

Diaphoresis: Excess or profuse sweating.

Dyspnea on exertion (DOE): Dyspnea that occurs with low level activity or during the usual activities of daily living.

Dressler's syndrome: Pericarditis occurring within the post MI period.

Dyspnea: The feeling of breathlessness that occurs when there is a higher demand for ventilation than can be met by comfortable breathing; air hunger; normally accompanies vigorous exercise.

Endothelium-derived relaxing factor (EDRF): Secreted by endothelial cells, relaxes vascular smooth muscle, which results in arteriolar dilation; nitric oxide is an example.

Ejection fraction (EF): The percent of LVEDV that was ejected from the LV during systole; expressed as the ratio of stroke volume to LVEDV (SV divided by LVEDV).

Exercise tolerance test (ETT, graded exercise or stress test): The measure of the efficiency of the cardiorespiratory system. The subject is placed on a treadmill and is monitored with an ECG and sometimes oxygen collection device. The workload is increased until the subject reaches exhaustion, or until signs of exertional intolerance and distress.

> **False negative ETT:** An ETT that does not detect the presence of ischemia when it exists.
>
> **False positive ETT:** An ETT that incorrectly detects the presence of ischemia when it does not exist.
>
> **Negative ETT:** No ischemia present during an ETT.
>
> **Positive ETT:** Ischemia present during an ETT.

Heart sounds: The auscultatory sounds of the cardiac cycle.

> **S_1:** The normal first heart sound, produced by the closure of the mitral and tricuspid valves; marks the beginning of systole.
>
> **S_2:** The normal second heart sound, produced by the closure of the aortic and pulmonic valves; marks the end of systole and the beginning of diastole.
>
> **S_3:** Ventricular gallop: Abnormal heart sound associated with the presence of CHF.
>
> **S_4:** Atrial gallop: Abnormal heart sound associated with an MI.

Intra-aortic balloon pump (IABP): A catheter with a large inflatable balloon that is placed within the aorta and is synchronized to the ECG, it inflates during diastole and increases perfusion of coronary arteries and deflates during systole thereby decreasing afterload and myocardial work.

Inotropy: Contractility.

Ischemia: A temporary decrease in oxygenated blood supply to the tissues.

Levine sign: A classic sign of angina, a clenched fist placed over the sternum.

Metabolic equivalents (METs): The amount of oxygen consumption at rest is referred to as 1 MET and corresponds to 3.5 mL O_2/kg/min.

Myocardial infarction (MI)

> **Non-Q wave (nontransmural) MI:** An MI that does not extend throughout the myocardium but rather remains in the subendocardial area; it does not have an abnormal Q wave on the ECG.
>
> **Transmural (Q wave) MI:** An MI through the full thickness of myocardial tissue, extending from the subendocardium to the subepicardium; most often associated with an abnormal Q wave on ECG.

MVo$_2$: Myocardial oxygen demand.

Nitrates: A category of anti-ischemic medications that vasodilates arteries and in particular veins resulting in a decrease in afterload and preload.

Normal sinus rhythm (NSR): Normal cardiac conduction beginning in the sinoatrial node.

Orthopnea: Dyspnea that occurs in the recumbent position and is relieved when upright.

> **Two pillow orthopnea:** Orthopnea that is relieved when the head is elevated on two pillows.

Orthostatic hypotension (postural hypotension): A prolonged drop in blood pressure that accompanies a position change from supine to upright.

Pallor: The absence of a pink, rosy color; paleness.

Premature atrial contraction (PAC): An ectopic beat originating in the atria.

Paroxysmal atrial tachycardia (PAT): A series of PACs occurring at a rate of 100 to 200 bpm.

Pulmonary capillary wedge pressure (PCWP): The pressure within a pulmonary capillary determined by a balloon catheter.

Pericardial friction rub: Abnormal auscultatory finding associated with pericardial inflammation.

Peripheral vascular resistance (PVR): The resistance to blood flow; a property primarily of arterial vascular system.

Persantine thallium: A non-exercise diagnostic test to detect the presence of ischemia.

Phases I, II, II, IV: Designations of levels of cardiac rehabilitation based on the time since the cardiac event, level of acuity, and need for supervision and monitoring.

Pitting edema: The indentation to the skin when pressure is applied; a measure of the severity of peripheral edema.

Point of maximal impulse (PMI): Located at the apex of the heart, the area of the strongest ventricular contraction; located in the fifth intercostal space, mid-clavicular line.

Paroxysmal nocturnal dyspnea (PND): Dyspnea that awakens a person suddenly from sleep.

Pre-renal failure: Altered kidney function due to a non-kidney cause (heart failure) occurring before the blood reaches the kidneys.

Preload: Venous return; a factor of stroke volume.

Pressure autoregulation: Autoregulation in response to a decrease in blood flow.

Primary prevention: A program of nutrition, exercise and counseling to decrease the impact of CAD risk factors with the goal of decreasing the initial occurrence of CAD.

Percutaneous transluminal coronary angioplasty (PTCA): Revascularization procedure to restore coronary blood by compressing the atherosclerotic plaque against the walls of the artery via an inflated balloon.

Pulmonary edema: Pulmonary congestion; may be due to an increase in capillary hydrostatic pressure (e.g., LV dysfunction), decreased plasma oncotic pressure, lymphatic insufficiency, altered alveolar-capillary membrane permeability, or other less common causes.

Premature ventricular contraction (PVC): An ectopic beat originating in the ventricles.

Rate pressure product (RPP): An estimation of myocardial oxygen demand; the product of heart rate and systolic blood pressure.

Rate of Perceived Exertion (RPE) scale: A scale that allows the exerciser to subjectively rate his or her feelings during exercise, taking into account fitness level, environmental conditions, and general fatigue levels; developed by Borg.[94, p 67]

Remodeling: The process of ventricular dilation and hypertrophy following an MI that results in alteration of LV function.

Retrograde flow: Opposite of the normal antegrade flow.

Starling's length-tension relationship: As muscle length increases, force production will also increase.

Stress echo: An echocardiogram that is taken at the time of an exercise tolerance test.

Stroke volume: The volume of blood ejected from the LV with each ventricular contraction, expressed in mL/min; the difference between LV end diastolic volume and LV end systolic volume.

Sudden death: Cardiac arrest; pulselessness and breathlessness.

Supraventricular beats: Ectopic beats originating above (supra) the ventricles.

Supraventricular tachycardia (SVT): Supraventricular ectopic beats occurring at a rate of 150 to 250 bpm.

Sympatholytics: Opposing or inhibiting the action of the sympathetic nervous system; some drugs may act as sympatholytics.

Sympathomimetics: Mimics the action of the sympathetic nervous system; some drugs may act as sympathomimetics.

Tachycardia: A heart rate greater than 100 bpm.

Thrombus: A blood clot that obstructs a blood vessel or a cavity of the heart.

Troponin I and T: An inhibitory protein in muscle fibers; elevated levels provide a marker for MI.

Uncomplicated MI: An MI that is not complicated by post-MI ischemia, LV dysfunction, or ventricular arrhythmias such as v-tach or v-fib.

APPENDIX A

The Minnesota LIVING WITH HEART FAILURE™ Questionnaire

These questions concern how your heart failure (heart condition) has prevented you from living as you wanted during the last *month*. The items listed below describe different ways some people are affected. If you are sure an item does not apply to you or is not related to your heart condition then circle "0" (No) and go on to the next item. If an item does apply to you, then circle the number rating how much it prevented you from living as you wanted.

Did your heart failure (heart condition) prevent you from living as you wanted during the last month by:

	No	Very Little				Very Much
1. Causing swelling in your ankles, legs, etc?	0	1	2	3	4	5
2. Making you sit or lie down during the day?	0	1	2	3	4	5
3. Making your walking or climbing stairs difficult?	0	1	2	3	4	5
4. Making your work around the house or yard more difficult?	0	1	2	3	4	5
5. Making your going places away from home more difficult?	0	1	2	3	4	5
6. Making your sleeping well at night more difficult?	0	1	2	3	4	5
7. Making your relating or doing things with your friends or family difficult?	0	1	2	3	4	5
8. Making your working to earn a living more difficult?	0	1	2	3	4	5
9. Making your recreational pastimes, sports, or hobbies more difficult?	0	1	2	3	4	5
10. Making your sexual activities more difficult?	0	1	2	3	4	5
11. Making you eat less of the foods you like?	0	1	2	3	4	5
12. Making you short of breath?	0	1	2	3	4	5
13. Making you tired, fatigued, or low on energy?	0	1	2	3	4	5
14. Making you stay in the hospital?	0	1	2	3	4	5
15. Costing you money for medical care?	0	1	2	3	4	5
16. Giving you side effects from medications?	0	1	2	3	4	5
17. Making you feel you are a burden to your family or friends?	0	1	2	3	4	5
18. Making you feel a loss of self-control in your life?	0	1	2	3	4	5
19. Making you worry?	0	1	2	3	4	5
20. Making it difficult for you to concentrate or remember things?	0	1	2	3	4	5
21. Making you feel depressed?	0	1	2	3	4	5

APPENDIX B

Suggested Answers to Case Study Guiding Questions

1. What is a reasonable presenting diagnosis? Identify each piece of information (and how you interpret it) that you used to make this diagnosis.

ANSWER: The differential diagnosis would be congestive heart failure versus ischemia versus infarction. SOB may be due to ischemia, which would explain his SOB with exertion for the months prior to today. The fact that he could not lie down, and that his symptoms improved with an upright position favors CHF at this time; however, CHF could result from either ischemia or an infarction.

- EKG: c/w an MI; the fact that the ST is normal, favors CHF and not ischemia or a new infarction.
- Heart sounds: S_3 is a typical finding with CHF.
- Lung sounds: in this setting, crackles supports the dx of CHF.
- Echo: suggests that there has been considerable myocardial damage and along with the dilated LV, there is the potential for CHF.
- JVD: abnormally elevated; c/w CHF.

2. Explain the pathophysiology of the patient's presenting symptoms.

ANSWER: SOB with exertion and rest. Perhaps because of LV remodeling following his large anterior MI, his LV has enlarged to the point of systolic dysfunction and has begun to fail. As a result of the LV failure, there is an increase in LVEDP/LVEDV, which is transmitted to the left atrium and pulmonary veins, which are likely engorged and fluid has leaked into the interstitial spaces of the lung. Venous return is greater in supine than in sitting, so there will be a higher LVEDV which will aggravate the symptoms; when the patient sits up, gravity assists in decreasing the filling volume somewhat and patient experiences temporary relief.

3. If the patient's symptoms and signs worsened and he was admitted to the CCU,
(a) What do you think his Swan-Ganz reading could reasonably look like?

ANSWER: Consistent with LV failure; PCWP above 20 mm Hg, RA and CVP above 10 mm Hg.

(b) What signs/symptoms would bring the patient to the CCU?

ANSWER:
- Hypotension.
- Worsening SOB.
- Increased signs of congestion on physical examination.
- Decreased arterial oxygenation.

(c) What might be a reasonable cause of his signs/symptoms worsening?

ANSWER: Ischemia.

(d) What other drugs/interventions might be given in the CCU?

ANSWER:
- IABP if patient unable to be stabilized with medications.
- Diuretics and ACE inhibitors to decrease preload.
- Supplemental oxygen to assist with arterial oxygenation.

4. What rhythm do you think the patient is in and why? What do you think might be a reason for this rhythm?

ANSWER: Atrial fibrillation is the classic irregular rhythm. The dilated LA, creates an opportunity for atrial arrhythmias to occur.

5. What do you think the CxR would look like and why?

ANSWER: Engorged vascular vessels, pulmonary edema, enlarged heart.

6. What is your assessment of his vital signs in response to PT intervention? What is your plan for your next session?

ANSWER: Flat BP response; adaptive HR response (i.e., he was able to increase HR with activity; however his HR appears to be too high for the limited work). The next session should include shorter distances, slower pace, more rests as well as sitting activities, restorator, and so forth.

7. What exercise prescription would you recommend for the patient at home (modality, intensity, duration, frequency)?

ANSWER: Slow ambulation, ambient conditions, stationary bike; the goal is to gradually increase duration and to keep intensity at a low-moderate level and never allowing HR to be above 115 bpm. Generally resting heart rate plus 10 to 15 bpm is a prudent prescription.

Susan B. O'Sullivan

LEARNING OBJECTIVES

1. Describe the etiology, pathophysiology, symptomatology, and sequelae of stroke.
2. Identify and describe the examination procedures used to evaluate patients with stroke to establish a diagnosis, prognosis, and plan of care.
3. Describe the role of the physical therapist in assisting the patient in recovery from stroke in terms of interventions, patient-related instruction, coordination, communication, and documentation.
4. Identify and describe strategies of intervention during acute (inpatient) rehabilitation.
5. Analyze and interpret patient data, formulate realistic goals and outcomes, and develop a plan of care when presented with a clinical case study.

Stroke is an acute onset of neurological dysfunction due to an abnormality in cerebral circulation with resultant signs and symptoms that correspond to involvement of focal areas of the brain.[1] The term **cerebrovascular accident** (CVA) is used interchangeably with stroke to refer to the cerebrovascular conditions that accompany either ischemic or hemorrhagic lesions. Clinically, a variety of deficits are possible, including changes in the level of consciousness, and impairments of sensory, motor, cognitive, perceptual, and language functions. To be classified as stroke, focal neurological deficits must persist for at least 24 hours. Motor deficits are characterized by paralysis **(hemiplegia)** or weakness **(hemiparesis),** typically on the side of the body opposite the site of the lesion. The term *hemiplegia* is often used generically to refer to the wide variety of problems that result from stroke. The location and extent of the lesion, the amount of collateral blood flow, and early acute care management determine the severity of neurological deficits in an individual patient. Impairments may resolve spontaneously with neurological recovery **(reversible ischemic neurological deficit)** generally within 3 weeks. Residual neurological impairments are those that persist longer than 3 weeks and may lead to permanent disability and dependence. Strokes may be categorized by etiological categories (thrombosis, embolus, or hemorrhage), management categories (transient ischemic attack, minor stroke, major stroke, deteriorating stroke, young stroke), and anatomical categories (specific vascular territory).

EPIDEMIOLOGY

Stroke is the third leading cause of death and the most common cause of disability among adults in the United States. It affects approximately 600,000 individuals each year with an estimated number of 4,000,000 stroke survivors. The incidence of stroke increases dramatically with age, doubling every decade after 55 years of age. For white men aged 65 to 74, the incidence is about 14.4 per 1000 population; for ages 75 to 84 it is 24.6 and for 85 and older it is 27.0. Twenty-eight percent of strokes occur in individuals under the age of 65. The incidence of stroke is about 19 percent higher for males than females. Compared to whites, African-Americans have a two to three-fold risk of ischemic stroke and are 2.5 times more likely to die of stroke.[2,3]

About 31 percent of individuals who have an initial stroke die within a year, a rate that is increased in individuals age 65 or older. At 12 years only 34 percent of patients are still alive.[2,4] The type of stroke is significant in determining survival. Patients with intracerebral hemorrhage account for the largest number of deaths following an acute episode (59 to 72% at 3 months) followed by subarachnoid hemorrhage (43% at 3 months) and thromboembolic stroke (30% at 3 months).[5] Survival rates are dramatically lessened by a number of medical comorbidities and patient characteristics, including age, hypertension,

heart disease, and diabetes. Loss of consciousness at stroke onset, lesion size, persistent severe hemiplegia, multiple neurological deficits, and history of previous stroke are also important predictors of mortality. Patients who suffer recurrent episodes of stroke usually experience the same type, and these are influenced by the same risk factors influencing survival.

Of survivors, an estimated 300,000 (30 to 40%) will have significant disability. Stroke survivors represent the largest group admitted to inpatient rehabilitation hospitals (34% of first admissions).[6]

Epidemiological studies reveal a steady decline in the incidence of stroke in the last 30 years and especially in the last decade. From 1985 to 1995 the stroke death rate fell 17.3 percent.[2] Similar downward trends have also been noted in the incidence of cardiovascular disease. Better diagnosis and treatment, and control of modifiable stroke risk factors have been implicated in contributing to the rates of decline.[7,8] Table 17–1 summarizes the epidemiology of stroke.

Table 17–1 EPIDEMIOLOGY OF STROKE

Vital statistics—United States (1989)

Incidence of stroke	500,000
Prevalence of stroke	2,980,000
Mortality due to stroke	147,470

Etiology of stroke (cerebral is used here to refer to the entire brain)

	Percent
Ischemic stroke	
Cerebral thrombosis	47–67
Cerebral embolus	14
Subtotal	61–81
Hemorrhagic stroke	
Intracerebral	8–16
Subarachnoid	4–8
Subtotal	12–24
Other or cause uncertain	0–25

Mortality rates (ranges from published reports)

30-day mortality	17–34
1-year mortality	25–40
3-year mortality	32–60

Risk factors for stroke

Potentially modifiable	**Not modifiable**
Transient ischemic attacks (TIA), especially in the presence of 70–99% carotid artery stenosis	Prior stroke Age Race Gender
Hypertension	Family history of stroke
Atrial fibrillation or other source of cardiac emboli	
Left ventricular hypertrophy	
Congestive heart failure	
Cigarette smoking	
Coronary artery disease	
Alcohol consumption	
Cocaine use	
Obesity	
Diabetes mellitus	
High serum cholesterol	

Note: The 1989 estimated incidence of stroke in the United States was 500,000; however, more recent data indicate that this estimate is closer to 550,000.

From Post-Stroke Rehabilitation Guideline Panel: Post-Stroke Rehabilitation Clinical Practice Guideline. Aspen, Gaithersburg, MD, 1996, p 24, with permission.

ETIOLOGICAL CATEGORIES

Atherosclerosis is a major contributory factor in cerebrovascular disease. It is characterized by plaque formation with an accumulation of lipids, fibrin, complex carbohydrates, and calcium deposits on arterial walls that leads to progressive narrowing of blood vessels. Interruption of blood flow by atherosclerotic plaques occurs at certain sites of predilection. These generally include bifurcations, constrictions, dilation, or angulations of arteries. The most common sites for lesions to occur are at the origin of the common carotid artery or at its transition into the middle cerebral artery, at the main bifurcation of the middle cerebral artery, and at the junction of the vertebral arteries with the basilar artery (Fig. 17-1).

Two main mechanisms result in stroke. Strokes can be *ischemic,* the result of a thrombus, embolism, or conditions that produce low systemic perfusion pressures. The resulting lack of cerebral blood flow (CBF) deprives the brain of needed oxygen and glucose, disrupts cellular metabolism, and leads to injury and death of tissues. A thrombus results from platelet adhesion and aggregation on plaques. **Cerebral thrombosis** refers to the formation or development of a blood clot or thrombus within the cerebral arteries or their branches. It should be noted that lesions of extracranial vessels (carotid or vertebral arteries) can also produce symptoms of stroke. Thrombi lead to ischemia, or occlusion of an artery with resulting infarction or tissue death **(atherothrombotic brain infarction [ABI]).** Thrombi can also become dislodged and travel to a more distal site in the form of an intra-artery embolus. **Cerebral embolus** (CE) are traveling bits of matter formed elsewhere that are released into the bloodstream and travel to the cerebral arteries where they lodge in a vessel, producing occlusion and infarction. The most common etiology results from cardiovascular disease (valvular disease, myocardial infarction, arrhythmias, congenital heart disease). Occasionally systemic disorders may produce septic, fat, or air emboli that affect the cerebral circulation. Ischemic strokes may also result from low systemic perfusion, the result of cardiac failure or significant blood loss with resulting systemic hypotension. The neurological deficits produced with systemic failure are global in nature with bilateral neurological deficits.[9]

Strokes can also be *hemorrhagic,* with abnormal bleeding into extravascular areas of the brain secondary to aneurysm or trauma. Hemorrhage results in increased intracranial pressures with injury to brain tissues and restriction of distal blood flow. **Intracerebral hemorrhage** (IH) is caused by rupture of a cerebral vessel with subsequent bleeding into the brain. Primary **cerebral hemorrhage** (non-traumatic spontaneous hemorrhage) typically occurs in small blood vessels weakened by atherosclerosis producing an **aneurysm. Subarachnoid hemorrhage (SH)** occurs from bleeding into the subarachnoid space typically from a saccular or **berry aneurysm** affecting primarily large blood vessels. Developmental defects that produce weakness in the blood vessel wall are major contributing factors to the formation of an aneurysm. Hemorrhage is closely linked to chronic hypertension. **Arteriovenous malformation (AVM)** is another congenital defect that can result in stroke. AVM is characterized by a tortuous tangle of arteries and veins with agenesis of an interposing capillary system. The abnormal vessels undergo progressive dilatation with age and eventually bleed in about 50 percent of cases. The resulting hemorrhage can be either subarachnoid or intracerebral. Sudden and severe cerebral bleeding can result in death within hours, because intracranial pressures rise rapidly and adjacent cortical tissues are displaced or compressed.[9] Ischemic stroke is the most common type of stroke, accounting for 61 to 81 percent of all strokes. Hemorrhagic strokes account for 12 to 24 percent of strokes.[3]

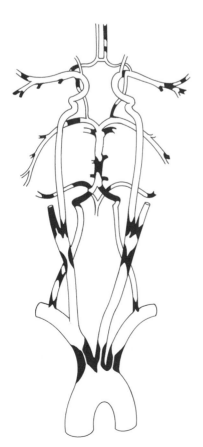

Figure 17-1. Preferred sites for atherosclerotic plaque. (From American Heart Association, Diagnosis and Management of Stroke, 1979, p 4, with permission.)

RISK FACTORS

Cardiovascular diseases affecting the brain and heart share a number of common risk factors important to the development of atherosclerosis. Major risk factors for stroke are hypertension, heart disease, and diabetes. In patients with ABI, 70 percent have hypertension, 30 percent coronary heart disease, 15 percent congestive heart disease, 30 percent peripheral arterial disease, and 15 percent diabetes. This coexistence of vascular problems increases significantly with the age of the patient. The risk for stroke is especially strong in patients with systolic and diastolic blood pressures elevated above 160/95 mmHg. Patients with marked elevations of hematocrits are also at an increased risk of occlusive stroke owing to a generalized reduction of CBF. Cardiac disorders such as rheumatic heart valvular disease, endocarditis, arrhythmias (particularly atrial fibrillation), or cardiac surgery significantly increase the risk of embolic stroke. Transient ischemic attacks (TIAs) are another important risk factor for stroke. Although only 10 percent of strokes are preceded by TIAs, about 36 percent of individuals who experience one or more TIAs will go on to develop a major stroke within 5 years.[3,10]

Stroke Prevention

Stroke is a preventable disease with risk factors that are potentially modifiable. Regulation of blood pressure is critical. Dietary adjustments include control of cholesterol and lipids. Cessation of cigarette smoking significantly decreases risk as does reducing physical inactivity and obesity. Control of associated diseases, especially diabetes and heart disease, is essential. As with a cardiac risk profile, the more risk factors present or the greater the degree of abnormality of any one factor, the greater the risk of stroke. Stroke risk factors considered nonmodifiable include increasing age, gender (male), race (African-American), prior stroke, and heredity. Less documented risk factors include excessive alcohol consumption and drug abuse.[10]

Effective stroke prevention also depends on improving public awareness concerning the **early warning signs of stroke.** Only about half of Americans can recognize even one warning sign. These include

- Sudden, severe headaches with no known cause
- Sudden weakness or numbness of the face, arm, or leg on one side of the body
- Loss of speech, or trouble talking or understanding speech
- Sudden dimness or loss of vision, particularly in only one eye
- Unexplained dizziness, unsteadiness or sudden falls, especially along with any of the previous symptoms.

The significance of recognizing early warning signs rests with prompt initiation of emergency treatment. Early computed tomography (CT) scans are used to differentiate between atherothrombotic stroke and hemorrhagic stroke. If the stroke is atherothrombotic, clot-dissolving enzymes, (e.g., tissue plasminogen activator [TPA]), can be administered. To be effective, the drug must be given within 3 hours after symptoms begin. TPA cannot be given with hemorrhagic stroke because the drug may worsen bleeding. Although this treatment has been available since 1996 and can dramatically reduce death and disability, current estimates indicate that only 1 in 20 individuals experiencing stroke receives the treatment. Patients who do receive TPA are one-third more likely to recover with no disability or minimal disability as compared to those who do not receive the treatment. Major heart and stroke organizations are currently promoting the use of the term **brain attack** to help individuals recognize the importance of calling 911 and seeking immediate emergency care.[11,12]

PATHOPHYSIOLOGY

Interruption of blood flow for only a few minutes sets in motion a series of pathoneurological events. Complete cerebral circulatory arrest results in irreversible cellular damage with a core area of focal infarction within minutes. The area surrounding the core is termed the ischemic prenumbra and consists of viable but metabolically lethargic cells. The ischemia triggers a number of damaging and potentially reversible events including the release of cascades of chemicals. The release of excess glutamate, an excitatory neurotransmitter, causes changes in calcium ion distribution with additional calcium influx and overload in intracellular calcium. This in turn results in the sustained activation of destructive calcium-sensitive enzymes producing additional cell death, generally within hours. There is an extension of the infarction into the prenumbra area. Research efforts are currently directed toward development of drugs that might reverse the metabolic changes of the ischemic brain following treatment with glutamate receptor antagonists.[12,13]

Ischemic brain edema, an accumulation of fluids, begins within minutes of the insult and reaches a maximum by 3 to 4 days. It is the result of tissue necrosis and widespread rupture of cell membranes with movement of water from the blood into brain tissues. The swelling then gradually subsides, generally disappearing by 3 weeks. Significant edema can elevate intracranial pressures, leading to secondary brain damage and neurological deterioration from contralateral and caudal shifts of brain structures **(brainstem herniation).** Clinical signs of elevating intracranial pressures (ICP) include decreasing level of consciousness (stupor and coma), widened pulse pressure, increased heart rate, irregular respirations (Cheyne-Stokes respirations), vomiting, unreacting pupils (cranial nerve III signs), and papilledema. Cerebral edema is the most frequent cause of death in acute stroke and is characteristic of large infarcts involving the middle cerebral artery.[14]

MANAGEMENT CATEGORIES

Transient ischemic attack (TIA) refers to the temporary interruption of blood supply to the brain. Symptoms of focal neurological deficit may last for only a few minutes or for several hours, but do not last more than 24 hours. After the attack is over there is no evidence of residual brain damage or permanent neurological dysfunction. TIAs may result from a number of different etiological factors including occlusive episodes, emboli, reduced cerebral perfusion (arrhythmias, decreased cardiac output, hypotension, overmedication with antihypertensive medications, **subclavian steal syndrome**) or cerebrovascular spasm. The major clinical significance of TIA is as a precursor to susceptibility for both cerebral infarction and myocardial infarction. Patients are classified as having a **major stroke** in the presence of stable, usually severe, deficits. The term **deteriorating stroke** is used to refer to the patient whose neurological status is deteriorating after admission to the hospital. This change in status may be due to cerebral or systemic causes (e.g., cerebral edema, progressing thrombosis). The category of **young stroke** is used to describe a stroke affecting persons below the age of 45. Younger individuals may have potential for better recovery.[14]

ANATOMICAL CATEGORIES

CBF varies with the patency of the vessels. Progressive narrowing secondary to atherosclerosis decreases blood flow. As in coronary heart disease, symptomatic changes generally result from a restriction of flow greater than 80 percent. The symptomatology of stroke is dependent on a number of factors, including (1) the location of the ischemic process, (2) the size of the ischemic area, (3) the nature and functions of the structures involved, and (4) the availability of collateral blood flow. Symptomatology may also depend on the rapidity of the occlusion of a blood vessel because slow occlusions may allow collateral vessels to take over, whereas sudden events do not.

Cerebral Blood Flow

CBF is controlled by a number of **autoregulatory mechanisms (cerebral)** that modulate a constant rate of blood flow through the brain. These mechanisms provide homeostatic balance, counteracting fluctuations in systolic blood pressure while maintaining a normal flow of 50 to 60 milliliters per 100 grams of brain tissue per minute. The brain has high energy requirements and very little metabolic reserves. It requires a continuous, rich perfusion of blood to deliver oxygen and glucose to the tissues. Cerebral flow represents approximately 17 percent of available cardiac output. Chemical regulation of CBF occurs in response to changes in blood concentrations of carbon dioxide or oxygen. Vasodilation and increased CBF are produced in response to an increase in $Paco_2$ or a decrease in Pao_2, while vasoconstriction and decreased CBF are produced by the opposite stimuli. Blood flow is also altered by changes in the blood pH. A fall in pH (increased acidity) produces vasodilation, and a rise in pH (increased alkalinity) produces a decrease in blood flow. Neurogenic regulation alters blood flow by vasodilating vessels in direct proportion to local function of brain tissue. Released metabolites probably act directly on the smooth muscle in local vessel walls. Changes in blood viscosity or intracranial pressures may also influence CBF. Changes in blood pressure produce minor alterations of CBF. As pressure rises, the artery is stretched, resulting in contraction of smooth muscle in the vessel wall. Thus, the patency of the vessel is decreased, with a consequent decrease in CBF. As pressure falls, contraction lessens and CBF increases. Following stroke, autoregulatory mechanisms may be impaired.[13,15]

Knowledge of cerebral vascular anatomy is essential to understand the symptomatology, diagnosis, and management of stroke. Extracranial blood supply to the brain is provided by right and left internal carotid arteries and by the right and left vertebral arteries. The internal carotid artery begins at the bifurcation of the common carotid artery and ascends in the deep portions of the neck to the carotid canal. It turns rostromedially and ascends into the cranial cavity. It then pierces the dura mater and gives off the ophthalmic and anterior choroidal arteries before bifurcating into the middle and anterior cerebral arteries. The anterior communicating artery communicates with the anterior cerebral arteries of either side, giving rise to the rostral portion of the **circle of Willis** (Fig. 17-2). The vertebral artery arises as a branch off the subclavian artery. It enters the vertebral foramen of the sixth cervical vertebra and travels through the foramina of the transverse processes of the upper six cervical vertebrae to the foramen magnum and into the brain. There it travels in the posterior cranial fossa ventrally and medially and unites with the vertebral artery from the other side to form the basilar artery at the upper border of the medulla. At the upper border of the pons, the basilar artery bifurcates to form the posterior cerebral arteries and the posterior portion of the circle of Willis. Posterior communicating arteries connect the posterior cerebral arteries with the internal carotid arteries and complete the circle of Willis.

Vascular Syndromes

ANTERIOR CEREBRAL ARTERY SYNDROME

The anterior cerebral artery (ACA) is the first and smaller of two terminal branches of the internal carotid artery. It supplies the medial aspect of the cerebral hemisphere (frontal and parietal lobes) and subcortical structures, including the basal ganglia (anterior internal capsule, inferior caudate nucleus), anterior fornix, and anterior four fifths of the corpus callosum (Fig. 17-3). Because the anterior communicating artery allows perfusion of the proximal anterior cerebral artery from either side, occlusion

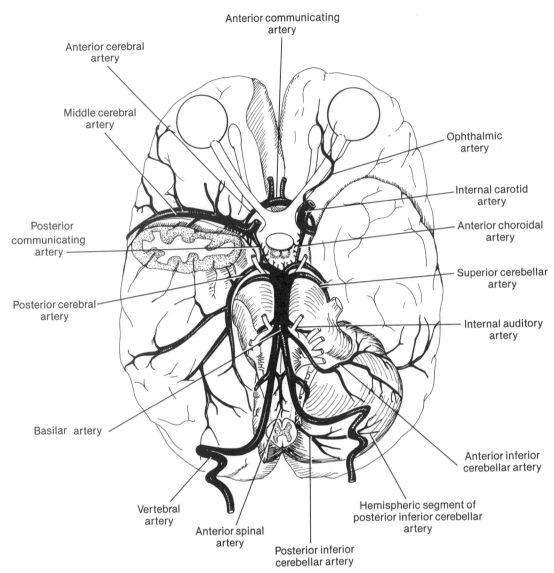

Figure 17-2. Cerebral circulation: Circle of Willis. (From DeArmond, S, et al: A Photographic Atlas—Structure of the Human Brain, ed 2. Oxford University Press, New York, 1976, p 171, with permission.)

proximal to this point results in minimal deficit. More distal lesions produce more significant deficits. Table 17–2 presents the clinical manifestations of ACA syndrome. The most common characteristic of ACA syndrome is contralateral hemiparesis and sensory loss with greater involvement of the lower extremity because the somatotopic organization of the medial aspect of the cortex includes the functional area for the lower extremity.

MIDDLE CEREBRAL ARTERY SYNDROME

The middle cerebral artery (MCA) is the second of the two main branches of the internal carotid artery and supplies the entire lateral aspect of the cerebral hemisphere (frontal, temporal, and parietal lobes) and subcortical structures, including the internal capsule (posterior portion), corona radiata, globus pallidus (outer part), most of the caudate nucleus, and the putamen (Fig. 17-4). Occlusion of the proxi-

mal MCA produces extensive neurological damage with significant cerebral edema. Increased intracranial pressures typically lead to loss of consciousness, brain herniation, and possibly death. Table 17–3 presents the clinical manifestations of MCA syndrome. The most common characteristics of MCA syndrome are contralateral spastic hemiparesis and sensory loss of the face, upper extremity (UE), and lower extremity (LE), with the face and UE more involved than the LE. Lesions of the parieto-occipital cortex of the dominant hemisphere (usually the left hemisphere) typically produce aphasia. Lesions of the right parietal lobe of the nondominant hemisphere (usually the right hemisphere) typically produce perceptual deficits (e.g., **unilateral neglect,** anosognosia, apraxia, and spatial disorganization). **Homonymous hemianopsia** (a visual field defect) is also a common finding. The MCA is the most common site of occlusion in stroke.

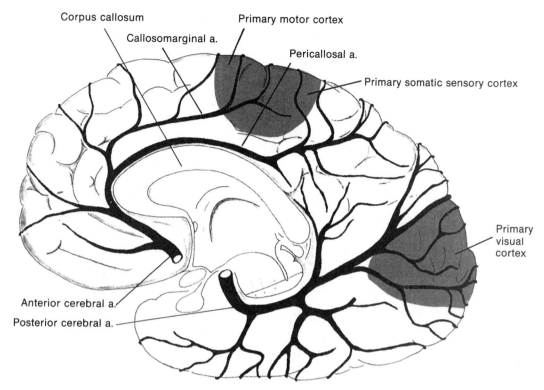

Figure 17-3. Cerebral circulation: A diagram of a midsagittal view of the brain illustrates the distribution of the anterior and posterior cerebral arteries. (From Willard F: Medical Neuroanatomy. Lippincott, Philadelphia, 1993, p 181, with permission.)

INTERNAL CAROTID ARTERY SYNDROME

Complete occlusion of the internal carotid artery produces massive infarction in both middle cerebral and anterior cerebral arterial territories. Extensive cerebral edema occurs and frequently leads to coma and death. Incomplete occlusions can produce a mixture of middle cerebral and/or anterior artery symptoms.

POSTERIOR CEREBRAL ARTERY SYNDROME

The two posterior cerebral arteries (PCAs) arise as terminal branches of the basilar artery and each supplies the corresponding occipital lobe and medial and inferior temporal lobe (see Fig. 17-3). It also supplies the upper brainstem, midbrain, and posterior diencephalon, including most of the thalamus. Table 17-4 presents the clinical manifestations of PCA syndrome. Occlusion proximal to the posterior communicating artery typically results in minimal deficits owing to the collateral blood supply from the posterior communicating artery (similar to ACA syndrome). Occlusion of thalamic branches may produce hemianesthesia (contralateral sensory loss) or **thalamic sensory syndrome (thalamic pain)** (a persistent and unpleasant hemibody sensation). Occipital infarction produces homonymous hemianopsia, visual **agnosia,** prosopagnosia (inability to recognize faces), or, if bilateral, cortical blindness. Temporal lobe ischemia results in an amnesic syndrome with memory loss. Involvement of subthalamic branches may involve subthalamic nucleus or its pallidal connections, producing a wide variety of deficits. Contralateral hemiplegia occurs with involvement of the cerebral peduncle.

VERTEBROBASILAR ARTERY SYNDROME

The vertebral arteries arise from the subclavian arteries and travel into the brain along the medulla where they merge at the inferior border of the pons to form the basilar artery. The vertebral arteries supply the cerebellum (via posterior inferior cerebellar arteries) and the medulla (via the medullary arteries). The basilar artery supplies the pons (via pontine arteries), the internal ear (via labyrinthine arteries),

Table 17-2 CLINICAL MANIFESTATIONS OF ANTERIOR CEREBRAL ARTERY SYNDROME

Signs and Symptoms	Structures Involved
Paresis of opposite foot and leg and to a lesser extent the arm	Primary motor area, medial aspect of cortex, internal capsule
Mental impairment (perseveration, confusion, and amnesia)	Localization unknown
Sensory impairments primarily in lower extremity	Primary sensory area, medial aspect of cortex
Urinary incontinence	Posteromedial aspect of superior frontal gyrus
Problems with imitation and bimanual tasks, apraxia	Corpus callosum
Abulia (akinetic mutism), slowness, delay, lack of spontaneity, motor inaction	Uncertain localization

From Fredericks, C, and Saladin, L: Pathophysiology of the Motor Systems. FA Davis, Philadelphia, 1996, p 504, with permission.

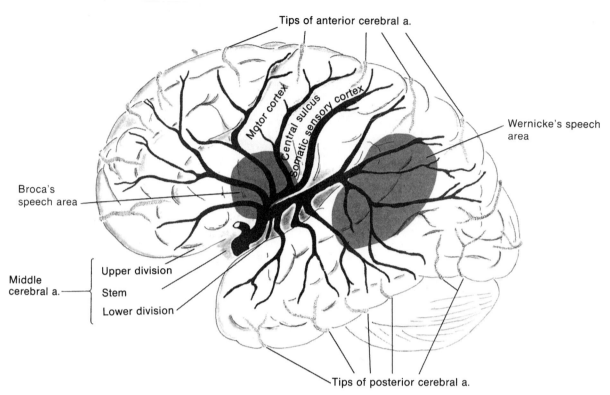

Figure 17-4. Cerebral circulation: Diagram of a lateral view of the brain illustrates the distribution of the middle cerebral artery. (From Willard F: Medical Neuroanatomy. Lippincott, Philadelphia, 1993, p 182, with permission.)

Table 17–3 CLINICAL MANIFESTATIONS OF MIDDLE CEREBRAL ARTERY SYNDROME

Signs and Symptoms	Structures Involved
Paresis of contralateral face, arm, and leg (leg is least affected)	Primary motor cortex and internal capsule
Sensory impairment over the contralateral face, arm, and leg (pain, temperature, touch, vibration, position, two-point discrimination, stereognosis)	Primary sensory cortex and internal capsule
Motor speech disorder (expressive-aphasia-telegraphic halting speech)	Broca's cortical area in the dominant hemisphere
Wernicke's or receptive aphasia (fluent but often jargon speech, poor comprehension)	Wernicke's cortical area in the dominant hemisphere
Perceptual problems such as unilateral neglect, apraxias, depth perception problems, spatial relation difficulties	Parietal sensory association cortex
Homonymous hemianopia	Optic radiation in internal capsule
Loss of conjugate gaze to the opposite side	Frontal eye fields or their descending tracts
Ataxia of contralateral limb(s) (sensory ataxia)	Parietal lobe

From Fredericks, C, and Saladin, L: Pathophysiology of the Motor Systems. FA Davis, Philadelphia, 1996, p 502, with permission.

and the cerebellum (via the anterior inferior and superior cerebellar arteries). The basilar artery then terminates at the upper border of the pons giving rise to the two posterior arteries (see Fig. 17-2).

Complete occlusion of the basilar artery is a catastrophic event. Patients typically experience occipital headache, diplopia, progressive quadriplegia, bulbar paralysis, coma, and frequently death. **Locked-in syndrome (LIS)** results from ventral pontine lesions and is defined as quadriplegia and anarthria with preserved consciousness and sensation. Thus the patient cannot move or speak but remains alert and oriented. Only one voluntary movement, vertical gaze, remains. Communication can be established via vertical eye movements. Mortality rates are high (59%), and those patients that do survive are usually left with severe impairments associated with brainstem dysfunction.[16–18]

Occlusions of the vertebrobasilar system can produce a wide variety of symptoms with both ipsilateral and contralateral signs, because some of the tracts in the brainstem will have crossed and others will not. Numerous cerebellar and cranial nerve abnormalities also typically occur. Table 17–5 presents the clinical manifestations of vertebrobasilar artery syndrome. Several different specific brain-

Table 17–4 CLINICAL MANIFESTATIONS OF POSTERIOR CEREBRAL ARTERY SYNDROME

Signs and Symptoms	Structures Involved
Peripheral Territory	
Contralateral homonymous hemianopia	Primary visual cortex or optic radiation
Prosopagnosia (difficulty naming people on sight)	Visual association cortex
Dyslexia (difficulty reading) without agraphia (difficulty writing), color naming (anomia), and color discrimination problems	Dominant calcarine lesion and posterior part of corpus callosum
Memory defect	Lesion of inferomedial portions of temporal lobe bilaterally or on the dominant side only
Topographic disorientation	Nondominant primary visual area, usually bilaterally
Central Territory	
Thalamic syndrome: sensory impairments (all modalities), spontaneous pain, and dysesthesias	Ventral posterolateral nucleus of thalamus
Involuntary movements; choreoathetosis, intention tremor, hemiballismus	Subthalamic nucleus or its pallidal connections
Contralateral hemiplegia	Cerebral peduncle—midbrain
Weber's syndrome: oculomotor nerve palsy and contralateral hemiplegia	Third nerve and cerebral peduncle of midbrain
Paresis of vertical eye movements, slight miosis and ptosis, and sluggish pupillary light response	Supranuclear fibers to third nerve

From Fredericks, C, and Saladin, L: Pathophysiology of the Motor Systems. FA Davis, Philadelphia, 1996, p 509, with permission.

stem syndromes may result, with lateral medullary (Wallenberg's) syndrome being one of the most common.

Extracranial injuries to the vertebral arteries as they travel through the cervical spine can also produce vertebrobasilar signs and symptoms. Forceful neck motions (e.g., whiplash or aggressive neck manipulations) are among the more common types of injuries.

HISTORY AND EXAMINATION

An accurate history profiling the timing of neurological events is obtained from the patient or from family members in the case of the unconscious or noncommunicative patient. Of particular importance are the pattern of onset and the course of initial neurological symptoms. An abrupt onset with rapid coma is suggestive of cerebral hemorrhage. Severe headache typically precedes loss of consciousness. An embolus also occurs rapidly, with no warning, and is frequently associated with heart disease and/or heart complications. A more variable and uneven onset is typical with thrombosis. The patient's past history including episodes of TIAs or head trauma, presence of major or minor risk factors, medications, pertinent family history, and any recent alterations in patient function (either transient or permanent) are thoroughly investigated.

The physical examination of the patient includes a general medical examination as well as a neurological examination. An investigation of vital signs (heart rate, respiratory rate, blood pressure) and signs of cardiac decompensation is essential. The neurological examination stresses function of the cerebral hemispheres, cerebellum, cranial nerves, eyes, and sensorimotor system. The presenting symptoms will help to determine the location of the lesion, and comparison of both sides of the body will reveal the side of the lesion. Bilateral signs are suggestive of brainstem lesions or massive cerebral involvement.

Neurovascular tests are performed. These include

1. Neck flexion. Meningeal irritation secondary to SH will produce resistance or pain with neck flexion.
2. Palpation of arteries. Both superficial and deep arteries are palpated including temporal, facial, carotid, subclavian, brachial, radial, abdominal aorta, and lower extremity arteries.
3. Auscultation of heart and blood vessels. Abnormal heart sounds, murmurs, or bruits may be present and indicate increased flow turbulence and stenosis in a vessel.
4. Ophthalmic pressures. Abnormal pressures in the ophthalmic artery may indicate problems in the internal carotid artery.

DIAGNOSTIC TESTS

A number of routine laboratory and diagnostic tests are performed. These include

1. Urinalysis: detects infection, diabetes, renal failure, or dehydration.
2. Blood analysis: provides a complete blood count (CBC), platelet count, prothrombin time, partial thromboplastin time, and erythrocyte sedimentation rate.
3. Blood sugar level.
4. Blood chemistry profile: indicates serum electrolytes and serum cardiac enzyme levels; elevation of the creatinine phosphokinase isoenzyme CPK MB is indicative of coincidental cardiac infarction.
5. Blood cholesterol and lipid profile.
6. Radiograph of the chest (heart size, lungs).
7. Electrocardiograph (ECG): used to detect arrhythmias as a source of emboli or coincidental heart disease; stroke may also cause ECG

Table 17–5 CLINICAL MANIFESTATIONS OF VERTEBROBASILAR ARTERY SYNDROME

Signs and Symptoms	Structures Involved
Medial medullary syndrome (occlusion of vertebral artery or branch of vertebral or lower basilar artery)	
Ipsilateral to lesion	
Paralysis with atrophy of half the tongue	CN XII, hypoglossal nucleus or nerve
Contralateral to lesion	
Paralysis of arm and leg	Corticospinal tract
Impaired tactile and proprioceptive sense over 50% of the body	Medial lemniscus
Lateral medullary syndrome (occlusion of vertebral, posterior inferior cerebellar, basilar)	
Ipsilateral to lesion	
Decreased pain and temperature sensation in face	Descending tract and nucleus of fifth nerve
Ataxia of limbs, falling to side of lesion	Vestibular nuclei and connections
Vertigo, nausea, vomiting	Vestibular nuclei and connections
Nystagmus	Vestibular nuclei and connections
Horner's syndrome (miosis, ptosis, decreased sweating)	Descending sympathetic tract
Dysphagia, hoarseness, paralysis of vocal cord, diminished gag reflex	CN IX and CN X nuclei or nerve fibers
Sensory impairment of ipsilateral arm, trunk, or leg	Cuneate and gracile nuclei
Contralateral to lesion	
Impaired pain and thermal sense over 50% of body, sometimes face	Spinothalamic tract
Basilar artery syndrome—combination of the various brainstem syndromes plus those arising in the posterior cerebral artery distribution	
Paralysis or weakness of all extremities, plus all bulbar musculature	Corticobulbar and corticospinal tracts bilaterally
Diplopia, paralysis of conjugate lateral or vertical gaze, internuclear ophthalmoplegia, horizontal or vertical nystagmus	Ocular motor nerves, apparatus for conjugate gaze, medial longitudinal fasciculus
Blindness, impaired vision, various visual field defects	Primary visual cortex
Bilateral cerebellar ataxia	Cerebellar peduncles and the cerebellar hemispheres
Coma	Reticular activating system
Sensation may be strikingly intact in the presence of almost total paralysis (locked in)	Sparing of tegmentum of pons
Thalamic pain syndrome	Thalamic nuclei
Medial inferior pontine syndrome (occlusion of paramedian branch of basilar artery)	
Ipsilateral to lesion	
Paralysis of conjugate gaze to side of lesion (preservation of convergence)	Pontine "center" for lateral gaze paramedian pentine reticular formation (PPRF)
Nystagmus	Vestibular nuclei and connections
Ataxia of limbs and gait	Middle cerebellar peduncle
Diplopia on lateral gaze	Abducens nerve or nucleus
Contralateral to lesion	
Paresis of face, arm, and leg	Corticobulbar and corticospinal tract in lower pons
Impaired tactile and proprioceptive sense over 50% of the body	Medial lemniscus
Lateral inferior pontine syndrome (occlusion of anterior inferior cerebellar artery)	
Ipsilateral to lesion	
Horizontal and vertical nystagmus, vertigo, nausea, vomiting	Vestibular nerve or nucleus
Facial paralysis	Seventh nerve or nucleus
Paralysis of conjugate gaze to side of lesion	Pontine "center" for lateral gaze (PPRF)
Deafness, tinnitus	Auditory nerve or cochlear nucleus
Ataxia	Middle cerebellar peduncle and cerebellar hemisphere
Impaired sensation over face	Main sensory nucleus and descending tract of fifth nerve
Contralateral to lesion	
Impaired pain and thermal sense over half the body (may include face)	Spinothalamic tract
Medial midpontine syndrome (paramedian branch of midbasilar artery)	
Ipsilateral to lesion	
Ataxia of limbs and gait (more prominent in bilateral involvement)	Middle cerebellar peduncle
Contralateral to lesion	
Paralysis of face, arm, and leg	Corticobulbar and corticospinal tract
Deviation of eyes	PPRF
Lateral midpontine syndrome (short circumferential artery)	
Ipsilateral to lesion	
Ataxia of limbs	Middle cerebellar peduncle
Paralysis of muscles of mastication	Motor fibers or nucleus of cranial nerve V
Impaired sensation over side of face	Sensory fibers or nucleus of cranial nerve V

Table 17–5 CLINICAL MANIFESTATIONS OF VERTEBROBASILAR ARTERY SYNDROME—*Continued*

Signs and Symptoms	Structures Involved
Ipsilateral to lesion—continued	
Medial superior pontine syndrome (paramedian branches of upper basilar artery)	
Cerebellar ataxia	Superior or middle cerebellar peduncle
Internuclear ophthalmoplegia	Medial longitudinal fasciculus
Contralateral to lesion	
Paralysis of face, arm, and leg	Corticobulbar and corticospinal tract
Lateral superior pontine syndrome (syndrome of superior cerebellar artery)	
Ipsilateral to lesion	
Ataxia of limbs and gait, falling to side of lesion	Middle and superior cerebellar peduncles, superior surface of cerebellum, dentate nucleus
Dizziness, nausea, vomiting	Vestibular nuclei
Horizontal nystagmus	Vestibular nuclei
Paresis of conjugate gaze (ipsilateral)	Uncertain
Loss of optokinetic nystagmus	Uncertain
Miosis, ptosis, decreased sweating over face (Horner syndrome)	Descending sympathetic fibers
Contralateral to lesion	
Impaired pain and thermal sense of face, limbs, and trunk	Spinothalamic tract
Impaired touch, vibration, and position sense, more in leg than arm (tendency to incongruity of pain and touch deficits)	Medial lemniscus (lateral portion)

From Fredericks, C, and Saladin, L: Pathophysiology of the Motor Systems. FA Davis, Philadelphia, 1996, p 505, with permission.

abnormalities, typically T-wave inversion, prolonged QT interval, and ST inversion.

8. Echocardiography: may reveal valvular disease (a source of emboli) or other heart conditions such as congestive heart failure, recent myocardial infarction.

Modern cerebrovascular imaging techniques have vastly improved the accurate diagnosis of stroke. These include

1. **Computerized tomography (CT)** scan is the most commonly used imaging technique. An intravenous iodinated contrast dye may be used to enhance the density of intravascular blood. CT resolution only allows identification of large arteries and veins, and venous sinuses. In the acute phase, the CT scans are used to rule out other brain lesions such as tumor or abscess and to identify hemorrhagic stroke. In the case of suspected stroke, an emergency CT is used to rule out hemorrhage if anticoagulants or clot-busting drugs are to be administered. Many times CT scans during the acute phase are negative with no clear abnormalities. In the subacute phase, CT scans can delineate the development of cerebral edema (within 3 days) and infarction (within 2 to 10 days) by showing areas of decreased density. It is important to remember that the extent of CT lesion does not necessarily correlate with clinical signs or changes in function (Fig. 17-5).

2. **Magnetic resonance imaging (MRI).** MRI measures nuclear particles as they interact with a powerful magnetic field. Greater resolution of the brain and its structural detail is obtained with MRI than with a CT scan. Magnetic resonance imaging is more sensitive in the diagnosis of acute strokes, allowing detection of cerebral infarction within 2 to 6 hours after stroke. It is also able to detail smaller lesions. The disadvantages of MRI are longer scanning times, higher cost, and limited availability.

3. **Positron emission tomography (PET).** Positron emission from an injected radionuclide is measured. The use of PET allows imaging of regional blood flow and localized cerebral metabolism. Early use of PET scanning can be used to determine lesion location. Scanning may also help to determine areas of tissue where ischemia is reversible. The high cost and limited accessibility of this diagnostic tool limit its use.

4. **Ultrasound transcranial Doppler.** This technique is used for imaging the neck and chest vessels (carotid, vertebral, and subclavian arteries).

5. **Cerebral angiography.** Cerebral angiography is invasive and involves the injection of radiopaque dye into blood vessels with subsequent radiography. It provides the best visualization of the vascular system and is often used when surgery is considered (carotid stenosis, arteriovenous malformations). It may also be used if CT or MRI scans are unavailable. There are risks to angiography; death or stroke occurs in 1 to 2 percent of cases, with minor complications in 5 to 6 percent of cases.[13,19]

DIRECT IMPAIRMENTS

Somatosensory Deficits

Sensation is frequently impaired but rarely absent on the hemiplegic side. Deficits are reported in about 53 percent of patients with stroke and can range from loss of superficial and/or deep sensations to impairments in the combined cortical sensations (see Chapter 6).[3] The type and extent of deficit is

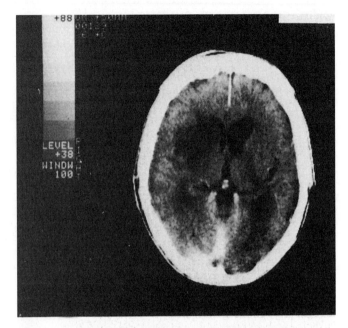

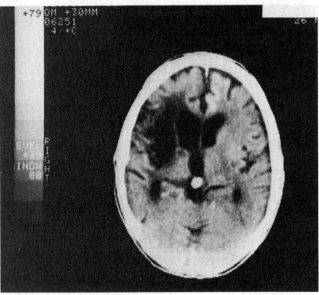

Figure 17-5. Computed tomography scan of a patient with infarction of the middle cerebral artery territory. (From Hackinski, W, and Norris, JW: The Acute Stroke. FA Davis, Philadelphia, 1985, p 194, with permission.)

related to the location and extent of the vascular lesion. Specific localized areas of dysfunction are common with cortical lesions, whereas diffuse involvement throughout the whole side suggests deeper lesions involving the thalamus and adjacent structures. The most common distribution of loss is a face-UE-LE pattern (reported in 55% of cases). Less frequently, impairments may be noted in face-UE (29 percent of cases) or UE-LE (7% of cases).[20] Symptoms of crossed anesthesia (ipsilateral facial impairments with contralateral trunk and limb deficits) typify brainstem lesions. Proprioceptive losses are common. In one study 44 percent of patients with stroke demonstrated significant proprioceptive loss with associated impairments noted

in motor control, postural function, and balance.[21] Loss of superficial touch, and pain and temperature sensation is also common. Profound hemisensory loss can contribute to unilateral neglect, difficulty with functional tasks, and increased risk of self-injury. The patient may also complain of abnormal sensations such as numbness, dyesthesias, or hyperesthesia.

Pain

Hemorrhagic or ischemic stroke can result in severe headache, or neck and face pain. Lesions of the PCA involving the ventral posterior-lateral thalamus can result in thalamic sensory syndrome, a neurogenic condition affecting the superficial sensations (touch, pain, and temperature). The syndrome is characterized by continuous severe pain and an exaggerated response to stimuli affecting the contralateral half of the body. Paroxysmal exacerbations (spasms) of pain may be triggered by simply stroking the skin, pinprick, contact with heat or cold, and pressure. Loud noises, bright lights, or other mild irritants may also trigger pain. Thalamic syndrome is typically delayed in onset, not appearing until weeks or months after the onset of stroke. Spontaneous recovery is rare and suffering may be intolerable. Patients may experience little relief from analgesic treatment. The debilitating nature of thalamic pain frequently prevents the patient from actively participating in rehabilitation.[22]

Pain may also result from indirect impairments such as muscle imbalances and improper movement patterns (movement adaptation syndrome), and poor alignment (postural stress syndrome). For example, knee pain is a common finding with prolonged or severe hyperextension during gait. The sequelae of pain are reduced function, impaired concentration, depression, and decreased rehabilitation potential.

Visual Deficits

Homonymous hemianopsia, a visual field defect, occurs with lesions involving the optic radiation in the internal capsule (MCA distribution) or to the primary visual cortex (PCA distribution). It occurs in about 26 percent of patients with stroke.[3] The patient experiences loss of vision in the contralateral half of each visual field; that is, the nasal half of one eye and temporal half of the eye corresponding to the hemiplegic side. Field defects contribute to the patient's overall lack of awareness of the hemiplegic side. Patients who are aware of the deficit can compensate with head turning movements. Patients may also experience impairments in **visual neglect** (visual inattention), depth perception, and other problems in spatial relationships. See Chapter 29 for a complete discussion of visual and perceptual deficits. Paralysis of conjugate gaze from involvement of frontal lobe eye field area, cranial nerve III, or gaze centers in the pontine reticular formation result in **forced gaze deviation.** Unopposed action of eye muscles causes the eyes to deviate in the direction of the intact musculature. Patients with hemispheric lesions may look away from the hemiplegic side, while patients with brainstem lesions may look toward the hemiplegic side.[23] Brainstem strokes may also produce signs of diplopia, vertigo, oscillopsia, or visual distortions.

Motor Deficits

SEQUENTIAL RECOVERY STAGES

During the early stages of stroke, flaccidity with no voluntary movement is common. Usually this is replaced by the development of spasticity, hyperreflexia, and mass patterns of movement, termed **synergies (mass).** Muscles involved in synergy patterns are often so strongly linked together that isolated movements outside the mass synergistic patterns are not possible. As recovery progresses, spasticity and synergies begin to decline and advanced movement patterns become possible. This general pattern of recovery was described in detail by Twitchell[24] and Brunnstrom[25,26] who elaborated the process into six distinct stages (Box 17-1). Bobath[27] collapsed the sequence into three main recovery stages: (1) the initial flaccid stage, (2) the stage of spasticity, and (3) the stage of relative recovery. Additional investigators have confirmed

---

Box 17-1 SEQUENTIAL RECOVERY STAGES IN HEMIPLEGIA

STAGE 1 Recovery from hemiplegia occurs in a stereotyped sequence of events that begins with a period of *flaccidity* immediately following the acute episode. *No movement of the limbs* can be elicited.

STAGE 2 As recovery begins, the basic limb synergies or some of their components may appear as associated reactions, or *minimal voluntary movement* responses may be present. At this time, *spasticity* begins to develop.

STAGE 3 Thereafter, the patient gains *voluntary control of the movement synergies,* although full range of all synergy components does not necessarily develop. *Spasticity* has further increased and may become *severe.*

STAGE 4 Some *movement combinations that do not follow the paths of either synergy* are mastered, first with difficulty, then with more ease, and *spasticity begins to decline.*

STAGE 5 If progress continues, *more difficult movement combinations* are learned as the basic limb synergies lose their dominance over motor acts.

STAGE 6 With the *disappearance of spasticity,* individual joint movements become possible and *coordination* approaches normal. From here on, as the last recovery step, normal motor function is restored, but this last stage is not achieved by all, for the recovery process can plateau at any stage.

From Brunnstrom, S: Movement Therapy in Hemiplegia. Harper & Row, New York, 1970, with permission.

---

this pattern of motor recovery following stroke.[28–30] Several important points merit consideration. Motor recovery occurs in a relatively predictable pattern. The recovery stages are viewed as sequential, although variability in the clinical picture at each stage is possible. Not all patients recover fully. Patients may plateau at any stage, depending on the severity of their involvement and their capacity for adaptation. Finally, recovery rates differ among patients and within patients. For example, the UE may be more involved and demonstrate less complete recovery than the LE (seen in MCA syndrome).

ALTERATIONS IN TONE

Flaccidity (hypotonicity) is present immediately after stroke and is due to cerebral shock. It is generally short-lived, lasting hours, days, or weeks. Flaccidity may persist in a small number of patients with lesions restricted to the primary motor cortex or cerebellum.[9] **Spasticity** (hypertonicity) emerges in about 90 percent of cases and occurs on the side of the body opposite the lesion predominately in antigravity muscles. In the UE, spasticity is frequently strong in scapular retractors; shoulder adductors, depressors, and internal rotators; elbow flexors and forearm pronators; and wrist and finger flexors. In the neck and trunk, spasticity may cause slumping (increased side flexion) to the hemiplegic side. In the LE, spasticity is often found in the pelvic retractors, hip adductors and internal rotators, hip and knee extensors, plantarflexors and supinators, and toe flexors.[27] The effects of spasticity include restricted volitional movement, static posturing of the limbs, and, in severe cases, the development of contractures. The automatic adjustment of muscle tension that occurs normally in preparation for and during a movement task, termed *automatic postural tone,* is also impaired.[31] Thus, patients with stroke may lack the ability to stabilize proximal joints and trunk appropriately, with resulting postural malalignment, balance impairments, and increased risk for falls. The relationship between residual muscle strength, synergistic movements, and spasticity is not well defined.

ABNORMAL SYNERGY PATTERNS

Abnormal synergistic patterns are typically present and are characterized as highly stereotyped and obligatory. Thus, the patient is unable to move an isolated segment of a limb without producing movements in the remainder of the limb. The patient is also limited in the ability to vary or adapt movements to varying task or environmental demands. Initially synergies may be elicited either reflexively, as associated reactions, or as minimal voluntary movements (stage 2). As recovery progresses into stage 3 they emerge more fully into the basic limb synergies and are strongly associated with spasticity and **associated reactions.** Two distinct abnormal synergy patterns have been described for each extremity: a flexion synergy and an extension synergy (Table 17-6). An inspection of the synergy com-

Table 17–6 SYNERGY PATTERNS OF THE EXTREMITIES

	Flexion Synergy Components	Extension Synergy Components
Upper extremity	Scapular retraction/ elevation or hyper- extension	Scapular protraction
	Shoulder abduction, external rotation	Shoulder adduction,[a] internal rotation
	Elbow flexion[a]	Elbow extension
	Forearm supination	Forearm pronation[a]
	Wrist and finger flexion	Wrist and finger flexion
Lower extremity	Hip flexion,[a] abduc- tion, external rotation	Hip extension, adduc- tion,[a] internal rotation
	Knee flexion	Knee extension[a]
	Ankle dorsiflexion inversion	Ankle plantarflexion,[a] inversion
	Toe dorsiflexion	Toe plantarflexion

[a]Generally the strongest components.

ponents reveals that certain muscles are not usually involved in either synergy. These muscles include the (1) latissimus dorsi, (2) teres major, (3) serratus anterior, (4) finger extensors, and (5) ankle evertors. These muscles, therefore, are generally difficult to activate. Loss of normal synergistic control has important functional implications. Activities of daily living (ADLs) and functional mobility skills (FMSs) are typically impaired. As recovery progresses into stage 4 and beyond, the basic limb synergies begin to disappear as more isolated (out-of-synergy) movements are possible and movement control begins to emerge.[26,32]

ABNORMAL REFLEXES

Reflexes are altered and vary according to the stage of recovery. Initially, stroke results in hypoflexia. During the middle stages of recovery, when spasticity and synergies are strong, **hyperreflexia** emerges. Stretch reflexes are hyperactive and patients typically demonstrate clonus, clasp-knife reflexes, and a positive Babinski.

Primitive or tonic reflex patterns may appear in a readily identifiable form similar to that seen in other types of neurological insult (e.g., traumatic brain injury, cerebral palsy). Thus, movement of the head may elicit an obligatory change in resting tone or movement of the extremities. Flexion of the neck may result in flexion of the UEs and extension of the LEs; extension of the neck produces the opposite responses **(symmetric tonic neck reflex [STNR])**. Head rotation to the left may cause extension of the left UE and LE (jaw limbs) with flexion of the right UE and LE (skull limbs); head rotation to the right causes the reverse pattern **(asymmetric tonic neck reflex [ATNR])**. Supine positioning may produce an increase in extensor tone, while prone positioning increases flexor tone **(symmetric tonic labyrinthine reflex [STLR])**. Rotation of the upper trunk with respect to the pelvis may also influence the extremities. Rotation toward the hemiplegic side results in flexion of the

hemiplegic UE and extension of hemiplegic LE. Rotation toward the uninvolved side produces the opposite responses **(tonic lumbar reflex [TLR])**. Finally, pressure on the bottom of the hemiplegic foot may produce a strong co-contraction response of LE extensors and flexors, resulting in a rigidly extended and fixed limb (positive support reaction).[26,27,33]

Associated reactions may also be present. These consist of unintentional movements of an involved limb resulting from an intended action of another limb (e.g., the sound limbs) or reflex stimulation (e.g., yawning, sneezing, coughing, or stretching). They are easier to elicit in the presence of spasticity and may be enhanced by tonic reflexes. Generally, although this is not true in every case, associated reactions elicit the same direction of movement in the contralateral UE (e.g., flexion evokes flexion), whereas in the LE opposite movements are elicited (e.g., flexion of one lower extremity evokes extension of the other). Elevation of the hemiplegic UE with the elbow extended above the horizontal may elicit an extension and abduction response of the fingers **(Souques' phenomenon)**. Resistance to abduction or adduction produces a similar response in the opposite limb (adduction elicits adduction) in both the upper and lower extremities **(Raimiste's phenomenon)**. **Homolateral limb synkinesis** is the term used to describe the mutual dependency that exists between hemiplegic limbs (flexion of the UE elicits flexion of the LE on the hemiplegic side). The presence of associated reactions precludes normal volitional movement and severely limits functional performance, especially in the UE.[26,27,32,34]

PARESIS AND ALTERED MUSCLE ACTIVATION PATTERNS

Paresis or weakness is found in 80 to 90 percent of all patients after stroke.[20] Patients are unable to generate tension or force necessary for initiating and controlling movement and posture. The degree of weakness may vary from a complete inability to achieve any visible contraction to measurable impairments in force production. The distribution is related to the location of the lesion. Common patterns include contralateral hemiparesis (opposite UE and LE) or monoparesis (opposite UE weakness). Owing to the high incidence of MCA strokes, the UE is frequently more affected than the LE. About 20 percent of individuals paralyzed by stroke fail to regain any functional use of the affected UE. Typically the distal muscles are more affected than proximal ones. Quadriparesis or quadriplegia may result from lesions of the brainstem. The amount of paresis experienced by the patient may also vary according to specific situational contexts. Thus, a patient may appear stronger in some functional tasks than in others. Paresis on the "supposedly normal" unaffected side has also been reported.[35,36] Increased fatigability is present in paretic muscles.[37]

Specific changes occur in both the motor unit and muscle. The number of functioning agonist motor units is decreased by as much as 50 percent at 6 months in some patients with stroke.[38] Abnormal recruitment of motor units with altered order and impaired firing rates has also been reported.[38–43] Thus patients demonstrate inefficient muscle activation, difficulties trying to maintain a constant level of force production, and increased effort while complaining of feelings of weakness. Denervation potentials are common; the result of denervation changes in the corticospinal tracts.[44] Overall reaction times are increased, a finding also reported for the unaffected extremities and for the elderly in general. Movement times are prolonged, a timing abnormality that contributes to impairment of coordinated motor sequences.[45,46] Changes in muscle composition include atrophy of muscle fibers with a greater loss of type II fast-twitch fibers (a finding also reported in the elderly). The selective loss of type II fibers results in difficulty with initiation and production of rapid, high-force movements.

Active restraint arising from spastic antagonist muscles has been suggested as a negative influence on agonist movement and a cause of agonist weakness. Bobath,[27] whose theories form the basis of neurodevelopmental treatment (NDT), suggested that strengthening techniques for agonists and excessive effort should be avoided in favor of inhibition techniques designed to reduce spasticity in spastic muscles. This conclusion has been challenged by a number of investigators who demonstrate that the problems clearly lie with inadequate motor unit recruitment and paresis of agonists.[39,47,48] Inappropriate co-activation of agonist-antagonist muscles has also been reported in patients with stroke and may be a significant factor in producing disordered timing and sequencing of muscle activity.

Paresis may also result from inactivity and limitations in mobility (an indirect impairment). Disuse atrophy is most apparent in weight-bearing muscles. If muscles are left unused over time, muscle stiffness and learned nonuse are the most likely results.[49] Early activation and forced use of the involved extremities is effective in counteracting these effects.[50] Patients recovering from stroke consistently demonstrate the strong negative impact of paresis on functional outcomes. Impairments in gait, balance, UE functional tasks, and manual dexterity have all been linked directly to impairments of strength.[51–53]

Incoordination can result from proprioceptive losses (sensory ataxia), cerebellar lesions (cerebellar ataxia), or motor weakness. Dyssynergia, the inappropriate timing and sequencing of muscles for purposeful movement, impairs function and limits adaptability to changing environmental demands. Basal ganglia involvement may lead to slow movements (bradykinesia) or adventitious movements (chorea or hemiballismus).

MOTOR PROGRAMMING DEFICITS

Hemispheric differences have been reported in the area of motor programming. The left dominant hemisphere has a primary role in the sequencing of movements. Thus individuals with left CVA (right hemiplegia) with frontal and posterior parietal lesions may present with deficits in motor planning or **apraxia.** They demonstrate difficulty initiating and performing purposeful movements that cannot be accounted for by inadequate strength, loss of coordination, impaired sensation, attention difficulties, abnormal tone, movement disorders, intellectual deterioration, poor comprehension, or uncooperativeness. Patients are unable to complete complex sequences of movements, and may take longer to learn a task. They also demonstrate slower movements overall, with more hesitancy. There are two main forms of apraxia: (1) **ideomotor,** where movement is not possible on command but may occur automatically, and (2) **ideational,** where purposeful movement is not possible, either automatically or on command. See Chapter 29 for a more complete discussion of apraxia.

The right hemisphere, on the other hand, may have an increased role in sustaining a movement or posture. Thus individuals with right CVA (left hemiplegia) characteristically demonstrate **motor impersistence,** an inability to sustain a movement or posture.[54,55] In a study of motor programming differences, Light et al.[56] found support for these conclusions and also noted deficits in motor programming in both involved and "uninvolved" upper extremities of patients with left CVA.

DISTURBANCES IN POSTURAL CONTROL AND BALANCE

Balance is frequently disturbed following stroke with impairments in steadiness, symmetry, and dynamic stability common.[57–60] Problems may exist when reacting to a destabilizing external force (reactive postural control) or during self-initiated movements (anticipatory postural control). Thus, the patient may be unable to maintain balance in sitting or standing or to move in a weight-bearing posture without loss of balance. Disruptions of central sensorimotor processing may lead to an inability to adapt postural movements to changing task and environmental demands and impair motor learning.[61] Patients with stroke typically demonstrate asymmetry with most of the weight in sitting or standing shifted to the nonparetic side. They also demonstrate increased postural sway in standing (a finding characteristic of the elderly in general). Delays in the onset of motor activity, abnormal timing and sequencing of muscle activity, and abnormal co-contraction result in disorganization of the postural synergies. For example, proximal muscles may be activated in advance of distal muscles or in some patients, very late (a finding also found in many elderly). Compensatory responses typically include excessive hip and knee movements. Corrective responses to perturbations or destabilizing forces are frequently inadequate and may result in loss of balance. Patients with hemiplegia typically fall in the direction of weakness.[62,63]

Speech and Language Disorders

Patients with lesions involving the cortex of the dominant hemisphere (typically the left hemisphere) demonstrate speech and language impairments. **Aphasia** is the general term used to describe an acquired communication disorder caused by brain damage and is characterized by an impairment of language comprehension, formulation, and use. Aphasia has been estimated to occur in 30 to 36 percent of all patients with stroke.[3] There are many different types of aphasias; major classification categories are fluent, nonfluent, and global. In **fluent aphasia (Wernicke's or receptive aphasia),** speech flows smoothly with a variety of grammatical constructions and preserved melody of speech. Auditory comprehension is impaired. Thus, the patient demonstrates difficulty in comprehending spoken language and in following commands. The lesion is located in the auditory association cortex in the left lateral temporal lobe. In **nonfluent aphasia (Broca's or expressive aphasia)** the flow of speech is slow and hesitant, vocabulary is limited, and syntax is impaired. Speech production is labored or absent while comprehension is good. The lesion is located in the premotor area of the left frontal lobe. **Global aphasia** is a severe aphasia characterized by marked impairments of both production and comprehension of language. It is often an indication of extensive brain damage. Severe problems in communication may limit the patient's ability to learn and often impedes successful outcomes in rehabilitation.

Patients with stroke commonly present with **dysarthria** with a reported incidence ranging from 48 to 57 percent.[3] This term refers to a category of motor speech disorders caused by impairment in parts of the central or peripheral nervous system that mediate speech production. Respiration, articulation, phonation, resonance, and/or sensory feedback may be affected. The lesion can be located in the primary motor cortex in the frontal lobe, the primary sensory cortex in the parietal lobe, or the cerebellum. Volitional and automatic actions such as chewing and swallowing and movement of the jaw and tongue may be impaired. In patients with stroke, dysarthria can accompany aphasia, complicating the course of rehabilitation. See Chapter 30 for a complete discussion of this topic.

Dysphagia

Swallowing difficulty, **dysphagia,** occurs in about 12 percent of patients with lesions affecting the medullary brainstem (cranial nerves IX and X), large vessel pontine lesions, as well as in acute hemispheric lesions (especially infarcts in the MCA and PCA).[3] Dysfunction of the lips, mouth, tongue, palate, pharynx, larynx, or proximal esophagus all contribute to dysphagia. The most frequent problem seen with dysphagia is delayed triggering of the swallowing reflex (86% of patients) followed by reduced pharyngeal peristalsis (58% of patients) and reduced lingual control (50% of patients).[64] Altered mental status, altered sensation, poor jaw and lip closure, impaired head control, and poor sitting posture also contribute to the patient's swallowing difficulties. Most patients demonstrate multiple problems that can include drooling, difficulty ingesting food, compromised nutritional status, and dehydration.

Aspiration, penetration of food, liquid, saliva, or gastric reflux into the airway, occurs in about one-third of patients with dysphagia. It is more common during the acute phase of recovery and can occur during any phase of swallowing. Aspiration is an important complication in that it can lead to acute respiratory distress within hours, aspiration pneumonia, and, if left untreated, death. Early assessment and treatment of dysphagia is essential to prevent aspiration. Videofluoroscopic examination (a modified barium swallow [MBS]) is the most commonly used technique to examine the preparatory, oral, pharyngeal, and esophageal phases of swallowing. Fiberoptic endoscopic examination of swallowing (FEES) provides information about laryngeal function, hypopharyngeal residue, and airway protection (aspiration).[65]

Dysphagia may be severe enough to require the use of tube feeding, either a nasogastric (NG) tube for short periods of time or an invasive gastrostomy (G) tube for more long-term care. Nutrition can also be provided through intravenous route (total parenteral nutrition [TPN]). There are numerous risks and complications associated with these feeding methods and difficult clinical decisions are made by the family in conjunction with the medical or dysphagia team.

Perceptual Dysfunction

Lesions of the cortex can produce visual-perceptual impairments, with a reported incidence ranging from 32 to 41 percent.[3] They occur most frequently with right-sided lesions and left hemiparesis. These may include disorders of **body scheme disorder** or **body image disorder,** spatial relation disorder, agnosias, and apraxia. Body scheme refers to a postural model of the body including the relationship of the body parts to each other and the relationship of the body to the environment. Body image is the visual and mental image of one's body that includes feelings about one's body. Both may be distorted. Specific impairments of body scheme/body image include unilateral neglect, anosognosia, somatoagnosia, right-left discrimination, finger agnosia, and anosognosia. **Spatial relations syndrome** refers to a constellation of impairments that have in common a difficulty in perceiving the relationship between the self and two or more objects in the environment. It includes specific impairments in figure-ground discrimination, form discrimination, spatial relations, position in space, and topographical disorientation. Agnosia is the inability to recognize or recognize incoming information despite intact sensory capacities. Agnosias can include visual object agnosia, auditory agnosia or tactile agnosia (astereognosis). Apraxia is a disorder of voluntary skilled learned movement, as discussed. The reader is referred to Chapter 29 for a more complete discussion of these deficits and their management.

Ipsilateral pushing, termed **Pusher Syndrome** by Davies,[66] is an unusual motor behavior characterized by the patient's strong lateral lean toward the hemiplegic side in all positions. During sitting, the lean is far over toward the hemiplegic side, often onto the wheelchair arm. During transfers and standing the strong lateral lean (push) creates an unstable situation with a high risk of falls because the hemiplegic LE typically cannot effectively support the body weight. The patient strongly resists any attempts to passively correct posture to mid-line or symmetrical weight-bearing. This pattern is totally opposite the expected postural pattern seen in most patients after stroke, that is, increased weight-bearing to the sound side to compensate for deficits on the affected side. The problem is more common in left hemiplegia than right and may be associated with hemisensory loss, and visual and perceptual difficulties. In one study, Pedersen et al.[67] identified the behavior in about 10 percent of 327 patients with stroke. These investigators found no significant association between ipsilateral pushing and hemineglect and anosognosia. They suggested the deficit may be more the result of impairment of subcortical sensory pathways. Functional mobility is impaired for patients with ipsilateral push. Typically the patient demonstrates severe problems in transfers, standing, and gait. The use of a cane during ambulation is problematic because patients use the cane to increase push to the hemiplegic side. Peterson et al. demonstrated that patients with ipsilateral pushing often have poorer rehabilitation outcomes (lower Barthel Index scores at discharge) with longer hospital stays and prolonged recovery times.

Cognitive Dysfunction

Cognitive deficits are present with lesions involving the brain and include impairments in attention, memory, or executive functions. Premorbid changes associated with pathological aging may also account for some of the dysfunction noted and should be carefully determined from interviews with family, significant others, or caregivers. The patient with stroke may be largely unaware of what is going on in the external environment, a deficit of impaired alertness. Attention is the ability to select and attend to a specific stimulus while simultaneously suppressing extraneous stimuli. **Attention disorders** include impairments in sustained attention, selective attention, divided attention, or alternating attention. Memory is defined as the ability to store experiences and perceptions for later recall. **Memory disorders** include impairments in immediate

recall and short-term or long-term memory. Immediate and short-term memory deficits are common, occurring in about 36 percent of patients with stroke while long-term memory typically remains intact.[3] Thus, the patient cannot remember the instructions for a new task given only minutes or hours ago but can easily remember things done 30 years ago. Memory gaps may be filled with inappropriate words or fabricated stories, a deficit termed **confabulation.** The patient may be confused, demonstrating disorientation to person, place, and/or time and an inability to understand the specific context of a conversation. Confusion is often the result of diffuse, bilateral lesions. **Perseveration** is the continued repetition of words, thoughts, or acts not related to current context. Thus the patient gets "stuck" and repeats words or acts without much success at stopping. Patients may also demonstrate decreased insight into disease or disability and impaired motivation.[68,69] Executive functions, defined as those capacities that enable a person to engage in purposeful behaviors, include volition, planning, purposeful action, and effective performance. Patients with impairments in executive functions demonstrate an inability to self-monitor and self-correct behaviors. Problems in impulsiveness, inflexibility, poor planning ability, lack of foresight, and impaired judgement may be typically evident. These in turn lead to an inability to make realistic appraisals of the environment and to learn, posing enormous safety risks. See Chapter 29 for a complete discussion of this topic.

Dementia can result from multiple infarcts of the brain, termed **multi-infarct dementia.** It is characterized by a generalized decline in higher brain functions with faulty judgement, impaired consciousness, poor memory, diminished communication, and behavioral or mood alterations. These changes are often associated with episodes of cerebral ischemia, focal neurological signs, and hypertension. The patient may fluctuate between periods of impaired function and periods of improved or normal function, demonstrating a step-wise progression of disease.[70]

Sensory losses coupled with an unfamiliar hospital environment and inactivity following acute stroke can lead to temporary symptoms such as irritability, confusion, restlessness, and sometimes psychosis, delusions, or hallucinations. Nighttime may be particularly problematic. Positioning the bed with the affected side toward the door may limit social interaction and increase disorientation. Some patients with diminished capacity are equally unable to deal with a sensory overload, produced by too much stimulation. Altered arousal levels are implicated.

Affective Disorders

Lesions to the right hemisphere tend to impair emotional functioning. The patient with stroke may demonstrate an emotional dysregulation syndrome termed **emotional lability (emotional dysregulation syndrome)**. It is characterized by pathological laughing and weeping in which the patient changes quickly from laughing to crying with only slight provocation. Such a patient is typically unable to inhibit the expression of spontaneous emotions.[71] Frequent crying may also accompany depression. Deficits in apathy produce a shallow affect and blunted emotional responses and can accompany lesions of the prefrontal cortex, posterior internal capsule, or basal ganglia. Lesions of the prefrontal cortex or hypothalamus can also lead to increased frustration levels. The patient may be irritable, agitated, hypercritical, and/or intolerant of his or her current situation or caregivers. Reactions may include verbal or physical outbursts. Changes in the ability to sense, move, communicate, think, or act as before are enormously frustrating by themselves and may produce behavioral responses. These behaviors along with a poor social perception of one's self and environment may lead to increasing isolation and stress.[72,73]

Depression is extremely common, occurring in about one-third of the cases.[3] Most patients remain significantly depressed for many months, with an average time of 7 to 8 months. The period from 6 months to 2 years after a CVA is the most likely time for depression to occur. Depression occurs in both mildly and severely involved patients and thus is not significantly related to the degree of impairment. Patients with lesions of the left hemisphere may experience more frequent and more severe depression than patients with right hemisphere or brainstem strokes.[74,75] These findings suggest that post-stroke depression is not simply a result of psychological reaction to disability but rather a direct impairment of the CVA. Prolonged depression may interfere with the success of rehabilitation goals and outcomes.

Behavioral Hemispheric Differences

Individuals with stroke differ widely in their approach to processing information and in their behaviors. Those with *left hemisphere damage* (right hemiplegia) demonstrate difficulties in communica-tion and in processing information in a sequential, linear manner. They are frequently described as cautious, anxious, and disorganized. This makes them more hesitant when trying new tasks and increases the need for feedback and support. They tend, however, to be realistic in their appraisal of their existing problems. Individuals with *right hemisphere damage* (left hemiplegia), on the other hand, demonstrate difficulty in spatial-perceptual tasks and in grasping the whole idea of a task or activity. They are frequently described as quick and impulsive. They tend to overestimate their abilities while acting unaware of their deficits. Safety is therefore a far greater issue with patients with left hemiplegia, where poor judgement is common. These patients also require a great deal of feedback when learning a new task. The feedback should be focused on slowing down the activity, checking steps, and relating it to the whole task. The patient with left hemiplegia frequently cannot attend to visuospatial cues effectively, especially in a cluttered or crowded environment.[54,76,77] Table 17–7 summarizes behaviors attributed to the left and right hemispheres.

Seizures

Seizures occur in a small percentage of patients with stroke and are slightly more common in occlusive carotid disease (17%) than in MCA disease (11%). Seizures can occur at the onset (e.g., with cerebral hemorrhage in about 15% of the cases), during the acute phase, or several months after stroke. They tend to be of the partial motor type.[78] Seizures are potentially life threatening if not controlled. Anticonvulsant medications may be given to individuals with a history of seizures.

Bladder and Bowel Dysfunction

Disturbances of bladder function are common during the acute phase, occurring in about 29 percent of cases.[3] Urinary incontinence can result from bladder hyperreflexia or hyporeflexia, disturbances of sphincter control, and/or sensory loss. A toileting schedule for prompted voiding is often

Table 17–7 BEHAVIORS ATTRIBUTED TO THE LEFT AND RIGHT HEMISPHERES

Behavior	Left Hemisphere	Right Hemisphere
Cognitive style	Processing information in a sequential, linear manner Observing and analyzing details	Processing information in a simultaneous, holistic, or gestalt manner Grasping overall organization or pattern
Perception/cognition	Processing and producing language	Processing nonverbal stimuli (environmental sounds, speech intonation, complex shapes, and designs) Visual-spatial perception Drawing inferences, synthesizing information
Academic skills	Reading: sound-symbol relationships, word recognition, reading comprehension Performing mathematical calculations	Mathematical reasoning and judgement Alignment of numerals in calculations
Motor	Sequencing movements Performing movements and gestures to command	Sustaining a movement or posture
Emotions	Expression of positive emotions	Expression of negative emotions Perception of emotion

implemented to reduce the incidence of incontinence and to accommodate for factors that cause functional incontinence such as inattention, mental status changes, or immobility. Generally this problem improves quickly. Persistent incontinence is often due to a treatable medical condition (e.g., urinary tract infection). Pads and special undergarments or external collection devices may be used if incontinence proves refractory. Urinary retention can be controlled pharmacologically and with intermittent or indwelling catheterization. Early treatment is desirable to prevent further complications such as chronic urinary tract infection and skin breakdown. Patients who are incontinent often suffer embarrassment, isolation, and depression. Persistent incontinence is associated with a poor long-term prognosis for functional recovery.

Disturbances of bowel function can include incontinence and diarrhea or constipation and impaction. Patients who are constipated may require stool softeners and dietary/fluid modifications to resolve this problem. Physical activity is also helpful to improve these problems.[3]

INDIRECT IMPAIRMENTS AND COMPLICATIONS

Venous Thromboembolism

Deep venous thrombosis (DVT) and pulmonary embolism are potential complications for all immobilized patients. The incidence of DVT in patients with stroke is as high as 47 percent with an estimated 10 percent of deaths attributed to pulmonary embolism.[3] The dangers are particularly high during the acute phase when venous stasis from bed rest, limb paralysis and decreased activity, hemineglect, and reduced cognitive status significantly elevate the risks. The hallmark clinical signs of DVT include rapid onset of unilateral leg swelling with dependent edema. The patient may report tenderness, a dull ache, or a tight feeling in the calf; pain is usually not severe. A positive *Homan's sign* (pain in the calf with passive dorsiflexion) may be seen during physical examination. However, this test lacks good sensitivity and specificity because a substantial number of patients with DVT do not demonstrate this sign. About 50 percent of the cases do not present with clinically detectable symptoms and can be identified only by radiocontrast venography (the gold standard), impedance plethysmography, or Doppler ultrasonography.

Prompt diagnosis and treatment of acute DVT are necessary to reduce the risk of fatal pulmonary embolism. Pharmacological management consists of anticoagulant therapy (blood thinners). Prophylactic use of low-dose heparin (LDH) or low-molecular-weight (LMW) heparin has been shown to reduce the incidence by 45 percent and 79 percent, respectively. Symptomatic treatment of DVT consists of bed rest and elevation of the limb until tenderness subsides (generally 3 to 5 days) to prevent pressure fluctuations within the venous system and emboli. Edema management may include intermittent pneumatic compression and compression stockings.[79] Careful daily monitoring of the lower limbs is essential. Early mobilization and ambulation are important primary prevention measures.

Skin Breakdown

Ischemic damage and subsequent necrosis of the skin may result in the development of pressure sores (decubiti). The incidence in patients with stroke is reported to be 14.5 percent.[80] The skin breaks down typically over bony prominences from pressure, friction, shearing, and/or maceration. Intense pressure for a short time or low pressure for a long time result in pressure sores. Friction occurs as the skin rubs against the surface, for example, when the patient slides down in bed or is pulled up. Spasticity and contractures can also contribute to increased friction. Shearing occurs when the two layers of skin move in opposite directions on each other, for example, during transfers from bed to stretcher without a pull sheet. Maceration is caused by excess moisture, for example, with urinary incontinence. Additional risk factors include reduced activity (bedfast or chairfast), immobility, decreased sensation, abnormal patterns of movement, poor nutrition, and decreased level of consciousness. The incidence of pressure sores is increased with comorbid medical conditions such as infections, peripheral vascular disease, edema, and diabetes.[3]

Daily systematic inspection of the skin, particularly over high-risk areas is essential in recognizing the early signs of breakdown. The skin needs to be kept clean, dry, and protected from injury. Proper techniques for positioning, turning, and transferring are essential. A positioning schedule is instituted and the time in each position is limited. Assumption of upright postures (sitting and standing) is promoted as soon as possible.

Pressure-limiting devices to minimize high concentrations of pressure are used. These may include foam pads, alternating pressure mattress, water mattress, air-fluidized bed, sheepskin, heel and elbow protectors, multipodus boots, and trapeze. Proper positioning (seating) in the wheelchair and use of pressure relieving devices (gel or air cushions) are also critical. Lubricants, protective dressings, and barrier sprays may also be used. Ensuring the patient has adequate nutrition and hydration will also protect against skin breakdown as will early mobilization by the rehabilitation team.

Decreased Flexibility

Decreasing range of movement (ROM), contracture, and deformity may result from loss of voluntary movement and immobilization. Flexibility of connective tissue is lost and muscles experience disuse atrophy. As contractures progress, edema and pain may develop and further restrict attempts to gain motion. In the UE, limitations in shoulder motions are common. Contractures also frequently develop at elbow flexors, wrist and finger flexors, and forearm pronators. In the lower extremity, plantarflexion contractures are common. Alterations in alignment coupled with decreased efficiency of muscles may lead to increased energy expenditure, altered patterns of movement, and excessive effort. Daily ROM exercises, positioning, and resting splints are important to maintain flexibility.

Shoulder Subluxation and Pain

Shoulder pain is extremely common following stroke, occurring in 70 to 84 percent of cases.[81,82] Pain is typically present with movement and, in more severe cases, at rest. Several causes of shoulder pain have been widely proposed. In the flaccid stage, proprioceptive impairment, lack of tone, and muscle paralysis reduce the support and normal seating action of the rotator cuff muscles, particularly the supraspinatus. The ligaments and capsule thus become the shoulder's sole support. The normal orientation of the glenoid fossa is upward, outward, and forward, so that it keeps the superior capsule taut and stabilizes the humerus mechanically. Any abduction or forward flexion of the humerus, or scapular depression and downward rotation, reduces this stabilization and causes the humerus to sublux. Initially the subluxation is not painful, but mechanical stresses resulting from traction and gravitational forces produce persistent malalignment and pain. Glenohumeral friction-compression stresses also occur between the humeral head and superior soft tissues during flexion or abduction movements in the absence of normal scapulohumeral rhythm (shoulder impingement syndrome). During the spastic stage, abnormal muscle tone may contribute to poor scapular position (depression, retraction, and downward rotation) and contributes to subluxation and restricted movement. Secondary tightness in ligaments, tendons, and joint capsule can develop quickly. Adhesive capsulitis is a common finding. Poor handling and positioning of the hemiplegic UE have been implicated in producing joint microtrauma and pain. Activities that traumatize the shoulder include passive range of motion (PROM) without adequate mobilization of the scapula (maintaining normal scapulohumeral rhythm), pulling on the UE during a transfer, or using reciprocal pulleys.[81,83] Pain can significantly impair the patient's ability to move and achieve independent status in functional tasks.

Reflex Sympathetic Dystrophy

Reflex sympathetic dystrophy (RSD; shoulder hand syndrome) occurs in approximately 12 to 25 percent of cases.[3] It develops in characteristic stages.

In *stage 1*, the patient reports severe pain and stiffness in the shoulder, which is worse with movement and in certain positions, for example, lying in bed at night. There is a loss of ROM in abduction, flexion, and external rotation movements. Pain is progressive, spreading to involvement of the wrist and hand. Edema develops primarily over the dorsum of the hand. The wrist tends to assume a flexed position with intense pain likely during wrist extension movements. The elbow is not involved. Early vasomotor changes include discoloration (pale and cool or pink) and alterations in temperature. The skin may be hypersensitive to touch, pressure, or temperature variations. The patient typically guards against movement attempts. *Stage 2* is characterized by subsiding pain and early dystrophic changes: muscle and skin atrophy, vasospasm, hyperhidrosis (increased sweating), and course hair and nails. There is radiographic evidence of early osteoporosis. In *stage 3*, the atrophic phase, pain and vasomotor changes are rare. There is progressive atrophy of the skin, muscles, and bones (severe osteoporosis is evident). Pericapsular fibrosis and articular changes become pronounced. The hand typically becomes contracted in a clawed position with metacarpophalangeal (MP) extension and interphalangeal (IP) flexion (similar to the intrinsic minus hand). There is marked atrophy of thenar and hypothenar muscles with flattening of the hand. Chances of reversal of signs and symptoms are high for stage 1 and variable for stage 2, while stage 3 changes are largely irreversible.[84]

Early diagnosis and treatment are critical in preventing or minimizing the late changes of RSD. Because of close daily contact with the patient, the therapist is frequently one of the first to recognize and report early signs and symptoms. Radionuclide bone scans (scintigraphy) can be used to reliably confirm early symptoms of RSD. Successful medical treatments of RSD may include use of nonsteroidal anti-inflammatory drugs (NSAIDs) or oral corticosteroids. Therapy for RSD typically includes proper handling of the upper extremity, including avoiding trauma and traction injuries (e.g., prolonged dangling). Additional interventions include proper shoulder mobilization, joint active assisted range of motion (AAROM) and active range of motion (AROM), and edema control with massage, exercise, and skin compression. Ice baths or contrast baths can be used to produce quick vasomotor restriction. This should be followed by AAROM or AROM of arm motions. Family/caregiver education is important to ensure proper extremity handling and transfer techniques. Persistent pain may be managed with sympathetic blockade using drugs such as reserpine and guanethidine or surgical sympathectomy.[85,86]

Deconditioning

Patients who suffer a stroke as a result of cardiac disease may demonstrate impaired cardiac output, cardiac decompensation, and serious rhythm disorders. If these problems persist, they can directly alter cerebral perfusion and produce additional focal signs (e.g., mental confusion). Cardiac limitations in exercise tolerance may restrict rehabilitation potential and require diligent monitoring and careful exercise prescription by the physical therapist.[87] Deconditioning is also a common finding in older adults with limited activity levels and may have been present prior to the stroke. Age-related changes in the cardiorespiratory systems (reduced cardiac output, decreased maximal oxygen uptake, decreased respiratory capacity) and musculoskeletal systems (decreased muscle mass, strength, lean body mass) all affect exercise tolerance and endurance levels.[88] Prolonged bed rest during the acute stroke phase further diminishes cardiovascular endurance and rehabilitation potential. Decreased activity levels may also be related to depression, a common finding in stroke.

FUNCTIONAL DISABILITIES

Functional mobility skills are typically impaired following stroke and vary considerably from individual to individual. During the acute stroke phase (within the first 3 weeks), 70 to 80 percent of patients demonstrate mobility problems in ambulation while 6 months to 1 year later the figures are reversed, with 70 to 80 percent of patients able to walk independently, with or without assistive devices.[86] Basic ADL skills such as feeding, bathing, dressing, and toileting are also compromised during acute stroke, with 67 to 88 percent of patients demonstrating partial or complete dependence. Independence in ADLs also improves with time with only 24 to 53 percent of survivors requiring partial or total assistance 6 months to 1 year later. The ability to perform functional tasks is influenced by a number of factors. Motor and perceptual impairments have the greatest impact on functional performance, but other limiting factors include sensory loss, disorientation, communication disorders, and decreased cardiorespiratory endurance.[89,90]

RECOVERY FROM STROKE

Recovery from stroke is generally fastest in the first weeks after onset, with measurable neurological and functional recovery occurring in the first 1 to 3 months after stroke. Patients continue to make functional gains at a reduced rate for up to 6 months or longer after insult. Some patients may demonstrate prolonged recovery with improvements occurring over a period of years, especially in the areas of language and visuospatial function.[3] Rates of improvement will vary across management categories: patients suffering minor stroke recover rapidly with few or no residual deficits whereas severely impaired individuals demonstrate more limited recovery. An important finding is that recovery has been demonstrated even in patients with extensive central nervous system (CNS) damage and advanced age.[29,30,91–94] Early recovery is generally thought to be the result of resolution of local vascular and metabolic factors. Thus the reduction of edema, absorption of damaged tissue, and improved local circulation allows intact neurons that were previously inhibited to regain function. CNS plasticity is thought to account for continuing recovery. In the presence of cell death, functional reorganization of the CNS (function-induced plasticity) occurs. The stimulation from active rehabilitation and an enriched environment plays an important part in brain repair and recovery.[95]

MEDICAL MANAGEMENT

Medical management of completed stroke includes strategies to[96,97]

1. Maintain circulation and oxygenation. Oxygen is delivered via mask or nasal cannula. Patients rarely require intubation or assisted ventilation.
2. Maintain adequate blood pressure. Hypotension or extreme hypertension is treated; hypertension agents have the added risk of inducing hypotension and decreasing cerebral perfusion.
3. Maintain sufficient cardiac output. If the causes of stroke are cardiac in origin, medical management focuses on control of arrhythmias and cardiac decompensation.
4. Restore fluid and electrolyte balance.
5. Maintain blood glucose levels within the normal range.
6. Control seizures and infections.
7. Control intracranial pressures and herniation using anti-edema agents. Ventriculostomy may be indicated to monitor and drain cerebrospinal fluid.

Pharmacological interventions to limit or reverse the degree of ischemic neuronal damage have not been shown to be effective in this regard. This is an area of active research. Neurosurgery may be indicated in cases where intracranial bleeding or compression causes elevated intracranial pressures, because death may result from brain herniation and brainstem compression. Generally superficial or lobar lesions (subdural hematoma, aneurysm, subarachnoid hemorrhage, and arteriovenous malformation) are more amenable to neurosurgery than large, deep lesions.

Current trends toward shorter hospital stays (average stay is about 7.5 days) and early discharge have resulted in an increase in the number of serious medical complications patients are presenting with while in the rehabilitation facility or receiving home care intervention. The rate of serious medical complications on rehabilitation admission ranges from 22 to 48 percent.[96] These complications in turn may result in delays in the start of rehabilitation therapies for some patients or in the temporary cessation of therapy while medical complications are resolved. About 7 percent of patients require transfer back to the acute hospital setting.[86] Therapists have to be vigilant in monitoring patients for potential medical problems (e.g., cardiac arrhythmias, wide variations in blood pressure).

REHABILITATION MANAGEMENT

Rehabilitation begun early in the acute stage optimizes the patient's potential for functional recovery. Early mobilization prevents or minimizes the harmful effects of deconditioning and the potential for secondary impairments. Functional reorganization is promoted through stimulation and use of the affected side. Learned nonuse of the hemiplegic extremities and maladaptive patterns of movement are prevented. Mental deterioration, depression, and apathy can be reduced through the fostering of a positive outlook on the rehabilitation process. Patients need to be presented early on with an organized plan of care that addresses their individual goals and stresses resumption of normal ADLs. It is equally important that patients receive adequate information and know that various forms of support are available, if they need them.

Rehabilitation can begin as soon as the patient is medically stabilized, typically within 72 hours. Patients may be admitted to a specific stroke unit or neurological unit with rehabilitation services. Evidence supports the benefits of such services in significantly improving functional outcomes when compared to patients not receiving those services.[98–102]

Patients with moderate or severe residual deficits generally require intensive rehabilitation services to assist them in functional recovery. Patients are referred to acute rehabilitation (inpatient hospital rehabilitation) if they can tolerate an intensity of services consisting of two or more rehabilitation disciplines, 5 days a week for a minimum of 3 hours of active rehabilitation per day. Less intensive services can be obtained from subacute rehabilitation programs, generally found in nursing facilities or in a subacute hospital unit. Services in subacute units are variable, ranging from 1 hour of services 2 to 3 times per week to daily, shorter duration services. Post acute rehabilitation services can also be delivered at home or in an outpatient facility. Generally the patient who benefits from these services demonstrates less severe involvement and more functional mobility than those requiring hospitalization.[3]

Optimal timing of rehabilitation based on individual patient readiness is an important consideration. A number of factors appear to be related to rehabilitation readiness, including the side of the lesion. There is some evidence to suggest that patients with right hemiplegia may respond more favorably to earlier comprehensive rehabilitation efforts. Patients with left hemiplegia who suffer more cognitive-perceptual deficits and generally have longer rehabilitation stays may benefit from additional preadmission time to allow for cognitive and perceptual-motor reorganization. Equally impor-

tant factors that influence the timing of rehabilitation efforts include medical stability, motivation, patient endurance, recovery, and ability to learn. In an era of time-limited payment for comprehensive rehabilitation services, selecting the optimal time for rehabilitation training may prevent unnecessary patient failures and improve long-term functional outcomes.[103,104]

Comprehensive services for the patient with stroke can best be provided by a team of rehabilitation specialists including the physician, nurse, physical therapist, occupational therapist, medical social worker, and case manager. Additional disciplines may also include a neuropsychologist, speech/language pathologist, dietician, ophthalmologist, or recreational therapist. One of the critical tasks of the team is the development of an integrated plan of care with unified goals and outcomes and treatments that are mutually reinforced by all team members.

Assessment Methods for Patients with Stroke

Assessments will be determined by the therapist based on each patient's unique needs, impairments, and disabilities. Assessments will vary by severity of the problem, stage of recovery, phase of rehabilitation, as well as other factors. The purposes of assessment are to document the diagnosis and monitor recovery from stroke, identify patients who are most likely to benefit from rehabilitation efforts and the most appropriate type of facility, develop a specific plan of care, monitor progress toward projected goals and outcomes, and plan for discharge. The neurological examination provides the main source of information for clinical decision making (Box 17–2). This section will also review instruments that are specific to the assessment of patients with stroke.

Level of Consciousness

Altered level of consciousness (coma, decreased arousal levels) may occur with extensive brain damage and can be assessed using the Glasgow Coma Scale.[105,106] The patient's spontaneous behaviors and responses to external stimuli are observed and documented. The Rancho Levels of Cognitive Functioning Scale (LCFS) can be used to observe the patient's ability to process information and resultant behaviors.[107] See Chapter 24 for a more complete discussion of these scales. Because the patient's behaviors can be expected to fluctuate widely, frequent repeat observations are necessary.

Speech and Language Deficits

Profound deficits in communication (aphasia) are common with lesions in the language-dominant hemisphere and will interfere with other assess-

Box 17–2 ELEMENTS OF THE NEUROLOGICAL EXAMINATION

General demographics: age, gender, primary language, race/ethnicity
Social history
   Family and caregiver resources
   Social interactions and support systems
Occupation/employment
Living environment: home and work barriers
History
   Current condition
   Past medical/surgical history
Medications
Other tests and measures
Level of consciousness, arousal, attention
Communication and language
Cognition and learning style
Cranial nerve integrity
Sensory integrity
Perception
Joint integrity and mobility
   Range of motion (ROM)
   Joint hypermobility/hypomobility
   Soft-tissue changes: swelling, inflammation, restriction
Pain
Integumentary integrity
Motor function (motor control and motor learning)
   Tone
   Reflexes
   Voluntary movement patterns: head, trunk, limbs
   Stereotypical movements
   Posture: sitting, standing, locomotor
   Coordination, dexterity, agility
   Sensorimotor integration
   Motor planning
Muscle performance
   Strength, power, and endurance
Postural control and balance
Gait and locomotion
   Wheelchair management and mobility
   With and without the use of assistive, orthotic, and supportive devices
Functional status and activity level
   Functional mobility skills
   Basic ADLs
   Instrumental ADLs
   Assistive and adaptive devices
Aerobic capacity and endurance

ments and rehabilitation efforts in general. Therefore the patient's communication abilities should be fully ascertained before proceeding with other assessments. It is not uncommon for family and staff to overestimate the patient's abilities to understand language, especially if the patient is cooperative. Close collaboration with the speech/language pathologist is important in making an accurate determination of the patient's communication deficits. Receptive language functions (auditory comprehension, reading comprehension) and expressive language function (word finding, fluency, writing) should be carefully assessed. Neuromotor disorders (dysarthria, apraxia) need to be clearly differentiated from aphasia. If communication is severely limited and alternate forms required (gestures, demonstra-tion, communication boards), therapists should be fully knowledgeable of such methods before further examination begins. Assessment of speech and language is discussed fully in Chapter 30.

Cranial Nerve Integrity

The presence of swallowing difficulties and drooling necessitates an assessment of the motor nuclei of the lower brainstem cranial nerves (IX, X, and XII) affecting the muscles of the face, tongue, larynx, and pharynx. This includes an examination of motor function of the lips, mouth, tongue, palate, pharynx, and larynx. The gag reflex should be assessed because hypoactivity may lead to aspiration into the airway. Adequacy of cough mechanisms should also be carefully examined. Detailed examination of swallowing is typically performed by specialists. Therapists need to be able to recognize the presence of swallowing difficulties and initiate prompt referral to the dysphagia team. Facial sensation and weakness (cranial nerve VII) and labyrinthine/auditory function (cranial nerve VIII) should be assessed.

Cognitive Dysfunction

It is important to assess cognition early because it may affect the validity of other assessments. An examination of recall (short- and long-term memory), orientation (to person, place, time, and situation), ability to follow instructions (one-, two-, and three-level commands), and attention span can be made from observations of the patient's interactions and responses to specific questions. Higher cortical functions can be assessed using tests of simple arithmetic and abstract reasoning. The Mini-Mental Status Examination (MMSE) provides a valid and reliable quick screen of cognitive function.[108] An assessment of learning deficits (retention and generalization) usually requires repeat sessions with the patient before a complete picture can be ascertained. Difficulties arise in reaching an accurate determination of cognition when the patient presents with deficits in communication. Close collaboration with the occupational therapist and speech/language pathologist is essential. See Chapter 29 for further discussion of this topic.

Sensory Integrity

A sensory examination should include testing of superficial sensations (e.g., touch, pressure, sharp or dull discrimination, temperature) and deep sensations (proprioception, kinesthesia, pallesthesia). Combined (cortical) sensations such as stereognosis, tactile localization, two-point discrimination, texture recognition should also be examined (see Chapter 6). Deficits may be apparent in one sensory modality and not in others. Differences can also be expected between the hemiplegic extremities. Comparisons with the intact side can be made, but the therapist should be cognizant that deficits may exist in the supposedly "normal" extremities secondary to effects of comorbid conditions (e.g., neuropathy) or aging. Profound sensory deficits will negatively impact on rehabilitation outcomes and goals.

Disorders of Vision

The visual system should be carefully investigated, including tests for acuity, pupillary responses, ocular mobility, and visual field defects (homonymous hemianopsia). Ocular motility disturbances may be present with brainstem strokes, such as diplopia, oscillopsia, visual distortions, or paralysis of conjugate gaze. Visual field defects need to be differentiated from visual neglect (an inattention to or neglect of visual stimuli presented on the involved side). The patient with pure hemianopsia is typically aware of the deficit and will spontaneously compensate by moving the eyes or head toward the side of deficit; the patient with visual neglect will be unaware (inattentive) of the deficit. See Chapter 29 for a detailed description of visual assessment procedures. The use of prescriptive eyeglasses should be determined prior to any testing; the therapist should ensure eyeglasses are worn and clean.

Perceptual Dysfunction

Significant information on sensory and perceptual deficits will be provided by close collaboration with the occupational therapist. Many tests and formalized test batteries have been developed to assess body scheme, body image, spatial relations, agnosia, and apraxia. These are discussed fully in Chapter 29. Because the patient with left hemiplegia may behave in ways that tend to minimize his or her disabilities, it is easy for staff to overestimate the patient's perceptual abilities. The use of gestures or visual cues may decrease this patient's ability to perform specific perceptual tests, whereas verbal cues may increase chances for success. Carefully structuring the environment to minimize clutter and activity, provide clear boundaries and reference points, as well as provide adequate lighting will also improve performance of the patient who exhibits significant visuospatial deficits.

Problems in unilateral neglect (lack of awareness of part of the body or the external environment) will limit movement and use of the involved extremities (usually the nondominant left side). The patient typically does not react to sensory stimuli (visual, hearing, or somatosensory) presented on the involved side. Careful observation of spontaneous use of affected limbs as well as specific responses to inquiries for movement on or toward the hemiplegic side will provide important information about

neglect. Persistent neglect may negatively impact rehabilitation outcomes.

Joint Integrity and Mobility

An assessment of joint integrity and mobility should include an assessment of ROM, joint hypermobility and hypomobility, and soft-tissue changes (swelling, inflammation, or restriction). The shoulder and wrist should be examined closely because joint malalignment problems are common. For example, edema of the wrist often produces malaligned carpal bones with resulting impingement during wrist extension. Problems with spasticity may result in inconsistent ROM findings, because fluctuations in tone may exist from one testing session to the next. Thus tonal abnormalities should be noted at the time of examination. AROM tests are invalid for the patient in early or middle recovery when paresis, tonal changes, or abnormal synergies influence performance and preclude the isolated movements required in standard AROM tests. ROM limitations and developing contracture should be carefully documented. The presence of pain should also be documented. The therapist needs to carefully identify the nature of the pain and how the pain relates to joint movement and limitation.

Motor Deficits

The patient with stroke typically exhibits a number of deficits in motor function (motor control and motor learning). For the patient in early and middle recovery, assessment of tone and reflexes is essential. Passive motion testing can be used to reveal either hypertonicity or hypotonicity. The position of the affected limbs at rest and with movement should be observed for tonal influences. An assessment of stretch reflexes and pathological reflexes (e.g., Babinski, tonic reflex activity) should be performed.

Voluntary movement patterns should be examined for synergy dominance (stereotypic movements). The therapist bases the assessment on a knowledge of the typical components of the synergies. It is possible for one limb to vary significantly from the other (e.g., the UE may demonstrate more synergistic dominance than the LE). Synergistic dominance versus isolated joint control may also vary within a limb (e.g., the shoulder may demonstrate more isolated control than the wrist and hand). The quality of movement pattern should also be observed. A determination is made of which muscles are functional and which are not (spatial organization of movement) as well as the timing of the components (temporal organization).

Paresis is a common finding. Although an assessment of strength is necessary, the traditional manual muscle test poses problems of validity in the presence of spasticity, reflex, and synergy dominance. An estimation of strength can be made from observation of active movements during functional tasks.[109]

Movements can be graded using the following ordinal scale[3]:
- No movement: a grade of 0
- Palpable contraction or flicker: a grade of 1
- Movement with gravity eliminated: a grade of 2
- Movement against gravity: a grade of 3
- Movement against some resistance but weaker than the other side: a grade of 4
- Normal strength: a grade of 5

Slower than normal movements (bradykinesia), or abnormal involuntary movements (chorea, hemiballismus) may also occur and should be carefully assessed.

The patient in late recovery demonstrates improving motor control. Movements are not bound by synergy and therefore can be examined for selective or isolated control. Manual muscle tests and dynamometry can be used to provide accurate information on residual deficits in strength, power, and endurance. Coordination and timing deficits may become more apparent in the absence of tone and synergy restrictions. Coordination tests can be used, for example, finger-to-nose, heel-to-shin, and rapid alternating movements (see Chapter 7). The ability to perform skilled movements (writing, dressing, feeding) should be examined.

Gait is altered following a stroke owing to a number of factors. Some of the more common problems in hemiplegic gait and their possible causes are summarized in Box 17–3. An assessment of gait typically includes an observational gait analysis (OGA), an examination of the movement patterns at the ankle, foot, knee, hip, pelvis, and trunk during walking (kinematic gait analysis). Gait is observed from the different planes of motion and deviations are identified.[110,111] Videotaping an OGA improves identification of gait deviations, provides a visual record of performance, and offers a useful teaching tool in assisting the patient in remediation of gait problems. Quantitative measures of distance and time, cadence, velocity, and stride times should also be obtained using measured walkways and a stopwatch. Kinetic gait analysis involves the forces involved in gait and requires sophisticated equipment (force plates) to obtain data. See Chapter 10 for a more complete discussion of this topic.

Disturbances in Postural Control and Balance

Postural control and balance are essential elements of a stroke assessment. Control can be assessed in sitting and standing. The patient's ability to maintain a steady position (steadiness) as well as postural alignment and position (symmetry) within the base of support are assessed. Dynamic stability control can be assessed by having the patient move within a given posture (weight shift) without losing balance. The patient should be encouraged to shift weight in all directions, especially to the paretic side where deficits are expected. Functional tasks that utilize moving from one posture to another (e.g., supine to sit, sit to stand) can also be used to assess dynamic postural control. Both reactive postural control (response to perturbations) and anticipatory postural control (response to voluntary extremity movements) should be documented.[112,113]

Standardized assessment instruments that can be used to measure balance function include the Berg Balance Scale,[114,115] the Functional Reach Test,[116] and the Tinetti Performance Oriented Mobility Assessment.[117] Sensory contributions to balance can be assessed by using the Clinical Test of Sensory Interaction and Balance.[118] Platform biofeedback systems have also been used to examine balance function in patients with stroke. Objective data concerning measures of sway and sway path excursion, symmetry, and limits of stability can be obtained.[119] See Chapter 8 for a more complete discussion of these instruments.

Standardized Stroke Assessment Instruments

Several standardized instruments are available for the assessment of motor function. The pioneering work of Signe Brunnstrom[25] led to the development of the **Fugl-Meyer Assessment of Physical Performance (FMA)**.[28,120] Test items are organized into five sequential recovery stages. A three-point ordinal scale is used to measure impairments of volitional movement with grades ranging from 0 (item cannot be performed) to 2 (item can be fully performed). Specific descriptions for performance accompany individual test items. Subtests exist for UE function, LE function, balance, sensation, ROM, and pain. The cumulative test score for all components is 226 with availability of specific subtest scores (e.g., UE maximum score is 66, LE score 34; balance score 14). This instrument has good validity and high reliability ($r = .99$) for assessing motor function and balance.[121] Quantifiable outcome data allow this instrument to be accurately used for research purposes. The instrument requires an estimated 30 to 40 minutes to administer (see Appendix A).

The **Motor Assessment Scale (MAS)** was developed by Carr and Shephard[122] to measure impairments and disability on a six-point ordinal scale. It includes eight items of motor function, including movement transitions (supine to sidelying, supine to sit, sit to stand), balanced sitting, walking, upper-arm function, hand movements, and advanced hand function. The ninth item assesses muscle tone. This instrument has been shown to be highly reliable ($r = 0.89$ to .99) with high concurrent validity (0.88 correlated with the Fugl-Meyer assessment).[123]

Functional Assessments

Functional measures are used to assess the impact of impairments, establish outcomes, goals, and plan of care, monitor progress and outcomes

---

Box 17–3 GAIT DEVIATIONS COMMONLY SEEN FOLLOWING STROKE

Stance Phase
Trunk/pelvis
Unawareness of affected side: poor proprioception
Forward trunk:
Weak hip extension
Flexion contracture
Hip
Poor hip position (typically adduction or flexion): poor proprioception
Trendelenburg limp: weak abductors
Scissoring: spastic adductors
Knee
Flexion during forward progression:
Flexion contracture combined with weak knee extensors and/or poor proprioception
Ankle dorsiflexion range past neutral, combined with weak hip and knee extension or poor proprioception at knee and ankle
Weakness in extension pattern or in selective motion of hip and knee extensors and plantarflexors
Slow contraction of knee extensors; knee remains flexed 20 to 30 degrees during forward progression
Hyperextension during forward progression:
Plantarflexion contracture past 90 degrees
Impaired proprioception: knee wobbles or snaps back into recurvatum
Severe spasticity in quadriceps
Weak knee extensors: compensatory locking of knee in hyperextension
Ankle/foot
Equinus gait (heel does not touch the ground): spasticity or contractures of gastroc-soleus
Varus foot (patient bears weight on the lateral surface of the foot): hyperactive or spastic anterior tibialis, post tibialis, toe flexors, and soleus
Unequal step lengths: hammer toes caused by spastic toe flexors prevent the patient from stepping forward onto the opposite foot because of pain/weight-bearing on flexed toes
Lack of dorsiflexion range on the affected side (approximately 10 degrees is needed)

Swing Phase
Trunk/pelvis
Insufficient forward pelvic rotation (pelvic retraction): weak abdominal muscles
Inclination to sound side for foot clearance: weakness of flexor muscles
Hip
Inadequate flexion:
Weak hip flexors, poor proprioception, spastic quadriceps, abdominal weakness (hip hikers), hip abductor weakness of opposite side
Abnormal substitutions include circumduction, external rotation/adduction, backward leaning of trunk/dragging toes; momentum/uncontrolled swing
Exaggerated hip flexion: strong flexor synergy
Knee
Inadequate knee flexion:
Inadequate hip flexion and poor foot clearance; spastic quadriceps
Exaggerated but delayed knee flexion: strong flexor synergy
Inadequate knee extension at weight acceptance: spastic hamstrings or sustained total flexor pattern
Weak knee extensors or poor proprioception
Ankle/foot
Persistent equinus and/or equinovarus: plantarflexor contracture or spasticity; weak dorsiflexors, delayed contraction of dorsiflexors; toes drag during midswing
Varus: spastic anterior tibialis, weak peroneals, and toe extensors
Equinovarus: spasticity of post tibialis and/or gastroc-soleus
Exaggerated dorsiflexion: strong flexor synergy pattern

Adapted from educational materials used at Rancho Los Amigos Medical Center, Downey, CA, and Spaulding Rehabilitation Hospital, Boston, MA.

of stroke rehabilitation efforts, and determine long-term placement. Instruments can include items to assess functional mobility skills (bed mobility, movement transitions, transfers, locomotion, stairs), basic ADL skills (feeding, hygiene, dressing), and instrumental ADL skills (communication, home chores). Information on functional disability following stroke is typically gained through performance-based assessment.[124] The *Barthel Index*[125] and the *Functional Independence Measure (FIM)*[126] have been extensively tested and demonstrate excellent reliability, validity, and sensitivity. Granger et al.[127] reported that a score of 60 on the Barthel Index (out of a possible 100) was pivotal in determining the attainment of assisted independence. Patients with stroke having scores below this level demonstrated marked dependence, whereas scores below 40 demonstrated severe dependence. These patients typically had longer rehabilitation stays and were less

likely to be discharged to home. Higher FIM scores have also been correlated to successful outcomes, discharge home and return to the community.[128] See Chapter 11 for a more detailed discussion of these instruments.

ACUTE REHABILITATION: GOALS AND OUTCOMES

Goals and outcomes of physical therapy during acute rehabilitation adapted from the *Guide to Physical Therapist Practice*[129] include the following:

1. Changes associated with recovery are monitored.
2. Tolerance to positions and activities is increased.
3. Upright (out of bed) and weight-bearing status is improved.

4. Risk of secondary impairments and reoccurrence of condition is reduced.
5. Joint integrity and mobility is maintained.
6. Awareness of the hemiplegic side and motor function (motor control and motor learning) are improved.
7. Trunk control, symmetry, and balance are improved.
8. Strength, power, and endurance are increased.
9. Functional independence in ADLs and functional mobility are increased.
10. Aerobic capacity and endurance are increased.
11. Patient, family, and caregiver knowledge and awareness of the diagnosis, prognosis, interventions, and goals and outcomes are increased.
12. Care is coordinated with patient, family, and caregivers, and other professionals.
13. Safety of patient, and family, caregivers is improved.
14. Placement needs are determined.
15. Self-management of symptoms is improved.
16. Sense of well-being is improved.
17. Awareness and use of community resources are improved.

ACUTE REHABILITATION: INTERVENTIONS

Motor Learning Strategies

Recovery from stroke and learning is based on the brain's capacity for reorganization and adaptation. An effective rehabilitation plan capitalizes on this potential and encourages functional use of the involved segments. Activities are selected that are meaningful and important to the patient. Optimal motor learning can be ensured through attention to a number of factors, most importantly, strategy development, feedback, and practice.

STRATEGY DEVELOPMENT

The therapist first assists the patient in learning the desired task (cognitive stage). More specifically, critical task elements and successful outcomes and goals are identified. The desired task is demonstrated at the ideal performance speeds. The patient then begins to practice. If the task has a number of interrelated steps, practice of component parts may precede practice of the whole task. It is important, however, not to delay practice of the integrated task because this may interfere with effective transfer of learning. The therapist should give clear, simple verbal instructions; do not overload the patient with excessive or wordy commands. Reinforce correct performance and intervene when movement errors become consistent. Manual guidance can be used to assist the patient through the activity especially for positioning or postural tasks. Active participation of the affected side should be encouraged early. Prac-

ticing the movements on the unaffected side first can yield important transfer effects to the affected side. Simultaneous practice of similar movements on both sides (bilateral activities) can also improve learning and promote integration of the two sides of the body. Visualization of the movement components (mental practice) can help some patients in initially organizing the movement.

As initial practice progresses, the patient is asked to assess performance and identify problems, specifically, what difficulties exist, what can be done to correct the difficulties, and what movements can be eliminated or refined. If a complex task is practiced, the patient is asked to identify if the correct components were performed, how the individual components fit together, and if they were appropriately sequenced. If the patient is unable to provide an accurate assessment of problems, the therapist can prompt the patient in decision making and utilize demonstration to help identify problems. For example, if the patient consistently falls to the right while standing, questions can be directed toward this problem (e.g., "In what direction did you fall?" "What do you need to do to prevent yourself from falling?"). The patient is thus actively involved in developing problem solving skills (self-monitoring and self-correction of movements). These skills are essential in ensuring independence and generalizability of learning to other environments and variations.

FEEDBACK

Feedback can be intrinsic (naturally occurring as part of the movement response) or extrinsic (provided by the therapist). During early motor learning the therapist will provide extrinsic feedback (e.g., verbal cueing, manual cueing) to shape performance. It is important to monitor performance carefully and provide accurate feedback. The patient's attention should be directed to naturally occurring intrinsic feedback. During early intervention visual inputs are critical for motor learning. This can be facilitated by having the patient watch the movement. If the patient needs glasses, make sure they are worn during therapy. Use of a mirror can be an effective adjunct for some patients to improve visual feedback, especially during postural and positioning activities. It is, however, contraindicated in patients with marked visuospatial perceptual impairments. During later learning (associative phase), proprioception becomes important for movement refinement. This can be encouraged by early and carefully reinforced weight-bearing (approximation) on the affected side during upright activities. Additional proprioceptive inputs (manual contacts, tapping, stretch, tracking resistance, antigravity postures, or vibration) can be used to improve feedback and stimulate learning. The patient should be encouraged to "feel the movement" while learning to distinguish correct movement responses from incorrect ones. Surface electromyography (EMG) can also be used to provide augmented proprioceptive feedback. Exteroceptive inputs (light rubbing, stroking) may be used to provide additional sources of sensory inputs, particularly where distortions of proprioception exist. As treatment progresses, the emphasis again shifts from extrinsic to intrinsic feedback and to self-monitoring and correcting movement responses. Great care must be taken to avoid sensory bombardment or feedback dependence. This requires careful assessment during each treatment session. Therapists should also limit use of immediate feedback to allow the patient adequate time for introspection. Pain and fatigue (either mental or physical) should also be avoided, because each will result in decreased performance.

PRACTICE

The therapist organizes the patient's schedule to ensure practice sessions are appropriate to foster learning. Repetition of the desired task will improve performance and motivation. This is important to ensure that the patient experiences success. Rest periods should be provided. Most hospitalized patients initially require a distributed practice schedule owing to limited endurance. Staff and family efforts should be coordinated to ensure consistency of practice during off-therapy times. The patient should be progressed and challenged with task variation or a new task as soon as the previous one has been mastered or almost mastered. Variable practice (practice of similar or related tasks) will improve learning, specifically retention and generalizability of skills, and should be instituted as soon as possible. The patient should be encouraged to self-monitor practice sessions and recognize when fatigue may be setting in and rest is required.

Careful attention to the learning environment will also yield important therapeutic gains. Distractions should be reduced and a consistent and comfortable environment provided in which the patient can exercise. Initially this will be a closed environment with no distractions. Later the environment can be varied, providing an appropriate level of contextual interference. Thus the patient is progressed toward performing the same skill in an open, variable environment. The patient should be assisted in transferring skills to real-life environments. The addition of "Easy Street Environments" to many rehabilitation centers provides important access to natural community environments.

Treatment sessions should begin and end on a positive note, ensuring the patient has success in treatment and continuing motivation. Family and caregivers should be taught supportive techniques. Finally, the therapist should communicate support and encourage the patient; recovery from stroke is an extremely stressful experience and will challenge the abilities of both patient and family.

MOTOR RELEARNING PROGRAMME FOR STROKE

Carr and Shephard[130] have developed a motor relearning programme for stroke that incorporates many aspects of motor learning theory and provides practical guidelines for retraining functional skills (e.g., balanced sitting and standing, transfer skills, gait, etc.). Their approach focuses on task-specific learning, and the development of active movement control through effective use of feedback and practice. Facilitation techniques are deemphasized in favor of verbal instruction, demonstration, and manual guidance. The approach is based on four distinct steps (Box 17–4):

1. Analysis of the task: The therapist carefully observes and analyses the patient's performance and identifies missing components.
2. Practice of the missing components: The therapist explains the missing components, their relationship to the task, and assists the patient in identification of the goal. Practice of the missing components occurs with emphasis on careful instruction, demonstration, verbal and visual feedback, and manual guidance to facilitate learning.
3. Practice of task: The task, outcomes, and goals are carefully explained and practiced. There is a continuing emphasis on use of instruction, demonstration, verbal and visual feedback, and manual guidance to facilitate learning of the required task. Flexibility is encouraged.
4. Transference of training: The task is practiced in varying environmental contexts, shifting learning from structured environments to more open real-life environments.

Motor Control Training

Training should focus on improving motor control by stressing selective (out-of-synergy) movement patterns. Movement combinations that allow

---

```
┌─────────────────────────────────────────┐
│      Box 17–4  THE FOUR STEPS IN THE     │
│      MOTOR RELEARNING PROGRAMME          │
├─────────────────────────────────────────┤
│ Step 1 Analysis of task                  │
│      Observation                         │
│      Comparison                          │
│      Analysis                            │
│ Step 2 Practice of missing components    │
│      Explanation—identification of goal  │
│      Instruction                         │
│      Practice + verbal and visual        │
│        feedback + manual                 │
│        guidance                          │
│ Step 3 Practice of task                  │
│      Explanation—identification of goal  │
│      Instruction                         │
│      Practice + verbal and visual        │
│        feedback + manual                 │
│        guidance                          │
│      Reevaluation                        │
│      Encourage flexibility               │
│ Step 4 Transference of training          │
│      Opportunity to practice in context  │
│      Consistency of practice             │
│      Organization of self-monitored      │
│        practice                          │
│      Structured learning environment     │
│      Involvement of relatives and staff  │
└─────────────────────────────────────────┘
```

From Carr, J, and Shephard, R: A Motor Relearning Programme for Stroke, 2nd ed. Aspen Pub, Rockville, MD, 1987, p 31, with permission.

success in functional tasks (e.g., feeding, dressing, gait) should be emphasized. Patients frequently respond to movement commands with gross or mass patterns of movement and excessive effort. The linking together of the proper components and the refinement of isolated control requires a great deal of mental concentration and volitional control. Inhibition of unwanted activity and excessive effort is crucial to the patient's success. Movements that are performed too quickly or with too much force will be ineffective in producing the control needed. Initially, the therapist should select postures that assist the desired motion through optimal biomechanical position and/or optimal point in the range. As control develops, postures can be changed to more difficult ones that challenge developing control. For example, initial extension can be first attempted in sidelying using isometric holding (shortened held resisted contraction). The posture can then be changed to sitting with the same holding in extension. Exercises may start out guided or assisted but should shift to active and lightly resisted as soon as possible. Often the resistance of gravity acting on the body, or slight manual resistance, is enough to initiate or facilitate the correct muscular responses through proprioceptive loading. If the patient's motor responses are weak and/or hypotonic, direct facilitation using a variety of different stimuli may be necessary to assist the patient in initiation of movement. For example, the patient who lacks adequate control of elbow extension can be positioned in sitting with the affected UE weightbearing. Tapping can be applied over the triceps to facilitate holding in extension.

Normal function implies variability in movement performance. Muscles need to be activated in a variety of patterns and types of contractions. Eccentric contractions are easier to perform than concentric ones and should therefore be selected first. All three types—eccentric, isometric, and concentric—are important to include in an exercise program. For the patient with stroke who demonstrates disordered control of movements, this may be problematic. However, because all types of contractions are necessary for normal function, practice in variations of contractions is necessary. Weak muscles (typically antagonistic to strong spastic muscles) should be activated first in unidirectional patterns. As control develops, exercises can shift to include slow active reciprocal contractions of agonist and antagonist muscles first in limited ranges, then in full range. This emphasis on balanced interaction of both agonists and antagonists is crucial for normal coordination and function. Proprioceptive neuromuscular facilitation (PNF) patterns using a technique of slow reversals are ideal for this. Finally, the exercise program needs to incorporate context-specific environments to ensure adaptability and generalizability of skills.

REMEDIATION/FACILITATION APPROACHES

Traditional remediation/facilitation approaches have as their primary focus the use of therapeutic exercises and neuromuscular facilitation techniques to reduce sensorimotor deficits and promote motor recovery and improved function. The affected body segments are targeted to prevent learned nonuse and overcompensation by intact segments. Thus, training using these approaches requires some degree of voluntary movement control. Developmental postures and activities are used to limit the degrees of freedom and focus functional training on specific body segments. The three approaches most commonly used include: neurodevelopmental treatment (NDT), movement therapy in hemiplegia, and proprioceptive neuromuscular facilitation (PNF).

Neurodevelopmental treatment (NDT), a treatment approach initially developed by Bobath,[27] identifies the essential problems of the patient with stroke as poor control of selective movement patterns and widespread abnormal tone and reflex activity. The validity of this strong emphasis on abnormal tone and reflexes as a primary cause of disordered control has been questioned in recent years.[131] In NDT the patient learns to control tone and movement through the use of patterns that promote "normal" selective movements (outof-synergy) during functional activities. Automatic reactions (righting, equilibrium, protective extension) are facilitated through the use of postural and sensory stimulation. Kinesthetic, proprioceptive, tactile, and vestibular feedback are used to facilitate normal movement experiences. Compensatory training strategies (use of the less involved segments) are avoided for fear that recovery and use of the involved segments will be suppressed. Movement control within the context of functional tasks is emphasized. Carryover is promoted through family and caregiver education.

Movement therapy in hemiplegia, developed by Brunnstrom,[26] is designed to promote recovery in patients with stroke. Patients relearn movement control through structured activities that promote normal function. Brunnstrom was one of the first to describe the stereotypic patterns of abnormal synergistic control and recovery. Many practical training activities are suggested to stimulate out-of-synergy combinations. Initially Brunnstrom suggested that patients with low-level recovery should be first encouraged to gain control of the basic limb synergies and then progress to out-of-synergy combinations. Because the repeated use of synergies may make isolated joint control more difficult to obtain, this concept is now viewed as inappropriate. Concepts of motor learning such as positive reinforcement and repetition are stressed.[132]

Coordinated movement can also be promoted using *proprioceptive neuromuscular facilitation (PNF)* patterns and techniques, developed by Kabat and Knott.[133] Patterns are selected to reinforce and develop selective movement control while avoiding synergistic patterns. For example, the therapist would select UE D1 extension with elbow straight instead of D2 patterns, which more closely resemble the synergistic patterns associated with stroke (UE D2 flexion with elbow flexing and D2 extension with elbow extending). Lower extremity D1 extension with the knee flexing would be an appropriate pattern to practice if the patient were experiencing incomplete knee flexion with hip extension at toe-off. Lower extremity D1 extension promotes the necessary combination of hip extension and abduction needed to regain stance phase stability and reduce a Trendelenburg gait pattern. Bilateral symmetrical (BS) patterns are also very useful to achieve overflow from the sound side to the affected side. For example, BS LE D2 flexion with knee extension enhances knee stability needed for transfers, standing, and gait. Appropriate PNF techniques include slow reversals, timing for emphasis with repeated contractions if components are weak. Rhythmic initiation works particularly well in assisting with motor learning. Hold-relax active movement can be used if initiation of movement is difficult. The technique of agonistic reversals is effective in developing the eccentric control necessary for normal function. Thus functional activities of bridging, stand to sit, or kneeling to heel-sitting might be practiced using an agonist reversal (AR) technique. In the PNF approach, there is a large emphasis on effective motor learning using strategies such as practice, repetition, visual guidance of movement, and so forth.[134]

COMPENSATORY TRAINING (FUNCTIONAL) APPROACH

The focus of a compensatory training approach is on the early resumption of functional independence using the uninvolved or less involved segments for function. For example, the patient with left hemiplegia is taught to dress using the right upper extremity. Central to this approach is the concept of substitution. The patient is first made aware of movement deficiencies (cognitive awareness is developed). Changes are then made in the patient's overall approach to functional tasks. Alternate ways to accomplish the task are suggested, simplified, and adopted. The patient practices and relearns the task using the new pattern. The patient then practices the new pattern in the environment in which the function is expected to occur. Energy conservation techniques are incorporated to ensure the patient can complete all daily tasks.

A second central tenet of this approach is modification of the environment (adaptation) to facilitate relearning of skills, ease of movement, and optimal performance. For example, the patient with unilateral neglect is assisted in dressing by color-coding of shoes (red tape on the left shoe, yellow tape on the right shoe). The wheelchair brake toggle is extended and color-coded to allow the patient easy identification.

One of the major criticisms of this approach is the focus on uninvolved segments that may suppress recovery and contribute to learned nonuse of impaired segments. For example, the patient with stroke fails to learn to use the involved extremities. Focus on task-specific learning may also lead to the development of *splinter skills* (skills that cannot be easily generalized to other environments or to

variations of the same task). However, a compensatory training approach may be the only realistic approach possible when the patient presents with severe impairments and functional losses. For example, the patient with severe Pusher syndrome may not be able to transfer from bed to wheelchair using a stand-pivot transfer. A slide-board generally permits a safe transfer with less assistance. Patients with severe sensorimotor deficits and extensive comorbidities (e.g., severe cardiac and respiratory compromise or Alzheimer's disease) may be limited in their ability to actively participate in rehabilitation and to relearn motor skills, and would also benefit from a compensatory training approach.

Efficacy of Approaches

Attempts have been made to validate the rehabilitation approaches through controlled research trials. Studies attempting to delineate differences between conventional exercise approaches (ROM, functional training) and neuromuscular facilitation approaches (NDT, movement therapy in hemiplegia, PNF, sensorimotor integrative treatment) have failed to show significant advantages of one approach over another.[135–139] Wagenaar et al.[140] compared the effectiveness of two neurological approaches, movement therapy and NDT, using functional recovery measures (Barthel index and Action Research Arm test). They found no significant difference between these methods in influencing functional recovery with the exception of one patient whose speed of walking improved with the movement therapy approach. Basmajian et al.[141] compared EMG biofeedback therapy and NDT on UE function and also failed to find a difference in outcome between these two therapies. As in the previous studies, improvements were noted in both groups.

Important conclusions to be drawn from these studies are that (1) collectively they provide consistent evidence for the beneficial effects of physical therapy, and (2) there is as yet no one optimal approach for patients with stroke. It should be pointed out that many of these studies were subject to serious methodological flaws.[142,143] For example, they included a small sample size, heterogenesis stroke population, poorly defined treatments, and/or inappropriate outcome measures. Because patients with stroke present with variable symptoms, attempts to group patients and rigidly apply any one approach or outcome measure can be expected to yield unsatisfactory results.

Therapists should consider a balanced or integrated approach, selecting interventions from the different approaches that have the greatest chance of successfully remediating impairments and promoting functional recovery. Compensatory strategies and interventions are important to consider early to improve the patient's abilities with functional tasks. They also provide an important early source of motivation for the patient and family as they see progress is being made. As recovery progresses, the interventions can be directed at improving motor control of the affected side and decreasing reliance on compensatory strategies. The choice of interventions must also take into consideration other factors, including cost effectiveness in terms of length of stay and number of allotted physical therapy visits, age of the patient and number of comorbidities, ease of delivering care, and potential discharge placement.

Positioning Strategies

Positioning of the patient is one of the first considerations during early rehabilitation. The room should be arranged to maximize patient awareness of the hemiplegic side. A bed positioned with the hemiplegic side toward the main part of the room, door, and source of interaction (nursing, family, TV) will stimulate the patient to turn toward and engage the affected side. The resulting sensory stimulation to the stroke side can be used to promote integration and symmetry of the two sides of the body. However, this may be contraindicated in cases of severe unilateral neglect or anosognosia because the arrangement may contribute to sensory deprivation and withdrawal. In the example given the patient would be unable to compensate for the deficits by turning the head toward the affected side.

Every consideration should be given to positioning the patient out of undesirable postures (e.g., those that promote abnormal synergies and postures that can lead to decubitus ulcers, contractures, or postural deformity). Correct positions encourage proper joint alignment, symmetry, and comfort. Because patients spend a considerable amount of "down time" in their room either in bed or in a chair, a positioning program can effectively address the risks associated with this inactive time. Variations in position can be effectively managed through the use of a positioning schedule. Prolonged static positioning in any one posture must be avoided. Emphasis should be on increasing out-of-bed time and correct upright positioning in armchair/wheelchair. Early standing in the parallel bars, standing frame, or on a tilt table is also important. Mobilization techniques and exercise are important early interventions.

The following malalignments are common and result from weakness or paralysis, disordered muscle tone, and/or visual-perceptual dysfunction. Prolonged positioning in these abnormal postures can result in shortening of muscles and soft tissues with elongation and loss of antagonist function and should be avoided.

1. Pelvic/trunk malalignment. An asymmetric pelvic position is assumed with more weight borne on the ischial tuberosity on the sound side. This results in lateral flexion of the trunk and head shifted toward the affected side. A posterior pelvic tilt is also common. This results in sacral sitting with a flattened lumbar curve and an exaggerated thoracic curve (kyphosis) and forward head.
2. Scapular malalignment. A position of scapular downward rotation is assumed. Scapular instability (winging) may also be present, especially in weight-bearing postures.
3. Glenohumeral malalignment. Lateral flexion of the trunk and downward rotation of the scapula result in humeral depression and subluxation.
4. Upper extremity malalignment. The limb is typically held in internal rotation and adduction with elbow flexion, forearm pronation, wrist flexion and ulnar deviation, and finger flexion. Thus the hand is commonly held tightly fisted across the chest.
5. Lower extremity malalignment. In standing, a position of pelvic retraction and elevation is assumed, with hip and knee extension and hip adduction/internal rotation (i.e., a scissoring position); in sitting the hip and knee are flexed with hip abduction and external rotation (i.e., a flexor synergy pattern). Ankle plantarflexion is common to both.

While each patient's positioning needs should be carefully determined, generic positioning strategies have been described in detail.[27,66,144,145] These include:

1. *Lying in the supine position.* The trunk should be positioned in midline with the head/neck in slight flexion. A small pillow or towel under the scapula will assist in scapular protraction. The affected upper limb rests on a supporting pillow externally rotated and abducted with elbow extension, wrist neutral, fingers extended. The affected lower limb is positioned with the hip forward (pelvis protracted) on a small pillow or towel roll. The lower extremity is in a neutral position relative to rotation. The affected knee can be positioned with a small towel roll to prevent hyperextension (Fig. 17-6). A plastic padded orthosis can be used to position the foot and ankle in neutral position. If spasticity is present, an inhibitory cast can be used (see Chapter 24, Figs. 24-8 through 24-10).
2. *Lying on the unaffected side.* The head/neck should be neutral and symmetrical with the

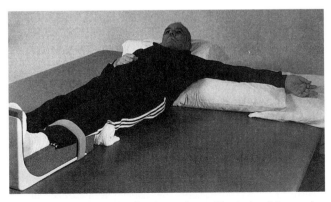

Figure 17-6. Positioning for the patient with stroke: lying supine.

trunk aligned straight. A small pillow under the rib cage can be used to elongate the hemiplegic side. The affected upper limb is protracted and placed well forward on a supporting pillow, elbow extended, wrist neutral, fingers extended, and thumb abducted. The affected lower limb is aligned with the hip forward (pelvis protracted), knee flexed and supported on a pillow (Fig. 17-7).

3. *Lying on the affected side.* The head/neck should be neutral and symmetrical with the trunk aligned straight. The affected upper limb is positioned well forward with the elbow extended, forearm supinated, wrist neutral, fingers extended, and thumb abducted. The affected lower limb is positioned in hip extension with knee flexion. An alternate position is slight hip and knee flexion with pelvic protraction. The unaffected LE is positioned in flexion on a supporting pillow (Fig. 17-8).

4. *Sitting in a bed or wheelchair.* The patient should sit with the head/neck and trunk in midline alignment. Symmetrical weight bearing on both buttocks should be encouraged. The LEs should be positioned in neutral with respect to rotation.

If the patient is receiving nutrition via a G-tube or NG-tube the bed must be elevated to at least 45 degrees to prevent aspiration. Pillows may be needed to bring the head/neck to the upright position. The affected UE is supported on a pillow.

When sitting in a wheelchair, the pelvis should be aligned in a stable neutral position as opposed to the more typical posterior tilt position. A wheelchair cushion with a solid base of support should be provided. The hips and knees should be positioned in 90 degrees of flexion, with weight-bearing on the posterior thighs and feet. Lateral flexion of the trunk should be avoided. Alignment may be improved with the addition of lateral trunk supports, lap tray, or an arm trough. Head and neck supports may be required for the patient with poor head control or weakness. The affected UE should be supported, either with an arm trough or lap tray. The trough is typically wedged to elevate the hand and decrease edema. The scapula should again be slightly protracted, humerus supported with wrist neutral, and fingers extended and abducted in a functional hand

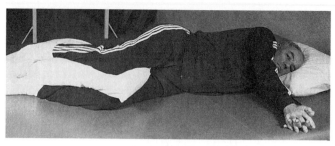

Figure 17-8. Positioning for the patient with stroke: on the affected side.

position. Positioning of the UE on a trough or lap tray is also important for the patient with neglect, visual field defects, or sensory loss because it helps to increase awareness of the affected limb, and avoids the problems of the affected arm dangling over the wheelchair armrest with resultant trauma.[146] Because most patients will propel their wheelchair using the unaffected arm and leg, the seat-to-floor height will need to be lower to allow the patient's foot to reach the floor (often referred to as a hemi chair). The affected foot should be supported on a footrest. Although an elevating leg rest may be necessary to control for edema in the affected foot, it may also contribute to poor sitting position by increasing stretch on hamstring muscles, resulting in an increased posterior tilt of the pelvis.

Range of Motion/Prevention of Limb Trauma

Soft tissue/joint mobilization and daily ROM exercises are initiated early to maintain joint integrity and mobility and prevent contracture. AROM exercises are always preferable to passive ROM (PROM). Edema may develop with the loss of voluntary movement and inactivity. In addition to ROM exercises, elevation, massage, icing, or compression wrapping may be necessary. If contracture is progressive, more frequent ROM (e.g., twice daily or more) and sustained stretching (e.g., 20 to 30 minutes) using positioning and/or splinting techniques will be necessary. Coordination with family and caregivers is essential if these impairments are to be successfully managed.

In the UE, correct PROM techniques include careful attention to external rotation and distraction of the humerus, especially as ranges approach 90 degrees of flexion or more. The scapula should also be mobilized in upward rotation on the thoracic wall to prevent soft tissue impingement in the subacromial space during all overhead movements (Fig. 17-9). The use of overhead pulleys for self-ROM is generally contraindicated because of failure to achieve the above requirements for scapula movement. Although full ROM should be performed in all motions, comparisons should be made to the unaffected side. Consideration should be given to age-related and other premorbid factors. Inadequate ROM of the UE can lead to the development of adhesive capsulitis and/or shoulder-hand syn-

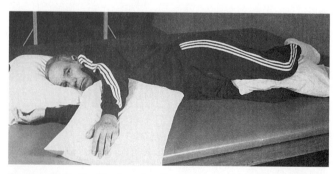

Figure 17-7. Positioning for the patient with stroke: on the unaffected side.

drome.[147,148] Full extension of the elbow is important because the majority of patients with stroke will develop tightness and spasticity in elbow flexors resulting in a resting posture of flexion. Normal length of wrist and finger extensors should also be maintained as tightness is typical in flexion. Edema and tonal changes may produce impingement with wrist extension. In this situation, the carpal bones should be mobilized prior to stretching at the wrist. Strategies to teach patients safe self-ROM techniques should be instituted early. These include:[149]

1. Shoulder ROM to 90 degrees using an arms cradled position: the affected extremity is supported and lifted by the unaffected extremity.
2. "Table-top polishing:" the affected extremity is positioned in humeral flexion with scapular protraction and elbow extension, hand open and positioned on the table; the sound hand guides movements of the affected hand forward and side-to-side.
3. Table-top positioning of the affected upper extremity, trunk movements: the trunk moves forward/backward, turns side-to-side.
4. Sitting, hands clasped together, reaching to the floor.
5. Supine, both hands are clasped together and placed behind the head, the elbows fall flat to the mat; this activity should only be considered if scapula upward mobility is present. This may be difficult for some patients.

Splinting the hand can also be considered. Either a dorsal or volar resting pan splint can be used. A resting hand (pan) splint positions the forearm, wrist, and fingers in a functional position (20 to 30 degrees of wrist extension, MP flexion 40 to 45 degrees, IP flexion 10 to 20 degrees, and thumb opposition). It is more appropriate for nighttime use

than daytime when spontaneous function is desired. In the presence of spasticity, tone-reducing devices should be considered (finger abduction splint, firm cone, spasticity reduction splint, or inflatable pressure splint).

During position changes, care must be taken not to pull on the UE or let it hang unsupported, because of the risk of a traction injury. A pouch sling or single strap hemisling with two cuffs that support the elbow and wrist can be used to mechanically support the humerus during activity and upright postures. Slings may prevent soft tissue stretching and relieve pressure on the neurovascular bundle but do little to prevent subluxation if scapular and trunk malalignment are not adequately addressed. They have the additional negative feature of positioning the arm close to the body in adduction, internal rotation, and elbow flexion. With prolonged use, contractures and increased flexor tone may develop. Slings also impair trunk mobility, balance, body image, and may increase body neglect and learned nonuse. An alternate approach to the traditional sling is a humeral cuff sling. This device has an arm cuff on the distal humerus supported by a figure-eight harness. It provides humeral support and slight external rotation while allowing elbow extension, and may also provide some reduction of subluxation (Fig. 17-10).[149] This style of sling can be worn for longer periods because it does not restrict the elbow in a flexed position or limit distal function.

Some rehabilitation centers recommend using a sling with subluxation greater than 1 inch (2.5 cm). Gillan[150] suggests the following guidelines are appropriate to consider when prescribing a sling:

1. Slings are appropriate for initial transfer and gait training, but overall use should be minimized during rehabilitation.
2. Slings that position the upper extremity in flexion are less desirable and should be used only for select upright activities and only for short time frames.
3. No one sling is appropriate for all patients; selection and use should be carefully monitored.
4. Scapular taping may provide an effective alternative to slings.

Activities that enhance trunk and scapular alignment, functional use of the UE during weight-bearing and reaching, and activate rotator cuff muscles are important in producing appropriate functional outcomes. A padded arm trough attached to the arm of a wheelchair may also be used to control for shoulder subluxation. As spasticity emerges, the use of a sling is generally contraindicated. Care must be taken to mobilize the arm and prevent prolonged posturing, especially in internal rotation and adduction with pronation, wrist, and finger flexion. Full ROM in shoulder elevation activities (stressing elongation of the pectoralis major and latissimus dorsi with scapular rotation) should be maintained.

Because most patients regain some use of their lower extremities early in recovery, ROM techniques

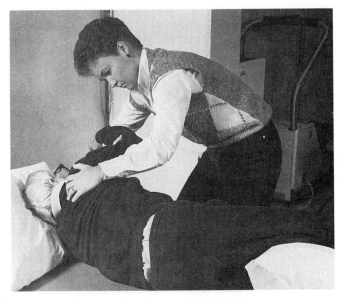

Figure 17-9. Range of motion exercises for the affected upper extremity. The therapist carefully mobilizes the scapula during arm elevation.

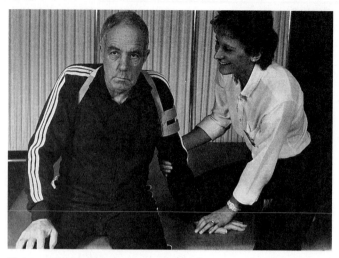

Figure 17-10. Sitting, with extended arm support. The patient is wearing a humeral cuff sling to prevent subluxation of the shoulder. The therapist assists in stabilizing the elbow and fingers in extension.

should focus on specific areas of deficit. For many patients, voluntary movement in the foot and ankle remains limited and tone quickly progresses from initial flaccidity to spasticity. Patients typically present with limitation of range in the plantar-flexors. Weight-bearing and rocking in modified plantigrade or prolonged static positioning using adaptive equipment (i.e., tilt table with toe wedges) can be used to gain range through the use of slow, maintained stretch. Facilitation of active contraction of dorsiflexors can also be used to provide reciprocal inhibition to plantarflexors. If synergistic influence is strong, the patient can be effectively positioned supine on a mat with the affected lower limb abducted off the side with knee flexed and foot flat on the floor or a stool. This position of hip abduction and extension with knee flexion serves to break up synergistic dominance and position the limb out of the typical spastic scissoring posture. Care should be taken to stretch hip flexors owing to increased sitting time in a wheelchair or elevated bed. If hip flexor contractures are allowed to develop, they can lead to increased difficulty with functional tasks such as transfers and ambulation.

Sensory Training Strategies

Patients who have significant sensory impairments may demonstrate impaired or absent spontaneous movement because of the lack of sensory input before and during movement. The more the patient can be encouraged to use the affected side, the greater the chance of increased awareness and function. Conversely, the patient who refuses to use the hemiplegic side contributes to the problems imposed by lack of sensorimotor experience. Without attention during treatment, this learned nonuse phenomenon can contribute to further deterioration.[49] Treatment should therefore involve the pa-

tient using the hemiplegic side in volitional motor tasks. The presentation of repeated sensory stimuli will maximize use of residual sensory function and capitalize on sensory recovery. Stretch, stroking, superficial and deep pressure, and weight-bearing with approximation can all be used during therapy to increase sensory inputs on the affected side. The selection of sensory inputs should be directly related to the functional task at hand and provided to those body surfaces directly used in the task (e.g., stroking the hand with different textured fabrics). Stimulation should be of sufficient intensity to engage the system but not produce adverse effects (e.g., withdrawal). The patient's attention should be focused directly on the task at hand.[151,152] Johnstone[145] suggests that inflatable pressure splints can be used during treatment to provide additional sensory stimulation (deep pressure, muscle, and joint sensations). In more severe cases, she suggests a program of intermittent pressure therapy to stimulate movement within the tissues and overcome problems of sensory accommodation.[145]

A safety education program should be instituted early for patients, family, and caregivers to improve awareness of sensory deficits and ensure protection of anesthetic limbs. This is particularly important for preventing upper limb trauma during transfer and wheelchair activities. Compensatory training strategies for patients with hemianopsia and unilateral neglect includes teaching scanning movements of the eyes and head to access the visual environment on the affected side.

Strategies for Tone Reduction

Patients who demonstrate the strong spasticity typically seen during the middle phases of recovery may benefit from a number of techniques designed to modify or reduce tone. These include elongation of spastic muscles through ROM and positioning techniques. The technique of rhythmic rotation (a passive manipulation technique) can be effective in achieving the lengthened range. The therapist slowly moves the limb into the lengthened range while gently rotating it back and forth through internal and external rotation. Once full range is achieved, the limb is placed in the lengthened position, for example, a weight-bearing posture in which the upper limb is extended, abducted, and externally rotated with elbow, wrist, and finger extension (see Fig. 17-10). Additional inhibitory effects can be attained from prolonged pressure, for example, on the long flexor tendons of the hand. Slow rocking movements (rocking the body over the elongated limb) also increase inhibitory effects through adding influences of slow vestibular stimulation. Spasticity in the quadriceps can be similarly inhibited through prolonged pressure and weight-bearing in kneeling or quadruped positions. A reduction in truncal tone can be promoted using techniques of rhythmic initiation or slow reversals and rotation within the trunk axis (segmental trunk patterns: upper and lower trunk rotation) (Fig. 17-11). Sidelying, sitting, or hooklying are frequently used to engage trunk rotation. PNF upper trunk patterns (chopping or lifting) that emphasize rotational movements of the trunk can also be effective in reducing trunk tone.[153]

Local facilitation techniques (muscle tapping, vibration) can be applied to activate antagonists and may prove successful in further reducing spasticity in some patients. However, as Bobath[27] points out, reciprocal relationships are not always within a normal range, particularly in the presence of strong spasticity. In this example, these techniques may serve to increase rather than decrease tone and produce spastic co-contraction. Cold in the form of ice wraps or ice packs can be used to temporarily decrease spasticity. Additional strategies that produce a generalized reduction in CNS activity and tone include soothing verbal commands, and cognitive relaxation techniques. Once inhibition and ROM are achieved, it is important to encourage active contraction of antagonists and functional movements to prolong the inhibitory effects. At all times the patient should be instructed to avoid excess effort and heavy resistance.

Johnstone suggests the use of inflatable pressure splints (air splints) to stabilize and maintain an extremity in an elongated position. Inhibition of tone, for example, spastic elbow flexors, is provided. Splints also help to control unwanted associated reactions, and assist in early weight-bearing.[145] Figure 17-12 demonstrates the use of an air splint to stabilize elbow extension in the quadruped position while Figure 17-13 demonstrates its use in the modified plantigrade position. Patients with a flaccid, hypotonic limb benefit from the use of pressure splints to provide increased sensory input. When used in conjunction with early weight-bearing, tone is facilitated. Long or full limb pressure splints also

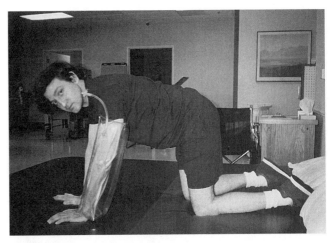

Figure 17-12. Use of a pressure splint applied to support the elbow in extension during weight-bearing in the quadruped position. Weight-bearing is on the hands and knees.

assist in controlling edema, a common problem of paralyzed limbs. Positioning with elevation is an important consideration.

Strategies to Reestablish Postural Control and Improve Functional Mobility

The loss of sensory and motor function on one side will present a tremendous challenge for the patient struggling to adjust and relearn functional movements. Initial treatment strategies should focus on trunk symmetry and using both sides of the body (bilaterally) rather than just the sound side. Guided and active assisted movements provide a good early base for learning postural control. The patient should be given only as much assistance as needed and should be encouraged to actively participate in movement as soon and as much as possible. Too much assistance on the part of the therapist can foster dependency and impede motor learning. Functional training activities should focus on rolling, supine-to-sit transitions, sitting, bridging, sit-to-stand transitions, standing, transfers, and walking.[153]

Rolling and sitting up should be encouraged in both directions, onto the sound side to promote early independence and onto the affected side to encourage functional reintegration of the hemiplegic side and symmetry. Extremity movement patterns (e.g., PNF D1 flexion of the UE or LE) can be used to facilitate improved rolling through overflow and momentum. Or both hands can be clasped together in a prayer position. Rolling onto the affected side (sidelying position or sidelying-on-elbow position) is important to promote early weight-bearing. The forearm-supported position also has the added benefit of elongating the lateral trunk flexors, which may be spastic. Rolling onto the unaffected side is more difficult and requires the patient use the affected body segments. Care must be take to ensure the patient does not leave the

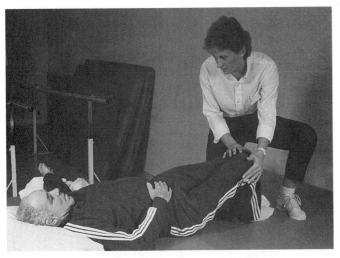

Figure 17-11. Inhibition of truncal tone through lower trunk rotation. The therapist uses the technique of rhythmic initiation to increase mobility.

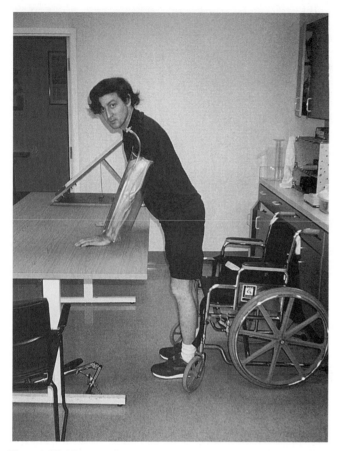

Figure 17-13. Use of a pressure splint applied to support the elbow in extension during weight-bearing in the modified plantigrade position. Weight-bearing is on the hands and feet.

ity), moving in the posture (controlled mobility), and finally challenges to dynamic balance (reaching). A common problem with hemiplegia is the inability of the upper trunk to move independently of the lower trunk (dissociate). Trunk mobility in balanced flexion/extension, lateral flexion, and rotation should therefore be stressed. Gentle resistance can be applied to assist in holding, using techniques of alternating isometrics and rhythmic stabilization. Weight shifts should incorporate moving forward-backward, side-to-side, and diagonally with upper trunk rotation. Lateral weight shifts to the affected side typically are the most difficult. Manual contacts in the direction of the movement combined with gentle resistance (slow reversals, slow reversal hold) can provide important early learning cues. UE activities that encourage shoulder ROM (arms cradled position, prayer position hands to floor, PNF chop/reverse chop) can also be incorporated. The patient should also practice scooting in sitting ("butt walking") to ensure mobility for dressing (putting pants on) and sit-to-stand transitions (coming to the edge of the seat to place the feet back and under the body).

The patient with Pusher syndrome will present with different problems. The patient will sit asymmetrically, but with most of the weight borne on the affected side. The patient will use the unaffected UE and LE to push over to the affected side. Efforts by the therapist to manually guide the patient to a more symmetrical position will often result in the patient pushing harder to the affected side. Intervention should consist of tapping the patient on the unaffected shoulder and asking the patient to shift toward that side. Active movements are more likely to be successful than active-assisted or passive movements. A mirror is another useful tool if the patient does not present with visual-perceptual deficits. The patient can be progressed to sitting with the affected LE crossed over the unaffected LE.

hemiplegic UE behind but rather brings it forward. This can be accomplished by clasping the hands together in a prayer position first. The affected LE can also be used to assist in rolling by pushing off from a flexed and adducted, hooklying position (Fig. 17-14). This encourages an important advanced limb pattern needed for gait (hip extension with knee flexion) and also facilitates early weight-bearing of the foot in the supine position. Finally the patient can be assisted in moving into the sitting position from sidelying on the affected side by shifting the LEs over the edge of the bed and pushing up to full sitting position using both UEs.

Early training in sitting should focus on the development of a symmetrical posture. The therapist can aid the patient by ensuring proper spine and pelvic alignment. The pelvis should be neutral, spine straight. Feet should be flat on the support surface. Typically patients with stroke will sit asymmetrically with weight borne more on the sound side, pelvis tilted posteriorly, and upper trunk flexed. Lateral flexion to the affected side is also common. The therapist should manually guide the patient into the correct sitting position. Early sitting can be assisted by having the patient use the UEs for bilateral support (at sides or in front: on table top, large ball, or therapist's shoulders). A progression that can be utilized includes first holding in the posture (stabil-

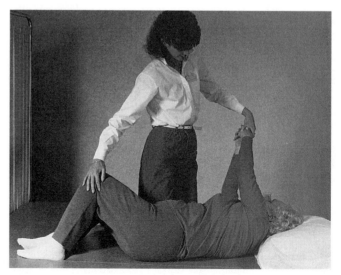

Figure 17-14. Early mobility activities: rolling onto the unaffected side. The therapist guides the movement and assists the upper extremity pattern of prayer position.

Sitting exercises on a Swiss ball can also be used to promote symmetrical sitting.

Bridging activities develop control in trunk and hip extensors for important functional tasks, including the use of a bedpan, reduction of pressure on the buttocks, and initial bed mobility (scooting). It also develops pelvic control, advanced limb control (hip extension with knee flexion), and stimulates early weight-bearing on the foot (Fig. 17-15). Bridging activities should include assisted and independent assumption of the posture, holding in the posture, and moving in the posture (lateral and rotational weight shifts, bridge and placing hips to one side). If the affected LE is unable to hold in a hooklying position, the therapist will need to assist by stabilizing the foot. Lifting the unaffected foot off the surface while maintaining the pelvis level significantly increases the difficulty and can be used to increase demands on the affected side. Difficulty can also be increased by varying the position of the UEs, from extended and abducted at sides, to arms across the chest or hands clasped together in a prayer position.

Sit-to-stand transitions should be practiced, with an emphasis on symmetrical weight-bearing and controlled responses of trunk (Fig. 17-16). Initially the patient must actively flex the trunk and use momentum to shift the weight forward (flexion-momentum phase).[154] The patient with hemiplegia tends to extend, pushing the trunk backward. The forward weight shift can be facilitated by having the therapist rock the patient forward on the count of three. The patient can be assisted to reach forward with both UEs, hands clasped together. Alternately the patient can push off with both hands off the support surface, a generally less effective strategy to encourage forward weight shift. The patient's movements are then directed into the extension or upward phase by recruiting hip and knee extensors. Weakness of these muscles may result in incomplete extension or the patient may collapse midway through the task. The height of the seat can be elevated at first to aid in ease of standing up.

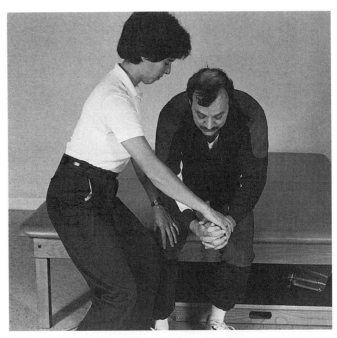

Figure 17-16. Sit-to-stand movement transitions. The therapist assists the patient in straightening his affected knee while he brings his center of mass forward. Hands are held together in a prayer position.

Progression is then to lower seat heights. Trunk rotation and side bending can be increased by having the patient stand up and shift the pelvis to one side or the other before sitting down (place to one side). By using a platform mat for this activity, the patient can move all the way around the mat first in one direction, then in the other. UEs should be clasped and held straight ahead (elbows extended) during this activity.

Modified plantigrade is an ideal early standing posture in which to develop control. The affected UE is extended and weight-bearing (out of synergy), while the affected LE is holding (also out of synergy in hip flexion with knee extension). In addition the posture has a wide (four-limb) base of support and is very stable (Fig. 17-17). The patient then moves into upright standing first with bilateral upper extremity support in the parallel bars or with light touch down on a high table. A wall can also be used to provide initial support. As soon as possible the patient should be encouraged to practice free standing. As in sitting, an appropriate progression in standing includes first holding in the posture (stability), moving in the posture (controlled mobility), and finally withstanding challenges to dynamic balance (e.g., reaching in all directions). The patient is assisted in proper alignment and in taking weight on the affected LE. Gentle resistance can be applied to assist in holding, using techniques of alternating isometrics, and rhythmic stabilization. Weight shifts should incorporate moving forward-backward, side-to-side, and diagonally (incorporating upper trunk rotation). Lateral weight shifts to the affected side typically are the most difficult. Manual contacts in the direction of the movement combined with gentle

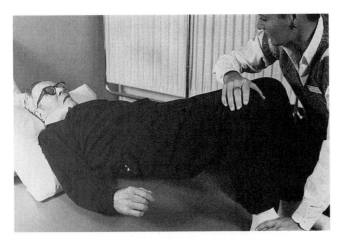

Figure 17-15. Early mobility activities: bridging. The patient combines hip extension with knee flexion. The therapist assists in stabilizing the affected knee in flexion with foot flat.

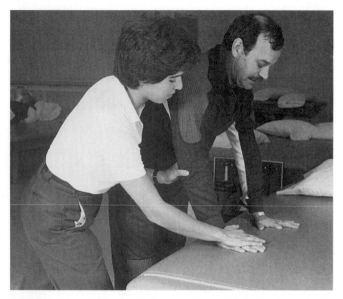

Figure 17-17. Early weight-bearing in modified plantigrade with extended arms. The therapist assists elbow and finger extension of the affected right upper extremity.

resistance (slow reversals, slow reversal hold) can provide important early learning cues.

During early transfers, the patient may be more or less a passive participant. Adjusting the hospital bed to the height of the chair or wheelchair will help to decrease the difficulty of the transfer. Staff often emphasize the sound side by placing the chair to that side and having the patient stand and pivot a quarter turn on the unaffected LE before sitting down. Although this technique promotes early and safe independence in transfers, it neglects the affected side and may make subsequent training more difficult. The patient should be taught to transfer to both sides. This is important from a functional standpoint as well. Most bathrooms are not large enough to position the wheelchair on both sides of a tub or toilet. Also, the patient is not likely to be able to reposition the wheelchair once he or she transfers into bed so that a transfer toward the unaffected side can be achieved when getting out of bed. Transferring to the hemiplegic side may be more difficult at first but will assist in overall reeducation and reintegration of the two sides of the body (Fig. 17-18). When transferring, the patient's affected arm can be stabilized in extension and external rotation against the therapist's body. Alternately, the patient's UEs (hands in prayer position) can be placed to one side on the therapist's shoulders. The therapist can then assist in the forward weight shift by using manual contacts, either at the upper trunk or pelvis. The affected LE may be stabilized by the therapist's knee exerting a counterforce on the patient's as needed. Transfer training should also include practice in transferring to various different surfaces (chair, toilet, tubseat, car, etc.).

Functional mobility training is begun early and continued throughout the course of rehabilitation. Training activities and postures are varied. Additional postures such as prone on elbows, quadruped,

sidesitting, kneeling, and half-kneeling may be appropriate and can be used to increase the level of difficulty and focus on specific body segments and deficiencies in control. Some postures may not be appropriate for all patients (e.g., prone-on-elbows for the client with cardiorespiratory compromise or a flaccid, subluxed UE, or kneeling for the client with osteoarthritis). Advanced training should include strategies for getting down to and up from the floor in the event of a fall.[153]

Training in ADLs is usually directed by the occupational therapist. Close coordination between therapists is important to ensure that skills are being learned in a consistent manner (e.g., compensatory versus remediation/facilitation strategy). Adaptive equipment may be necessary to assist the patient in independence. The reference should be the patient's home environment and expected daily activity. Energy conservation techniques will need to be incorporated into the patient's daily plan to ensure adequate functional reserves.

Strategies to Improve Upper Extremity Control

UE training should first focus on pelvic/trunk and scapular alignment. Early mobilization, ROM, and positioning are important elements and have been

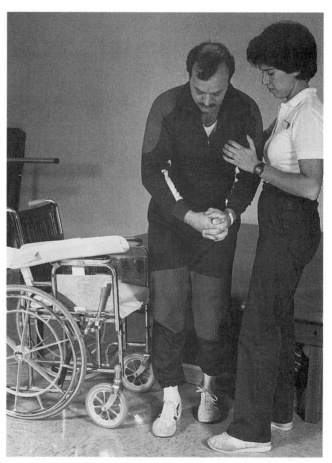

Figure 17-18. Transferring to the affected side. The patient learns to control standing up and pivoting with the affected leg leading. The therapist assists in balance.

previously discussed. Relearning of movement patterns is typically limited by weakness, spasticity, and synergies as well as sensory loss.

UE weight-bearing is an important early activity. The stimulation of shoulder stabilizers and elbow extensors will serve to strengthen these muscles and counteract the effects of excess flexor hypertonus and a dominant flexion synergy. The affected extremity can also participate in functional activities that require additional postural support (e.g., standing, stabilizing with the affected extremity while the sound extremity performs ADLs). Weight-bearing activities can be performed in sitting (see Fig. 17-10), modified plantigrade (see Fig. 17-17), or standing positions. The quadruped posture provides the greatest challenge for UE weight-bearing but may be too difficult for some patients. Control should progress from initial holding in the posture to controlled mobility (weight shifting and reaching movements with the unaffected UE).

Activities to retrain reach patterns are important components of UE training. Patients with stroke have the greatest difficulty regaining control of scapular upward rotation and protraction, elbow extension, and wrist and finger extension. Shoulder protraction with external rotation should be practiced early. Initially, this can be performed in a sidelying or supine position, where the patient's UE is supported by the therapist in shoulder flexion with elbow extension. The UE is mobilized forward and the patient is asked to hold this position. If holding is successful, then eccentric and reciprocal movements are attempted (using techniques of hold-after positioning, push-pull, modified hold-relax active movement, or slow reversals). Once initial control is achieved, the posture can be altered to a more challenging one. The patient sits with UE supported by a tabletop and is encouraged to slide hand over tabletop, recruiting shoulder flexors, scapular protractors, and elbow extensors. A cloth can be used to decrease friction effects. In sitting, the patient can also practice reaching forward and downward, picking up objects off the floor. This activity also promotes the desired shoulder components of protraction and flexion, with elbow extension. Progression is then to sitting, reaching forward, overhead, or sideward, elevating the UE while maintaining elbow extension. This is a very difficult activity and may need to be guided or resisted (tracking resistance) to facilitate the desired pattern.[150] A PNF D1 thrust pattern can also be used. Push-ups in modified plantigrade or prone-on-elbows are also effective strategies. Functional movements should be stressed, including hand to mouth and hand to opposite shoulder, because these motions are important for feeding, bathing, and dressing.

Training should also emphasize wrist and finger movements independent of shoulder and elbow motions. The patient practices wrist extension, finger extension, opposition, and manipulation in combination with reach movements. Voluntary release is generally much more difficult to achieve than voluntary grasp, and inhibitory techniques may

be necessary before extension movements are successful. Manipulation of common objects (e.g., cup, fork, toothbrush, pencil) in combination with functional tasks of daily living should be practiced. Forks, toothbrushes, and pens may need to have built-up handles for grasp. The therapist must observe these movements carefully and assist in eliminating those aspects of performance that interfere with effective control.

Strategies to Improve Lower Extremity Control

Training of the LE essentially prepares the patient for gait. Specific impairments such as decreased ROM or strength need to be addressed. Pregait mat activities should concentrate on strengthening muscles in the appropriate movement patterns needed for gait while breaking up the obligatory synergy patterns. For example, hip and knee extensors need to be activated with hip abductors and dorsiflexors for stance. Hip extension with knee flexion is needed to allow for toe-off at the end of stance. A variety of activities can be used to promote knee flexion with hip extension, including bridging, supine knee flexion with hip extension over the side of the mat, or standing modified plantigrade with knee flexion. Hip adduction should be stressed during flexion movements of the hip and knee, while abduction should be stressed during extension movements (e.g., supine, PNF LE D1 flexion and extension; sitting, crossing and uncrossing the affected LE over the unaffected).

Pelvic control is important and can be promoted through lower trunk rotation activities that emphasize forward pelvic rotation (protraction) in a number of postures (e.g., sidelying; supine, modified hooklying with the affected LE pushing off; kneeling; standing, or sitting on a Swiss ball, pelvic shifting). An effective progression increases the challenge to the patient gradually by modifying postures until synergy influence is completely lacking (e.g., hip abduction can be performed first in hooklying, then supine, sidelying, modified plantigrade, and standing positions). To vary contraction patterns, dorsiflexors can be activated in sitting by first having the patient hold and slowly let the foot move down, then pull the foot up. This simulates the functional expectations of the normal gait cycle as the foot goes from swing phase through stance. The sequence can then be repeated in standing, a much more difficult position in which to control dorsiflexors. Voluntary control of eversion is often difficult to achieve because these muscles do not function in either synergy. The application of stretch and resistance to these muscles during an activity that recruits dorsiflexors and evertors may be effective in initiating a response (e.g., in bridging, the patient moves both the knees laterally to the affected side).

Control of knee function is often problematic. Reciprocal action (smooth reversals of flexion and extension movements) should be stressed early, beginning first in sitting, then in partial sitting (Fig.

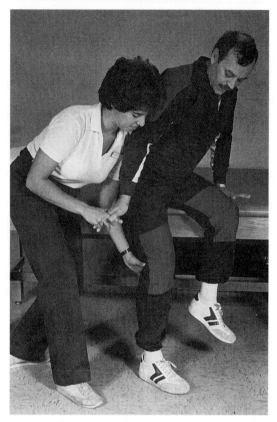

Figure 17-19. Early weight-bearing on the affected leg. The therapist assists controlled, small-range flexion and extension movements of the knee. The affected arm is maintained in an inhibitory position.

17-19), modified plantigrade, or supported standing positions, and progressing to standing and walking. Disassociation of UE movements during LE training is also an important consideration and can be achieved through positioning and voluntary holding (e.g., having the patient hold clasped hands together in a prayer position overhead during a LE activity; see Fig. 17-16).

Strategies to Improve Balance

Once initial stability control of body segments is achieved in upright postures, the patient is ready to practice dynamic balance activities. The patient is instructed to explore his or her limits of stability (LOS) through low-frequency weight shifting. The patient learns how far in any one direction he or she can move and how to align the center of gravity (COG) within their base of support (BOS) to maintain upright stability. Patients with stroke typically demonstrate reduced voluntary sway, with more weight-bearing directed to the sound side than the affected side. The therapist will therefore need to stress symmetrical weight-bearing, as well as activities that overcompensate, shifting the weight more onto the affected extremities. Postural perturbations can be used to displace the patient's center of mass (COM) and stimulate normal synergies required for balance (e.g., in standing ankle, hip, or stepping

strategies).[154] Patients with stroke typically exhibit delayed, varied, or absent responses. Latency, amplitude, and timing of muscle activity are all characteristically disturbed. It is therefore important to proceed slowly in training and to select challenges appropriate for the patient's level of control. The patient's attention should be directed to the appropriate strategy needed to maintain balance.[155]

The therapist can also have the patient sit or stand on a moveable support surface (Fig. 17-20), thereby stimulating adjustments through displacement of the BOS. For example, the patient sits on a gymnastic ball or equilibrium (wobble) board. The patient learns to actively control posture while the device is moved (therapist-initiated, reactive responses), or while the patient actively moves the device (patient-initiated, anticipatory responses). Anticipatory postural adjustments can also be challenged by having the patient perform voluntary movements that have a destabilizing effect. For example, in kneeling the patient can perform reaching and cone stacking (Fig. 17-21). Functional activities that typically provide destabilizing influences include sit-to-stand transitions, turning 360°, and floor-to-standing transitions. Dual task training tasks such as standing while catching or kicking a ball or walking while carrying an object (e.g., glass of water) are excellent choices. They redirect the patient's attention to the task at hand rather than allowing the patient to focus on the task of balance. The patient's attention can also be diverted by carrying on a conversation with the therapist during the training session. This strategy introduces a level of cognitive interference and can be effective in both evaluating and training automaticity of balance. Sensory conditions should also be varied to challenge the adequacy of balance.[153]

Force platform biofeedback (center-of-pressure biofeedback) provided to the patient while standing on a computerized force-plate system has been shown to be effective in improving balance.[156] Improvements have been found in steadiness (reduced sway),[157] postural symmetry,[157,158] and dynamic

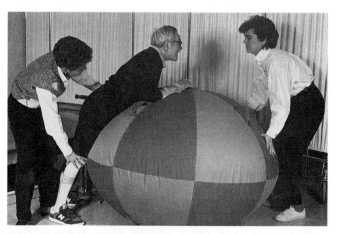

Figure 17-20. Standing, balance training in a modified plantigrade position. One therapist stimulates medial-lateral weight shifts while the other therapist supports the patient on the ball.

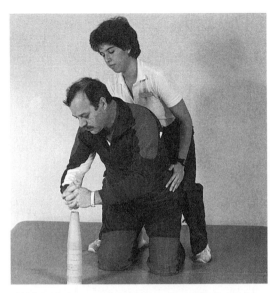

Figure 17-21. Balance training in kneeling. The therapist assists in maintenance of the kneeling posture while encouraging the patient in the weight shift and cone-stacking task.

stability.[158–160] Nichols[119] points out that the evidence is stronger and more consistent for the latter two parameters than for changes in steadiness. Improved balance from platform training has also been positively correlated with improved function, specifically transfer skills, endurance,[160] functional reach,[161] and measures of ADLs and home mobility.[158] Evidence of carryover to improved locomotor performance is conflicting.[157,160,161] Failure to find significant correlations to gait may be reflective of the dissimilarity between testing and training modes.

Safety education about fall prevention is a critical factor in ensuring maintenance of the patient's hard-won functional independence. Balance training should encourage active problem solving. The patient is presented with challenges, is able to identify potential problems, and recruits safe strategies to maintain balance.

Strategies to Improve Gait

Gait training is optimally initiated early.[163] Walking is an important motivational activity for most patients. Early walking also prevents or minimizes the development of indirect impairments (e.g., DVT, deconditioning). On the negative side, early walking increases the risk of falls. Although parallel bars and ambulation aids (e.g., hemi walkers, quad canes, canes) assist in early gait stability and safety, prolonged use of these devices can be problematic. These devices fail to challenge and develop balance. They also promote asymmetry and stimulate excessive weight shift and dependence on the unaffected side. Gait is typically slower with assistive devices. It is important to progress patients as quickly as possible to the least restrictive device and to practice

gait without the assistive device. The patient's safety is paramount and proper guarding techniques should be maintained at all times.

Specific gait activities should continue to focus on the selective movements needed and on appropriate timing. Movement deficiencies will vary from patient to patient and should be carefully identified (Box 17–2). Critical areas of stance phase control that will need to be addressed during gait training include initial weight acceptance, midstance control, and forward weight advancement during end stance on the hemiplegic limb. During swing, a drop foot or decreased hip and knee flexion may result in excessive limb length and compensatory gait changes (e.g., circumducted gait). Finally persistent posturing of the UE in flexion and adduction during gait must be also addressed. This latter problem can be effectively controlled through positioning the hemiplegic UE in extension and abduction with the hand open (Fig. 17-22) or with the use of an air splint.

The patient should practice functional, task-specific locomotor skills: walking forward, backward, sideward, and in a crossed pattern (sidestepping, braiding). Elevation activities (stepping up; stair climbing, step over step; over and around obstacles) and community activities (ramps, curbs, crossing the street, uneven terrain) should also be practiced. Initially gait will be slow and deliberate.

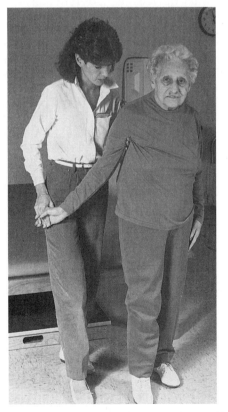

Figure 17-22. Assisted ambulation. The therapist provides support and assists in the lateral weight transfer onto the affected side. The arm is maintained in an inhibitory position (extension abduction and external rotation).

As control develops the patient should be encouraged to improve gait speed while maintaining safety. Timing and reciprocity of movements can be improved with the use of a treadmill, cycle ergometer, and Kinetron isokinetic device.[163] The therapist initially presets the movements to utilize slower speeds; progression is then to more rapid speeds as control improves. For example, a rate of movement approaching 1 cycle per second, which is within normal parameters for heel-strike to heel-strike, is the desired end point of isokinetic training.

An important goal of training is to have the patient be able to monitor his or her performance and recognize and initiate corrective actions. The patient should be able to vary walking speed and direction, navigate changes in the support surface and the environment, and be able to carry on a conversation while walking. Functional practice in real-life environments will assist the patient in developing the confidence needed for meeting the demands of everyday life.

ORTHOTICS

An orthosis may be required when persistent problems prevent safe ambulation. Prescription will depend on the unique gait problems each patient presents. The pattern of instability and weakness at the ankle and knee, and the extent and severity of spasticity and sensory deficits of the limb are major factors to be considered when prescribing an orthosis. Temporary devices (e.g., dorsiflexor assists) may be used during the early stages while recovery is proceeding to allow the patient to practice standing and walking. Permanent devices are prescribed once the patient's status stabilizes. It is often useful to consult with a certified orthotist if a permanent orthosis is needed.

An ankle-foot orthosis (AFO) is commonly prescribed to control deficient knee and ankle/foot function. These may include a custom molded AFO (posterior leaf spring, modified AFO, or solid ankle AFO [Fig. 17-23]), or conventional double upright/dual channel AFO. The most commonly used AFO is a posterior leaf spring (PLS) to control for drop foot. A modified AFO has a slightly wider lateral brim and can provide additional control of calcaneal and forefoot inversion and eversion. A solid ankle molded AFO provides maximum stabilization through its wide lateral trim lines. Movement in all planes (dorsiflexion, plantarflexion, inversion, and eversion) is limited. The conventional double upright metal orthosis may be ordered for patients who cannot tolerate plastic AFOs owing to sensory impairments or diabetic neuropathy, or who require additional controls. A posterior stop can be added to limit plantarflexion while a spring assist can be added to assist dorsiflexion (Klenzak joint). Disadvantages of metal devices include heavier weight, less cosmetic appearance, and increased difficulty in putting it on. An air-stirrup ankle brace has also been used to provide medial-lateral stability at the

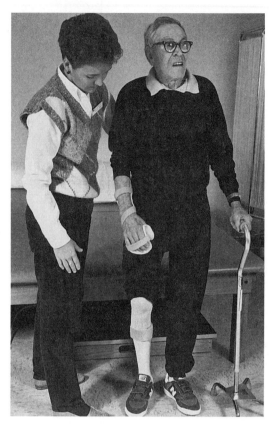

Figure 17-23. Assisted ambulation using a plastic ankle-foot orthosis and a quad cane. A resting pan splint supports the patient's affected hand.

subtalar joint while allowing dorsiflexion and plantar flexion.[164]

Knee problems in hemiplegia can usually be controlled by adjusting the position of the ankle. An ankle set in 5 degrees dorsiflexion limits knee hyperextension, while an ankle set in 5 degrees plantarflexion stabilizes the knee during midstance and prevents knee buckling.[165] A patient with knee hyperextension without foot and/or ankle instability may benefit from the application of a Swedish Knee Cage to protect the knee. Extensive bracing using a knee-ankle-foot orthosis (KAFO) is rarely indicated or successful. The added weight and restrictions in normal knee joint motion significantly increase energy costs and limit independent function.

The therapist must frequently reassess the patient's motor function and recovery. The need for an orthosis or a particular type of orthosis may change with continuing recovery. The therapist may need to recommend a change in prescription or discontinuing the use of a device. With limited reimbursements, ordering a new orthosis may prove problematic and speaks to the need to anticipate changes when ordering the initial device. For example, a good option for the patient who needs a custom molded solid AFO is to order a hinged AFO with a plantarflexion stop. As the patient regains sufficient knee and dorsiflexor control, the device can be adjusted to remove the stop and allow the hinges to work. Orthotic training includes donning and doffing instructions, skin inspections, and education in safe use of the device during gait. See Chapter 31 for a more complete description of these devices.

Strategies to Improve Feeding and Swallowing

Dysphagia is typically managed by a multidisciplinary team, including the speech/language pathologist, occupational therapist, physical therapist, nutritionist, and physician. The outcomes/goals of dysphagia management are to (1) improve strength, coordination, and range of oral musculature, (2) promote normal feeding through graduated resumption of activities, (3) promote volitional control through effective verbal coaching, and (4) provide effective education and support.

Patients on prolonged bed rest with marked deconditioning, marked paralysis, or dysarthria may experience impaired or shallow breathing patterns. Improved chest expansion can be achieved by effective use of manual contacts, resistance, and stretch to various chest wall segments. Diaphragmatic, basal, and lateral costal expansion should be stressed. An important prespeech activity consists of having the patient maintain a vocal expression (e.g., "ah") during the entire expiratory phase, because poor breath control often contributes to soft or vacillating sound production. Respiratory activities can be combined with movement patterns whenever possible (e.g., inspiration with PNF bilateral symmetrical D2 flexion patterns and expiration with D2 extension). During any sustained activity (isometric holding), breath control should be emphasized; the Valsalva maneuver should always be avoided. This is especially important in patients with documented concomitant hypertension.

A critical component of dysphagia management is the attainment of appropriate postural position. The head should be held in a chin-down position rather than extended or tipped back. This reduces the chances of aspiration or choking and promotes normal swallowing through appropriate alignment of the necessary structures. If the patient lacks adequate head control, the head should be supported either manually or with supports. Head rotation movements can be used to move the bolus of food away from the direction of rotation. This is an effective compensatory strategy to enhance swallowing in unilateral disorders. Additional swallowing maneuvers (e.g., supraglottic swallow) can also be taught.[65]

Facial exercises including movements of the lips, tongue, cheeks, and jaw should be practiced. The patient is instructed to purse lips and hold a tongue depressor between the lips. Tongue movements in all directions are practiced and can be resisted manually (using a sterile gauze or glove to cover finger) or with a moist tongue depressor. Firm pressure to the anterior third of the tongue can be used to stimulate the posterior elevation of the tongue by pushing the tongue against a tongue depressor. Cheek exercises include practice in puffing, blowing bubbles, and drinking thick liquids through a straw. Jaw movements can be stimulated by vibrating or pressing above the upper lip for closure and under the lower lip for opening. Jaw closure can also be assisted when necessary during feeding by holding the jaw firmly closed using a *jaw control technique* (e.g., thumb on jaw line, index finger between lower lip and chin, and middle finger under chin applying firm pressure). Stretch, resistance, or quick ice are used to facilitate the desired movements as necessary. The use of a mirror may also be helpful during facial exercises, provided the patient does not have visuospatial dysfunction.[65,166]

Food presentation is an important part of dysphagia management. Food should be positioned at an appropriate height and distance from the patient and in the patient's visual field. Adapted utensils, plate guards, and nonslip mats can be used to assist in the transfer of food to the mouth. Food should be at first semimoist (e.g., pureed food, pasta, boiled chicken) progressing to foods rich in taste, smell, and texture, qualities that assist in facilitating the swallowing reflex. Favorite foods should be employed whenever possible. Sucking control and saliva production can be stimulated using small amounts of ice water or an ice cube. The therapist can also apply deep pressure on the neck above the thyroid notch to stimulate sucking. Resisted sucking can be promoted using a straw and very thick liquids (slushes, shakes), or by holding the open end of the straw against the finger. As sucking control proceeds, thinner liquids can be substituted. Patients with a hypoactive gag reflex may be stimulated briefly with a cotton swab to develop this response. Modification of the eating environment is also an important consideration. Every effort should be made to ensure that the environment is pleasant, free from distraction, devoid of unpleasant sights and smells, and provides adequate lighting. The patient's full attention should be directed to the task at hand by using appropriate and consistent verbal cues. The importance of mealtime for social interaction should not be overlooked.[166]

Conditioning Strategies

Patients with stroke demonstrate decreased levels of physical conditioning following periods of prolonged immobility and reduced activity. The energy costs to complete many functional tasks are higher than normal owing to the abnormal ways in which the activities are performed.[167–170] Many patients also demonstrate concomitant cardiovascular disease and may be recovering from acute cardiac events at the same time.[87,171,172] These patients require careful assessment of cardiopulmonary responses during exercise and appropriate monitoring. Vital signs, heart rate, and ratings of perceived exertion (RPE) are all important measures of cardiopulmonary adaptation to exercise. Signs and symptoms of exertional intolerance (i.e., excessive fatigue, dyspnea, dizziness, diaphoresis, nausea, vomiting, chest pain) should be monitored closely and can signal an inappropriate level of exercise intensity and cardiac decompensation.[88,173] Occasionally, patients will require electrocardiographic telemetry to ensure safety during rehabilitation activities.

Individuals recovering from stroke can benefit from exercise intervention to improve cardiovascular fitness. During acute inpatient rehabilitation, functional activities are appropriate for training. Improving sitting and standing tolerance, and functional mobility activities such as transfers and walking can be used for initial low level training. During postacute outpatient rehabilitation, stroke survivors may be able to engage in a more traditional exercise training program such as treadmill walking or stationary bicycling. To ensure safety, patients should receive a thorough examination before starting a program.[174] Considerations for prescription should be based on individual abilities and interests. Prescriptive elements include mode (type of exercise), frequency, intensity, and duration (see Chapter 16).[175,176] The use of a training log or exercise diary is an excellent way to keep track of prescriptive elements, objective measurements (heart rate, blood pressure), and subjective reactions (RPE, perceived enjoyment). Adequate supervision, monitoring, and safety education about warning signs for impending stroke and heart attack are critical components.[177] Conditioning programs for patients with stroke can yield significant improvements in physical fitness, functional status, psychological outlook, and self-esteem.[178,179] Regular exercise may also have the additional benefit of reducing risk from recurrent stroke or heart attack. Finally, patients who participate in a regular conditioning program may be more successful in adopting continuing, life-long exercise habits and in moving beyond the disability of stroke.

Electrotherapeutic Modalities

BIOFEEDBACK

Electromyographic biofeedback (EMG-BFB) has been used to improve motor function in patients with hemiplegia. This technique allows patients to alter motor unit activity based on augmented audio and visual feedback information. Thus, firing frequency can be decreased in spastic muscles, or increased, along with recruitment of additional motor units, in weak, hypoactive muscles (see Chapter 33 for a more complete description of this topic). Patients in the chronic stage (typically defined as 1 year post stroke) or patients in late recovery for whom spontaneous recovery is more or less complete (6 months post stroke) have demonstrated positive results that have been attributed to biofeedback therapy.[180–186] Reported benefits include improvements in ROM, function, gait speed,

and voluntary control. Other studies[141,187,188] have failed to yield significant differences over conventional therapy. Most researchers indicate that effectiveness of biofeedback neuromuscular reeducation is greatest when used as an adjunct to conventional therapy in a combined approach.

Limb load devices that provide feedback about the amount of loading or weight-bearing on the hemiplegic limb have been effective in improving gait. Patients receiving this training demonstrate more normal weight-bearing and stance times on their affected limb and increased swing times on their unaffected limb.[186]

FUNCTIONAL ELECTRICAL STIMULATION

Neuromuscular electrical stimulation (NMES) has been used with patients recovering from stroke to facilitate gains in voluntary motor control, muscle strength, and reduction of spasticity. NMES has been shown to increase the ability of muscle to exert force by preferentially activating the fast-contracting motor units.[189] Effective treatment results in stroke rehabilitation have been reported using NMES to improve dorsiflexor function and prevent drop foot,[190–191] wrist extension function,[192–193] and spasticity reduction associated with antagonist muscle activation.[194]

The term functional electrical stimulation (FES) refers to the use of electrical stimulation to assist in functional tasks. FES to the posterior deltoid and supraspinatus muscles has been used in patients with stroke to reestablish glenohumeral alignment and reduce subluxation,[195] and to restore upper extremity volitional control.[196] It has also been used during gait to assist dorsiflexor function as an orthotic aid.[182] Multichannel FES (MFES) uses a program developed from individual profiles of EMG and anthropometric measurements to stimulate antagonistic groups of muscles. Significant improvements of gait in patients with stroke have been reported.[197–202] Because the patients had limbs that had been paralyzed for more than 6 months, the results suggest a significant motor learning effect. As with the biofeedback research, optimal results have been obtained when combined with conventional therapy.[197]

Patient and Family Education

Stroke represents a major health crisis for patients and their families. Ignorance about the cause of the illness or the recovery process and misconceptions concerning the rehabilitation program and potential outcomes can negatively influence coping responses and progress in rehabilitation. Frequently the problems seem unmanageable and overwhelming for the family, especially when faced with alterations in the patient's behavior, cognition, and emotion. Patients may feel depressed, isolated, irritable, or demanding. Families often demonstrate reactions that include initial relief and hope for full recovery, followed by feelings of entrapment, depression, anger, or guilt when complete recovery does not occur. These changes and feelings can strain even the best of relationships. Therapists can often have a dramatic influence on this situation because of the high frequency of contact and the often close relationships that develop with patients and their families. There are a number of important guidelines to follow when planning educational interventions:[3]

1. Give accurate, factual information; counsel family members about the patient's capabilities and limitations; *avoid* predictions that categorically define expected function or future recovery.

2. Structure interventions carefully, giving only as much information as the patient or family need or can assimilate; provide reinforcement and repetition.

3. Adapt interventions to ensure they are appropriate to the educational and cultural background of the patient and family. A variety of educational interventions should be considered: didactic sessions, books, brochures, and videotapes, and family participation in therapy.

4. Provide a forum for open discussion and communication.

5. Be supportive, sensitive, and maintain a positive, hopeful manner.

6. Assist patients and families in confronting alternatives and developing problem solving abilities.

7. Motivate and provide positive reinforcement in therapy; enhance patient satisfaction and self-esteem.

8. Refer patients and families to support and self-help groups such as the following national associations and local stroke clubs:

   American Heart Association Stroke
   Connection
   7272 Greenville Avenue
   Dallas, TX 75231-4569
   1–800–AHA–USA1 (1–800–242–8721)
   www.americanheart.org

   National Stroke Association
   8480 East Orchard Road
   Suite 1000
   Englewood, CO 80111-5015
   1–800–STROKES (1–800–787–6537)

9. Psychotherapy and counseling (e.g., sexual, leisure, vocational) can assist in improving overall quality of life and should be recommended as needed.

DISCHARGE PLANNING

Planning for discharge begins early in rehabilitation and intimately involves the patient and family. Potential placement (safe place of residence), level of family and community support, and need for continued medical and rehabilitation services should all be explored. Family members should regularly participate in therapy sessions to learn exercises and activities designed to support the patient's independence. Discharge should be considered when reasonable treatment outcomes/goals are attained. Indication of the attainment of a functional ceiling can be assumed when there is lack of evidence of progress at two successive evaluations over a period of 2 weeks (4 weeks for subacute rehabilitation).[3] Home visits should be made prior to discharge to determine the home's physical structure and accessibility. Potential problems can be identified and corrective measures initiated. Home adaptations, assistive devices, and supportive services should be in place before the patient is discharged to home. Several trial home stays may be helpful in smoothing the transition from rehabilitation center to home. Patients with residual stroke deficits who will be receiving outpatient or home therapy should be given all the necessary information concerning these services. Community services should be identified and information provided to the patient and family. Long-term follow-up at regularly scheduled intervals should be initiated in order to maintain patients at their highest possible functional level.

POSTACUTE REHABILITATION

The patient may be referred for continuing rehabilitation either through outpatient or home care services. A complete record of medical and rehabilitation services should be made available to these agencies. The intensity of services provided is considerably less than that of acute rehabilitation, generally limited to a few hours per week spread over 2 to 3 visits. Many of the outcomes/goals and interventions begun during acute rehabilitation are continued and progressed during the postacute phase to sustain the gains made and maintain or improve the patient's functional performance. The challenges of being home provide additional daily stresses for the patient and family. Difficulties should be assessed and addressed promptly as they arise. The therapist needs to maintain a continuing emphasis on the development of problem-solving skills to ensure successful adaptation and independent function. Interventions should focus on health promotion, fall prevention, and safety in the home and community environments. Fall risk factors (weakness, restricted ROM, balance or gait problems, inappropriate use of assistive devices, orthostatic hypotension, medication side effects) should be eliminated or minimized as appropriate or possible. Environmental assessment and modification is an important part of a fall prevention program. Finally, the patient should be assisted in the resumption of social and recreational activities. With increasing activity levels, it is important to monitor the patient's endurance levels carefully and instruct in energy conservation techniques. A small number of stroke survivors can be evaluated and assisted in return to work. As the patient becomes successful in the home and community environment, services should be gradually phased out. Follow up visits at periodic intervals are recommended to identify problems as they develop and to ensure long-term maintenance of function.[3]

STROKE REHABILITATION OUTCOMES

Rehabilitation programs for patients with stroke have been shown to improve functional outcomes and allow patients to regain independence.[142,203-204] Between 75 and 85 percent of patients are discharged to home, and of these 70 to 80 percent are independent in ambulation with and without assistive devices. Between 50 and 66 percent are independent in ADLs and only 17 percent require assistance in bowel and bladder care.[86] Health care costs are also minimized when compared to long-term placement in nursing homes.[205]

Some patients demonstrate spontaneously good recovery without the benefits of rehabilitation, whereas other patients demonstrate poor recovery of function regardless of rehabilitation efforts. Current recommendations from the World Health Organization suggest that rehabilitation efforts should be directed toward the middle band of patients who can make satisfactory recovery only through intensive rehabilitation.[1] Major difficulties in stroke outcome studies appear to be the lack of uniform criteria in the selection of patients for rehabilitation, as well as differences in duration, type, and onset of rehabilitation programs.[206,207] Patients who generally do poorly in rehabilitation demonstrate (1) advanced age and profound neurological impairments (paresis, loss of proprioception), (2) decreased alertness, poor attention span, judgement, memory, and an inability to learn new tasks or follow simple commands, (3) severe visuospatial hemineglect, (4) persistent medical problems (e.g., bowel and bladder incontinence, cardiovascular disease), (5) serious language disturbances, and (6) less well defined social and economic problems.[86,208,209]

Most patients are able to maintain their independent living status following discharge. The severity of physical disability, age, and persistent psychological and/or emotional problems (depression, irritability) are the primary factors that determine continuing success in independent living and quality of life. Other key factors identified include marital status (the presence of a helpful, caring spouse), elimination of home barriers, and transportation.[210,211]

SUMMARY

Stroke can result from a number of different vascular events that interrupt cerebral circulation and impair brain function. These include cerebral thrombosis, emboli, or hemorrhage. The location and size of the ischemic process, the nature and functions of the structures involved, the availability of collateral blood flow, and effectiveness of early emergency medical management all influence the symptomatology that evolves. For many patients, stroke represents a major cause of disability, with diffuse problems affecting widespread areas of function. From a practical standpoint, patients with stroke present a tremendous challenge for clinicians. Effective rehabilitation should take advantage of spontaneous recovery. Rehabilitation interventions seek to promote recovery and independence through remediation, compensatory, and functional training strategies. Interventions also focus on the prevention of secondary impairments. The utilization of effective motor learning strategies with a focus on real-life environments is critical for the successful attainment of functional outcomes.

QUESTIONS FOR REVIEW

1. Differentiate between each of the following vascular syndromes: anterior cerebral artery, middle cerebral artery, internal carotid artery, posterior cerebral artery, and vertebrobasilar artery. What are the differences that can be expected between hemispheric lesions?

2. What are the major causes of stroke? Define and explain each.

3. What diagnostic measures are used to confirm stroke? Describe the role of the CT scan in the implementation of emergency medical measures.

4. Describe the normal recovery process in stroke including expected stages of recovery. Give an example of how this knowledge will influence your selection of interventions.

5. What are the major sensory, motor, language, perceptual, and cognitive impairments produced with stroke?

6. Describe the dynamics and causative factors of shoulder dysfunction in hemiplegia. How should this knowledge influence your selection of assessment procedures and interventions?

7. Differentiate between two standardized stroke assessment instruments: the Fugl-Meyer Assessment of Physical Performance and the Motor Assessment Scale.

8. What are the key strategies that can be used in positioning the patient with stroke during the acute stage?

9. Identify critical motor learning strategies for treating the patient with stroke.

10. Identify four strategies that could be used during acute rehabilitation to reestablish postural control and improve functional mobility.

11. What are the essential elements of interventions designed to improve upper extremity function? Lower extremity function? Identify three strategies for each.

12. How can timing deficits in ambulation be overcome? Identify two strategies.

13. Identify and describe common orthotic devices used for the patient with stroke. What are the major indications and contraindications for each?

14. List the possible uses of EMG-BFB and NMES in the rehabilitation of patients with stroke.

15. Differentiate between the focus of rehabilitation efforts during the acute and postacute phases of stroke rehabilitation.

16. What are the essential elements included in an educational program for the patient with stroke and family members?

17. What are the major factors affecting stroke outcome?

CASE STUDY

HISTORY: The patient/client is a 41 year-old male admitted to an acute care hospital with a diagnosis of CVA with R hemiparesis (L MCA). Admitted to a rehabilitation facility 10 days later.

PAST MEDICAL HISTORY
- Seizure disorder since childhood. Dilantin was discontinued 5 years ago.
- History of mild hypertension well controlled with medication.
- Smokes 1 pack/day; 20 year history.

MEDICATIONS
Persantine 50 mg po tid
Tenormin 25 mg po qd
Aspirin 10 grains po bid

TESTS
- Carotid angiography: complete occlusion of left internal carotid artery.
- Cardiac ultrasound: intermittent mitral valve prolapse.
- EKG: nonspecific ST wave changes.
- CT scan: initial scan unremarkable; repeat CT scan consistent with a large left middle cerebral artery ischemic infarction.

SOCIAL HISTORY: Patient lives with his wife and three teenage children and was independent and active prior to CVA. He has a college education and has worked for 20 years as a computer programmer. There is a two-stair access to a rented, single family house.

COGNITION
- Disoriented to time.
- Good attention span for 30- to 45-minute treatment session.
- Difficult to assess further owing to language impairment but cognitive deficits are probably due to severity of comprehension deficits.
- Patient has difficulty following directions for motor responses; two or three step commands.

LANGUAGE-COMMUNICATION
a. Auditory comprehension: moderate to severe decrease in understanding words and simple concrete sentences; unreliable yes/no responses.
b. Verbal expression: severely decreased to nonfunctional; limited to only occasional automatic words.
c. Reading comprehension: severely decreased to nonfunctional at a word level. Unable to match word to object.
d. Written expression: to be assessed.
e. Gestures: spontaneous use of gestures not evident.

PHYSICAL THERAPY ASSESSMENT
  PROM
    BUEs WNL; R shoulder pain at end ranges
    BLEs WNL except R dorsiflexion 0 to 5 degrees.
  Tone
    RUE increased tone (moderate to severe) in elbow flexors; shoulder adductors and internal rotators.
    RLE increased tone (moderate) in hip and knee extensors, plantar flexors.
  Motor Control
    RUE: partial motion (1/2 range) in extensor synergy pattern (shoulder and elbow extension); no voluntary motion of hand.
    Cannot perform flexor synergy pattern at all.
    Demonstrates RUE neglect and often lets UE drop off the wheelchair.
    RLE: full motion in both extensor and flexor synergy patterns with extensor pattern dominating;
      Extensor synergy achieved with associated reaction of RUE (extensor synergy).
    LUE and LLE: full isolated movement with G+ to N strength.
  Sensory
    RUE: impaired, severity difficult to determine due to communication deficits.
      No apparent sensation to sharp/dull stimuli.
      Moderate decrease in light touch sensitivity.
    RLE: few consistent responses to sharp/dull stimuli proximally;
      Moderate to severe decrease distally;
      No sensation noted on dorsum of foot.
    Patient reports pain in both RUE and RLE.
      Proprioception: non-appropriate responses; difficult to assess owing to patient's difficulty with understanding of questions being asked.
  Coordination
    LUE and LLE intact.
    RUE and RLE unable to test.
  Postural Reactions/Balance
    Head control: good
    Sitting:
      Static control: good, able to maintain balance without support.
      Maintains centered alignment (COM) for 5 minutes.

Continued

Continued

Dynamic control: fair, able to maintain balance

Weight shifting with reduced limits of stability (LOS).

Shifts to R are reduced 50 percent; shifts to L are normal.

Standing: in parallel bars

Static control: fair, able to maintain independent standing in parallel bars for up to 1 minute with LUE hand hold.

Dynamic control: poor

Unable to weight shift to R without loss of balance.

Weight shifts to L are reduced 50 percent.

Motor Planning

Appears to have mild motor apraxia; difficult to assess owing to communication deficits.

Endurance

Tolerates ¾-hour treatment session with occasional rests.

Functional Assessment: Functional Independence Measure (FIM)

Functional mobility skills:

Rolls to R: Independent with bed rail (FIM 6)

Rolls to L: Min Assist (FIM 4)

Scoots up in bed: with Supervision (FIM 5)

Supine-to-sit: Min Assist (FIM 4)

Sit-to-supine: Min Assist (FIM 4)

Transfers bed-to-chair: Stand pivot transfer, mod assist (FIM 3)

W/C mobility: Ambulates 150 feet with supervision (FIM 5); uses L UE and foot for propulsion

Gait

Locomotion: Ambulates short distances in parallel bars only; requires max assist of one (FIM 2).

Requires assist in initiation of movement of RLE.

Requires assist with R knee control for extension.

R foot is plantarflexed and supinated during stance, foot drop during swing.

AFO ordered

Stairs: NA; to be evaluated at a later date.

ADLs

Eating: Supervision (FIM 5)

Bathing: Min assist RLE, mod assist RUE (FIM 4/3)

Dressing: Min assist RLE, mod assist RUE (FIM 4/3)

Patient Is Very Motivated and Cooperative: He appears anxious about his future and exhibited a brief episode of crying during the initial assessment. Family is supportive and anxious to have him home again.

Case Study Guiding Questions

1. Identify/categorize this patient's problems in terms of:
   a. Direct impairments
   b. Indirect impairments
   c. Composite impairments: combined effects of both direct and indirect impairments
   d. Functional limitations/disabilities
2. Identify your goals (remediation of impairments) and outcomes (remediation of functional limitations/disability) for this patient.
3. Formulate five treatment interventions with one progression that could be used during the first 3 weeks of therapy. Provide a brief rationale that justifies your choice.
4. Identify relevant teaching/motor learning strategies appropriate for the initial physical therapy sessions with this patient.

REFERENCES

1. World Health Organization: Stroke: 1989. Recommendations on stroke prevention, diagnosis, and therapy: Report of the WHO Task Force on Stroke and Other Cerebrovascular Disorders, 1989. 20:1407, 1989.
2. American Heart Association: 1998 Heart and Stroke Statistical Update. American Heart Association, Dallas, 1998.
3. Post-Stroke Rehabilitation Guideline Panel: Post-Stroke Rehabilitation Clinical Practice Guideline. Aspen, Gaithersburg, MD, 1996 (formerly published as AHCPR Publication No. 95-0662, May 1995).
4. Wolf, PA, et al: Secular trends in stroke incidence and mortality. The Framingham Study. Stroke 23:1551, 1992.
5. Solzi, J, et al: Hemiplegics after a first stroke: Late survival and risk factors. Stroke 14:703, 1983.
6. Granger, C, and Hamilton, B: The Uniform Data System for Medical Rehabilitation report of first admissions for 1992. Am J Phys Med Rehabil 73:51, 1994.
7. McGovern, PG, et al: Trends in mortality, morbidity, and risk factor levels for stroke from 1960 through 1990. JAMA 268:753, 1992.
8. Broderick, JP, et al: Incidence of rates of stroke in the eighties: The end of the decline in stroke. Stroke 20:577, 1989.
9. Saladin, L: Cerebrovascular Disease: Stroke. In Fredericks,

CM, and Saladin, LK: Pathophysiology of Motor Systems. FA Davis, Philadelphia, 1996, p 486.
10. American Heart Association: Heart Stroke Facts. American Heart Association, Dallas, 1996.
11. Donnarumma, R, et al: Overview: Hyperacute rt-PA stroke treatment. The NINDS rt-PA Stroke Study Group. J Neurosci Nurs 29:351, 1997.
12. Zivin, J, and Choi, D: Stroke therapy. Sci Am July:56, 1991.
13. Guberman, A: An Introduction to Clinical Neurology. Little, Brown and Co., Boston, 1994.
14. Hachinski, V, and Norris, J: The Acute Stroke. FA Davis, Philadelphia, 1985.
15. Curtis, S, and Porth, C: Disorders of brain function. In Porth, C: Pathophysiology, 5th ed. Lippincott, Philadelphia, 1998, p 879.
16. Haig, A, et al, V: Locked-in syndrome: A review. Curr Concepts Rehabil Med 2:12, 1986.
17. Haig, A, et al: Mortality and complications of the locked-in syndrome. Arch Phys Med Rehabil 68:24, 1987.
18. Bauby, J: The Diving Bell and the Butterfly. Alfred A. Knopf, New York, 1997.
19. Glick, T: Neurologic Skills: Examination and Diagnosis. Blackwell Scientific, Boston, 1993.
20. Bogousslavsky, J, et al: The Lausanne stroke registry:

Analysis of 1,000 consecutive stroke patients. Stroke 19: 1083, 1988.

21. Smith, D, et al: Proprioception and spatial neglect after stroke. Age Ageing 12:63, 1983.

22. Fields, H: Pain. McGraw-Hill, New York, 1987.

23. Haerer, A: Clinical manifestations of occlusive cerebrovascular disease. In Smith, R (ed): Stroke and the Extracranial Vessels. Raven, New York, 1984.

24. Twitchell, T: The restoration of motor function following hemiplegia in man. Brain 47:443, 1951.

25. Brunnstrom, S: Motor testing procedures in hemiplegia based on recovery stages. J Am Phys Ther Assoc 46:357, 1966.

26. Brunnstrom, S: Movement Therapy in Hemiplegia. Harper & Row, New York, 1970.

27. Bobath, B: Adult Hemiplegia: Evaluation and Treatment, ed 2. Heinemann, London, 1978.

28. Fugl-Meyer, A, et al: The post stroke hemiplegic patient, 1. A method for evaluation of physical performance. Scand J Rehabil Med 7:13, 1976.

29. Gray, C, et al: Motor recovery following acute stroke. Age Ageing 19:179, 1990.

30. Wade, D, et al: Recovery after stroke: The first 3 months. J Neurol Neurosurg Psychiatry 48:7, 1985.

31. Schenkman, M, and Butler, R: Automatic postural tone in posture, movement, and function. Forum on physical therapy issues related to cerebrovascular accident. American Physical Therapy Association, Alexandria, VA, 1992.

32. Michels, E: Synergies in Hemiplegia. Clin Management 1:9, 1981.

33. Bobath, B: Abnormal Postural Reflex Activity Caused by Brain Lesions, ed 3. Heinemann, London, 1985.

34. Mulley, G: Associated reactions in the hemiplegic arm. Scand J Rehabil Med 14:17, 1982.

35. Mizrahi, E, and Angel, R: Impairment of voluntary movement by spasticity. Ann Neurol 5:594, 1979.

36. Watkins, M, et al: Isokinetic testing in patients with hemiparesis: A pilot study. Phys Ther 64:184, 1984.

37. Bourbonnais, D, and Vanden Noven, S: Weakness in patients with hemiparesis. Am J Occup Ther 43:313, 1989.

38. Dattola, R, et al: Muscle rearrangement in patients with hemiparesis after stroke: An electrophysiological and morphological study. Eur Neurol 33:109, 1993.

39. Gowland, C, et al: Agonist and antagonist activity during voluntary upper-limb movement in patients with stroke. Phys Ther 72:624, 1992.

40. Tang, A, and Rymer, W: Abnormal force: EMG relations in paretic limbs of hemiparetic human subjects. J Neurol Neurosurg Psychiatry 44:690, 1981.

41. Rosenfalck, A, and Andreassen, S: Impaired regulation of force and firing pattern of single motor units in patients with spasticity. J Neurol Neurosurg Psychiatry 43:907, 1980.

42. Knutsson, E, and Martensson, C: Dynamic motor capacity in spastic paresis and its relationship to prime mover dysfunction, spastic reflexes and antagonistic coordination. Scand J Rehabil Med 12:93, 1980.

43. McComas, A, et al: Functional changes in motoneurons of hemiparetic patients. J Neurol Neurosurg Psychiatry 36:183, 1973.

44. Spaans, F, and Wilts, G: Denervation due to lesions of the central nervous system: An EMG study in cases of cerebral contusion and cerebrovascular accidents. J Neurol Sci 57:291, 1982.

45. Dickstein, R, et al: Reaction and movement times in patients with hemiparesis for unilateral and bilateral elbow flexion. Phys Ther 73:37, 1993.

46. Buonocore, M, et al: Psychomotor skills in hemiplegic patients: Reaction time differences related to hemispheric lesion side. Neurophysiol Clin 20:203, 1990.

47. Sahrmann, S, and Norton, B: The relationship of voluntary movement to spasticity in the upper motor neuron syndrome. Ann Neurol 2:460, 1977.

48. Bohannon, R, and Smith, M: Relationship between static muscle strength deficits and spasticity in stroke patients with hemiparesis. Phys Ther 67:1068, 1987.

49. Taub, E: Somatosensory deafferentation research with monkeys. In Ince, L (ed): Behavioral Psychology in Rehabilitation Medicine: Clinical Applications. Williams & Wilkins, Baltimore, 1980, p 371.

50. Wolf, S, et al: Forced use of hemiplegic upper extremities to reverse the effect of learned nonuse among chronic stroke and head-injured patients. Exp Neurol 104:125, 1989.

51. Bohannon, R: Selected determinants of ambulation capacity in patients with hemiplegia. Clin Rehab 3:47, 1989.

52. Bohannon, R: Correlation of lower limb strengths and other variables in standing performance in stroke patients. Physiother Can 41:198, 1989.

53. Hamrin, E, et al: Muscle strength and balance in post stroke patients. Ups J Med Sci 87:11, 1982.

54. Murray, E: Hemispheric specialization. In Fisher, A, et al (eds): Sensory Integration Theory and Practice. FA Davis, Philadelphia, 1991, p 171.

55. Kimura, D: Acquisition of a motor skill after left-hemisphere damage. Brain 100:527, 1977.

56. Light, K, et al: Motor programming deficits of patients with left versus right CVAs. Forum on Physical Therapy Issues Related to Cerebrovascular Accident. American Physical Therapy Association, Alexandria, VA, 1992.

57. Horak, F, et al: The effects of movement velocity, mass displaced and task certainty on associated postural adjustments made by normal and hemiplegic individuals. J Neurol Neurosurg Psychiatry 47:1020, 1984.

58. Dickstein, R, et al: Foot-ground pressure pattern of standing hemiplegic patients: Major characteristics and patterns of movement. Phys Ther 64:19, 1984.

59. Mizrahi, J, et al: Postural stability in stroke patients: Vectorial expression of asymmetry, sway activity, and relative sequence of reactive forces. Med Bio Eng Comput 27:181, 1989.

60. Badke, M, and DiFabio, R: Balance deficits in patients with hemiplegia: Considerations for assessment and treatment. In Duncan, P, (ed): Balance: Proceedings of the APTA Forum. American Physical Therapy Association, Alexandria, VA, 1990, p 73.

61. DiFabio, R, and Badke, M: Relationship of sensory organization to balance function in patients with hemiplegia. Phys Ther 70:543, 1990.

62. Shumway-Cook, A, and Woollacott, M: Motor Control Theory and Practical Applications. Williams & Wilkins, Baltimore, 1995.

63. Duncan, P, and Badke, M: Determinants of abnormal motor control. In: Duncan, P, and Badke, M (eds): Stroke Rehabilitation: The Recovery of Motor Control. Year Book, Chicago, 1987, p 135.

64. Veis, S, and Logemann, J: Swallowing disorders in persons with cerebrovascular accident. Arch Phys Med Rehabil 66:372, 1985.

65. Skvarla, AM, and Schroeder-Lopez, RA: Dysphagia Management. In Gillen, G, and Burkhardt, A: Stroke Rehabilitation. A Function-Based Approach. Mosby, St. Louis, 1998, p 407.

66. Davies, P: Steps to Follow—A Guide to Treatment of Adult Hemiplegia. Springer-Verlag, New York, 1985.

67. Pedersen, P, et al: Ipsilateral pushing in stroke: Incidence, relation to neuropsychological symptoms, and impact on rehabilitation. The Copenhagen stroke study. Arch Phys Med 77:25, 1996.

68. Arnadottir, G: Impact of Neurobehavioral Deficits on Activities of Daily Living. In Gillen, G, and Burkhardt, A: Stroke Rehabilitation. A Function-Based Approach. Mosby, St. Louis, 1998, p 285.

69. Starkstein, S, and Robinson, R: Neuropsychiatric aspects of stroke. In Coffey, C, and Cummings, J (eds): Textbook of Geriatric Neuropsychiatry. American Psychiatric Press, Washington, DC, 1994, p 457.

70. Hibbard, MR, and Gordon, WA: The comprehensive psychological assessment of individuals with stroke. J Neurol Rehabil 2:9, 1992.

71. Robinson, R, et al: Pathological laughing and crying following stroke: Validation of a measurement scale and a double-blind study. Am J Psychiatry 150:286, 1993.

72. Binder, L: Emotional problems after stroke. Stroke 15:174, 1984.

73. Robinson, R, et al: A two-year longitudinal study of post-stroke mood disorders: Diagnosis and outcome at one and two years. Stroke 18:837, 1987.

74. Robinson, R, and Price, T: Post-stroke depressive disorders: A follow-up study of 103 patients. Stroke 13:635, 1982.

75. Robinson, R, and Benson D: Depression in aphasic patients: Frequency, severity, and clinical-pathological correlations. Brain Lang 14:282, 1981.

76. Diller, L: Perceptual and intellectual problems in hemiplegia: Implications for rehabilitation. Med Clin North Am 53:575, 1969.

77. American Heart Association: How Stroke Affects Behavior. American Heart Association, Dallas, 1994.

78. Cocito, L, et al: Epileptic seizures in cerebral arterial occlusive disease. Stroke 13:189, 1982.

79. Clagett, GP, et al: Prevention of venous thromboembolism. Chest 102(suppl):391, 1992.

80. Roth, EJ: Medical complications encountered in stroke rehabilitation. Phys Med Rehabil Clin North Am 2:563, 1991.

81. Bruton, J: Shoulder pain in stroke: Patients with hemiplegia or hemiparesis following cerebrovascular accident. Physiotherapy 71:2, 1985.

82. Roy, C: Shoulder pains in hemiplegia: A literature review. Clin Rehabil 2:35, 1988.

83. Calliet, R: The Shoulder in Hemiplegia. FA Davis, Philadelphia, 1980.

84. Tepperman, P, et al: Reflex sympathetic dystrophy in hemiplegia. Arch Phys Med Rehabil 65:442, 1984.

85. Brandstater, M, and Basmajian, J: Stroke rehabilitation. Williams & Wilkins, Baltimore, 1987.

86. Dobkin, B: Neurologic Rehabilitation. FA Davis, Philadelphia, 1996.

87. Buck, L: The coincidence of heart disease and stroke: Pathogenesis and considerations for therapy. Neurology Report 18:29, 1994.

88. Mol, V, and Baker, C: Activity intolerance in the geriatric stroke patient. Rehabil Nursing 16:337, 1991.

89. Mills, V, and DiGenio, M: Functional differences in patients with left or right cerebrovascular accidents. Phys Ther 63:481, 1983.

90. Bernspang, B, et al: Motor and perceptual impairments in acute stroke: Effects on self-care ability. Stroke 18:1081, 1987.

91. Dombovy, M, and Bach-y-Rita, P: Clinical observations on recovery from stroke. Adv Neurol 47:265, 1988.

92. Dombovy, M, et al: Disability and use of rehabilitation services following stroke in Rochester, Minnesota, 1975–1979. Stroke 18:830, 1987.

93. Kelly-Hayes, M, et al: Time course of functional recovery after stroke: The Framingham Study. J Neurol Rehabil 3:65, 1989.

94. Ferrucci, L, et al: Recovery of functional status after stroke: A postrehabilitation follow-up study. Stroke 24:200, 1993.

95. Stein, D, et al: Brain Repair. Oxford Univ Pr., New York, 1995.

96. Kalra, L, et al: Medical complications during stroke rehabilitation. Stroke 26:990, 1995.

97. Adams H, et al (eds): Management of Patients with Acute Ischemic Stroke. American Heart Association, Dallas, 1994.

98. Langhorne, P, et al: Do stroke units save lives? Lancet 342:395, 1993.

99. Hayes, S, and Carroll, S: Early intervention care in the acute stroke patient. Arch Phys Med Rehabil 67:319, 1986.

100. Strand, T, et al: A non-intensive stroke unit reduces functional disability and the need for long-term hospitalization. Stroke 16:29, 1985.

101. Hamrin, E: Early activation in stroke: Does it make a difference? Scand J Rehabil Med 14:101, 1982.

102. McCann, B, and Culbertson, R: Comparisons of two systems for stroke rehabilitation in a general hospital. J Am Geriatr Soc 24:211, 1976.

103. Johnston, M, and Keister, M: Early rehabilitation for stroke patients: A new look. Arch Phys Med Rehabil 65:437, 1984.

104. Novack, T, Satterfield, W, and Connor, M: Stroke onset and rehabilitation: Time lag as a factor in treatment outcome. Arch Phys Med Rehabil 65:316, 1984.

105. Teasdale, G, and Jennett, B: Assessment of coma and impaired consciousness. Lancet ii:81, 1974.

106. Teasdale, G, and Jennett, B: Assessment and prognosis of coma after head injury. Acta Neurochir 34:45, 1976.

107. Rehabilitation of the Head Injured Adult: Comprehensive Physical Management. Professional Staff Association, Rancho Los Amigos Hospital, Downey, CA, 1979.

108. Folstein, MF, et al: Mini mental state: A practical method for grading the cognitive state of patients for the clinician. J Psychiatr Res 12:189, 1975.

109. Bohannon, R: Measurement and treatment of paresis in the geriatric patient. Top Geriatr Rehabil 7:15, 1991.

110. Turnbull, G, and Wall, J: The development of a system for the clinical assessment of gait following a stroke. Physiotherapy 71:294, 1985.

111. Holden, M, et al: Clinical gait assessment in the neurologically impaired: Reliability and meaningfulness. Phys Ther 64:35, 1984.

112. Badke, M, and DiFabio, R: Balance deficits in patients with hemiplegia: Considerations for assessment and treatment. Balance: Proceedings of the APTA Forum. American Physical Therapy Association, Alexandria, VA, 1990.

113. Badke, M, and Duncan, P: Patterns of rapid motor responses during postural adjustments when standing in healthy subjects and hemiplegic patients. Phys Ther 63:13, 1983.

114. Berg, KO, et al: Measuring balance in the elderly: Preliminary development of an instrument. Physiother Can 41:304, 1989.

115. Berg, KO, et al: Measuring balance in the elderly: Validation of an instrument. Canadian Journal of Public Health 83(suppl):7, 1992.

116. Duncan, P, et al: Functional reach: A new clinical measure of balance. J Gerontol 45:192, 1990.

117. Tinetti, ME: Performance-oriented assessment of mobility problems in elderly patients. J Am Geriatr Soc 34:119, 1986.

118. Shumway-Cook, A, and Horak, F: Assessing the influence of sensory interaction on balance: Suggestion from the field. Phys Ther 66:1548, 1986.

119. Nichols, D: Balance retraining after stroke using force platform biofeedback. Phys Ther 77:553, 1997.

120. Fugl-Meyer, A: Post-stroke hemiplegia assessment of physical properties. Scand J Rehabil Med 7:85, 1980.

121. Duncan, P, et al: Reliability of the Fugl-Meyer Assessment of Sensorimotor Recovery following cerebrovascular accident. Phys Ther 63:1606, 1983.

122. Carr, J, et al: Investigation of a new motor assessment scale for stroke patients. Phys Ther 65:175, 1985.

123. Pool, J, and Whitney, S: Motor Assessment Scale for stroke patients: Concurrent validity and interrater reliability. Arch Phys Med Rehabil 69:195, 1988.

124. Collen, C, et al: Mobility after stroke: Reliability of measurements of impairment and disability. Int Disabil Stud 12:6, 1990.

125. Mahoney, F, and Barthel, D: Functional evaluation: Barthel Index. Md State Med J 14:61, 1965.

126. Keith, RA, et al: The Functional Independence Measure. Advances in clinical rehabilitation 1:6, 1987.

127. Granger, C, et al: Stroke rehabilitation: Analysis of repeated Barthel Index measures. Arch Phys Med Rehabil 60:14, 1979.

128. Uniform Data Service, Data Management Service: UDS Update. State Univ of New York at Buffalo, 1993.

129. American Physical Therapy Association: Guide to Physical Therapist Practice. American Physical Therapy Association, Alexandria, VA, 1999.

130. Carr, J, and Shepherd, R: A Motor Relearning Programme for Stroke, ed 2. Aspen, Rockville, MD, 1987.

131. Sahrmann, SA, and Norton, BJ: The relationship of voluntary movement to spasticity in the upper motor neuron syndrome. Ann Neurol 2:460, 1977.

132. Sawner, K, and LaVigne, J: Brunnstrom's Movement Therapy in Hemiplegia, ed 2. Lippincott, New York, 1992.

133. Voss, D, et al: Proprioceptive Neuromuscular Facilitation, ed 3. Harper & Row, Philadelphia, 1985.

134. Adler, S, et al: PNF in Practice. Springer-Verlag, Berlin, 1993.

135. Logigian, M, et al: Clinical exercise trial for stroke patients. Arch Phys Med Rehabil 64:364, 1983.
136. Stern, P, et al: Effects of facilitation exercise techniques in stroke rehabilitation. Arch Phys Med Rehabil 51:526, 1970.
137. Lord, J, and Hall, K: Neuromuscular reeducation versus traditional programs for stroke rehabilitation. Arch Phys Med Rehabil 67:88, 1986.
138. Dickstein, R, et al: Stroke rehabilitation: Three exercise therapy approaches. Phys Ther 66:1233, 1986.
139. Jongbloed, L, et al: Stroke rehabilitation: Sensorimotor integrative treatment versus functional treatment. Am J Occup Ther 43:391, 1989.
140. Wagenaar, R, et al: The functional recovery of stroke: A comparison between neuro-developmental treatment and the Brunnstrom method. Scand J Rehabil Med 22:1, 1990.
141. Basmajian, J, et al: Stroke treatment: Comparison of integrated behavioral physical therapy vs traditional physical therapy programs. Arch Phys Med Rehabil 68:267, 1987.
142. Ernst, E: A review of stroke rehabilitation and physiotherapy. Stroke 21:1082, 1990.
143. Ashburn, A, et al: Physiotherapy in the rehabilitation of stroke: A review. Clin Rehabil 7:337, 1993.
144. Johnstone, M: Therapy for Stroke. Churchill Livingstone, New York, 1991.
145. Johnstone, M: Restoration of Normal Movement after Stroke Patient. Churchill Livingstone, New York, 1995.
146. Johann, C: Seating and wheeled mobility prescription. In Gillen, G, and Burkhardt, A: Stroke Rehabilitation: A Function Based Approach. Mosby, St. Louis, 1998, p 437.
147. Kumar, R, et al: Shoulder pain in hemiplegia: The role of exercise. Am J Phys Med Rehabil 69:205, 1990.
148. Bohannon, R, et al: Shoulder pain in hemiplegia: Statistical relationship with five variables. Arch Phys Med Rehabil 67:514, 1986.
149. Brooke, M, et al: Shoulder subluxation in hemiplegia: Effects of three different supports. Arch Phys Med Rehabil 72:582, 1991.
150. Gillen, G: Upper extremity function and management. In Gillen, G, and Burkhardt, A: Stroke Rehabilitation. A Function-Based Approach. Mosby, St. Louis, 1998, p 109.
151. Dannenbaum, R, and Dykes, R: Sensory loss in the hand after sensory stroke: Therapeutic rationale. Arch Phys Med Rehabil 69:833, 1988.
152. Weinberg, J, et al: Training sensory awareness and spatial organization in people with right brain damage. Arch Phys Med Rehabil 60:491, 1979.
153. O'Sullivan, S, and Schmitz, T: Physical Rehabilitation Laboratory Manual Focus on Functional Training. FA Davis, Philadelphia, 1999.
154. Horak, F, et al: Postural perturbations: New insights for treatment of balance disorders. Phys Ther 77:517, 1997.
155. Hocherman, S, and Dickstein, R: Postural rehabilitation in geriatric stroke patients. Top Geriatr Rehabil 7:60, 1991.
156. Shumway-Cook, A, et al: Postural sway biofeedback: Its effect on reestablishing stance stability in hemiplegic patients. Arch Phys Med Rehabil 69:395, 1988.
157. Winstein, C, et al: Standing balance training: Effect on balance and locomotion in hemiparetic adults. Arch Phys Med Rehabil 70:755, 1989.
158. Sackley, C, and Baguley, B: Visual feedback after stroke with the balance performance monitor: Two single-case studies. Clin Rehabil 7:189, 1993.
159. Hamman, R, et al: Training effects during repeated therapy sessions of balance training using visual feedback. Arch Phys Med Rehabil 73:738, 1992.
160. McRae, J, et al: Rehabilitation of hemiplegia: Functional outcomes and treatment of postural control. Phys Ther 74(suppl):S119, 1994.
161. Fishman, M, et al: Comparison of functional upper extremity tasks and dynamic standing. Phys Ther 76(suppl):79, 1996.
162. Seeger, B, and Caudrey, D: Biofeedback therapy to achieve symmetrical gait in children with hemiplegic cerebral palsy: Long-term efficacy. Arch Phys Med Rehabil 64:160, 1983.
163. Richards, C, et al: Task-specific physical therapy for optimization of gait recovery in acute stroke patients. Arch Phys Med Rehabil 74:612, 1993.
164. Burdett, R, et al: Gait comparison of subjects with hemiplegia walking unbraced, with ankle-foot orthosis, and with air-stirrup brace. Phys Ther 68:1197, 1988.
165. Lehmann, J, et al: Knee movements: Origin in normal ambulation and their modification by double-stopped ankle-foot orthoses. Arch Phys Med Rehabil 63:345, 1982.
166. Carr, E: Assessment and treatment of feeding difficulties after stroke. Top Geriatr Rehabil 7:35, 1991.
167. Corcoran, P, et al: Effects of plastic and metal braces on speed and energy cost of hemiparetic ambulation. Arch Phys Med Rehabil 5:69, 1970.
168. Hirschberg, G, and Ralston, H: Energy cost of stairclimbing in normal and hemiplegic subjects. Am J Phys Med 44:165, 1965.
169. Bard, G: Energy expenditure of hemiplegic subjects during walking. Arch Phys Med Rehabil 44:368, 1963.
170. Roth, E, et al: Cardiovascular response to physical therapy in stroke rehabilitation. Neurorehabilitation 2:7, 1992.
171. Roth, E, et al: Stroke rehabilitation outcome: Impact of coronary artery disease. Stroke 19:41, 1988.
172. Buck, L: The coincidence of heart disease and stroke: Pathogenesis and considerations for therapy. Neurology Report 18:29, 1994.
173. Monga, T, et al: Cardiovascular response to acute exercise in patients with cerebrovascular accidents. Arch Phys Med Rehabil 69:937, 1988.
174. King, M, et al: Adaptive exercise testing for patients with hemiparesis. J Cardiopulmon Rehabil 9:237, 1989.
175. American College of Sports Medicine: Guidelines for Exercise Testing and Prescription, ed 5. Lea & Febiger, Philadelphia, 1995.
176. American Association of Cardiovascular and Pulmonary Rehabilitation: Guidelines for Cardiac Rehabilitation Programs. Human Kinetics, Champaign, IL, 1991.
177. Gordon, N: Stroke: Your Complete Exercise Guide. Human Kinetics, Champaign, IL, 1993.
178. Brinkmann, J, and Hoskins, T: Physical conditioning and altered self-concept in rehabilitated hemiplegic patients. Phys Ther 59:859, 1979.
179. Tangeman, P, et al: Rehabilitation of chronic stroke patients: Changes in functional performance. Arch Phys Med Rehabil 71:876, 1990.
180. Mandel, A, et al: Electromyographic versus rhythmic positional biofeedback in computerized gait retraining with stroke patients. Arch Phys Med Rehabil 71:649, 1990.
181. Wolf, S, et al: Comparison of motor copy and targeted biofeedback training techniques for restitution of upper extremity function among patients with neurological disorders. Phys Ther 69:719, 1989.
182. Cozean, C, et al: Biofeedback and functional electric stimulation in stroke rehabilitation. Arch Phys Med Rehabil 69:401, 1988.
183. Wolf, S, and Binder-Macleod, S: Electromyographic biofeedback applications to the hemiplegic patient—changes in lower extremity neuromuscular and functional status. Phys Ther 63:1404, 1983.
184. Prevo, A, et al: Effect of EMG feedback on paretic muscles and abnormal co-contraction in the hemiplegic arm, compared with conventional physical therapy. Scand J Rehabil Med 14:121, 1982.
185. Glantz, M, et al: Biofeedback therapy in post-stroke rehabilitation: A meta-analysis of the randomized controlled trials. Arch Phys Med Rehabil 76:508, 1995.
186. Binder, S, et al: Evaluation of electromyographic biofeedback as an adjunct to therapeutic exercise in treating the lower extremities of hemiplegic patients. Phys Ther 61:886, 1981.
187. Mulder, T, et al: EMG feedback and the restoration of motor control. A controlled group study of 12 hemiparetic patients. Am J Phys Med 65:173, 1986.
188. Inglis, J, et al: Electromyographic biofeedback and physical therapy of the hemiplegic upper limb. Arch Phys Med Rehabil 65:755, 1984.
189. Trimble, M, and Enoka, R: Mechanisms underlying the

training effects associated with neuromuscular electrical stimulation. Phys Ther 71:273, 1991.

190. Cranstam, B, et al: Improvement of gait following functional electrical stimulation. Scand J Rehabil Med 9:7, 1977.

191. Merlitte, R, et al: Clinical experience of electronic peroneal stimulators in 50 hemiparetic patients. Scand J Rehabil Med 11:111, 1979.

192. Bowman, B, et al: Positional feedback and electrical stimulation: An automated treatment for the hemiplegic wrist. Arch Phys Med Rehabil 60:497, 1979.

193. Packman-Braun, R: Relationship between functional electrical stimulation duty cycle and fatigue in wrist extensor muscles of patients with hemiparesis. Phys Ther 68:51, 1988.

194. Levine, M, et al: Relaxation of spasticity by electrical stimulation of antagonist muscles. Arch Phys Med 33:668, 1952.

195. Baker, L, and Parker, K: Neuromuscular electrical stimulation of the muscles surrounding the shoulder. Phys Ther 66:1930, 1986.

196. Smith, L: Restoration of volitional limb movement in hemiplegia following patterned functional electrical stimulation. Percept Mot Skills 71:851, 1990.

197. Bogataj, U, et al: The rehabilitation of gait in patients with hemiplegia: A comparison between conventional therapy and multichannel functional electrical stimulation therapy. Phys Ther 75:490, 1995.

198. Jacobs-Daly, J, et al: Electrically induced gait changes post stroke, using an FNS system with intramuscular electrodes and multiple channels. J Neurol Rehab 7:17, 1993.

199. Marsolais, E, et al: FNS application for restoring function in stroke and head-injury patients. J Clinical Engineering 15:489, 1990.

200. Bogataj, U, et al: Restoration of gait during two to three weeks of therapy with multichannel electrical stimulation. Phys Ther 69:319, 1989.

201. Malezic, M, et al: Multichannel electrical stimulation of gait in motor disabled patients. Orthopedics 7:1187, 1984.

202. Stanic, U, et al: Multichannel electrical stimulation for the correction of hemiplegic gait. Scan J Rehabil Med 10:75, 1978.

203. Davidoff, G, et al: Acute stroke patients: Long-term effects of rehabilitation and maintenance of gains. Arch Phys Med Rehabil 72:869, 1991.

204. Tangeman, P, et al: Rehabilitation of chronic stroke patients: Changes in functional performance. Arch Phys Med Rehabil 71:876, 1990.

205. Johnston, M, and Keith, R: Cost-benefits of medical rehabilitation: Review and critique. Arch Phys Med Rehabil 64:147, 1983.

206. Johnston, M, et al: Prediction of outcomes following rehabilitation of stroke patients. Neurorehabilitation 2:72, 1992.

207. Dombovy, M, et al: Rehabilitation for stroke: A review. Stroke 17:363, 1986.

208. Galski T, et al: Predicting length of stay, functional outcome, and aftercare in the rehabilitation of stroke patients. Stroke 24:1794, 1993.

209. Granger, C, and Hamilton, B: Measurement of stroke rehabilitation outcome in the 1980s. Stroke 1990 21(suppl II):1146, 1990.

210. DeJong, G, and Branch, L: Predicting the stroke patient's ability to live independently. Stroke 13:648, 1982.

211. Ahlsio, B, et al: Disablement and quality of life after stroke. Stroke 15:886, 1984.

SUPPLEMENTAL READINGS

Carr, J, and Shephard, R: A Motor Relearning Programme for Stroke, ed 2. Aspen, Rockville, MD, 1987.

Carr, J, and Shephard, R: Neurological Rehabilitation Optimizing Motor Performance. Butterworth Heinemann, Woburn, MA, 1998.

Charness, A: Stroke/Head Injury—A Guide to Functional Outcomes in Physical Therapy Management. Aspen, Rockville, MD, 1986.

Davies, P: Steps to Follow—A Guide to the Treatment of Adult Hemiplegia. Springer-Verlag, New York, 1985.

Davies, P: Right in the Middle—Selective Trunk Activity in the Treatment of Adult Hemiplegia. Springer-Verlag, New York, 1990.

Duncan, P, and Badke, M: Stroke Rehabilitation: The Recovery of Motor Control. Year Book, Chicago, 1987.

Gillen, G, and Burkhardt, A: Stroke Rehabilitation—A Function-Based Approach. Mosby, St. Louis, 1998.

Johnston, M: Restoration of Normal Movement after Stroke. Churchill Livingstone, New York, 1995.

Reyerson, S, and Levit, K: Functional Movement Reeducation. Churchill Livingstone, New York, 1997.

Zoltan, B: Vision, Perception and Cognition, ed 3. Slack, Thorofare, NJ, 1996.

GLOSSARY

Agnosia: The inability to recognize or make sense of incoming information despite intact sensory capacities.

Aneurysm: Localized abnormal dilatation of a blood vessel, usually an artery. Due to congenital defect or weakness of the wall of the vessel.

  Berry aneurysm: A small saccular congenital aneurysm of a cerebral vessel.

Aphasia: An acquired communication disorder caused by brain damage and characterized by an impairment of language comprehension, formulation, and use.

  Fluent aphasia: A type of aphasia in which speech flows smoothly, with a variety of grammatical constructions and preserved melody of speech; paraphasias and circumlocutions may be present. Auditory comprehension may be impaired (e.g., Wernicke's aphasia).

  Nonfluent aphasia: A type of aphasia in which the flow of speech is slow and hesitant; vocabulary is limited, and syntax is impaired; articulation may be labored (e.g., Broca's aphasia).

  Global aphasia: A severe aphasia characterized by marked impairments of both production and comprehension of language; often an indication of extensive brain damage.

Aneurysm: Localized abnormal dilatation of a blood vessel, usually an artery; due to a congenital defect or weakness in the wall of the vessel.

Apraxia: A disorder of voluntary skilled learned movement characterized by an inability to initiate and perform purposeful movements that cannot be accounted for by inadequate strength, loss of coordination, impaired sensation, attention deficits, abnormal tone, movement disorders, intellectual deterioration, poor comprehension or un-cooperativeness.

Ideational: Purposeful movement is not possible, either automatically or on command.

Ideomotor: Purposeful movement is not possible upon command but may occur automatically.

Arteriovenous malformation (AVM): An abnormality in embryonic development leading to a skein of tangled arteries and veins, usually without an intervening capillary bed. It commonly occurs along the distribution of the middle cerebral artery and its rupture produces cerebral hemorrhage.

Aspiration: Penetration of food, liquid, saliva, or gastric reflux into the airway; common in dysphagia patients.

Associated reactions: Automatic responses of the limbs as a result of action occurring in some other part of the body, either by voluntary or reflex stimulation. In hemiplegia, these reactions are stereotyped and abnormal.

Asymmetric tonic neck reflex (ATNR): Head rotation to the left causes extension of the left arm and leg (skull limbs) with flexion of the right arm and leg (jaw limbs); head rotation to the right causes the reverse pattern.

Ataxia: A general term used to describe uncoordinated movement; may influence gait, posture, and patterns of movements.

Atherosclerosis: Thickening of the walls of the arteries due to plaque formation with loss of elasticity and contractility.

Atherothrombotic brain infarction (ABI): Infarction or death of brain tissue resulting from a thrombus.

Attention disorders: Impaired ability to select and attend to a specific stimulus while simultaneously suppressing extraneous stimuli; includes impairments in sustained attention, selective attention, divided attention, or alternating attention.

Autoregulatory mechanisms (cerebral): Mechanisms that modulate a constant rate of blood flow through the brain.

Brain attack: The term used to denote acute stroke; used to help individuals understand the need for early emergency care of stroke.

Brainstem herniation: Secondary brain damage and neurological deterioration resulting from significant edema, elevated intracranial pressures, with resulting contralateral and caudal shifts of brain structures.

Body image disorder: A disturbed perception in the visual and mental image of one's body, including the feelings about one's body, especially in relation to health and disease.

Body scheme disorder: A disturbed perception in the postural model of one's body, including the relationship of the body parts to each other and the relationship of the body to the environment.

Cerebral embolus: Traveling bits of matter formed elsewhere and released into the bloodstream; emboli travel to cerebral vessels where they lodge, producing occlusion and infarction; emboli may be dislodged plaque, or less commonly septic, fat or air molecules.

Cerebral hemorrhage: Abnormal bleeding into the extravascular areas of the brain secondary to aneurysm or trauma.

Intracerebral hemorrhage (IH): Rupture of a cerebral vessel with subsequent bleeding into the cerebral hemispheres.

Subarachnoid hemorrhage (SH): Rupture and bleeding into the subarachnoid space typically from a berry or saccular aneurysm.

Cerebral thrombosis: Formation of a blood clot or thrombus within the cerebral arteries or their branches.

Circle of Willis: Union of the anterior, middle, and posterior cerebral arteries (branches of the carotid and vertebralbasilar arteries), forming an anastomosis at the base of the brain.

Confabulation: The patient fills in memory gaps with inappropriate words or fabricates stories.

Dysarthria: Term for a category of motor speech difficulties caused by impairment in the parts of the central or peripheral nervous system that mediate speech production; respiration, articulation, phonation, resonance, and/or sensory feedback may be affected.

Dysphagia: Inability to swallow or difficulty in swallowing; the result of dysfunction of the lips, mouth, tongue, palate, pharynx, larynx, and/or proximal esophagus.

Early warning signs of stroke: Include sudden and severe headache with no known cause; weakness or numbness of the face, arm, or leg on one side of the body; difficulty speaking or trouble understanding speech; sudden loss or dimming of vision, particularly in one eye; unexplained dizziness, unsteadiness or sudden falls.

Emotional lability (emotional dysregulation syndrome): Unstable or changeable emotional state characterized by pathologic laughing and weeping in which the patient changes quickly from laughing to crying with only slight provocation.

Flaccidity: Deficient or absent muscle tone.

Forced gaze deviation: Deviation of the eyes secondary to unopposed action of eye muscles.

Fugl-Meyer Assessment of Physical Performance (FMA): A stroke assessment instrument organized into five sequential recovery stages; utilizes specific subtests for upper extremity and lower extremity function, balance, sensation, range of motion, and pain; items are scored on a 3-point ordinal scale.

Hemiparesis: Motor weakness (partial paralysis) affecting one half of the body.

Hemiplegia: Motor paralysis of one half of the body.

Homonymous hemianopsia: Loss of vision in the contralateral half of each visual field, the nasal half of one eye and the temporal half of the other eye corresponding to the hemiplegic side.

Homolateral limb synkinesis: An associated reaction between the hemiplegic limbs; flexion of the arm elicits flexion of the leg on the hemiplegic side, or vice versa.

Hyperreflexia: Hyperactive, brisk stretch reflexes; associated with clonus, spasticity and clasp-knife phenomena, and a positive Babinski (upper motor neuron signs).

Ipsilateral pushing (Pusher syndrome): An unusual motor behavior characterized by the patient's strong lateral lean toward the hemiplegic side in all positions.

Locked-in syndrome (LIS): Quadriplegia and anarthria with preserved consciousness; secondary to a ventral pontine lesion.

Memory disorders: An inability to store experiences and perceptions for later recall; commonly includes impairments in immediate recall, short-term memory, or less commonly long-term memory.

Motor impersistence: An inability to sustain a movement or a posture.

Motor Assessment Scale (MAS): A stroke assessment scale that measures impairments and disability using 8 items of motor function and 1 item to assess muscle tone; items are scored using a 6 point ordinal scale.

Multi-infarct dementia: Deteriorative mental state characterized by reduction in intellectual faculties; the result of multiple small strokes.

Perservation: The continued repetition of words, thoughts, or acts not related to current context.

Raimiste's phenomenon: An associated reaction in which abduction or adduction of the normal limb produces a similar response in the affected limb.

Reflex sympathetic dystrophy ([RSD], shoulder-hand syndrome): Pain develops first in the shoulder then hand, followed by the development of sympathetic vasomotor symptoms of the hand. Late stage changes include progressive atrophy of the skin, muscles, and bones; the result of trauma, traction injuries or prolonged immobility of the shoulder or hand.

Reversible ischemic neurological deficit: Impairments resolve spontaneously with neurological recovery, generally within 3 weeks.

Souques' phenomenon: An associated reaction in which elevation of the hemiplegic arm above the horizontal may elicit an extension and abduction response of the fingers.

Spatial relations syndrome: A constellation of perceptual deficits that have in common a difficulty in perceiving the relationship between the self and two or more objects in the environment.

Spasticity: Increased tone of muscle causing stiff, awkward movements; the result of an upper motor lesion.

Stroke (cerebrovascular accident, CVA): Acute onset of neurological dysfunction due to an abnormality in cerebral circulation with signs and symptoms that correspond to involvement of focal areas of the brain.

Deteriorating stroke: Neurological status deteriorates after admission to the hospital.

Major stroke: Stable, usually severe neurological deficit.

Young stroke: Affecting persons below the age of 45.

Subclavian steal syndrome: Shunting of blood, which was destined for the brain, away from the cerebral circulation. This occurs when the subclavian artery is occluded. Blood then flows from the opposite vertebral artery across to and down the vertebral artery on the side of the occlusion.

Symmetric tonic labyrinthine reflex (STLR): A response to positioning in which the supine position produces an increase in extensor tone and the prone position increases flexor tone.

Symmetric tonic neck reflex (STNR): A response to flexion of the neck that results in flexion of the arms and extension of the legs; extension of the neck produces the opposite responses.

Synergies (mass): Stereotyped, mass movement patterns associated with neurological deficit; movements are primitive, automatic, reflexive, and highly stereotyped; characteristic of patients with stroke in the early and middle stages of recovery.

Thalamic sensory syndrome (thalamic pain): A neurogenic condition affecting the superficial sensations (touch, pain, and temperature); continuous, unpleasant sensation or pain on the hemiplegic side.

Tonic lumbar reflex (TLR): Rotation of the upper trunk toward the affected side produces flexion of the upper limb and extension of the lower limb. Rotation towards the sound side produces the opposite response.

Transient ischemic attack (TIA): Temporary interruption of blood supply to the brain. Symptoms of neurological deficit may last for only a few minutes or hours but do not last over 24 hours. After the attack no evidence of residual brain damage or neurological damage remains.

Unilateral neglect: The inability to register and to integrate stimuli and perceptions from one side of the environment (usually the left). As a result, the patient ignores stimuli occurring in that side of personal space.

Visual neglect (visual inattention): Decreased awareness of the body and environment on the side of the body opposite to the cerebral lesion; occurs in the absence of specific sensory deficit.

APPENDIX A

FUGL-MEYER ASSESSMENT OF PHYSICAL PERFORMANCE[1]

Name _____ History Number _____

Age _____ Address _____

Date of CVA _____ Phone _____

Diagnosis _____

Aphasis _____

Sex _____

Handedness _____

Significant Medical History _____

Test Number _____ Tester _____

General Instructions:
Utilize a quiet testing area, free of distractions. Select a time that the patient is optimally alert. Give clear and concise instructions. Utilize demonstration as well as verbal instructions. Motor: instruct the patient to perform the required movement with the non-affected extremity first. Each movement should be repeated three times; scoring is based on the best performance. Verbal encouragement is allowed; direct facilitation of movement is not. Balance: use a firm, unexpected push to test for parachute reactions. Sensation, Joint Motion and Joint Pain: compare responses to the non-affected side. Equipment needed: low plinth or bed, chair, table, reflex hammer, cotton ball, pencil, small peice of cardboard, small jar, tennis ball, stop watch, and blindfold.[63,p216]

---

[1]Fugl-Meyer, A, et al. The post-stroke hemiplegic patient. A method for evaluation of physical performance. Scand J Rehab Med 7:213, 1975, with permission.

Continued

APPENDIX A *Continued*

FUGL-MEYER ASSESSMENT OF PHYSICAL PERFORMANCE

SUMMARY OF SCORES

MOTOR

Upper arm _____   Maximum Score ___36___

Wrist & hand _____   Maximum Score ___30___

    TOTAL UPPER EXTREMITY SCORE _____   MAXIMUM   SCORE ___66___

    TOTAL LOWER EXTREMITY SCORE _____   MAXIMUM   SCORE ___34___

_____   _____   PERCENTAGE
TOTAL MOTOR SCORE _____   TOTAL MAXIMUM SCORE 100   OF RECOVERY
                                                                     _____

BALANCE
       TOTAL SCORE _____   MAXIMUM SCORE ___14___

SENSATION
       TOTAL SCORE _____   MAXIMUM SCORE ___24___

JOINT RANGE OF MOTION
       TOTAL SCORE _____   MAXIMUM SCORE ___44___

PAIN
       TOTAL SCORE _____   MAXIMUM SCORE ___44___

_____   _____   PERCENTAGE
TOTAL FUGL-MEYER SCORE _____   TOTAL MAXIMUM SCORE 226   OF RECOVERY
                                                                     _____

FUGL-MEYER ASSESSMENT OF PHYSICAL PERFORMANCE

Area	Test	Scoring Criteria	Maximum Possible Score	Attained Score
UPPER EXTREMITY (sitting)	*Motor*			

	I. Reflexes
	  a. biceps ____
	  b. triceps ____
		0—No reflex activity can be elicited.
		2—Reflex activity can be elicited.
			4	

	II. Flexor Synergy
	  elevation ____
	  shoulder retraction ____
	  abduction (at least 90°) ____
	  external rotation ____
	  elbow flexion ____
	  forearm supination ____
		0—Cannot be performed at all.
		1—Performed partly.
		2—Performed faultlessly.
			12	

	III. Extensor Synergy
	  shoulder adduction/internal rotation ____
	  elbow extension ____
	  forearm pronation ____
		0—Cannot be performed at all.
		1—Performed partly.
		2—Performed faultlessly.
			6	

	IV. Movement Combining Synergies
	  a. Hand to lumbar spine ____
	
	  b. Shoulder flexion to 90° elbow at 0° ____
	
	  Pronation/supination of forearm with elbow at 90° and shoulder at 0° ____
		0—No specific action performed.
		1—Hand must pass anterior superior iliac spine.
		2—Action is performed faultlessly.
		0—Arm is immediately abducted or elbow flexes at start of motion.
		1—Abduction or elbow flexion occurs in later phase of motion.
		2—Faultless motion.
		0—Correct position of shoulder and elbow cannot be attained, and/or pronation or supination cannot be performed at all.
		1—Active pronation or supination can be performed even within a limited range of motion, and at the same time the shoulder and elbow are correctly positioned.
		2—Complete pronation and supination with correct positions at elbow and shoulder.
			6	

	V. Movement Out of Synergy
	  a. Shoulder abduction to 90° elbow at 0° and forearm pronated ____
	
	  b. Shoulder flexion, 90–180° elbow at 0° and forearm in mid position ____
	
	  c. Pronation/supination of forearm elbow at 0° and shoulder between 30–90° of flexion ____
		a. 0—*Initial* elbow flexion occurs or any deviation from pronated forearm occurs.
		  1—Motion can be performed partly, or if during motion, elbow is flexed or forearm cannot be kept in pronation.
		  2—Faultless motion.
		b. 0—Initial flexion of elbow or shoulder abduction occurs.
		  1—Elbow flexion or shoulder abduction, occurs during shoulder flexion.
		  2—Faultless motion.
		c. 0—Supination and pronation cannot be performed at all or elbow and shoulder positions cannot be attained.
		  1—Elbow and shoulder properly positioned and pronation and supination performed in a limited range.
		  2—Faultless motion.
			6	

Continued

FUGL-MEYER ASSESSMENT OF PHYSICAL PERFORMANCE *Continued*

Area	Test	Scoring Criteria	Maximum Possible Score	Attained Score
UPPER EXTREMITY	*Motor* VI. Normal Reflex Activity ____ biceps and/or finger flexors and triceps ____	(This stage, which can render the score of two, is included only if the patient has a score of 6 in stage V.) 0—At least 2 of the 3 phasic reflexes are markedly hyperactive. 1—One reflex markedly hyperactive or at least 2 reflexes are lively. 2—No more than one reflex is lively and none are hyperactive.	2	
WRIST	VII. a. Stability, elbow at 90°, shoulder at 0° b. Flexion/extension, elbow at 90°, shoulder at 0° ____ c. Stability, elbow at 0°, shoulder at 30° ____ d. Flexion/extension, elbow at 0°, shoulder at 30° ____ e. Circumduction ____	a. 0—Patient cannot dorsiflex wrist to required 15°. 1—Dorsiflexion is accomplished, but no resistance is taken. 2—Position can be maintained with some (slight) resistance. b. 0—Volitional movement does not occur. 1—Patient cannot actively move the wrist joint throughout the total ROM. 2—Faultless, smooth movement. c. Scoring is the same as for item a. d. Scoring is the same as for item b. e. 0—Cannot be performed. 1—Jerky motion or incomplete circumduction. 2—Complete motion with smoothness.	10	
HAND	VIII. a. Finger Mass Flexion ____ b. Finger Mass Extension ____ c. Grasp #1—MP joints extended and PIPS & DIPS are flexed. Grasp is tested against resistance. d. Grasp #2—Patient is instructed to adduct thumb, 1st carpometacarpophalangeal and interphalangeal joint at 0° e. Grasp #3—Patient opposes the thumb pad against the pad of index finger. A pencil is interposed ____ f. Grasp #4—The patient should grasp a cylinder shaped object (small can), the volar surface of the 1st and 2nd finger against each other ____ g. Grasp #5—A spherical grasp.	a. 0—No flexion occurs. 1—Some flexion, but not full motion. 2—Complete active flexion (compared with unaffected hand). b. 0—No extension occurs. 1—Patient can release an active mass flexion grasp. 2—Full active extension. c. 0—Required position cannot be acquired. 1—Grasp is weak. 2—Grasp can be maintained against relatively great resistance. d. 0—Function cannot be performed. 1—Scrap of paper interposed between the thumb and index finger can be kept in place, but not against a slight tug. 2—Paper is held firmly against a tug. e. Scoring procedures are the same as for Grasp #2. f. Scoring procedures are the same as for Grasp #2 and #3. g. Scoring procedures are the same as for Grasp #2, 3, and 4.	14	
HAND	IX. Coordination/Speed—Finger to nose (five repetitions in rapid succession). a. Tremor ____ b. Dysmetria ____ c. Speed ____	a. 0—Marked tremor. 1—Slight tremor. 2—No tremor. b. 0—Pronounced or unsystematic dysmetria. 1—Slight or systematic dysmetria. 2—No dysmetria. c. 0—Activity is more than 6 seconds longer than unaffected hand. 1—2 to 5 seconds longer than unaffected hand. 2—Less than 2 seconds difference.	6	
		TOTAL MAXIMUM SCORE OF UPPER EXTREMITY	66	

FUGL-MEYER ASSESSMENT OF PHYSICAL PERFORMANCE

Area	Test	Scoring Criteria	Maximum Possible Score	Attained Score
LOWER EXTREMITY (supine)	I. Reflex activity—tested in supine position. Achilles ____ Patellar ____	0—No reflex activity 2—Reflex activity	4	
Supine	II. A. Flexor Synergy Hip flexion ____ Knee flexion ____ Ankle dorsiflexion ____	A. 0—Cannot be performed 1—Partial motion 2—Full motion	6	
	B. Extensor synergy—(motion is resisted) Hip extension ____ Adduction ____ Knee extension ____ Ankle plantarflexion ____	B. 0—No motion 1—Weak motion 2—Almost full strength compared to normal	8	
SITTING (knees free of chair)	III. Movement Combining Synergies A. Knee flexion beyond 90° ____ B. Ankle dorsiflexion ____	A. 0—No active motion 1—From slightly extended position knee can be flexed but not beyond 90° B. 0—No active flexion 1—Incomplete active flexion 2—Normal dorsiflexion	4	
STANDING	IV. Movement out of Synergy Hip at 0° A. Knee flexion ____ B. Ankle dorsiflexion ____	A. 0—Knee cannot flex without hip flexion 1—Knee begins flexion without hip flexion, but doesn't get to 90°, or hip flexes during motion 2—Full motion as described B. 0—No active motion 1—Partial motion 2—Full motion	4	
SITTING	V. Normal Reflexes Knee flexors ____ Patellar ____ Achilles ____	0—2 of the 3 are markedly hyperactive 1—One reflex is hyperactive or 2 reflexes are lively 2—No more than 1 reflex lively	2	
(SUPINE)	VI. Coordination/Speed Heel to opposite knee (5 repetitions in rapid succession) A. Tremor ____ B. Dysmetria ____ C. Speed ____	A. 0—Marked tremor 1—Slight tremor 2—No tremor B. 0—Pronounced or unsystematic 1—Slight or systematic 2—No dysmetria C. 0—Six seconds slower than unaffected side 1—Two to 5 seconds slower 2—Less than 2 seconds difference	6	
		TOTAL MAXIMUM LOWER EXTREMITY SCORE	34	

Continued

FUGL-MEYER ASSESSMENT OF PHYSICAL PERFORMANCE *Continued*

Area	Test	Scoring Criteria	Maximum Possible Score	Attained Score
BALANCE	1. Sit without support ____	0—Cannot maintain sitting without support 1— Can sit unsupported less than 5 minutes 2— Can sit longer than 5 minutes		
	2. Parachute reaction, non-affected side ____	0— Does not abduct shoulder or extend elbow 1— Impaired reaction 2— Normal reaction		
	3. Parachute reaction, affected side ____	Scoring is the same as #2		
	4. Supported standing	0— Cannot stand 1— Stands with maximum support of others 2— Stands with minimum support of one for 1 minute		
	5. Stand without support	0— Cannot stand 1— Stands less than 1 minute or sways 2— Stands with good balance more than 1 min.		
	6. Stand on unaffected side ____	0— Cannot be maintained longer than 1–2 sec. 1— Stands balanced 4–9 seconds 2— Stands balanced more than 10 sec.		
	7. Stand on affected side ____	0— Scoring is the same as #6		
		MAXIMUM BALANCE SCORE	14	
UPPER AND LOWER EXTREMITIES	*Sensation* I. Light Tough a. Upper arm ____ b. Palm of hand ____ c. Thigh ____ d. Sole of foot ____	0— Anesthesia 1— Hyperaesthesia/dyesthesia 2— Normal	8	
	II. Proprioception a. Shoulder ____ b. Elbow ____ c. Wrist ____ d. Thumb ____ e. Hip ____ f. Knee ____ g. Ankle ____ h. Toe ____	0— No sensation 1— Three quarter of answers are correct, but considerable difference in sensation compared with unaffected side. 2— All answers are correct, little or no difference	16	

FUGL-MEYER ASSESSMENT OF PHYSICAL PERFORMANCE

Area	Test		Scoring Criteria	Maximum Possible Score	Attained Score
	Joint Pain/Motion Motion	Pain			
SHOULDER	Flexion		Motion Scoring	Motion	
	Abduction to 90°		0— Only a few degrees of motion	44	
	External rotation		1— Decreased passive range of motion		
	Internal rotation		2— Normal passive range of motion		
ELBOW	Flexion				
	Extension		Pain Scoring	44	
WRIST	Flexion		0— Marked pain at end of range or pain through range		
	Extension		1— Some pain		
FINGERS	Flexion		2— No pain		
	Extension				
FOREARM	Pronation				
	Supination				
HIP	Flexion				
	Abduction				
	External rotation				
	Internal rotation				
KNEE	Flexion				
	Extension				
ANKLE	Dorsiflexion				
	Plantarflexion				
FOOT	Pronation				
	Supination				

APPENDIX B

Suggested Answers to Case Study Guiding Questions

1. Identify/categorize this patient's problems in terms of: direct impairments, indirect impairments, composite impairments, and functional limitations/disabilities.

ANSWER

Direct	Indirect	Composite	Functional Limitations
dec. cognition	RUE/LE pain	dec. dynamic sitting balance	dec. bed mobility
aphasia, receptive & expressive	dec. ROM R. ankle	dec static/ dynamic standing balance	dec. transfers
mild motor apraxia		gait deviations	dec. w/c mobility
R unilateral neglect		dec. safety awareness	dec. ambu- lation
dec. RUE/LE sensation			dec. BADL's
RUE/LE hemiparesis			
RUE/LE hypertonicity			
Impaired voluntary movement			
RUE/LE synergy patterns			
associated reactions			

2. Identify your goals (remediation of impairments) and outcomes (remediation of functional limitations/disability) for this patient.

ANSWER

1. Goals (immediate, short-term goals):
   a. Patient will be independent in bed mobility: rolling onto the R side and supine-to-sit from the R 100% of the time within 2 weeks.
   b. Patient will be independent in bridging while maintaining RUE in an inhibitory prayer position, 100% of the time within 2 weeks.
   c. Patient will be independent and safe in sit-to-stand transfers 100% of time within 2 weeks.
   d. Patient will demonstrate symmetrical weight shifting in sitting, BUEs in a prayer position, with supervision, 4 out of 5 trials, within 2 weeks.
   e. Patient will maintain a symmetrical position in kneeling, with BUEs in a prayer position, for 2 minutes, within 2 weeks.
2. Outcomes:
   a. Patient will be I and safe in functional mobility skills (bed mobility, transfers, w/c mobility).
   b. Patient will be I and safe in ambulation for community distances with a right AFO and cane on all surfaces and stairs.
   c. Patient will be I and safe in all basic and instrumental ADLs.

d. Patient and family will understand and verbalize safety precautions during all functional mobility skills.

3. Formulate five treatment interventions with one progression that could be used during the first 3 weeks of therapy. Provide a brief rationale that justifies your choice.

ANSWER

TREATMENT INTERVENTION 1:

Bed mobility: Rolling onto the affected side, sidelying on R elbow, progressing to sitting from the R side, using BUE for support, active assistive movement.

Rationale: Promotes independent bed mobility, use of the affected side and integration.

TREATMENT INTERVENTION 2:

Bridging: assumption of the bridge position with BUE in prayer position, active assisted movements progressing to agonist reversals.

Rationale: Bridging breaks up LE synergy pattern, strengthens hip extensors, knee flexors, and ankle stabilizers, promotes early weight-bearing through the foot and ankle. Important as a lead-up skill for bed mobility, sit-to-stand transitions, and gait (end stance and toe-off).

TREATMENT INTERVENTION 3:

Sitting: Weight shifts in all directions with emphasis on increasing range of shifts to the R side, BUE extended hands in a prayer position, progressing to sitting, chop/reverse chop PNF patterns.

Active assisted movement to slow reversals (PNF pattern).

Rationale: Improves postural control (trunk rotation), promotes dynamic balance control in sitting, decreases unilateral neglect (BUEs in prayer position).

TREATMENT INTERVENTION 4:

Kneeling: Holding, symmetrical weight-bearing, BUE extended, hands in prayer position, alternating isometrics/rhythmic stabilization.

Progressing to kneeling, weight shifts with emphasis on increasing range to the R side, active assisted movement to slow reversals.

Rationale: Provides inhibitory influence to spastic knee extensors while promoting hip extensor and trunk control in upright, antigravity position, decreases unilateral neglect (BUEs in prayer position).

TREATMENT INTERVENTION 5:

Sit-to-stand movement transitions, BUEs extended with hands in a prayer position.

Active assisted movement, high seat progressing to low seat.

Rationale: Promotes independence in functional mobility, strengthens hip and knee extensors, promotes postural control and dynamic balance.

4. Identify relevant teaching/motor learning strategies appropriate for the initial rehabilitation sessions with this patient.

ANSWER

1. Communication: Maintain eye contact, speak slowly and directly to patient. Use one-step commands.
2. Demonstration: Carefully demonstrate all training activities to patient. Be sure to demonstrate ideal performance of desired skill. Utilize manual guidance as appropriate to assist early learning.
3. Emphasize use of visual feedback to facilitate early learning; have the patient look at movements to improve movement control.
4. Bilateral transfer: Have the patient practice the desired skill using the L extremities first. Then practice the desired task using the affected extremities.
5. Promote reintegration of the two sides of the body. Emphasize/utilize the R extremities in all tasks as appropriate.
6. Utilize a distributed practice schedule to improve initial performance. Frequent rests minimize stress and fatigue and promote ease of movement.
7. Utilize a closed environment, free of distractions to maximize early learning.
8. Include patient and family in decision making. Encourage active participation of family members early in rehabilitation.
9. Carefully monitor signs of frustration and fatigue. Provide encouragement and positive feedback. Reward successes while providing a realistic appraisal of performance.

Peripheral Vascular Disease and Wound Care

C. Alan Knight

LEARNING OBJECTIVES

1. Identify risk factors that contribute to peripheral vascular disease.
2. Understand the physiology and pathophysiology of the peripheral vascular system.
3. Recognize the characteristic features commonly associated with different peripheral vascular diseases.
4. Identify the components of a comprehensive examination of a patient with peripheral vascular disease.
5. Describe physical therapy interventions for patients with peripheral vascular disease.
6. Explain the role of physical therapy in wound care.

INTRODUCTION

The human circulatory system is a uniquely designed tubular delivery system in which blood, the fluid that sustains life, is distributed throughout the body via a four-chambered muscular pump and a maze of highly organized pathways called the *peripheral vascular system*. The primary function of the circulatory system is to transport and deliver oxygen, nutrients, and waste products through the arterial, capillary, venous, and lymphatic systems. This chapter focuses on the peripheral vascular system and the major disease processes associated with the arterial and venous structures as well as pathology of the lymphatic system. Physical therapists are among the primary team members involved in management of peripheral vascular disease (PVD). PVD is often associated with an underlying cause such as cerebral vascular accident (CVA), amputation, or aneurysm. Management of PVD also includes wound care. Upon completion of a thorough examination of the patient, the physical therapist can determine which system is involved and can manage the disease appropriately.

ANATOMY AND PHYSIOLOGY OF THE PERIPHERAL VASCULAR SYSTEM

The human body is a magnificent creation with remarkable systems that produce movement, create thought, and sustain life. But there are times when even the most advanced systems begin to fail. Attention to normal anatomical and physiological function is essential to understanding the pathology associated with the peripheral vascular system.

General Blood Vessel Structure

The peripheral vascular system can be divided into two distinct systems: the *arterial system* and the *venous system*. Many experts include a third system, the *lymphatic system*. The lymphatic system works in conjunction with the venous system, to assist uptake of excessive extracellular fluid and waste products in the tissues. It also provides a defense against pathogens that enter the body.

The framework of the peripheral vascular system is the blood vessels. Vessel structure is dependent on

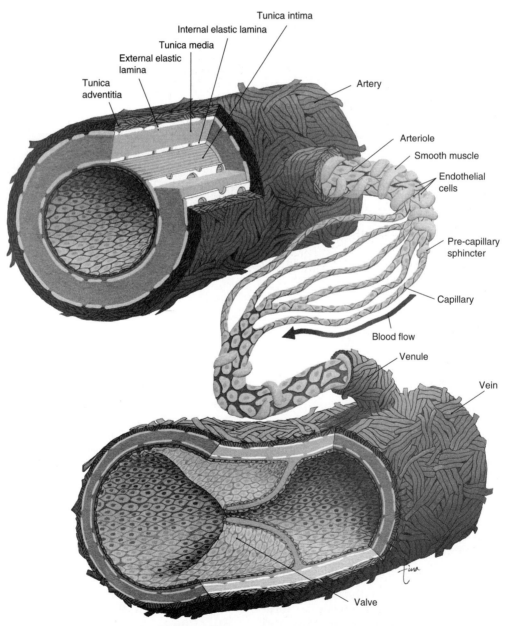

Figure 18-1. Structure of an artery, arteriole, capillary network, venule, and vein. (From Scanlon, VC, and Sanders, T: Essentials of Anatomy and Physiology, ed 2. FA Davis, Philadelphia, p 283, with permission.)

the type of vessel as well as its required function. The basic design of all vessels is the presence of three layers of tissue called *tunics* (Fig. 18-1). The *tunica intima* is the innermost layer of the vessel, and is composed of three layers: endothelium, connective tissue, and a basement membrane. The endothelial layer is the only layer present in all vessels and is a continuous layer with the endocardium of the heart.[1] The next layer is the *tunica media*, composed mainly of smooth muscle. This layer makes up the bulk of the arterial vessel wall. The outermost layer is the *tunica adventitia*, which contains both elastic and collagenous fibers that embody the vessel wall. This layer is the thickest in the vein.

The Arterial System

Arteries are the elastic, muscular, tubular extensions of the heart that carry oxygen-rich blood at high pressures to all parts of the body. Pressures within the vessel vary according to the type of organ supplied and the distance from the heart. Pressures are greater in the major arteries near the heart compared to the pressures in smaller, more distal arteries, especially during ventricular contraction. The vessels close to the heart are more elastic in nature. The distal vessels tend to be more muscular to propel the blood to the outermost regions of the body. Because of the contractile nature of the vessels, the arterial system operates without the assistance of valves. The arterial vasculature has the ability to vasoconstrict and vasodilate secondary to impulses sent via the sympathetic branches of the autonomic nervous system (which stimulates the vasomotor fibers of the vessel).[2]

The artery branches off into smaller arteries called **arterioles,** which eventually lead to the smallest of all the vessels known as **capillaries.** This is the level at which exchange of gases, nutrients, and waste occur between the cells and the capillary complex to maintain cellular survival.

The Venous System

The veins, which receive the deoxygenated blood, are structured similarly to the arteries. However, the tunica media is poorly developed and has an insignificant supply of elastic or smooth muscle fibers. Because of the inability to contract, the vein relies on a system of valves that assist the return of blood to the heart. The valves are formed from the tunica intima layer and are designed to allow only a one-way flow of blood. As blood circulates toward the heart, the valves are open and allow for smooth passage of blood proximally through the vein. When blood attempts to flow back, the flaps fill with blood, closing the valves and preventing reflux of blood (Fig. 18-2). The valves of the venous system are more common in the lower limbs where the forces of gravity are the greatest.

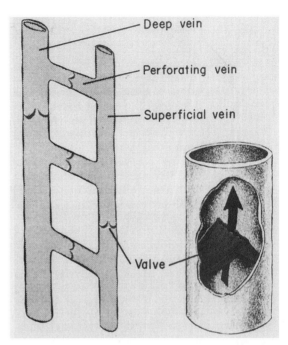

Figure 18-2. The venous valves of the legs. (From Textbook of Medical Physiology, ed 7. WB Saunders, Philadelphia, with permission.)

As blood moves through the peripheral vascular system, pressures decrease as it moves through the arterial vessels toward the veins. Therefore, movement of blood through veins is not as dependent on heart function as in the arteries. Blood flow now is contingent on valvular competency and skeletal muscle contraction.[3] For example, when the skeletal muscle surrounding a vein contracts, it presses on the vessel causing a squeezing or milking effect. This propels the blood through the vein toward the heart (Fig. 18-3).

The venous system has divisions that are unique to the lower extremity. They are classified as the superficial veins, perforating veins, and deep veins. The superficial system is composed of the subcutaneous veins that are sometimes visible through the skin. The perforating or communicating veins provide a connection between the superficial and deep veins. The deep veins are larger in size and usually follow their corresponding arteries.

The Lymphatic System

To thoroughly understand the peripheral vascular system, a third vessel system will be briefly reviewed. The lymphatic system, a system closely related to the cardiovasculature of the body, assists in circulating body fluids and providing a mechanism of defense against pathogens. The lymphatics of the human body include extensive networks of capillaries, collecting vessels, lymph nodes, and lymph organs such as the tonsils, spleen, and thymus. One of the major tasks of the lymph system is to serve as a transport channel for fluid and proteins from the interstitium to return back to the blood stream. The lymphatics

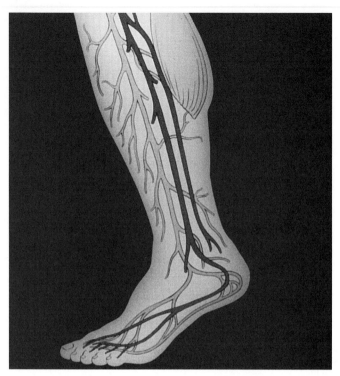

Figure 18-3. Calf muscle pump function.

also serve as an immunological surveillance system of peripheral antigens and circulating leukocytes. The lymph vessels have a similar design as the venous system in that they rely on peristaltic motion and valvular closure to move fluid toward the central ducts that empty into the venous system.[4]

DISEASES OF THE PERIPHERAL VASCULAR SYSTEM

Vascular disease ranks as an important cause of morbidity and mortality. Clinical diagnosis and selection of interventions are key issues in management of this disease process. Careful attention to patient history and physical examination data is essential to determine the type of peripheral vascular disease and course of action to treat the condition. Of all the peripheral vascular diseases, a majority of the cases are diagnosed with chronic venous insufficiency (CVI). Usually associated with CVI is the presence of a leg ulcer. Among patients with leg ulcerations aged 65 or older, venous insufficiency was found in 82 percent, arterial insufficiency in 38 percent, and diabetes in 38 percent.[5]

Diseases of the Artery

Four major risk factors are associated with development of arterial insufficiency. These include *smoking, diabetes,* a *high-fat diet,* and *hypertension.*

ACUTE ARTERIAL OCCLUSIVE DISEASE
Arterial Thrombosis and Embolism

A sudden cessation of blood flow to an extremity, usually requiring emergency surgical intervention, is the most common presentation of acute arterial occlusive disease. Etiology of this disease is not completely understood, but frequently the occlusion is the result of a thrombus or embolus. Symptoms are usually an abrupt onset of pain, deathlike **pallor,** and lack of pulses. As **ischemia** progresses, paresthesias can develop. Cutaneous sensations are the first to be disrupted followed by complete loss of sensation. Further advancement of the ischemic condition leads to decreased motor function, **gangrene,** and even paralysis.[6]

Cases of arterial thrombosis, in which a clot, plaque, or foreign body blocks the vessel, are often associated with a preexisting atherosclerotic condition that leads to turbulent flow of blood in the lumen. The turbulence can activate platelet collection against the preexisting plaque material resulting in a blockage. This causes partial or complete blockage from a *thrombus*.

In formation of an arterial *embolism,* portions of the previously formed thrombus can break away. The embolism then courses through the vascular system until it becomes lodged in a smaller diameter artery. This results in an ischemic condition at another portion of the artery.[7]

CHRONIC ARTERIAL INSUFFICIENCY
Atherosclerosis

It is estimated that approximately 50 percent of all deaths in the United States associated with arterial disease are caused by **atherosclerosis.**[8] This condition is characterized by nodular deposits of fatty material that can line the wall of the artery (Fig. 18-4). These deposits, known as *plaques,* gradually decrease the size of the lumen, impede the flow of blood through the vessel, and can potentially cause complete blockage of the vessel. As a result, ischemia and tissue necrosis can occur, which ultimately lead to development of gangrene. Atherosclerosis not only affects vascular structures but also impairs vascular reactivity. Normal endothelium-dependent mechanisms of vascular relaxation are impaired, which predisposes the vessel to excessive vasoconstriction.[9]

The vessel walls of the arterial system may develop degenerative changes in which they lose their elasticity and become *sclerotic,* otherwise known as "hardening of the arteries" or **arteriosclerosis** obliterans, a peripheral manifestation of atherosclerosis. Arteriosclerosis obliterans is responsible for 95 percent of cases of chronic occlusive arterial disease.[10] Because of the inability to expand and constrict with changing pressures, the vessel may rupture.

Clinically, a patient typically presents with the symptom of **intermittent claudication.** This symptom is related to the supply and demand of blood needed during muscle activity. During episodes of

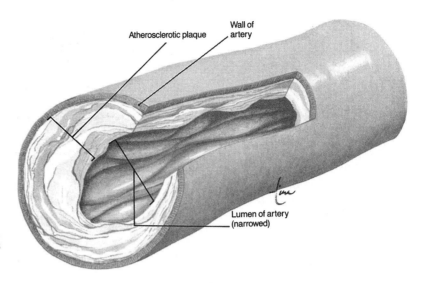

Figure 18-4. Atherosclerosis obstructing blood flow in an artery. (From Scanlon, VC, and Sanders, T: Essentials of Anatomy and Physiology, ed 2. FA Davis, Philadelphia, p 284, with permission.)

intermittent claudication, the supply of blood is less than the muscle's demand, which produces pain and cramping in the involved muscles. The calf musculature is most often affected. Typically, the symptomatic threshold of intermittent claudication is associated with approximately 50 percent occlusion of the affected vessel. Another common symptom associated with arterial insufficiency is *rest pain*. Rest pain, an expression of reduced basal blood flow, is manifested when the occlusion of the vessel is greater than 80 to 90 percent.[11] Patient complaints of rest pain are usually noted when the patient is sedentary or attempting to sleep at night. The pain is usually severe and unrelenting at times. Distal structures are deprived of blood when the extremity is elevated even in a supine position because of the occlusive disease. Other components of the clinical picture include diminished or absent pulses, pallor of the skin, **trophic changes,** an extremity cool to the touch, and possibly the presence of a wound (Fig. 18-5).

Thromboangiitis Obliterans

Thromboangiitis, also known as Burger's Disease, is another cause of occlusive arterial disease of the extremities. This disease is relatively rare yet clinically similar to atherosclerosis except that it occurs primarily in young men who smoke heavily. It affects the small vessels of the extremities beginning distally and moving proximally. Etiology is still not completely understood, but there appears to be a direct correlation between cigarette smoking and manifestation of the disease. Symptoms are exacerbated with smoking and cease when smoking is stopped.[12] The inflammatory reaction appears owing to an increased sensitivity to nicotine, which prompts an invasion of lymphocytes. The arterial occlusion is usually the result of a thrombus.

As mentioned, the symptoms of thromboangiitis obliterans parallel those of atherosclerosis but are typically more severe. Rest pain is usually the initial symptom followed by intermittent claudication.

However, the claudication affects the foot more than the calf.[13]

FUNCTIONAL ARTERIAL DISORDERS

The arterial diseases in this classification of peripheral vascular disease are caused by vasospasms or excessive dilation of the affected vessels. These include such disorders as **Raynaud's syndrome, acrocyanosis,** and **erythromelalgia.**

Raynaud's phenomenon, a hallmark of Raynaud's syndrome, refers to spasm of arterioles affecting the digits, along with intermittent pallor of

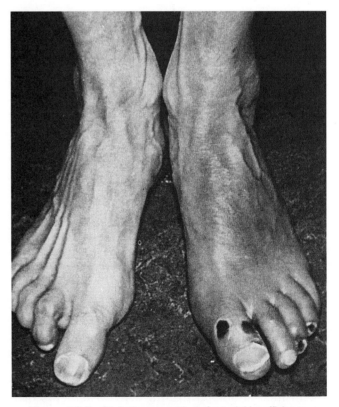

Figure 18-5. Clinical presentation of arterial insufficiency.

the skin. Exact etiology may be idiopathic or secondary to other conditions such as **scleroderma,** rheumatoid arthritis, systemic lupus erythematosus (SLE), or some other arterial occlusive disease.[14] Clinical manifestation of Raynaud's syndrome consists of intermittent attacks of **cyanosis** of the digits when exposed to cold or emotional upset. Warming usually restores color to the hands. The thumb is rarely involved. Pain is usually not present but the individual may report paresthesia. Small ulcerations at the tips of the fingers may occur. There is usually no report of intermittent claudication and the distal pulses are usually palpable.

Acrocyanosis is cyanosis of the distal extremities. It typically affects hands and fingers or the feet and toes. Erythromelalgia is bilateral vasodilation affecting the extremities, especially the feet. It is marked by redness, burning, and throbbing sensations and increased skin temperature.

Diseases of the Vein

Peripheral vascular diseases related to dysfunction of the venous system are more prevalent than those of an arterial origin. It is estimated that 24 million people are afflicted with varicose veins and approximately 7 million experience venous insufficiency.[15] This higher incidence of venous involvement is not well understood. Unlike the arterial diseases that have several major risk factors contributing to their development, venous disease has only family history as a major risk factor.[16]

ACUTE VENOUS DISEASE

When a patient is diagnosed with a venous disease such as thrombosis or thromboembolism, a referral to physical therapy is postponed. Those at increased risk include patients on bed rest (e.g., following surgical intervention) and patients using drugs that promote clotting.

Venous thrombosis is defined as an obstruction of the blood flow in the vein secondary to a collection of coagulated blood. Pain associated with the thrombus is related to the periphlebitis (inflammation of tissues around the vein), a symptom relieved by recumbence. The pain is usually described as a deep ache in the muscle such as a "Charlie horse."[17]

Superficial venous thrombosis (SVT) or true phlebitis is somewhat different from deep venous thrombosis (DVT) seen clinically. The major defining feature of SVT is the conspicuous cordlike nodules that can be palpated along the affected vein. The more prevalent of the two is DVT. Clinical manifestation of DVT includes the presentation of *Homans' signs.* These signs include an increase in edema or girth of the affected limb, painful palpation or painful passive stretch of the vein, and an extremity that is significantly warmer when compared to the unaffected limb.

Thromboembolism occurs when fragments of a thrombus detach and lodge in smaller vessels and obstruct blood flow. The common sites for a lower extremity embolism to lodge are the lungs and the brain. In both cases death can occur.

VARICOSE VEINS

A condition of the veins that affects approximately 15 percent of all adults is *varicose veins.* Causes of varicose veins or varicosities can be linked to a family history and an occupation that requires prolonged standing in one position. Obesity and pregnancy can contribute to the problem.[18]

Treatment is discontinued if the condition develops during the course of physical therapy intervention.

The pathology of varicose veins is usually attributed to prevalence of incompetent valves, which produce increased venous pressure and eventually lead to an overstretched vein. The varicosities are characterized by large, bulbous enlargements of the veins beneath the skin, especially in the lower extremities.

CHRONIC VENOUS INSUFFICIENCY

CVI is a frequently diagnosed vascular disease. This disease is largely confined to the lower extremities and is usually unilateral. It is characterized by both *macrocirculatory* and *microcirculatory* dysfunction of the venous system. This dysfunction results in increased venous hypertension, which can eventually progress to a chronic condition and become physically, emotionally, and socially debilitating.

The macrocirculatory components to the pathophysiology of venous insufficiency have several manifestations. Normal valvular function begins to fail and the valve loses its ability to properly close. Leaflet destruction or vein distention are significant findings with a poorly functioning valve. Because the valve or valves do not close properly, this leads to a condition known as **venous reflux.** This is described as the backward flow of blood through a diseased vein.

The macrocirculatory component known as the calf muscle pump, an important mechanism for the movement of blood through the venous system, can also be affected. This results in a diminished ability to eject venous blood flow from the calf back to the heart. Another macrocirculatory mechanism that plays an important role in the movement of venous blood is the venous plexus of the foot. This sensitive plexus, located at the arch of the foot, is activated with each step and shunts blood through the venous system toward the heart. Individuals with poor mobility and decreased ambulatory status begin to lose both of these valuable hemodynamic controls.

Pressure in the venous system has been studied by Browse[19] in both normal and abnormal vessels. At rest, the venous system has a pressure of approximately 90 mmHg. During contraction of the calf muscles, the pressure increases to around 200 mmHg in the deep venous system. After contraction, the pressure drops to 10 mmHg in the deep system and to 30 mmHg in the superficial system. The blood now moves from higher pressure to lower pressure, which means blood flows from the superficial to the deep venous system. With venous insufficiency, the pressure will remain higher in the deep system owing to the pathology described and can result in blood moving in the wrong direction in the venous system, and therefore increased venous hypertension. Owing to the increased venous hypertension and congestion that occurs with CVI, clinical presentation includes an edematous lower extremity as well as erythema, dermatitis, and stasis pigmentation termed *hemosiderin* (a dark staining pigment by-product of lysed red blood cells that causes an internal stain of the affected limb).

The development of a leg ulceration in the presence of CVI can also occur. The largest number of lower extremity ulcerations (80%) result from venous insufficiency.[20] The microcirculatory components of venous disease are not completely understood, but several theories do exist to explain the sequelae of this disease process and subsequent breakdown in the integumentary system.

The *Fibrin-cuff Theory* was first described by Browse and Burnand.[21] It postulates that a leakage of fibrinogen occurs through the pores created from the distended vein secondary to the elevated venous pressures. The fibrinogen develops into a fibrin cuff around the vessel producing a cascade of events in which tissue oxygenation and tissue repair decreases. The skin begins to develop **lipodermatosclerosis.**

The *Leukocyte Trapping Theory*, which is associated with the Fibrin-cuff Theory, was proposed by Coleridge-Smith et al.[22] It identifies the trapping of neutrophils (a granular leukocyte) in the endothelial lining. These neutrophils then become activated and release cytokines (proteins produced primarily in the white blood cells) that damage the vessel wall. Figure 18-6 represents the sequence of events that may occur with CVI.

Another microcirculatory event that may lead to venous ulceration is the most recent theory described by Greenwood et al.[23] known as the

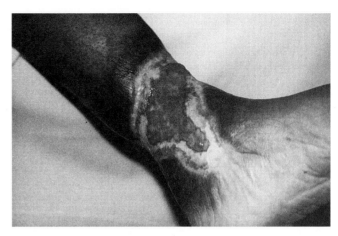

Figure 18-7. Venous insufficiency with leg ulcer.

ischemia-reperfusion injury. This condition can be most easily described by the presence of free radicals that can develop in the body. Free radicals are highly reactive molecules that can become chemically active under certain conditions, such as a condition of ischemia-reperfusion. When tissues are deprived of blood and then reperfused, free radicals are released and result in damage or death of tissues. The endothelial lining of capillaries are affected, resulting in increased leakage from the vessel.

A common characteristic of CVI leg ulcers is the location of the wounds on the affected extremity (Fig. 18-7). An overwhelming majority of leg ulcers develop along the medial aspect of the lower extremity. Several different theories attempt to explain this anatomical predilection for ulcer development. The most common explanation is associated with dysfunction of the perforating or communicating veins. The formation of venous ulcers along the medial aspect of the lower leg may be related to the location of the perforating veins (found along the medial aspect of the lower extremity). If valvular incompetence develops in the perforators and reflux is significant, high pressure can develop at the junction of the superficial vein and the perforating vein. This leads to tissue ischemia and ultimately a skin ulceration along the medial aspect of the leg at the medial maleollar area.[21]

Lymphedema: Clinical Picture, Classification, and Causes

The clinical picture seen in lymphedematous skin is caused by a pathophysiological process that precedes the failure of the lymphatic system. The decreased transport capacity of the lymph system leads to an increase in protein-rich fluid. This lymphostatic condition can affect the dermal microcirculation in which the artery and venous system become damaged. This condition is known as *lymphostatic hemangiopathy*. The surrounding tissues are then infiltrated by a number of inflammatory cells. This inflammatory response releases cytokines that act on epidermal and dermal struc-

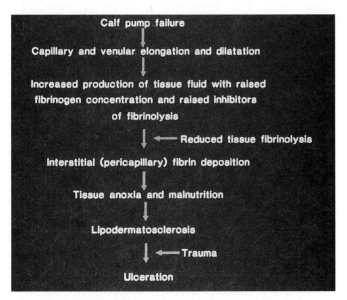

Calf pump failure

↓

Capillary and venular elongation and dilatation

↓

Increased production of tissue fluid with raised fibrinogen concentration and raised inhibitors of fibrinolysis

↓ ← Reduced tissue fibrinolysis

Interstitial (pericapillary) fibrin deposition

↓

Tissue anoxia and malnutrition

↓

Lipodermatosclerosis

↓ ← Trauma

Ulceration

Figure 18-6. Cascade of events of venous insufficiency.[19]

tures such as the connective tissue, collagen, and elastic fibers. Vascular proliferation, angiosarcomas, and fibrosis occur, which ultimately lead to chronic lymphedema.[24]

The first clinical classification system for lymphedema was devised by Kinmonth et al.[25] in 1957, which divided all cases into secondary and primary lymphedema. Secondary lymphedemas are classified as those caused by a recognized extrinsic disease process. Secondary lymphedema is more common than primary. These types of lymphedema result from obstruction, obliteration, or functional insufficiency of the lymphatics secondary to some identifiable pathological process. These processes include lymphedema associated with infection, inflammation (with no evidence of infection), trauma, malignancies, or underlying venous disease. Primary lymphedemas include those in which no other disease process or intrinsic abnormalities can be identified. Considerable confusion surrounds the pathophysiology of primary lymphedema, and has resulted in a variety of classification systems. An age-related classification with no reference to etiology was developed by Kinmouth et al.[25] that divided lymphedema into the following three subgroups:
- Congenital (lymphedema at birth)
- Praecox (presenting before age 35)
- Tarda (after age 35)

In the 1950s, Kinmonth[26] developed another system based on the following three major categories of lymphographic findings:
- **Aplasia** (no formed lymph pathways) (e.g. Milroy's disease)
- Hypoplasia (lymphatics present but less than normal)
- Hyperplasia (lymphatics larger and more numerous)

A third classification system that includes both clinical and lymphographic abnormalities was developed by Browse and Stewart:[27]
- Distal obliteration, which constitutes approximately 80 percent of the primary lymphedemas, is described as total absence or reduction in number of distal lymphatics; usually presents as mild edema of both ankles and lower leg.
- Proximal obliteration (approximately 10%) usually involves the entire limb and is unilateral.
- Congenital lymphedema (approximately 10%) usually presents at birth or an early age and can be either unilateral or bilateral in presentation.

EXAMINATION AND TREATMENT OF PERIPHERAL VASCULAR DISEASE

A thorough examination of a patient with the diagnosis of PVD can differentiate *arterial dysfunction* from *venous dysfunction*. By gathering data from the history and performing the tests and measures discussed in this chapter, the therapist can establish a diagnosis and develop a plan of care to meet the needs of the individual patient. The content of this chapter is reflective of the current elements of patient management, which are schematically presented in the physical therapy algorithm of care (Fig. 18-8).

Examination

The examination is the initial component in the management of the patient and includes patient history, review of systems, and data collection using specific tests and measures.

PATIENT HISTORY

As with any patient examination, the initial step is to obtain a complete history. If available, prior to the patient interview, requisition of medical records can be useful in understanding the patient's previous medical condition. The interview with the patient should include questions concerning past medical history (e.g., history of diabetes mellitus, hypertension, or any cardiac condition). Information should be gathered about medications and any prior treatment for the current problem(s), as well as history of relevant surgical or medical treatment procedures involving the vascular system. A social history can reveal details of life-style patterns such as use of tobacco, dietary habits, and use of alcohol. A history of onset of symptoms and mechanism of injury should be included. Information should also be gathered about the individual's work environment and job skills required that may contribute to the pathology and impairments.

SUBJECTIVE EXAMINATION

The subjective examination addresses the current symptoms including presentation, behavior, and factors that either increase or decrease symptoms.

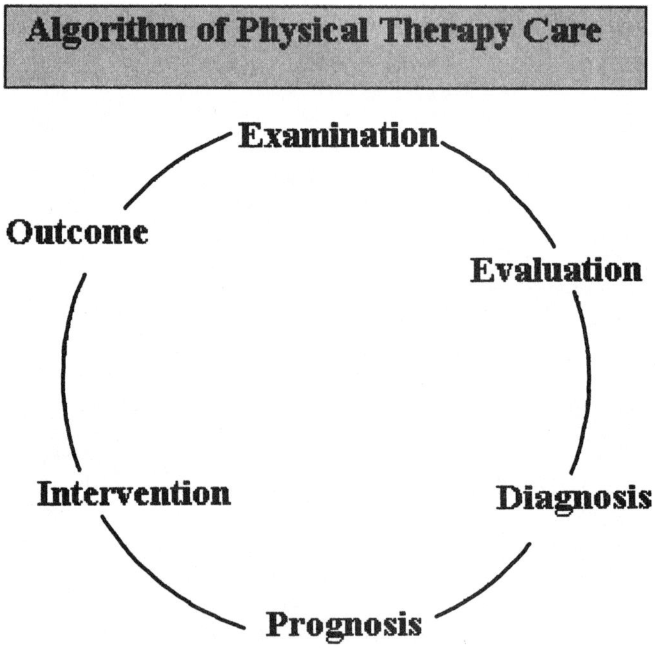

Figure 18-8. Algorithm of physical therapy care.

Questions concerning intermittent claudication, rest pain, and how positioning of the lower extremity affects pain can provide valuable information about the vascular status of the patient.

OBJECTIVE EXAMINATION
Observation

The objective section of the initial examination should begin with observation of the patient. Any evidence of cellulitis or edema should be noted. Presence of discolorations of the skin such as hemosiderin staining should be documented. Cyanosis or pallor, loss of hair, evidence of a wound or a previous amputation need also to be recorded. Characteristics of the gait pattern should be observed and can provide clues into areas that need to be addressed during treatment.

Motor-Sensory Status

A gross motor examination to assess range of motion (ROM) and strength should be included in the initial examination. These tests can provide information about the effectiveness of muscular activity in promoting blood flow as well as general mobility of the patient. Sensory testing using light touch and pressure should be included as well as the use of the *Semmes-Weinstein monofilaments* (Fig. 18-9). These monofilaments can detect different cutaneous sensory levels. The instrument consists of a handle with nylon projections of various thickness that require different forces to bend the material. The 5.07 monofilament indicates protective sensation if felt by the patient.

Temperature

Temperature of the skin can be assessed with a variety of tools such as a **radiometer, thermistor,** test tubes, or basic palpation skills. Altered temperatures of the affected limb versus the uninvolved side or more proximal body part can provide important insight into vascular dysfunction. In cases of arterial insufficiency, skin temperature will be reduced

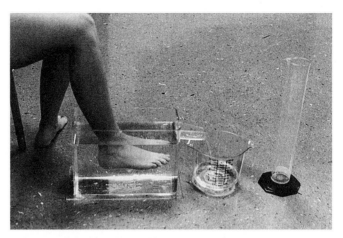

Figure 18-10. Volumetric examination for edema.

according to severity of disease. With venous insufficiency, there may be little or no change in temperature of the affected limb. The radiometer or thermistor provides quantitative data and can be compared to information gained from palpation of the extremity.

Circumferential (Girth) Measurements

Circumferential measurements of an extremity are essential to identifying and monitoring the extent of, and documenting changes in, edema. Girth measurements should be taken in reference to bony prominences to allow consistency for tracking changes during subsequent measurements. **Volumetrics,** a quantitative system to measure edema, can also be used (Fig. 18-10). This process can be time consuming and cumbersome but is a very accurate method of determining changes in edema.

Vascular Examination

The vascular examination allows the therapist to determine which vascular system is involved.

Pulses

The presence or absence of pulses should be addressed. With PVD, palpation of the distal arteries is typically more important that monitoring the larger vessels of the neck and chest. Palpation should focus on the more distal arteries such as the brachial and radial arteries along with the femoral, popliteal, dorsalis pedis, and posterior tibial arteries.

Auscultation

Auscultation is performed by listening to the vessel with a stethoscope. This assessment is useful in identifying turbulent blood flow in the vessel (a **bruit**). Detection of a bruit may indicate the possibility of partial blockage of that artery.

Doppler Ultrasound

One of the most useful diagnostic tools for assessment of the vascular system is the Doppler ultrasound. The Doppler can provide the therapist a quick assessment of both the arterial and venous

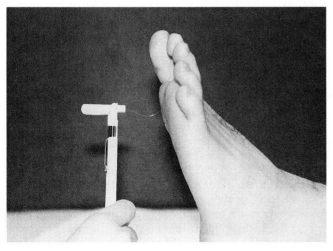

Figure 18-9. Use of Semmes-Weinstein monofilament.

system. The units are compact and easy to operate. These ultrasound units operate according to the Doppler principle in which a 5-, 8-, or 10-MHz frequency is transmitted into the desired vessel. The signal is then reflected off moving red cells back toward the Doppler's probe at a different frequency, which is known as a *frequency shift*. This event is converted into a sound that is heard by the examiner.

The most common test performed with Doppler ultrasound is the **ankle-brachial index (ABI).** This procedure provides valuable information regarding the arterial system. Initially, the examiner must locate the dorsalis pedis or posterior tibial artery with the Doppler. Next, a blood pressure cuff is placed around the calf and is inflated until cessation of the audible signal occurs. The cuff is then slowly released until the signal is heard. At this point, the examiner reads the gauge of the cuff and the pressure reading is recorded (Fig. 18-11). The same procedure is repeated at the upper extremity with the cuff placed on the arm over the brachial artery, and the Doppler placed at the radial artery (Fig. 18-12). The lower extremity pressure is divided by the upper extremity pressure and a ratio or index is calculated. Normal values for the ABI are 1.0 or slightly higher. Table 18–1 provides ranges of ABI values and possible vascular complications. Segmental pressures can also be assessed to determine different pressures and levels of vascular flow.

Falsely elevated indices of an ABI, or an ABI greater than 1.2 with a history of claudication and/or rest pain, can be indicative of arterial disease. Pressure in an atherosclerotic vessel can be elevated by the plaques along the vessel wall that have decreased the opening of the lumen. The resultant increase in the blood flow resistance elevates dopplerable pressure. If pressure readings during cuff inflation exceed 200 mmHg or the sound cannot be cessated, arteriosclerosis or calcified vessels are suspected. In some situations blood flow cannot be occluded when using the blood pressure cuff because of the noncompressibility of a diseased vessel. The ABI is recorded as unattainable secondary to a

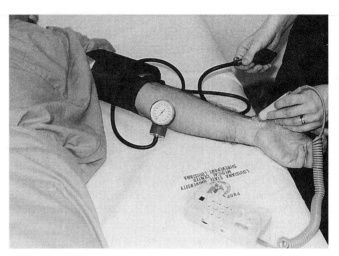

Figure 18-12. ABI set-up to test the upper extremity.

noncompressible artery. The Pole Test (described below) has been devised to determine an ABI value in these situations.

Pole Test (For Falsely Elevated ABI). The presence of a falsely elevated ABI from partially calcified distal arteries can occur and can be accompanied by severe leg ischemia. In patients with leg ischemia, the level of elevation at which the foot takes on significant pallor correlates to the level at which the Doppler signal disappears over a distal artery. In a calcified artery, this level represents systolic blood pressure. Using a pole that is calibrated to convert height of ankle elevation into mmHg, the systolic blood pressure can be assessed. Calibrations on the pole are marked at 13-centimeter intervals, which correspond to 10 mmHg.[29] The procedure for the pole test is similar to the ABI examination except that a blood pressure cuff is not needed. The upper extremity value is determined as usual. The dorsalis pedis pulse is then located and the foot is slowly elevated until the audible signal disappears. A reading is taken on the pole at the level when the sound stops. An alternative method, if a pole is not available, involves the distance, in centimeters, between the ankle and the bed at which the sound disappears. This value can be multiplied by 0.735 to give systolic pressure (Pole ABI elevated leg systolic pressure/arm systolic pressure).

Reflux Test. Assessment of the venous system can also be performed with the use of Doppler ultrasound. The Doppler is used to listen for reflux over major veins in the lower extremity. The easiest and most common vessel to assess is the greater saphenous vein that runs along the medial aspect of calf and thigh. The probe is placed over the saphenous vein to detect an audible signal of venous blood flow. The vessel sound can be augmented by squeezing the extremity distal to the probe to detect for obstructions as well as determine proper placement of the probe (Fig. 18-13). To listen for reflux, the extremity should be squeezed proximal to the probe (Fig. 18-14). No audible signal should occur unless there is valvular incompetence; then an audible signal will be heard.

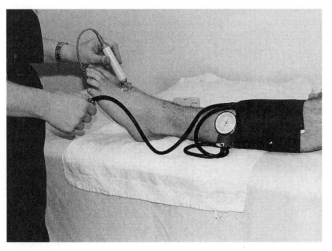

Figure 18-11. ABI set-up to test the lower extremity.

Table 18–1 ANKLE-BRACHIAL INDICES WITH CORRESPONDING INDICATIONS

ABI Ranges	Possible Indication
>1.2	Falsely elevated, arterial disease, diabetes
1.19–0.95	Normal
0.94–0.75	Mild arterial disease, + intermittent claudication
0.74–0.50	Moderate arterial disease, + rest pain
<0.50	Severe arterial disease

SPECIAL TESTS
Venous Filling Time

This test in the past has primarily been used to assess venous circulation but can also provide valuable information about the arterial system. The patient is positioned supine and the affected extremity is elevated to empty blood from superficial veins of the limb. Next, the patient hangs the extremity over the edge of the treatment table into a dependent position. Time is recorded when the veins on top of the foot have refilled. Normal filling time is approximately 15 seconds. A time greater than 15 seconds is indicative of potential arterial disease whereas a time below 15 seconds would suggest venous insufficiency.

Rubor of Dependency

The rubor of dependency test can provide information concerning the state of both the arterial and venous systems. The test is performed in similar fashion to the venous filling test. The patient is positioned supine and the color of both feet is examined. The affected limb is then elevated for several seconds, and lowered back to the original position. The time is recorded for color of the tested foot to match the stationary foot. If arterial disease is present, it may take longer than 20 to 30 seconds for color to return and will usually be bright red. If the color returns immediately, this may denote the presence of venous insufficiency.

Claudication Test

The claudication test provides information about arterial involvement. One of the earliest signs of arterial disease is intermittent claudication. As discussed, claudication is a painful cramping most

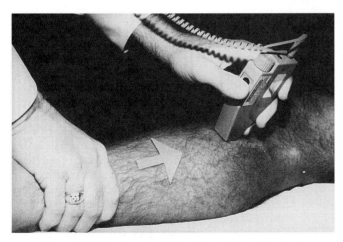

Figure 18-13. Augmentation of a vein for reflux test.

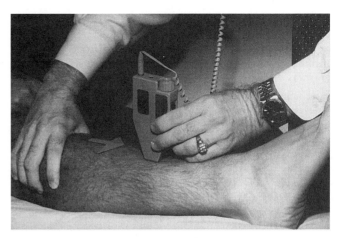

Figure 18-14. Hand position to test for reflux.

often occurring in the lower leg muscle owing to an insufficient supply of blood to working muscles. The patient begins to ambulate using a treadmill or an unobstructed level surface. The claudication test is recorded as the time or distance at which this painful symptom occurs.

Cuff Test

Whenever a patient is referred to physical therapy with a vascular disease, it is important to assess for the presence of a DVT. Usually a thorough work up by a physician should detect the potential for development of a DVT, but occasionally it can be overlooked as wound or musculoskeletal pain. This test is performed by placing a blood pressure cuff around the lower leg and inflating the cuff. If the patient is unable to tolerate cuff pressure greater than 40 mmHg, there is a high probability of an active DVT. The test can be augmented with a forceful squeeze of the calf region or passive dorsiflexion of the calf by the examiner. A positive result is severe pain expressed by the patient (+ Homan's sign).

Percussion Test

Percussion of a major superficial vein of the lower extremity can be useful in determining valve competency. With the lower extremity in a dependent position, the greater saphenous vein is palpated distal to the knee with one hand while the vein is tapped approximately 6 to 8 inches proximal to the knee with the other. If a wave of fluid is detected under the distal palpation site, this indicates an incompetent valve or valves.

Trendelenburg Test

The Trendelenburg test is a simple way to assess if the valves are functioning properly, especially within the perforation system. The patient is positioned supine and the lower extremity is elevated to approximately 75 degrees to allow venous blood to empty. A tourniquet is placed around the thigh to prevent superficial venous backflow. The lower extremity is then placed in a dependent position. The process of venous filling is observed. Should the superficial veins fill quickly, the valves of the perforator vein have become incompetent. If immediate filling is noted with release of the tourniquet, the superficial system has incompetent valves. Normal venous filling would demonstrate neither situation, and the veins would fill approximately 25 to 30 seconds after the lower extremity is placed in a dependent position.

Air Plethysmography

Air plethysmyography (APG) is a noninvasive vascular examination of both the arterial and venous systems (Fig. 18-15). This clinical tool has the capability to detect minute changes in leg volume and can be performed during static or postural changes as well as during light exercise. It is also a reliable predictor of the presence or reoccurrence of venous ulcers. The APG provides a quantitative measure of venous reflux, calf pump function, and residual venous volume after exercise. Venous obstruction as well as arterial inflow can also be studied. The APG can differentiate between the superficial and deep venous systems and provide data that may help identify the system of dysfunction. Other similar devices exist such as *photoplethysmography* (PPG), *light refection rheography* (LPR), and a more invasive measure known as the *ambulatory venous pressure* (AVP) examination. The APG is fundamentally different, more versatile and less painful than PPG, LRR, and AVP studies. Prior to 1997, a physical therapist could administer the test and be reimbursed for this service. Currently the test can only be performed by a certified vascular technician if Medicare reimbursement is an issue. The primary use of the APG in physical therapy is for research purposes.

Stemmer's Test

This test can be performed to clarify the presence or evidence of lymphedema or lymphostasis. **Stemmer's sign** is the inability to pick up a fold of skin at the base of the second toe of the affected extremity.

ADDITIONAL VASCULAR STUDIES

Venography and arteriography are two common contrast dye studies that may be ordered by a physician to further examine a patient's vascular system. There are also several diagnostic imaging studies that are utilized for examination of the lymphatics. These include tests known as interstitial lymphangiography and conventional lymphography as well as lymphoscintigraphy and fluorescence-microlymphography. The results from these tests are very accurate and the therapist should request the findings or interpretations of these tests, if available, to correlate with findings from tests and measures described in this chapter.

Evaluation, Diagnosis, and Prognosis

The evaluation process calls for the physical therapist to make clinical judgements from the data gathered during the examination. The data should reveal a cluster of signs and symptoms that guide the therapist in determining a diagnosis.

PHYSICAL THERAPY FINDINGS OF ARTERIAL INSUFFICIENCY

The major findings consistent with arterial insufficiency will incorporate many of the following conditions. The patient history may be significant for hypertension and/or diabetes. Previous surgical history may include bypass grafts or amputations of the lower extremity. The patient will often have a significant smoking habit. *Subjectively*, the patient may present with complaints of pain on ambulation and rest pain, as well as pain in the lower extremity with elevation. The patient may report coldness of the feet and hands and may describe color changes in the digits. *Objectively*, the examiner may observe a pale appearance to the extremity, and temperature of the distal aspect of the extremities will be decreased. Edema may or may not be present in the affected extremity. The vascular examination will yield absent or diminished pulses, possibly the presence of a bruit, and the ABI will be decreased or falsely elevated. If the ABI is falsely elevated the pole test results will presumably be decreased. The special tests, such as *rubor of dependency* and *venous filling time*, will have extended time frames. The Trendelenburg test, percussion examination, and the cuff test should all be negative.

PHYSICAL THERAPY FINDINGS OF CHRONIC VENOUS INSUFFICIENCY

The principal findings consistent with venous insufficiency should include many of the following. During history taking, the patient may report the presence of diabetes, hypertension, and/or congestive heart failure. The occurrence of a previous leg ulcer or DVT may be reported as well as the prevalence of varicosities. *Subjectively*, the patient rarely reports evidence of intermittent claudication or rest pain. Edema, if present, can be decreased with elevation with no painful side effects. The patient may report the skin on the affected lower extremity as darker than normal. *Objectively*, there should be no evidence of a pale appearance of the extremity, but

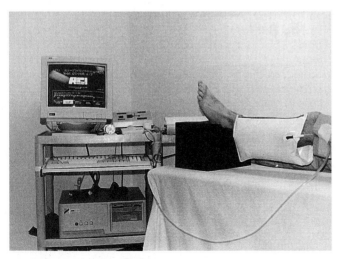

Figure 18-15. APG set-up to test affected extremity.

hemosiderin staining of the lower extremities may be present. All involved extremities will be warm to the touch and may be significant for edema. Findings from the vascular examination are typically the opposite of arterial insufficiency. Distal pulses should be strong. Reflux may be detected with the Doppler and further Doppler examination should reveal a normal ABI. **Rubor** of dependency and venous filling time results will indicate immediate filling of the veins. There may be positive percussion and Trendelenburg tests. The cuff test is usually negative except in the presence of active DVT. If an APG is performed, it will reveal an elevated venous filling index, which correlates to reflux, decreased ejection fraction (poor calf function), and increased residual volume in the affected extremity.

There are times when a patient may present with *mixed etiologies*. That is, the patient demonstrates a combination of both *arterial insufficiency* and *venous insufficiency*. In these cases, the patient should be carefully assessed to provide safe and effective care. A general rule of thumb is to treat the more severe pathology, but each case is unique and all findings must be considered.

DIFFERENTIAL DIAGNOSIS OF LYMPHEDEMA

The diagnosis of **lymphedema** can be achieved most reliably by standard diagnostic procedures including a thorough history, physical examination (which includes inspection and palpation), and the results of imaging studies. *Subjectively*, the patient typically reports similar information found with the venous insufficiency diagnosis. There may be a history of malignant disorders reported in the patient history. One major distinction that differentiates venous disease from lymphedema is the rate at which edema resolves. With venous insufficiency, edema resolves within several hours of elevation but may require several days to resolve in a patient with lymphedema. *Objectively*, inspection of the extremities and trunk for generalized aberrations from normal skin texture and color can reveal deepened natural skin creases, thickened cutaneous folds, pronounced soft local swelling, as well as fibrosis of the skin. There is usually no evidence of a skin ulceration, which is a common finding with venous insufficiency. A positive Stemmer's sign and columnar deformation of the legs can also be seen. Another way to differentiate between lymphedema and venous insufficiency is to use Doppler ultrasound to rule out venous reflux. Palpation can be used to identify local or generalized swelling, including subcutaneous lymph node enlargement.

PROGNOSIS OF PERIPHERAL VASCULAR DISEASE

Prognosis involves the projected level of improvement associated with a pathology as well as the severity and chronicity of impairments. A plan of care is developed from evaluation of data collected during the initial examination. This plan includes prognostic predictions, types of intervention, goals and projected outcomes, and time frames required to accomplish desired outcomes.

With respect to PVD, prognosis can be favorable with physical therapy intervention. The major goals and desired interventions focus on patient education and exercise programs. When wound care is required, the goals and interventions are expanded.

OUTCOMES

Outcomes are related to functional limitations, disabilities, prevention strategies, and patient satisfaction. General outcomes of physical therapy intervention for *peripheral vascular disease* include the following:

1. The patient understands the disease process.
2. The patient can restore desired level of function (if diminished because of the PVD).
3. The patient can improve his or her quality of life.
4. The patient can prevent further progression of the disease.
5. The patient can achieve resolution of an acute or chronic wound (if applicable).

General outcomes of physical therapy intervention for *arterial insufficiency* include the following:

1. The patient understands the disease process and the appropriate foot and skin care protocol (see Appendices A and B).
2. The patient demonstrates understanding of the indications and contraindications of a home exercise and walking program.

General outcomes of physical therapy intervention for *chronic venous insufficiency* include the following:

1. The patient understands the disease process, techniques to control edema, and proper skin care.
2. The patient demonstrates an understanding of a home exercise and walking program.
3. The patient can properly manage the use of appropriate vascular compression garments.

Intervention

Intervention is the purposeful and skilled interaction between the therapist and the patient using various procedures and techniques to produce changes that relate to goals and outcomes.

ACUTE ARTERIAL AND VENOUS DISEASE

Physical therapy intervention with acute arterial or venous disease is frequently not needed, may even be contraindicated. The treatment of either disease process requires immediate medical attention and usually surgical intervention. Once the acute arterial occlusive disease is discovered, immediate intravenous heparinization is indicated to prevent further progression of the thrombosis. Surgical intervention frequently includes procedures such as a thrombectomy, bypass grafts for revascularization, and embolectomy, as well as **endarterectomy.** Physical therapy intervention for patients who underwent surgery may be provided postoperatively in the form of passive range of motion for DVT prophylaxis. In

Table 18–2 SAMPLE VASCULAR REHABILITATION PROGRAM: EXERCISE AND WALKING

A. Sample Exercise and Walking Program for Arterial Insufficiency

Week	Exercises	Intensity	Ambulation
1–3	Isometrics: quadriceps and hamstring sets AROM: ankle pumps, heel slides, heel and toe raises in sitting	3 sets, 15 reps, 2–3 times daily (monitor pain)	⅛–½ mile or just prior to point of claudication (1–2 times a day)
4–6	AROM and resistive exercise: add to above exercises—standing toe raises, straight leg raises, wall squats; hip, knee, and ankle exercises with 2–3 lb weights	3 sets, 20 reps, 2–3 times daily	½–1 mile or to point of claudication
7–10	Continue resistive exercises, increase resistance as tolerated	3 sets, 20 reps, 3 times daily	1+ miles or distance as tolerated

B. Sample Exercise and Walking Program for Venous Insufficiency

Types of Exercises	Walking Program
Isometric exercise: quadriceps and hamstring sets AROM and resistive exercise: ankle pumps, short arc quadriceps exercise, heel cord stretches (PROM), sitting and standing toe and heel raises	Ambulating 2–3 times per day for 15–30 minutes each time Taking frequent breaks at a desk job or short breaks to walk for a job that entails standing in place.

acute venous disease, such as a DVT, bed rest and anticoagulants are immediately introduced. Surgical interventions may call for the implantation of antiembolism devices such as the Greenfield filter, which is placed in the affected vessel to trap a potential embolus from moving to life-threatening areas. As the patient's condition improves and the clot has resolved, physical therapy invention addresses restoration of patient mobility. It may also require measuring and fitting the patient for compression garments for reduction of residual edema and educating the patient about the risk of developing other venous complications.

CHRONIC ARTERIAL DISEASE

Intervention for chronic arterial disease is beginning to expand. Patient education and exercise are the cornerstone of physical therapy intervention, but recently the introduction of new modalities have emerged to improve circulation and decrease the risk of amputation.

Patient education should incorporate foot and skin care instructions (see Appendices A and B), limb protection, explanation of the disease process, and risk factor modification. The literature indicates that abstinence from smoking is associated with reduction of the painful symptoms of Beuger's disease as well as reductions in elevated serum cholesterol levels. Lipid-lowering therapy can induce atherosclerotic regression in the diseased arteries.[30]

The patient should also be introduced to a vascular rehabilitation program. Several studies examining the effects of supervised exercise and ambulation programs for patients with arterial insufficiency indicate that such programs improve function, relieve pain, promote a greater sense of well-being, and ultimately decrease the risk of further complications of arterial insufficiency.[31–33] It has also been reported that pain-free walking distance can be expected to double after 3 months of exercise train-

ing.[34] A recent study examining the effects of a vascular rehabilitation program on walking distances for subjects with lower extremity arterial occlusive disease found significant improvement in walking distances and intermittent claudication. Fifty-five percent of the subjects had documented increases in walking distance ranging from 122 to 450 percent, as well as smoking cessation and improved participation in a daily home exercise program.[35] The vascular rehabilitation program should also incorporate patient education addressing risk factor modification and stress reduction techniques together with the exercise and walking programs. Table 18–2 presents a sample vascular rehabilitation program.

A unique modality used in the treatment of PVD, especially arterial insufficiency, is a therapeutic device called Vasotrain 447 (Enraf-Nonius, Delft, Holland). This vacuum compression therapy (VCT) device (Fig. 18-16) provides alternating cycles of positive and negative pressure in which the affected

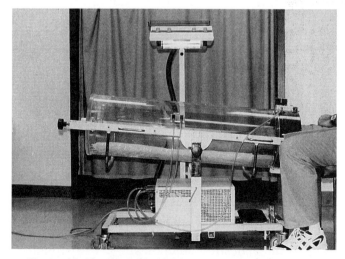

Figure 18-16. Vasotrain 447 (vacuum-compression device).

extremity rests inside an airtight cylinder. In the negative pressure cycle, the vessels of the extremity are dilated and blood flows into the extremity; the positive pressure cycle applies gentle compression to push blood out of the extremity. This device has been shown to improve wound condition in the ischemic limb and allow for complete wound resolution.[36] Further research is warranted to examine the effects of VCT on diminished ABIs.

A new modality has recently become available that has been effective in the nonsurgical treatment of arterial insufficiency. One manufactured system is called ArtAssist (ACI Medical, San Marcos, CA), a variation of an intermittent compression pump system. It delivers high pressures at quick bursts that can empty the venous system. This seems to trigger an arteriovenous reflex that results in greater arterial inflow.[37]

CHRONIC VENOUS INSUFFICIENCY

Physical therapy plays a vital role in the treatment of CVI. Conservative management of CVI usually focuses on decreasing edema, preventing or resolving leg ulcerations, patient education, and an exercise and walking program. Patient education should include understanding the disease process, management of edema, skin care, and wound care if needed. All patients with CVI should be encouraged to participate in a walking program. Ambulation facilitates calf muscle pump action and assists with venous blood return. The exercise program should address the lower extremities to improve muscle function (see Table 18–2).

The most common clinical feature of CVI is edema. To address the edema, compression therapy and compression garments are often incorporated into the plan of care if there is no arterial disease present. Intermittent pneumatic compression (IPC) therapy has proven effective in reducing edema (Fig. 18-17). It mimics calf pump action and has been shown to facilitate wound healing.[38–41] Anytime compression therapy is initiated, it is important to obtain a current blood pressure reading. Inflation pressures should never exceed the patient's diastolic pressure. This can create complications during treatment such as chest pain or headaches. An ABI assessment should also be performed on a patient with CVI to

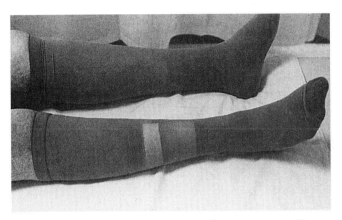

Figure 18-18. Patient wearing custom fitted support stockings.

rule out any arterial disease. If an ABI ranges from 0.95 to 0.75, caution should be taken and the patient monitored closely. With an ABI above 0.75, compression therapy should be avoided.

Once limb girth has stabilized after several treatments of IPC, the patient should be fitted with appropriate vascular compression garments such as a class II (30 to 40 mmHg) custom-fitted or prefabricated stocking[42] (Fig. 18-18). Interim stockings can be used, for example, an elastic tubular stocking known as Tubigrip (Convatec, Princeton, NJ), until edema has resolved.

When a wound accompanies the diagnosis of CVI, compression therapy is an effective intervention for promoting healing. Stockings may not be appropriate because of wound size and amount of drainage, yet proper vascular support after IPC should be provided by use of compressive dressings. The *Unna boot* (Fig. 18-19), is an inelastic paste-impregnated gauze bandage. It is the traditional compressive dressing used for treatment of wounds associated with CVI. The primary action of the Unna boot is to prevent further swelling of the leg and improve

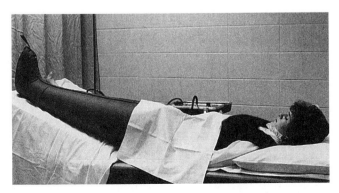

Figure 18-17. Intermittent pneumatic compression pump.

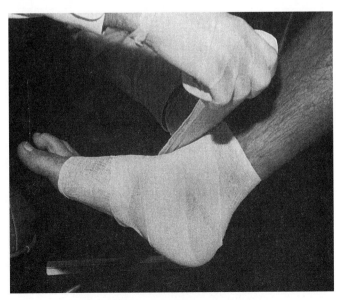

Figure 18-19. Unna's boot application.

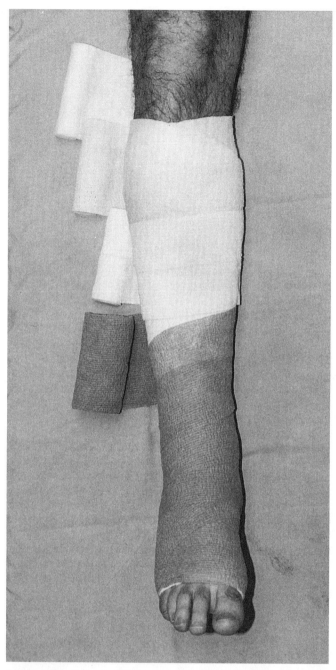

Figure 18-20. Profore™ is a four layer bandage system consisting of a cotton, crepe, and two compression layers (top-bottom).

muscle pump function. It is intended for use with patients who are ambulatory and not indicated for those confined to bed or a wheelchair. Variations of the compressive dressing include other *short stretch* bandages such as Comprilan (Beiersdorf, Inc., Charlotte, NC), *long stretch* bandages such as an ACE (Becton, Dickinson Co., Franklin Lakes, NY), wrap and Setopress (Convatec, Princeton, NJ), as well as the *bandage systems* like Profore (Smith & Nephew, Largo, FL) (Fig. 18-20) and Dynaflex (Johnson & Johnson, Arlington, TX). Any of these compressive dressings can be effective for wound management in the presence of venous insufficiency.

The most common surgical interventions for the patient with CVI are **ligation,** a surgical cutting of diseased perforated veins, as well as vein stripping, **sclerotherapy,** and **valvuloplasty.**

LYMPHEDEMA

Physical therapy intervention for treatment of lymphedema may include the use of intermittent pneumatic compression devices, **combined physical decongestive therapy (CPDT),** as well as the use of compression garments and monitoring the impact of drug management. If conservative management is not effective, surgical intervention is considered.

As with venous insufficiency, pneumatic compression devices have been used to successfully treat lymphedema since the 1980s.[43–44] Intermittent pneumatic compression systems with multiple gradient, sequential chambers have been developed to provide a more effective movement of fluid from the distal aspect to the proximal region of the affected extremity.

Techniques have been developed to augment or replace the compression pump. CPDT is a recognized method of treatment for lymphedema, especially in Europe, and is becoming more and more popular in the United States. CPDT has been perfected and utilized effectively during the past 25 years and several studies have supported its effectiveness for treating lymphedema.[45–47] The therapeutic goal of CPDT is to normalize the volume and consistency of the edematous, swollen extremity. CPDT includes the following treatments:[48] (1) manual lymph drainage, (2) compressive bandages (after manual lymph drainage has been performed to avoid new fluid collection in the treated area), (3) hygienic measures, and (4) decongestive exercise (for the bandaged extremities).

When performing CPDT, the therapist begins with *manual lymph drainage* at the nonedematous quadrants adjacent to the trunk quadrant of the edematous extremity. The result is a "sucking" effect on the lymphatics of the edematous trunk quadrant. The interstitial fluid of the obstructed quadrants is then drained into the neighboring edema-free quadrants. The swollen extremity is treated only after drainage of the trunk (treatment always progresses from proximal to distal). Exclusions or barriers to manual lymph drainage techniques include the presence of scar tissue, radiogenic fibrosis, or a skin ulcer.[48] Manual lymph drainage is performed on a once or twice daily basis for approximately 45 minutes over a 4- to 6-week period.

After manual lymph drainage has been performed, bandaging is essential to optimize effectiveness of treatment. Short-stretch bandages are typically the most beneficial type of bandaging for CPDT. These compression bandages preserve the gains of manual lymph drainage treatments and are worn constantly except during treatment and for purposes of hygiene. CPDT has achieved approximately a 70 percent edema reduction in most cases of lymphedema.[48] Contributing factors to unsuccessful intervention include lack of patient compliance, incorrect diagnosis, or incomplete treatment or understanding of the techniques.

Once lymphedema has been controlled and girth measurements have plateaued, compression garments become an integral part of treatment. The indicated pressure or grade of compression for these garments is 40 to 50 mmHg, or greater than 50 mmHg if lymphedema is severe. Classes of compression garments have been established. Table 18–3 presents the recommended pressure and indications for the use of each class of stocking. For the lower extremity, compression garments range from knee high to thigh high to full length for unilateral or bilateral involvement. The upper extremity garments range from a glove or gauntlet to full-length sleeves with shoulder and/or trunk attachments. Several companies provide quick fit or off-the-shelf garments such as JUZO (Cuyahoga, Ohio) or JOBST (Toledo, Ohio), but also provide custom fabricated garments.

Table 18–3 VASCULAR/LYMPHEDEMA COMPRESSION GARMENT CLASSIFICATION

Class	Pressure (mm Hg)	Indications
Class I	20–30	Varicose veins, phlebitis, edema during pregnancy
Class II	30–40	Venous insufficiency, mild lymphedema
Class III	40–50	Lymphedema, postthrombotic syndrome
Class IV	>50	Severe lymphedema

Numerous surgical methods for lymphedema are available to correct the pathological component. These procedures include resection, drainage, and reconstruction.

WOUND MANAGEMENT

Wound care has become an integral part of physical therapy practice. Major advances in wound care have developed over the past 15 to 20 years and physical therapy has contributed to these advances through evidence-based practice. The role of the physical therapist in treatment of PVD frequently involves the management of a wound that is associated with the diseased extremity. A brief discussion of the phases of healing, wound assessment, and treatment interventions follows.

Physiology of Normal Wound Healing: A Three-Phase Process

Once homeostasis has occurred, wounds progress through three overlapping phases of healing (Fig. 18-21).

PHASE I: INFLAMMATORY PHASE: DAYS 0 TO 10

This phase, also known as the phagocytic phase, is characterized by vasodilation, migration of leukocytes, release of histamine, and stimulation of nociceptive receptors. These characteristics correlate with the cardinal signs of inflammation: *redness*, *heat*, *swelling*, and *pain*. Inflammation is the immune system's reaction to injury and is the building block essential for healing. This phase sets into motion a cascade of events that continues the healing process. During this phase, platelets that have been activated during homeostasis release substances known as platelet-derived growth factors (PDGF) and epidermal growth factors.[49] These two factors facilitate migration of granulocytes and macrophages. Other cellular events occur to prevent the spread of **infection** and promote the perfusion of blood to the injured area (increasing nutrition to damaged tissues). One primary nutrient carried to the wound that is essential for healing and controlling infection is oxygen. Oxygen has been described

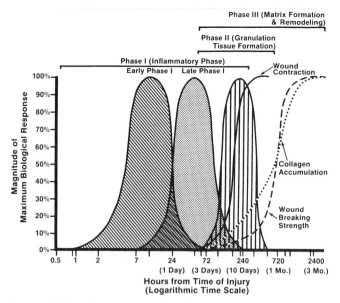

Figure 18-21. Three overlapping phases of wound healing. (From McCulloch, JM, Kloth, LC, and Feedar, JA: Wound Healing Alternatives in Management, FA Davis, Philadelphia, p 33, with permission.)

as a natural antibiotic for preventing wound infections.[50] The presence of neutrophils, mast cells, and macrophages facilitate the healing process. Macrophages are the key cells that bridge the gap between the inflammatory phase and the proliferative phase of healing.[51]

PHASE II: PROLIFERATIVE PHASE: DAYS 3 TO 20

This phase is characterized by formation of granulation tissue, **wound contraction,** and reepithelialization. The accumulation of **fibroblasts** in the wound develops into a collagen matrix. This matrix, along with a vascular network, forms a delicate healing tissue known as **granulation tissue.** The presence of myofibroblasts assist with wound contraction to decrease the size of the wound opening and facilitate epidermal cell migration from the wound edges. A phenomenon known as *contact inhibition* occurs when migration of the epidermal cells meet at the center of the wound. At this time, epidermal cell migration ends and stratification of these cells occur, leading into the third and final phase of healing.[52]

PHASE III: MATURATION PHASE: DAY 9 UP TO 2 YEARS

During this phase, remodeling of the newly formed epithelium occurs. Newly formed skin has only approximately 15 percent the strength of normal skin.[51] The collagen structure becomes more organized and tensile strength of the scar increases. The maturation phase is an ongoing process, even after wound closure, and can take months to even years to complete. Physical therapy intervention for wound care typically occurs during this phase. Frequently the wound is in a chronic healing state and can be "stuck" in this phase for extended periods of

time, from weeks to months to years. Examples of chronic wounds are presented in Box 18-1.

Usually, a wound follows the normal progression of repair. However, several factors can delay this process precipitating development of a chronic wound. These factors are classified as either *intrinsic* (e.g., patient age), *extrinsic* (e.g., cytotoxic topical agents), or *iatrogenic* (e.g., poor wound management). A thorough evaluation of examination data will guide the physical therapist in developing a plan of care to optimize wound healing.

Wound Examination

HISTORY

When examining a patient who presents with a wound, the interview is vital in determining the primary problem, the nature of the wound, and other underlying pathological processes. The history should include questions concerning the mechanism of injury, date of onset, and progression of the wound since onset. Questions should address the patient's previous medical and surgical history, and previous treatment for the condition. Life-style patterns should be investigated, especially with regard to smoking, use of alcohol, and eating habits.

SUBJECTIVE EXAMINATION

The subjective examination is required to gain information about the current symptoms. The patient should be questioned about both the behavior and characteristics of the symptoms (e.g., "Is there any pain associated with the wound or the extremity?" "Are there certain positions that make the symptoms better or worse?").

OBJECTIVE EXAMINATION

The objective examination provides the practitioner with quantitative data about the patient's integumentary integrity and wound status. Observation is an important component of data gathering and will assist in providing a clear description of the status, characteristics, and location of the wound. Characteristics of the wound that are typically assessed include the (1) type of lesion (either primary or secondary), (2) stage of the wound, (3) type and amount of drainage, and (4) colors in the wound (which relate to the types of tissues). The presence of edema or odor and a description of the skin area adjacent to the wound are pertinent details

---

Box 18-1 TYPES OF CHRONIC WOUNDS

• Ischemic arterial ulcers
• Pressure ulcers
• Venous insufficiency ulcers
• Neuropathic ulcers
• Rheumatoid ulcers
• Vasculitis ulcers

Table 18–4 WOUND CLASSIFICATIONS

Stage	Description	Tissue Involvement or Loss
I	Nonblanchable erythema, epidermis and dermis intact	None
II	Complete loss of epidermis, partial disruption of the dermis (blister)	Partial thickness wound
III	Complete loss of epidermis and dermis, extends down to but not through underlying fascia	Full thickness wound (superficial involvement)
IV	Complete loss of epidermis and dermis with destruction of fascia with muscle, bone, or joint involvement	Full thickness wound (deep involvement)

included in the objective examination. *Primary lesions* include **macules, papules,** or **vesicles** that may be present on the skin. *Secondary lesions* develop as a result of a primary lesion and include a common wound known as an *ulcer.*

Standard systems for classification of wounds have been developed. The National Pressure Ulcer Advisory Panel (NPUAP) has developed a system to describe the stage of tissue destruction of pressure ulcers that has been used successfully to describe a variety of other types of wounds. New terminology is available to better describe all types of wounds. Table 18–4 presents the NPUAP staging system and level of tissue loss. A description of the size and depth of the wound is also included in the objective assessment. Several techniques are available for determining the size of the wound and include (1) use of a tape measure to obtain the length and width, (2) tracing films that provide the exact shape and surface area, and (3) photographic documentation to secure a precise, visual depiction of the wound. To measure the volume of the wound, if appropriate, volumetric measurements can be obtained. This technique is performed by filling a large syringe with saline to a known volume and slowly injecting the fluid until it is level with the surrounding skin. The amount of fluid injected is determined by subtracting the quantity remaining in the syringe from the starting amount. New technologies are continuously being developed and allow for such

assessments as computer digitization of wounds that provide exact surface areas and volumes. Performed at regular intervals, these assessment techniques provide objective data to quantify the rate of wound healing.

An important component of the objective tests and measures are the vascular examination and the special tests presented earlier in this chapter. These tests and measures provide the therapist with valuable information about wound healing potential and/or type of vascular involvement. In addition, any evidence of wound infection or contamination should be documented. Table 18–5 provides common descriptors used in documenting types of drainage as well as the associated wound condition. Table 18–6 provides a comparison of the typical arterial versus venous insufficiency wound characteristics. Owing to its vital role in wound healing, a nutritional assessment should also be included in the objective examination. A sample patient data collection form is provided in Appendix C.

Outcomes and Goals of Treatment

Wound management should incorporate the following outcomes and goals of physical therapy intervention:

1. The patient understands self-care of the wound and management of the PVD (if applicable) such as identification of signs of infection, and so forth.
2. Provide a moist wound healing environment (Box 18–2 summarizes the benefits of a moist healing environment).
3. Promote granulation tissue formation and decrease necrotic tissue at the wound site.
4. Promote wound reepithelialization or resolution.
5. Decrease pain associated with the wound as well as with dressing changes.
6. Decrease risk of wound infections.
7. Improve physical function (if decreased secondary to the wound) and return to previous level of participation in activities of daily living.

Table 18–5 TYPES OF WOUND DRAINAGE

Type	Description	Wound State
Serous	Clear, shiny exudate; can have a slightly yellow appearance	Healthy
Sanguineous	Red, bloody drainage	Healthy
Serosanguineous	Pinkish-red colored exudate	Healthy
Seropurulent	Brighter yellow drainage, slightly thicker exudate than serous; slightly malodorous	Contaminated/infected
Purulent/pus	Thick, cloudy, or opaque exudate; malodorous	Infected

Table 18–6 COMPARISON OF ARTERIAL VERSUS VENOUS INSUFFICIENCY WOUND CHARACTERISTICS

Characteristic	Arterial Insufficiency	Venous Insufficiency
Granulation tissue	Pale red	Bright red
Drainage	Minimal	Moderate to heavy
Location	Toes, feet, anterior tibial area	Medial malleolus
Pain	Moderate to severe	Mininal
Edema	(+)/(−)	(+)/(−)
Shape	Well-circumscribed or "punched out" appearance	Irregular
Hemisiderin staining	(−)	(+)

Box 18–2 BENEFITS OF A MOIST WOUND HEALING ENVIRONMENT

Facilitates autolysis or autolytic debridement
Promotes angiogenesis
Bathes cells in a naturally protein- and enzyme-rich environment
Enhances epidermal cell migration
Optimizes immune system function
Increases patient comfort and compliance with dressing changes
Decreases the number of dressing changes

Intervention

Physical therapy intervention for wound management may include a variety of modalities and/or the use of appropriate wound dressing to promote optimal healing conditions.

MODALITIES

The following modalities are effective in treatment of a variety of wounds, and in facilitating wound healing.

Hydrotherapy

Hydrotherapy is a common tool used in the care of wounds. Variations in application of hydrotherapy include use of whirlpools, pulsed lavage, and syringe irrigation. The major indication for hydrotherapy is for mechanical **debridement** of nonviable tissue and to promote development of granulation tissue. The primary contraindications for whirlpool treatments include venous insufficiency, because whirlpool can increase venous congestion and hypertension in the dependent extremity. Caution must be exercised with use of the whirlpool in the presence of arterial insufficiency because heat dissipation will be compromised.

Ultrasound

Ultrasound is a modality used commonly in physical therapy for pain management has shown success in the treatment of wounds. Ultrasound is delivered directly into the wound by use of a coupling medium such as an amorphous hydrogel or hydrogel sheet. Ultrasound is more effective when performed during the inflammatory phase. Both thermal and nonthermal settings promote wound healing. Nonthermal ultrasound is indicated for acute wounds and arterial insufficiency. For chronic wounds, thermal settings may be effective.[53–55]

Compression Therapy

The use of intermittent pneumatic compression pumps discussed previously is an important component of intervention for CVI. The compression assists with venous return and stimulates the release of cellular factors that facilitate wound healing.

Electrical Stimulation

Electrical stimulation has demonstrated effectiveness in facilitating healing of both acute and chronic wounds. Electrical stimulation has a galvanotoxic effect on the cells needed for healing. By using high-volt pulsed (direct) current (HVPC) directly in the wound, the following can occur: (1) attraction of neutrophils, macrophages, and epidermal cells, which facilitate debridement and reepithelialization of the wound; this can be advanced by using the *anodal (+) pole*; and (2) the *cathodal (–) pole* facilitates an increased fibroblastic activity as well as attraction of neutrophils. Therefore, negative polarity is recommended to fight infection and promote granulation and has been shown to decrease inflammation and reduce edema.[56–58]

Ultraviolet Radiation

Ultraviolet (UV) light has been effective in treatment of chronic wounds to decrease the bacterial load and initiate an inflammatory response secondary to erythema created when using this modality.[59] It has been used effectively in the treatment of acne vulgaris, eczema, atopic dermatitis, and psoriasis.[59–60] UV-C, a variation of ultraviolet light, is most effective for decreasing the bacterial load in the wound, whereas UV-B is most successful in treatment of skin diseases such as psoriasis, and eczema. Treatment doses range from 15 to 30 seconds, 2 to 3 times a week or until superficial wound contamination has resolved.[61] Contraindications include herpes simplex, lupus erythematosus, *acute* psoriasis, and eczema.

Radiant Heat

Infrared radiation increases local wound and skin temperatures facilitating higher metabolic rates and improving circulatory activity to the wound.[62] Warm-Up (Augustine Medical, Eden Prairie, MN) therapy (Fig. 18-22), is a radiant heat system that normalizes the temperature within the wound, and provides localized heat and humidity. It has been effective in treating chronic wounds even in the presence of vascular compromise.[63]

Vacuum Assisted Closure

Vacuum Assisted Closure (V.A.C.™; KCI Medical, San Antonio, TX) is effective for a variety of wounds. It includes a special surgical foam and an occlusive drape connected to a programmable pump. It has been shown to promote rapid wound edge approximation, formation of granulation tissue, and reepithelialization. This modality is used to hasten wound contraction and reepithelialization, enhance surgical intervention, and increase success rates of a split thickness skin graft.[64] Current research is directed toward determining if use of this modality decreases length of hospitalization by facilitating a more rapid closure of the wound with fewer complications. Contraindications for use of V.A.C.™ therapy include untreated osteomyelitis and fistulas of unknown origin.

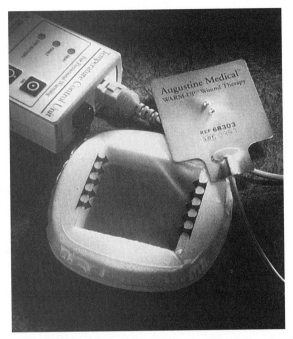

Figure 18-22. Warm-Up™ radiant heating unit (Augustine Medical, Eden Prairie, MN).

WOUND DRESSINGS

To guide the decision-making process, major categories of dressings will be discussed. Some controversy continues to exist about the use of gauze dressings versus microenvironmental dressings. Gauze dressings can be detrimental to healing tissues and should be avoided by substituting a more "wound-friendly" dressing. However, gauze dressings are particularly useful with less than 50 percent granulation at the wound site. Gauze dressing can be cost effective in this situation, primarily for mechanical debridement of the devitalized tissue from the wound.

The selection of a specific dressing is guided chiefly by the amount of exudate and the status of the wound. There are literally hundreds of commercially available dressings. The classification of microenvironmental dressings according to their actions are described in the following section. Appendix D includes a list of dressing types with product name and manufacturers (this list is not exhaustive). Appendix E presents considerations to guide the decision-making process for dressing choice relative to the amount of wound exudate.

Absorbent dressings are used for moderate to highly exudating wounds and include semipermeable foams, calcium alginate dressings, hydrophilic fiber dressings, absorbent antimicrobial dressings, and collagen dressings.

Semipermeable Foams

Foam dressings are ordinarily developed from an absorbent polyurethane material. They are hydrophilic in nature and allow for rapid uptake of fluid to control heavily exudating wounds. The foam dressings absorb excess drainage and provide a moist wound environment. Foam dressings are not indicated for dry or desiccated wounds.

Calcium Alginate Dressings

Calcium alginate dressings, which are manufactured from a seaweed derivative, are indicated for highly exudating wounds and in some instances can be used with wounds with low exudate. Primary use of alginate dressings is for wounds that have a high output of exudate. As the wound exudate reacts with the dressing a gel matrix is formed. Therefore, these dressings control wound exudate and provide a moist healing environment. The alginate dressings usually require a secondary dressing to secure them in place. When wound exudate is minimal, the alginate dressing can be moistened with saline to provide moisture to the wound.

Hydrophilic Fiber Dressings

These synthetic dressings, such as Aquacel (Convatec, Princeton, NJ) and Dynaflex (Johnson & Johnson, Arlington, TX), are highly absorbent. They are similar to the calcium alginate dressings in that they absorb high amounts of wound exudate, provide a moist healing environment, and decrease the risk of maceration to tissues adjacent to the wound. These dressings are not indicated for dry wounds unless the dressing is activated by saline prior to application.

Absorbent Antimicrobial Dressings

Iodosorb (Healthpoint, Fort Worth, TX) is an absorbent ointment with antimicrobial benefits. It is designed to be highly absorbent while providing a moist healing environment. Each gram of the cadexomer hydrophilic bead absorbs up to approximately 6 mL of fluid. The ointment contains a small amount of elemental iodine (0.9%). As the wound exudate reacts with the gel, the iodine is released to decrease the bacterial load in the wound.

Collagen Dressings

Collagen provides the structural foundation of tendon, bone, and skin. It is the most abundant protein found in the body and plays an integral role in wound healing. Many of the collagen dressings are developed from bovine (ox) hide and have demonstrated effective wound healing properties. Because collagen can absorb 40 to 50 times its weight in fluid, these dressings are used for moderate to high exudating wounds. When placed into a wound it acts as a hemostatic agent, but with continued use may accelerate the wound healing process.

Hydrocolloid Dressing

Hydrocolloids are developed from a gel-forming polymer material combined with an impermeable backing to create an occlusive environment over the wound. These dressings are indicated for low to moderate exudating wounds. The colloid material reacts with the exudate to form a gel matrix but has only minimal absorptive capabilities. The benefits of the occlusive environment include the development of a moist healing environment, promotion of **autolytic debridement,** and the creation of new capillaries in the wound known as **angiogenesis.**

Hydrogel Dressing

Hydrogels are composed of amorphous gels or incorporated into sheet or island dressings. They are intended to hydrate a dry, desiccated wound bed. Hydrogels have no absorptive capabilities and should be avoided with moderate to heavy exudating wounds. They are also indicated for wounds with **eschar.** The gel is applied to the eschar after being scored or cut and can aid in eschar removal upon the next dressing change. Most hydrogel dressings require a secondary dressing to secure them in place.

Semipermeable Film Dressing

Transparent or clear films were devised primarily as a secondary dressing or for use in conjunction with other dressings. They are typically adhesive in nature and the dressings have a high moisture permeability vapor rate (MPVR). The MVPR indicates the "breathability" of the dressing. This feature allows the transfer and exchange of important gases through the dressing while providing a fluid-proof barrier for the wound. If used alone, the dressing traps moisture against the wound and has no absorptive capabilities.

CONSIDERATIONS FOR THE INSENSITIVE WOUND

In cases of the neuropathic (diabetic) wound, the ulcer or lesion is usually associated with the foot and located on the plantar aspect of the foot. The plantar location of the wound is associated with loss of protective sensation, which is characteristic of peripheral neuropathy experienced by patients with diabetes. Treatment for the plantar wound should include the wound management techniques previously described. Pressure reduction to the affected foot must be achieved either by strict bed rest (ideal but not practical in the outpatient setting) or by use of a non-weight-bearing (NWB) gait pattern using a walker or crutches. Partial weight-bearing (PWB) gaits are usually not ideal but may be more practical for some patients. PWB allows the patient to protect the wound and continue to be functional in accomplishing activities of daily living.

The most effective technique for midfoot and forefoot neuropathic foot ulcers is the **total contact walking cast** (Fig. 18-23). For rearfoot ulcers the posterior walking splint (a modification of the total contact walking cast) is most effective. Other less effective alternatives to the cast and splint are customized or specialized footwear such as the Orthowedge (Alimed, Inc., Dedham, MA), which can decrease the weight at the forefoot owing to its unique design (Fig. 18-24) especially when used with an assistive device.

DEBRIDEMENT

There are two basic categories of debridement, nonselective and selective. *Nonselective debridement* effects all tissues exposed in the wound. This technique can be effective in liberating the wound of nonviable tissue but can be harmful to delicate healing tissue. These techniques include hydrotherapy, wet-to-dry dressings, as well as radical surgical debridement. *Selective debridement* is the more conservative of the two categories because these techniques protect the healing tissue while effectively eliminating necrotic tissue. Selective techniques include

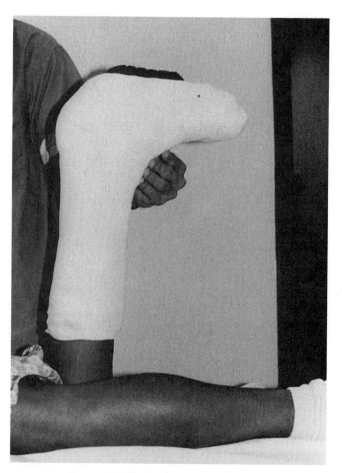

Figure 18-23. Total contact walking cast.

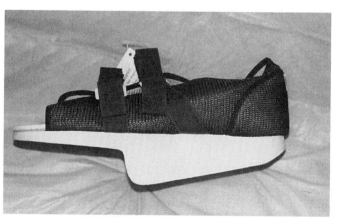

Figure 18-24. Orthowedge™ healing shoe (Alimed, Inc., Dedham, MA).

sharp, autolytic, and enzymatic debridement. **Sharp debridement** is accomplished by use of a scalpel, scissors, or tweezers to remove necrotic tissue. Autolytic debridement involves use of synthetic dressings, which provide a moist healing environment and allow the patient's own body to cleanse the wound. **Enzymatic debridement** utilizes topical ointments impregnated with enzymes placed directly in the wound to assist with debridement. Enzymatic debridement requires a prescription from a physician.

SUMMARY

PVD is a prevalent pathological process with a variety of clinical presentations. An overview of the more commonly encountered PVDs has been presented together with suggested assessment procedures and interventions. A thorough examination of the patient's vascular status will allow the physical therapist to establish a diagnosis, prognosis, and plan of care to achieve desired outcomes.

The role of the physical therapist in wound care has expanded dramatically in recent years. Knowledge of normal tissue repair and chronic healing states, administration of selected modalities, application of appropriate wound covers, and debridement techniques allow the physical therapist to provide safe and effective wound management for patients with a variety of diagnoses. General guidelines have been presented for developing an algorithm of care to achieve improved patient function and quality of life.

QUESTIONS FOR REVIEW

1. Describe the anatomical differences between the arterial system and vascular systems.

2. A patient presents to you with a chief complaint of pain in the lower extremity. The patient has a history of diabetes and hypertension. What questions would you ask to rule out vascular insufficiency or arterial insufficiency?

3. A patient presents with a diagnosis of venous insufficiency with an edematous right lower extremity. Upon examination, you note the extremity is very warm to the touch with the presence of a positive cuff test. Do you continue with the examination and provide IPC treatment? Provide a rationale for your answer.

4. Compare and contrast two interventions for arterial insufficiency and two interventions for venous insufficiency.

5. When examining a patient with arterial insufficiency, what type of objective information would you expect to find?

6. A patient presents to physical therapy with large medial leg ulcers and all test results point toward venous insufficiency. There is a large wound with approximately 80 percent beefy red granulation, 20 percent yellow slough, and a moderate amount of drainage. Describe appropriate treatment interventions for this patient.

CASE STUDY

A 62 year-old male is referred to physical therapy for evaluation and management of a left lower extremity wound. The patient reports no history of diabetes, but is mildly hypertensive. He smokes two packs of cigarettes per day and drinks one or two beers per week. Previous management with gauze dressing and use of growth factors have been unsuccessful. The patient states the wound started from hitting his leg on a bedpost approximately 3 months ago. The wound has progressively worsened since initial injury. The patient also reports mild pain in feet at night while sleeping. He is able to ambulate nearly ½ mile before leg cramps begin. This patient presents with a large, painful, anterior tibial wound on his left lower extremity that has limited his normal activity. The wound has approximately 25 percent granulation tissue and little or no drainage. The majority of the wound is covered with adherent slough and there is a small area of eschar. The injured lower extremity is cool to the touch; the pulses are dopplerable but not palpable. The ABI examination on the left lower extremity was 115/160 ≥0.72. Mild edema is present and both the rubor and venous filling times are delayed.

Guiding Questions

1. What are the precipitating factors associated with this patient's condition?

2. What signs and symptoms are significant from the examination?

3. Are the signs and symptoms consistent with findings for arterial or venous insufficiency?

4. What interventions would be appropriate for this patient?

5. What would be an appropriate wound dressing? Provide a rationale for your selection.

6. Identify outcomes of physical therapy intervention for this patient.

7. Identify goals of treatment for this patient.

8. Establish a plan of care for this patient.

REFERENCES

1. Spence, A: Basic Human Anatomy, ed 3. Benjamin/Cummings Publishing, Menlo Park, CA, 1990.
2. Guyton, A, and Hall, JE: Human Physiology and Mechanisms of Disease, ed 6. Saunders, Philadelphia, 1997.
3. Hole, JW (ed): Human Anatomy and Physiology, ed 4. William C. Brown Publishers, Dubuque, Iowa, 1987.
4. Ikomi, F, and Schnid-Schonbein, GW: Lymph transport in the skin. Clin Dermatol 13:419, 1995.
5. Hannson, C: Optimal treatment of venous ulcers in elderly patients. Drugs Aging 5:324, 1994.
6. Cranley, JJ: Vascular Surgery, vol 1: Peripheral Arterial Disease. Harper & Row, Philadelphia, 1972.
7. Fairbain, JF, et al: Acute Arterial Occlusion of the Extremities. In Juergans, JL, et al (eds): Peripheral Vascular Disease. Saunders, Philadelphia, 1980, p 381.
8. McCulloch, JM, et al: Wound Healing: Alternatives in Management, ed 2. FA Davis, Philadelphia, 1995.
9. Cooke, J: Endothelial function and peripheral vascular disease. In Spittell, JA (ed): Contemporary Issues in Peripheral Vascular Disease. Philadelphia, FA Davis, 1992, p 1.
10. deWolfe, VG: Chronic Occlusive Arterial Disease of the Lower Extremity. In Spittell, JA (ed): Clinical Vascular Disease. FA Davis, Philadelphia, 1983, p 15.
11. Rockson, SG, and Cooke, J: Peripheral arterial insufficiency: Mechanisms, natural history, and therapeutic options. Adv Intern Med 43:255, 1998.
12. Correlli, F: Beurger's disease: Cigarette smoker disease may always be cured by medical therapy. J Cardiovasc Surg 14:28, 1973.
13. Hirai, M, and Shionoya, S: Intermittent claudication of the foot and Buerger's disease. Br J Surg 65:210, 1978.
14. Berkow, R, and Fletcher, AJ (eds): Merck Manual, ed 16. (Section 3, Number 12) Merck Research Laboratories, Rahway, NJ, 1992, p 583.
15. Cook, WW, et al: Venous thromboembolism and other venous disease in the Tecumseh community health study. Circulation 48:839, 1973.
16. Burton, C (1995): Practical Leg Ulcer Management. Excerpt from Symposium on Advanced Wound Care, San Diego, CA, 1995.
17. Hume, MH: Acute venous thrombosis. In Spittel, JA (ed): Clinical Vascular Disease. FA Davis, Philadelphia, 1983, p 121.
18. Marieb, E, and Mallatt, J: Blood vessels. In Spence, AP (ed); Human Anatomy. Benjamin/Cummings Publishing, Menlo Park, CA, 1992, p 309.
19. Browse, NL: Venous ulcerations. British Journal of Medicine 226:1920, 1983.
20. Gjores, JE: Symposium on venous leg ulcers: Opening comments of the symposium. Acta Chir Scand Suppl 544:7, 1988.
21. Browse, NL, and Burnand, KG: The cause of venous ulceration. Lancet 2:243, 1982.
22. Coleridge-Smith, PD, et al: Causes of venous ulceration: A new hypothesis. BMJ 296:1726, 1988.
23. Greenwood, JE, et al: The possible role of ischemia-reperfusion in the pathogenesis of chronic venous ulceration. Wounds 7:211, 1995.
24. Daroczy, J: Pathology of lymphedema. Clin Dermatol 13:433, 1995.
25. Kinmonth, JB, et al: Primary lymphedema: Clinical and lymphangiographic studies of a series of 107 patients in which lower limbs were affected. Br J Surg 45:1, 1957.
26. Kinmonth, JB, and Taylor, GW: Primary lymphedema: Classification and other studies based on oleolymphography and clinical features. J Cardiovasc Surg 15:8, 1969.
27. Browse, NL, and Stewart, G: Lymphedema: Pathophysiology and classification. J Cardiovasc Surg 26:91, 1985.
28. Harwood, CA, and Mortimer, PS: Causes and clinical manifestations of lymphatic failure. Clin Dermatol 13:459, 1995.
29. Smith, F, et al: Falsely elevated ankle pressures in severe leg ischemia. Surgery 172:130, 1996.
30. Blankenhorn, D, and Hodis, H: Arterial imaging and atherosclerosis reversal. Arteriosclerotic Thrombosis 14:177, 1994.
31. Vogt, M, et al: Lower extremity arterial disease and the aging process: A review. J Clin Epidemiol 45:529, 1992.
32. Cooke, J: Medical management of chronic arterial disease. In Cook, J, and Frohlicj, E (eds): Current Management of Hypertensive and Vascular Disease. Mosby, St. Louis, 1992, p 203.
33. Duprez, D, and Clement, D: Medical treatment of peripheral vascular disease: Good and bad. Eur Heart J 13:149, 1992.
34. Ernst, E, and Fialka, V: A review of the clinical effectiveness of exercise therapy for intermittent claudication. Arch Intern Med 113:135, 1990.
35. Williams, LR, et al: Vascular rehabilitation: Benefits of a structured exercise and risk modification program. J Vasc Surg 14:320, 1991.
36. McCulloch, JM, and Kemper, CC: Vacuum-compression therapy for the treatment of an ischemic ulcer. Phys Ther 73:165, 1993.
37. Christen, Y, et al: Effects of pneumatic compression on venous hemodynamics and fibrinolytic activity. Blood Coagul Fibrinolysis 8:185,1997.
38. Eze, AR, et al: Intermittent calf and foot compression increases lower extremity blood flow. Am J Surg 172:130, 1996.
39. Gaylarde, PM, et al: The effect of compression on venous stasis. Br J Dermatol 128:255, 1993.
40. Coleridge-Smith, et al: Sequential gradient pneumatic compression enhances venous ulcer healing: A randomized trial. Surgery 108:871, 1990.
41. McCulloch, J: Intermittent compression in the treatment of a chronic stasis ulceration. Phys Ther 61:1452, 1981.
42. Lippman, HI, and Briere, JP: Physical basis of external supports in chronic venous insufficiency. Arch Phys Med Rehabil 52:555, 1971.
43. Richmand, DM, et al: Sequential pneumatic compression for lymphedema. Arch Surg 120:1116, 1985.
44. Zelikovski, A, et al: Lympha-press: A new pneumatic device for the treatment of lymphedema of the limbs. Lymphology 13:68, 1980.
45. Casley-Smith, JR: The pathophysiology of lymphedema. In Heim, LR (ed): IXth International Congress of Lymphedema (Tel-Aviv, Israel). Immunology Research Foundation, Inc. Newburgh, NY, 1983, p 125.
46. Foldi, E, et al: Conservative treatment of lymphedema of the limbs. Angiology 36:171, 1985.
47. Foldi, M, and Casley-Smith, JR: Lymphangiology. Schattauer, New York, 1983.
48. Weissleder, H, et al: Therapy concepts. In Weissleder, H, and Schuchhardt, C (eds): Lymphedema: Diagnosis and Treatment, ed 2. Kagerer Kommunikation, Bonn, Germany, 1997, p 263.
49. Deuel, TF, et al: Chemotaxis of monocytes and neutrophils to platelet-derived growth factor. J Clin Invest 69:1064, 1982.
50. Knighton, DR, et al: Oxygen as an antibiotic: The effects of inspired oxygen on infection. Arch Surg 119:199, 1984.
51. Peacock, EE: Wound Repair, ed 3. Saunders, Philadelphia, 1984.
52. Krawczyk, WS: A pattern of epidermal cell migration during wound healing. J Cell Biol 49:247, 1971.
53. Ferguson, NH: Ultrasound in the treatment of surgical wounds. Physiotherapy 67:12, 1981.
54. Roch, C, and West, J: A controlled trial investigating the effects of ultrasound on venous ulcers referred from general practitioners. Physiotherapy 70:475, 1984.
55. McDiarmid, T, et al: Ultrasound in the treatment of pressure sores. Physiotherapy 71:66, 1985.
56. Brown, M, and Gogia, PP: Effects of high voltage stimulation on cutaneous wound healing in rabbits. Phys Ther 67:662, 1987.
57. Dunn, MG, et al: Wound healing using a collagen matrix: Effect of dc electrical stimulation. J Biomed Mater Res 22:191, 1988.

58. Bourguignon, GJ, and Bourguignon, LYW: Electrical stimulation of protein and DNA synthesis in human fibroblasts. FASEB J 1:398, 1987.

59. Licht, S: History of ultraviolet therapy. In Stillwell, GK (ed): Therapeutic Electricity and Ultraviolet Radiation, ed 3. Williams & Wilkins, Baltimore, 1983, p 1.

60. Scott, BO: Clinical uses of ultraviolet radiation. In Licht, E (ed): Therapeutic Radiation and Ultraviolet Radiation, ed 2. Waverly, Baltimore, 1967, p 335.

61. Scott, BO: Clinical uses of ultraviolet radiation. In Stillwell, GK (ed): Therapeutic Radiation and Ultraviolet Radiation, ed 3. Williams & Wilkins, Baltimore, 1983, p 228.

62. Michlovitz, SL: Biophysical principles of heating and superficial heat agents. In Michlovitz, SL (ed): Thermal Agents in Rehabilitation, ed 2. FA Davis, Philadelphia, 1990, p 88.

63. Doe, PT, et al: A new method of treating venous ulcers with topical radiant warming. Journal of Wound Care 4:87, 1997.

64. Argenta, LC, and Morykwas, MJ: Vacuum assisted closure: A new method for wound control and treatment: Clinical experience. Ann Plast Surg 38:563, 1997.

SUPPLEMENTAL READINGS

Ellis, H: Varicose Veins: How They are Treated and What You Can Do to Help. Arco, New York, 1982.

Barker, WF: Peripheral Arterial Disease, ed 2. Saunders, Philadelphia, 1975.

Holling, HE: Peripheral Vascular Diseases: Diagnosis and Management. Lippincott, Philadelphia, 1972.

Kappert, A, and Winsor, T: Diagnosis of Peripheral Vascular Disease. FA Davis, Philadelphia, 1972.

Krasner, D (ed): Chronic Wound Care: A Clinical Source Book for Health Care Practitioner. Health Management Publication, King of Prussia, PA, 1990.

Spittell, JA: Contemporary issues in peripheral vascular disease. Cardiovasc Clin 22:3, 1992.

Spittell, JA (ed): Clinical Vascular Disease. FA Davis, Philadelphia, 1983.

Sussman, C, and Bates, BM (eds): Wound Care: A Collaborative Practice manual for Physical Therapists and Nurses. Aspen, Gaithersburg, MD, 1998.

Weissleder, H, and Schuchhardt, C (eds): Lymphedema: Diagnosis and Therapy, ed 2. Kagerer Kommunikation, Bonn, Germany, 1997.

GLOSSARY

Acrocyanosis: Cyanosis of the extremities due to a vasomotor disturbance. It is seen in catatonia or hysteria.

Agenesis: The failure of an organ or part of an organ to develop or grow.

Anastomotic: Pertaining to the natural communication between two vessels.

Angiogenesis: The formation of new blood vessels.

Ankle-brachial index (ABI): Test designed to assess the vascular system; the lower extremity pressure is divided by the upper extremity pressure and a ratio or index is calculated; segmental pressures can also be assessed to determine different pressures and levels of vascular flow.

Aplasia: The failure of an organ or tissue to develop normally.

Arteriole: The smallest subunit of the arterial system.

Arteriosclerosis: A condition whereby there is hardening of the walls of arteries. This may involve the intima and media.

Arteriovenous fistula: An abnormal connection between the arterial and venous systems.

Atherosclerosis: A form of arteriosclerosis in which yellowish plaques (atheromas) form within the vessel walls. The plaques consist of lipids and other blood-borne substances.

Autolytic debridement: Use of synthetic dressings that provide a moist healing environment; allows the patient's own body to cleanse the wound.

Bifurcation: A point of branching or forking of a vessel.

Bruit: An adventitious sound heard in a blood vessel during auscultation that is caused by the turbulent flow of blood.

Capillary: A small blood vessel that connects arterioles to venules.

Combined physical decongestive therapy (CPDT): A specialized form of massage, bandaging, and exercise used to open collateral lymphatics and remove excess fluid from an affected limb so that the proper drainage can occur.

Cyanosis: A slightly bluish-gray or purple discoloration of the skin caused by a decreased hemoglobin content in the blood.

Debridement: Removal of dead or damaged tissue from a wound.

Endarterectomy: An excision or removal of the thickened, atheromatous intimal layer of an artery.

Enzymatic debridement: Removal of tissue by use of topical ointments impregnated with enzymes placed directly in the wound.

Erythromelalgia: Bilateral vasodilation affecting the extremities, especially the feet; marked by redness, burning, throbbing, and increased skin temperature.

Eschar: A dark, thick leathery scab or covering of a full-thickness wound.

Fibrin: A whitish-yellow protein formed by the action of thrombin on fibrinogen.

Fibroblast: Any cell or corpuscle from which connective tissue is developed.

Fistula: An abnormal connection between two areas.

Gangrene: Tissue death or necrosis; usually due to impaired or absent blood supply.

Granulation tissue: A matrix of collagen, hyaluronic acid, and fibronectin in a newly formed vascular network.

Hemosiderin: A pigment released from hemoglobin owing to red cell lysis.

Indurated: Hardened.

Infection: The presence of bacteria or microorganisms is $>10^5$ per gram of tissue determined by a quantitative culture.

Intermittent claudication: A severe pain in the lower extremity that occurs with activity but subsides with rest. It is the result of inadequate arterial blood supply to the exercising muscles.

Ischemia: A restriction in blood supply to a body part; usually local and temporary in nature.

Ligation: The surgical clipping and tying off of a diseased vein.

Lipodermatosclerosis: The progressive replacement of skin and subcutaneous tissue by fibrous tissue as a result of calf pump failure.

Lymphedema: The reduced transport capacity of the lymphatic system with normal volume of lymph transported waste.

Maceration: The process of softening a solid (skin) by saturating it with fluid or drainage.

Macule: Discolored spot on the skin, neither raised nor depressed.

Milroy's disease: The autosomal dominant, congenital form of lymphedema resulting in the aplasia or hypoplasia of the lymphatic system.

Pallor: Paleness or absence of coloration in the skin.

Papule: Red elevated area on the skin.

Radiometer: A temperature-measuring device designed to measure infrared radiation.

Raynaud's phenomenon: A process initiated by exposure to cold or emotional disturbance. It results in intermittent episodes of pallor followed by cyanosis, then redness of the digits, before a return to normal.

Rubor: Redness of the skin caused by inflammation.

Scleroderma: A chronic disease of unknown etiology that causes a sclerosis or hardening of the skin and other internal organs.

Sclerotherapy: The use of sclerosing agent injected into varices such as varicose veins in the extremities, hemorrhoids, and for superficial varicosities of the skin.

Sharp debridement: Use of a scalpel, scissors, or tweezers to remove necrotic tissue.

Slough: Wound description of nonviable tissue, fibrin, and pus.

Stemmer's sign: The inability to pick up a fold of skin at the base of the second toe; reliable evidence of lymphedema.

Stasis dermatitis: An inflammatory condition of the skin caused by pooling of venous blood.

Thermistor: A temperature-measuring device designed to gauge the contact temperature of the skin.

Total contact walking cast: A specialized closed toe walking cast that is fabricated for precise conforming fit to reduce the pressure on the foot sustained during ambulation.

Trophic changes: Observable alterations of the skin and digits owing to poor arterial nutrition.

Valvuloplasty: Plastic repair of a valve, especially a valve of the heart.

Vascular prosthesis: Any artificial component placed into the vascular system to perform a function previously performed by a unit of the system. An example is an artificial heart valve.

Venous reflux: The back flow of blood through a vein that has valvular incompetence.

Venule: The smallest subunit of the venous system.

Vesicle: A small fluid filled blister on the skin.

Volumetrics: A system that uses a calibrated cylinder for determining the amount of water displaced from a specialized container for quantitatively measuring edema.

Wound contraction: Process in which a full thickness wound decreases in size by centripetal movement of the entire thickness of the surrounding skin.

APPENDIX A

Foot Care Instructions

- Wash your feet daily.
- Dry between your toes after bathing.
- Wear clean socks.
- Test the temperature of the bath water with a part of your body that feels things properly. If that is not possible, use a thermometer. Temperature should be 85° to 90°.
- Inspect your feet, using a mirror if necessary, every day (look for cuts, scratches, cracks, redness, swelling, discoloration, and bruises).
- Report unusual changes in your feet immediately.
- If you have diabetes, follow your doctor's plan.
- Wear shoes that fit properly.
- Do not walk barefoot.
- Do not sit with your legs crossed.
- Do not wear stockings with elastic tops.
- Do not wear round elastic garters.
- Do not smoke.
- Do not expose yourself to cold weather.
- Do not use a hot water bottle or heating pad.
- Do not get sunburned.
- Do not put medicine on corns or cut them without supervision.
- Do not wear run-down shoes.
- Do not wear worn-out socks.
- Do not dig into corners of toes.

APPENDIX B

Patient Education: Skin Care and Footwear Instructions

SKIN CARE

1. Wash gently every day using lukewarm water and mild soap.
2. Dry thoroughly, especially between the toes.
3. Use a lanolin lotion or petroleum jelly to soften the dry skin. Do not apply lotion between the toes.
4. Use powder or cornstarch between the toes.
5. To increase air circulation through the toes, wisps of lamb's wool may be used between the toes. The lamb's wool should be changed daily. (Cotton or cotton balls should not be used, because the fibers are irritating to the skin.)

INSPECTION

1. Inspect your feet daily.
2. Look for blisters, sores, corns, calluses, redness, swelling, pain, and drainage (these may be signs of ill-fitting shoes).
3. Call your doctor about any problems with sores that do not heal.
4. Check your shoes daily for stones, tacks, and nails, which can cause blisters, sores, and ulcers.

SAVE YOUR SOLES

1. Use a pumice stone to treat corns and calluses. No sharp instruments or home remedies should be used! Store-bought "cures" contain an acid that can harm the skin tissue.
2. Wear clean, non-elastic cotton socks and change them daily.
3. Say "goodbye" to going barefoot.
4. Wear comfortable leather shoes. Alternate shoes each day to allow them to breathe and dry.
5. Cold feet? Wear warm, cotton, nonconstricting socks to bed; do not use hot water bottles or heating pads.
6. Cut toenails straight across even with the ends of the toe. Do not cut into the corners. Use an emery board or nail file for sharp edges.
7. Break in shoes gradually. Shop for shoes in the afternoon when your feet are the largest.

APPENDIX C

Sample Patient Data Collection Form

Patient Name: _____ I.D. _____

Admit Date: _____ Age: _____ Sex: ( ) M   ( ) F

Occupation: _____ Problem: _____

When did problem first develop? _____
      Developed spontaneously ( )
      Developed from injury   ( ) _____

Has problem gotten ( ) better   ( ) worse   ( ) remained same

Medical/Social History

	Self	Family
Diabetes	( )	( ) _____
PVD	( )	( ) _____
HTN	( )	( ) _____
CHF	( )	( ) _____
Other _____	( )	( ) _____

Medications: _____
                _____

Allergies: _____

Does patient use any tobacco products?   ( ) Yes   ( ) No

Subjective:

Is pain present?   ( ) Yes   ( ) No   Paresthesia ( )   Anesthesia ( )

Type of Pain?   ( ) sharp/burning   ( ) dull aching
              ( ) constant   ( ) intermittent

How does pain change with position? _____
_____

Has a culture been taken?   ( ) Yes   ( ) No
      Results? _____

Have radiographs been taken?   ( ) Yes   ( ) No
      Results? _____

Continued

APPENDIX C Continued

Have any other special tests been performed? ( ) Yes   ( ) No

    Results? _____

Objective:

Wound Locations:	Stage	Color/Tissue	Exudate
1)	I-Reddened, Intact	R-Red-Granulation	O-None
	II-Partial Thickness	Y-Yellow-Slough	S-Serous
2)	III-Full Thickness	B-Black-Eschar	SA-Sero-sanguinous
	IV-Vasc/Bone Involved	M-Mixed (specify)	P-Purulent
3)			

Status:

Wnd # | Stage | Color/Tissue | Exudate | Undermining | Dimensions

Other Objective Tests

Temperature: _____

        _____

Girth: _____

        _____

Volumetrics: _____

        _____

Point of Measurement

( ) Right ( ) Left _____

( ) Right ( ) Left _____

( ) Right ( ) Left _____

( ) Right ( ) Left _____

( ) Right ( ) Left _____

( ) Right ( ) Left _____

Pulses: Good = 2+   Dorsalis Pedis   (R) _____ (L) _____

        Weak = 1+   Posterior Tibial (R) _____ (L) _____

        Absent = 0   Popliteal (R) _____ (L) _____

                  Femoral (R) _____ (L) _____

                  Other _____ (R) _____ (L) _____

Bruits: ( ) Yes   ( ) No _____

Percussion Test: Right ( ) Positive ( ) Negative

                  Left   ( ) Positive ( ) Negative

Trendelenburg Test: Right ( ) Positive ( ) Negative

                  Left   ( ) Positive ( ) Negative

Cuff Test: Right ( ) Positive ( ) Negative
               Left ( ) Positive ( ) Negative

Doppler Index: Dorsalis Pedis   Right _____   Left _____

               Posterior Tibial Right _____   Left _____

Rubor of Dependency: Right ( ) Positive ( ) Negative
                      Left ( ) Positive ( ) Negative

Venous Filling Time: Right ( ) Positive ( ) Negative
                      Left ( ) Positive ( ) Negative

Claudication Time: _____

Semmes-Weinstein Monofilament Testing

Location	Rating
_____ _____	( ) Normal ( ) Abnormal
_____ _____	( ) Normal ( ) Abnormal
_____ _____	( ) Normal ( ) Abnormal
_____ _____	( ) Normal ( ) Abnormal

Other Findings:

Assessment:

Plan:

APPENDIX D

Wound Product Names and Manufacturer

Category	Product Name	Manufacturer
Calcium Alginates	Algiderm	ConvaTec
	Sorbsan	Bertek Pharmaceuticals
	Curasorb	Kendall
Semipermeable Foams	Allevyn	Smith & Nephew
	Curafoam	Kendall
	Flexzan	Bertek Pharmaceuticals
	Lyofoam	ConvaTec
Hydrocolloid	Comfeel	Coloplast
	Curaderm	Kendall
	Cutinova Hydro	Beirsdorf
	DuoDerm	ConvaTec
	Restore	Hollister
	Replicare	Smith & Nephew
	Tegasorb	3M
Hydrogel Sheet	Clear Site	New Dimensions in Medicine
	Curagel	Kendall
	Aquasorb	DeRoyal
	Second Skin	Spenco
	Flexderm	Bertek Pharmaceuticals
Amorphous Gels	Carusym	Carrington Lab
	Restore	Hollister
	Curasol	Healthpoint
	Panaflex	Sage
Transparent Films	Bioclusive	Johnson & Johnson
	Blister film	Sherwood Medical
	IV3000	3M
	Polyskin	Kendall

APPENDIX E

Dressing Decision Tree

Moderate to High Exudating Wound

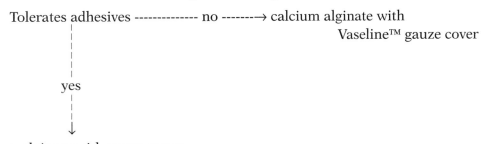

Tolerates adhesives ------------- no -------→ calcium alginate with

Vaseline™ gauze cover

yes

↓

calcium alginate with gauze cover

calcium alginate with adhesive foam

calcium alginate with hydrocolloid

hydrophillic fiber dressing

Minimal Exudating Wound

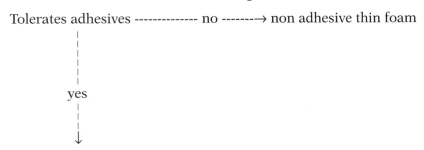

Tolerates adhesives ------------- no -------→ non adhesive thin foam

yes

↓

hydrocolloid, alginate with clear film,

adhesive thin foam dressing

Dessicated or Dry Wound

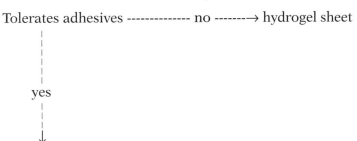

Tolerates adhesives ------------- no -------→ hydrogel sheet

yes

↓

hydrogel with clear film, moistened alginate

with clear film, hydrogel covered with hydrocolloid

APPENDIX F

Suggested Answers to Case Study Guiding Questions

1. What are the precipitating factors that are associated with this patient's condition?

ANSWER: The patient is a regular smoker with a poorly healing wound that is painful. Therefore, his overall level of function will likely be reduced.

2. What signs and symptoms are significant from the examination?

ANSWER
- Mild rest pain, intermittent claudication.
- Left lower extremity is cool to the touch.
- Pulses are not palpable but are dopplerable.
- ABI is decreased (0.72).
- Rubor of dependency and venous filling times are delayed.

3. Are the signs and symptoms consistent with findings for arterial or venous insufficiency?

ANSWER: Arterial insufficiency.

4. What interventions would be appropriate for this patient?

ANSWER
- A vascular rehabilitation program.
- Initiate use of the Vasotrain or the ArtAssist.

5. What would be an appropriate wound dressing? Provide a rationale for your selection.

ANSWER: An occlusive dressing that can maintain a moist healing environment, promote autolysis, and the formation of granulation.

6. Identify outcomes of physical therapy intervention for this patient.

ANSWER
- Patient education (instruction in disease process, home exercise and walking program).
- Improve granulation to 100 percent in 6 weeks.
- Complete wound resolution in 3 months.
- Increase patient's walking distance by one-third.

7. Identify goals of treatment for this patient.

ANSWER
- Decrease pain in wound with use of appropriate dressing.
- Increase granulation by 50 percent in 2 weeks.
- Increase walking distance by 25 percent in 3 weeks.
- Provide a moist wound healing environment.

8. Establish a plan of care for this patient.

ANSWER: Patient will be seen 3 to 5 times per week for appropriate modalities to facilitate wound healing, use of occlusive dressing to manage wound, and establish a vascular rehabilitation program to address mobility.

APPENDIX G

World Wide Web

PVD and Wound Care Internet addresses of interest:

www.veinsonline.com
www.venousinfo.com

www.woundcarenet.com
www.smtl.co.uk/world-wide-wounds/.com
http://members.aol.com/woundnet
www.woundcare.org

Assessment and Treatment of Individuals Following Lower Extremity Amputation

19

Bella J. May

LEARNING OBJECTIVES

1. Identify major etiological factors leading to amputation surgery.
2. Describe the major concepts involved in amputation surgery.
3. Describe the major components of postoperative management.
4. Identify components of the examination for an individual with a lower extremity amputation.
5. Properly position a person with a lower extremity amputation postoperatively.
6. Describe and demonstrate a method of proper residual limb bandaging.
7. Develop an exercise program to prepare an individual for eventual prosthetic fitting.
8. Be aware of the psychological impact of lower extremity amputation.
9. Analyze and interpret patient data, formulate realistic goals and outcomes, and develop a plan of care when presented with a clinical case study.

As you enter the physical therapy department this Monday morning, you note several new referrals coming out of the computer printer. You reflect that it is almost a year since you graduated from school. The time has gone by so fast and you have learned so much. You are pleased you took this position in a large regional hospital because you have had the opportunity to rotate through various services. You are currently working with general medical and surgical patients including those who have had vascular surgery.

You reach for the printout of new referrals and see one for a 72 year-old woman with diabetes and atherosclerosis. You treated her several months ago for an ulcer on the plantar surface of her right first metatarsal and know she had some problems with diabetic control. The patient had a right transtibial (below knee) amputation Sunday afternoon and is now referred for therapy. You are a little sad. The patient is a widow and lives alone although she has three grown children and six grandchildren in town. You remember how she talked about her garden and her other activities and wonder what her prognosis will be for rehabilitation.

The major cause of lower extremity amputation today continues to be **peripheral vascular disease (PVD),** particularly when associated with smoking and diabetes.[1-3] Major improvements in noninvasive diagnosis, revascularization, and wound healing techniques have lowered the overall incidence of amputations for vascular disease.[4-6] However, it has been reported that between 2 to 5 percent of individuals with PVD without diabetes and 6 to 25 percent of those with PVD and diabetes come to amputation.[6-11] Perioperative mortality has been variously reported between 7 and 13 percent and is usually associated with other medical problems such as cardiac disease and strokes.[12-14]

The second leading cause of amputation is trauma, usually from motor vehicle accidents or gunshots. Individuals with traumatic amputations are usually young adults and more frequently men.[14-15] Improved imaging techniques, more effective chemotherapy, and better limb salvage procedures have reduced the incidence of amputation from osteogenic sarcoma. In many instances, the tumor can be removed along with the involved section of bone. The limb is then reconstructed using bone grafts or metal implants. The reconstructed limb frequently provides as functional an extremity as a prosthesis and does not appear to affect 5-year survival rates, which have increased from about 20 percent in the 1970s to 60 to 70 percent in the 1980s.[16-20] Regardless of the cause of amputation, physical therapists have a major role in the rehabilitation program. Early onset of appropriate treatment influences the eventual level of rehabilitation.

LEVELS OF AMPUTATION

Traditionally, levels of amputation have been identified by anatomical considerations such as below knee and above knee. In 1974, the Task Force on Standardization of Prosthetic-Orthotic Terminology developed an international classification system to define amputation levels. Table 19–1 describes the major terms in common use today.

Traumatic amputations may be performed at any level; the surgeon tries to maintain the greatest bone length and save all possible joints. A variety of surgical techniques may be necessary to create a functional residual limb. Guillotine amputations may precede secondary closure with skin flaps; occasionally, free tissue flaps, taken from some other area of the body, may be used to cover deformities. Amputations for vascular diseases are generally performed at partial foot, transtibial, or transfemoral levels. The limited vascular supply mitigates against effective residual limb healing at the Symes level in most instances.

Patients with unilateral transtibial amputations regardless of age are quite likely to become functional prosthetic users; many individuals with bilateral transtibial amputations can be successfully rehabilitated. Elderly people with unilateral transfemoral amputations have more difficulty becoming prosthetically independent and most patients with bilateral transfemoral amputations do not become functional prosthetic users.[21,22] Generally, hip disarticulation, hemipelvectomies, and hemicorporectomies are performed either for tumors or for severe trauma and represent a small percentage of the population of individuals with amputations.

As you prepare to go see the patient, you mentally review what you know about amputation surgery

Table 19–1 LEVELS OF AMPUTATION

Partial toe	Excision of any part of one or more toes.
Toe disarticulation	Disarticulation at the metatarsal phalangeal joint.
Partial foot/ray resection	Resection of the 3rd, 4th, 5th metatarsals and digits.
Transmetatarsal	Amputation through the midsection of all metatarsals.
Syme's	Ankle disarticulation with attachment of heel pad to distal end of tibia. May include removal of malleoli and distal tibial/fibular flares.
Long transtibial (below knee)	More than 50% tibial length.
Transtibial (below knee)	Between 20 and 50% of tibial length.
Short transtibial (below knee)	Less than 20% tibial length.
Knee disarticulation	Amputation through the knee joint; femur intact.
Long transfemoral (above knee)	More than 60% femoral length.
Transfemoral (above knee)	Between 35 and 60% femoral length.
Short transfemoral (above knee)	Less than 35% femoral length.
Hip disarticulation	Amputation through hip joint; pelvis intact.
Hemipelvectomy	Resection of lower half of the pelvis.
Hemicorporectomy	Amputation both lower limbs and pelvis below L4–L5 level.

and the healing process. You are pleased that her amputation was at a transtibial level but are concerned about the potential for primary healing. You think about the effects of surgery and the factors that will influence healing.

Surgical Process

The specific type of surgery is at the discretion of the surgeon and is often determined by the status of the extremity at the time of amputation. The surgeon must remove the part of the limb that must be eliminated, allow for primary or secondary wound healing, and construct a residual limb for optimal prosthetic fitting and function. Numerous factors affect the selection of level of amputation. Conservation of residual limb length is important, as is uncomplicated wound healing. Surgical techniques vary with the level and cause of amputation, and a description of each type of surgical procedure is beyond the scope of this book. Interested readers may consult specific textbooks of surgical procedures. However, the physical therapist needs to understand some of the basic principles of amputation surgery.

Skin flaps are as broad as possible and the scar should be pliable, painless, and nonadherent. For most transfemoral and nondysvascular transtibial amputations, equal length anterior and posterior flaps are used, placing the scar at the distal end of the bone (Figs. 19-1 and 19-2). Long posterior flaps are often used in dysvascular transtibial amputations because the posterior tissues have a better blood supply than anterior skin. This places the scar anteriorly over the distal end of the tibia; care must be taken to ensure that the scar does not become adherent to the bone (Fig. 19-3A and B). Stabilization of major muscles allows for maximum retention of function. Muscle stabilization may be achieved by **myofascial closure, myoplasty, myo-**

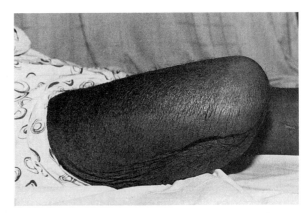

Figure 19-2. Transfemoral residual limb with incision from equal length flaps.

desis, or **tenodesis.** In most transtibial and transfemoral amputations, a combination of myoplasty (muscle to muscle closure) and myofascial closure is used to ensure that the muscles are properly stabilized and do not slide over the end of the bone. In some centers, myodesis (muscle attached to periosteum or bone) is employed particularly in transtibial amputations. More rarely, a tenodesis (tendon attached to bone) may be used for muscle stabilization. Whatever the technique, muscle stabilization under some tension is desirable at all levels where muscles must be transected.

Severed peripheral nerves form **neuromas** (a collection of nerve ends) in the residual limb. The neuroma must be well surrounded by soft tissue so as not to cause pain and interfere with prosthetic wear. Surgeons identify the major nerves, pull them down under some tension then cut them cleanly and sharply and allow them to retract into the soft tissue of the residual limb. Neuromas that form close to scar tissue or bone generally cause pain and may require later resection or revision.

Hemostasis is achieved by ligating major veins and arteries; **cauterization** is used only for small bleeders. Care is taken not to compromise circulation to distal tissues, particularly the skin flaps, which are important to uncomplicated wound healing.

Bones are sectioned at a length to allow wound closure without excessive redundant tissue at the end of the residual limb and without placing the incision under great tension. Sharp bone ends are smoothed and rounded; in transtibial amputations, the anterior portion of the distal tibia is **beveled** to reduce the pressure between the end of the bone and the prosthetic socket. Care is taken to ensure that the bone is physiologically prepared for the pressures of prosthetic wear.

Tissue layers are approximated under normal physiological tension and the incision is closed, usually with regular sutures. A drainage tube may be inserted as necessary.

In a traumatic amputation, the surgeon attempts to save as much bone length and viable skin as possible and preserve proximal joints while providing for appropriate healing of tissues without

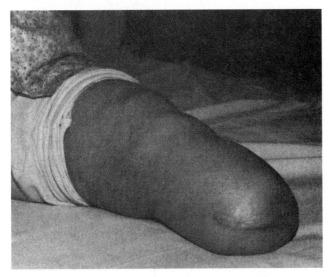

Figure 19-1. Transtibial residual limb with incision from equal length flaps.

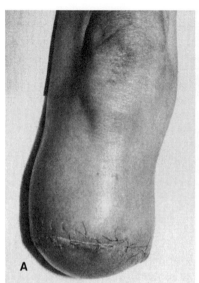

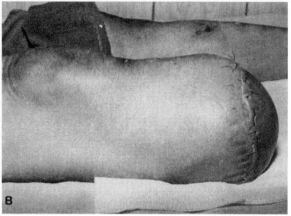

Figure 19-3. *A* and *B.* Transtibial residual limb with anterior incision from a long posterior flap.

secondary complications such as infection. In potentially "dirty" (involving foreign substances) amputations, the incision may be left open with the proximal joint immobilized in a functional position for 5 to 9 days to prevent invasive infection. **Secondary closure** also allows the surgeon to shape the residual limb appropriately for prosthetic rehabilitation.

Amputation for vascular disease is generally considered an elective procedure; the surgeon determines the level of amputation by assessing tissue viability through a variety of measures. Segmental limb blood pressures can be determined by Doppler systolic blood pressure measurement, Transcutaneous oxygen measurement, and skin blood flow by radioisotope or plethysmography are also determined. Doppler systolic blood pressure measures have been reported to be quite accurate in predicting viable level of amputation, but have not been as accurate in predicting amputations that do not heal.[23] Improvements in noninvasive assessment techniques have greatly reduced the use of **arteriography** to determine amputation level.

Healing Process

The surgeon's goal is to amputate at the lowest possible level compatible with healing.[24–26] There are a number of factors that may affect healing. Postoperative infection, whether from external or internal sources, is a major concern. Individuals with contaminated wounds from injury, infected foot ulcers, or other causes are at greater risk. Research indicates that smoking is a major deterrent to wound healing; one study reported that cigarette smokers had a 2.5 percent higher rate of infection and reamputation than nonsmokers.[27] There is some indication that failed attempts at limb revascularization may negatively influence healing at transtibial levels.[25–28] Other factors influencing wound healing are the severity of the vascular problems, diabetes, renal disease, and other physiological problems such as cardiac disease.[28–30]

REHABILITATION OUTCOMES

What will be the most appropriate outcomes for the patient at this time, you ask yourself. You wish you had seen her just before the amputation so you could have begun preparing her for the rehabilitation program. You know you will have only a few days before she is discharged to go home and need to develop outcomes that are as functional as possible. You also wonder if a home health referral will be possible after she leaves the hospital.

The earlier the onset of rehabilitation, the greater the potential for success. The longer the delay, the more likely the development of complications such as joint contractures, general debilitation, and a depressed psychological state. The postoperative program can be arbitrarily divided into two phases: (1) the postsurgical phase is the time between surgery and fitting with a definitive prosthesis or until a decision is made not to fit the patient, and (2) the prosthetic phase starts with delivery of a permanent replacement limb. The goal of the total rehabilitation program is to help the patient regain the presurgical level of function. For some, it will mean return to gainful employment with an active recreational life. For others, it will mean independence in the home and community. For still others, it may mean living in the sheltered environment of a retirement center or nursing home. If the amputation resulted from long-standing chronic disease, the goal may be to help the person function at a higher level than immediately before surgery.[31] The major outcomes of the postsurgical period are to:

1. Promote as high a level of independent function as possible.
2. Guide the development of the necessary physical and emotional level for eventual prosthetic rehabilitation.

3. Independence in mobility and self-care.
4. Independence in bed mobility and basic transfers.
5. Supervised or independent mobility with crutches or walker.
6. Demonstrate knowledge of proper residual limb positioning, bandaging, and care.

If the cause of amputation was PVD, an additional general outcome would be to teach the individual proper care of the remaining lower extremity and ensure adequate understanding of the disease process.

The major outcomes (short-term goals) of the postsurgical program generally are to:

1. Reduce (prevent) postoperative edema and promote healing of the residual limb.
2. Prevent contractures and other complications.
3. Maintain or regain strength in the affected lower extremity.
4. Maintain or increase strength in the remaining extremities.
5. Assist with adjustment to the loss of a body part.
6. Demonstrate knowledge of basic residual limb exercises.
7. Learn proper care of the remaining extremity.
8. Determine the feasibility of prosthetic fitting.

The success of the rehabilitation program is determined to some extent by the individual's psychological and physiological status and the physical characteristics of the residual limb. The longer the residual limb, the better potential for successful prosthetic ambulation regardless of level of amputation. A well-healed, cylindrical limb with a nonadherent scar is easier to fit than one that is conical or has redundant tissue distally or laterally. The vascular status of the remaining extremity will affect the rehabilitation program as will the physiological age of the individual. The presence of conditions such as diabetes, cardiovascular disease, visual impairment, limitation of joint motion, and muscle weakness may affect the eventual level of function. In the final analysis, a cooperative patient who takes an active part in the rehabilitation program is necessary for achievement of rehabilitation goals. If the patient appears noncompliant, it behooves the therapist to try to understand what is driving the patient's motivation and to make sure the patient understands the relationship between the postsurgical program and eventual prosthetic rehabilitation.

THE CLINIC TEAM

The majority of amputations today are performed by vascular surgeons who may or may not be knowledgeable about prosthetic rehabilitation. Referral to an amputation clinic or to physical therapy may be delayed for many weeks as the surgeon waits until the residual limb heals completely and the postoperative edema has been absorbed. Such delays are undesirable and may limit the eventual level of function. Ideally, the clinic team should become involved before surgery, or at least immediately after. Unfortunately, many amputations are performed in hospitals without the services of an amputation clinic or a well-trained team that can develop and supervise the program. The physical therapist may be the only person with competence in prosthetic rehabilitation. Close communication between the vascular surgeon and the physical therapist may serve to increase the likelihood of early referrals.

Members

The clinic team plans and implements comprehensive rehabilitation programs designed to meet the physical, psychological, and economic needs of the patient. Most clinic teams are located in rehabilitation facilities or university health centers. The team generally includes a physician, physical therapist, occupational therapist, prosthetist, and social worker. Other health professionals who often contribute to the team are the nurse, vocational counselor, dietitian, psychologist, and, possibly, administrative coordinator. Table 19–2 outlines the major functions of team members. The clinic team may meet monthly, bimonthly, or weekly depending on the caseload; patients are seen regularly and decisions are made using input from all team members. A screening clinic held by the physical and occupational therapists prior to the actual clinic allows for the careful evaluation of each person to be seen and improves the effectiveness of the clinic function.[32]

Table 19–2 AMPUTATION CLINIC TEAM FUNCTIONS

Physician	Clinic chief; coordinates team decision making; supervises patient's general medical condition; orders appliances.
Physical therapist	Assesses and treats patients through postsurgical and prosthetic phases; makes recommendations for prosthetic components and whether or not to fit the patient. May be clinic coordinator.
Prosthetist	Fabricates and modifies prosthesis; recommends prosthetic components; shares data on new prosthetic developments.
Occupational therapist	Assesses and treats patients with amputations of the upper extremities; makes recommendation for components.
Social worker	Financial counselor and coordinator, liaison with third-party payers and community agencies; helps family cope with social and financial problems.
Dietician	Consultant for patients with diabetes or those needing diet and nutritional guidance.
Vocational counselor	Assesses patient's employment potential; provides education and training; assists with placement.

In centers without an amputation clinic, close communication between the patient, surgeon, and physical therapists with the later addition of the prosthetist, is important to ensure an optimum level of decision making.

POSTOPERATIVE DRESSINGS

Reading the chart before going to see the patient, you note that the surgeon did not use a rigid postoperative dressing but rather applied a soft dressing covered with an elastic wrap. This information raises your concerns about edema control. Reviewing the chart, you note that the surgery went well, that the patient is afebrile, that vital signs are within normal limits, that she is not spilling sugar, and that she is voiding appropriately. The incision is reported to look clean and the drain is to be removed tomorrow morning. The nursing staff had her out of bed twice yesterday. You also check the patient's medications finding that she is on medication for diabetes, hypertension, and pain as needed. She had pain medication about an hour ago.

Surgeons have several options regarding the postoperative dressing including (1) immediate postoperative fitting or **rigid dressing,** (2) semirigid dressing, or (3) soft dressing. It is important for some sort of edema control to be used because excessive edema in the residual limb can compromise healing and cause pain.

Rigid Dressings

In the early 1960s, orthopedic surgeons in the United States started experimenting with a technique developed in Europe that consisted of fitting the person with a plaster of Paris socket made in the configuration of the definitive prosthesis. An attachment incorporated at the distal end of the dressing allows the later addition of a foot and pylon allowing limited weight-bearing ambulation within a few days or a week of surgery **(immediate postoperative prosthesis).**[33–35] Use of immediate postoperative rigid dressings vary greatly and are more prevalent in some areas of the country than others. Generally, orthopedic surgeons use the technique more than vascular surgeons. The advantages of the techniques are:
1. It greatly limits the development of postoperative edema in the residual limb, thereby reducing postoperative pain and enhancing wound healing.
2. It allows for earlier ambulation with the attachment of a pylon and foot.
3. It allows for earlier fitting of the permanent prosthesis by reducing the length of time needed for shrinking the residual limb.
4. It is configured to each individual residual limb.
The major disadvantages are:
1. It requires careful application by an individual

knowledgeable about prosthetic principles, often a prosthetist and occasionally a physical therapist.
2. It requires close supervision during the healing stage.
3. It does not allow for daily wound inspection and dressing changes.

Semirigid Dressings

There are a number of **semirigid dressings** that have been reported in the literature and may or may not be used in a particular center. All provide better control of edema than the soft dressing but each has some disadvantage that limits its use. **Unna's dressing,** gauze impregnated with a compound of zinc oxide, gelatin, glycerin, and calamine, may be applied in the operating room. Its major disadvantage is that it may loosen easily and is not as rigid as the plaster of Paris dressing. Little[36–39] first reported the use of an *air splint* to control postoperative edema as well as aid in early ambulation (Fig. 19-4). The air splint is a plastic double wall bag that is pumped to the desired level of rigidity. It has a zipper and encases the entire extremity, which is covered with an appropriate postsurgical dressing. While allowing improved visual wound inspection, the constant pressure does not intimately conform to the shape of the residual limb. The environment of the plastic is hot and humid, requiring frequent cleaning. The *Controlled Environment Treatment (CET)* was developed at the National Biomechanical Research and Development Unit of Roehampton, England, and has been used in some centers in the United States.[38,39] The CET is composed of a console that controls pressure, temperature, and humidity, sterilizes the air in the unit, and a polyvinyl transparent bag, which encases the residual limb. The bag's flexibility allows active exercises of the involved extremity as well as standing at bedside but the hose and machine limit bed mobility and ambulation.

Soft Dressings

The **soft dressing** is the oldest method of postsurgical management of the residual limb. Currently there are two forms of soft dressings: the elastic wrap and the elastic **shrinker.** The major advantages are that it is:
1. relatively inexpensive.
2. lightweight and readily available.
3. able to be laundered.
The major disadvantages are:
1. Relatively poor control of edema.
2. The elastic wrap requires skill in proper application.
3. The elastic wrap needs frequent reapplication.
4. Either can slip and form a tourniquet.
5. New shrinkers must be purchased as the residual limb gets markedly smaller.

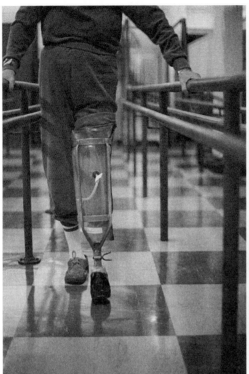
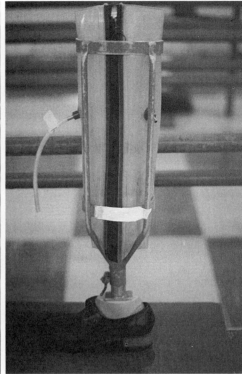

Figure 19-4. Air splint.

6. Shrinker cannot be used until the sutures have been removed and primary healing has occurred.

ELASTIC WRAPS

The elastic wrap may be applied over the postsurgical dressing if care is taken to ensure proper compression. A dressing is applied to the incision followed by some form of gauze pad, then the compression wrap. The soft dressing is indicated in cases of local infection, but is not the treatment of choice for the majority of individuals. The patient or a family member should learn to apply the wrap as soon as possible after wound care is no longer necessary. Many elderly individuals with transfemoral amputations do not have the necessary balance and coordination to wrap effectively.

Some surgeons prefer delaying elastic wrap until the incision has healed and the sutures have been removed. Leaving the residual limb without any pressure wrap allows for full development of postoperative edema, which may be quite uncomfortable and interfere with circulation in the many small vessels in the skin and soft tissue, thereby potentially compromising healing. The therapist can discuss the benefits of early wrapping if no other form of rigid dressing is used.

One of the major drawbacks of the elastic wrap is that it needs frequent rewrapping. Movement of the residual limb against the bedclothes, bending and extending the proximal joints, and general body movements will cause slippage and changes in pressure. Covering the finished wrap with a stockinet helps to reduce some of the wrinkling. However, careful and frequent rewrapping is the only effective way to prevent complications. Nursing staff, family members, and the patient as well as the physical therapist or physical therapist assistant need to assume responsibility for frequent inspection and rewrapping of the residual limb. Residual limb wrapping is described in detail later in this chapter.

SHRINKERS

Shrinkers are socklike garments knitted of heavy rubber reinforced cotton; they are conical in shape and come in a variety of sizes (Fig. 19-5). Shrinkers come in different sizes so it is not economical to purchase a shrinker while the residual limb is still covered with gauze dressings. Elastic wrap and shrinkers will be discussed in greater detail later in this chapter.

EXAMINATION

As you enter the patient's room you find her laying in bed, alert and awake. An incentive spirometer is on the bedside table. The patient looks tired and you realize you will not be able to gather all the information you need during this one visit. You think through the data that must be collected and begin to set priorities, deciding what needs to be done today and what can be put off for another time. Because the patient will probably not be in the hospital long, information regarding the status of the residual limb, her postsurgical cardiopulmonary and general physiological function, her ability to be mobile, the condition of the remaining lower extremity, and her feelings about the amputation may be the most important data to obtain.

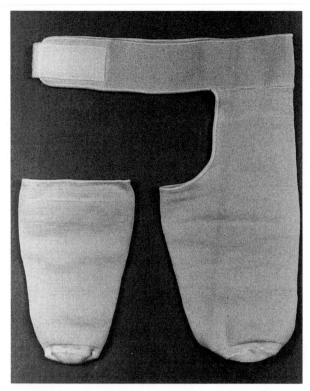

Figure 19-5. (*Left*) Transtibial shrinker. (*Right*) Transfemoral shrinker.

Careful examination of each individual is an integral part of physical therapy management. Examination data are obtained continuously throughout this period as the incision heals and the person's tolerance improves. Table 19–3 outlines the typical data needed during a postsurgical evaluation. The availability of some of these data will depend in part on the treatment of the residual limb by the surgeon.

Range of Motion

Gross range of motion estimations are adequate for examination of the uninvolved extremity but specific goniometric measurements are necessary for the amputated side. Hip flexion, extension, abduction, and adduction measurements are taken early in the postoperative phase following transtibial amputation. Measurement of knee flexion and extension are taken, if the dressing allows, after some incisional healing has occurred. Hip flexion, extension, abduction, and adduction range of motion measurements are taken several days after surgery when the dressing allows, following transfemoral amputation. Measurement of internal and external hip rotation is difficult to obtain and unnecessary if no gross abnormality or pathology is evident. Joint range of motion is monitored throughout the postsurgical period.

Muscle Strength

Gross manual muscle testing of the upper extremities and uninvolved lower extremity is performed early in the postoperative period. Manual muscle testing of the involved lower extremity must usually wait until most healing has occurred. With a transtibial amputation, good strength in the hip extensors and abductors as well as the knee extensors and flexors are needed for satisfactory prosthetic ambulation. For the patient with a transfemoral amputation, good strength of the hip extensors and abductors is a requirement. The strength of these muscles should be monitored throughout the postsurgical program.

Residual Limb

Residual limb measurements are generally taken and reported in centimeters for uniformity with others involved in the care of individuals who have had an amputation. Circumferential measurements of the residual limb are taken as soon as the dressing will allow, then regularly throughout the postsurgical period. Measurements are made at regular intervals over the length of the residual limb. Circumferential measurements of the transtibial or Symes residual limb are started at the medial tibial plateau and taken every 5 to 8 centimeters depending on the length of the limb. Length of the residual limb is measured from the medial tibial plateau to the end of the bone.

Circumferential measurements of the transfemoral or through knee residual limb are started at the ischial tuberosity or the greater trochanter, whichever is most palpable, and taken every 8 to 10 centimeters. Length is measured from the ischial tuberosity or the greater trochanter to the end of the bone. If there is considerable excess tissue distal to the end of the bone, then length measurements are taken to both the end of the bone and the incision line. For accuracy of repeat measurements, exact landmarks are carefully noted. If the ischial tuberosity is used in transfemoral measurements, hip joint position is noted as well.

Other information gathered about the residual limb includes its shape (conical, bulbous, redundant tissue), skin condition, sensation, and joint proprioception.

The Phantom Limb

The majority of individuals will encounter a **phantom limb** following amputation. In its simplest form, the phantom is the sensation of the limb that is no longer there. The phantom, which usually occurs initially immediately after surgery, is often described as a tingling, pressure sensation, sometimes a numbness. The distal part of the extremity is most frequently felt although, on occasion, the person will feel the whole extremity. The sensation is responsive to external stimuli such as bandaging or rigid dressing; it may dissipate over time or the person may have the sensation throughout life. Phantom sensation may be painless and usually

Table 19–3 POSTSURGICAL ASSESSMENT GUIDE

General medical information	• Cause of amputation (e.g., disease, tumor, trauma, congenital) • Associated diseases/symptoms (e.g., neuropathy, visual disturbances, cardiopulmonary disease, renal failure, congenital anomalies) • Current physiological state (e.g., postsurgical cardiopulmonary status, vital signs, shortness of breath, pain) • Medications
Skin	• Scar (e.g., healed, adherent, invaginated, flat) • Other lesions (e.g., size, shape, open, scar tissue) • Moisture (e.g., moist, dry, scaly) • Sensation (e.g., absent, diminished, hyperesthesia) • Grafts (e.g., location, type, healing) • Dermatological lesions (e.g., psoriasis, eczema, cysts)
Residual limb length	• Bone length (transtibial limbs measured from medial tibial plateau; transfemoral limbs measured from ischial tuberosity or greater trochanter) • Soft tissue length (note redundant tissue)
Residual limb shape	• Cylindrical, conical, bulbous end, etc. • Abnormalities (e.g., "dog ears," adductor roll)
Vascularity (both limbs if amputation cause is vascular)	• Pulses (e.g., femoral, popliteal, dorsalis pedis, posterior tibial) • Color (e.g., red, cyanotic) • Temperature • Edema (circumference measurement, water displacement measurement, caliper measures) • Pain (type, location, duration) • Trophic changes
Range of motion (ROM)	• Residual limb (specific for remaining joints) • Other lower extremity (gross for major joints)
Muscle strength	• Residual limb (specific for major muscle groups) • Other extremities (gross for necessary function)
Neurological	• Pain (phantom [differentiate sensation or pain], neuroma, incisional, from other causes) • Neuropathy • Cognitive status (e.g., alert, oriented, confused) • Emotional status (e.g., acceptance, body image)
Functional status	• Transfers (e.g., bed-to-chair, to toilet, to car) • Mobility (e.g., ancillary support, supervision) • Home/family situation (e.g., caregiver, architectural barriers, hazards) • Activities of daily living (e.g., bathing, dressing) • Instrumental activities of daily living (e.g., cooking, cleaning)
Other	• Preamputation status (e.g., work, activity level, degree of independence, life-style) • Prosthetic goals (desire for prosthesis, anticipated activity level and life-style) • Financial (e.g., available payment for prosthesis) • Prior prosthesis (if bilateral)

does not interfere with prosthetic rehabilitation. It is important for the patient to understand that the feeling is quite normal.

Phantom pain, on the other hand, is usually characterized as either a cramping or squeezing sensation, or a shooting or a burning pain. Some individuals report all three. The pain may be localized or diffuse; it may be continuous or intermittent and triggered by some external stimuli. It may diminish over time or may become a permanent and often disabling condition. In the first 6 months following surgery, phantom pain has been found to be related to preoperative limb pain in location and intensity. However, that relationship does not last and preoperative pain is not believed to be related to long-term phantom pain.[40] There is little agreement about the cause or treatment of either phantom sensation or pain and the literature is replete with studies of the phenomena.[41–45] Melzack[46] suggested that at least 70 percent of patients with amputations suffer from phantom pain. He indicated that patients view the phantom as part of themselves re-

gardless of where it is felt in relation to the body. Melzack suggests that phantom sensation and pain originate in the cerebrum.

"I postulate that the brain contains a neuromatrix, or network of neurons, that, in addition to responding to sensory stimulation, continuously generates a characteristic pattern of impulses indicating that the body is intact and unequivocally one's own."[46p123]

He reputes the general belief that phantom sensation and pain only occur with acquired amputations after the age of 5 or 6, indicating that all individuals who are missing a limb from whatever cause, as well as individuals who lose the use of their limbs through spinal cord injury, feel the missing limbs. Melzack believes that the brain not only responds to stimuli, but can generate perceptual experiences without external stimuli. "We do not need a body to feel a body."[46p126] Although management of phantom pain continues to be problematic, Melzack states:

". . . phantom limbs are a mystery only if we assume the body sends sensory messages to a passively receiving brain. Phantoms become comprehensible once we recognize that the brain generates the experience of the body. Sensory inputs merely modulate that experience; they do not directly cause it."[46p126]

The residual limb should be carefully examined to differentiate phantom pain from any other condition such as a neuroma. Sometimes, wearing a prosthesis will ease the phantom pain. Noninvasive treatments such as ultrasound, icing, TENS, or massage have been used with varying success. Mild non-narcotic analgesics have been of limited value with some individuals and no particular narcotic analgesic has proven effective. On occasion, in the presence of trigger points, injection with steroids or local anesthetic has reduced the pain temporarily. A variety of surgical procedures such as chordotomies, **rhizotomies,** and peripheral **neurectomies** have been tried with limited success. In some instances, hypnosis has been useful in carefully selected patients. The treatment of phantom pain can be very frustrating for the clinic team and the patient.[41–46]

Other Data

The vascular status of the uninvolved lower extremity is determined and its condition noted. Data gathered include condition of the skin, presence of pulses, sensation, temperature, edema, pain on exercise or at rest, presence of wounds, ulceration, or other abnormalities.

Activities of daily living and functional mobility skills including transfer and ambulatory status are examined and documented. Information on the patient's home situation, including any constraints or special needs, is valuable in establishing an individually relevant treatment program. Data regarding presurgical activity level and the person's own long-range goals are obtained through interview.

The person's apparent emotional status and degree of adjustment are noted. Exploration of the patient's suitability and desire for a prosthesis is begun and continues throughout the postsurgical period. Any other problems that may affect the rehabilitation program and outcomes are evaluated and documented.

EMOTIONAL ADJUSTMENT

As you perform the initial examination of the patient and talk with her about the amputation, you realize that she is quite depressed. Although losing the limb did not come as a shock because she had been struggling with a foot ulcer that would not heal, she verbalizes concern about her ability to return to her own home. She keeps saying, "I don't want to go to one of those places."

Initial reaction to the loss of a limb is usually grief and depression. If the amputation was traumatic, the immediate reaction may include disbelief. The person may experience insomnia, restlessness, and have difficulty concentrating. Some individuals may actually mourn the possible loss of a job or the ability to participate in a favorite sport or other activities rather than the lost limb per se. In the early stages, the person's grief may alternate with feelings of hopelessness, despondency, bitterness, and anger. Socially the patient may feel lonely, isolated, and the object of pity. Concerns about the future, about body image and sexual function, about the responses of family and friends, and about employment all affect the individual's reactions.

Long-term adjustment depends to a great extent on the individual's basic personality structure, sense of accomplishment, and place in the family, community, and world. In general, many individuals with amputations make a satisfactory adjustment to the loss and are reintegrated into a full and active life. In achieving final acceptance, the individual may go through a number of stages including denial, anger, euphoria, and social withdrawal.

Some individuals may try to avoid distressing thoughts of the lost limb through conscious self-control or by avoiding situations or people that remind them of the lost limb. Some may display temper tantrums or irrational resentment. Some may revert to childlike states of helplessness and dependence.

Many individuals are not fully aware of the consequences of amputation and may fear other physical limitations as a result of the surgery. Fear of impotence or sterility may lead some men to make grandiose statements or display reckless behavior to mask the fear. Thorough explanations of the amputation process and implications by the surgeon or other health worker may alleviate many of these fears.

Generally, people who have had an amputation may dream about themselves as having an intact limb. This image may be so vivid that they fall as they get up at night and attempt to walk to the bathroom without a prosthesis or crutches. Individuals who have lost their leg through injury may dream about the battle or accident in which they were injured. Such reenactments may lead to insomnia, trembling fits, speech impediments, and difficulty with concentration. In general, individuals with congenital amputations or acquired amputations before the age of 5 do not have some of the problems mentioned above because their amputation is a part of their developed self-image.

Psychological Support

The patient needs to receive reassurance and understanding from the entire rehabilitation team. The staff should create an open and receptive environment and be willing to listen. The patient should know what to expect during the entire process. The surgeon and therapists should carefully explain the steps and expectations of rehabilitation. Audiovisual media, such as films or slides, may be helpful.

Others with amputations who have made satisfactory adjustments in their lives and successfully completed rehabilitation may provide support, information on life-style changes, and encouragement in private or group sessions. Professionals skilled in group dynamics and patient education are helpful, especially for medical or technical advice regarding such issues as diabetes, medications, or PVD. Family and friends are often included. A nonthreatening atmosphere helps individuals express their feelings and frustrations.

Patients have various attitudes toward the prosthesis. Some are particularly concerned about its appearance, hoping that it will conceal their disability and give the illusion of an intact body. Others claim to be concerned primarily with the restoration of function. When the artificial limb is fitted, the patient must face the fact that the natural limb has been lost irrevocably. If individuals with amputations have been told that the prosthesis will replace their own limb, they may have unrealistic expectations that appearance and function will be as good as in the nonamputated extremity. Realistic adjustment will be necessary as the person learns to use the artificial substitute. Good predictors for adjustment to the prosthesis are motivation to master the prosthesis and to return to an active life-style.

The Elderly

The elderly individual with a lower extremity amputation is not content to sit in a wheelchair or limp with a walker, but seeks effective rehabilitation services and a meaningful life-style. The immediate reaction to amputation is no different than that of any other individual except that the amputation will usually not come as a surprise. The reaction may depend in part on the severity of preoperative pain and the extent of attempts to save the limb. Individuals who have suffered considerable pain may be grateful that the pain has ended. Patients who underwent extensive medical and surgical procedures to save the limb may have a sense of failure that the efforts were not successful. In general, the reactions of an elderly person will be similar to that of any other adult individual with an amputation. Some may feel a sense of hopelessness and despair, and have a preoccupation with impending death. Some may have insomnia, anorexia, and be withdrawn. Some elderly individuals may experience a loss of self-esteem and be afraid of becoming dependent. In some instances, the person may express that he or she has nothing to live for and desires death. Occasionally suicide may be contemplated or attempted. The elderly person seldom uses denial because the functional and anatomical deficit is obvious. Elderly persons are more likely to dream that the amputation has taken place as compared to younger individuals. The elderly person may view the amputation as impending death because the rest of the body is vulnerable.

If preoperative attitudes are unrealistically hopeful, postoperative disturbances may be more severe. The elderly person should not be led to expect a total cure. Learning to use an artificial limb may be a slow and discouraging ordeal and the patient may not express distress or depression in front of the optimism of others. Sharing and support from other elderly patients can be quite helpful as can a realistic attitude by rehabilitation team members.

Rehabilitation includes not only preparation of the individual physically and psychologically for the community, but preparation of the community for individuals with amputations. Public education media are useful means of information, particularly for prospective employers. As with other physically challenged individuals, those with amputations need to be accepted and integrated into the community because of their abilities and not their disabilities.

INTERVENTIONS

If the patient is to return to her own home, she will need to be ambulatory and able to take care of her residual limb. If she goes to her own home rather than a rehabilitation center, she will need some homemaking help as well as home health care for continued nursing and physical therapy. On the other hand, transfer to a rehabilitation center might help her reach an adequate level of independence to be able to function at home with minimal support until she can be fitted with a prosthesis. You decide to discuss this further with the physician and social worker. In the meantime, you realize that your treatment program will need to focus on functional mobility skills, residual limb care, and care of the intact leg.

Residual Limb Care

Individuals not fitted with a rigid dressing or a **temporary prosthesis** use elastic wrap or shrinkers to reduce the size of the residual limb. The patient, family member, or professional staff member applies the bandage, which is worn 24 hours a day, except when bathing.

Removable rigid dressings for use with transtibial amputations are available and may be an important alternative to the elastic wrap. Regretfully, there are fewer alternatives for the person with a transfemoral amputation; rigid dressings and inexpensive temporary prostheses are more difficult to fabricate and elastic wraps or shrinkers are only minimally effective. It may be advisable to fit the individual following transfemoral amputation with a definitive prosthesis early and then adjust it for shrinkage by using additional socks or a liner.

Edema in the residual limb is often difficult to

control owing to complications of diabetes, cardiovascular disease, or hypertension. An intermittent compression unit can be used to reduce edema on a temporary basis. Transfemoral and transtibial sleeves are commercially available.

Proper hygiene and skin care are important. Once the incision is healed and the sutures removed, the person can bathe normally. The residual limb is treated as any other part of the body; it is kept clean and dry. Individuals with dry skin may use a good skin lotion. Care must be taken to avoid abrasions, cuts, and other skin problems. Friction massage, in which layers of skin, subcutaneous tissue, and muscle are moved over the respective underlying tissue, can be used to prevent or mobilize adherent scar tissue. The massage is done gently, after the wound is healed and when no infection is present. Patients can learn to properly perform a gentle friction massage to mobilize the scar tissue and help decrease hypersensitivity of the residual limb to touch and pressure. Early handling of the residual limb by the patient is an aid to acceptance and is encouraged, particularly for individuals who may be repulsed by the limb.

The patient is taught to inspect the residual limb with a mirror each night to make sure there are no sores or impending problems, especially in areas not readily visible. If the person has diminished sensation, careful inspection is particularly important. Because the residual limb tends to become a bit edematous after bathing as a reaction to the warm water, nightly bathing is recommended, particularly once a prosthesis has been fitted. The elastic bandage, shrinker, or removable rigid dressing is reapplied after bathing. If the person has been fitted with a temporary prosthesis, the residual limb is wrapped at night and any time the prosthesis is not worn. Sometimes, individuals fitted in surgery with a rigid dressing then transferred immediately into a temporary prosthesis do not know how to bandage, and encounter difficulties with edema after they remove the prosthesis at night. Learning proper bandaging is part of the therapy program because most people will need to wrap the limb at one time or another.

Patients have been known to apply a variety of "home and folk remedies" to the residual limb. Historically, it was believed that the skin had to be toughened for prosthetic wear by beating it with a towel-wrapped bottle. Various ointments and lotions have been applied; residual limbs have been immersed in substances such as vinegar, salt water, and gasoline to harden the skin. Although the skin does need to adjust to the pressures of wearing an artificial limb, there is no evidence to indicate that "toughening" techniques are beneficial. Such methods may actually be deleterious; research indicates that soft pliable skin is better able to cope with stress than tough dry skin. Patient education regarding proper skin care can reduce the use of home remedies.

The skin of the residual limb may be affected by a variety of dermatological problems such as eczema, psoriasis, or radiation burns. Some of these conditions may mitigate against fitting or wrapping. Treatment may include ultraviolet irradiation, whirlpool, reflex heating, hyperbaric oxygen, or medication. Care must be taken in using ultraviolet or heat in the presence of **dysvascular** disease. The whirlpool may not be the treatment of choice because it increases circulation and edema in the part under treatment. The advantages of the whirlpool as a cleansing agent for skin problems, infected wounds, or incidence of delayed healing must be balanced against its disadvantages before effectiveness can be determined for any individual person.

Residual Limb Wrapping

There are several effective methods of wrapping the residual limb. Patients tend to wrap their own residual limb in a circular manner, often creating a tourniquet, which may compromise healing and foster the development of a bulbous end. Although the transtibial residual limb can be effectively wrapped in a sitting position, it is difficult to properly wrap and anchor the transfemoral limb while sitting. Elderly patients often cannot balance themselves in the standing position while wrapping. An effective bandage is smooth and wrinkle free, emphasizes angular turns, provides pressure distally, and encourages proximal joint extension. The ends of bandages are fastened with tape, safety pins, or Velcro rather than clips, which can cut the skin and do not anchor well. A system of wrapping that uses mostly angular or figure-of-eight turns was developed specifically to meet the needs of the elderly patient and has been in use for the past 30 years.[47] Figures 19-6 and 19-7 illustrate the techniques.

THE TRANSTIBIAL BANDAGE

Two 4-inch elastic bandages are usually enough to wrap most transtibial residual limbs. Very large residual limbs may require three bandages. The transtibial bandages should not be sewn together so that the weave of each bandage can be brought in contraposition to the other to provide more support. Although an elastic wrap does not provide as much pressure as a rigid dressing, the development of postsurgical edema must be detered as much as possible; therefore, a firm, even pressure against all soft tissues is desirable. If the incision is placed anteriorly, then an attempt should be made to bring the bandages from posterior to anterior over the distal end.

The first bandage is started at either the medial or lateral tibial condyle and brought diagonally over the anterior surface of the limb to the distal end. One edge of the bandage should just cover the midline of the incision in an anterior-posterior plane. The bandage is continued diagonally over the posterior surface then back over the beginning turn as an anchor. At this point, there is a choice; the bandage may be brought directly over the beginning point as indicated in step 2, or it may be brought across the

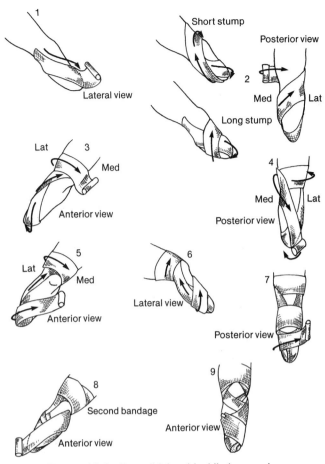

Figure 19-6. Transtibial residual limb wrapping.

front of the residual limb in an "X" design. The latter is particularly useful with long residual limbs and aids in bandage suspension. An anchoring turn over the distal thigh is made making sure that the wrap is clear of the patella and is not tight around the distal thigh.

After a single anchoring turn above the knee, the bandage is brought back around the opposite tibial

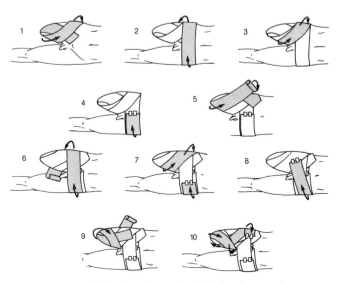

Figure 19-7. Transfemoral residual limb wrapping.

condyle and down to the distal end of the limb. One edge of the bandage should overlap the midline of the incision and the other wrap by at least ½ inch to ensure adequate distal end support. The figure-of-eight pattern is continued as depicted in steps 4 through 7 until the bandage is used up. Care should be taken to completely cover the residual limb with a firm and even pressure. Semicircular turns are made posteriorly to bring the bandage in line to cross the anterior surface in an angular line. This maneuver provides greater pressure on the posterior soft tissue while distributing pressure anteriorly where the bone is close to the skin. Each turn should partially overlap other turns so the whole residual limb is well covered. The pattern is usually from proximal to distal and back to proximal, starting at the tibial condyles and covering both condyles as well as the patellar tendon. Usually, the patella is left free to aid in knee motion, although with extremely short residual limbs, it may be necessary to cover it for better suspension.

The second bandage is wrapped like the first, except that it is started at the opposite tibial condyle from the first bandage (step 8). Bringing the weave of each bandage in contraposition exerts a more even pressure. With both bandages, an effort is made to bring the angular turns across each other rather than in the same direction.

THE TRANSFEMORAL BANDAGE

For most residual limbs, two 6-inch and one 4-inch bandages will adequately cover the limb. The two 6-inch bandages can be sewn together end-to-end taking care not to create a heavy seam; the 4-inch bandage is used by itself. The patient is depicted sidelying in Figure 19-7, which allows a family member or therapist easy access to the residual limb. The patient with good balance on the remaining limb can bandage the residual limb in the standing position, but it is difficult for the patient to self-bandage correctly in the sitting position.

The 6-inch bandages are used first. The first bandage is started in the groin and brought diagonally over the anterior surface to the distal lateral corner, around the end of the residual limb, and diagonally up the posterior side to the iliac crest and around the hips in a spica. The bandage is started medially so that the hip wrap will encourage extension. After the turn around the hips, the bandage is wrapped around the proximal portion of the residual limb high in the groin, then back around the hips. Although this is a proximal circular turn, it does not create a tourniquet as long as it is continued around the hips. Going around the medial portion of the residual limb high in the groin ensures coverage of the soft tissue in the adductor area and reduces the possibility of an adductor roll, a complication that can seriously interfere with comfortable prosthetic wear. In most instances, the first bandage ends in the second spica and is anchored with tape or pin.

The second 6-inch bandage is wrapped like the first but is started a bit more laterally. Any areas not covered with the first bandage must be covered at this time. The second bandage is also anchored in a hip spica after the first figure-of-eight and after the second turn high in the groin. While more of the first two bandages are used to cover the proximal residual limb, care must be taken that no tourniquet is created. Bringing the bandage directly from the proximal medial area into a hip spica helps to keep the adductor tissue covered and prevents rolling of the bandage to some degree.

The 4-inch bandage is used to exert the greatest amount of pressure over middle and distal areas of the residual limb. It is usually not necessary to anchor this bandage around the hips because friction with the already applied bandages and good figure-of-eight turns limit slippage. The 4-inch bandage is generally started laterally to bring the weave across the weave of previous bandages. Regular figure-of-eight turns in varied patterns to cover the entire residual limb are the most effective.

Bandages are applied with firm pressure from the outset. Elastic bandages can be wrapped directly over a soft postsurgical dressing so that bandaging can begin immediately after surgery. The elastic wrap controls edema more effectively if minimal gauze coverage is used over the residual limb. Several gauze pads placed just over the incision are usually adequate protection without compromising the effect of the wrap. Care must be taken to avoid any wrinkles or folds that can cause excessive skin pressure particularly over a soft dressing.

Shrinkers

The transtibial shrinker is rolled over the residual limb to midthigh and is designed to be self-suspending. Individuals with heavy thighs may need additional suspension with garters or a waist belt. Currently available transfemoral shrinkers incorporate a hip spica, which provides good suspension except with obese individuals (Fig. 19-5). Care must be taken that the patient understands the importance of proper suspension; any rolling of the edges or slipping of the shrinker can create a tourniquet around the proximal part of the residual limb. Shrinkers are easier to apply than elastic bandages and may be a better alternative, particularly for the transfemoral residual limb. Shrinkers are more expensive to use than elastic wrap; the initial cost is greater, and then new shrinkers of smaller sizes must be purchased as the limb volume decreases. However, shrinkers are a viable option for individuals who are not able to properly wrap the residual limb.

Positioning

One of the major outcomes of the early postoperative program is to prevent secondary complications such as contractures of adjacent joints. Contractures can develop as a result of muscle imbalance or fascial tightness, from a protective withdrawal reflex into hip and knee flexion, from loss of plantar stimulation in extension, or as a result of faulty positioning such as prolonged sitting. The patient should understand the importance of proper positioning and regular exercises in preparing for eventual prosthetic fit and ambulation.

With the transtibial amputation, full range of motion in the hips and knee, particularly in extension, is needed. While sitting, the patient can keep the knee extended by using a posterior splint or a board attached to the wheelchair. The patient with a transfemoral amputation needs full range of motion in the hip, particularly in extension and adduction. Prolonged sitting is to be avoided, especially for individuals who have difficulty walking with crutches. Some time each day should be spent in the prone position. Elevation of the residual limb on a pillow following either transfemoral or transtibial amputation can lead to the development of hip flexion contractures and should be avoided (Figs. 19-8 and 19-9). The early postoperative period is critical in establishing positive patterns of activity that will aid the patient throughout the rehabilitative period. Taking the time to teach the patient to assume responsibility for her or his own care can reap later benefits.

Contractures

Some individuals will present with hip or knee flexion contractures. Mild contractures may respond to manual mobilization and active exercises but it is almost impossible to reduce moderate to severe contractures by manual stretching, especially hip flexion contractures. There are some who advocate holding the extremity in a stretched position with weights for a considerable length of time. There is

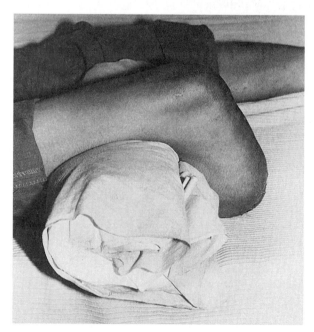

Figure 19-8. Improper positioning of residual limb on a pillow.

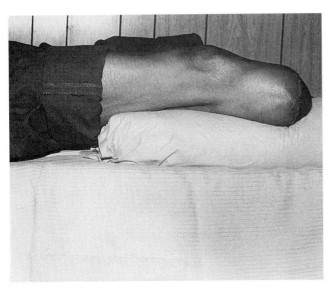

Figure 19-9. Improper positioning of residual limb over a pillow.

little evidence that this traditional approach is successful. Facilitated stretching techniques (PNF) are more effective than passive stretching; hold-relax and hold-relax active contraction that utilizes resisted contraction of antagonist muscles may increase range of motion, particularly of the knee. One of the more effective ways of reducing a knee flexion contracture is to fit the patient with a patellar-tendon-bearing (PTB) prosthesis aligned in a manner that places the hamstrings on stretch with each step. Such prosthetic alignment provides an active stretch that is quite effective. Hip flexion contractures are more frequently found in persons with transfemoral amputations. It is difficult to walk out a hip flexion contracture with the transfemoral prosthesis. In some instances, depending on the severity of the contracture and the length of the residual limb, the contracture can be accommodated in the alignment of the prosthesis. A hip or knee flexion contracture of less than 15 degrees is not usually a problem. Prevention, however, continues to be the best treatment for contractures.

Exercises

The exercise program is individually designed and includes strengthening, balance, and coordination activities. The postsurgical dressing, degree of postoperative pain, and healing of the incision will determine when resistive exercises for the involved extremity can be started. The postoperative exercise program can take many forms and a home exercise program (HEP) is desirable. The hip extensors and abductors, and knee extensors and flexors are particularly important for prosthetic ambulation. Figures 19-10 and 19-11 depict a series of exercises particularly well designed to strengthen key muscles around the hip and knee. These exercises can be adapted for a HEP because they are simple to perform and require no special equipment.

A general strengthening program that includes the trunk and all extremities is often indicated, particularly for the elderly person who may have been quite sedentary prior to surgery. Proprioceptive neuromuscular exercise routines are also beneficial. The exercise program needs to be individually developed and emphasize those muscles that are most active in prosthetic function. Isometric exercises as depicted in Figures 19-10D and 19-11A may be contraindicated for some individuals with cardiac disease or hypertension. Both exercises can be modified by having the patient actually lift the buttocks off the treatment table in a modified bridging movement.

The younger, more active person with a traumatic amputation does not usually lose a great deal of muscle strength. Many elderly individuals, however, are relatively sedentary after surgery and need encouragement to develop good strength, coordination and cardiopulmonary endurance for later ambulation.

Ideally, the exercise program should be sequenced for progressive motor control and increasing coordination and function. The patient should progress from bed to mat activities using exercises that emphasize coordinated functional mobility. The postoperative status will be determined to a great extent by the preoperative activity level, length of time of disability, and other medical problems as well as the effects of the surgery itself. Because many patients are discharged from the hospital as early as a week after surgery, referral to a rehabilitation center or home health agency is important to provide the necessary continuity of care.

Early mobility is important to total physiological recovery. The patient needs to resume independent activities as soon as possible. Movement transitions (supine-to-sit, sit-to-stand) are preliminary to ambulation activities. Care must be taken during early bed and transfer movements to protect the residual limb from any trauma. The patient must be advised not to push on or slide the residual limb against the bed or chair. The patient also needs to be cautioned against spending too much time in any one position to prevent the development of joint contractures or skin breakdowns.

Most individuals with unilateral amputations have little difficulty adjusting to the change in balance that results from the loss of a limb. Sitting and standing balance activities are a useful part of the early postsurgical program. Upper extremity strengthening exercises with weights or elastic bands are important in preparation for crutch walking. Shoulder depression and elbow extension are particularly necessary to improve the ability to lift the body in ambulation. Individuals with bilateral amputations who have one healed residual limb will often use that limb as a prop for bed activities and transfers. Often a debilitated person with bilateral amputations who is unable to lift the body with the arms will be able to transfer when allowed to use the old prosthesis to push on.

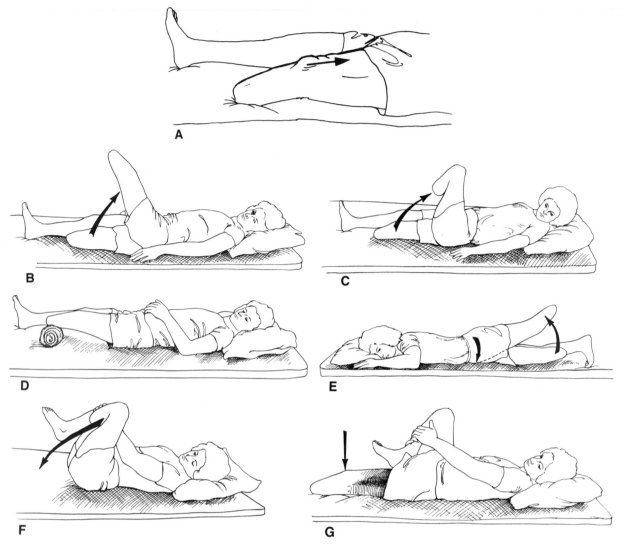

Figure 19-10. (A–G). Exercises for individuals with transtibial amputations to maintain or increase muscle strength and flexibility.

Mobility

Walking is an excellent exercise and necessary for independence in daily life. Gait training can start early in the postoperative phase, and the person with a unilateral lower extremity amputation can become quite independent using a three-point gait pattern on crutches. Many elderly individuals have difficulty learning to walk on crutches. Some are afraid, some lack the necessary balance and coordination, and others lack endurance. Walking with crutches without a prosthesis requires a greater expenditure of energy than walking with a prosthesis.

Independence in crutch walking is an outcome worthy of considerable therapy time. The individual who can ambulate with crutches will develop a greater degree of general fitness than the person who spends most of the time in a wheelchair. Crutch walking is good preparation for prosthetic ambulation and the person who can learn to use crutches generally will not have difficulty learning to use a prosthesis. However, the individual who cannot

learn to walk with crutches independently may still become a very functional prosthetic user. It may take considerable time for an elderly person to learn to use crutches, but the benefits are worth the efforts. Even if the individual can only use crutches in the sheltered environment of the home, such ambulation should be encouraged. An early graduated mobility program is also important for cardiovascular training and the development of endurance. Cardiovascular endurance is necessary for effective prosthetic ambulation, particularly at the transfemoral level.

There are advantages and disadvantages to using a walker for support during the postsurgical period. Certainly, walking with a walker is physiologically and psychologically more beneficial than sitting in a wheelchair, but it should be used only if the person cannot learn to walk with crutches. A walker is sturdier than crutches but cannot be used on stairs and curbs. It is sometimes difficult for the person who has used a walker during the postsurgical period to switch to crutches or a cane when fitted

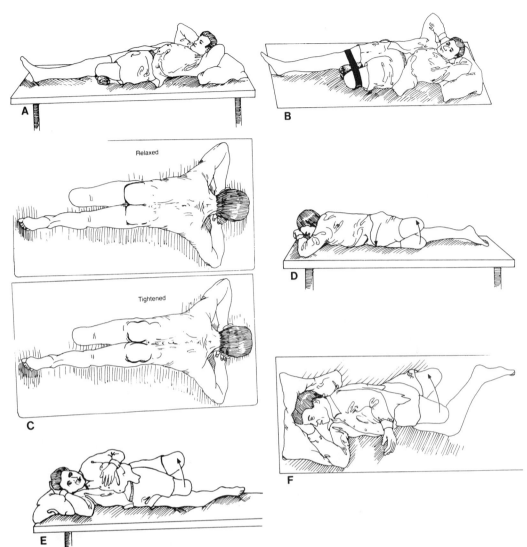

Figure 19-11. (A–F). Exercises for individuals with transfemoral amputations to maintain or increase muscle strength and flexibility.

with a prosthesis, because the gait pattern used with a walker is not appropriate with a prosthesis. A walker encourages a step-to gait pattern whereas efficient prosthetic use requires a step-through gait pattern. A reciprocal walker is not safe during the postsurgical period when the individual is using a three-point gait pattern. All individuals with an amputation need to learn some form of mobility without a prosthesis for use at night or when the prosthesis is not worn for some reason.

Temporary Prostheses

Many individuals are not fitted with any type of prosthetic appliance until the residual limb is free from edema and much of the soft tissue has shrunk, a process that can take many months of conscientious limb wrapping and exercises. During this period, the patient is limited to a wheelchair or to ambulation with crutches or a walker. Most individuals cannot return to work or fully participate in activities of daily living while waiting for the residual limb to mature. Once fitted with a definitive

prosthesis, the residual limb continues to change in size and a second prosthesis is often required within the first 2 years. Early fitting with a temporary prosthesis can greatly enhance the postsurgical rehabilitation program. A temporary prosthesis includes a socket designed and constructed according to regular prosthetic principles and attached to some form of pylon, a foot, and some type of suspension. Figures 19-12 and 19-13 depict two different temporary transtibial prostheses, both suspended by a sleeve. Figure 19-13 shows the socket itself with the sleeve removed. (See Chapter 20 for more details on prosthetic components.) Individuals fitted with a temporary prosthesis are taught to use the prosthesis correctly and, depending on physiological status, use little if any external support.

A temporary prosthesis can be fitted as soon as the wound has healed. There are many advantages to using a temporary prosthesis:

1. It shrinks the residual limb more effectively than the elastic wrap.
2. It allows early bipedal ambulation.
3. Many elderly people can walk safely with a temporary prosthesis and a cane who other-

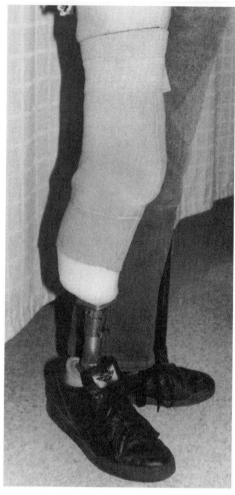

Figure 19-12. Transtibial temporary prosthesis.

distribute the forces transmitted from the floor to the end of the residual limb and is now contraindicated, particularly for the person with vascular disease. Many temporary sockets today are made of lightweight thermoplastic materials that can be formed over a positive cast of the residual limb; some are constructed of a fiberglass material that can be formed directly over the residual limb. The prosthesis is usually suspended by a Neoprene sleeve or a supracondylar cuff. The prosthesis is worn with a wool sock of appropriate thickness; when the residual limb has shrunk so that three wool socks are needed to maintain socket fit, a new socket needs to be constructed. The temporary prosthesis is usually fabricated by a prosthetist but can be fabricated by a therapist, physician, or any individual who is skilled in the application of prosthetic principles and socket design and who has access to the appropriate materials. Prosthetic components such as feet of various sizes, suspension straps, knee joints, and pylons are now generally available.

It is easier to fabricate a transtibial socket, but the use of a temporary prosthesis is very important in the rehabilitation of patients with transfemoral amputations.[48] The temporary prosthesis should incorporate the regular socket, articulated knee

wise would not be ambulatory during the postsurgical period.
4. Some individuals can return to work.
5. It provides a means of evaluating the rehabilitation potential of individuals with a questionable prognosis.
6. It is a positive motivating factor, providing a replacement for the missing part of the body.
7. It reduces the need for a complex exercise program because many people can return to full active daily life.
8. It can be used by individuals who may have difficulty obtaining payment for a definitive prosthesis.

The transtibial temporary socket may be simply constructed of reinforced plaster of Paris or it may be prosthetically fabricated from plastic materials. Fabricating the socket of plastic is preferable because the plaster of Paris socket is not particularly sturdy and needs to be changed frequently. In all instances, the socket design should follow regular prosthetic principles and should incorporate the use of a regular prosthetic foot attached to the socket with an aluminum pipe or pylon for proper gait pattern and weight distribution. A crutch tip, frequently used in the early days, does not adequately

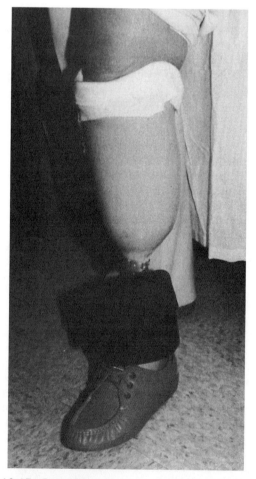

Figure 19-13. Transtibial temporary prosthesis with suspension sleeve lowered to show socket.

joint, foot, and pylon. Suspension may be with Silesian bandage or pelvic band.

PATIENT EDUCATION

As you work with the patient, you are glad that you started teaching her about PVD and the care of her legs when you were initially treating her. If she is to return home from the hospital, she needs to learn and understand enough to be a partner in the rehabilitation process rather than a passive recipient of information. You know that teaching is not telling and that you have to devise ways to actively involve the patient in learning important concepts and activities. From experience you have learned that the better patients understand the care of their own bodies, the greater the compliance with home programs.

Patient education is an integral and ongoing part of the rehabilitation program. Information on the care of the residual limb, proper care of the uninvolved extremity, positioning, exercises, and diet, if the patient has diabetes, are necessary for the patient to be a full participant in the rehabilitation program.

Many individuals with vascular disease who lose one leg will be concerned about the other leg and receptive to learning proper care. An understanding of the physiological and functional implications of PVD helps the individual assume responsibility for care of the residual limb and remaining extremity. The education program must be individually designed to be relevant and may include:

1. A discussion of the disease process, the physiological effects of the symptoms, and life-style changes to reduce risk factors.
2. Information on the benefits of exercises, lower extremity cleanliness, proper foot care, and proper shoe fitting.
3. Methods of edema control.
4. The use of exercise to improve circulatory status.

Edema, pain, and changes in skin color or temperature may indicate impending problems. If the person is ambulatory on the remaining extremity, the symptoms may reflect too much stress; if the person spends considerable time sitting with the leg in a dependent position, it may be necessary to elevate the extremity. Intermittent claudication (cramping of the calf) during activity indicates the need to stop at least temporarily. The collateral circulation of the remaining extremity is developed slowly through a progressive program of exercises and ambulation. It is important to remember that too much activity may be as harmful as too little.

Care must be taken not to overwhelm the patient with too much information at one time; information overload leads to forgetfulness. It is more effective to prioritize the information and ask the person to remember one new thing each session rather than try to teach a complex program at one time. Written materials are necessary to supplement the teaching and help the patient remember what is required. It is also important for the program to be tailored to the individual's life-style. Involving the patient in establishing priorities and timing enhances compliance. Compliance is also increased if the program meets the person's own desired outcomes. The same approach can be used for the HEP. Once the patient is discharged, either weekly clinic visits or home health supervision throughout the postsurgical phase provide a check on home activities, on the condition of the residual limb, and is supportive to the patient and family.

BILATERAL AMPUTATION

The postsurgical program for the person with bilateral lower extremity amputations is similar to the program developed for someone with a unilateral amputation except possibly ambulation. If the individual was fitted and ambulated after unilateral amputation, the prosthesis is useful for transfer activities and limited ambulation in the home. Some individuals may be able to use the prosthesis with external support to get around the house more easily, particularly for bathroom activities. Fitting with a temporary prosthesis, as mentioned, is advisable, particularly if the amputations are at transtibial levels. The higher the initial level of amputation, the more difficult ambulation becomes.

All individuals with bilateral amputations need a wheelchair on a permanent basis. The chair should be as narrow as possible with removable desk arms and removable leg rests. Amputee wheelchairs with offset rear wheels and no leg rests are not recommended unless the therapist is sure that the person will never be fitted with prostheses, even cosmetically. It is easier to add anti-tipping devices to the rear of the wheelchair or attach small weights to the front uprights for use when the foot rests are removed.

The postsurgical program includes mat activities designed to help the person regain a sense of body position and balance, upper extremity and residual limb strengthening exercises, and regular range of motion exercises. Functional mobility training should stress independence in bed mobility, transfers, and wheelchair use. With bilateral amputations, individuals spend considerable time sitting and are therefore more prone to develop flexion contractures, particularly around the hip joints. The patient should be encouraged to sleep prone if possible, or at least spend some time in the prone position each day. The therapy program also emphasizes range of motion of the residual limbs. Some people move about their homes on their knees, or the buttocks. Knee pads made of heavy rubber used by field workers are effective protectors for the residual limbs. Protectors can also be fabricated of foam or felt.

Temporary prostheses are of great value in the rehabilitation of patients with bilateral transtibial amputations. Temporary prostheses are used to evaluate ambulation potential and as an aid to

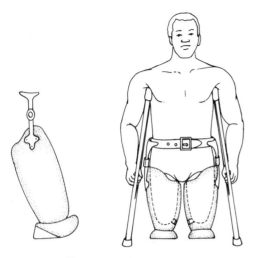

Figure 19-14. Stubbies.

balance and transfer activities. If the individual was initially fitted following the first amputation, the temporary prosthesis will allow resumption of general mobility. The ambulatory potential of patients with bilateral transfemoral amputations is uncertain, particularly among the elderly. Some individuals may be fitted with bilateral transfemoral temporary prostheses for use in cardiovascular training but continue to use a wheelchair for functional activities.

The person with bilateral transfemoral amputations can be fitted with shortened prosthesis called **"stubbies"** (Fig. 19-14). Stubby prostheses have regular sockets, no articulated knee joints or shank, and modified rocker bottoms turned backward to prevent the person from falling backward. Because the patient's center of gravity is much lower to the ground and the prostheses are nonarticulated, they are relatively easy to use. Stubbies allow the individual with bilateral transfemoral amputations to acquire erect balance and participate in ambulatory activities quickly and with only moderate expenditures of energy. Their acceptance, however, is quite variable; some like to use them for activities of daily living in the home but rely on a wheelchair outside the home. Although prescribed rather rarely, they are most effective for individuals with short residual limbs or who will not be able to ambulate with regular prostheses. Temporary prostheses of different heights can be used to determine ambulatory potential, but care must be taken to ensure that the temporary limbs are constructed well enough to tolerate the stresses generated in walking.

NONPROSTHETIC MANAGEMENT

The postsurgical period is designed to determine the individual's suitability for prosthetic replacement. Not all people with amputations are candidates for a prosthesis, regardless of personal desire. The cost of the prosthesis and the energy demands of prosthetic training require that the clinic team

use some judgement in selecting individuals for fitting.

There is no general rule that can safely be applied to all patients in making the decision to fit or not to fit. The patient is part of the decision-making process but the fact that the individual wants a prosthesis is not enough. Many people are not aware of the physiological demands of prosthetic ambulation, particularly at transfemoral levels. The development of lightweight prostheses, stance control knees, hydraulic mechanisms, and energy conserving feet have made it possible to successfully fit many more individuals than in the past; however, some consideration for nonfitting is necessary.

Transtibial Levels

Most individuals amputated at any transtibial level can be successfully fitted with a prosthesis. Flexion contractures, scars, poorly shaped residual limbs, and adherent skin are not necessarily contraindications for fitting even though such problems create difficulty with socket fit. Circulatory problems in the nonamputated extremity, unless so severe as to preclude any ambulation, are indications for fitting at the earliest possible time because bipedal ambulation reduces stress on the remaining extremity. Additionally, the individual who has learned to ambulate with one prosthesis is more likely to be able to ambulate with two. There are few contraindications to fitting someone with a transtibial amputation other than contraindications to ambulation itself. Individuals who were not ambulatory prior to surgery for reasons other than the problems leading to the amputation will probably not be ambulatory with an amputation. However, individuals who were nonambulatory and debilitated because of infection, lack of diabetic control, and ulcers will probably regain the necessary strength and coordination for ambulation after the diseased limb has been removed. Generally, individuals requiring nursing or custodial care will not be able to use a prosthesis; often equipment sent to a nursing home becomes lost and fitting such individuals may be an inappropriate use of limited resources.

Transfemoral Levels

Many patients can become relatively functional prosthetic users with or without external support. The physiological demands of walking with a transfemoral prosthesis are considerably higher than walking with a transtibial prosthesis and not all individuals have the necessary balance, strength, and energy reserves.[49] Severe hip flexion contractures, obesity, weakness or paralysis of hip musculature, and poor balance and coordination may mitigate against successful ambulation. The person's level of activity and participation in the postsurgical program helps in determining potential for prosthetic ambulation. A temporary prosthesis is a good assessment tool.

Most individuals amputated at hip levels are younger and learn to use a prosthesis relatively easily. Although early fitting is physically and psychologically beneficial, active involvement in chemotherapy or radiation therapy will delay fitting. Radiation therapy often burns the skin making fitting impossible until the skin has healed. Patients undergoing chemotherapy are often ill, lose weight, and usually do not have the energy to participate in a prosthetic training program. The postsurgical program is individually adjusted and supportive until the therapy is complete. If the person has lost considerable weight, fitting may have to be delayed because it is difficult to adjust a prosthesis for increases in weight.

Bilateral Amputations

Fitting or not fitting someone with bilateral amputations is a difficult decision. Young, agile individuals are generally good candidates for prosthetic fitting. Most patients with bilateral transtibial amputations can become quite functional with prostheses. Most individuals with bilateral transfemoral amputations have considerable difficulty learning to use two prostheses. Patients with one transfemoral and one transtibial amputation generally can learn to use two prosthesis if the first amputation was at the transfemoral level, and if the person successfully used a transfemoral prosthesis before losing the other leg.

The person who has lost portions of both lower extremities needs more strength, better coordination, better balance, and greater cardiorespiratory reserves than the person who has lost a portion of

one lower extremity. Obesity makes fitting of bilateral prostheses more difficult. The decision to fit or not to fit is made after careful, individual evaluation of the person's total potential and needs.

Individuals who are not fitted with a prosthesis need to become as independent as possible in a wheelchair. The therapy program includes training in all transfers, wheelchair mobility, and activities of daily living. The program emphasizes sitting balance, moving safely in and out of the wheelchair, and other activities to support as independent a life-style as the person's physical and psychological condition allows. Education in the proper care of the residual limb is also important, although wrapping the residual limb is no longer necessary unless the person is more comfortable with the limb covered.

SUMMARY

Most individuals with lower extremity amputations can be helped to return to a full and useful life following the loss of a limb. A program of postoperative care that includes consideration of the physical and emotional needs will enable most patients to become functional prosthetic users. Many prosthetic problems can be avoided by properly preparing the individual for prosthetic wear. In this chapter, concepts related to the postoperative management of the individual with a lower extremity amputation have been presented. Through a process of careful assessment and open communication, a comprehensive program designed to meet the needs of an individual patient can be achieved. The individuality of each person presenting for rehabilitation is one of the challenges of physical therapy practice.

QUESTIONS FOR REVIEW

1. Discuss the advantages and disadvantages of the following methods of postsurgical residual limb management:
   a. Rigid dressing
   b. CET
   c. Air splint
   d. Soft dressing
2. Discuss the proper method of wrapping the transtibial and the transfemoral residual limb.
3. A 72 year-old man with a history of diabetes, cardiovascular disease, and PVD has been referred for physical therapy 24 hours post right transtibial amputation for gangrene. What examination data

are needed to plan an appropriate treatment program? Which are the most critical to obtain on the first visit?
4. Design an exercise program for an 82 year-old individual with a left transfemoral amputation who is referred 2 weeks post amputation.
5. Discuss the advantages and disadvantages of teaching an elderly person to walk with crutches versus walking with a walker following a unilateral amputation.
6. Which postsurgical activities are more important with bilateral amputations than unilateral amputations? How might you teach these activities?

CASE STUDY

REFERRAL: The patient is a 72 year-old female status post right transtibial amputation yesterday secondary to arteriosclerotic gangrene.

Current Medical History: Diabetes type II since age 48 controlled by insulin 20 units bid. Arteriosclerosis; hypertension controlled by medication;

treated for ulcer plantar surface of right first metatarsal area for past 3 months. Ulcer did not heal leading to amputation.

PAST MEDICAL HISTORY: Hysterectomy at age 42, otherwise unremarkable.

SOCIAL: Widow who lives alone. Three grown children and six grandchildren in the area.

PHYSICAL THERAPY EVALUATION (INITIAL)

Chart Review: Pt alert and awake in no apparent distress. Right residual limb wrapped in soft gauze dressing covered with an elastic wrap. Drain in place. Incision clean on dressing change.

BP: 142/70, pulse 66, respiration normal.

Respiratory care reports patient using spirometer properly, normal cough, no evidence of respiratory problems.

Pt c/o of some pain in residual limb; pain medication given.

Pt has been sitting at the side of the bed × 2/day.

EXAMINATION DATA: (Obtained initially then prior to discharge from hospital)

Gross muscle strength of left lower extremity and both upper extremities grossly within functional limits (WFL).

Right hip flexion, abduction and adduction grossly WFL; hip extension tested sidelying and graded a 3+. Demonstrates active motion of right knee flexion and extension with no resistance given at this time.

Residual limb measurements deferred until initial healing has taken place.

Gross range of motion of left lower extremity and both upper extremities grossly WFL. Left hip extension measurements deferred until patient can lie prone or on right side. Gross range of motion of the right hip grossly WFLs except hip extension to 0 degrees measured sidelying. Right knee flexion and extension grossly functional. Specific measurement deferred until dressing can be removed.

Left lower extremity is hairless below the ankle. Skin is warm to touch. Popliteal pulse palpable but not dorsalis pedis pulse. Toes are warm to touch. Proprioceptive sensation intact. Diminished sensation over plantar surface of left foot and dorsum or first metatarsal. No evidence of edema in left lower extremity. Sensation testing of right residual limb deferred secondary to dressing.

Bed Mobility: rolling to left: FIM level 7; rolling to right and prone: not tested.

Supine-to-sit and return: FIM level 6.

Transfers: Sit-to-stand with walker: FIM level 3. Stand-to-sit in chair or bed: FIM level 3.

Ambulation: Ambulation with walker: FIM level 3 for 5 feet.

OUTCOMES OF PHYSICAL THERAPY TO DISCHARGE FROM HOSPITAL

1. Independent in bed mobility and all transfers.
2. Independent in mobility with crutches or walker for 40 feet.
3. Demonstrate a knowledge of proper residual limb positioning, bandaging, and care.
4. Demonstrate a knowledge of basic residual limb exercises.
5. Demonstrate a knowledge of proper care of the left lower extremity.

ADDITIONAL EXAMINATION FINDINGS: Obtained following discharge from hospital by home health physical therapist.

Residual Limb: Sutures in place, incision healing well, no drainage; length 13.6 centimeters from medial tibial plateau (MTP).

Circumferential measurements from MTP
    5 cm below MTP = 35 centimeters
    l0 cm below MTP = 38 centimeters
    12 cm below MTP = 37 centimeters
    Sensation intact.

ROM knee in flexion and extension = WNL.
ROM right hip in extension to 0 degrees.

ADDITIONAL PHYSICAL THERAPY OUTCOMES FOR TOTAL POSTSURGICAL PERIOD

1. Independent in care of residual limb including bandaging or using shrinker.
2. Independent in crutch (walker) ambulation within home environment.
3. Demonstrate home exercise program as outlined.

Guiding Questions

1. The patient's residual limb was wrapped in a soft dressing after amputation. Compare the advantages and disadvantages of the rigid dressing, the semirigid dressing, and soft dressings. What problems might the patient incur with a soft dressing?

2. Review the examination data given for the patient. What data would be important to obtain on the first postoperative visit and what can be deferred? What other data would you obtain and when?

3. Describe your initial treatment program for the patient.

4. What would be the focus of follow-up care after discharge?

REFERENCES

1. Levy, LA: Smoking and peripheral vascular disease. Clin Podiatr Med Surg 9:165, 1992.
2. Ritz, G, et al: Diabetes and peripheral vascular disease. Clin Podiatr Med Surg 9:125, 1992.
3. McCollum, PT, and Walker, MA: Major limb amputation for end-stage peripheral vascular disease: Level selection and alternative options. In Bowker, JH, and Michael, JW (eds): Atlas of Limb Prosthetics: Surgical, Prosthetic and Rehabilitation Principles. Mosby-Year Book, St. Louis, 1992, p 25.
4. Quigley, FG, et al: Impact of femoro-distal bypass on major lower limb amputation rate. Aust N Z J Surg 68:35, 1998.
5. Hallett, JW Jr., et al: Impact of arterial surgery and balloon angioplasty on amputation: A population bases study of 1155 procedures between 1973 and 1992. J Vasc Surg 25:29, 1997.
6. Cuson, TM, and Bongiorni, DR: Rehabilitation of the older lower limb amputee: A brief review. J Am Geriatr Soc 44:1388, 1996.
7. Yeager, RA, et al: Surgical management of severe acute lower extremity ischemia. J Vasc Surg 15:385, 1992.
8. Taylor, LM, et al: Limb salvage vs. amputation for critical ischemia. Arch Surg 126:1251, 1991.
9. Edelman, D, et al: Prognostic value of the clinical examination of the diabetic foot ulcer. J Gen Intern Med 12:537, 1997.
10. Moss, SE, et al: The prevalence and incidence of lower extremity amputation in a diabetic population. Arch Intern Med 152:610, 1992.
11. Knighton, DR, et al: Amputation prevention in an independently reviewed at-risk diabetic population using a comprehensive wound care protocol. Am J Surg 160:466, 1990.
12. Krajewski, LP, and Olin, JW: Atherosclerosis of the aorta and lower extremities arteries. In Young, JR, et al (eds): Peripheral Vascular Diseases. Mosby-Year Book, St. Louis, 1991, p 179.
13. Harris, KA, et al: Rehabilitation potential of elderly patients with major amputations. J Cardiovasc Surg (Torino) 32:463, 1991.
14. Ebskov, LB: Relative mortality in lower limb amputees with diabetes mellitus. Prosthet Orthot Int 20:147, 1996.
15. Kay, HW, and Newman, JD: Relative incidence of new amputations: Statistical comparisons of 6,000 new amputees. Prosthet Orthot Int 29:3, 1975.
16. Lane, JM, et al: New advances and concepts in amputee management after treatment for bone and soft-tissue sarcomas. Clin Orthop 256:22, 1990.
17. Link, MP, et al: Adjuvant chemotherapy of high-grade osteosarcoma of the extremity. Clin Orthop 270:8, 1991.
18. Simon, M: Limb salvage for osteosarcoma in the 1980s. Clin Orthop 270:264, 1990.
19. Springfield, DS: Introduction to limb-salvage surgery for sarcomas. Orthop Clin North Am 22:1, 1991.
20. Yaw, KM, and Wurtz, LD: Resection and reconstruction for bone tumors in the proximal tibia. Orthop Clin North Am 22:133, 1991.
21. Waters, RL, et al: Energy cost of walking of amputees: The influence of level of amputation. J Bone Joint Surg 58A:42, 1976.
22. Steinberg, FU, et al: Prosthetic rehabilitation of geriatric amputee patients: A follow-up study. Arch Phys Med Rehabil 66:742, 1985.
23. Moore, TJ: Planning for optimal function in amputation surgery. In Bowker, JH, and Michael, JW (eds): Atlas of Limb

Prosthetics: Surgical, Prosthetic and Rehabilitation Principles. Mosby-Year Book, St. Louis, 1992, p 59.
24. Michaels, JA: The selection of amputation level: An approach using decision analysis. Eur J Vasc Surg 5:451, 1991.
25. Sarin, S, et al: Selection of amputation levels: A review. Eur J Vasc Surg 5:611, 1991.
26. Spence, VA, et al: Assessment of tissue viability in relation to selection of amputation level. Prosth Orthot Int 8:67, 1984.
27. Lind, J, et al: The influence of smoking on complications after primary amputations of the lower extremity. Clin Orthop 267:211, 1991.
28. Evans, WE, et al: Effect of a failed distal reconstruction on the level of amputation. Am J Surg 160:217, 1990.
29. Tsang, GMK, et al: Failed femorocrural reconstruction does not prejudice amputation level. Br J Surg 78:1479, 1991.
30. Ljungman, C, et al: Risk factors for early lower limb loss after embolectomy for acute arterial occlusion: A population-based case-control study. Br J Surg 78:1482, 1991.
31. May, BJ: Amputations and Prosthetics: A case study approach. FA Davis, Philadelphia, 1996.
32. May, BJ: A statewide amputee rehabilitation programme. Prosthet Orthot Int 2:24, 1978.
33. Burgess, EM: Amputations of the lower extremities. In Nickel, VL (ed): Orthopedic Rehabilitation. Churchill-Livingston, New York, 1982, p 377.
34. Sarmiento, A, et al: Lower-extremity amputation: The impact of immediate postsurgical prosthetic fitting. Clin Orthop 68:22, 1967.
35. Harrington, IJ, et al: A plaster-pylon technique for below-knee amputation. J Bone Joint Surg (Br) 73:76, 1991.
36. Little, JM: A pneumatic weight-bearing prosthesis for below-knee amputees. Lancet 1:271, 1971.
37. Little, JM: The use of air splints as immediate prosthesis after below-knee amputation for vascular insufficiency. Med J Aust 2:870, 1970.
38. Burgess, EM: Wound healing after amputation: Effect of controlled environment treatment, a preliminary study. J Bone Joint Surg 60A:245, 1978.
39. Kegel, B: Controlled environment treatment (CET) for patients with below-knee amputations. Phys Ther 56:1366, 1976.
40. Jensen, TS, et al: Immediate and long-term phantom limb pain in amputees: Incidence, clinical characteristics and relationship to pre-amputation limb pain. Pain 21:267, 1985.
41. Iacono, RP, et al: Pain management after lower extremity amputation. Neurosurgery 20:496, 1987.
42. Fisher, A, and Meller, Y: Continuous postoperative regional analgesia by nerve sheath block for amputation surgery: A pilot study. Anesth Analg 72:300, 1991.
43. Malawer, MM, et al: Postoperative infusional continuous regional analgesia. Clin Orthop Rel Res 266:227, 1991.
44. Mouratoglou, VM: Amputees and phantom limb pain: A literature review. Physiotherapy Practice 2:177, 1986.
45. Sherman, RA, et al: Phantom Pain: A lesson in the necessity for careful clinical research on chronic pain problems. J Rehabil Res Dev 25:vii, 1988.
46. Melzack, R: Phantom limbs. Sci Am 266:120, 1992.
47. Parry, M, and Morrison, JD: Use of the Femurett adjustable prosthesis in the assessment and walking training of new above-knee amputees. Prosthet Orthot Int 13:36, 1989.
48. Perry, J: Gait Analysis: Normal and pathological function. Slack Inc., Thorofare, NJ, 1992.

SUPPLEMENTAL READINGS

Andrews KL: Rehabilitation in limb deficiency. 3. The geriatric amputee. Arch Phys Med Rehabil 1996 Mar;77(3 Suppl): S14–7. Review.

Cohen-Sobel E, et al: Prosthetic management of a Chopart amputation variant. J Am Podiatr Med Assoc 1994 Oct;84(10): 505-10.

Condie E, et al: Slow rehabilitation of a traumatic lower limb amputee. Physiother Res Int 1998;3(4):233–8.

Cottrell-Ikerd V, et al: The Syme's amputation: a correlation of surgical technique and prosthetic management with an historical perspective. J Foot Ankle Surg 1994 Jul-Aug;33(4): 355–64.

Esquenazi A: Geriatric amputee rehabilitation. Clin Geriatr Med 1993 Nov;9(4):731–43. Review.

Kennedy MJ: Am I better off with out it?: a case study of a patient having a trans-tibial amputation after 52 years of chronic lower limb ulceration and pain. Prosthet Orthot Int 1997 Dec;21(3):187–8.

Pinzur MS, et al: Functional outcome of below-knee amputation in peripheral vascular insufficiency. A multicenter review. Clin Orthop 1993 Jan;(286):247–9.

Stewart CP, et al: Cause of death of lower limb amputees. Prosthet Orthot Int 1992 Aug;16(2):129–32.

Tuel SM, et al: Interdisciplinary management of hemicorporectomy after spinal cord injury. Arch Phys Med Rehabil 1992 Jul;73(7):669–73.

Tyre TE, et al: The outcome status of chronic pain patients 4 years after multidisciplinary care. Wis Med J 1994 Jan;93(1): 9–12.

GLOSSARY

Arteriography: Radiographic visualization of an artery following insertion of a radiopaque material.

Beveled (bone): The process of smoothing the cut ends of bone to prevent rough edges that could cause skin irritations from pressure against the prosthetic socket.

Cauterization: Destruction of tissue by use of a caustic agent such as heat, cold, electricity, or corrosive chemicals.

Dysvascular: Decreased peripheral vascular circulation; usually applied to arterial diseases.

Hemostasis: Arrest of bleeding.

Immediate postoperative prosthesis: Application of a temporary prosthesis immediately following amputation; usually consists of a plaster of Paris socket, pylon, and foot.

Myodesis: Method of muscle stabilization following amputation in which the cut muscle is sutured to periosteum or bone.

Myofascial closure: Method of muscle stabilization following amputation in which muscle is sutured to fascia; often used in combination with myoplasty.

Myoplasty: Method of muscle stabilization following amputation in which muscle is sutured to muscle; the cut flexor and extensor muscles are surgically attached; often used in combination with myofascial closure.

Neurectomy: Partial or total excision or resection of a nerve.

Neuroma: Collection of nerve cells that develop following transection of a nerve.

Peripheral vascular disease (PVD): A general term used to describe any disorder that interferes with arterial or venous blood flow of the extremities.

Phantom limb: The sensation that a part of the body that has become desensitized or has been amputated is still there.

Phantom pain: Pain originating from the desensitized or amputated body part.

Rhizotomy: Division or severance of a nerve root.

Rigid dressing: Plaster of Paris postoperative prosthetic socket made in the configuration of the permanent socket.

Secondary closure: Surgical closure performed several days after the initial amputation.

Semirigid dressing: Postoperative dressing made of a semirigid material and designed to contain edema.

Shrinker: Commercially made socklike garment of heavy rubber-reinforced cotton; designed to fit a residual limb.

Soft dressing: Postoperative dressing of soft materials such as gauze.

Stubbies: Short, transfemoral prosthetic sockets set on modified rocker feet; used to help individuals with bilateral transfemoral amputations move around outside of a wheelchair.

Temporary prosthesis: Prosthesis constructed and aligned like the permanent appliance but not cosmetically completed.

Tenodesis: Surgical attachment of a tendon to a bone.

Unna's dressing: A semirigid dressing consisting of gauze impregnated with zinc oxide, gelatin, glycerin, and calamine which is wrapped on the foot and lower limb; used in the management of venous ulcers primarily and occasionally with arterial foot ulcers.

APPENDIX

Suggested Answers to Case Study Guiding Questions

1. The patient's residual limb was wrapped in a soft dressing after amputation. Compare the advantages and disadvantages of the rigid dressing, the semirigid dressing, and soft dressings. What problems might the patient incur with a soft dressing?

ANSWER

Rigid Dressings

The advantages of the *rigid dressing* are:

1. It greatly limits the development of postoperative edema in the residual limb thereby reducing postoperative pain and enhancing wound healing.
2. It allows for earlier ambulation with the attachment of a pylon and foot.
3. It allows for earlier fitting of the permanent prosthesis by reducing the length of time needed for shrinking the residual limb.
4. It is configured to each individual residual limb.

The major disadvantages of the *rigid dressing* are:

1. It requires careful application by an individual knowledgeable about prosthetic principles, often a prosthetist, and occasionally a physical therapist.
2. It requires close supervision during the healing stage.
3. It does not allow for daily wound inspection and dressing changes.

Semirigid Dressings

The advantage of all *semirigid dressings* is that they provide better control of edema than the soft dressing but each has some disadvantage that limits its use.

Major disadvantages of *semirigid dressings*:

1. The Unna dressing: It may loosen easily and is not as rigid as the plaster of Paris dressing.
2. The air splint: While allowing visual wound inspection, the constant pressure does not intimately conform to the shape of the residual limb. The environment of the plastic is hot and humid requiring frequent cleaning.
3. The Controlled Environment Treatment (CET): The bag's flexibility allows active exercises of the involved extremity as well as standing at bedside but the hose and machine limit bed mobility and ambulation.

Soft Dressings

The advantages of the *soft dressings* are:

1. Relatively inexpensive
2. Lightweight and readily available
3. Can be laundered

The major disadvantages of the *soft dressings* are:

1. Relatively poor control of edema.

2. The elastic wrap requires skill in proper application.
3. The elastic wrap needs frequent reapplication.
4. Dressings can slip and form a tourniquet.
5. New shrinkers must be purchased as the residual limb gets markedly smaller.
6. Shrinker cannot be used until the sutures have been removed and primary healing has occurred.

Problems the patient might incur with a soft dressing include the following. As identified above, one of the major drawbacks of the elastic wrap is that it needs frequent rewrapping. Movement of the residual limb against the bedclothes, bending and extending the proximal joints, and general body movements will cause slippage and changes in pressure.

2. Review the examination data given for the patient. What data would be important to obtain on the first postoperative visit and what can be deferred? What other data would you obtain and when?

ANSWER: Initial data: Information regarding the status of the residual limb, the patient's postsurgical cardiopulmonary and general physiological function, her ability to be mobile, the condition of the remaining lower extremity, and her feelings about the amputation are likely the most important data to obtain.

Other data include:

- Associated diseases/symptoms (e.g., neuropathy, visual disturbances, cardiopulmonary disease, renal failure, congenital anomalies).
- Current physiological state (e.g., postsurgical cardiopulmonary status, vital signs, OOB, pain).
- Medications
- Skin integrity
  - Scar (e.g., healed, adherent, invaginated, flat)
  - Other lesions (e.g., size, shape, open, scar tissue)
  - Moisture (e.g., moist, dry, scaly)
  - Sensation (e.g., absent, diminished, hyperesthesia)
  - Grafts (e.g., location, type, healing)
  - Dermatological lesions (e.g., psoriasis, eczema, cysts)
- Residual limb length
- Vascularity (both limbs if amputation cause is vascular)
- Range of motion
- Muscle strength
- Neurological status
  - Pain (phantom [differentiate sensation or pain], neuroma, incisional, from other causes)

Continued

APPENDIX *Continued*

- Neuropathy
- Cognitive status (e.g., alert, oriented, confused)
- Emotional status (e.g., acceptance, body image)
- Functional status
  - Transfers (e.g., bed-to-chair, to toilet, to car)
  - Mobility (e.g., ancillary support, supervision)
  - Home/family situation (e.g., caregiver, architectural barriers, hazards)
  - Activities of daily living (e.g., bathing, dressing)
- Instrumental activities of daily living (e.g., cooking, cleaning)
- Other
  - Preamputation status (e.g., work, activity level, degree of independence, life-style)
  - Prosthetic goals (desire for prosthesis, anticipated activity level and life-style)

- Financial (e.g., available payment for prosthesis)
- Prior prosthesis (if bilateral)
- Data would be obtained continuously throughout the postoperative period.

3. Describe your initial treatment program for the patient.
ANSWER: The general areas of initial treatment intervention might logically include: residual limb care, positioning, exercise, mobility (ambulation) training, and patient education.

4. What would be the focus of follow-up care after discharge?
ANSWER: Follow-up treatment will need to focus on functional mobility, residual limb care, and the care of the intact limb.

Joan E. Edelstein

LEARNING OBJECTIVES

1. Relate various levels of amputation to prosthetic restoration.
2. Describe the major components of transtibial and transfemoral prostheses, including advantages and disadvantages of alternative components and materials.
3. Describe the distinctive features of partial foot, Syme's, and knee and hip disarticulation prostheses.
4. Outline the maintenance program for each prosthetic component.
5. Identify the principal features of transtibial and transfemoral prosthetic assessment.
6. Describe the physical therapist's role in management of individuals with lower-limb amputation.
7. Analyze and interpret patient data, formulate realistic goals and outcomes, and develop a plan of care when presented with a clinical case study.

A *prosthesis* is a replacement of a body part. A *prosthetist* is a health care professional who designs, fabricates, and fits prostheses. In the broadest sense, prostheses include dentures, wigs, and plastic heart valves. The physical therapist, however, is concerned primarily with limb prostheses (i.e., artificial legs and arms) and the management of individuals with lower- and upper-limb amputation.

Lower-limb amputation is much more prevalent than loss of the upper limb. The major causes of amputation are peripheral vascular disease, trauma, malignancy, and congenital deficiency. Vascular disease accounts for most leg amputations in individuals older than 50.[1,2] Trauma is responsible for the majority of amputations in younger adults and adolescents. Trauma and vascular disease are more common among men. Bone and soft tissue tumors are sometimes treated by removal of the limb, and adolescence is the period of peak incidence. Congenital deficiency refers to absence or abnormality of a limb evident at birth.

This chapter focuses on the lower limb because more individuals have lost a portion of the leg, as compared with the arm. Physical therapists are members of the rehabilitation team, working with occupational therapists and others to foster the patient's welfare. For patients with lower-limb amputation, physical therapists have the major role in assisting the patient to regain function. For those with upper-limb amputation, physical therapists may play a lesser role, cooperating with occupational therapists, depending on the administrative organization of the health care facility. Lower-limb prostheses will be described, together with a program for training patients in their use.

The concept of replacing a missing limb is very old. Prostheses, such as a forked stick forming a peg leg to support a **transtibial** (below-knee) amputation limb, were known in antiquity. Today, most individuals with lower-limb amputation are provided with a prosthesis. Function with one leg is very different from maneuvering with two legs; in contrast, most daily activities and vocational tasks are performed with a single upper limb.

The principal lower-limb prostheses are partial foot, Syme's, transtibial, and transfemoral (above-knee), as well as knee and hip disarticulation. The physical therapist should be familiar with their characteristics and their maintenance.

PARTIAL FOOT PROSTHESES

The purposes of partial foot prostheses are (1) to restore, as much as possible, foot function, particularly in walking, and (2) to simulate the shape of the missing foot segment. The patient who has lost one or more toes may simply pad the toe section of the shoe to improve the appearance of the upper portion of the shoe. Standing will not be affected, assuming the metatarsal heads remain. Late stance will be less forceful, particularly if the phalanges of the great toe are absent. An arch support helps to maintain alignment of the amputated foot.[3]

Transmetatarsal amputation disturbs foot appearance more noticeably. A prosthesis prevents the shoe from developing an unnatural crease in the forefoot area. The patient bears most weight on the heel and reduces the amount of time spent on the affected foot during walking. A particularly useful prosthesis consists of a plastic socket for the remainder of the foot. The socket is affixed to a rigid plate that extends the full length of the inner sole of the shoe. The plate has a cosmetic toe filler. The socket protects the amputated ends of the metatarsals, while the rigid plate restores foot length so that the person can spend more time during the stance phase of gait on the affected side than would otherwise be the case. To aid late stance, the bottom of the prosthesis or the sole of the shoe may have a convex rocker bar.

Amputation or disarticulation through the tarsals poses the additional problem of retaining the small foot segment in the shoe during swing phase. Foot length is apt to be diminished further by an equinus deformity of the amputated limb, resulting from unbalanced contraction of the triceps surae. Consequently, the prosthesis described for the transmetatarsal amputation may be augmented with a plastic calf shell, which is strapped around the leg.

TRANSTIBIAL (BELOW-KNEE) PROSTHESES

The transtibial level refers to an amputation in which the tibia and fibula are transected. The patient retains the anatomical knee and its motor and sensory functions. This is the predominant site of amputation, particularly for individuals with vascular disease. From a functional and prosthetic viewpoint, the **Syme's amputation** is similar; amputation is just above the malleoli, with all foot bones removed and the calcaneal fat pad retained. The Syme's amputation limb is longer than the transtibial amputation limb, improving prosthetic control; in addition, the individual with a Syme's amputation may be able to tolerate significant weight through the end of the limb. Prostheses for both the Syme's and transtibial levels include a foot-ankle assembly and socket; the transtibial prosthesis also has a shank and a suspension component.[4]

FOOT-ANKLE ASSEMBLY

The prosthetic foot restores the general contour of the patient's foot, absorbs shock at heel contact, plantarflexes in early stance, and simulates metatarsophalangeal hyperextension (toe-break action) in the latter part of stance phase (Fig. 20-1). Many foot-ankle assemblies also provide slight motion in the frontal and transverse planes.[5–9]

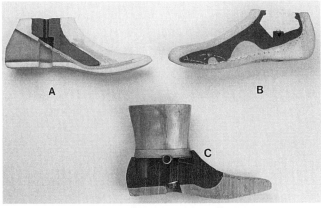

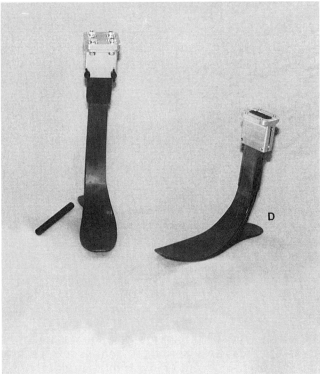

Figure 20-1. Cross-section of foot-ankle assemblies. (*A*) SACH. (*B*) SAFE. (*C*) Single-axis. (*D*) Springlite with adjustment rod.

Nonarticulated Feet

Most feet prescribed in the United States are nonarticulated, presenting a one-piece external appearance, without a cleft between the foot and lower portion of the shank. As compared with articulated feet, nonarticulated components are lighter in weight, more durable, and more attractive; some versions are made to suit high-heeled shoes.

SACH FOOT

The **solid ankle cushion heel (SACH)** assembly is the most commonly prescribed foot in current practice. It consists of a wooden **keel,** which terminates at a point corresponding to the joints. The rigid section is covered with rubber; the posterior portion is resilient, to absorb shock and permit

plantarflexion in early stance. Anteriorly, the junction of the keel and rubber toe allows the foot to hyperextend in late stance. The SACH foot is manufactured in a wide range of sizes to accommodate infants, adolescents, and adults, and with heel cushions of varying degrees of compressibility for those who strike the foot with different amounts of force, as well as in several plantarflexion angles to fit shoes with diverse heel heights. The heel cushion allows a very small amount of medial-lateral and transverse motion.

OTHER NONARTICULATED FEET

A version of the SACH foot is the **stationary attachment flexible endoskeleton (SAFE) foot.**[10] It has a rigid ankle block joined to the posterior portion of the keel at a 45-degree angle, which is comparable to that of the anatomical subtalar joint. The junction permits the SAFE foot wearer to maintain contact with moderately uneven terrain, because of the greater range of medial-lateral motion permitted in the rear-foot. The SAFE foot, however, is somewhat heavier, more expensive, and less durable than the SACH foot. Feet that have a springy sole store energy in early and midstance as the wearer moves along the foot, bending it slightly. In late stance, as the wearer transfers loading to the opposite foot, the spring in the prosthetic foot recoils, returning some of the stored energy. Such feet are described as energy storing/energy releasing, or dynamic.[11–15] For example, the Carbon Copy II foot has two carbon fiber longitudinal flexible plates. When the wearer walks at regular speed, the distal plate bends, then springs back to its resting shape. When the wearer runs, both plates bend, then straighten.[16,17] The Seattle foot incorporates a slightly flexible plastic keel, which bends somewhat at heel contact, storing energy.[18] At late stance, the keel recoils as the wearer unloads the foot, releasing energy for a springy termination to stance. Both the Flex-Foot and the Springlite foot include a long band of carbon fiber material, which extends from the toe to the proximal shank, as well as a posterior heel section. The long band acts as a leaf spring, enabling the foot to store considerable energy in early and midstance, and then to release energy at the end of stance phase. Active wearers, such as those who play basketball or run, utilize the energy-storing and energy-releasing capacity of these feet.[19,20] Although energy storing/releasing feet are flexible, the amount of energy stored is negligible.[21] They are also more expensive than alternative assemblies.

Articulated Feet

These components are manufactured with separate foot and lower shank sections, joined by a metal bolt or cable. The ease of foot motion is controlled by the use of rubber. In the rear is a resilient bumper to absorb shock and control plantarflexion excursion; it is easy for the prosthetist to substitute a firmer or softer bumper, depending on the patient. A heavy or very active client requires a firm bumper, whereas a frail individual needs a bumper that is soft enough to permit the foot to plantarflex with minimal loading. At early stance, slight loading of the heel causes the foot to plantarflex, ensuring that the wearer achieves the stable foot-flat position. Anterior to the ankle bolt is firmer rubber, the dorsiflexion stop, which resists dorsiflexion as the wearer moves forward over the foot. Articulated feet are subject to eventual loosening, which may be signaled by a squeaking noise.

SINGLE-AXIS FEET

The most common example of an articulated foot is the **single-axis foot.** It permits plantarflexion and dorsiflexion, as well as toe-break action, but does not allow medial-lateral or transverse motion. Some people prefer this simplicity of control.

MULTIPLE-AXIS FEET

These components move slightly in all planes to aid the wearer in maintaining maximum contact with the walking surface, even if the surface slopes or presents slight irregularities. **Multiple-axis feet** are heavier and less durable than single-axis or nonarticulated feet.

The clinician can select from a wide array of foot-ankle assemblies, in addition to the representative components described here.

Rotators

A rotator is a component placed above the prosthetic foot to absorb shock in the transverse plane. This action protects the user from chafing, which would otherwise occur if the socket were permitted to rotate against the skin. Rotators are most often used with single-axis feet and by very active individuals with transfemoral amputations.

Shank

Adjacent to the foot-ankle assembly (or rotator) in a transtibial prosthesis is the shank. It restores leg length and shape, and transmits the wearer's body weight from the socket to the foot. Two types of shank are used: exoskeletal and endoskeletal. The Syme's prosthesis does not have a shank because the socket encasing the amputated limb extends to the foot-ankle assembly.

EXOSKELETAL SHANK

In contrast, the **exoskeletal shank** (Fig. 20-2) is usually made of wood. It presents a rigid exterior, shaped to simulate the contour of the leg. The shank is finished with plastic tinted to match the wearer's skin color; some individuals opt for a multicolored or patterned shank. The exoskeletal shank, sometimes called **crustacean,** is very durable and, with

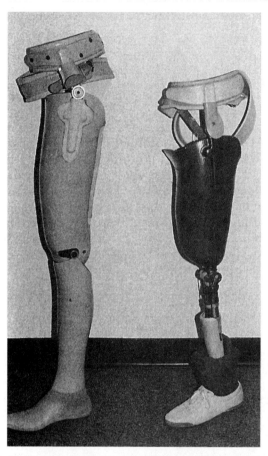

Figure 20-2. (Left) Exoskeletal transfemoral prosthesis with stance control mechanical knee mechanism. (Right) Endoskeletal transfemoral prosthesis with cosmetic cover rolled down. (From May, BJ: Amputations and Prosthetics: A Case Study Approach. FA Davis, Philadelphia, 1996, p 110, with permission.)

the plastic finish, impervious to liquids and most abrasives. Because exoskeletal shanks are less lifelike and do not permit changes in angulation of the prosthesis, they are less frequently prescribed.

ENDOSKELETAL SHANK

The **endoskeletal shank** (Fig. 20-3) consists of a central aluminum or rigid plastic pylon covered with foam rubber and a sturdy stocking or similar finish. The endoskeletal, or **modular,** shank is more lifelike than the shiny exoskeletal shank. In addition, the pylon has a mechanism that permits making slight adjustment of the angulation of the prosthesis; this may contribute to comfort and ease of walking. A few prosthetic foot-ankle assemblies, such as the Flex-Foot, incorporate an endoskeletal shank.

Socket

The amputated limb fits into a receptacle called the socket (Fig. 20-4). Although the original name for the modern transtibial socket was the **patellar-tendon-bearing (PTB)** socket,[22] the socket is designed to contact all portions of the amputated limb

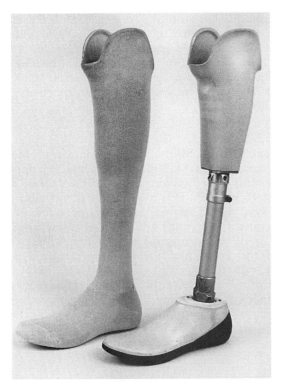

Figure 20-3. Transtibial (below-knee) prosthesis with SACH foot, endoskeletal shank, patellar-tendon-bearing socket, and supracondylar suspension with and without foam rubber covering.

for maximum distribution of load, as well as to assist venous blood circulation and provide tactile feedback. A more accurate name is total contact. Sockets are custom-molded of plastic, which is shaped over a model of the amputated limb. The prosthetist alters the model to improve comfort. Socket fabrication may be achieved by hand or by **computer-aided design/computer-aided manufacture (CAD-CAM)** involving an electronic sensor, which transmits a detailed map of the patient's limb to a computerized program consisting of socket-shape variations. The prosthetist selects the most appropriate shape, which is transmitted to an electronic carver that creates the model over which the plastic is shaped. Whether the model is made by hand or by computer, it provides **reliefs** in the socket; these are concavities in the socket over areas contacting sensitive structures, such as bony prominences; reliefs are located over the fibular head, tibial crest, tibial condyles, and anterior-distal tibia. The posterior brim is trimmed to provide adequate room for the medial and lateral hamstring tendons, so that the patient is comfortable when sitting. **Build ups** are convexities in the socket over areas contacting pressure-tolerant tissues, such as the belly of the gastrocnemius; the patellar tendon; proximalmedial tibia, corresponding to the pes anserinus; and the tibial and fibular shafts.

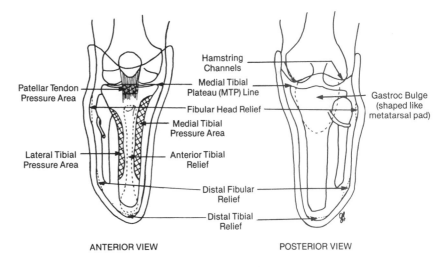

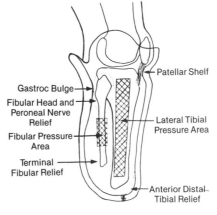

Figure 20-4. Patellar-tendon-bearing socket. (From Sanders, GT: Lower Limb Amputations: A Guide to Rehabilitation. FA Davis, Philadelphia, 1986, p 176, with permission.)

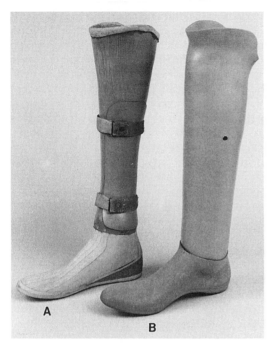

Figure 20-5. Syme's prostheses. (A) Socket with medial opening. (B) Socket with continuous walls and flexible liner.

When viewed from above, the socket resembles a triangle, the apex of which is formed by the relief for the tibial tubercle and crest, and the base angles of which are the hamstring reliefs. The anterior wall terminates at the midpatella, or above. The medial and lateral walls extend at least to the femoral epicondyles. The posterior wall lies across the popliteal fossa.

The socket is aligned on the shank in slight flexion to enhance loading on the patellar tendon, prevent genu recurvatum, and resist the tendency of the amputated limb to slide down the socket. Flexion also facilitates contraction of the quadriceps muscle. The socket is also aligned with a slight lateral tilt to reduce loading on the fibular head.

LINED SOCKET

The transtibial prosthetic socket generally includes a resilient **polyethylene** foam liner. In addition to cushioning the amputated limb, the removable liner facilitates alteration of socket size; the prosthetist can add material to the outside of the liner, reducing the volume of the socket while preserving smooth interior contours. The liner, however, adds to the bulk of the prosthesis and is a heat insulator, which the wearer may find uncomfortable in the summer. The Syme's prosthesis has a liner that assists entry of the bulbous distal end of the amputated limb, enabling the wearer to don the prosthesis easily.

UNLINED SOCKET

Although the unlined socket is sometimes referred to as a hard socket, that term is a misnomer, because the wearer has a soft interface provided by socks or a sheath worn with the unlined socket.

Occasionally, a resilient pad is placed in the bottom of the unlined socket to cushion the distal end of the amputated limb. The unlined socket is a more satisfactory choice for the individual whose limb has stabilized in volume, because it is harder to alter the shape of the unlined socket in comparison to the lined socket.

SYME'S SOCKET

Because the patient with a Syme's amputation can usually bear significant weight through the distal end of the amputated limb, the Syme's socket (Fig. 20-5) does not need to provide proximal loading. The socket trimlines are slightly lower, and the frontal and sagittal plane alignment less tilted, as compared to the transtibial socket. Relief for the tibial crest remains an important feature of the socket. If the distal end of the Syme's limb is markedly bulbous, the lower part of the medial wall can be made removable; the patient dons the socket, and then fastens the wall section in place.

Suspension

During the swing phase of walking, or whenever the wearer is not standing on the prosthesis, such as when climbing stairs or jumping, the prosthesis requires some form of suspension.[10]

CUFF VARIANTS

The modern transtibial prosthesis originated with a supracondylar cuff (Fig. 20-6), which is still widely used. The cuff, a leather strap encircling the thigh immediately above the femoral epicondyles, permits the user to adjust the snugness of suspension easily. Some individuals, however, object to the profile of the distal thigh created by the cuff. Others who have severely arthritic hands or limited vision have difficulty engaging the buckle or pressure loop closure on the cuff.

The cuff may be augmented by a **fork strap** and waist belt. The elastic fork strap extends from the outside of the anterior portion of the socket to the waist belt. The fork strap and waist belt may be indicated for individuals who climb ladders or engage in other activities during which the prosthesis is unsupported by the ground for long periods. An alternate to the cuff is a rubber sleeve, a tubular component that covers the proximal socket and the distal thigh. The sleeve provides excellent suspension and a streamlined silhouette when the wearer sits. Donning the sleeve, however, requires two strong hands and a thigh that does not have excessive subcutaneous tissue.

DISTAL ATTACHMENT

Very secure suspension is achieved with the use of a silicone sheath and special hardware. The sheath clings to the patient's skin during the swing and stance phases of walking. At the end of the sheath is

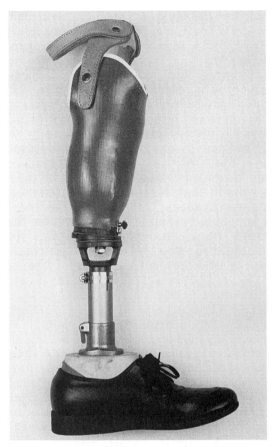

Figure 20-6. Transtibial (below-knee) temporary prosthesis with cuff suspension. Socket is mounted on an adjustable pylon shank with SACH foot.

a small fixture. The user inserts a rod that passes through the shank just below the socket, continues through the fixture on the sheath, and terminates at the other side of the shank. During the swing phase, the rod prevents the prosthesis from slipping away from the sheath.[23,24]

BRIM VARIANTS

The prosthesis may be suspended by its socket walls extended proximally.

Supracondylar Suspension

With **supracondylar (SC) suspension** (Fig. 20-7), the medial and lateral walls extend above the femoral epicondyles. The medial wall has a plastic wedge, which the client removes to don the prosthesis; the wedge is then placed between the socket and the medial epicondyle to retain the prosthesis on the limb. Alternatively, the wedge can be incorporated in a liner; for donning, the patient applies the liner, and then inserts the limb, with liner, into the socket. Supracondylar suspension increases medial-lateral stability of the prosthesis, presents a pleasing contour at the knee, and eliminates the need to engage a buckle or pressure loop on a cuff. It is more difficult to fabricate (and, hence, more expensive), and it is not readily adjustable.

Supracondylar/Suprapatellar Suspension

Presenting a contour of medial and lateral walls similar to the supracondylar suspension, the **supracondylar/suprapatellar (SC/SP) suspension** (Fig. 20-8) also features an anterior wall, which terminates above the patella. The short amputated limb is accommodated by SC/SP suspension. The high anterior wall may interfere with kneeling and presents a conspicuous appearance when the wearer sits.

THIGH CORSET

Some individuals with very sensitive skin on the amputated limb may benefit from thigh corset suspension (Fig. 20-9). Metal hinges attach distally to the medial and lateral aspects of the socket and proximally to a leather corset. Corset heights vary and may reach the ischial tuberosity for maximum weight relief on the amputated limb. The hinges increase frontal plane stability, and the corset leather increases area for load distribution. The resulting prosthesis, however, is heavier and apt to foster **piston action** because the hinges have a single pivot

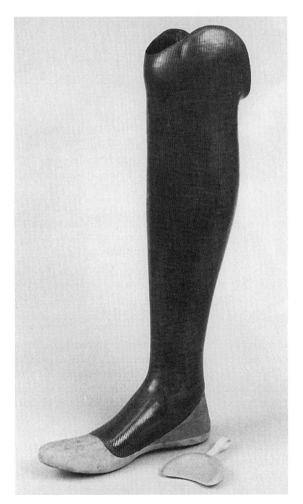

Figure 20-7. Transtibial (below-knee) prosthesis with SACH foot, exoskeletal shank, patellar-tendon-bearing socket, and supracondylar wedge suspension.

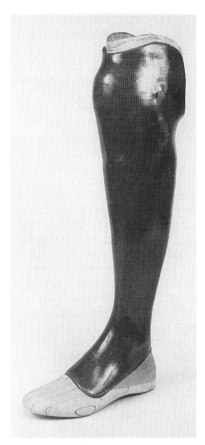

Figure 20-8. Transtibial (below-knee) prosthesis with supracondylar/suprapatellar suspension.

joint that does not articulate colinearly with the anatomical knee. Prolonged use of a thigh corset causes pressure atrophy of the thigh. A corset suspension is more difficult to don because the wearer must fasten laces or series of pressure-loop straps.

Syme's Suspension

The Syme's prosthesis is generally suspended by the contour of its brims and socket walls, without a cuff or other suspension mechanism.

TRANSFEMORAL (ABOVE-KNEE) PROSTHESES

Individuals with amputation between the femoral epicondyles and greater trochanter are fitted with **transfemoral** prostheses. Those whose limbs include the distal part of the femur can wear a knee disarticulation prosthesis, which differs from the transfemoral prosthesis in the type of knee unit and socket. If the amputation is proximal to the trochanter, the patient cannot retain or control a transfemoral prosthesis and is therefore a candidate for a hip disarticulation prosthesis. The transfemoral prosthesis consists of (1) foot-ankle assembly, (2) shank, (3) knee unit, (4) socket, and (5) suspension device.

The SACH foot is most commonly used for transfemoral prostheses. Because the single-axis

foot reaches the foot-flat position with minimal application of load, it is somewhat more frequently prescribed for transfemoral than for transtibial prostheses. Any foot, including the energy storing/ releasing designs such as the Seattle and Flex-Foot, can be incorporated in a transfemoral prosthesis. As compared with wearers of transtibial prostheses, however, most wearers of transfemoral prostheses do not load the prosthesis as vigorously. Consequently, less energy can be stored and released in a prosthetic foot.

Either the sturdy exoskeletal shank or the endoskeletal shank may be used. The latter creates a pleasing appearance, particularly in the knee area, and is adjustable; in addition, it is lighter than an exoskeletal shank. Problems of durability remain, particularly at the knee, where constant bending of the joint accelerates deterioration of the rubber cover.

Knee Unit

The prosthetic knee enables the user to bend the knee when sitting or kneeling and, in most instances, also permits knee flexion during the latter portion of the stance phase and throughout the swing phase of walking. Commercial knee units may be described according to four features: (1) **axis,**

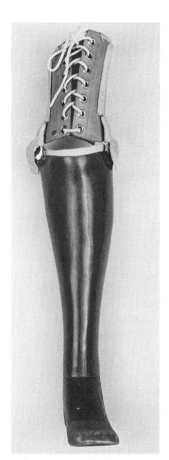

Figure 20-9. Transtibial (below-knee) prosthesis with thigh corset suspension.

(2) **friction mechanism,** (3) **extension aid,** and (4) **mechanical stabilizer.** Many combinations of features are available; not every knee unit has all four components.

AXIS SYSTEM

The thigh piece can be connected to the shank either by a simple **single-axis hinge** (Fig. 20-10), which is the usual arrangement, or by **polycentric linkage** (Fig. 20-11). Polycentric systems provide greater stability to the knee, inasmuch as the momentary center of knee rotation is posterior to the wearer's weight line during most of stance phase;[25] this style is less common because of its greater complexity and because other means are available to stabilize the knee.

FRICTION MECHANISMS

In the simplest sense, the leg of the transfemoral prosthesis is a pendulum swinging about the knee. For the elderly individual who walks slowly for short distances, a basic pendulum is adequate. For more energetic walkers, however, adjustable friction mechanisms that modify the pendular action of the knee are desirable to reduce the asymmetry between the motions of the sound and prosthetic legs. If the knee does not have sufficient friction to retard its natural pendular action, the individual who walks rapidly experiences high heel rise at the beginning of swing phase and terminal impact of the knee (abrupt, often noisy, extension) at the end of swing phase. Friction mechanisms change the knee swing by modifying the speed of knee motion during

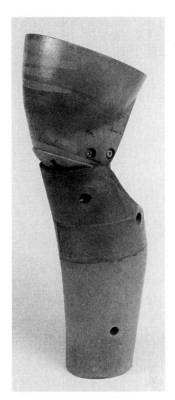

Figure 20-11. Polycentric knee unit.

various parts of swing phase and by affecting knee swing according to walking speed.

Time

The most popular knee unit has **constant friction** (Fig. 20-12), generally including a clamp that grasps the knee bolt. Throughout a given swing phase, the amount of friction is unvarying. It is easy to loosen or tighten the clamp to change the ease of knee motion. A more sophisticated device applies **variable friction,** in which the amount of friction changes during a given swing phase. At early swing, high friction is applied to retard heel rise; during midswing, friction diminishes to permit the knee to swing easily; at late swing, friction increases to dampen impact.

Medium

The medium through which friction is applied influences performance. The usual medium is **sliding friction,** such as when a clamp slides about the knee bolt. This method is simple, but it does not accommodate automatically to changes in walking speed. A more complex approach is **fluid friction,** either oil (hydraulic friction)[12] (Fig. 20-13) or air (pneumatic friction). Unlike sliding friction, fluid friction varies directly with velocity. Thus with a hydraulic or pneumatic unit, if the wearer suddenly walks faster, the knee increases friction instantly to prevent high heel rise and terminal impact. Consequently, the movements of the prosthetic and sound limbs are more symmetrical than would be the case with sliding friction.[26] Oil or air is contained in a

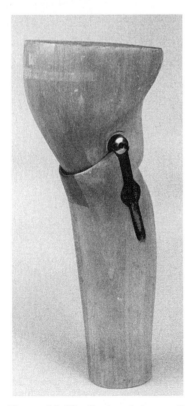

Figure 20-10. Single-axis knee unit.

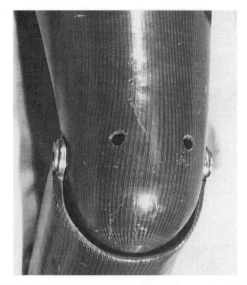

Figure 20-12. Single-axis constant friction knee unit. Note the two screws that permit adjusting the friction.

cylinder in the knee unit. A piston descends in the cylinder during early swing, causing the knee to flex. The speed of piston descent depends on the type of fluid and the walking speed. Later, the piston ascends, extending the knee. Hydraulic units provide more friction than do pneumatic devices. Both types are more expensive than the simpler sliding friction designs. Various combinations of friction designs are manufactured, such as constant sliding friction, variable sliding friction, and variable fluid friction.

EXTENSION AID

Many knee units have a mechanism to assist knee extension during the latter part of swing phase. The simplest type is an external aid, consisting of elastic webbing located in front of the knee axis. The elastic stretches when the knee flexes in early swing and recoils to extend the knee in late swing. Webbing tension is easily adjusted, but tends to pull the knee into extension when the wearer sits. The internal extension aid is an elastic strap or coiled spring within the knee unit. It functions identically to the external aid during walking, but unlike the external aid, the internal type keeps the knee flexed when the individual sits. Acute knee flexion causes the strap or spring to pass behind the knee axis, maintaining the flexed attitude.

STABILIZERS

Most knee units do not have a special device to increase stability. The patient controls knee action by hip motion, aided by the alignment of the knee in relation to other components of the prosthesis. The prosthetic knee joint is usually aligned posterior to a line extending from the trochanter to the ankle (TKA line). The patient who has excellent balance and muscular control may have the knee bolt placed

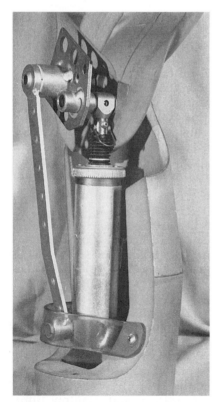

Figure 20-13. Mauch Swing 'N Stance single-axis hydraulic knee unit, which provides both brake and lock options, depending on the position of the "U"-shaped fixture at the back of the unit. The unit is attached to half a thigh-shank component to expose the knee bolt.

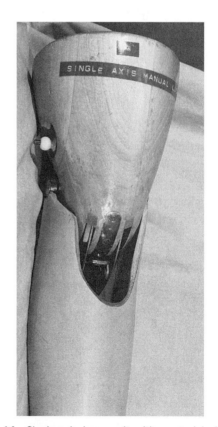

Figure 20-14. Single-axis knee unit with manual lock. Note the white knob that the wearer uses to disengage the lock.

on the TKA line, thus creating TKA alignment. Elderly or debilitated patients may benefit from additional mechanical security.

Manual Lock

The simplest mechanical stabilizer is a manual lock (Fig. 20-14), in which a pin lodges in a receptacle and is released only when the wearer manipulates an unlocking lever. When engaged, the manual lock prevents knee flexion. The user is secure not only during early stance, but through the rest of the gait cycle, when knee flexion would be desirable. To compensate for difficulty in advancing the locked prosthesis, the shank should be shortened approximately ½ inch (1 cm). Another problem inherent with the manual lock is the need to disengage it when the wearer sits.

Friction Brake

A more elaborate stabilizing system, the **friction brake** (Fig. 20-15), provides very high friction during early stance, resisting any tendency of the knee to flex. One design, incorporated in a sliding friction unit, involves the mating of a wedge and groove upon loading, assuming the knee is flexed less than 25 degrees. Another version of friction brake is found in several hydraulic units; during early stance, additional fluid resistance markedly retards piston descent and thus stabilizes the knee.

From midstance through heel contact, friction brakes do not interfere with knee motion. In addition, they do not impede the patient who transfers from standing to sitting. Such devices add to the cost

of the prosthesis and, if improperly used, may not protect the patient from falling.

SOCKET

As is the case with all prosthetic sockets, the transfemoral socket should be a total-contact device to distribute load over the maximum area, thereby reducing pressure. Total-contact fitting also provides counterpressure to assist venous return and prevent distal edema, and it enhances sensory feedback to foster better control of the prosthesis.

Most transfemoral sockets are made of a combination of plastics. A flexible socket (Fig. 20-16) of thin polyethylene thermoplastic encompasses the entire amputated limb. The plastic can be spotheated to facilitate alteration of socket fit. It adheres to the skin better than does rigid plastic, thereby improving suspension; it also dissipates body heat more effectively and affords the wearer sensory input from external objects, such as chairs. The socket is encased in a rigid frame so that the wearer may transmit weight through the distal components of the prosthesis to the ground.

Transfemoral sockets are designed to emphasize loading on pressure-tolerant structures, such as the ischial tuberosity, gluteal musculature, sides of the thigh, and, to a lesser extent, distal end of the amputated limb. The socket must avoid excessive pressure on the pubic symphysis and perineum.

Quadrilateral Socket

The traditional transfemoral socket is quadrilateral in shape when viewed from above (Fig. 20-17). The socket features a horizontal posterior shelf for the ischial tuberosity and gluteal musculature, a medial brim at the same level as the posterior shelf, an anterior wall 2½ to 3 inches (6–8 cm) higher to apply a posteriorly directed force to the thigh to retain the tuberosity on its shelf, and a lateral wall the same height as the anterior wall to aid in medial-lateral stabilization. Concave reliefs are (1) anterior-medial, for the pressure-sensitive adductor longus tendon; (2) posterior-medial, for the sensitive hamstring tendons and sciatic nerve; (3) posterior-lateral, to permit the gluteus maximus to contract and bulge without being crowded; and (4) anterior-lateral, to allow adequate room for the rectus femoris. The anterior wall has a convexity, Scarpa's bulge, to maximize pressure distribution in the vicinity of the femoral triangle. The lateral wall may have reliefs for the greater trochanter and the distal end of the femur.

Ischial Containment Socket

An alternate design (Fig. 20-18) is sometimes called the contoured adducted trochanter-controlled alignment method.[27–29] Its walls cover the ischial tuberosity and part of the ischiopubic ramus to augment socket stability. To increase frontal plane stability and minimize bulk between the thighs, the medial-lateral width of the socket is narrower than that of the quadrilateral socket. The anterior wall is lower than in the quadrilateral socket, whereas the

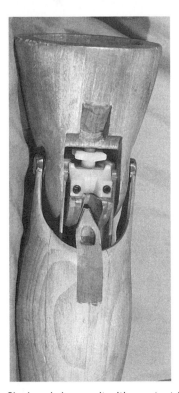

Figure 20-15. Single-axis knee unit with constant friction, internal spring extension aid, and brake.

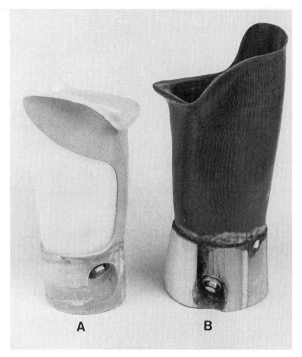

Figure 20-16. Quadrilateral total suction sockets. (*A*) Flexible socket in rigid frame. (*B*) Rigid polyester laminate socket.

lateral wall covers the greater trochanter. Weight-bearing occurs on the sides and bottom of the amputated limb.

Both the ischial containment and quadrilateral sockets can be made of a combination of flexible and rigid plastic, or entirely of rigid material.

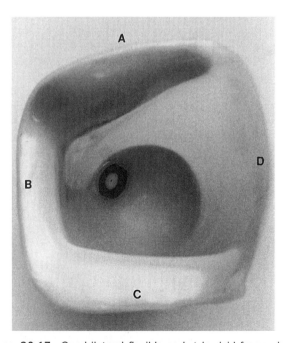

Figure 20-17. Quadrilateral flexible socket in rigid frame viewed from above. (*A*) Anterior wall. (*B*) Medial wall. (*C*) Posterior wall. (*D*) Lateral wall.

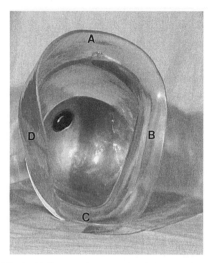

Figure 20-18. Ischial containment flexible transfemoral (above-knee) socket. Note the relatively narrow medial-lateral dimension. (*A*) Anterior brim. (*B*) Medial brim. (*C*) Posterior brim. (*D*) Lateral brim.

Fit and Alignment

Regardless of socket shape and materials, the socket should fit snugly to minimize the risk of chafing and maximize the wearer's control of the prosthesis. Slight socket flexion is desirable for several reasons: (1) to facilitate contraction of the hip extensors, (2) to reduce lumbar lordosis, and (3) to provide a zone through which the thigh may be extended to permit the wearer to take steps of approximately equal length. For wearers of quadrilateral sockets, socket flexion also enhances positioning the ischial tuberosity on the posterior brim.[30]

Suspension

Three means are used to suspend the transfemoral prosthesis: (1) total suction, (2) partial suction, and (3) no suction.

SUCTION SUSPENSION

Suction refers to the pressure difference inside and outside the socket. With suction suspension, internal socket pressure is less than external pressure; consequently, atmospheric pressure causes the socket to remain on the thigh. The socket brim must fit snugly, and a one-way air-release valve is located at the bottom of the socket.

Total Suction

Maximum control of the prosthesis, without any encumbering auxiliary suspension, can be achieved only if the socket fits very snugly to give total suction (Fig. 20-19); if the patient experiences changes in amputated limb volume, suction will be lost.

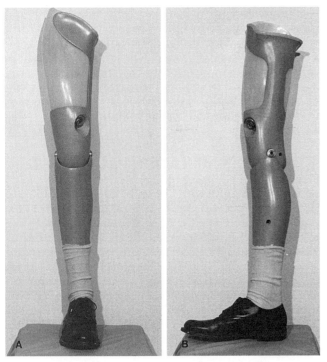

Figure 20-19. Transfemoral (above-knee) prosthesis with SACH foot, exoskeletal shank, single-axis constant friction knee unit, and quadrilateral flexible socket with suction suspension. (*A*) Anterior view. (*B*) Medial view.

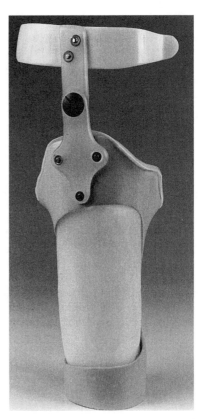

Figure 20-21. Quadrilateral partial suction socket with rigid plastic pelvic band attachment.

Partial Suction

A socket that is slightly loose may enable partial suction suspension. The patient wears a sock. Because socket fit is looser, an auxiliary suspension aid is needed, either a fabric Silesian bandage (Fig. 20-20), or a rigid plastic or metal hip joint and pelvic band (Fig. 20-21). These aids encircle the pelvis. The Silesian bandage also controls the transverse plane orientation of the prosthesis on the thigh, while the hip joint restricts transverse and frontal motion at the hip. The pelvic band adds weight to the prosthesis and may impose uncomfortable pressure against the torso when the wearer sits.

NO SUCTION

If the socket has a distal hole but no valve, then there is no pressure difference between inside and outside the socket. The client wears one or more socks and requires a pelvic band. The relatively loose socket makes donning easy, but hinders control of the prosthesis and sitting comfort.

DISARTICULATION PROSTHESES

Individuals with knee or hip disarticulation wear prostheses that include the same distal components as prostheses for lower levels. Any prosthetic foot can be used with either an endoskeletal or exoskeletal shank. The major distinction, therefore, is in the proximal portion of the prostheses.

KNEE DISARTICULATION PROSTHESES

When amputation is at or distal to the femoral epicondyles, the patient should have excellent prosthetic control because (1) thigh leverage is at a

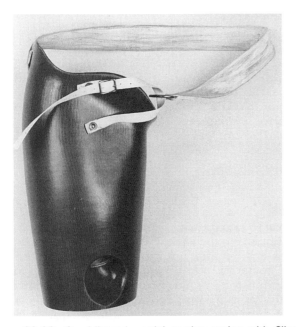

Figure 20-20. Quadrilateral partial suction socket with Silesian bandage.

maximum, (2) most of the body weight can be borne through the distal end of the femur, and (3) the broad epicondyles provide rotational stability. The problem presented by knee disarticulation is primarily cosmetic; when the individual sits, the thigh on the amputated side may protrude slightly. The knee disarticulation prosthesis (Fig. 20-22) has a streamlined knee that minimizes protrusion, as well as a specially designed socket.

Socket

Two types of sockets are currently in use. Both are made of plastic and usually terminate below the ischial tuberosity. Generally, no additional suspension aids are needed. One version features an anterior opening to accommodate a bulbous amputated limb. After the limb is inserted, the wearer closes the socket with lacing or pressure-loop tapes. The other design has no anterior opening and is suitable for limbs that are not bulbous.

Knee Unit

Several units are specifically manufactured for knee disarticulation. All have a thin proximal attach-

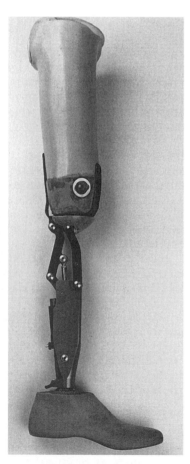

Figure 20-22. Knee disarticulation prosthesis with SACH foot, endoskeletal shank, polycentric hydraulic friction knee unit, and quadrilateral socket with suction suspension.

ment plate to minimize added thigh length. One may choose among hydraulic, pneumatic, and sliding friction units, with or without polycentric linkage. Even with a special knee unit, the thigh will be slightly longer. Consequently, the shank is shortened equivalently, so that when the person stands, the pelvis is level. When the individual sits, the thigh on the prosthetic side will project slightly.

HIP DISARTICULATION PROSTHESES

A hip disarticulation prosthesis (Fig. 20-23) is fitted to a person with amputation above the greater trochanter (very short transfemoral), removal of the femoral head from the acetabulum (hip disarticulation), or removal of the femur and some portion of the pelvis (hemipelvectomy). Prostheses for proximal levels share common hip, knee, and foot assemblies and alignment, but differ with regard to socket design. The endoskeletal thigh and shank predominate because they afford appreciable weight saving in these massive prostheses.

Socket

The basic socket is plastic molded to provide weight-bearing on the ipsilateral ischial tuberosity and both iliac crests. The person with a hemipelvectomy who does not retain the ipsilateral tuberosity or crest has a socket with a higher proximal trimline, sometimes encompassing the lower thorax. This individual supports weight on the remainder of the pelvis, on the abdomen, and perhaps on the lower ribs.

Hip Unit

Various joints provide hip flexion. They have an extension aid to bias the prosthesis toward the stable neutral position. Positioning the mechanical hip anterior to a point corresponding to the anatomical hip also contributes to hip stability. The joint is below the normal hip, so that with sitting, the prosthetic thigh will not protrude unattractively.

Stability

Several attributes combine to make the hip disarticulation prosthesis very stable, namely the hip extension aid, anterior placement of the hip joint, posterior placement of the knee unit, and a knee extension aid. The prosthesis may be shortened slightly, primarily to aid clearance during swing phase, but also to encourage the wearer to apply maximum weight to the prosthesis and to increase stability.

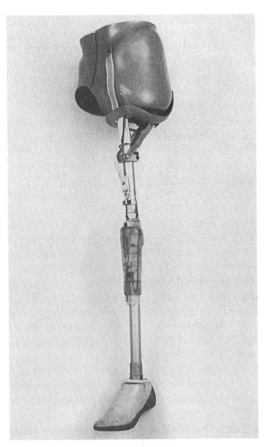

Figure 20-23. Hip disarticulation prosthesis with SACH foot, endoskeletal shank, single-axis knee and extension aid, single-axis hip with extension aid, and rigid socket.

Socks and Sheaths

All individuals with lower-limb amputations, except those wearing transfemoral prostheses suspended by total suction or those using a sheath, require a supply of clean socks of appropriate material, size, and shape. It is expeditious to include an order of at least a dozen socks at the time the prosthesis is ordered, so that third-party payment may cover this relatively inexpensive but important accessory.

Fabric socks are woven in various thicknesses, referred to as *ply*, designating the number of threads knitted together. Cotton socks absorb perspiration readily and are the least allergenic; they are made in two-, three-, and five-ply, the last being the thickest. Wool socks provide good cushioning, woven in three-, five-, and six-ply; they are expensive and must be laundered carefully. Orlon/Lycra socks are manufactured in two- and three-ply thicknesses. They can be washed easily without shrinking. This synthetic fabric combination affords considerable resilience, but does not absorb much perspiration.

A nylon sheath creates a smooth surface over the skin, thereby reducing the risk of chafing, especially in hot weather and among those with much scarring. Some transtibial prosthesis wearers are able to use a woman's knee-high nylon stocking if the amputated limb is slender. Because nylon does not absorb perspiration, liquid passes through the weave to be absorbed by an outer sock of cotton, wool, or Orlon/Lycra. Silicone, urethane, and other synthetic sheaths provide excellent shock absorption and abrasion resistance; they also can aid in suspending the socket on the patient's limb, and are designed to be worn next to the skin. They are, however, more expensive than fabric socks or sheaths.

Regardless of material, the shape of the sock or sheath is important for comfort. An interface of proper size fits smoothly without wrinkling or undue stretching. The sock or sheath should be long enough to terminate above the most proximal part of the socket or thigh corset.

It is common practice to add more socks as the amputated limb shrinks. Nevertheless, when the patient requires a total of 15-ply of socks to achieve snug fit, the socket should be altered or replaced by the prosthetist. Excessive sock padding distorts the weight-bearing characteristics of the socket, losing the effect of strategically placed build-ups and reliefs.

PROSTHETIC MAINTENANCE

Optimal function depends on proper care of socks or sheaths, prosthesis, amputated limb, and intact limb, as well as general health maintenance. Guidelines for personal hygiene are presented in Chapter 19. In addition to ensuring cleanliness, the individual should wear a well-fitting sock and shoe on the sound foot and the mate to the shoe on the prosthesis. Both shoes should be in excellent condition.

As with any appliance, the prosthesis benefits from simple regular maintenance, which generally avoids costly, time-consuming repairs. Printed instructions pertaining to the prosthesis and socks or sheath are helpful for patient education.

Socket and Suspension

Plastic sockets should be washed with a cloth dampened in warm water that has a very small amount of mild soap dissolved in it. The socket is then wiped with a damp, soap-free cloth, and dried with a fresh towel. In warm climates, the socket should be washed every evening so that it will be completely dry when the patient dresses the following morning.

The transfemoral suction valve should be brushed daily to remove talcum and lint, which might clog the tiny aperture. The valve should be inserted and removed only with one's fingers, because tools are apt to damage the internal mechanism or outer threads.

Leather corsets should be kept dry. Use of saddle soap will keep leather clean. If the patient is incontinent, the thigh corset should be made of flexible **polyester laminate** or polypropylene, which are impervious to urine.

Socket liners made of polyethylene foam can be washed by hand in tepid water with mild soap, rinsed, and air-dried overnight. They should not be subjected to direct sunlight when removed from the prosthesis.

Knee Unit

Sliding friction mechanisms tend to loosen with walking and thus require periodic tightening to retain the original adjustment. The frequency of tightening depends on how much the wearer walks. Most units have a pair of screws in front or in the rear of the knee unit that can be turned clockwise with an Allen wrench or common screwdriver. After turning each screw a quarter turn, the client should walk for at least 5 minutes to ascertain the effectiveness of the adjustment.

Squeaking at the knee or articulated ankle indicates the need for oil. The rubber or felt extension bumper in the knee unit will erode after prolonged vigorous use, and the wearer will then notice that the knee begins to hyperextend. The bumper, visible when the knee is flexed, must be replaced by the prosthetist.

The external kick strap extension aid gradually loses its elasticity. The user will then experience high heel rise in early swing and slow knee extension at the end of swing phase. The simplest approach is to tighten the strap through its buckle. Eventually, the prosthetist will need to replace the elastic webbing. Internal elastic extension aids are not subject to rubbing from the trouser leg or skirt and thus do not lose elasticity as readily. Steel spring internal aids retain their effectiveness for the life of the prosthesis.

Pneumatic and hydraulic units must be protected against tears of the rubber shield protecting the piston. The piston must not be scratched, because this would allow air and debris to enter the cylinder. Air bubbles in the unit will cause a spongy feeling, and possibly noise with walking. At night, the prosthesis should be stored upright, with the knee extended to exclude air from the cylinder.

Foot-Ankle Assembly

One should avoid getting the prosthetic foot wet, especially if the foot is an articulated model. If this happens, the shoe and sock should be removed to allow the foot to dry completely, away from direct heat. The wearer should also avoid stepping into sand and similar materials that might enter the cleft between the foot and shank section and restrict the excursion of the foot. The prosthetist would have to disassemble the foot to clean it.

The client should inspect the foot periodically to spot cracking at the toe-break or tip of the keel; such a crack will curl the toes and prevent smooth transi-tion during late stance. A deteriorated heel cushion or plantar bumper will cause one to appear to be walking in a hole. Although most feet are now molded to simulate toes, the patient should not walk barefoot because the sole of the prosthetic foot is not intended to resist much abrasion.

Foot socks wear much more quickly on the prosthetic side, because the hard foot-ankle assembly and shank rub against the fabric. Stair risers also scuff the sock. Some people find that wearing two socks helps cushion the outer one against premature formation of holes.

The individual must be instructed regarding wearing shoes of the same heel height as was the case when the prosthesis was aligned. Too low a heel interrupts late stance; an unduly high heel makes the knee less stable. If the prosthesis has the usual foot designed for low-heeled shoes, and the wearer wishes to wear flat-heeled shoes, a ½ inch (1 cm) shim should be placed inside both shoes at the heel. High-heeled shoes require that the foot be changed, either by unbolting it and replacing it with a foot with an appropriate plantarflexion angle, or by adjusting a heel-height screw found in certain models of feet. Boots and other footwear with stiff upper sections restrict the action of any foot assembly that is designed to provide substantial dorsiflexion and plantarflexion.

Removing the shoe is easier if the prosthesis is not worn. With the shoe unlaced completely, one grasps the counter, then pushes the heel of the shoe off the back of the foot. Finally, pull the shoe upward off the forefoot. The shoe should be put on the prosthetic foot with the aid of a shoehorn.

Exterior Finish

The usual finish of exoskeletal shanks is polyester laminate, which is impervious to most liquids. It needs only to be wiped periodically with a cloth dampened with dilute detergent to remove surface soil. Marks can be scoured gently with kitchen cleanser; excessive abrasion will dull the finish.

The soft foam cover of the endoskeletal prosthesis requires reasonable caution against exposure to direct heat, penetrating objects, and solvents. The outer covering will need replacement whenever it becomes unacceptably soiled or torn. The transfemoral version tends to deteriorate at the knee, especially if the wearer kneels a great deal.

PHYSICAL THERAPY MANAGEMENT

Physical therapists participate in the management of patients with amputation at several key stages: (1) preoperative, (2) postoperative-preprosthetic, (3) prosthetic prescription, (4) prosthetic assessment, and (5) prosthetic training.

The first two stages are described in Chapter 19. The following discussion emphasizes the responsibilities of the physical therapist with regard to the patient and prosthesis. Ideally, the therapist works as a member of a **clinic team,** together with the physician and prosthetist. Others, such as a social worker, vocational counselor, and psychologist may participate in the team on a regular basis or as needed. The clinic team provides the best environment for exchange of information and viewpoints regarding the patient and fosters efficient treatment. The team meets to formulate the prospective prescription, assess the newly delivered prosthesis, and reassess the patient and prosthesis upon completion of prosthetic training. The therapist, therefore, has an integral part to play in these critical points in rehabilitation, as well as conducting prosthetic training. If a formal clinic team is not established in the therapist's work setting, then one must coordinate the recommendations of the physician and prosthetist.

With either administrative situation, the physical therapist:
1. Performs preprescription assessment.
2. Contributes to prosthetic prescription.
3. Assesses the prosthesis.
4. Facilitates prosthetic acceptance.
5. Trains the patient to don, use, and maintain the prosthesis.

Preprescription Assessment

Successful prosthetic rehabilitation depends on matching the individual's physical and psychosocial characteristics to a prosthesis composed of carefully selected components. Although everyone who wears a prosthesis has an amputation or comparable limb deficiency, the reverse is not true. That is, some people with amputations are not candidates for prostheses or prefer not to use prostheses. Prostheses are contraindicated for patients with severe dementia or depression, or advanced cardiopulmonary disease. If the person displays significant changes associated with organic brain syndrome, then prosthetic fitting is contraindicated. Individuals with bilateral amputations who are unable to transfer independently or don underwear by themselves are most unlikely to benefit from definitive prostheses. Similarly, the patient with bilateral amputations who had sustained unilateral amputation previously and was unable to don and walk with a prosthesis is not a candidate for prostheses. Some people with high amputations, especially hip disarticulation, find that a prosthesis is unduly cumbersome; they prefer to ambulate with a pair of crutches or depend on a wheelchair. Several sports, particularly swimming, are easier to perform without a prosthesis.

Physical Examination

The physical therapist should measure and record the patient's physical attributes, such as active and passive range of motion of all lower-limb joints on both lower extremities. Knee and hip flexion contractures compromise prosthetic alignment and appearance. A knee lock may be needed in a transfemoral prosthesis, and an alternative socket design for a transtibial prosthesis. Severe contractures preclude fitting with conventional components, or may contraindicate provision of any prosthesis. The deleterious effects of contractures are especially serious with bilateral amputations.

The length of the amputated limb is measured. The individual with a short transtibial amputation may require SC/SP suspension. Every attempt should be made to fit the patient with a short transfemoral amputation with suction or partial-suction suspension to retain the prosthesis on the thigh.

Muscle strength of all limbs and trunk should be assessed. Frequently, the elderly patient with vascular disease experiences reduced physical activity as leg pains and foot ulceration develop. Such an individual may present with marked debility, which would interfere with prosthetic use or necessitate use of a unit with a knee lock.

The therapist should inspect the skin, noting any lesions. The patient may require a nylon or silicone sheath to provide a smooth interface between socket and skin to avoid irritating tender or grafted skin.

Sensory function is another factor requiring assessment. For example, an individual with impaired proprioception at the knee will need extra prosthetic stability in the form of higher medial and lateral walls, or side joints attached to a thigh corset, on the transtibial prosthesis. Blindness does not preclude fitting, but it does pose problems with regard to selecting components that are easy to don, as well as altering the training program. If the patient complains of a neuroma, the problem must be addressed surgically or conservatively before fitting can proceed.

Physical therapists assess the ability of patients to learn and retain new information, as well as short- and long-term memory. Other neurological changes, such as cerebrovascular accident, complicate fitting and training. Ipsilateral hemiplegia is not as detrimental to prosthetic rehabilitation as contralateral paralysis. In both instances, the prosthesis should be designed for maximum stability. Patients with mild neurological impairments often respond favorably to altered training strategies, which the therapist designs on an individualized basis.

The circulatory status of the amputated and sound limbs requires careful scrutiny. The physical therapist should teach the patient to inspect the intact foot, using a hand mirror to visualize the plantar surface. Inspection aims to identify incipient areas of abrasion so that corrective measures may be instituted before ulceration or infection ensues. In addition, the patient should be taught to keep the sound foot clean and should wear clean hose and a well-fitting shoe (see Chapter 18 for additional guidelines for managing the patient with peripheral vascular disease). Sequential measurements of amputated limb circumference as well as palpation will indicate whether the patient has edema. Measures should be instituted to stabilize limb volume so that the patient can retain the fit of the prosthetic socket. The patient with vascular impairment may benefit from prosthetic fitting, which transfers some stress from the contralateral limb. In addition, should the person come to bilateral amputation, previous experience with donning and controlling a unilateral prosthesis is invaluable in adjusting to a pair of prostheses.

Prosthetic prescription also hinges on the patient's cardiopulmonary condition. The clinic team must formulate a realistic goal based on the individual's physical capacity, particularly as related to exercise tolerance and endurance. The person who is not expected to walk rapidly is an unlikely candidate for an energy-storing/releasing foot or a fluid-controlled knee unit. Nevertheless, a fluid-controlled knee unit that incorporates a braking mechanism is appropriate for selected patients with generalized weakness.

Obesity is another factor to be considered in the preprescription assessment. The obese individual is more apt to fluctuate in body weight, necessitating provision of socket liners and several socks to compensate for changing limb circumference. Similarly, those who have renal disease, especially if requiring dialysis, experience volume changes that need prosthetic accommodation.

Arthritis affects prosthesis prescription. Diminished lower-limb mobility or deformity compromises prosthetic alignment. Patients with hip or knee arthroplasty, however, function quite well in the prosthesis. Hand and wrist stiffness and malalignment affect the mode of donning; a laced corset should be avoided. Canes and crutches may require modification.

One of the most useful assessment procedures involves observing the patient's ability to transfer from bed to wheelchair. To accomplish this maneuver, the individual must have reasonable strength, balance, and coordination, as well as adequate comprehension. Functional assessment is an essential component of physical therapy management (see Chapter 11 for a detailed discussion).

Psychosocial Assessment

The physical therapist ordinarily treats the patient more frequently than any other member of the clinic team and thus is more likely to be attuned to the individual's attitudes. The patient who is excessively fearful will be served best by prosthetic rehabilitation beginning with a **temporary (provisional) prosthesis.** Motivation is a cardinal determinant of prosthetic outcome. Again, strong motivation demonstrated through use of a temporary prosthesis and compliance with other elements of the rehabilitation program are reliable predictors of prosthetic success. One should guard against unrealistic expectations. Involving the patient and family in group situations with other persons with amputation, in the physical therapy department, and in social environments fosters constructive attitudes.

The therapist should also weigh the likelihood that the individual will be able to care for complex mechanisms and have the financial resources to obtain prosthetic servicing, especially of components, such as the foam rubber covering of the endoskeletal shank, which is less durable.

Prosthetic Prescription

Because no prosthetic component is ideal for all clients, it is necessary to select components that are most apt to meet the individual's needs. Alternatives to every element of the prosthesis have advantages and disadvantages. The task of the physical therapist, in conjunction with other team members, is to judge the relative merits of various feet, shanks, and other components in light of objective and subjective information pertaining to the prosthetic candidate.

Some people can be expected to function best with a sophisticated prosthesis that enhances the wearer's ability to engage in vigorous walking and athletics. Others are best served by a simple, inexpensive device. The most accurate predictor of future function is the patient's performance with a previous prosthesis. For the wearer who seeks a replacement prosthesis, the clinic team should consider the extent of use of the previous limb, together with any changes in the patient's physique and life-style. For example, if the person fitted with one prosthesis now returns with bilateral amputation, never having used the original prosthesis, that patient is a very poor candidate for bilateral prosthetic fitting. In contrast, another person who had been fitted with a simple transfemoral prosthesis expresses the wish to participate in sports. By demonstrating good use of the original prosthesis, that individual is likely to derive considerable benefit from a new prosthesis with a fluid-controlled knee unit and an energy-storing/releasing foot.

Prescription for the new patient is more difficult. Depending on the interval between amputation surgery and prescription, the amputated limb may not have stabilized in volume; the patient may not have achieved the maximum benefit from the preprosthetic program. The best criterion for prosthetic prescription in such an instance is performance with a temporary (provisional) prosthesis. This appliance includes a well-fitting socket, suitable suspension, pylon, and foot; with the transfemoral model, it usually has a knee unit. The temporary prosthesis allows preliminary gait and activities training. The major difference between the temporary and definitive (permanent) prosthesis is appearance. The temporary socket is designed for easy alteration to accommodate change in amputated limb volume. Ordinarily, little attention is paid to the color and shape of the temporary prosthesis.

Transtibial (Below-Knee) Temporary Prosthesis

Most transtibial temporary prostheses have sockets made of thermoplastic material that becomes malleable at temperatures low enough to permit forming directly on the patient. One can also obtain mass-produced adjustable sockets; it is necessary to pad the socket bottom so that the amputated limb does not develop distal edema. Some temporary prostheses have a plaster socket molded to the amputated limb. Plaster is inexpensive, readily available, and easy to use. The resulting socket, however, is rather heavy and bulky. Suspension is usually by a cuff or thigh corset. The pylon can be an aluminum component manufactured for this purpose; such a pylon has a proximal fixture that permits small changes in prosthetic alignment. A simpler pylon can be made with polyvinylchloride piping, such as used for plumbing. The pipe is lightweight and can be spot-heated to enable slight alteration in alignment. A SACH foot is customarily used on temporary prostheses.

Transfemoral (Above-Knee) Temporary Prosthesis

The easiest approach is to use a polypropylene socket (Fig. 20-24), which is manufactured in several sizes and has straps for circumferential adjustment. The socket can be suspended with a Silesian bandage or pelvic band, and is mounted on a knee unit, which may include a manual lock. Alternatively, a custom-fabricated socket of plaster or low-temperature thermoplastic can be used. Some individuals with bilateral transfemoral amputations use a pair of stubbies (see Chapter 19, Fig. 19-14). These are nonarticulated prostheses; the sockets are mounted on short platforms, drastically reducing the wearer's height in order to increase balance stability. The platforms each have a rearward projection to protect the patient from a backward fall.

Prosthetic Assessment

The prosthesis should be assessed before the patient engages in prosthetic training and should be reassessed at the conclusion of training. The procedure is intended to determine the adequacy of prosthetic fit and function, as well as the wearer's opinion of appearance and overall satisfaction. Assessment typically follows a sequence of examining the prosthesis while the patient stands (static assessment), examining the patient's gait (dynamic assessment), and finally examining the prosthesis off the patient (additional static assessment). In many institutions, the physical therapist assesses the prosthesis and presents a summary of findings to the clinic team. The team makes the final determination regarding the acceptability of the prosthesis. At

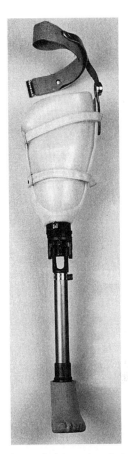

Figure 20-24. Transfemoral (above-knee) temporary prosthesis with adjustable polypropylene socket, pelvic band, and adjustable pylon shank with SACH foot.

initial examination, the team has three options: (1) pass, (2) provisional pass, and (3) fail. Pass indicates that no changes are needed in the prosthesis and the patient can proceed to training. Provisional pass signals that one or more minor problems require correction, none of which would interfere with training. Failure is the team's judgement that the prosthesis has a major fault that should be corrected to the team's satisfaction before commencement of prosthetic training. For example, poor finishing of the prosthetic foot merits a provisional pass, whereas a socket that abrades the amputated limb should be graded as fail.

If the therapist intends to train a patient who is not managed by a formal clinic team, it is especially critical that one examine the prosthesis prior to initiating training to discover any problems that would negate the future program.

At the final assessment, two ratings are available: pass indicates that no problems exist and the patient uses the prosthesis in a manner commensurate with that individual's physical capacity; fail means that major or minor problems remain.

No special materials are needed to assess the prosthesis, except for a checklist and a straight chair. For final assessment, stairs and a ramp are needed. Appendices A and B contain the checklists referred to in the following sections.

Transtibial (Below-Knee) Assessment

Most items on the checklist in Appendix A are self-explanatory. Each contributes to forming an accurate judgement of the adequacy of the prosthesis.

STATIC ASSESSMENT

The prosthesis is assessed while the wearer stands and sits. In addition, the amputated limb and details of the prosthesis are examined. The prosthesis should be compared with the prescription. Departures from the original specifications must be approved by the individual who authorized the prescription.

The new wearer should stand in the parallel bars or other secure environment, attempting to bear equal weight on both feet. The therapist should solicit subjective comments about comfort. Estimates of anterior-posterior and medial-lateral alignment are aided by slipping a sheet of paper under various parts of the shoe. Ideally, the patient should stand with both heels and soles flat on the floor. Malalignment, indicated by excessive weight-bearing on one portion of the shoe, may be confirmed by subsequent analysis of gait.

Most prostheses are constructed so that when the individual stands, the pelvis is level. If the pelvis tilts, the therapist should place lifts under the foot on the shorter side to restore a level pelvis. If the total lift measures ½ inch (1 cm) or less, no attention is needed. For greater discrepancy, one should seek causative factors. An amputated limb that sinks too far into the socket will make the prosthetic side appear short, and the wearer will probably complain of discomfort.

Piston action refers to vertical motion of the socket when the patient elevates the pelvis. Socket slippage is caused by looseness, inadequate suspension, or both. Socket walls should fit snugly, as should the thigh corset if it is part of the prosthesis.

Comfortable sitting is a primary need for all people. The posterior brim should not impinge into the popliteal fossa, and hamstring reliefs should be adequate, especially on the medial side where the semitendinosus and semimembranosus insert relatively distally. Placement of the tabs of the cuff or the joints of the corset also influences sitting comfort.

DYNAMIC ASSESSMENT

Appraisal of the gait pattern and performance of other ambulatory activities is an essential part of rehabilitation. For most patients, a major reason for being fitted with a prosthesis is to resume walking. Nevertheless, no prosthesis eradicates entirely the anatomical and physiological changes produced by amputation. When walking, the person who wears a prosthesis compensates for anatomical and prosthetic deficiencies. Some are inherent to amputation; others are abnormalities of the body or the prosthesis. Because virtually all people walk with a prosthesis in a manner different from the nondisabled walking pattern, prosthetic gait represents compensation for the patient's altered locomotor apparatus. The term "gait compensation" may be a more accurate descriptor than the more commonly used "gait deviation" inasmuch as the patient with amputation is most unlikely ever to walk exactly like a nondisabled person.

No prosthesis replaces the lost sensation, skeletal continuity, muscle integrity, and weight loss caused by amputation. Anatomical deficiencies are aggravated in the presence of pain, contracture, weakness, instability, or incoordination. Similarly, prosthetic components do not replace every function of the missing limb. For example, most prosthetic feet do not move through the full excursion of the human counterpart. Inadequacies in the prosthesis compel the wearer to adopt gait compensations. Such problems include a poorly fitted socket, prosthetic malalignment, malfunctioning components, and improper height of the prosthesis. Compounding the problem are incorrect donning of the prosthesis and wearing inappropriate shoes. The physical therapist must determine when a gait compensation exists and what its cause is likely to be so that remedial action may be taken. Otherwise, the patient is compelled to expend more energy walking and to exhibit a more conspicuously abnormal gait. The new wearer will have had brief experience walking in the prosthesis during the course of prosthetic fabrication. Although a smooth gait is unlikely on the day of the initial examination, gross departure from the usual gait exhibited by others with similar prostheses should be noted and causes sought.

Transtibial analysis focuses on action of the knee on the amputated side during stance phase. Both knees should flex in a controlled manner during early and late stance phase. Excessive flexion indicates that the socket is aligned too far anterior in relation to the foot, or is excessively flexed; this deviation may cause the patient to fall. If the knee flexes too much only during early stance, the cause may be a heel cushion that is too firm for that wearer. Conversely, insufficient knee flexion results from posterior displacement of the socket or inadequate socket tilting. When viewed in the frontal plane, the socket brim should maintain reasonable contact with the leg; excessive lateral thrust of the prosthetic brim suggests that the prosthetic foot has been positioned too far medially. Table 20–1 summarizes the prosthetic and anatomical causes of gait compensations and deviations.[33–37]

At the initial assessment, performance on stairs and inclines may be omitted because the patient has not had training in these activities.

Assessment with the Prosthesis off the Patient

After conducting the dynamic assessment, the therapist should examine the amputated limb for signs of proper loading. The posterior wall should be at the same level as the build-up for the patellar ligament when the patient stands. Because one cannot ascertain this relationship when the prosthesis is being worn, a substitute check is performed.

Table 20–1 TRANSTIBIAL (BELOW-KNEE) PROSTHETIC GAIT ANALYSIS

Compensation/ Deviation	Prosthetic Causes	Anatomical Causes
EARLY STANCE		
1. Excessive knee flexion	High shoe heel Insufficient plantarflexion Stiff heel cushion Socket too far anterior Socket excessively flexed Cuff tabs too posterior	Flexion contracture Weak quadriceps
2. Insufficient knee flexion	Low shoe heel Excessive plantarflexion Soft heel cushion Socket too far posterior Socket insufficiently flexed	Extensor hyperreflexia Weak quadriceps Anterior-distal pain Arthritis
MIDSTANCE		
1. Excessive lateral thrust	Excessive foot inset	
2. Medial thrust	Foot outset	
LATE STANCE		
1. Early knee flexion: drop off	High shoe heel Insufficient plantarflexion Keel too short Dorsiflexion stop too soft Socket too far anterior Socket excessively flexed Cuff tabs too posterior	Flexion contracture
2. Delayed knee flexion: walking uphill	Low shoe heel Excessive plantarflexion Keel too long Dorsiflexion stop too stiff Socket too far posterior Socket insufficiently flexed	Extensor hyperreflexia

Stand the prosthesis on a table; place the end of a long pencil or ruler on the anterior socket bulge and rest the ruler on the posterior brim. In a well-constructed prosthesis, the ruler will slant upward toward the rear, indicating that when the individual stands in the prosthesis and compresses the heel cushion, the wall will be at the proper height.

Any straps or cuff should provide reasonable adjustability. Construction is a guide to future durability, as well as contributing to acceptable appearance of the prosthesis.

Transfemoral (Above-Knee) Assessment

A similar checklist is used to assess the transfemoral prosthesis (Appendix B). It is most important to recognize that seldom is one item of major significance. The therapist and entire team should look for patterns that might herald future difficulty. For example, malalignment detected in static analysis should be confirmed during gait.

STATIC ASSESSMENT

The patient who has a flesh roll above the socket either did not don the socket properly or has a thigh that is larger than that for which the socket was made. Perineal pressure results from sharpness of the medial brim or insufficiency of the adductor longus relief in a quadrilateral socket.

The knee unit should be stable enough to withstand a blow delivered by the therapist to the posterior aspect of the unit. Stability is influenced by the **alignment** of the knee in relation to the hip and prosthetic ankle. The farther posterior the knee bolt, the more stable the knee will be. Polycentric linkage and mechanical stabilizers also contribute to stability. If the socket is opaque, the only way to judge its snugness is by palpating tissue protruding through the valve hole when the valve is removed.

The checklist is designed to help the clinician assess the fit of the socket, regardless of shape or material. If the prosthesis has a quadrilateral socket, proper location of the adductor longus tendon and ischial tuberosity ensures that the patient has donned the socket correctly. A horizontal posterior brim allows weight to be borne on the gluteal musculature as well as the ischial tuberosity. The **ischial containment socket** is intended to cover the ischial tuberosity, yet allow the client to move the hip in all directions comfortably, without socket gapping.

The lateral attachment of the Silesian bandage should be superior and posterior to the greater trochanter for best control of prosthetic rotation. Anteriorly, the attachment should be at the level of the ischial seat, or slightly below, to aid in adducting the prosthesis.

The pelvic joint and band should fit the torso snugly for optimum control of the prosthesis and to minimize bulkiness.

The patient should be able to sit comfortably with the prosthesis. Posterior discomfort may indicate inadequate hamstring relief, or a sharp or thick posterior brim.

DYNAMIC ASSESSMENT

Gait analysis gives the clinic team members the opportunity to assess the adequacy of socket fit, and of prosthesis alignment and adjustment. The patient also influences the walking pattern by the timing and force of muscular contraction and the presence or absence of contractures. The goal of walking with a transfemoral prosthesis is a comfortable, safe, efficient gait, rather than duplicating the gait of someone wearing a transtibial prosthesis or one who does not have amputation. Table 20–2 summarizes transfemoral prosthetic gait compensations.

Compensations/Deviations Best Viewed from Behind

Many individuals with transfemoral amputation abduct the prosthesis to improve frontal plane balance. Hip abduction contracture predisposes patients to this deviation, which is seen in stance phase. Inadequate socket adduction, socket looseness, or medial discomfort causes the fault. Circumduction is a displacement exhibited in swing phase if the prosthesis is too long or if the patient is reluctant to allow the knee to bend. Socket looseness also may result in circumduction. The patient may shift the

Table 20–2 TRANSFEMORAL (ABOVE-KNEE) PROSTHETIC GAIT ANALYSIS

Compensation/Deviation	Prosthetic Causes	Anatomical Causes
LATERAL DISPLACEMENTS		
1. Abduction: stance	Long prosthesis	Abduction contracture
	Abducted hip joint	Weak abductors
	Inadequate lateral wall adduction	Laterodistal pain
	Sharp or high medial wall	Adductor redundancy
		Instability
2. Circumduction: swing	Long prosthesis	Abduction contracture
	Locked knee unit	Poor knee control
	Loose friction	
	Inadequate suspension	
	Small socket	
	Loose socket	
	Foot plantarflexed	
TRUNK SHIFTS		
1. Lateral bend: stance	Short prosthesis	Abduction contracture
	Inadequate lateral wall adduction	Weak abductors
	Sharp or high medial wall	Hip pain
		Instability
		Short amputation limb
2. Forward flexion: stance	Unstable knee unit	Instability
	Short walker or crutches	
3. Lordosis: stance	Inadequate socket flexion	Hip flexion contracture
		Weak extensors
ROTATIONS		
1. Medial (lateral) whip: heel off	Faulty socket contour	With sliding friction unit; fast pace
	Knee bolt externally (internally) rotated	
	Foot malrotated	
	Prosthesis donned in malrotation	
2. Foot rotation at heel contact	Stiff heel cushion	
	Malrotated foot	
EXCESSIVE KNEE MOTION		
1. High heel rise: early swing	Inadequate friction	
	Slack extension aid	
2. Terminal impact: late swing	Inadequate friction	Forceful hip flexion
	Taut extension aid	
REDUCED KNEE MOTION		
1. Vault: swing	See above: circumduction	With sliding friction unit; fast pace
2. Hip hike: swing	See above: circumduction	
UNEVEN STEP LENGTH	Uncomfortable socket	Hip flexion contracture
	Insufficient socket flexion	Instability

trunk excessively. Lateral trunk bending toward the prosthetic side during stance phase generally accompanies abducted gait. It should be noted, however, that all individuals with transfemoral amputation have an incomplete abductor mechanism, and tend to compensate by bending toward the prosthetic side. Although the hip joint and gluteus medius are usually in good condition, lack of skeletal continuity to the ground compromises the effectiveness of abductor contraction. If the prosthesis is too long, the patient is apt to abduct; if it is too short, the patient will bend laterally without abducting.

Whips refer to rotation of the heel at late stance. If the socket does not fit well, contraction with bulging of the thigh musculature will cause the prosthesis to rotate abruptly as it is being unloaded at the end of stance phase. Although less likely, malrotation of the knee unit or foot-ankle assembly may contribute to whipping. Rotation of the foot on heel contact is a much more serious deviation. It indicates inadequate compression of the heel cushion or plantar bumper and can result in a fall.

Compensations/Deviations Best Viewed from the Side

Forward trunk shifting in stance phase is a compensation that some patients use to cope with knee instability. If the walker or crutches are too short, the individual will lean forward. Lumbar lordosis results from inadequate socket flexion and is aggravated by a hip flexion contracture.

Improper adjustment of the knee unit gives rise to uneven heel rise and terminal swing impact. If both deviations are present, the probable cause is insufficient friction. If the knee exhibits impact without undue heel rise, it is more likely that the extension aid is too tight.

To compensate for reduced knee motion, the vigorous walker may vault, excessively plantarflexing the sound ankle to afford extra room to clear the prosthesis during prosthetic swing phase. A less strenuous compensation for actual or functional prosthesis length is hip hiking, when the patient elevates the pelvis on the prosthetic side.

Step lengths will be unequal if the patient has a

hip flexion contracture or inadequate balance; a longer step is taken with the prosthesis. The longer prosthetic step gives the person more time on the sound limb. A flexion contracture prevents the sound limb from passing the prosthetic side during swing phase on the sound side.

ASSESSMENT WITH THE PROSTHESIS OFF THE PATIENT

Following the static assessment, the therapist should examine the prosthesis and amputated limb as indicated on the checklist. A resilient back pad enables the patient to sit quietly without undue trouser or skirt abrasion. The pad is unnecessary with a flexible socket.

Facilitating Prosthetic Acceptance

Amputation generally is regarded as a grievous occurrence, with its visibility a constant reminder of the individual's abnormality.[38,39] The physical therapist can help the patient and family accept the reality of amputation and the prosthesis by verbal and nonverbal communication. One's calm respect for the patient as a worthy human being, regardless of limb condition, should set a model for the attitudes of others. Clinic team management accords not only the benefits of better prosthetic provision but also brings the individual in contact with clinicians who convey experience and confidence in dealing with problems that the person may have considered unique.

As soon as possible, the hospitalized patient should be treated in the physical therapy department, rather than on the ward. The bustle of the department should help dispel despondency. Although postoperative mourning is expected, prolonged depression is not constructive. Peer support groups are often very effective in aiding acceptance of the prosthesis and in learning special procedures for accomplishing activities. Observation and eventual participation in sports programs for the physically challenged is another way people learn to cope and gain the most from rehabilitation. The physical therapist, by virtue of close daily contact with the patient, is also in a position to recommend to the clinic those who might profit from psychological counseling and psychiatric services.

Prosthetic Training

Learning to use a prosthesis effectively involves being able to don it correctly, develop good balance and coordination, walk in a safe and reasonably symmetrical manner, and perform other ambulatory and self-care activities. Treatment goals and outcomes depend on the patient's physical status, preprosthetic experience, and quality of prosthesis. Using the prosthesis only to assist in transferring from the wheelchair to the toilet may be an appropriate outcome for an elderly person with multiple disabilities, whereas the program for the youngster with traumatic amputation might extend to a full range of sports.

DONNING

Correct application of the prosthesis and frequent inspection of the amputated limb are very important, especially for the beginner and those with poor circulation. Patients with partial foot, Syme's, and transtibial amputations can don the prosthesis while seated, after having applied the correct number and sequence of socks or sheath. Then, in most instances, the individual simply inserts the amputated limb into the socket. With SC/SP suspension, one applies the liner to the amputated limb, then inserts the limb and liner into the socket. The initial entry into the socket with corset suspension may be made while sitting; however, final tightening of laces or straps should be done in the standing position to ensure that the limb is lodged suitably in the socket.

Those with transfemoral amputation also can begin the donning process while seated. Total suction wearers may use either a pulling or pushing method. To pull oneself into the socket, the patient applies a light dusting of talcum powder to the thigh to reduce friction. Then one applies a pulling sock, a tubular cotton stockinette approximately 30 inches (76 cm) long, a roll of elastic bandage wound around the thigh, or a nylon stocking. Whatever the donning aid, it should be placed high in the groin to pull in proximal tissues. After placing the sock-encased thigh into the socket, one draws the distal end of the aid through the valve hole. Although it is possible to complete the donning process while seated, most people prefer to stand while pulling the sock or other aid out through the valve hole. By leaning forward, the body's weight line will prevent the prosthetic knee from flexing inadvertently. The patient alternately flexes and extends the sound hip and knee while tugging downward on the donning aid until it slips from the prosthesis. Finally, one inserts the valve.

To push into the socket, one should coat the thigh with a lubricating lotion, push it into the socket, then install the valve. Patients who use partial suction apply a sock, making certain the proximal margin of the sock extends to the inguinal ligament. The patient then introduces the amputated limb into the socket, taking care that the thigh is correctly oriented; pulls the distal end of the sock down through the valve hole enough to ensure that the skin is smooth; tucks the sock back into the socket; and inserts the valve. Finally, one secures the pelvic band or Silesian bandage. If suction is not used, donning is similar to the method used with partial suction, except that there is no valve.

BALANCE AND COORDINATION

Exercises are similar for all patients with lower-limb amputations, although the individual with a transfemoral or hip disarticulation prosthesis may be expected to encounter more difficulty controlling the mechanical knee, as compared to those who need only deal with two anatomical knees. All must learn to bear weight on the amputated side. A graduated program for increasing prosthetic tolerance minimizes the danger of skin abrasion, particularly if the amputated limb presents skin grafts, poor circulation, or diminished sensation. The patient should alternately exercise and rest, with cardiopulmonary monitoring a routine part of the program, especially for high-risk individuals.[40]

Some clinicians eschew parallel bars because the fearful patient pulls on them, which will be fruitless when progressing to a cane. When bars are used, the therapist should encourage the patient to rest the open hand on the bar for support, rather than using a viselike grip. A plinth or sturdy table offers the dual advantages of providing good support on only one side, ordinarily the contralateral side, and unidirectional control, because the patient can only push, never pull, for balance.

Static erect balance reintroduces the novice to bipedal posture. The patient should strive for level pelvis and shoulders, vertical trunk without excessive lordosis, and equal weight-bearing. The therapist should guard and assist the patient as necessary. When the physical therapist stands near the prosthesis, this encourages the patient to shift his or her weight onto it. To suggest symmetrical performance, refer to the limbs as "right" and "left," or "sound" and "prosthetic," rather than discouraging the patient with "good" and "bad." The client must learn to utilize proximal sensory receptors to maintain balance and perceive the position of the prosthesis without looking at the floor. Some patients respond well to increased use of visual feedback (e.g., using a mirror).

Dynamic exercises improve medial-lateral, sagittal, and rotary control. The patient learns that hip flexion causes the knee to bend, and hip extension stabilizes the knee during stance phase. Placing the sound foot ahead of the prosthesis makes the prosthetic knee more stable. Patients should be instructed in weight shifting in both symmetrical and stride positions and in stepping movements. Stepping on a low stool or step platform with the sound leg obliges the patient to shift weight onto the prosthesis and increases stance phase duration on the prosthesis.[41] Symmetrical performance is fostered by having all exercises performed rhythmically with both the right and left legs.

GAIT TRAINING

Walking is a natural progression from dynamic balance exercises as the patient takes successive steps. Some people respond well to viewing themselves on videotape.[42] The cassettes also form a valuable record of performance and progress. Videotapes are useful reinforcements of instruction for the patient who has a home rehabilitation program. Rhythmic counting and walking in time with music in 2/4 time also improves gait symmetry and speed. In the physical therapy department, an apparatus that includes a suspension harness provides a protected environment for the patient to learn gradual weight bearing on the prosthesis.[43]

A cane or pair of forearm crutches are appropriate aids for the client who is unable to achieve a safe gait without undue fatigue. Sometimes the cane is used only outdoors to aid in negotiating curbs and other ground irregularities and to signal oncoming traffic. Ordinarily the cane is used on the contralateral side to enhance frontal plane balance. If bilateral assistance is required, a pair of forearm crutches is preferable to two canes. The crutches remain clasped around the forearms when the user opens a door. Axillary crutches tempt the patient to lean on the axillary bars, risking impingement of the radial nerves; they are also inconvenient when climbing stairs. An aluminum walker provides maximum stability, which is particularly useful for patients with generalized weakness. The walker should be adjusted so that the user does not lean too far forward.

FUNCTIONAL ACTIVITIES

The prosthesis wearer who is learning to walk also should gain experience in performing a wide variety of functional mobility skills. Activities such as transferring to various chairs add interest to the program and, for some patients, may be more important than long-distance ambulation. The training program for vigorous individuals includes stair climbing, negotiating ramps, retrieving objects from the floor, kneeling, sitting on the floor, running, driving a car, and engaging in sports. The fundamental difference between these activities and walking is the way each leg is used. Walking implies symmetrical usage, but the other activities are done asymmetrically, with greater reliance on the strength, agility, and sensory control of the sound limb.

Generally, the patient should have the opportunity to analyze each new situation and arrive at a solution to the problem, rather than depending on directions from the therapist. Most tasks can be accomplished safely in several ways. The learner profits from observing other prosthesis wearers as well as from professional instruction.

TRANSFERS

Rising from different chairs, the toilet, and car are primary skills even for people who are elderly or debilitated. Most patients enter the physical therapy department in a wheelchair. Initially, the patient can park the chair at the parallel bars or at a plinth. After locking the wheelchair and raising the footrests, the patient should sit forward and transfer weight to the intact leg, then push down on the chair armrests. The individual will find that placing the sound foot close to the chair enables rising by extending the knee and hip on the sound side. Sitting is accomplished by placing the sound foot close to the chair and lowering oneself by controlled hip and knee flexion on the sound side.

For both standing and sitting, the beginner should

have the advantage of a chair with armrests that enable use of the hands to control and assist trunk movement. Later the person should practice sitting in deep upholstered sofas and low chairs, as well as benches, the toilet, and other seats that do not have armrests. Transfer into an automobile should be an integral part of the training regimen; otherwise, the patient faces a gloomy future, confined to home or dependent on special transportation systems. To enter the right (passenger) side of an automobile, the prosthetic wearer faces toward the front of the car. The person with a right prosthesis puts the right hand on the door post and the left hand on the back of the front seat, then swings the left leg into the car, slides onto the car seat, and finally places the prosthesis in the car. The individual with a left prosthesis may find that sitting sideways with both feet out the car door is easiest. One then pivots on the seat while swinging the prosthesis into the car, then puts the intact right foot inside the car.

CLIMBING

Patients with Syme's and transtibial amputations generally ascend and descend stairs and inclines with steps of equal length in step-over-step progression.[44] Those with unilateral transfemoral amputation, in contrast, ascend by leading with the sound foot and learn to descend by first placing the prosthesis on the lower step. A few individuals with transfemoral amputation subsequently learn to control prosthetic knee flexion in order to descend step-over-step. Curbs present a slightly different problem, because there is no handrail. The techniques are basically the same, however. If the stairs, ramp, or curb are too steep, the individual may climb diagonally or sidestep with the prosthesis kept on the downhill side.

Final Examination and Follow-up Care

Economic strictures may compel the therapist to conclude the training program after the patient is able to walk and to negotiate basic transfers and stair climbing but before the full range of training activities is completed. Before discharge, the patient and prosthesis should be reassessed to make certain that socket fit, prosthetic appearance, and function are acceptable. The checklist used for initial examination can be used. The physical therapist should instruct the patient with regard to the patient's responsibility for reporting skin redness and any loose or missing parts from the prosthesis.

The new prosthesis wearer should return to the training site at regular intervals so that the clinic team may assess socket fit. Most will require major socket revision or replacement during the first year to accommodate shrinkage. Follow-up visits are good opportunities to augment training and to encourage the individual to engage in the widest possible range of activities.

Functional Capacities

Functional capacities refer to the individual's ability to walk, transfer from chairs, climb stairs, and perform other ambulatory activities, including recreational endeavors. A primary responsibility of the clinic team is to predict the probable function of the person with a new amputation, to determine whether the individual would benefit from a prosthesis, and what degree of activity is likely.[45–49] Because many people with lower-limb amputation are elderly with several medical problems, the need for accurate forecasting and ongoing monitoring is especially critical.

Walking with a prosthesis increases energy cost.[50–52] Compared with those people with two sound limbs, the individual with a unilateral transtibial prosthesis requires slightly more oxygen when walking at a comfortable speed; the person wearing a transfemoral prosthesis consumes nearly 50 percent more oxygen than normal. The prosthesis wearer chooses a comfortable pace, because at a speed that is natural for the individual, the energy cost per minute is similar to that of the person who does not require a prosthesis, although speed is slower.[53–55] The lower the amputation level, the less the metabolic disadvantage. Among persons with transtibial amputations older than 40, those with long amputated limbs average minimal increase in energy, but persons with shorter limbs work harder. Those with bilateral transtibial amputations expend less energy than those with unilateral transfemoral amputations. Individuals whose amputation was traumatic perform more efficiently than those whose amputation was caused by vascular disease at every amputation level. People who sustained trauma walk faster and use less oxygen than their dysvascular counterparts.

The metabolic toll results in part from the socket, which surrounds semifluid tissue, giving imperfect anchorage. The resulting pseudoarthrosis is more difficult to control than in an intact limb. The foot-ankle assembly transmits no plantar tactile or proprioceptive sensation, does not move through as large an excursion as the normal foot, and does not initiate the dynamic propulsion characteristic of normal gait. The transfemoral prosthesis also incorporates a knee unit that provides no proprioception to the wearer. The problem is aggravated by the fact that a prosthesis is operated by remotely located muscles that contract longer and more forcefully than in normal gait. With transfemoral amputation, for example, the prosthetic foot is placed by hip motion. The resulting alteration of motion is reflected in asymmetry of timing, further disturbing gait smoothness. Individuals with prostheses walk with greater vertical movement, inasmuch as the knee, whether prosthetic for the transfemoral prosthesis wearer or anatomical in the transtibial wearer, does not flex as much as the contralateral knee during stance phase.

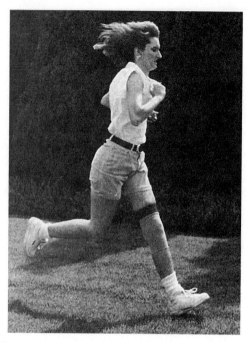

Figure 20-25. Patient running with a left transtibial prosthesis. (From May, BJ: Amputations and Prosthetics: A Case Study Approach. FA Davis, Philadelphia, 1996, p 200, with permission.)

Sports participation is an excellent extension of rehabilitation for patients of all ages. Older adults may enjoy fishing, golfing, dancing, Tai Chi Chuan, and shuffleboard, and younger people may add basketball, tennis, archery, and track events (Fig. 20-25) to their range of activities. Most sports do not require any adaptation to the prosthesis. Horseback riding is a superb activity that fosters trunk control and seated balance. The hiker should pack extra amputated limb socks or a sheath to protect the skin; a well-fitting, comfortable hiking boot is essential. Bowling and participating in shot put are facilitated by emphasizing balance on the intact leg. For sports that involve running, an energy storing/releasing foot is most suitable. The socket should fit snugly with very secure suspension to minimize abrasion of the amputated limb. Clients with Syme's or transtibial amputations usually run with reasonably symmetrical step lengths, although they will favor the sound limb, which has greater propulsive

ability.[56,57] Those with a knee disarticulation or transfemoral amputation will derive most of the propulsive force from the sound leg and use the prosthesis as a momentary prop. Many marathon competitions have a category for people with disabilities. Jumping, as in basketball, requires the athlete to generate a substantial upward force with the sound leg; landing is more comfortable on the sound leg, particularly for those who wear transfemoral prostheses. Some activities are facilitated by minor modification of the equipment, such as a toe loop on a bicycle pedal. Other activities are generally performed without a prosthesis, such as swimming and skiing. The skier will probably use ski poles equipped with small rudders, in a "three-track" manner. Soccer is usually played without a prosthesis, with the player using a pair of crutches. Some individuals enjoy playing tennis and field events in a wheelchair. Equipment and techniques developed for individuals with paraplegia usually can be adapted for people with amputations. Recreational programs designed for children and adults with amputations help the participants to return to active life-styles. The physical therapist should be able to refer patients to convenient recreational clubs, camps, and sporting events. The desired outcome is to maximize each person's functional capacity and zest for life.

SUMMARY

This chapter has focused on management of people with lower-limb amputations. Characteristics and function of the principal lower-limb prostheses and prosthetic components have been discussed. In addition, the responsibilities of the physical therapist in prosthetic management have been emphasized. Successful prosthetic rehabilitation depends on close collaboration among the patient, physical therapist, physician, prosthetist, and other team members. This will provide an environment for information exchange and will foster coordinated management. The result will be an optimum match between the patient's physical and psychosocial characteristics and a prosthesis capable of fulfilling its intended purposes.

QUESTIONS FOR REVIEW

1. What are the principal causes of amputation in the elderly? In the young?
2. Describe appropriate prostheses for individuals with various partial foot amputations.
3. Distinguish between the Syme's and the transtibial amputation limbs and prostheses.
4. What prosthetic feet are especially suitable for geriatric patients? Why?
5. Name the reliefs and build-ups in the transtibial socket.
6. Contrast the modes of suspension for the

transtibial prosthesis. Which suspension is indicated for an individual with a short amputated limb?
7. Classify knee units according to friction mechanisms.
8. Compare the quadrilateral and the ischial containment transfemoral sockets.
9. Describe the modes of suspension of the transfemoral prosthesis. In which type(s) does the client wear a sock?

10. How is the wearer of a hip disarticulation prosthesis prevented from inadvertently flexing the hip and knee?

11. Outline a maintenance program for a transfemoral prosthesis with hydraulic knee unit and endoskeletal shank.

12. What factors should be assessed prior to formulating a prosthetic prescription?

13. How can the physical therapist assess and improve the patient's psychological status?

14. What features of the transtibial prosthesis are considered in static assessment? In dynamic assessment?

15. Delineate the training program for a patient with a transfemoral prosthesis.

CASE STUDY

CURRENT PROBLEM: The patient is a 67 year-old man with diabetic arteriosclerosis. He sustained a right transtibial amputation 5 months ago. He was treated in the inpatient physical therapy department for 3 weeks. The wound healed satisfactorily. His physical therapist taught him to transfer independently and ambulate using a temporary prosthesis and a walker. He was discharged with a home program consisting of exercises to promote strength, joint mobility, and endurance. He was also told to keep an elastic shrinker sock on his amputated limb whenever he was not wearing the temporary prosthesis. In addition, the physical therapist instructed the patient in care of the left foot, including thorough foot washing every evening; inspecting all surfaces of the foot, using a mirror; wearing a clean sock and well-fitting shoe each day; and careful nail trimming. He was fitted with a permanent prosthesis 3 months after surgery. The prosthesis consisted of a SACH foot, endoskeletal shank, total contact socket, and cuff suspension. He returned to the rehabilitation department today complaining of difficulty keeping his balance on the irregular terrain on the golf course where he had gone for the first time since his surgery. He also mentioned that his golf score was poorer than it had ever been.

PAST MEDICAL HISTORY: The patient was in fairly good health until 6 months ago, when he went on a long-awaited trip to Europe. On the trip he did much more walking than usual, even though he had to stop every 50 feet because of cramping pain in his legs. His wife noticed that the hallux and second toe on his right foot were discolored. The discolored area became painful. On his return home he was examined by his primary care physician, who diagnosed gangrene and adult-onset diabetes. Despite aggressive wound care, the gangrene progressed to involve the entire foot. An amputation was required. His diabetes is now stabilized with diet.

SOCIAL HISTORY: The patient is a retired accountant who lives with his wife. For years, he played golf on vacations. Upon retirement last year, he had looked forward to more frequent golfing.

PHYSICAL THERAPY ASSESSMENT FINDINGS
REVIEW OF SYSTEMS
- Cognitive status: Alert, oriented, memory intact.
- Endurance: Fair, tolerance to activity is approximately 30 minutes (with some fluctuation); occasional rest periods required.
- Vision: Intact with corrective lens
- Blood pressure: 140/86
- Respiratory rate: WFL

RANGE OF MOTOR ASSESSMENT
Goniometric assessment (ROM) of both lower limbs: WNL

Gait: The patient is a functional ambulator using a transtibial prosthesis. Gait is slow, with longer steps on the right side; without the cane he leans to the right side. When outdoors he uses a cane in the left hand. He can climb stairs slowly, using the handrail. On uneven surfaces, he widens his walking base and walks slowly.

OBSERVATIONAL ANALYSIS (GENERAL FINDINGS)
- Overall decrease in speed of movement
- Diminished, awkward weight transfer

Hip/Pelvis (Bilateral)
- Decreased pelvic rotation
- Diminished hip flexion

Knee: Diminished knee flexion on right

Foot/Ankle: Minimal medial-lateral motion on right

Sensation
- Lower limbs: sharp/dull, light touch, temperature, proprioception: WFL bilaterally
- Sensation in both upper limbs: WFL

STRENGTH:

Manual Muscle Test (MMT) Grades

	Right	Left
HIP		
• Flexion	G	G
• Extension	G	G
• Abduction	G	G
• Adduction	G	G
• External Rotation	G–	G–
• Internal Rotation	G–	G–
KNEE		
• Flexion	G–	G
• Extension	F+	G–
FOOT/ANKLE		
• Dorsiflexion	N/A	G
• Plantarflexion	N/A	G
• Inversion	N/A	G
• Eversion	N/A	G
• Upper limb strength: WFL		

N/A, not applicable owing to amputation; WFL, within functional limits.

PROSTHETIC ASSESSMENT: Socket is loose, as indicated by piston action

BALANCE
- Standing
  Static: Good; able to maintain static position for unlimited period
  Dynamic: Fair+; difficulty maintaining balance on uneven terrain
- Sitting: WFL

FUNCTION
1. Transfers, sit to stand: FIM level = 7 with the exception of floor to stand transfers.
2. Patient is independent in all BADL (FIM levels = 6 and 7).
3. Patient is independent in approximately 80 percent of IADL; FIM level = 7 (limitations imposed by fatigue and low ambulatory tolerance).

PATIENT DESIRED OUTCOME (GOALS)
- Play golf at previous level of proficiency
- Walk without depending on cane when outdoors
- Improve endurance

GUIDING QUESTIONS
1. Formulate a clinical problem list.
2. Formulate a patient asset list.
3. Establish goals and outcomes and formulate a plan of care.

REFERENCES

1. Torres, MM: Incidence and causes of limb amputations. Phys Med Rehabil 8:1, 1994.
2. Roth, EJ, et al: Cardiovascular disease in patients with dysvascular amputation. Arch Phys Med Rehabil 79:205, 1992.
3. Mueller, MJ, and Strube, MJ: Therapeutic footwear: Enhanced function in people with diabetes and transmetatarsal amputation. Arch Phys Med Rehabil 78:952, 1997.
4. Doyle, W, et al: The Syme prosthesis revisited. Journal of Prosthetics and Orthotics 5:95, 1993.
5. Edelstein, JE: Current choices in prosthetic feet. Clin Rev Phys Rehab Med 2:213, 1991.
6. Gitter, A, et al: Biomechanical analysis of the influence of prosthetic feet on below-knee amputee walking. Am J Phys Med 70:142, 1991.
7. Barth, DG, et al: Gait analysis and energy cost of below-knee amputees wearing six different prosthetic feet. Journal of Prosthetics and Orthotics 4:63, 1992.
8. Czerniecki, JM, and Gitter, AJ: Prosthetic feet: A scientific and clinical review of current components. State of the Art Reviews in PM&R 8:109, 1994.
9. Powers, CM, et al: Influence of prosthetic foot design on sound limb loading in adults with unilateral below-knee amputations. Arch Phys Med Rehabil 75:825, 1994.
10. Campbell, JW, and Childs, CW: The SAFE foot. Orthotics and Prosthetics 34:3, 1980.
11. Menard, MR, et al: Comparative biomechanical analysis of energy-storing prosthetic feet. Arch Phys Med Rehabil 73:451, 1992.
12. Perry, J, and Shanfield, S: Efficiency of dynamic elastic response prosthetic feet. J Rehabil Res Dev 30:137, 1993.
13. Alaranta, H, et al: Subjective benefits of energy-storing prostheses. Prosthet Orthot Int 18:92, 1994.
14. Snyder, RD, et al: The effect of five prosthetic feet on the gait and loading of the sound limb in dysvascular below-knee amputees. J Rehabil Res Dev 32:309, 1995.
15. Torburn, L, et al: Energy expenditure during amputation in dysvascular and traumatic below-knee amputees: A comparison of five prosthetic feet. J Rehabil Res Dev 32:111, 1995.
16. Arbogast, R, and Arbogast, CJ: The Carbon Copy II—from concept to application. Journal of Prosthetics and Orthotics 1:32, 1988.
17. Barr, AE, et al: Biomechanical comparison of the energy-storing capabilities of SACH and Carbon Copy II prosthetic feet during the stance phase of gait in a person with below-knee amputation. Phys Ther 72:344, 1992.
18. Arya, AP, et al: A biomechanical comparison of the SACH, Seattle and Jaipur feet using ground reaction forces. Prosthet Orthot Int 19:37, 1995.
19. Lehmann, JF, et al: Comprehensive analysis of energy storing prosthetic feet: Flex Foot and Seattle foot versus standard SACH foot. Arch Phys Med Rehabil 74:1225, 1993.
20. Macfarlane, PA, et al: Transfemoral amputee physiological requirements: Comparisons between SACH foot walking and Flex-Foot walking. Journal of Prosthetics and Orthotics 9:138, 1997.
21. Ehara, Y, et al: Energy storing property of so-called energy-storing prosthetic feet. Arch Phys Med Rehabil 74:68, 1993.
22. Radcliffe, C: The biomechanics of below-knee prostheses in normal, level bi-pedal walking. Artificial Limbs 6:16, 1962.
23. Kristinsson, O: The ICEROSS concept: A discussion of philosophy. Prosthet Orthot Int 17:49, 1993.
24. Datta, D, et al: Outcome of fitting an ICEROSS prosthesis: Views of transtibial amputees. Prosthet Orthot Int 20:111, 1996.
25. Radcliffe, CW: Four-bar linkage prosthetic knee mechanisms: Kinematics, alignment and prescription criteria. Prosthet Orthot Int 18:159, 1994.
26. Murray, MP, et al: Gait patterns in above-knee amputee patients: Hydraulic swing control vs. constant friction knee components. Arch Phys Med Rehabil 64:339, 1983.
27. Gottschalk, FA, et al: Does socket configuration influence the position of the femur in above-knee amputation? Journal of Prosthetics and Orthotics 2:94, 1989.
28. Pritham, CH: Biomechanics and shape of the above-knee socket considered in light of the ischial containment concept. Prosthet Orthot Int 14:9, 1990.
29. Gailey RS, et al: The CAT-CAM socket and quadrilateral socket: A comparison of energy cost during ambulation. Prosthet Orthot Int 17:95, 1993.
30. Gottschalk, FA, and Stills, M: The biomechanics of transfemoral amputation. Prosthet Orthot Int 8:12, 1994.
31. Lilja, M, and Oberg, T: Proper time for definitive transtibial prosthetic fitting. Journal of Prosthetics and Orthotics 9:90, 1997.
32. Isakov, E, et al: Influence of prosthesis alignment on the standing balance of below-knee amputees. Clin Biomech 9:258, 1994.
33. Edelstein, JE: Prosthetic and orthotic gait. In Smidt, GL (ed): Gait in Rehabilitation. Churchill Livingstone, New York, 1990, pp. 281–300.
34. Lemaire, ED, et al: Gait patterns of elderly men with transtibial amputations. Prosthet Orthot Int 17:27, 1993.
35. Isakov, E, et al: Double-limb support and step-length asymmetry in below-knee amputees. Scand J Rehabil Med 29:75, 1996.
36. Powers, CM, et al: The influence of extremity muscle force on gait characteristics in individuals with below-knee amputations secondary to vascular disease. Phys Ther 76:369, 1996.
37. Sanderson, DJ, and Martin, PE: Lower extremity kinematic and kinetic adaptation in unilateral below-knee amputees during walking. Gait & Posture 6:126, 1997.
38. Ryarczyk, BD, et al: Social discomfort and depression in a sample of adults with leg amputations. Arch Phys Med Rehabil 73:1169, 1992.
39. Breakey, JW: Body image: The lower-limb amputee. Journal of Prosthetics and Orthotics 9:58, 1997.
40. Adler, JC, et al: Treadmill training program for a bilateral below-knee amputee with cardiopulmonary disease. Arch Phys Med Rehabil 68:858, 1987.

41. Gailey, RS, and McKenzie, A: Prosthetic Gait Training Program for Lower Extremity Amputees. University of Miami School of Medicine, Miami, 1989.
42. Netz, P, et al: Videotape recording: A complementary aid for the walking training of lower limb amputees. Prosthet Orthot Int 5:147, 1981.
43. Hunter, D, and Smith-Cole, E: Energy expenditure of below-knee amputees during harness-supported treadmill ambulation. J Orthop Sports Phys Ther 21:268, 1995.
44. Power, CM, et al: Stair ambulation in persons with trans-tibial amputation: An analysis of the Seattle LightFoot. J Rehabil Res Dev 34:9, 1997.
45. Medhat, A, et al: Factors that influence the level of activities in persons with lower extremity amputation. Rehabil Nurs 15:13, 1990.
46. Siriwardena, GA, and Bertrand, PV: Factors influencing rehabilitation of arteriosclerotic lower limb amputees. J Rehabil Res Dev 28:35, 1991.
47. Muecke, L, et al: Functional screening of lower-limb amputees: A role in predicting rehabilitation outcome? Arch Phys Med Rehabil 73:851, 1992.
48. Nissen, SJ, and Newman, WP: Factors influencing reintegration to normal living after amputation. Arch Phys Med Rehabil 73:548, 1992.
49. Greive, AC, and Lankhorst, GJ: Functional outcome of lower-limb amputees: A prospective descriptive study in a general hospital. Prosthet Orthot Int 20:79, 1996.
50. Water, RL: The energy expenditure of amputee gait. In Bowker, JH, and Michael, JW (eds): Atlas of Limb Prosthetics: Surgical, Prosthetic and Rehabilitation Principles, ed. 2. Mosby-Year Book, St. Louis, 1992, p 381.
51. Gailey, RS, et al: Energy expenditure of trans-tibial amputees during ambulation at self-selected pace. Prosthet Orthot Int 18:84, 1994.
52. Boonstra, AM, et al: Energy cost during ambulation in transfemoral amputees: A knee joint with a mechanical swing-phase control vs. a knee joint with a pneumatic swing-phase control. Scand J Rehabil Med 27:77, 1995.
53. Jaegers, SMHJ, et al: The relationships between comfortable and most metabolically efficient walking speed in persons with unilateral above-knee amputation. Arch Phys Med Rehabil 74:521, 1993.
54. Hermodsson, et al: Gait in transtibial amputees: A comparative study with healthy subjects in relation to walking speed. Prosthet Orthot Int 18:68, 1994.
55. Jones, ME, et al: Weight-bearing and velocity in transtibial and transfemoral amputees. Prosthet Orthot Int 21:183, 1997.
56. Czerniecki, JM, and Gitter, A: Insights into amputee running: A muscle work analysis. Am J Phys Med Rehabil 71:209, 1992.
57. Prince, F, et al: Running gait impulse asymmetries in below-knee amputees. Prosthet Orthot Int 16:19, 1992.

SUPPLEMENTAL READING

Bowker, JH, and Michael, JW (eds): Atlas of Limb Prosthetics, ed 2. Mosby, St. Louis, 1992.
Burgess, EM, and Rappoport, A: Physical Fitness: A Guide for Individuals with Lower Limb Loss. Department of Veterans Affairs, Washington, DC, 1992.
Engstrom, B, and Van de Van, C: Physiotherapy for Amputees: The Roehampton Approach. Churchill Livingstone, New York, 1985.
Ham, R, and Cotton, L: Limb Amputation: From Aetiology to Rehabilitation. Chapman & Hall, London, 1991.
Karacoloff, LA, et al: Lower Extremity Amputation: A Guide to Functional Outcomes in Physical Therapy Management, ed 2. Aspen, Gaithersburg, MD, 1992.
Kegel, B: Sports for the Leg Amputee. Medic, Redmond, WA, 1986.
May, BJ: Amputations and Prosthetics: A Case Study. FA Davis, Philadelphia, 1996.
Mensch, G, and Ellis, PM: Physical Therapy Management of Lower Extremity Amputations. Aspen, Gaithersburg, MD, 1986.
Moore, WS, and Malone, JM (eds): Lower Extremity Amputation. WB Saunders, Philadelphia, 1989.
Murdoch, G, et al (eds): Amputation: Surgical Practice and Patient Management. Butterworth Heinemann, Oxford, 1996.
Palmer, ML, and Toms, JE: Manual for Functional Training, ed 3. FA Davis, Philadelphia, 1992.
Sanders, GT: Lower Limb Amputations: A Guide to Rehabilitation. FA Davis, Philadelphia, 1986.

GLOSSARY

Alignment: Position of one component relative to another; alignment refers to both angular and linear positions.

Axis (prosthetic): Component of the prosthetic knee unit; creates the connection between the thigh piece (socket) and shank; may be either a single-axis hinge or polycentric linkage.

Build-ups: Convexities within a socket to increase loading on pressure-tolerant tissues.

Clinic team: Group of health care professionals that conducts prosthetic (and/or orthotic) rehabilitation. The basic team consists of a physician who serves as chief, physical and/or occupational therapists, and prosthetist (and/or orthotist). Others may participate on a regular or specific basis, such as a social worker, vocational counselor, or psychologist.

Computer-aided design/computer-aided manufacturer (CAD-CAM): Prosthetic construction that involves electronic mapping of the amputated limb, relating the limb shape to socket designs, and automatic carving of a positive model over which plastic is molded to create the socket.

Endoskeletal (modular, pylon) shank: Prosthetic shank in which the support consists of a rigid pipe usually covered with resilient material to simulate the contour of the contralateral leg. Modular refers to the ease of interchanging foot and knee units. Pylon is the pipe itself, although "pylon" is also used to signify a temporary prosthesis.

Exoskeletal (crustacean) shank: Prosthetic shank in which the support consists of rigid material at the periphery, usually covered with a thin layer of polyester laminate. Crustacean refers to the placement of the supporting structure externally, as is the case with animals such as the lobster.

Extension aid: Mechanism designed to assist prosthetic knee extension during the latter part of swing phase; may consist of elastic webbing placed externally across the knee unit, or an elastic strap or metal spring within the knee unit.

Fork strap: Prosthetic suspension and knee extension aid; consists of a fork-shaped elastic strap extending from the anterior portion of the transtibial prosthetic shank to a waist belt.

Friction brake: Device in a prosthetic knee unit that resists knee flexion during early stance phase, commonly a spring-loaded wedge that is forced into a groove upon transfer of body weight to the prosthesis.

Friction mechanisms: Devices that permit adjusting the resistance to swing of the prosthetic knee unit.

    Constant friction: Mechanism that applies uniform resistance throughout swing phase; may be incorporated in sliding or hydraulic friction mechanisms.

    Variable friction: Mechanism that applies greater friction at early and late swing; may be incorporated in sliding, hydraulic, or pneumatic friction mechanisms.

    Sliding friction: Mechanism consisting of solid structures that resist motion by moving against each other, such as a clamp on the knee bolt.

    Fluid friction: Mechanism consisting of a cylinder (hydraulic, oil-filled; or pneumatic, air-filled) in which a piston connected to the knee hinge moves up and down. Fluid friction knee units automatically compensate for changes in walking speed, increasing friction when the wearer walks faster.

Ischial containment socket: Transfemoral socket that covers the ischial tuberosity and is relatively narrow in width.

Keel: Rigid longitudinal portion of a prosthetic foot terminating distally at a point corresponding to the metatarsophalangeal joints.

Mechanical stabilizer: A device that increases stability of the prosthetic knee unit, such as a manual lock or friction brake.

Multiple axis foot: A mechanism in an articulated prosthetic foot that permits sagittal, frontal, and transverse plane motion.

Patellar-tendon-bearing (PTB): Refers to the modern total-contact transtibial socket that places moderate load on the patellar tendon.

Piston action: Vertical motion of the prosthetic socket on the amputated limb; evident during gait as an up-and-down movement of the prosthesis. Pistoning is caused by looseness of the socket or inadequate suspension, or both.

Polycentric linkage: Mechanism in a knee unit that permits the momentary axis of knee flexion to change through the arc of motion; a common design is the four-bar linkage, consisting of two pairs of two bars of unequal length, pivoting on both ends, on the medial and lateral sides of the knee unit. Polycentric linkage increases knee stability.

Polyester laminate: Thermosetting plastic used for rigid prosthetic sockets and for finishing the exterior of exoskeletal shanks. Polyester resin saturates layers of fabric, producing a hard, durable material.

Polyethylene: Thermoplastic material used for flexible sockets; the plastic becomes malleable when heated, permitting its contour to be changed.

Relief: Concavity within a socket to decrease loading on pressure-sensitive tissue.

Single-axis: Prosthetic articulation that permits motion only in the sagittal plane about a fixed bolt.

Single-axis foot: Prosthetic foot that provides plantarflexion and dorsiflexion at a point corresponding to the anatomical ankle.

Single-axis hinge: Prosthetic unit that permits flexion and extension at a point corresponding to the epicondylar level.

Solid ankle cushion heel (SACH) foot: Prosthetic foot in which the posterior-superior portion of the keel is attached to the shank, without a definite ankle joint, and a posterior-inferior compressible wedge permits plantarflexion during early stance. The distal end of the keel permits hyperextension of the foot during late stance.

Stationary attachment flexible endoskeleton (SAFE) foot: Prosthetic foot that has a rigid ankle block attached to the shank, without a definite ankle joint; the anterior portion of the block terminates at a 45 degree angle, abutting a somewhat more flexible keel, to permit inversion and eversion. The distal end of the keel permits hyperextension of the foot during late stance. The posterior-inferior surface has compressible material to permit plantarflexion during early stance.

Suction: Mode of prosthetic suspension in which an airtight socket is held on the amputated limb by atmospheric pressure. Pressure is greater on the outside than on the inside of the socket. Commonly, suction suspension is used on transfemoral prostheses, in which the snug socket has an air-release valve.

Supracondylar (SC) suspension: Mode of transtibial prosthetic suspension in which the socket is held on the amputated limb by snug contact immediately above the femoral epicondyles; a plastic wedge is inserted between the medial epicondyle and the proximal-medial socket wall.

Supracondylar/suprapatellar (SC/SP) suspension: Mode of transtibial prosthetic suspension in which the socket is held on the amputated limb by supracondylar suspension augmented by a high anterior socket margin that terminates immediately above the patella.

Syme's amputation: Amputation at the supramalleolar level, in which all foot bones are removed and the calcaneal fat pad is attached to the anterior skin flap to cushion the distal end of the limb.

Temporary (provisional) prosthesis: Device consisting of a socket designed to accept full weight-bearing, attached to a pylon and foot. Unlike a definitive (permanent) prosthesis, the temporary one may not be cosmetically finished. For the transfemoral prosthesis, the pylon usually is surmounted by a knee unit.

Transfemoral: Above-knee.

Transtibial: Below-knee.

APPENDIX A

Transtibial (Below-Knee) Prosthetic Assessment

1. Is the prosthesis as prescribed?
2. Can the client don the prosthesis easily?

Standing

3. Is the client comfortable when standing with the heel midlines 6 in (15 cm) apart?
4. Is the anterior-posterior alignment satisfactory?
5. Is the medial-lateral alignment satisfactory?
6. Do the contours and color of the prosthesis match the opposite limb?
7. Is the prosthesis the correct length?
8. Is piston action minimal?
9. Does the socket contact the amputation limb without pinching or gapping?

Suspension

10. Does the suspension component fit the amputation limb properly?
11. Does the cuff, fork strap, or thigh corset have adequate provision for adjustment?

Sitting

12. Can the client sit comfortably with hips and knees flexed 90 degrees?

Walking

13. Is the client's performance in level walking satisfactory?
14. Is the client's performance on stairs and ramps satisfactory?
15. Can the client kneel satisfactorily?
16. Does the suspension function properly?
17. Does the prosthesis operate quietly?
18. Does the client consider the prosthesis satisfactory as to comfort, function, and appearance?

Prosthesis off the Client

19. Is the skin free of abrasions or other discolorations attributable to this prosthesis?
20. Is the socket interior smooth?
21. Is the posterior wall of the socket of adequate height?
22. Is the construction satisfactory?
23. Do all components function satisfactorily?

APPENDIX B

Transfemoral (Above-Knee) Prosthetic Assessment

1. Is the prosthesis as prescribed?
2. Can the client don the prosthesis easily?

Standing

3. Is the client comfortable when standing with the heel midlines 6 in (15 cm) apart?
4. Is any flesh roll above the socket minimal?
5. Is the client free from vertical pressure in the perineum?
6. Do the contours and color of the prosthesis match the opposite limb?
7. Is the prosthesis the correct length?
8. Is the knee stable?
9. When the socket valve is removed, is the distal tissue firm?

Quadrilateral Socket

10. Does the ischial tuberosity rest on the posterior brim?
11. Is the posterior brim approximately parallel to the floor?
12. Is the adductor longus tendon located in the anterior-medial corner?

Ischial Containment Socket

13. Does the posterior-medial corner of the socket cover the ischial tuberosity?
14. Can the client hyperextend the hip on the amputated side comfortably?
15. Can the client flex the hip 90 degrees comfortably, without socket gapping?
16. Can the client abduct the hip on the amputated side comfortably, without socket gapping?

Suspension

17. Does the Silesian bandage control prosthetic rotation and adduction adequately?
18. Does the pelvic band conform to the torso?

Sitting

19. Can the client sit comfortably with hips and knees flexed 90 degrees?
20. Does the socket remain securely on the thigh, without gapping or rotating?
21. Are both thighs approximately the same length and height from the floor?
22. Can the client lean forward to touch the shoes?

Walking

23. Is the client's performance in level walking satisfactory?
24. Is the client's performance on stairs and ramps satisfactory?
25. Does the suspension function properly?
26. Does the prosthesis operate quietly?
27. Does the client consider the prosthesis satisfactory as to comfort, function, and appearance?

Prosthesis off the Client

28. Is the skin free of abrasions or other discolorations attributable to this prosthesis?
29. Is the socket interior smooth?
30. With the prosthesis fully flexed on a table, can the thigh piece be brought to at least the vertical position?
31. If the socket is totally rigid, is a back pad attached?
32. Is the construction satisfactory?
33. Do all components function satisfactorily?

APPENDIX C

Suggested Answers to Case Study Guiding Questions

1. Formulate a clinical problem list.
ANSWER
a. Loose prosthetic socket
b. Asymmetrical gait
c. Poor walking endurance
d. Difficulty balancing, especially on uneven terrain
e. Less-than-normal muscle power

2. Formulate a patient asset list.
ANSWER
a. Well-healed amputation wound
b. Diabetes is under control
c. Stable marriage
d. Motivated to golf

3. Establish goals and outcomes and formulate a plan of care.
ANSWER: GOALS AND OUTCOMES
a. Increase motor power, especially in right lower limb.
b. Increase endurance, especially in walking.
c. Adjust socket to improve fit.
d. Provide a silicone sheath to reduce skin abrasion.
e. Substitute a foot that provides more excursion than the SACH. For example, the SAFE foot or a multiple axis foot would improve balance on uneven terrain.
f. Increase right quadriceps strength to at least good plus.
g. Increase aerobic endurance.

4. Formulate a physical therapy plan of care.
ANSWER: PLAN OF CARE
a. Make appointment for patient with the prosthetist to obtain new foot, silicone sheath, and socket adjustment.
b. Cybex exercise for quadriceps, bilaterally.
c. Stationery bicycle for aerobic conditioning.
d. Instruction in postural control while walking with particular emphasis on trunk rotation.
e. Balance training activities.
f. Home program to include Theraband resistance exercises for quadriceps, bilaterally; use of stationery bicycle; graduated walking program with his wife; trunk rotational exercises; increase frequency of golfing.

Arthritis 21

Andrew A. Guccione
Marian A. Minor

LEARNING OBJECTIVES

1. Describe the epidemiology, pathology, pathogenesis, disease course, and common clinical manifestations of arthritis.
2. Identify the medical diagnostic procedures commonly used in the examination of arthritis, including laboratory tests and radiography.
3. Describe the medical management of the individual with arthritis.
4. Differentiate between rheumatoid arthritis and osteoarthritis.
5. Explain the procedures commonly used in assessing the individual with rheumatoid arthritis or osteoarthritis.
6. Discuss the rehabilitation management of the individual with arthritis.
7. Describe responses to psychosocial factors associated with arthritis that affect achievement of rehabilitation goals.
8. Explain the importance of a team approach for the individual with arthritis.
9. Analyze and interpret patient data, formulate realistic goals and outcomes, and develop a plan of care when presented with a clinical case study.

The terms "arthritis" and **"rheumatism"** are generic references to an array of over 100 diseases that are divided into 10 classification categories. Two major forms of arthritis will be considered in this chapter. **Rheumatoid arthritis (RA),** a **systemic** inflammatory disease, will be presented in detail; **osteoarthritis (OA),** a localized process that has been known in the past as **degenerative joint disease (DJD),** will also be discussed. Taken together, these two forms of arthritis account for most of the cases of arthritis that a physical therapist is likely to encounter in clinical practice.

RHEUMATOID ARTHRITIS

RA is a major subclassification within the category of diffuse connective tissue diseases that also includes juvenile arthritis, **systemic lupus erythematosus (SLE),** progressive systemic sclerosis or scleroderma, polymyositis, and dermatomyositis. The first clinical description of the disease is attributed to A.J. Landré-Beauvais in 1800, although analysis of pictorial art of the late Renaissance has provided some evidence for the existence of RA in earlier times. Early descriptive comparisons of patient symptomatology were complicated by the lack of uniform agreement about the distinguishing characteristics of the disease, a difficulty that persists even today given the wide spectrum of clinical presentations associated with this disease. Although the term "rheumatoid arthritis" was first used by Garrod in 1858, it was not accepted by the American Rheumatism Association (ARA) as the official terminology until 1941. The American College of Rheumatology (ACR), formerly the ARA, has revised the diagnostic terminology and criteria for RA several times in the last 40 years and continues to monitor them for accuracy and validity.[1]

Classification Criteria

Clinically, the differential diagnosis of RA is predicated upon the patient's signs and symptoms and careful exclusion of other disorders. When conducting epidemiological and other kinds of research studies, it is often necessary to identify homogeneous groups of individuals with relatively similar signs and symptoms of RA given the wide spectrum of clinical presentations seen in this disease. Although other sets of criteria exist for this purpose, the ACR classification criteria are most often used to determine whether an individual's clinical presentation should be counted as a case of RA. Previous criteria allowed four classifications of RA: classical, definite, probable, and possible. The latter two designations were problematic because many patients with probable or possible RA often were discovered to have another disease when reexamined at a later time. Therefore, new criteria were tested and established in 1987 based on a combination of signs, symptoms and laboratory findings that have persisted for a specified period of time (Table 21–1).[2] A diagnosis of RA is now established upon the presentation of four of the seven listed criteria. The joint signs and symptoms described in criteria one through four must have lasted for at least 6 weeks.[1,2]

Epidemiology

The calculation of prevalence rates can be complicated by the "type" of RA a person had at the time the epidemiological survey was conducted as well as the criteria used. When the prevalence of RA in Sudbury, Massachusetts, was studied using both the 1958 ARA criteria and the more stringent New York criteria, remarkable differences at follow-up were reported, emphasizing the difficulty with prevalence studies that used less stringent inclusion criteria, such as those that had been previously accepted for probable and possible RA.[3] It has been estimated that the prevalence rate of definite RA among adults in the United States is approximately 10 cases per 1000 people, or approximately 2.1 million persons.[4] RA affects women two to three times more often than men in the typical years of onset between the ages of 20 and 60 years. Men and women over the age of 65 appear to be affected at the same rate. There is a general increase in prevalence for both sexes as age increases. Although RA is found around the world, there are some differences in the prevalence of RA in certain subpopulations, a fact that suggests a possible role for genetic or environmental factors in the etiology of the disease. For example, black Americans may have a lower prevalence of RA than whites, whereas several Native American

Table 21–1 THE 1987 REVISED CRITERIA FOR THE CLASSIFICATION OF RHEUMATOID ARTHRITIS[a]

Criterion	Definition
1. Morning stiffness	Morning stiffness in and around the joints, lasting at least one hour before maximal improvement.
2. Arthritis of three or more joint areas	At least three joint areas simultaneously have had soft tissue swelling or fluid (not bony overgrowth alone) observed by a physician. The 14 possible areas are right or left PIP, MCP, wrist, elbow, knee, ankle, and MTP joints.
3. Arthritis of hand joints	At least one area swollen (as defined above) in a wrist, MCP, or PIP joint.
4. Symmetric arthritis	Simultaneous involvement of the same joint areas (as defined in 2) on both sides of the body (bilateral involvement of PIPs, MCPs, or MTPs is acceptable without absolute symmetry).
5. Rheumatoid nodules	Subcutaneous nodules, over bony prominences, or extensor surfaces, or in juxtaarticular regions, observed by a physician.
6. Serum rheumatoid factor	Demonstration of abnormal amounts of serum rheumatoid factor by any method for which the result has been positive in < 5% of normal control subjects.
7. Radiographic changes	Radiographic changes typical of rheumatoid arthritis on posteroanterior hand and wrist radiographs, which must include erosions or unequivocal bony decalcification localized in or most marked adjacent to the involved joints (osteoarthritis changes alone do not qualify).

From Arnett,[2] p 319 with permission.
[a]For classification purposes, a patient shall be said to have rheumatoid arthritis if he or she has satisfied at least four of these seven criteria. Criteria 1 through 4 must have been present for at least 6 weeks. Patients with two clinical diagnoses are not excluded. Designation as classic, definite, or probable rheumatoid arthritis is *not* to be made.

groups demonstrate higher prevalence rates. There also is a lower prevalence of RA in native Japanese and native Chinese peoples compared to whites.[1,4,6]

Etiology

Like many other chronic diseases, the etiology of RA is unknown. Current research into the causes of RA is based on a complex, but as yet incomplete, appreciation of the functions of the immune system. Briefly, an **antigen** is a substance, usually foreign to the host, that provokes the immune system into action. The immune system may respond to the antigen directly (cellular immunity) or by the production of **antibodies** that circulate in the serum (humoral immunity). These responses involve two general kinds of lymphocytes: T cells, which are responsible for cellular immunity, and B cells, which produce circulating antibodies specific to the antigen. Antibodies are immunoglobulins, a type of serum protein.[1]

Based on the fact that individuals with RA produce antibodies to their own immunoglobulins, there is some reason to believe that RA is an *autoimmune* disorder. It is not clear, however, whether this antibody production is a primary event or results as a response to a specific antigen from an external stimulus. Current theory and research on the cellular basis of autoimmunity suggest that aberrant functioning of cell-mediated immunity and defective T lymphocytes may trigger the autoimmune response that underlies RA.[7,8] A specific etiological agent for RA has not been identified even though investigators have been able to identify that specific external etiological agents may produce an inflammatory arthritis, for example, **Lyme disease.** The disease that is finally manifested may be more dependent on the host's manner of response than on the agent or the mechanism involved.[9]

Current evidence suggests that a variety of agents may initiate an arthritis through a number of different mechanisms. A number of bacterial organisms have been suggested including streptococcus, clostridia, diphtheroids, and mycoplasmas, but no connections have been definitively proven. There has also been discussion of a viral etiology for RA, particularly surrounding the evidence that the serum of patients with RA reacts with cells infected by the Epstein-Barr virus (EBV). The EBV can initiate lymphoid proliferation, which suggests that it has the ability to alter the regulation of the immune system. As with other investigations that seek to identify a viral etiology for RA, research in this area remains speculative.[9–11]

Rheumatoid factors (RF) have received considerable attention in the search for a causative agent in RA because they are found in the sera of approximately 70 percent of all patients with RA. RF are antibodies specific to IgG. Current theory suggests that RF arise as antibodies to "altered" autologous (the patient's own) IgG. Some modification of IgG changes its configuration and renders it an autoimmunogen, stimulating the production of RF. IgM is the first class of immunoglobulins formed after contact with an antigen and most RF are of this class, although RF may be of any immunoglobulin class.[1] The exact biological role of RF is unknown, and is given less weight in current theories on the pathogenesis of RA.[8] RA occurs in the absence of RF in a substantial number of individuals. Individuals with RA, however, who do have RF, or seropositive disease, have increased frequency of subcutaneous nodules, vasculitis, and polyarticular involvement.[1,11]

Recent studies have also sought to establish a genetic predisposition to the development of RA. Human leukocyte antigens (HLA) are found on the cell surface of most human cells, and are capable of generating an **immune response** when genetically incompatible tissues are grafted to each other, for example, during organ transplants. Genes controlling these HLA are found on the sixth chromosome. Four loci have been described: HLA-A, HLA-B, HLA-C, and HLA-D. RA has been associated with increased HLA-D and HLA-DR (D related) antigens, suggesting that certain genes determine whether a host is prone to an immunological response that leads to RA.[6,9,11] HLA-DR4 is associated with more aggressive disease, especially among seronegative patients (in individuals with RA but without RF).[1,12]

Pathology

Long-standing RA is characterized by the grossly edematous appearance of the **synovium** with slender villous or hairlike projections into the joint cavity. There are distinctive vascular changes including venous distention, capillary obstruction, neutrophilic infiltration of the arterial walls, and areas of thrombosis and hemorrhage. Synovial proliferation of vascular granulation tissue, known as **pannus,** dissolves collagen as it extends over the joint cartilage. Eventually, if RA continues, the granulation tissue will result in adhesions, **fibrosis** or bony **ankylosis** of the joint. Chronic inflammation can also weaken the joint capsule and its supporting ligamentous structures, altering joint structure and function. Tendon rupture and fraying tendon sheaths may produce imbalanced muscle pull on these pathologically altered joints resulting in the characteristic musculoskeletal deformities seen in advanced RA.[1]

Pathogenesis

The key features that differentiate synovial joints from other kinds of joints are exactly those features that make them susceptible to persistent inflammation. Rapid changes in the cellular content and volume of the synovial fluid following alterations in blood flow are possible owing to low pressure in the joint space and the lack of a limiting membrane between the joint space and the synovial blood vessels. High molecular weight substances such as macroglobulins and fibrinogens can pass through the synovial capillaries during periods of inflammation and are not easily cleared.[1] Because the cartilage is avascular, antigen-antibody complexes may be sequestered within the joint cavity and may facilitate a process of phagocytosis and further development of pannus. Although it is accepted that sustained **synovitis** requires the proliferation of new blood vessels, the exact mechanism of capillary growth is not currently understood. One attractive hypothesis is that activated macrophages, responding to antigen-antibody complexes, may stimulate this development.

In established synovitis, polymorphonuclear (PMN) leukocytes are chemotactically drawn into the joint cavity and contribute to the inflammatory destruction of the synovium, although the exact mechanism of this destruction is unknown. It is known that the lysosomal enzymes, which are released from these leukocytes, can directly injure synovial tissues.[1,11,13]

Clinical Diagnostic Criteria

The clinical diagnosis of RA is based on careful consideration of three factors: the clinical presentation of the patient, which is elucidated through history-taking and physical examination; the corroborating evidence gathered through laboratory tests and radiography; and the exclusion of other possible diagnoses.[1,5]

SIGNS AND SYMPTOMS
Systemic Manifestations
Morning stiffness lasting more than 3 minutes is a hallmark symptom of RA. Difficulty in moving upon awakening and generalized stiffness despite morning activity help to differentiate this sign from the stiffness of a particular joint seen in DJD following inactivity.[2] Morning stiffness can be qualified in terms of its severity and duration, both of which are directly related to the degree of disease activity. As with other systemic diseases, anorexia, weight loss, and fatigue also may be present.[1,2,14]

Joint Involvement
RA is marked by a bilateral and symmetrical pattern of joint involvement. Clinically, the patient presents with immobility and the cardinal signs of inflammation: pain, redness, swelling, and heat.[1] The term **arthralgia** is used to refer to pain in a joint. The joint examination also may reveal **crepitus,** which is audible or palpable grating or crunching as the joint is moved through its range of motion (ROM). Crepitus is the result of uneven degeneration of the joint surface.

Cervical Spine
The cervical spine is often involved in RA.[15,16] The atlantoaxial joint and the midcervical region are the most common sites of inflammation, which leads to decreased ROM, particularly in rotation, 50 percent of which takes place at the C1 to C2. Involvement of these two vertebrae may produce life-threatening situations if the transverse ligament of the atlas should rupture or if the odontoid process should fracture or herniate through the foramen magnum. Cervical involvement may also produce radiating pain and nerve and cord compression, which is most likely to be seen in the lower cervical spine where the cervical lordosis is greatest.[1] Although neurological involvement is not inevitable in individuals with cervical subluxations, it has been estimated that 1-year mortality reaches 50 percent in patients who do have cord compression. Magnetic resonance imaging (MRI) is particularly useful for visualizing both the spinal column and the cord in these cases.[5]

Ankylosing spondylitis is an inflammation of one or more vertebrae of the spine that may accompany rheumatoid disease. It primarily affects the sacroiliac, spinal facet, and costovertebral joints, and progresses to eventual fusion (ankylosis) of the involved joints.

Temporomandibular Joint
Involvement of this synovial joint results in an inability to open the mouth fully (approximately 2 inches) with normal side-to-side gliding and protrusion. In resting position, the normal approximation of the upper and lower teeth may be altered following persistent inflammation.[1,5]

Shoulders
Shoulder involvement may be seen in the glenohumeral, sternoclavicular, or acromioclavicular joints. These joints may demonstrate degeneration, pain, and loss of ROM. The scapulothoracic articulation may secondarily exhibit a loss of ROM as well. Chronic inflammation of the shoulders causes the capsule and the ligaments to become distended and thinned. Joint surfaces may be eroded until the shoulder eventually becomes unstable. Additionally, **tendinitis** and **bursitis** may complicate management.[1,14,17]

Elbows
Inflammation, capsular and ligamentous distension, and joint surface erosion may lead to elbow instability and irregular or catching movements. Flexion contractures frequently develop, the outcome of persistent spasm secondary to pain.[1,14]

Wrists
Early synovitis between the eight carpal bones and the ulna leads to a fairly rapid development of a flexion contracture, which ultimately diminishes the individual's ability to execute power grasp. Chronic inflammation of the proximal row of carpals can lead to a volar **subluxation** of the wrist and hand on the radius, accentuating the normal 10 to 15 degrees of volar inclination of the carpus on the distal radius (Fig. 21-1). Chronic inflammation leads to the loss of radial ligamentous support and destruction of the extensor carpi ulnaris and the fibrocartilage on the distal side of the ulna. The attenuation of these restraining structures allows the proximal carpals to slide down the distal radius toward the ulna, creating a radial deviation of the distal row of carpals in the wrist relative to the two bones of the forearm, where normally there are 5 to 10 degrees of ulnar deviation (Fig. 21-2).[14] Stenosing tenosynovitis of the first dorsal compartment of the wrist **(deQuervain's disease)** may also occur.

Hand Joints
Metacarpophalangeal. Soft-tissue swelling around the metacarpophalangeal (MCP) joints is very common. The volar subluxation and ulnar drift of the MCPs frequently seen in RA are thought to result from accentuation of the normal structural shapes of these joints that tilt the proximal phalanges in an ulnar direction. The anatomical placement

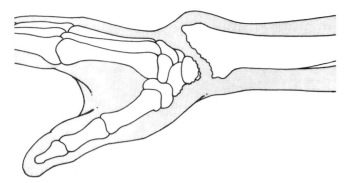

Figure 21-1. Volar subluxation of the carpus on the radius as a result of erosive synovitis of the radiocarpal joint. (From Melvin, J,[14] p 280 with permission.)

and length of the collateral ligaments, which are most stretched during MCP flexion, and the insertions of the intrinsics, which also pull from an ulnar direction, also contribute to ulnar drift at the MCPs during hand motion. Weakened ligaments cannot resist a pull toward volar subluxation during power pinch or grasp when flexor tendons "bowstring" across MCPs through frayed tendon sheaths damaged by long-term synovitis.[14] The bowstring effect

results from moving the fulcrum of the flexor tendons distally which places an ulnar and volar pull on the proximal phalanges (Fig. 21-3). Radial deviation of the carpals will further enhance MCP ulnar drift as the phalanges try to compensate for the loss of normal ulnar deviation at the wrist. This is known as the **zigzag effect,** where forces in the hand try to move the index finger back into its normal functional position in line with the radius (see Fig. 21-2).[14,18–22]

Proximal Interphalangeal. Swelling of the proximal interphalangeal (PIP) joints produces a fusiform or "sausage"-like appearance in the fingers. There are two characteristic deformities seen at the PIP in individuals with RA. The first of these is known as **swan neck deformity** and consists of PIP hyperextension and distal interphalangeal (DIP) flexion. Swan neck deformities arise in three distinct ways, depending on the site of initial involvement.[14,22] Most commonly, swan neck deformity follows from initial synovitis of the MCP, where the pain of chronic synovitis leads to reflex muscle spasm of the intrinsics (Fig. 21-4). The biomechanical force of the intrinsics then combines with the hypermobility found in the chronically inflamed and structurally changed PIP resulting in volar subluxation and PIP hyperextension. Swan neck deformity may also result when the volar capsule of the PIP is stretched, the lateral bands move dorsally, and tension placed on the flexor digitorum profundis by the PIP flexes the DIP (Fig. 21-5). In these instances, a rupture of the flexor digitorum sublimus further predisposes an individual to swan neck deformity. A third mechanism for developing swan neck defor-

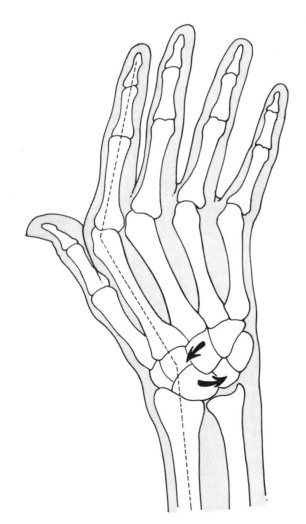

Figure 21-2. Relationship between wrist and metacarpophalangeal joint deformity. (From Melvin, J,[14] p 281 with permission.)

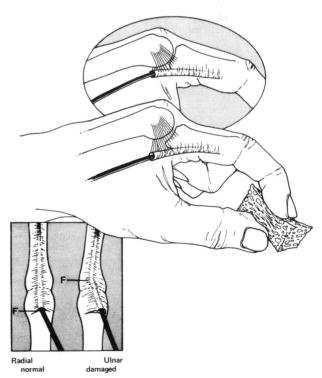

Figure 21-3. Influence of the long flexors in metacarpophalangeal drift deformity. (From Melvin, J,[14] p 283 with permission.)

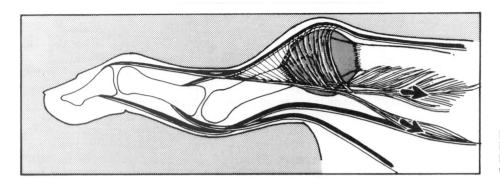

Figure 21-4. Swan neck deformity with initial synovitis at the metacarpophalangeal joint. (From Melvin, J,[14] p 285 with permission.)

mity involves a rupture of the extensor digitorum communis at its insertion on the DIP resulting in DIP flexion and PIP hyperextension owing to unrestrained pull by the flexor digitorum profundis (Fig. 21-6).[14]

The other characteristic deformity of the PIP is known as a **boutonniere deformity** and consists of DIP extension with PIP flexion (Fig. 21-7). As a result of chronic synovitis, the insertion of extensor digitorum communis into the middle phalanx known as the central slip lengthens and the lateral bands slide volarly to force the PIP into flexion. Bony formation or outgrowths around the end of a joint are termed **osteophytes.** Those found at the PIP are known as **Bouchard's nodes,** and may be seen in OA. They are unrelated to RA, although an individual may have both kinds of arthritis at the same time.[14]

Distal Interphalangeal. The distal interphalangeal (DIP) joints are most often uninvolved in RA. Osteophytes are, however, common in OA and are called **Heberden's nodes.** Occasionally, the tendon of the extensor digitorum communis will rupture, and the unopposed pull of the flexor digitorum profundis will pull the DIP into flexion. This condition is known as **mallet finger** deformity.[14]

Thumb. As in the other digital joints, the primary cause of deformity in the thumb is synovial swelling. The fibers of the dorsal hood mechanism over the MCP, the joint capsule and the collateral ligaments, and the tendons of extensor pollicis brevis and extensor pollicis longus are particularly affected. The exact mechanism of thumb deformities depends on the particular combination of affected structures and may be classified according to the criteria elaborated by Nalebuff.[23] Similar to other hand deformities, the actual presentation depends on the site of initial synovitis, the direction of imbalanced

muscle forces, and the integrity of the surrounding joint structures. A type I deformity, consisting of MCP flexion with IP hyperextension without involvement of the carpometacarpal (CMC) joint, is most commonly seen. Type II deformity is assigned when the CMC is subluxed and the IP is held in hyperextension. CMC subluxation and MCP hyperextension is classified as a type III deformity, and is more commonly found in RA than a type II deformity.[14,23]

Mutilans Deformity (Opera-glass Hand). Grossly unstable thumbs and severely deformed phalanges are indicative of **mutilans-type deformity.** Also known as opera glass hand, the transverse folds of the skin of the thumb and fingers resemble a folded telescope. Radiographic study of the bones of the hand reveals severe bone resorption, erosion, and shortening of the MCP, PIP, radiocarpal, and radioulnar joints especially. The negative impact of this deformity on hand function and activities of daily living (ADL) is significant.[14]

Hip

Although patients may present with complaints of pain in the groin, often owing to trochanteric bursitis, the hip is less commonly involved in RA than in other kinds of arthritis. Radiographic hip disease is seen in about half of all patients with RA. Severe inflammatory destruction of the femoral head and the acetabulum may push the acetabulum into the pelvic cavity, a condition known as **protrusio acetabuli.**[1,5,14]

Knees

Because of the relatively large amount of synovium in the knee, it is one of the most frequently affected joints in RA. Chronic synovitis results in

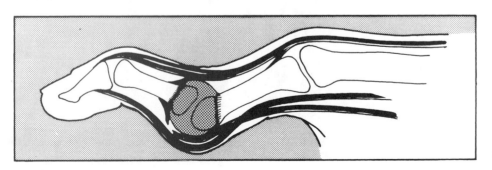

Figure 21-5. Swan neck deformity with initial synovitis at the proximal interphalangeal joint. (From Melvin, J,[14] p 286 with permission.)

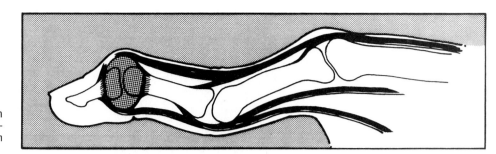

Figure 21-6. Swan neck deformity with initial synovitis at the distal interphalangeal joint. (From Melvin, J,[14] p 287 with permission.)

distension of the joint capsule, attenuation of the collateral and cruciate ligaments, and destruction of the joint surfaces. Painful knees may be held in slightly flexed positions ultimately resulting in flexion contractures.[1,5,14]

Ankles and Feet

Chronic synovitis accentuates the natural tendency of the talus to glide medially and plantarward resulting in pressure on the calcaneus and leading to hindfoot pronation. The spring ligament is also stretched by these occurrences flattening the medial longitudinal arch (Fig. 21-8). The calcaneus may erode or develop bony **exostoses** known as spurs. As synovitis weakens the transverse arch, the metatarsals spread and a splayed forefoot **(splayfoot)** may develop (Fig. 21-9). Synovitis of the metatarsophalangeal (MTP) joints is extremely common and **metatarsalgia** (pain over the metatarsal heads) may develop. A **hallux valgus** and **bunion** (a painful bursitis over the medial aspect of the first MTP joint) may also be present. When volar subluxation of the MTP combines with flexion of the PIP and hyperextension of the DIP joints, this condition is commonly referred to as **hammer toes** (Fig. 21-10). The MTPs may also exhibit volar subluxation of the metatarsal head with flexion of the PIP and DIP joints, known as **cock-up** or **claw toes** (Fig. 21-11). As the capsule and intertarsal ligaments are weakened and stretched, the proximal phalanges move dorsally on the metatarsal head (Fig. 21-12). Similar to conditions observed in the hand, the long toe extensors "bowstring" over the PIP joints while the flexors are displaced into the intertarsal spaces.[1,5,14,24,25]

Muscle Involvement

Muscle atrophy around affected joints may be present early. It is not definitively known, however, whether this atrophy is the result simply of disuse or selective attrition of muscles owing to some unknown mechanism specifically related to the disease itself. Atrophy in the intrinsic muscles of the hand and the quadriceps are particularly evident in long-standing disease, although the mechanisms for these changes may not be the same. It appears that individuals with RA experience selective attrition of type II (phasic) muscle fibers through some unknown mechanism.[26,27] There is also some evidence that type I (tonic) muscle fibers of the quadriceps will undergo selective atrophy following anterior cruciate damage.[28] Loss of muscle bulk may also be the result of a peripheral neuropathy, **myositis,** or steroid-induced myopathy. Muscle weakness may be due to either reflex inhibition secondary to pain or atrophy.[26–28]

Tendons

Inflammation of the synovial lining of the tendon sheaths results in a tenosynovitis that interferes with the smooth gliding of the tendon through the sheath and may directly damage the tendon itself. Eventually the tendon may rupture. A patient with tendon damage or muscle weakness may exhibit a **lag phenomenon,** which refers to a substantial differ-

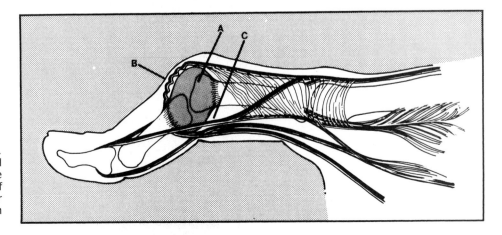

Figure 21-7. Boutonniere deformity. *A.* Synovitis of the proximal interphalangeal joint; *B.* Osteophytes at the end of the joint (Bouchard's nodes); *C.* Repture of the central tendenous slip of the extensor hood. (From Melvin, J,[14] p 287 with permission.)

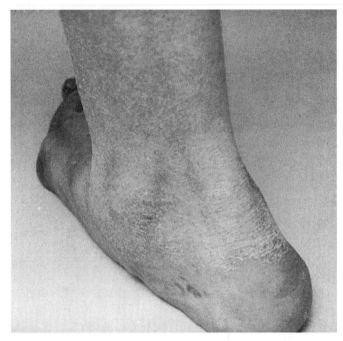

Figure 21-8. Posterior-medial view of the foot and ankle showing calcaneal valgus, pes planus (flatfoot) and hallux valgus. (Used by permission of the Arthritis Foundation.)

ence in passive versus active ROM. This is a nonspecific finding that therapists need to examine carefully to determine its cause and design appropriate treatment.[5,14]

LABORATORY TESTS

Two concepts are essential to a full understanding of the use of laboratory tests in the detection of RA. The first is the concept of the *sensitivity* of a test, which indicates the proportion of truly diseased individuals who have a positive test. The clinical value of sensitive tests is particularly evident in those instances when a negative misdiagnosis would be deleterious to the health of the patient. In research terms, sensitivity is equivalent to the laboratory test's ability to avoid a false negative result. The

concept of *specificity*, on the other hand, refers to the proportion of truly nondiseased individuals who have a negative test. In other words, the specificity of a laboratory test is a measure of its ability to avoid false positives. The clinical diagnostician will usually choose a mix of both sensitive and specific tests to confirm clinical impressions during the diagnostic process.

Elevated erythrocyte sedimentation rate (ESR) or C reactive protein (CRP), acute phase reactants, indicate the presence of active inflammation. Although it is characteristic that patients with RA have active inflammation, up to 40 percent of patients with RA have normal values for these tests despite marked clinical evidence of inflammation. Normal ESR and CRP values do not exclude a diagnosis of RA; nor do elevated levels signify a diagnosis of RA. Rheumatoid factor (RF) is the result of the binding of two immunoglobulins. The presence or absence of RF neither confirms nor rules out a diagnosis of RA. Up to 25 percent of people with RA do not have a positive RF (seronegative RA), whereas a positive RF is seen in a number of other diseases with an immunological component (e.g., leprosy, tuberculosis, chronic hepatitis), and occasionally in individuals with no disease. A positive RF cannot confirm a diagnosis of RA; however, in combination with clinical criteria, positive RF may help to confirm a clinical impression.

A complete blood count (CBC) is routinely ordered because a number of findings are commonly associated with RA. Red blood cell counts are often decreased, indicating the anemia of chronic disease found in approximately 20 percent of individuals with RA. By comparison, the white blood cell count is generally normal. Thrombocytosis, a high platelet count, is not uncommon in active RA.

HLA-DR4 typing for presence of the *0401 or *0101 haplotype has demonstrated that people with these haplotypes have a fivefold higher likelihood of developing RA, and 70 percent of people with RA have these haplotypes. On the other hand, 30 percent of individuals with RA do not have these

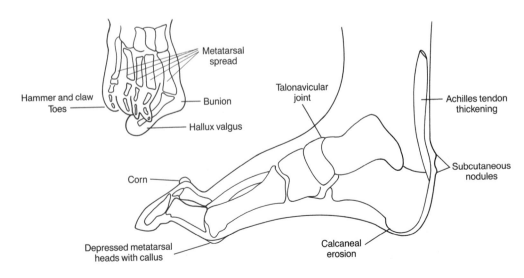

Figure 21-9. Major foot and ankle deformities seen in rheumatoid arthritis. (From Dimonte, P, and Light, H,[79] p 1149 with permission of the American Physical Therapy Association.)

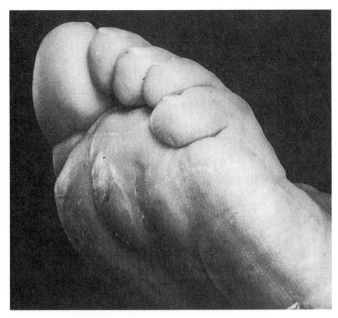

Figure 21-10. Metatarsophalangeal subluxation. (Used by permission of the American College of Rheumatology.)

haplotypes. However, most people who have these haplotypes do not have RA. Therefore, it is of interest in genetics-related research, but is not clinically useful in the diagnosis or management of RA.

A synovial fluid analysis can greatly enhance the process of differential diagnosis. Normal synovial fluid is transparent, yellowish, viscous, and without clots. Synovial fluid from inflamed joints is cloudy, less viscous owing to a change in hyaluronate proteins, and will clot. Significant inflammation will also increase the number of proteins in the fluid. A culture can be done to identify potential bacterial agents as the cause of the joint inflammation. If the joint is inflamed, there will be

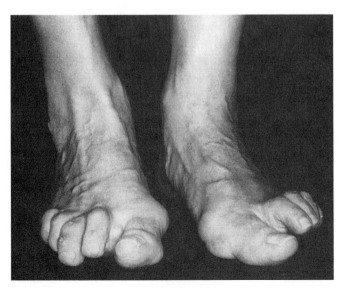

Figure 21-11. Common deformities of the rheumatoid foot. (Used by permission of the American College of Rheumatology.)

an elevation of white blood cells in the fluid, 90 percent of which may be PMN leukocytes. Normal fluid has a low cell count with only 25 percent PMN representation. The presence of crystals may confirm the diagnosis of **gout** (urate crystals) or **pseudogout** (calcium pyrophosphate crystals). A mucin clot is formed in synovial fluid by mixing it with acetic acid. If the synovial fluid is normal, a ropelike mass will form in a clear solution after mixing. Shredding indicates fair mucin clotting, and the formation of small masses with shreds is indicative of a poor mucin clot. Poor clotting accompanies acute infectious arthritis. Inflammatory arthritis, such as RA, produces fair mucin clotting. Good mucin clotting of the synovial fluid is found in a joint that presents with a noninflammatory arthritis.[1,5]

RADIOGRAPHY

Radiographic assessment is an essential component of the diagnostic work up for RA. Physical therapists working in rheumatology should be avid consumers of the radiographic information available in a patient's record. They should also develop a basic proficiency in identifying abnormalities in joint structure and the surrounding soft tissues that influence the course and outcome of rehabilitation. The ability to identify abnormalities assumes that the therapist has a firm notion of how a normal joint appears on a radiograph. Therapists can orient themselves to a radiograph by considering three parameters: alignment, bone density and surface, and cartilaginous spacing (Figs. 21-13 and 21-14). In assessing alignment, the therapist should note whether the long axes of the proximal and distal bones of the joint are in their normal spatial relationships and whether the convex surface of one fits well with the concavity of the other. Bone density, in the absence of **osteoporosis,** should be somewhat opaque and milky and appear evenly distributed throughout. The cortices of each bone should be distinct, appropriately thick, and well defined. The soft tissues surrounding the joints should conform to known anatomical shape. The therapist should note any soft tissue swelling evident on the radiograph that might limit function. Finally, the therapist should note whether there is even spacing between the joint surfaces. Uneven, reduced, or absent spacing suggests loss of cartilage or erosion of the joint surfaces. Overall, the joint surface should be smooth and conform to known anatomical shape without osteophytes. The progression of the disease can be characterized along four stages following periodic radiographic assessment (Box 21–1). The radiographic changes seen early in the disease are nonspecific, and usually limited to swelling in the surrounding soft tissues, joint **effusions,** and periarticular demineralization. Diagnostic confirmation is available only later in the disease process when the typical joint space narrowing and erosions in the hands and feet are seen in the characteristic bilateral distribution.[29]

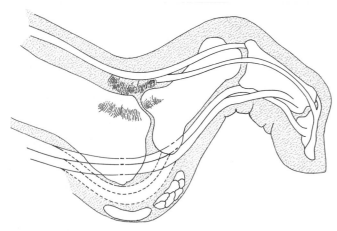

Figure 21-12. Relationship of structures to the metatarsal heads in metatarsalgia. (From Moncur, C, and Shields, M,[24] p 10 with permission of American Physical Therapy Association.)

Indirect Impairments and Complications

DECONDITIONING

People with RA are less physically fit (cardiorespiratory status, muscular strength and endurance, flexibility, and body composition) than their peers without arthritis. Rheumatologic research in conditioning exercise has demonstrated that this situation is not entirely due to the disease process, but is compounded by inadequate levels of regular physical activity.[30,31] In addition to the deconditioning of inactivity, studies of body composition in individuals with RA have shown a marked degree of *cachexia* (wasting of lean body mass) and elevated resting energy expenditure. It appears that immune system activity and inflammation even in individuals with ostensibly well-controlled disease, create an increased metabolism with subsequent loss of lean body tissue.[32]

RHEUMATOID NODULES

Rheumatoid nodules are the most common extra-articular manifestations of RA and occur in approximately 25 percent of patients. They are most commonly found in the subcutaneous or deeper connective tissues in areas subjected to repeated mechanical pressure such as the olecranon bursae, the extensor surfaces of the forearms, and the Achilles tendons. Nodules are usually asymptomatic, although they can be tender and may cause skin breakdown or become infected.[1,5]

VASCULAR COMPLICATIONS

Most forms of vascular lesions associated with RA are silent, although the fulminant form of rheumatoid arteritis can be life threatening, and accompanied by malnutrition, infection, congestive heart failure, and gastrointestinal bleeding. Foot or wrist drop may occur as a result of vasculitis of the vasa arteriosum to the nerve supply of the radial or superficial peroneal nerves.[1,5]

NEUROLOGICAL MANIFESTATIONS

Mild peripheral neuropathies are often seen in RA, particularly in elderly patients and are unrelated to vasculitis. Most neuropathies result from nerve compression or entrapment such as **carpal tunnel** or **tarsal tunnel syndromes.**[1,5]

CARDIOPULMONARY COMPLICATIONS

Pericarditis can be demonstrated at autopsy in about 4 percent of patients, but clinically detectable heart disease from RA is rare. Similarly, pleuropulmonary manifestations are most commonly asymptomatic, although pleuritis is commonly found on autopsy.[1,5]

OCULAR MANIFESTATIONS

Ocular lesions are usually associated with the dry eyes of **Sjogren's syndrome,** which is an inflammatory disorder of the lacrimal and salivary glands. Scleritis and the relatively more benign episcleritis can also be present, and require careful medical treatment.[1,33]

Clinical Manifestations

DISEASE ONSET AND COURSE

Disease onset in RA is most usually insidious with complaints of generalized joint pain and stiffness. Men who develop RA past the age of 60 typically present without stiffness and swelling in the upper extremities.[5] The question of whether elderly-onset RA represents a distinct disease remains controversial. Comparisons of elderly-onset RA with early-onset RA have revealed that abrupt onset and large

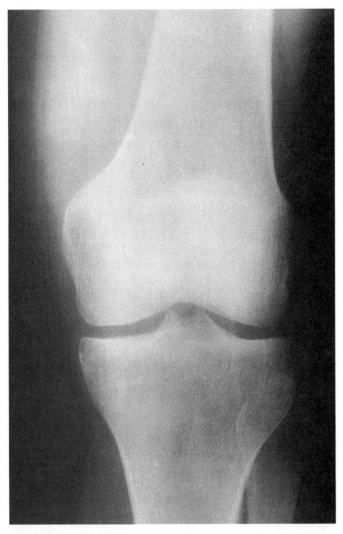

Figure 21-13. Frontal view of the normal knee. (Used by permission of the American College of Rheumatology.)

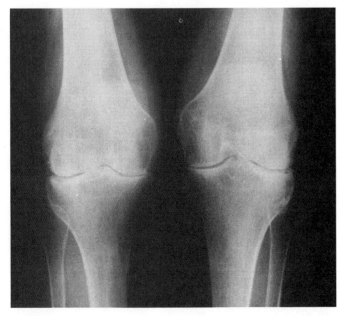

Figure 21-14. Frontal view of the knee with characteristics of rheumatoid arthritis. (Used with permission of the American College of Rheumatology.)

joint involvement, particularly of the shoulder girdle, were more common in the older group. The elderly-onset group also more commonly had features of **polymyalgia rheumatica,** a distinct disease affecting the shoulder and pelvic girdles, with which elderly-onset RA can be confused.[34] Older adolescent females may present with a chronic erosive arthritis of the knees without other joint involvement or systemic manifestations. It is not known whether this presentation is a variation of juvenile arthritis, adult-onset RA, or a distinct form of arthritis involving only a few joints.[5]

Acute onset is seen in 8 to 15 percent of patients. Onset is intermediate in approximately 15 to 20 percent of patients. Most often, the onset is insidious lasting weeks to months. Disease progression is highly variable. High titers of RF can indicate a more severe disease course. Spontaneous remissions can occur, although it often remains unclear if the individual had an accurately diagnosed case of RA or some other disease. Fifteen to 20 percent of patients experience an intermittent course characterized by partial to complete remissions longer than the periods of exacerbations. A third group of patients experience the full destructive process of progressive RA.[1,5]

PROGNOSIS

The question of mortality associated with RA is highly controversial. Previously it was widely believed that RA itself was not usually a cause of death, although conditions such as systemic vasculitis and atlantoaxial subluxation could be fatal. Now there is a growing body of evidence that individuals with RA may not live as long as their counterparts without disease, especially if the early years of RA were marked by aggressive disease and poor functional status. Causes of death occurring more frequently in patients with RA as compared to the general population are infections and renal, respiratory, and gastrointestinal disease.[35,36] Even in patients with milder forms of RA, long-term inflammation ultimately results in joint destruction and significant functional loss. Almost 50 percent of individuals with RA will eventually have marked restrictions in ADL or will be incapacitated.[1] Individuals with late-onset RA appear to have a better functional outcome than those with early onset, but it is unclear whether this finding is the result of having the disease for a shorter period of time or of having a different form of the disease itself.[34] A broad classification of functional disability has been developed by the ARA to characterize the progressive impacts of the disease (Table 21–2). Loss of income is the most severe loss and is directly attributable to work disability secondary to loss of physical function.[37–41]

OSTEOARTHRITIS

OA is marked by two localized, pathological features: the progressive destruction of articular cartilage and the formation of bone at the margins

---

Box 21–1 CLASSIFICATION OF PROGRESSION OF RHEUMATOID ARTHRITIS

Stage I, Early
[a]1. No destructive changes on radiographic examination.
2. Radiographic evidence of osteoporosis may be present.

Stage II, Moderate
[a]1. Radiographic evidence of osteoporosis, with or without slight subchondral bone destruction; slight cartilage destruction may be present.
[a]2. No joint deformities, although limitation of joint mobility may be present.
3. Adjacent muscle atrophy.
4. Extra-articular soft tissue lesions, such as nodules and tenosynovitis may be present.

Stage III, Severe
[a]1. Radiographic evidence of cartilage and bone destruction, in addition to osteoporosis.
[a]2. Joint deformity, such as subluxation, ulnar deviation, or hyperextension, without fibrous or bony ankylosis.
3. Extensive muscle atrophy.
4. Extra-articular soft tissue lesions, such as nodules and tenosynovitis may be present.

Stage IV, Terminal
[a]1. Fibrous or bony ankylosis
2. Criteria of stage III

From Schumacher, Klippel, and Robinson (eds.): Primer on Rheumatic Diseases, ed 9, Arthritis Foundation, Atlanta, 1988, p 318, with permission.

[a]These criteria must be present to permit classification of a patient in any particular stage or grade.

of the joint.[1,42] The disease process of OA confines itself to the affected joint. However, the impairment, functional limitation, and disability related to OA can reach far beyond the perimeters of articular cartilage and subchondral bone. Research documenting the personal and socioeconomic impact of OA increasingly recognizes its importance in both personal and socioeconomic terms.

Table 21–2 AMERICAN COLLEGE OF RHEUMATOLOGY REVISED CRITERIA FOR CLASSIFICATION OF FUNCTIONAL STATUS IN RHEUMATOID ARTHRITIS[a]

Class I	Completely able to perform usual activities of daily living (self-care, vocational, and avocational)
Class II	Able to perform usual self-care and vocational activities, but limited in avocational activities
Class III	Able to perform usual self-care activities, but limited in vocational and avocational activities
Class IV	Limited in ability to perform usual self-care, vocational, and avocational activities

From Hochberg, MC, et al: The American College of Rheumatology 1991 revised criteria for the classification of global functional status in rheumatoid arthritis. Arthritis Rheum 35:498, 1992, with permission of the American College of Rheumatology.

[a]Usual self-care activities include dressing, feeding, bathing, grooming, and toileting. Avocational (recreational and/or leisure) and vocational (work, school, homemaking) activities are patient-desired and age- and sex-specific.

Classification

Although joint inflammation is implied by the "-itis" in osteoarthritis, inflammation is typically found only after there has been substantial articular degeneration. The synovium of an osteoarthritic joint, however, can demonstrate marked changes, similar to those seen in RA in some joints.[43] In epidemiological studies, OA is often graded on radiographs according to the criteria of Kellgren and Lawrence, an ordinal scale of 5 levels:

1. grade 0, normal radiograph;
2. grade 1, doubtful narrowing of the joint space and possible osteophytes;
3. grade 2, definite osteophytes and absent or questionable narrowing of the joint space;
4. grade 3, moderate osteophytes and joint space narrowing, some sclerosis, and possible deformity; and
5. grade 4, large osteophytes, marked narrowing of joint space, severe sclerosis and definite deformity.

Most studies have used grade 2 (the presence of definite osteophytes) as the criterion for defining disease, although a few others have required evidence of joint space narrowing (grade 3), corresponding to clinically identified disease, to designate OA.[44] Although radiographic evidence of joint space narrowing and osteophytes may help confirm the diagnosis and classify the stage of OA, the clinical criteria for hip and knee OA are described in terms of pain and limitation of motion (Box 21–2).[45,46] Radiography adds little to the accuracy of the clinical diagnosis, and there is no clear association between radiographic findings and function or pain. In OA of the knee, muscle strength and pain are

---

Box 21–2 CLINICAL CLASSIFICATION CRITERIA FOR KNEE AND HIP OSTEOARTHRITIS (95% SENSITIVITY, 69% SPECIFICITY)

Knee Osteoarthritis
1. Knee pain
2. Joint stiffness ≤ 30 minutes
3. Crepitus
4. Bony enlargement
5. Bony tenderness
6. No palpable warmth

Hip Osteoarthritis
1. Hip internal rotation ≥ 15 degrees with pain, morning stiffness ≤ 60 minutes, and age > 50 years, *or*
2. Hip internal rotation < 15 degrees, and hip flexion ≤ 155 degrees

---

From Altman, R, et al: Development of criteria for the classification and reporting of osteoarthritis: Classification of osteoarthritis of the knee. Arthritis Rheum 29:1039, 1986; and Altman, R, et al: The American College of Rheumatology criteria for the classification and reporting of osteoarthritis of the hip. Arthritis Rheum 34:505, 1991.

more explanatory of functional loss than radiographic findings.[47]

Patients with OA can be further differentiated in two ways. Some cases of OA are classified as *idiopathic*, when the etiology of the disease is unknown. Idiopathic OA may be localized to a specific joint, or generalized, affecting three or more joints. OA is classified as *secondary*, when the etiology (e.g., trauma, congenital malformation, or other musculoskeletal disease) can be identified.[14]

Epidemiology

OA is an extremely common condition after 40 years of age, although it may not always be symptomatic when present. It is widespread in adults over 60, and affects men more than women.[48,49] It is likely that more than 60 million adults in the United States have OA. Severe or moderate hip OA occurs in 3.1 percent of persons 55 to 74 years of age and knee OA affects 13.8 percent of persons 65 to 74.[43] Studies concerning racial predisposition to OA have yielded conflicting data, depending on the joint studied.

Etiology

Similar to RA, no single factor that predisposes an individual to OA has been identified. Although aging is indeed strongly associated with OA, it must be emphasized that aging in itself does not cause OA, nor should OA be considered a "normal" aging process.[42,50] Several factors related to aging may, however, contribute to its development. Trauma prior to adulthood may initiate a remodeling of bone that alters joint mechanics and nutrition in a way that becomes problematic only later in life. The role of repetitive "microtrauma" in the etiology of OA has also received attention.[1,42] Specifically, occupational tasks such as repetitive knee bending have been linked to the development of OA.[51] Finally, obesity has been shown to be a risk factor for the development of OA in later life.[1,52]

Pathology

Animal models involving knee trauma have provided much of the basis for what we now know about the earliest changes associated with OA in humans. Thus, it is possible that subtle, crucial, and as yet undiscovered differences in humans may alter our understanding of OA in the future. The first osteoarthritic change in articular cartilage, which has been confirmed in humans, is an increase in water content. This increase suggests that the proteoglycans have been allowed to swell with water far beyond normal, although the mechanism by which this occurs is unknown.[1,42] Additionally, there are changes in the composition of newly synthesized proteoglycan. In later stages of disease progression, proteoglycans are lost, which diminishes the water content of cartilage. As proteoglycans are lost, articular cartilage loses its compressive stiffness and elasticity, which in turn, results in the transmission of compressive forces to underlying bone. Changes in cartilage proteoglycans will also negatively affect the ability of the cartilage to form a squeeze film over its surface during joint loading. Collagen synthesis is increased initially, although there is a shift from type II collagen fibers to a larger proportion of type I collagen, the kind found in skin and fibrous tissue. As the articular cartilage is destroyed, the joint space narrows.[53]

One of the first noticeable changes in cartilage is the mild fraying or "flaking" of superficial collagen fibers. Deeper fraying or "fibrillation" of the upper third of the cartilage follows, and occurs in areas of greater weight bearing. The cartilage may degenerate to the point that subchondral bone is exposed. Subchondral bone in turn can then become sclerotic and stiffer than normal bone.[53] These changes in cartilage and bone result in increased friction, decreased shock absorption, and greater impact loading of the joint. The traditional view of OA is that the disease process starts with an unrepaired injury to articular cartilage; however, there is also evidence that reduced compliance in bone and periarticular structures may initiate the degenerative processes.[54,55]

The process of osteophyte formation in OA is not well understood. Current hypotheses have implicated increased vascularity in degenerated cartilage, venous congestion from subchondral cysts and thickened subchondral trabeculae, and the continued sloughing of articular cartilage. Each of these hypotheses may explain how this bony growth contributes to the pain and loss of motion that accompany OA.

Pathogenesis

Unlike the synovium in RA, the major pathological changes of OA are found in the articular cartilage, particularly the concentration of proteoglycan, which diminishes according to the severity of the disease. Furthermore, there are metabolic changes in the rate of enzyme production that facilitate the destruction of cartilage. Even though proteoglycan concentration decreases with OA, it is also true that proteoglycan and collagen synthesis increases until the later stages of the disease. This seeming paradox has given rise to several hypotheses concerning the pathogenesis of OA, which have yet to be proven. Given that proteoglycan synthesis increases with OA, it is possible that the quality of this newly synthesized product may not be equal to meeting the biomechanical load normally placed on an adult joint.[42]

Clinical Diagnostic Criteria

SIGNS AND SYMPTOMS

Clinically, a diagnosis is often made on the basis of symptoms, and signs (e.g., pain and swelling, loss of ROM, and bony deformity). Not all joints are equally affected by OA. In the upper extremity, the DIPs, PIPs, and CMC of the thumb are commonly involved. The cervical and lumbar spine, hips, knees, and first MTP are also sites for OA. The MCPs, wrists, elbows, and shoulders are usually spared in primary OA.[49] Unlike RA, OA does not have a bilateral, symmetrical presentation. A single joint or any combination of joints on one individual may be affected.[48] OA is not a systemic disease, and is therefore not associated with systemic complaints such as generalized morning stiffness, fever, or loss of appetite. Individuals with OA may experience some stiffness in particular joints upon awakening that is similar to the stiffness felt when mobilizing the same joints after inactivity during the day, but this stiffness does not last nearly as long as in individuals with RA nor is it generalized to the entire body.[49] Crepitus is a common clinical finding in OA as well as in RA.[1,43,49]

Although cartilage degeneration is the primary manifestation of OA, cartilage is aneural, and therefore not the cause of a person's pain. Pain in OA may be attributed to incongruent articulations of joint surfaces, periosteal elevation secondary to bone proliferation at the joint margin, abnormal pressures on subchondral bone, trabecular microfractures, and distention of the joint capsule. Many patients will also experience a secondary synovitis, especially when the knee is involved.[49]

Symptoms do not always match the severity of the disease on radiographs. Some patients may magnify the pain they experience.[14] More importantly, unlike individuals with RA who report pain on motion and at rest, the pain associated with OA is likely to occur or worsen only with motion, except in the later stages of the disease.[49]

OA of the hip commonly results in decreased ROM with a tendency for the hip to be held in a somewhat flexed, abducted, and externally rotated position and the knee in flexion. Decreased hip ROM is clearly associated with decreased walking speed, decreased stride length, and increased energy expenditure. Maximum walking speed of 1.8 miles per hour is not uncommon in older persons with hip OA and decreased hip motion.[56] Moreover, decreased hip ROM is commonly associated with pain, loss of function, and limitations in physical activity.[43]

Patients with the most severe disease may not move their joints as often or in the ways that exacerbate their symptoms. Therefore, pain and disease severity in individuals with OA are potentially related to functional loss, although not in the same way. Among elders, it has been shown, for example, that the functional loss associated with severe radiographic OA without symptoms is more likely than the loss associated with the presence of symptoms but milder disease.[57] One explanation of this finding is that individuals with OA limit their functional activities to avoid movements that are painful. In the clinical examination of the patient with OA one might assume that pain is a primary factor in limiting function as is the case in patients with RA. A clinical examination predicated on this assumption could lead to the hasty conclusion that the patient's functional status is normal if pain is absent. Given that individuals with OA may reduce or eliminate their symptoms by avoiding certain activities, clinicians should explore functional limitations in patients with OA separately from the evaluation of symptoms.

MEDICAL MANAGEMENT

Pharmacological Therapy in Rheumatoid Arthritis

In RA, joint destruction and irreversible damage are most pronounced in the first years after disease onset. Therefore, medical management includes an aggressive approach to stop or retard the disease process as well as to control pain and inflammation. It is currently believed that adequate pharmacological therapy initiated in the early stages of the disease results in less joint damage and functional loss. There are three major classifications of drugs used in RA management: nonsteroidal anti-inflammatory drugs (NSAIDs), corticosteroids, and disease-modifying antirheumatic drugs (DMARDs).[1,58,59]

NONSTEROIDAL ANTI-INFLAMMATORY DRUGS

NSAIDs are a basic element in long-term treatment of RA, having both **analgesic** and anti-inflammatory actions. At lower doses, the NSAID effect is analgesic, through the peripheral inhibition of pro-inflammatory prostaglandin synthesis. At higher doses, the effect is anti-inflammatory probably through both prostaglandin inhibition and alteration in macrophage and neutrophil function. Although NSAIDs provide symptomatic relief, they do not alter the underlying disease process. There are a great many NSAIDs available over the counter and by prescription. The major differences are dosing parameters, cost, and potential side effects; all have similar rates of discontinuance for toxicity. The major serious and most common side effects are gastrointestinal complaints ranging from nausea to gastrointestinal bleeding and ulcers. Individuals at increased risk for gastrointestinal complications are the elderly, smokers, those taking corticosteroids, and those with severe arthritis or comorbidities. If NSAID use is essential, some products may be found to have less toxicity than others, and prophylactic therapy is available. Other possible side effects include dizziness, headache, drowsiness or **tinnitus,** kidney dysfunction, and elevation of liver enzymes. Patients taking NSAIDS should be monitored every 3 to 4 months with CBC and biochemical profiles, as well as stool guaiac assessment for occult blood.

The original NSAID was aspirin, which is still comparable in effectiveness, but requires up to 35 tablets a day to achieve an anti-inflammatory effect. The decision of which NSAID to prescribe is based on known toxicities, dosing preferences, and cost. Individual response to an NSAID is extremely variable in terms of both effectiveness and tolerance. Therefore, it often requires several month-long trials to find the best product. Taking more than one NSAID increases the risk of toxicity with no increase in benefit. NSAIDs are prescribed for patients with RA at the onset of symptoms to provide rapid pain relief and control of inflammation while waiting for the slower-acting DMARD to become effective. Table 21–3 lists the NSAIDs currently available.

DISEASE-MODIFYING ANTIRHEUMATIC DRUGS

DMARDs are a heterogenous group of drugs exhibiting a wide range of chemical structures, modes of actions, clinical indications, and toxicities. To be classified as a DMARD, a drug must show evidence of changing the course of RA for at least 1 year (improved function, reduced inflammation, and slowing or prevention of structural damage). DMARDs are slow acting, requiring from 3 weeks to 3 months to become effective. Currently prescribed DMARDs include gold compounds (oral and parenteral), penicillamine, antimalarial drugs, sulfasalazine, methotrexate, azathioprine, cyclophosphamide, and cyclosporin. These drugs once were known as "second-line agents," denoting their late introduction in treatment for fear of serious toxicity. However, evidence shows that these drugs are no more toxic than NSAIDs, and current philosophy is to initiate DMARDs early and attempt to maintain treatment for at least 2 to 5 years. Individuals taking DMARDs should be monitored regularly for the toxicities accompanying the specific drug.

Methotrexate has demonstrated outstanding effectiveness, safety and long-term acceptability, as well as exhibiting a fairly rapid onset of action (3 to 6 weeks). Common side effects are nausea, vomiting, diarrhea, and mouth ulcers. Potentially more serious, but less common, are liver toxicity and pulmonary interstitial inflammation. Individuals taking methotrexate should be monitored for toxicity and cautioned to avoid alcohol. Table 21–3 lists the most common DMARDs.

CORTICOSTEROIDS

Corticosteroids are analogs of the naturally occurring hormone cortisone, and are the most powerful anti-inflammatory drugs available. Corticosteroids may be given systemically via oral or intravenous routes, or locally via intra-articular or periarticular injection. After the discovery of cortisone in the 1940s, until the serious, life threatening side effects of long-term use were recognized in the late 1950s, cortisone was thought to be a "wonder drug." Side effects of long-term, high-dose systemic corticosteroids are now known to include osteoporosis, muscle wasting, adrenal suppression, increased susceptibility to infections, impaired wound healing, cataracts, glaucoma, hyperlipidemia, and aseptic bone necrosis. The use of systemic corticosteroids to halt inflammation is still indicated in cases where there is unremitting disease and severe extra-articular inflammation. However, the drug is administered in as low a dose as possible for as short a period of time as possible to maximize benefit and minimize adverse effects. Monitoring should include blood counts, serum potassium and glucose levels, and observation for side effects.

Local injection into a joint, bursa, tendon, or tendon sheath may be used when inflammation is localized. Generally it is agreed that intra-articular injections provide benefit for local inflammation with minimal systemic effect, but should be limited to no more than 2 to 4 per year to reduce the risk of osteonecrosis and soft tissue damage.

Pharmacological Therapy in Osteoarthritis

Drug therapy in OA has no effect on disease progression and is ancillary to the more general measures of pain control, which include patient-related instruction, joint protection, and exercise. The goals of drug therapy in patients with OA are to relieve pain and decrease inflammation when it is present. Oral analgesics, NSAIDs, and corticosteroid injections are the primary medications used in OA management.[58]

Acetaminophen, an oral analgesic, is usually the drug of first choice. Acetominophen-containing compounds (Tylenol, Panadol, Anacin-3) have almost no toxicity in recommended doses and do not cause GI bleeding. However, there is no anti-inflammatory effect and acetaminophen cannot be substituted for NSAIDs in this regard. Clinical studies in OA demonstrate that acetaminophen (3 to 4 g/d) provides similar symptom relief to NSAIDs. Acetaminophen may be taken episodically as needed for pain or regularly when symptoms are more severe and long lasting.[60] Liver and kidney toxicity can occur with acetaminophen use. Hepatoxicity most often occurs after a drug overdose, but also may appear with therapeutic use, especially in individuals who drink excessive amounts of alcohol. Kidney toxicity is less common.

NSAIDs have a place in the management of persons with OA who do not respond to acetaminophen and nonpharmacological measures. NSAIDs may be used in combination with acetaminophen, and should be kept to the lowest effective dose to minimize GI toxicity. Intra-articular corticosteroid injections are often used for acute episodes with an expected modest response of 1 to 4 weeks duration.[61] The knee is the most common site; however, soft tissue injections for subacromial, anserine, and trochanteric bursitis also may be effective.

Topical analgesics may be either rubifacients, which contain methylsalicilate, chemical compounds that produce a counter-irritant effect, or capsaicin compounds, which reduce pain through depletion of the neurotransmitter substance P in

Table 21–3 DRUGS IN THE MANAGEMENT OF OSTEOARTHRITIS AND RHEUMATOID ARTHRITIS

Drug	Common Brand Names	Side Effects	Cautions and Contraindications
Analgesics			
Acetaminophen	Tylenol, Excedrin caplets, Panadol, Anacin-3	Potential for renal and liver toxicity	Not recommended with high alcohol consumption
NSAIDs	**OTC:** Advil, Motrin IB, Nuprin, Actron, Orudis KT, Aleve **Prescription:** Voltaren, Lodine, Nalfon, Ansaid, Indocin, Motrin, Ordis, Meclomen, Relafen, Naprosyn, Anaprox, Daypro, Feldene, Clinoril, Tolectin	Gastrointestinal bleeding, ulcers, nausea, diarrhea, indigestion, rash, dizziness, drowsiness, slowed blood clotting, tinnitus, uid retention	Sensitivity or allergy to similar drugs; kidney, liver or heart disease; hypertension; asthma; ulcers; anticoagulant therapy
Corticosteroids			
Systemic: oral or intravenous	Prednisone, Prednisolone, Methylprednisolone, Triamcinolone, Cortisone, Hydrocortisone, Dexamethasone	With long-term/high-dose: Cushing syndrome, osteoporosis, cataracts, insomnia, hypertension, immune suppression, elevated blood sugar, mood changes, restlessness, increased appetite	Diabetes, infection, hypothyroidism, hypertension, osteoporosis, gastric ulcer
Injection	Triamcinolone, Prednisolone, Methylprednisolone, Dexamethasone, Hydrocortisone, Betamethasone	Post-injection are (424 h), transient systemic reaction, increased diabetic symptoms, soft tissue disruption from direct injection	Presence of infection, previous failure to respond
DMARDs			
Methotrexate	Rheumatrex	Common side effects: decreased appetite, abdominal discomfort, nausea, diarrhea, skin rash, itching, oral ulcers, photosensitivity, infection, unusual bleeding/bruising, bone marrow suppression	Liver or lung disease, alcoholism, immune system or bone marrow suppression, infection, pregnancy
Injectable gold	Myochrisine, Solganol		Kidney disease, bone marrow suppression, colitis
Oral goldAuranon	Ridaura		Previous adverse reaction to gold compound, kidney, liver or inammatory bowel disease
Azathioprine	Imuran	Individual drugs may also have other specic toxicities and increase risk for other conditions	Kidney or liver disease, pregnancy
Cyclophosphamide	Cytoxan		Kidney or liver disease, pregnancy, infection
Cyclosporin	Sandimmune Neoral		Kidney or liver disease, pregnancy, infection
Hydroxychloroquine	Plaquenil		Antimalarial drug allergy, retinal abnormality, pregnancy
Penicillamine	Cuprimine Depen		Penicillin allergy, blood disease, kidney disease
Sulfasalazine	Azuldine		Sulfa or aspirin allergy, kidney or liver disease, blood disease, bronchial asthma
Minocycline	Minocin		Tetracycline or sun sensitivity

peripheral nerves. To date, the only topical analgesic to show consistent efficacy in controlled clinical trials is capsaicin.[62] Capsaicin is an alkaloid derived from red chili peppers and is available in topical analgesic creams in varying concentrations (Zostrix, Capsaicin-P, Dolorac). It has been shown to decrease pain approximately 40 percent when applied to specific joints four times daily. The initial stinging or burning sensation disappears after several days of use; however, the need for frequent daily applications may limit the acceptability of this therapy for some patients.[58]

SURGICAL MANAGEMENT

Surgery represents one of the greatest advances in the management of arthritis in the last 35 years. Surgery is not appropriate, however, for every individual with either RA or OA, and the careful selection of the patient and the timing of the procedure are critical. The primary indications for surgery are pain, loss of function, and progression of deformity, although the last two are not always correlated. Surgical outcomes are greatly affected by the personal characteristics of the individual patient such as motivation and the quality of postoperative rehabilitation. Postoperative rehabilitation goals are to restore mobility to the affected joint, promote stability within the joint, and regain active control of joint motion.

In general there are three procedures that may be performed on soft tissues: **synovectomy,** soft tissue release, and tendon transfers. Similarly, there are three general bone and joint procedures: **osteotomy,** prosthetic **arthroplasty,** and **arthrodesis.** The choice of specific postoperative physical therapy procedures will depend on the particular surgical intervention, the extent of joint involvement prior to surgery, individual characteristics of the patient, and manifestations of the disease. It is particularly important to remember that the patient with RA, compared to a peer with OA, will have multiple joint involvement, which will ultimately affect the functional outcome of the procedure. The patient with RA is also likely to be a surgical candidate at a much younger age than the patient with OA.[1,63]

Over 500,000 total joint arthroplasty (TJA) surgeries of the hip or knee are performed annually, the majority of which are for patients with OA.[64] These highly successful procedures have revolutionized the management of disabling arthritis in the lower extremity. The physical therapist is an important member of an interdisciplinary team involved in preoperative education, postoperative management, and rehabilitation. The primary goals following TJA are to restore function, decrease pain, and gain muscle control to enable the individual to return to previous, or improved, levels of functioning. Immediate postoperative and rehabilitation management is shaped by a variety of factors, including the type of prosthesis, as well as surgical technique and approach. Initial treatment includes therapeutic exercise, transfer and gait training, and instruction in ADLs.[64] Once the individual has achieved an adequate level of function and release from surgical precautions, instruction in establishing a routine of regular exercise and physical activity to support musculoskeletal and cardiovascular fitness is crucial to long-term outcomes and quality of life. A study investigating knee joint motion, strength, and gait in older persons who had undergone unilateral TJA knee arthroplasty 1 year previously, and who were considered to be "rehabilitation successes," found significant differences between the OA subjects and control subjects without arthritis in lower extremity range of motion, muscle performance, and gait. During walking, active knee ROM was less than expected, ROM and angular velocity of knee and hip were less on the side with the arthroplasty and greater on the unaffected side, and joint loading was less at heel strike on the side with the arthroplasty and greater and more rapid on the unaffected side. Push off was diminished bilaterally, as were gait velocity and stride length.[65]

REHABILITATIVE MANAGEMENT

Because arthritis is a chronic, progressive disease, care providers must always concern themselves with the long-range trajectory of the illness beyond the particular point in time that the care is provided. RA is a systemic disease with multiple impacts on all facets of the individual's life. OA can significantly alter a person's function and quality of life. Although each professional regards the individual as a whole person, the expertise of each professional addresses only certain aspects of the complex and interconnected problems faced by that individual. Without a broad range of expertise, none of these problems can be adequately solved. Therefore, the rehabilitation of the individual with arthritis requires the intense and coordinated efforts of a variety of health professionals including physical therapists. Although a therapist may provide services to assist a person in adjusting to the effects of a medical condition, it is the individual who must live within the constraints imposed by the illness each day and who is the ultimate authority on the goals of therapy in whatever setting services are provided.

The objectives of treatment of OA and RA are similar: to maximize function and impede or remediate musculoskeletal impairment. Owing to the global effects of RA on function, the remainder of this chapter will concentrate on the patient with RA, assuming that similar goals and treatment will apply to the individual with OA and can be adapted whenever appropriate. The overall rehabilitation goals in RA are specific to the three stages of inflammation: acute, subacute, and chronic. During the acute stage, the primary goal is to reduce pain and inflammation by resting affected joints and applying pain relief modalities. Other goals are to maintain ROM, strength, and endurance, and assist independence in ADLs. As the inflammation subsides and the individual enters the subacute stage, efforts should be directed toward increasing ROM, strength, and endurance and regaining independence in a broader range of ADLs. Affected joints should continue to be protected through proper positioning and reduced biomechanical stress. Once the inflammatory process has been controlled, the goals of rehabilitative management will change. Expanded goals will include the independent resumption of previous levels of ADL including work. The rehabilitation program will also seek to maintain optimal levels of physical, psychological, and social functioning with particular emphasis on patient education that enables the individual to reestablish a sense of control over one's life despite chronic illness.[14,66,67]

Physical Therapist Examination

The primary functional limitations of the individual with RA result from impairment of the musculoskeletal system. Therefore, an extensive and careful examination of the musculoskeletal system as it contributes to the overall functional disability of the patient is imperative. Because quality care of the individual with RA involves an entire team of professionals, the physical therapist must carefully review the chart, if one is available in the setting in which the services will be provided, and consult with all other caregivers to ascertain their proposed plans and goals of intervention.

The physical therapist should begin an examination by taking a patient history that will orient the therapist to the nature and extent of the current problem and relate that problem to the patient's past medical history. During the interview the therapist should elicit from the patient that individual's understanding of the disease and what is personally seen as the major problem at hand. In particular, the therapist should be concerned with identifying "red flag" signs and symptoms that indicate the need for immediate medical follow up (Table 21–4).[68] In the acute and subacute stages, the patient is most often concerned with pain, which should be assessed in terms of its location, duration, and intensity along with the other signs of inflammation (heat, **erythema,** and swelling). In the chronic stages, individuals are usually more concerned with loss of function, deformity, and the prevention of further deterioration. Specific information on joint symptoms, morning stiffness, previous level of activity, pattern and degree of fatigue, and current medication regimen should also be gathered. Although the majority of tests and measures used in examining the individual with RA are generic to the practice of physical therapy, many of these procedures require particular adaptations owing to the nature of joint involvement. Following the history, a review of the cardiopulmonary, integumentary, and neuromuscular systems should be undertaken before performing more definitive examination of the musculoskeletal system.

Table 21–4 "RED FLAGS" SUGGESTING THE NEED FOR URGENT EVALUATION AND MANAGEMENT

Flag	Differential Diagnosis
History of significant trauma	Soft tissue injury, internal derangement, or fracture
Hot, swollen joint	Infection, systemic rheumatic disease, gout, pseudogout
Constitutional signs (e.g., fever, weight loss, malaise)	Infection, sepsis, systemic rheumatic disease
Weakness	
Focal	Focal nerve lesion (compartment syndrome, entrapment neuropathy, mononeuritis multiplex, motor neuron disease, radiculopathy[a])
Diffuse	Myositis, metabolic myopathy, paraneoplastic syndrome, degenerative neuromuscular disorder, toxin, myelopathy,[a] transverse myelitis
Neurogenic pain (burning, numbness, parathesia)	
Asymmetric	Radiculopathy,[a] reflex sympathetic dystrophy, entrapment neuropathy
Symmetric	Myelopathy,[a] peripheral neuropathy
History of significant trauma	Soft tissue injury, internal derangement, or fracture
Claudication pain pattern	Peripheral vascular disease, giant cell arteritis (jaw pain), lumbar spinal stenosis

[a]Radiculopathy and myelopathy may be due to infectious, neoplastic, or mechanical processes.

RANGE OF MOTION

Goniometric measurement of passive ROM is indicated at all affected joints following a gross ROM assessment. Common wisdom suggests that a complete goniometric baseline is useful for documenting the progression of a chronic disease. Unless the method of measurement for each joint has been standardized in the clinical setting and used in every assessment, the potential variations in intrarater and interrater reliability of goniometry call this practice into question, particularly given the considerable time that gathering such a database requires.[69] Although such a database may be useful in terms of a particular physical therapy episode of care, it is of questionable value when compared to data collected by another therapist using a different instrument and method of measurement. If joint pain or poor activity tolerance prohibit measurement of passive ROM, the therapist may consider substituting a functional ROM test by asking the patient to touch various body parts (e.g., the top of the head and small of the back) to determine the ROM available for performing self-care activities. During the ROM examination, the therapist should note any tenderness, crepitus, or pain on movement.

A number of studies demonstrate that arthritis in "only" one joint is more typically a multijoint problem. A consistent finding regarding lower extremity ROM in the presence of OA of the knee is decreased ROM in the hip, knee, and ankle of the involved side, as well as significantly limited motion in all three joints of the uninvolved limb. When older persons with knee OA are compared to nonarthritic controls, ROM in both limbs and at all joints is diminished.[70]

When there is OA in a hip or knee, active motion in functional positions should be examined in all joints of both lower extremities. It is important to observe motion for symmetry and smoothness during gait, stair climbing, and arising from a chair. Ascending stairs requires the greatest amount and velocity of knee flexion and may be one of the best activities for assessment of knee function.[65] Decreased ROM at the hip and knee increases the risk for injury and falls. Nearly 50 degrees hip flexion and 90 degrees knee flexion are required to recover balance from a stumble during walking.[71]

STRENGTH

Application of standard manual muscle tests to assess strength in RA may be inappropriate because of pain at various points in the range. A patient may be strong in the pain-free portion of range, but weak secondary to reflex inhibition in the very portion of the range that is essential to a functional activity. Joint effusions also inhibit muscle contraction.[72] Individuals with severe deformity and deranged joints are inappropriate candidates for traditional tests of strength. A functional test of strength, therefore, is more indicative of rehabilitation needs and will identify the anticipated goals of strengthening programs prior to initiating treatment. An additional complicating factor in the application of conventional muscle tests is the frequent display of the lag phenomenon. Because the patient is able to move only partway through the available range, traditional grading systems are not sensitive to recording changes, because the gap between active and passive ROM narrows as a result of treatment. A therapist may want to comment specifically on the degrees of active motion and the grade of strength exhibited in that arc of motion. If a traditional testing method is used, therapists should also document the particular approach to testing used (e.g., break testing, isometric holding at the end of range, or resistance throughout the ROM), which will clarify the meaning of the grade assigned. Break testing generally yields higher grades than would be received if full range testing were done. It is also important to record whether the patient was receiving any medications that might alter performance or exercise tolerance. The therapist also may wish to document the time of day to account for the effects of morning stiffness.

The functional threshold for lower extremity strength has yet to be determined. However, reports from studies that have assessed knee strength as a percentage of body weight suggest that isokinetic strength measured at velocities between 60 and 180 degrees per second should be 20 and 30 percent body weight for knee extension and 20 to 25 percent for knee flexion.[65,70] Isometric knee extension below 10 kg of force (measured with the hip at neutral and knee at 90 degrees) corresponded to marked disability in a study of persons with OA of the knee.[47]

JOINT STABILITY

The ligamentous laxity of any affected joint should be fully investigated. Ligamentous instability of upper and lower extremity joints may be a significant deterrent to ADL and ambulation. Improper loading of an unstable joint may also further contribute to its deformation.

ENDURANCE

Fatigue is one of the systemic manifestations of RA and should be carefully examined both during the course of a single day and over several days to obtain a full understanding of its pattern. The decreased cardiovascular fitness of individuals with RA demands specific attention.[30] Heart rate, respiratory rate, and blood pressure should all be measured during a functional activity that is reasonably stressful for the patient's current level of fitness. Excessive increases may indicate the need for more extensive and sophisticated tests and measures. Because the costosternal and costovertebral articulations are synovial joints, chest expansion, breathing, and coughing may be compromised in the patient with RA and should be examined.

FUNCTIONAL ASSESSMENT

As with any long-term disease process, a number of different functional tests may be indicated. Functional assessments may include ADL, work, and leisure activities (see Chapter 11). The choice of a functional assessment instrument is influenced by several factors including the characteristics and needs of the individual patient, the level and depth of information required, and its predictive value in gauging the efficacy of treatment.[73–75] As with goniometric measurement, the reliability and validity of the instrument should be known if the data are to be used for comparative purposes. The Functional Status Index, which was designed expressly to be used in outpatient rheumatologic settings, is an instrument known to be reliable and valid as well as provide enough baseline data to be an effective screen of patient performance (see Appendix A).[76,77] This instrument is used to establish an individual's function in a representative sample of typical ADL along the parameters of pain, difficulty, and dependence experienced by the individual in performing these activities. Another arthritis-specific instrument, the revised Arthritis Impact Measurement Scales (AIMS2), expands the concept of function to include performance in psychological and social domains as well as physical function. The AIMS2 also measures the patient's satisfaction with current functional status and individual preferences for outcome.[78]

MOBILITY AND GAIT

A complete examination of bed mobility and transfers is essential, particularly in the initial acute stage or later recurrence of multiple joint inflammation. A complete and detailed gait examination is one of the most important contributions of the physical therapist to the rehabilitation team's understanding of the individual's functional abilities and serves to identify additional areas for examination and intervention (Table 21–5).[79] Substantial differences in knee ROM and gait velocity between patients with either OA or RA and their peers without arthritis have been demonstrated.[80]

SENSORY INTEGRITY

Any indication of peripheral neuropathy or nerve involvement should be investigated using standard examination procedures (see Chapter 6). Sensory changes that are concomitant with other conditions such as diabetes or normal processes such as aging should be considered when appropriate.

PSYCHOLOGICAL STATUS

There is no personality type specific to individuals with RA or any other kind of arthritis that has been demonstrated in any scientifically acceptable way. Individuals with chronic arthritis experience years of functional and social loss that would stress any person's ability to cope and adapt.[81] Reports of pain are, however, significantly correlated with self-reports of depression but not correlated with functional level.[82] The overall psychological status of the individual with RA is generally similar to those individuals with other chronic diseases that threaten a severe change in body image and disruption of social integration. Individuals respond to these threats with various coping strategies to maintain psychological equilibrium. No single strategy is better than another, although some strategies ultimately facilitate the achievement of positive outcomes whereas others hinder an individual's progress toward self-chosen goals. Assessment of the patient's attitude toward rehabilitation as well as that of family members can assist the therapist in achieving the goals of treatment as well as instill a

Table 21–5 ANALYSIS OF GAIT DEVIATIONS, PHYSICAL EXAMINATION FINDINGS, AND TREATMENT GOALS

Gait Deviations	Physical Examination Findings	Treatment Goals
Pronated foot		
Shuffled progression	Tenderness over subtalar midtarsal area	Relieve subtalar and midtarsal joint stresses
Decreased step length	Limited inversion range	Increase ankle inversion
Initial contact with medial border of foot	Weak and painful posterior tibialis muscle	Strengthen posterior tibialis muscle
Decreased single-limb balance	Pronated weight-bearing posture of foot	Stabilize hypermobile joints with rigid orthosis
Prolonged double-support phase	Lax medial collateral ligament of knee	Maintain neutral alignment in stance by foot positioning
Late heel rise		
Plantarflexion of ipsilateral ankle in swing		
Genu valgus with weight-bearing		
Hallux valgus		
Lateral and posterior weight shift	Lateral deviation of great toe	Accommodate foot with wide toe box shoe
Late heel rise	Swelling of first MTP joint	Increase extension of great toe
Decreased single-limb balance	Shortening of flexor hallucis brevis muscle	Relieve weight-bearing stresses
	Tenderness of great toe	
	Weakness of great toe abduction	
Metatarsophalangeal joint subluxation		
Diminished roll off	Painful MTP heads with weight-bearing	Redistribute pressure with metatarsal bar
Decreased single-limb stance	Callus formation over MTP heads	Relieve pressure with soft cutout shoe insert
Apropulsive progression	Ulcerations over MTP heads	Increase flexion mobility of MTP joints
Decreased single-limb balance	Limited MTP flexion	Accommodate foot with extra-depth shoe
	Prominent MTP heads	
Hammer or claw toes		
Diminished roll off	Posture of MTP joint hyperextension with proximal and distal interphalangeal joint flexion	Improve toe alignment with metatarsal bar
Decreased single-limb stance		Accommodate foot with extra-depth shoe
Apropulsive progression	Posture of MTP and distal interphalangeal joint hyperextension with proximal interphalangeal flexion	
Decreased single-limb balance		
	Callus formation at plantar tips and dorsum of proximal interphalangeal joint	Diminish pressure with soft insert
	Limited MTP flexion	Increase toe mobility
Painful heel		
Toe-heel pattern	Painful active plantar flexion	Decrease inflammation with steroid injection or modalities
No heel contact in stance	Painful passive and active dorsiflexion	Relieve weight-bearing stress
Decreased stride length	Swelling and pain at Achilles insertion	Decrease pressure over spur with soft shoe insert
Decreased velocity	Tenderness over spur	
Plantarflexion of ankle in swing	Decreased ankle dorsiflexion range	Maintain ankle mobility
Increased hip flexion in swing		
Decreased step length of contralateral limb		

From Dimonte and Light,[79] with permission.
MTP, metatarsal-phalangeal.

realistic, yet positive, orientation to future functional ability. The individual with RA is requested to implement a series of changes in daily life with respect to medications, exercise, and self-care. Failure to comply with professional recommendations is often interpreted as a rejection of the care provider's assistance or psychologically maladaptive behavior. The physical therapist must avoid using one's professional authority as a reason to exert control over another person. Allowing the individual to set the direction of treatment and to use the expertise of the care provider to attain these self-chosen goals offers the greatest opportunity for responsible and humane care.

ENVIRONMENTAL BARRIERS

The therapist should be aware of physical barriers in the home and work environments that might require specific examination and recommendations for change (see Chapter 12). A discussion about the home and work environments may reveal conditions that impede regaining complete independence and make the individual aware of the possibilities for altering these environments. The costs of such changes may be a limiting factor for implementing these recommendations.

Goals and Outcomes

Specific goals and outcomes of physical therapist intervention for the individual with arthritis include the following:
1. Decrease pain.
2. Increase or maintain the ROM of all joints sufficient for functional activities.
3. Increase or maintain muscle strength sufficient for the patient's level of function.
4. Increase joint stability and decrease biomechanical stress on all affected joints.
5. Increase endurance for all functional activities.
6. Promote independence in all ADLs, including bed mobility and transfers.
7. Improve efficiency and safety of gait pattern.
8. Establish patterns of adequate physical activity or exercise to maintain or improve musculoskeletal and cardiovascular fitness.
9. Educate the patient, family and other personnel to promote the individual's capacity for self-management.

The particular goals and outcomes identified for each patient will depend on the type of arthritis, the clinical presentation, and individual circumstances. Although programs for individuals with chronic diseases usually stress self-reliance, therapists must be accountable for their own professional actions. This includes determining the plan of care, implementing that plan safely and effectively, and delegating responsibility appropriately. One component of professional accountability is documentation of anticipated goals and outcomes that allow an outside party to determine the purposes of intervention and the degree to which the therapist realized these objectives. The therapist should also be able to ensure that these objectives are attained in the most expedient manner. Goals and outcomes should be specifically tailored to meet the needs of the patient and should be stated clearly in terms of measurable criteria and the time period proposed for achievement (e.g., increase ROM of the left shoulder in 3 weeks, and independent ambulation with platform crutches for at least 250 feet without fatigue within 1 month). Stating time frames for achievement of goals and outcomes serves as a check for the therapist. Failure to achieve a certain goal in a proposed period of time suggests that the therapist needs to reevaluate the nature of the problem or reformulate the plan of care along different lines to produce the desired effect. Goals and outcomes should be revised to reflect changes owing to other factors that may affect progress or alter the proposed time frames.

Direct Interventions

MODALITIES FOR PAIN RELIEF

Therapists may choose from a variety of physical agents that provide superficial and deep heat as well as superficial cold to affected joints. The primary purpose of using any of these modalities is to suppress and control the symptoms of inflammation. Superficial heat is used to produce localized analgesia and increase local circulation in the area to which it is applied. It penetrates only a few millimeters, however, and does not enter the depth of the synovial cavity. Superficial heat can be delivered through a number of means: moist hot pack, dry heating pads and lamps, paraffin, and hydrotherapy. There is no conclusive evidence that any method of application achieves a significantly better therapeutic effect, but patients often report clinically a greater tolerance for and comfort derived from moist heat. Paraffin is particularly useful in delivering superficial heat to irregularly shaped joints or to individuals who cannot tolerate the weight of a moist hot pack. Although paraffin mixtures can be concocted at home by the patient, instructions for their use should be provided cautiously because of the high flammability of the wax. Although hydrotherapy is one of the most expensive and time-consuming methods for delivering superficial heat, it does have the added advantage that the therapist can combine heat with exercise. It may also orient the patient to the value of a therapeutic swimming program that can be undertaken in conjunction with or following treatment.

Deep heating modalities may affect the viscoelastic properties of collagen and increase the plastic stretch of ligaments. Their use in treating individuals with RA during the acute stage of inflammation is contraindicated in that they may stimulate collagenase activity within the joint furthering its destruction.[83–85]

Local applications of cold will also produce local analgesia and increase superficial circulation at the site of application following an initial period of vasoconstriction. It is particularly useful around joints that are swollen, a condition that usually worsens with the application of superficial heat modalities. Therapists may use either wet or dry application techniques. Superficial cold is contradicted in patient's with **Raynaud's phenomenon** or *cryoglobulinemia,* an abnormal protein in the blood that forms gels at low temperatures. Both may be associated with RA.[67]

Therapists may also wish to consider using other modalities for pain relief in treating the individual with RA including relaxation training and transcutaneous electrical nerve stimulation (TENS), although the value of TENS as reported in the literature is controversial.[86,87] Splints may be used to immobilize specific joints and help reduce pain and swelling by providing local rest. They may also negatively impact function during the times they are worn and should be used judiciously for this purpose.[14] Complete bed rest may similarly be beneficial but should be weighed against the deleterious systemic effects on the musculoskeletal and cardiopulmonary systems that its overuse can produce.[67,88–90]

JOINT MOBILITY

A major factor affecting joint mobility in individuals with RA is the position in which they are kept when not in motion. Patients should be taught proper positioning when resting and should be encouraged to perform self-ROM to the extent possible, especially when any joint has been immobilized. In the acute stage, joint motion should be kept to a minimum because repetitive motion aggravates inflammation and delays recovery.[91] Therapists may apply neurophysiological principles of therapeutic exercise to lengthen shortened muscles.[92] Patients should be given the opportunity to rest frequently when performing these exercises. Pain should be respected at all times and should be minimal after exercise. Common wisdom recommends that exercise-induced pain should subside within 1 hour. If the patient reports discomfort in excess of 1 hour, it is a good indicator that either the intensity or the duration of the exercise was too great and should be reduced at the next treatment session. Patients should be encouraged to exercise on their own during those times of the day when they feel best. Therapists should coordinate their treatment sessions with a patient's medication schedule so that treatment will be administered during a period of maximum analgesia. Local pain relief modalities prior to or following treatment are important considerations and should be used as indicated. Splints and casts may be used to maintain newly gained ROM following treatment.[67]

STRENGTHENING

Decreased muscle function (strength, endurance, power) in persons with arthritis arises from a number of sources: intra-articular and extra-articular inflammatory disease processes, side effects of medication, disuse, reflex inhibition in response to pain

and joint effusion, impaired proprioception, and loss of mechanical integrity around the joint. A variety of muscle conditioning programs can be effective for improving strength, endurance, and function without exacerbation of pain or disease activity.[93]

Initially, isometric exercise may be indicated to improve muscle tone, static endurance, and strength and to prepare joints for more vigorous activity. Isometric contractions performed at 70 percent of the maximal voluntary contraction, held for 6 seconds and repeated 5 to 10 times per day, can increase strength significantly. Successful isometric regimens have included contractions at several combinations of muscle length and joint angles.[94] Although isometric exercise does avoid the concern of joint motion and mechanical irritation, it can produce other unwanted effects. Isometric exercise at more than 40 percent maximal voluntary contraction constricts blood flow through the exercising muscle. Restricted circulation in the muscle can produce unnecessary postexercise muscle soreness, and the increased peripheral vascular resistance produces increased blood pressure. In the knee and hip, high-intensity isometric contraction has been shown to significantly increase intra-articular pressure.[95,96]

Instructions to a patient for isometric exercise should include the cautions to (1) maintain the contraction for no more than 6 seconds, (2) avoid maximal effort because it is neither necessary nor desirable, (3) exhale during the contraction and inhale during a similar time period of relaxation, (4) and not contract more than two muscle groups at a time.

Dynamic exercise includes both shortening (concentric) and lengthening (eccentric) contractions. Strength and endurance may be improved through resistance (physiological overload) supplied by weight of the body part or external resistance in the form of free weights, elastic bands, or a variety of resistive exercise equipment. A cautious approach to resistance training is recommended to protect unstable or inflamed joints from damage. Strengthening exercise should be performed within the pain-free range. Maximum benefit and maintenance can be achieved by incorporating functional movements and body positions in the recommended exercise routine. The patient should learn to perform exercises rhythmically with well-controlled movement toward the outer part of the range and to modify resistance, repetitions, or frequency as needed. Gradual progression of resistance and repetition is recommended. Reduction in intensity, frequency, or motion should be made if increased joint swelling or pain occurs. Loads of up to 70 percent one repetition maximum (1RM) used in a circuit resistance training program of persons with controlled RA demonstrated no exacerbation in joint symptoms and significant improvements in strength and function.[32] In persons with knee osteoarthritis, 16 weeks of progressive muscular training including isometric and isotonic exercise of increasing loads and speeds resulted in improved function, independence, and decreased pain.[94] Table 21–6 summarizes major considerations in selecting isometric or dynamic strengthening.

JOINT STABILITY

Splints may be used to relieve pain, reduce inflammation, protect weak joints, preserve anatomical alignments, and enhance function. There is no conclusive evidence, however, that they prevent deformities beyond the degree they help to relieve inflammation during acute periods.[14] Therapists should target functional activities that require specific techniques of joint protection.[97] Patients should be encouraged to incorporate joint care into all ADL to minimize pain and conserve energy (see Appendix B).

Splinting of the lower extremity joints may also provide relief during periods of acute inflammation and pain.[98] When the patient is ready to resume functional activities and ambulation, foot orthotics can serve the dual purpose of relieving biomechanical stresses and enhancing function.[24,99–101] For example, a **metatarsal bar** or **metatarsal pad** may be used to relieve metatarsal pain and pressure. Finding the proper shoe can be a vexing problem for the individual with arthritic foot deformities, particularly as cosmesis evaporates with each additional recommendation for a shoe modification. The cost of special shoes may be formidable for some individuals and may not be reimbursable under many insurance programs. A good shoe will provide support and eliminate unnecessary joint motion in the talocalcaneal joint with a firm and wide heel counter. It should also help to maintain normal bony alignment and accommodate all existing foot deformities within a toe box of adequate dimensions. Pressure should be evenly distributed along the plantar surface of the foot during weight bearing. The latter goal may require the fabrication of orthoses. A **rocker sole** or shoe sole that is curved at the toe can be used to facilitate pushoff for limited ankle motion.

ENDURANCE TRAINING

The cardiovascular fitness of individuals with RA or OA may be compromised. Several studies have attested to the ability to improve this impairment through regular cardiovascular conditioning without aggravating joints. Programs similar to those designed for patients with cardiac conditions can be instituted for individuals with arthritis by adapting the method of conditioning to a non-weight-bearing apparatus such as a bicycle ergometer or aquatic program. Furthermore, patients who have engaged in such a program often report an increase in self-esteem and psychological outlook.[102–109]

FUNCTIONAL TRAINING

Functional training for the individual with RA proceeds in the same fashion as it would be accomplished for other individuals with similar deficits. Therapists may choose to reduce the functional demands of an activity either temporarily, such as under conditions of acute inflammation, or permanently by incorporating a variety of aids into ADL that substitute for lost ROM and strength. These modifications can include long-handled appliances and devices with built-up handles for easier grasp. There are aids for dressing and grooming as well as personal hygiene.

Upper extremity involvement, particularly of the wrist and hands, may complicate the choice of an ambulation aid by precluding any weight-bearing on these affected joints. In these instances, platform attachments can be used to transform the forearm into a weight-bearing surface. Rearranging the home or work environment also can improve a person's functional abilities. Raising beds or chairs can reduce the effort needed to stand up. Railings placed around the bed, bath, and along stairways also can help increase an individual's independence.

Table 21–6 PURPOSES, PARAMETERS AND PRECAUTIONS FOR ISOMETRIC AND DYNAMIC EXERCISES FOR STRENGTHENING

Isometric	Dynamic
Purpose	
• Minimize atrophy • Prepare for dynamic and weight-bearing activity • Improve muscle tone • Maintain/increase static strength and endurance	• Increase muscle power • Improve function • Promote strength of bone and cartilage • Maintain/increase dynamic strength and endurance • Enhance synovial blood flow
Parameters	
• Perform at functional joint angles • Intensity: ≤ 70% one MVC • Duration: 6 second contraction • Frequency: 5–10 repetitions daily	• Perform in pain-free range • Use functional activities/movement patterns • Intensity: Progress to ≤ 70% one RM • Capable of 8–10 repetitions of motion against gravity before additional resistance • Duration: Progress to 8–10 exercises, 8–10 repetitions • Frequency: 2–3 times/week on alternate days
Precautions	
• May increase blood pressure • Exhale during contraction; avoid valsalva maneuver • May increase intra-articular pressure • Decreased muscle blood flow	• May increase biomechanical stress on unstable or malaligned joints • Avoid forces on involved hands and wrists • May increase intra-articular pressure

MVC, maximal voluntary contraction; RM, repetition maximum.

GAIT TRAINING

Specific deviations will be evident throughout the gait cycle. These will include decreased velocity, cadence and stride length, prolonged period of double support, inadequate heel strike and toe off, and diminished joint excursion through both swing and stance. Gait deviations in the patient with RA specifically owing to progressive foot deformities will also be evident (see Table 21–5).[79] Therapists should address the underlying joint and muscle impairments that contribute to these deviations prior to initiating gait training with persons with any type of arthritis.

The degree to which the gait of an individual with arthritis should, or can, approximate normal gait is one of the most difficult questions in designing a therapeutic program. Some "abnormalities" such as antalgic limping may in fact reduce joint loading. Joint destruction may necessitate the introduction of ambulation aids as cumbersome as platform crutches or rolling walkers with platform attachments. The gait of the individual with RA or OA should be safe, functional, and cosmetically acceptable to the patient rather than an unattainable idealized version of the norm.

Decreased walking speed in arthritis is common and there is general agreement that increased speed is a meaningful measure of functional improvement. For example, a person's ability to walk fast enough to cross the street with the timing of the traffic light is important for functional community locomotion. However, increased walking speed without attention to joint biomechanics may be undesirable. In a clinical trial of a nonsteroidal drug for persons with knee OA, all with a varus deformity, gait variables were included as outcome measures. The researchers found that self-reported pain diminished and walking speed increased in the active therapy group. At the same time, kinetic analysis of joint forces showed the increased speed was accompanied by increased adductor moment at the knee and greater loading of the medial compartment.[110] This additional loading of the joint and increased stress on lateral supporting tissue may not be worth the gains of increased speed. Attention to biomechanical factors thus should be considered in comprehensive management, even when drug therapy decreases pain and improves gait speed.

EDUCATION

Patient education in the rheumatic diseases has been shown to result in positive changes in knowledge, health behaviors, beliefs, and attitudes that affect health status, quality of life, and health care utilization.[111] As in any chronic illness, education should include tasks needed to deal with the condition (taking medications, exercise), tasks necessary to carry out important social and vocational roles, and tasks needed to deal with the emotional consequences of chronic illness such as depression, fear, and frustration. The evidence is overwhelming that education designed to teach self-management skills and increase client self-efficacy for these tasks is the most effective.[112] The Arthritis Foundation (1330 West Peachtree Street, Atlanta, Georgia 30309, 404/872-7100), can supply the clinician or the individual with a variety of educational materials, pamphlets, and self-help courses that will increase cognitive understanding of the disease process and self-management skills. Many local chapters of the Foundation hold individual and family support groups to increase psychosocial adaptation as well as run aquatic and land exercise programs in public facilities. The Arthritis Health Professions Association, the professional section of the Arthritis Foundation, can provide the therapist with scientific and clinical enrichment for enhanced practice as well as a network of professional colleagues who work in rheumatology.

SUMMARY

RA and OA are the two kinds of arthritis that a physical therapist is likely to see in clinical practice. The primary functional limitations of the individual with RA or OA result from musculoskeletal impairments. Irregularities on the bone surface, loss of joint mobility, muscle weakness, and atrophy contribute directly to limitations in ADL and the ability to work. Pain secondary to changes in normal joint structure and function often limits function as well. Musculoskeletal impairments related to arthritis may also lead to impairments of other systems, such as decreased cardiovascular endurance for functional activities. The physical therapist is well suited to evaluate and treat these impairments and remediate the functional limitations they cause. Rehabilitation of the individual with arthritis is most often directed toward restoring or maintaining joint mobility and strength and emphasizes functional retraining. Patient education promotes the highest possible level of functional independence.

QUESTIONS FOR REVIEW

1. What epidemiological factors are related to RA?

2. What are the major pathological changes seen in RA?

3. State two hypotheses concerning the pathogenesis of RA.

4. Describe three factors that may predispose an individual to osteoarthritis.

5. Describe two changes in articular cartilage associated with OA.

6. Name at least two laboratory tests used in the diagnosis of RA and state their purposes.

7. Explain three parameters for orienting to radiographs.

8. Describe the typical joint changes seen with RA for the following joints: atlantoaxial, temporomandibular, carpals, knees, and talocalcaneal.

9. Define the following deformities: ulnar drift, swan neck, boutonniere, hammer toes, claw toes, and hallux valgus.

10. Describe the overall goals of medical management for RA and OA.

11. What are the primary indications for surgery in RA?

12. Discuss the psychosocial impacts of arthritis and suggest how the physical therapist may assist development of patient-centered coping strategies.

13. Describe the key points in taking a history for the individual with arthritis.

14. What adaptations of standard examination procedures should be made in assessing the individual with RA?

15. What are the general goals of physical therapy in treating individuals with RA or OA?

16. Explain the progression of a strengthening program and the purpose of each kind of exercise.

17. Discuss treatment alternatives for increasing ROM.

18. Design a cardiovascular conditioning program for an individual with lower extremity joint involvement.

19. State at least four principles of joint protection and give a practical application of each.

20. What criteria guide the selection of shoes for the individual with RA?

21. What are the purposes of splints?

22. Describe gait deviations commonly associated with RA.

23. Describe what kinds of assistive devices and ambulation aids are most suited to the individual with RA.

CASE STUDIES

Case #1 – Rheumatoid Arthritis

The patient is a 35 year-old married woman who has two children in elementary school and is a tax accountant. At this time she works about 20 hours a week. She has been referred to physical therapy by her rheumatologist whom she has just seen for the third time. Her history indicates a 2-year period of complaints of joint swelling and pain, fatigue, and increasing weakness. She had been diagnosed over this time with carpal tunnel syndrome, knee osteoarthritis, fibromyalgia, and Lyme disease; however, her symptoms continued to worsen on NSAIDs and anti-depressants, and she was referred to the rheumatologist 3 months ago. History, physical examination, laboratory, and radiographic evidence have confirmed a diagnosis of seronegative RA. She began a course of methotrexate and NSAIDs 1 month ago.

At the initial examination by a physical therapist, she reports that her morning stiffness is now less than 30 minutes (high of 3 hours); pain and swelling in hands, feet, and elbows is markedly less, and she is feeling more energetic. Systems review of the integumentary system is nonremarkable except for a slight edema and redness of the distal joints of the upper extremity. Her blood pressure and respiratory rate are within normal limits. Her resting heart rate is 72 but increases to 96 with modest exertion.

ROM is limited at the shoulder, elbows, wrists and MCPs. She lacks 10 degrees of knee extension and has no ankle dorsiflexion or hip extension beyond neutral. Strength is good minus to fair. She exhibits a forward head, rounded shoulder posture, with the beginning of a marked kyphosis. She complains of the most pain in wrists, elbows, and ankles, and general weakness. She is relieved that at last she has been diagnosed with a condition for which there is effective treatment and she trusts

her rheumatologist. Her immediate goals are to regain comfortable motion, strength and stamina and to avoid deformity. Eventually she expects to be able to return to full time employment.

Guiding Questions: Case #1

1. What are the anticipated goals and desired outcomes of intervention in this case?

2. Formulate a physical therapy plan of care.

3. What resources are available to her in the community as part of her program of patient-related instruction?

4. What supportive devices might be used to decrease symptoms and increase function?

5. How would her physical therapist optimally schedule her return visits to clinic?

Case #2 – Osteoarthritis

The patient is a 68 year-old African-American woman whose bilateral knee pain has increased over the past 6 months. She is 5 feet 2 inches tall and weighs 180 pounds. She has type II diabetes, hypertension, and hypercholesterolemia for which she takes prescribed medication. She lives with her daughter's family, takes care of the two elementary school-age grandchildren, and helps with housework during the day while the parents are at work. She is having trouble getting up and down from sitting, using stairs, getting in and out of the car, bathing the children, or walking for more than 10 minutes at a time. She has had intermittent knee pain and stiffness for the past 5 years and has treated symptoms with over-the-counter medications including aspirin, acetaminophen, and NSAIDs. She also has used topical agents and a number of alternative therapies.

She recently visited her primary care physician because the increased knee pain and stiffness has made it extremely difficult for her to continue her work in the home. Radiographs show bilateral joint space narrowing, more in the medial compartments, and greater on the right. There is evidence of bony sclerosis and osteophytes. Joint alignment is good on the left, but there is slight genu varum on the right. Her physician has suggested a course of conservative measures at this time and a consult with a physical therapist. The patient and her doctor have agreed to discuss surgical options if she is not satisfied with her condition in 3 to 6 months.

Beginning with a history and systems review at the initial examination by the physical therapist, the patient reports that she no longer goes out to shop, visit, or eat out with the family because she is so slow, tires quickly and requires help to get in and out of the car and up curbs and steps without rails. She admits to feeling low and blue much of the time. Her pain is usually relieved by rest, and wakes her up only occasionally at night. Her concerns are being able to stay active and to continue her role in the family. She has heard about glucosamine and chondroitin sulfate and asks about their effectiveness and safety. Her heart rate is 84, her blood pressure is 140/80, and her respiratory rate is 16. There is no appreciable increase of her vital signs with increased activity owing to the slow pace at which she moves.

The integumentary integrity of all four extremities is unremarkable. Sensory integrity of the distal extremities is intact.

Selected tests and measures reveal weakness and loss of motion in hips, knees, and ankles bilaterally, an antalgic and slow gait, left knee pain of 7 out of 10 while walking and 9 out of 10 while climbing stairs, and right knee pain at 6 out of 10 for all activities on a visual analog scale (VAS). She is wearing house slippers and shows marked ankle pronation on the right. Weight-bearing calcaneal valgus is under 10 degrees on the right; 5 degrees on the left.

Guiding Questions: Case #2

1. What kinds of goals should the physical therapist discuss with the patient as the anticipated goals of intervention?

2. Formulate a plan of care for this patient and determine an optimal schedule for follow-up by the physical therapist.

3. What kind of orthotic device would reduce this patient's impairments and increase her function?

4. What should be included in patient-related instruction to maximize this patient's function?

5. What strategies would maximize this patient's adherence to her home program?

REFERENCES

1. Klippel, JH (ed): Primer on the Rheumatic Diseases, ed 9. Arthritis Foundation, Atlanta, 1997.
2. Arnett, FC, et al: The American Rheumatism Association 1987 revised criteria for the classification of rheumatoid arthritis. Arth Rheum 31:315, 1988.
3. O'Sullivan, JB, and Cathcart, ES: The prevalence of rheumatoid arthritis. Followup evaluation of the effect of criteria on rates in Sudbury, Massachusetts. Ann Intern Med 76:573, 1972.
4. Lawrence, RC, et al: Estimates of the prevalence of arthritis and selected musculoskeletal disorders in the United States. Arthritis Rheum 41:778, 1998.
5. Harris, ED, Jr: The clinical features of rheumatoid arthritis. In Kelley, WN, et al (eds): Textbook of Rheumatology, ed 3. Saunders, Philadelphia, 1989, p 943.
6. Spector, TD: Rheumatoid arthritis. Rheum Dis Clin North Am 16:513, 1990.
7. Crow, MK, and Friedman, SM: Microbial superantigens and autoimmune response. Bull Rheum Dis 41:1, 1992.
8. Carpenter, AB: Immunology and inflammation. In Wegener, ST, et al (eds): Clinical Care in the Rheumatic Diseases. American College of Rheumatology, Atlanta, 1996, p 9.
9. Bennett, JC: The etiology of rheumatic diseases. In Kelley, WN, et al (eds): Textbook of Rheumatology, ed 3. Saunders, Philadelphia, 1989, p 138.
10. Fox, RI, et al: Epstein Barr virus in rheumatoid arthritis. Clin Rheum Dis 11:665, 1985.
11. Harris, ED, Jr: Pathogenesis of rheumatoid arthritis. In Kelley, WN, et al (eds): Textbook of Rheumatology, ed 3. Saunders, Philadelphia, 1989, pp 905–942.
12. Goldstein, R, and Arnett, FC: The genetics of rheumatic disease in man. Rheum Dis Clin North Am 13:487, 1987.
13. Firestein, GS, and Zvaifler, NJ: The pathogenesis of rheumatoid arthritis. Rheum Dis Clin North Am 13:447, 1987.
14. Melvin, JL: Rheumatic Disease: Occupational Therapy and Rehabilitation, ed 3. FA Davis, Philadelphia, 1989.
15. Moncur, C, and Williams, HJ: Cervical spine management

in patients with rheumatoid arthritis. Phys Ther 68:509, 1988.
16. Kramer, J, et al: Rheumatoid arthritis of the cervical spine. Rheum Dis Clin North Am 17:757, 1991.
17. Gibson, KR: Rheumatoid arthritis of the shoulder. Phys Ther 66:1920, 1986.
18. Hakstian, RW, and Tubiana, R: Ulnar deviation of the fingers. J Bone Joint Surg 49:299, 1967.
19. Pahle, JA, and Raunio, P: The influence of wrist position on finger deviation in the rheumatoid hand. J Bone Joint Surg 51:664, 1969.
20. Swezey, RL, and Fiegenberg, DS: Inappropriate intrinsic muscle action in the rheumatoid hand. Ann Rheum Dis 30:619, 1971.
21. Smith, EM, et al: Role of the finger flexors in rheumatoid deformities of the metacarpophalangeal joints. Arthritis Rheum 7:467, 1964.
22. English, CB, and Nalebuff, EA: Understanding the arthritic hand. Am J Occup Ther 7:352, 1971.
23. Nalebuff, EA: Diagnosis, classification and management of rheumatoid thumb deformities. Bull Hosp Jt Dis 24:119, 1968.
24. Moncur, C, and Shields, M: Clinical management of metatarsalgia in the patient with arthritis. Clin Mngmnt Phys Ther 3:7, 1983.
25. Kirkup, JR, et al: The hallux and rheumatoid arthritis. Acta Orthop Scand 48:527, 1977.
26. Edstrom, L, and Nordemar, R: Differential changes in Type I and Type II muscle fibers in rheumatoid arthritis. Scand J Rheum 3:155, 1974.
27. Nordemar, R, et al: Changes in muscle fiber size and physical performance in patients with rheumatoid arthritis after 7 months physical training. Scand J Rheum 5:233, 1976.
28. Edstrom, L: Selective atrophy of red muscle fibers in the quadriceps in longstanding knee-joint dysfunction. J Neurol Sci 11:551, 1970.

29. Forrester, DM, and Brown, JC: The radiographic assessment of arthritis: The plain film. Clin Rheum Dis 9:291, 1983.

30. Ekblom, B, et al: Physical performance in patients with rheumatoid arthritis. Scand J Rheum 3:121, 1974.

31. Minor, MA, et al: Exercise tolerance and disease related measures in patients with rheumatoid arthritis and osteoarthritis. J Rheumatol 15:905, 1988.

32. Rall, LC, and Roubenoff, R: Body composition, metabolism, and resistance exercise in patients with rheumatoid arthritis. Arthritis Care Res 9:151, 1996.

33. Tessler, HH: The eye in rheumatic disease. Bull Rheum Dis 35:1, 1985.

34. Deal, CL, et al: The clinical features of elderly-onset rheumatoid arthritis. Arthritis Rheum 28:987, 1985.

35. Pincus, T, and Callahan, LF: Early mortality in RA predicted by poor clinical status. Bull Rheum Dis 41:1, 1992.

36. Callahan, LF, and Pincus, T: Mortality in the rheumatic diseases. Arthritis Care Res 8:229, 1995.

37. Yelin, EH, et al: The work dynamics of the person with rheumatoid arthritis. Arthritis Rheum 30:507, 1987.

38. Yelin, E, and Felts, WR: A summary of the impact of musculoskeletal conditions in the United States. Arthritis Rheum 33:750, 1990.

39. Lubeck, DP: The economic impact of arthritis. Arthritis Care Res 8:304, 1995.

40. Yelin, EH: Musculoskeletal conditions and employment. Arthritis Care Res 8:311, 1995.

41. Allaire, SH, et al: Reducing work disability associated with rheumatoid arthritis: Identification of additional risk factors and persons likely to benefit from intervention. Arthritis Care Res 9:349, 1996.

42. Mankin, HJ, and Brandt, KD: Pathogenesis of osteoarthritis. In Kelley, WN, et al (eds): Textbook of Rheumatology, ed 3. Saunders, Philadelphia, 1989, p 1469.

43. Mankin, HJ: Clinical features of osteoarthritis. In Kelley, WN, et al (eds): Textbook of Rheumatology, ed 3. Saunders, Philadelphia, 1989, p 1480.

44. Kellgren, JH, and Lawrence, JS: Atlas of Standard Radiographs: The Epidemiology of Chronic Rheumatism, vol 2. Oxford, Blackwell Scientific, 1963.

45. Altman, R, et al: Development of criteria for the classification and reporting of osteoarthritis: Classification of osteoarthritis of the knee. Arthritis Rheum 29:1039, 1986.

46. Altman R, et al: The American College of Rheumatology criteria for the classification and reporting of osteoarthritis of the hip. Arthritis Rheum 34:505, 1991.

47. McAlindon TE, et al: Determinants of disability in osteoarthritis of the knee. Ann Rheum Dis 52:258, 1993.

48. Felson, DT: Osteoarthritis. Rheum Dis Clin North Am 16:499, 1990.

49. Moskowitz, RW: Osteoarthritis—Signs and symptoms. In Moskowitz, RW, et al (eds): Osteoarthritis: Diagnosis and Medical/Surgical Management, ed 2. Philadelphia, Saunders, 1992, p 255.

50. Brandt, KD, and Fife, RS: Ageing in relation to the pathogenesis of osteoarthritis. Clin Rheum Dis 12:117, 1986.

51. Anderson, JJ, and Felson, DT: Factors associated with knee osteoarthritis (OA) in the HANES I survey: Evidence for an association with overweight, race and physical demands of work. Am J Epidemiol 128:179, 1988.

52. Felson, DT, et al: Obesity and knee osteoarthritis: The Framingham Study. Ann Intern Med 109:18, 1988.

53. Threlkeld, AJ, and Currier, DP: Osteoarthritis: Effects on synovial joint tissues. Phys Ther 68:364, 1988.

54. Radin, EL, and Paul, IL: Does cartilage compliance reduce skeletal impact loads? The relative force-attenuating properties of articular cartilage, synovial fluid, periarticular soft tissues and bone. Arthritis Rheum 13:139, 1970.

55. Radin, EL, and Paul, IL: Response of joints to impact loading. I. In vitro wear. Arthritis Rheum 14:356, 1971.

56. Gussoni, M, et al: Energy cost of walking with hip joint impairment. Phys Ther 70:295, 1990.

57. Guccione, AA, et al: Defining arthritis and measuring functional status in elders: Methodological issues in the study of disease and disability. Am J Public Health 80:945, 1990.

58. Miller, DR: Pharmocologic interventions. In Wegener, ST, et al (eds): Clinical Care in the Rheumatic Diseases. American College of Rheumatology. Atlanta, 1996, p 65.

59. Moncur, C, and Williams, HJ: Rheumatoid arthritis: Status of drug therapies. Phys Ther 75:511, 1995.

60. Stein, CM, et al: Osteoarthritis. In Wegener, ST, et al (eds): Clinical Care in the Rheumatic Diseases. American College of Rheumatology. Atlanta, 1996, p 177.

61. Meinke, CJ: Intrarticular treatment of osteoarthritis and guidelines to its assessment. J Rheumatol 21(suppl 41):74, 1994.

62. Zhang, WY, and Li Wan Po, A: The effectiveness of topically applied capsaicin: A meta-analysis. Eur J Clin Pharmacol 46:517, 1994.

63. Sledge, CB: Reconstructive surgery in rheumatic diseases. In Kelley, WN, et al (eds): Textbook of Rheumatology, ed 3. Saunders, Philadelphia, 1989, p 1927.

64. Ganz, SB, and Viellion, G: Pre- and post-surgical management of the hip and knee. In Wegener, ST, et al (eds): Clinical Care in the Rheumatic Diseases. American College of Rheumatology, Atlanta, 1996, p 103.

65. Jesevar, DS, et al: Knee kinematics and kinetics during locomotor activities of daily living in subjects with knee arthroplasty and in healthy controls. Phys Ther 73:229, 1993.

66. Minor, MA: Exercise in the management of osteoarthritis of the hip and knee. Arthritis Care Res 7:169, 1994.

67. Gerber, LH: Rehabilitation of patients with rheumatic diseases. In Kelley, WN, et al (eds): Textbook of Rheumatology, ed 3. Saunders, Philadelphia, 1989, p 1904.

68. American College of Rheumatology Ad Hoc Committee on Clinical Guidelines: Guidelines for the initial evaluation of the adult patient with acute musculoskeletal symptoms. Arthritis Rheum 39:1, 1996.

69. Miller, PJ: Assessment of joint motion. In Rothstein, JM (ed): Measurement in Physical Therapy. Churchill Livingstone, New York, 1985, p 103.

70. Messier, SP, et al: Osteoarthritis of the knee: Effects on gait, strength, and flexibility. Arch Phys Med Rehabil 73:29, 1992.

71. Grabiner, MD, et al: Kinematics of recovery from a stumble. J Gerontol 48:M97, 1993.

72. Geborek, P, et al: Joint capsular stiffness in knee arthritis. Relationship to intraarticular volume, hydrostatic pressures, and extensor muscle function. J Rheumatol 16:1351, 1989.

73. Liang, MH, et al: Comparative measurement efficiency and sensitivity of five health status instruments for arthritis research. Arthritis Rheum 28:542, 1985.

74. Guccione, AA, and Jette, AM: Assessing limitations in physical function in patients. Arthritis Care Res 1:120, 1988.

75. Guccione, AA, and Jette, AM: Multidimensional assessment of functional limitations in patients with arthritis. Arthritis Care Res 3:44, 1990.

76. Jette, AM: Functional capacity evaluation: An empirical approach. Arch Phys Med Rehabil 61:85, 1980.

77. Jette, AM: Functional Status Index: Reliability of a chronic disease evaluation instrument. Arch Phys Med Rehabil 61:395, 1980.

78. Meenan, RF, et al: AIMS2: The content and properties of a revised and expanded Arthritis Impact Measurement Scales health status questionnaire. Arthritis Rheum 35:1, 1992.

79. Dimonte, P, and Light, H: Pathomechanics, gait deviations, and treatment of the rheumatoid foot. Phys Ther 62:1148, 1982.

80. Brinkmann, JR, and Perry, J: Rate and range of knee motion during ambulation in healthy and arthritic subjects. Phys Ther 65:1055, 1985.

81. Parker, JC, and Wright, GE: Psychological assessment. In Wegener, ST, et al (eds): Clinical Care in the Rheumatic Diseases. American College of Rheumatology, Atlanta, 1996, p 41.

82. Bradley, LA: Psychological aspects of arthritis. Bull Rheum Dis 35:1, 1985.

83. Harris, ED, Jr, and McCroskery, PA: The influence of temperature and fibril stability on degradation of cartilage collagen by rheumatoid synovial collagenase. New Engl J Med 290:1, 1974.

84. Feibel, A, and Fast, A: Deep heating of joints: A reconsideration. Arch Phys Med Rehabil 57:513, 1976.

85. Oosterveld, FGJ, et al: The effect of local heat and cold therapy on the intraarticular and skin surface temperature of the knee. Arthritis Rheum 35:146, 1992.

86. Griffin, JW, and McClure, M: Adverse responses to transcutaneous electrical nerve stimulation in a patient with rheumatoid arthritis. Phys Ther 61:354, 1981.

87. Mannheimer, C, and Carlsson, C: The analgesic effect of transcutaneous electrical nerve stimulation (TENS) in patients with rheumatoid arthritis: A comparative study of different pulse patterns. Pain 6:329, 1979.

88. Partridge, REH, and Duthie, JJR: Controlled trial of the effects of complete immobilization of the joints in rheumatoid arthritis. Ann Rheum Dis 22:91, 1963.

89. Gault, SJ, and Spyker, JM: Beneficial effects of immobilization of joints in rheumatoid arthritis and related arthritis. Arthritis Rheum 12:34, 1969.

90. Mills, JA, et al: The value of bedrest in patients with rheumatoid arthritis. New Engl J Med 284:453, 1971.

91. Michelsson, JE, and Riska, EB: The effect of temporary exercising of a joint during an immobilization period: An experimental study on rabbits. Clin Orthop Rel Res 144:321, 1979.

92. Cherry, DB: Review of physical therapy alternatives for reducing muscle contracture. Phys Ther 60:877, 1980.

93. Rall, LC, et al: The effect of progressive resistance training in rheumatoid arthritis. Arthritis Rheum 39:415, 1996.

94. Fisher, NM, et al: Muscle rehabilitation: Its effect on muscular and functional performance of patients with knee arthritis. Arch Phys Med Rehabil 72:367, 1991.

95. James, MJ, et al: Effect of exercise on 99mTc-DPTA clearance from knees with effusions. J Rheumatol 21:501, 1994.

96. Krebs, DE, et al: Exercise and gait effects on in vivo hip contact pressures. Phys Ther 71:301, 1990.

97. Cordery, JC: Joint protection, a responsibility of the occupational therapist. Am J Occup Ther 19:285, 1965.

98. Nicholas, JJ, and Ziegler, G: Cylinder splints: Their use in arthritis of the knee. Arch Phys Med Rehab 58:264, 1977.

99. Locke, M, et al: Ankle and subtalar motion during gait in arthritic patients. Phys Ther 64:504, 1984.

100. Marks, RM, and Myerson, MS: Foot and ankle issues in rheumatoid arthritis. Bull Rheum Dis 46:1, 1997.

101. Fransen, M, and Edmonds, J: Off-the-shelf footwear for people with rheumatoid arthritis. Arthritis Care Res 10:250, 1997.

102. Harkcom, TM, et al: Therapeutic value of graded aerobic exercise training in rheumatoid arthritis. Arthritis Rheum 28:32, 1985.

103. Ekblom, B, et al: Effect of short-term physical training on patients with rheumatoid arthritis I. Scand J Rheum 4:80, 1975.

104. Ekblom, B, et al: Effect of short-term physical training on patients with rheumatoid arthritis II. Scand J Rheum 4:87, 1975.

105. Nordemar, R, et al: Physical training in rheumatoid arthritis: A controlled long-term study. I. Scand J Rheum 10:17, 1981.

106. Nordemar, R: Physical training in rheumatoid arthritis: A controlled long-term study. II. Functional capacity and general attitudes. Scand J Rheum 10:25, 1981.

107. Minor, MA, et al: Efficacy of physical conditioning exercise in patients with rheumatoid arthritis and osteoarthritis. Arthritis Rheum 32:1396, 1989.

108. Kovar, PA, et al: Supervised fitness walking in patients with osteoarthritis of the knee. Ann Intern Med 116:529, 1992.

109. Melton-Rogers, S, et al: Cardiorespiratory responses of patients with rheumatoid arthritis during bicycle riding and running in water. Phys Ther 76:1058, 1996.

110. Schnitzer, TJ, et al: Effect of piroxicam on gait in patients with osteoarthritis of the knee. Arthritis Rheum 36:1207, 1993.

111. Boutaugh, ML, and Lorig, KR: Patient education. In Wegener, ST, et al (eds): Clinical Care in the Rheumatic Diseases. American College of Rheumatology, Atlanta, 1996, p 53.

112. Lorig, K, and Gonzalez, V: The integration of theory and practice: A 12-year case study. Health Educ Q 19:355, 1992.

GLOSSARY*

Analgesic: Medication or modality used to relieve pain.

Ankylosing spondylitis: Chronic bone and joint disease in which the inflammatory process primarily affects the sacroiliac, spinal facet, and costovertebral joints.

Ankylosis: Immobility or fixation of a joint.

Antibody: A protein developed in response to an antigen, belonging to one of the immunoglobulin classes.

Antigen: Any substance that induces the formation of antibodies that will react specifically to that antigen.

Arthralgia: Pain in a joint.

Arthrodesis: Surgical procedure designed to produce fusion of a joint.

Arthroplasty: Any surgical reconstruction of a joint; may or may not involve prosthetic replacement.

Avascular necrosis: Necrosis of part of a bone secondary to ischemia; most commonly seen in the femoral or humeral head.

Bouchard's nodes: Osteophyte formation around the proximal Boutonniere deformity. Finger deformity with flexion of the proximal interphalangeal joint and hyperextension of the distal interphalangeal joint.

Boutonniere deformity: Contracture of hard musculature marked by proximal interphalangeal joint flexion and distal interphalangeal joint extension.

Bunion: Hallux valgus with a painful bursitis over the medial aspect of the first metatarsophalangeal joint.

Bursitis: Inflammation of a bursa that can be due to frictional forces, trauma, or rheumatoid diseases.

Carpal tunnel syndrome: Compression of the median nerve in the carpal flexor space; commonly seen in patients with flexor tenosynovitis.

Cock-up (claw) toe: Deformity with hyperextension of the metatarsophalangeal joint and flexion of the proximal and distal interphalangeal joints.

Crepitus: A grating, crunching, or popping sensation (or sound) that occurs during joint or tendon motion.

Degenerative joint disease (DJD): A name sometimes used for osteoarthritis.

deQuervain's disease: Stenosing tenosynovitis of the first dorsal compartment of the wrist involving the abductor pollicis longus and the extensor pollicis brevis.

Edema: Perceptible accumulation of excess fluid in the tissues.

Effusion: Excess fluid in the joint indicating irritation or inflammation of the synovium; escape of fluid into a body cavity.

Erythema: Redness.

Exostoses: Ossifications of muscular or ligamentous attachments.

Fibrosis: Abnormal formation of fibrous tissue.

Gout: Disease characterized by acute episodes of arthritis with the presence of sodium urate crystals in the synovial fluid or deposits of urate crystals in or about the joints and other tissues.

Hammer toe: Deformity with hyperextension of the metatarsophalangeal joint, flexion of the proximal interphalangeal, and hyperextension of the distal interphalangeal joints.

Hallux valgus: Valgus deformity at the first metatarsophalangeal joint.

Heberden's nodes: Bony enlargement of the distal interphalangeal joint; characteristic of primary degenerative joint disease.

Immune response: The reaction of the body to substances that are foreign or interpreted as foreign. A cell-mediated immune response involves the production of lymphocytes by the thymus (T cells) in response to an antigen. A humoral immune response involves the production of plasma lymphocytes (B cells) in response to an antigen and results in the formation of antibodies.

Lag phenomenon: Difference between active and passive range of motion.

Lyme disease: An epidemic, systemic inflammatory disorder characterized by recurrent episodes of polyarthritis, skin lesions, and involvement of the cardiac and nervous systems following a tick bite. Named after the Connecticut town where it was first discovered in 1975.

Mallet finger deformity: Deformity involving only flexion of the distal interphalangeal joint; secondary to disruption of the insertion of the extensor tendon into the base of the distal phalanx.

Metatarsal bar: Ridge on the sole of the shoe to relieve metatarsal pressure and pain.

Metatarsal pad: Pad placed inside the shoe proximal to the metatarsal heads to relieve metatarsal pressure and pain.

Metatarsalgia: Pain over the metatarsal heads on the plantar aspect of the foot.

Morning stiffness: This term describes the prolonged generalized stiffness that is associated with inflammatory arthritis upon awakening. The stiffness is indicative of systemic involvement. The duration of the stiffness correlates with the intensity of the disease. This generalized stiffness is in contrast to the localized stiffness seen in osteoarthritis which results from inactivity.

Mutilans-type deformity (Opera-glass Hand): Severe bony destruction and resorption in a synovial joint. In the fingers it results in a telescopic shortening.

Myositis: Inflammatory disease of striated muscle.

Osteoarthritis (OA): The most common rheumatic disease characterized by the progressive loss of articular cartilage and the formation of bone at the joint margin.

Osteophytes: Bone growths at joint margins.

Osteoporosis: Condition characterized by a loss of bone cells. It can be a primary condition or associated with other diseases, drug therapies (steroids), or disuse; can be improved or minimized with exercise.

Osteotomy: Surgical cutting of a bone.

Pannus: Excessive proliferation of synovial granulation tissue that invades the joint surfaces.

Polymyalgia rheumatica: Relatively common condition most typically found over the age of 50 and in females. Characterized by marked pain of the shoulder and pelvic girdle muscles, elevated sedimentation rate, and absence of muscle disease.

Protrusio acetabuli: Condition in which the head of the femur pushes the acetabulum into the pelvic cavity.

Pseudogout: Similar to gout clinically but a condition in which the synovitis is due to deposits of pyrophosphate crystals.

Raynaud's phenomenon: Intermittent attacks of pallor followed by cyanosis, then redness of digits, before return to normal.

Rheumatism: General term for acute and chronic conditions characterized by inflammation, muscle stiffness and soreness, and joint pain.

Rheumatoid arthritis (RA): A systemic disease characterized by a bilateral, symmetrical pattern of joint involvement and chronic inflammation of the synovium.

Rheumatoid factor (RF): An immunoglobulin found in the blood of a high percentage of adults with rheumatoid arthritis. A person may be described as seronegative or positive. A latex fixation or sheep cell agglutination test is used to determine if the factor is present.

Rocker sole: Shoe sole, curved at the toe to facilitate push off for limited ankle motion.

Sjogren's syndrome: Disease of the lacrimal and parotid glands, resulting in dry eyes and mouth; frequently occurs with rheumatoid arthritis, systemic lupus erythematosus, and systemic sclerosis.

Splayfoot: Transverse spreading of the forefoot.

Subluxation: Incomplete or partial dislocation.

Swan neck deformity: Finger deformity involving hyperextension of the proximal interphalangeal joint and flexion of the distal interphalangeal joint.

Synovectomy: Surgical procedure to remove the synovial lining of joints or tendon sheaths.

Synovium: Tissue lining synovial joints, tendon sheaths, and bursa. In the joint it produces fluid to lubricate the joint and is the part of the joint that becomes inflamed in inflammatory joint disease.

Synovitis: Inflammation of the synovium.

Systemic: A condition that affects the body as a whole.

Systemic lupus erythematosus (SLE): Systemic inflammatory disease characterized by small vessel vasculitis and a diverse clinical picture.

Tarsal tunnel syndrome: Neuropathy of the distal portion of the tibial nerve at the ankle caused by chronic pressure on the nerve at the point it passes through the tarsal tunnel.

Tendinitis: Inflammation of a tendon.

Tinnitus: Subjective ringing or buzzing sensations in the ear; used as an indicator of aspirin toxicity.

Zigzag effect: Ulnar drift at the metacarpophalangeal joints associated with radial deviation of the wrist.

---

*Adapted from Melvin, JL: Rheumatic Disease: Occupational Therapy and Rehabilitation, ed 3. FA Davis Co., Philadelphia, 1989; and Thomas, CL (ed): Taber's Cyclopedic Medical Dictionary, ed 18. FA Davis, Philadelphia, 1997.

APPENDIX A

Functional Status Index

KEY: ASSISTANCE: 1 = independent; 2 = uses devices; 3 = uses human assistance;
4 = uses devices and human assistance; 5 = unable or unsafe to do the activity

PAIN: 1 = no pain; 2 = mild pain; 3 = moderate pain; 4 = severe pain

DIFFICULTY: 1 = no difficulty; 2 = mild difficulty; 3 = moderate difficulty; 4 = severe difficulty

Time frame: On the average during the past 7 days

ACTIVITY	ASSISTANCE (1–5)	PAIN (1–4)	DIFFICULTY (1–4)	COMMENTS
Mobility				
Walking inside	_____	_____	_____	
Climbing up stairs	_____	_____	_____	
Rising from a chair	_____	_____	_____	
Personal care				
Putting on pants	_____	_____	_____	
Buttoning a shirt/blouse	_____	_____	_____	
Washing all parts of the body	_____	_____	_____	
Putting on a shirt/blouse	_____	_____	_____	
Home chores				
Vacuuming a rug	_____	_____	_____	
Reaching into low cupboards	_____	_____	_____	
Doing laundry	_____	_____	_____	
Doing yardwork	_____	_____	_____	
Hand activities				
Writing	_____	_____	_____	
Opening container	_____	_____	_____	
Dialing a phone	_____	_____	_____	
Social activities				
Performing your job	_____	_____	_____	
Driving a car	_____	_____	_____	
Attending meetings/appointments	_____	_____	_____	
Visiting with friends and relatives	_____	_____	_____	

Used by permission of Alan M. Jette.

APPENDIX B

Joint Protection, Rest, and Energy Conservation

JOINT PROTECTION

Why Is Joint Protection Important?

Overuse and abuse of arthritic joints may lead to progressive deterioration of the joint and its surrounding tissues. Positive action is necessary to protect joints, conserve energy, and preserve function.

During activity, a normal joint is protected by the muscles around it that absorb the forces on the joint, preventing undue strain on the tendons, ligaments, and cartilage. A diseased joint is mechanically weak and poorly stabilized, which can contribute to the overstretching of the tendons and ligaments and damage to the cartilage. This increased stress can increase the destruction of the joint and cause increased pain.

How Can Joints Be Protected?

The main idea in joint protection is to minimize the strain on joints in daily activities. Joint protection techniques try to reduce the force on the joint, to slow down the joint damage. Good posture and positioning, changing the method of an activity, and pacing all help to protect the joint.

Which Joints Need Protection?

People with a local type of arthritis, like osteoarthritis, need to pay close attention to the joints that are involved with the arthritis. People with a systemic or whole-body type of arthritis, like rheumatoid arthritis, need to reduce the stress on all their joints. In addition to the joint protection principles and examples listed below, people with rheumatoid arthritis should look at the section below entitled Care of Rheumatoid Arthritis in the Hands.

In planning your joint protection, start by concentrating on the joints that are currently giving you the most trouble. Check off the principles that apply most strongly to you, and list several examples of how you can apply that principle to your problem joints.

JOINT PROTECTION PRINCIPLES

Your Examples

☐ 1. *Respect Pain*
   a. It is important to distinguish between discomfort and pain. _____
   b. Pain that lasts for more than 1 to 2 hours after an activity indicates that the activity is too stressful and needs to be modified. _____
   c. If there is a sharp increase in pain during activity, stop and rest, then modify the activity. _____
   d. If there is unusual pain or stiffness the next day, look back at the previous day's activities to see if they were too strenuous. _____

☐ 2. *Avoid Positions of Deformity*
   The foremost position of deformity for most joints is flexion, bending of the joint. Maintaining a bent position increases the possibility of deformity.
   a. Stand erect, with weight evenly divided on both feet. _____
   b. Lay as flat as possible in bed; do not curl up or prop yourself up on several pillows. _____
   c. Work with your hands flat. _____
   d. Avoid tight grip or squeezing. _____

☐ 3. *Avoid Awkward Positions*
   Use each joint in its most stable and functional position: Extra strain is placed on a joint when it is twisted or rotated.
   a. Rise straight up from sitting, rather than leaning to one side for support. _____
   b. Reposition feet rather than twisting trunk or knees. _____
   c. Stand on a stool to reach overhead. _____
   d. Reposition yourself closer to object rather than stretch your reach. _____
   e. Sit to clean or garden, rather than squatting or kneeling down. _____
   f. Use good posture when you stand, sit, and lie down. _____

☐ 4. *Use Strongest Joints or Distribute the Force over Several Joints*
   The stress on each individual joint is less if it is divided over several joints. The larger joints have greater muscles surrounding them to absorb the stress.
   a. Use two hands whenever possible. _____
   b. Carry packages in both arms rather than in one. _____
   c. Carry a shoulder purse, or purse handle over forearm rather than in fingers. _____
   d. Use knapsack to carry packages on back. _____
   e. Lift objects from underneath, using wrist and elbow, rather than pinch gripping the sides. _____
   f. Lift objects with your knees bent, your back straight. _____
   g. Move large objects with body weight behind it, the push coming from the legs. _____
   h. Push with open palm or forearm rather than fingers. _____

☐ 5. *Use Adapted Equipment*
   Find equipment that will reduce the stress on the joint or make the job easier.
   The Self-Help Manual for People with Arthritis is a catalog of adapted equipment available from the local Arthritis Foundation. _____
   a. Equipment can be modified by:
      1. Building up the handle so it is easier to grasp. _____
      2. Extending the handle so it is easier to reach. _____
   b. Equipment available:
      Walking aids
      Self-care aids
      Bathroom safety
      Homemaking equipment
      Job modification equipment

Joints that need protection: _____

Activities to be modified: _____
_____
_____

ADDITIONAL REMINDERS FOR THE PROTECTION OF THE RHEUMATOID HAND

1. Through exercise, maintain wrist extension (ability to pick hand up off table) to ensure power grip.
2. Through exercise, maintain supination (ability to turn palm up) to ensure ability to hold and to carry objects.
3. Avoid positions of deformity.
   a. Finger flexion
      1. Avoid making fist or tight grip—use built-up handles.
      2. Work with hand flat—use dust mitts, sponges.
      3. Avoid prolonged holding of objects: pen, book, pan, needle.
      4. Avoid putting any pressure on bent knuckles.
   b. Ulnar deviation (tendency of fingers to slide to little finger side)
      1. Avoid pressure toward little finger side of hand.
      2. Any twisting of hand, open door knobs, jars, etc., should be turned toward thumb.
      3. Grip objects parallel across palm, not diagonal; for example, hold utensil like dagger to cut food, stir with wooden spoon.
4. Avoid stress on small joints of hand.
   a. Use two hands whenever possible.
   b. Substitute larger stronger joints: for example, lift or carry with palms or forearm, not small finger joints; carry bag over elbow or shoulder, not in fingertips.
   c. Avoid activities involving pinching motions.
   d. Avoid twisting and squeezing motions with hands.

GETTING ADDITIONAL REST

Rest is important because it reduces the pain and fatigue that accompany arthritis. In addition, it aids the body's healing process and helps control the inflammation. Rest also may reduce the stress on joints and protect them from further damage. All of these benefits are important in managing arthritis.

Each day you need to make sure you get enough whole body rest, local joint rest, and emotional rest. There are many options: Mark off the options that may be possible for you.

☐ 1. *Plenty of Nightly Rest*
   Get the usual 8 to 10 hours of nightly rest. It is not as important that you sleep for that length of time, but make sure you stretch out with your joints supported, so that your body can rest.

☐ 2. *Daily Rest Periods*
   Ideally, several times a day you can stretch out for 15 to 60 minutes with your joints supported. Again, it is the body rest, not sleep, that is most important.

☐ 3. *Five-Minute "Breathers"*
   Partway through a task, sit back and take it easy for a few minutes. This will allow you to finish the task almost as quickly but more comfortably and with less fatigue.

☐ 4. *Local Joint Rest*
   When a joint hurts, stop and rest. If your hip or knee hurts while walking, sit down for a few minutes with your legs supported; if your hand hurts while writing, stop and lay

it flat for a few minutes. Splints can be used to rest painful wrists or fingers. If your neck hurts, lay down with just a small pillow supporting the curve of your neck. Any painful joint can be given extra rest.

☐ 5. *Take Time for Relaxing Activities*
   Listening to music, reading, playing cards, or other light leisure activities all can be a pleasant change of pace and can be restful and refreshing for you.

There are unlimited options for getting additional rest. It takes creativity to find ways to fit extra rest into your schedule; then it takes self-discipline to make sure you follow through, incorporating the additional rest in your activities. Making the effort to get more rest can pay off in a reduction of pain and fatigue.

Ways to get more rest:

Systemic, whole body rest _____

Local joint rest _____

Emotional rest _____

ENERGY CONSERVATION TO REDUCE FATIGUE

Why is Energy Conservation Important?

One of the major symptoms of arthritis may be fatigue—getting tired very easily. In the inflammatory types of arthritis, fatigue may be part of the disease process. In all types of arthritis, pain and difficult movement may use up energy, so you tire more easily.

It is important to avoid getting overtired. Fatigue may increase the possibility of a flare-up in inflammatory types of arthritis like rheumatoid arthritis. In all types of arthritis, fatigue may make the pain and stiffness seem worse, and it will make activities more difficult. We hope to reduce this fatigue by conserving energy and using it carefully.

How Can You Reduce Fatigue?

Some people try to conserve energy and reduce fatigue by staying in bed all day. Others stop doing anything that is not absolutely necessary each day. Unfortunately, the activities that are usually cut out are the leisure activities—the enjoyable things people do for themselves or for fun. These are not good ideas.

You can conserve energy and reduce fatigue by modifying and simplifying your activities, pacing yourself, getting additional rest, and using adapted equipment.

Energy Conservation

By conserving your energy, you may be able to do as much or more activity with less pain and fatigue. We are trying to avoid both overactivity and underactivity. Conserving your energy and simplifying your work is *not* being lazy. It is not sensible to overtire yourself. Overwork will not keep your joints mobile, but it may damage your joints further.

It is not so much *what* you do, but *how* you do it that can help control your fatigue. An attempt should be made to modify any activities that leave you overly tired or cause pain that continues for more than 1 to 2 hours.

You will need to identify ways that your own daily activities can be simplified. As you read through the energy conservation strategies, check off strategies that may work for you, and list several of your own examples.

Continued

APPENDIX B *Continued*

☐ 1. *Plan the Task*   Your Examples
    a. Think the task through.   _____
    b. Decide when and where the job is best done.   _____
    c. Plan out the simplest approach to the job.   _____
    d. Gather all supplies before you begin.   _____
    e. Arrange step sequence so that it moves in one direction (usually left to right).   _____
    f. Use fewer, more efficient movements to complete task.   _____
☐ 2. *Eliminate Extra Trips*
    a. Organize your shopping list according to how the store is laid out.   _____
    b. Stay in the laundry room until your laundry is finished.   _____
    c. Clean one area at a time.   _____
☐ 3. *Use Good Posture and Body Mechanics*
    a. Sit to work; you will be more stable and use your strength more efficiently.   _____
    b. Use large strong muscle groups, rather than straining individual muscles and joints.   _____
    c. Lift with your knees bent, your back straight.   _____
    d. Carry objects close to your body.   _____
    e. Push objects, with body weight behind it, rather than pulling or carrying.   _____
    f. Avoid awkward bending, reaching, and twisting.   _____
☐ 4. *Don't Fight Gravity*
    a. Slide, rather than lift objects.   _____
    b. Use wheeled cart.   _____
    c. Use lightweight equipment.   _____
    d. Stabilize pitcher on surface and tilt to pour, rather than picking it up.   _____
☐ 5. *Pace Yourself*
    a. Get plenty of nightly rest.   _____
    b. Plan several rest periods during the day.   _____
    c. Rest before you get tired.   _____
    d. Avoid a rush.   _____
    e. Work at a steady rate with rest period.   _____
    f. Develop a rhythm to your movements.   _____
☐ 6. *Use Energy-Saving Devices*
    a. Convenience foods.   _____
    b. Adapted equipment.   _____

Strategies to be tried: _____   Activities to be modified: _____
_____   _____
_____   _____
_____   _____
_____   _____

Excerpted from Brady, TJ: Home Management of Arthritis: Developing Your Own Plan. Arthritis Foundation, Minnesota Chapter, Minneapolis, 1983. Used by permission of the author.

APPENDIX C

Suggested Answers to Case Study Guiding Questions
Case #1—Rheumatoid Arthritis

1. What are the anticipated goals and desired outcomes of intervention in this case?

ANSWER: The anticipated goals of treatment for this patient are to increase her endurance, self-manage her symptoms, maintain her upper and lower extremity range of motion and strength, protect her joints, and increase her independence in basic and instrumental ADLs. Her desired outcome is to return to work.

2. Formulate a physical therapy plan of care.

ANSWER: The initial plan of care includes 15 minutes of general range of motion exercises to be performed at home twice a day (after a warm shower in the morning and at night before retiring).

3. What resources are available to her in the community as part of her program of patient-related instruction?

ANSWER: She is referred to the 6-week arthritis self-management course offered by the local chapter of the Arthritis Foundation.

4. What supportive devices might be used to decrease symptoms and increase function?

ANSWER: She is fitted with resting and work splints for the wrists, semirigid foot orthotics, and supportive footwear. She is given oral and written instructions for proper posture and positioning while seated and in bed. She is encouraged to begin a walking routine in her neighborhood by beginning with a 10-minute walk at a comfortable pace in the morning and again in the afternoon, 3 days a week.

5. How would her physical therapist optimally schedule her return visits to clinic?

ANSWER: To achieve her desired outcome, the intervention was progressed to three 10-minute sessions a day, 5 days a week in addition to the home program. Eventually, she hopes to be able to return to her prior exercise habit of working out at the fitness club 4 days a week and is going to investigate the possibilities for attending aquatic aerobics and performing lap swimming. She will return to physical therapy every 2 weeks for four visits to assess her progress and revise her home exercise program as needed.

Case #2—Osteoarthritis

1. What kinds of goals should the physical therapist discuss with the patient as the anticipated goals of intervention?

ANSWER: The patient and her therapist agree that increased flexibility and strength in her lower extremities will help her achieve her functional goals and manage pain. Greater general endurance for walking and daily activities will help promote a more positive attitude about her ability to be useful and to participate in family activities. They also agree that being able to exercise with other people outside the home would help her maintain an exercise program and she would enjoy the company of other adults.

2. Formulate a plan of care for this patient and determine an optimal schedule for follow-up by the physical therapist.

ANSWER: The patient was given a 15-minute home program for lower extremity range of motion and strengthening to be done every day. She also enrolled in an Arthritis Foundation aquatic exercise program twice a week at the local YMCA.

3. What kind of orthotic device would reduce this patient's impairments and increase her function?

ANSWER: Examination of ankle and foot posture had indicated that a semirigid foot orthosis with a medial heel wedge on the right could decrease calcaneal valgus to less than 5 degrees, reduce pronation, and reduce load on the medial compartment of the knee. The patient was fitted with an orthosis and supportive walking shoes.

4. What should be included in patient-related instruction to maximize this patient's function?

ANSWER: She was instructed in proper use of a cane to use when she goes out in public and taught problem-solving strategies to minimize stair climbing at home. She also was provided a written copy of her home exercise program and other informational pamphlets from the local Arthritis Foundation on living with arthritis. She returned to the therapist weekly for four visits to review and revise the exercise program as needed.

5. What strategies would maximize this patient's adherence to her home program?

ANSWER: Her return to her physician was scheduled 4 months after she began physical therapy. At that time, she reported that she enjoys the aquatics class and performs her home program 3 to 4 times a week. Her son-in-law drops her off at the Y on his way to work in the morning and she gets a ride home with a class member or takes a taxi.

Range of motion and strength have increased at hips, knees, and ankles. She is able to transfer to and from the car and manage curbs independently. She used the cane for 2 months, but does not use it now. She reports that her knee pain is a 3 on the 0 to 10 VAS. She believes her greatest gains have been in reduction of knee pain, increased stamina

Continued

APPENDIX C *Continued*

for working around the house, and increased walking speed, which allows her to shop and make trips with her family. She states she will continue her exercise program and is interested in adding a daily walk in the neighborhood. She has decided not to use glucosamine/chondroitin supplements now, because the cost is more than what she is spending for her exercise class and taxi fare.

Multiple Sclerosis 22

Susan B. O'Sullivan

LEARNING OBJECTIVES

1. Describe the etiology, pathophysiology, symptomatology, and sequelae of multiple sclerosis (MS).
2. Identify and describe the examination procedures used to evaluate patients with MS to establish a diagnosis, prognosis, and plan of care.
3. Describe the role of the physical therapist in assisting the patient with MS in terms of direct interventions and patient-related instruction to maximize function.
4. Describe appropriate elements of the exercise prescription for patients with MS.
5. Identify the neuropsychological and social effects of MS and describe appropriate interventions to maximize quality of life.
6. Analyze and interpret patient data, formulate realistic goals and outcomes, and develop a plan of care when presented with a clinical case study.

OVERVIEW

Multiple sclerosis (MS) is a chronic, often disabling, demyelinating disease of the central nervous system (CNS). It affects largely young adults between the ages of 20 and 40, and is often referred to as the "great crippler of young adults." It was described as early as 1822 in the diaries of an English nobleman and further depicted in an anatomy book in 1858 by a British medical illustrator. Dr. Jean Cruveibier, a French physician, first used the term "islands of sclerosis" to describe areas of hardened tissue discovered on autopsy. However it was Dr. Jean Charcot in 1868 who defined the disease by its characteristic clinical and pathological findings: paralysis, and the cardinal symptoms of intention **tremor,** scanning speech, and nystagmus, later termed **Charcot's triad.** Using autopsy studies he identified areas of hardened plaques and termed the disease *sclerosis in plaques*.[1]

MS is an unpredictable disease that varies greatly from one individual to another in terms of clinical presentation and the severity of symptoms presented. The onset typically occurs between the ages of 15 and 50 years, with a peak in the third decade. The disease is rare in children, as is the onset of symptoms in adults over the age of 50 years. It affects an estimated 30 to 80 per 100,000, or 250,000 to 350,000 individuals in the United States.[2] The incidence in females is twice that in males. Clinically MS is characterized by multiple signs and symptoms and fluctuating periods of exacerbation and remission. An **exacerbation** involves a relapse or period of symptom flare up, whereas a **remission** is a period free of evolving symptoms. The course of the disease is highly unpredictable. In the early stages, relatively complete remission of initial symptoms may occur; however, as the disease progresses, the remissions may become less complete with increased neurological dysfunction and complications that affect multiple body systems.[3]

ETIOLOGY

The precise etiology of MS is unknown. Available research indicates that a number of factors may be involved. It is now generally accepted that MS is an **autoimmune disease** in which the body's own defenses attack the CNS. Although the trigger has not been clearly identified, mounting evidence suggests that viral infection initiates the immunological insult. Exposure to common viruses (Rubeola, rubella, canine distemper) has been investigated and generally discounted. The herpes HHV-6 virus is under current investigation. The presence of increased immunoglobulin (IgG) and oligoclonal bands in the cerebrospinal fluid (CSF) of 65 to 95 percent of MS patients provides convincing evidence of viral infection eliciting the autoimmune response. Genetic factors can also play a role in the acquisition of MS. Approximately 15 percent of patients have a positive family history (first-degree relative, such as a parent or sibling with MS). Genetic studies have revealed multiple markers in multiplex families, defined as families in which several members have MS. In particular, MHC proteins, encoded on chromosome 6, have been linked to antibody production (class I antigens) and MS.[4] It appears that although individuals do not inherit the disease, they may inherit a genetic susceptibility to immune system dysfunction.

Epidemiological studies have revealed a worldwide distribution of MS with areas of high, medium, and low frequency. High-frequency areas include the northern United States, Scandinavian countries, northern Europe, southern Canada, New Zealand, and southern Australia, with the incidence reported at rates of 30 to 80 (or more) per 100,000 population. Areas of medium frequency (southern United States and Europe, and the rest of Australia) have a reported incidence of 10 to 15 per 100,000. Low-frequency areas (Asia and Africa) have reported rates of less than 5 per 100,000. MS affects predominately white populations; blacks demonstrate approximately half the risk of acquiring the disease. Low rates are also reported in Asians and Native Americans living in high-risk areas. Migration studies indicate the geographic risk of an individual's birthplace is retained if migration occurs after the age of 15 years. Individuals migrating before this age assume the risk of their new location. Two epidemics of MS have been reported in the literature, one in the Faroe Islands off the coast of Scotland and one in Iceland after occupation by soldiers during World War II. These epidemiological studies lend support to a theory that exposure to an environmental agent before puberty, such as a slow-acting virus that can remain latent in the nervous system, may predispose a person to the development of MS later on.[5,6]

PATHOPHYSIOLOGY

Viral infection triggers the production of lymphocytes (T cells, B cells) and macrophages, which in turn appear to produce cytotoxic effects within the CNS. Reactive astogliosis results in destruction of *oliogodendrocytes* (myelin-producing cells) and the myelin sheath that surrounds the nerve. **Myelin** serves as an insulator, speeding up the conduction along nerve fibers from one node of Ranvier to another (termed *saltatory conduction*). It also serves to conserve energy for the nerve because depolarization occurs only at the nodes.[7] Disruption of the myelin sheath **(demyelination)** slows neural transmission and causes nerves to fatigue rapidly. With severe disruption, conduction block occurs with resulting disruption of function. Local inflammation, edema, and infiltrates surround the acute lesion and can cause a mass effect, further interfering with the conductivity of the nerve fiber. Conceivably, this inflammation (which gradually subsides) may, in part, account for the pattern of fluctuations in function that characterize this disease. During the early stages of MS, remaining oligodendrocytes may survive the initial insult and produce remyelination. As the disease becomes more chronic, no oligodendrocytes are preserved, and remyelination does not occur. The demyelinated areas eventually become filled with fibrous astrocytes and undergo a process called gliosis. **Gliosis** refers to the proliferation of neuroglial tissue within the CNS that results in glial scars **(plaques).** At this stage, the axon itself may become impaired. In advanced cases, there are both acute and chronic lesions of varying size scattered throughout the brain and spinal cord. They primarily affect white matter, although lesions of gray matter have also been identified in advanced disease. There are certain areas of predilection, such as the optic nerve, subcortical (especially periventricular) white matter, corticospinal tracts, posterior white columns of the spinal cord, and cerebellar peduncles.[8–10]

CLINICAL MANIFESTATIONS: DIRECT IMPAIRMENTS

Signs and symptoms of MS vary considerably, depending on the location of specific lesions. Early symptoms often include minor visual disturbances, paresthesias, incontinence, weakness, and fatigability. In advanced stages, patients demonstrate severe involvement; common symptoms including spastic paraplegia, neurogenic bladder, visual impairment, dysarthria, intention tremor, ataxia, nystagmus, and emotional lability (Box 22–1).[3] In severe cases, patients can become completely disabled. The onset of symptoms can develop rapidly over a course of minutes or hours; less frequently, onset is insidious, occurring over a period of weeks or months.

Sensory Impairments

Complete loss of any single sensation (anesthesia) is rare. Focal deficits can produce limited areas of sensory loss. Altered sensations are far more common and can include **paresthesias** (pins and needles sensation) or numbness of the face, body, or extremities. Disturbances in position sense are

From: Lechtenberg, R[11], p 40–41, with permission.

also frequent, as are lower extremity impairments of vibratory sense.[11]

Approximately 80 percent of patients with MS experience pain, with clinically significant pain occurring in about 20 percent.[12] **Dysesthesias,** abnormal burning or aching, are the most common type of pain in MS. **Hyperpathia,** a hypersensitivity to minor sensory stimuli, can occur. For example, a light touch or light pressure stimulus elicits a severe pain reaction. **Trigeminal neuralgia** results from demyelination of the sensory division of the trigeminal nerve and is characterized by stabbing, short attacks of severe facial pain. Eating, shaving, or simply touching the face may trigger painful episodes. A common sign of posterior column damage in the spinal cord is **Lhermitte's sign.** Flexion of the neck produces a sensation like an electric shock running down the spine and into the lower extremities. Chronic *neuropathic pain* can result from demyelinating lesions in spinothalamic tracts or in sensory roots. Pain can also develop with prolonged posturing (often the result of powerful spasticity), persistent forceful muscle spasms, and muscle and ligament strain. Anxiety and fear can worsen pain symptoms.

Visual Impairments

Visual symptoms are common with MS and are found in approximately 80 percent of patients. Involvement of the optic nerve can produce altered visual acuity; blindness is rare. **Optic neuritis,** inflammation of the optic nerve, is a common problem, and can produce blurring or graying of vision, or blindness in one eye. A **scotoma** or dark spot may occur in the center of the visual field. Pain may or may not be present; it is localized behind the eye and worsened by eye movements. Neuritis rarely affects both eyes, and is usually self-limiting. Vision generally improves within 4 to 12 weeks. Damage to the optic nerve will also affect light reflexes. Marcus Gunn pupil often develops with MS in individuals who have had an episode of optic neuritis. Shining a bright light into the healthy eye will produce reflex contraction in both eyes (consensual light reflex). If the light is then shone in the affected eye, there occurs a paradoxical widening (dilation) of both pupils.

Eye movements can be disturbed in a variety of ways. **Nystagmus** is common in patients with MS and results from lesions affecting the cerebellum or central vestibular pathways. This involves involuntary cyclical movements of the eyeball (horizontal or vertical) that develop when the patient looks to the sides or vertically (gaze-induced nystagmus) or when the patient moves the head. **Internuclear ophthalmoplegia (INO)** produces incomplete eye adduction (lateral gaze palsy) on the affected side and nystagmus of the opposite abducting eye with gaze to one side. It is caused by demyelination of the pontine medial longitudinal fasciculus (MLF). Additional impairments in conjugate gaze and control of eye movements may also be present with brainstem lesions affecting cranial nerves III, IV, and VI or the MLF. **Diplopia,** double vision, occurs when the muscles that control the eyes are not well coordinated. Visual disturbances frequently remit and are seldom the primary cause of disability.[11] The effects of impaired vision on balance and movement should be carefully assessed.

Motor Impairments

Patients with MS demonstrate signs and symptoms of **upper motor neuron (UMN) syndrome** secondary to damage of the corticospinal tracts or motor cortex. Paresis, spasticity, brisk tendon reflexes, involuntary flexor and extensor spasms, clonus, Babinski's sign, exaggerated cutaneous reflexes, and loss of precise autonomic control all characterize UMN syndrome[13] (see Chapter 8 for detailed descriptions). Movements are slow, stiff, and weak, the result of loss of orderly recruitment and reduced firing rate modulation of motoneurons. Impaired force production results in dyssynergic patterns of movement and disturbed agonist-antagonist relationships. Muscle weakness can vary from a mild paresis, often transient at first, to total paralysis of the involved extremities. Weakness as an indirect impairment secondary to disuse atrophy and prolonged inactivity must also be considered.

Spasticity is an extremely common problem in patients with MS, occurring in 90 percent of all cases. Spasticity can range from mild to severe, depending on the progression of the disease, and is typically more pronounced in the lower extremities than the upper. Spasticity can interfere with volitional movement, sleep, and functional activities of daily living (ADL). Spasticity can also cause pain, disabling contractures, abnormal posturing, and problems in maintaining skin integrity. Spasticity fluctuates on a daily basis and can be exacerbated by certain factors, such as extremes of temperature, humidity, infections, or noxious stimuli (e.g., tight clothing). Certain antidepressant agents (serotonin-reuptake inhibitors such as fluoxetine, sertraline, and paroxetine) can also exacerbate spasticity and should be used cautiously.[14] Spasticity does not typically abate during spontaneous remissions.[11] In patients with advanced disease, spasticity can be quite disabling and difficult to manage.

Fatigue, defined as a sense of physical tiredness and lack of energy distinct from sadness or weakness,[15] is one of the most common complaints reported by patients with MS. Patients consistently report that fatigue interferes with physical functioning (79% of patients), and overall role performance (67% of patients).[15,16] Fatigue is a daily event for most patients, with over half of patients reporting that fatigue is their most serious symptom.[15] Although fatigue can come on abruptly and severely at any time of the day, patients often report waking relatively refreshed but experiencing worsening fatigue by early afternoon and evening. Patients who experience fatigue demonstrate reduced overall activity levels and perceived health status.[17] Severity of disease does not seem to be related to fatigue severity; that is, individuals mildly affected by disease (ambulatory patients) report disabling fatigue as often as more severely disabled patients.[13,18] Both patients with MS and normal healthy individuals report that fatigue is worsened by vigorous exercise, stress, and depression.[13] Individuals with MS who reported being depressed also reported more fatigue. Environmental mastery (sense of control) is a strong psychosocial predictor of fatigue. Individuals with a low sense of environmental mastery reported significantly more fatigue and fatigue-related distress.[19] Fatigue is aggravated by heat and humidity, reported by 92 percent of patients.[15] Improvement has been reported with rest, sleep, relaxation/prayer, moderate exercise, and cool water.[16]

Demyelinating lesions in the cerebellum and cerebellar tracts are common in MS, producing cerebellar symptoms. Clinical manifestations include ataxia, postural and intention tremors, hypotonia, and truncal weakness. **Ataxia** is a general term used to describe uncoordinated movements characterized by **dysmetria, dyssynergia,** and **dysdiadochokinesia.** Progressive ataxia of the trunk and lower limbs is often apparent. During sitting or standing, when a limb or the body must be supported against gravity, the patient typically presents with **postural tremor** (shaking, back-and-forth oscillatory movements). During gait, ataxia is demonstrated by a staggering, wide-based pattern with poor foot placement and slow, uncoordinated progression of reciprocal lower extremity movement. Severe numbness of the feet may contribute to difficulty with standing or walking (sensory ataxia). An intention (action) tremor occurs when purposeful movement is attempted, and they result from the inability of the cerebellum to dampen motor movements. Intention tremors vary in severity from slight, barely perceptible quivering (fine tremor) to wide oscillations (gross tremors). Severe tremors impose significant limitations in performance of functional activities, particularly in such areas as personal hygiene, eating, and dressing (see Chapter 7 for a complete discussion of coordination deficits).

Dizziness is a common symptom of MS and results from lesions affecting the cerebellum (archicerebellum) or central vestibular pathways. Patients may also experience difficulties with balance (dysequilibrium), **vertigo,** nausea (motion sickness), and so forth. Symptoms are precipitated or made worse by movements of the head or eyes. Patients can also experience a paroxysmal attack or sudden onset of symptoms. This can be brought on by a period of hyperventilation.[20]

Cerebellar and brainstem involvement produces **dysarthria.** Speech is slowed with long pauses and disrupted melody, referred to as **scanning speech.** Words are slurred and speech volume is low, affecting clarity. These changes are the result of incoordination of the tongue and oral muscles. Poor coordination of the tongue and oral muscles can also result in **dysphagia** or difficulty in swallowing. Signs of swallowing dysfunction include difficulty chewing and maintaining a lip seal, inability to swallow (ingest food), and spitting or coughing during or after meals. Aspiration pneumonia can develop if foods or liquids are inhaled into the trachea. Signs of this include a wet voice quality with gurgling or sounds of congestion, and fever. The patient is also at risk for poor nutritional intake and dehydration and may experience weight loss. Poor coordination of breath control and posture contributes to speech and feeding difficulties.[11]

Cognitive and Behavioral Dysfunction

Cognitive deficits in MS are common, seen in approximately 50 percent of patients. The deficits typically range from mild to moderate impairment, with only 10 percent of patients experiencing problems severe enough to interfere with daily activities. Cognitive deficits are related to the specific distribution of the lesions rather than to the overall severity of the disease, its course, or the patient's disability status. Impairments in cognitive function can include deficits in memory, attention and concentration, learning, conceptual reasoning, speed of information processing and reaction time, and executive functions (e.g., planning, sequencing, problem solving, self-monitoring, and self-correcting). Focal frontal lobe lesions can produce cognitive inflexibility. Significant mental deterioration (global dementia) is relatively rare and may be seen in rapidly progressing disease (malignant MS) or in patients with significant cerebral lesions. Level of cognitive dysfunction is a major factor in determining quality of life, social functioning, employment status, and function in ADL.[21-23]

Depression is common in patients with MS, and has been reported in 25 to 55 percent of cases.[25] It can occur as a direct result of MS lesions, as a side effect of some drugs (e.g., steroids, adrenocorticotrophic hormone [ACTH], interferon medications), or as a psychological reaction to the stresses of this far-reaching and unpredictable disease.[23] Anxiety, denial, anger, aggression, or dependency can also occur. Patients with MS face enormous issues related to the ambiguity of their health status, the unpredictable course of disease activity, unpredictable future status, and the loss of effective functioning during the prime of their lives. Feelings of learned helplessness and low self-efficacy are common and have been linked to depression.[24] Moreover, many of the symptoms of MS (tremor, scanning speech, incontinence) are embarrassing or humiliating, causing additional emotional distress.

Affective disorders occur in about 10 percent of cases and can include changes in mood, feelings, emotional expression, and control. **Euphoria** consists of an exaggerated feeling of well-being, a sense of optimism incongruent with the patient's incapacitating disability. It is found primarily in patients with advanced disease.[23] **Emotional dysregulation syndrome** (lack of control with uncontrollable laughing or crying) and/or bipolar affective disorders (alternating periods of depression and mania) can also occur. The incidence of these symptoms is significantly higher in patients with MS than in patients with other chronic neurological conditions and has been linked to disseminated disease and demyelinating lesions in the frontal lobes, diencephalic, and limbic centers.[25]

Bladder and Bowel Dysfunction

Urinary bladder dysfunction occurs at some time during the course of the disease in about 80 percent of patients.[26] Losses in volitional and synergistic control of the micturition reflex is produced by demyelinating lesions affecting the lateral and posterior spinal tracts unmasking the sacral reflex arc. Types of bladder dysfunction can include a small, spastic bladder (a failure to store problem), a flaccid or big bladder (a failure to empty problem), or a dyssynergic bladder. The dyssynergic or conflicting bladder represents a problem with coordination between the bladder contraction and sphincter relaxation.[6] Common symptoms include urinary urgency, urinary frequency, hesitancy in starting urination, nocturia (frequency at night), dribbling, and incontinence. The severity of bladder symptoms is associated with severity of other neurological symptoms, particularly pyramidal tract involvement. Progressive loss of functional mobility (e.g., hand skills, sitting balance and transfer skills, ambulation) contributes to personal hygiene problems, emotional distress, and the development of secondary complications. These can include large residual urine volume after voiding (retention), and a tendency for recurrent urinary tract infections. Renal disease and renal failure are uncommon complications.[26]

Bowel function may also be impaired and can be directly influenced by CNS lesions affecting control of the gastrocolic reflex. Constipation is also a frequent consequence of inactivity, lack of fluid intake, and medication side effects. Incontinence can also occur as a result of drugs used to manage symptoms.

Sexual dysfunction is common, affecting as many as 91 percent of men and 72 percent of women. In women symptoms can include changes in sensation, vaginal dryness, trouble reaching orgasms, and loss of libido. In men symptoms can include impotence, decreased sensation, difficulty or inability to ejaculate, and loss of libido. Sexual activity is also affected by the appearance of other symptoms such as spasticity, uncontrollable spasms, pain, weakness and fatigue, bladder or bowel incontinence, losses in functional mobility, and changes in self-image. Psychological factors have a large impact on function. Sexual dysfunction has tremendous functional and pschyosocial implications for both patient and partner.[5,11]

DISEASE COURSE

The course of the disease is highly variable and unpredictable. At one end of the continuum, there is **benign MS,** defined as disease in which the patient remains fully functional in all neurological systems 15 years post onset, affecting about 20 percent of cases. At the other end of the continuum, there is **malignant MS,** a relatively rare disease course that is rapidly progressing, leading to significant disability in multiple neurological systems and death within a relatively short time. Exacerbations (relapses) and remissions (periods of stability or recovery) are the rule. In an attempt to clarify categories of MS, an international survey of professionals reached consensus on the definitions and terminology to describe the categories of MS (Box 22–2).[27] Because the course of the disease may alter, clinicians need to be alert to changes in signs or symptoms in terms of severity and frequency.

EXACERBATING FACTORS

New clinical signs and symptoms can occur at any time and without provocation. However several factors have been identified with worsening of symptoms in MS and/or relapses. Avoiding these aggravating factors is important in ensuring the patient's optimal function.[11]

Box 22–2 DEFINITIONS AND TERMINOLOGY USED TO DESCRIBE CATEGORIES OF MULTIPLE SCLEROSIS[27]

1. **Relapsing-remitting MS:** characterized by relapses with either full recovery or some remaining neurological signs/symptoms and residual deficit upon recovery. The periods between relapses are characterized by lack of disease progression.
2. **Primary-progressive MS:** characterized by disease progression from onset, without plateaus or remissions or with occasional plateaus and temporary minor improvements.
3. **Secondary-progressive MS:** characterized by initial relapsing-remitting course, followed by progression at a variable rate that may also include occasional relapses and minor remissions.
4. **Progressive-relapsing MS:** characterized by progressive disease from onset but without clear acute relapses that may or may not have some recovery or remission. It is commonly seen in people who develop the disease after 40 years of age.

An individual whose overall health deteriorates is more likely to have a relapse than one who remains healthy. Viral or bacterial infections (e.g., cold, flu, bladder infection) and diseases of major organ systems (e.g., hepatitis, pancreatitis, asthma attacks) are associated with exacerbations of disease. Stress has also been associated with worsening of symptoms and relapses. Both major life stress events (divorce, death, losing a job) and minor stresses can affect the immune system and the course of MS.[23]

Individuals with MS demonstrate an adverse reaction to heat, known as **Uthoff's symptom.** External heat, either in the form of climatic conditions (a hot room) or warm bath causes a temporary worsening of the symptoms of MS. The effect is usually immediate and dramatic in terms of reduced function and increased fatigue. Internal elevations in temperature (fever, increased body temperature following prolonged exercise) also produce similar effects. Heat is thought to interfere with already impaired transmission of affected nerves.

Hyperventilation is also associated with temporary worsening of MS symptoms. Changes in the chemical composition of blood are sufficient to interfere with normal brain and spinal cord function. Additional factors that contribute to transient symptom worsening include exhaustion, dehydration, malnutrition, and sleep deprivation. All provide additional stress on an already compromised nervous system. Their effects are completely reversible with resolution of the precipitating factors.[11]

DIAGNOSIS

The diagnosis of MS is based on history, clinical findings, and supportive laboratory tests. Criteria used to establish the diagnosis include two or more attacks of neurological symptoms reflecting predominant involvement of white matter lesions (e.g., optic nerve or corticospinal tracts). Two time patterns are identified: (1) two or more attacks, each lasting more than 24 hours and separated by no less than 1 month; or (2) chronically progressive deficits persisting for at least 6 months. For example, the patient may present with blurred vision and tingling in the arms occurring sporadically over several months. A detailed history helps to pinpoint episodic bouts as well as other positive factors (e.g., young adult, northern European Caucasian descent, positive family history). The neurological examination confirms the presence of symptoms (Box 22–1) and rules out other identifiable etiologies.

Various diagnostic tests are used to assist in the diagnosis:

1. *CSF examination:* Cell count and protein count are normal or slightly elevated. Patients with MS show elevated gamma globulin (IgG) more than 15 percent of total protein (seen in 70% of patients), and oligoclonal bands of IgG on agarose electrophoresis (seen in 85 to 90% of patients).[11] These changes are not unique to MS, however, and may be seen with other infections. Elevated levels of myelin basic protein or myelin proteolytic fragments in higher than normal concentrations indicate active demyelination and are useful diagnostic indicators during acute episodes.[28,29]
2. *Magnetic resonance imaging (MRI):* MRI is a sensitive tool for confirming disease when used along with other clinical and CSF data. Demyelinating plaques are seen as areas of increased signal intensity in 95 percent of patients with clinically defined MS. MRI is able to detect both small and large lesions with high resolution. The appearance of multiple lesions scattered throughout the brain and spinal cord is highly suggestive of MS. Lesions revealed on MRI do not always correlate with clinical disability, because lesion formation can be far greater than the clinical presentation of symptoms. Serial MRIs can be used to document disease progression. Computed tomography (CT) can be helpful in detecting large lesions but is limited in its ability to detect the smaller plaques that occur with MS. Contrast enhancement techniques can be used to increase sensitivity.[4]
3. *Evoked Potential Testing:* The presence of demyelinating lesions on sensory pathways can be confirmed by visual, auditory, or somatosensory evoked potentials. Prolonged latencies and conduction disturbances can reveal the presence of silent lesions (e.g., optic nerve involvement), and offer confirmation of disease when considered with other presenting symptoms.[4] See Table 22–1 for a summary of diagnostic tests.

Table 22–1 DIAGNOSTIC TESTS

Test	Finding
Cerebrospinal fluid	Usually abnormal protein composition
Visual evoked potentials	Latency prolonged (same changes with all causes of optic neuritis, optic nerve compression, and other causes of visual loss)
Computed tomography (CT) of the brain	Scattered areas of increased density (white patches on high-contrast CT)
Magnetic resonance imaging (MRI)	Scattered areas of abnormal nerve tissue

Cerebrospinal Fluid in Multiple Sclerosis	
Pressure	Normal
Appearance	Normal
Cell count	Normal or slightly increased white blood cells
Protein content	Normal or slightly elevated
Gamma globulin	More than 15% of total protein
Oligoclonal bands	Positive in 85–90% with MS
	False positive in 4% of all patients
	IgG typically increased

From Lechtenberg, R[11], p 68–69, with permission.

PROGNOSIS

MS is a disease of variable severity. Only a very small percentage of patients actually die as a consequence of the disease. For most individuals, life expectancy is not reduced, with 74 percent of patients surviving 25 years after onset of symptoms. If numerous complications evolve (e.g., pneumonia, bladder infection, recurrent skin ulcers), life span may be reduced.[11] Several prognostic indicators have been identified in predicting outcomes.

1. *Onset with only one symptom:* This is one of the strongest indicators of a favorable prognosis.
2. *Course of disease:* **Progressive (chronic) MS** is generally considered more ominous, whereas benign and **relapsing-remitting MS** are usually associated with a more favorable prognosis.
3. *Onset before the age of 40:* Onset after 40 is frequently associated with a progressive-relapsing course and increased disability.
4. *Neurological status at 5 years:* Significant pyramidal and cerebellar signs with involvement at multiple sites at 5 years is associated with a poorer prognosis and more severe disability.

It is important to remember that these remain general guidelines and may not necessarily describe the outcome for individual patients.

MEDICAL MANAGEMENT

Medical management of the patient with MS is directed at the overall disease process itself and at management of specific symptoms. There is currently no treatment that can prevent or cure MS. The establishment of comprehensive care centers for patients with MS has enhanced ongoing treatment. Careful assessment of multisystem function coupled with prompt management of flare-ups and symptomatic and supportive treatment are essential elements of care.[30,31]

Immunosuppressant drugs such as ACTH and steroids (prednisone, dexamethasone, betamethasone, methylprednisolone) are used to treat acute flare-ups and shorten the duration of the episode. These drugs exert a powerful anti-inflammatory effect, diminishing swelling within the CNS. Methylprednisolone may also have a long-term protective effect against new relapses. Initially, high-dose corticosteroids are given intravenously for a brief course (e.g., 4 days), followed by a gradual tapering off of dosage over a period of 10 days to 5 to 6 weeks. The drugs are associated with major side effects, which can include fluid retention, acne, ulcers, bone loss (osteoporosis), cataracts, and cognitive changes.[6] General drugs that can provide long-term suppression of the immune system and prevent relapse and disease progression include cyclophosphamide, azathioprine, cyclosporin, and methotrexate. They may be used alone or in combination with steroids (e.g., cyclophosphamide and ACTH). Potentially serious adverse effects can occur with these powerful immunosuppressant drugs, including suppression of blood production by bone marrow, bleeding disorders, and increased risk of infection.[11]

Recent advances in pharmacotherapy have produced synthetic interferon drugs (interferon beta-1a [Betaseron], interferon beta 1-b [Avonex]) that have substantial immunomodulating properties. Two-thirds of patients receiving these drugs have significantly reduced rates of relapse and slower disease progression. Clinical trials have primarily included ambulatory patients with relapsing-remitting MS.[32–34] Adverse effects can include initial fever and malaise with occasional nausea and depression.[6] An additional disadvantage of these drugs is cost, estimated at $11,000.00 a year for weekly doses. Glatiramer acetate (Copaxone [COP]I) is a synthetic drug that has also been shown to reduce the frequency of attacks in patients with relapsing-remitting MS and appears to have fewer side effects. Weekly plasma exchange has been used in combination with drugs to treat relapse and disease progression, with limited effectiveness. It can produce adverse side effects, including hypotension and deep venous thrombosis.[11,34]

Symptomatic treatment is a mainstay of medical management of patients with MS. A variety of drugs are used to alleviate such MS symptoms as spasticity, weakness, fatigue, urinary symptoms, visual symptoms, sensory symptoms, pain, and depression.[6,11] The clinician should have a thorough understanding of the medications the patient is taking, the expected benefit, and potential adverse reactions.

Management of spasticity and spasms includes the use of skeletal muscle relaxants[6,34] (Table 22–2). Use of agents such as lioresal (Baclofen), tizanidine (Zanaflex), dantrolene (Dantrium), clonidine (Catapress), and diazepam (Valium) is common. The

Table 22–2 MEDICATIONS FOR THE MANAGEMENT OF SPASTICITY

Medication	Notes
Baclofen (Lioresal)	May produce weakness at higher dose
Tizanidine (Zanaflex)	Often combined with baclofen; may produce drowsiness
Sodium dantrolene (Dantrium)	May produce weakness
Diazepam (Valium)	Highly sedating; most often used at night; may become addictive
Clonazepam (Klonopin)	Sedating; most often used at night
Cyproheptadine HCl (Periactin)	Sedating; used primarily as an "add on" medication
Cyclobenzaprine HCl (Flexeril)	Used for back spasms; most often combined with other medications
Gabapentin (Neurontin)	May ease spasms that are difficult to manage
L-dopa (Sinemet)	Especially useful for nighttime spasms
Selegiline (Eldepryl)	Especially useful for nighttime spasms
Carbamazepine (Tegretol)	Used for flexor spasms of the arm or leg
Cortisone	Effective for paroxysmal spasms; should only be used on short-term basis

From Schapiro, R[6], p 37, with permission.

reduction in spasticity must be balanced with the possibility of adverse effects with overdosing. These typically include sedation (drowsiness), weakness, and decreased function. The therapist needs to be alert to these changes and communicate with the physician to achieve optimal dosing for rehabilitation. The therapist must also recognize that spasticity can be used to enhance function, substituting for lack of strength. For example, if extensor spasticity can be used to stand during a stand-pivot transfer, significant reduction of spasticity with medications might only serve to produce loss of function. Carbamazepine (Tegretol) can be effective in reducing paroxysmal (sudden, sharp onset) spasms. Patients who do not adequately respond to conservative drug treatment (e.g., those with intractable spasticity or spasms) may benefit from intrathecal administration of baclofen directly into the lumbar spinal cord via a catheter. A programmable implanted pump controls the dosage. Significant reduction in spasticity and spasms has been reported in the lower extremities and trunk with less improvement reported in the upper extremities.[34,35] There are relatively few adverse effects.

Surgical interventions for spasticity management include tendonotomies and neurosurgical ablative procedures.[6,13] Tendonotomy may be indicated for fixed contractures to enhance function and facilitate nursing care. The typical surgical candidate has had spastic paralysis for many years resulting in a nonfunctional limb and serious complications (e.g., contractures and skin breakdown).[32] Phenol, a chemical used to decrease severe spasticity, can be injected into muscle, causing a motor point block.[12] Botulism toxin (Botox) is a paralytic agent that can cause a temporary blockage of a nerve and muscle. Repeat injections are required (see Chapter 24 for a more complete description of the medical management of spasticity).

Urinary problems are almost universal and require a complete urodynamic assessment to identify the specific cause of the problem and to arrive at the appropriate course of treatment (Table 22–3). Treatment for a spastic bladder typically involves pharmacological management with anticholinergic drugs (e.g., imipramine [Tofranil] and oxybutynin chloride [Ditropan]) to regulate bladder emptying. Adverse effects can include dry mouth, tachycardia, and accommodation disturbances. A flaccid bladder is managed with alternate techniques for emptying, including instruction in the *Crede maneuver* (the application of manual downward pressure over the lower abdomen) or intermittent self-catharization. A dyssynergic bladder is typically managed with alpha-blockers (e.g., phenoxybenzamine, clonidine, terozosin). If the bladder problem cannot be controlled with medication and/or intermittent or continuous catheterization (indwelling or Foley catheter; condom or Texas catheter), then a surgical urinary diversion (suprapubic catheter) may be necessary. For example, the patient with advanced disease and significant ataxia of the upper extremities may be unable to manually perform self-catheterization. Urinary tract infections result from retention of urine in the bladder and from catheterization procedures. Antibiotic therapy is the mainstay of treatment. Dietary modifications are also important and typically include reducing fluids that stress the bladder (e.g., caffeinated drinks, alcohol) and increasing agents that improve urine acidity (e.g., cranberry or prune juice).[6,11]

Constipation is a common problem and is typically managed with dietary changes. These include increased fluid intake, high-fiber foods and unprocessed fruits, bulk laxative (Metamucil), or dioctyl sodium sulfosuccinate (Colace). Regular or continu-

Table 22–3 TYPES OF BLADDER DYSFUNCTION

Problem	Symptoms	Treatment
Small, spastic bladder ("failure to store")	Increased frequency, urgency, dribbling, and/or incontinence	Oxybutynin (Ditropan) Hyoscyamine (Levsinex, Levbid) Tolterodine tartrate (Detrol) Flavoxate HCl (Urispas) Imipramine (Tofranil) Antihistamines
Flaccid ("big") bladder ("failure to empty")	Frequency, urgency, dribbling, hesitancy, incontinence	Credé technique Intermittent self-catheterization
Dyssynergic bladder ("conflicting")	*Either* (a) urgency followed by hesitation in beginning to void; *or* (b) dribbling or incontinence	Alpha blockers

From Schapiro, R[6], p 70, with permission.

ous use of irritating laxatives and enemas is not recommended.[11]

Pain is managed according to the pathogenesis. Carbamazepine (Tegretol), phenytonin (Dilantin), and amitriptyline (Elavil) are standard drugs used for pain in patients with MS.[12] The discomfort and pain associated with spasticity and spasms may be managed with over-the-counter or prescription anti-inflammatory drugs. Pain and numbness can sometimes be successfully managed with a brief course of corticosteroids. Trigeminal neuralgia is commonly treated with carbamazepine (Tegretol) or diphenyl-hydantoin (Dilantin). Chronic pain can be managed with behavioral approaches and medications. Sometimes antidepressants such as amitriptyline (Elavil) are used, or pain is managed with mild painkillers (acetaminophen [Tylenol] or ibuprofen [Motrin]). Narcotic analgesics are problematic and not typically prescribed.[11]

Symptomatic treatment of fatigue can include the use of the drugs. Amantadine (Symmetrel) and pemoline (Cylert) are the most commonly prescribed. Patients may become less responsive to these medications over the course of a few months, necessitating an intermittent course of treatment.[11] Adverse effects can include peripheral edema, diminished concentration, nervousness, and insomnia.[34] Weakness is sometimes improved with the administration of 4-aminopyridine and 3,4-diaminopyridine.[12] Agents to improve tremor (e.g., isoniazid [INH], clonazepam [Klonopin]) have been used with varying degrees of success (Table 22–4). Dizziness and vertigo can be managed with antimotion drugs (Meclizine [Antivert, Bonine] or with scopolamine patches). Severe cases may require the administration of a short course of corticosteroids.

Depression can be managed with antidepressant medications (e.g., fluoxetine [Prozac], Paxil, sertraline [Zoloft]). These antidepressants can also decrease fatigue. Stimulant medications (e.g., methylphenidate [Ritalin], pemoline (Cylert), dextroamphetamine] Dexedrine) can also be used but may be habit forming. Patients with emotional lability can be treated with amitriptyline (Elavil).[11] Professional counseling and participation in support groups often help the patient cope with the stresses of this unpredictable disease. An active life-style also helps reduce depression and anxiety.

REHABILITATION MANAGEMENT

The chronicity of this disease, along with its unpredictable course, may lead some to view individuals with MS as poor rehabilitation candidates. This view is contradicted by available research, which demonstrates that patients with MS can make significant functional gains from rehabilitation.[37–44] A coordinated interdisciplinary team is necessary to oversee the comprehensive care needed to address the patient's complex and multifaceted problems. The team typically includes the physician, nurse, physical therapist, occupational therapist, speech/language pathologist, nutritionist, and social worker. As with any team, the patient is the central figure, with family and caregivers being key members. The ideal rehabilitation program considers the patient's disease history, course and symptoms, and areas of deficit, including impairments, functional limitations, disability, and handicap. Of equal importance are the patient's abilities (assets), priorities, and resources (e.g., family, home, community). A focus on long-range planning is critical for effective management. An organized continuum of care is necessary with provisions for anticipated hospital-based, outpatient, and home/community-based episodes of care.

Restorative rehabilitation involves intervention that is focused on improvement of strength, endurance, reduction of spasticity, and so forth. An intensive, time-limited inpatient rehabilitation episode of care may be indicated for a patient with unstable or relapsing MS with the emergence of new symptoms and functional limitations. The desired outcome is to restore or maximize function, using remedial and compensatory training strategies.

Many individuals with MS also require a **functional maintenance program** designed to manage the effects of progressive disease. An ongoing rehabilitation program is indicated (e.g., home program, outpatient program). Strategies are developed to prevent or slow decline of function, and promote regular exercise, good health, and self-management skills. The enhancement of quality of life may in fact be the most meaningful outcome for patients in the face of persistent chronic disease. Shifting reimbursement trends have significantly altered the services that clinicians can provide. Therapists are being allotted fewer visits that are spread over longer time periods (e.g., one to two times per month over the course of several months). Functional maintenance programs are typically not well funded by private insurance. Medicare, which covers services for the elderly and the disabled, will cover functional maintenance if the skills of a therapist are needed to manage a patient because of identified dangers (e.g.,

Table 22–4 MEDICATIONS FOR THE MANAGEMENT OF TREMOR

Medication	Notes
Hydroxyzine (Atarax, Vistaril)	May settle a minor tremor that has been worsened by stress
Clonazepam (Klonopin)	May decrease tremor through sedative effect
Propranolol (Inderal)	May provide modest relief
Buspirone (Buspar)	An antianxiety agent that has some antitremor effect
Ondansetron (Zofran)	May significantly decrease tremor with few side effects; cost is prohibitive
Primidone (Mysoline)	An anti-epileptic drug that may help tremor in low doses; highly sedating
Acetazolamide (Diamox)	A diuretic that may help some people; may alleviate tremors influenced by posture

From Schapiro, R[6], p 48, with permission.

risk of secondary impairments, loss of functional capabilities). The therapist initially evaluates the patient, designs a program appropriate to the capacity and tolerance of the patient and the objectives of medical management, implements the plan, and periodically reevaluates the plan as required by the patient's condition. A variety of interventions are used to achieve goals and outcomes, including direct interventions, patient-related instruction, environmental modification, and supportive counseling. The primary emphasis, however, is to teach patients, family, and caregivers the management skills necessary to carry out the maintenance program.[45,46] Careful documentation is required to ensure adequate reimbursement of functional maintenance programs.

Assessment and Evaluation

Because many different areas of the CNS may be affected, it is imperative that a careful examination be performed to determine the extent of neurological and functional involvement. Subsequent reexamination at specified intervals should attempt to distinguish change in status as well as effects of treatment. It may not always be possible to differentiate change in status associated with remission of symptoms from treatment outcomes. Considering the variability of symptoms of any individual patient, it is often beneficial to perform the initial examination over a period of a few days to obtain a representative sample of baseline functioning. Fatigue and exacerbating factors should be taken into account when scheduling the examination.

Data can be obtained through the patient's history, systems review, and relevant tests and measures. The selection of examination procedures and level of inquiry are determined by the patient's unique status. The severity of problems, stage of disease (acute, subacute, chronic), age, phase and setting of rehabilitation, and other factors must all be taken into account in structuring the assessment.

The following are specific areas of assessment and relevant tests and measures that can be used to examine function in patients with MS (for more detailed descriptions, see earlier assessment chapters):

1. *Cognitive assessment:* Examine memory function, attention, concentration, conceptual reasoning, problem solving, speed of information processing; effects of fatigue on cognitive performance; and the ability to self-monitor and self-correct. A useful instrument is the Mini Mental Status Exam (MMSE).[47]
2. *Assessment of affective and psychosocial functioning:* Determine emotional stability; presence of emotional lability, euphoria, emotional dysregulation; depression (severity, length, effect on functional performance, feelings of helplessness); level of stress and anxiety, coping strategies; and presence of sleep disorders.
3. *Assessment of sensory integrity:* Examine superficial and deep sensations (touch, pressure, temperature, pain, proprioceptive) and combined or cortical sensations (stereognosis, tactile localization, two-point discrimination); presence of Lhermitte's sign.
4. *Visual assessment:* Examine acuity, tracking, accommodation; presence of visual deficits (blurred vision, field defects [scotoma], diplopia).
5. *Pain assessment:* Determine pain behaviors and reactions during specific movements and provoking stimuli, subjective appraisal; presence of hyperpathia, dysesthesias. Instruments can include the McGill Pain Questionnaire[48] and the visual analog scale.
6. *Assessment of cranial nerve integrity:* Examine motor and sensory cranial nerve function; presence of deficits (optic pain [optic neuritis], oculomotor dyscontrol, dysphagia, impaired gag reflex, trigeminal neuralgia).
7. *Assessment of range of motion (ROM):* Examine functional ROM; specific ROM deficits (AROM, PROM) using goniometers.
8. *Postural assessment:* Examine resting posture, static and dynamic control; presence of postural abnormalities (postural tremor, dyssynergia, deformity). Instruments can include posture grids/plumb lines, still photography or videotape, platform posturography.
9. *Assessment of muscle performance:* Examine functional strength and endurance; specific deficits in strength, power, and endurance can be measured by manual muscle tests and isokinetic dynamometry; strong spasticity may be a contraindication.
10. *Fatigue assessment:* Determine the frequency, duration, and severity of fatigue; precipitating factors and factors associated with cessation of fatigue; activity levels and efficacy of rest attempts. The Modified Fatigue Impact Scale (MFIS) was developed by the National Multiple Sclerosis Society Fatigue Guidelines Development Panel.[49]
11. *Assessment of temperature sensitivity:* Examine the degree of temperature sensitivity and its effect on fatigue and weakness. A tympanic membrane thermometry (ear thermometer) can be used before, during, and after moderate-intensity exercise. A determination of the correlation between temperature changes and worsening of neurological symptoms can be made.
12. *Assessment of motor function:*
    a. *Assessment of corticospinal signs:* Examine for paresis, spasticity, hyperactive DTRs, positive Babinski's sign, involuntary spasms (flexor or extensor); determine level or severity of hypertonicity, hyperreflexia in both the extremities and trunk

using modified Ashworth scale. Determine differences between lower limbs versus upper limbs, right and left sides; factors that influence tone.

b. *Assessment of cerebellar signs:* Examine for ataxia, intention tremor, nystagmus, postural imbalance, dysarthria; observe effects of position change (e.g., sitting-to-standing); note any increase in ataxic movements with increased demands for postural stability.

c. *Assessment of vestibular dysfunction:* Examine for dizziness, vertigo, nystagmus, blurred vision with head and body movements, and postural imbalance.

d. The Amended Motor Club Assessment (AMCA) has been developed to assess the nature and degree of motor and functional deficits in patients with MS.[50]

13. *Assessment of gait, locomotion, and balance:*

a. *Assessment of gait:* Determine gait parameters and characteristics: examine stability, safety, endurance; with significant ataxia, consider videotaped performance. Useful instruments include the Dynamic Gait Index,[51] the Ambulation Index (AI),[52] and the Rivermead Visual Gait Assessment (RVGA).[53]

b. *Assessment of orthotic and assistive devices:* Determine alignment and fit, safety, practicality and ease of use, and energy conservation and expenditure.

c. *Assessment of wheelchair skills:* Examine functional mobility, management, safety, transfer skills, and energy conservation and expenditure.

d. *Assessment of balance:* Examine static and dynamic balance, reactive and anticipatory balance, sensory organization, and synergistic strategies. Useful instruments include the Clinical Test for Sensory Interaction in Balance,[54] dynamic posturography,[55,56] the Berg Balance Scale,[57] and the Tinetti Performance Oriented Mobility Assessment (POMA).[58]

14. *Assessment of aerobic capacity and endurance:* Determine resting vital signs (heart rate, blood pressure, respiratory rate), breathing patterns; exertional symptoms (dyspnea, elevated blood pressure, heart rate, respiratory rate) during and after activity; perceived exertion. Useful instruments include the Rating of Perceived Exertion Scale (RPE scale)[59] and the dyspnea scale.[60]

15. *Assessment of skin integrity and condition:* Examine for areas of insensitivity, bruising, and skin breakdown; determine level of continence (dryness); bed and wheelchair positions, effectiveness of pressure relieving compensatory strategies and pressure-relieving devices (PRDs); cognitive status and safety awareness.

16. *Functional assessment:* Examine functional mobility skills, basic activities of daily living (BADLs), instrumental activities of daily living (IADLs); social functioning; community and work adaptive skills. A useful instrument is the Functional Independence Measure (FIM).[61,62]

17. *Environment assessment (home, community, and work):* Examine physical space for barriers, access, safety; a specific task-analysis (patient performance-based assessment) in relevant environments (home, work) may be included.

18. *General Health Measures:* General health measures can be used to assess individual outcomes across a broad spectrum. Instruments typically include items that assess ability to perform routine daily activities and quality of life (e.g., physical and social function, general health and vitality, emotional well-being, bodily pain, etc.). They are most useful in determining global or long-term health outcomes and may lack the sensitivity needed to document short-term outcomes of treatment. Measures of general health status that can be used include the Rand 36-Item Health Survey SF-36,[63] the Sickness Impact Profile,[64] and the Assessment of Motor and Process Skills (AMPS).[65]

19. *Disease-specific measures:* Disease-specific measures are designed to assess attributes unique to a specific disease entity. Items are included to provide information about the disease process and outcomes, and ideally document clinically meaningful change over time. Thus these instruments have greater responsiveness or sensitivity to change than general health measures. Examples of instruments developed specifically for the assessment of patients with MS include the **Expanded Disability Status Scale (EDSS)** and the **Minimum Record of Disability (MRD).**

a. *Expanded Disability Status Scale (EDSS):* In 1955, Kurtzke[66] developed a 10-point scale for rating overall disability in MS (the Disability Status Scale or DSS). This scale was expanded in 1983 to increase its clinical sensitivity by including half-point increments, becoming the EDSS.[67] This scale has been widely adopted by clinicians and has been used to standardize patient samples in MS research. Patients are graded on the basis of presenting symptoms in eight different functional systems (FS), including pyramidal, cerebellar, brainstem, sensory, bowel and bladder, visual, mental, and other functions (see Appendix A). Scoring of the EDSS uses a 0 to 10, 20-step scale, with 0 equal to normal neurological function and 10.0 equal to death owing to MS. The final score is based on grades obtained in the FS assessment. For example, patients classified in EDSS step 2.5 demonstrate minimal disability in two FS (two FS grade 2, others 0 or 1). The EDSS focuses on ambulation as the primary indicator of disability (see scores 3.0 through 6.5 for levels of ambulation; patients with scores 7.0 or greater are unable to walk). Criticisms of the EDSS include its lack of sensitivity to changes that do not include functional mobility (ambulation) and problems in interrater reliability with patients whose performance is less impaired (scores in the lower ranges, ambulation less impaired).[68]

b. *The Minimum Record of Disability (MRD):* The MRD was developed by the International Federation of Multiple Sclerosis Societies in 1985.[69] This instrument includes three subscales: the EDSS with FS, the Incapacity Status Scale (ISS), and the Environmental Status Scale (ESS). It is widely used and includes classification of dysfunction according to World Health Organization terminology (1980). Thus, measurement addresses impairments (the FS and EDSS), disability (ISS), and handicap (ESS). The ISS includes 16 items to assess functional disability in ADL. The ESS measures social performance including work status, financial and economic status, place of residence, personal assistance, transportation, community assistance, and social activity. Solari et al.[70] examined the validity of the self-administered version of the MRD and found that assessment of ambulatory ability, ADL skills, and social activities was both accurate and cost-effective. A copy of the MRD can be obtained from the National Multiple Sclerosis Society.

c. *Multidimensional quality of life measures:* Advances in pharmacological treatments for relapses and symptom management can be expected to prolong life and lessen symptoms for many individuals. Quality of life issues therefore become increasingly important. Multidimensional quality of life measures have been developed for use with individuals who have MS. These include the Functional Assessment of Multiple Sclerosis quality of life instrument by Cella et al.;[71] Quality of Life in MS by Pfenning et al.;[72] and the Multiple Sclerosis Quality-of-Life questionnaire (MS-QPL-54) by Vickrey et al.[73] The Fatigue Impact Scale (FIS)[74] was developed to measure the impact of fatigue on quality of life. DiFabio et al.[75] used health-related quality of life to compare a group of patients with chronic, progressive MS receiving weekly outpatient rehabilitation (defined as a maintenance program) for 1 year with a matched, wait-listed control group not receiving rehabilitation. The researchers found the treatment group improved on several measures of health status, including energy/fatigue, social function, social support, and change in general health when compared to the control group. Moreover, the rate of decline for the control group was greater than for the treatment group. For this group of patients with chronic progressive involvement, reducing the overall rate of decline and improving quality of life provided an appropriate focus for functional maintenance programs.

Setting Realistic Goals and Outcomes

The determination of appropriate goals and outcomes, as well as interventions, should be based on careful assessment and evaluation of the patient's individual abilities and needs. Full involvement of the patient and family in all stages of planning will help to ensure success. Goals and outcomes of physical therapy for patients with MS, adapted from the *Guide to Physical Therapist Practice*,[76] include:

1. Ability to perform self-care and home management (ADLs and IADLs) is increased.
2. Performance levels in physical tasks and employment, recreational, or leisure activities are improved.
3. Disability associated with acute or chronic stages of MS is reduced.
4. Care is coordinated with patient/client, family, caregivers, and other professionals.
5. Intensity of care is decreased.
6. Self-management of symptoms is improved.
7. Behaviors that foster health habits, wellness, and prevention are enhanced.
8. Risk of secondary impairments and flare ups is reduced.
9. Joint integrity and mobility is maintained.
10. Strength, power, and endurance are increased.
11. Postural control is improved.
12. Motor function is improved.
13. Pain is decreased.
14. Gait, locomotion, and balance are improved.
15. Aerobic capacity and endurance are increased.
16. Safety of patient, family, and caregivers is improved.
17. Patient, family, and caregiver knowledge and awareness of the diagnosis, prognosis, goals and outcomes, and interventions are increased.
18. Patient knowledge of personal and environmental factors associated with exacerbation of MS or its symptoms is increased.
19. Patient knowledge of activity pacing and energy conservation is increased.
20. Decision making is enhanced regarding the

use of rehabilitation and community resources.

21. Level of stress is decreased and psychological adjustment of patient and family is enhanced.

Interventions

Interventions are discussed by general areas of deficit, and address both direct and indirect impairments (Fig. 22-1). Interventions that focus on reducing functional limitations, preventing disability, and improving quality of life will be discussed.

SENSORY DEFICITS AND SKIN CARE

Strategies should be instituted to increase awareness of sensory deficits, compensate for sensory loss, and promote safety. It is important to remember that sensory deficits may remit, so ongoing assessment is necessary. The success of compensatory training strategies depends on the availability of other intact sensory systems. For example, visual compensation techniques can be instituted when deficits in proprioception produce imbalance and place the patient at risk for falls. If multiple sensory systems are involved (e.g., vision is also impaired), compensatory strategies are not likely to be successful.

Patients with proprioceptive losses demonstrate impairments in movement control and motor learning. They require increased use of other sensory systems, especially vision. Tapping, verbal cueing, and/or biofeedback can all be effective forms of augmented feedback. Proprioceptive loading (through exercise, resistance, weights, or pool) may heighten residual proprioceptive function and improve movement awareness.

Visual loss will interfere with movement and postural control. Blurred vision may be improved by the use of tinted glasses that reduce glare. Safety can be improved by reducing clutter and increasing the contrast between items in the environment (e.g., stair markings). Vision may be reduced in dim light, so adequate night lighting is necessary. Double vision is frequently controlled by placing a patch over one eye, especially for reading, driving, or watching television. However, eye patches will prevent possible adaptation of the CNS and therefore are not recommended for continuous use. Eye patches also interfere with depth perception. Prism eyeglasses can be used to correct double images.[6] If low vision persists, the patient should be referred to a low-vision clinic or one of the national service organizations that provide help to individuals with vision impairments (National Association for Visually Handicapped, National Federation of the Blind, American Foundation for the Blind).

Patients with deficits in superficial sensations risk damage to insensitive areas of skin. The development of decubitus ulcers becomes a major concern with severe involvement. Changes in skin turgor, static posturing, and prolonged pressure over bony prominences increase the likelihood of skin breakdown. Patients may not feel the discomfort of prolonged positioning or may be unable to shift position because of weakness or spasticity. In addition, spasticity and/or spasms may cause friction effects between the skin and supporting surfaces. Awareness, protection, and care of desensitized parts should be taught early in the rehabilitation process and consistently reinforced by all members of the team. The patient and family should be educated in the following principles of skin care:

1. The skin should be kept clean and dry. Soiled skin should be cleansed and dried promptly.
2. The skin should be inspected regularly (at least once a day) and carefully, with particular attention to persistent areas of redness and over bony prominences.
3. Clothing should be breathable and comfortable (soft, not too loose or wrinkled, or too tight). Seams, buttons, and pockets should not press on the skin, particularly in weight-bearing areas.
4. Regular pressure relief is essential. Patients should be instructed to change their position or be changed frequently, typically every 2 hours in bed and every 15 minutes when sitting in a wheelchair. Wheelchair push-ups or repositioning maneuvers should be taught to relieve pressure.
5. Pressure relieving devices (PRDs) may be necessary to protect insensitive areas and should be used regularly. These can include mattresses (water, gel, air, or alternating pressure) to distribute body weight and reduce shear and friction in bed. Sheepskins, air or

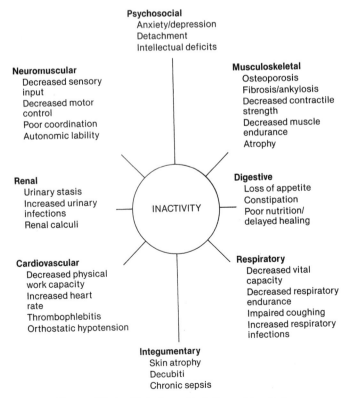

Figure 22-1. Clinical manifestations of inactivity.

foam cushions, cuffs, and/or boots may be necessary to protect body areas prone to breakdown (shoulder blades, elbows, ischial tuberosities, sacrum, trochanters, knees, malleoli, or heels). Cushions (foam; pressure-relieving cushions, either fluid or air) are necessary for patients who spend prolonged periods of time sitting in their wheelchair.

6. Prevention is the best strategy. The patient must be cautioned against activities that might traumatize the skin. Dragging, bumping, or scraping body parts during a transfer or bed mobility activities can injure the skin. Thermal injury can result from contact with hot water or hot objects. If skin redness develops (lasting longer than 30 minutes) patients should be instructed to stay off the area until the redness disappears. Blisters, blue areas, or open sores indicate more serious injury and require immediate attention. This may include systemic antibiotic therapy for infection, wound management techniques (cleansing and debridement, topical antibiotic agents, and protective dressings), and plastic surgery.[77]

7. Important preventive measures for maintaining skin integrity and function include maintaining good nutrition and drinking plenty of fluids.

PAIN

The management of pain depends on an accurate assessment of the causes of pain. Musculoskeletal strain or joint malalignment from chronically weakened muscles are important considerations and are responsive to physical therapy intervention. Patients may experience relief of pain with regular stretching or exercise, massage, and ultrasound. Postural retraining and correction of faulty movement patterns along with orthotic and/or adaptive seating devices can reduce malalignment and pain. Stabbing pain from Lhermitte's sign may be relieved with a soft collar to limit neck flexion. Hydrotherapy or pool therapy using *lukewarm* water may have a beneficial effect on painful paresthesias.[8] Pressure stockings or gloves can also be used to relieve pain, converting the sensation of pain to one of pressure. Neutral warmth may also be a factor in the pain relief experienced. Patients with long-standing pain will benefit from referral to a total management approach for chronic pain, for example, the multidisciplinary pain clinic (see Chapter 28). Stress management techniques, relaxation training, meditation, and so forth are often helpful in reducing both anxiety and pain. The use of transcutaneous electrical nerve stimulation (TENS) to modulate pain in patients with MS has had conflicting results, with some patients experiencing a worsening of symptoms.[11]

SPASTICITY

Spasticity, with its resultant fixed postures and contractures, may be responsive to a variety of physical therapy interventions, including modalities, therapeutic exercise, positioning, or any combination thereof. Topical cold (ice packs or wraps, cold bath or spray) can reduce spasticity by decreasing tendon reflex excitability and clonus, and by slowing conduction of impulses in nerves and muscles. The effects of cryotherapy are relatively short-lived, although some patients may experience enhanced ability to move that lasts for minutes or hours. It is important to remember that some patients, particularly those with intact sensation, may react to the unpleasant sensation of cold with fight or flight (autonomic nervous system) responses, such as increased heart rate, respiratory rate, or nausea. Cryotherapy is contraindicated in these patients.

Stretching exercises begun early in the course of the disease and continued daily can help patients maintain joint integrity and mobility in the face of unremitting spasticity. Thus patients are taught self-stretching exercises as part of their home exercise program. Family members and/or caregivers are also instructed in proper stretching exercises. Caution must be used to prevent fast, ballistic stretching movements, because spasticity is velocity sensitive. Stretching movements need to proceed slowly to gradually achieve the desired range. Each stretched position should be maintained for at least 30 to 60 seconds to allow the muscle to adjust to the new position. Combining stretching movements with rhythmic rotation (gentle rotation of the limb) is often an effective strategy in gaining new range. Stretching should be well timed with the middle of the dosing schedule of anti-spasticity medications to ensure optimal results. Typically the lower extremities demonstrate stronger spasticity than the upper extremities, especially in the extensor antigravity muscles. Although spasticity varies greatly from person to person, muscles that require particular emphasis during stretching include the quadriceps, adductors, and plantarflexors. For patients who spend prolonged times sitting in a wheelchair, stretching should also address the hamstrings and hip flexors. Prolonged static stretching of these muscles can be achieved through the use of a tilt table.

Active exercises should focus on contraction of the antagonist muscles to maintain tone reduction through mechanisms of reciprocal inhibition. Movements that encourage or utilize spasticity should be discouraged. When exercise was combined with low doses of baclofen, patients with MS who had minimal to moderate spasticity demonstrated significant improvements in overall levels of tone.[78]

Functional mat activities aimed at reducing tone should concentrate on trunk and proximal movements, because many patterns of hypertonus seem to be fixed from the action of the stronger proximal muscles. Extensor tone seems to predominate, so activities that stress lower extremity flexion with trunk rotation are generally the most effective. For example, lower trunk rotation (LTR) in sidelying or hooklying, can be effective in reducing extensor tone. One very effective strategy is to position the patient in hooklying with a Swiss ball under the flexed legs and gently rock the ball back and forth.

Moving from quadruped position to side-sitting can also be effective in reducing extensor tone in some patients as the activity combines LTR with prolonged inhibitory pressure on the quadriceps.[79] Specific techniques that may be effective in reducing tone include neurodevelopmental treatment (NDT) handling techniques,[80,81] and the proprioceptive neuromuscular facilitation (PNF) technique of rhythmic initiation.[82] A more generalized decrease in tone may be achieved through techniques aimed at decreasing overall CNS central set and tone (e.g., slow rocking, soothing verbal commands. Cognitive relaxation techniques (e.g., progressive relaxation exercises) can also aid in generalized tone reduction. Finally, it is important to reduce or eliminate all factors that can aggravate spasticity, (e.g., heat, humidity, stress).

Positioning out of abnormal or spastic postures is an important component of the rehabilitation program. In general, prolonged or static positioning in any fixed posture can be deleterious to the patient with strong spasticity and should be avoided. For example, the patient with moderate to severe lower extremity tone who lies in bed all day with the lower extremities positioned in extension, adduction, and plantarflexion may be unable to flex enough at the hips and knees to sit in a wheelchair. Similarly, the feet will remain fixed in plantarflexion and cannot be positioned on the footpedals. A positioning schedule using varied positions (in bed, in a chair or wheelchair) will help keep the patient from getting stuck in any one posture. Mechanical devices (e.g., splints, casts, toe spreader, finger spreader) can be helpful in maintaining position and preserving joint structures. Inhibitory casts that position the limb at end range also have the added effect of reducing stretch reflex sensitivity and tone, and may be a necessary short-term intervention.[83,84]

FATIGUE

Fatigue is a common problem in MS and can be quite debilitating. Chronic fatigue is characterized by ineffective task performance, excessive tiredness, sense of weakness, feelings of discomfort, and less complete recovery after rest. Aversion to activity for fear of bringing on fatigue is also common.[17,85] The resultant lowered activity levels have important implications for diminished health status and the development of secondary impairments related to deconditioning and disuse. Therapists are faced with a balancing act, on one hand prescribing exercise, while on the other hand cautiously avoiding overwork and the development of fatigue.[86]

Patients need to be taught strategies of energy conservation and activity pacing. **Energy conservation** refers to the adoption of strategies that reduce overall energy requirements. These can include modifying the task or modifying the environment to ensure successful completion of daily activities. Thus the patient learns new ways to perform a task that conserves energy. For example, a motorized scooter can be considered for community mobility to help conserve energy and maintain independence.

Activities that are difficult or have high energy needs can be broken down into component parts. **Activity pacing** refers to the balancing of activity with rest periods interspersed throughout the day. For the patient with chronic fatigue, periodic rest periods often need to be planned in advance, when patients are considering their daily schedule. Time-outs should be instituted if an activity becomes exhaustive. Overall levels of energy can be improved if patients learn to limit their activities, saving their energy for those activities that are truly important to them (e.g., activities that are enjoyable and meaningful in terms of the individual's life-style). The occupational therapist can give valuable suggestions in terms of planning, work simplification, and developing energy-efficient activities.

During an acute exacerbation, the patient will fare better if he or she is allowed to rest for a few days. Allowing the patient to continue the same level of exercise or ambulation is not helpful. Therapy can be reinstituted when the deterioration has stabilized and no new symptoms are appearing. The focus and pace of therapy must be readjusted according to the patient's specific abilities and needs at that time.[11]

PARESIS

Muscle weakness varies considerably from patient to patient. Patients with corticospinal lesions demonstrate reduced muscle strength, power, and endurance, and impaired reciprocal relationships in association with spasticity and other UMN signs. Patients with cerebellar lesions may demonstrate asthenia or generalized muscle weakness. Patients also typically experience weakness secondary to prolonged inactivity and generalized deconditioning. Improving strength and endurance through regular exercise are therefore important goals of therapy. Strengthening of residual function allows maximum use of affected extremities for as long as possible. Strengthening of unaffected muscles allows effective use of compensatory strategies (e.g., upper extremity strengthening for push-up transfers and wheelchair use). Strengthening should also focus on muscles needed for effective use of assistive devices (e.g., shoulder and elbow extensors necessary for crutch gaits). Setting realistic goals and selecting exercises the patient finds enjoyable will ensure improved motivation and compliance.[87]

Strengthening exercises have been used with patients with MS and are safe and effective when used in moderation. Individuals with minimal impairments and stable disease appear to have the best exercise tolerance and therefore achieve optimal benefit. This finding speaks to the need to institute exercises early in the course of the disease before secondary impairments develop.[86] It is important to consider the following general guidelines. Submaximal exercise intensities (low to moderate intensities) are tolerated, whereas maximal exercise is not. More frequent repetitions are necessary to achieve a training effect. At the same time, exercise must be carefully balanced with adequate rest periods. The patient with MS will progress more slowly through the training program. Prior to strengthening exercises, stretching exercises may be necessary to decrease spasticity and ensure adequate flexibility.[87] Precautions should be taken to prevent the deleterious effects of overwork and overheating. Exercising to the point of fatigue is contraindicated and can result in worsening of symptoms, most notably weakness. This may have additional adverse effects on the continuing motivation of the patient. Exercise sessions should be scheduled during optimal times, such as in the morning, when body core temperatures tend to be at their lowest and before fatigue sets in. Environmental temperatures should be controlled. Air conditioning is a medical necessity in many climates. Additional cooling can be achieved through the use of fans, pool exercises,[88] or a personal cooling suit (e.g., Mark VII Personal Cooling System[89]).

Resistance training modes can include isokinetic dynamometry or progressive resistance exercises. Significant improvements have been reported in patients with MS on measures of strength and endurance,[88,90] fatigability (percentage of peak torque decline),[88] and perception of peripheral fatigue.[88] Strengthening can also be achieved using a functional training approach.[79] PNF patterns[82] are ideal because of their emphasis on diagonal movement (often helpful in reducing tone) and on combining the actions of major synergistic muscle groups (helpful when the patient fatigues easily). Because the patient typically has a limited amount of energy to expend, PNF patterns are more economical than exercising individual muscles. Training using functional activities focuses on strengthening of proximal muscles. This has important carry over for improved function and reduced energy expenditures. Patterns and activities can be resisted with weight cuffs, elastic resistance bands (e.g., Theraband), or manual resistance.

The use of group classes and self-paced exercises can be a valuable component of a rehabilitation program. The therapist's primary role in this approach is one of educator and group leader. Successful management of group classes requires careful, individualized assessment of group members to determine specific goals and exercises. Significant improvement in functional mobility, balance, and ADL skills have been demonstrated in a group of 40 patients with MS not in active exacerbations.[91]

ATAXIA

Ataxia is common in MS and can be difficult to manage. The patient typically presents with incoordination, tremor, and disturbances of posture, balance, and gait. Therapy is directed at promoting postural stability, accuracy of limb movements, and functional balance and gait. Postural stability can be improved by focusing on static control (holding) in a number of different weight-bearing, antigravity postures (e.g., prone on elbows, sitting, quadruped, kneeling, plantigrade, and standing). Progression through a series of postures is used to gradually increase postural demands by varying the base of support (BOS), raising the center of mass (COM), and increasing the number of body segments (degrees of freedom) that must be controlled.[79] Specific exercise techniques designed to promote stability include joint approximation applied through proximal joints (shoulders or hips) or head and spine, alternating isometrics (PNF), and rhythmic stabilization (PNF). Patients with significant ataxia will not be able to hold steady and may benefit from the application of the technique of slow reversal-hold (PNF), progressing through decrements of range. The desired end point is steady midrange holding.

Dynamic postural responses can be challenged by incorporating controlled mobility activities (weight shifting or rocking, moving in and out of postures or movement transitions). The patient should practice important functional movement transitions, such as supine-to-sit, sit-to-stand, and scooting. Distal extremity movements can be superimposed on proximal stability to further challenge dynamic postural control. For example, resisted PNF chop or lift patterns combine upper extremity movements with trunk movements (flexion with rotation or extension with rotation).

An important goal of therapy is to promote safe and functional balance. Static balance control can be improved using force platform training. The patient with ataxia learns to reduce postural sway (frequency and amplitude) and control center of alignment position. The added biofeedback from visual and/or auditory feedback displays can improve control in some patients. Somatosensory, visual, and vestibular inputs can be varied, as appropriate, to assist in sensory compensation by sensory systems less involved (e.g., standing eyes open to eyes closed, standing on a flat surface to a foam surface). Prolonged latencies (onset of responses) should be expected.[52,53] Dynamic balance control can be challenged using self-initiated movements (e.g., reaching, turning, bending). A moveable surface can also be used. For example, sitting activities on a Swiss ball are an excellent way to promote dynamic balance control.

Control of dysmetric limb movements can be promoted through the use of PNF extremity patterns using light resistance to modulate force output and reciprocal actions of muscles (e.g., slow reversals or slow-reversal-hold). **Frenkel's exercises** were originally developed in 1889 to treat patients with tabes dorsalis and problems of sensory ataxia owing to a loss of proprioception. These exercises can be applied in the treatment of MS to remediate problems of dysmetria. The exercises are performed in supine, sitting, and standing. Each activity is performed slowly with the patient using vision to guide correct movement. The exercises require a high degree of mental concentration and effort and are, therefore, not appropriate for all patients with MS. For those patients with the prerequisite abilities, they may be helpful in regaining some control of Ataxic movement through cognitive processes. Patients with partial sensation can progress to practicing exercises with eyes closed. Frenkel's exercises are presented in Box 22–3.

Ataxic movements have sometimes been helped by the application of light weights to provide additional proprioceptive loading and stabilize movements. Velcro weight cuffs (wrist or ankle) or a weight belt or weighted jacket can reduce dysmetric movements and tremors of the limbs or trunk. The extra weights will also increase energy expenditure, and must therefore be used cautiously in order not to bring about increased fatigue. Weighted canes or walkers can be used to reduce ataxic upper extremity movements during ambulation. For patients with significant tremor, this may mean the difference between assisted and independent ambulation. Elastic resistance bands (e.g., Theraband) can also be used to provide resistance and reduce ataxic movements. For example, upper extremity reaching movements such as those used for feeding can be improved with Theraband resistance. Air splints can also be used to stabilize limb movements. A soft neck collar can stabilize head and neck tremors. All these strategies, however, should be viewed as compensatory. Once the devices are removed, ataxic movements will return or in some cases may actually temporarily worsen.

The pool is an important therapeutic medium to practice static and dynamic postural control in sitting and standing. Water provides graded resistance that slows down the patient's ataxic movements, while the buoyancy aids in upright balance. Swimming and shallow water calisthenics have been shown effective in improving strength, decreasing muscular fatigability, and increasing endurance in a group of patients with MS.[88] In addition, the use of moderate or cool water temperatures (no greater than 85° F) may help moderate spasticity.

In general, patients with ataxia do better in a low-stimulus environment that allows them to concentrate more fully on control of their movements. They benefit from augmented feedback (verbal cueing of knowledge of results, knowledge of performance; biofeedback) and repetition to improve motor learning. The patient with MS is often restricted in practice by neuromuscular fatigue and neurological deficits that impair sensory feedback, attention, memory, and concentration. The successful therapist will need to carefully identify the patient's resources and abilities and capitalize on them to maximize learning.

FUNCTIONAL TRAINING

Functional training should focus on the development of problem solving skills and appropriate compensatory strategies to ensure that ADL tasks can be performed. The overall goal is to maintain independence or improve functional status. Training in functional skills of bed mobility, transfers, wheelchair use, and ambulation is directed by the physical therapist. ADL training sequences for dressing, personal hygiene, bathing, toileting, and feeding are typically directed by the occupational therapist, whereas training in communication skills is directed by the speech/language pathologist. Close communication among team members is necessary to ensure that training methods are consistently applied and successful. Full participation of the patient in all phases of planning will increase personal involvement, while decreasing dependency and passivity.[92]

The majority of patients with MS will use multiple adaptive devices.[93] This requires careful attention to appropriate prescription of devices and environmental modifications to assist the patient in conserving energy and maintaining function. Mobility aids may include the use of bed or toilet grab bars, an overhead trapeze, raised seats, transfer board, or hydraulic lift. Adapted or weighted feeding utensils

---

Box 22–3 FRENKEL'S EXERCISES

General instructions: Exercises can be performed with the part supported or unsupported, unilaterally or bilaterally. They should be practiced as smooth, timed movements, performed to a slow, even tempo by counting out loud. Consistency of performance is stressed and a specified target can be used to determine range. Four basic positions are used; they are lying, sitting, standing, and walking. The exercises progress from postures of greatest stability (lying, sitting) to postures of greatest challenge (standing, walking). As voluntary control improves, the exercises progress to stopping and starting on command, increasing the range, and performing the same exercises with eyes closed. Concentration and repetition are the keys to success. A similar progression of exercises can be developed for the upper extremities. Examples:

1. Half-lying: hip and knee flexion and extension of each limb, foot flat on plinth.
2. Half-lying: hip abduction and adduction of each limb with the foot flat, knee flexed; then with knee extended.
3. Half-lying: hip and knee flexion and extension of each limb, heel lifted off plinth.
4. Half-lying: heel of one limb to opposite leg (toes, ankle, shin, patella).
5. Half-lying: heel of one limb to opposite knee, sliding down crest of tibia to ankle.
6. Half-lying: hip and knee flexion and extension of both limbs, legs together.
7. Half-lying: reciprocal movements of both limbs—flexion of one leg during extension of the other.
8. Sitting: knee extension and flexion of each limb; progress to marking time.
9. Sitting: hip abduction and adduction.
10. Sitting: alternate foot placing to a specified target (using floor markings or a grid).
11. Standing up and sitting down: to a specified count.
12. Standing: foot placing to a specified target (floor markings or grid).
13. Standing: weight shifting.
14. Walking: sideways or forward to a specified count. (A Frenkel mat, parallel lines or floor markings may be used as targets to control foot placement, stride length and step width.)
15. Walking: turning around to a specified count. (Floor markings can be helpful in maintaining a stable base of support.)

and plate guards can assist the patient in feeding. Long-handled shoe horns, reachers, button hooks, sock aids, or Velcro closures can assist in dressing. Effective communication may require built-up writing utensils or a universal cuff for written communication or more sophisticated computerized devices.[94] The clinician needs to (1) recognize when a device is indicated, and (2) assist the patient in acceptance and in learning how to use the device *before* significant deterioration of function occurs.[95]

AMBULATION

Ambulation is frequently impaired. However, at least 65 percent of patients with MS are still walking after 20 years.[6] Early gait problems often include poor balance and heaviness of one or more limbs. Patients frequently report difficulty lifting their legs (hip flexor weakness). Weak dorsiflexors are also common, resulting in foot drop. Problems with foot clearance may result in a circumducted gait pattern. Later problems center on developing clonus, spasticity, sensory loss, and/or ataxia. Weakness generally extends to include the quadriceps and hip abductors. Quadriceps weakness typically results in hyperextension of the knee and forward flexion of the trunk with increased lumbar lordosis. Hip abductor weakness results in a Trendelenburg gait pattern with a strong lateral lean to the weak side.

A well-designed exercise program of tone reduction, stretching, and strengthening exercises can assist in improving gait and balance. See Chapter 14 for specific preambulation and gait training activities. Standing and walking activities should stress safety, adequate weight transfer with trunk rotation, a stable base of support, and controlled progression. Pool walking can assist in reducing tone and fatigue and controlling ataxia.

Patients with MS may require assistive devices. In one study of 1145 patients with MS, 4 percent were using crutches, 6 percent leg braces, and 12 percent walkers or canes.[96] Ankle-foot stability can be achieved by the addition of an ankle-foot orthosis (AFO). The most common type prescribed is the standard polypropylene AFO, prescribed for foot drop, poor knee control (hyperextension), minimal to moderate spasticity, and poor somatosensation.[87] An AFO with an articulated joint can be used to provide more rigid control for the ankle (e.g., plantarflexion stop). Rocker shoes (modified Danish clogs) have also been successful with selected patients with MS in compensating for lost ankle mobility. Gait patterns appeared more normal, with a significant savings in energy cost (150% over ambulation without rocker shoes).[97] Although knee-ankle-foot orthoses may be required for additional control, they rarely provide significant functional gains because of the increased energy expenditure required. Canes, forearm crutches, or a walker may be necessary to compensate for deficits in balance or strength. For the patient with increasing fatigue levels, a large-wheeled walker with locking hand brakes and a seat may prove helpful by allowing him or her to take rests. The addition of weights to an ambulatory aid may help stabilize the device and diminish the excursion of limb ataxia.

As the disease progresses, many patients benefit from a wheeled mobility device (powered scooter or wheelchair). The course and progression of the disease and presenting symptoms should be taken into consideration when deciding on a device. For patients with adequate trunk stability, upper extremity function, and appropriate visual, perceptual, and cognitive skills, a scooter provides needed mobility while conserving energy. Scooters also do not carry the same negative stigma that a wheelchair does.[6] Both three- and four-wheel scooters are available. Four-wheel scooters have superior outdoor and uneven terrain performance, but are not as easily transported. Features that should be recommended include a seat that rotates for easy mounting and dismounting, easy dismantling for loading into the car, and steering mechanisms that minimize the work of the upper extremities. One disadvantage of scooters is that seating cannot be customized. They are not designed for prolonged sitting or for patients with moderate to severe neurological impairment. Scooters also have a wider turning radius than wheelchairs and are generally not suitable for in-home use. A wheelchair should be considered when postural demands necessitate increased support. A standard wheelchair is often not much help to patients with MS because of fatigue and the coordination it takes to propel it. A power wheelchair should be considered when these impairments prevent manual propulsion. Power wheelchairs are more costly, more difficult to repair, and require transportation by a wheelchair-accessible van or bus.

Wheelchair seating should ensure proper alignment of the pelvis, trunk and head, and limbs while enhancing function. Common malalignments include posterior tilting of the pelvis (sacral sitting) with kyphosis, typically the result of spasticity in the hamstring muscles. This can be improved with the addition of a cushion with a solid base of support (solid seat or wood insert) to prevent hammocking of the wheelchair upholstery. Postural alignment can also be assisted by the addition of contoured seating (custom built) or a contoured wheelchair cushion (e.g., contoured cushion with gel). A solid back support and adjustable lateral trunk supports may be needed to enhance postural alignment and upright sitting. Footrests should be positioned to ensure that the thighs are parallel to the floor. If extensor spasms are strong, they can actually result in throwing the patient out of the chair. A strong lap belt that secures firmly around the pelvis is necessary for safety. For patients who present with strong adductor spasticity, a medial knee block (pommel) may be necessary. Patients who no longer demonstrate adequate trunk and head stability require an alternate seating design. For some patients, the tilt-in-space wheelchair with head/neck support may be a better option than a reclining wheelchair with high back and elevating leg rests. The former maintains the normal hip sitting angle; the latter produces extension of the hips and may feed into strong extensor spasticity. Elevating leg rests tend to stretch hamstring muscles and may cause posterior pelvic tilting when spasticity is present. The reclining wheelchair with elevating leg rests also creates greater environmental access problems. Motorized control of the seat back (available in either tilt-in-space or reclining wheelchairs) will allow the patient to make easy adjustments in position, thus preventing skin breakdown.

One of the constraints the therapist will have to deal with is limited financial resources to accommodate the changing wheelchair needs of the patient with progressive disease. Many third-party payers will not reimburse for new wheelchairs prescribed within specified time intervals or may be hesitant to finance expensive specialty wheelchairs such as the tilt-in-space chair or a second lightweight chair for traveling. The therapist needs to provide careful documentation of the patient's functional limitations and potential outcomes to justify the cost of the new chair. For example, a likely deleterious outcome for a patient who is denied reimbursement for a tilt-in-space chair may be skin breakdown. The costs of nursing and surgical care for decubitus ulcers can then be compared to the cost of the new wheelchair, which can be justified as a preventive measure. It is equally important to anticipate future needs as they relate to rate of disease progression when ordering a wheelchair.

Patients should be instructed in transfer and wheelchair mobility/management skills. A transfer board or hydraulic lift may be necessary as upper extremity function deteriorates. Attention to good sitting posture and pressure relief techniques is essential to maintain alignment and prevent skin breakdown. Patients should be encouraged to balance time in the wheelchair with other activities, such as walking or exercising, and should be extra diligent in stretching muscles that tend to contract as a result of prolonged sitting (e.g., hip and knee flexors).

CARDIORESPIRATORY FITNESS

Chronic disease is associated with decreased levels of physical activity and reduced cardiorespiratory fitness. Changes that can be expected include decreased physical work capacity, decreased vital capacity, increased heart rate at rest and in response to exercise, decreased muscular strength, increased fatigue, increased anxiety, and depression. Patients with MS can also exhibit abnormalities in autonomic nervous system function, including abnormal heart rate and blood pressure responses during Valsalva maneuver or exercise stress.[98–100] Reported incidence of these changes has been as high as 50 percent of patients with MS. A direct relationship exists between the duration and extent of disease and the likelihood of autonomic cardiovascular dysfunction. Patients with mild disease typically do not exhibit changes, whereas patients with significant long-standing disease are much more likely to demonstrate autonomic dysfunction.[101] Patients with MS can also demonstrate respiratory muscle

dysfunction (weakness, dyssynergia), which contributes to reduced exercise tolerance.[102]

Individuals with stable MS appear to be good candidates for exercise training.[86] Research is limited but accumulating. Ponichtera-Mulcare et al.[103] assessed the effects of aerobic training on nine individuals with MS compared to nondisabled, matched controls and found no significant differences in training effects during discontinuous, submaximal training using recumbent cycling. However, final maximal oxygen effort (Vo_{2max}) was found to be significantly lower in the MS group. Gappamier et al.[104] examined the effects of a 15-week aerobic training program on 46 individuals with mild to moderate MS. A cycle ergometer was used for the exercise program, which included sessions three times a week for 40 minutes. Training intensities were high, approaching maximum levels at 73 to 82 percent of predicted heart rate maximum. The researchers found a significant improvement in exercise capacity following exercise training, evidenced by an improvement in maximum oxygen uptake (Vo_{2max}) of 20 percent. Gehlsen et al.[88] investigated the relationship between strength training and an aquatic training program (freestyle swimming and calisthenics) on a group of 10 patients with MS. Submaximal training intensities were used (60 to 75% heart rate maximum). The researchers found significant improvement on measures of muscle performance and fatigability. Kirsch and Myslinki[105] reported on two individual case reports. Aerobic fitness programs were individualized for both patients. Positive effects with training were reported, including improvements in aerobic capacity and a positive functional effect on their daily lives.

Safety is an important consideration for individuals with such a complex disorder as MS. Aerobic fitness programs should be designed to run within a healthcare environment where professionals can monitor changes rather than at a fitness gym. Individualized exercise prescription is essential and should be based on careful assessment of cardiovascular responses during a measured exercise challenge. Thus, a medically supervised exercise tolerance test should be given (e.g., submaximal treadmill or bike test). Prescription is based on four interrelated elements: frequency of exercise, intensity of exercise, type of exercise, and time or duration (the FITT equation). Frequency will depend on the overall level of fitness of the individual and on the intensity and duration of exercise used. Daily exercise at lower levels of intensity is recommended for individuals with limited exercise capacities (e.g., 3 to 5 metabolic equivalent [METs]); individuals with capacities greater than five METs can engage in frequencies of three times a week.[60] Submaximal levels of exercise have been shown to be safe and are recommended,[86] whereas maximal exercise risks producing undesirable effects (e.g., abnormal autonomic nervous system responses, heat intolerance, fatigue). Type or training mode can include swimming or pool calisthenics, cycle ergometry (upper or lower extremity, recumbent), step aerobics, and/or walking. Careful attention must be given to safety in selecting the exercise mode. For example, the patient with balance instability may have difficulty with a walking program, but may do much better with either pool walking or cycle ergometry. A suitable environment in which temperature is tightly controlled is also important and has been previously discussed. A discontinuous training sequence that carefully balances exercise with rest time is indicated; continuous training is contraindicated. Circuit training, in which improved work capacity is developed through the use of various different stations that alternate work between upper and lower extremities, may also prove best for reducing the likelihood of fatigue. Progression through the stations should depend on the individual's recovery of heart rate after a specified rest period.[105] Outcome measures should include measures of cardiorespiratory performance: heart rate and blood pressure measures before, during, and after exercise. Electrocardiographic monitoring can be used initially to ensure that the patient is safe, and to ensure accurate measurements of pulse. Perception of exertion using Borg's RPE scale is also an important measure. Finally functional improvement and quality of life measures are important outcome measures. The overall success of a fitness program may be best assessed by determining the individual's level of understanding of the basic principles of conditioning and independence in self-monitoring and decision-making relative to safety, exercise progression, and home exercises.[105]

Prolonged inactivity (bed rest) can result in significant deconditioning and the development of numerous secondary impairments (see Fig. 22-1). Shallow respiratory patterns may contribute to speech difficulties and recurrent respiratory infections. Thus, respiratory muscle strengthening is an important component of treatment, and should be combined with activities to improve trunk stability, head control, and sitting balance. Breathing can be facilitated through proper placement of manual contacts and resistance. The therapist must focus on diaphragmatic breathing, effective coughing, and segmental expansion. Incentive spirometry can also improve respiratory control.

SPEECH AND FEEDING DIFFICULTIES

When speech or feeding difficulties are apparent, physical therapy efforts should be closely coordinated with those of the speech/language pathologist. A detailed assessment is necessary, including videofluoroscopy for dysphagia. The physical therapist can assist in reducing speech and feeding difficulties by improving sitting position, head control, and oral-motor coordination. An upright posture with a slightly flexed head position is necessary to achieve good swallowing and avoid aspiration. Oral-motor exercises can improve mouth function and include specific exercises for lip closure, tongue movements, and jaw control. Stretch and resistance can be used to facilitate and strengthen muscle actions. Sucking reflexes and saliva production can be stimulated by using an ice cube or a water popsicle. Resistive sucking through a straw can also be helpful. Brief icing of the tongue, back of the mouth, and laryngeal area of the neck may stimulate swallowing as can pressure on the neck and thyroid notch. Thicker liquids, which provide some resistance and therefore some facilitation of muscle action, are generally easier to swallow than thin liquids. Gradually, semisoft, moist foods are introduced (pasta, mashed potatoes, squash, jello). Alternating liquid with solid food can also assist passage of food. Crumbly or stringy foods are avoided (cake, cookies, chips, celery, cheeses). The patient should not attempt to talk during eating. Fatigue can also affect feeding, and patients may benefit from eating their main meal in the morning and from eating multiple small meals throughout the day. The speech/language pathologist also teaches swallowing techniques, including the power swallow. This involves having the person first inhale and then hold his or her breath, thereby closing the airway. The person then swallows, exhales, and swallows again. Feeding tubes may be necessary with severe dysphagia. Family members and caregivers should be taught the Heimlich maneuver.[6,106,107]

COGNITIVE TRAINING

Cognitive deficits can present major difficulties for the patient and for rehabilitation efforts in general. Compensatory strategies for memory deficits should be considered. These include the use of memory aids, timing devices, and environmental strategies. A posted schedule, memory book, audiotapes, or pill dispenser can assist the patient in completing daily tasks. Training should include how to use the device, when and where to use it, and practice adapting its use to new or novel situations. Cueing devices such as an alarm clock, bell timer, or watch alarm can help patients remember when to do certain tasks (e.g., taking medications, performing pressure relief). Structuring and labeling the environment can also be an effective strategy in assisting memory (e.g., labeled drawers, cabinets). Directions for functional tasks (e.g., transfers) should be carefully written down for patients and caregivers. Complex tasks can be broken down with clear written directions provided for each step. Directions can be posted in different areas of the home (e.g., steps for toilet or tub transfer posted in the bathroom).[108] Additional cognitive strategies that may be helpful include mental rehearsal, requesting assistance, maximizing alertness, avoidance of difficult situations, immediate action, and mental exercise.[23] Poor follow-through should be expected among patients with significant cognitive deficits. The efforts of family and caregivers need to be fully maximized.

Psychosocial Issues

Individuals with MS and their families may show a variety of psychosocial adaptations. These can be similar to the stages of grief associated with death and dying: anger, bargaining, depression, and finally acceptance. Depression is extremely common. Reactions do not necessarily relate to the severity of the disease. For example, a person with mild disease can be severely depressed, whereas the person with severe disability is not. The unique feature of a relapsing-remitting disease course is that it requires continual readjustment every time a new set of symptoms appears. Patients who appear well adjusted at one stage may regress as the disease worsens. The uncertainty of MS produces both cognitive and emotional stresses; patients feel out of control and unsure of themselves. Matson and Brooks point out that living with MS requires not only initial acceptance, but also a tremendous flexibility to deal with this lack of closure.[109] Patients also experience the cumulative effects of smaller, everyday stresses that are associated with inability to perform ADL, dependency on others, architectural barriers, and so forth.[110] Many factors play a role in determining how an individual reacts to MS. These include the overall effect of the disease on daily life functioning, previous coping skills, perceived self-efficacy, extent of social support, and spiritual well-being. Patients are typically dealing with multiple losses: loss of social functioning, interpersonal relationships, employment status, independence, and ADL skills. Patients may experience attitudes of "wait and see" or "nothing can be done." The longer they are exposed to these attitudes, the less likely they are to seek help.[111] Learned helplessness, low self-efficacy, and lack of environmental mastery have been identified as major factors contributing to depression and fatigue.[19] **Self-efficacy** is the belief that an individual will be able to deal with particular situations that may contain novel, unpredictable, and stressful elements.[113]

The primary roles of the clinician can be categorized as caring professional, teacher expert, and competent professional.[114] A positive, affirming attitude can effectively influence patient attitudes. Clinicians should be sensitive, respectful, accepting, compassionate, and positive, relaying to their patients a strong belief that treatment can be beneficial. This maintenance of therapeutic hope is extremely important. As teacher, the therapist assists the patient and family in their understanding of the disease, the importance of life-style modification, and the rehabilitation process and specific treatments. A great deal of information is needed in the beginning that should be reinforced throughout the course of rehabilitation. Personal and family counseling should be provided early in the course of the disease and continued with later episodes of care as needed.

Timely referral to neurorehabilitation services is important, beginning at the time of diagnosis. Too often, services are not begun until the individual becomes severely disabled. The overall focus of rehabilitation should be to keep the individual with MS as active as realistically possible and promote compensatory strategies to alleviate problems.[46] Plans of care should emphasize meaningful functional activities, remaining abilities, and desired outcomes. Activities that prove attainable ensure patient success and build self-efficacy. The promotion of self-management skills is also an important strategy to improve self-efficacy.[113] Many patients with MS report that they lack the knowledge and skills needed to exercise safely.[115] Promoting environmental mastery can be achieved with techniques such as time management, activity pacing, energy conservation, and work simplification.[19] The use of stress reduction techniques (e.g., progressive relaxation techniques, meditation) are helpful in promoting effective coping.

Referral to a support group can provide a necessary psychological base for patients and their families. Within this environment individuals can gain accurate and useful information about the disease, discuss common problems and methods of coping, and share anxieties. Thus, it provides a necessary forum to assist in the continual adjustment process. The National Multiple Sclerosis Society is a valuable resource for patients and their families.

A significant number of patients with MS (one out of every two patients) will require the assistance of another person at some point in the course of their disease.[116] This places an extra burden on family members and/or on the financial resources of the patient if outside attendants must be utilized. The majority of caregivers experience moderate levels of stress associated with their care-giving duties. As the level and duration of physical care increases, caregivers may experience additional stresses, including exhaustion, confinement and loss of personal freedom, and financial pressures. The clinician will need to be sensitive to these issues. Considerable time and energy will be devoted to counseling and educating caregivers and coordinating home management. Cultural, religious, and personal values and beliefs should be respected. Conflicts, problems, and tensions should be carefully examined. A positive attitude and an honest, open approach generally prove most helpful.

SUMMARY

MS is a chronic, often disabling progressive disease of the CNS, characterized by widespread demyelinating lesions in the brain and spinal cord. The severity and progress of specific symptoms are varied and unpredictable. Most individuals with MS are diagnosed between the ages of 20 and 40. It is generally accepted that MS involves an abnormal autoimmune reaction that may be triggered by exposure to viruses. Environmental studies indicate that risk or exposure occurs during childhood. The diagnosis is usually based on clinical findings. Evidence of two or more episodes of symptoms associated with distinct CNS lesions occurring over time or progressing over time is used to establish the diagnosis. Laboratory and electrophysiological tests and MRI are used to confirm the diagnosis.

MS is an unpredictable disease, typically presenting with an exacerbating-remitting course. A progressive course or combination of the two may also be seen. Common clinical findings include disturbances in sensation, vision, motor function (including spasticity), fatigue, ataxia, cognitive and behavioral function, and bladder and bowel function. Numerous secondary impairments can arise from prolonged inactivity and deconditioning. Survival and disability rates are variable, with life expectancies approaching normal.

Medical management is primarily symptomatic, although treatments are available to reduce acute flare-ups and slow disease progression. There is no specific preventive or curative treatment.

Rehabilitation efforts are restorative, directed toward improving functional status and managing impairments. Functional maintenance programs are also necessary to manage the effects of progressive disease. Strategies to promote regular exercise, good health, and self-management skills are key elements. The therapist as a caring professional, expert teacher, and competent professional examines and evaluates the patient and develops an appropriate plan of care. Important outcomes of treatment include the promotion of successful psychosocial adjustment and quality of life. Comprehensive efforts of an interdisciplinary team are needed to provide coordinated and continuing care with anticipated hospital-based, outpatient, and home/community episodes of care.

QUESTIONS FOR REVIEW

1. What are the primary areas of the CNS involved in MS? What are the most common signs and symptoms?

2. How is the diagnosis of MS established? What tests and measures are used to confirm the diagnosis?

3. Differentiate between the different clinical courses MS can take. How will they influence overall intervention strategies?

4. What are the clinical effects of prolonged inactivity for the patient with chronic, progressive MS? Identify three strategies that can be used to counteract these effects.

5. Discuss Uthoff's symptom and how this will influence the design of an exercise program for the patient with MS.

6. What components should be included in a physical therapy examination? Identify four standardized measures that would be appropriate to use with the patient with MS.

7. What therapeutic exercises and techniques can be used to moderate spasticity?

8. What therapeutic exercises and techniques can be used to modify paresis? Ataxia?

9. What therapeutic strategies can be used to improve cardiorespiratory fitness? Precautions?

10. Differentiate between a rehabilitation program with restorative focus versus one with a functional maintenance focus. Consider goals/outcomes and overall training approach.

11. What are the major considerations in ordering a wheelchair for a person with chronic progressive MS?

12. What psychosocial issues in adjustment does the patient with relapsing-remitting MS face? How can adjustment and self-efficacy be facilitated?

CASE STUDY

HISTORY: The patient is a 27 year-old graduate student who was admitted with a chief complaint of double vision for 2 weeks. She reported that both lower extremities (LEs) seem weaker recently. Three months earlier, she had noticed persistent tingling of her fingers on the left hand and some numbness on the left side of her face.

Neurological examination showed a scotoma in the upper field of the left eye, weakness of the left medial rectus muscle, horizontal nystagmus on left lateral gaze, and mild weakness of the left central facial muscles. All other muscles had normal strength. The deep tendon reflexes were normal on the right and brisk on the left, and there was a left extensor plantar response. The sensory system was unremarkable.

The patient was discharged a few days later, seemingly improved after corticosteroid treatment. She was readmitted 4 months later, however, because she noticed difficulty in walking and her speech had become thickened.

NEUROLOGICAL EXAMINATION FINDINGS
- Wide-based ataxic gait.
- Minor slurring of speech.
- Bilateral tremor in the finger-to-nose test.
- Dysdiadochokinesia.
- CT scan was within normal limits.
- MRI scan revealed numerous white areas indicative of lesions.
- Lumbar puncture showed 56 milligrams of protein with increased level of gamma globulin. All other CSF findings were normal.

Treatment with high doses of intravenous corticosteroids seemed to improve the neurological symptoms. Patient was discharged home with a referral for outpatient rehabilitation. Two months later the patient's symptoms worsened and she is now admitted for intensive rehabilitation.

MEDICAL MANAGEMENT
- Prednisone 20 mg PO QID
- Maalox 30 cc PO QID
- Valium 10 mg QID

SOCIAL HISTORY: Patient has been living on her own for several years until her recent illness. She has taken a medical leave from graduate school and plans on returning home to live with her parents. They are both supportive of this idea and would like some advice as to how to modify their two-story home. There are five entry stairs with a handrail on both sides. There is a first floor bathroom, and they plan to convert the first floor study into a bedroom.

They are both in their early 60s, in good health, and very anxious about their daughter's rapidly deteriorating condition.

EXAMINATION FINDINGS

Mental Status:
Alert, oriented
Memory intact
At times lacks insight, seems unaware of the seriousness of her condition
Euphoric at times; other times she is depressed and cries easily

Communication:
Speech is dysarthric, difficult to understand

Vision:
Transient double vision
Gaze-evoked nystagmus to both left and right
Ocular dysmetria
Upper field defect of left eye

Endurance/Fatigue:
Moderate to severe impairment
Tolerance to activity is approximately 10 minutes before rest is required

Skin:
WNL except for small bruise on right lateral malleolus

ROM:
WNL except for 0 degrees right dorsiflexion; 0–5 degrees left dorsiflexion

Tone:
Moderate extensor spasticity both lower extremities (BLEs), left greater than right
Occasional extensor spasms, which are a major safety risk when they occur during transfers

Sensation:
Paresthesias BLEs with moderate proprioceptive losses, ankle joints greater than proximal joints
Both upper extremities (BUEs): mild decrease in light touch, left greater than right

Strength:
Moderate paraparesis
BLEs: generally functional muscle grades (able to move against gravity) with the greatest weakness noted at the hips
Standard MMT positions not used owing to spasticity
BUEs fair+ to good-strength

Coordination:
Intention tremors BUEs with moderate limb ataxia
RAMs are severely impaired
Voluntary movements BUEs are hypermetric
BLEs: movements restricted by spasticity and spasms

Balance:
Sitting balance
Static: with eyes open, able to maintain position independently up to 3 minutes with moderate postural tremor; with eyes closed, truncal ataxia is pronounced
Dynamic: with eyes open, able to weight shift to left and right to about 40 percent of limits of stability (LOS); with eyes closed, experiences loss of balance (LOB) with minimal weight shifts
Standing balance
Static: Able to maintain standing position in parallel bars with moderate assistance × 1 for up to 1 minute; during standing, patient is unable to maintain centered alignment; demonstrates moderate postural tremor; with eyes closed, sway is in- creased dramatically and patient quickly loses her balance
Fixates: tends to keep her hips and knees stiff in extension/hyperextension
Dynamic: unable to weight shift with LOB

Functional:
Bed mobility:
ModA × 1 for supine-to-sit
Independent (I) in rolling to right and left
Transfers:
MaxA × 1 for stand pivot transfers and sit to stand transfers
Gait:
Patient has used a walker in the past
Current: walks in the parallel bars with MaxA × 2 × 5 feet
Wheelchair:
Propels self independently in standard wheelchair for short distances only (15 feet)
Requires a lap belt due to extensor spasms, which can cause her to fling out of the chair
Posture in w/c: sacral sitting

BADLs:
MinA × 1 for bathing and dressing
I in eating with proper positioning, set ups, and adaptive equipment

PATIENT'S GOALS: Would like to regain ambulation skills and independent living status. She recognizes the need to live with her parents for the time being but sees this as only temporary.

Continued

Guiding Questions

1. Identify/categorize this patient's problems in terms of:
    a. Direct impairments
    b. Indirect impairments
    c. Composite impairments: combined effects of both direct and indirect impairments
2. Identify two outcomes (the remediation of functional limitations and disability) and two goals (remediation of impairments) for this patient.
3. Formulate four treatment interventions that could be used at the start of therapy to achieve the stated outcomes and goals. Provide a brief rationale for each.
4. What strategies would you use to develop self-management skills and promote self-efficacy and quality of life?

REFERENCES

1. Dean, G: The multiple sclerosis problem. Sci Am 223:40, 1970.
2. Anderson, D, et al: Revised estimate of the prevalence of multiple sclerosis in the United States. Ann Neurol 31:333, 1992.
3. Gorelick, P: Clues to the mystery of multiple sclerosis. Postgrad Med J 85:125, 1989.
4. Guberman, A: An Introduction to Clinical Neurology. Little, Brown and Co., Boston, 1994.
5. Guyton, A: Basic Neuroscience, ed 2. Saunders, Philadelphia, 1991.
6. Shapiro, RT: Symptom Management in Multiple Sclerosis, ed 3. Demos Publishing, New York, 1998.
7. Matthews, WB, et al: McAlpine's Multiple Sclerosis. Churchill Livingstone, Edinburgh, 1991.
8. Goodman, C, and Boissonnault, W: Pathology: Implications for the Physical Therapist. Saunders, Philadelphia, 1998.
9. Kurtzke, J: Epidemiological contributions to multiple sclerosis: An overview. Neurology 30:61, 1980.
10. McFarlin, D, and McFarland, H: Multiple sclerosis. N Engl J Med 307:1183, 1982.
11. Lechtenberg, R: Multiple Sclerosis Fact Book, ed 2. FA Davis, Philadelphia, 1995.
12. Shapiro, R: Symptom management in multiple sclerosis. Ann Neurol 36:S1230, 1994.
13. Katz, R, and Rymer, Z: Spastic hypertonia: Mechanisms and measurement. Arch Phys Med Rehabil 70:144, 1989.
14. Stolp-Smith, K, et al: Management of impairment, disability, and handicap due to multiple sclerosis. Mayo Clin Proc 72:1184, 1997.
15. Krupp, L, et al: Fatigue in multiple sclerosis. Arch Neurol 45:435, 1988.
16. Freal, J, et al: Symptomatic fatigue in multiple sclerosis. Arch Phys Med Rehabil 65:135, 1984.
17. Packer, T, et al: Fatigue secondary to chronic illness: Postpolio syndrome, chronic fatigue syndrome, and multiple sclerosis. Arch Phys Med Rehabil 75:1122, 1994.
18. Fisk, J, et al: The impact of fatigue on patients with multiple sclerosis. Le Journal Canadien Des Sciences Neurologiques 21:9, 1994.
19. Schwartz, C, et al: Psychosocial correlates of fatigue in multiple sclerosis. Arch Phys Med Rehabil 77:165, 1996.
20. Herrera, W: Vestibular and other balance disorders in multiple sclerosis. Neurol Clin 5:407, 1990.
21. Petersen, R, and Kokmen, E: Cognitive and psychiatric abnormalities in multiple sclerosis. Mayo Clin Proc 64:657, 1989.
22. Franklin, G, et al: Cognitive loss in multiple sclerosis. Arch Neurol 46:162, 1989.
23. Brassington, J, and Marsh, N: Neuropsychological Aspects of Multiple Sclerosis. Neuropsychol Rev 8:43, 1998.
24. Shnek, Z, et al: Helplessness, self-efficacy, cognitive distortions and depression in multiple sclerosis and spinal cord injury. Ann Behav Med 19:287, 1997.
25. Minden, S, and Schiffer, R: Affective disorders in multiple sclerosis. Arch Neurol 47:98, 1990.
26. Andrews, K, and Husmann, D: Bladder dysfunction and management in multiple sclerosis. Mayo Clin Proc 72:1176, 1997.
27. Lublin, F, and Reingold, S: Defining the clinical course of multiple sclerosis: Results of an international survey. Neurology 46:907, 1996.
28. Dick, G, and Gay, D: Multiple sclerosis: Autoimmune or bicrobial? A critical review with additional observations. J Infect 16:25, 1988.
29. Johnson, K: Cerebrospinal fluid and blood assays of diagnostic usefulness in multiple sclerosis. Neurology 30:106, 1980.
30. Tindall, R: Therapy of acute and chronic multiple sclerosis. Compr Ther 17:18, 1991.
31. DiFabio, R, et al: Extended outpatient rehabilitation: Its influence on symptom frequency, fatigue, and functional status for persons with progressive multiple sclerosis. Arch Phys Med Rehabil 79:141, 1998.
32. Noseworthy, J: Therapeutics of multiple sclerosis. Clin Neuropharmacol 14:49, 1991.
33. Goodin, D: The use of immunosuppressive agents in the treatment of multiple sclerosis: A critical review. Neurology 41:980, 1991.
34. van Oosten, B, et al: Multiple sclerosis therapy: A practical guide. Drugs 49:201, 1995.
35. Azouvi, P, et al: Intrathecal Baclofen administration for control of severe spinal spasticity: Functional improvement and long-term follow-up. Arch Phys Med Rehabil 77:35, 1996.
36. Abel, N, and Smith, R: Intrathecal Baclofen for treatment of intractable spinal spasticity. Arch Phys Med Rehabil 75:54, 1994.
37. Freeman, J, et al: The impact of inpatient rehabilitation on progressive multiple sclerosis. Ann Neurol 42:236, 1997.
38. Aisen, ML, et al: Inpatient rehabilitation for multiple sclerosis. J Neurol Rehabil 10:43, 1996.
39. Kidd, D, et al: The benefit of inpatient neurorehabilitation in multiple sclerosis. Clin Rehabil 9:198, 1995.
40. Francabandera, FL, et al: Multiple sclerosis rehabilitation: Inpatient versus outpatient. Rehabilitation Nursing 13:251, 1988.
41. Carey, R, and Seibert, J: Who makes the most progress in inpatient rehabilitation? An analysis of functional gain. Arch Phys Med Rehabil 69:337, 1988.
42. Reding, MJ, and La Rocca, NG: Acute-hospital care versus rehabilitation hospitalization for management of nonemergent complications in multiple sclerosis. Journal of Neurol Rehabil 1:13, 1987.
43. Greenspun, B, et al: Multiple sclerosis and rehabilitation outcome. Arch Phys Med Rehabil 68:434, 1987.
44. Feigenson, JS, et al: The cost-effectiveness of multiple sclerosis rehabilitation: A model. Neurology 31:1316, 1981.
45. Moffa-Trotter, M, and Anemaet, W: Addressing functional maintenance programs in home care. Advance, August 24, 1998.
46. Mertin, J: Rehabilitation in multiple sclerosis. Ann Neurol 36:S130, 1994.
47. Folstein, M: Mini-mental state: A practice of method for grading the cognitive state of patients for the clinician. J Psychiatr Res 12:189, 1975.
48. Melzack, R: The McGill Pain Questionnaire: Major properties and scoring methods. Pain 1:227, 1975.
49. Multiple Sclerosis Council for Clinical Practice Guidelines: Fatigue and Multiple Sclerosis Evidence-Based Manage-

ment Strategies for Fatigue in Multiple Sclerosis. Paralyzed Veterans of America, New York, 1998.

50. De Souza, L, and Ashburn, A: Assessment of motor function in people with multiple sclerosis. Physiother Res Int 1:98, 1996.

51. Shumway-Cook, A, and Woollacott, M: Motor Control Theory and Practical Applications. Williams & Wilkins, Baltimore, 1995.

52. Schwid, S, et al: The measurement of ambulatory impairment in multiple sclerosis. Neurology 49:1419, 1997.

53. Lord, SE, et al: Visual gait analysis: The development of a clinical assessment and scale. Clin Rehabil 12:107, 1998.

54. Shumway-Cook, A, and Horak, F: Assessing the influence of sensory interaction on balance. Phys Ther 66:1548, 1986.

55. Nelson, S, et al: Vestibular and sensory interaction deficits assessed by dynamic platform posturography in patients with multiple sclerosis. Ann Otol Rhinol Laryngol 104:62, 1995.

56. Jackson, R, et al: Abnormalities in posturography and estimations of visual vertical and horizontal in multiple sclerosis. Am J Otol 16:88, 1995.

57. Berg, K, et al: Measuring balance in the elderly: Preliminary development of an instrument. Physiotherapy Canada 41:304, 1989.

58. Tinetti, M: Performance-oriented assessment of mobility problems in elderly patients. J Am Geriatr Soc 34:119, 1986.

59. Borg, G: Psychophysical bases of perceived exertion. Med Sci Sports Exerc 14:377, 1982.

60. American College of Sports Medicine: ACSM's Guidelines for Exercise Testing and Prescription, ed 5. Williams & Wilkins, Baltimore, 1995.

61. Guide for the Uniform Data Set for Medical Rehabilitation including the FIM instrument, Version 5.0. State University of New York at Buffalo, Buffalo, 1996.

62. Granger, C, et al: Functional assessment scales: A study of persons with multiple sclerosis. Arch Phys Med Rehabil 71:870, 1990.

63. Kurtin, P, et al: Patient-based health status measures in outpatient dialysis: Early experiences in developing an outcomes assessment program. Med Care 30(suppl 5):136, 1992.

64. Gilson, B, et al: The Sickness Impact Profile: Development of an outcome measure of health care. Am J Public Health 65:1304, 1975.

65. Doble, S, et al: Functional competence of community-dwelling persons with multiple sclerosis using the Assessment of Motor and Process Skills. Arch Phys Med Rehabil 75:843, 1994.

66. Kurtzke, J: On the evaluation of disability in multiple sclerosis. Neurology 11:686, 1961.

67. Kurtzke, J: Rating neurological impairment in multiple sclerosis: An expanded disability status scale (EDSS). Neurology 33:1444, 1983.

68. Noseworthy, J, et al. and Canadian Cooperative MS Study Group: Interrater variability with the Expanded Disability Status Scale (EDSS) and Functional Systems (FS) in a multiple sclerosis clinical trial. Neurology 40:971, 1990.

69. Haber, A, and LaRocca, N (eds): M.R.D. Minimal Record of Disability for Multiple Sclerosis. National Multiple Sclerosis Society, New York, 1985.

70. Solari, A, et al: Accuracy of self-assessment of the minimal record of disability in patients with multiple sclerosis. Acta Neurol Scand 87:43, 1993.

71. Cella, D, et al: Validation of the Functional Assessment of Multiple Sclerosis quality of life instrument. Neurology 47:129, 1996.

72. Pfenning, L, et al: Quality of life in multiple sclerosis. MS Management 2:26, 1995.

73. Vickrey, BG, et al: A health-related quality of life measure for multiple sclerosis. Qual Life Res 4:187, 1995.

74. Fisk, J, et al: The impact of fatigue on patients with multiple sclerosis. Le Journal Canadien Des Sciences Neurologiques 21:9, 1994.

75. DiFabio, R, et al: Health-related quality of life for patients with multiple sclerosis: Influence of rehabilitation. Phys Ther 77:1704, 1977.

76. American Physical Therapy Association: Guide to Physical Therapist Practice. APTA, Alexandria, VA, 1999.

77. McCulloch, J, et al: Wound Healing: Alternatives in Management, ed 2. FA Davis, Philadelphia, 1995.

78. Brar, S, et al: Evaluation of treatment protocols on minimal to moderate spasticity in multiple sclerosis. Arch Phys Med Rehabil 72:186, 1991.

79. O'Sullivan, S, and Schmitz, T: Physical Rehabilitation Laboratory Manual: Focus on Functional Training. FA Davis, Philadelphia, 1999.

80. Bobath, B: The treatment of neuromuscular disorders by improving patterns of co-ordination. Physiotherapy 55:18, 1969.

81. Davies, P: Right in the Middle. Springer-Verlag, New York, 1990.

82. Voss, D, et al: Proprioceptive Neuromuscular Facilitation, ed 3. Harper & Row, Philadelphia, 1985.

83. Carlson, S: A neurophysiological analysis of inhibitive casting. Phys Occup Ther Pediatr 4:31, 1984.

84. Cusick, B: Serial Casts: Their use in the Management of Spasticity Induced Foot Deformity. Words at Work, Lexington, KY, 1987.

85. McComas, A, et al: Fatigue brought on by malfunction of the central and peripheral nervous systems. In Simon, C, et al (ed): Fatigue. Plenum Press, New York, 1995, p 495.

86. Costello, E, et al: Exercise prescription for individuals with multiple sclerosis. Neurology Report 20:24, 1996.

87. Shapiro, R: Multiple Sclerosis: A Rehabilitation Approach to Management. Demos, New York, 1991.

88. Gehlsen, G, et al: Effects of an aquatic fitness program on the muscular strength and endurance of patients with multiple sclerosis. Phys Ther 64:653, 1984.

89. Erland, C, et al: Effects of the Mark VII personal cooling system on selected symptoms of multiple sclerosis. (Abstract.) Neurology Report 19:23, 1995.

90. Svensson, B, et al: Endurance training in patients with multiple sclerosis: Five case studies. Phys Ther 74:1017, 1994.

91. DeSouza, L: A different approach to physiotherapy for multiple sclerosis patients. Physiotherapy 70:428, 1984.

92. Kottke, F: Philosophic consideration of quality of life for the disabled. Arch Phys Med Rehabil 63:60, 1982.

93. Baum, H, and Rothschild, B: Multiple sclerosis and mobility restriction. Arch Phys Med Rehabil 64:591, 1983.

94. Frankel, D: Multiple Sclerosis. In Umpred, D (ed): Neurological Rehabilitation, ed 3. Mosby, St. Louis, 1995, p 588.

95. Wolf, B: Occupational therapy for patients with multiple sclerosis. In Maloney, F, et al (eds): Interdisciplinary Rehabilitation of Multiple Sclerosis and Neuromuscular Disorders. Lippincott, Philadelphia, 1985, p 103.

96. Baum, H, and Rothschild, B: Multiple sclerosis and mobility restriction. Arch Phys Med Rehabil 64:591, 1983.

97. Perry, J, et al: Rocker shoe as walking aid in multiple sclerosis. I. Arch Phys Med Rehabil 62:59, 1981.

98. Ponichtera-Mulcare, J: Exercise and multiple sclerosis. Med Sci Sports Exerc 25:451, 1993.

99. Anema, J, et al: Cardiovascular autonomic function in multiple sclerosis. J Neurol Sci 104:129, 1992.

100. Sterman, A, et al: Disseminated abnormalities of cardiovascular autonomic functions in multiple sclerosis. Neurology 35:1665, 1985.

101. Pentland, B, and Ewing, D: Cardiovascular reflexes in multiple sclerosis. Eur Neurol 26:46, 1987.

102. Foglio, K, et al: Respiratory muscle function and exercise capacity in multiple sclerosis. Eur Respir J 7:23, 1994.

103. Ponichtera-Mulcare, J, et al: Maximal aerobic exercise in persons with multiple sclerosis. Clinical Kinesiology 46:12, 1993.

104. Gappmaier, E, et al: Aerobic exercise in multiple sclerosis (abstract). Neurology Report 19:41, 1995.

105. Kirsch, N, and Myslinski, MJ: The effect of a personally designed fitness program on the aerobic capacity and function for two individuals with multiple sclerosis. Phys Ther Case Reports 2:19, 1999.

106. Ruttenberg, N: Assessment and treatment of speech and swallowing problems in patients with multiple sclerosis. In Maloney, F, et al (eds): Interdisciplinary Rehabilitation of

Multiple Sclerosis and Neuromuscular Disorders. Lippincott, Philadelphia, 1985, p 129.
107. Simmons-Mackie, N: Disorders in oral, speech, and language functions. In Umpred, D (ed.): Neurological Rehabilitation, ed 3. Mosby, St. Louis, 1995, p 747.
108. Zoltan, B: Vision, Perception, and Cognition, ed 3. Slack Inc., Thorofare, NJ, 1996.
109. Matson, R, and Brooks, N: Adjusting to multiple sclerosis: An exploratory study. Soc Sci Med 11:245, 1977.
110. Pulton, T: Multiple sclerosis social psychological perspective. Phys Ther 57:170, 1977.
111. Kraft, G, et al: Disability, disease duration, and rehabilitation services needs in multiple sclerosis: Patient perspective. Arch Phys Med Rehabil 67:164, 1986.

112. Cervera-Deval, J, et al: Social handicaps of multiple sclerosis and their relation to neurological alterations. Arch Phys Med Rehabil 75:1223, 1994.
113. Shnek, Z, et al: Helplessness, self-efficacy, cognitive distortions, and depression in multiple sclerosis and spinal cord injury. Ann Behav Med 19:287, 1997.
114. Leino-Kilpi, H, et al: Elements of empowerment and MS patients. J Neurosci Nurs 30:116, 1998.
115. Stuifbergen, A, and Roberts, G: Health promotion practices of women with multiple sclerosis. Arch Phys Med Rehabil 78(suppl 5):S-3, 1997.
116. Price, G: The challenge to the family. Am J Nurs 80:283, 1980.

SUPPLEMENTAL READINGS

Cook, S (ed): Handbook of Multiple Sclerosis. Marcel Dekker, New York, 1990.
Dittmar, S, and Gresham, G: Functional Assessment and Outcome Measures for the Rehabilitation Health Professional. Aspen, Gaithersburg, MD, 1997.
Halper, J, and Holland, N: Comprehensive Nursing Care in Multiple Sclerosis. Demos Vermande, New York, 1997.
Kalb, RC, and Scheinberg, LC (eds): Multiple Sclerosis and the Family. Demos, New York, 1992.

Matthews, WB, et al: McAlpine's Multiple Sclerosis, ed 2. Churchill Livingstone, New York, 1991.
National Multiple Sclerosis Society, 733 Third Ave., New York, NY 10017; http://www.nmss.org/
Reader, AT (ed): Interferon Therapy of Multiple Sclerosis. Marcel Dekker, New York, 1997.

GLOSSARY

Activity pacing: The balancing of activity with rest periods interspersed throughout the day.

Ataxia: A general term used to describe uncoordinated movement, especially that manifested when voluntary muscular movements are attempted; may influence gait, posture, and patterns of movement.

> **Sensory ataxia:** Ataxia resulting from interference in conduction of sensory responses, especially proprioceptive impulses from muscles. The condition becomes aggravated when the eyes are closed (+Romberg's sign).

Autoimmune disease: A disease produced when the body's normal tolerance of its own antigenic markers on cells disappears. Autoantibodies are produced by B lymphocytes and attack normal cells.

Benign MS: A disease course in which the patient remains fully functional in all neurological systems 15 years post onset.

Charcot's triad: Cardinal symptoms of multiple sclerosis including intention tremor, scanning speech, and nystagmus.

Demyelination: Destruction or removal of the myelin sheath of nerve tissue by a disease process.

Diplopia: Double vision that occurs when the muscles that control the eyes are not well coordinated.

Dysarthria: A motor-speech disorder caused by impairment in parts of central or peripheral nervous system that mediate speech production. Respiration, articulation, phonation, resonance, and/or prosody may be affected; chewing, swallowing, and movements of the tongue may also be deviant.

Dysesthesias: Abnormal burning or aching sensations.

Dysdiadochokinesia: Impaired ability to perform rapid alternating movements (RAM).

Dysmetria: Impaired ability to judge the distance or range of a movement.

Dysphagia: Inability to swallow or difficulty in swallowing.

Dyssynergia: Impaired ability to associate muscles together for complex movement; decomposition of movement.

Emotional dysregulation syndrome: Lack of emotional control with uncontrollable laughing and crying.

Energy conservation: Life-style suggestions and techniques designed to minimize fatigue and avoid exhaustion by conserving energy.

Euphoria: An exaggerated feeling of well-being, a sense of optimism incongruent with the patient's incapacitating disability.

Exacerbation: Acute worsening or flare-up of neurological signs and symptoms, usually associated with inflammation and demyelination in the brain and spinal cord.

Expanded Disability Status Scale (EDDS): A functional assessment scale used to measure the severity of functional impairment in multiple sclerosis.

Fatigue: A sense of physical tiredness and lack of energy distinct from sadness or weakness.

Frenkel's exercises: Exercises designed to improve incoordination and ataxia resulting from a loss of proprioception.

Functional maintenance program: A program designed to manage the effects of progressive disease; rehabilitation is ongoing (home program or outpatient program) and focused on strategies to prevent or slow decline of function, promote regular exercise, good health, and self-management skills.

Gliosis: Proliferation of neuroglial tissue within the central nervous system that results in glial scars (plaques).

Hyperpathia: A hypersensitivity to minor sensory stimuli.

Internuclear ophthalmoplegia (INO): Incomplete eye adduction (lateral gaze palsy) on the affected side and nystagmus of the opposite abducting eye with gaze to one side.

Lhermitte's sign: A sensation like an electric shock running down the spine and into the lower extremities and produced by flexing the neck.

Malignant MS: A relatively rare disease course that is rapidly progressing, leading to significant disability in multiple neurological systems and death within a relatively short time.

Minimum Record of Disability (MRD): A functional assessment scale that measures the physical incapacity (Incapacity Status Scale, ISS) and environmental handicaps (Environmental Status Scale, ESS) experienced by persons with MS.

Myelin: The phospholipid-protein of the cell membranes of Schwann cells and oligodendrocytes (CNS) that forms the myelin sheath of neurons. It acts as an electrical insulator and increases the velocity of impulse transmission.

Nystagmus: Involuntary, cyclical movement of the eyeball; movement may be in any direction. Develops in response to lesions affecting the cerebellum or vestibular system.

Optic neuritis: Inflammation of the optic nerve that may produce blurring or graying of vision, or blindness in one eye; often associated with pain in the eye.

Paresthesias: Abnormal sensations such as numbness, prickling, or tingling without apparent cause.

Plaques: Sclerosed (hardened) and scarred myelin in areas of the brain and spinal cord, causing a short-circuiting of electrical transmission.

Progressive (chronic) MS: Characterized by progressive onset of symptoms and disability with no apparent or significant respite from disease.

Relapsing-remitting MS: Characterized by relapses with either full recovery or some remaining neurological signs/symptoms and residual deficit upon recovery. The periods between relapses are characterized by lack of disease progression.

Remission: A period free of evolving symptoms.

Restorative rehabilitation: Rehabilitation that is focused on the remediation of impairments, functional limitations, and disability.

Scanning speech: A speech pattern characterized by slowed speech with long pauses and disrupted melody; volume is low and clarity is affected.

Scotoma: Island-like blind gap in the visual field.

Self-efficacy: The belief that an individual will be able to deal with particular situations that may contain novel, unpredictable, and stressful elements.

Tremor: A quivering or continuous shaking; an involuntary movement of a part or parts of the body resulting from alternate contractions of opposing muscles.

> **Intention (action) tremor:** A tremor exhibited or intensified when attempting coordinated movement.
>
> **Postural tremor:** A tremor affecting postural muscles and control.

Trigeminal neuralgia (tic douloureux): Degeneration (demyelination) of the sensory division of CN V (trigeminal nerve), resulting in severe, paroxysmal pain in the face.

Upper motor neuron (UMN) syndrome: Motor dysfunction observed in patients with lesions of the corticospinal or pyramidal tract in the brain or spinal cord. Characterized by spasticity, abnormal reflex behaviors, loss of precise autonomic control, impaired muscle activation, paresis, decreased dexterity, and fatigability.

Uthoff's symptom: Individuals with MS exhibit an adverse reaction to heat; the effect is usually immediate and dramatic in terms of reduced function and increased fatigue.

Vertigo: Sensation of movement of one's body or of objects moving about or spinning.

APPENDIX A

An Expanded Disability Status Scale (EDSS) for Evaluating Patients with Multiple Sclerosis

Functional Systems.

Pyramidal Functions
0. Normal.
1. Abnormal signs without disability.
2. Minimal disability.
3. Mild or moderate paraparesis or hemiparesis; severe monoparesis.
4. Marked paraparesis or hemiparesis; moderate quadriparesis; or monoplegia.
5. Paraplegia, hemiplegia, or marked quadriparesis.
6. Quadriplegia.
V. Unknown.

Cerebellar Functions
0. Normal.
1. Abnormal signs without disability.
2. Mild ataxia.
3. Moderate truncal or limb ataxia.
4. Severe ataxia, all limbs.
5. Unable to perform coordinated movements due to ataxia.
V. Unknown.
X. Is used throughout after each number when weakness (grade 3 or more on pyramidal) interferes with testing.

Brainstem Functions
0. Normal.
1. Signs only.
2. Moderate nystagmus or other mild disability.
3. Severe nystagmus, marked extraocular weakness, or moderate disability of other cranial nerves.
4. Marked dysarthria or other marked disability.
5. Inability to swallow or speak.
V. Unknown.

Sensory Functions (revised 1982)
0. Normal.
1. Vibration or figure-writing decrease only, in one or two limbs.
2. Mild decrease in touch or pain or position sense, and/or moderate decrease in vibration in one or two limbs; or vibratory (c/s figure writing) decrease alone in three or four limbs.
3. Moderate decrease in touch or pain or position sense, and/or essentially lost vibration in one or two limbs; or mild decrease in touch or pain and/or moderate decrease in all proprioceptive tests in three or four limbs.
4. Marked decrease in touch or pain or loss of proprioception, alone or combined, in one or two limbs; or moderate decrease in touch or pain and/or severe proprioceptive decrease in more than two limbs.
5. Loss (essentially) of sensation in one or two limbs; or moderate decrease in touch or pain and/or loss of proprioception for most of the body below the head.
6. Sensation essentially lost below the head.
V. Unknown.

Bowel and Bladder Functions (revised 1982)
0. Normal.
1. Mild urinary hesitancy, urgency, or retention.
2. Moderate hesitancy, urgency, retention of bowel or bladder, or rare urinary incontinence.
3. Frequent urinary incontinence.
4. In need of almost constant catheterization.
5. Loss of bladder function.
6. Loss of bowel and bladder function.
V. Unknown.

Visual (or Optic) Functions
0. Normal.
1. Scotoma with visual acuity (corrected) better than 20/30.
2. Worse eye with scotoma with maximal visual acuity (corrected) of 20/30 to 20/59.
3. Worse eye with large scotoma, or moderate decrease in fields, but with maximal visual acuity (corrected) of 20/60 to 20/99.
4. Worse eye with marked decrease of fields and maximal visual acuity (corrected) of 20/100 to 20/200; grade 3 plus maximal acuity of better eye of 20/60 or less.
5. Worse eye with maximal visual acuity (corrected) less than 20/200; grade 4 plus maximal acuity of better eye of 20/60 or less.
6. Grade 5 plus maximal visual acuity of better eye of 20/60 or less.
V. Unknown.
X. Is added to grades 0 to 6 for presence of temporal pallor.

Cerebral (or Mental) Functions
0. Normal.
1. Mood alteration only (does not affect DSS score).
2. Mild decrease in mentation.
3. Moderate decrease in mentation.
4. Marked decrease in mentation (chronic brain syndrome—moderate).
5. Dementia or chronic brain syndrome—severe or incompetent.
V. Unknown.

Other Functions.
0. None.
1. Any other neurologic findings attributed to MS (specify).
V. Unknown.

Expanded Disability Status Scale (EDSS)
0 = Normal neurologic exam (all grade 0 in functional systems [FS]; cerebral grade 1 acceptable).
1.0 = No disability, minimal signs in one FS (i.e., grade 1 excluding cerebral grade 1).
1.5 = No disability minimal signs in more than one FS (more than one grade 1 excluding cerebral grade 1).
2.0 = Minimal disability in one FS (one FS grade 2, others 0 or 1).
2.5 = Minimal disability in two FS (two FS grade 2, others 0 or 1).
3.0 = Moderate disability in one FS (one FS grade 3, others 0 or 1), or mild disability in three or four FS (three/four FS grade 2, others 0 or 1) though fully ambulatory.
3.5 = Fully ambulatory but with moderate disability in one FS (one grade 3) and one or two FS grade 2; or two FS grade 3; or five FS grade 2 (others 0 or 1).
4.0 = Fully ambulatory without aid, self-sufficient, up and about some 12 hours a day despite relatively severe disability consisting of one FS grade 4 (others 0 or 1), or combinations of lesser grades exceeding limits of previous steps. Able to walk without aid or rest some 500 meters.
4.5 = Fully ambulatory without aid, up and about much of the day, able to work a full day, may otherwise have some limitation of full activity or require minimal assistance; characterized by relatively severe disability, usually consisting of one FS grade 4 (others 0 or 1) or combinations of lesser grades exceeding limits of previous steps. Able to walk without aid or rest for some 300 meters.
5.0 = Ambulatory without aid or rest for about 200 meters; disability severe enough to impair full daily activities (e.g., to work full day without special provisions). (Usual FS equivalents are one grade 5 alone, others 0 or 1; or combinations of lesser grades usually exceeding specifications for step 4.0.)
5.5 = Ambulatory without aid or rest for about 100 meters; disability severe enough to preclude full daily activities. (Usual FS equivalents are one grade 5 alone, others 0 or 1; or combinations of lesser grades usually exceeding those for step 4.0.)
6.0 = Intermittent or unilateral constant assistance (cane, crutch, or brace) required to walk about 100 meters with or without resting. (Usual FS equivalents are combinations with more than two FS grade 3+.)
6.5 = Constant bilateral assistance (canes, crutches, or braces) required to walk about 20 meters without resting. (Usual FS equivalents are combinations with more than two FS grade 3+.)
7.0 = Unable to walk beyond about 5 meters even with aid, essentially restricted to wheelchair; wheels self in standard wheelchair and transfers alone; up and about in wheel-

chair some 12 hours a day. (Usual FS equivalents are combinations with more than one FS grade 4+; very rarely, pyramidal grade 5 alone.)

7.5 = Unable to take more than a few steps; restricted to wheelchair; may need aid in transfer; wheels self but cannot carry on in standard wheelchair a full day; may require motorized wheelchair. (Usual FS equivalents are combinations with more than one FS grade 4+.)

8.0 = Essentially restricted to bed or chair or perambulated in wheelchair, but may be out of bed itself much of the day; retains many self-care functions; generally has effective uses of arms. (Usual FS equivalents are combinations, generally grade 4+ in several systems.)

8.5 = Essentially restricted to bed much of the day; has some effective use of arm(s); retains some self-care functions. (Usual FS equivalents are combinations, generally 4+ in several systems.)

9.0 = Helpless bed patient; can communicate and eat. (Usual FS equivalents are combinations, mostly grade 4+.)

9.5 = Totally helpless bed patient; unable to communicate effectively or eat/swallow. (Usual FS equivalents are combinations, almost all grade 4+.)

10.0 = Death due to MS.

From Kurtzke,[67] with permission.

APPENDIX B

Modified Fatigue Impact Scale (MFIS)

Fatigue is a feeling of physical tiredness and lack of energy that many people experience from time to time. But people who have medical conditions like MS experience stronger feelings of fatigue more often and with greater impact than others.

Following is a list of statements that describe the effects of fatigue. Please read each statement carefully, then *circle the one number* that best indicates how often fatigue has affected you in this way during the *past 4 weeks*. (If you need help in marking your responses, *tell the interviewer the number* of the best response.) *Please answer every question.* If you are not sure which answer to select, choose the one answer that comes closest to describing you. Ask the interviewer to explain any words or phrases that you do not understand.

Name: _____   Date: _____ / _____ / _____

ID#: _____   Test: 1   2   3   4

Because of my fatigue during the past 4 weeks . . .

	Never	Rarely	Sometimes	Often	Almost always
1. I have been less alert.	0	1	2	3	4
2. I have had difficulty paying attention for long periods of time.	0	1	2	3	4
3. I have been unable to think clearly.	0	1	2	3	4
4. I have been clumsy and uncoordinated.	0	1	2	3	4
5. I have been forgetful.	0	1	2	3	4
6. I have had to pace myself in my physical activities.	0	1	2	3	4
7. I have been less motivated to do anything that requires physical effort.	0	1	2	3	4
8. I have been less motivated to participate in social activities.	0	1	2	3	4
9. I have been limited in my ability to do things away from home.	0	1	2	3	4
10. I have trouble maintaining physical effort for long periods.	0	1	2	3	4
11. I have had difficulty making decisions.	0	1	2	3	4
12. I have been less motivated to do anything that requires thinking.	0	1	2	3	4
13. My muscles have felt weak.	0	1	2	3	4
14. I have been physically uncomfortable.	0	1	2	3	4
15. I have had trouble finishing tasks that require thinking.	0	1	2	3	4
16. I have had difficulty organizing my thoughts when doing things at home or at work.	0	1	2	3	4
17. I have been less able to complete tasks that require physical effort.	0	1	2	3	4
18. My thinking has been slowed down.	0	1	2	3	4
19. I have had trouble concentrating.	0	1	2	3	4
20. I have limited my physical activities.	0	1	2	3	4
21. I have needed to rest more often or for longer periods.	0	1	2	3	4

Instructions for Scoring the MFIS

Items on the MFIS can be aggregated into three subscales (physical, cognitive, and psychosocial), as well as into a total MFIS score. All items are scaled so that higher scores indicate a greater impact of fatigue on a person's activities.

Physical Subscale

This scale can range from 0 to 36. It is computed by adding raw scores on the following items:
4 + 6 + 7 + 10 + 13 + 14 + 17 + 20 + 21.

Cognitive Subscale

This scale can range from 0 to 40. It is computed by adding raw scores on the following items:
1 + 2 + 3 + 5 + 11 + 12 + 15 + 16 + 18 + 19.

Psychosocial Subscale

This scale can range from 0 to 8. It is computed by adding raw scores on the following items: 8 + 9.

Total MFIS Score

The total MFIS score can range from 0 to 84. It is computed by adding scores on the physical, cognitive, and psychosocial subscales.

From: Multiple Sclerosis Council for Clinical Practice Guidelines,[49] with permission.

APPENDIX C

Suggested Answers to Case Study Guiding Questions

1. Identify/categorize this patient's problems in terms of

ANSWER

a. Direct impairments:

Transient diplopia, scotoma, nystagmus with left lateral gaze; paresthesias left hand, BLEs; trigeminal neuralgia; paresis BLEs; spasticity BLEs, hyperactive DTRs; intention tremor, hypermetria BUEs; ataxic gait; dysarthria; emotional dysregulation.

b. Indirect impairments:

Decreased ROM dorsiflexion BLEs; bruising left lateral malleolus.

c. Composite impairments: combined effects of both direct and indirect impairments

Moderate to severe decrease in endurance; decreased strength BLEs; decreased balance in sitting and standing.

d. Functional limitations and disabilities
- Dependent bed mobility
- Dependent transfers
- No independent sitting or standing
- Dependent ambulation and wheelchair mobility
- Decreased BADLs
- Difficulty with communication secondary to dysarthria

2. Identify two outcomes (the remediation of functional limitations and disability) and two goals (remediation of impairments) for this patient.

ANSWER:

Outcome: Patient will be independent in bed mobility within 6 weeks.

Goal: Patient will move from supine-to-sit with Min S (verbal cues) within 2 weeks.

Goal: Patient will perform bridging with Min A × 1 within 2 weeks.

Outcome: Patient will be independent and safe in all transfers within 6 weeks.

Goal: Patient will perform sit-to-stand transfers with Min A × 1 within 3 weeks.

Goal: Patient will perform pivot transfer bed-to-chair with Mod A × 1 within 3 weeks.

3. Formulate four treatment interventions that could be used at the start of therapy to achieve the stated outcomes and goals. Provide a brief rationale of each.

a. Hooklying, lower trunk rotation with both legs on a Swiss ball

Rationale: This is an initial mobility procedure that should reduce spasticity in BLEs.

b. Bridging, elevation, lightly resisted movement.

Rationale: This exercise will strength hip extensors, needed for sit-to-stand transfers; BLEs are in a position of flexion (hooklying), necessary to break up LE extensor spasticity.

c. Quadruped, over Swiss Ball, weight shifting in small decrements of range progressing to holding steady; alternating isometrics (light resistance) can be applied to facilitate postural muscles.

Rationale: This is a stable posture (low COG, wide BOS); inhibitory pressure to quadriceps helps to break up extensor spasticity BLEs.

d. Sit-to-stand transfers, moving to a position of modified plantigrade (BUEs weight-bearing); an elevated seat can be used to decrease the range of motion and work.

Rationale: Strengthens hip and knee extensors while providing stabilization of initial standing posture with BUEs; the hip is slightly flexed while the knees are extending (helps to break up extensor spasticity).

4. What strategies would you use to develop self-management skills and promote self-efficacy and quality of life?

ANSWER: Self-management and self-efficacy can be achieved by using strategies that promote mastery of important (meaningful) functional tasks and the environment. These can include energy conservation, activity pacing and time management, and work simplification strategies. Stress reduction techniques (e.g., progressive relaxation techniques, meditation) are important to enhance coping skills. It is also important to select activities that the patient can master (or almost master) to allow the patient to experience success. General health measures and exercises that counteract deconditioning also promote mastery and self-efficacy.

LEARNING OBJECTIVES

1. Describe the etiology, pathophysiology, clinical manifestations, and sequelae of Parkinson's disease.
2. Identify and describe the examination procedures used to evaluate patients with Parkinson's disease to establish a diagnosis, prognosis, and plan of care.
3. Describe the role of the physical therapist in assisting the patient with Parkinson's disease in terms of direct interventions and patient-related instruction to maximize function.
4. Describe appropriate elements of the exercise prescription for patients with Parkinson's disease.
5. Identify the neuropsychological and social effects of Parkinson's disease and describe appropriate interventions to maximize quality of life.
6. Analyze and interpret patient data, formulate realistic goals and outcomes, and develop a plan of care when presented with a clinical case study.

Parkinson's disease (PD) is a chronic, progressive disease of the nervous system characterized by the cardinal features of rigidity, akinesia, bradykinesia, tremor, and postural instability. In addition the disease may cause a variety of indirect impairments and complications, some of which are produced by various combinations of the cardinal signs, including movement and gait disturbances, masked face, cognitive and perceptual disturbances, communication and swallowing dysfunction, autonomic dysfunction, and so forth (Table 23–1). Onset is insidious with a slow rate of progression. Disruption in daily functions, roles and activities, and depression are common in individuals with Parkinson's disease.

EPIDEMIOLOGY

Parkinson's disease (PD) occurs in about 1 percent of the population older than 55 years of age and becomes increasingly common with advancing age, reaching proportions of 2.6 percent of the population by age 85 years. In the United States there are 1.5 million individuals with PD, with 50,000 new

Table 23–1 MANIFESTATIONS OF PARKINSON'S DISEASE

Cardinal manifestations of Parkinson's disease
Tremor
Rigidity
Bradykinesia
Postural instability

Secondary manifestations of Parkinson's disease

Incoordination	Edema
Micrographia	Scoliosis
Blurred vision	Kyphosis
Impaired upgaze	Pain and sensory symptoms
Blepharospasm	Seborrhea
Glabellar reflex	Constipation
Dysarthria	Urinary urgency, hesitancy, and frequency
Dysphagia reflex	Loss of libido
Sialorrhea	Impotence
Masked facies	Freezing
Hand and foot	Dementia
deformities	Depression
Dystonia	

From Stern, M, and Hurtig, H: The Comprehensive Management of Parkinson's Disease. PMA, New York, 1988, p 4, with permission.

cases appearing annually. This number is expected to rise with the aging of the population. The mean age of onset is between 58 and 62 years, with the majority of cases having their onset between the ages of 50 and 79. A small percentage—as many as 10 percent—develop young-onset PD, which is defined by the appearance of initial symptoms before the age of 40. These individuals usually have a more benign long-term course. Males are slightly more at risk for developing PD than females.[1,2]

ETIOLOGY

The term **parkinsonism** is used to refer to a group of disorders that produce abnormalities of basal ganglia (BG) function. Parkinson's disease, or primary parkinsonism, is the most common cause affecting approximately 78 percent of patients. Secondary parkinsonism results from a number of different causes, including inherited and acquired neurodegenerative disorders. The term parkinsonism-plus syndromes refers to those conditions with symptoms of multiple system degeneration (Box 23–1).

1. *Parkinson's disease (primary parkinsonism).* Etiology is idiopathic or unknown. True PD or paralysis agitans was first described as "the shaking palsy" by James Parkinson in 1817.[3] Two distinct clinical subgroups have been identified. One group includes individuals whose dominant symptoms include postural instability and gait disturbances (postural instability gait disturbed [PIGD]). Another group includes individuals with tremor as the main feature (tremor predominant). Patients who are tremor predominant typically demonstrate few problems with bradykinesia or postural instability.[4]

2. *Postinfectious parkinsonism (secondary parkinsonism).* The influenza epidemics of encephali-

tis lethargica that occurred from 1917 to 1926 affected large numbers of individuals. The onset of parkinsonian symptoms typically occurred after many years, giving rise to the theory that a slow virus was infecting the brain. There has been no recent recurrence of this influenza and the incidence of this type of parkinsonism is slowly decreasing in frequency.[5] Moving case histories of these individuals are portrayed in the book *Awakenings* by Oliver Sacks.[6] The development of parkinsonism with other encephalitic conditions is rare. Parkinsonism has also been reported with cryptococcal meningitis and Jacob-Creutzfeldt disease.[7]

3. *Toxic parkinsonism (secondary parkinsonism).* Parkinsonian symptoms occur in individuals exposed to certain industrial poisons and chemicals (manganese, carbon disulfide, carbon monoxide, cyanide, methanol). The most common of these toxins is manganese, which represents a serious occupational hazard to

Box 23–1 CAUSES OF PARKINSONISM

Idiopathic Parkinson's disease
Drugs
    Phenothiazines
    Butyrophenones
    Metoclopramide
    Reserpine
    Flunarizine
    Alpha-methyldopa
    Lithium
    Amiodarone
Toxins
    Manganese
    MPTP
    Carbon monoxide
    Carbon disulfide
    Amyotrophic lateral sclerosis–parkinsonism-dementia of Guam (cycad)
Brain tumors
Trauma (dementia pugilistica)
Encephalitis
    Von Economo's encephalitis
    Venezuelan
    Japanese B
    Western equine
Cerebrovascular disease: lacunar state
Akinetic/rigid syndromes with parkinsonian features (Parkinson's plus)
    Progressive supranuclear palsy
    Huntington's disease
    Striatonigral degeneration
    Corticobasal ganglionic degeneration
    Olivopontocerebellar degeneration
    Normal-pressure hydrocephalus
    Alzheimer's disease
    Wilson's disease
    Hallervorden-Spatz disease
    Shy-Drager syndrome
    Familial calcification of the basal ganglia (Fahr's disease)

From Guberman, A: Introduction to Clinical Neurology. Little, Brown, and Co., Boston, 1994, p 195, with permission.

many miners.[3] Severe and lasting classic parkinsonian has been inadvertently produced in individuals who injected a synthetic heroin containing the chemical MPTP.[8]

4. *Pharmacological parkinsonism (secondary parkinsonism).* A variety of drugs can produce extrapyramidal dysfunction that mimics the signs of PD. These drugs are thought to interfere with dopaminergic mechanisms either presynaptically or postsynaptically. They include (1) *neuroleptic drugs* such as chlorpromazine (Thorazine), haloperidol (Haldol), thioridazine (Mellaril), and thiothizene (Navane); (2) *antidepressant drugs* such as amitriptyline (Triavil), amoxapine (Asendin), and trazodone (Desyrel), and (3) *antihypertensive drugs* such as methyldopa (Aldomet) and reserpine. High doses of these medications are particularly problematic in the elderly and the severity of effects noted may be related to subclinical PD. Withdrawal of these agents usually reverses the symptoms within a few weeks, although in some cases the effects can be long lasting.[7]

5. *Metabolic causes (secondary parkinsonism).* Parkinsonism can be caused in rare cases by metabolic conditions, including disorders of calcium metabolism that result in BG calcification. These include hypothyroidism, hyperparathyroidism, hypoparathyroidism, and Wilson's disease.[5]

6. *Akinetic/rigid syndromes with parkinsonian features (Parkinson-plus syndromes).* A group of neurodegenerative diseases can affect the substantia nigra and produce parkinsonian symptoms along with other neurological signs. These diseases include striatonigral degeneration (SND), Shy-Drager syndrome, progressive supranuclear palsy (PSPO), olivopontocerebellar atrophy (OPCA), cortical-basal ganglionic degeneration, and so forth. Many of these conditions are rare and affect relatively small numbers of individuals. In addition, parkinsonian symptoms can be exhibited in atherosclerosis, Alzheimer's disease, Wilson's disease, and Huntington's disease. Early in their course these diseases may present with rigidity and bradykinesia indistinguishable from PD. However, other diagnostic symptoms eventually appear (e.g., cognitive impairment in Alzheimer's disease). Another diagnostic feature is that Parkinson-plus syndromes typically do not show measurable improvement from the administration of anti-Parkinson medications such as levodopa (L-dopa) therapy (termed the *apomorphine test*).[9,10]

PATHOPHYSIOLOGY

The basal ganglia (BG) are a collection of interconnected gray matter nuclear masses deep within the brain. It is now considered to be composed of the caudate and putamen (collectively termed the striatum) plus the globus pallidus, subthalamic nucleus, and the substantia nigra (Fig. 23-1). The BG play an important role in the production of voluntary movements and control of postural adjustments associated with voluntary movements. Activity is initiated by input to the main input nuclei, caudate and putamen, from the cerebral cortex and thalamus. Widespread cortical areas are involved in sending signals to the BG, including sensory, motor, and association areas. The striatum also receives input from the substantia nigra and the pedunculopontine tegmental nucleus of the midbrain. Output is channeled primarily through the globus pallidus and substantia nigra via thalamocortical projections to prefrontal and premotor cortex areas. Within the BG, information is integrated and modulated from the cerebral cortex and thalamus through multiple parallel circuits. These complex circuits are divided into *direct* and *indirect* anatomical pathways that have opposing actions (Fig. 23-2). The direct pathway facilitates flow of signals to the thalamus activating some movements while the indirect pathway inhibits information flow and suppresses other movements.

Damage to the BG results in motor disturbances that can be hyperkinetic or hypokinetic. Hyperkinetic disturbances are characterized by excessive or abnormal movements (e.g., chorea, dyskinesias, dystonia). Hypokinetic disturbances are characterized by slowness or lack of movement (e.g., akinesia and bradykinesia seen in PD; Table 23–2 a and b). The substantia nigra pars compacta (SNpc) works to facilitate movement through both direct and indirect pathways of the motor loop.

PD is associated with degeneration of dopaminergic neurons that produce **dopamine.** They have their cell bodies in the SNpc and send their axons to the striatum (caudate nucleus and putamen). A degeneration of 80 percent of neurons is estimated to occur before signs of the disease become clinically evident. Nigral cell loss is more prevalent in the ventral cell group and loss of the melanin-containing neurons produces characteristic changes in depigmentation (Fig. 23-3). There are other deficiencies in neurotransmitters as well (e.g., serotonin, norepinephrine). The effects of these depletions are less well understood. As the disease progresses and neurons degenerate, they develop characteristic cytoplasmic inclusion bodies, called Lewy's bodies. Other sites of predilection include the dorsal motor nucleus of the vagus, the hypothalamus, the locus ceruleus, the cerebral cortex, and the autonomic ganglia.[12]

Loss of dopaminergic neuron influence leads to a reduction in spontaneous movement. Thus the patient wants to move but cannot. Tremor and rigidity are viewed as release phenomena, representative of loss of inhibitory influences within the BG. Significant changes in striatal dopamine receptors may also occur, resulting in decreased binding sites for dopamine in the BG. This may explain the loss of clinical effectiveness of L-dopa (a dopamine [DA]

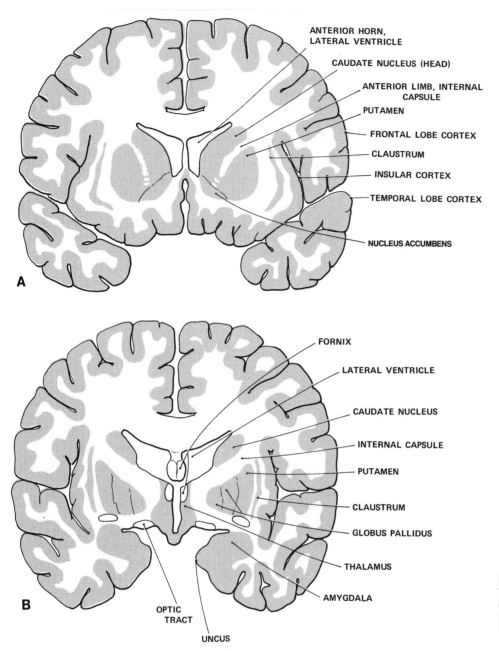

ANTERIOR HORN,
LATERAL VENTRICLE

CAUDATE NUCLEUS (HEAD)

ANTERIOR LIMB, INTERNAL
CAPSULE

PUTAMEN

FRONTAL LOBE CORTEX

CLAUSTRUM

INSULAR CORTEX

TEMPORAL LOBE CORTEX

NUCLEUS ACCUMBENS

A

FORNIX

LATERAL VENTRICLE

CAUDATE NUCLEUS

INTERNAL CAPSULE

PUTAMEN

CLAUSTRUM

GLOBUS PALLIDUS

THALAMUS

AMYGDALA

B   OPTIC
       TRACT

UNCUS

Figure 23-1. The major structures of the basal ganglia. (Adapted from Cote L, and Crutcher MD. The basal ganglia. (From Kandel E, et al [eds]: Principles of Neuroscience, ed 3. Elsevier, New York, 1991, p 80, with permission.)

substitution treatment) during later stages of the disease.[13–15]

CLINICAL MANIFESTATIONS

Rigidity

Rigidity is one of the clinical hallmarks of PD. Patients frequently complain of "heaviness" and "stiffness" of their limbs. **Rigidity** is defined as resistance to passive motion that is not velocity dependent. It is felt uniformly in muscles on both sides of the joint and in movements in both directions. Spinal stretch reflexes are normal, and long latency reflexes are enhanced. Rigidity is present regardless of the task, amplitude, or speed of

movement. Two types are identified: cogwheel or leadpipe. **Cogwheel rigidity** is a jerky, ratchetlike resistance to passive movement as muscles alternately tense and relax. **Leadpipe rigidity** is a constant, uniform resistance to passive movement, with no fluctuations. Rigidity is typically unequal in distribution. It affects proximal muscles first, especially the shoulders and neck. It progresses to involve muscles of the face and extremities. Rigidity may initially affect the left or right side, eventually spreading to involve the whole body.[18] As the disease progresses, rigidity becomes more severe. Rigidity decreases the ability of patients to move easily. For example, loss of bed mobility or loss of reciprocal arm swing during gait are often related to the degree of truncal rigidity. Active movement, mental concentration, or emotional tension may all increase the amount of rigidity present. Prolonged rigidity re-

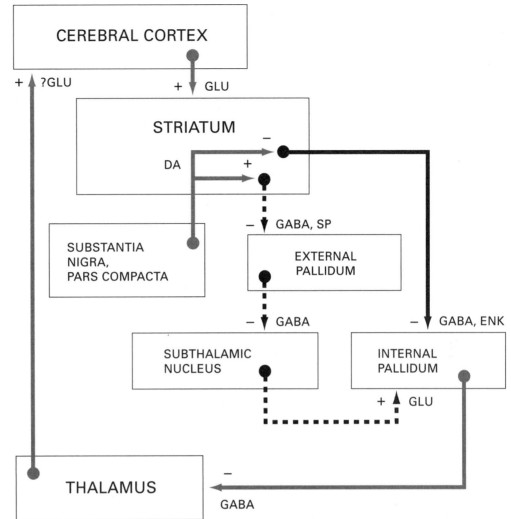

Figure 23-2. Schematic diagram of some connections of the basal ganglia, showing excitatory (+) and inhibitory (–) synapses and neurotransmitters. The direct striopallidal projection is bold shaded and the indirect projection is dashed. Corticonigral and corticosubthalamic projections, which are excitatory, are not shown in the diagram. (From Kiernan, JA: Barr's The Human Nervous System: An Anatomical Viewpoint, ed 7. Lippincott-Raven, Philadelphia, 1998, p 255, with permission.)

sults in decreased available range of motion (ROM) and serious secondary complications of contracture and postural deformity. Rigidity also has a direct impact on increasing resting energy expenditure and fatigue levels.[17,18]

Akinesia and Bradykinesia

Patients with PD demonstrate problems with voluntary movement. **Akinesia** refers to difficulty initiating movement. Moments of **freezing** may occur and are characterized by a sudden break or block in movement. Akinesia represents a deficit in the preparatory phase of movement control and can be directly influenced by the degree of rigidity as

well as stage of disease and fluctuations in drug action. Disturbances in attention and depression can also compound problems with akinesia. **Bradykinesia** refers to slowness and difficulty maintain-

Table 23–2a MOTOR DISTURBANCES PREDICTED FROM THE BASAL GANGLIA MODEL

Disordered Process	Clinical Result
1. Overactive indirect pathway	Akinesia, rigidity
2. Underactive indirect pathway	Chorea, hemiballismus
3. Overactive direct pathway	Dystonia, athetosis, or tic
4. Underactive direct pathway	Bradykinesia

Table 23–2b MOVEMENT DISORDERS AS EXPLAINED BY THE BASAL GANGLIA MODEL

Disorder	Pathophysiology	Disordered Process (from Table 23–2a)
Parkinson's disease	Decreased dopamine from SNpc	1 and 4
L-Dopa dyskinesia	Increased exogenous dopamine	2 and 3
Early Huntington's disease	Decreased putaminal activity of the GABA-enk neurons	2
Late Huntington's disease	Decreased putaminal activity of both types of GABA neurons	2 and 4
Hemiballismus	Subthalamic nucleus lesion	2
Dystonia	Overactivity of the putamen	3 (and 1)
Tic	Overactivity of the putamen	3

From Hallett, M[15], p 181, with permission.

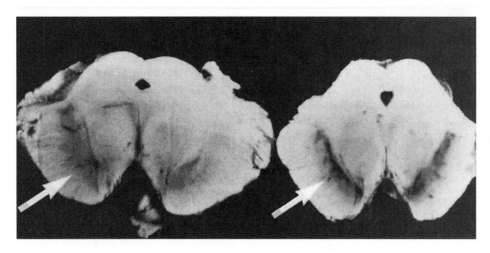

Figure 23-3. The substantia nigra in PD. The upper layer (zona compacta) of the substantia nigra normally has many melanin-containing neurons. In the transverse section through the midbrain (*left*), the substantia nigra of a patient with PD shows a marked depletion of melanin-containing nerve cells. This produces a characteristic pallor (depigmentation) compared with a normal control (*right*). (From Rowland, LP [ed]: Merritt's Textbook of Neurology, ed 8. Copyright Lea & Febiger, Philadelphia, 1989, p 659, with permission.)

ing movement. Movements are typically reduced in speed, range, and amplitude, termed **hypokinesia.** Rigidity and depression can also influence bradykinesia. Often, it is the most disabling symptom of parkinsonism, with the slowness and prolonged movement times leading to increased dependence in daily tasks.[16]

Motor planning deficits are present with this disease. Overall control is impaired in routine actions representative of ingrained motor programs (e.g., handwriting). Patients with PD typically demonstrate **micrographia,** an abnormally small handwriting that is difficult to read (see Fig. 23-4). Patients also have more difficulty performing simultaneous and sequential tasks. Thus, they experience difficulty in integrating two motor programs at the same time and in maintaining ongoing activity. For example, the patient "freezes up" when carrying out another motor task while walking. Or the patient is slow and hesitant or unable to switch from one movement to another during a transfer sequence. Freezing episodes may also be triggered by confrontation of competing stimuli. For example, the patient slows or stops walking when exposed to a narrowed space or an obstacle. To compensate for impaired control, individuals with PD may resort to slower, visually guided movements to ensure movement accuracy. Motor learning may also be impaired, particularly for sequential tasks and procedural learning.

Torque production is decreased at all speeds resulting in functional difficulties and muscle weakness.[19–21] It is thought to be caused by insufficient neural activation of muscles. Electromyographic studies reveal that motor unit recruitment is delayed and that once initiated is characterized by asynchronization; that is, pauses and an inability to smoothly increase firing rate as contraction continues.[22,23] These difficulties are compounded during the production of complex movements.[24] As the disease progresses, disuse weakness evolves and contributes to movement difficulties.[24,25] Movements that appear jerky may indicate influence of underlying tremor.

A common perception among patients is an increased sense of effort associated with movement that is manifested by difficulty activating and sustaining responses.

Tremor

Tremor is the initial symptom of PD in about 50 percent of patients. It is an involuntary oscillation of a body part occurring at a slow frequency of about 4 to 7 cycles per second. The parkinsonian tremor is described as a resting tremor, because it is typically present at rest and disappears with voluntary movement. This is usually manifest as a pill-rolling tremor of the hand, although resting tremors may also be seen in the feet, lips, tongue, and jaw. Some individuals demonstrate **postural tremor** when muscles are used to maintain a position against

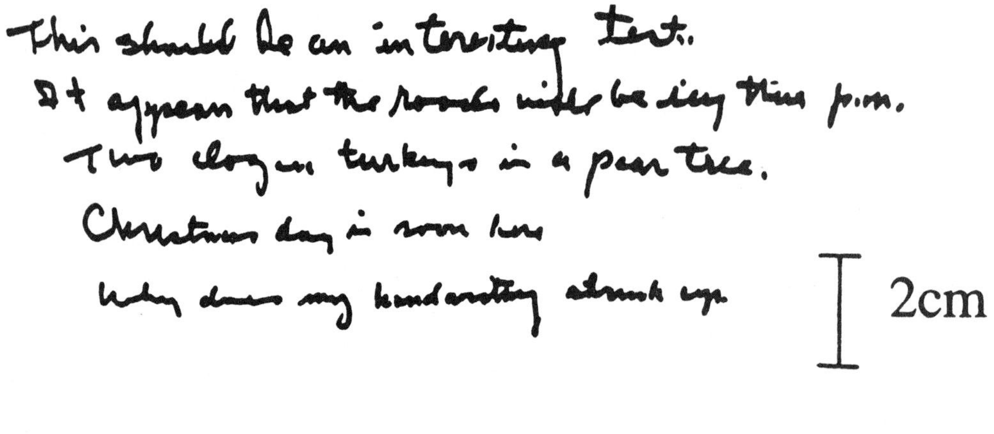

Figure 23-4. Micrographia in PD. Patients with PD may have problems maintaining the scale of their movements. (From Phillips, JG, et al: What can indices of handwriting quality tell us about parkinsonian handwriting? Hum Movt Sci 10: 301, 1991, with permission.)

gravity. Tremor tends to be less severe when the patient is relaxed and unoccupied; it is diminished by voluntary effort, and disappears completely during sleep. It is aggravated by emotional stress or fatigue. In the early stages, tremor is usually unilateral, quite mild and occurs for only short periods, whereas in later stages tremor can become severe, interfering with daily function. Fluctuations in frequency and intensity are common.[27]

Postural Instability

Patients with PD demonstrate abnormalities of posture and balance. The ability to maintain steady posture may be unimpaired under conditions of undisturbed stance and full attention. As the base of support narrows (tandem stance or single-limb stance) or as attention demands vary (divided attention situations), postural instability increases. Patients experience increasing difficulty during dynamic destabilizing activities such as self-initiated movements (e.g., functional reach, walking, turning). Patients also perform poorly under conditions of perturbed balance.[29] Frequent falls and fall injury are the result of progressive loss of balance reactions, with about one-third of patients experiencing falls and 13 percent falling more than once a week.[30,31] Patients tend to respond to instability with an abnormal pattern of coactivation, resulting in a rigid body and an inability to utilize normal postural synergies to recover balance.[32] Patients also demonstrate difficulty in regulating

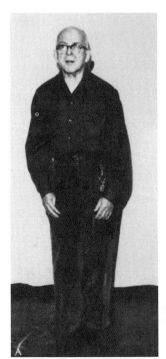
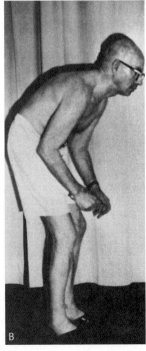

Figure 23-5. Posture and PD. The body posture of a patient with PD. (*A*) Front view. (*B*) Side view. (From Rowland, LP [ed]: Merritt's Textbook of Neurology, ed 8. Copyright Lea & Febiger, Philadelphia, 1989, p 529, with permission.)

feed-forward, anticipatory adjustments of postural muscles during voluntary movements.[33,34] Postural reactions become increasingly impaired as the disease progresses. Contributing factors include rigidity, decreased muscle torque production, loss of available ROM particularly of trunk motions, and weakness. Extensor muscles of the trunk demonstrate greater weakness than flexor muscles, contributing to the adoption of a flexed, stooped posture with increased flexion of the neck, trunk, hips, and knees.[19,28] This results in a significant change in the center-of-alignment position, positioning the individual at the forward limits of stability (Fig. 23-5). Patients with PD also demonstrate an inability to adapt movement strategies to changing sensory conditions, a problem in sensorimotor adaptation.[32] Visuospatial impairment has been identified in patients with PD and correlated with lower scores in mobility.[35] Some patients are unable to perceive the upright or vertical position, which may indicate an abnormality in processing of vestibular, visual, and proprioceptive information contributing to balance.

INDIRECT IMPAIRMENTS AND COMPLICATIONS

A variety of indirect impairments and complications are possible (see Table 23–1).

Poverty of Movement

Poverty of movement characterizes patients with PD. There is an overall decrease in the total number and excursion of movements. As task complexity increases, movement difficulty increases. This provides evidence of a central deficit in motor planning in patients with PD.[36] Rotation movements are reduced, resulting in movements that are basically uniplanar (in one plane of motion). Automatic or unconscious movements are impaired or lost. An example of this is the loss of reciprocal arm swing during gait. As a result of the loss of automatic movements, there are high cortical demands on the patient who is required to think about each aspect of movement to execute it successfully. Constantly combating the effects of bradykinesia, rigidity, and movement impoverishment can lead to mental fatigue and loss of motivation.

Fatigue

In patients with fully developed PD, fatigue is one of the most common symptoms reported. The patient has difficulty in sustaining activity and experiences increasing weakness and lethargy as the day progresses. Repetitive motor acts may start out strong but decrease in strength as the activity progresses. Thus, the first few words spoken may be loud and strong but diminish rapidly as speech progresses. Performance decreases dramatically with great physical effort or mental stress. Rest or sleep may restore mobility. When L-dopa therapy is initiated, the patient may notice a dramatic improvement initially and feel significantly less fatigued. In long-standing disease and drug therapy, fatigue typically reappears.[37]

Masked Face

Facial expression is described as **masked face** with infrequent blinking and lack of expression. Smiling may be possible only on command or with volitional effort. This can have a significant impact on social interaction and social disability.

Musculoskeletal Changes

Most patients with PD are elderly and show the effects of generalized musculoskeletal deconditioning. The more chronic and generalized the disease becomes, the greater the level of muscle weakness and fatigue. Patients demonstrate loss of flexibility. Lack of movement in any body segment leads to contracture development of both contractile and noncontractile tissue. Contractures commonly develop in hip and knee flexors, hip rotators and adductors, plantarflexors, dorsal spine and neck flexors, shoulder adductors and internal rotators, and elbow flexors. Function becomes progressively more limited by these musculoskeletal constraints. **Kyphosis** is the most common postural deformity (Fig. 23-5). Some patients may develop **scoliosis** from leaning consistently to one side when sitting or walking. This generally results from unequal distribution of rigidity in the trunk. Older individuals with reduced activity levels and poor diet are likely to develop osteoporosis. Loss of automatic movement and poor balance reactions result in frequent falls and fracture of osteoporotic bone. Fracture healing may also be delayed or disordered.

Gait Disturbances

The gait pattern of the patient with PD is characterized by impoverished movement and decreased velocity. Hip, knee, and ankle motions are reduced with a generalized lack of extension at all three joints. Trunk and pelvic motions are also diminished, resulting in decreased stride length and reciprocal arm swing. Patients characteristically walk with small, shuffling steps. There is a loss of normal heel-toe progression. Stance phase and double support are lengthened while the period of single-limb support is shortened. Asymmetries of gait are common. Abnormal stooped posturing can contribute to development of a **festinating gait,** characterized by a progressive increase in speed with a shortening of stride. Thus, the patient takes multiple short steps to catch up with his or her center of mass (COM) and avoid falling, and may eventually break into a run or trot. A **propulsive**

gait has a forward accelerating quality, whereas the less common **retropulsive gait** has a backward accelerating one. Some patients are able to stop only when they come in contact with an object or a wall. Patients who are toe-walkers owing to plantarflexion contractures exhibit an additional postural instability from narrowing of their base of support. Turning or changing direction is particularly difficult and typically accomplished by taking multiple small steps. Problems with controlling posture and balance also directly impact on gait and safety.[26,38]

Swallowing and Communication Dysfunction

Dysphagia, impaired swallowing, is present in an estimated 50 to 95 percent of patients. Dysphagia can lead to choking or aspiration pneumonia and impaired nutrition with significant weight loss. Nutritional inadequacy can contribute to the fatigue and exhaustion that patients experience. Dysphagia is the result of rigidity, reduced mobility, and restricted range of movement. Individuals with PD experience problems in all four phases of swallowing: oral preparatory, oral, pharyngeal, and esophageal. Thus the patient demonstrates abnormal tongue control, and problems with chewing, bolus formation, delayed swallow response, and peristalsis. Patients also typically experience excessive drooling **(sialorrhea)** as a result of increased salivary production and decreased spontaneous swallowing. Drooling is particularly problematic while sleeping or initiating speech and in advanced cases increases the risk of aspiration. Excessive drooling has important social implications.[39-42]

Speech is impaired in 50 to 73 percent of patients. Patients with PD experience **hypokinetic dysarthria,** which is characterized by decreased voice volume, monotone/monopitch speech, imprecise or distorted articulation, and uncontrolled speech rate. In addition, patients have difficulty initiating speech and in maintaining speech. Speech difficulties are also the result of rigidity and bradykinesia. Patients experience reduced mobility, restricted range of movement, and uncontrolled rate of movement of muscles controlling respiration, phonation, resonation, and articulation. In advanced cases, the patient may speak in whispers or not at all, demonstrating **mutism.** Speech difficulties contribute to social isolation and social disability.[41,42]

Visual and Sensorimotor Disturbances

Visual disturbances are common in PD. These can include blurring of vision and difficulty in reading, which is not corrected by glasses. Impaired vision can be made worse by some anticholinergic medications. Conjugate gaze and saccadic eye movements may also be impaired. Eye pursuit movements may have a jerky, cogwheeling quality. Decreased blinking can produce bloodshot, irritated eyes that burn and itch. Pupillary abnormalities are also possible with decreased reflex responses to light and nociceptive stimuli.[44]

Although patients with PD do not suffer from primary sensory loss, as many as 50 percent experience paresthesias and pain. These can include sensations of numbness, tingling, abnormal temperature, and pain that is cramplike and poorly localized. These symptoms are most commonly intermittent, and vary in intensity and location. Although the cause is unknown, some of the discomfort these patients experience may result from lack of movement, muscle rigidity, faulty posture, or ligamentous strain **(postural stress syndrome).** For example, low back pain may occur as a result of a stooped posture. Some patients also experience extreme motor restlessness, or **akathisia,** which affects as many as 25 percent of patients. Akathisia is often described as painful and interferes with relaxation and sleep.[44,45]

Cognitive and Behavioral Dysfunction

Dementia occurs in approximately one third of the patients with PD. Older patients appear to be at greatest risk for dementia, with rates as high as 60 percent reported for individuals 80 years or older. Dementia is associated with increased mortality rates.[46] Coexisting Alzheimer's disease or multi-infarct dementia secondary to atherosclerotic disease are also common in the elderly and may be contributory factors in some patients with dementia. Deficits may include loss of executive functions (reasoning, abstract thinking, judgement, and so forth) and memory impairment. Patients can also demonstrate deficits with memory and visuospatial skills without dementia. **Bradyphrenia,** a disorder of intellectual function, is common in patients with PD. It is characterized by a slowing of thought processes with lack of concentration and attention. Patients typically demonstrate problems with selective attention and in shifting attention. Patients may also demonstrate learning deficits, especially with procedural learning required to learn a new motor skill. Increased practice time may be required for learning.[46,47]

Perceptual deficits are also present in this disease. Patients demonstrate significantly more errors than normal on visual perception tasks involving spatial organization. The BG, in association with the frontal lobe, appear to play an important role in the integration of sensory information. Deficits have been reported in vertical perception, topographic orientation, body scheme, and spatial relations. Motor tasks involving gestural movements, delayed double tasks, tracking, and constructional ability may be impaired.[35,45]

Depression is common, occurring in 25 to 40 percent of patients. A significant number of patients develop depression prior to or just after onset of motor symptoms, suggesting an endogenous cause that may be related to underlying changes in the serotoninergic system.[47] Patients may demonstrate symptoms of major depression, including apathy, passivity, loss of ambition or enthusiasm, and changes in appetite, sleep, and dependency. Suicidal thoughts may be present. Patients may also demonstrate a **dysthymic disorder** characterized by variability in dysphoric mood, or atypical depression characterized by intermittent episodes of severe anxiety.[46]

In severe cases, behavioral changes may also result from the sensory deprivation caused by the marked paucity of movement. Drug-related psychoses can occur. For example, hallucinations and delusions are common complications owing to L-dopa toxicity.[46] Insomnia may occur as a result of muscular discomfort or as a result of drug toxicity.

Autonomic Dysfunction

Autonomic nervous system dysfunction (dysautonomia) occurs with PD. Common problems include excessive perspiration, greasy skin, increased salivation, thermoregulatory abnormalities (including uncomfortable sensations of heat or cold), bladder dysfunction (urinary frequency, urgency, and nocturia), and impotence. Patients have low appetites and decreased motility of the gastrointestinal (GI) tract. Constipation is a common problem for most patients with PD.

Cardiopulmonary Dysfunction

Cardiovascular abnormalities can include orthostatic hypotension and low resting blood pressure (BP). Cardiac arrhythmias can also occur as a result of L-dopa toxicity.[40]

Patients with PD typically demonstrate pulmonary functional impairments, reported in as many as 84 percent of patients. Airway obstruction (e.g., air trapping, lung insufflation) is the most frequently reported pulmonary problem (56% of patients) and has been linked to episodes of pulmonary failure. The etiology remains unknown but may be linked to bradykinetic disorganization of respiratory movements. Restrictive dysfunction is also common (28% of patients) and has been linked to the decreased chest expansion that occurs as a result of rigidity of the trunk muscles, loss of musculoskeletal flexibility, and kyphotic posture. Patients with PD demonstrate lower forced vital capacity (FVC), lower forced expiratory volume (FEV_1), and higher residual volume (RV) and airway resistance (RAW) values when compared to age-matched controls. Function in daily living activities is decreased in patients with pulmonary dysfunction.[48–50]

A sedentary life-style with decreased activity levels contributes to cardiopulmonary deconditioning. Limited research suggests that patients with mild to moderate PD do not appear to demonstrate significantly different exercise capacity (maximal heart rate, maximal oxygen consumption) when compared to age-matched controls.[51,52] However these patients did demonstrate decreased peak power, and higher submaximal heart rates and oxygen consumption rates than controls.[52] Patients with moderate to severe disease do demonstrate decreased maximal oxygen consumption.[53,54]

In long-standing disease, the lower extremities may exhibit circulatory changes owing to venous pooling as a result of decreased mobility and prolonged sitting. Thus, patients can present with mild to moderate edema of the feet and ankles, which usually subsides during sleep.

DIAGNOSIS

Early diagnosis of PD is difficult. There is no single definitive test or group of tests used to diagnose the disease. The diagnosis is usually made on the basis of history and clinical examination. Handwriting samples, speech analysis, interview questions that focus on developing symptomatology, and physical examination are used in the preclinical stage to detect early manifestations of the disease. A diagnosis of PD can be made if at least two of the four cardinal features are present. Exclusion of Parkinson-plus syndromes is necessary (see Box 23–1). The presence of extrapyramidal signs that are bilateral symmetrical and do not respond to L-dopa and dopamine agonists (apomorphine test) is suggestive of these syndromes, not PD.[10] Laboratory tests and neuroimaging procedures are usually normal. Computed tomography (CT) or magnetic resonance imaging (MRI) scans may be used to identify other pathologies in individuals with poor L-dopa response, dementia, or pyramidal signs.[55]

DISEASE COURSE

The disease is slowly progressive, with a long subclinical period, estimated at 20 to 30 years. Before L-dopa therapy, 28 percent of patients became severely disabled (functionally dependent) or died within 5 years of diagnosis, 61 percent within 10 years, and 83 percent within 15 years. Following L-dopa therapy, only 9 percent had become disabled or had died at 5 years, 21 percent at 10 years, and 37.5 percent at 15 years. Overall the mean survival has increased by about 5 years since the introduction of L-dopa.[56] Patients who are tremor predominant typically have an earlier onset with less functional impairment and more benign progression. Patients in the PIGD group tend to have more pronounced functional and mental status deterioration with more rapid disease progression and poor prognosis. Neurobehavioral disturbances and dementia are also more common in this group.[4]

An estimate of the stage and severity of the disease can be made using a staging scale. The most widely used is the **Hoehn-Yahr Classification of Disability Scale** (Table 23–3).[56] It provides a useful measure for charting the progression of the disease.

Table 23–3 HOEHN AND YAHR CLASSIFICATION OF DISABILITY

Stage	Character of Disability
I	Minimal or absent; unilateral if present.
II	Minimal bilateral or midline involvement. Balance not impaired.
III	Impaired righting reflexes. Unsteadiness when turning or rising from chair. Some activities are restricted, but patient can live independently and continue some forms of employment.
IV	All symptoms present and severe. Standing and walking possible only with assistance.
V	Confined to bed or wheelchair.

From Hoehn and Yahr[56], p 433, with permission.

Stage I is used to indicate minimal disease involvement, whereas stage V is indicative of severe deterioration in which the patient is confined to bed or wheelchair. Mortality is usually due to the development of secondary complications, for example, pneumonia, or thromboembolism.

MEDICAL MANAGEMENT

There is no cure for PD. Medical therapy is symptomatic and individualized. Most anti-parkinsonian medications became available in the 1960s and have become the mainstay of management. Nutritional management is also an important consideration. Some patients benefit from surgical intervention. With effective management, the effects of the disease and indirect impairments and complications are minimized.[57]

Pharmacological Management

Medications are prescribed to manage the direct effects of the disease as well as some of the indirect effects and adverse side affects of the mainstay drugs. Drug management can be divided into early protective therapy and symptomatic treatment in the middle and late stages of the disease (Table 23–4).

Patients in the early stages of PD may be given the drug selegiline or deprenyl (Eldepryl), a monamine oxidase-B (MAO-B) inhibitor. This drug appears to inhibit the action of a putative toxin or reduce oxidative stress on neurons. Clinically, selegiline has been shown to delay the primary endpoint at which patients need to start taking L-dopa by about 9 months and may slow the normal progression of the disease. Selegiline also appears to have a mild direct treatment effect, improving performance on measures of disability and motor impairment (a 10% improvement in bradykinesia).[57] Individuals are typically given selegiline in the early stages of the disease, at the time of diagnosis or soon after. There are few adverse effects but high costs of the medication may limit its use.[58]

Dopamine replacement is the mainstay of therapy for PD. **Levodopa (L-dopa)** was first introduced

Table 23–4 PHARMACOLOGY OF PARKINSON'S DISEASE

Drug Class	Example	Average Dosage[a]	Cost (AWC)[b]	Side Effects
Anticholinergics	Trihexyphenidyl	2 mg tid	2-mg tablets $19.65/100	Dry mouth, dizziness, blurred vision
	Bentropin	1 mg bid	1-mg tablets $23.56/100	Tachycardia, dry mouth, nausea, vomiting, confusion
Dopamine replacement	Levodopa/carbidopa	10/100 tid/qid	$63.88/100	Dystonia
		25/100 tid/qid	$68.81/100	Abnormal, involuntary movements
	(Sinemet)	25/250 tid	$88.19/100	Nausea, vomiting
	(Sinemet CR)	25/100 tid	$72.10/100	Confusion
		25/200 bid	$144.19/100	Dreams, hallucinations
Dopamine agonists	Pergolide	1 mg tid	$244.68/100 (1-mg tablets)	Nervousness, dyskinesias, insomnia, hallucinations, nausea, confusion, erythromelalgia
	Bromocriptine	5 mg bid	$219.24/100 (5-mg tablets)	Nausea, headache, dizziness, fatigue, cramps/constipation, confusion, pulmonary/peritoneal fibrosis
Amantadine		100 mg bid	$30.00/100 (generic)	Lightheadedness, livedo reticularis, edema
MAOI-B[c]	Seligiline	5 mg bid	$128.19/60	Nausea, dreams, hallucinations, confusion, dyskinesias

[a]bid, twice a day; tid, three times a day; qid, four times a day.
[b]AWC, average wholesale cost.
[c]MAOI-B, monoamine oxidase inhibitor, type B.
From Cutson, T et al.[62], p 367, with permission.

in 1961 as an experimental drug and came into widespread clinical use in 1967. It is a metabolic precursor of dopamine that is able to cross the blood-brain barrier and raise the level of striatal dopamine in the basal ganglia; thus, administration of the drug represents an attempt to correct the essential neurochemical imbalance. Most of L-dopa (almost 99%) is metabolized before reaching the brain, requiring administration of high doses that can produce numerous side effects. Today, L-dopa is commonly administered with carbidopa, a decarboxylase inhibitor that allows a higher percentage of L-dopa to enter the CNS. Thus, lower doses of L-dopa can be used with fewer adverse side effects. Sinemet is the most common carbidopa/L-dopa medication. Its primary benefit is in alleviating bradykinesia and rigidity with less effect on tremor. It does not appear to have a direct impact on postural instability.[57] The initial functional improvement is often dramatic. This is sometimes referred to as the honeymoon period, in which there is clear-cut drug effectiveness and long-term L-dopa response. Sinemet is available in immediate-release (IR) and controlled-release (CR) formulations. The IR form has a short half-life requiring multiple oral dosing throughout the day. The CR form is a long-acting, sustained release preparation that is associated with better outcome (improved ADL scores, improved quality of life) and fewer chronic complications.[59]

There are numerous adverse side effects to L-dopa therapy, but these usually do not present as serious problems. Most can be managed by adjusting the dosage and administering the medication in combination with other drugs to manage symptoms. The most common disturbances are (1) gastrointestinal (anorexia, nausea, vomiting, constipation), (2) mental restlessness, general overactivity, anxiety or depression, (3) cardiovascular (orthostatic hypotension and arrhythmias), (4) genitourinary (dysuria), (5) neuromuscular (choreiform and involuntary movements), and (6) sleep disturbances (insomnia, sleep fragmentation).[57] During the initial dosing, patients may feel so much better that they may engage in sudden heavy physical activity, seriously overtaxing their musculoskeletal and/or cardiovascular systems. The therapist needs to watch for this and to pace the patient accordingly.

Long-term use of L-dopa therapy results in a deterioration of the drug's overall therapeutic effectiveness. For many patients the therapeutic window is 5 to 7 years before the benefit wears off and symptoms recur sooner between doses. This is thought to result from a progressive decrease in responsiveness of the dopamine receptors and diminution in central dopamine storage capacity. Thus, the drug is usually reserved for individuals who experience symptoms in the middle and late stages of the disease and is not recommended in the initial stages for mildly affected patients.[57] Wearing-off or **end-of-dose deterioration** is a worsening of symptoms during the expected time-frame of medication effectiveness. *Off episodes*, or sudden episodes of immobility, may appear. Fluctuations in motor performance, termed **on-off phenomenon,** occur in about 50 percent of patients treated for more than 2 years. Involuntary movements, **dyskinesias,** often emerge in tandem with end-of-dose deterioration. Initially these may appear as facial grimacing with twitching of the lips and tongue protrusion. With time the involuntary movements become more prevalent, vigorous, and more extensive, involving the limbs, trunk and neck. The presence of disabling dyskinesias is often timed with peak dose and alternates with end-of-dose wearing off. Patients may also experience disabling psychiatric toxicity (visual hallucinations, delusions, and paranoia), depression, anxiety, abnormal sleep patterns, early morning akinesia, and pain. These changes are dose related and indicate the need for drug modification. Deprenyl can be administered with L-dopa to control mild wearing-off phenomena.[57] Unsupervised reduction or sudden discontinuation of L-dopa is contraindicated and may produce dangerous, life-threatening adverse effects. Although drug holidays (a weaning off medications) are no longer recommended, they may be necessary for patients with severe L-dopa–induced psychiatric toxicity. These patients require hospitalization and close monitoring during this period.[7]

Anticholinergic agents are used to block cholinergic function and moderate tremor; they have little or no effect on rigidity, bradykinesia, and postural instability. They may also be given in conjunction with L-dopa to smooth motor fluctuations. Trihexyphenidyl (Artane), benztropine (Cogentin), ethopropazine (Parsidol), and procyclidine (Kemadrin) are commonly prescribed drugs in this group. Adverse effects include blurred vision, dizziness, dry mouth, constipation, and urinary retention. Central toxicity is indicated by impaired memory, confusion, hallucinations, and delusions.[7,57]

Amantadine (Symadine) is an anti-viral agent that has anti-parkinson effects. Its exact mechanism is unclear but it appears to have both dopaminergic and anticholinergic properties. Patients taking amantadine demonstrate modest improvement in tremor, rigidity, and bradykinesia. A major benefit is its limited adverse effects, which can include ankle edema, mottled skin (livedo reticularis), confusion, and nightmares.[7]

Patients with moderate to advanced PD who demonstrate declining responses to L-dopa therapy may benefit from dopamine agonist drugs such as bromocriptine (Parlodel), and pergolide (Permax). They are thought to improve the function of dopamine receptors, allowing lower doses of Sinemet to be administered (L-dopa–sparing) with prolonged effectiveness. Their greatest benefit is on rigidity and bradykinesia and can also be used to reduce motor fluctuations later in the disease. Adverse effects are similar to those of L-dopa, with orthostatic lightheadedness and nausea being the most common. Additional treatment options include new generation dopamine agonists (ropinirole, pramipexole, and cabergoline) and COMPT inhibitors (tolcapone [Tasmar]).[60,61]

The therapist needs to be fully aware of each of the medications the patient is taking and potential adverse effects. It is important to remember that patients on L-dopa therapy may demonstrate fluctuations related to medication cycle. Optimal performance can be expected at peak dosage whereas worsening performance is associated with end-of-dose cycle and medication depletion. Therapists are involved in monitoring drug effectiveness. This includes functional assessments of physical performance, self-report functional measures, and clinical examination of impairments.[63] As the disease progresses, patients may develop a tolerance for a particular medication, necessitating a change in prescription. Often, it is the therapist who first notices a change in the patient's status as the patient's system adapts to either the amount or type of drug prescribed. Accurate observation, examination, and reporting of these changes greatly assists the physician in modifying a drug prescription. Therapists may also be involved during clinical drug trials as new medications or combinations are developed.

Nutritional Management

A high-protein diet can block the effectiveness of L-dopa. The dietary amino acids in protein compete with L-dopa absorption. This is particularly problematic in patients with chronic disease who exhibit fluctuations in motor performance. Thus patients are generally advised to follow a high-calorie, low-protein diet. Generally no more than 15 percent of calories should come from protein. Dietary recommendations may also include shifting the intake of daily protein to the evening meal when patients are less active. These modifications minimize motor fluctuations and maximize responsiveness to L-dopa therapy. The patient is also encouraged to eat a variety of foods and may be advised to take dietary supplements to ensure adequate intake of vitamins and minerals. Patients are also advised to increase their daily intake of water and dietary fiber to alleviate problems of constipation.[63–65]

Rigidity and bradykinesia can limit upright posture and upper extremity feeding movements. Learned motor plans, for example, using a cup or eating utensils, may also be difficult. Occupational therapy to improve feeding and recommended adaptive eating devices are of considerable importance in helping to maintain nutrition and general health status. The speech/language pathologist also has an important role in the evaluation of dysphagia and the recommendation of strategies to assist with swallowing dysfunction. Education should focus on the importance of maintaining good nutritional intake.

Surgical Management

Stereotaxic surgery, the surgical lesioning of the brain, was pioneered in the 1950s but fell out of favor with the advent of L-dopa therapy.[66] More recently it has become an accepted treatment for patients with advanced PD who respond poorly to medication. Advances in neuroimaging and microelectrode recording techniques have improved precise localization of the deep-brain targets. Better understanding of the functional organization of the BG has also been an important factor in its increasing use. Bilateral surgery is not performed because it has been associated with an unacceptable level of complications.[67]

Pallidotomy involves producing a destructive lesion in the BG (globus pallidus internus [Gpi]). The lesion reduces excessive Gpi inhibitory activity that results in tonic thalamic hypoactivity.[71] It has primary effects on alleviating symptoms on the opposite side of the body, including tremor and L-dopa–produced dyskinesias and motor fluctuations.[68,69] Significant improvement has also been reported in bradykinesia, and functional performance; some improvement in ipsilateral signs (tremor and bradykinesia) has also been reported.[71] **Thalamotomy** involves producing a destructive lesion within the thalamus (ventral intermediate nucleus [VIN]). It has been shown to effectively reduce contralateral tremor in about 85 percent of patients, and to a lesser extent rigidity and L-dopa–induced dyskinesias. Bradykinesia, ipsilateral tremor, and postural instability are not improved.[67]

Deep brain stimulation (DBS) involves the implantation of electrodes in the brain (VIN of the thalamus) where they block nerve signals that cause symptoms. A pacemaker is implanted in the chest, with a thin wire that goes under the skin to the brain electrodes. High-frequency stimulation is provided. The patient can control the pacemaker's on-off switch while the physician determines the amount of stimulation it delivers, tailoring it to the individual's needs. Thalamic DBS was first approved in 1997 and is used to control disabling tremor. Total suppression is observed in 68 percent of patients and major improvement in 26 percent. Chronic stimulation may also improve rigidity. The major advantage of DBS is its potential to alter symptoms without producing an irreversible brain lesion. Subthalamic implants are still regarded as experimental.[71] DBS has also been shown to significantly improve patient performance on instrumental activities of daily living (IADL), with the greatest improvement noted when control is for tremor in the dominant hand.[72]

Transplantation of cells capable of delivering dopamine into the striatum of patients with advanced PD is an experimental treatment and currently under investigation. Studies include the grafting of fetal cells or autotransplantation with the patient's own adrenal medullary cells. Ethical problems are posed with the use of human embryonic tissue. There is also low availability of fetal tissue. Only modest improvements have been observed with greater improvements noted with fetal implants as opposed to adrenal implants. Much of the reported benefit is lost by the end of 2 years. Adverse side effects and deaths have been reported. Patients usually undergo immunosuppression following surgery to reduce the risks of graft rejection. Currently under investigation are techniques to expand cell production and use genetically engineered cells. Availability of these surgical procedures is very limited.[73–75]

REHABILITATIVE MANAGEMENT

Rehabilitation can have an important impact on reducing functional limitations and disability, and promoting optimal health. The enhancement of quality of life is perhaps the most important outcome for individuals with a chronic disease. Optimal management involves a coordinated team of health professionals, including the physician, nurse, physical therapist, occupational therapist, speech/language pathologist, psychologist, and social worker. Consultation to other specialists may also be necessary, for example, nutritionist, gastroenterologist, urologist, pulmonologist, and so forth. The patient and family member (caregiver) are key members of the team who should be fully involved in all aspects of the treatment planning process. The team provides a supportive environment and counseling to assist patients and their family members in the difficult adjustment to living with a chronic disease.

The ideal rehabilitation program considers the patient's disease history, course and symptoms, and areas of deficit including impairments, functional limitations, disability, and handicap. Of equal importance are the patient's abilities (assets), priorities, and resources including family, home, and community resources. Deterioration of condition and medication-induced fluctuations in performance should be expected. A focus on long-range planning is critical for effective management. An organized continuum of care is optimal, with coordination between hospital-based, outpatient, and home/community-based episodes of care.

Restorative rehabilitation is focused on improvement of strength, ROM, functional performance, endurance, and so forth using remedial and compensatory training strategies. Individuals with PD also benefit from **functional maintenance programs** designed to manage the effects of progressive disease. Strategies are developed to prevent or slow decline of function, and promote regular exercise, good health, and self-management skills. Shifting reimbursement trends have significantly altered the services that clinicians can provide, limiting the number of visits spread over longer time periods (e.g., one to two times per month over the course of several months). Functional maintenance programs are typically not well funded. Medicare, which covers services for the elderly and the disabled, will cover functional maintenance if the skills of a therapist are needed to manage a patient because of identified dangers (e.g., risk of secondary impairments, loss of functional capabilities). The therapist initially evaluates the patient, designs a program appropriate to the capacity and tolerance of the patient and the objectives of medical management, implements the plan, and periodically reevaluates the plan as required by the patient's condition. A variety of interventions are used to achieve goals and outcomes of functional maintenance, including direct interventions, supervision of assistive personnel, patient-related instruction, environmental modification, and supportive counseling. The primary emphasis is, however, to teach patients, family and caregivers management skills to carry out the maintenance program. Careful documentation is required to ensure adequate reimbursement of a functional maintenance program.

Assessment and Evaluation

Data can be obtained from the patient's history, systems review, and relevant tests and measures. The selection of examination procedures and level of inquiry are determined by the patient's unique status. The severity of problems, stage of disease, age, phase and setting of rehabilitation, and other factors must all be taken into account in structuring assessment. An evaluation of the results of assessment data must take into account stage and chronicity of disease. During the early and middle stages of PD, measures of impairment and physical performance appear to be relatively stable.[74] During late stages of the disease and under conditions of fluctuating symptoms with pharmacological instability, measures can be expected to be less stable.

Specific areas of assessment and relevant tests and measures that can be used to examine function in patients with PD are presented. A description of the unique problems presented by this patient group follows. For a complete description of tests and measures, see earlier assessment chapters.

COGNITION

An assessment of memory function, orientation, conceptual reasoning, problem solving, and judgement should be made. Speed of information processing, attention, and concentration are particularly important to assess if bradyphrenia is suspected. A useful instrument is the Mini Mental Status Exam (MMSE).[75]

AFFECTIVE AND PSYCHOSOCIAL FUNCTIONING

The therapist should determine overall levels of stress and anxiety, and available coping strategies. It is important to assess for depressive symptoms such as sadness, apathy, passivity, insomnia, anorexia, weight loss, inactivity and dependency, inability to concentrate and impaired memory, or suicidal ideation. Useful assessment instruments include the Geriatric Depression Scale[76] or the Beck Depression Inventory.[77] It is equally important to determine the patient's premorbid interests, abilities, and daily activities to translate them into a treatment program that will engage the patient's full cooperation.

SENSORY INTEGRITY

A screening examination of sensory integrity is indicated (superficial and deep sensations, combined cortical sensations). Sensory changes can be expected with aging (blunting of touch sensations and proprioception with greater losses in lower extremities than upper, distal extremities than proximal). Patients with PD may experience paresthesias (sensations of numbness or tingling). Specific deficits may be indicative of comorbid pathology, for example, stroke, diabetic neuropathy, and so forth.

PAIN

An assessment of the presence of pain is indicated. Mild aching and cramplike sensations are common in patients with PD and are often poorly localized. It is important to examine for postural stress syndrome (pain linked to lack of movement, faulty movements or posture, and ligamentous strain). Frequent pain or excruciating pain are not common but may also occur. Useful assessment instruments include The McGill Pain Questionnaire[78] and the visual analog scale.

VISUAL FUNCTION

An assessment of vision should include a determination of acuity, peripheral vision, tracking, accommodation, light and dark adaptation, and depth perception. Visual changes can be expected with aging such as loss of visual acuity, inability to focus on printed word (presbyopia), decreased adaptation to light, sensitivity to light and glare, and loss of color discrimination. Patients with PD may experience blurring of vision and difficulty reading not corrected by glasses as well as problems with eye pursuit (cogwheeling). Specific deficits may be indicative of comorbid pathologies that are common in the elderly, such as cataracts (clouding of central vision first, then peripheral), glaucoma (early loss of peripheral vision), senile macular degeneration or diabetic retinopathy (early loss of central vision), and cerebrovascular accident (CVA; homonymous hemianopsia). Medications may also produce impaired or fuzzy vision, for example, antidepressants and anticholinergics.

RANGE OF MOTION

An assessment of musculoskeletal ROM and flexibility is important. The therapist can measure specific ROM deficits (AROM, passive ROM [PROM]) using goniometers and so forth. Patients with PD are likely to present with losses in hip and knee extension, dorsiflexion, shoulder flexion, elbow extension, dorsal spine and neck extension, and axial rotation. To a lesser extent, many of these changes are also experienced by the elderly in general and are characteristic of senile posture. It is particularly important to examine spinal ROM (ability to rotate, flex, and extend the spine) because patients with PD have been shown to exhibit deficits in this area.[79] All segments of the spine should be examined, including cervical, thoracic, and lumbar segments. Hamstring length can be assessed using a straight leg test.

POSTURE

An assessment of resting posture and changes in posture that occur with movement is indicated. The therapist can use posture grids/plumb lines, still photography, or videotape to document changes. Patients with PD typically assume a flexed, stooped posture (kyphosis with forward head) with the center of mass placed forward within the limits of stability. The mobility of the spine should be examined during a series of movements, such as functional axial rotation (looking behind) and walking.

MUSCLE PERFORMANCE

An assessment of functional strength and endurance is indicated. The therapist can measure specific strength deficits using manual muscle testing (MMT). Hand-held and isokinetic dynamometry can be used to quantify peak force (torque output). Patients with PD have been shown to exhibit deficits in the rate of force development[19,21] and in maximum torque production capability.[19,79] Isokinetic dynamometry can also be used to document muscle endurance and has been suggested for documenting tremor, using slow speeds of movement (25 mm/s) and low torques.[80]

MOTOR FUNCTION

Motor function should be examined for the presence of BG signs.

Rigidity

Distribution of rigidity is very often unequal. It is therefore important to determine which body segments are affected and the severity of involvement. Tone changes in the neck and shoulders are suggestive of early disease, whereas tone changes in the trunk and extremities are typically present with more extensive disease. Deficits in functional mobility and postural reactions should be suspected in the presence of significant trunk rigidity. The patient should be examined for facial immobility (hypomimia or masked face); the ability to smile or use the muscles of facial expression should also be examined. A determination of severity of rigidity can be made based on criteria of ease of passive movement and availability of ROM. For example, a determination of severe rigidity is made if ROM can only be achieved with difficulty (see Appendix A). An inspection of active and automatic movements should be performed to determine the limitations imposed by rigidity.

Bradykinesia

A stopwatch can be used to quantify detectable slowing of movement. Patients with PD may demonstrate considerable movement hesitancy, with time lapses between the patient's desire to move and the actual movement response (slowed **reaction time**). Similarly, **movement time**—the time it takes to complete an activity—is also prolonged. The therapist should examine overall amplitude and poverty of movement. As the disease progresses, marked slowness, poverty, and small amplitude of movement should be expected. Timed tests for rapid alternating movements (RAM) can also be used to assess the effects of bradykinesia. These include pronation-supination movements, opening and closing of hands, and tapping (finger or foot tapping).

Motor planning ability can be assessed by observing performance during a complex movement sequence, for example, a transfer from bed to chair.

More sophisticated methods have been used to study movement in patients with parkinsonism, largely in the research setting. Electromyography (EMG) has been used to quantify the effects of rigidity and bradykinesia on motor performance. Long latency EMG responses (50 to 120 msec) have been observed when muscles are subjected to sudden stretch. Abnormal patterns of motor unit recruitment have also been observed.[37,81] Tests for reaction time (RT, the interval between the presentation of a stimulus and the start of movement) and movement time (MT, the interval between the beginning and end of movement) have also been used to study upper extremity motoric slowing. Patients with PD demonstrate both prolonged RTs and MTs, with larger increases reported in movement time. These results suggest that bradykinesia may represent a deficit of autoevoked arousal mechanisms (individual will) rather than exoevoked mechanisms (response to external stimuli).

Tremor

The location, persistence, and severity (amplitude) of tremor should all be recorded. The therapist should also determine if tremor is present at rest (the typical pattern) or if it is present with action and interferes with function. This latter pattern may occur in severe, long-standing disease. Upper extremity functional skills such as writing, feeding, and dressing should be closely examined for effects of tremor.

Postural Instability

A thorough assessment of balance is indicated. There are a large variety of clinical balance tests from which to choose. Therapists should include tests that assess static control (sitting or standing) under conditions of varying base of support (e.g., feet apart, feet together, tandem). The ability to maintain sitting or standing while under conditions of perturbation should also be examined. This includes both self-initiated challenges such as reaching or lifting and unexpected postural perturbations such as a push or pull. The influence of individual sensory systems (e.g., eyes open to eyes closed) and the ability to integrate visual, somatosensory, and vestibular inputs should be examined (e.g., standing on foam, eyes closed). Available postural strategies and reactions to challenges should be carefully documented (e.g., ankle, hip, and stepping strategies). Responses to perturbation may include instability with recovery (typically delayed in PD) or absence of postural responses (patient would fall if not caught by examiner). The patient may also exhibit development of a propulsive or retropulsive gait as he or she attempts to regain the base of support under the center of gravity.

Functional tests of balance are also important. Many of these instruments have been developed for use with the elderly and correlate well with frequency of falls (e.g., Performance Oriented Mobility Assessment by Tinetti). Individuals with PD have been shown to exhibit greater problems with tandem stance, single-limb stance, and reactive balance tests including functional reach and external perturbation.[82] Tests in which there are competing attentional demands (dual-task demands) would also be very difficult for these patients because they would be unable to use cognitive attentional mechanisms to override the deficits produced by the BG. Useful instruments include:

- Clinical Test for Sensory Interaction in Balance (CTSIB)[83]
- Force platform (dynamic) posturography[84]
- Functional Reach (FR)[85]
- Berg Balance Scale[86]
- Tinetti's Performance Oriented Mobility Assessment (POMA)[87]
- Timed Up and Go Test[88]

The Timed Up and Go Test is a particularly useful instrument for patients with PD because it includes tasks that are typically problematic. The individual rises from a chair, walks 10 feet, turns, and then returns to the chair. It uses time as an outcome measure. Scores within 10 seconds are normal for most adults; scores of 11 to 20 seconds are within normal limits for frail elderly or disabled patients; scores greater than 20 seconds are considered abnormal and indicate need for further assessment.

GAIT

An assessment of gait is indicated. Parameters and characteristics of gait that should be examined include stride length, step width, speed, stability, safety, and distance (endurance). The patient with PD typically exhibits decreased velocity, and a shuffling gait pattern with short steps and loss of heel strike. There is also a loss of trunk rotation and reciprocal arm swing. Gait should be examined during all movement directions: forward, backward, and sideward. A complex gait pattern like braiding can be used to examine difficulties in motor planning. The therapist should document freezing episodes (gait blocks) that appear during walking, including how often freezing episodes occur (frequency) and how long they last (duration). Also important is a determination of fall history and any fall injuries that may have occurred. The use of assistive devices, the need for contact guarding from family members or caregivers during walking, or triggering cues should be carefully documented.

DYSPHAGIA AND SPEECH IMPAIRMENTS

An examination of swallowing function, feeding, and speech is important. Referral to a speech/language pathologist is indicated if the patient demonstrates functional limitations in any of these areas.

AUTONOMIC CHANGES

The therapist should examine for problems with autonomic dysfunction. Excessive drooling (salivation) or sweating, greasy skin, and abnormalities in thermoregulation should be noted. Episodes of orthostatic hypotension should be carefully documented, with blood pressures taken at rest and after position change.

CARDIORESPIRATORY ENDURANCE

Cardiorespiratory endurance may be reduced from impaired respiratory function and long-standing inactivity, both common problems in chronic PD. An examination of respiratory function should include inspection of rib cage compliance, chest wall mobility, and thoracic expansion. Visual inspection of breathing patterns and an assessment of the influence of posture on breathing should be performed. Ventilation variables (respiratory rate, minute ventilation, inspiratory time) should be determined. Changes in breathing pattern with activity should also be noted. Objective measurements can include circumferential measurements of the chest and abdomen. Relevant pulmonary function tests include spirometry: flow-volume, lung volumes, and airway resistance (e.g., forced vital capacity [FVC], forced expiratory volume [FEV], maximal expiratory flow [MEF], maximal inspiratory flow [MIF], total lung capacity [TLC], residual volume [RV], and airway resistance [RAW].[50,89]

The therapist should assess resting vital signs (heart rate, blood pressure, and respiratory rate). Comparison can then be made to those same variables following exercise or a physical performance test. Reduced maximal heart rate and maximal oxygen consumption along with higher submaximal heart rates should be expected with deconditioning. Exertional symptoms (dyspnea, dizziness or confusion, excessive fatigue, pallor, etc.) should be carefully documented. Perceived exertion can be documented using Borg's Rating of Perceived Exertion Scale (RPE scale).[90] The patient should be questioned regarding knowledge and use of energy conservation and activity pacing strategies. Useful tests for this group of patients include the 6-Minute Walk Test[91] or 10-meter Walk Test.[92] An incremental exercise tolerance test (cycle ergometry exercise, treadmill test) can also be used.[51]

SKIN INTEGRITY AND CONDITION

The therapist should examine the patient closely for areas of bruising and skin breakdown. Patients who are severely disabled may be restricted to bed, a wheelchair, or both. Incontinence may occur during late stage disease. The effect of these problems on skin integrity should be carefully documented. Use and effectiveness of pressure-relieving strategies and devices should also be documented.

FUNCTIONAL STATUS

An assessment of functional status is indicated. Specific functional mobility skills are examined. Basic activities of daily living (BADLs) and IADLs along with the need for and appropriate use of adaptive equipment are typically assessed by the occupational therapist.

During functional performance tests, each skill

should be analyzed to determine the influence of direct and indirect impairments. For example, a problem in gait may be due to a primary impairment of severe rigidity or it may be due to secondary impairments of decreased ROM and poor posture.[93] The approach used in treatment to remediate the problem will be very different depending on the source of the problem. Patients with PD will most likely demonstrate difficulties in those activities having a rotational component, such as rolling or turning in bed or sitting up. Standing up, gait and fine motor skills, such as feeding or dressing, will also be difficult. The time it takes to initiate and to complete an activity should be recorded. Because these patients experience increased fatigue with resultant fluctuations in performance, examination sessions should be kept brief. Repeat assessments should be taken at the same time of day and at the same time in the medication cycle. An accompanying videotape of functional performance can provide an objective record of problems. An assessment of functional performance in the home (or work) environment is also indicated as part of a functional maintenance program. The patient's physical environment is examined for barriers, access, and safety.

Measures of functional ability that can be used include:
- The Functional Independence Measure (FIM)[94]
- Katz Index of Independence in Activities of Daily Living[95]

GENERAL HEALTH MEASURES

General health measures can be used to assess individual outcomes across a broad spectrum. Instruments typically include items that assess ability to perform routine daily activities and quality of life (e.g., physical and social function, general health and vitality, emotional well-being, bodily pain, etc.). General health measures have also been used to study large populations. They are most useful in determining global or long-term health outcomes and may lack the sensitivity needed to document short-term outcomes of treatment.[96]

Measures of general health status that can be used include:
- Rand 36-Item Health Survey SF-36[97,98]
- Sickness Impact Profile[99]

DISEASE-SPECIFIC MEASURES

Disease-specific measures are designed to assess attributes unique to a specific disease entity. Items are included to provide information about the disease process and outcomes, and ideally document clinically meaningful change over time. Thus these instruments have greater responsiveness or sensitivity to change than general health measures. Examples of instruments developed specifically for the assessment of patients with PD include the Unified Parkinson's Disease Rating Scale and Parkinson's Disease Questionnaire (PDQ-39).

The *Unified Parkinson's Disease Rating Scale*[100] was devised in the late 1980s to document the overall effects of the disease and is presented in Appendix A. It includes an assessment of the direct and indirect effects of PD and the effect of drug-related fluctuations. It is divided into three parts: mental status, activities of daily living, and the motor scale. Items are graded on a scale of 0 to 4, with 0 being normal and 4 being the most severe. Scored performances are frequently used to measure disease progression and the patient's response to drug therapy.

The *Parkinson's Disease Questionnaire (PDQ-39)* is a 39-item questionnaire that was developed from in-depth interviews with patients with PD.[101] It focuses on the subjective report of the impact of PD on daily life and addresses eight health-related quality of life dimensions (mobility, ADLs, emotional well-being, stigma, social support, cognitions, communication, and bodily discomfort). The PDQ-39 produces a profile of scores on the eight individual dimensions. A summary score (the Parkinson's disease summary index [PDSI]) can also be determined, with scores that range from 0 (perfect health) to 100 (worst health). It provides a useful indication of the global impact of PD on health status. Internal and test-retest reliability were found to be high with reported ranges from 0.68 to 0.96. Construct validity was assessed by comparing the PDSI with other measures of health. Significant and high correlations were found between the PDQ-39 and the SF-36 and the Hoehn and Yahr staging score.[102,103]

Setting Realistic Goals and Outcomes

A determination of appropriate goals and outcomes, and interventions should be based on careful assessment and evaluation of the patient's individual abilities, impairments, and functional limitations. Goals and outcomes of physical therapy for patients with PD adapted from the *Guide to Physical Therapist Practice*[104] include:

1. Ability to perform self-care and home management (ADLs and IADLs) is increased.
2. Performance levels in physical tasks and employment, recreational, or leisure activities are improved.
3. Disability associated with PD is reduced.
4. Care is coordinated with patient, family, caregivers, and other professionals.
5. Intensity of care is decreased.
6. Self-management of symptoms is improved.
7. Behaviors that foster health habits, wellness, and prevention are enhanced.
8. Risk of secondary impairments is reduced.
9. Joint integrity and mobility are maintained.
10. Strength, power, and endurance are increased.
11. Postural control is improved.
12. Motor function is improved.
13. Pain is decreased.
14. Gait, locomotion, and balance are improved.
15. Aerobic capacity and endurance are increased.

16. Safety of patient, family, and caregivers is improved.
17. Patient, family, and caregiver knowledge and awareness of the diagnosis, prognosis, goals and outcomes, and interventions are increased.
18. Patient knowledge of activity pacing and energy conservation is increased.
19. Decision making is enhanced regarding use of rehabilitation and community resources.
20. Level of stress is decreased and psychological adjustment of patient and family is enhanced.

The attainment of these goals and outcomes is dependent on a realistic understanding of the disease, impairments, functional limitations, and resultant disability.

Interventions

Because each patient is unique and presents a different set of problems, interventions will vary accordingly. Early intervention is critical in preventing the devastating musculoskeletal impairments these patients are so prone to develop. Interventions also focus on improvement of motor competencies and functional performance. Education of patients, family members, and caregivers is critical to attaining optimal outcomes. In general, the therapist encourages as much activity and movement as possible to overcome the effects of immobility and deconditioning. However, movement must be carefully balanced with adequate rest periods to ensure the patient does not fatigue or become exhausted.

RELAXATION EXERCISES

Gentle rocking and rotational exercises can be used to produce generalized relaxation of excessive muscle tension due to rigidity. This effect was described almost 100 years ago in Paris by Professor Charcot, who noted dramatic improvement in patients with PD following rides in bumpy, horse-drawn carriages. Following this observation he constructed a vibrating chair to use with his patients.[105] Although the exact mechanism underlying rigidity has not been identified, the beneficial effects of slow repetitive vestibular stimulation on excess tone have been demonstrated.[106,107]

Relaxation exercises should precede all other interventions, for example, ROM and stretching, balance activities, gait training, and so forth. Slow, rhythmic, rotational movements through small ranges of motion are effective in temporarily reducing rigidity.[108] Exercises should initially be performed in fully supported positions. Examples include:

1. Supine, slow side-to-side head rotations
2. Supine, bilateral symmetrical proprioceptive neuromuscular facilitation (PNF) D2F pattern (flexion, abduction, external rotation) and its reverse D2E pattern (extension, adduction, internal rotation)
3. Hooklying, lower trunk rotations
4. Sidelying, upper and lower trunk rotations
5. Sidelying trunk rotations combined with scapular patterns (shoulder protraction with elevation and retraction with depression)

The PNF technique of *rhythmic initiation (RI)*, in which movement progresses from passive to active-assistive to lightly resisted or active movement was specifically designed to overcome the crippling effects of immobility in PD.[110] The goal of treatment should be to have the patient actively participate in the exercises and to eventually be able to independently use them as part of a home exercise program (HEP). The patient with cognitive impairments will require the assistance of family members or caregivers.

Additional strategies and techniques to promote relaxation can be considered. Deep breathing exercises can be incorporated into rotational exercises to enhance relaxation. For example, bilateral symmetrical D2F patterns can be combined with inspiration while expiration is combined with bilateral symmetrical (BS) D2E patterns. A determination of the patient's ability to attend to dual-task demands should be made prior to combining exercises. A rocking chair can be an effective aid in reducing muscle tone. Some patients may benefit from cognitive imaging or meditation techniques (e.g., the relaxation response of Benson[111]) or Jacobson's progressive relaxation techniques.[112] Relaxation audiotapes can be used at home as part of the HEP. Some gentle positions of yoga can be effective for patients with PD because of the emphasis on combining relaxation with deep breathing and slow, steady stretching.[113] Additionally, some of the techniques of Feldenkrais, which focus on relaxation techniques to promote mobility can be of value.[109]

Stress management techniques are an important adjunct to relaxation exercises. A daily schedule needs to be planned to accommodate the restrictions of the disease and the functional needs of the patient. Life-style modifications and time management techniques reduce anxiety associated with movement difficulties and prolonged times required to complete basic functional tasks.

FLEXIBILITY EXERCISES

Both active and passive ROM exercises are used to improve flexibility. Ideally ROM exercises emphasize active motions that are performed two to three times a day. Exercises should focus on strengthening the patient's weak, elongated extensor muscles, while ranging the shortened, tight flexor muscles. Passive ROM exercises work within the patient's available ROM to maintain range. Because these patients have a minimum of energy to expend and multiple clinical problems, they benefit from ROM exercises in physiological patterns of motion. For example, PNF patterns combine several motions at once while emphasizing rotation, a movement component that is typically lost early in PD.[110] In the upper extremities, bilateral symmetrical D2 flexion patterns are ideal in promoting upper trunk extension and in counteracting kyphosis. In the lower extremities, hip and knee extension should be emphasized, ideally in a D1 extension pattern (hip extension, abduction, internal rotation) to counteract the typical flexed, adducted position of the lower extremities. Specific muscle contractures may respond to active muscle inhibition techniques such as the PNF hold-relax (HR) or contract-relax (CR) techniques.[110] Of the two, CR is the preferred technique because it combines autogenic inhibition from isometric contraction of the tight agonist muscle with active rotations of the limb. ROM exercises should also emphasize restoring range in the neck and trunk and can be performed in combination with rotational exercises to promote relaxation.

Traditional stretching techniques can also be used to elongate muscles. Special consideration should be given to the gentle stretching of elbow flexors, hip and knee flexors, and ankle plantarflexors. Stretching can be combined with joint mobilization techniques to reduce tightness of the joint capsule or of ligaments around a joint. By using selected grades of accessory movement, both improved ROM and decreased pain can be achieved.[115] Stretching techniques are an important component of the HEP. The patient or caregiver should be instructed in the appropriate stretching exercises and the importance of maintaining the stretch force for at least 15 to 30 seconds. Ideally the stretches are repeated at least three to five times. Ballistic stretches (high-intensity bouncing stretches) should be avoided because they are linked to increased injury. Muscle tears or ruptures of weakened tissues are especially prevalent in elderly, sedentary individuals.[116] The therapist should also avoid aggressive stretching (forcing a joint beyond its normal range). Vigorous stretching can stimulate pain receptors and cause rebound muscle contraction. Excessive stretching also causes tearing and weakness of tissues, scar formation, and more shortening. Patients with PD who are elderly and have long-standing disease must be considered at risk for osteoporosis and therefore must be stretched accordingly. The therapist should also use caution when stretching edematous tissue, a common lower extremity problem associated with immobility. Risk of injury is increased in this situation.[116]

Passive positioning, a long duration technique to improve flexibility, can also be used to stretch tight muscles and soft tissues. Patients in late-stage PD are likely to demonstrate severe flexion contractures of the trunk and limbs. The "phantom pillow" posture may develop in supine; that is, the head and shoulders are flexed as if there were a pillow present. Early on the patient may benefit from daily positioning in pronelying. As the disease progresses and significant postural deformity and cardiorespiratory impairments develop, the patient may not tolerate this position. The patient with a developing lateral curvature can be positioned in sidelying with a small pillow under the lateral trunk. Mechanical low load stretching can also be used. For example, the patient who is bedridden may benefit from weights applied to reduce hip and knee flexion contractures. This approach utilizes a weighted pulley and traction setup with low load weights (e.g., 5 to 15 lbs or 5 to 10% of body weight). The stretch is prolonged, with times ranging from 20 to 30 minutes to several hours. Additional mechanical stretching can be achieved through the use of a tilt table, for example, the patient is positioned with fixed leg straps to reduce hip and knee flexion contractures or toe wedges to reduce plantarflexion contractions.[116]

MOBILITY EXERCISES

An exercise program for patients with PD should be based on functional movement patterns that engage several body segments at once. The overall focus is on improving mobility/controlled mobility function with specific emphasis on improving segmental mobility of the head, trunk, and proximal segments (hips and shoulders). For example, prone-on-elbows and prone-extension activities can be used to improve thoracic and neck extension. However, some patients will not be able to tolerate these positions. Standing with elbows extended and hands weight bearing on a wall can alternately be used to promote upper trunk extension (e.g., standing wall push-ups or corner push-ups). Relaxation exercises are important prerequisites to all mobility training. Progression to more difficult motor activities should be gradual so the patient maintains relaxation as much as possible. The patient will benefit initially from assisted movements progressing to active movements (e.g., the PNF technique of RI) to improve initial motor performance. Movements should be rhythmic and reciprocal, and should progress toward increasing ROM.

Bed mobility activities (rolling, supine-to-sit transitions) are essential skills that are often problematic owing to truncal rigidity. Transitions that utilize sidelying on elbow as an interim posture improve the level of trunk rotation and lateral flexion and should be practiced. Sitting control can be facilitated first through exercises designed to improve pelvic mobility (anterior and posterior tilts, side-to-side tilts, pelvic clock exercises). The Swiss ball provides an excellent tool to facilitate these motions. Pelvic mobility exercises should also be practiced while sitting on a stationary surface such as a mat table. Upper extremity weight-bearing while sitting can be used to lock up the upper trunk and focus movements at the pelvis and lower trunk.[109] Progression can then be to weight shifting and UE reaching activities. Reaching should be practiced in all directions, with particular emphasis on promoting rotational movements of the trunk. Static-dynamic control can be enhanced by incorporating PNF extremity patterns with sitting. For example, bilateral symmetrical upper extremity D2F and D2E patterns are ideal because they expand the restricted chest while promoting upper trunk extension. Or a lift/reverse lift pattern or chop/reverse chop pattern can be used to promote upper trunk extension with rotation while in sitting. Static-dynamic activities for the lower trunk and pelvis in sitting can include crossing one leg over the other or scooting. Sit-to-stand transfers are also difficult for many patients with PD. Initial rocking forward and backward can be used to promote relaxation and enhance the patient's ability to move weight forward over the feet. At home a rocking chair can be an effective compensatory aide to facilitate independent sit-to-stand transfers. Practice from a raised seat may help promote independent movement. Standing up to a modified plantigrade position with the upper extremities extended (shoulders flexed to 90 degrees) and hands weight-bearing on a wall or on a high treatment table can improve initial stability in standing. Progression is from supported standing to unsupported. Tactile cueing or light resistance to hip extensors on the anterior pelvis can be used to promote full extension in standing. Once standing, rotational movements of the trunk should be practiced. For example, reciprocal arm swings or reaching movements can be used to promote trunk rotation. Weight shifting and stepping movements should be incorporated to promote pelvic rotation. Lateral side steps or step ups using a low platform step can be used to improve abductor function. Patients with PD typically experience a high number of falls and should be taught how to get up after a fall. To that end, skills in quadruped creeping should be practiced so the patient is able to move to a nearby stable chair or couch at home. The patient should also practice transitions moving from quadruped to kneeling to half-kneeling and finally to standing using UE support.[117]

Adequate strength and ROM are essential components needed for the performance of functional tasks. Weakness can result from both direct neurally induced factors as well as indirect disuse from inactivity. Although concerns have been expressed about using strength training in patients with PD, this area has not been well researched. The likelihood of increasing rigidity, bradykinesia, or fatigue may well depend on the specific status of the individual and on the exercise prescription. Published studies that have systematically looked at these factors are lacking.[118] However, the benefits of strength training in the frail elderly have been well documented by the Frailty and Injuries: Cooperative Studies of Intervention Techniques (FICSIT) trials.[119] Collectively these studies have shown that the frail elderly improve on measures of strength, functional mobility, balance, gait, fall risk, and quality of life following interventions that include strength training.[120–123] It is reasonable to assume that some patients with PD could demonstrate similar benefits. Patients in the early stages of the disease with mild to moderate impairments would most likely benefit from this type of training. As with any exercise, individualized prescription and proper monitoring by the physical therapist are required.[118]

Mobilizing facial muscles is another important goal of exercise, because the patient will have limited social interaction and poor feeding skills in the presence of marked rigidity and bradykinesia. These factors can greatly influence the patient's overall psychological state, motivation, and social isolation. Use of massage, stretch, manual contacts, and verbal commands can be used to enhance facial movements. Reciprocal motions should be stressed. The patient can be instructed to practice lip pursing, movements of the tongue, swallowing, and facial movements such as smiling, frowning, and so forth. A mirror can be used to provide visual feedback. In cases where eating is impaired by immobility, the movements of opening and closing the mouth and chewing should be combined with neck stabilization in a neutral position. Verbal skills should be practiced in association with breath control.

BALANCE ACTIVITIES

A number of positions and activities can be used to improve balance. Training should begin with weight shifts in both sitting and standing in order to help the patient develop an appreciation of his or her limits of stability. The therapist can assist by verbally cueing for postural and safety awareness and by using light tactile cues to facilitate the desired responses. The complexity of the activity can be altered by increasing the range of the weight shift or adding upper extremity tasks (e.g., reaching, cone stacking, picking up an object off the floor, tying shoes, and so forth). Movement transitions such as sit-to-stand or half-kneeling-to-standing, and stepping and walking can also be used to challenge the postural control system. The focus should be on appropriate timing of the activity, evidenced by smooth reciprocal motions within normal time constraints. Sitting activities on the gymnastic ball can be very helpful in promoting automatic balance reactions (e.g., stepping or marching with reciprocal arm swings, upper trunk rotation patterns with arm swings). Externally induced perturbations in the form of gentle manual displacements of the patient's center of gravity can be used but should be monitored carefully. They are contraindicated if an increase in postural tone and fixation is noted.[117]

It is important to remember that learning is task-specific. Thus practice of a variety of balance activities is essential to ensure motor learning. Practice should be expanded to include varying sensory and environmental conditions. Whenever possible the therapist should try to duplicate the conditions the patient will encounter in everyday life. The level of challenge is important. A therapist should know the limitations of the patient and the specific demands of the task and choose tasks accordingly.

Adequate strength and ROM are important components needed to withstand the challenges of balance. The patient can be instructed in standing heel-rises and toe-offs, partial wall squats and chair rises, single-limb stance with side-kicks or back-kicks, and marching in place, all while maintaining light touch-down support of the hands. Collectively these are sometimes referred to as the "kitchen sink exercises" and are important components of the HEP for patients with balance deficiencies.[117]

GAIT TRAINING

Gait training focuses on primary gait deficits which, typically include slowed speed, shuffling gait pattern, diminished arm swing and trunk movements, and an overall attitude of flexion while walking.[124] Specific goals are to lengthen stride, broaden base of support, improve stepping, improve heel-toe gait pattern, increase contralateral trunk movement and arm swing, and provide a program of regular walking. The patient can practice marching in place, emphasizing high stepping to strengthen hip flexors. Weight transference can be practiced using stepping movements forward and back. The therapist can ensure there is adequate pelvic rotation to initiate stepping by placing the hands on the pelvis and using light stretch and resistance to facilitate the desired motions. Sidestepping and crossed-step walking can be practiced. The PNF activity of braiding, which combines sidestepping with alternate crossed-stepping, is an ideal training activity for the patient with PD because it emphasizes lower trunk rotation with stepping movements. It can be practiced with the patient holding on lightly to the therapist's hands or as a free walking pattern. The patient should also practice stopping, starting, changing direction, and turning. Turns of 180 or 360 degrees should be practiced emphasizing small steps and a wide base of support. Two wands or sticks (held by the patient and therapist, one in each hand) can be used to facilitate reciprocal arm swing during gait. The therapist uses his or her arm swing to assist the patient's.

Visual cues can improve the gait of patients with PD. The problem of a shuffling gait can oftentimes be remedied by using small blocks of about 2 to 3 inches (5 to 7.5 cm) to provide a target for the patient to step over. Alternately, brightly colored transverse lines can be effective in initiating and controlling stepping. Other triggering cues that have been used successfully with patients with PD include the use of an inverted walking stick[125,126] and virtual reality lenses that provide a stepping target. Bagley et al.[127] found the use of visual cues in the form of yellow, triangular tubes placed at regular intervals on the floor significantly improved step length, velocity, and cadence in patients with PD. Improvements were also noted in time parameters (stride time, and durations of single- and double-limb support). Once the cues were removed however, the changes did not persist. One of the more recent approaches to improve the gait of individuals who experience frequent freezing episodes has been the use of trained assistance dogs. The movements of the dogs appear to act as triggers to stimulate stepping movements in individuals with PD.

Auditory cues can be effective in improving gait and reducing episodes of freezing (gait blocks). Patients respond positively to brisk march music or other similar types of rhythmic music.[128] Selection of music can be assisted by a certified music therapist. During treatment the patient can be instructed to sing along with the music while marching in place or walking in time with the music. Auditory stimulation in the form of brisk music provided by a portable cassette or compact disc player has been shown to enhance gait parameters, including step length, velocity, and cadence.[129] Platz et al.[130] found significant improvements in the speed of aimed movements with training using rhythmic auditory cues. Moreover, the effects transferred to an untrained limb and were partially maintained after a time delay. The metronome has also been shown to stimulate walking in patients with PD. In one study comparing free walking with walking using march music, tactile stimulation, and metronome stimulation at a rate of 96 beats per minute, the metronome stimulation was found to significantly reduce the number of freezing episodes and lengthen stride. March music was also effective, but less so; tactile stimulation actually produced negative results.[131]

MOTOR LEARNING STRATEGIES

There is evidence to suggest that motor learning is impaired in PD.[132–134] Overall procedural learning is slower. The planning of complex movements is particularly problematic. The patient will demonstrate more difficulty carrying out simultaneous movements (dual tasks) owing to an inability to integrate two motor programs at the same time.[135] The resultant interference of one movement with the other will result in difficulty maintaining the activity and slowing of movement. Planning sequences of movement is also problematic for the same reasons. For example, freezing episodes are common when the patient rises from a chair and then attempts to walk.[136] In situations where attention is divided, learning of activities is also typically more difficult. The therapist will need to structure treatment sessions accordingly to minimize these problems. For patients in the early stages of the disease, training has been shown to improve learning and performance.[130] In long-standing disease, training will likely be less successful and compensatory strategies should become the focus of training.

As discussed, the patient with PD exhibits impairments in the use of self-initiated, internal triggers for movement while external cues are generally successful. External cues appear to facilitate movement by utilizing additional cerebellar and cortical brain areas.[137] The cues may have a common mode of action, hypothesized by Ferrandez and Blin[138] as tapping into motivational and arousal processes to influence motor behavior. Selection of the right type of cues and specificity of cues will depend on the individual patient. Dietz et al.[126] found that the predicted long-term benefit of a particular type of cue was dependent on its initial success.

There are negative aspects to using sensory cues to trigger desired behaviors. Cues are clearly not practical for continuous everyday use. The home environment can more easily be modified to include cues, whereas the community environment cannot. The requirements for cognitive attention are high and thus cueing would not be suitable for patients with cognitive impairments. Schenkman[139] suggests that the effort required to pay conscious attention to triggering cues to stimulate walking may be functionally limiting. For example, the patient might be unable to perform another functional task while walking such as carrying an object. Community ambulation would also likely be more difficult as attention might be diverted. These difficulties are especially apparent for patients in the late middle stages of PD when deficits in simultaneous and sequential performance of motor tasks are present. Methods of cueing are not likely to be effective when medication instability and disease fluctuations are present. For example, the patient in a full-blown off period would have a difficult time moving at all and is not likely to respond to external cueing. However, for many patients, using cues is a valid treatment strategy and one in which a learning effect should be anticipated.[136]

FUNCTIONAL ADAPTATIONS

The patient should be carefully assessed in terms of needs for adaptations and assistive devices that can improve function. Loose-fitting clothing with Velcro closures can be used to facilitate dressing. To promote bed mobility, the patient can be helped to assume a sitting position by elevating the head of the bed with blocks of approximately 4 inches (10 cm), or by using an electronic hospital bed. A simpler solution might include attaching a knotted rope to the end of the bed to pull on. The bed should be stable and the mattress firm to facilitate rolling and ease of getting in and out. Satin sheets and pajamas may enhance bed mobility. If patients have problems in standing up, they should avoid soft, deep upholstered chairs. A firm chair with arm rests (captain's chair) should be used instead. The chair can be raised about 4 inches (10 cm) and secured with blocks, or tilted forward by elevating only the back legs about 2 inches (5 cm). Chairs that have spring-loaded seats that push the patient into standing are heavily marketed to the geriatric population but should be used with caution. The patient is propelled into standing but may have difficulty getting his or her balance within an appropriate time frame when first reaching the standing position.

If the patient demonstrates a shuffling gait, shoes should have leather or hard composition soles, because shoes with crepe or rubber soles will not slide easily. A festinating gait can sometimes be alleviated by the addition of modified heel or shoe wedges. A flat heel or toe wedge may slow down a propulsive gait, whereas a raised heel or heel wedge may diminish a retropulsive gait pattern. The use of assistive devices can be problematic owing to movement difficulties. A cane or walker may be helpful with some patients with mild disease, either to restrict a propulsive gait or to assist in balance. It is important that the height of the device not promote increased flexion of the trunk. Patients with more pronounced movement difficulties and poor balance are not likely to benefit from assistive devices. Walkers with wheels are particularly hazardous, and are likely to increase a festinating gait. Patients with a retropulsive gait would likely fall over backwards, carrying the assistive device with them.

Most patients utilize devices to assist in ADLs. Reachers can be used to provide assistance in dressing as well as for other activities. Eating can be facilitated in a number of ways. The patient should be seated properly, close to the table, with good posture. Specially adapted utensils, plate guards, and enlarged handles can aid the patient's efforts. Because eating time will be prolonged, heated plates may help keep food warm and palatable. Drooling and/or spills should be anticipated and clothing protected. Extra time should be planned, and the patient should not feel rushed.

RESPIRATORY EXERCISES

Respiratory dysfunction is linked to morbidity and mortality in patients with PD. Both obstructive and restrictive ventilatory deficits are present.[50,51,140] A comprehensive pulmonary rehabilitation program should be instituted. Components include diaphragmatic breathing exercises, air-shifting techniques, and exercises that recruit neck, shoulder, and trunk muscles. The patient should be instructed in deep breathing exercises to improve chest wall mobility and vital capacity. Air shifts are promoted to lesser-ventilated areas of the lung. For example, basal expansion can be promoted using manual stretch and resistance to those segments. Upper body resistance training exercises are indicated. These can include raising and lowering a dowel with light weights added to increase resistance (e.g., 500 g or 1 lb). Weights are increased as function improves. As previously mentioned, chest wall mobility can be improved by using PNF upper extremity bilateral symmetrical D2 flexion and extension patterns. Light weights (wrist cuffs) can also be added to these exercises. Patients are encouraged to coordinate breathing with upper extremity movement. Exercises are performed in unsupported sitting to promote trunk stabilization. A focus on improving trunk extension is especially important in improving breathing patterns in patients with postural kyphosis. Koseoglu et al.[141] utilized a similar pulmonary rehabilitation program in a group of nine patients with PD. They found improved upper extremity endurance and pulmonary function (oxygen consumption [Vo_2], minute ventilation (V_E), and respiratory rate) when compared to a group of age-matched healthy controls.

AEROBIC CONDITIONING

Deconditioning and decreased endurance are evident in individuals with PD. Standardized exercise testing can be used to safely measure level of fitness prior to commencing an aerobic exercise program.[52] Submaximal intensities (e.g., 50 to 70% of heart rate reserve) are indicated to improve cardiovascular and metabolic responses in this patient group. A conservative approach with careful monitoring is indicated. Training modes can include upper and lower extremity ergometry and walking. Selection will depend on the specific abilities of the patient; for example, postural instability and increased risk of falls will require use of a stationary or seated ergometer. For most patients a program of regular walking is recommended. The duration, speed, and terrain covered can be modified, based on individual ability. Accessibility to indoor walking is important in case of inclement weather (e.g., shopping mall walking). The minimum recommended frequency is 3 to 5 days per week. Daily walking with short bouts throughout the day are recommended for individuals with lower functional capacity. Intermittent exercise with repetitive exercise-rest periods is indicated for these patients who are elderly and deconditioned, and who present with pulmonary dysfunction.[142] Swimming, although an excellent aerobic activity, should not be done without supervision because it may be too risky for the patient with moderate disease who experiences episodes of freezing.[143]

GROUP AND HOME EXERCISES

Group exercise classes are often organized for patients with PD. Patients benefit from the positive support, camaraderie, and communication the group situation offers. Careful assessment of each patient prior to admission into a group is essential. Patients should be able to perform the therapeutic core of the class. Selecting patients with similar levels of disability is often advisable because the sense of competition can frequently be a key factor in motivating groups. The ratio of staff to patients should be kept small (ideally 1:8 or 1:10), and extra staff should be added if patients are unable to work on their own. A variety of activities can be used to stimulate and motivate patients. The patients can begin in the seated position and progress to standing, using light, touch-down support of the back of the chair. Warm-up activities or calisthenics involving large joints should be used to help patients limber up and get going. Progression is to combination movements (upper and lower extremities with trunk rotation). Well-structured, low-impact aerobics are an appropriate focus for a group class. For example, patients can march in place, first in sitting, then in standing. The group can then practice walking with an emphasis on taking large, high steps. Music is used to provide necessary stimulation to movement and movement pacing. Exercise stations (e.g., stationary bicycle, mats, pulleys, etc.) can also be used. Exercises done by the whole group together should focus on important exercise goals (e.g., improving ROM, mobility, etc.). Dancing and other games can follow the aerobic portion, with such activities as line dancing, ball activities, beanbag toss, and so forth. The activities selected should be interesting and varied. Finally, relaxation training should be incorporated into each class.[144]

The HEP includes many of the interventions already discussed, with exercises designed to improve relaxation, flexibility, strength, and cardiorespiratory function. A key element is stressing the importance of regular daily exercise and the avoidance of prolonged periods of inactivity. The HEP should be realistic and of moderate duration and intensity. The patient should be cautioned against overdoing activity, which could result in excessive fatigue. Early morning warm-up calisthenics are often helpful in reducing the increased stiffness patients may experience upon arising. Patients and families can be taught compensatory techniques or triggering maneuvers to overcome the crippling effects of bradykinesia and freezing. Home ROM exercises can often be assisted by the use of adaptive equipment. For example, wall pulleys can be used to improve upper extremity ROM, provided episodes of freezing are not common. Hanging from an overhead bar can also be used to provide a maintained stretch on the upper trunk and extremity flexors. Use of a wand or cane can also be effective in promoting overhead motions. In standing, a countertop or sturdy chair should be used to assist in stabilization during calisthenics and balance activities.[145]

PATIENT AND FAMILY EDUCATION

Patients, family members, and caregivers need to be educated about PD, what the disease entails, and how symptoms are managed. They should be informed about medications, including purpose, dosage, and possible adverse side effects. Patients are also taught to recognize signs of either over- or under-medication. They need to understand what preventative measures can be taken to minimize the secondary complications and impairments that typically result. They need to learn how PD affects normal movement and possible strategies to solve movement problems. It is important to discuss everyday situations that might pose problems in the home or work environments. The patient and family should be assisted in developing decision making and behavioral skills to promote optimal self-care. A satisfactory time schedule for completion of daily tasks should be established. Patients cannot be hurried because performance will suffer. Caregivers should be encouraged not to provide too much assistance because this will foster dependence. Interventions can take the form of direct one-on-one instruction, group sessions, printed materials, and video or computer presentations. The therapist's approach needs to be enthusiastic and supportive. Teaching style should incorporate careful observation, gentle corrections, and a stimulating voice.[145,146]

Community support groups are available for many patients and their families. They disseminate information and offer a chance to discuss common issues, problems, and management tips. They also can provide a stabilizing influence, assisting patients and families to focus on healthy behaviors, coping skills, and acceptance. For some patients in the early stages of the disease, participation in a support group may increase levels of distress as they observe more disabled patients. Groups particularly targeted to patients with early stage disease and similar ages may be more helpful.[147]

Educational pamphlets, newsletters, and location of support groups can be obtained through national Parkinson's disease associations:

1. National Parkinson Foundation (NPF)
   1501 N.W. 9th Ave., Bob Hope Road
   Miami, FL 33136
   (800) 327-4545   www.parkinson.org
2. Parkinson's Disease Foundation (PDF)
   William Black Research Building
   640 West 168th St., New York, NY 10032
   (800) 457-6676   www.pdf.org
3. The United Parkinson Foundation and International Tremor Foundation
   833 Washington Blvd.
   Chicago, IL 60610
   (312) 733-1893
4. The American Parkinson Disease Association (APDA)
   60 Bay Street
   Staten Island, NY 10301
   (800) 223-2732   www.apdaparkinson.com

Psychosocial Issues

The progressive nature of PD necessitates frequent personal and social adjustments, and affects all aspects of life for both the patient and family. Disruption in daily functions, roles, and activities are experienced. Some of the changes associated with PD are socially isolating (masked face, progressive immobility, and unintelligible speech) whereas other changes (increased salivation, perspiration, decreased sexual function) are distressing and socially embarrassing.[148] The patient may feel increasingly isolated and family relationships may suffer. Depression is extremely common. A comprehensive assessment is needed to determine each individual's unique situation and emotional resources.[147]

The principle goal for team members is to assist the patient and family in their understanding of the disease and in developing insights and adjustments that lead to more effective living. Some individuals are able to successfully deal with the changes associated with the disease; others are not. Coping skills can be facilitated. First and foremost education is the key to assisting patients and family members assume responsibility. Feelings of hopelessness and dependency are reduced as the patient develops a sense of control over his or her own life. Self-management skills that should be promoted include advanced planning of activities, effective time management strategies, and stress management techniques. It is equally important to ensure that patients do not become isolated and that appropriate services are available. Team members must be vigilant regarding their assumptions and expectations. A condescending or pessimistic and limiting attitude can become a self-fulfilling prophecy. Patients and family members need reassurances and encouragement.

An overall emphasis on what patients can do rather than what they cannot do helps to empower patients. Therapists need to provide a message of hope tempered with realism.

Management Considerations by Stage of Disease

In the early stages of the disease, patients are functional and independent. They are typically seen on an outpatient basis. Medical therapies may include the administration of Seligiline to stay the need for L-dopa and other drugs designed to provide symptomatic relief (e.g., anticholinergics for tremor).[62] A referral for physical therapy is often not initiated at this stage, although benefits could clearly be obtained. Interventions that focus on prevention or reversal of musculoskeletal and cardiorespiratory impairments and improvement of general health status would benefit the patient. Early education for patient and family can provide meaningful assistance in understanding the disease and its ramifications. Early referral to support groups is also helpful (Table 23–5).

During the middle stages of the disease, symptoms are more readily apparent and functional limitations emerge. The patient is still independent in gait and many ADLs, although performance is slowed and less efficient. Some assistance may be required. Treatment with L-dopa is typically delayed until the middle stages, although individual differences exist. Once placed on L-dopa patients may exhibit a dramatic improvement in symptoms, most notably in rigidity and bradykinesia. The alleviation of these symptoms does not always produce a similar amount of improvement in their function, however; poor habits and faulty posture may have developed. These patients will usually respond quite well to a rehabilitation program designed to correct musculoskeletal impairments and promote mobility and independent function. Training in compensatory techniques and energy-conserving strategies is indicated.[62] Family and caregiver instruction is intensified to assist the patient in remaining functionally mobile. For some patients day treatment programs are a viable option. Some are structured to provide a variety of recreational activities and general health measures. Other day programs are more treatment oriented. Both focus on providing social interaction.[147]

Patients with late-stage disease typically demonstrate a number of complications including pharmacological intolerance, increased primary symptoms, fixed musculoskeletal impairments, a decline in cognitive functioning, sleep disturbances, incontinence, malnutrition, significant cardiopulmonary compromise, and severe immobility. Patients are dependent in many or most of their daily functional mobility skills and ADLs. They may be wheelchair bound or bedridden. Family and community resources are vital in maintaining the patient in the

Table 23–5 OVERVIEW OF PARKINSON'S DISEASE MANAGEMENT

| Stage | Characteristics | Treatment Considerations | | |
		Pharmacological Agents	Physical	Psychosocial
Early	Fully functional May have unilateral tremor, rigidity	Anticholinergics (tremor) Seligiline (possible neuro-protection)	Preventative exercise program	Education information
Early middle	Symptoms bilateral, brady-kinesia, rigidity Mild speech impairment Axial rigidity, stooped posture, stiffness Gait impairment begins	Levodopa/carbidopa Seligiline	Corrective exercise program	Counseling Support group Monitor for depression
Late middle	All symptoms worse but independent in ADL[a] May need minor assistance Balance problems	Levodopa/carbidopa Dopamine agonists Seligiline Antidepressants	Compensatory and corrective exercise Speech/language therapy Occupational therapy	Caregiver issues (medications, mobility) Monitor for dementia
Late	Severely disabled, impaired Dependent with ADLs	Levodopa/carbidopa Dopamine agonists Antidepressants	Compensatory exercise Dietary concerns Skin care Hygiene Pulmonary function	Dementia Depression

[a]ADLs, activities of daily living.
From Cutson, T et al.[62] p 370, with permission.

home. Some patients may require placement in a chronic care facility. At this stage of disease, patients generally do not respond as well to medical management and experience decreasing effectiveness of pharmacological interventions, fluctuations in performance, and adverse side effects of chronic dopaminergic medication. These changes can be a source of great frustration to the patient and family. Goals and expectations need to be restructured. During late-stage disease, the therapist needs to focus on skin care to avoid breakdown and pressure wounds, pulmonary hygiene to avoid pneumonia, and assistance in positioning and feeding to avoid malnutrition, aspiration, and pneumonia.[62] Caregiver training becomes increasingly important. Safety for both the caregiver and the patient becomes a primary concern as patients are assisted in position changes in bed or during transfers. Patients should be encouraged and assisted to move as much as possible and not let everything be done for them. Often, environmental adaptations may mean the difference between total dependence and partial independence. The rehabilitation team should be supportive of the patient's efforts no matter how small they may be. Patients in late-stage PD demonstrate extremely limited skills to interact with their environment, with increasing social isolation and withdrawal. Families also suffer from the increasing demands of care, burnout, and social isolation. Therapists need to maximize psychosocial support and be readily available for consultation.

A limited number of clinical reports have demonstrated that physical therapy can be beneficial in the management of PD. Comella et al.[127] reported that repetitive exercises for ROM, endurance, balance, and gait resulted in improvements in scores for rigidity and bradykinesia as measured by the United Parkinson's Disease Rating Scale. Schenkman et al.[128] demonstrated improvements in balance, gait, and functional movement following physical therapy in a small number of patients. It is clear that more research is needed to demonstrate the benefits for patients at each stage of the disease.

SUMMARY

PD is a chronic, progressive disorder of the BG characterized by the cardinal features of rigidity, bradykinesia, tremor, and postural instability. Secondary impairments include the development of abnormal fixed postures, poverty of movement, fatigue, masked face, contractures, a festinating gait pattern, swallowing and communication difficulties, visual and sensorimotor disturbances, cognitive and behavioral dysfunction, autonomic dysfunction, and cardiopulmonary changes. Pharmacological interventions have become the mainstay of treatment and provide early protective therapy and symptomatic treatment. Effective rehabilitation focuses on the patient's history, stage of disease and symptoms, areas of functional deficit, and residual abilities and assets. Interventions can be restorative; that is, rehabilitation is focused on the improvement of strength, ROM, functional skills, endurance, and so forth using remedial and compensatory training strategies. Individuals with PD also benefit from functional maintenance programs designed to manage the effects of progressive disease. Strategies are developed to prevent or reduce indirect impairments, and promote regular exercise, good health, and self-management skills. A comprehensive team approach including active involvement of patient and family can provide optimal benefits. Team members need to be active during all stages of the disease, directing the patient and family toward maintenance of function and providing psychosocial support as needed.

QUESTIONS FOR REVIEW

1. What are the major CNS structures involved in PD? How is the function of these structures altered?

2. What are the cardinal features of PD? Secondary impairments and complications?

3. What components should be included in a physical therapy examination? Identify four standardized measures that would be appropriate to use with the patient with PD.

4. Describe the drug therapy used in PD. How might a physical therapy program be influenced by drug management?

5. What are the major goals and outcomes of physical therapy intervention? How might they vary by stage of disease?

6. What are the effects of prolonged inactivity for the patient with PD? Identify three strategies that can be used to counteract these effects.

7. Identify three activities/techniques that can be used to relax the patient and improve ROM.

8. What therapeutic strategies can be used to improve cardiorespiratory fitness? Precautions?

9. Describe the gait deficits common in patients with PD. What interventions can be used to remediate or compensate for the expected gait deficits?

10. What types of interventions are appropriate for the patient with advanced disease who is relatively unresponsive to pharmacological management?

11. Differentiate between a rehabilitation program with a restorative focus versus one with a functional maintenance focus. Consider goals/outcomes and overall training approach.

12. What are the major considerations in patient and family education? Psychosocial counseling?

CASE STUDY

The patient is a 60 year-old woman with a 7-year history of PD. Lately she has experienced increasing severity of symptoms and is referred for outpatient physical therapy and a home exercise program.

HISTORY: She first presented with tremor of her left hand that progressed to include stiffness and awkwardness of her left arm and leg. Her family physician referred her to a neurologist who found moderate tremor and rigidity on the left side. He prescribed Artane, which was helpful for a while. Eventually the tremor became worse, especially under conditions of stress when she was unable to use her left arm at all. She was then started on Sinemet and referred for an initial episode of physical therapy as an outpatient. Once Sinemet began to work and her symptoms dramatically lessened, she stopped doing her home exercise program. Over the next few years when her symptoms increased, her dose of Sinemet was increased.

CURRENT STATUS: She is currently taking Sinemet and bromocriptine. She reports bouts of dyskinesia about 45 minutes into taking her Sinemet that involve involuntary writhing movements of her shoulders and neck. Her chief complaints are:

1. Difficulty walking, especially when she has to go through a narrow doorway, or walk in a crowded place.

2. Episodes of gait blocks; if she tries to do something while walking like take a tissue out of her pocket, she stops abruptly in her tracks. The harder she tries to move, the worse it gets. Episodes of freezing have lasted up to 20 minutes.

3. Postural instability: over the past month she has experienced occasional bouts of uncontrolled or unsteady balance. This is particu-

larly disturbing to her because if it occurs while she is walking, it causes her to fall. She has fallen nine times in the past month, with no residual fall injury. Because of her increased fear of falling, she has stopped going out by herself.

4. She is experiencing increased difficulty rolling over in bed, getting out of bed, and standing up from a chair. Her husband now has to provide assistance 90 percent of the time to accomplish these activities.

5. She reports having trouble sleeping at night. She has stopped drinking coffee but this has not helped. She wakes four to five times a night, and requires assistance from her husband to go to the bathroom at night. She also has hallucinated at night, claiming to see insects on the wall. During these periods she becomes extremely frightened.

6. Her medication seems to be helping less and less. If she plans to go out, she takes an extra Sinemet. She revisted her neurologist in hopes that he would increase her dosage. Instead he told her the symptoms were most likely the result of excess medication. He instructed her not to take the extra Sinemet and has adjusted her dosage.

PHYSICAL EXAMINATION FINDINGS: Mental status: alert, oriented × 3; she is displaying mild deficits in short-term memory.

She is showing signs of depression: she is less interested in going out, socializing, and reports frequent insomnia.

Speech: Mild dysarthria, hypophonia

Sensation: Slightly decreased proprioception bilaterally in both ankles; otherwise intact

Tone: Rigidity (cogwheel type) moderate in extremities L > R

Marked rigidity throughout neck and trunk
Masklike face

ROM: Decreased due to moderate rigidity; limitations noted in:

Bilateral elbow extension (10–140 degrees)
Bilateral hip extension (0–10 degrees)
Bilateral knee extension (10–120 degrees)
Bilateral ankle dorsiflexion (0–15 degrees RLE; 0–10 degrees LLE)

Strength: Generally fair (3/5) to good (4/5).

Poor (2/5) muscle grades noted in ankle dorsiflexors.

Motor: Moderate to severe resting tremors, L hand > R hand.

Bradykinesia: marked slowness, poverty of movement.

Hesitation on initiation of movement; frequent arrests of ongoing movement.

Posture: Overall body alignment is forward and flexed; kyphotic spine with forward head.

Gait: Ambulates independently with a shuffling gait pattern with decreased step length and arm, trunk, hip and knee motions; tendency for propulsive gait.

Balance: Decreased limits of stability; patient's forward alignment increases her tendency to fall forward.

She has slow reactions to loss of balance with decreased rotational movements of trunk and minimal use of ankle, hip, and stepping strategies.

Timed Up & Go score is 36 seconds.

Patient is fearful of falling.

Functional Mobility: Generally decreased.

Requires moderate assist: rolling in bed, supine-to-sit transfers, sit-to-stand transfers.

Can sit and stand independently; demonstrates minimal weight shifting abilities.

Unable to bridge secondary to hip flexion contractures.

Patient has good safety awareness.

Self-Care: Requires minimal assistance to supervision for feeding; minimal assist for dressing.

Cardiopulmonary: Shallow (upper respiratory) breathing pattern.

Generally decreased functional capacity (estimated FWC is 6 metabolic equivalents [METs]).

Patient fatigues easily and requires frequent rest periods.

Mild edema both ankles.

Skin: Intact, no areas of breakdown.

Experiences bouts of increased perspiration.

Guiding Questions:

1. Identify/categorize this patient's problems in terms of:
   a. Direct impairments
   b. Indirect impairments
   c. Composite impairments: combined effects of both direct and indirect impairments
   d. Functional limitations
2. Identify two outcomes (the remediation of functional limitations and disability) and two goals (remediation of impairments) for this patient.
3. Formulate four treatment interventions that could be used at the start of therapy to achieve the stated outcomes and goals. Provide a brief rationale for each.
4. What strategies would you use to develop self-management skills and promote quality of life?

REFERENCES

1. Marttila, R: Parkinson's disease: Epidemiology. In Koller, W (ed): Handbook of Parkinson's Disease. Marcel Dekker, New York, 1987, p 35.
2. Stern, M, et al: The epidemiology of Parkinson's disease: A case control study of young onset and old onset patients. Arch Neurol 48:903, 1991.
3. Parkinson, J: An Essay on the Shaking Palsy. Sherwood Neely & Jones, London, 1817.
4. Zetusky, W, et al: The heterogeneity of Parkinson's disease: Clinical and prognostic implications. Neurology 35:522, 1985.
5. Koller, W: Classification of Parkinsonism. In Koller, W (ed): Handbook of Parkinson's Disease. Marcel Dekker, New York, 1987, p 51.
6. Sacks, O: Awakenings. HarperCollins, New York, 1990.
7. Pfeiffer, R, and Ebadi, M: Pharmacologic management of Parkinson's disease. In Cohen, A, and Weiner, W (eds): The Comprehensive Management of Parkinson's Disease. Demos, New York, 1994, p 9.
8. Langston, JW, and Ballard, P: Chronic parkinsonism in humans due to a product of meperidine-analog synthesis. Science 219:976, 1983.
9. Burns, S: Atypical Parkinsonism: The Many Faces of Parkinsonism. Parkinson Report. National Parkinson Foundation, Miami, 1989.
10. Bakheit, AMO: Early diagnosis of Parkinson's disease. Postgrad Med J 71:151, 1995.
11. Hornykiewicz, O: Biochemical aspects of Parkinson's disease. Neurology 51(suppl 2):S2, 1998.
12. Forno, L: Neuropathology of Parkinson's disease. J Neuropathol Exp Neurol 55:259, 1996.
13. Snell, R: Clinical Neuroanatomy for Medical Students, ed 4. Lippincott-Raven, Philadelphia, 1997.
14. Ma, TP: The Basal Ganglia. In Haines, D (ed): Fundamental Neuroscience. Churchill Livingstone, New York, 1997, p 364.
15. Hallett, M: Physiology of basal ganglia disorders: An overview. Can J Neurol Sci 20:177, 1993.
16. Weinrich, M, et al: Axial versus distal motor impairment in Parkinson's disease. Neurology 38:540, 1988.
17. Jankovic, J: Pathophysiology and clinical assessment of motor symptoms in Parkinson's disease. In Koller, W (ed): Handbook of Parkinson's disease. Marcel Dekker, New York, 1987, p 99.
18. Melnick, M: Management of motor manifestations. In Cohen, A, and Weiner, W (eds): The Comprehensive Management of Parkinson's Disease. Demos, New York, 1994, p 39.
19. Corcos, D, et al: Strength in Parkinson's disease: Relationship to rate of force generation and clinical status. Ann Neurol 39:79, 1996.
20. Pedersen, S, and Oberg, B: Dynamic strength in Parkinson's disease: Quantitative measurements following withdrawal of medication. Eur Neurol 33:97, 1993.
21. Stelmach, G, et al: Force production characteristics in Parkinson's disease. Exp Brain Res 76:165, 1989.
22. Milner-Brown, H, et al: Electrical properties of motor units in parkinsonism and a possible relationship

with bradykinesia. J Neurol Neurosurg Psychiatry 42:35, 1979.

23. Dengler R, et al: Behavior of motor units in parkinsonism. Adv Neurol 53:167, 1990.

24. Bennett, K, et al: A kinematic study of the reach to group movement in a study with hemi-Parkinson's disease. Neuropsychologia 31:713, 1993.

25. Yanagawa, S, et al: Muscular weakness in Parkinson's disease. Adv Neurol 53:259, 1990.

26. Pederson, S, et al: Gait analysis, isokinetic muscle strength measurement in patients with Parkinson's disease. Scand J Rehabil Med 29:67, 1997.

27. Cohen, A: Tremors and the Parkinson Patients. Parkinson Report. National Parkinson Foundation, Miami, 1991.

28. Bridgewater, K, and Sharpe, M: Trunk muscle performance in early Parkinson's disease. Phys Ther 78:566, 1998.

29. Smithson, F, et al: Performance on clinical tests of balance in Parkinson's disease. Phys Ther 78:577, 1998.

30. Koller, W, et al: Falls and Parkinson's disease. Clin Neuropharmacol 12:98, 1989.

31. Paulson, G, et al: Avoiding mental changes and falls in older Parkinson's patients. Geriatrics 41:59, 1986.

32. Horak, F, et al: Postural instability in Parkinson's disease: Motor coordination and sensory organization. Neurology Report 12:54, 1988.

33. Traub, M, et al: Anticipatory postural reflexes in Parkinson disease and other akinetic-rigid syndromes and in cerebellar ataxia. Brain 103:393, 1980.

34. Rogers, M: Disorders of posture, balance, and gait in Parkinson's disease. In Studenski, S (ed): Clinics in Geriatric Medicine. Gait and Balance Disorders 12:825, 1996.

35. Maeshima, S, et al: Visuospatial impairment and activities of daily living in patients with Parkinson's disease. Am J Phys Med Rehabil 76:383, 1997.

36. Rogers, M, and Chan, C: Motor planning is impaired in Parkinson's disease. Brain Res 438:271, 1988.

37. Marsden, CD: "On-off phenomena" in Parkinson's disease. In Rinne, UK, et al (eds): Parkinson's Disease: Current Progress, Problems and Management. Elsevier/North-Holland Biomedical Press, New York, 1980.

38. Murray, P, et al: Walking patterns of men with Parkinsonism. Am J Phys Med 57:278, 1978.

39. Berger, J: Impaired swallowing and excessive drooling in Parkinson's disease. Parkinson Report. National Parkinson Foundation, Miami, 1985, p 1.

40. Tanner, C, et al: ANS disorders. In Koller, W (ed): Handbook of Parkinson's Disease. Marcel Dekker, New York, 1987, p 145.

41. Parris, R: Swallowing Dysfunction. In Cohen, A, and Weiner, W (eds): The Comprehensive Management of Parkinson's Disease. Demos, New York, 1994, p 89.

42. Robbins, J, et al: Swallowing and speech production in Parkinson's disease. Ann Neurol 19:282, 1986.

43. DePippo, K: Communication dysfunction. In Cohen, A, and Weiner, W (eds): The Comprehensive Management of Parkinson's Disease. Demos, New York, 1994, p 75.

44. Weiner, W: Non-motor Symptoms in Parkinson's Disease. Parkinson Report. National Parkinson Foundation, Miami, 1990.

45. Koller, W: Sensory Symptoms in Parkinson's Disease. Parkinson Report. National Parkinson Foundation, Miami, 1985.

46. Mayeux, R: Behavioral and cognitive dysfunction. In Cohen, A, and Weiner, W (eds): The Comprehensive Management of Parkinson's disease. Demos, New York, 1994, p 119.

47. Levin, B, and Reisman, S: The Psychological Aspects of Parkinson's Disease. Parkinson Report. National Parkinson Foundation, Miami, 1989.

48. Hovestadt, A, et al: Pulmonary function in Parkinson's disease. J Neurol Neurosurg Psychiatry 52:329, 1989.

49. Vinchen, W, et al: Involvement of upper-airway muscles in extrapyramidal disorders. N Engl J Med 311:438, 1984.

50. Sabate, M, et al: Obstructive and restrictive pulmonary dysfunction increases disability in Parkinson disease. Arch Phys Med Rehabil 77:29, 1996.

51. Canning, C, et al: Parkinson's disease: An investigation of exercise capacity, respiratory function, and gait. Arch Phys Med Rehabil 78:199, 1997.

52. Protas, E, et al: Cardiovascular and metabolic responses to upper- and lower-extremity exercise in men with idiopathic Parkinson's disease. Phys Ther 76:34, 1996.

53. Saltin, B, and Landin, S: Work capacity, muscle strength, and SDH activity in both legs of hemiparetic patients and patients with Parkinson's disease. Scand J Clin Lab Invest 35:531, 1975.

54. Carter, J, et al: The effect of exercise on levodopa absorption. Neurology 42:2042, 1992.

55. Tetraud, J: Preclinical detection of motor and nonmotor manifestations of Parkinson's disease. Geriatrics 46:43, 1991.

56. Hoehn, M, and Yahr, M: Parkinsonism: Onset, progression and mortality. Neurology 17:427, 1967.

57. Golbe, L, and Sage, J: Medical Treatment of Parkinson's disease. In Kurlan, R: Treatment of Movement Disorders. Lippincott, Philadelphia, 1995, p 1.

58. Ward, C: Does selegiline delay progression of Parkinson's disease? A critical re-evaluation of the DATATOP study. J Neurol Neurosurg Psychiatry 57:217, 1994.

59. Wasielewski, P, and Koller, W: Quality of life and Parkinson's disease: The CR FIRST Study. J Neurol 245(suppl 1):S28, 1998.

60. Lewitt, P: New options for treatment of Parkinson's disease. Bailliere's Clinical Neurology 6:109, 1997.

61. Kuntzer, T: Treatment of Parkinson's disease. Eur Neurol 36:396, 1996.

62. Cutson, T, et al: Pharmacological and nonpharmacological interventions in the treatment of Parkinson's disease. Phys Ther 75:363, 1995.

63. Mantero-Atienza, E, et al: Nutritional Considerations of Parkinson's disease. National Parkinson Foundation, Miami, 1990.

64. National Parkinson Foundation: The Parkinson Handbook. National Parkinson Foundation, Miami, 1990.

65. Burns, B, and Carr-Davis, E: Nutritional management. In Cohen, A, and Weiner, W (eds): The Comprehensive Management of Parkinson's Disease. Demos, New York, 1994, p 103.

66. Cooper, I, et al: Bilateral parkinsonism: Neurosurgical rehabilitation. J Am Geriatr Soc 16:11, 1968.

67. Pollak, P, et al: New surgical treatment strategies. Eur Neurol 36:396, 1996.

68. Favre, J, et al: Pallidotomy: A survey of current practice in North America. Neurosurgery 39:883, 1996.

69. Iacono, R, et al: The results, indications, and physiology of posteroventral pallidotomy for patients with Parkinson's disease. Neurosurgery 36:1118, 1995.

70. Ondo, W, et al: Assessment of motor function after stereotactic pallidotomy. Neurology 50:266, 1998.

71. Hauser, R, et al: Surgical therapies for Parkinson's disease. In Kurlan, R: Treatment of Movement Disorders. Lippincott, Philadelphia, 1995, p 57.

72. Hariz, G, et al: Assessment of ability/disability in patients treated with chronic thalamic stimulation for tremor. Mov Disord 13:78, 1998.

73. Zurn, A, et al: Symptomatic cell therapies: Cells as biological minipumps. Eur Neurol 36:396, 1996.

74. Schenkman, M, et al: Reliability of impairment and physical performance measures for persons with Parkinson's disease. Phys Ther 77:19, 1997.

75. Folstein, M, et al: Mini-Mental Status: A practical method for grading the cognitive state of patients for the clinician. J Psychiatr Res 12:189, 1975.

76. Yesavage, J, and Brink, T: Development and validation of a geriatric depression screening scale: A preliminary report. J Psychiatr Res 17:41, 1983.

77. Gallagher, D: The Beck Depression Inventory and older adults review of its development and utility. In Brink, T (ed): Clinical Gerontology: A Guide to Assessment and Intervention. Haworth Press, New York, 1986, p 149.

78. Melzack, R: The McGill Pain Questionnaire: Major properties and scoring methods. Pain 1:277, 1975.

79. Bridgewater, K, and Sharpe, M: Trunk muscle performance in early Parkinson's disease. Phys Ther 78:566, 1998.

80. Bohannon, R: Documentation of tremor in patients with central nervous system lesions. Phys Ther 66:229, 1986.

81. Dengler, R, et al: Behavior of motor units in parkinsonism. Adv Neurol 53:167, 1990.

82. Smithson, F, et al: Performance on clinical tests of balance in Parkinson's disease. Phys Ther 78:577, 1998.

83. Shumway-Cook, A, and Horak, F: Assessing the influence of sensory interaction on balance. Phys Ther 66:1548, 1986.

84. Goldie, et al: Force platform measures for evaluating postural control: Reliability and validity. Arch Phys Med Rehabil 70:510, 1989.

85. Duncan, P, et al: Functional reach: A new clinical measure of balance. J Gerontol 45:M192, 1990.

86. Berg, K, et al: Measuring balance in the elderly: Preliminary development of an instrument. Physiotherapy Canada 41:304, 1989.

87. Tinetti, M: Performance-oriented assessment of mobility problems in elderly patients. J Am Geriatr Soc 34:119, 1986.

88. Podsiadlo, D, and Richardson, S: The timed "up and go": A test of basic functional mobility for frail elderly patients. J Am Geriatr Soc 39:142, 1991.

89. Deutsch, J: Speech breathing and Parkinson's disease: Abstract and commentary. Neurology Report 18:43, 1994.

90. Borg, G: Psychophysical bases of perceived exertion. Med Sci Sports Exerc 14:377, 1982.

91. Guyatt, G, et al: The 6-minute walk: A new measure of exercise capacity in patients with chronic heart failure. Can Med Assoc J 32:919, 1985.

92. Weiner, D, et al: Does functional reach improve with rehabilitation? Arch Phys Med Rehabil 74:796, 1993.

93. Schenkman, M, and Butler, R: A model for multisystem evaluation treatment of individuals with Parkinson's disease. Phys Ther 69:932, 1989.

94. Guide for the Uniform Data Set for Medical Rehabilitation including the FIM instrument, Version 5.0 Buffalo: State University of New York at Buffalo, 1996.

95. Katz, S, et al: Studies of illness in the aged, The Index of ADL: A standardized measure of biological and psychological function. JAMA 185:914, 1963.

96. Dittmar, S, and Gresham, G: Functional Assessment and Outcome Measures for the Rehabilitation Professional. Aspen, Gaithersburg, MD, 1997.

97. Kurtin, P, et al: Patient-based health status measures in outpatient dialysis: Early experiences in developing an outcomes assessment program. Med Care 30(suppl 5):136, 1992.

98. McHorney, C, et al: The MOS 36-Item Short-Form Health Survey (SF-36). II. Psychometric and chemical and clinical tests of validity in measuring physical and mental health constructs. Med Care 31:247, 1993.

99. Gilson, B, et al. The Sickness Impact Profile: Development of an outcome measure of health care. Am J Public Health 65:1304, 1975.

100. Fahn, S, et al: Unified Parkinson's Disease Rating Scale. In: Fahn, S, et al (eds): Recent Developments in Parkinson's Disease, vol 2. Macmillan Health Care Information, Florham Park, NJ, 1987.

101. Petro, V, et al: The development and validation of a short measure of functioning and well being for individuals with Parkinson's disease. Qual Life Res 4:241, 1995.

102. Jenkinson, C, et al: Self-reported functioning and well-being in patients with Parkinson's disease: Comparison of the Short-form Health Survey (SF-36) and the Parkinson's Disease Questionnaire (PDQ-39). Age Ageing 24:505, 1995.

103. Fitzpatrick, R, et al: Health-related quality of life in Parkinson's disease: A study of outpatient clinic attenders. Mov Disord 12:916, 1997.

104. American Physical Therapy Association: Guide to Physical Therapist Practice. APTA, Alexandria, VA, 1999.

105. Tyler, W: History of Parkinson's Disease. In Koller, W (ed): Handbook of Parkinson's Disease. Marcel Dekker, New York, 1987.

106. Pederson, D: The soothing effects of rocking as determined by the direction and frequency of movement. Can J Behav Sci 7:237, 1975.

107. Peterson, B, et al: Changes in response of medial pontomedullary reticular neurons during repetitive cutaneous, vestibular, cortical and fectal stimulation. J Neurophysiol 39:564, 1976.

108. Schenkman, M, et al: Management of individuals with Parkinson's disease: Rationale and case studies. Phys Ther 69:944, 1989.

109. Schenkman, M: Physical therapy intervention for the ambulatory patient. In Turnbull, G (ed): Physical Therapy Management of Parkinson's Disease. Churchill Livingstone, New York, 1992, p 137.

110. Voss, D, et al: Proprioceptive Neuromuscular Facilitation, ed 3. Harper & Row, New York, 1985.

111. Benson, H: The Relaxation Response. Avon, New York, 1975.

112. Jacobson, E: Progressive Relaxation. University of Chicago Press, Chicago, 1938.

113. Vishnudenananda, S: The Complete Illustrated Book of Yoga. Pocket Books, New York, 1972.

114. Feldenkrais, M: Awareness Through Movement: Health Exercises for Personal Growth. Harper & Row, New York, 1972.

115. Kaltenborn, F: Mobilization of the Extremity Joints: Examination and Basic Treatment Techniques. Olaf Norlis Bokhandel, Oslo, 1989.

116. Kisner, C, and Colby, L: Therapeutic Exercise Foundations and Techniques, ed 3. FA Davis, 1996.

117. O'Sullivan, S, and Schmitz, T: Physical Rehabilitation Laboratory Manual. FA Davis, Philadelphia, 1999.

118. Glendinning, D: A rationale for strength training in patients with Parkinson's disease. Neurology Report 21:132, 1997.

119. Ory, M, et al: Frailty and injuries in later life: The FICSIT trials. J Am Geriatr Soc 41:283, 1993.

120. Fiatarone, M, et al: High-intensity strength training in nonagenarians. JAMA 263:3029, 1990.

121. Judge, J, et al: Effects of resistive and balance exercises on isokinetic strength in older persons. J Am Geriatr Soc 42:937, 1994.

122. Tinnetti, M, et al: A multifactorial intervention to reduce the risk of falling among elderly people living in the community. N Engl J Med 331:821, 1994.

123. Wolfson, L, et al: Balance and strength training in older adults: Intervention gains and Tai Chi maintenance. J Am Geriatr Soc 44:498, 1996.

124. Wall, J, and Turnball, G: The kinematics of gait. In Turnball, G: Physical Therapy Management of Parkinson's disease. Churchill Livingstone, New York, 1992, p 49.

125. Dunne, J, et al: Parkinsonism: Upturned walking stick as an aid to locomotion. Arch Phys Med Rehabil 68:380, 1987.

126. Dietz, M, et al: Evaluation of a modified inverted walking stick as a treatment for Parkinsonian freezing episodes. Mov Disord 5:243, 1990.

127. Bagely, S, et al: The effect of visual cues on the gait of independently mobile Parkinson's patients. Physiotherapy 77:415, 1991.

128. Eni, G: Gait improvements in parkinsonism: The use of rhythmic music. Int J Res 11:272, 1988.

129. Thaut, M, et al: Rhythmic auditive stimulation in gait training for Parkinson's disease patients. Mov Disord 11:193, 1996.

130. Platz, T, et al: Training improves the speed of aimed movements in Parkinson's disease. Brain 121:505, 1998.

131. Enzensberger, W, and Fischer, P: Metronome in Parkinson's disease. Lancet 347:1337, 1996.

132. Harrington, D, et al: Procedural memory in Parkinson's disease: Impaired motor but not visuoperceptual learning. J Clin Exp Neuropsychol 12:323, 1990.

133. Jackson, G, et al: Serial reaction time learning and Parkinson's disease: Evidence for a procedural learning deficit. Neuropsychologia 33:577, 1995.

134. Soliveri, P, et al: Learning manual pursuit tracking skills in patients with Parkinson's disease. Brain 120:1325, 1997.

135. Brown, R, and Marsden, C: Dual task performance and processing resources in normal subjects and patients with Parkinson's disease. Brain 114:215, 1991.

136. Nieuwboer, A, et al: Is using a cue the clue to the treatment of freezing in Parkinson's disease. Physiother Res Int 2:125, 1997.

137. Jahanshahi, M, et al: Self-initiated versus externally trig-

gered movements. 1. An investigation using measurement of regional cerebral blood flow with PET and movement-related potentials in normal and Parkinson's disease subjects. Brain 118:913, 1995.

138. Ferrandez, A, and Blin, O: A comparison between the effect of intentional modulations and the action of L-dopa on gait in Parkinson's disease. Behavioral Brain Research 45:177, 1991.

139. Schenkman, M: Invited commentary to: Temporal stability of gait in Parkinson's disease. Phys Ther 76:763, 1996.

140. Tzelepis, G, et al: Respiratory muscle dysfunction in Parkinson's disease. Am Rev Respir Dis 138:266, 1988.

141. Koseoglu, F, et al: The effects of a pulmonary rehabilitation program on pulmonary function tests and exercise tolerance in patients with Parkinson's disease. Funct Neurol 12:319, 1997.

142. American College of Sports Medicine: ACSM's Guidelines for Exercise Testing and Prescription, ed 5. Baltimore, Williams & Wilkins, 1995.

143. Wroe, M, and Greer, M: Parkinson's disease and physical therapy management. Phys Ther 53:631, 1973.

144. Pedersen, S, et al: Group training in parkinsonism: Quantitative measurements of treatment. Scand J Rehabil Med 22:207, 1990.

145. Hurwitz, A: The benefit of a home exercise regimen for ambulatory Parkinson's disease patients. J Neurosci Nurs 21:180, 1989.

146. Davis, J: Team management of Parkinson's disease. Am J Occup Ther 31:300, 1977.

147. Feldman, R, et al: Psychosocial factors in the treatment of Parkinson's disease: A contextual approach. In Cohen, A, and Weiner, W (eds): The Comprehensive Management of Parkinson's Disease. Demos, New York, 1994, p 193.

148. Abuli, S, et al: Parkinson's disease symptoms: Patient's perceptions. J Adv Nurs 25:54, 1997.

149. Comella, C, et al: Physical therapy and Parkinson's disease: A controlled clinical trial. Neurology 44:376, 1994.

SUPPLEMENTAL READINGS

Cohen, A, and Weiner, W (eds): The Comprehensive Management of Parkinson's Disease. Demos, New York, 1994.

Huber, S, and Cummings J (eds): Parkinson's Disease: Neurobehavioral Aspects. Oxford University Press, New York, 1992.

Koller, WC (ed): Handbook of Parkinson's Disease. Marcel Dekker, New York, 1987.

Jankovic, J, and Tolosa, E (eds): Parkinson's Disease and Movement Disorders. Urban and Schwarzenberg, Baltimore, 1993.

Turnbull, G (ed): Physical Therapy Management of Parkinson's Disease. Churchill Livingstone, New York, 1992.

GLOSSARY

Akathisia (acathisia): Extreme motor restlessness.

Akinesia: Inability to initiate or execute movement.

Anticholinergic agents: Drugs used to block excessive cholinergic activity in patients with PD. Commonly used drugs include Artane, Cogentin, or Akineton.

Basal ganglia (BG): A collection of interconnected gray matter nuclear masses deep within the brain; located beneath the cerebral cortex and just lateral to the dorsal thalamus; composed of the caudate nucleus and putamen (collectively termed the striatum) plus the globus pallidus, subthalamic nucleus, and the substantia nigra.

Bradykinesia: Extreme slowness and difficulty maintaining movement.

Bradyphrenia: A disorder of intellectual function characterized by a slowing of thought processes with lack of concentration and attention.

Deep brain stimulation (DBS): The implantation of electrodes in the brain (VIN of the thalamus) where they block nerve signals that cause symptoms; the pacemaker is implanted within the chest.

Dopamine: An inhibitory neurotransmitter secreted by neurons that are located in the substantia nigra and terminate in the striate region of the basal ganglia.

Dyskinesias: Involuntary movements; often associated with long-term use of L-dopa therapy.

Dysphagia: Inability to swallow or difficulty in swallowing.

Dysthymic disorder: Variability in dysphoric mood or atypical depression characterized by intermittent episodes of severe anxiety.

End-of-dose deterioration (wearing off): A worsening of symptoms during the expected time-frame of medication effectiveness; seen with long-term use of L-dopa therapy.

Festinating gait: Abnormal gait characterized by an involuntary progressive increase in the speed with a shortening of stride.

    Propulsive gait: A festinating gait that has a forward accelerating quality.

    Retropulsive gait: A festinating gait that has a backward accelerating quality.

Freezing: A sudden episode of immobility or block in movement.

Functional maintenance program: A rehabilitation program designed to manage the effects of progressive disease; includes strategies to prevent or slow decline of function, and promote regular exercise, good health, and self-management skills.

Hoehn-Yahr Classification of Disability Scale: A scale used to classify the stage and severity of PD.

Hypokinesia: Movements that are reduced in speed, amplitude, and range.

Hypokinetic dysarthria: Difficult and defective speech characterized by decreased voice volume, monotone/monopitch speech, imprecise or distorted articulation, and uncontrolled speech rate.

Kyphosis: An exaggeration or angulation of the posterior curve of the spine; usually found in the dorsal spine.

Levodopa (L-dopa): A drug used in the treatment of PD to raise the level of striatal dopamine in the basal ganglia; the mainstay of therapy for PD.

Masked face: Masklike expression with infrequent blinking and lack of facial expression.

Micrographia: An abnormally small handwriting that is difficult to read.

Movement time: The time it takes to complete a movement or activity.

Mutism: Condition of being unable to speak or speaking only in whispers.

On-off phenomenon: Fluctuations in motor performance and response; seen with long-term use of L-dopa therapy.

Parkinsonism: Refers to a group of disorders that produce abnormalities of basal ganglia function, with PD or idiopathic parkinsonism being the most common.

Postural stress syndrome: Discomfort and stress associated with lack of movement, muscle rigidity, faulty posture, or ligamentous strain.

Postural tremor: Oscillation of a body part (usually proximal segments) that occurs when a limb is maintained against gravity.

Reaction time (RT): The interval between the presentation of a stimulus and the start of movement.

Restorative rehabilitation: Rehabilitation that is focused on the improvement of impairments and functional limitations using remedial and compensatory training techniques.

Rigidity: Muscle stiffness or resistance to passive motion that is not velocity dependent; sustained contraction of muscle resulting in an inability to bend or be bent.

Cogwheel rigidity: A jerky, ratchetlike resistance to passive movement as muscles alternately tense and relax.

Leadpipe rigidity: A constant, uniform resistance to passive movement, with no fluctuations.

Scoliosis: A lateral curvature of the spine.

Sialorrhea: Excessive drooling.

Stereotaxic surgery: Surgical lesioning of the brain.

Pallidotomy: A destructive lesion is produced in the BG, the globus pallidus internus (Gpi).

Thalamotomy: A destructive lesion is produced within the thalamus, the ventral intermediate nucleus (VIN).

Transplantation: The surgical transplantation of cells capable of delivering dopamine into the striatum of patients with advanced PD; grafts may involve fetal cells or the patient's own adrenal medullary cells; an experimental procedure not in widespread use.

Tremor: An involuntary oscillation of a body part occurring at a slow frequency of about 4 to 7 oscillations per second; in PD typically present at rest, resting tremor.

APPENDIX A

Unified Rating Scale for Parkinsonism Version 3.0: February 1987*

I. Mentation, behavior and mood
  1. *Intellectual impairments:*
    0 = None.
    1 = Mild. Consistent forgetfulness with partial recollection of events and no other difficulties.
    2 = Moderate memory loss, with disorientation and moderate difficulty handling complex problems. Mild but definite impairment of function at home with need of occasional prompting.
    3 = Severe memory loss with disorientation for time and often to place. Severe impairment in handling problems.
    4 = Severe memory loss with orientation preserved to person only. Unable to make judgments or solve problems. Requires much help with personal care. Cannot be left alone at all.
  2. *Thought disorder* (due to dementia or drug intoxication):
    0 = None.
    1 = Vivid dreaming.
    2 = "Benign" hallucinations with insight retained.
    3 = Occasional to frequent hallucinations or delusions; without insight; could interfere with daily activities.
    4 = Persistent hallucinations, delusions, or florid psychosis. Not able to care for self.
  3. *Depression:*
    0 = Not present.
    1 = Periods of sadness or guilt greater than normal, never sustained for days or weeks.
    2 = Sustained depression (1 week or more).
    3 = Sustained depression with vegetative symptoms (insomnia, anorexia, weight loss, loss of interest).
    4 = Sustained depression with vegetative symptoms and suicidal thoughts or intent.
  4 *Motivation/initiative:*
    0 = Normal.
    1 = Less assertive than usual; more passive.
    2 = Loss in initiative or disinterest in elective (nonroutine) activities.
    3 = Loss of initiative or disinterest in day-to-day (routine) activities.
    4 = Withdrawn, complete loss of motivation.

II. Activities of daily living (determine for "on/off")
  5. *Speech:*
    0 = Normal.
    1 = Mildly affected. No difficulty being understood.
    2 = Moderately affected. Sometimes asked to repeat statements.
    3 = Severely affected. Sometimes asked to repeat statements.
    4 = Unintelligible most of the time.
  6. *Salivation:*
    0 = Normal.
    1 = Slight but definite excess of saliva in mouth; may have nighttime drooling.
    2 = Moderately excessive saliva; may have minimal drooling.
    3 = Marked excess of saliva with some drooling.
    4 = Marked drooling, requires constant tissue or handkerchief.
  7. *Swallowing:*
    0 = Normal.
    1 = Rare choking.
    2 = Occasional choking.
    3 = Requires soft food.
    4 = Requires nasogastric tube or gastrotomy feeding.
  8. *Handwriting:*
    0 = Normal.
    1 = Slightly slow or small.
    2 = Moderately slow or small; all words are legible.
    3 = Severely affected; not all words are legible.
    4 = The majority of words are not legible.
  9. *Cutting food and handling utensils:*
    0 = Normal.
    1 = Somewhat slow and clumsy, but no help needed.
    2 = Can cut most foods, although clumsy and slow; some help needed.
    3 = Food must be cut by someone, but can still feed slowly.
    4 = Needs to be fed.
  10. *Dressing:*
    0 = Normal.
    1 = Somewhat slow, but no help needed.
    2 = Occasional assistance with buttoning, or with getting arms in sleeves.
    3 = Considerable help required, but can do some things alone.
    4 = Helpless.
  11. *Hygiene:*
    0 = Normal.
    1 = Somewhat slow, but no help needed.
    2 = Needs help to shower or bathe; or very slow in hygienic care.
    3 = Requires assistance for washing, brushing teeth, combing hair, going to bathroom.
    4 = Foley catheter or other mechanical aids.

12. *Turning in bed and adjusting bed clothes:*
0 = Normal.
1 = Somewhat slow and clumsy, but no help needed.
2 = Can turn alone or adjust sheets, but with great difficulty.
3 = Can initiate, but not turn or adjust sheets alone.
4 = Helpless.

13. *Falling (unrelated to freezing):*
0 = None.
1 = Rare falling.
2 = Occasionally falls, less than once per day.
3 = Falls on average of once daily.
4 = Falls more than once daily.

14. *Freezing when walking:*
0 = None.
1 = Rare freezing when walking; may have start-hesitation.
2 = Occasional freezing when walking.
3 = Frequent freezing. Occasionally falls from freezing.
4 = Frequent falls from freezing.

15. *Walking:*
0 = Normal.
1 = Mild difficulty; may not swing arms or may tend to drag leg.
2 = Moderate difficulty, but requires little or no assistance.
3 = Severe disturbance of walking, requiring assistance.
4 = Cannot walk at all, even with assistance.

16. *Tremor:*
0 = Absent.
1 = Slight and infrequently present.
2 = Moderate; bothersome to patient.
3 = Severe; interferes with many activities.
4 = Marked; interferes with most activities.

17. *Sensory complaints related to parkinsonism:*
0 = None.
1 = Occasionally has numbness, tingling, or mild aching.
2 = Frequently has numbness, tingling, or aching; not distressing.
3 = Frequent painful sensations.
4 = Excruciating pain.

III. Motor examination

18. *Speech:*
0 = Normal.
1 = Slight loss of expression, diction, and/or volume.
2 = Monotone, slurred but understandable; moderately impaired.
3 = Marked impairment, difficult to understand.
4 = Unintelligible.

19. *Facial expression:*
0 = Normal.
1 = Minimal hypomimia, could be normal "poker face."
2 = Slight but definitely abnormal diminution of facial expression.
3 = Moderate hypomimia; lips parted some of the time.
4 = Masked or fixed facies with severe or complete loss of facial expression; lips parted ¼ in or more.

20. *Tremor at rest:*
0 = Absent.
1 = Slight and infrequently present.
2 = Mild in amplitude and persistent; or moderate in amplitude, but only intermittently present.
3 = Moderate in amplitude and present most of the time.
4 = Marked in amplitude and present most of the time.

21. *Action or postural tremor of hands:*
0 = Absent.
1 = Slight; present with action.
2 = Moderate in amplitude, present with action.
3 = Moderate in amplitude with posture holding as well as action.
4 = Marked in amplitude; interferes with feeding.

22. *Rigidity* (judged on passive movement of major joints with patient relaxed in sitting position; cogwheeling to be ignored):
0 = Absent.
1 = Slight or detectable only when activated by mirror or other movements.
2 = Mild to moderate.
3 = Marked; but full range of motion easily achieved.
4 = Severe; range of motion achieved with difficulty.

23. *Finger taps* (patient taps thumb with index finger in rapid succession with widest amplitude possible, each hand separately):
0 = Normal.
1 = Mild slowing and/or reduction in amplitude.
2 = Moderately impaired; definite and early fatiguing; may have occasional arrests in movement.
3 = Severely impaired; frequent hesitation in initiating movements or arrests in ongoing movement.
4 = Can barely perform the task.

24. *Hand movement* (patient opens and closes hands in rapid succession with widest amplitude possible, each hand separately):
0 = Normal.
1 = Mild slowing and/or reduction in amplitude.
2 = Moderately impaired; definite and early fatiguing; may have occasional arrests in movement.
3 = Severely impaired; frequent hesitation in initiating movements or arrests in ongoing movement.
4 = Can barely perform the task.

Continued

APPENDIX A *Continued*

25. *Rapid alternating movements of hands* (pronation-supination movements of hands, vertically or horizontally, with as large an amplitude as possible, both hands simultaneously):
    0 = Normal.
    1 = Mild slowing and/or reduction in amplitude.
    2 = Moderately impaired; definite and early fatiguing; may have occasional arrests in movement.
    3 = Severely impaired; frequent hesitation in initiating movements or arrests in ongoing movement.
    4 = Can barely perform the task.

26. *Leg agility* (patient taps heel on ground in rapid succession, picking up entire leg; amplitude should be about 3 inches):
    0 = Normal.
    1 = Mild slowing and/or reduction in amplitude.
    2 = Moderately impaired; definite and early fatiguing; may have occasional arrests in movement.
    3 = Severely impaired; frequent hesitation in initiating movements or arrests in ongoing movement.
    4 = Can barely perform the task.

27. *Arising from chair* (patient attempts to arise from a straight-backed wood or metal chair with arms folded across chest).
    0 = Normal.
    1 = Slow; or may need more than one attempt.
    2 = Pushes self up from arms of seat.
    3 = Tends to fall back and may have to try more than one time, but can get up without help.
    4 = Unable to arise without help.

28. *Posture:*
    0 = Normal erect.
    1 = Not quite erect, slightly stooped posture; could be normal for older person.
    2 = Moderately stopped posture, definitely abnormal; can be slightly leaning to one side.
    3 = Severely stooped posture with kyphosis; can be moderately leaning to one side.
    4 = Marked flexion with extreme abnormality of posture.

29. *Gait:*
    0 = Normal.
    1 = Walks slowly, may shuffle with short steps, but no festination or propulsion.
    2 = Walks with difficulty, but requires little or no assistance; may have some festination, short steps, or propulsion.
    3 = Severe disturbance of gait, requiring assistance.
    4 = Cannot walk at all, even with assistance.

30. *Postural stability* (response to sudden posterior displacement produced by pull on shoulders while patient is erect with eyes open and feet slightly apart; patient is prepared):
    0 = Normal.
    1 = Retropulsion, but recovers unaided.
    2 = Absence of postural response; would fall if not caught by examiner.
    3 = Very unstable, tends to lose balance spontaneously.
    4 = Unable to stand without assistance.

31. *Body bradykinesia and hypokinesia* (combining slowness, hesitancy, decreased arm-swing, small amplitude, and poverty of movement in general):
    0 = None.
    1 = Minimal slowness, giving movement a deliberate character; could be normal for some persons. Possibly reduced amplitude.
    2 = Mild degree of slowness and poverty of movement that is definitely abnormal. Alternatively, some reduced amplitude.
    3 = Moderate slowness, poverty, or small amplitude of movement.
    4 = Marked slowness, poverty, or small amplitude of movement.

IV. Complications of therapy (in the past week)
    A. Dyskinesias
    32. *Duration: What proportion of the waking day are dyskinesias present?* (historical information)
        0 = None
        1 = 1–25% of day.
        2 = 25–50% of day.
        3 = 51–75% of day.
        4 = 76–100% of day.
    33. *Disability: How disabling are the dyskinesias?* (historical information; may be modified by office examination)
        0 = Not disabling.
        1 = Mildly disabling.
        2 = Moderately disabling.
        3 = Severely disabling.
        4 = Completely disabled.
    34. *Painful dyskinesia: how painful are the dyskinesias?*
        0 = No painful dyskinesias.
        1 = Slight.
        2 = Moderate.
        3 = Severe.
        4 = Marked.
    35. *Presence of early morning dystonia* (Historical information):
        0 = No
        1 = Yes
    B. Clinical fluctuations
    36. *Are any "off" periods predictable as to timing after a dose of medication?*
        0 = No
        1 = Yes

37. *Are any "off" periods unpredictable as to timing after a dose of medications?*
    0 = No
    1 = Yes
38. *Do any of the "off" periods come on suddenly, for example, over a few seconds?*
    0 = No
    1 = Yes
39. *What proportion of the waking day is the patient "off" on average?*
    0 = None
    1 = 1–25% of day.
    2 = 26–50% of day.
    3 = 51–75% of day.
    4 = 76–100% of day.
  C. Other complications
40. *Does the patient have anorexia, nausea, or vomiting?*
    0 = No
    1 = Yes
41. *Does the patient have any sleep disturbances, for example, insomnia or hypersomnolence?*
    0 = No
    1 = Yes
42. *Does the patient have symptomatic orthostasis?*
    0 = No
    1 = Yes
Record the patient's blood pressure, pulse and weight on the scoring form.
V. Modified Hoehn and Yahr staging
Stage 0   = No signs of disease.
Stage 1   = Unilateral disease.
Stage 1.5 = Unilateral plus axial involvement.
Stage 2   = Bilateral disease, without impairment of balance.
Stage 2.5 = Mild bilateral disease, with recovery on pull test.
Stage 3   = Mild to moderate bilateral disease;

some postural instability; physically independent.
Stage 4   = Severe disability; still able to walk or stand unassisted.
Stage 5   = Wheelchair bound or bedridden unless aided.
VI. Schwab and England activities of daily living scale
100%—Completely independent. Able to do all chores without slowness, difficulty, or impairment. Essentially normal. Unaware of any difficulty.
90%—Completely independent. Able to do all chores with some degree of slowness, difficulty, and impairment. Might take twice as long. Beginning to be aware of difficulty.
80%—Completely independent in most chores. Takes twice as long. Conscious of difficulty and slowness.
70%—Not completely independent. More difficulty with some chores. Three to four times as long in some. Must spend a large part of the day with chores.
60%—Some dependency. Can do most chores, but exceedingly slowly and with much effort. Errors; some impossible.
50%—More dependent. Help with half, slower, and so forth. Difficulty with everything.
40%—Very dependent. Can assist with some chores, but does few alone.
30%—With effort, now and then does a few chores alone, or begins alone. Much help needed.
20%—Nothing done alone. Can be a slight help with some chores. Severe invalid.
10%—Totally dependent, helpless. Complete invalid.
0%—Vegetative functions, such as swallowing, bladder and bowel functions, not functioning. Bedridden.

From Stern and Hurtig,[4] pp 36–41, with permission.
*Definitions of 0–4 scale.

APPENDIX B:

Suggested Answers to Case Study Guiding Questions

1. Identify/categorize this patient's problems in terms of:

ANSWER

a. Direct impairments:

Tremor; moderate rigidity: L > R; bradykinesia; akinesia: frequent arrests of movement; postural instability: unsteady balance; decrease proprioception bilaterally both ankles; cognitive changes: mild memory loss; speech changes: mild dysarthria, hypophonia; dysautonomia: increased perspiration

b. Indirect impairments:

Decreased ROM (flexion contractures): both elbows, hips, knees and ankles; decreased strength: generally fair to good; poor ankle dorsiflexors

c. Composite impairments:

Postural abnormalities: flexed, stooped posture
Gait changes: shuffling gait pattern
Decreased endurance: FWC of 6 METs
Depression

d. Functional limitations:

Dependent bed mobility; dependent transfers
Dependent BADLs
Gait instability/frequent falls
Difficulty with communication secondary to dysarthria

2. Identify two outcomes (the remediation of functional limitations and disability) and two goals (remediation of impairments) for this patient.

ANSWER

Outcome: Patient will be independent in bed mobility with minimal cueing within 4 weeks.

Goal: Patient will move supine-to-sidelying on elbows to sitting with minimal assist within 2 weeks.

Goal: Patient will be independent in upper trunk and head rotation movements in sitting with minimal cueing within 2 weeks.

Outcome: Patient will be independent and safe in gait with minimal cueing within 4 weeks.

Goal: Patient will increase ROM in trunk and LE extension both hips and knees by 5 degrees within 3 weeks.

Goal: Patient will stand with shoulders in vertical alignment over hips (no forward lean) with minimal cueing and self-monitoring.

3. Formulate four treatment interventions that could be used at the start of therapy to achieve the stated outcomes and goals. Provide a brief rationale of each.

ANSWER

1. Sidelying, upper and lower trunk rotation progressing to trunk counterrotation using rhythmic initiation.
   Rationale: this is an initial mobility procedure that should help to relax rigidity in the trunk. Assisted movement can be progressed to active movements (self-relaxation).

2. Sitting, upper trunk and head rotation with reaching for an object placed out to the side and slightly behind; verbal cueing and cone stacking to trigger movements.
   Rationale: this is a controlled mobility activity that should assist in relaxing rigidity of the trunk and enhancing movement of the upper trunk; functional carry-over is expected in promoting the upper trunk rotation needed in supine for initial rolling.

3. Standing, corner push-ups; active stretches of anterior shoulder muscles and dorsal spine.
   Rationale: this stretching activity will improve ROM in dorsal spine and anterior shoulders, and enhance postural extension.

4. Standing, modified plantigrade with BUEs extended and weight-bearing in the forward position on a wall, marching in place; marching music will be used to cue the patient's movements.
   Rationale: the modified plantigrade position reduces the risk of falls while the patient practices high stepping movements. BUEs extended and forward on the wall encourages flexion of both shoulders and extension of elbows. The music provides the triggering cues to pace the movements.

4. What strategies would you use to develop self-management skills and promote self-efficacy and quality of life?

ANSWER: Self-management and self-efficacy can be achieved by using strategies that promote mastery of important (meaningful) functional tasks and the environment. These include energy conservation, activity pacing, and time management strategies. Stress reduction techniques (e.g., meditation) are important to enhance coping skills. It is also important to select activities that the patient can master (or almost master) in order to allow the patient to experience success. General health measures and exercises that counteract deconditioning also promote mastery.

Traumatic Brain Injury 24

George D. Fulk
Aaron Geller

LEARNING OBJECTIVES

1. Describe the pathophysiology of traumatic brain injury.
2. Describe the interdisciplinary team concept employed in the rehabilitation of individuals with traumatic brain injury.
3. Identify the different team members involved in the management of the patient with traumatic brain injury and differentiate their respective roles.
4. Describe two clinical rating scales and their usefulness.
5. Describe commonly seen deficits that result from traumatic brain injury.
6. Describe the role of the physical therapist in the different episodes of care of the patient with traumatic brain injury.
7. Explain cognitive considerations required during physical therapy examination and intervention.
8. Identify the components of a physical therapy examination for the patient with traumatic brain injury.
9. Describe treatment interventions available to the physical therapist in working with the patient with traumatic brain injury at the various stages of rehabilitation.
10. Analyze and interpret patient data, formulate realistic goals and outcomes, and develop a plan of care when presented with a clinical case study.

The traumatic brain injury population is among the most challenging of all patient populations that a physical therapist may encounter. Because of the multiple body systems affected by a brain injury and the strong likelihood of secondary impairments, a physical therapist must be proficient in a wide variety of examination and intervention techniques. Owing to behavioral difficulties encountered on the road to recovery, a physical therapist working with this population must also possess strong interpersonal skills, be able to react quickly and effectively to suddenly changing situations, and have keen observation skills. These factors and others can make working with this population challenging and exhausting, both emotionally and physically. However, the rewards of assisting a patient with a severe brain injury return home or to school vastly outweigh the challenges of rehabilitation.

The patient with a brain injury is treated across a wide continuum of care, which includes acute hospitalization, rehabilitation centers, community re-entry programs, outpatient therapy, schools, vocational rehabilitation, and assisted living centers.[1] Because of the wide variety of impairments and complications arising from a brain injury, it is vital that a strong team concept be employed when treating this population. A physical therapist is an important member of this team in any setting. It is crucial that there be open communication between all team members to ensure safe, timely, and consistent treatment. Regardless of the setting you work in, it is important to remember that the patient is the key member of the team.

Traumatic brain injury is a common and devastating occurrence in American society. It is the number one killer of children and young adults. On average, one person is hospitalized with a brain injury for every minute of every day, totaling more than 500,000 such hospitalizations per year. Of those, approximately 70,000 people will develop intellectual, behavioral, and/or physical disabilities that will prevent return to a normal, independent life-style and 2000 people will exist in a **persistent vegetative state (PVS)**. Motor vehicle accidents cause one half of all traumatic brain injuries, with falls accounting for 21 percent, assaults and violence 12 percent, and sports and recreation 10 percent. Men are injured more often than women. The typical patient is between the ages of 15 and 24 years at the time of injury.[2] It is estimated that traumatic brain injuries cost the United States $48.3 billion per year. Fatal brain injuries account for $16.6 billion a year and hospitalizations $31.7 billion a year.[3]

Because there is no "cure" for a brain injury, it is important that healthcare professionals become involved in preventative measures. This may involve community outreach and educating high-risk groups, particularly teenagers. One example is *Think First*, an association that educates students on the devastating effects of a brain injury or spinal cord injury. Students are taught the basics about how the brain and spinal cord work. They are also instructed on preventative measures such as wearing bike helmets and seat belts, the dangers of driving while intoxicated, and the importance of using proper protective equipment during athletics. Perhaps the most effective tool used by the *Think First* program is having brain injury survivors accompany the therapists. They are able to tell the students firsthand about the debilitating effects of a brain injury. Seeing and hearing their stories has a much more profound effect on the students than listening to a lecture on the dangers of drinking and driving.

CLASSIFICATION AND PATHOPHYSIOLOGY

Traumatic brain injuries are classified as *mild, moderate,* or *severe* based on the **Glasgow Coma Scale** (Table 24–1). They may also be classified according to numerous other factors. These include open or closed injury (depending on whether or not the skull is fractured and if there is an open wound);

Table 24–1 GLASGOW COMA SCALE

Activity	Score
EYE OPENING	
Spontaneous	4
To speech	3
To pain	2
No response	1
BEST MOTOR RESPONSE	
Follows motor commands	6
Localizes	5
Withdraws	4
Abnormal flexion	3
Extensor response	2
No response	1
VERBAL RESPONSE	
Oriented	5
Confused conversation	4
Inappropriate words	3
Incomprehensible sounds	2
No response	1

From Jennett and Teasdale,[7] p 78, with permission.

high-velocity or low-velocity impact (depending on whether it resulted from high-speed trauma such as a motor vehicle accident or low-speed trauma such as a blow from a blunt object or a fall from 6 ft or less); or as diffuse or focal. To an experienced clinician, each of these factors provides information that can be used in planning treatment and establishing a prognosis. Given such information, it is possible to make meaningful predictions about outcome. For example, a patient with an open brain injury has a much greater risk of infection than a patient with a closed brain injury. High-velocity injuries are more likely to involve diffuse axonal injury than low-velocity injuries. Furthermore, the location of the brain injury provides a wealth of clues as to what specific deficits are likely to be encountered. For example, nondominant parietal lobe lesions are likely to result in spatial relation problems, frontal lobe damage is likely to produce deficits in executive functioning such as judgement and reasoning, and so forth. Much can be gleaned from information about the patient's injury. However, because traumatic brain injury is often multifocal and the effects are cumulative, it is very difficult even for the most experienced clinician to precisely predict outcome. The following is a discussion of some of the most important factors to consider.

FACTORS THAT INFLUENCE OUTCOME

Three main factors influence the final outcome for individuals with brain injury. They are the *premorbid status* of the patient, the amount of immediate damage to the brain from the impact of the brain injury (the *primary injury*), and the cumulative effect of secondary brain damage produced by systemic and intracranial mechanisms that occur after the initial injury (*secondary injury*).

Premorbid Status

When a brain injury occurs in a person who has already lost a sizeable number of neurons because of previous brain disease or injury, the result of that brain injury is usually much worse than it would have been without prior brain damage. This is true even with a good recovery from the prior insult.[4] Thus, in a patient who has previously experienced a traumatic brain injury, stroke, or encephalitis, a relatively minor brain injury can be very disabling. Similarly, older patients with some preexisting loss of neurons may do poorly after traumatic brain injury. Therefore, when assessing potential for recovery, it is important to establish the pre-injury status of the patient. This can be derived from previous medical records, academic records, job history, and information gathered from the patient's family.

Primary Injury

Depending on the nature, direction, and magnitude of the forces applied to the skull, brain, and body, primary damage to the brain may be of any or all of the following types.[5] **Local brain damage** is localized to the area of the brain that is under the site of impact on the skull. The damage may be in the form of a clot, contusion, or laceration, or a combination of the three. It may be mild, moderate, or severe. More severe damage may result in localizing neurological signs, depending on the location of the injury.

A severe blow to the head may result in brain damage not only directly under the site of impact, but also directly opposite the site of impact. This results from the brain "bouncing" and making contact with the skull at a site opposite from the site of impact. Such injuries are referred to as **coup-contrecoup injuries.**

Polar brain damage occurs when the head is subjected to acceleration and deceleration forces, such as in a head-on collision. The damage results when the brain moves forward inside the skull and then suddenly stops due to impact with the skull. Damage to the tips (poles) and undersurface of the temporal and frontal lobes are most common. Damage to the occipital pole can also occur, but is much less common.

Diffuse axonal injury (DAI) refers to widely scattered shearing of subcortical axons within their myelin sheaths that is not isolated to any one location, but causes a dramatic cumulative effect. DAI may occur in isolation or in association with local or polar damage. It is apparent in subcortical white matter in moderate injuries. With increasing severity, lesions extend downward and inward to include the midbrain and brainstem. With this type of injury, the patient is deeply comatose from the time of injury, usually with abnormal posturing of the extremities and autonomic dysfunction.[2]

Secondary Injury

The energy requirements of the brain are extremely high. Following severe brain injury, numerous conditions conspire to decrease the energy supply, causing secondary injury to the brain. A major pathological process seen with patients with traumatic brain injury is **hypoxic-ischemic injury (HII).** Such an injury may result in infarction of a particular vascular territory in the brain owing to compromise of circulation secondary to shifting brain structures. A more diffuse form of HII, resulting in secondary brain injury, is caused by arterial hypoxemia.[2] The causes of arterial hypoxemia range from obstruction of the airway to myocardial infarction, pericardial effusion, arrhythmia, congestive heart failure, pulmonary embolus, and pneumothorax. These systemic injuries may result in any number of respiratory impairments that deprive the brain of much-needed oxygen. Arterial hypotension, often the result of massive blood loss, may also contribute to HII.

Late-occurring **intracranial hematomas** are another source of secondary brain damage. This complication can transform a seemingly mild injury into a life-threatening situation within hours. Intracranial hematomas are often associated with patients who "talk and die," that is those who are lucid for a period of time after the initial injury but who later lapse into coma and die. This late-appearing loss of consciousness is due to compression of the brain by the expanding hematoma (mass effect). This "lucid interval" occurs in only a portion of patients with traumatic brain injury. Many are in coma from the initial injury and the hematoma may go undetected and untreated, causing an avoidable death. These hematomas are usually classified according to their site **(epidural, subdural, or intracerebral)** and by the time after injury in which they develop: acute within 3 days; subacute; or chronic, more than 2 to 3 weeks.

Because the rigid skull surrounds the brain, swelling or abnormality of brain fluid dynamics often results in increased **intracranial pressure (ICP).** Normal ICP is 5 to 10 mmHg. Even mildly increased ICP is associated with increased morbidity in survivors. Severely increased ICP may result in **herniation** of the brain. Figure 24-1 and Table 24–2 present various types of herniation syndromes and their effects. Other causes of secondary brain damage include intracranial infection, cerebral artery vasospasm, tumors, **obstructive hydrocephalus,** and **post-traumatic epilepsy.** Clearly, the early medical management of patients with traumatic brain injury can have a major impact on the eventual outcome.

Recent research findings indicate that neurochemical changes also contribute to brain damage after trauma. Diffuse axonal injury is accompanied by **autodestructive cellular phenomena** that involve surges in levels of excitatory neurotransmitters.[6] These neurochemical changes set up a cas-

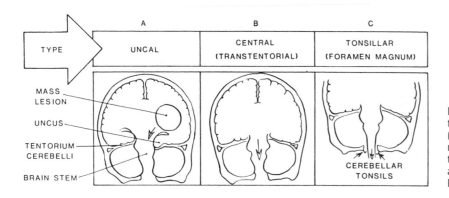

Figure 24-1. Herniations of the brain. (*A*) Herniation of uncus of temporal lobe through tentorial notch. (*B*) Herniation of midbrain and pons through tentorial notch. (*C*) Herniation of medulla and cerebellar tonsils through foramen magnum. (Adapted from Plum, F, et al: The Diagnosis of Stupor and Coma, ed 2. FA Davis, Philadelphia, 1972, with permission.)

cade of intracellular events that impede neuronal function and may go on to destroy neurons. These phenomena render cells extremely sensitive to other insults such as hypoxia. Several treatments to counter these neurochemical changes are currently under investigation. These include the delivery of anticholinergic medication, free radical scavengers, cooling, and hyperbaric oxygen.

COMMONLY ASSOCIATED INJURIES

Because of the high velocity, traumatic nature of most brain injuries, many survivors will present with associated injuries that can be just as devastating as the primary brain injury. Box 24–1 identifies the more predominant associated injuries. These can have a profound impact on the treatment plan for the individual with brain injury. For example, a patient who suffered a moderate to severe brain injury in addition to a spinal cord injury, at any level, will present with unique challenges for the rehabilitation team.

CLINICAL RATING SCALES

Clinical rating scales have been developed in an effort to standardize the description of patients who have sustained traumatic brain injuries and to facilitate research in establishing outcomes. The most commonly used scales are briefly described. Information regarding reliability is provided where it is available.

Glasgow Coma Scale

The Glasgow Coma Scale, developed by Jennett and Teasdale, is used to document level of consciousness and define the severity of injury.[7] It relates consciousness to motor response, verbal response, and eye opening (see Table 24–1). The Glasgow Coma Scale (GCS) has been extensively tested for interrater reliability and shown to be reliable (*r* = 0.92).[8] Patients scoring a total of 8 or less are identified as having coma and severe brain injuries. Patients with moderate brain injuries score from 9 to

Table 24–2 HERNIATIONS OF THE BRAIN

Type	Location	Cause	Anatomic Structures Involved	Clinical Effects
Uncal	Tentorial notch, midbrain	Mass lesion in temporal lobe or middle fossa	Hippocampal gyrus and uncus	
			Oculomotor nerve	
			Cerebral peduncle	Paresis of nerve III
			Midbrain ascending reticular activating system	Hemiparesis Coma
			Posterior cerebral artery	Homonymous hemianopia
Central (transtentorial)	Tentorial notch, midbrain	Mass lesion in frontal, parietal, or occipital lobe	Midbrain and pons	Decerebrate rigidity
		Progression of uncal herniation	Ascending reticular activating system	Coma
Tonsillar (foramen magnum)	Foramen magnum, medulla	Mass lesion in posterior fossa	Cerebellar tonsils	Neck pain and stiffness
		Progression of uncal or transtentorial herniation	Indirect activation pathways	Flaccidity
			Ascending reticular activating system	Coma
			Vasomotor centers	Alteration of pulse, respiration, blood pressure

From Daube, JR, et al: Medical Neurosciences, ed 2. Little, Brown, & Co., Boston, 1986, p 368, with permission.

Box 24–1 INJURIES ASSOCIATED WITH TRAUMATIC BRAIN INJURY

Open wounds
Fractures, open and/or closed
    Skull
    Long bones
    Ribs
Spinal cord injury
Peripheral nerve damage
Internal organ injuries (e.g., collapsed lung)
Soft tissue injury

12, and those with mild brain injuries score from 13 to the maximum of 15 points on the GCS. The GCS and the next rating scale are the most commonly used clinical rating scales.

Ranchos Los Amigos Level of Cognitive Functioning

The **Rancho Los Amigos Level of Cognitive Functioning (LOCF)** is a descriptive scale that outlines a predictable sequence of cognitive and behavioral recovery seen in individuals with traumatic brain injury (Box 24–2).[9] A patient may

plateau at any level. This scale does not address specific cognitive deficits, but is useful for communicating general cognitive and/or behavioral status and using that information for treatment planning. Although this scale is used frequently, no published data are available regarding its reliability.

Rappaport's Disability Rating Scale

Rappaport's Disability Rating Scale (DRS) covers a wide range of functional areas and is used to classify levels of disability ranging from death to no disability (Table 24–3). It is used serially to document patient progress over time. The DRS has demonstrated a high level of interrater reliability ($r = 0.97$).[10]

Glasgow Outcome Scale

The Glasgow Outcome Scale (GOS) has been expanded from its original three categories to eight. The categories are dead, vegetative, and two levels each of severely and moderately disabled and good recovery (Table 24–4). This scale is used primarily for research purposes so that outcome can be quantified. In a reliability study with two raters and 150 patients, agreement was high ($r = 0.95$).[11]

Box 24–2 RANCHO LOS AMIGOS LEVELS OF COGNITIVE FUNCTIONING (LOCF)[a]

I. NO RESPONSE
Patient appears to be in a deep sleep and is completely unresponsive to any stimuli.

II. GENERALIZED RESPONSE
Patient reacts inconsistently and nonpurposefully to stimuli in a nonspecific manner. Responses are limited and often the same regardless of stimulus presented. Responses may be physiological changes, gross body movements, and/or vocalization.

III. LOCALIZED RESPONSE
Patient reacts specifically but inconsistently to stimuli. Responses are directly related to the type of stimulus presented. May follow simple commands such as closing eyes or squeezing hand in an inconsistent, delayed manner.

IV. CONFUSED-AGITATED
Patient is in a heightened state of activity. Behavior is bizarre and nonpurposeful relative to immediate environment. Does not discriminate among persons or objects; is unable to cooperate directly with treatment efforts. Verbalizations frequently are incoherent and/or inappropriate to the environment; confabulation may be present. Gross attention to environment is very brief; selective attention is often nonexistent. Patient lacks short- and long-term recall.

V. CONFUSED-INAPPROPRIATE
Patient is able to respond to simple commands fairly consistently. However, with increased complexity of commands or lack of any external structure, responses are nonpurposeful, random, or fragmented. Demonstrates gross attention to the environment but is highly distractible and lacks ability to focus attention

on a specific task. With structure, may be able to converse on a social automatic level for short periods of time. Verbalization is often inappropriate and confabulatory. Memory is severely impaired; often shows inappropriate use of objects; may perform previously learned tasks with structure but is unable to learn new information.

VI. CONFUSED-APPROPRIATE
Patient shows goal-directed behavior but is dependent on external input or direction. Follows simple directions consistently and shows carryover for relearned tasks such as self-care. Responses may be incorrect due to memory problems, but they are appropriate to the situation. Past memories show more depth and detail than recent memory.

VII. AUTOMATIC-APPROPRIATE
Patient appears appropriate and oriented within the hospital and home settings; goes through daily routine automatically, but frequently robotlike. Patient shows minimal to no confusion and has shallow recall of activities. Shows carryover for new learning but at a decreased rate. With structure is able to initiate social or recreational activities; judgement remains impaired.

VIII. PURPOSEFUL-APPROPRIATE
Patient is able to recall and integrate past and recent events and is aware of and responsive to environment. Shows carryover for new learning and needs no supervision once activities are learned. May continue to show a decreased ability relative to premorbid abilities, abstract reasoning, tolerance for stress, and judgement in emergencies or unusual circumstances.

[a]Condensed form. From Professional Staff Association, Rancho Los Amigos Hospital,[9] pp 87–88, with permission.

Table 24–3 DISABILITY RATING SCALE

Category	Item
Arousability, awareness and responsivity	Eye opening[1]
	Verbalization[2]
	Motor response[3]
Cognitive ability for self-care	Feeding[4]
	Toileting[4]
	Grooming[4]
Dependence on others	Level of functioning[5]
Psychosocial adaptability	"Employability"[6]

[1]Eye Opening		[2]Best Verbal Response		[3]Best Motor Response		[4]Cognitive ability for self-care (Does patient know how and when? Ignore motor disability.)	
Spontaneous	0	Oriented	0	Obeying	0	Complex	0
To speech	1	Confused	1	Localizing	1	Partial	1
To pain	2	Inappropriate	2	Withdrawing	2	Minimal	2
None	3	Incomprehensive	3	Flexing	3	None	3
		None	4	Extending	4		
				None	5		

[5]Level of Functioning		[6]"Employability"		Disability Categories	
				Total DR Score	Level of Disability
Completely independent	0	Not restricted	0	0	None
Independent in special environment	1	Selected jobs	1	1	Mild
Mildly dependent[a]	2	Sheltered workshop	2	2–3	Partial
Moderately dependent[b]	3	Not employable	3	4–6	Moderate
Markedly dependent[c]	4			7–11	Moderately severe
Totally dependent[d]	5			12–16	Severe
				17–21	Extremely severe
				22–24	Vegetative state
				25–29	Extreme vegetative state
				30	Death

Condensed form. From Rappaport,[10] p 119, with permission.
[a]Needs limited assistance (nonresident helper).
[b]Needs moderate assistance (person in home).
[c]Needs assistance with all major activities at all times.
[d]24-hour nursing care required.

Table 24–4 GLASGOW OUTCOME SCALE

Extended Scale		Original Scale	Contracted Scales			
Dead		Dead	Dead			Dead
				Dead or vegetative	Dead or vegetative	
Vegetative		Vegetative				
Degree of disability:			Dependent			
	5	Severely disabled		Severely disabled		
	4					Survivors
	3				Conscious	
	2	Moderately disabled	Independent	Independent		
	1					
	0	Good recovery				
Total Categories	8		5	3		2

From Jennett and Teasdale,[7] p 306, with permission.

DIAGNOSTIC PROCEDURES

To aid in diagnosis and establishing a prognosis, patients with brain injury often receive numerous special tests in addition to the standard neurological examination. Following is a brief description of these tests.

Electroencephalograms and Evoked Potentials

Measures of central nervous system (CNS) activity from electroencephalograms (EEGs) have been made for over 60 years, but advances in computer technologies are revolutionizing the ways in which EEGs are used. EEGs are easily obtained, noninvasive, and inexpensive. They can be repeated as often as needed. Information provided by EEG is both qualitative and quantitative in nature. EEGs are most useful with gray matter injuries. As new ways to quantify the information are developed, the usefulness of EEG increases. A particular form of quantified EEG activity is the *evoked potential* (EP). In EP testing, the EEG signals from subcortical and primary sensory areas of the cortex are averaged in response to repetitive presentations of sensory stimuli. This type of electrophysiological testing has proven very useful in the assessment of sensory function and has been used with some success to predict clinical outcomes from the early stages of moderate to severe brain injury.[12] Virtually all patients with traumatic brain injury present with abnormal EEGs. They are of limited value in determining whether patients should have their anticonvulsant medication adjusted.

Computed Tomography

Introduced in 1973, computed tomography (CT) scanning revolutionized the acute management of traumatic brain injury.[13] In particular, CT scans are successful in identifying hematomas, ventricular enlargement, and atrophy. However, comparisons of CT and MRI confirm that CT is relatively insensitive to many of the lesions present after trauma. Professionals and family members should be warned that a lack of significant abnormalities on CT does not rule out the presence of extensive brain damage. In particular, DAI is virtually undetectable on CT or magnetic resonance imaging (MRI).

Magnetic Resonance Imaging

Introduced in the early 1980s, MRI is more sensitive than CT to lesions after brain injury, particularly to nonhemorrhagic lesions. Patients with normal CT scans may have evidence of abnormality on MRI.

Cerebral Blood Flow Mapping

The measurement of cerebral blood flow (CBF) is used to clarify dynamic relationships between physiology and behavior. Positron emission tomography (PET) is the method of choice for measurement of CBF, but is of limited clinical value owing to the scarcity of PET centers. There are only approximately 60 centers worldwide. PET clearly shows disturbances in cerebral metabolism beyond the structural abnormalities demonstrated by MRI or CT.[14,15] Another type of CBF mapping, called single photon emission computed tomography (SPECT) is available in the routine hospital nuclear medicine department. The major limitation of SPECT, in comparison with PET, is that it measures relative rather than absolute perfusion. This can lead to difficulties in interpreting results. For example, an area of high blood flow may truly be hyperemic, or may actually have normal blood flow that is only relatively high due to generally reduced flow in other regions.[16] In the future, SPECT and PET may be used to document the regional metabolism of specific neurotransmitters and receptors.

MANAGEMENT OF PATIENTS WITH TRAUMATIC BRAIN INJURY

Management of the individual with traumatic brain injury will be discussed in two sections. First, the acute medical management of this population and medications commonly used will be presented. This is followed by rehabilitative management as classified by the Ranchos Los Amigos LOCF. Common impairments associated with brain injury are included.

ACUTE MEDICAL MANAGEMENT

Early medical management focuses on determination of the severity of the injury, preservation of life, and prevention of further damage. Because it is impossible to make a valid assessment of neurological function in a patient who is hypoxemic or shocked, the very first step is to ensure that the patient has an adequate airway, is adequately oxygenated, and has satisfactory arterial blood pressure and peripheral circulation. Level of consciousness is determined using the GCS. Following a brief but thorough neurological examination, the patient usually undergoes radiographic examination of the cervical spine. X-rays must exclude fractures, but they should also be performed with dynamic flexion and extension views to rule out ligamentous instability, which could lead to increased risk of subluxation and subsequent secondary quadriplegia. The patient usually then undergoes more specialized tests, as previously described. ICP is monitored. This can be done via a catheter in the lateral ventricle, a screw in the skull inserted into the subarachnoid space, or a transducer placed directly in the epidural space. If the ICP becomes elevated over a mean value of 25 mmHg, measures are taken to reduce the pressure. Increased ICP limits the perfusion of blood in the brain tissues. This can lead to secondary injury. If the ICP is consistently below 20 mmHg for 24 hours, the monitoring system can be discontinued.[4]

MEDICATIONS

The physical therapist typically spends more time with the patient as compared to the medical doctor. As such, the therapist assumes an advantageous team position to alert the physician regarding a host of varied medical problems that can be treated with medications. This serves to enhance the patient's medical status, which in turn maximizes the patient's ability to participate in therapy sessions. Areas that the therapist might logically provide recommendations include pain management, spasticity, motor restoration, and cognitive issues including level of consciousness, awareness, attention quality including hemispatial neglect, speech, memory, and disinhibited emotional, physical, and sexual behaviors. The physician has a similar responsibility to inform the rehabilitation team when doses are increased or when new medications are started. Because patients with brain injury are often on several medications at one time, all team members typically take an active role in monitoring side effects and determining the impact of the medications.

The first step that must be embraced prior to treating disorders of cognition include identification of medical dyshomeostasis. Hyponatremia, infection, hydrocephalus, and a host of medical sequelae of traumatic brain injury, stroke, or other CNS events may compromise cognition and proceed to endanger the patient's life if untreated. Similarly, a host of cognitively offensive medications should be discontinued or substituted for safer agents. A general rule is that highly lipophilic drugs, which cross the blood-brain barrier, should be substituted for hydrophilic drugs, which poorly penetrate into the brain. For example, both tolterodine (Detrol) and oxybutynin (Ditropan) will relax a spastic bladder, but oxybutynin also crosses into the brain to exert sedating anticholinergic effects. Similarly, the highly lipophilic beta-blocker propranolol (Inderal) controls blood pressure, but also causes mood depression and sedation, unlike atenolol (Trenomin), which is lipophobic and exhibits the same cardioactivity. Because impaired cognition impacts all areas of function, consideration for substitution or discontinuation of cognitively offensive medications must be assessed within the context of the management of the spectrum of rehabilitation conditions. Refer to Appendix A for commonly prescribed medications with comments and side effects for each medication.

Pain

Pain can profoundly impair a patient's ability to participate in therapies. Intruding thoughts of pain may compromise the patient's attention. Spasticity, disinhibited behavior, as well as the spectrum of cognitive dysfunction issues are often exacerbated by pain. Pain management must be initially addressed in a prophylactic manner. In particular, if it is expected that therapy sessions will entail application of noxious stimuli as with stretching contracted tissues, then premedication with ibuprofen or other nonsteroidal anti-inflammatory drugs, or weak narcotics such as codeine or propoxyphene an hour prior to therapies may markedly enhance tolerance and participation.

Prophylaxis for painful constipation may be achieved through the delivery of medications. Lactulose, colace, and fiber compounds such as psyllium (Konsyl) are nonaddictive agents that are safe for long-term use. Stimulants may adversely destroy the intrinsic neural network in the intestines, a particular concern in a young patient with traumatic brain injury who may use the medication for decades, eventually culminating in the need for a colostomy. Stress ulcer prophylaxis with famotidine (Pepcid), sucralfate (Carafate), lansoprazole (Prevacid), or similar agents can prevent painful gastric ulcers. Early identification and treatment of oral thrush Candida infection with nystatin or fluconazole may prevent this common infection from causing pain. Urinary retention and overflow incontinence may be identified and treated with tamsulosin (Flomax) or terazosin (Hytrin) to relax the internal smooth muscle sphincter, baclofen to relax the external striated muscle sphincter, and bethanechol (Urecholine) to enhance or tolterodine to diminish bladder contractility.

Pain from fractures, decubiti, or other slowly healing conditions should be managed in the individual with brain injury with minimal use of cognitively offensive medications. The first interventions utilized should be physical modalities, including topical application of ice and heat, ultrasound, transcutaneous electrical nerve stimulation (TENS), and massage. If unresponsive to acetaminophen (Tylenol), nonsteroidal anti-inflammatories, and weak narcotics, then nasal calcitonin (Miacalcin), oral baclofen, oral gabapentin, and a host of other agents are often profoundly better tolerated than narcotics with respect to slowing of the rate of thought processing and other cognitive issues. In particular, topical analgesics such as Ben-Gay, lidocaine cream (Emla cream), Aspercream, and capsaicin cream should be considered. Appendix A lists some common medications used for pain with comments and side effects.

Arousal, Awareness, Attention, and Initiation

Level of consciousness has been described as a continuum of awake, lethargic, stuporous, obtunded, and coma. The GCS defines **coma** as patients with GGS score less than or equal to 8. Vegetative patients are awake, but exhibit no objective signs of awareness of their internal or external environments. The term persistent vegetative state must be discarded, because patients may ascend from this state years following the event, and the nomenclature "persistent" implies that therapy and medical interventions should not be pursued. A host of medications may be utilized to enhance level of consciousness, increase awareness, and improve rate of thought processing and attention quality such that the patient is able to maximally participate in therapy sessions. Noradrenergics such as methylphenidate (Ritalin), dextroamphetamine (Dexedrine), and protryptyline may be prescribed. Methylphenidate has been described as reversing coma[17,18] and levodopa/carbidopa (Sinemet) has facilitated reversal of vegetative state.[19] Treatment trials with all psychostimulants should be attempted to enhance duration and quality of life. Individual uniqueness at the biochemical receptor mandates trials with multiple stimulants to facilitate arousal and awareness. Dopaminergics such as amantadine, bromocriptine, pergolide (Permax), Sinemet, and selegiline (Eldepryl) may also be highly efficacious. The attention deficit of hemineglect has been described as being responsive to dopaminergics.[20] New agents to treat narcolepsy continue to be developed, and all of these medications may be tried to maximize cognition after traumatic brain injury, stroke, encephalitis, multiple sclerosis, or dementing processes. Modafinil (Provigil) was approved for the treatment of narcolepsy by the Food and Drug Administration (FDA) in December of 1998, and its mechanism of psychostimulation is different from all preceding agents.

Memory, Aphasia, and Motor Restoration of Strength and Function

Memory is required for patients to benefit from learning new skills. After cognitively offensive medications that cause increased lethargy, slowed mental processing, and other potentially negative side effects are discontinued, memory often markedly improves, as exemplified by anticholinergic substitution of lipophilic oxybutinin for hydrophilic tolterodine, to treat spastic bladders. Medications that can be prescribed to enhance memory include the aforementioned noradrenergics. In addition, donepezil (Aricept) and other cholinergic agonists[21] may be delivered to improve memory. The intracranial bleeds that have been reported in association with Ginko biloba[22] suggests the merit of caution in prescribing the potential multiple active ingredients in this herb. Should a pharmaceutical company isolate the ingredient that is responsible for Ginko's memory-enhancing attributes, and should this agent prove safe, then it may serve as a valuable treatment option at that time. Research with naloxone, nootropics such as piracetam, and other agents suggest

options may be available in the future to address impaired memory.

Patients who are aphasic are less able to optimally participate in therapies. Expressive language deficits prevent the patient from making his or her needs known. These language deficits may respond favorably to dopaminergics such as bromocriptine,[23] amphetamines,[24] and piracetam.[25]

Motor restoration of strength and function can be maximized through the avoidance of potentially detrimental agents such as benzodiazepines, phenytoin (Dilantin), alpha blockers such as prazosin, and dopamine blockers such as haloperidol (Haldol).[26] In addition, hemiplegia and hemiparesis secondary to cortical, subcortical white matter, and brainstem stroke have been reported as improving with sympathomimetics such as methylphenidate and dextroamphetamine. Basic science and clinical research supports a greater improvement with physical therapy when patients are taking these medications than when taking medications alone or physical therapy without medications.[27]

Disinhibited Behavior

Disinhibited behavior, along with fecal incontinence, constitutes the most frequent reason why young patients with brain injury cannot return home to their families in the community. The enormous compromise to quality of life that accompanies institutionalization of these young people is inestimable. Disinhibited behavior may manifest in several different forms, including emotional, sexual, and physical behaviors. *Emotional disinhibition* includes spontaneous crying or laughing episodes that are inappropriate to the situation. This means that a patient may be free of mood depression, sad feelings, and not be in a distressing situation, yet spontaneously burst into tears. The disinhibition is often quite disconcerting to the patient, as he or she is often aware of the disinhibition but unable to control the behavior. Aggressive disinhibition may vary in intensity, ranging from calling names to punching. Sexual disinhibition ranges from inappropriate comments to masturbation to sexual attacks.

Antipsychotic medications are occasionally used to treat disinhibition. However, these proconvulsant agents globally suppress cognition, and should be reserved for individuals with psychotic delusions or hallucinations. Treating a physically disinhibited young patient with brain injury with haloperidol may unnecessarily cause excessive lethargy or sleep. Instead, use of agents that selectively extinguish the aggression without compromising other preserved components of cognition may afford return to the community, productivity, and a high quality of life. Aggression may respond to noradrenergic psychostimulants, lithium, anticonvulsants, beta blockers,[28] or a host of other medications.[29] Levodopa, tricyclic antidepressants,[30] and seratonergic antidepressants[31] are successfully utilized to treat emotional disinhibition. Sexual disinhibition may respond to buspirone, lithium, clonazepam, clomipramine, clozapine, or hormonal agents such as medroxyprogesterone or cyproterone.[32]

The delineation between medical and functional sequelae following brain injury is indistinct, and there exists considerable overlap of many different conditions. The team environment of traumatic brain injury neurorehabilitation affords numerous opportunities for interaction between the physical therapist and other team members. These interactions provide an atmosphere of information exchange that can be used to vastly improve the medical and functional status of the patient.

REHABILITATION MANAGEMENT

Interdisciplinary Team

As mentioned in the introduction, the basis for rehabilitation of the patient with a brain injury is an *interdisciplinary team*. No one person could possibly have the knowledge and skills necessary to treat all of the aspects of a brain injury. An interdisciplinary team approach is essential to providing the most comprehensive care that will lead to maximizing the patient's functional recovery.[33–36] Within the context of the team, individual members collaborate, contributing their expertise in a specific area, thereby enhancing everyone's skills. Communication and open mindedness are the key to any team. The different team members must share their skills and findings with the whole team, and be willing to learn from other team members to promote optimal return of function. The physical therapist must be willing to share a unique knowledge of motor control, but be open to learning from other team members such as the speech/language pathologist about cognitive deficits. All team members should take what they have learned from other team members and incorporate it into their treatment. This will lead to a more extensive, consistent, and complete approach to care.

Some members may play more prominent roles depending on which setting the client is in. For example, a recreational therapist will not likely be involved with a patient in the acute hospital, but would play a vital role in a community re-entry setting. The following sections describe some of the team members involved in the care of brain injury survivors and their roles in an acute rehabilitation hospital.

PATIENT AND FAMILY

It cannot be stressed enough that the most important members of the team are the patient and his or her family. Both the patient's and the family's lives are likely to be dramatically changed as a result of the injury. Familial roles may change. The patient who previously took care of the children may be on the receiving end of care now. The team examination must garner information regarding the patient's work, school, financial status, and social history. Family members should be questioned to obtain information on the patient's life-style, favorite hobbies, and other likes and dislikes. Information about the family dynamics should be ascertained. Who is the head of the household? Who is the breadwinner in the family? Is the patient responsible for taking care of the children? All of these and many other similar questions should be answered to develop a comprehensive plan of care.

Education is another essential aspect of care that should begin as soon as possible with the family, and patient when appropriate. The great majority of lay people are unaware of the implications of a brain injury. They may think their loved one will wake up from a coma and return to his or her previous life-style with little difficulty, like in a television movie. Unfortunately, this is rarely the case. It is the job of the entire interdisciplinary team to begin educating the family and patient on the affects of a brain injury and the long, arduous road to recovery. The family should be introduced to the Ranchos Los Amigos LOCF Scale and what to expect at the different stages. It is often beneficial to provide educational material for the patient and family.[34] The physical therapist should begin education on simple things such as how to perform passive range of motion to more complex issues such as how the brain controls movement and spasticity. Family members often ask if the patient will return to a "normal" life, or how much function he or she will regain. During the initial stages of recovery in the acute hospital and acute rehabilitation hospital, this question is impossible to answer. Every patient recovers differently and at different rates. The best way to help answer family questions and concerns is through education.

PHYSICIAN

In the acute rehabilitation hospital the physician overseeing the rehabilitation of the individual with a brain injury is usually a physiatrist or neurologist. The physiatrist has expertise and training in physical medicine rehabilitation and function. A neurologist's skills lay in the realm of the brain and the rest of the nervous system. A neurologist will have particular knowledge related to how the brain may recover and what impairments are likely to be seen given the location and the extent of the injury. Both a physiatrist and neurologist have vast knowledge in neuropharmacology, an extremely important part of management with this patient population.[33] Certain medications may have harmful side effects that may not be readily apparent. For example, a physiatrist or neurologist may be able to prescribe a less sedating drug than would normally be used in a different patient population to treat a certain clinical problem.

SPEECH/LANGUAGE PATHOLOGIST

Due to the nature of a brain injury the speech/language pathologist (SLP) plays an important and diverse role in the rehabilitation of the individual with brain injury. The SLP examines, evaluates, and treats communication, swallowing, and cognitive impairments in this patient population. As can be seen from the list of impairments in Box 24–3 this can be a challenging task. It is important for the physical therapist to be in close communication with the SLP to provide consistency of care for the communication, swallowing, and communication impairments. With the guidance of the SLP, the team will be able to devise the most effective and consistent way to communicate with the patient. He or she will also be able to instruct the team in how the patient's cognitive deficits may impede new learning, which in turn will affect everyone's interactions with the patient and treatment plans.

OCCUPATIONAL THERAPIST

The occupational therapist (OT) examines, evaluates and treats the patient's ability to perform activities of daily living (ADLs), visual/perceptual impairments, upper extremity function, sensory integration, and will often work with the SLP in treating cognitive impairments. Basic ADLs (BADLs) include dressing, self-feeding, bathing, and grooming. Instrumental ADLs (IADLs) include home management, housekeeping, grocery shopping, driving, and telephone use. In the rehabilitation hospital the occupational and physical therapist often work very closely together. A useful treatment approach is co-treatments with the OT. Having two

---

Box 24–3 DIRECT IMPAIRMENTS ASSOCIATED WITH TRAUMATIC BRAIN INJURY

Cognitive deficits
    Altered level of consciousness/alertness
    Post traumatic amnesia/ memory deficits
    Altered orientation
    Attention span deficits
    Problem solving/ reasoning deficits
    Perseveration
    Impaired safety awareness
    Impaired insight
    Impaired executive functioning
Neuromuscular deficits
    Abnormal tone
    Sensory deficits
    Motor control deficits
    Impaired balance/ataxia/nystagmus
    Paresis/paralysis
Visual deficits
Perceptual deficits
Swallowing deficits/dysphagia
Behavioral disinhibition
Communication deficits
    Receptive aphasia
    Expressive aphasia
    Motor speech/dysarthria
    Auditory deficits
    Impaired reading comprehension
    Impaired written expression
    Impaired pragmatics
    Impaired language skills

---

trained professionals working at the same time with the patient can be very productive. Many times two sets of experienced and trained hands are needed to effectively treat the patient. This is especially true with patients that have severe motor control and cognitive deficits. The OT will also work closely with the nursing staff to educate them on the best ways to assist the patient with ADLs.

REHABILITATION NURSE

The nurse is responsible for dispensing medications and closely monitoring their effects. The nurse will initiate a bowel and bladder retraining program to assist the patient in learning to become continent again. Bowel and bladder control is extremely important for self-esteem. The nurse performs daily monitoring of vital signs to make sure the patient remains medically stable. The nurse will inspect the patient's skin daily to ensure there are no signs of skin breakdown. The nurse also has the difficult task of consistently following through with the team's treatment plan throughout the day. For example, the third nursing shift needs to continue to follow splinting schedules established by the physical and occupational therapists. The nurse often has the most interactions on a regular basis with the patient's family.

CASE MANAGER/TEAM COORDINATOR

The case manager acts as the coordinator for the team. The case manager is often a nurse, medical social worker, or other health professional. The case manager will run team meetings, schedule family meetings, and act as a liaison with third-party payers. He or she must ensure that there is good communication among all team members in order to ensure that the rehabilitation care being provided is truly team oriented. The case manager will also be in constant communication with the patient and family to ensure that their needs are being met and that questions and concerns are adequately addressed. The case manager will coordinate payment and insurance benefit issues with the case manager from the patient's insurance company. In addition, the case manager is responsible for setting up follow-up and discharge services for the patient and family.

MEDICAL SOCIAL WORKER

The medical social worker (MSW) provides much needed support to both the family and patient. During the first few days after the initial injury, the family is in a state of crisis. They are thrown into a world that they, most likely, never knew existed. The MSW can support the family with education and counseling. As the patient progresses with recovery the MSW will also provide counseling for the patient. This is very important as the patient begins to have more awareness and insight into his or her deficits. If the patient has behavioral impairments the MSW can be pivotal in assisting both the patient and family. By providing counseling to both the family and patient, the MSW helps them cope with what may be a lifelong disability.

NEUROPSYCHOLOGIST

The neuropsychologist plays an important role on the team. He or she will often perform neuropsychological testing when it is appropriate to determine the patient's baseline cognitive functioning. He or she will also assist the team in developing a behavioral management program. When the patient with a brain injury has severe behavioral impairments the neuropsychologist assumes the role of the team leader.

OTHER MEMBERS

Many individuals with severe brain injury will require ventilatory support.[37] The *respiratory care practitioner* plays a vital role in the evaluation and treatment of respiratory impairments. In the rehabilitation hospital, the respiratory care practitioner monitors the patient's pulmonary status and provides appropriate treatment. A primary goal is to decannulate the patient at this stage of rehabilitation.

A *recreational therapist* assists the patient's return to activities enjoyed prior to the accident, or in helping identify new activities that the patient will find rewarding. This is an extremely important part of rehabilitation. Being able to perform in some type of leisure or recreational activities is a significant step in returning to a fulfilling life-style. Unfortunately, many insurance companies no longer reimburse for the services of a recreational therapist.

Direct and Indirect Impairments

Traumatic brain injury is associated with a wide variety of impairments, both direct and indirect, functional limitations, and disabilities that may lead to handicap. Box 24–3 identifies some of the prevalent impairments following traumatic brain injury. A single patient may not display all of the listed impairments.

COGNITIVE IMPAIRMENTS

Altered level of consciousness occurs consistently with acceleration-deceleration type injuries and may occur with some focal injuries. Consistent use of terminology in dealing with altered consciousness is important. According to Jennett and Teasdale, coma is defined as "not obeying commands, not uttering words, and not opening the eyes."[7] Sometimes the GCS score is used to define coma, with a score of 8 or less defining coma. It is important to note that coma usually lasts only a few weeks at most. Patients with a continuing decreased level of awareness with intact eye opening and sleep-awake cycles, but no ability to follow commands or speak, are described as vegetative or akinetic mute. These patients may have an alert level of consciousness, but may be misdiagnosed as being in a coma because of restricted interactions with the external environment.

Post-traumatic amnesia (PTA) describes the time between the injury and the time when the patient is again able to remember ongoing events, such as what was eaten for breakfast or what happened the day before. While the patient has PTA, it is as though each moment exists in isolation. There is no carry-over of information from hour to hour or day to day. The implications on functional training are obvious. It is interesting to note, though, that there appears a difference between *declarative* and *procedural memory*. Whereas the patient with PTA is unable to describe memories (declarative memory), he or she may, at times, show carry-over of skills that do not require verbal explanation (procedural memory). For example, a patient may improve in his or her ability to play a game that was played prior to the injury without any memory of having previously played the game. This is often accompanied by improvement in automatic activities such as gait.

Orientation and memory deficits are common cognitive impairments. The patient is often disoriented to person, place, and time. This, coupled with ongoing memory deficits, makes learning new skills and relearning old ones very difficult. The patient many times presents with a decreased attention span. He or she is easily distractible. The distraction can be external, or in some cases, internal. This can also contribute to the difficulty in forming new memories. The patient may not be able to focus on a task for a long enough period of time to be able to form a memory. The patient may also lack insight into his or her impairments and safety awareness. This can be especially problematic with the patient that has fair to good physical skills, but still requires some physical assistance. The patient may not realize that he or she cannot transfer out of bed or ambulate across a street without supervision or physical assistance. *Perseveration* is a phenomenon where a patient will repeat a task or word over and over without knowing they are doing it. As the patient progresses through the later stages of recovery, more high level executive functioning and problem solving deficits will be noticeable. The patient will have difficulty planning tasks and problem solving his or her way through difficulties encountered while performing a task. Owing to the wide range of potential cognitive deficits and their impact on ability to function, frequent communication among team members is warranted.

NEUROMUSCULAR IMPAIRMENTS

The patient with traumatic brain injury often presents with abnormal tone. This may range from spasticity that severely affects the entire body and greatly inhibits normal, functional movement to lesser tone that affects individual muscle groups and may not impair function. Because spasticity is an impairment that physical therapists often treat and is fairly common in individuals with brain injury, a separate section devoted to this topic is presented later in the chapter.

Sensory deficits commonly exist with the patient with traumatic brain injury. Proprioception and kinesthesia are of particular concern to the physical therapist. Ambulation and other mobility skills can be secondarily impaired if the individual does not know where his or her body is in space. Impaired proprioception, visual deficits, or vestibular losses will affect balance skills.

Motor control deficits are the primary concern of the physical therapist. Chapter 8 provides an in-depth discussion of motor control deficits and examination. Almost all patients that experience a traumatic brain injury will have some balance deficits, even if they are subtle. As balance control is mainly centered in the cerebellum and brainstem, nystagmus and ataxia sometimes accompany deficits in balance. Individuals that experience traumatic brain injury can also exhibit hemiparesis. See Chapter 17 for an in-depth discussion on the impairments following cerebral vascular accident (CVA) for further details on hemiparesis. The motor impairments may be similar to a person who has had a CVA, but the overall disability is often much more complicated owing to the multiple body systems affected.

VISUAL PERCEPTUAL IMPAIRMENTS

Damage to cranial nerves or the occipital lobes can cause visual deficits. This can include hemianopsia or on rare occasions cortical blindness. Perceptual impairments can include spatial neglect, apraxia, spatial relations syndrome, somatagnosia, and right-left discrimination deficits. As mentioned, the occupational therapist is the expert in assessing and treating impairments in these areas. See Chapter 29 for a discussion of perceptual deficits.

SWALLOWING IMPAIRMENTS

Following traumatic brain injury, many individuals commonly experience *dysphagia*. Swallowing deficits can be caused by damage to cranial nerves, motor control impairments, apraxia, and poor postural control. The speech/language pathologist is the primary team member in treating this impairment (see Chapter 30). However, the physical therapist may assist the SLP with proper positioning and improving motor control.

BEHAVIORAL DEFICITS

Research and clinical experience have established that behavioral disorders are the most enduring and socially disabling of any of the impairments commonly seen after traumatic brain injury.[38] Long-term changes in behavior such as sexual disinhibition, emotional disinhibition, apathy, aggressive disinhibition, low frustration tolerance, and depression often lead to a life of seclusion and loneliness. Factors to be considered in the evaluation and management of behavior are the person's premorbid personality; the physical, cognitive, and emotional effects of the injury; and the nature of the social

environment. Typically, neuropsychologists skilled in the evaluation and treatment of behavioral disorders play a leading role in determining behavioral programs. However, to achieve a successful outcome, behavior programs need to be generalized across all treatment settings.

COMMUNICATION IMPAIRMENTS

Numerous types of communication deficits are noted with patients following brain injury, and these can have a significant impact on rehabilitation. Expressive or receptive aphasia, reading comprehension and written expression, language skill deficits, and dysarthria may be present to varying degrees. See Chapter 30 for a discussion of these deficits.

Indirect Impairments

Due to the complex nature of traumatic brain injury and often prolonged bed rest, patients are likely to suffer from a variety of indirect impairments. The following is a list of the more commonly seen indirect impairments:

1. Contractures
2. Mobility deficits
3. Skin breakdown
4. Heterotropic ossification
5. Decreased endurance
6. Infection
7. Pneumonia
8. Impaired speech, owing to tracheotomy
9. Deep venous thrombosis

Many of the impairments can be avoided, or at least minimized, if a proactive treatment approach is adopted. If not treated early, the indirect impairments can be more debilitating than the direct ones. The section devoted to management according to Ranchos Los Amigos levels I, II, and III will discuss treatment techniques to decrease the likelihood of indirect impairments

Role of the Physical Therapist

The patient with brain injury is involved in rehabilitation throughout a wide continuum of care, experiencing many episodes of care. Physical therapists are likely to treat the patient in all the phases of rehabilitation. This next section will address how the physical therapist examines and treats this patient population in the different settings. Because of the diverse and complex impairments, it is difficult to categorize assessment and treatment techniques from a physical therapy standpoint. The following sections will break down the physical therapy management according to the Ranchos Los Amigos LOCF Scale. However, it must be emphasized that physical return does not mirror the Ranchos Los Amigos Scale of Cognitive and Behavioral Recovery. For example, just because an individual is moving from level IV to level V does not mean that he or she will begin to show a similar gain in physical function. Two patients with brain injury may be in stage IV of recovery, but one may have severe physical impairments and be confined to a wheelchair, while the other may be able to ambulate independently and have minimal physical impairments. Also, patients often move from one Ranchos Los Amigos level to the next in stages. A patient beginning to enter stage V will have periods where he or she still demonstrates stage IV behaviors. This is commonly seen during more stressful situations. For example, if a patient who is just starting to enter stage V enters a crowded and noisy room, he or she may become agitated and aggressive due to over-stimulation. The patient's recovery may plateau at any point along the Ranchos Los Amigos Scale.

RANCHOS LOS AMIGOS LEVELS I, II, AND III: DECREASED OR LOW-LEVEL RESPONSE LEVELS

Examination

At these low-level stages of recovery, the individual is usually in the acute hospital. In level I the patient is unresponsive to stimuli. In level II the patient reacts inconsistently to any stimuli. The response may be total body movements, vocalizations, or physiological changes. The response is often the same regardless of the stimuli. Level III is characterized by localized response to stimuli that is directly related to the type of stimuli presented (see Box 24–2). With changes in the healthcare delivery system, more and more patients who are at levels II and III may be seen in a rehabilitation hospital. The first step in beginning an examination of a patient at these stages of recovery is to conduct a comprehensive chart review. Because of the strong likelihood of various precautions and complications seen in this patient population, it is important to obtain all of the critical information from the chart before actually seeing the patient. The patient may be on a ventilator; he or she may have weight-bearing precautions and range of motion restrictions owing to orthopedic injuries, open wounds, or external fixators present. By doing a complete chart review the therapist can begin to form a picture of the patient. This will assist in preparation for the initial examination. Because the patient's status is so dynamic at these stages it is important to check with the patient's primary nurse before beginning any session.[39] The therapist should ascertain what the patient's vital signs are, if the patient is running a temperature, how alert the patient is, and if there are any contact precautions in effect. Due to the likelihood of various infections, team members may need to wear gowns, gloves, and/or masks when treating the patient.

The initial part of the examination should focus on observation of the patient. Key questions to address include:

1. What posture is the patient in? Is there evidence of primitive postures or reflexes?
2. Are the patient's eyes open or closed?
3. Is the patient able to track to auditory or visual stimulation?
4. Is the patient able to vocalize?
5. Does the patient exhibit any active movement? Is the movement purposeful or nonpurposeful?
6. Does the patient react to tactile/painful stimulation?
7. Do the patient's vital signs change when external stimulation is presented?

Primitive postures may include those associated with **decorticate** or decerebrate rigidity. In decorticate rigidity, the upper extremities are in a flexed posture and the lower extremities are extended. This is indicative of a lesion at or above the upper brainstem (above the superior colliculus). With **decerebrate** rigidity, both the upper and lower extremities are positioned in extension. The lesion is located in the brainstem between the vestibular nucleus and the superior colliculus.[40]

The initial examination should also include assessment of tone and passive range of motion. Because of the strong possibility of developing secondary impairments such as contractures it is extremely important to precisely document tone and passive range of motion measurements. There are a variety of measurement scales used to assess tone. One is the Modified Ashworth Scale (Table 24–5). If it is not medically contraindicated, the examination should include an attempt to sit the patient up on the side of the bed with assistance. The therapist should monitor vital signs and document any changes in tone or head and trunk control. When it is appropriate the patient should be transferred into a wheelchair. The patient will usually require the assistance of two to three people to transfer at this stage. In most cases, a reclining wheelchair or tilt-in-space wheelchair is the best option for positioning, with a specialized pressure-reducing cushion. Often it may take a few treatment sessions to complete the examination. Even then the examination will be ongoing. Whenever the therapist is working with the patient he or she should prudently look for signs of progress or regression.

Table 24–5 MODIFIED ASHWORTH SCALE FOR GRADING SPASTICITY

Grade	Description
0	No increase in muscle tone.
1	Slight increase in muscle tone, manifested by a catch and release or by minimal resistance at the end of the ROM when the affected part(s) is moved in flexion or extension.
1+	Slight increase in muscle tone, manifested by a catch, followed by minimal resistance throughout the remainder (less than half) of the ROM.
2	More marked increase in muscle tone through most of the ROM, but affected part(s) easily moved.
3	Considerable increase in muscle tone, passive movement difficult.
4	Affected part(s) rigid in flexion or extension.

From Bohannon and Smith,[65] p 207, with permission.

Intervention

Following is a list of anticipated goals of treatment at these stages of recovery adapted from the American Physical Therapy Association's *Guide to Physical Therapist Practice.*[42]

1. Physical function and level of alertness are increased.
2. The risk of secondary impairments is reduced.
3. Motor control is improved.
4. The effects of tone are managed.
5. Postural control is improved.
6. Tolerance of activities and positions is increased.
7. Joint integrity and mobility are improved or remain functional.
8. Family and caregivers are educated on patient's diagnosis, physical therapy interventions, goals, and outcomes.
9. Care is coordinated between all team members.

Several goals can be addressed whenever the physical therapist interacts with the patient. Goals are not achieved in isolation.[39] For example, when passive range of motion is performed, the patient's level of alertness is increased, joint mobility and integrity are improved, risk of secondary impairments is reduced, and tolerance to position is increased. Treatment sessions should be in a highly structured and stable, closed environment. Therapists should also strive for consistency in the time and length of treatment, and the same therapist should strive to treat the patient the majority of the time.

Improving Arousal through Sensory Stimulation

Whenever the therapist treats the patient he or she is providing stimulation in a variety of ways. When performing passive range of motion the therapist should talk to the patient explaining what he or she is doing and provide orientation. It is important to tell the patient where they are, what the date it is, who you are, and why the patient is in the hospital. The therapist should explain and demonstrate treatment techniques to the patient before performing them. This will provide tactile, auditory, painful, proprioceptive, and visual stimulation. Early mobilization such as sitting on the edge of the bed, transferring to a wheelchair, or using a tilt table for early standing will all increase the patient's level of alertness. The therapist should attempt to engage the patient by asking him or her to attempt to move the limb when performing passive range of motion, or to track the movement of the limb with the eyes when it is being ranged.

Sensory stimulation is an intervention used to increase the level of arousal and elicit movement. The theory is that by providing stimulation in a controlled, multisensory manner, with a balance of stimulation and rest, the reticular activating system may be stimulated causing a general increase in arousal. The value of sensory stimulation for patients who are slow to recover remains unproven. Theoretical support for such programs comes from research in four areas: (1) effects of sensory deprivation on neurological recovery; (2) effects of "enriched" environments on behavior and nervous system structure and function; (3) nervous system plasticity; and (4) effects of environmental input during sensitive periods of neurodevelopment. For a thorough review of these findings, see Ansell.[43] Stimulation is most effectively administered for short treatment sessions (15 to 30 min). It is important to present stimuli in an orderly manner via one or two modalities at a time to prevent overstimulation. Some recent research has suggested that providing multimodal, familiar sensory stimulation is effective. This means that sensory stimulation is provided in a discrete manner to each of the senses using familiar objects or sensations. The stimuli could be photographs of family members, favorite music, or food tastes.[44] The importance of carefully structuring the sensory experiences has led one author to prefer the term "sensory regulation" to sensory stimulation.[45] One must allow sufficient time for processing delays that are likely to exist, and repetition of the same stimulus is necessary for the documentation of response consistency.

Although the treatment is referred to as sensory stimulation, it is actually the response that is of greatest interest. During this type of treatment, the patient must be closely monitored for subtle responses such as changes in heart rate, blood pressure, rate of respiration, or diaphoresis. Various motor responses, such as eye movements, facial grimacing, changes in posture, head turning, or vocalization should be recorded. In monitoring a response, it is important to note the following characteristics:

1. *Latency:* The time delay between stimulus and response.
2. *Consistency:* The number of times within a given number of stimuli presentations that the patient responds in the same manner.
3. *Intensity:* The response should be proportionate to the stimulation. For example, a gentle squeezing of the Achilles tendon may normally cause a subtle withdrawal, but should not result in a massive movement of the entire lower extremity.
4. *Duration:* Brief forms of stimuli should result in brief forms of response.

Auditory stimulation is the most obvious place to begin. Normal conversational tones should be used and the therapist should begin by identifying him- or herself and explaining what is to be done. Discussions of topics that have meaning to the patient seem to be the most logical. Intermittent use of the radio or television may be therapeutic, but constant background noise is undesirable. Habituation to background noise is likely to occur and provides competition for meaningful stimuli.

Visual stimulation is provided by the use of familiar objects such as photographs of family and friends. It is important to systematically stimulate all areas of the visual field, to compensate for visual field deficits that may exist, and to document varying responses in different parts of the visual field. Visual attentiveness (how long the patient can maintain visual attention on an object) and visual tracking should also be documented.

Olfactory stimulation can be provided by placing scents under the patient's nose for 10 to 15 seconds during quiet breathing. Patients with a tracheotomy are not likely to respond because they do not breathe through their noses. Personal experience indicates that favorable results are most likely using patients' own favorite smells, such as freshly brewed coffee or a mate's favorite cologne.

Gustatory stimulation may involve the application of a cotton swab dipped in a flavored solution to the lips and gums, or may involve the use of flavored ice chips, Popsicles, and so forth. A therapist skilled in dysphagia management should be involved in this treatment due to the increased risk of aspiration and the need to assess complex swallowing responses. Often it is the speech/language pathologist that provides this type of treatment.

Tactile stimulation is provided during most functional activities such as turning, bathing, dressing, and so forth. Whereas most of us will note that different parts of our bodies are often in contact with one another (such as when crossing our legs, resting our head on our hands, crossing our arms), patients with brain injuries are usually positioned in ways that prevent this. Tactile stimulation might include using the patient's own hands, for example, by placing a washcloth in the hand and guiding him or her through the motions of face washing.

Vestibular stimulation can be provided by neck range of motion, rolling on a mat, rocking, or pushing the patient in a wheelchair.

A particularly important aspect of a sensory stimulation program is developing the patient's potential to perform a consistent, reliable response, with minimal latency, which can be applied to a simple yes/no communication system. Eye blinks or finger tapping may provide a viable yes/no response system through which the patient can communicate. Of course, this requires the cognitive ability to interact meaningfully with the environment and is not feasible for all patients.

Preventing Secondary Impairments

Because of the patient's inability to move at these stages, he or she is susceptible to many secondary impairments. If these are not addressed early in rehabilitation, they are likely to impede future progress, and can even be life threatening. Proper positioning both in bed and in a wheelchair is essential. Good positioning will assist in preventing skin breakdown, contractures, and assist with pulmonary hygiene. It can also help in normalizing tone. When in bed the head should be kept in neutral. This will help prevent neck contractures and lessen the effects of tonic neck reflexes (Fig. 24-2.) The hips and knees should be slightly flexed, but range of motion should

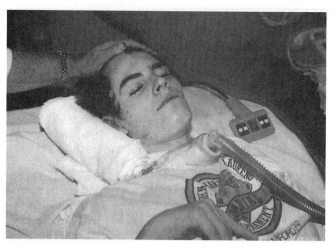

Figure 24-2. Head and neck positioned in neutral using towels. (From Mackay et al.,[39] p 286, with permission.)

be monitored to make sure that contractures do not develop. The therapist should instruct the nurses and family members in how to properly position and turn the patient. Turning will help prevent skin breakdown as well as pneumonia. Patients should be turned every 2 hours when in bed. Air mattresses are an effective way to prevent pressure sores. Table 24–6 presents strategies for positioning and handling.

Proper wheelchair positioning is important. Because of reduced postural control at these stages, a reclining wheelchair or a tilt-in-space wheelchair is commonly used. Proper pelvic and head positioning are the key elements in promoting good posture in a wheelchair (Fig. 24-3.) Refer to Chapter 32 for further discussion on wheelchairs. Splints can be used to assist in positioning. Multi podus boots can be used to position the foot to prevent foot drop and skin breakdown on the heel (Fig. 24-4.) However, these devices should not be used when the patient has increased plantarflexor tone because the splint may cause an increase in tone.

Postural drainage, percussion, and vibration are often used cooperatively by respiratory care, physical therapy, and nursing staffs. Percussion should be deferred in the presence of increased ICP.

Passive range of motion will help prevent contractures and deep venous thrombosis; may decrease hypertonicity; and provides sensory stimulation. When moving the upper extremities during range of motion, care should be taken to mobilize the scapula, and to maintain proper joint mechanics at the glenohumeral joint. If this is not done, the humerus is likely to impinge in the glenoid fossa, causing pain and destabilizing the joint capsule. With the lower extremities it is essential to maintain the range of motion at all joints. However, the ankle and toes are especially important as decreased range at the foot can greatly impact on functional activities such as transfers, sitting, wheelchair positioning, ambulation, and stair climbing. When performing range of motion, forceful or aggressive motions should be avoided. There is some indication that

Table 24–6 TECHNIQUES TO DECREASE ABNORMAL POSTURING AND PRIMITIVE REFLEXES

Area	Positioning	Handling
Head	1. Neutral position 2. Roll placed behind neck to support head and neck curvature 3. Roll parallel to head to prevent lateral flexion and rotation	1. Gentle range of motion when ICP and cerebral perfusion stable 2. Hands at base of skull or on sides of head
Trunk	1. Rolls behind shoulders 2. Roll behind hip if rotation is occurring 3. Normal alignment needs to be maintained	1. Hand on scapula, arm supported, rhythmical protraction/retraction, elevation/depression 2. Hand on posterior pelvis, leg supported, rhythmical elevation and depression (rotation) 3. When patient stable: rolling segmentally
Upper extremity	1. Roll behind shoulder 2. Cone in hand if fingers in flexion 3. Wedges between fingers if adducted 4. When stable: turn onto side for weight-bearing into arm	1. Relaxation of scapula (1 above) 2. Hand placed in patient's hand from ulnar side to help decrease flexor tone of elbow, wrist, and hand 3. Range of motion of fifth finger or thumb to help break up flexor tone 4. Hand placed over biceps when increased extensor tone and over the triceps when increased flexor tone
Lower extremity	1. Hips and knees supported in a slightly flexed position 2. No pressure on ball of foot medially 3. Roll between legs if strong adduction or internal rotation	1. Hand on lateral side sole of foot for range of motion of foot, knee, and hip 2. Hands placed above and below knee, medially for external rotation, hip and knee flexion 3. Hand behind knee for flexion and external rotation of hip, flexion of knee

From MacKay, L, et al[39], with permission.

forceful passive range of motion may be a causative factor for **heterotopic ossification,** especially when spasticity and increased tone are present. Heterotopic ossification is the formation of bone in muscle and other soft tissue. It usually occurs at the more proximal joints (shoulders, hips, and knees).[35,46]

Managing the Effects of Tone and Spasticity

Spasticity is a common problem throughout the continuum of care with many patients. There are a wide variety of methods available to the therapist and entire rehabilitation team to treat the adverse affects of tone. Interventions used to manage tone are discussed below.

Early Mobilization

Mobilization is extremely important because it addresses many of the goals of treatment in these early stages of recovery. As soon as the patient is medically stable, the patient should be transferred to a sitting position and out of bed to a wheelchair or chair. All precautions should be observed. The patient's head should be properly supported, as the patient is not likely to have adequate neck and head control to maintain an upright posture without support. Often it is beneficial to perform co-treatments with an occupational therapist when first

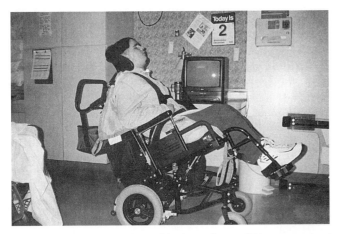

Figure 24-3. Wheelchair positioning using a tilt-in-space wheelchair. The wheelchair is tilted to assist in maintaining the patient's posture. The headrest maintains his head in an upright and neutral position. The straps on his chest will keep him sitting upright when the seat is tilted forward. The tilt-in-space aspect allows for pressure relieving when the angle of tilt is changed. The pad underneath the patient is used with a lift to transfer the patient. Also, in the background against the wall in the lower right-hand corner, is a lap tray that can be used to better position his upper extremities. Photographs of his family and friends are taped to the tray.

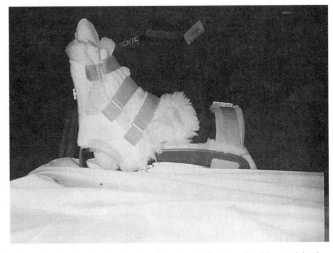

Figure 24-4. Multi-podus boot used for foot and ankle positioning and to prevent skin breakdown on the heel. This type of positioning device may not be beneficial for the patient with moderate to severe tone at the ankle; it is not strong enough to prevent the ankle from plantarflexing and may even increase tone.

sitting and transferring the patient. This way there are two skilled professionals to assist the patient, as maximal assistance is often required. Use of a tilt table is also advantageous because it allows early weight-bearing through the lower extremities while the upright position improves overall level of alertness.

When attempting early functional tasks, such as sitting and grooming activities, *therapeutic guiding* techniques described by Davies[35] are effective. The therapist aims to assist the patient in interacting with the environment because the patient is unable to do so. The goal is to aid the patient in learning by guiding the patient's body in the performance of a functional task. Guiding provides tactile, proprioceptive, and kinesthetic stimulation when performing a task. It also allows the therapist to continually assess the patient's abilities as the therapist's hands and body can directly feel the patient.[35]

Documentation

Documentation for the patient with a brain injury can be very challenging. The patient often progresses at a slower rate than other patient populations and the changes are often more difficult to quantify. With the increase of managed care, it is important for the therapist to be able to effectively document changes to show that the patient is moving along the road to recovery. Examples of documentation at these stages of recovery include:

- Patient's neck postured in left rotation with left upper extremity abducted, elbow extended in possible asymmetric tonic neck reflex posture (ATNR).
- Patient inconsistently tracks to right to auditory stimulation.
- Patient exhibits active, nonpurposeful movement in right upper and lower extremities.
- Patient withdraws to painful stimuli on right side of body.
- No reaction to painful stimuli on left side of body.

Patient and Family Education

The goal of patient and family education is to teach the family about the stages of recovery and what can be expected in the future. By becoming informed, the family often does not feel so helpless. Although it is impossible to predict long-term outcome at this early stage, families should be informed of possible outcomes. The therapist should be realistic but provide hope for the family. It is often beneficial to have a medical social worker consult with the family to provide support and guidance. The therapist should try to involve family members in treatment sessions when appropriate and the patient is medically stable. Family members should be instructed in how to perform passive range of motion exercises and appropriate sensory stimulation. They should also be trained in how to properly position the patient. It is often useful for family members to be given packets or worksheets with pictures and instructions in how to perform these interventions,

so they can effectively perform them when the therapist is not there.

RANCHOS LOS AMIGOS LEVEL IV: CONFUSED-AGITATED

Examination

It is extremely challenging to examine the individual who is in the confused-agitated stage of recovery. The patient can be markedly agitated, to the point of physically acting out. The patient is confused. He or she will have poor memory, usually both short- and long-term. The patient will have a decreased attention span and be easily distracted. The patient may be emotionally disinhibited and prone to emotional outbursts. These may range from verbally acting out to physically attempting to hurt themselves or others to sexually inappropriate behaviors. Refer to Box 24–2 for further description of this stage. Again, it is often helpful to have another therapist to assist in the examination. This could be another physical therapist, an occupational therapist, or a speech/language pathologist.

It is difficult to make formal measurements of such things as range of motion or strength because the patient will often be unable to cooperate; therefore, the therapist must again have keen observation skills and the ability to estimate. The therapist should examine functional mobility, balance both in sitting and standing if the patient is able, range of motion, strength, motor control, tone, sensation, and reflexes. The physical therapist should also begin to assess the patient's cognitive abilities in this stage. This will include orientation, attention span, memory, insight, safety awareness, and alertness. Is the patient able to follow commands: one-step, two-step, or multi-step commands? Is the patient oriented to person, place, or time? Do they recognize family members? It is beneficial to consult with other team members, especially the speech/language pathologist, to garner their opinion on the patient's cognitive status.

Intervention

Following is a list of expected goals adapted from the American Physical Therapy Association's *Guide to Physical Therapist Practice*.[42]

1. Patient's endurance is improved.
2. Joint mobility and integrity are maintained.
3. Risk of secondary impairments is reduced.
4. Tolerance of activities is increased.
5. Patient's family is educated regarding patient's diagnosis, prognosis, physical therapy interventions, and outcomes.
6. Care is coordinated between all team members.

The overall goals of physical therapy at this stage of recovery are to maintain the functional capabilities of the patient. This will include range of motion, strength, and endurance. Generally, the therapist should work near the patient's physical level of function and attempt to improve endurance rather than attempt to progress to more challenging skills that would require new learning. The most important goal the whole team strives to achieve in this stage of recovery is to prevent the agitated outbursts that occur, and to help the patient control his or her behavior. It is important to provide a highly structured and stable, closed environment for the patient. The neuropsychologist can assist the team by providing insight into different ways to manage the patient's agitated behavior. Different medications may be effective in helping the patient control outbursts. The neuropsychologist may set up a behavioral program that will provide additional external structure and aid the patient in learning to control his or her behavior.

The therapist must be extremely creative and flexible during the examination and subsequent treatment in this stage of recovery. The following special considerations will help in the management of patients at this level of recovery.

Remember that the patient is confused. To help decrease confusion, the patient should be seen by the same person at the same time and in the same place every day. Establishing a daily routine is very important. It is calming and reassuring to have a sense of familiarity. Consistency is important. Additionally, orientation should be provided frequently and in a non-threatening manner. At this stage, it is often better to provide orientation information than to challenge the patient to provide it, particularly if the patient is not expected to succeed.

Expect No Carryover

Teaching new skills in this stage is unrealistic. The patient may begin to perform a functional task, such as brushing teeth or ambulating. However, this does not indicate a general learning ability, as brushing your teeth and especially walking are automatic skills with an ingrained neural network. The use of charts or graphs may be useful to help the patient progress each day. Without the use of such aids, the patient is likely to have no recall of the previous day's performance and therefore will be unable to build on it.

Model Calm Behavior

The patient is likely to perceive and reflect the demeanor of the caregiver. Therefore, it is important for the therapist to assume a calm and focused affect. The patient often is unable to control his or her behavior. The patient's behavior is impulsive. He or she may not feel safe. To help the patient feel safe, it is important for the therapist to be perceived as in control of his or her emotions and behavior.

The individual will have a limited attention span. Because of the limited attention span, the patient may not be able to concentrate on any given activity for a very long time. It is important to be prepared with numerous activities. If the patient cannot be redirected to the selected task, it is appropriate to attempt to engage him or her in another.

Expect Egocentricity

At this point in recovery, the patient cannot be expected to see another's point of view. He or she will tend to think only of themselves and, at this point, it is unwise to stress the patient with attempts to do otherwise.

Offer Options

Treat the patient at an appropriate age level. Give control to the patient when it is appropriate. Control can be given while maintaining therapeutic intervention by phrasing questions as "Would you rather play ball or go for a walk?" This prevents situations where the patient chooses an undesirable or unrealistic activity if asked, "What would you like to do?" or the case where the patient simply answers "No" when asked, "Would you like to . . . ?" Provide safe choices for the patient, but always give him or her an option. It lets the patient feel like he or she has some control over the situation. This is extremely important as the patient often feels out of control because of the situation. By providing the patient with some sense of control you are treating him or her like another human.

Documentation

Documentation may read like:
- Passive range of motion appears to be within functional limits in bilateral lower extremities except for right dorsiflexion, which appears to be −10 degrees from neutral.
- Patient exhibits active range of motion at all muscle groups, except for right dorsiflexion.
- Active range of motion in all four extremities is non-purposeful and uncoordinated.
- Patient exhibits impaired safety awareness and is disoriented to place and time.
- Unable to assess formally due to patient's decreased ability to follow commands and behavioral outbursts.

Patient and Family Education

As mentioned, it is difficult to provide education for the patient at this stage as the patient has very little, if any, ability for new learning. However, it is extremely important to provide education for the patient's family. Above all the family should understand that the patient does not have control of his or her behavior at this stage. The patient is not striking out or swearing at others because of an intent to hurt others, but because of agitation and confusion. Many times families do not understand why a patient is performing these unruly behaviors. They must be told that these behaviors are a symptom of the brain injury just as the patient's inability to walk or eat is. It is important to educate the family that entering this stage is a good sign because it indicates that the patient is moving into the next phase of recovery. It is usually short lived, typically lasting only a few weeks at most.[1] Family members should also be taught to use the above strategies when interacting with their loved one. Consistency is important for everyone, including family members. If a behavioral plan is being implemented, the family should be a part of devising it and carrying it out.

RANCHOS LOS AMIGOS LEVELS V AND VI: CONFUSED-INAPPROPRIATE AND CONFUSED-APPROPRIATE

Examination

At these stages of recovery, a more formal and accurate physical therapy examination should be done. Refer to Box 24–2 for a description of patient behavior at these stages of recovery. The patient is confused, but with structure is able to follow simple commands. The examination methods may need to be modified, because the patient will still have difficulty with more complex tasks and an open environment. The examination may need to be done over a number of treatment sessions. It is important to obtain concise and objective data at this point. Prior to these stages it is difficult to acquire precise measurements when assessing the patient. The examination should include range of motion, both passive and active, of all four extremities and the neck and trunk; and sensation, including kinesthesia, proprioception, light touch, deep pressure, and pin prick. Examination of the patient's neuromuscular status includes tone and reflexes; strength, which may be difficult to assess accurately owing to abnormal tone and motor control; coordination; motor control; and balance, both in sitting and standing. It is important to closely observe the patient's movements for ataxia, postural instability, and nystagmus with changes in position.

The patient's functional status should be examined. Bed mobility skills, including rolling to both sides and moving to and from sitting and supine, should be assessed. Transfer skills should be assessed. The patient with decreased lower extremity strength and poor balance and trunk control may benefit from use of a transfer board to assist with the transfer. Additional functional mobility skills (ambulation, stairs, and wheelchair mobility) should also be assessed as appropriate. Functional skills should also be assessed in varying environments (closed to open) to determine how the patient performs in a more stressful environment. Many times the patient will not perform as well in an open, variable environment as in a closed one.

Intervention

The following goals are adapted from the American Physical Therapy Association's *Guide to Physical Therapist Practice*.[42]

1. Performance of functional mobility and ADLs is increased.
2. Gait, mobility, and balance are improved.
3. Motor control and postural control are increased.
4. Risk of secondary impairments is reduced.
5. Strength and endurance are increased.
6. Safety with functional mobility tasks and ADLs is improved.
7. Patient and family are educated on diagnosis, prognosis, physical therapy interventions, and goals.
8. Tolerance of activities is improved.
9. Care is coordinated between all team members.

It should be restated that the patient's physical recovery does not mirror the cognitive recovery of the Ranchos Los Amigos scale. The goal of treatment at these stages is to maximize the patient's functional mobility skills. This would necessitate improvements in motor control, strength, endurance, and balance. Safety should also be emphasized at all times in these stages. The ultimate goal of all treatment is to return the individual with brain injury to the community and home. It is during levels V and VI that the brain injury survivor must begin to learn the necessary safety skills that will allow him or her to return to the community, if possible.

Some of the same strategies used in level IV should be employed when working with individuals in levels V and VI. As has been noted throughout this chapter, patients have multiple cognitive deficits that can impede new learning. Treatment sessions should be thoughtfully planned to maximize the patient's motor learning capabilities. Practice should be distributed and variable. This allows for sufficient rest time due to the patient's decreased endurance, concentration, and attention span. Feedback is also very important. Because this patient population often has sensory and perceptual impairments, augmented feedback is necessary as opposed to intrinsic feedback. Again, consistency is very important, not only as a tool to improve motor learning capacity, but to improve cognition and behavior as well. Refer to Chapter 13 for an in-depth discussion of motor learning.

A *memory book* can be a useful tool during these levels of recovery. Typically it is a notebook containing a calendar that can be updated daily by any team member. It also has the names and pictures of all of the different team members that work with the patient. The patient's daily schedule is placed in the notebook. The patient, or therapist, writes what the patient did during that therapy session in the book. It contains different sections into which independent exercise programs or cognitive worksheets are placed. When able, the patient can begin to record information in the memory book. It also serves as a way to pass information to the family and caregivers if they are not able to be with the patient during therapy sessions. Family members can read the book to learn what the patient did in therapy. Overall, the book serves as a mechanism for the patient to compensate for his or her memory deficits.

There are a plethora of treatment techniques that are effective in treating the patient with a brain injury who has neuromuscular impairments. Survivors of brain injury present with such a wide range of impairments and disabilities that it is impossible to say that one technique is better than another. Traditional techniques in neurorehabilitation all take a motor learning approach. Because of the varying impairments, therapists should be well versed in a variety of treatment options, not just one approach. There is no empirical evidence definitively stating that one treatment method is better than another when working with this population.

Many treatment approaches utilize the developmental sequence and muscle facilitation techniques to some extent in their treatment methods.[47] Using developmental postures to facilitate movement and inhibit abnormal movement patterns is an excellent treatment foundation to help restore normal movement and maximize functional mobility. Employing the developmental sequence in a logical, sequential manner will help improve the functional skills of the patient.[48] Working on static control and progressing to controlled mobility and finally skill level tasks is an appropriate progression in each developmental posture. Table 24–7 identifies the different postures in the developmental sequence and what benefits are derived from working in each posture. Refer to the *Physical Rehabilitation Laboratory Manual: Focus on Functional Training* for a more in-depth and detailed discussion on treatment techniques and treatment modifications using the functional developmental sequence.[48] It is not necessary to progress through each lower posture to move on to the next. It is important, however, to link each treatment activity to improved function. For example, if the patient has poor lower trunk control in standing and the treatment includes practicing static control in quadruped, the therapist should include functional standing at the sink at the end of the treatment session. This will help educate the patient on why it was beneficial to get on all fours and how it will help him or her functionally. Figures 24-5, 24-6, and 24-7 depict sample treatment activities with a patient using modifications in the developmental postures. Because of secondary impairments and accessory injuries such as long bone fractures, it may be necessary to adapt activities. A Swiss ball can be a useful tool to improve balance, modify tone, and improve trunk control.

Documentation

Examples of documentation include:
- Patient able to ambulate 75 feet with minimal assistance in a closed environment, without device. However, in an open environment, the physical therapy gym, patient requires moderate assistance and multiple verbal cues to ambulate 75 feet.
- Patient able to transfer wheelchair to and from bed with minimal assistance with two to three verbal cues for brake management and safety techniques. However, in an open environment, patient requires moderate assistance to transfer wheelchair to and from bed and multiple verbal cues for safety techniques.
- Patient exhibits increased extensor tone in R LE, 3 on modified Ashworth scale.
- Patient presents with decreased safety awareness and is highly distractible, both internally

Table 24–7 DEVELOPMENTAL SEQUENCE POSTURES AND TREATMENT BENEFITS

Posture	Treatment Benefits
1. Prone-on-elbows	• Improve upper trunk, UE and neck/head control. • Facilitate flexor tone. • Increase ROM at hip extensors. • Improve shoulder stabilizers strength. • Wide BOS, low COG.
2. Quadruped	• Improve upper trunk, lower trunk, LE, UE, and neck/head control. • Weight-bearing through hips. • Increase hip stabilizers strength. • Decrease extensor tone at knees by weight-bearing. • Increase shoulder stabilizers strength. • Weight-bearing through shoulders, elbows, and wrists. • Increase extensor ROM at wrists and fingers. • Wide BOS, low COG.
3. Bridging	• Improve lower trunk and LE control. • Increase hip stabilizers strength. • Weight-bearing through feet and ankles. • Lead up activity for bed mobility. • Wide BOS, low COG.
4. Sitting	• Improve upper trunk, lower trunk, LE, and head/neck control. • Weight-bearing through UE. • Functional posture. • Improve balance reactions. • Medium BOS, medium COG.
5. Kneeling and half-kneeling	• Improve head/neck, upper trunk, lower trunk, and LE control. • Weight-bearing through hips. • Inhibit extensor tone at knees. • Increase hip stabilizers strength. • Improve balance reactions. • Weight-bearing through ankle in half-kneeling. • Narrow BOS, high COG (kneeling). • Wide BOS, high COG (half-kneeling).
6. Modified plantigrade	• Improve head/neck, upper trunk, lower trunk, UE, and LE control. • Weight-bearing through UE and LE. • Improve balance reactions. • Functional posture. • Increase extensor ROM at wrists and fingers. • Wide BOS, high COG.
7. Standing	• Improve head/neck, upper trunk, lower trunk, and LE control. • Weight-bearing through LE. • Improve balance reactions. • Functional posture. • Narrow BOS, high COG.

BOS, base of support; COG, center of gravity; LE, lower extremity; ROM, range of motion; UE, upper extremity.

and externally. These traits are increased in an open environment.

Patient and Family Education

During levels V and VI, it is important to emphasize safety education with the patient. The individual is, hopefully, beginning to exhibit improved mobility skills at these stages but often lacks the insight to recognize that he or she may not be safe to ambulate or transfer by themselves yet. The above-

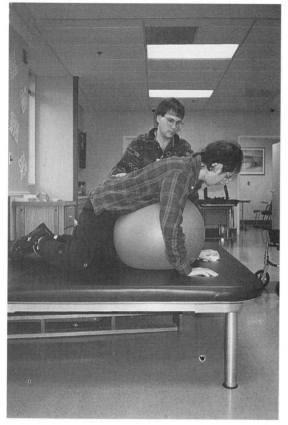

Figure 24-5. Modification of quadruped using a Swiss ball and weight under left hand. The Swiss ball is assisting the patient in maintaining the quadruped posture. Due to long bone fractures in his upper and lower extremities and increased tone, he would be unable to maintain this beneficial posture without the use of the ball. The ankle cuff weight under his left hand prevents his wrist from fully extending. Because of the previously mentioned fractures he does not have sufficient PROM at the wrist to maintain this posture without the ankle cuff weight under his left hand.

mentioned memory book is a good way to educate the patient and it acts as a good orientation guide. Videotaping the patient during treatment sessions is also an effective technique. It allows the patient to see how he or she is performing a task. The patient is then better able to correct or compensate for impairment. When used over a period of time, the patient can also see improvement. This is especially important when the patient feels like little progress is being made. With memory deficits, the patient will have a hard time recalling that he or she could not move as easily only a few days or weeks ago. A videotape can clearly document ease of movement and level of impairment.

Family members can learn how to assist the patient with functional mobility. They should be instructed in proper body mechanics when assisting with functional mobility so as to avoid risking injury to the patient or themselves. This typically includes training in bed mobility, transfers, ambulation, and wheelchair mobility skills. Family members should also be educated on how to assist the patient with strengthening exercises and passive range of motion. All of these skills are important for family members

to learn how to render, as they may become a care-giver for the patient if the patient requires physical assistance upon discharge to home.

RANCHOS LOS AMIGOS LEVELS VII AND VIII: APPROPRIATE RESPONSE LEVELS

It is usually in the late confused-appropriate stage and early automatic-appropriate stages that the patient is discharged from inpatient rehabilitation. Box 24–2 provides a description of the patient's behavior at these stages. Prior to discharge, it is crucial to wean the patient from the structure that was so important in the early stages of recovery. As the patient becomes better able to control him- or herself, control of environment should be lessened. Therapy is often delivered in a day treatment setting, with the emphasis of all disciplines on community re-entry and return to work or school. In this setting the patient goes to therapy throughout the day and returns home in the late afternoon.

Examination and Intervention

At these levels, the restoration of physical function is not significantly different than for patients without brain injury. The same examination techniques discussed in levels V and VI should be used. The following goals have been adapted from the

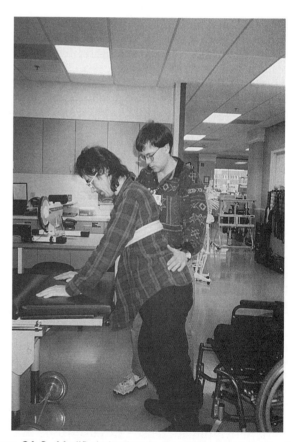

Figure 24-6. Modified plantigrade. Due to the long bone fractures and increased tone, the patient is not able to maintain this posture in good alignment. However, it is still a beneficial posture because it allows for weight-bearing on all four extremities and will improve his trunk and extremity control.

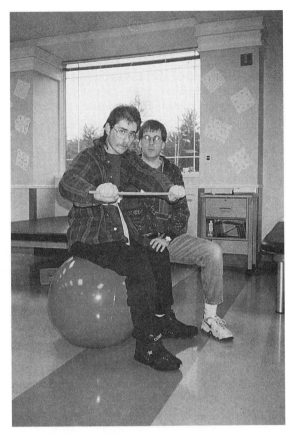

Figure 24-7. Sitting on Swiss ball and rotating to either side will improve the patient's balance, upper trunk rotation, trunk control, and posture. The dowel is used to isolate upper trunk rotation.

American Physical Therapy Association's *Guide to Physical Therapist Practice*.[42]

1. Patient and family educated on diagnosis, prognosis, physical therapy intervention, and goals.
2. Safety of patient and family is improved.
3. Ability to perform physical tasks related to ADLs, community and work reintegration, and leisure activities is increased.
4. Functional mobility is improved.
5. Motor control, balance, and postural control is improved.
6. Self-management of symptoms is increased.
7. Strength and endurance are increased.
8. Level of supervision and assistance for task performance is decreased.

The major goal of treatment at these stages is to assist the patient in integrating the cognitive, physical, and emotional skills that are necessary to function in the real world. Judgement, problem solving, and planning are emphasized.

For the demands of treatment to approximate the demands of the real world, treatment focuses on advanced activities such as community skills, social skills, and daily living skills. For examples of these skills, see Table 24–8. The interdisciplinary team emphasizes use of compensatory strategies and the patient assumption of self-responsibility. Because the patient now has some insight into his or her own

strengths and weaknesses, it is important to involve the individual in decision making as much as possible. The patient at this level is working to reintegrate back into home and community. Therefore, the focus of treatment is to maintain performance while decreasing structure and supervision. Independent work and cooperative work with others are encouraged. Many times group treatment sessions are beneficial. Honest feedback from the therapist and support group is crucial for the patient to learn how to function in society with his or her present abilities and limitations. Teaching the patient to give as well as receive feedback is an important aspect of therapy at this point.

Almost all patients who have incurred a moderate to severe brain injury will experience some degree of difficulty with sensorimotor integration. Even those without focal motor deficits will have subtle problems with activities that require speed, flexibility, interlimb coordination, rhythm, and timing. Therapists at Rancho Los Amigos coined the term *robot syndrome* to describe a characteristic set of problems observed in patients 6 months to 1 year after brain injury.[49] The robot syndrome is characterized by robot-like motion, excessive eating, and sedentary avocational activities. No one factor is thought to cause the syndrome. Rather, residual sensorimotor, cognitive, and psychosocial deficits contribute.

Documentation

Examples of documentation include:
- Patient requires 3 to 4 verbal cues to safely ambulate across a street at stop light with R AFO.
- Patient requires minimal assistance and 2 to 3 verbal cues to locate two objects in grocery store aisle; patient exhibits nystagmus in bilateral eyes when turning head upward and to right to look for objects.
- Patient requires three verbal cues to safely find way from hospital entrance to physical therapy gym.

Patient and Family Education

At these stages of recovery the patient should be educated in how to best compensate for residual impairments or disabilities. The patient and family should contact local support groups. Being able to talk to another survivor of brain injury or family member who has gone through some of the same difficulties can be of great benefit. If necessary, the

Table 24–8 COMPONENTS OF COMMUNITY SKILLS, SOCIAL SKILLS, AND DAILY LIVING SKILLS PROGRAMS

Daily Living	Social Skills	Community Skills
Food preparation	Introductions	Shopping
Housekeeping	Nonverbal communication	Public transport
Money management	Assertiveness	Map reading
Meal planning	Listening skills	Leisure planning
Telephone use	Giving/receiving feedback	Community resources
Time management		

patient and family members should continue with regular counseling provided by a medical social worker or neuropsychologist. The World Wide Web is a great place for family members or patients to find information and support groups. The national organization is:

Brain Injury Association, Inc.
105 N. Alfred St.
Alexandria, VA 22314
(800) 444-6443
http://www.biausa.org.

Most states have local chapters that can provide information and support.

Beginning around level VII, patients should be involved in a regularly scheduled program of physical activity that strives to expand their movement capabilities and make movement an enjoyable experience. The goal of such treatment is to encourage an active life-style to avoid future complications. It is important to help the patient develop a realistic fitness program that can be followed independently after physical therapy is discontinued. Even for the patient who has significant focal motor deficits, a program designed to promote overall fitness is an important aspect of therapy and should not be neglected. Research has shown that survivors of brain injuries who participate in a regular exercise program have better self-esteem and lead healthier lives.[41]

SPECIAL CONSIDERATIONS
Abnormal Tone

The patient with traumatic brain injury often presents with abnormalities in muscle tone. In most cases the patient has increased tone, hypertonia, or spasticity. *Spasticity* is a clinical triad of mass spasms, spastic hypertonus, and hyperreflexia. Although usually the phenomenon presents with all three components, any can exist in isolation or with different severities of expression at different joints. Each component can have medically and functionally beneficial or detrimental aspects. Mass spasms can be painful and predispose to falls during transfers, but also serve to maintain muscle bulk to prevent decubiti. Spastic hypertonus may cause contractures, which will prevent sitting in a wheelchair for freedom of mobility. However, biceps hypertonus may cause elbow flexion at 90 degrees that can be utilized to carry grocery bags. Knee extension hypertonus may be used for standing to assist with transfers and gait. Ankle plantarflexion hypertonus during ambulation may cause effective leg lengthening, contributing to falls, but may also enhance venous return, decreasing the risks for deep venous thrombosis. Each patient must be assessed individually with attention directed toward both medical stability and functional enhancement.

The physical therapist has a great many interventions at his or her disposal to assist in managing the patient's hypertonicity. The foundations of spasticity management are therapeutic stretching and strengthening exercises with adjunctive modalities and functional retraining. Passive range of motion

and selective strengthening of the antagonist muscles can help to decrease spasticity. Positioning is an important adjunct in the management of tone abnormalities. Maintaining the head and neck in a neutral position is important for minimizing the effects of primitive postures that may cause an increase in tone. Keeping the whole body in proper alignment is also important. Refer to Table 24–6 for positioning strategies.

Splints and **serial casting,** or inhibitive casting, are other interventions that can assist in decreasing hypertonicity. These devices maintain a constant stretch on the hypertonic muscle, thereby increasing the range of motion and decreasing tone. Serial casting is often used with the patient that presents with plantarflexor or biceps contractures. These may be due to either increased tone or prolonged shortening of the muscle. In a patient who presents with a plantarflexion contracture, the ankle is stretched into as much dorsiflexion as possible and then a short leg cast is applied. In approximately 1 week the cast is removed. The muscle is stretched again and another cast applied (Figs. 24-8, 24-9, and 24-10.) This procedure is repeated until satisfactory gains in range of motion have been achieved, or there is no further progress made. Precise range of motion measurements should be taken between each casting. Because the individual with brain injury is likely to have impaired sensation and communication, and behavioral deficits, there is a risk of skin breakdown or the patient hurting him or herself or others with the cast. The decision to use casts should be made carefully. The benefits and possible side effects should be thoroughly discussed with input from appropriate team members. Hands-on experience under the supervision of a skilled clinician is recommended before attempting to cast patients.[50–52]

Positioning splints and air casts will temporarily inhibit tone. Wrist and hand splints are effective. When using these devices, the therapist should set up a schedule of use, and slowly increase the time they are on, as the patient's tolerance improves. The team should carefully monitor for signs of skin breakdown. Air casts can be used to help modify abnormal tone.

Neuromuscular electrical stimulation will cause temporary inhibition of abnormally high tone. The electrical stimulation can be applied to either the agonist or antagonist muscle.[53] Other interventions that have temporary inhibitive effects on hypertonicity are increased weight-bearing on the affected limb, rhythmic rotation, and aquatic therapy.

Similarly, botulinum toxin (Botox) and phenol **nerve blocks** are synergistic antispasticity interventions. These injections have no cognitive sequelae associated with their delivery. In addition, the amount of medication delivered can be titrated to remove a portion of detrimental spasticity, and leave sufficient spastic hypertonus for functional use. Spastic hypertonus of a muscle can be eliminated to unmask volitional strength in the antagonist muscle, which can subsequently be trained for functional

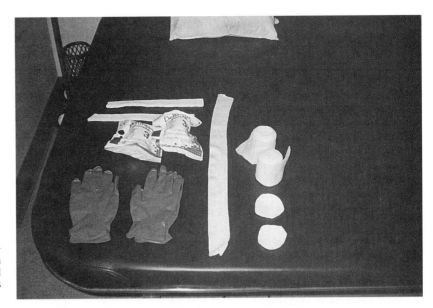

Figure 24-8. Materials used for serial casting: fiberglass casting material, rubber gloves, stockinette, a layer of padding to wrap around the lower leg, and padding for the malleoli and proximal and distal ends of the cast.

use. For example, injections to weaken a spastic biceps muscle may unmask volitional elbow extension strength of the triceps for transfer mobility tasks.

Botulinum toxin is a medication that paralyzes the muscle into which it is injected. It prevents the presynaptic nerve from releasing acetylcholine into the synaptic cleft such that a hyperactive CNS can-

not effect a muscle contraction. Phenol demyelinates nerve in lower concentrations and denatures axonal protein at higher concentrations.[54] As such, phenol prevents the hyperactive CNS from activating the muscle by interrupting the connecting nerve transmission between the CNS and muscle. Botox is best delivered to highly innervated sites such as the intrinsic hand muscles, paraspinals, pectoralis major,

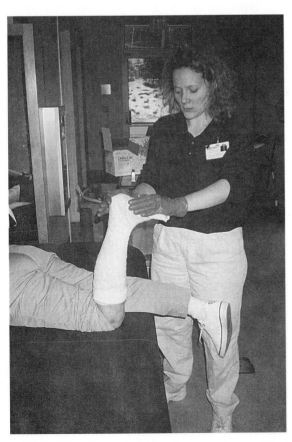

Figure 24-9. First a layer of padding is wrapped around the lower leg and foot.

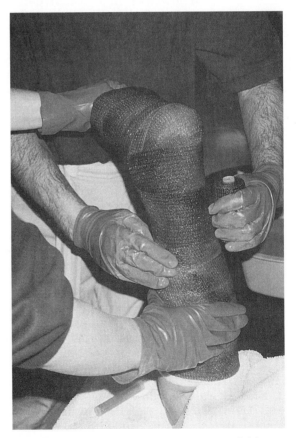

Figure 24-10. Then the fiberglass casting material is wrapped around the lower leg and foot. One clinician does the wrapping while another holds the leg and foot in the proper position.

and rectus abdominus as well as muscles surrounded by tight fascial compartments, such as the long finger flexors in the forearm and the tibialis posterior in the deep compartment in the leg.[55]

The technique of delivery of injected antispasticity agents is quite simple, though technically demanding to execute. After the appropriate nerve or muscle is identified, the skin is cleansed and a needle is inserted through the skin. Electricity is delivered via a connecting wire, and transmitted only to the tip of the needle. When the tip is close enough to the nerve (approximately .5 mm) only 1 milliamp of current is required to stimulate the nerve and observe muscle contraction. The medication is subsequently injected. The presynaptic nerve must absorb Botox, so maximal onset of effect is delayed 1 to 3 weeks. Phenol works immediately, and so additional medication can be delivered to titrate the desired antispasticity effect.

Medications prescribed to treat spasticity include dantrolene (Dantrium), baclofen (Lioresal), tizanidine (Zanaflex), clonidine (Catapress), and diazepam (Valium). All of these agents have sedating properties, and so they are most commonly used in the treatment of mass spasms and clonus, but less so for spastic hypertonus. Dantrolene is characteristically described as the preferred antispasticity agent in traumatic brain injury. However, it also has dose- and duration-dependent toxicity, a concern in a young person who may require the medication for decades. Baclofen given at night often decreases spasms and pain in the patient with stroke and brain injury, and it is safe for chronic use. Tizanidine is similar to baclofen in its side effect profile, and should be tried with patients who cannot tolerate the latter medication. The team should be informed when dosing changes are made, as all antispasticity agents weaken muscles, including those of deglutition, predisposing to swallowing difficulties and aspiration pneumonia. All team members are responsible for alerting the physician that dosing changes may be needed to achieve an optimal balance between spasticity treatment and side effects from excessive dosing. Refer to Appendix A for further information on specific medications used to treat spasticity.

Surgical interventions for spasticity management include orthopedic tenotomies as well as neurosurgical ablative and nondestructive procedures. Rhizotomy was commonly performed to treat severe spasticity refractory to therapies, nerve blocks, and medications, but is more and more frequently being supplanted by baclofen pump implantation. This pump is implanted in the abdominal wall without the need to destroy healthy tissue, and a catheter delivers baclofen to the lumbar spinal cord to decrease lower extremity spasticity. Some drug may ascend to decrease upper extremity spasticity, but excessive rostral delivery may compromise respiratory function. A "generalization phenomenon" noted with Botox and phenol injections in which sites remote from the treated site may exhibit remission of spasticity via segmental spinal cord interaction

may also explain the mechanism by which upper extremity spasticity is occasionally decreased with baclofen pump technology. Adjunctive nerve blocks to the upper extremities are often required, and continual physical therapy treatment to maximize independent function is mandatory.

In cases where the patient has severe spasticity that continues to impede functional progress, the individual can be referred to a spasticity clinic. The team working in a spasticity clinic usually consists of a physiatrist, physical therapist, and occupational therapist. They will evaluate the effectiveness of existing interventions and systematically try new ones in an effort to improve the patient's function and pain relief.

Adaptive Equipment

Due to the wide variety of impairments and resulting functional limitations and disability that the patient with brain injury may have, he or she is likely to benefit from the use of adaptive equipment to enhance abilities and increase independence. With today's advanced computer technology, adaptive equipment can range from a simple letter board used for communication to a complex *environmental control unit (ECU)* that will allow the individual to open doors, answer the telephone, and turn on the television from his or her wheelchair. A wheelchair is a form of adaptive equipment that the physical therapist is likely to prescribe to enhance functional mobility. Wheelchairs can range from manual to power. With today's technology, a power wheelchair can be controlled in a variety of ways. These include a joystick, sip and puff, head control, tongue control, or even a single switch. Seating systems can be adapted so the patient can perform independent pressure reliefs using a power system. It must be kept in mind, however, that using a power wheelchair, especially one controlled with just one switch, requires a great deal of cognitive skill. Refer to Chapter 32 for further discussion on wheelchairs.

Goal Setting and Outcome Prediction

This is probably the most difficult aspect of working with the patient with traumatic brain injury. From the acute stage through rehabilitation, there are very few reliable indicators of eventual outcome. Nevertheless, it is important to attempt to set realistic goals and outcomes, and modify them as necessary. Hopefully, with experience, therapists learn to identify trends and make more accurate predictions. For this to occur, therapists need to make concentrated attempts to look for such trends. Likelihood of success is increased with interdisciplinary cooperation and interactions with senior staff or clinical specialists. Of particular interest is the possibility of combining the results of formal neuropsychological testing with functional information gathered by the physical therapist, occupational therapist, and speech/language pathologist to predict learning potential and functional outcome. Efforts to set goals and plan treatments for a patient with a brain injury are strengthened by a thorough understanding of his or her learning capacity. Ideally, the goal is for patients to be able to perform a wide variety of tasks consistently, automatically, and in a variety of situations. However, if it were determined that a particular patient had very little ability to generalize information from one situation to another, then it might be reasonable to practice very specific skills in the environment in which the patient would need to use them. Although this might be considered to be a very low level of functioning, it may optimize that particular patient's potential.

There is much to be learned about physical therapy interventions for patients with brain injury. There are a great many studies on the cognitive aspects and interventions with this population, but there is very little research on motor control and motor learning. Most studies examining motor learning have not included subjects with brain injury. Most studies examining learning in the patient with brain injury have not focused on motor skills. Guidelines for the application of motor learning principles to patients with brain injury are available, but further research is needed.[56]

Issues related to outcome in brain injury rehabilitation are extremely complex. Although we are able to identify early recovery patterns in a very general sense, it is significantly more difficult to characterize long-term outcome. Researchers at the University of Virginia studied brain injury survivors at 3 months post injury and found that 4 percent were vegetative, 8 percent were severely disabled, 22 percent were moderately disabled, and 66 percent had made a good recovery.[57] It is important to note, however, that studies such as this tend to look at recovery from a point of view that reflects a medical perspective of recovery. In this age of competition for the health care dollar, the availability of lengthy and expensive rehabilitation can no longer be taken for granted,

even for those with health insurance. A central question in the administration of brain injury services today is, "Who is the customer?" Payers, families, professionals, and survivors of brain injury may have different perceptions about what constitutes a successful outcome. Being able to live independently, have earned income, and manage daily activities and affairs are usually outcomes that survivors strive for. Many are able to reach this level of independence, and many are not. At this point, our ability to predict who will and who will not is limited. The field of brain injury rehabilitation provides a wealth of challenging questions for researchers from many fields.

SUMMARY

A traumatic brain injury is a devastating and life-changing event for the individual and his or her family. The resulting impairments make working with the patient with brain injury extremely rewarding and challenging. There are a multitude of issues to consider. The physical therapist must adapt traditional physical therapy examination and intervention techniques to the unique motor control, cognitive, and behavioral challenges that are presented. The interdisciplinary team offers a unique opportunity for the physical therapist to learn and grow. By working together with a team, the physical therapist is able to provide appropriate care that will help the brain injury survivor reach maximum potential.

The authors and editors gratefully acknowledge the contributions of Patricia Leahy, PT, NCS. Her expertise and commitment to excellence have enriched this chapter and the profession.

QUESTIONS FOR REVIEW

1. Discuss how premorbid status, primary brain injury, and secondary brain injury influence the final outcomes for patients with traumatic brain injury.

2. Describe local, polar, and diffuse brain injury in terms of areas commonly affected and the most common mechanisms of injury. Is it possible for one patient to have more than one type?

3. What is meant by secondary injury? Give three examples of secondary brain injury.

4. Describe how each of the following rating scales is utilized: Glasgow Coma Scale, Rancho Los Amigos Levels of Cognitive Functioning Scale, Rappaport's Disability Rating Scale, Glasgow Outcome Scale.

5. List and describe three procedures that augment the standard neurological examination in diagnosing and establishing a prognosis for patients with brain injury.

6. Describe the role of the physical therapist in the management of the patient with brain injury who is in the no response, generalized response, and localized response levels of recovery (LOCF).

7. How would a physical therapy plan of care need to be modified for a patient with post-traumatic amnesia?

8. What is the significance of a patient's cognitive and behavioral status in relation to his or her physical therapy goals and outcomes?

9. List and describe key elements in planning interventions appropriate for the patient in the confused-inappropriate and confused-appropriate stages of recovery.

10. How does knowledge of a patient's ability or inability to learn new information affect a physical therapist's plan of care?

11. Describe the importance of the team approach in treating the patient with brain injury. Describe the roles of key members of the team in the acute rehabilitation setting.

12. List the important aspects of patient and family education in the low, middle, and high levels of recovery.

13. Why is it especially important to monitor the effects of different medications in this patient

population? Describe the difference between lipophobic and lipophilic medications. Why is one more appropriate for the patient with brain injury than the other?

14. List and describe key elements in planning interventions appropriate for the patient in the confused-agitated stage of recovery.

CASE STUDY

Part A. The patient is a 34 year-old female who was involved in a motor vehicle accident (MVA). She was struck by another car as she exited her car. The patient suffered a severe closed brain injury. She was taken to a local hospital. CT scan revealed a right temporal parietal hemorrhage, a left parietal hemorrhage, diffuse edema, and multiple contusions. At the acute hospital, the patient underwent a ventriculostomy, gastrostomy tube placement, and tracheostomy. Her ICP was slightly elevated. The ventriculostomy was removed approximately 2 weeks after her initial injury. Approximately 6 weeks after her initial injury, the patient was transferred to an acute rehabilitation hospital.

PAST MEDICAL HISTORY: Healthy, 34 year-old female with no significant past medical history.

SOCIAL HISTORY: Patient worked as an administrative assistant at a college. She was very active in the community. She enjoyed outdoor activities and was president of the local Sierra Club chapter. She has a very supportive fiancé (who was at the scene of the accident) and mother. Patient is right handed.

PHYSICAL THERAPY EXAMINATION FINDINGS

Arousal/Consciousness
- Patient's eyes are open with random eye movements, but not able to track to auditory or visual stimuli. Patient does blink eyes when startled.
- Patient does not respond to verbal commands.
- Patient not able to vocalize, or make any attempt at communication.

Vital Signs
- Heart rate: 72
- Blood pressure: 124/72
- Respiratory rate: 12

Motor Control
- Patient presents with decorticate posturing.
- Nonpurposeful movement in bilateral upper and lower extremities, more movement on right side than left.
- No active dorsiflexion exhibited on either side.
- Increased extensor tone bilateral lower extremities, 3 on left and 2 on right (modified Ashworth scale).
- Increased flexor tone in bilateral upper extremities, 3 on left and 2 on right (modified Ashworth scale). Multi-beat continuous clonus left plantarflexors, and 2 to 3 beat clonus right plantarflexors.

Joint Integrity and Passive Range of Motion (PROM)
- Bilateral lower extremities WNL except right DF: −14 degrees from neutral and left DF: −24 degrees from neutral.
- Right upper extremity WNL.

- Left upper extremity WNL except shoulder abduction: 0–86 degrees, flexion: 0–94 degrees, external rotation: 0–45 degrees, elbow extension: −18 degrees. One finger subluxation left shoulder.

Postural Control and Balance
- Patient requires maximal assistance of one to sit on edge of bed.
- Requires minimal to moderate assistance to maintain head control in sitting.
- Patient inconsistently exhibits delayed equilibrium and protective reactions in sitting.
- Patient tolerated sitting for approximately 5 minutes, and then patient exhibited increase in tone and respiratory rate.

Functional Mobility
- Patient is dependent for all mobility. This includes rolling, moving to and from supine and sitting, transfers, and wheelchair mobility.
- Patient is not able to stand.
- FIM scores: bed/chair transfers: 1, walk: 1, w/c: 1, stairs: 1.

OTHER FINDINGS
- Patient has tracheostomy intact.
- She exhibits dysphagia and is NPO except for trial feedings with the speech/language pathologist.
- Patient has stage three decubiti on bilateral heels.
- She also has an infection, methicillin-resistant *Staphylococcus aureus* (MRSA), in lungs. As a result of this, patient is on contact precautions. Gown, gloves, and mask should be worn when working with the patient.

MEDICATIONS
- Vancomyacin: 250 mg via IV q 12 hours for 5 days, for the infection.
- Heparin: 5000 U, subcutaneous q 12 hours, to prevent DVT.
- Ativan: 1 mg via G-tube, PRN, q 6 hours, in case of any increased agitation.

Guiding Questions

1. Categorize the patient's level of consciousness upon admission to the acute rehabilitation hospital based on the Glasgow Coma Scale and level of cognitive functioning based on the Ranchos Los Amigos LOCF.

2. Categorize her problems in terms of direct impairments, indirect impairments, and functional limitations.

3. Describe three physical therapy interventions that would be appropriate for this patient at this time. Include at least one related to family education.

Part B. The patient described above has continued to progress. She is still in the acute rehabilitation hospital and it is now 7 weeks later, 13 weeks post-injury.

PHYSICAL THERAPY EXAMINATION FINDINGS

Motor Control
- Increased extensor tone left lower extremity, 2 on modified Ashworth scale. Left upper extremity flexor tone, 2 on modified Ashworth scale. Right upper and lower extremity tone WNL.
- Patient exhibits full AROM at all muscle groups in right upper and lower extremity.
- Strength is in G/G–(4/4–) range at all muscle groups on right except dorsiflexion is F–(3–) and hip abduction is F+(3+).
- Patient exhibits ½ to ¾ AROM against gravity in left upper and lower extremity at all muscle groups except trace dorsiflexion.
- Patient exhibits impaired coordination in all four extremities, worse on left than right. Delayed initiation, dysdiadochokinesia, and slower speed of movement on left. Accuracy decreases with increase in speed of movement with all four extremities. Minimally ataxic gait pattern.

PROM: WNL all four extremities except right dorsiflexion: 0 degrees, left dorsiflexion: –10 degrees from neutral (patient has on a short leg serial cast on left), left elbow extension: –5 degrees.

Sensation: Intact throughout to light touch, pin prick, deep pressure, hot/cold, and proprioception.

Postural Control/Balance
- Sitting: static, patient able to maintain sitting balance with moderate challenges; dynamic, patient able to reach moderately outside BOS and maintain balance.
- Standing: static, patient able to stand for 3 to 5 minutes with minimal assistance; dynamic, patient requires moderate assistance to ambulate 35 feet. Decreased weight-bearing on left lower extremity.

Patient exhibits protective reactions in sitting, delayed to both left and right, slower to left than right. Patient also exhibits righting reactions both in sitting and standing. Both are moderately delayed, greater delay in standing than sitting.

Functional Mobility
- Bed mobility: rolling to left, independent; rolling to right, minimal assistance; supine-to-sit, minimal to moderate assistance; sit-to-supine, supervision. Patient requires two to three verbal cues with all the above, except for rolling to left, for technique.
- Transfers: Bed to and from w/c, moderate assistance; stand pivot to left or right. Patient requires two to three verbal cues to correctly position w/c and to lock brakes.
- Wheelchair mobility: Patient able to propel w/c

150 feet with supervision and verbal cues. Patient uses bilateral lower extremities to propel w/c.
- Ambulation: Patient able to ambulate 35 feet with moderate assistance, forearm crutch in right upper extremity, and hinged AFO with plantarflexion block set at 0 degrees on right lower extremity.
- Stairs: Unable to perform at this time.
- FIM score: Bed/chair transfers: 3, walk: 1, w/c: 1, stairs: 1.

OTHER DISCIPLINES FINDINGS

Cognition: Patient exhibits short-term memory impairments. She is inconsistently disoriented to place and time. Oriented to person 100 percent of the time. Patient able to follow two- to three-step commands when in a closed environment. When in an open environment, the patient is only able to follow one-step commands. Patient exhibits decreased insight into deficits and impaired safety awareness. Patient is easily distracted, able to attend to task for only 5 minutes at best.

Communication: Patient exhibits expressive aphasia. She is able to make basic needs known using verbal language and gestures. She exhibits severe word retrieval deficits. Her receptive language skills are WNL.

Vision and Perception: WNL.

OTHER INFORMATION: Patient's tracheostomy has been removed, and her infection is cleared. The only medication the patient is taking is bromocriptine. She has a custom-fit hinged AFO with a plantarflexion block for her right foot, and her left foot and ankle are casted in a short leg serial cast. She wears a bivalve elbow extension brace on her left elbow at night. She had previously undergone serial casting at her left elbow. Her skin on both heels is now intact.

Guiding Questions
4. Describe how this patient's memory impairments will affect physical therapy interventions and how the physical therapist should tailor interventions to maximize the patient's motor learning abilities.
5. List five possible goals and outcomes for this patient.
6. Describe two interventions that would be appropriate for this patient.

Part C. It is now approximately 5 months after the initial accident. The same patient is now discharged home with her husband. She married her fiancé during the last week of her stay in the rehabilitation hospital. She returns to the rehabilitation hospital to participate in the day treatment program from 8:30 to 3:30 Monday through Friday. The patient requires 24-hour supervision due to continuing cognitive, communication, and mobility impairments.

PHYSICAL THERAPY EXAMINATION FINDINGS

Motor Control

- Tone: WNL all four extremities.
- Coordination: Impaired in both upper and lower extremities. Slowed movement, accuracy decreases with increase in speed, worse on left than right. Minimally ataxic gait pattern.
- Strength: Right upper extremity WNL. Right lower extremity WNL except dorsiflexion: F+. Left upper extremity G at all muscle groups. Left lower extremity G at all muscle groups except dorsiflexion: F– and hip abduction: F–.

PROM: WNL all four extremities except right dorsiflexion, 0–8 degrees; left dorsiflexion, 0 degrees.

Postural Control

- Sitting: static, WNL; dynamic, WNL. Balance reactions WNL.
- Standing: Static, able to maintain balance with minimal challenges; dynamic balance reactions minimally delayed.

Functional Mobility

- Bed mobility: Rolling to left and right, independent. Moving to and from sit and supine, independent.
- Transfers: W/c to and from bed, supervision with one to two verbal cues for safety and locking brakes. Floor-to-stand, moderate assistance.
- Wheelchair mobility: Independent in the home.
- Ambulation: Supervised 300 feet in a closed environment (home or in the hospital) with bilateral hinged AFOs with plantarflexion blocks. The right one is set at 5 degrees of plantarflexion, and the left one is set at neutral. She uses a forearm crutch in the right upper extremity. In an open environment, the patient requires contact guard to minimal assistance to ambulate.
- Stairs: Contact guard up and down one flight with bilateral AFOs and one railing.
- FIM scores: Bed/chair transfers: 5, walk: 5, wheelchair: 5, stairs: 4.

Cognition: Patient oriented to person, place, and time 100 percent of the time. Patient has shown improvement in short-term memory and new learning; however, she is still impaired in this area. She is able to follow four- to five-step commands in a closed environment. Patient performs best in a highly structured environment. In an open environment, patient becomes easily distracted, needing verbal cues to complete a task. Patient's insight and safety awareness have improved, but they are still impaired. For example, she requires verbal reminders not to transfer or ambulate independently.

Communication: Patient exhibits moderate word finding deficits and anomia (inability to remember names of objects).

Guiding Questions

7. List and prioritize the patient's direct impairments, indirect impairments, and functional limitations.

8. Describe two interventions appropriate for this patient. At least one intervention should focus on community re-entry.

REFERENCES

1. Dobkin B: Neurological Rehabilitation. FA Davis, Philadelphia, 1996, p 257.
2. Interagency Head Injury Task Force Report, National Institute of Neurological Disorders and Stroke. National Institutes of Health, Bethesda, MD, 1989.
3. Rubin, R, et al: The Cost of Disorders of the Brain. Foundation for Brain Research, Washington, DC, 1992.
4. Miller, J, et al: Early evaluation and management. In Rosenthal M, et al. (eds): Rehabilitation of the Adult and Child with Traumatic Brain Injury, ed 2. FA Davis, Philadelphia, 1990, p 21.
5. Adams J: Head injury. In Adams, J, et al (eds): Greenfield's Neuropathology, ed 4. Edward Arnold, London, 1984, p 85.
6. Katz D: Neuropathology and neurobehavioral recovery from closed head injury. J Head Trauma Rehabil 7:1, 1992.
7. Jennett, B, and Teasdale, G: Management of Head Injuries. FA Davis, Philadelphia, 1981.
8. Teasdale, G, et al: Observer variability in assessing impaired consciousness and coma. J Neurol Neurosurg Psychiatr 41:603, 1978.
9. Rehabilitation of the Head Injured Adult. Professional Staff Association, Ranchos Los Amigos Hospital, Downey, CA, 1979.
10. Rappaport, M, et al: Disability rating scale for severe head trauma coma to community. Arch Phys Med Rehabil 63:118, 1982.
11. Jennett, B, et al: Disability after severe head injury: Observations on the use of the Glasgow Outcome Scale. J Neurol Neurosurg Psychiatr 44:285, 1981.
12. Thatcher, R, et al: Comparisons between EEG, CT scan, and Glasgow Coma Scale predictors of recovery of function in neurotrauma patients. In Zappulla R, (ed): Windows on the Brain: Neuropsychology's Technological Frontiers. New York Academy of Science, New York, 1991.
13. French, B, and Dublin, A: The value of computerized tomography in the management of 1000 consecutive head injuries. Surg Neurol 7:171, 1977.
14. Jenkins, A, et al: Brain lesions detected by magnetic resonance imaging in mild and severe head injury. Lancet ii:445, 1986.
15. Langfitt, T, et al: Computerized tomography, magnetic resonance imaging, and positron emission tomography in the study of brain trauma: Preliminary observations. J Neurosurg 64:760, 1986.
16. Wilson, J, and Wyper, D: Neuroimaging and neuropsychological functioning following closed head trauma: CT, MRI, and SPECT. J Head Trauma Rehabil 7:29, 1992.
17. Lichtigfeld, FJ, and Gillman, MA: Methylphenidate for reversal of drug-induced coma. Clin Neuropharmacol 13:459, 1990.
18. Worzniak, M, et al: Methylphenidate in the treatment of coma. J Fam Pract 44:495, 1997.
19. Haig, AJ, and Ruess, JM: Recovery from vegetative state six months duration associated with Sinemet (Levodopa/Carbidopa). Arch Phys Med Rehabil 71:1081, 1990.
20. Fleet, WS, et al: Dopamine agonist therapy for neglect in humans. Neurology 37:1765, 1987.
21. Cardenas, DD, et al: Oral physostigmine and impaired memory in adults with brain injury. Brain Inj 8:579, 1994.
22. Rowin, J, and Lewis, SL: Spontaneous bilateral subdural hematomas associated with chronic Ginko biloba ingestion. Neurology 46:1775, 1996.

23. Gupta, SR, and Mlcoch, AG: Bromocriptine treatment of nonfluent aphasia. Arch Phys Med Rehabil 73:373, 1992.
24. Walker-Baston, D, et al: Use of amphetamine in the treatment of aphasia. Restorative Neurology and Neuroscience 4:47, 1992.
25. Huber, W, et al: Piracetam as an adjuvant to language therapy for aphasia: A randomized double-blind placebo-controlled pilot study. Arch Phys Med Rehabil 78:245, 1997.
26. Goldstein, LB: Potential effects of common drugs on stroke recovery. Arch Neurol 55:454, 1998.
27. Feeney, DM: From laboratory to clinic: Noradrenergic enhancement of physical therapy for stroke or trauma patients. Brain Plasticity, Advances in Neurology 383, 1997.
28. Jenkins, SC, and Maruta, T: Therapeutic use of propranolol for intermittent explosive disorder. Mayo Clin Proc 62:204, 1987.
29. Horn, LJ: Atypical medications for the treatment of disruptive, aggressive behavior in the brain-injured patient. J Head Trauma Rehabil 2:18, 1987.
30. Schiffer, RD, et al: Treatment of pathologic laughing and weeping with amitryptyline. N Engl J Med 312:1480, 1985.
31. Sloan, RL, et al: Fluoxetine as a treatment for emotional lability after brain injury. Brain Inj 6:315, 1992.
32. O'Connor, M, and Baker, W: Depo-medroxyprogesterone acetate as an adjunctive treatment in three aggressive schizophrenic patients. Acta Psychiatr Scand 67:399, 1983.
33. Mackay, L, et al: Team-focused intervention within critical care. In Mackay, L, et al (eds): Maximizing Brain Injury Recovery Integrating Critical Care and Early Rehabilitation. Aspen, Gaithersburg, MD, 1997, p 56.
34. Senelick, R, and Ryan, C: Living with Brain Injury: A Guide for Families. HealthSouth Press, Birmingham, AL, 1998.
35. Davies, P: Starting Again Early Rehabilitation After Traumatic Brain Injury or Other Severe Brain Lesion. Springer-Verlag, Berlin, 1994.
36. Semlyen, J, et al: Traumatic brain injury: Efficacy of multidisciplinary rehabilitation. Arch Phys Med Rehabil 79:678, 1998.
37. Morgan, A, et al: Respiratory management of the brain-injured patient. In Mackay, L, et al (eds): Maximizing Brain Injury Recovery Integrating Critical Care and Early Rehabilitation. Aspen, Gaithersburg, MD, 1997, p 331.
38. Rappaport, M, et al: Head injury outcome up to ten years later. Arch Phys Med Rehabil 70:885, 1989.
39. Chapman, P: Physical Therapy in the Intensive Care Unit. In Mackay, L, et al (eds): Maximizing Brain Injury Recovery Integrating Critical Care and Early Rehabilitation. Aspen, Gaithersburg, MD, 1997, p 271.
40. Griffith, E, and Mayer, N: Hypertonicity and movement disorders. In Rosenthal, M, et al (eds): Rehabilitation of the Adult and Child with Traumatic Brain Injury, ed 2. FA Davis, Philadelphia, 1990, p 127.
41. Gordon, W, et al: The benefits of exercise in individuals with traumatic brain injury: A retrospective study. J Head Trauma Rehabil 13:58, 1998.
42. American Physical Therapy Association: Guide to Physical Therapist Practice. APTA, Alexandria, VA, 1999.
43. Ansell, B: Slow-to-recover brain-injured patients: Rationale for treatment. J Speech Hear Res 34:1017, 1991.
44. Wilson, S, et al: Vegetative state and response to sensory stimulation: An analysis of 24 cases. Brain Inj 10:807, 1996.
45. Wood, R: Critical analysis of the concept of sensory stimulation for patients in vegetative states. Brain Inj 5:401, 1991.
46. Horn, H, and Garland, D: Medical and orthopedic complications associated with traumatic brain injury. In Rosenthal, M, et al (eds): Rehabilitation of the Adult and Child with Traumatic Brain Injury, ed 2. FA Davis, Philadelphia, 1990, p 107.
47. Rinehart, M: Strategies for improving motor performance. In Rosenthal, M, et al (eds): Rehabilitation of the Adult and Child with Traumatic Brain Injury, ed 2. FA Davis, Philadelphia, 1990, p 331.
48. O'Sullivan, SB, and Schmitz, TJ: Physical Rehabilitation Laboratory Manual: Focus on Functional Training. FA Davis, Philadelphia, 1999.
49. Mercer, L, and Boch, M: Residual sensorimotor deficits in the adult head-injured patient. Phys Ther 63:1988, 1983.
50. Leahy, P: Precasting worksheet: An assessment tool. Phys Ther 68:72, 1988.
51. Carlson, S: A neurophysiological analysis of inhibitive casting. Physical and Occupational Therapy in Pediatrics 4:31, 1984.
52. Cusick, B: Serial Casts: Their Use in the Management of Spasticity Induced Foot Deformity. Words at Work, Lexington, KY, 1987.
53. Baker, LL: Clinical uses of neuromuscular electrical stimulation. In Nelson, RM, and Currier, DP, (eds): Clinical Electrotherapy, ed 2. Appleton & Lange, Norwalk, CN, 1991, p 143.
54. Glenn, MB: Nerve blocks for the treatment of spasticity. Phys Med and Rehabil: State of the Art Rev 8:481, 1994.
55. Geller, AG: Botulinum toxin [versus phenol for spasticity]. Arch Phys Med Rehabil 78:233, 1997.
56. Riolo-Quinn, L: Motor learning considerations in treating brain injured patients. Neurology Reports 14:12, 1990.
57. Rimel, RW, et al: Characteristics of the head-injured patient. In Rosenthal, M, et al (eds): Rehabilitation of the Adult and Child with Traumatic Brain Injury, ed 2. FA Davis, Philadelphia, 1990, p 8.
58. Kaplitz, SE: Withdrawn, apathetic geriatric patients responsive to methylphenidate. J Am Geriatr Soc 28:271, 1975.
59. Clark, ANG, and Mankikar, GD: d-Amphetamine in elderly patients refractory to rehabilitation procedures. J Am Geriatr Soc 27:174, 1979.
60. Wroblewski, BA, et al: Methylphenidate and seizure frequency in brain injured patients with seizure disorders. J Clin Psychiatr 53:86, 1992.
61. Andrews, DG, et al: A comparative study of the cognitive effects of phenytoin and carbamazepine in new referrals with epilepsy. Epilepsia 27:128, 1986.
62. Dodrill, CB, and Troupin, AS: Psychotropic effects of carbamazepine in epilepsy: A double blind comparison with phenytoin. Neurology 27:1023, 1977.
63. Miller, LG, and Jankovic, J: Metoclopramide-induced movement disorders. Arch Intern Med 149:2486, 1989.
64. Samie, MR, et al: Life-threatening tardive dyskinesia caused by metoclopramide. Movement Disorders 2:125, 1987.
65. Bohannon, R, and Smith, M: Interrater reliability of a modified Ashworth scale of muscle spasticity. Phys Ther 67:206, 1987.

SUPPLEMENTAL READINGS

Bergen, A, and Colangelo, C: Positioning the Client with Central Nervous System Dysfunction. Valhalla Rehab Publications, Valhalla, New York, 1985.
Eames, P: Management of behavior disorders. Journal of Head Trauma Rehabilitation 3, 1988.
Finger, S, et al (eds): Brain Injury and Recovery. Plenum, New York, 1988.
Friedman, WA: Head injuries. Ciba Clinical Symposia 35, 1983.
Griffith, E, and Lemberg, S: Sexuality and the Person with Traumatic Brain Injury. FA Davis, Philadelphia, 1993.
Horn, LJ, and Cope, DN (eds): Traumatic brain injury. Phys Med Rehabil 3, 1989.

Katz, DI, and Alexander, MP (eds): The neurology of head injury. Journal of Head Trauma Rehabilitation 7, 1992.
Kreutzer, JS, and Wehman, P (eds): Community Integration Following Traumatic Brain Injury. Paul H Brookes, Baltimore, 1990.
Kreutzer, JS, and Wehman, PH (eds): Cognitive Rehabilitation for Persons with Traumatic Brain Injury: A Functional Approach. Paul H Brookes, Baltimore, 1991.
Levin, HS, et al: Neurobehavioral Consequences of Closed Head Injury. Oxford University Press, New York, 1982.
Zasler, ND, et al: Coma stimulation and coma recovery: A critical review. Neuro Rehabil 1:3340, 1991.

GLOSSARY

Autodestructive cellular phenomena: A series of events that occur in the brain due to trauma-induced changes in cellular membranes.

Coma: A state of unconsciousness in which there is no eye opening (even to pain), failure to obey commands, and inability to utter recognizable words.

Coup-contrecoup injury: Coup contusions occur at the site of contact while contrecoup contusions occur in brain tissue opposite the point of contact.

Decerebrate rigidity: Tonic posturing of the limbs in extension.

Decorticate rigidity: Tonic posturing of the upper limbs in flexion and the lower limbs in extension.

Diffuse axonal injury (DAI): Widely scattered shearing of axons which, although not intense in any one location, causes dramatic disability as a result of its cumulative effect.

Glascow Coma Scale (GCS): A scale that documents level of consciousness and severity of brain injury; based on best motor response, verbal response, and eye opening.

Herniation: Protrusion of an organ or part of an organ through a surrounding wall or cavity. In the brain, several types of herniation occur. The following herniations are listed in order of progressing severity.

    Central herniation: Protrusion of the midbrain and pons through the tentorial notch.

    Tonsillar herniation: Protrusion of the medulla and cerebellar tonsils through the foramen magnum.

    Uncal herniation: Protrusion of the uncus and hippocampal gyrus of the brain through the tentorial notch.

Heterotopic ossication: Abnormal bone growth in soft tissue that may result in loss of range of motion. The most common locations are the shoulder, elbow, and hip.

Hypoxic-ischemic injury (HII): Brain damage that results from arterial hypotension and hypoxemia and is complicated by raised intracranial pressure, cerebral vasospasm, brain edema, and combinations of these, as well as an impaired ability of the vessels of the brain to autoregulate.

Intracranial hematoma: A collection of blood within the cranium that results from leakage from a blood vessel.

    Epidural hematoma: Extravascular blood mass located between the dura and the skull.

    Intracerebral hematoma: Extravascular blood mass located within the brain tissue.

    Subdural hematoma: Extravascular blood mass located beneath the dura.

Intracranial pressure (ICP): Measure of pressure inside the cranium. Normal ICP is 5 to10 mmHg.

Local brain damage: Injury localized to the area of the brain underlying the site of impact. Produces predictable neurological signs according to the specific location.

Nerve block: Administration of a local anesthetic to a peripheral nerve for the purpose of decreasing spasticity.

Obstructive hydrocephalus: Enlargement of the ventricles of the brain caused by an impairment of flow and absorption of cerebrospinal fluid.

Persistant vegetative state (PVS): Failure to evolve out of vegetative state by 12 months (in trauma) or 3 months (in anoxia).

Polar brain damage: Injury that results from contact between the surfaces of the brain and the cranium. Most commonly affects the frontal and temporal lobes.

Post-traumatic amnesia (PTA): State during the time between injury and when the patient is able to form memories of ongoing events.

Post-traumatic epilepsy: Seizure disorder that develops following head trauma.

Rancho Los Amigos Scale of Level of Cognitive Function (LOCF): A descriptive scale that outlines a predictable sequence of cognitive and behavioral recovery seen in individuals with traumatic brain injury.

Serial casting: Repeated application and removal of casts for the purpose of increasing passive range of motion, and decreasing tone.

Vegetative state (VS): A state of unconsciousness marked by the return of irregular sleep/wake cycles and normalization of so-called vegetative functions: respiration, digestion, blood pressure control. The cortex is permanently damaged.

APPENDIX A

Pharmacology: Pain

Agent	Side Effects, Comments
Ben-Gay	Ben-Gay is a topical medication whose only dangers are inadvertent application to the eyes if the hands are not thoroughly cleansed after self-application. No cognitive side effects occur with Ben-Gay, and so it is a preferred analgesic in the brain-injured population.
Acetaminophen (Tylenol)	This medication is a more potent analgesic than most people realize. However, it is antipyretic, so fever is extinguished and fewer alerting signs are present to suggest infection. This is why topical modalities such as ice and heat as well as topical medications are often preferred.
Calcitonin (Miacalcin)	Miacalcin is calcitonin, an endogenous hormone. It frequently reduces neuropathic as well as somatic pain without any cognitive sequelae.
NSAIDs	Aspirin and other NSAIDs are extremely effective to decrease pain. Patients taking concomitant anticoagulants should receive choline magnesium trisalicylate (Trilisate) or salsalate (Disalcid), the only NSAIDs, that do not affect platelet aggregation and bleeding. Any patient with a history of a GI bleed, and most post-traumatic patients, should receive ulcer prophylaxis medications such as ranitidine (Zantac), misoprostol (Cytotec), or omeprazole (Prilosec).
Narcotics	Weak analgesics such as propoxyphene and codeine have limited cognitive side effects, but in the patient with a brain injury, slowed thought processing and exacerbation of impaired memory, attention, and orientation may occur. Meperidine (Demerol) should be avoided, because its active metabolite may cause seizures. Combination medications such as Darvocet and Percocet must be monitored, as high dosing of these narcotics and acetaminophen combination drugs may cause liver toxicity from excess acetaminophen.

Pharmacology: Insomnia

Agent	Side Effects, Comments
Melatonin	This endogenous hormone is produced in decreasing quantities as people age. It is extremely safe, and may promote natural re-establishment of sleep wake cycles.
Trazodone	Priapism may occur in males with the need for emergent urosurgical reduction, but it is extremely safe and effective in females
Zolpidem (Ambien)	Half-life is only 2.5 hours, so daytime sedation is less common than with benzodiazepines.
Temazepam (Restoril)	As with all benzodiazepines, long-term use causes mood depression, irritability, physical and psychogenic addiction, and memory dysfunction. However, this agent has an 8-hour half-life and may promote restful sleep during the inpatient stay, allowing optimal participation during the following day's therapy session.
Amitriptyline (Elavil)	Undesirable, because potent anticholinergic-mediated side effects include cardiac arrhythmias, urinary retention, acute glaucoma, confusion, constipation, and xerostomia.

Pharmacology: Mood Depression

Agent	Side Effects, Comments
Methylphenidate (Ritalin)	Reversal of depression is often achieved much faster than with conventional tricyclic antidepressants such as amitriptyline (Elavil), nortriptyline (Pamelor), and desipramine. Ritalin is safe even with patients over 90 years of age[58,59] and has been suggested to have anticonvulsant properties.[60]
Paroxetine (Paxil)	Generally extremely well tolerated, but mania, seizures, and extrapyramidal side effects may be seen at high doses. Similar agents include sertraline (Zoloft) and fluoxetine (Prozac).

Note: Patients must be monitored for appetite suppression from methylphenidate or seratonergic antidepressants, because megesterol (Megace), oxandrolone, cyproheptadine, dronabinol, and several other agents may be used to stimulate appetite to allow patients to tolerate the antidepressant. Tricyclic antidepressants such as amitriptyline are often less well tolerated than methylphenidate or seratonergic agonist antidepressants.

Continued

APPENDIX A Continued

Pharmacology: Seizures

Agent	Side Effects, Comments
Carbamazepine (Tegretol)	Confusion, tachycardia, bone marrow suppression, hepatotoxicity, and hyponatremia may occur. However, cognitive side effects are often less than those identified with phenytoin (Dilantin).[61,62]
Valproic acid	Confusion, bone marrow suppression, and hepatotoxicity may occur with valproic acid, but cognitive sequelae may be less than with phenytoin and slightly more than carbamazepine.
Phenytoin (Dilantin)	Confusion, bone marrow suppression, hepatotoxicity, cerebellar degeneration, anemia, and peripheral neuropathy occur with phenytoin, making it less desirable than carbamazepine or valproate. Confusion is far less than with phenobarbitol or primidone, more than carbamazepine.
Phenobarbitol	This medication is extremely sedating, especially after brain injury. Like phenytoin, it has the advantage of being able to be delivered via IV access for rapid loading in the emergency room, but should be tapered to off when carbamazepine or valproate have been added and are therapeutic.
Gabapentin (Neurontin)	Confusion may be seen at higher doses, but this medication is extremely safe, and far less sedating than phenobarbitol or primidone, but not FDA approved for tonic-clonic seizure prophylaxis.

Note: Often, anticonvulsants can be tapered 1–3 months after TBI or stroke, especially if the patient is still in the inpatient setting and can be closely monitored. This often profoundly improves cognition.

Pharmacology: Antipsychotics

Agent	Side Effects, Comments
Haloperidol (Haldol)	Irreversible tardive dyskinesia after even a single dose, seizures, confusion, and fatal neuroleptic malignant syndrome may occur with haloperidol and other antipsychotics. It is a potent antipsychotic to treat delusions and hallucinations. If the goal of treatment is sedation to treat dangerous disinhibited aggressive behavior, however, then chlorpromazine (Thorazine) may be a better antipsychotic selection.
Chlorpromazine (Thorazine)	This drug has the same side effects as haloperidol, but less risk for tardive dyskinesia because it is a less potent antipsychotic. However, it has more sedating side effect properties as well as greater risk for orthostatic hypotension.
Clozapine	Seizures, bone marrow suppression, and sedation occur with clozapine, but this is the only antipsychotic without risk for tardive dyskinesia. In addition, it may also improve the amotivational signs of schizophrenia, which are exacerbated with any other antipsychotics.
Risperidone	As with other new "atypical" antipsychotics such as nefazodone (Serzone) and olanzepine, it has far less risk of tardive dyskinesia relative to older agents such as haloperidol.

Pharmacoloay: Nausea, Gastric Stasis

Agent	Side Effects, Comments
Cisapride (Propulsid)	Gastric ulcers as well as arrhythmias may occur if this medication is given with other drugs that increase the Q-T interval. Gastric ulcers can be prevented by concomitantly delivering antacids, pump inhibitors. Cisapride is a cholinergic agonist, and so it does not negatively affect cognition.
Metoclopramide (Reglan)	Sedation, seizures, and irreversible tardive dyskinesia may occur after even a single dose,[63] and tardive dyskinesia can be life threatening.[64] As such, metoclopramide is universally a second-line agent to cisapride unless concomitant delivery of Q-T prolongation drugs precludes delivery of cisapride. Metoclopramide improves gastric emptying and is anti-emetic.
Prochlorperazine (Compazine)	This agent has the same considerable side effects as metoclopramide, as both are antipsychotic derivatives. In light of its side effect profile, it is always a third line drug relative to trimethobenzanide, ondansterone (Zofran), and dronabinol to control nausea.
Trimethobenzanide (Tigan)	This agent is only rarely associated with extrapyramidal or cognitive side effects. It is an inexpensive first line choice for nausea, but less potent than other agents.
Ondansterone (Zofran)	Ondansterione is an extremely safe anti-emetic, but expensive. Its mechanism is via the seratonergic system and it does not have negative cognitive side effects.

Continued

Pharmacology: *Arousal, Awareness, Memory, Aphasia, Motor Restoration*

Agent	Side Effects, Comments
Donepezil (Aricept)	Donepezil is a cholinergic agonist, which may improve memory.
Dextroamphetamine (Dexedrine)	This medication is a dopamine and norepinephrine agonist and may improve cognitive parameters. Patients may develop nausea or appetite suppression, similar to methylphenidate, which has a similar mechanism of action, although dextroamphetamine is often felt to be somewhat more potent.
Bromocriptine	This agent is a post-synaptic dopamine agonist, and has been described as improving hemispatial neglect, expressive aphasia, and awareness in vegetative state. It may lower blood pressure, cause nausea, or very rarely cause cardiac or retroperitoneal fibrosis. It has anticonvulsant properties.
Pergolide (Permax)	Similar to bromocriptine, except that pergolide also has dopamine agonist properties at dopamine-1 receptor, and so may be a more potent psychostimulant in vegetative patients.
Levodopa-carbidopa (Sinemet)	Sinemet is dopamine, so patients who cannot synthesize their own dopamine may benefit from this agent to reverse the vegetative state or promote awakening from coma.
Modafinil	This medication was recently approved as a psychostimulant for narcolepsy. It has a different mechanism relative to conventional stimulants, and may prove effective in cognitive enhancement.

Pharmacology: *Disinhibited Behavior*

Agent	Side Effects, Comments
Atenolol	As with all beta blockers, this medication may selectively extinguish aggression.
Propranolol	This highly lipophilic beta blocker may extinguish aggression but also predisposes to mood depression, delayed rate of thought processing, and other cognitive sequelae.
Lithium	Lithium may extinguish aggression, but also has a narrow therapeutic window and may cause renal and other organ toxicity, as well as seizures.
Paroxetine (Paxil)	This seratonergic antidepressant may extinguish pathological disinhibited laughing and crying, as can sertraline, fluoxetine, or the tricyclic antidepressants such as amitriptyline. Seratonergic antidepressants have far less toxicity than tricyclic agents.
Buspirone	Usually used to treat anxiety without the amnesic, mood depression, and irritability problems associated with lorazepam (Ativan), alprazolam (Xanax), and other benzodiazepines, buspirone may selectively extinguish sexual disinhibition.

Spasticity

Agent	Side Effects, Comments
Botulinum toxin (Botox)	Injected medication which decreases spasticity by paralyzing the muscle at the level of the neuromuscular junction. It lasts only 3 to 4 months, and cannot be titrated during the office visit as onset of antispasticity effect is delayed 1 to 2 weeks. There are no cognitive side effects. Botulinum toxin weakens the injected muscle but unmasks strength in the antagonist. As with phenol, injected medications are best for spastic hypertonus, and oral agents are preferred for body mass spasms.
Phenol	Phenol is an injected medication that decreases spasticity by paralyzing the muscle at the level of the peripheral nerve. It lasts weeks to years, as defined by the selected technique of delivery. Onset is immediate, and no cognitive side effects occur. The agonist as well as the antagonist may reveal unmasked strength. It is inexpensive. Phenol is relatively contraindicated in small as well as deep muscles.
Tizanidine (Zanaflex)	Sedation is the most common side effect, and it often resolves after 3 to 7 days. Tizanidine cannot be co-prescribed with dantrolene. Tizanidine can be taken for long-term management without ill effects, and has analgesic properties.
Baclofen (Lioresol)	Sedation is the most common side effect, and resolves in days. If the patient abruptly discontinues the medication, seizures or psychosis may result. As with tizanidine, baclofen is safe with long-term use and has analgesic properties.
Dantrolene (Dantrium)	This agent has the least cognitive side effects of all antispasticity agents. It has dose- and duration-dependent hepatotoxicity, so it is not favored in young patients, especially if greater than 200 mg a day is required on a continued basis.
Clonidine (Catapress)	Similar mechanism as tizanidine, but more sedating and more likely to decrease blood pressure.
Diazepam (Valium)	This agent is highly sedating, has considerable addictive potential, and adversely affects attention, memory, and mood. It is contraindicated after stroke and brain injury, but very helpful after spinal cord injury to afford adjustment to impairment and disability.

APPENDIX B

Suggested Answers to Case Study Guiding Questions

1. Categorize the patient's level of consciousness upon admission to the acute rehabilitation hospital based on the Glasgow Coma Scale and her level of cognitive functioning based on the Ranchos Los Amigos Levels of Cognitive Functioning, (LOCF).

ANSWER: The patient's eye opening score is a 4, her best motor response is a 4, and her verbal response is a 1, for a total score of 9 on the Glasgow Coma Scale. This indicates that she is out of coma at this time. The patient presents with inconsistent and nonpurposeful movement to stimuli. This indicates that she is in level II, Generalized Response, (LOCF).

2. Categorize her problems in terms of direct impairments, indirect impairments, and functional limitations.

ANSWER:

Direct Impairments:
1. Altered level of consciousness
2. Impaired communication
3. Impaired motor control
4. Abnormal tone
5. Impaired swallowing
6. Impaired balance

Indirect Impairments:
1. Decreased PROM/contractures
2. Skin breakdown
3. Infection
4. Impaired voice, possibly due to tracheostomy
5. Impaired endurance

Functional limitations:
1. Dependent for all functional mobility

3. Describe three physical therapy interventions that would be appropriate for this patient. Include at least one related to family education.

ANSWER: There are a wide variety of interventions that are appropriate for the patient at this level of functioning. Sensory stimulation is important. Auditory stimulation is provided whenever interacting with the patient. Consistent orientation and describing the intervention to the patient should be done during the treatment session. Tactile stimulation is provided when performing passive range of motion. Asking the patient to attempt to track a limb while it is being ranged provides visual stimulation. Photographs of family members and favorite things in the patient's room will provide visual stimulation. These can also be used during treatment sessions. The patient can be asked to track the photographs, or to identify who is in the photograph. Gustatory stimulation cannot be performed at this time because the patient has dysphagia and is NPO.

Assisting the patient into upright postures is another intervention that is beneficial at this stage of recovery. Being in an upright posture will help stimulate the arousal centers in the brain. This can include using a tilt table. The tilt table will also provide weight-bearing through the lower extremities and stretch her contracted plantarflexors. Sensory stimulation can also be provided while the patient is on the tilt table. Assisted sitting will also bring the patient to an upright posture. Therapeutic guiding techniques can be done in this posture. For example, the therapist can perform guiding to assist the patient with washing her face, or grooming. This will provide a multitude of sensory stimulation as well.

The patient's fiancé and mother can be taught how to perform PROM and sensory stimulation. Her family should be educated regarding her prognosis and taught about the Ranchos Los Amigos Scale of Level of Cognitive Functioning. This is extremely important, because the patient is likely to need some level of assistance when she is discharged from the rehabilitation hospital.

4. Describe how this patient's memory impairments will affect physical therapy interventions and how the physical therapist should tailor interventions to maximize the patient's learning abilities.

ANSWER: The patient's impaired short-term memory will make learning new skills very difficult. There will be very little carryover when teaching her new tasks. The following steps should be taken in order to maximize the patient's learning abilities. Consistency is very important. The same therapist should strive to treat the patient at the same times every day. A memory book should be started with the patient. Treatment sessions should begin and end with a functional task that is relevant to the patient. Tasks that are meaningful for the patient should be employed in the treatment session. Appropriate feedback should be given. Videotaping treatment sessions and reviewing them with the patient is also appropriate.

5. List five possible goals and outcomes for this patient.

ANSWER
1. The patient will be supervised for all aspects of bed mobility.
2. The patient will transfer wheelchair to and from bed with contact guard/supervision with appropriate orthosis.
3. The patient will ambulate 150 feet with contact guard/minimal assistance in a closed environment i.e., in the home, with appropriate assistive device and orthosis.
4. The patient will ambulate up and down four steps with one rail with minimal assistance and appropriate orthosis.

5. The patient will perform a functional task in standing for 10 minutes with supervision and appropriate orthosis.

6. Describe two interventions that would be appropriate for this patient at this time.

ANSWER: Using the developmental postures for functional training would be beneficial for this patient. Quadruped, kneeling, and half-kneeling would improve balance, trunk control, gluteus medius strength, and inhibit her extensor tone at the knees. These postures are safe as they all have a low center of gravity and wide base of support. Half-kneeling would increase ROM and strength in dorsiflexion. Modified plantigrade and standing activities would improve her balance, trunk control, and lower extremity strength. Modified plantigrade would also improve the ROM in dorsiflexion, and increase her upper trunk stability.

Swiss ball activities in sitting, supine, and prone would help improve her balance, trunk control, lower extremity strength, and modify her tone.

When her short leg cast is removed, aquatic therapy would be particularly beneficial. This would help improve her balance, trunk control, and upper and lower extremity strength. Using a pool with the water temperature between 90° and 94°F will help modify her tone.

7. List and prioritize the patient's direct impairments, indirect impairments, and functional limitations.

ANSWER

Direct Impairments
1. Impaired cognition
   a) Memory deficits
   b) Attention span deficits
   c) Problem solving/reasoning deficits
      • Impaired safety awareness
      • Impaired insight
      • Impaired executive functioning
2. Impaired communication
   a) Expressive aphasia
3. Neuromuscular impairments
   a) Motor control deficits
      • Impaired strength
      • Impaired coordination
      • Ataxia
   b) Impaired balance

Indirect Impairments
1) Decreased PROM
2) Decreased endurance
Functional Limitations
1) Supervised ambulation in the home, minimal assistance/contact guard ambulation in an open environment with device and orthosis.
2) Contact guard on stairs with rail and orthoses.
3) Moderate assistance with floor-to-stand transfers.

8. Describe two interventions appropriate for this patient. At least one intervention should focus on community re-entry.

ANSWER: Physical therapy intervention should focus on enhancing the patient's mobility skills in the community. Appropriate treatments include ambulating in a supermarket and having the patient search for different items in an aisle, ambulating in a busy mall and searching for specific stores, and ambulating across a busy intersection.

It is important to include the patient in the decision making process when planning community based trips. The patient is likely to perform better if it is an activity that is important to her. Many times a community outing is a group activity involving other patients. Having all of the patients participate in planning the outing is also therapeutic. The patients learn to interact in a group setting and can practice important social skills.

Many of the same interventions mentioned earlier would still be appropriate for the patient. Kneeling, half-kneeling, modified plantigrade, and standing would all be beneficial developmental postures. Swiss ball activities and aquatic therapy would help improve balance, strength, and coordination.

At this level of recovery it is important to have the patient begin an independent exercise program. Simple ROM, strengthening exercises, and walking for cardiovascular fitness are appropriate at first. Then progress to a more comprehensive fitness program. Endurance training on a stationary bike or treadmill and weight training are appropriate. This can be done at a local health club. In some cases rehabilitation hospitals have fitness programs where discharged patients can use the available exercise equipment for a nominal fee. It is important to include the patient in designing the exercise program. If the patient is not invested in the program then she is not likely to follow through with it.

Michael C. Schubert
Susan J. Herdman

LEARNING OBJECTIVES

1. Identify and differentiate vestibular symptom pathology from other manifestations of vertigo, dizziness, and disequilibrium.
2. Identify and describe the examination procedures used to evaluate patients with vestibular dysfunction to establish a diagnosis, prognosis, and plan of care.
3. Describe appropriate elements of the rehabilitation program for patients with vestibular dysfunction.
4. Analyze and interpret patient data and determine appropriate interventions for the clinical problems presented.

Physical therapists are likely to encounter patients with vestibular disorders in a variety of clinical settings. Vestibular disorders occur following head trauma, viral insults, and antibiotic ototoxicity. Dizziness is the third most common complaint reported to physicians behind chest pain and fatigue.[1] Among the adult population, 42 percent report experiencing dizziness or vertigo at some time.[2] It is estimated that 76 million Americans will suffer from a vestibular disorder of some sort.[2] A teaching hospital reported peripheral vestibular disorders accounted for greater than 50 percent of persistent dizziness among outpatients whose primary complaint was dizziness.[3]

Cawthorne[4] and Cooksey[5] were the first clinicians to advocate exercises for persons suffering from dizziness and vertigo. It has only been within the last two decades, however, that our knowledge of vestibular function and related disorders has profoundly changed the approaches toward rehabilitation. As with most disorders of the human body, if vestibular dysfunction can be diagnosed and treated early, functional limitations are minimized, and the progression toward disability can be prevented.

The peripheral vestibular system will serve as the primary focus of this chapter because it is the most common origin for patient signs and symptoms. The physical therapist, however, must recognize patterns of signs and symptoms from a central pathology as well. To appreciate the complexity of the vestibular system and its vital role in human function, a brief synopsis of anatomy and physiology is provided. Once the normally functioning vestibular system is understood, the reader will be able to discern anomalies of the system and begin to formulate effective rehabilitation strategies.

ANATOMY

Peripheral Vestibular System

There are three primary functions of the peripheral vestibular system: (1) to stabilize visual images on the fovea of the retina during head movement to allow clear vision; (2) to maintain postural stability, especially during movement of the head, and (3) to provide information used for spatial orientation.

Within the temporal bone on each side of the skull lies a membranous structure called the labyrinth. The labyrinth contains two different types of movement sensors: **semicircular canals (SCC)** and the **otolith organs** (Fig. 25-1). There are three SCCs, the anterior or superior, posterior or inferior, and horizontal or lateral. The SCC are filled with a fluid, called **endolymph,** which moves freely within each canal in response to the direction of angular head movement. As the endolymph moves, it bends the sensory receptor cells (hair cells) located in the cupula (Fig. 25-2). Each of the SCCs responds best to movement in its own plane. For example, the

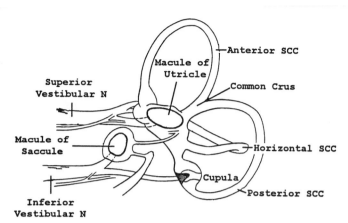

Figure 25-1. The three semicircular canals (SCCs) lie 90 degrees from each other. Each SCC is filled with endolymphatic fluid, which moves within each of the SCC in response to angular head motion. The two otolith structures, the utricle and saccule, respond to linear acceleration. Note the labyrinth contribution to the vestibular nerve is comprised of both a superior and inferior division. This is a left vestibular labyrinth. (From Schuknecht, HF: Pathology of the Ear, Lea & Febiger, Philadelphia, 1993, p 534, with permission.)

horizontal SCC has its greatest firing rate when the head is moving horizontally.

The otoliths, comprised of the saccule and the utricle, respond to linear acceleration and to the pull of gravity. Calcium carbonate crystals (otoconia) are embedded in a gelatinous matrix within

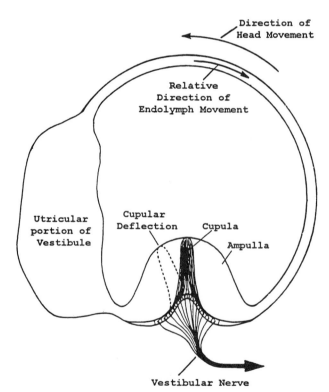

Figure 25-2. Cross-section of a semicircular canal with arrows to illustrate the relationship between direction of head movement and direction of endolymph. As the endolymph moves within the semicircular canal, it deflects off the cupula and distorts the hair cells. (From Melvill-Jones, G: Organization of Neural Control in the Vestibulo-Ocular Reflex Arc. The Control of Eye Movements. Academic Press, New York, 1971, with permission.)

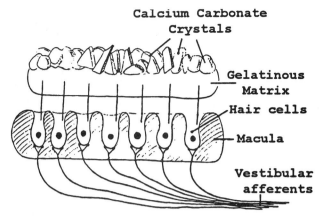

Figure 25-3. The calcium carbonate crystals (otoconia) provide weight to the gel matrix, serving as an inertial mass allowing linear motion to excite the hair cells in the macula of the utricle and saccule. (Adapted from Baloh and Hornrubia,[13] p 4, with permission.)

the utricle and saccule. The sensory receptors, or hair cells, project into this gelatinous matrix. As the head moves linearly, as in an elevator, the calcium carbonate crystals shift, distorting the hair cells, which generates a receptor potential in the hair cell (Fig. 25-3).

Information about angular and linear velocity is sent to the vestibular nuclei in the brainstem and to the cerebellum for processing (Fig. 25-4). The vestibular signals interact in the central nervous system (CNS) with visual and somatosensory cues. The CNS integrates the three sensory inputs and produces an appropriate motor plan for gaze and postural stability. Signals from the three SCCs are primarily used for gaze stability, whereas signals from the utricle and saccule are primarily used for postural stability.

Central Vestibular System

The vestibular nuclei have extensive connections with the cerebellum, reticular formation, thalamus, and cerebral cortex (vestibular cortex). Connections with the reticular formation, thalamus, and the vestibular cortex* enable the vestibular system to contribute to the integration of arousal and conscious awareness of the body, as well as discerning between movement of self and the environment.[10,11] The cerebellar connections help to modulate the vestibulo-ocular reflex (VOR), maintain posture during active and static activities, and coordinate limb movements. Lesions in the central lower brainstem structures can mimic peripheral vestibular pathology. For example, an infarct in the vestibular nuclei may have symptomology consistent with a unilateral vestibular lesion (UVL). Central lesions in the cortex and upper brainstem result in perceptual

---

*Monkey studies have identified the junction of the parietal and insular lobes as the location of the primary vestibular cortex.[6–9]

disorders such as the abnormal perception of visual vertical.[12]

PHYSIOLOGY AND MOTOR CONTROL

To understand the signs and symptoms of vestibular dysfunction, basic physiology and motor control theory of the vestibular system is reviewed, enabling the reader to recognize the mechanisms responsible for disorders. Important principles of the vestibular system include the tonic firing rate, VOR, push-pull mechanism, inhibitory cut off, and the velocity storage system (VSS).

Tonic Firing Rate

The normal vestibular system has a tonic firing rate of 80 pulses per second.[13] This means that even when the head is stationary, as in sleep, the vestibular system is still active. Angular or linear movement of the head can increase or decrease the firing rate of the vestibular system.

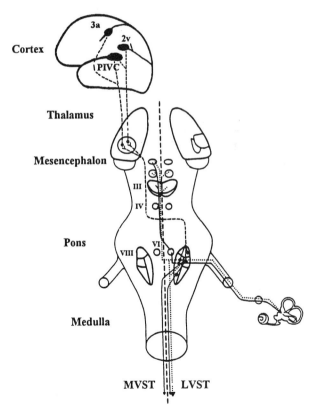

Figure 25-4. The semicircular canal (angular) and otolith (linear) input is sent to the vestibular nuclei, primarily the medial and superior. From there, the information is sent to the ocular motor nuclei (VI, IV, III) for mediation of the vestibulo-ocular reflex. For arousal and conscious awareness of the head and body in space, the information is further sent to the thalamus and cortex. For maintenance of postural control, the vestibular signal is sent distally as the medial and lateral vestibulo-spinal tracts (MVST, LVST), PIVC, parieto-insular vestibular cortex. (Adapted from Brandt and Dieterich,[10] p 343, with permission.)

Vestibulo-Ocular Reflex and Vestibulo-Ocular Reflex Gain

Gaze stability during rapid head movement is maintained by the **vestibulo-ocular reflex (VOR).** The input from the SCCs goes to the vestibular nuclei and from there to the oculomotor nuclei. The SCC afferent synapses with the oculomotor nuclei producing a slow-phase eye movement (VOR) in the opposite direction of the head movement. For example, when the head is moved down, the anterior SCCs are stimulated. The input from the anterior SCC causes both eyes to slowly move in the direction opposite the angular head movement, or up, as can be seen in Figure 25-5.

Normally, as the head moves in one direction, the eyes will move in the opposite direction with equal velocity. This relationship of eye velocity to head velocity is expressed as the **vestibular gain** (eye velocity/head velocity = 1).

When the head is moving at velocities less than 60 degrees per second, gaze stability can be maintained using **smooth pursuit.**[14] In situations where the head moves greater than 60 degrees per second, the vestibular system generates eye movement in the direction opposite the head movement to maintain gaze on the target. The VOR operates at head velocities as great as 350 to 400 degrees per second.[13] Beyond velocities of 400 degrees per second, the gain of the VOR decreases and gaze stability degrades.

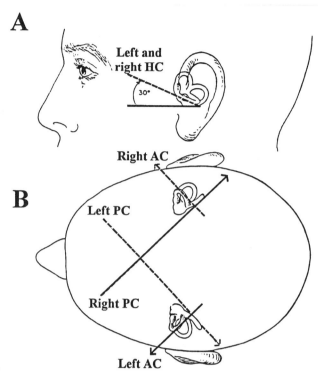

Figure 25-6. *(A)* Orientation of the horizontal semicircular canals (SCC) in situ, with the head neutrally aligned. *(B)* The semicircular canals (anterior and posterior) work in pairs. The arrows indicate the angular pitch direction of individual SCC stimulation. The dashed and continuous lines illustrate each SCC has an equally opposing SCC, sensitive to the opposite angular pitch direction of the head, for example, the right anterior canal (right AC) is paired with the left posterior canal (left PC). (Adapted from Baloh and Hornrubia,[13] p 27, with permission.)

Push-Pull Mechanism

This concept is very important to the understanding of the effect of a UVL on the VOR. The brain detects head movement through comparison of inputs from the two vestibular systems. The SCCs all work in pairs; the right anterior SCC is paired with the left posterior SCC and vice versa, and the two horizontal canals are a pair. As the head is turned to the right, the right horizontal SCC will have an increased firing rate (depolarized) while the left horizontal SCC has a decreased firing rate (hyperpolarized). This is called the **push-pull mechanism.** The CNS is then responsible for recognizing the difference and interpreting movement. A faulty interpretation will lead to difficulties with gaze stabilization, motion perception, and postural stability. Figure 25-6 illustrates the push-pull mechanism.

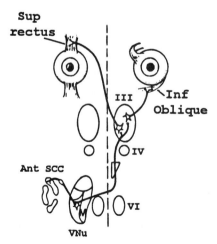

Figure 25-5. From the anterior semicircular canal (Ant SCC), the signal travels to the vestibular nuclei (VNu). The signal continues to the contralateral oculomotor nuclei (III). From there, synapses are made with the superior rectus, which moves the eye upward and the inferior oblique, which moves the eye upward and torsionally. Also shown are the oculomotor nuclei IV, and VI. (Adapted from Baloh and Hornrubia,[13] p 52, with permission.)

Inhibitory Cut Off

Rotation of the head to the side depolarizes the hair cells of that labyrinth and causes an increase in the firing rate of the vestibular neurons for head velocities of up to 350 to 400 degrees per second.[13] A concomitant hyperpolarization of the opposite labyrinth also occurs. However, the hyperpolarization of the hair cells in the opposite labyrinth can only decrease the firing rate to zero, at which point the inhibition is cut off **(inhibitory cut off).** The response to head movements that hyperpolarize the hair cells is limited to a velocity range up to 80 degrees per second. Therefore, with a rotation to the right of 120 per second, the right ear increases its firing rate from 80 (tonic firing rate) to 200 degrees per second. The left ear will decrease from 80 to zero, not to negative 40.*

Velocity Storage System

The signal generated by movement of the cupula is brief, lasting only as long as the cupula is deflected. The response is sustained, however, by a circuit of neurons in the medial vestibular nucleus and lasts longer than 10 seconds in the normal vestibular system. The purpose of sustaining the vestibular input may be to signal the brain that movement is still occurring even though the cupula is no longer reporting it.

ASSESSMENT

History

The history is a particularly important part of the examination and can expedite the physical examination. Three key items to taking the history are the symptoms, tempo, and circumstances.

SYMPTOMS

It is essential to determine what the patient is experiencing when he or she uses the term **dizziness.** Unfortunately "dizziness" is an imprecise term; it is difficult for patients and clinicians to describe, and is vaguely defined as the sensation of whirling or feeling a tendency to fall. Ideally, patients should be directed away from using the word. However, most complaints of "dizziness" can be categorized as vertigo, lightheadedness, or disequilibrium.

Many patients use the term "vertigo" incorrectly and thus the clinician must inform the patient of the definition. **Vertigo** is defined as an illusion of movement, most commonly a sense of spinning. It is due to an asymmetry in the tonic firing rate of the two vestibular systems. Vertigo is most common during the acute stage of a UVL, but may also manifest itself with acute unilateral brainstem lesions affecting the root entry zone of the peripheral vestibular neurons or the vestibular nuclei.

Lightheadedness is vague and less localizing than vertigo. It can be caused by other nonvestibular factors such as hypotension, hypoglycemia, or anxiety. Typically, lightheadedness is defined as a sense of feeling as if about to faint.

Disequilibrium is defined as the subjective sensation that a person is off balance. Typically, acute and chronic vestibular lesions will produce disequilibrium. Often, however, this symptom is associated with nonvestibular problems such as decreased somatosensation or weakness in the lower extremities (Table 25–1).

When a patient complains of visual blurring with head motion, he or she is experiencing oscillopsia. **Oscillopsia** is a visual instability with head movement in which images appear to move or bounce. It is due to decreased VOR gain.

Assessment of Subjective Complaints

Visual Analog Scale

Use of a visual analog scale (VAS) is an effective technique to obtain subjective intensity ratings of disequilibrium, dizziness, vertigo, and oscillopsia. The patient is asked to answer a question and mark on a 10-centimeter line where their symptoms exist at that moment. The clinician then measures the line and obtains a quantified value.[15]

Dizziness Handicap Inventory

The Dizziness Handicap Inventory (DHI) is a popular tool used to measure a patient's self-perceived handicap as a result of vestibular disorders (Table 25–2).[16] The DHI has excellent test-retest reliability ($r = 0.97$) and good internal consistency reliability ($r = 0.89$). Patients respond to 25 questions, which are subgrouped into functional, emotional, and physical components. The DHI provides quantification of the patient's perception of disequilibrium and its impact on daily activities. It is useful to establish subjective improvement. Robertson and Ireland[17] found that the DHI did not correlate with functional balance ability as measured with computer dynamic posturography (CDP). Although patients had perceptions of handicap, they did not manifest a physical balance disorder. The authors concluded that anxiety and differing coping abilities of patients were the reasons for the poor correlation.

Functional Disability Scale

Telian and Shepard[18] developed a Functional Disability Scale to determine a patient's response to physical therapy (Table 25–3). The scale is administered before and after therapy. Analysis revealed patients with greater subjective belief that their vestibular disorders were disabling did not improve as much as those patients who perceived themselves to be less disabled.

Table 25–1 POSSIBLE CAUSES OF SYMPTOMS

Symptom	Possible Cause
Vertigo	BPPV, unilateral peripheral hypofunction, unilateral central lesion affecting the vestibular nuclei
Lightheadedness	Orthostatic hypotension, hypoglycemia, anxiety, panic disorder
Dysequilibrium	Bilateral vestibular lesion, chronic unilateral vestibular lesion, lower extremity somatosensation loss, upper brainstem/vestibular cortex lesion, motor pathway lesions

BPPV, benign paroxysmal positional vertigo.

---

*For each degree per second head velocity, there is an approximate 1 pulse per second change in firing rate.

Table 25–2 FINAL α VERSION OF DIZZINESS HANDICAP INVENTORY WITH CORRECTED ITEM-TOTAL CORRELATION COEFFICIENTS

Dizziness Handicap Inventory[a]

Instructions: The purpose of this scale is to identify difficulties that you may be experiencing because of your dizziness or unsteadiness. Please answer "yes," "no," or "sometimes" to each question. *Answer each question as it pertains to your dizziness or unsteadiness problem only.*

Item	Item Total
P1. Does looking up increase your problem?	.54
E2. Because of your problem, do you feel frustrated?	.34
F3. Because of your problem, do you restrict your travel for business or recreation?	.76[b]
P4. Does walking down the aisle of a supermarket increase your problem?	.39
F5. Because of your problem. do you have difficulty getting into or out of bed?	.50
F6. Does your problem significantly restrict your participation in social activities such as going out to dinner, going to movies, dancing, or to parties?	.69
F7. Because of your problem, do you have difficulty reading?	.44
P8. Does performing more ambitious activities like sports, dancing, or household chores such as sweeping or putting dishes away increase your problem?	.54
E9. Because of your problem, are you afraid to leave your home without having someone accompany you?	.43
E10. Because of your problem, have you been embarrassed in front of others?	.46
P11. Do quick movements of your head increase your problem?	.51
F12. Because of your problem, do you avoid heights?	.49
P13. Does turning over in bed increase your problem?	.43
F14. Because of your problem, is it difficult for you to do strenuous housework or yardwork?	.58
E15. Because of your problem, are you afraid people may think you are intoxicated?	.30
F16. Because of your problem, is it difficult for you to go for a walk by yourself?	.62
P17. Does walking down a sidewalk increase your problem?	.58†
E18. Because of your problem, is it difficult for you to concentrate?	.49†
F19. Because of your problem, is it difficult for you to walk around your house in the dark?	.48
E20. Because of your problem, are you afraid to stay home alone?	.27
E21. Because of your problem, do you feel handicapped?	.41
E22. Has your problem placed stress on your relationships with members of your family or friends?	.46
E23. Because of your problem, are you depressed?	.41
F24. Does your problem interfere with your job or household responsibilities?	.56
P25. Does bending over increase your problem?	.57

[a]A "yes" response is scored 4 points. A "sometimes" response is scored 2 points. A "no" response is scored 0 points.

[b]Questions with the highest corrected item-total correlation for each subscale. F indicates functional subscale; E, emotional subscale; P, physical subscale.

From Jacobsen, GP, and Newman, CW.[16] p 424, with permission.

Motion Sensitivity Quotient

Smith-Wheelock et al.[19] developed the Motion Sensitivity Quotient (MSQ), which provides a subjective score of the patient's dizziness. The test involves placing patients into positions incorporating head or entire body motion to assess whether the movement reproduces dizziness (Fig. 25-7). If the patient reports an increased symptom intensity moving into a provoking position, the intensity is assigned a point, graded by the patient between 1 (mild) and 5 (severe). The duration of symptoms are also assigned points from 0 to 3 (0–4 seconds = 0; 5–10 seconds = 1; 11–30 seconds = 2; >30 seconds = 3). The symptom intensity and duration values are then added together for a score. The MSQ is calculated by multiplying the number of positions that provoked symptoms by the score, and dividing by 2048. An MSQ score of zero means no symptoms and 100 means severe dizziness in all positions.

TEMPO

The clinician must determine if the patient has had an acute attack of vertigo (within 3 days), chronic disequilibrium, or if the patient is having episodes of dizziness. If the patient is suffering from episodic vertigo, the clinician must attempt to determine the average duration of the episodes in seconds, minutes, or hours. This information is critical in determining the diagnosis and providing the appropriate treatment.

CIRCUMSTANCES

The physical therapist must also determine under what circumstances the patient experiences symptoms. This will eventually help to determine the most effective form of treatment. It is important to discern whether the patient has the symptoms with particular movements, positions, or at rest. Perhaps the patient is sensitive to motion as the passenger in a car though the body is still. Maybe moving the head into certain positions leads to a vigorous vertigo.

Table 25–3 FUNCTIONAL DISABILITY SCALE

0	No disability-negligible symptoms
1	No disability-bothersome symptoms
2	Mild disability-performing usual duties
3	Moderate disability-disrupts usual duties
4	Recent severe disability-medical leave
5	Established severe disability

Note: The physical therapist assigns the patient a score before and after treatment, based on interview history (from Telian et al[18]p90 with permission).

Name: _____ Age: _____ Sex: _____ Date: _____

	INTENSITY	DURATION	SCORE
Baseline Symptoms			
1. Sitting-to-supine			
2. Supine-to-left side			
3. Left-to-right side			
4. Supine-to-sit			
5. Left hallpike			
6. Return from hallpike			
7. Right hallpike			
8. Return from hallpike			
9. Sitting: nose □ left knee			
10. Return to sit			
11. Sitting: nose □ right knee			
12. Return to sit			
13. Sitting: head rotation 5×			
14. Sitting: head flex. and ext. 5×			
15. Standing: turn right			
16. Standing: turn left			
Intensity: rated from 0 to 5 (0 = no SX, 5 = severe SX)			
Duration: rated from 0 to 3 (5-10 sec = 1 point, 11-30 sec = 2 points, ≥30 sec = 3 points)			

Motion sensitivity quotient: $\dfrac{\text{\#Provoking positions} \times \text{score} \times 100}{2048}$ = _____ Total

Note: An MSQ score of zero means no symptoms and 100 means severe dizziness in all positions. (Adapted from Smith-Wheelock, et al,[19] p 221, with permission.)

Figure 25-7. Motion sensitivity quotient. (Adapted from Smith-Wheelock et al,[19] p 221, with permission.)

PHYSICAL EXAMINATION

The oculomotor tests are the most localizing and diagnostic means to examine the vestibular system. The key tests include observation for nystagmus, examination of the VOR at high acceleration (head thrust test), head-shaking–induced nystagmus (HSN), positional testing, and the clinical dynamic visual acuity (DVA) test.

Nystagmus is the primary diagnostic indicator used in identifying most peripheral and central vestibular lesions. An involuntary eye movement, nystagmus due to a **peripheral vestibular lesion** is composed of both slow and fast phase eye movements. The direction of the nystagmus is named by the direction of fast phase of the eye movement.

In a vestibular lesion, the slow-phase eye movement is due to relative excitation of one side of the vestibular system. The fast phase is simply a resetting eye movement. For example, in left-beating nystagmus, the eyes move slowly to the right (VOR), and the resetting eye movement is to the left (quick phase). Therefore, the direction opposite the quick phase of the nystagmus localizes the side of the vestibular lesion.

Nystagmus due to a vestibular lesion is most commonly seen after an acute unilateral insult, **spontaneous** (at rest) **nystagmus.** This type of nystagmus occurs in the absence of motion because of the asymmetry between the functioning and nonfunctioning sides of the vestibular systems. The brain perceives the asymmetry as active stimulation from the uninvolved side. Spontaneous nystagmus in the light due to peripheral lesions typically resolves after 7 days.[20,21] The resolution of the spontaneous nystagmus is in part due to visual suppression as well as the adaptive capabilities of the CNS.

Observation for Nystagmus

Nystagmus can be suppressed in light and when a person fixates on a target.[22] As a result, the observation of nystagmus should be performed under conditions in which the person cannot visualize the surrounding environment. This can be achieved with Frenzel lenses or an infrared camera system. Frenzel lenses are goggles that have magnifying lenses enabling the clinician to observe for nystagmus by preventing the patient from fixating on a target. An infrared camera uses infrared light to illuminate the eye though the patient is unable to see.

Head Thrust Test

The VOR is examined using both slow (<60 degrees/sec) and rapid head rotations[23] in a horizontal direction (Fig. 25-8). The head thrust test is performed by having the patient first fixate on a near target (e.g., the clinician's nose). The patient's head is moved slowly through a small amplitude while the patient attempts to maintain fixation on the target. Then the patient is advised that the head will be moved quickly. The normal individual will be able to maintain gaze on the target during head movement. In a patient with a vestibular loss, the head movement will cause the eyes to move off the target (no VOR) and the patient will make a saccade to refixate on the target. A **saccade** is a fast eye movement. A patient who has a unilateral peripheral or central vestibular lesion will not be able to maintain gaze when the head is rotated quickly toward the side of the lesion. Similarly, a patient with a bilateral peripheral vestibular lesion will make refixation saccades when the head is thrust to either side. The test is then repeated with the patient fixating on a distant target approximately 6 feet away.

Head-Shaking–Induced Nystagmus

The **head-shaking–induced nystagmus (HSN)** test is useful in the diagnosis of a unilateral peripheral vestibular defect. The patient must wear Frenzel lenses or use a video infrared camera to avoid suppression of nystagmus. The patient is instructed to close his or her eyes. The clinician flexes the head 30 degrees (to place the horizontal SCC parallel with the ground) and oscillates the head horizontally 20 times at a frequency of 2 hertz. Upon stopping the oscillation, the patient opens the eyes and the clinician checks for nystagmus. In normal subjects, there will be no nystagmus. An asymmetry in the vestibular system, however, may result in HSN. Typically, a unilateral peripheral vestibular lesion will result in a horizontal nystagmus with the quick phase toward the normal side and the slow phase directed toward the lesioned side. Not all patients with a UVL will have HSN. Patients with a bilateral vestibular hypofunction will not have HSN because there is no asymmetry between the vestibular systems; neither system is contributing input. The presence of vertical nystagmus after either horizontal or vertical head shaking suggests a central lesion.

Positional Testing

Positional testing is used to identify vertigo and nystagmus. The most common cause of positional vertigo is a disorder called **benign paroxysmal positional vertigo (BPPV)** in which otoconia are dislodged and float into the SCC, causing an abnormal signal when the person changes head position. The abnormal signal results in brief vertigo and nystagmus. The direction of the nystagmus is specific for which canal is involved. In the **Hallpike-Dix test**[24] the patient is moved from sitting with the head rotated 45 degrees to one side, to a supine position with the head extended 30 degrees beyond horizontal, head still rotated 45 degrees (Fig. 25-9). The maneuver places the posterior SCC in a plane parallel with the pull of gravity. The test can also be performed by having the patient move into a sidelying position (Fig. 25-10). In both versions illustrated, the ear toward the ground is the labyrinth being tested. When the patient is placed into the Hallpike-Dix position, the clinician should observe the eyes for nystagmus. The direction of the nystagmus and its duration help to determine whether the patient has BPPV or a central lesion. Table 25–4 is useful to help discern which SCC is involved with the BPPV.

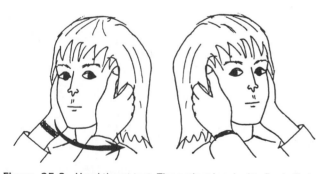

Figure 25-8. Head thrust test. The patient is asked to fixate first on a near and then distant target. The clinician then rapidly moves the patient's head to the left (large arrow) through a small amplitude. The patient is able to maintain focus on the distant target. A positive head thrust test would display the patient's eyes falling away from the target. In such a case the patient must use a refixation saccade to refocus eyes on the target. (From Baloh, RW, et al: Dizziness, Hearing Loss and Tinnitus. FA Davis, Philadelphia, 1998, p 62, with permission.)

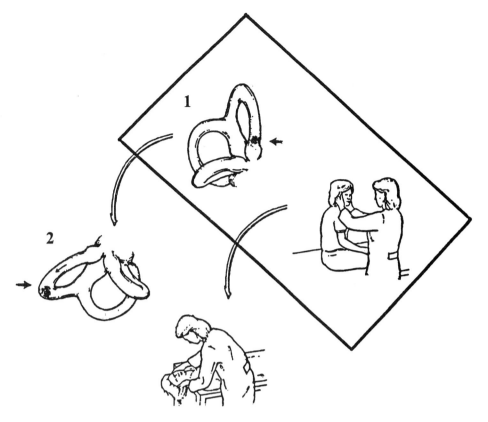

Figure 25-9. The Hallpike-Dix test. *(1)* The patient sits on the examination table and the clinician turns the head horizontally 45 degrees. *(2)* As the examiner maintains the 45-degree rotation, the patient is quickly brought straight back so that the neck is extended 30 degrees beyond the horizontal. The examiner must look for nystagmus and ask the patient if vertigo is being experienced. The patient is then slowly brought back to the starting position, and the other side is tested. The side that reproduces nystagmus and vertigo is the side that has the benign paroxysmal positional vertigo (BPPV). Shown here for testing right posterior or right anterior semicircular canal BPPV. (Adapted from Tusa, RJ: Canalith Repositioning for Benign Positional Vertigo. Education Program Syllabus. American Academy of Neurology, Minnesota, 1998, p 6, with permission.)

Clinical Dynamic Visual Acuity Test

This clinical test measures visual acuity during head movement. In patients with vestibular deficits, the eyes will not be stable in space during head movements. This results in a decrement in visual acuity. The clinical dynamic visual acuity (DVA) test has been shown to reliably measure functional VOR.[25] Static acuity is determined first. The patient is asked to "Read the lowest line you can see" on a wall-mounted acuity chart. The Lighthouse EDTRS wall chart is appropriate for this test. The patient then attempts to read the chart while the clinician horizontally oscillates the patient's head at a frequency of 2 hertz. A metronome is useful to ensure correct frequency of oscillation. In normal subjects, head movement results in little or no change in visual acuity (<1 line). A three or more line decrement in visual acuity during head movement is suggestive of vestibular hypofunction.[26]

Gait and Balance Testing

The assessment of gait and balance problems is important for determination of a patient's functional status. Testing should consist of a range of assessments including static balance, weight shifting, automatic postural responses, and ambulation. The balance tests are not specific to the vestibular system. Table 25–5 includes some common balance tests and expected results.

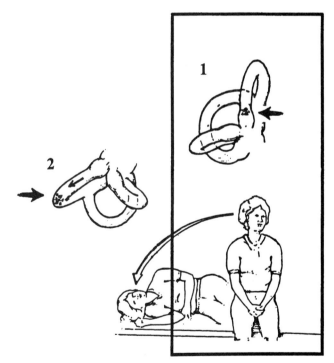

Figure 25-10. The Seated Hallpike-Dix test. *(1)* The patient sits on the edge of the examination table. The clinician turns the head horizontally 45 degrees. *(2)* As the examiner maintains the 45-degree rotation, the patient is quickly brought down to the side opposite the head rotation (pictured here as the right side). The examiner checks for nystagmus and vertigo, then slowly brings the patient to the starting position. The other side is then tested. (Adapted from Tusa, RJ: Canalith Repositioning for Benign Positional Vertigo. Education Program Syllabus. American Academy of Neurology, Minnesota, 1998, p 6, with permission.)

Table 25–4 IDENTIFICATION AND INCIDENCE[a] OF BENIGN PAROXYSMAL POSITIONAL VERTIGO IN THE SEMICIRCULAR CANALS BASED ON NYSTAGMUS

SCC Involvement	Nystagmus	Incidence (%)[a]
Posterior canal	Up-beating and torsional[b]	63
Anterior canal	Down-beating and torsional[b]	12
Horizontal canal	Horizontal	1
Vertical canal	Torsion only	24

[a]Twenty-four percent of cases were indistinguishable between posterior and anterior SCC BPPV.[36]

[b]The torsional[58] component occurs because of the oblique muscle attachments the vertical SCCs synapse with.

VESTIBULAR FUNCTION TESTS

The more common vestibular function tests include caloric testing and rotary chair tests. **Caloric testing** involves infusing the external auditory canal with air or water. This stimulus introduces a temperature gradient causing movement of the endolymph within the horizontal SCC. The stimulated canal generates a horizontal nystagmus response, which can then be quantified. This test is particularly useful for determining the side of the deficit, because each labyrinth is stimulated separately. A variation with ice water is useful to determine whether any function exists in the vestibular system for patients with severe loss. However, the caloric test is limited in the information provided because only the horizontal SCC is being stimulated.

The rotary chair test stimulates the vestibular system by rotating subjects in the dark. The VOR is measured during rotation and compared to normal responses. The rotary chair test can actively stimulate both vestibular systems. The test, although it provides information across the lower frequency range of the vestibular system, only assesses vestibular function at frequencies up to 1 hertz.

VESTIBULAR SYSTEM DYSFUNCTION

Mechanical

The most common cause of vertigo, benign paroxysmal positional vertigo or BPPV, can be considered a biomechanical disorder. Symptoms of BPPV include vertigo with change in head position, nausea with or without vomiting, and disequilibrium. In the most common form, a latency of onset of the vertigo once the head is in the provoking position is less than 15 seconds and the duration is usually less than 60 seconds. The vertigo and nystagmus are direct impairments caused by the misplaced otoconia. Indirect impairments include the symptoms of nausea, vomiting, and imbalance. BPPV is believed to occur via one of two mechanisms: **cupulolithiasis** and **canalithiasis.** Both of the theories involve the otoliths becoming dislodged from the utricle and falling into the SCCs. Schuknecht[27] first theorized that fragments of otoconia break away and adhere to the cupula of one of the SCCs (cupulolithiasis). When the head is moved into certain positions, the weighted cupula is deflected by the pull of gravity. This abnormal signal results in vertigo and nystagmus, which persists as long as the patient is in the provoking position. Cupulolithiasis, therefore, does not explain the brief duration of the vertigo common in BPPV. Hall et al.[28] proposed a second theory, canalithiasis, in which the otoconia are floating freely in one of the SCCs. When a patient changes head position, the pull of gravity causes the freely floating otoconia to move inside the SCC resulting in endolymph movement and deflection of the cupula. Figure 25-11 illustrates BPPV occurring from cupulolithiasis or canalithiasis.

Decreased Receptor Input

The most common causes of unilateral vestibular pathology leading to decreased or eliminated receptor input are viral insults, trauma, and vascular

Table 25–5 COMMON BALANCE TESTS AND EXPECTED RESULTS RELATED TO SPECIFIC DIAGNOSIS

Test	BPPV	UVL	BVL	Central Lesion
Romberg	Negative	Acute: positive Chronic: negative	Acute: positive Chronic: negative	Often negative
Tandem Romberg	Negative	Positive, eyes closed	Positive	Positive
Single-legged stance	Negative	May be positive	Acute: positive Chronic: negative	May be unable to perform
Gait	Normal	Acute: wide-based, slow, decreased arm swing and trunk rotation Compensated: normal	Acute: wide-based, slow, decreased arm swing and trunk rotation Compensated: mild gait deviation	May have pronounced ataxia
Turn head while walking	May produce slight unsteadiness	Acute: may not keep balance Compensated: normal	May not keep balance or slows cadence to perform	May not keep balance, increased ataxia

BPPV, benign paroxysmal postural vertigo; BVL, bilateral vestibular lesion; UVL, unilateral vestibular lesion.

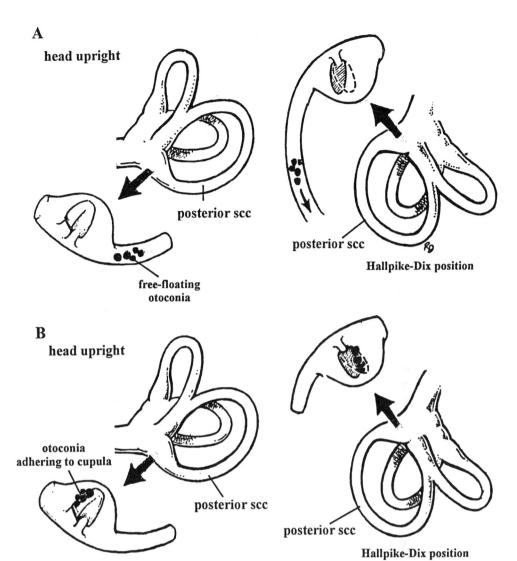

Figure 25-11. Illustrated is benign paroxysmal positional vertigo of the posterior SCC, note the cupular deflection. *(A)* Canalithiasis indicates free-floating otoconia within the SCC. When the head is moved into a position which places the SCC parallel to the pull of gravity, the free-floating otoconia move to the dependent position within the canal. The movement of the free-floating otoconia results in deflection of the cupula. *(B)* Cupulolithiasis indicates otoconia adhering to the cupula. When the head is moved to a position placing one of the SCC parallel to the pull of gravity, the cupula is continually displaced. Illustrated is BPPV of the posterior SCC, also note the cupular deflection.

events. Patients who sustain a UVL will experience direct impairments of vertigo, spontaneous nystagmus, oscillopsia with head movements, postural instability, and disequilibrium. Initially, the patient will experience the vertigo and nystagmus impairments due to the asymmetry created when one vestibular system is no longer functioning. This resolves within 3 to 7 days assuming the patient is exposed to common daylight conditions.[20] Spontaneous nystagmus beyond this time period should alert the clinician to a possible central lesion or an unstable peripheral vestibular lesion. The direct impairments of visual blurring, postural instability, and disequilibrium respond to physical therapy intervention. Because vertigo owing to asymmetry will resolve within 7 days, symptoms of vertigo beyond 2 weeks should be considered an indirect impairment, also necessitating vestibular rehabilitation techniques.

The most common cause of a bilateral vestibular lesion (BVL) is **ototoxicity.** Certain aminoglycosides (gentamycin, streptomycin) are readily taken up by the hair cells of the vestibular apparatus and continue to build in the system even after the person has stopped using the antibiotic. The primary complaint is disequilibrium. Oscillopsia and gait ataxia are clinical signs common with a BVL diagnosis, all direct impairments. Unless the BVL is asymmetric, the patient will not experience nausea or vertigo, because there is no asymmetry in the tonic firing rate of the vestibular neurons. Halmaygi et al.[29] reported that patients with gentamycin ototoxicity have posture and gait abnormalities, decreased visual acuity with head movement, and reduced VOR gains resulting in a positive head thrust test. These impairments are likely permanent though patients with BVL can return to high levels of activity.

Head trauma is another method of sustaining a peripheral vestibular lesion. Decreased receptor input occurs with damage to the vestibule within its protective encasement, the bony labyrinth. Patients who have sustained a traumatic brain injury (TBI) commonly suffer from vertigo.[30] Tuohimaa[31] reported 78 percent of patients sustaining a mild head injury had acute complaints of vertigo, and 20 percent still experienced the vertigo 6 months later. The central processing of the vestibular input may also be the cause of the vertigo reported in patients with TBI.

Central Nervous System Lesions

Injury to the CNS can affect the vestibular system through a variety of diagnoses.[11] These include:
1. Cerebrovascular insult particularly of the anterior-inferior cerebellar artery (AICA), posterior-inferior cerebellar artery (PICA), and vertebral artery
2. Traumatic brain injury
3. Vertebrobasilar insufficiency
4. Demyelinating diseases such as multiple sclerosis (MS)

Nystagmus is also helpful to diagnose CNS pathology. Nystagmus from a cerebellar lesion may be in a pure vertical direction.[32] The nystagmus may not have a slow component and the eyes therefore oscillate at equal speeds, called **pendular nystagmus.** Pendular nystagmus is often indicative of congenital disorders, such as the absence of central vision. Another clue to discern a central versus a peripheral vestibular pathology is the recovery time. Unlike nystagmus following a peripheral vestibular lesion, nystagmus from a central vestibular lesion may never resolve.

Vertigo can be a symptom with central pathology but is uncommon and if present, it is often much less intense than with a peripheral vestibular lesion. Patients with lesions of the vestibular nuclei can present with vertigo, nystagmus, and disequilibrium similar to the patient with a peripheral vestibular lesion. However, central lesions above the level of the vestibular nuclei will manifest lateropulsion, head tilt, and visual perceptual difficulties as well as oculomotor signs. **Lateropulsion** refers to the person's tendency to fall to one side.

Brandt et al.[12] classify central vestibular syndromes from a clinical consensus of establishing perceptual, ocular motor, and postural signs. They report that the most sensitive signs of unilateral brainstem infarct are tilt of the patient's subjective visual vertical (SVV) and ocular torsion. A positive SVV is described as the patient's perception of vertical being tilted (the axes of the eyes and head are not horizontal). **Ocular torsion** refers to both eyes rotating downward toward the direction of tilt.

Ocular torsion combined with head tilting and skew deviation encompass a triad of signs termed a complete **ocular tilt reaction (OTR).**[33] In a study of patients with Wallenberg syndrome, one-third of these patients demonstrated a complete OTR[34] (Fig. 25-12). **Skew deviation** of the eyes appears as one eye being superiorly displaced in comparison with the other eye.

"Red flags" that should alert the clinician to a central vestibular etiology include horizontal or

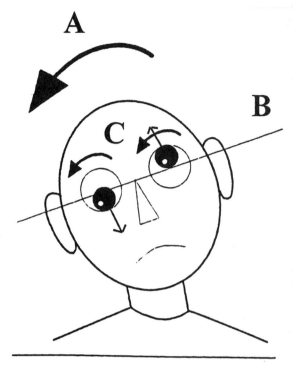

Figure 25-12. The ocular tilt reaction (OTR) consists of a triad of symptoms: *(A)* Head tilting to the right, indicated with the large bolded arrow. *(B)* Skew deviation of the eyes (right eye is down, left eye is up), indicated with the line drawing and straight arrows. *(C)* Torsion of the eyes to the right, indicated with the two smaller bolded arrows. (Adapted from Brandt and Dieterich,[10] p 339, with permission.)

vertical **diplopia** lasting longer than 2 weeks after the onset of a unilateral vestibular loss, persistent pure vertical positional nystagmus (anterior canal cupulolithiasis should be ruled out), and a spontaneous up beating nystagmus (rare). The therapist should refer a patient with these manifestations to a neurologist.

It is not within the scope of this chapter to expand on the differential diagnosis within the CNS, identifying the site of lesion. However, the physical therapist must recognize the difference between central and peripheral vestibular dysfunction because this guides the treatment strategy. Table 25–6 is to be used as a guide to discern central vestibular pathology from peripheral vestibular pathology.

INTERVENTIONS

Benign Paroxysmal Positional Vertigo

Goals and outcomes of physical therapy for the treatment of BPPV include the following:
1. Replace the otoconia into the vestibule.
2. Reduce the vertigo associated with head motion.
3. Improve balance.
4. Educate the patient about self-treatment strategies in the advent of reoccurrence.
5. Return to daily activity involving head motion.

Table 25–6 COMMON SYMPTOMS ASSOCIATED WITH CENTRAL VERSUS PERIPHERAL VESTIBULAR PATHOLOGY

Central Nervous System	Peripheral Nervous System
Abnormal smooth pursuit and abnormal saccadic eye movement tests.	Smooth pursuit and saccades usually normal; positional testing may reproduce nystagmus.
SX usually do not include hearing loss.	SX may include hearing loss, fullness in ears, tinnitus.
SX might include diplopia, altered conscious, lateropulsion.	
SX of acute vertigo not usually suppressed by visual fixation.	SX of acute vertigo usually suppressed by visual fixation.
	SX of acute vertigo usually intense (more than central vestibular pathology).
Pendular nystagmus (eyes oscillate at equal speeds).	Nystagmus will incorporate slow and fast phases (jerk nystagmus).
Pure persistent vertical nystagmus persists regardless of positional testing (persistent downbeat nystagmus in Hallpike-Dix may indicate anterior canal BPPV).	Spontaneous persistent horizontal nystagmus will resolve within 7 days in a patient with UVL.

BPPV, benign paroxysmal postural vertigo; SX, symptoms; UVL, unilateral vestibular lesion.

Because BPPV is the most common peripheral vestibular pathology, physical therapists should be familiar with treatment of this disorder. Three different treatment approaches have been developed, each based on the pathophysiology of this disorder. The techniques include canalith repositioning treatment, the liberatory procedure, and Brandt-Daroff exercises.

The *canalith repositioning treatment*[35] (CRT) is based on the canalithiasis theory of free-floating debris in the SCC. The patient's head is moved into different positions in a sequence that will move the debris out of the involved SCC and into the vestibule (general term for the location of the utricle and saccule; see Fig. 25-1). Once the debris is in the vestibule, the symptoms resolve. The positions used in the treatment of posterior and anterior SCC canalithiasis are the same. CRT has also been adapted for application to the horizontal SCC, although BPPV is much less common in either the horizontal or anterior SCC.[36] Figure 25-13 illustrates the CRT as applied to either the left posterior or left anterior SCC. After the treatment, the patient is fitted with a soft collar as a reminder to avoid vertical head movements that may again dislodge the otoconia. The patient is instructed to remain upright for 1 to 2 nights (sleep in a recliner chair) and then to avoid sleeping on the involved side for 5 additional nights. It is important to instruct the patient that horizontal movement of the head should be performed to prevent stiff neck muscles.

The *Liberatory*[37] *(Semont) maneuver* is based on the cupulolithiasis theory. It involves rapidly moving the patient through positions designed to dislodge the debris from the cupula (Fig. 25-14). Similar to CRT, the patient must avoid the provoking position and keep the head in an upright position for 1 to 2 nights after the treatment.

Brandt-Daroff[38] *exercises* were originally designed to habituate the CNS to the provoking position, but they may act by dislodging debris from the cupula or by causing debris to move out of the canal. Figure 25-15 illustrates the exercises. The exercise should be performed for 10 to 20 repetitions, three times a day until the patient has no vertigo for 2 consecutive days. If the patient has severe vertigo or complaints of nausea, the exercise protocol can be altered by decreasing the number of repetitions to five, again performed three times a day. It is important to

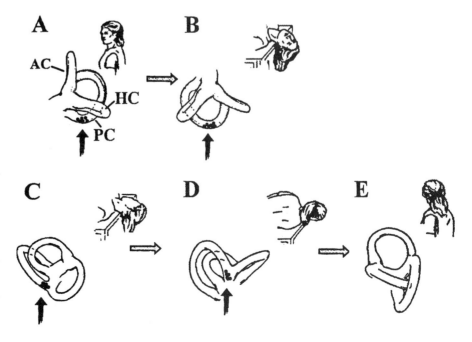

Figure 25-13. Canalith Repositioning Treatment (CRT). *(A)* The patient's head is first rotated toward the involved side, pictured here as the left. *(B)* The patient is then moved into the Hallpike-Dix position with the affected left ear toward the ground. *(C)* Next, the head is rotated 180 degrees to the right side. It is important to maintain the 30-degree neck extension during this step. *(D)* The patient is rolled onto the right shoulder and *(E)* slowly brought up to sitting position, head still rotated to the right. The patient may then be fitted with a soft collar. Note the orientation of the labyrinth for each stage. The arrow points to the free-floating debris and shows its movement through the canal into the common crus *(D)*. AC, anterior SCC; PC, posterior SCC; HC, horizontal SCC. *Between each step, the clinician must wait 1 to 2 minutes or until the vertigo and nystagmus has stopped to ensure replacement of the otoconia.* (From Tusa, RJ: Canalith Repositioning for Benign Positional Vertigo. Education Rehabilitation Program Syllabus. American Academy of Neurology, Minnesota, 1998, p 13, with permission.)

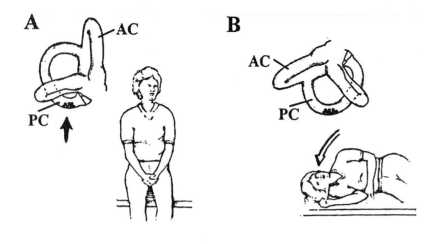

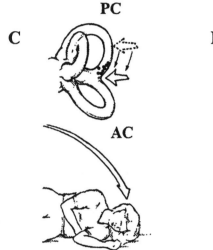

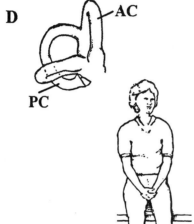

Figure 25-14. Liberatory (Semont) maneuver for posterior SCC BPPV. *(A)* The patient starts in a sitting position, then turns the head 45 degrees to one side (left) then quickly lies down on the opposite shoulder (right). *(B)* The patient should be instructed to remain in this position for 30 seconds or until the vertigo stops. The patient then slowly returns to the starting position *(A)*, maintaining the head rotation (left) until sitting upright. Next, the patient turns the head to the opposite direction (right) and lies down on the other shoulder (left) *(C)*, observing the similar 30 second time guidelines. The exercise should be done 10 to 20 times, three times per day until the patient is without vertigo for two consecutive days. (Adapted from Johnson and Griffen,[39] p 10, with permission from Mosby, Inc.)

explain to the patient that the movements must be performed rapidly and that this will probably provoke the patient's vertigo. Patient education should also include informing the patient that it is normal to have some residual symptoms of disequilibrium and nausea upon completing the exercise. The residual symptoms are usually temporary and patients need to continue the exercises.

The physical therapy goal of performing CRT and liberatory procedures are to replace the otoconia into the vestibule, where the calcium crystals can be reabsorbed. The Brandt-Daroff exercises, although originally designed to habituate the peripheral vestibular response, have also led to a complete remission of symptoms, sometimes after the first exercise session.[38] Physical therapy outcomes should also include teaching the patient how to use the appropriate techniques at home, because BPPV has a recurrence rate of 30 percent.[39] See Table 25–7 for suggested guidelines for use of the CRT, the liberatory procedure, or Brandt-Daroff exercises.

Unilateral Vestibular Lesion

Goals and outcomes of physical therapy for the treatment of UVL include the following:
1. Improve stability of gaze during head movement.
2. Decrease sensitivity to motion.
3. Improve static and dynamic postural stability.
4. Establish a home exercise program (HEP) that includes walking.

Patients with UVL should be informed that recovery time upon initiating vestibular rehabilitation averages 8 weeks. To ensure compliance with the vestibular rehabilitation exercises, patients should be encouraged frequently and informed of the outcomes and goals.

GAZE STABILITY

The purpose of these exercises is to improve the VOR and other systems that are used to assist gaze stability with head motion. The two primary para-

Figure 25-15. Brandt-Daroff treatment for posterior SCC BPPV. The physical therapist should be assisting the patient through this positioning procedure. *(A)* The head is rotated 45 degrees to the left. *(B)* The patient moves from sitting to right sidelying and stays in this position for 1 minute. *(C)* The patient is then rapidly moved 180 degrees, from right sidelying to left sidelying. The head should be in the original starting position, left rotated in this illustration. After 1 minute in this position, *(D)* the patient returns to sitting and may be fitted with a soft collar. AC, anterior SCC; PC, posterior SCC; HC, horizontal SCC. (Adapted from Johnson and Griffen,[39] p 10, with permission from Mosby, Inc.)

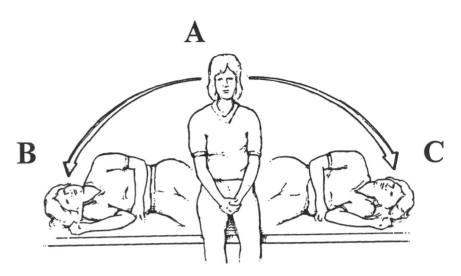

digms are X1 (times 1) and X2 (times 2) exercises.[40] In the X1 exercise the patient is asked to move the head horizontally (and vertically if appropriate) as quickly as possible while maintaining focus on a stable target. Trying to keep the target in focus is very important because a small amount of retinal slip is the signal to improve the response of the remaining vestibular system. **Retinal slip** occurs when the image of an object moves off the fovea of the retina, resulting in visual blurring. The patient must learn to slow the head movement if the target becomes blurred. A good target to use is a business card, asking the patient to focus on a word or a letter within a word. The starting target distance should be an arm's length away. The X2 paradigm requires the patient to move the head and target in opposite directions (Fig. 25-16). Both paradigms should be made increasingly more difficult as the patient improves. Examples of increasing difficulty include the use of a distracting background while the patient attempts to read the letter or word (checkerboard, venetian blinds), varying the distance from which the patient performs the exercises, moving the head more rapidly, and performing the exercise while standing.

POSTURAL STABILITY

The purpose of postural stability exercises is to improve balance by encouraging the development

Table 25–7 BENIGN PAROXYSMAL POSITIONAL VERTIGO TREATMENT TECHNIQUES

Treatment Procedure	Diagnosis/Symptoms
CRT	BPPV due to canalithiasis
	Posterior SCC canalithiasis is the most common
Liberatory maneuver	BPPV due to cupulolithiasis
	Posterior SCC cupulolithiasis is the most common
Brandt-Daroff exercises	Persistent/residual or mild vertigo (even after CRT)
	For the patient who may not tolerate CRT

BPPV, benign paroxysmal positional vertigo; CRT, canalith repositioning treatment; SCC, semicircular canal.

of balance strategies within the limitations of the patient, be they somatosensory, visual, or vestibular. The exercises should challenge the patient and be safe enough to perform independently (Table 25–8). It is important to incorporate head movement into the exercises because most patients with vestibular loss tend to decrease their head movement.

MOTION SENSITIVITY

Habituation training is warranted when a patient with a UVL has continual complaints of dizziness. *Habituation* is defined as the reduction in response to a repeatedly performed movement. These exercises were the first successful methods used to treat persons with vestibular disorders. Shumway-Cook and Horak[41] and others[19] have developed versions of positional tests based on the original work of Cawthorne,[4] Cooksey,[5] Norre and DeWeerdt,[42] and Dix.[43,44] As our knowledge of the vestibular system improves, however, we are able to provide more specific exercises than what habituation offers. Clinicians should not treat all vestibular patients with habituation exercises. For example, habituation exercises for a patient with a BVL is inappropriate.

The physical therapist instructs the patient in positions that provoke the symptoms. When a position elicits a mild to moderate dizziness, the patient remains in the provoking position for 30 seconds or until the symptoms abate, whichever comes first.[41] The patient is provided with a home exercise program (HEP) based on the results of the positional evaluation.[19,41] The provoking exercises are performed from three to five times each, two to three times a day. Figure 25-17 gives an example of an HEP using vestibular habituation training. The exercises are designed to reproduce the dizziness and the patient should be encouraged that the symptoms normally decrease within 2 weeks. If after 2 weeks the symptoms are no better, the habituation exercises should first be changed. If this is not helpful, the patient should be referred to either a physical therapist with training in vestibular

A
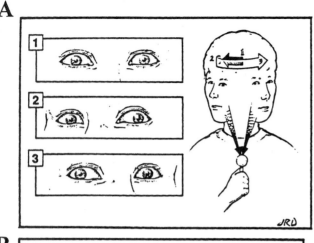

B
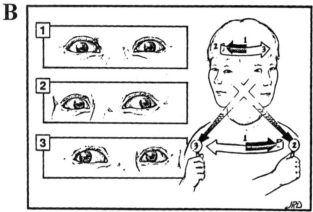

Figure 25-16. Gaze stability exercises. *(A)* X1 paradigm: The patient is instructed to focus their eyes on a near target. While maintaining focus on the target, the patient horizontally rotates the head keeping the target still. *(B)* X2 paradigm: The patient is instructed to focus the eyes on a near target. While the focus is maintained, the patient horizontally rotates the head and the target in *opposite* directions. Both X1 and X2 paradigms require vigilance of the patient to ensure clear vision during the motions. Both exercises are typically performed for 1 to 2 minutes, five times a day. It can be repeated using vertical head movements. (From Johnson and Griffen,[39] p 12, with permission.)

rehabilitation* or to a physician for further evaluation.

Bilateral Vestibular Lesion

Goals and outcomes of physical therapy for the treatment of BVL include the following:
1. Reduce subjective complaints of gaze instability.
2. Improve static and dynamic balance.
3. Instruct the patient in a HEP that includes walking.

---

*The Vestibular Disorders Association (VEDA) has a list of physical therapists in each state, interested in treating patients with vestibular disorders. The VEDA phone number is 1-503-229-7705.

4. Educate the patient in activities that may be more difficult owing to the disorder.

Treatment of patients with a BVL is designed to address the primary complaints of **gaze instability** during head motion, disequilibrium, and gait ataxia. Gaze stability exercises can be similar to the X1 paradigm described in treatment for UVL. Use of the X2 paradigm is not recommended for a patient with a BVL because this exercise may cause excessive retinal slip in patients with BVL. Instead, exercises that incorporate sequenced eye and head movements and the use of imaginary targets may improve gaze stability by enhancing central preprogramming of eye movements (Table 25–9).

Patients with BVL depend on somatosensation and/or vision to maintain postural stability. Balance exercises should enhance the use of these cues. Care must be taken that the exercises are performed safely because people with BVL are more likely to fall. It is imperative to begin the patient on a walking program, daily if tolerated. This can be progressed to ambulating on different surfaces (grass, gravel, sand) and in different environments (grocery store, mall). Recovery from a lesion involving both vestibular systems takes much longer than a unilateral lesion. Patients should be informed that as long as 2 years will be necessary to ensure as complete a recovery as possible. For this reason, patient education emphasizing daily activity is a high priority. Daily activity must continue beyond the course of vestibular rehabilitation. Other recommended activities include exercises in a pool and Tai Chi. The pool provides an environment of reduced gravity, allowing the patient to move safely without the risk of falling quickly to the ground. Tai Chi incorporates slow, controlled motions used to improve balance, flexibility, and increase strength. In most cases, a person with a bilateral vestibular loss will incur a functional disability. Certain activities may always be limited, such as walking in the dark, night driving, or sports involving quick movements of the head.[45] Older patients may have to use an assistive device such as a cane for safe ambulation at night or on uneven surfaces. It should be noted that habituation exercises do not work for the patient with a bilateral vestibular loss.[18]

Central Vestibular Lesion

Goals and outcomes of physical therapy for the treatment of central vestibular lesions include the following:
1. Ensure fall prevention strategies and necessary safety precautions are in place to allow safe functioning within the home and community.
2. Educate patient in compensatory strategies to assist in gaze stability.
3. Instruct the patient in a HEP that includes walking.

Once an accurate diagnosis of central vestibular pathology is made, the physical therapist must be

Table 25–8 BALANCE EXERCISES AND PROGRESSIONS

Begin With	Progress To	Purpose
1. Stand with feet shoulder-width apart, arms across the chest.	Bring feet closer together. Close eyes. Stand on a sofa cushion/pillow.	Enhance the use of vestibular signal for balance by decreasing base of support. Eyes closed increases reliance on vestibular signals for balance.
2. Practice ankle sways: anterior-posterior and medial-lateral.	Doing circle sways. Close eyes.	Teaches the patient to use a correct ankle strategy.
3. Attempt to walk with heel touching toe on firm surface.	Do the same exercise on carpet.	Enhance the use of vestibular signal for balance by decreasing base of support. Doing the exercise on carpet decreases proprioception, increasing difficulty.
4. Practice walking and turning around.	Making smaller turns. Close eyes.	The turning stimulates and challenges the vestibular system.
5. Walk and move your head side-to-side.	Counting backwards from 100 by threes.	Challenge balance and stimulate both vestibular systems.

Note: These exercises represent a limited number of exercises which are effective at improving functional balance. Each of the balance exercises should be performed three times a day for 1–2 minutes each repetition.

careful in choosing rehabilitation strategies. Expectations for recovery should be described initially to the patient. Generally, the time to recover will be 6 months or more, and may be incomplete.[46] Many of the adaptive mechanisms thought responsible for recovery of the vestibular system are central processes that may have been damaged in the initial central lesion. In patients with TBI, vestibular rehabilitation may not be the treatment of choice because of its irritating nature, further disorienting the patient.

The examination described previously will be essential in discerning a peripheral versus central vestibular pathology. The physical therapy intervention for a **central vestibular lesion** at the level of the brainstem (vestibular nuclei) likely will be similar to a unilateral vestibular lesion, with the same expectations for recovery. Vestibular cortical lesions may also recover, similar to the process a cerebral vascular accident might.

PATIENT EDUCATION

The vestibular system requires movement to recover from most lesions. This premise should be the primary operative when educating patients about returning to daily activity, exercising independently at home, and as a general guideline for their recovery. The vestibular system will not improve maximally without stimulation. The challenge for both the outpatient and inpatient physical therapist is determining the amount of exertion the patient can tolerate, creating the effective form of vestibular stimulation without causing deleterious effects.

Instructions for the Patient:
Once in the provoking position, wait for 10 seconds to determine if the dizziness will occur. If you experience symptoms of dizziness, remain in the position for an additional 20 seconds (30 seconds total) or until the dizziness abates, whichever comes first. If you do not experience any symptoms you may return to your starting position. Now that you have returned to your starting position, remain here for 10 seconds to monitor your dizziness. If you are dizzy, remain in the return position for an additional 20 seconds (30 seconds total) or until the symptoms abate, whichever comes first. Repeat five times.

Example of Exercises:
1.) Quickly move from sitting upright to bending at the trunk as if to touch your nose to your knee.
2.) Quickly move from sitting at the edge of the bed to lying flat.
3.) In supine, roll onto your left then right side.

Guidelines for the Therapist:
Often, the patient may complain of a certain movement that provokes the symptoms which the evaluation does not incorporate. This movement can be adapted to be a part of the patient s home exercise program. The patient

	Mon	Tues	Wed	Thur	Fri	Sat	Sun
Duration (0—30 seconds)							
Intensity (0—5)							

Figure 25-17. Example of a home exercise program using habituation therapy.

Table 25–9 BILATERAL VESTIBULAR LESION EXERCISES TO IMPROVE CENTRAL PREPROGRAMMING OF EYE MOVEMENTS

Begin With	Progress To
1. Hold two targets at arm's length from your head. Look with your eyes first, then turn your head toward the target. Attempt to do this for 60 seconds.	Progress to increasing the distance used to see the target. Use a busy background (checkerboard, venetian blinds).
2. Perform exercise 1 in the vertical direction.	Same as horizontal exercise.
3. Hold one target at arm's length from your head. Close your eyes and turn your head away from the target, attempting to keep your eyes focused on the target. Open your eyes only after having turned your head.	Progress to doing this standing. Progress to decreasing base of support.

COMMON VESTIBULAR DIAGNOSES

Ménière's Disease

Ménière's disease is diagnosed by a documented low frequency hearing loss and episodic vertigo. The patient may also complain of a sense of fullness in the ear and **tinnitus.** The symptoms gradually increase in severity and then last 1 to 2 hours per episode. Chronic Ménière's disease, however, can result in unilateral peripheral vestibular hypofunction, for which rehabilitation is appropriate. The pathophysiology of Ménière's disease probably involves an increase in endolymphatic fluid causing distension of the membranous tissues.[47] Medical treatment is therefore directed toward reducing or preventing fluid buildup. Many patients can manage the symptoms well with a controlled diet. Patients with Ménière's disease should be placed on a 2 g/d or less sodium diet. This is the most important dietary restriction to follow. Other substances to avoid are caffeine and alcohol. Sometimes medical management includes use of a diuretic to control the amount of water in the body. Surgery to either prevent the fluid buildup in the inner ear (endolymphatic shunt placement) or to stop the abnormal vestibular signal (vestibular nerve section) may be indicated if the episodes are frequent enough to disturb daily function. Physical therapy is most beneficial in treating the effects of a unilateral vestibular hypofunction owing to chronic Ménière's disease, although the therapy will not stop the episodes of vertigo. Gaze and postural stability exercises may be appropriate. Physical therapy is also useful in the treatment of disequilibrium occurring after a vestibular neurectomy.

Perilymphatic Fistula

Perilymphatic fistula (PLF) is most commonly caused by a rupture of the oval or round windows, membranes that separate the middle and inner ear.

A rupture of these membranes results in leakage of the perilymph into the middle ear. The result is vertigo and hearing loss. Perilymph bathes the SCC, serving as a protective barrier between the bony and membranous labyrinth. PLF usually is caused from a traumatic event, such as excessive pressure changes as in deep-water diving, blunt head trauma without skull fracture, or extremely loud noise.[48] This diagnosis is much debated and the treatment for PLF is similarly ambiguous. Patients often are treated first with bed rest in hopes of allowing the membrane to heal. Surgical patches of the fistula are also performed. Physical therapy is contraindicated for most patients with PLF; however, it can be beneficial in those patients who have continual disequilibrium postoperatively. Medical management will likely include strict limitations on activities, warranting good communication between physical therapist and physician.

Acoustic Neuroma

Acoustic neuroma, also called vestibular schwannomma, is a benign tumor located on cranial nerve VIII. Complaints include progressive hearing loss, tinnitus, and disequilibrium. Treatment usually involves surgical excision of the tumor. Preoperatively, vertigo is present in less than 20 percent of cases.[49] Postoperatively, many patients experience vertigo because the procedure often requires sacrificing all or part of the vestibular nerve. Optimally, physical therapy is initiated during the early postoperative period to help the patient resolve symptoms of disequilibrium and oscillopsia.[50] Outpatient treatment should be considered similar to the treatment for a unilateral vestibular loss.

Motion Sickness

Motion sickness is a normal sensation but in some people becomes debilitating. The predominate explanation for motion sickness is the **sensory conflict theory.**[51] The three sensory inputs of proprioception, vestibular, and visual information do not match stored neural patterns the brain expects to recognize. As a result, persons experience pallor, nausea, emesis, diaphoresis, and motion sensitivity. Currently the most successful methods reported to combat motion sickness include the use of cognitive-behavioral management, medications, biofeedback, and habituation training using ground and flight situations.[52–55]

COMMON NONVESTIBULAR DIAGNOSES

Migraine-Related Dizziness

Migraine related dizziness can be deceptively similar to a peripheral vestibular lesion. The reason being is the vascular event occurs in a vestibular structure such as the vestibular nuclei. Migraine related symptoms include vertigo, dizziness, and motion sickness. Women between the ages of 35 and 45 have been found particularly prone to migraine-related dizziness.[56] The clinical examination will provide the differential diagnosis between vestibular pathology and migraine. If the therapist suspects migraine the patient should be referred to a neurologist, preferably one with a special interest in headache. Migraine is often well controlled with medication and diet.

Multiple Sclerosis

MS can affect cranial nerve VIII where it enters the brainstem and causes identical symptoms to a unilateral vestibular pathology. A magnetic resonance image (MRI) scan will need to be performed to ensure an accurate diagnosis of MS.

Cervical Vertigo

Cervical vertigo is a diagnosis commonly used in Europe yet controversial in the United States. A large percentage of persons suffering from motor vehicle accidents, however, do report symptoms of dizziness warranting further investigation into the source. The mechanisms of involvement are believed to be from at least two sources. First, the upper cervical spine sends proprioceptive input to the contralateral vestibular nucleus. Soft tissue injury and joint dysfunction might alter the afferent input contributing to spatial orientation. Second, a patient might have **vertebrobasilar insufficiency (VBI).** If VBI is suspected, vascular compromise must first be ruled out as a cause of the patient symptoms. The VBI test can be performed while the subject is seated. The patient leans forward and extends the neck. The neck is then rotated 45 degrees to the suspicious side. Symptoms of VBI include diplopia, dysarthria, syncope, headache, and visual field deficits as well as vertigo and nystagmus. Persons suspected of having VBI should be referred to a neurologist immediately. Repeated episodes of vertigo without the associated VBI symptoms usually suggests a peripheral vestibular diagnosis.[57]

CONTRAINDICATIONS

Physical therapy is not appropriate for unstable vestibular disorders such as Ménière's disease and PLF. Other contraindications the clinician should be alert to include sudden loss of hearing, increased feeling of pressure or fullness to the point of discomfort in one or both ears, and severe ringing in one or both ears. When treating patients who have had a surgical procedure, the clinician must be observant for discharge of fluid from the ears or nose, which may indicate cerebrospinal fluid leak. Patients with acute neck injuries may not be able to tolerate either the CRT or some of the gaze stability exercises.

SUMMARY

Physical therapists must recognize signs and symptoms associated with vestibular disorders because of the prevalence in medicine today. It is essential to differentiate a central pathology from a peripheral pathology. The central and peripheral lesions have separate manifestations and may require different intervention strategies. Additionally, vestibular disorders should not be treated similarly. The most common form of vertigo, BPPV, is a biomechanical problem readily treated with a single maneuver. This is in stark contrast to a patient with a bilateral vestibular lesion, which requires a greater rehabilitation effort.

The supplemental reading list contains other excellent literature for the reader interested in pursuing a greater depth of knowledge in vestibular rehabilitation.

QUESTIONS FOR REVIEW

1. Differentiate the two movement sensors of the vestibular system.

2. Describe how a poor vestibular gain explains the clinical sign of a refixation saccade, seen in a positive head thrust test.

3. Why does the patient with an acute unilateral vestibular lesion experience spontaneous nystagmus?

4. What is the pathology of BPPV due to cupulolithiasis?

5. What are the key elements in taking a history?

6. Explain inhibitory cut off.

7. Differentiate the X1 exercise paradigm from the X2 exercise paradigm.

8. In a patient with vestibular nystagmus, which part of the eye movement (slow or fast) is from the vestibular system? Why?

9. Describe how the Hallpike-Dix test would elicit nystagmus for posterior SCC BPPV.

10. What is meant by subjective visual vertical?

CASE STUDIES

Case Study 1

You are performing an initial examination of a patient with complaints of imbalance and dizziness. In a sitting position, at rest, the patient is observed to have a pure vertical nystagmus with head tilting to the left. The nystagmus is not altered with any change in head position, and the head-shaking–induced nystagmus test (HSN) is negative.

Guiding Questions

1. How will you differentiate between central or peripheral pathology as a cause of dizziness?
2. Is physical therapy appropriate at this time?

Case Study 2

After treating your patient with posterior canalithiasis using the canalith repositioning treatment (CRT), the patient is complaining of some neck pain and a vague sense of dizziness. The vertigo is gone.

Guiding Questions

3. How will you assess the benign paroxysmal positional vertigo (BPPV)?
4. Following treatment for BPVV, the patient continues to complain of neck pain and dizziness. Is it possible you made the symptoms worse?
5. Can you prescribe any other forms of exercise for the remaining dizziness?

Case Study 3

A patient with a unilateral vestibular lesion (UVL) complains of feeling worse after 7 days of starting a vestibular rehabilitation program. The patient has had no falls. The complaints consist of increased dizziness with head motion, nausea, and fatigue.

Guiding Questions

6. Is your rehabilitation program making the patient worse?
7. How can you modify the program?
8. What information will you tell your patient with a unilateral vestibular lesion regarding time to recover? BPPV? Bilateral vestibular lesion (BVL)? Central nervous system pathology?

Case Study 4

Three weeks after initiating vestibular rehabilitation for a patient with a bilateral vestibular loss your patient falls at home but is not injured.

Guiding Questions

9. Will you modify the physical therapy intervention?
10. Was your home exercise program too rigorous?

REFERENCES

1. Kroenke, K, and Mangelsdorf, D: Common symptoms in ambulatory care: Incidence, evaluation, therapy, and outcome. Am J Med 86:262, 1989.
2. Watson, MA, and Sinclair, H: Balancing Act: For People with Dizziness and Balance Disorders. Vestibular Disorders Association, Portland, 1992.
3. Kroenke, K, et al: Causes of persistent dizziness: A prospective study of 100 patients in ambulatory care. Ann Intern Med 117:898, 1992.
4. Cawthorne, T: The physiological basis for head exercises. Journal of the Chartered Society of Physiotherapy 30:106, 1944.
5. Cooksey, FS: Rehabilitation in vestibular injuries. Proc R Soc Med 39:273, 1946.
6. Grusser, OJ, et al: Localization and responses of neurones in the parieto-insular vestibular cortex of awake monkeys (macaca fascicularis). J Physiol 430:537, 1990.
7. Thier, P, and Erickson, G: Vestibular input to visual-tracking neurons in area MST of awake rhesus monkeys. Ann NY Acad Sci 656:960, 1992.
8. Buttner, U, and Buettner, UW: Parietal cortex (2v) neuronal activity in the alert monkey during natural vestibular and optokinetic stimulation. Brain Res 153:392, 1978.
9. Odkvist, LM, et al: Projection of the vestibular nerve area 3a arm field in the squirrel monkey (saimiri sciureus). Exp Brain Res 21:97, 1974.
10. Brandt, T, and Dieterich, M: Vestibular syndromes in the roll plane: Topographic diagnosis from brainstem to cortex. Ann Neurol 36:337, 1994.
11. Cooke, D: Central vestibular disorders. Neurology Report 20:22, 1996.
12. Brandt, T, et al: Vestibular cortex lesions affect the perception of verticality. Ann Neurol 35:403, 1994.
13. Baloh, RW, and Honrubia, V: Clinical neurophysiology of the vestibular system. FA Davis, Philadelphia, 1990.
14. Demer, JL: Evaluation of vestibular and visual oculomotor function. Otolaryngol Head Neck Surg 2:16, 1995.
15. Dixon, JS, and Bird, HA: Reproducibility along a 10 cm vertical visual analog scale. Ann Rheum Dis 40:87, 1981.
16. Jacobsen, GP, and Newman, CW: The development of the dizziness handicap inventory. Arch Otolaryngol Head Neck Surg 116:424, 1990.
17. Robertson, D, and Ireland, D: Dizziness handicap inventory correlates of computerized dynamic posturography. J Otolaryngol 24:118, 1995.
18. Telian, SA, et al: Habituation therapy for chronic vestibular dysfunction: Preliminary results. Otolaryngol Head Neck Surg 103:89, 1990.
19. Smith-Wheelock, M, et al: Physical therapy program for vestibular rehabilitation. Am J Otol 12:218, 1991.
20. Fetter, M, and Dichgans, J: Adaptive mechanisms of VOR compensation after unilateral peripheral vestibular lesions in humans. J Vestib Res 1:9, 1990.
21. LaCour, M, et al: Modifications and development of spinal reflexes in the alert baboon (papio papio) following an unilateral vestibular neurectomy. Brain Res 113:255, 1976.
22. Collins, WE: Habituation of vestibular responses with and without visual stimulation. In Kornhuber, HH (ed): Handbook of Sensory Physiology, vol I/2. Springer-Verlag, Berlin, 1974, p 369.
23. Halmagyi, GM, et al: The Human vestibulo-ocular reflex after unilateral vestibular deafferentation: The results of high acceleration impulsive testing. In Sharpe, JA, and Barber, HO (eds): The Vestibulo-Ocular Reflex and Vertigo. Raven Press, New York, 1993, p 45.
24. Dix, R, and Hallpike CS: The pathology, symptomatology and diagnosis of certain common disorders of the vestibular system. Ann Otol Rhinol Laryngol 6:987, 1952.
25. Venuto, P, et al: Inter-rater reliability of the clinical dynamic visual acuity test. Phys Ther 78:S21, 1998.
26. Sharpe, JA: Assessment and management of central vestibular disorders. In Herdman, SJ (ed): Vestibular Rehabilitation. FA Davis, Philadelphia, 1994, p 206.
27. Schuknecht, HF: Cupulolithiasis. Arch Otolaryngol 90:765, 1969.
28. Hall, SF, et al: The mechanisms of benign paroxysmal vertigo. J Otolaryngol 8:151, 1979.
29. Halmagyi, GM, et al: Gentamicin vestibulotoxicity. Otolaryngol Head Neck Surg 111:571, 1994.
30. Berman, J, and Frederickson, J: Vertigo after head injury: A five year follow-up. J Otolaryngol 7:237, 1978.
31. Tuohimma, P: Vestibular disturbances after acute mild head injury. Acta Otolaryngol Suppl (Stockh) 359:7, 1978.
32. Halmagyi, GM: Central Eye Movement Disorders. In Albert, DM, and Jakobiec, FA (eds): Principles and Practice of Ophthalmology, vol 4. Saunders, Philadelphia, 1994.

33. Brandt, T, et al: Plasticity of the vestibular system: Central compensation and sensory substitution for vestibular deficits. Brain Plasticity Adv in Neurol 73:297, 1997.

34. Dieterich, M, and Brandt, T: Wallenberg's syndrome: Lateropulsion, cyclorotation, and subjective visual vertical in thirty-six patients. Ann Neurol 31:399, 1992.

35. Epley, JM: The canalith repositioning procedure: For treatment of benign paroxysmal positional vertigo. Otolaryngol Head Neck Surg 107:399, 1992.

36. Herdman, SJ, et al: Eye movement signs in vertical canal benign paroxysmal positional vertigo. In Fuchs, AF, et al (eds). Contemporary Ocular Motor and Vestibular Research: A Tribute to David A. Robinson. George Thieme Verlag, Stuttgart, 1994, p 385.

37. Semont, A, et al: Curing the BPPV with a liberatory maneuver. Adv Oto-Rhino-Laryngol 42:290, 1988.

38. Brandt, T, and Daroff, RB: Physical therapy for benign paroxysmal positional vertigo. Arch Otolaryngol 106:484, 1980.

39. Herdman, SJ: Personal communication, 1998.

40. Johnson, R, and Griffin, J: Current Therapy in Neurologic Disease. Mosby Year-Book, St. Louis, 1993, p 12.

41. Shumway-Cook, A, and Horak, FB: Vestibular rehabilitation: An exercise approach to managing symptoms of vestibular dysfunction. Seminars in Hearing 10:196, 1989.

42. Norre, ME, and DeWeerdt, W: Treatment of vertigo based on habituation. J Laryngol Otol 94:971, 1980.

43. Dix, MR: The rationale and technique of head exercises in the treatment of vertigo. Acta Otorhinolaryngol Belg 33:370, 1979.

44. Dix, MR: The physiological basis and practical value of head exercises in the treatment of vertigo. The Practitioner 217:919, 1976.

45. Herdman, SJ (ed): Vestibular Rehabilitation. FA Davis, Philadelphia, 1994.

46. Shepard, NT, et al: Vestibular and balance rehabilitation therapy. Ann Otol Rhinol Laryngol 102:198, 1993.

47. Arenberg, IK: Ménières disease: Diagnosis and management of vertigo and endolymphatic hydrops. In Arenberg, IK (ed): Dizziness and Balance Disorders. Kugler Publications, New York, 1993, p 503.

48. Goodhill, V: Ear Diseases, Deafness and Dizziness. Harper and Row, Hagerstown, MD, 1979.

49. Clendaniel, RA: Unpublished material, 1998.

50. Herdman, SJ, et al: Vestibular adaptation exercises and recovery: Acute stage after acoustic neuroma resection. Otolaryngol Head Neck Surg 113:77, 1995.

51. Reason, JT: Motion sickness adaptation: A neural mismatch model. J R Soc Med 71:819, 1978.

52. Dobie, TG, and May, JG: Cognitive-behavioral management of motion sickness. Aviat Space Environ Med 65(suppl 10):C1, 1994.

53. Bagshaw, M, and Stott, JR: The desensitisation of chronically motion sick aircrew in the Royal Air Force. Aviat Space Environ Med 56:1144, 1985.

54. Golding, JF, and Stott, JR: Objective and subjective time courses of recovery from motion sickness assessed by repeated motion challenges. J Vestib Res 7:421, 1997.

55. Banks, RD, et al: The Canadian forces airsickness rehabilitation program, 1981–1991. Aviat Space Environ Med 63:1098, 1992.

56. Tusa, RJ: Personal communication, November 1997.

57. Baloh, R: The Essential of Neuro-otology. FA Davis, Philadelphia, 1984.

58. Herdman, SJ: Physical therapy in the treatment of patients with benign paroxysmal positional vertigo. Neurology Report 20:46, 1996.

SUPPLEMENTAL READINGS

Baloh, RW, and Honrubia, V: Clinical neurophysiology of the vestibular system. FA Davis, Philadelphia, 1990.

Epley, JM: The canalith repositioning procedure: For treatment of benign paroxysmal positional vertigo. Otolaryngol Head Neck Surg 107:399, 1992.

Fetter, M, and Dichgans, J: Adaptive mechanisms of VOR compensation after unilateral peripheral vestibular lesions in humans. J Vestib Res 1:9, 1990.

Hall, SF, et al: The mechanisms of benign paroxysmal vertigo. J Otolaryngol 8:151, 1979.

Herdman, SJ: Vestibular Rehabilitation. FA Davis, Philadelphia, 1994.

Herdman, SJ: Physical therapy in the treatment of patients with benign paroxysmal positional vertigo. Neurology Report 20:46, 1996.

Shumway-Cook, A, and Horak, FB: Vestibular rehabilitation: An exercise approach to managing symptoms of vestibular dysfunction. Seminars in Hearing 10:196, 1989.

Smith-Wheelock, M, et al: Physical therapy program for vestibular rehabilitation. Am J Otol 12:218, 1991.

GLOSSARY

Acoustic neuroma: Benign tumor of the vestibulo-cochlear cranial nerve.

Benign paroxysmal positional vertigo (BPPV): Vertigo owing to otoconia in the SCCs displaced from the utricle.

Caloric testing: Test infusing the external auditory canal with air or water causing movement of the endolymph within the horizontal SCC, allowing quantification; useful for determining the side of deficit.

Canalithiasis: Fragments of otoconia floating freely in the endolymph of the SCC; associated with positional vertigo.

Central vestibular lesion: A lesion in a vestibular pathway located in the CNS.

Cupulolithiasis: Fragments of otoconia gravitate to and become attached to the cupula of the SCC; associated with positional vertigo.

Diplopia: Double vision.

Dizziness: Sensation of lightheadedness, whirling or feeling a tendency to fall.

Disequilibrium: Subjective sensation that one is off balance.

Endolymph: Fluid within the SCCs.

Gaze instability: Difficulty maintaining visual focus, usually associated with motion.

Habituation training: Training using repeated movements to reduce the provocative stimulus.

Hallpike-Dix test: Positional test used to reproduce vertigo and nystagmus.

Head-shaking–induced nystagmus (HSN): Test used to discern vestibular asymmetry.

Inhibitory cut off: The velocity (80°/second) at which inhibition (hyperpolarization) of the hair cells in the labyrinth opposite head rotation no longer occurs.

Lateropulsion: Tendency to fall to one side.

Lightheadedness: Sense of feeling as if about to faint.

Ménière's disease: Recurrent group of symptoms including episodic vertigo, tinnitus, sensation of fullness in the ear, and hearing loss.

Nystagmus: Involuntary cyclical movement of the eyeball in any direction. It usually has clearly defined fast and slow components beating in opposite directions.

> **Gaze-evoked nystagmus:** Nystagmus induced by change in eye position.
>
> **Pendular nystagmus:** Nystagmus characterized by movement that is approximately equal in both directions.
>
> **Positional nystagmus:** Nystagmus induced by change in head position.
>
> **Spontaneous nystagmus:** Nystagmus from acute vestibular pathology; generally resolves within 7 days.

Ocular torsion: The superior pole of the eyes rotate in a clockwise or counterclockwise direction.

Ocular tilt reaction (OTR): Triad of signs including skew deviation, ocular torsion, and head tilt.

Oscillopsia: Visual blurring during head motion.

Otolith organs: Linear movement sensor of the vestibular system.

Ototoxicity: Toxicity of cranial nerve VIII or the vestibular system; caused by certain antibiotics (aminoglycosides [gentamycin, streptomycin]).

Peripheral vestibular lesion: A lesion in the peripheral vestibular organ or cranial nerve VIII.

Perilymphatic fistula (PLF): A rupture of the oval or round windows, causing an opening between the middle and inner ear.

Push-pull mechanism: A mechanism the brain uses to assess movement through comparison of inputs from the two vestibular systems.

Retinal slip: When the visual image falls off the fovea of the retina.

Saccade: Fast, involuntary eye movement.

Semicircular canals (SCCs): Angular movement sensors of the vestibular system.

Sensory conflict theory: Predominate explanation for motion sickness, which describes sensory inputs of proprioception, vestibular, and visual information not matching stored neural patterns.

Skew deviation: When one eye is superiorly displaced in comparison with the other eye.

Smooth pursuit: Voluntary eye movement used to follow a moving target.

Tinnitus: Ringing of the ears, commonly indicative of high frequency hearing loss.

Vertebrobasilar insufficiency (VBI): Ischemia in the region of the vertebral and basilar artery junction.

Vertigo: An illusion of movement, most commonly a sense of spinning.

> **Cervical vertigo:** Vertigo believed to arise from a cervical pathology.

Vestibular gain: Ratio of eye velocity to head velocity.

Vestibulo-ocular reflex (VOR): Reflex responsible for generating eye movements, which enable clear vision while the head is in motion.

Vestibulo spinal reflex (VSR): Reflex responsible for generating compensatory body movements in order to maintain head and postural stability, thereby preventing falls.

APPENDIX A

Suggested Answers to Guiding Questions

1. How will you differentiate between central or peripheral pathology as a cause of dizziness?

ANSWER:

1. The vertical nystagmus at rest can only be caused by a central nervous system lesion. If the lesion were peripheral you would likely see positive HSN and vertigo if the lesion is acute (asymmetry). The head tilt is usually suspicious of a central lesion though some patients with acute and subacute UVL may tilt the head (seldom).

2. Is physical therapy appropriate at this time?

ANSWER: Until the patient is medically cleared for physical therapy, the clinician should defer treatment.

3. How will you reassess for benign paroxysmal positional vertigo (BPPV)?

ANSWER: The patient will need to be retested for BPPV using the sidelying Hallpike-Dix testing position or using a tilt table, protecting the neck and back from injury.

4. Following treatment for BPPV, the patient continues to complain of neck pain and dizziness. Is it possible you may have made the symptoms worse?

ANSWER: The complaint of neck pain is most likely muscle spasm and should be addressed as a separate issue. It is not unusual for patients to have persistent disequilibrium, floating sensations, or dizziness after successful treatment of the BPPV. This may be due to a small residual amount of debris in the canal. These symptoms typically resolve in 2 or 3 weeks.

5. Can you prescribe any other forms of exercise for the remaining dizziness?

ANSWER: Brandt-Daroff exercises would be an appropriate follow up treatment option for the residual symptoms.

6. Is your rehabilitation program making the patient worse?

ANSWER: Subjective complaints of increased intensity are not uncommon following the exercises for a unilateral vestibular lesion and does not suggest a worsening of the vestibular condition. In most cases, it is because the patient had been limiting head movements as a way of avoiding feeling dizzy. Because the exercises involve significant head movement, the patient experiences an increase in dizziness.

7. How can you modify the program?

ANSWER: If necessary, patients can be instructed to modify their home exercise program to ensure compliance. This can be done in many different ways. The number of repetitions and duration of each exercise can be limited, the number of times per day the exercises are performed can be reduced from five to three or four, and the patient can rest for longer periods between performing the exercise session. It is imperative the clinician educate the patient that movement stimulates the vestibular system and is required to ensure the greatest possible recovery.

8. What information will you tell your patient with a unilateral vestibular lesion regarding time to recover? BPPV? Bilateral vestibular lesion (BVL)? Central nervous system pathology?

ANSWER

EXPECTATIONS FOR RECOVERY TIMES

Diagnosis	Recovery Time
UVL	6–8 weeks
BPPV	Remission in one/few treatment (85% of patients)
BVL	6 months–2 years
CNS pathology	6 months–2 years

9. Will you modify the physical therapy intervention?

ANSWER: A reevaluation of the exercise program is appropriate. The patient may not be able to perform the exercise safely or may not be performing the exercise correctly.

10. Was your home exercise program too rigorous?

ANSWER: The primary concern for the patient with a BVL is safety. The therapist must ensure the patient's home environment is not a balance hazard. Common recommendations include eliminating throw rugs, adding night lights to darkened hallways and rooms, using grab bars in bathrooms, and instructing persons in appropriate shoe wear. A home evaluation may be appropriate and can be an essential component promoting safe home environments and preventing falls.

Marlys J. Staley
Reg Richard

LEARNING OBJECTIVES

1. Describe the anatomy and physiology of the skin as an organ in the healthy state and damaged condition that occurs with a burn injury.
2. Describe the pathology, symptoms, and sequela of burn injuries.
3. Explain the treatment for a patient with various depths and extent of burn injury in relation to medical, surgical, and rehabilitation management.
4. Describe the consequences of contracture formation after burn injury and the treatment of this condition.
5. List the guidelines for management of hypertrophic scars.
6. State the type of skin care necessary after burn wound healing.
7. Analyze and interpret patient data, formulate realistic goals and outcomes, and develop a plan of care when presented with a clinical case study.

Burn injuries are one of the major health problems of the industrial world, and the United States annually records the highest incidence of burn injury.[1] Survey data have indicated that more than 2 million persons are burned each year. One-fourth of these require medical attention, and approximately 5000 deaths are related to burn injury.[2,3] In addition, it has been estimated that there is a 1 in 70 chance of an American being burned in his or her lifetime seriously enough to require hospitalization.[1]

Although these data report the extent of the health care problem caused by burn injury, recent medical advances have significantly reduced the number of deaths from burn injuries and have improved the prognosis and functional abilities of surviving patients.[4,5] The survival rate has improved annually owing to improved resuscitation techniques, the acute medical and surgical care that are now available, and continued research into the management and care of the patient with burns. As a result of improvement in care, treatment, and survival of burned patients, more physical therapists will become responsible for treating these patients for a significant portion of their rehabilitation in settings other than a hospital burn unit (e.g., outpatient clinics, community hospitals).

This chapter introduces the problems that occur with the different depths of burn injury and the complications that can result from thermal destruction of the skin. Current techniques used in the medical, surgical, and rehabilitative management of the patient who has been burned will be described. For more in-depth information regarding the assessment and treatment of the patient with a burn injury, the reader is referred to additional sources.[6–9]

EPIDEMIOLOGY OF BURN INJURIES

Although the morbidity and mortality of patients with burns has dramatically decreased in recent years, the epidemiology of burns remains basically the same. There is a peak incidence of burn injury in children 1 to 5 years of age, primarily from scalds from hot liquids.[2,3] The primary cause of burn injury in adolescents and adults is accidents with flammable liquids. Men between the ages of 16 and 40 have the highest incidence of injury.[1,2] Fires that occur in homes and other structural dwellings are responsible for less than 5 percent of the hospital admissions for burn injuries, but account for nearly 12 percent of the burn-related deaths in this country.[1,2] Most of these deaths are due to inhalation injury. The number of burn-related accidents has decreased presumably because of better preventative measures, such as smoke detectors, education, and more stringent fire codes.[10]

A major reason for the improved prognosis and survival of patients with severe burn injury is the availability of specialized burn centers.[4] The advent of the burn center and the concentrated care and research that has been generated by these facilities has improved the prognosis and survival of the most severely burned patient, as well as reduced the average hospital stay in most cases.

The American Burn Association* has established criteria for admission to a designated burn center:[11]

1. Partial and full-thickness burns greater than 10 percent of total body surface area (TBSA) in patients under 10 or over 50 years of age.
2. Partial and full-thickness burns greater than 20 percent TBSA in other age groups.
3. Full-thickness burns greater than 5 percent TBSA in any age group.
4. Partial and full-thickness burns involving the hands, feet, face, perineum, or skin overlying major joints.
5. Electrical burns including lightning injury.
6. Chemical burns.
7. Patients with inhalation injury.
8. Burn injury in patients with preexisting illness that could complicate management.
9. Any patient with a burn in whom concomitant trauma poses an increased risk of morbidity or mortality may be treated initially in a trauma center until stable before transfer to a burn center.
10. Burn injury in patients who will require special social and emotional or long-term rehabilitative support, including cases involving suspected child abuse.

Twenty-five years ago, there were only 12 specialized burn centers. Today there are 135 specialized centers for the care of patients with burn injuries and other skin disorders. This accounts for approximately 1700 beds in this country.[12] Furthermore, burn centers recently have begun to undergo the process of verification (voluntary quality assurance review) through the American Burn Association.[13]

A burn center is staffed by specialists—physicians, nurses, physical therapists, occupational therapists, dieticians, psychiatrists, psychologists, social workers, child life therapists, chaplains, pharmacists, vocational rehabilitation specialists, and other support personnel—who direct all their energies toward the care, treatment, and rehabilitation of the patient with a burn injury. Each member is an integral part of the team, and the most effective burn centers are successful because of their team approach to the care of each patient.[4]

SKIN ANATOMY AND BURN WOUND PATHOLOGY

The skin is the largest organ of the body, comprising approximately 15 percent of body weight. Anatomically, the skin consists of two distinct layers of tissue: the **epidermis,** which is the outermost layer exposed to the environment, and the deeper layer, termed the **dermis.**[14] Although not part of the skin per se, a third layer involved in the anatomical consideration of the skin is the subcutaneous fat cell layer directly under the dermis and above muscle fascial layers. These layers can be seen in Figure 26-1. The epidermis is avascular, but it performs several vital functions. The stratum corneum gives the skin its waterproof characteristic and serves the role of protection from infection. The stratum granulosum is the layer responsible for water retention and heat regulation. The stratum spinosum adds a layer of protection to the underlying stratum basale layer. Cells in the basal layer enable the epidermis to regenerate. This layer also contains melanocytes, which determine the coloration of the epidermis. The interface between the epidermis and the dermis is termed the *rete peg region*. This area consists of an extensive series of epidermal-dermal ridges and valleys that serve to increase the surface area between the epidermis and the dermis. These ridges act as a reservoir of skin and are needed to overcome frictional forces that skin is exposed to in daily activity. Lack of these ridges in the healed burn wound will result in blisters from abrasion and poor

---

*American Burn Association, 625 N. Michigan Ave., Chicago, IL, 60611; phone number: (800) 548–2876.

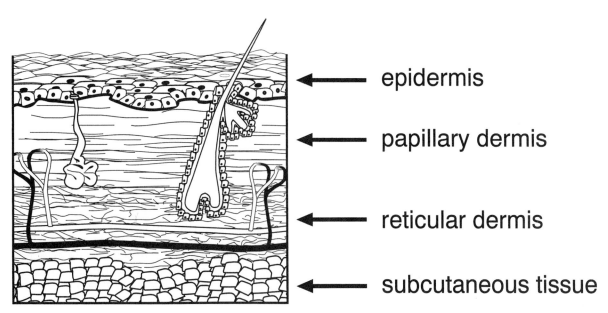

Figure 26-1. Cross-section of skin.

adherence of the new epidermal tissue when it comes in contact with clothing or other surfaces.

The dermis is considered the "true skin," because it contains blood vessels, lymphatics, nerves, collagen and elastic fibers. It also encloses the epidermal appendages (sweat and sebaceous glands, and hair follicles), which provide a deep source of epidermal cells. The dermis is 20 to 30 times thicker than the epidermis. It is comprised primarily of interwoven collagen and elastic fibers, which provide the skin with its tensile strength and elasticity to resist deformation. The predominantly parallel orientation of normal collagen in the dermis is different than the whorls of collagen typically seen in scar tissue that result from burn injury.[15] The hierarchical location of nerves in the skin is an important consideration to determine depth of burn injury (Table 26–1). The dermis can be subdivided into two layers: the superficial papillary layer and the deep reticular layer.[14] The papillae of the papillary layer project upward and interdigitate with the epidermis. The papillae contain vascular plexuses that serve, in part, to nourish the epidermis through osmosis. Morphologically, this layer is composed of a loose basket-weave network of collagen fibers. The reticular dermis lies below the papillary dermis and is composed of densely interwoven collagen fibers. The reticular dermis attaches to the subcutaneous tissue by an irregular interlacing network of fibrous connective tissue.

In addition to the functions mentioned already, the skin is important in temperature regulation through the excretion of sweat and electrolytes, secretion of oils that lubricate the skin, vitamin D synthesis, sensation, and cosmetic appearance and identity. As the result of a burn injury, some or all of these functions may be impaired and/or lost, and the patient's defense mechanisms will be compromised.

One basic pathophysiological consideration in a burn injury is the alteration of vascular integrity, which results in the formation of edema in the interstitial spaces. Edema formation occurs in the area of burn as well as in adjacent tissues. An initial concern of the physical therapist on the burn team is a decrease in patient range of motion (ROM) due to swelling.

The amount of skin destruction is based on temperature and length of time the tissue is exposed to heat.[16] The type of insult (i.e., flame, liquid, chemical, or electrical) also will affect the amount of tissue destruction. A tremendous amount of heat is not required to cause damage. At temperatures below 111°F (44°C), local tissue damage will not occur unless the exposure is for prolonged periods. In the temperature range between 111°F and 124°F (44°C to 51°C), the rate of cellular death doubles with each degree rise in temperature, and short exposures will lead to cell destruction.[16,17] At temperatures in excess of 124°F (51°C), exposure time needed to damage tissue is extremely brief.

CLASSIFICATIONS OF BURN INJURY

Until recently, burn injuries were classified according to their severity as first, second, and third

Table 26–1 LOCATION OF NERVES IN THE LAYERS OF THE SKIN

Structure	Location	Function
Free nerve ending	Epidermis	Pain, itch
Free nerve ending	Dermis	Pain
Merkel's disks	Stratum spinosum	Touch
Meissner's corpuscle	Papillary dermis	Touch
Ruffini's corpuscle	Papillary dermis	Warm
Krause's end bulb	Papillary dermis	Cold
Pacinian corpuscle	Reticular dermis	Pressure, vibration

degree. Although the lay public may still use these classifications, most medical literature now classifies burn injuries by the depth of skin tissue destroyed.[17] The degree to which a burn causes skin damage depends on many factors, including the duration and intensity of heat, skin thickness and area exposed, vascularity, and age.

The different classifications of burn wounds will present different clinical pictures, and each can change dramatically during the course of treatment. In addition to the amount of direct tissue damage from a burn, a patient's metabolic, physiological, and psychological condition will greatly affect the patient's clinical status. This section will present general clinical signs and symptoms seen in each of the burn wound classifications (Table 26–2).

Superficial Burn

A **superficial burn** causes cell damage only to the epidermis (Fig. 26-2). The classic "sunburn" is the best example of a superficial burn. Clinically, the skin appears red or erythematous.[18] The erythema is a result of epidermal damage and dermal irritation, but there is no injury to the dermal tissue. There is diffusion of inflammatory mediators from sites of epidermal damage and release of vasoactive substances from mast cells. The surface of a superficial burn is dry. Blisters will be absent, but slight edema may be apparent. After a superficial burn, there is usually a delay in the development of pain, at which point the area becomes tender to the touch.

The inflammatory reaction will cease, and the injured epidermis will peel off or desquamate in 2 to 3 days. Healing is spontaneous; that is, the skin will heal on its own, and no scar will be present.

Superficial Partial-Thickness Burn

With a superficial **partial-thickness burn** (Fig. 26-3) damage occurs through the epidermis and into the papillary layer of the dermis. The epidermal layer is destroyed completely, but the dermal layer sustains only mild to moderate damage. The most common sign of a superficial partial-thickness burn is the presence of intact blisters over the area that has been injured.

Although the internal environment of a blister is felt to be sterile, it has been shown that blister fluid contains substances that increase the inflammatory response and retard the healing process, and it is recommended that blisters be evacuated.[19-22] Healing will occur more rapidly if the skin is removed and an appropriate wound dressing applied.

Once blisters have been removed, the surface appearance of the burn area will be moist. The wound will be bright red because the dermis is inflamed. The wound will **blanch,** which means that if pressure is exerted against the tissue with a finger, a white spot appears as a result of displacement of blood in the capillaries under pressure. On release of pressure, the white area will demonstrate brisk capillary refill. Edema can be moderate.

This type of burn is extremely painful secondary to irritation of the nerve endings contained in the dermis. When the wound is open, the patient will be highly sensitive to temperature changes, exposure to air, and light touch. In addition to pain, fever may be present if areas become infected.

Some topical antimicrobial creams will cause the wound to develop a gelatin-like film that eventually will peel off, similar to the **desquamation** that occurs with a sunburn. This exudate is a coagulum of the topical antibiotic used to prevent infection and serum that seeps from the wound as a result of the insult to capillary integrity.

Table 26–2 BURN INJURY DIFFERENTIAL DIAGNOSIS

Depth of Burn	Wound Color/Vascularity	Surface Appearance/Pain	Swelling/Healing/Scarring
Superficial	Erythematous, pink or red; irritated dermis	No blisters, dry surface; delayed pain, tender	Minimal edema; spontaneous healing; no scars
Superficial partial-thickness	Bright pink or red, mottled red; inflamed dermis; erythematous with blanching and capillary refill	Intact blisters, moist surface, weeping or glistening; painful; sensitive to changes in temperature, exposure to air currents, light touch	Moderate edema; spontaneous healing; minimal scarring (discoloration)
Deep partial-thickness	Mixed red, waxy white; blanching with slow capillary refill	Broken blisters, wet surface; sensitive to pressure but insensitive to light touch or soft pin prick	Marked edema; slow healing; excessive scarring
Full-thickness	White (ischemic), charred, tan, fawn, mahogany, black, red; hemoglobin fixation; no blanching; thrombosed vessels; poor distal circulation	Parchment-like, leathery, rigid, dry; anesthetic; body hairs pull out easily	Area depressed; heals with skin grafting; scarring
Subdermal	Charred	Subcutaneous tissue evident; anesthetic; muscle damage; neurological involvement	Tissue defects; heals with skin grafting; scarring

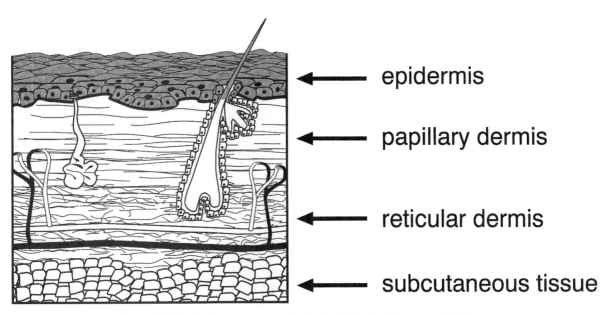

Figure 26-2. Shading represents depth of skin involved in a superficial burn.

Superficial partial-thickness burns heal without surgical intervention, by means of epithelial cell production and migration from the wound's periphery and surviving skin appendages. Coverage by new epithelium resumes the barrier function of the skin, and complete healing should occur in 7 to 10 days. There may be some residual skin color change due to destruction of melanocytes, but scarring is minimal.

Deep Partial-Thickness Burn

A deep partial-thickness burn injury (Fig. 26-4) involves destruction of the epidermis with damage of the dermis down into the reticular layer. Most of the nerve endings, hair follicles, and sweat glands

will be injured because most of the dermis is destroyed.

Deep partial-thickness burns appear as a mixed red or waxy white color. The deeper the injury, the more white it will appear. Capillary refill will be sluggish after the application of pressure on the wound.

The surface usually is wet from broken blisters and alteration of the dermal vascular network, which leaks plasma fluid. Marked edema is a hallmark sign of this burn depth. There is a large amount of evaporative water loss (15 to 20 times normal) because of tissue and vascular destruction.[16,23] An area of deep partial-thickness burn has diminished sensation to light touch or soft pin-prick, but retains the sense of deep pressure due to the

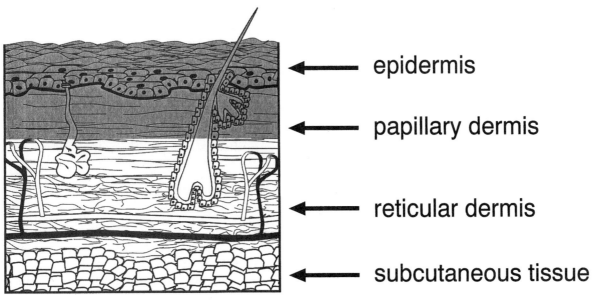

Figure 26-3. Shading represents depth of skin involved in a superficial partial-thickness burn.

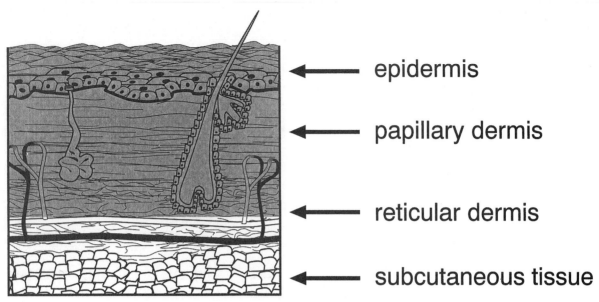

epidermis

papillary dermis

reticular dermis

subcutaneous tissue

Figure 26-4. Shading represents depth of skin involved in a deep partial-thickness burn.

location of the Pacinian corpuscle deep in the reticular dermis. Healing occurs through scar formation and re-epithelialization. By definition, the dermis is only partially destroyed; therefore, some viable epidermal cells may remain within the surviving epidermal appendages and serve as a source for new skin growth.

The depth of a deep partial-thickness injury is difficult to determine, so allowing the wound to demarcate during the first few days is necessary. Demarcation becomes evident after several days as the dead tissue begins to slough. Hair follicles that penetrate into the deeper dermal regions below the burn level remain viable. Preservation of hair follicles and new hair growth will indicate a deep partial-thickness burn rather than a full-thickness injury, and there is a corresponding greater potential for spontaneous healing. Factors that determine which epidermal structures survive and which die include the thickness of the skin in a particular location and/or the distance of the area from the source of heat.

Deep partial-thickness burns that are allowed to heal spontaneously will have a thin epithelium and may lack the usual number of sebaceous glands to keep the skin lubricated. New tissue usually appears dry and scaly, is itchy, and is easily abraded. Creams are necessary to artificially lubricate the new surface. Sensation and the number of active sweat glands will be diminished.

A deep partial-thickness burn generally will heal in 3 to 5 weeks if it does not become infected. It is critical to keep the wound free of infection, because infection can convert a deep partial-thickness burn into a deeper injury. The development of **hypertrophic** and **keloid scars** are a frequent consequence of a deep partial-thickness burn.

Full-Thickness Burn

In a **full-thickness burn** (Fig. 26-5) all of the epidermal and dermal layers are destroyed completely. In addition, the subcutaneous fat layer may be damaged to some extent.

A full-thickness burn is characterized by a hard, parchment-like eschar covering the area. **Eschar** is devitalized tissue consisting of desiccated coagulum of plasma and necrotic cells. Eschar feels dry, leathery, and rigid. The color of eschar can vary from black to deep red to white; the latter indicates total ischemia of the area. Frequently, thrombosis of superficial blood vessels is apparent and no blanching of the tissue is observed. The deep red color of the tissue is due to hemoglobin fixation liberated from destroyed red blood cells.

Hair follicles are completely destroyed, so bodily hair will pull out easily. All nerve endings in the dermal tissue are destroyed, and the wound will be *insensible* (without feeling); however, a patient may experience a significant amount of pain from the adjacent areas of partial-thickness burn that usually surround a full-thickness injury.

Another major problem that arises from deep burns is the damage to the peripheral vascular system. Because of large amounts of fluid leaking into the interstitial space beneath unyielding eschar, the pressure in the extravascular space increases, potentially constricting the deep circulation to the point of occlusion of blood flow. Because eschar does not have the elastic quality of normal skin, edema that forms in an area of circumferential burn can cause compression of the underlying vasculature. If this compression is not relieved, it may lead to eventual occlusion with possible necrosis of tissue distal to the site of injury. To maintain vascular flow, an **escharotomy** may be necessary. An escharotomy is a midlateral incision of the eschar.[24,25] Figure 26-6 shows an escharotomy and the result of pressure that forces the incision line open. Following an escharotomy, pulses are monitored frequently. If the escharotomy is successful, there will be an immediate improvement in the peripheral blood flow, demonstrated by normal pulses distal to the wound, and by return of normal temperature, sensation, and capillary refill of the distal extremity.

Although it may be difficult to differentiate a deep-partial from a full-thickness burn in the early postburn period, the differences will become evident after several days. With a full-thickness burn, there are no sites available for re-epithelialization of the wound. All epithelial cells have been destroyed, and skin grafting of tissue over the wound will be necessary. Grafting will be discussed in detail in the section on surgical intervention in the treatment of burns.

Subdermal Burn

An additional category of burn, the **subdermal burn,** involves complete destruction of all tissue from the epidermis down to and through the subcutaneous tissue (Fig. 26-7). Muscle and bone may be damaged. This type of burn occurs with prolonged contact with a flame or hot liquid and routinely occurs as a result of contact with electricity. Extensive surgical and therapeutic management is necessary to return a patient to some degree of function.

ELECTRICAL BURN

The signs and symptoms of an **electrical burn** may vary according to the type of current, intensity of the current, and the area of the body the electric current passes through.[26] A burn results from the passage of an electric current through the body after the skin has made contact with an electrical source. Electric current follows the course of least resistance offered by various tissue. Nerves, followed by blood vessels, offer the least resistance. Bone offers the most resistance.

Usually, there is an entrance and an exit wound. The *entrance wound* is located where the current came in contact with the body. The entrance wound is charred and depressed, and many times, is smaller than the *exit wound*. The skin appears yellow and ischemic. An exit wound typically appears as though there was an explosion out of the tissue at the site. It is dry in appearance. Tissues underlying the pathway of the current may be damaged as a result of the heat that developed. An extremity or area that appears viable after an injury may become necrotic and gangrenous in a few days. Arteries may undergo spasm, and there may be necrosis of the vascular wall. The blood supply to the surrounding tissues, including muscle, may be altered. Damaged muscle will feel soft. Because the course of tissue destruction is unpredictable, there may be unequal and uneven muscle damage. Time will be required to determine which tissues will remain viable and which will not.

There are other consequences of electricity passing through the body. One of the cardiac effects is arrhythmias, and possible causes of death from electrical burns are ventricular fibrillation or respiratory arrest. There also may be renal consequences leading to renal failure as a result of excessive protein breakdown and the shock to the kidney that follows a major trauma. One of the most severe complications of electric current damage is acute spinal cord damage or vertebral fracture. Clinically, these patients will have spastic paresis but may or may not have any sensory pathway changes over concomitant areas of spasticity.

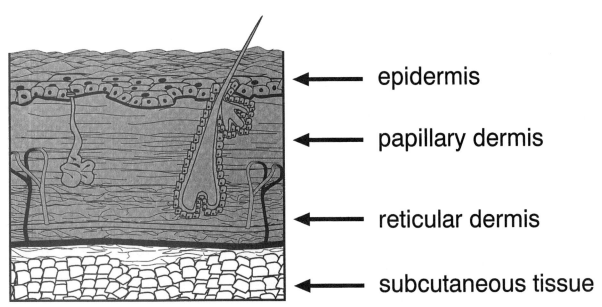

epidermis

papillary dermis

reticular dermis

subcutaneous tissue

Figure 26-5. Shading represents depth of skin involved in a full-thickness burn.

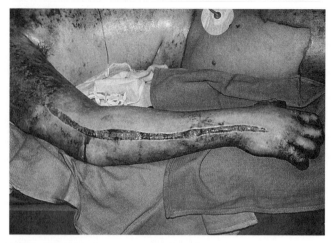

Figure 26-6. Escharotomy of the right upper extremity. (From Richard and Staley,[6] p 113, with permission.)

Burn Wound Zones

The burn wound consists of three zones (Fig. 26-8).[17] In the **zone of coagulation** cells are irreversibly damaged and skin death occurs. Because of the lack of viable tissue and the amount of eschar, the risk of infection is increased. If infection is not controlled, a full-thickness burn can convert to a deeper injury with additional cell death and necrosis of the underlying tissue. This potential complication emphasizes the need for careful monitoring of infection, the use of antibiotics, and the treatment of a burned patient in a specialized burn center. The **zone of stasis** contains injured cells that may die within 24 to 48 hours without specialized treatment. It is in this zone of stasis that infection, drying, and/or inadequate perfusion of the wound will result in conversion of potentially salvageable tissue to completely necrotic tissue. Splints or compression bandages, if applied too tightly, can

compromise this area. Finally, the **zone of hyperemia** is the site of minimal cell damage, and the tissue should recover within several days with no lasting effects.[27]

Extent of Burned Area

In addition to depth of burn, another major factor to assess when determining the severity of a burn injury is the extent of body burn. To allow for a rapid estimate of the percentage of total body surface area burned, Pulaski and Tennison[28] developed the **rule of nines.** The rule of nines divides the body surface into areas that are 9 percent, or multiples of 9 percent, of the total body surface. Figure 26-9 shows the percentages using the rule of nines for adults. Lund and Browder[29] modified the percentages of body surface area to account for age and to accommodate for growth of the different body segments. This method is the more accurate means of the two methods to determine the extent of burn injury. Figure 26-10 shows the relative percentages of burned area for children and adults according to the Lund and Browder formula. Although this formula provides an accurate assessment of TBSA, the use of the rule of nines is more practical in the emergent triage of a burned patient.

INDIRECT IMPAIRMENTS AND COMPLICATIONS OF BURN INJURY

Depending on the extent of burn injury, the depth of the burn, and the type of burn, there may be secondary systemic complications.[30] In addition, the health, age, and psychological status of a patient who is burned will affect these complications. This section will highlight some systemic complications

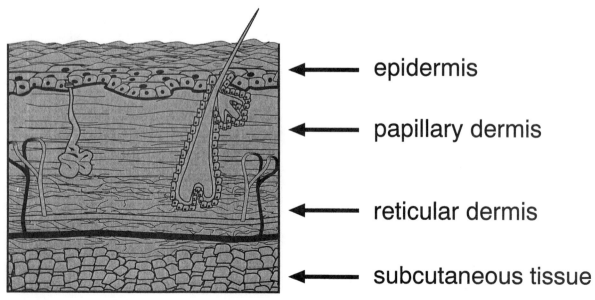

Figure 26-7. Shading represents depth of skin involved in a subdermal burn.

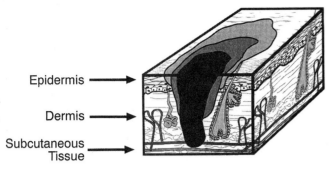

Epidermis →

Dermis →

Subcutaneous → Tissue

Figure 26-8. Zones of tissue damage as the result of a burn injury.

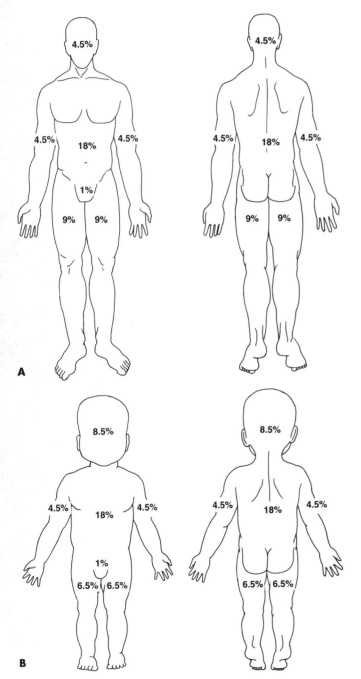

Figure 26-9. Rule of Nines to determine percentage of body surface area burn in adults *(A)* and children *(B)*.

a patient may experience after a significant burn injury.

Infection

Infection, in conjunction with organ system failure, is a leading cause of mortality from burns.[31] Some virulent strains of *Pseudomonas aeruginosa* and *Staphylococcus aureus* are resistant to antibiotics and have been responsible for epidemic infections in burn centers.[1,31] Systemic antibiotics are used to treat both burn and general system infections once they have been documented.[31,32] A bacterial count in excess of 10^5 per gram of tissue constitutes burn wound infection and levels of 10^7 to 10^9 are usually associated with lethal burns. Most wounds are treated with topical antibiotics, and these will be discussed in the section on medical care of burns.

Pulmonary Complications

Any patient who has been burned in a closed space should be suspected of having an **inhalation injury.**[33] Among patients with burns, the incidence of smoke inhalation may be in excess of 33 percent,[34] and this rises to 66 percent in patients with facial burns.[35] Several studies have indicated that the incidence of pulmonary complications is extremely high after severe burns, and that death due to pneumonia alone is attributed to a majority of the deaths following burn injury.[36]

Signs of an inhalation injury include:
• Any facial burns
• Singed nasal hairs
• Harsh cough
• Hoarseness
• Abnormal breath sounds
• Respiratory distress
• Carbonaceous sputum and/or hypoxemia.[36]

The primary complications associated with this injury are carbon monoxide poisoning, tracheal damage, upper airway obstruction, pulmonary edema, and pneumonia. Lung damage from inhaling noxious gases and smoke may be lethal. To determine the extent of inhalation injury, several diagnostic procedures can be performed. The most helpful diagnostic procedure is bronchoscopy.[36]

Metabolic Complications

Thermal injury causes a great metabolic and catabolic challenge to the body. Most of the recent advances in burn treatment and rehabilitation have come directly from the increased understanding of the metabolic demands of a burn injury and from the ability to improve the patient's nutritional status to meet these demands.[37] The consequences of the increased metabolic and catabolic activity following a burn are a rapid decrease in body weight, negative

Burn Estimate and Diagram
Age vs Area

Initial Evaluation

Cause of burn_____

Date of Burn_____

Time of Burn_____

Age_____

Sex_____

Weight_____

Date of Admission _____

Signature _____

Date_____

Burn Diagram

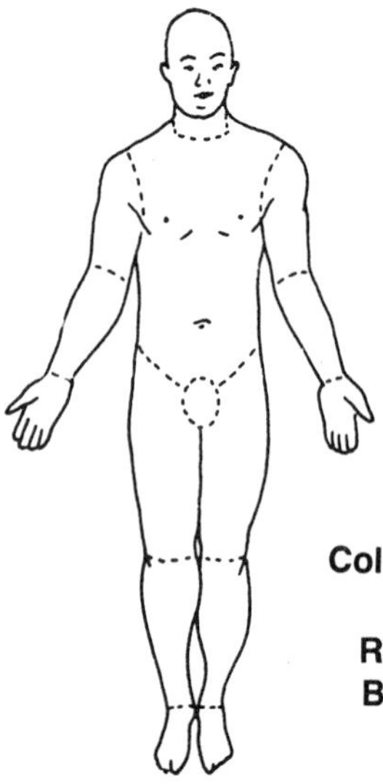

Color Code

Red - FT
Blue - PT

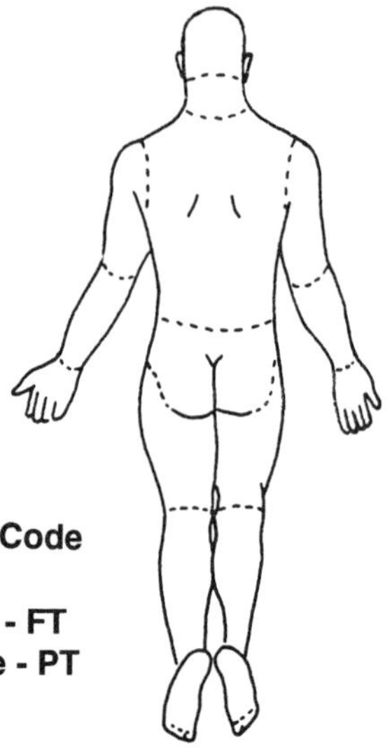

Area	Birth 1 yr.	1-4 yrs.	5-9 yrs.	10-14 yrs.	15 yrs.	Adult	PT	FT	Total	Donor Areas
Head	19	17	13	11	9	7				
Neck	2	2	2	2	2	2				
Ant. Trunk	13	13	13	13	13	13				
Post. Trunk	13	13	13	13	13	13				
R. Buttock	2 1/2	2 1/2	2 1/2	2 1/2	2 1/2	2 1/2				
L. Buttock	2 1/2	2 1/2	2 1/2	2 1/2	2 1/2	2 1/2				
Genitalia	1	1	1	1	1	1				
R.U. Arm	4	4	4	4	4	4				
L.U. Arm	4	4	4	4	4	4				
R.L. Arm	3	3	3	3	3	3				
L.L. Arm	3	3	3	3	3	3				
R. Hand	2 1/2	2 1/2	2 1/2	2 1/2	2 1/2	2 1/2				
L. Hand	2 1/2	2 1/2	2 1/2	2 1/2	2 1/2	2 1/2				
R. Thigh	5 1/2	6 1/2	8	8 1/2	9	9 1/2				
L. Thigh	5 1/2	6 1/2	8	8 1/2	9	9 1/2				
R. Leg	5	5	5 1/2	6	6 1/2	7				
L. Leg	5	5	5 1/2	6	6 1/2	7				
R. Foot	3 1/2	3 1/2	3 1/2	3 1/2	3 1/2	3 1/2				
L. Foot	3 1/2	3 1/2	3 1/2	3 1/2	3 1/2	3 1/2				
						Total				

Key: FT - Full Thickness
　　　PT - Part Thickness

Figure 26-10. Modified Lund and Browder chart for determination of percentage of body surface area burn for various ages. (Courtesy Shriners Burns Hospital, Cincinnati.)

nitrogen balance, and a decrease in energy stores that are vital to the healing process.[38]

As a result of the increased metabolic activity, there will be an increase of 1.8°F to 2.6°F (1°C to 2°C) in core temperature that seems to be due to a resetting of the hypothalamic temperature centers in the brain.[1] Wilmore et al.[39] hypothesized that there is a significant relationship between the increased evaporative heat loss from the impaired skin barrier over a burn and the hypermetabolic state. In any event, if individuals with burns are placed in a room with normal ambient temperature, excessive heat loss will be exhibited, and this will further exaggerate the stress response seen in these patients.[1,39] Therefore, it is recommended that room temperature be kept at 86°F (30°C), which will significantly reduce the metabolic rate.

As part of the patient's altered metabolism, muscle tissue is preferentially used as a source of energy. This situation, coupled with the effects of bed rest, causes muscles to atrophy and renders patients weak from both their burn injury and hospitalization.

Much of the improved management of burns has been attributed to the greater focus of research on the nutritional needs of patients. It is beyond the scope of this chapter to detail nutritional supplementation, and the interested reader is referred to several excellent reviews of advances in burn nutrition.[40–42]

Cardiac Function and Circulatory Complications

Hemodynamic changes result from a shift in fluid to the interstitium, which subsequently reduces the plasma and intravascular fluid volume in a patient with a burn. After these changes, there will be a tremendous initial decrease in cardiac output, which may reach 15 percent within the first hour after injury.[43,44]

Hematological and circulatory changes also occur after a severe burn injury. These changes include alterations in platelet concentration and function, clotting factors, and white blood cell components; red blood cell dysfunction; and decreases in hemoglobin and hematocrit.[45] These physiological alterations, coupled with cardiac changes and injured vascular beds, will significantly impact initial resuscitation efforts and, if the patient survives, how rapidly he or she will recover. Additionally, patients will exhibit decompensation from an endurance standpoint.

Heterotopic Ossification

Patients with burns are highly susceptible to the development of **heterotopic ossification (HO),** as shown by prospective studies demonstrating a very high reported incidence.[46–49] However, the actual number of cases that progress on to becoming clinically problematic is relatively low.[48,49] Why HO occurs in patients with burn injuries is uncertain. Suspected etiologies include greater than 20 percent TBSA burn, immobilization, microtrauma, high protein intake, and sepsis. The most common areas affected are the elbows, followed by the hips and shoulders; however, HO can appear anywhere throughout the body.[48,49] Usually HO occurs in areas of full-thickness injury or sites that remain unhealed for prolonged periods of time. Symptoms appear late in a patient's course of recovery and include decreased ROM, point-specific pain, and a quality of reported pain that differs from that experienced by patients with generalized burn.

Neuropathy

Peripheral neuropathy in patients with burns can take two forms: **polyneuropathy** or local neuropathy.[50] The cause of polyneuropathy is unknown. As with patients with HO, patients with peripheral neuropathy generally have a large TBSA burn, and the condition may be associated with sepsis. Fortunately, most neuropathies resolve over time.

Local neuropathies can be caused by a number of factors, most of which center around burn treatment issues, such as compression bandages applied too tightly, poorly fitted splints, or prolonged and inappropriate positioning of a patient.[50] The most common sites of involvement are the brachial plexus, ulnar nerve, and common peroneal nerve.

Pathological Scars

Burn scars occur in areas of deep partial-thickness burn that are allowed to heal spontaneously and in full-thickness burns that have been skin grafted, but where graft coverage is incomplete. Scars become pathological when they take on the form of **hypertrophy,** contracture or both. Each of these scar conditions is unique and should not be viewed as synonymous. A patient can have a hypertrophic scar that does not interfere with movement or a scar contracture band that is not hypertrophied. However, both conditions can exist simultaneously, and specific treatment for each is discussed later in this chapter.

BURN WOUND HEALING

The burn wound has been described and the causes and complications of burn injury have been reviewed. The remaining sections of this chapter will concentrate on the various types of medical and surgical therapeutic interventions and physical rehabilitation of the patient with a burn. First, however, it is necessary to outline the healing process of a burn wound.[51]

The two layers of the skin—the epidermis and dermis—differ morphologically, and they heal by separate mechanisms. In the following sections, the physiology of each component is described, and the clinical implications of burns to these areas are addressed.

Epidermal Healing

When a burn injures just the epidermis, or if there are viable cells lining the skin appendages, **epithelial healing** can occur on the surface of a wound. The stimulus for epithelial growth is the presence of an open wound exposing subepithelial tissue of the body to the environment. The intact epithelium attempts to cover an exposed wound through the ameboid movement of cells from the basal layer of the surrounding epidermis into the wound. The epithelial cells stop migration when they are completely in contact with other epithelial cells. After this **contact inhibition,** cells can begin to divide and multiply through mitosis. While epithelial cells move about the wound site, they maintain a connection with the normal epithelium at the wound margin. To continue migration and proliferation, a suitable base for the epithelial cells must be provided by adequate nutrition and blood supply, or else the new cells will die.

The process of epithelialization is most evident clinically in the partial-thickness wound that has intact hair follicles and glands. The epithelial cells from the skin appendages provide islands from which the wound may heal. The cells migrate peripherally from these **epithelial islands** into the wound. Skin growth and coverage actually can be seen over time from these epithelial islands.

Damage to sebaceous glands may cause dryness and itching of a healing wound. Lubrication can be a problem, and the new skin is characteristically dry and may split. Dryness may continue for a long time, because many of the sebaceous glands do not return to their normal function after a wound is epithelialized. Therapists need to educate patients about the type, frequency, and techniques of moisturizing cream application to lubricate newly healed tissue.

Dermal Healing

When an injury involves tissue deeper than the epidermis, **dermal healing,** or scar formation occurs. Scar formation can be divided into three phases: inflammatory, proliferative, and maturation. Although these phases will be described separately, they occur on a continuum and one phase often overlaps another.

INFLAMMATORY PHASE

The primary reaction of viable tissue to a burn wound is inflammation, which prepares the wound for healing through hemostatic, vascular, and cellular events. Inflammation begins at the time of injury, ends in about 3 to 5 days, and is characterized by redness, edema, warmth, pain, and decreased ROM. Initially, when a blood vessel is ruptured, the wall of the vessel contracts to decrease blood flow. Platelets aggregate, and fibrin is deposited to form a clot over the area. Fibrin serves a threefold function: it (1) partially retains body fluids, (2) protects the underlying cells from desiccation, and (3) provides a firm coagulum substance from which cells can infiltrate. Therefore, fibrin can be thought of as forming a lattice network, from which cells can climb and work themselves into the healing structure.

After a transient vasoconstriction of the vasculature, which lasts about 5 to 10 minutes, vessels vasodilate to increase blood flow to the area. There is increased permeability of the blood vessels, with leaking of plasma into the interstitial space and subsequent edema formation. Leukocytes infiltrate the area and begin to rid the site of contamination. Of particular importance is the presence of the macrophage, which is responsible for attracting fibroblasts into the area.

PROLIFERATIVE PHASE

During this phase, re-epithelialization is occurring at the surface of the wound, while deep within the wound, fibroblasts are migrating and proliferating. **Fibroblasts** are the cells that synthesize scar tissue, which is composed of collagen and protein polysaccharides. In addition, the fibroblasts produce a viscous ground substance that surrounds the collagen strands. The collagen is deposited with a random alignment and no true architectural arrangement of fibers. Stress (e.g., a force intended to

elongate the scar) applied to the developing tissue during this time causes the fibers to align along the direction of force.[52] During this period of fibroplasia, the tensile strength of the wound increases at a rate proportional to the rate of collagen synthesis.

In conjunction with collagen deposition, granulation tissue is formed during this phase. Granulation tissue consists of macrophages, fibroblasts, collagen, and blood vessels.[51] These newly formed blood vessels bring a rich blood supply to the area and encourage further wound healing. However, granulation tissue formation is not necessary for skin graft adherence, and excess granulation tissue may lead to increased hypertrophic scarring.

During the proliferative phase, **wound contraction** occurs. Wound contraction is an active process in which the body attempts to close a wound where a loss of tissue has occurred. The amount of contraction is determined by the amount of available mobile skin around the defect. It involves movement of existing tissue at the wound edge toward the center, not formation of new tissue. Wound contraction is stopped when (1) the edges of the wound meet, or (2) tension in the surrounding skin equals or exceeds the force of contraction. Skin grafting may decrease contraction, with thick grafts causing less contraction.

MATURATION PHASE

A wound is considered closed at the time epithelium covers the surface; however, wound healing involves remodeling of the scar tissue. During the maturation phase, there is a reduction in the number of fibroblasts, a decrease in vascularity due to a lesser metabolic demand, and remodeling of collagen, which becomes more parallel in arrangement and forms stronger bonds. The ratio of collagen breakdown to production determines the type of scar that forms. If the rate of breakdown equals or slightly exceeds the rate of production, maturation results in a pale, flat, and pliable scar. If the rate of collagen production exceeds breakdown, then a hypertrophic scar may result. This scar is characterized by being red and raised in appearance, and firm in texture; it stays within the boundary of the original wound. A keloid is a large, firm scar that overflows the boundaries of the original wound; it is more common in blacks and Asians. Both of these scars take a prolonged period of time to mature and can lead to both functional and cosmetic deformities.

MEDICAL MANAGEMENT OF BURNS

Advances in the medical management of burns have resulted in the survival of thousands of patients who 15 or 20 years ago would have died of their injuries. The research base and techniques available today at modern burn centers have enabled patients to receive better care through the use of more sophisticated techniques for the treatment of major burn injuries. This section will discuss the initial treatment of burn injuries and the surgical procedures associated with excision and grafting of new skin onto a burn wound.

Initial Management and Wound Care

The goals in the initial management of a patient with a burn are to address the major life-threatening problems and stabilize the patient through procedures designed to (1) establish and maintain an airway; (2) prevent cyanosis, shock, and hemorrhage; (3) establish baseline data on the patient, such as extent and depth of burn injury; (4) prevent or reduce fluid losses; (5) clean the patient and wounds; (6) assess injuries; and (7) prevent pulmonary and cardiac complications. Triage using these procedures applies to major burn trauma.

Initially, a patient must be transported from the site of injury to a treatment facility. If possible, transportation will be directly to a burn center, rather than to a hospital emergency room. The goals of treatment in transit are to stabilize the patient and maintain an airway. During the initial transportation phase, patient history and personal data are gathered when possible. The type of agent causing the burn is noted, and initial assessment of the burn injury takes place. Emergency medical personnel may use the rule of nines to estimate the percent of burn injury. Furthermore, they will prepare the individual for triage at the burn center by removing all burned clothing and jewelry and initiating the administration of fluid through an intravenous line.

One of the major advances in burn care has been in fluid volume replacement initially and throughout a patient's treatment. Research has led to an improved understanding of the physiological changes that occur in a patient after a burn injury and of the fluid volumes necessary to improve the chance for survival.[44] Information about the physiological changes responsible for the shifts in body fluids and protein has led to the use of intravenous solutions in an amount necessary to replace vital fluid and electrolytes.[54]

After a patient arrives at a burn center and adequate fluid resuscitation has been initiated, the burn team assesses the extent and depth of injury, and begins initial wound cleansing. Wound cleansing may be performed in a variety of settings, although the majority of burn centers still perform hydrotherapy in the care of patients.[55–57] The initial wound care session allows the team to establish body weight, examine a patient fully, remove hair where necessary, and start the **débridement** process by removing any loose skin. The goals of wound cleansing and débridement are to remove dead tissue, prevent infection, and promote revascularization and/or epithelialization of the area. Depending on the facility, physical therapists may be involved in the wound cleaning procedure.[56,58,59]

A large hydrotherapy tank or whirlpool tub usually will have some form of disinfectant in the water to assist in infection control.[55,60,61] Water temperature should be between 98.6°F and 104°F (37°C to 40°C). While a patient is in the water, adherent dressings are removed. Care must be taken when removing the dressings to ensure minimal or no bleeding. The removal of dressings in the water is less painful than dry removal. Some burn units have converted to the use of showers, spraying, or "bed baths" for the removal of dressings and daily cleaning of wounds.[62] Regardless of the wound cleansing approach, most patients require pain medication prior to wound care.

After dressings are removed, the wound should be inspected carefully. The appearance, depth, size, exudate, and odor are noted. *Infection* is characterized by thick purulent drainage, odor, fever, a brownish-black discoloration, rapid separation of eschar, boils in adjacent tissue, or conversion of a deep partial-thickness burn to a full-thickness injury.

Wound care is carried out using clean technique and sterile instruments. If **sharp débridement** (the use of surgical scissors or scalpel and forceps to remove eschar) is performed, sloughed epidermis and loose eschar are removed and pockets of pus are drained. The procedure needs to be performed carefully so that bleeding is minimal.

After the wounds have been cleaned, the patient should be kept warm to reduce any further metabolic demands due to additional heat loss. Topical medications and/or dressings are then reapplied. Table 26–3 presents common topical medications used in the treatment of burns. The technique of applying a topical cream or ointment without dressings is called the **open technique** and allows for ongoing inspection of the wound and assessment of the healing process. With this technique, the topical medication must be reapplied throughout the day.

The **closed technique** consists of applying dressings over a topical agent. Dressings serve several purposes: (1) they hold topical antimicrobial agents on the wound, (2) they reduce fluid loss from the wound, and (3) they protect the wound. Dressings are changed once or twice a day, depending on the size and type of wound, and the type of topical antimicrobial used.

Dressings consist of several layers. The first layer is nonadherent to protect the fragile healing surface from disruption. This may be followed by cotton padding to absorb wound drainage. The final layer consists of roll gauze or elastic bandages, which hold the other layers in place but allow movement.

Surgical Management of the Burn Wound

Primary excision is surgical removal of eschar. Much of the increased survival rate of patients with extensive burns has been due to the early primary excision of burn wounds.[63] Normally, a patient is taken to surgery after successful resuscitation, usually within 1 week of injury. As much of the eschar is removed at one time as possible. Proponents of early

Table 26–3 COMMON TOPICAL MEDICATIONS USED IN TREATMENT OF BURNS

Medication	Description	Method of Application
Silver sulfadiazine	Most commonly used topical antibacterial agent; effective against *Pseudomonas* infections.	White cream applied with sterile glove 2–4 mm thick directly to wound or impregnated into fine mesh gauze.
Mafenide acetate (Sulfamylon)	Topical antibacterial agent; effective against gram-negative or gram-positive organisms; diffuses easily through eschar.	White cream applied directly to wound with thin 1–2 mm layer twice daily; may be left undressed or covered with thin layer of gauze.
Silver nitrate	Antiseptic germicide and astringent; will penetrate only 1–2 mm of eschar; useful for surface bacteria; stains black.	Dressings or soaks used every 2 hours; also available as small sticks to cauterize small open areas.
Bacitracin/Polysporin	Bland ointment; effective against gram-positive organisms.	Thin layer of ointment applied directly to wound and left open.
Nitrofurazone (Furacin)	Antibacterial cream used in less severe burns; indicated to decrease bacterial growth.	Applied directly to wound or impregnated into gauze dressing.
Gentamycin (Garamycin)	Antibiotic used against gram-negative organism and staphylococcal and streptococcal bacteria.	Cream or ointment applied with sterile glove and covered with gauze.
Collagenase, Accuzyme	Enzymatic debriding agent selectively debrides necrotic tissue; no antibacterial action.	Ointment applied to eschar and covered with moist occlusive dressing with or without an antimicrobial agent.

primary excision believe that this approach is easier on a patient than repeated débridements, and that it promotes more rapid healing, reduces infection and scarring, and is more economical in terms of staff and hospital time.[63]

In many burn centers, a burn wound is closed with a graft at the time of primary excision. There are many types of grafts that can be used to close a wound. An **autograft** is a patient's own skin, taken from an unburned area and transplanted to cover a burned area. Autografts are desirable because they provide permanent coverage of the wound. An **allograft (or homograft)** is skin taken from an individual of the same species, usually cadaver skin. The skin can be kept frozen in skin banks for prolonged periods. Allografts are temporary grafts used to cover large burns when there is insufficient autograft available. **Xenograft (or heterograft),** is skin from another species, usually a pig. Allografts or xenografts are used until there is sufficient normal skin available for an autograft.

Perhaps the most progressive advancement in the care of patients with burns in recent years is the use of **skin substitutes** for coverage of an excised wound.[64–69] Skin substitutes consist of cultured autologous skin, which is grown in a laboratory from a biopsy of a patient's own tissue, the use of altered cadaver skin, or other biologically engineered tissues. Skin substitutes are used when large areas of burn exist and coverage is necessary for a patient's survival. Cultured autologous skin takes several weeks to grow and is highly susceptible to infection. Other biologically engineered tissues are more readily available and have demonstrated more reliable adherence than in the past. With the use of most skin substitutes, ROM exercises may be delayed and shearing forces must be avoided. Although skin substitutes are an expensive intervention for wound coverage, they are useful and have proved effective in managing patients with large burn wounds. A few types of skin substitutes include:

1. *Cultured epidermal autografts (CEA):* A skin biopsy is obtained from a patient, and only the epidermal cells are cultured.[64,65]
2. *Cultured autologous composite grafts:* A skin biopsy is obtained from a patient, and both epidermal and dermal cells are cultured. This forms a bilayer structure.
3. *Allogenic skin substitute:* The epidermal layer of skin and all immune cells are removed from cadaver skin. This tissue is applied to the graft bed and once adhered, a thin epidermal autograft or CEA is applied (e.g., Alloderm[66]).
4. *Cultured dermis (temporary):* Cultured dermal matrix is seeded with human neonatal fibroblasts and used as a temporary covering in place of cadaver skin. This substitute eventually is removed and replaced with an autograft (e.g., Dermagraft TC[67,68]).
5. *Cultured dermis (definitive):* This skin substitute is composed of cultured bovine collagen with a silicone outer layer. Pores in the material allow for controlled growth of a neodermis. After approximately 14 days, the silicone layer is removed and a very thin skin graft or CEA is applied (e.g., Integra[69]).

SKIN GRAFTING PROCEDURE

The removal of skin to graft onto a burn wound is done surgically under anesthesia. The skin used for a graft usually is removed with a **dermatome.** This instrument not only allows the surgeon to obtain a large amount of skin, but a more consistent thickness of skin can be obtained. The dermatome is adjusted to remove a predetermined thickness of skin for a **split-thickness skin graft.** A split-thickness skin graft contains epidermis and only the superficial layers of the dermis, as opposed to a **full-thickness skin graft,** which consists of the full dermal thickness.

The site from which a skin graft is taken is called a **donor site.** Common donor sites include the thighs, buttocks, and back. These wounds heal by re-epithelialization, like a partial-thickness burn, and require appropriate care to prevent additional dermal damage with resultant scar formation. A full-thickness skin graft has the disadvantage of leaving a full-thickness wound that will require either primary closure or grafting with a split-thickness skin graft.

Generally, the thinner the skin graft, the better the adherence, and the thicker the graft, the better the cosmetic result. Additionally, a thin graft will contract more than a thick skin graft once it has adhered to the wound bed. Selection of depth depends on many factors, including whether or not the donor site needs to be used again for another skin graft. Taking a thicker graft adversely affects the possibility of taking another graft from the same site for a prolonged period of time. Harvesting from split-thickness skin graft sites may be repeated in 10 to 14 days, depending on the amount of time the donor site takes to heal.

A **sheet graft** is a skin graft that is applied to a recipient bed without alteration following harvesting from a donor site (Fig. 26-11). The face, neck, and hands are covered with this type of graft for optimal cosmesis and function. When limited donor skin is available, most areas are covered with a **mesh graft** (Fig. 26-12). The meshing of a graft consists of processing the sheet graft through a device that makes tiny parallel incisions in a linear arrangement. This process permits the skin graft to be expanded before it is applied to the wound bed.[69] This technique allows coverage of a larger area, and once the graft adheres, the interstices heal through re-epithelialization.

A skin graft usually is held in place with sutures, staples, or steri-strips. Once a graft is fixed in position, any blood or serum that might have become located between the graft and the recipient site should be removed. Application of a pressure dressing facilitates contact between the graft and recipient site.

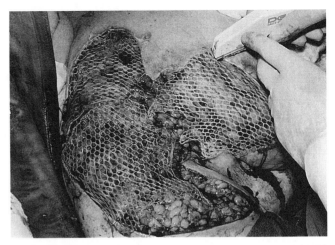

Figure 26-12. Meshed split-thickness skin graft applied to freshly excised wound and secured with staples.

One of the basic necessities for successful adherence of a graft is sufficient vascularity within the wound bed. Grafts will not adhere to nonvascularized areas, such as tendon. Once a skin graft has been applied, separation of a graft from its bed must be prevented. Separation may result from excessive motion, mechanical trauma, or hematoma formation. Initially, an area is immobilized with a dressing that provides firm, even compression on the wound. Other reasons for graft failure include inadequate excision of necrotic tissue and infection.

Survival of a skin graft depends on several factors: (1) circulation, which provides a nutritive supply to the graft; (2) inosculation, or the process by which a direct connection is established between a graft and the host vessels; and (3) penetration of the host vessels into a graft site. Except in darkly pigmented persons, grafts are white in color at the time of transplantation and begin to show a pinkish hue within a matter of hours after their placement on an adequate vascular bed.

The re-establishment of circulation in a skin graft will take place through the formation of direct anastomosis between respective vessels, invasion from the host bed forming new channels, or both. Twenty-four hours after grafting, numerous host vessels will have penetrated the graft.[51] The invasion of new capillaries seems to be the most important consideration in vascularization. Normally, within 72 hours, inosculation has proceeded to the point where the skin graft is secure. Initially, structural connections are fibrous. Collagen is then laid down to secure the attachment of the graft.

SURGICAL CORRECTION OF SCAR CONTRACTURE

If physical therapy interventions are unsuccessful in averting scar contracture formation, and limitations are noted in ROM and function, surgery may be required. In the past, reconstructive surgery usually was postponed while a burn wound was in the active, immature phase of scar formation.[71] More recently, however, successful release of scar contractures before scar maturation has been docu-

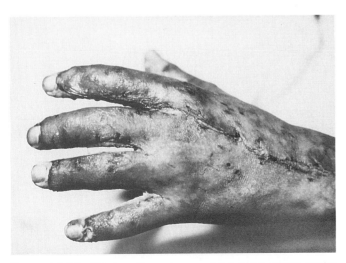

Figure 26-11. Sheet graft on dorsum of left hand, postoperative day 7. (From Richard and Staley,[6] p 183, with permission.)

mented.[72] Each patient's scar will require an individualized evaluation and treatment. Surgical treatment options are beyond the scope of this chapter, but common procedures to eliminate scar contractures are skin grafts and Z-plasties. A **Z-plasty** is shown in Figure 26-13. The Z-plasty serves to lengthen a scar by interposing normal tissue in the line of the scar. Skin grafts are used for more severe contractures.

PHYSICAL THERAPY MANAGEMENT

Rehabilitation of a patient with burns begins the moment he or she arrives at the hospital and is an ever-changing process that may need to be modified daily.[7–9,73] The previous sections of this chapter have discussed the pathophysiological changes and alterations of the skin that occur in the burn wound and the closure of that wound, including various types of skin graft materials. While the skin is healing, it is imperative that a patient's physical rehabilitation occurs concurrently. The physical rehabilitation consists of prevention of scar contracture, preservation of normal ROM, prevention or minimization of hypertrophic scar and cosmetic deformity, maintenance or improvement in muscular strength and cardiovascular endurance, return to function, and performance of activities of daily living (ADL).[6] The physical therapist interacts with other members of the burn team to assist patients in obtaining these outcomes. A patient can expect to return to a normal, productive life provided he or she complies with the treatment plan. For many patients, the most difficult phase of rehabilitation occurs after the wounds have healed and the scar tissue begins to contract. If a physical therapist is actively involved in the burn team, and can establish a program of movement rehabilitation in conjunction with the wound healing process, rehabilitation after healing will be much less problematic and more successful. The remainder of this chapter will address the physical therapist's role in the rehabilitation program of a patient who has sustained a burn injury.

Physical Therapy Assessment

After the initial assessment of the depth of burn and amount of TBSA involved, a physical therapist needs to assess a patient's ability to perform active movement of all extremities. Active or passive ROM may be limited as a result of edema, restrictive eschar, or pain, but an initial baseline measure should be obtained. In addition, the therapist needs to obtain an accurate history from the patient and family members regarding any preexisting limitations or previous injuries that may affect a patient's rehabilitation potential.

Other examination procedures discussed in this text can be included in the initial assessment and ongoing reassessments of a patient following burn injury (e.g., strength, ambulation, functional activities). Because healing of a burn wound is a dynamic process and changes may occur daily, the physical therapist needs to assess and monitor patients routinely for changes in skin integrity, ROM, and mobility. Frequent assessments will keep the therapist and other members of the burn care team abreast of potential problems so that intervention can occur before a potential problem becomes a real one.

In addition to the physical damage a burn has on a patient, there also may be an enormous psychological impact.[74,75] The physical therapist should be cognizant of a potential problem during ongoing assessments, because psychological trauma may affect the patient's progress and outlook toward his or her future and rehabilitation. Referral to an appropriate professional for intervention may be necessary.

Burn Injury Goals and Outcomes

Based on the assessment, the extent and depth of burn, and the patient's current health status, age, and physical and mental condition, the patient's prognosis can be estimated by the burn care team. Goals and outcomes for rehabilitation and physical

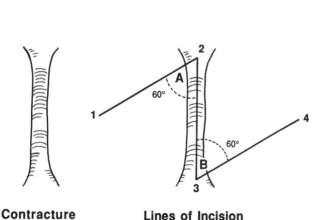

Contracture   **Lines of Incision**   **Result of Z-plasty**

Figure 26-13. Schematic diagram of Z-plasty procedure. (From Richard and Staley,[6] p 192, with permission.)

Table 26–4 POSITIONING STRATEGIES FOR COMMON DEFORMITIES

Joint	Common Deformity	Motions to Be Stressed	Suggested Approaches
Anterior neck	Flexion	Hyperextension	Use double mattress—position neck in extension (Fig. 26-14); with healing—rigid cervical orthosis
Shoulder-axilla	Adduction and internal rotation	Abduction, flexion and external rotation	Position with shoulder flexed and abducted Airplane splint
Elbow	Flexion and pronation	Extension and supination	Splint in extension
Hand	Claw hand (also called intrinsic minus position)	Wrist extension; metacarpophalangeal flexion, proximal interphalangeal and distal interphalangeal extension; thumb palmar abduction	Wrap fingers separately. Elevate to decrease edema. Position in *intrinsic plus* position, wrist in extension, metacarpophalangeal in flexion, proximal interphalangeal and distal interphalangeal in extension, thumb in palmar abduction with large web space
Hip and groin	Flexion and adduction	All motions, especially hip extension and abduction	Hip neutral (0°), extension with slight abduction
Knee	Flexion	Extension	Posterior knee splint
Ankle	Plantarflexion	All motions—especially dorsiflexion	Plastic ankle-foot orthosis with cutout at Achilles tendon and ankle positioned in 0° dorsiflexion

therapy management are contingent on the patient's prognosis and current medical status. It is difficult to list specific outcomes because of the varied nature of each burn injury; however, The Guide to Physical Therapist Practice (American Physical Therapy Association, Alexandria, VA, 1999) suggests that goals and outcomes for physical therapy intervention might include:

1. Wound and soft tissue healing is enhanced
2. Risk of infection and complications is reduced
3. Risk of secondary impairments is reduced
4. Attainment of full ROM
5. Restoration of preinjury level of cardiovascular endurance
6. Good to normal strength
7. Independent ambulation is achieved
8. Independent function in ADL and IADL is increased
9. Minimal scar formation
10. Patient, family, and caregivers understanding of expectations and goals and outcomes is increased
11. Aerobic capacity is increased
12. Self management of symptoms is improved

The optimal outcome of rehabilitation is the return of a patient to normal, preinjury function and life-style.

Physical Therapy Intervention

Patients with burns usually will begin physical therapy on the day of admission, following assessment and evaluation. The initial assessment of a patient will determine which areas need to be addressed first. Control and resolution of edema and preserving ROM usually are the first priorities of physical therapy treatments. Elevating the extremities and encouraging active movement, especially of the hands and ankles, help to minimize edema formation. Preventing scar contractures can be accomplished through positioning, splinting, and exercise. Exercise and ambulation also will help to minimize the deleterious effects of bed rest. Following wound closure, massage and compression therapy will assist with minimizing contracture formation and management of burn scars.

The scar that forms across a joint skin crease while a burn wound is healing is composed of immature collagen. A scar will shorten as a result of the contractile or pulling forces in scar tissue and limit ROM and function unless interventions are taken against this process. Although measures to prevent a contracture are undertaken in expectation of the best result, there will be patients who develop scar contractures. There are several methods available to the physical therapist to aid in the prevention and/or treatment of scar contracture.

As stated, positioning, splinting, and exercise are three relatively simple procedures effective in halting the scar contracture process. Active exercise and patient participation in functional activities are the best treatments to prevent or minimize contractures. However, owing to the relentless forces of scar tissue and pain associated with exercising a burned area, additional interventions may be necessary. Early and ongoing patient and/or family education is needed to help these individuals understand the necessity of the burn rehabilitation process.

POSITIONING AND SPLINTING

A patient's positioning program should begin on the day of admission.[8,9,58,76] Goals of a positioning program are to (1) minimize edema, (2) prevent tissue destruction, and (3) maintain soft tissues in an elongated state. General guidelines and some examples of proper positioning are provided in Table 26–4 and Figures 26-14 through 26-17. Burned areas should be positioned in an elongated state or neutral position of function.

Splinting can be viewed as an extension of the positioning program. There are certain "antideformity" positions in which patients generally are splinted; however, the therapist needs to assess the location of the burn and which movements are

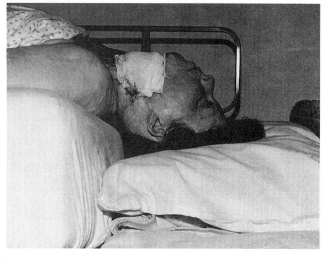

Figure 26-14. Positioning in bed of patient with burns of the anterior neck. (From Richard and Staley,[6] p 225, with permission.)

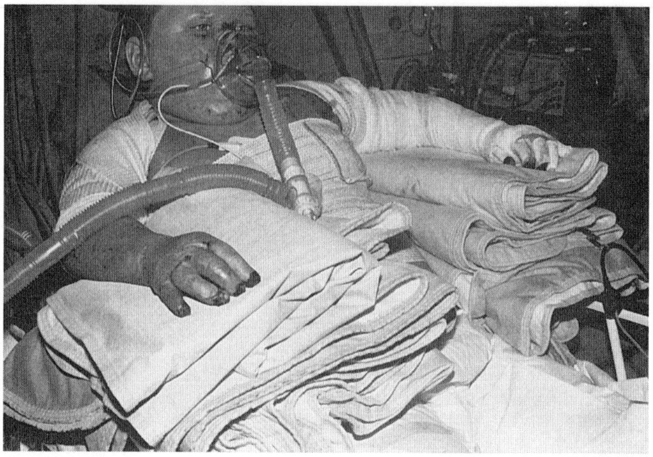

Figure 26-16. Proper positioning of upper extremities to reduce edema while seated. (From Richard and Staley,[6] p 231, with permission.)

difficult for the patient to achieve. With the exception of immobilizing a skin graft after surgery, splints should be fabricated for patients only if ROM or function would be lost without them. General indications for the use of splints include (1) prevention of contractures, (2) maintenance of ROM achieved during an exercise session or surgical release, (3) correction of contractures, and (4) protection of a joint or tendon.[77] Splint design should be kept simple so that a splint is easy to apply, remove, and clean. Splints usually are worn at night, when a patient is resting, or continuously for several days following skin grafting. Splints should conform to the body part, and care must be taken to ensure that there are no pressure points that may cause a breakdown in healing or normal skin. Splints should be checked routinely for proper fit and revised if necessary. Active motion is important, and splints and positioning are intended to serve as adjuncts to the therapy program until full active motion can be achieved.

Most splints used for burn injuries are static. The splint has no moveable parts, and maintains a position or immobilizes an area following skin grafting (Fig. 26-18). Dynamic splints also have been used successfully in the care of patients with a burn injury (Fig. 26-19).[78–80] These splints have moveable parts that allow joint movement. Dynamic splints apply a low-load, prolonged stress that can be adjusted to a patient's tolerance. They offer great potential for correcting a developing contracture and the early return of active function in areas of extensive burn and grafting. The use of continuous passive motion devices also is appropriate for certain patients with burn injuries.[81–85]

ACTIVE AND PASSIVE EXERCISE

Active exercise begins on the day of admission.[7–9,58,86] Any patient who is alert and able to follow commands is encouraged to perform active exercises of involved body parts frequently throughout the day. A patient should perform active exercise

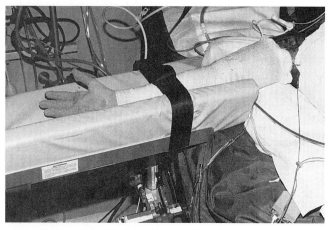

Figure 26-15. Positioning in bed of patient with burns of the axilla. (From Richard and Staley,[6] p 228, with permission.)

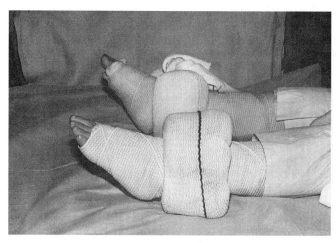

Figure 26-17. Elevation of heels off bed, with use of foam rolls encased in elastic netting. Note: this technique would not be used with burns to Achilles tendon area.

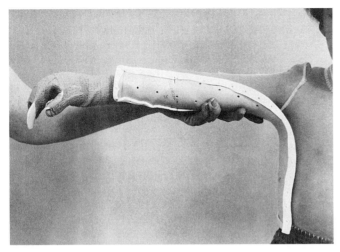

Figure 26-18. Static splint that immobilizes the shoulder in abduction and the elbow in extension.

of all extremities and trunk, including unburned areas. Dressing changes are an opportune time for an exercise session because the burn wound is visible, and the therapist can monitor the wound during the session. If a patient has just received a skin graft, active and passive exercise of the area may be discontinued for 3 to 5 days to allow the graft to adhere.[72,87,88] After the surgeon determines it is safe to begin exercise again, gentle ROM—first active and then passive, if needed—is reinstituted.

Active-assistive and passive exercise should be initiated if a patient cannot fully achieve active ROM. To keep the healed burned area moist, it should be lubricated before exercise is initiated. Care should be taken around areas of skin grafts, and stress should be applied in a gentle, prolonged, and gradual fashion. If the burn wounds are well healed, heating modalities (e.g., paraffin, ultrasound) may be used to increase the pliability of the tissue before exercise therapy.[89,90]

ROM in the area of unhealed burns is extremely painful, and most patients will indicate they would rather lose their motion than be subjected to the additional pain that occurs with movement. It usually is difficult and mentally draining on the physical therapist to push patients to exercise in and

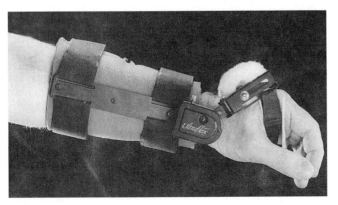

Figure 26-19. Dynamic splint used to provide a low-load, prolonged stress to scar tissue.

through pain, but it is critical that the therapist be persistent. Coordinating an exercise session with the administration of pain medication will lessen the painful experience for the patient.[74,86] Physical therapists should elicit the assistance of the family in keeping the patient motivated and mobile as much as possible.

RESISTIVE AND CONDITIONING EXERCISE

As a patient continues to recover, the rehabilitation program can be progressed to include strengthening exercises.[7,58,86] Patients with major burns may lose body weight, and lean muscle mass can decrease rapidly. Exercise may consist of isokinetic, isotonic, or other resistive training devices. General principles of exercise training and strength improvement should be followed, but they may need to be modified on the basis of a patient's condition and stage of wound healing. Resistive devices such as free weights and pulleys can be used to prevent loss of strength in areas not burned.

When a patient initially begins strengthening or endurance exercises, the physical therapist should monitor vital signs to assess cardiovascular and respiratory responses to treatment. In addition, overexertion may occur. Monitoring of pulse, blood pressure, and respiratory rate before, during, and after exercise, particularly in the recovery period after exercise, will yield valuable information as to the status of the cardiorespiratory system.

Patients should be encouraged to participate in exercises that will stress the cardiovascular system, such as walking from the burn unit to the physical therapy department. Cycling or rowing ergometry, treadmill walking, stair climbing, and other forms of aerobic exercise should be encouraged. These devices will not only work to increase cardiovascular endurance, but can have the added benefit of improving strength and ROM of the extremities. In addition, they introduce variety into the rehabilitation program. The physical therapist needs to be creative and innovative to motivate patients to increase their exercise capacity.

AMBULATION

Ambulation should be initiated at the earliest appropriate time. If the lower extremities are skin grafted, ambulation may be discontinued until it is safe to resume.[92–95] When ambulation is initiated, the lower extremities should be wrapped in elastic bandages in a figure-of-eight pattern to support the new grafts and promote venous return. If a patient cannot tolerate the upright position because of orthostatic intolerance or pain from the lower extremities in a dependent position, gradual increases in tilt-table treatment time will assist in preparing the patient for standing.[96,97] Initially, a patient may require an assistive device to ambulate. However, independent ambulation without a device should be achieved as soon as possible.

The physical therapist will spend a great deal of time with an individual patient during each exercise session. The rewards of a successful treatment program are tremendous when a patient who has suffered a life-threatening burn is able to walk out of the hospital and return to productive community involvement.

SCAR MANAGEMENT

Following wound closure, a skin graft or healed burn wound is vascular, flat, and soft. During the following 3 to 6 months, dramatic changes may occur. The newly healed areas may become raised and firm. Pressure has been used successfully to hasten scar maturation and minimize hypertrophic scar formation.[98] However, no one study validates the mechanism by which pressure alters scar tissue. Pressure may exert control over hypertrophic scarring by (1) thinning the dermis, (2) altering the biochemical structure of scar tissue, (3) decreasing blood flow to the area, (4) reorganizing collagen bundles, or (5) decreasing tissue water content. Constant pressure dressings or garments exerting pressure exceeding 25 mmHg will decrease the vascularity, decrease the amount of mucopolysaccharides, decrease collagen deposition, and significantly lessen localized edema.[7,98,99] The early hypertrophic scar is readily influenced by compressive forces and thus will respond to pressure therapy. The earlier the scar tissue is exposed to pressure, the better the result.[100,101] Usually, if the scar is less than 6 months old, it will respond to pressure therapy by conforming to the pressure, remaining flat on the surface, and not developing into a hypertrophic scar.[101] However, if the scar is still active or shows evidence of vascularity (red color), pressure therapy may be successful, even if the scar is 1 year old.

In general, if a patient's wounds heal in less than 10 to 14 days, which would be indicative of a superficial partial-thickness burn, pressure may not be needed. If wound healing takes longer than 10 to 14 days (as in a deep partial-thickness burn) or is skin grafted, pressure usually is indicated.[102]

Pressure Dressings

Elastic wraps can be used to provide vascular support of skin grafts and donor sites as well as to control edema and scarring. Elastic wraps should be used until a patient's skin or scars can tolerate the shearing force of pressure garment application, and open areas are minimal. Elastic wraps are applied in a figure-of-eight pattern on the lower extremities. A spiral wrap can be used on the upper extremities and a circular wrap on the trunk.[98]

A self-adherent elastic bandage can be used for the hand and toes.[98,103] This bandage adheres only to itself and can be used over dressings before the wounds have healed. It helps to minimize edema and control scar formation. It may be used before application of a glove or as definitive pressure on an infant's hand.

Tubular support bandages come in various circumferences and garment styles. They provide a moderate amount of compression and may be used as interim garments before a custom-made garment is fit.[98,104] The tubular support bandage is especially useful for small children who grow rapidly and require frequent alterations in garment size.

Several companies manufacture pressure garments. Some are ready made and come in several sizes to fit most patients; others are custom made for the individual patient. For the custom-made garments, a physical therapist uses tapes to measure the circumference of each limb every 1½ inches of its length to fit the garment exactly to the limb with the proper pressure. Garments are measured when a patient has only a few remaining open areas. The garments are very tight, and difficult to apply, but the pressure is necessary to prevent scar hypertrophy. Garments can be ordered for any or all body parts, including the face and head, and they come in many styles, options, and colors (Fig. 26-20).[98] Garments can be worn when the skin or scars can tolerate the shearing force of application. Pantyhose may be used under waist-height pressure garments to assist with donning. Garments usually are worn 23 hours a day (removed for bathing) for as long as 12 to 18 months to assist with scar remodeling. Garments should be washed daily to prevent buildup of perspiration and moisturizing cream, which may lead to scar maceration. The patient usually receives two sets of garments, one to wear and one to wash.

Adequate pressure may not be obtained with elastic wraps or pressure garments over concave surfaces, such as the sternum or axilla, and an insert may be necessary.[105] Inserts can be made of many materials including foam, silicone elastomer, elastomer putty, and gel pads.[98,106,107] These items need to be removed and cleaned regularly to prevent maceration of the underlying tissue.

Early, consistent use of pressure will result in flat, pliable scars, desensitization and protection of scars, and relief of itching. Pressure is necessary until scar maturation, when the scars are pale, flat, and soft.

Massage

Massage is an intervention that clinically appears useful to assist with ROM exercise by making the tissue more pliable. Deep friction massage may loosen scar tissue by mobilizing cutaneous tissue from underlying tissue and act to break up adhesions.[7,108] When massage is used in conjunction with ROM exercise, the immature scar can be elongated more easily, and contracture can be corrected. Although no study has validated the use of massage for patients with burn injuries,[109] in the long term, skin pliability and texture appear improved by the use of massage. Firm scars that are routinely massaged tend to soften. Edges or seams of grafts or any area that is raised and firm may benefit from massage. Scars should be massaged in a slow, firm manner for 5 to 10 minutes, 3 to 6 times daily.

Camouflage Make-up

For scars of the face, neck, and hands, camouflage make-up can be used.[9,98] This type of make-up may the actual ROM and movement pattern used in each exercise. A video facilitates education of those involved in the patient's rehabilitation program and helps to ensure consistency of treatment after discharge.[110]

The splinting schedule and pressure program that was followed in the hospital just before the patient's discharge should be continued at home. Before discharge, the patient and/or his or her family members should be able to apply and remove all splints and pressure appliances independently.

Proper skin care requires specifying the type of soap and cream a patient is to use. In general, soap should be mild without perfumes or other irritants. A moisturizing soap can be used after all open areas are healed. Moisturizing creams should be applied 2 to 3 times daily and should not contain perfumes or have a significant alcohol content. Patients should be instructed to massage the cream completely into their skin to avoid buildup on the surface. If a patient will be exposed to the sun, a sunscreen with a skin protection factor of at least 15 should be used and reapplied frequently.[106] Patients should be cautioned to avoid the sun if at all possible and to use hats or clothing to help protect their skin against the sun's rays.

Small, superficial open areas may plague a patient for many months after wound closure because of the fragility of a healed burn wound. The patient should be instructed to wash these areas twice daily, apply a small amount of antibiotic ointment, and cover the areas with a nonadherent dressing. Further irritation or maceration can be prevented by avoiding shearing forces, improper fit of clothing, brisk cleansing and soaking in water too long, or application of too much cream.

Itching may intensify when wounds have healed. A patient should be instructed to pat, rather than scratch, the irritated areas. Application of cream may help decrease itching; however, some patients may require oral medication to help control this problem.

Some patients with burn injury may require outpatient therapy to supplement the HEP and monitor and adjust their splinting and pressure program. Frequency of outpatient therapy is based on each patient's needs. Regardless of whether or not a patient receives outpatient therapy, he or she should be monitored at regular intervals through an outpatient clinic so burn team members can assess the patient's adjustment back into society and alter the rehabilitation program according to the patient's physical abilities and extent of scar maturation. When an adult patient's burns have matured and full ROM is achieved, further follow-up care is unnecessary. However, a child will need to be monitored until he or she is fully grown, because burn scars may not keep pace with a child's growth; surgical release of scar tissue may be necessary.

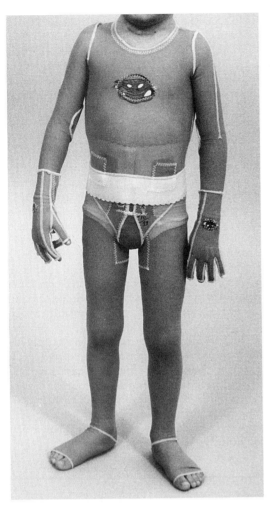

Figure 26-20. Pressure garments such as gloves, vest, and waist-height pants are worn to minimize hypertrophic scar formation.

be useful when a person has either hyperpigmentation or hypopigmentation of the skin due to the burn injury. In addition, make-up can be used before scar maturation, when the scar is still red, and a patient wants to go out in public without his/her pressure garments or devices for short periods of time. The cosmetics are opaque, color correct burn scars, and are available in multiple shades to accommodate various skin colors. They also are waterproof and can be worn during all activities. These products can be purchased in larger department stores or where theatrical products are sold.

FOLLOW-UP CARE

Before patients are discharged from the hospital, a therapist should provide them with information regarding a home exercise program (HEP), splinting and positioning program, and skin care.

A HEP should continue to stress frequent ROM exercises in combination with massaging areas involved in the burn injury. In addition, patients should be encouraged to perform as many ADL skills as possible independently. Therapists can videotape the patient's exercise program to provide the patient, family, and outpatient therapist with

COMMUNITY PROGRAMS

There are various community programs available to individuals who have survived a burn injury. The therapist should be aware of those in the patient's home community so that an appropriate referral can be made. If programs are not available, someone in the hospital or community may want to initiate a program. Programs may include:

1. Burn prevention programs: The American Burn Association, 625 N. Michigan Ave., Chicago, IL 60611; (800) 548-2876, has a Burn Prevention Committee with a myriad of printed materials.
2. School re-entry programs: Provided by the hospital staff for the students and staff in the child's school.[9,112]
3. Burn camp: Weekend- to week-long camp for children to interact in a controlled, outdoor environment with peers who have sustained a similar injury.[9,112] The American Burn Association has a Burn Camp Special Interest Group with readily available information about camps throughout the United States and Canada.
4. Adult support group: Provides an opportunity for individuals with or without their families to share experiences and gain support from others who have had similar injuries.[112]

SUMMARY

Burn injuries represent a major health problem in terms of management and care of surviving patients. Specific impairments and complications vary according to the extent and depth of thermal destruction of the skin. The classification of burn injuries is based on the depth of tissue destroyed and includes superficial burn, superficial partial-thickness burn, deep partial-thickness burn, full-thickness burn, and subdermal burn. The rule of nines and the Lund and Browder formula were developed to assist with the initial assessment of the extent of burn injury. The specific clinical signs and symptoms that result from a burn injury vary according to the different classifications. Indirect impairments can include infection, pulmonary, metabolic, skeletal, muscular, neurological, and cardiac/circulatory complications. Medical management addresses life-threatening problems and stabilization of the patient. Dressings with topical medications, débridement, surgical excision, and skin grafting are primary treatment measures. Skin substitutes are slowly becoming a practical alternative to skin grafting. Physical therapy management focuses on the prevention of scar contracture, maintenance of normal ROM, development of muscular strength and endurance, improvement of cardiovascular conditioning, independence in functional activities, and prevention of hypertrophic scarring. Although burn trauma and subsequent recovery can be a devastating life occurrence, there are treatment facilities and medical professionals to assist patients with burn injuries and their families return to as normal a life-style as possible.

QUESTIONS FOR REVIEW

1. Name the two primary layers of skin and list two functions of each.
2. Describe the differences between superficial, partial-thickness, and full-thickness burns.
3. Explain how a deep partial-thickness burn can convert to a full-thickness burn.
4. Compare the treatments for deep partial-thickness and full-thickness burns.
5. Describe the primary complications of the pulmonary system due to extensive burns.
6. What are the major metabolic complications associated with burns, and how are they treated?
7. List the three phases that occur in the healing of a burn wound.
8. What are the goals of the initial management and resuscitation of a patient with an acute burn injury?

9. Describe the various types of skin grafts.
10. Differentiate between a split-thickness and full-thickness skin graft.
11. List three essential factors for successful skin graft adherence.
12. List five goals and outcomes of a rehabilitation program for a patient with a burn injury.
13. Discuss the types of exercise that are useful in a patient's rehabilitation program.
14. What interventions can be used to prevent burn scar contractures?
15. What interventions can be used to prevent hypertrophic scar formation?
16. What information should be included in patient and family education before discharge from the hospital?

CASE STUDY

A 29 year-old male sustained a 30 percent TBSA burn 6 weeks before this outpatient assessment and evaluation. Patient was burned at home while he was refueling a lawnmower with gasoline, which ignited. Areas of the body affected by the burn included the right upper extremity, portions of the posterior and anterior trunk, lateral neck, right side of face, and thigh. Areas skin grafted included the right dorsal hand, forearm, and arm up to the axillary crease. The remaining burn wounds healed secondarily. The neck, face, and thigh burns were superficial. Patient was initially treated at a regional burn center and now is referred to the local hospital for follow-up outpatient physical therapy due to decreased right elbow extension, decreased shoulder flexion, and inability to reach overhead. The right upper extremity lacks 15 degrees (15 to 120 degrees) elbow extension and flexion of the shoulder is limited to 0 to 155 degrees. Scar contracture bands are noted at both locations at the end of available range with movement. The patient states he has some difficulty donning shirts and his jacket. All other movements are within functional limits (WFL). The patient's strength overall is considered WFL, as are other physical parameters. His wounds are all closed. The patient lives with his girlfriend and has medical benefits through his employer.

One week after his discharge from the hospital, the patient presented for his initial outpatient assessment wearing interim pressure garments, as instructed. He also brought the static elbow splint that had been issued to him during his acute hospitalization, but which "doesn't fit right anymore." The expected outcome for this patient is to regain full right upper extremity ROM and function.

Guiding Questions

1. Describe how you would approach the clinical problems presented. Your answer should address positioning, splinting, exercise, and scar-management interventions.

2. What patient education would you provide? Would this differ if the patient is compliant versus noncompliant with the therapy program?

3. What is the anticipated rehabilitation potential for this patient? Your thought process should include time from burn injury and stage of healing.

REFERENCES

1. Demling, RH: Medical progress: Burns. N Engl J Med 313:1389, 1986.
2. Pruitt Jr, BA, and Mason Jr, AD: Epidemiological, demographic and outcomes characteristics of burn injury. In Herdon, DN: Total Burn Care. Saunders, Philadelphia, 1996, p 5.
3. Baker, SP, et al: Fire, burns and lightning. In: The Injury Fact Book. Oxford University Press, New York, 1992, p 161.
4. Herndon, DN, et al: Teamwork for total burn care: Achievements, directions and hopes. In Herdon, DN (ed): Total Burn Care. Saunders, Philadelphia, 1996, p 1.
5. Saffle, JR, et al: Recent outcomes in the treatment of burn injury in the United States: A report from the American Burn Association patient registry. J Burn Care Rehabil 16:219, 1995.
6. Richard, RL, and Staley, MJ (eds): Burn Care and Rehabilitation: Principles and Practice. FA Davis, Philadelphia, 1994.
7. Ward, RS: Physical rehabilitation. In Carrougher, GJ (ed): Burn Care and Therapy. Mosby, St. Louis, 1998, p 293.
8. Moore, M: The burn unit. In Campbell, SK, et al (eds): Physical Therapy for Children. Saunders, Philadelphia, 1994, p 763.
9. Grigsby de Linde, L: Rehabilitation of the child with burns. In Tecklin, JS (ed): Pediatric Physical Therapy. Lippincott, Philadelphia, 1994, p 208.
10. Shani, E, and Rosenberg, L. Are we making an impact? A review of a burn prevention program in Israeli schools. J Burn Care Rehabil 19:82, 1998.
11. Committee on Trauma. American College of Surgeons: Guidelines for Operation of Burn Units. In: Resources for Optimal Care of the Injured Patient. American College of Surgeons, Chicago, IL, 1999, p 55.
12. Burn Care Resources in North America 1996–1997. American Burn Association, Chicago, 1996.
13. Supple, KG, et al: Preparation for burn center verification. J Burn Care Rehabil 18:58, 1997.
14. Holbrook, KA, and Wolff, K: The structure and development of skin. In Fitzpatrick, TB, et al (eds): Dermatology In General Medicine. McGraw-Hill, New York, 1993, p 97.
15. Lanir, Y: The fibrous structure of the skin and its relation to mechanical behavior. In Marks, R, and Payne, PA (eds): Bioengineering and the Skin. MIT Press, Massachusetts, 1981, p 93.
16. Moncrief, JA: The body's response to heat. In Artz, CP, et al (eds): Burns: A Team Approach. Saunders, Philadelphia, 1979, p 24.
17. Johnson, C: Pathologic manifestations of burn injury. In Richard, RL, and Staley, MJ (eds): Burn Care and Rehabilitation: Principles and Practice. FA Davis, Philadelphia, 1994, p 31.
18. Norris, PG, et al: Acute effects of ultraviolet radiation on the skin. In Fitzpatrick, TB, et al (eds): Dermatology in General Medicine. McGraw-Hill, New York, 1993, p 1651.
19. Heggers, JP, et al: Evaluation of burn blister fluid. Plast Reconst Surg 65:798, 1980.
20. Rockwell, WB, and Ehrlich, HP: Fibrinolysis inhibition in human burn blister fluid. J Burn Care Rehabil 11:1, 1990.
21. Garner, WL, et al: The effects of burn blister fluid on keratinocyte replication and differentiation. J Burn Care Rehabil 14:127, 1993.
22. Ono, I, et al: A study of cytokines in burn blister fluid related to wound healing. Burns 21:352, 1995.
23. Lund, T, et al: Pathogenesis of edema formation in burn injuries. World J Surg 16:2, 1992.
24. Mozingo, DW: Surgical management. In Carrougher, GJ (ed): Burn Care and Therapy. Mosby, St. Louis, 1998, p 233.
25. Miller, SF, et al: Triage and Resuscitation of the Burn Patient. In Richard, RL, and Staley, MJ (eds): Burn Care and Rehabilitation: Principles and Practice. FA Davis, Philadelphia, 1994, p 107.
26. Wittman, MI: Electrical and chemical burns. In Richard, RL, and Staley, MJ (eds): Burn Care and Rehabilitation: Principles and Practice. FA Davis, Philadelphia, 1994, p 603.
27. Williams, WG, and Phillips, LG: Pathophysiology of the burn wound. In Herndon, DN (ed): Total Burn Care. Saunders, Philadelphia, 1996, p 65.
28. Polaski, GR, and Tennison, AC: Estimation of the amount of burned surface area. JAMA 103:34, 1948.
29. Lund, CC, and Browder, NC: Estimation of area of burns. Surg Gynecol Obstet 79:352, 1955.
30. Sheridan, RL, and Tompkins, RG: Etiology and prevention of multisystem organ failure. In Herndon, DN (ed): Total Burn Care. Saunders, Philadelphia, 1996, p 302.
31. Heggers, J, et al: Treatment of infections in burns. In Herndon, DN (ed): Total Burn Care. Philadelphia, Saunders, 1996, p 98.
32. Weber, JM: Epidemiology of infections and strategies for control. In Carrougher, GJ (ed): Burn Care and Therapy. Mosby, St. Louis, 1998, p 185.
33. Moylan, JA: Smoke inhalation and burn injury. Surg Clin North Am 60:1530, 1980.
34. Greenberg, MI, and Walter, J: Axioms on smoke inhalation. Hosp Med 19:13, 1983.
35. Chu, CS: New concepts of pulmonary burn injury. J Trauma 21:958, 1981.
36. Cioffi Jr, WG: Inhalation injury. In Carrougher, GJ (ed): Burn Care and Therapy. Mosby, St. Louis, 1998, p 35.
37. Mancusi-Ungaro, HR, et al: Caloric and nitrogen balances as predictors of nutritional outcome in patients with burns. J Burn Care Rehabil 13:695, 1992.

38. Demling, RH, and DeSanti, L: Increased protein intake during the recovery phase after severe burns increases body weight gain and muscle function. J Burn Care Rehabil 19:161, 1998.

39. Wilmore, DW, et al: Effect of ambient temperature on heat production and heat loss in burn patients. J Appl Physiol 38:593, 1975.

40. Alexander, JW, et al: Beneficial effects of aggressive protein feeding in severely burned children. Ann Surg 192:505, 1980.

41. Dominioni, L, et al: Enteral feeding in burn hypermetabolism: Nutritional and metabolic effects on different levels of calorie and protein intake. J Parenter Enteral Nutr 9:269, 1985.

42. Matsuda, T, et al: The importance of burn wound size in determining the optimal calorie:nitrogen ratio. Surgery 94:562, 1983.

43. Demling, RH, et al: The study of burn wound edema using dichromatic absorptiometry. J Trauma 18:124, 1978.

44. Kramer, GC, and Nguyen, TT: Pathophysiology of burn shock and burn edema. In Herndon, DN: Total Burn Care. Saunders, Philadelphia, 1996, p 44.

45. Gordon, MD, and Winfree, JH: Fluid resuscitation after a major burn. In Carrougher, GJ (ed): Burn Care and Therapy. Mosby, St. Louis, 1998, p 107.

46. Munster, AM, et al: Heterotopic calcification following burns: A prospective study. J Trauma 12:1071, 1972.

47. Schiele, HP, et al: Radiographic changes in burns of the upper extremity. Diagnostic Radiology 104:13, 1971.

48. Rubin, MM, and Cozzi, GM: Heterotopic ossification of the temporomandibular joint in a burn patient. J Oral Maxillofac Surg 44:897, 1986.

49. Edlich, RF, et al: Heterotopic calcification and ossification in the burn patient. J Burn Care Rehabil 6:363, 1985.

50. Dutcher, K, and Johnson, C: Neuromuscular and musculoskeletal complications. In Richard, RL, and Staley, MJ (eds): Burn Care and Rehabilitation: Principles and Practice. FA Davis, Philadelphia, 1994, p 576.

51. Greenhalgh, DG, and Staley, MJ: Burn wound healing. In Richard, RL, and Staley, MJ (eds): Burn Care and Rehabilitation: Principles and Practice. FA Davis, Philadelphia, 1994, p 70.

52. Arem, AJ, and Madden, JW: Is there a Wolff's law for connective tissue? Surg Forum 25:512, 1974.

53. Staley, MJ, and Richard, RL: Scar management. In Richard, RL, and Staley, MJ (eds): Burn Care and Rehabilitation: Principles and Practice. FA Davis, Philadelphia, 1994, p 380.

54. Warden, GD: Fluid resuscitation and early management. In Herdon, DN (ed): Total Burn Care. Saunders, Philadelphia, 1996, p 53.

55. Thomson, PD, et al: A survey of burn hydrotherapy in the United States. J Burn Care Rehabil 11:151, 1990.

56. Saffle, JR, and Schnebly, WA: Burn wound care. In Richard, RL, and Staley, MJ (eds): Burn Care and Rehabilitation: Principles and Practice. FA Davis, Philadelphia, 1994, p 119.

57. Shankowsky, HA, et al: North American survey of hydrotherapy in modern burn care. J Burn Care Rehabil 15:143, 1994.

58. Ward, RS: The rehabilitation of burn patients. Crit Rev Phys Rehab Med 2:121, 1991.

59. Neville, C, and Dimick, AR: The trauma table as an alternative to the Hubbard tank in burn care. J Burn Care Rehabil 8:574, 1987.

60. Heggers, JP, et al: Bactericidal and wound-healing properties of sodium hypochlorite solutions. J Burn Care Rehabil 12:420, 1991.

61. Richard, RL: The use of chlorine bleach as a disinfectant and antiseptic in whirlpools. Physical Therapy Forum 7:7, 1988.

62. Carrougher, GJ: Burn wound assessment and topical treatment. In Carrougher, GJ (ed): Burn Care and Therapy. Mosby, St. Louis, 1998, p 142.

63. Miller, SF, et al: Surgical management of the burn patient. In Richard, RL, and Staley, MJ (eds): Burn Care and Rehabilitation: Principles and Practice. FA Davis, Philadelphia, 1994, p 180.

64. Cuono, C, et al: Use of cultured epidermal autografts and dermal allografts as skin replacement after burn injury. Lancet 8490:1123, 1986.

65. Munster, AM: Cultured epidermal autographs in the management of burn patients. J Burn Care Rehabil 13:121, 1992.

66. Lattari, V, et al: The use of a permanent dermal allograft in full-thickness burns of the hand and foot: A report of three cases. J Burn Care Rehabil 18:147, 1997.

67. Hansbrough, J et al: Clinical trials of a biosynthetic temporary skin replacement, Dermagraft-Transitional Covering, compared with cryopreserved human cadaver skin for temporary coverage of excised burn wounds. J Burn Care Rehabil 18:43, 1997.

68. Purdue, G, et al: A multicenter clinical trial of a biosynthetic skin replacement, Dermagraft-TC, compared with cryopreserved human cadaver skin for temporary coverage of excised burn wounds. J Burn Care Rehabil 18:52, 1997.

69. Heimbach, D, et al: Artificial dermis for major burns: A multicenter, randomized clinical trial. Ann Surg 208:313, 1988.

70. Richard, R, et al: A comparison of the Tanner and Bioplasty skin mesher systems for maximal skin graft expansion. J Burn Care Rehabil 14:690, 1993.

71. Larson, D, et al: Prevention and treatment of burn scar contracture. In Artz, CP, et al (eds): Burns: A Team Approach. Saunders, Philadelphia, 1979, p 466.

72. Greenhalgh, DG, et al: The early release of axillary contractures in pediatric patients with burns. J Burn Care Rehabil 14:39, 1993.

73. Richard, RL, and Staley, MJ: Burn patient evaluation and treatment planning. In Richard, RL, and Staley, MJ (eds): Burn Care and Rehabilitation: Principles and Practice. FA Davis, Philadelphia, 1994, p 201.

74. Moss, BF, et al: Psychologic support and pain management of the burn patient. In Richard, RL, and Staley, MJ (eds): Burn Care and Rehabilitation: Principles and Practice. FA Davis, Philadelphia, 1994, p 475.

75. Adcock, RJ, et al: Psychologic and emotional recovery. In Carrougher, GJ (ed): Burn Care and Therapy. Mosby, St. Louis, 1998, p 329.

76. Apfel, L, et al: Approaches to positioning the burn patient. In Richard, RL, and Staley, MJ (eds): Burn Care and Rehabilitation: Principles and Practice. FA Davis, Philadelphia, 1994, p 221.

77. Daugherty, M, and Carr-Collins, J: Splinting techniques for the burn patient. In Richard, RL, and Staley, MJ (eds): Burn Care and Rehabilitation: Principles and Practice. FA Davis, Philadelphia, 1994, p 242.

78. Richard, RL: Use of Dynasplint to correct elbow flexion burn contracture: A case report. J Burn Care Rehabil 7:151, 1986.

79. Richard, R, and Staley, M: Dynamic splinting: Basic science + modern technology. Physical Therapy Forum, 11:21, 1992.

80. Richard, RL, et al: Dynamic versus static splints: A prospective case for sustained stress. J Burn Care Rehabil 16:284, 1995.

81. Covey, MH, et al: Efficacy of continuous passive motion (CPM) devices with hand burns. J Burn Care Rehabil 9:397, 1988.

82. McAllister, LP, and Salazar, CA: Case report on the use of CPM on an electrical burn. J Burn Care Rehabil 9:401, 1988.

83. McGough, CE: Introduction to CPM. J Burn Care Rehabil 9:494, 1988.

84. Covey, MH: Application of CPM devices with burn patients. J Burn Care Rehabil 9:496, 1988.

85. Richard, RL, et al: The physiologic response of a patient with critical burns to continuous passive motion. J Burn Care Rehabil 11:554, 1990.

86. Humphrey, C, et al: Soft tissue management and exercise. In Richard, RL, and Staley, MJ (eds): Burn Care and Rehabilitation: Principles and Practice. FA Davis, Philadelphia, 1994, p 324.

87. Herndon, DN, et al: Management of the pediatric patient with burns. J Burn Care Rehabil 14:3, 1993.
88. Schwanholt, C, et al: A comparison of full-thickness versus split-thickness autografts for the coverage of deep palm burns in the very young pediatric patient. J Burn Care Rehabil 14:29, 1993.
89. Ward, RS: The use of physical agents in burn care. In Richard, RL, and Staley, MJ (eds): Burn Care and Rehabilitation: Principles and Practice. FA Davis, Philadelphia, 1994, p 419.
90. Ward, RS, et al: Evaluation of therapeutic ultrasound to improve response to physical therapy and lessen scar contracture after burn injury. J Burn Care Rehabil 15:74, 1994.
91. Black, S, et al: Oxygen consumption for lower extremity exercises in normal subjects and burn patients. Phys Ther 60:1255, 1980.
92. Schmitt, P, et al: Lower Extremity Burns and Ambulation. In Richard, RL, and Staley, MJ (eds): Burn Care and Rehabilitation: Principles and Practice. FA Davis, Philadelphia, 1994, p 361.
93. Schmitt, MA, et al: How soon is safe? Ambulation of the patient with burns after lower extremity skin grafting. J Burn Care Rehabil 12:33, 1991.
94. Burnsworth, B, et al: Immediate ambulation of patients with lower-extremity grafts. J Burn Care Rehabil 13:89, 1992.
95. Grube, BJ, et al: Early ambulation and discharge in 100 patients with burns of the foot treated by grafts. J Trauma 33:662, 1992.
96. Temmen, HJ, et al: Tilt table exercise guidelines for burn patients: Are cardiac exercise parameters appropriate? Proceedings of the American Burn Association 30:221, 1998.
97. Boyea, BL, et al: Use of the tilt table for postural reconditioning of burn patients prior to ambulation. Proceedings of the American Burn Association 30:233, 1998.
98. Staley, MJ, and Richard, RL: Scar management. In Richard, RL, and Staley, MJ (eds): Burn Care and Rehabilitation: Principles and Practice. FA Davis, Philadelphia, 1994, p 380.
99. Johnson, CL: Physical therapists as scar modifiers. Phys Ther 64:1381, 1984.
100. Kischer, CW, and Shetlar, MR: Microvasculature in hypertrophic scars and the effects of pressure. J Trauma 19:757, 1979.
101. Leung, PC, and Ng, M: Pressure treatment for hypertrophic scars. Burns 6:224, 1980.
102. Deitch, EA, et al: Hypertrophic burn scars: Analysis of variables. J Trauma 23:895, 1983.
103. Ward, RS, et al: Use of Coban self-adherent wrap in management of postburn hand grafts: Case reports. J Burn Care Rehabil 15:364, 1994.
104. Kealey, GP, et al: Prospective randomized comparison of two types of pressure therapy garments. J Burn Care Rehabil 11:334, 1990.
105. Cheng, JCY, et al: Pressure therapy in the treatment of post-burn hypertrophic scar: A critical look into its usefulness and fallacies by pressure monitoring. Burns 10:154, 1984.
106. Alston, DW, et al: Materials for pressure inserts in the control of hypertrophic scar tissue. J Burn Care Rehabil 2:40, 1981.
107. Perkins, K, et al: Current materials and techniques used in a burn scar management programme. Burns 13:406, 1987.
108. Miles, WK, and Grigsby, L: Remodeling of scar tissue in the burned hand. In Hunter, JM, et al (eds): Rehabilitation of the Hand. Mosby, St. Louis, 1984, p 841.
109. Patino, O, and Novick, C: Massage on hypertrophic scars. Proceedings of the American Burn Association 29:18, 1997.
110. Gallagher, J, et al: Discharge videotaping: A means of augmenting occupational and physical therapy. J Burn Care Rehabil 11:470, 1990.
111. Braddom, RL, et al: The physical treatment and rehabilitation of burn patients. In Hummel, RP (ed): Clinical Burn Therapy. John Wright PSG, Boston, 1982, p 297.
112. Leman, CJ, and Ricks, N: Discharge planning and follow-up burn care. In Richard, RL, and Staley, MJ (eds): Burn Care and Rehabilitation: Principles and Practice. FA Davis, Philadelphia, 1994, p 447.

SUPPLEMENTAL READINGS

Herdon, DN: Total Burn Care. Saunders, Philadelphia, 1996.
Richard, RL, and Staley, MJ (eds): Burn Care and Rehabilitation: Principles and Practice. FA Davis, Philadelphia, 1996.
Ward, RS: Physical rehabilitation. In: Carrougher, GJ (ed): Burn Care and Therapy. Mosby, St. Louis, 1998.
Burnsworth, B, Krob, MJ, and Langer-Schnepp, M: Immediate ambulation of patients with lower extremity grafts. J Burn Care Rehabil 13:89, 1992.
Heimbach, D, et al: Burn depth: A review. World J Surg 16:10, 1992.
Pruitt, B, and McManus, A: The changing epidemiology of infection in burn patients. World J Surg 16:57, 1992.

Cohen, IK, Diegelmann, RF, and Lindblad, WJ (eds): Wound Healing: Biochemical and Clinical Aspects. WB Saunders, Philadelphia, 1992.
Trofino, RB (ed): Nursing Care of the Burn-Injured Patient. FA Davis, Philadelphia, 1991.
Thompson, PD, et al: A survey of burn hydrotherapy in the United States. J Burn Care Rehabil 11:151, 1990.
Hutchinson, JJ, and McGuckin, M: Occlusive dressings: A microbiologic and clinical review. Am J Infect Control 18:257, 1990.

GLOSSARY

Allograft (or homograft): Skin used for temporary coverage of a burn wound; the skin is taken from the same species (usually cadaver skin).

Autograft: Skin taken from an unburned area of a patient, which is then transplanted to cover a wound.

Blanch: A white spot seen in the skin when pressure is applied. This is an indication of the presence of viable capillary beds; and the blanched area will become pink when pressure is released if the capillary bed is perfused.

Closed technique: The wound-care technique of covering a wound from the outside environment with an appropriate dressing.

Contact inhibition: Inhibition of the migration of epithelial cells when they are in contact with other epithelial cells on all sides.

Débridement: The removal of eschar and/or any loose tissue from a burn wound.

    Sharp débridement: Use of sterile scissors and forceps to remove eschar.

Dermal healing: The process whereby the dermis is repaired via scar formation.

Dermatome: Device used to harvest thin slices of skin for skin grafting.

Dermis: Deep layer of skin that contains blood vessels, lymphatics, nerve endings, collagen, and elastin, and that encloses the sweat glands, sebaceous glands, and hair follicles.

Desquamation: Peeling of the outer layers of the epidermis.

Donor site: Site from which a skin graft is taken.

Electrical burn: Injury sustained from the passage of electric current through the tissues of the body.

Epidermis: The outermost layer of the skin, which provides the body with a barrier to the environment.

Epithelial healing: The process of regeneration of the epidermis through epithelial cell migration, proliferation, and differentiation.

Epithelial islands: Surviving tissue from which new epithelial cell growth will originate.

Eschar: The dead, necrotic tissue from a burn wound.

Escharotomy: Midlateral incision of the burned eschar used to relieve pressure in an extremity or on the trunk.

Fibroblasts: A connective tissue cell that forms the fibrous tissues in the body.

Full-thickness burn: Burn involving the entire dermis.

Full-thickness skin graft: Graft containing epidermis and full dermal thickness.

Heterotopic ossification (HO): Abnormal bone growth in soft tissues.

Hypertrophic scar: Raised scar that stays within the boundaries of the burn wound and is characteristically red, raised, and firm.

Hypertrophy: Increase in size or bulk.

Inhalation injury: Injury sustained by the lungs due to breathing hot and/or toxic gases. Usually occurs when individual is burned in a closed space.

Keloid scar: Raised scar that extends beyond the boundaries of the original burn wound.

Mesh graft: Process whereby the donor skin is placed through a device that increases the surface area of the graft.

Open technique: Absence of dressings. Often used after skin grafting to the face.

Partial-thickness burn: Burn involving the epidermis and part of the dermis. Subcategories are superficial partial-thickness and deep partial-thickness burns, depending on the amount of dermis involved.

Peripheral neuropathy: Pathological condition of the peripheral nerves in which muscle weakness, paresthesias, impaired reflexes, and autonomic symptoms in the hands and feet are common.

  Polyneuropathy: Pathological condition of multiple nerves.

Primary excision: Surgical removal of eschar.

Rule of nines: Estimation used to determine the amount of total body surface area that has been burned. It divides the body into segments that are approximately 9 percent of the total.

Sheet graft: Autograft that is applied in a single sheet without alteration. May be split-thickness or full-thickness in depth.

Skin substitutes: Tissues engineered in a laboratory which are used to restore the essential functions of the skin, provide a barrier to the environment, and control evaporative water loss.

Split-thickness skin graft: Graft containing epidermis and only the superficial layers of the dermis.

Subdermal burn: Injury that involves complete destruction of all tissues from the epidermis down to and through the subcutaneous tissue.

Superficial burn: Burn involving only the epidermal layer; e.g., sunburn.

Wound contraction: Movement of the wound margins toward the center of the defect. Thought to be caused by the active movement of the fibroblasts in the wound bed.

Xenograft (or heterograft): Skin used as a temporary wound cover, which is harvested from another species of animal, usually a pig.

Z-plasty: Procedure used to surgically lengthen a burn scar contracture to allow for greater ROM.

Zone of coagulation: Cells are irreversibly damaged, and skin death occurs.

Zone of hyperemia: Site of minimal cell damage. Tissue should recover within several days.

Zone of stasis: Site of injured cells that may die without specialized treatment.

APPENDIX

Suggested Answers to Case Study Guiding Questions

1. Describe how you would approach the clinical problems presented. Your answer should address positioning, splinting, exercise, and scar-management interventions.

ANSWER: A positioning program will need to be continued at home during the night. This program will emphasize right shoulder abduction to at least 90 degrees and elbow extension. The shoulder may be positioned out on a nightstand with pillows or blankets on top. The patient had worn a static splint for the right elbow during his acute hospital stay; however, he may now benefit from the use of a dynamic splint to provide a prolonged stress into elbow extension. Overhead exercises and activities should stress the combined movements of shoulder flexion and elbow extension. Isolated passive elongation of the scar tissue overlying the shoulder and elbow joints should be followed by a combined upper extremity stretch. The scar management program should be progressed to the point where the patient is wearing customized pressure garments with insert material in the right antecubital and right axilla for increased pressure and softening of the scar tissue.

2. What patient education would you provide? Would this differ if the patient is compliant versus noncompliant with the therapy program?

ANSWER: Patient education would include information on the scar maturation process after a burn injury and how the different interventions of positioning, splinting, exercise, and scar management affect the healing tissue. In addition, information on postinjury skin care will be necessary. It should be stressed to the patient that burn rehabilitation is a long, ongoing process that requires patience and persistence for an optimal outcome. If the patient has concerns regarding his appearance or ability to return to work, support groups or vocational counseling may be appropriate. If the patient has family members who will be involved in his care, they should also attend some of the therapy sessions and be involved in the actual therapy program. The patient should be informed that therapy sessions will be more frequent early in the rehabilitation phase and, with follow-through at home, the frequency of these sessions will decrease. Patient compliance should be stressed, because the consequences of noncompliance are an extended rehabilitation time or even reconstructive surgery.

3. What is the anticipated rehabilitation potential for this patient? Your thought process should include time from burn injury and stage of healing.

ANSWER: The rehabilitation potential for this patient is excellent. He is young and was in a previously healthy state before the burn injury occurred. His scar tissue difficulties fall in the early phase of wound maturation, which is a time when scar tissue contracture is easily corrected.

Thomas J. Schmitz

LEARNING OBJECTIVES

1. Identify the major etiological factors associated with traumatic spinal cord injury.
2. Describe the clinical presentation following damage to the spinal cord.
3. Describe the indirect impairments and complications associated with spinal cord injury.
4. Identify the anticipated functional outcomes for patients with spinal cord injury at various lesion levels.
5. Identify and explain the relevant systems review and tests and measures included in the examination process.
6. Describe appropriate treatment interventions for both the acute and chronic phases of management.
7. Analyze and interpret patient data, formulate goals and outcomes, and develop a plan of care when presented with a clinical case study.

Spinal cord injury (SCI) is a low-incidence, high-cost disability requiring tremendous changes in an individual's life-style. It is estimated that approximately 10,000 new cases of SCI occur in the United States annually. A gross estimate indicates that there are between 183,000 and 203,000 individuals with SCI currently living in the United States. This represents approximately 721 to 906 per million population.[1,2]

DEMOGRAPHICS

Statistics from the National Spinal Cord Injury Database (NSCID) provide important demographic information about traumatic spinal cord injury. The NSCID was established in 1973 and contains information on over 18,100 individuals who sus-tained traumatic SCIs. Twenty-four federally funded Model SCI Care Systems have provided data to the NSCID. Information from the NSCID provide the statistical references reported in the following sections.[2]

Etiology

Spinal cord injuries can be grossly divided into two broad etiological categories: *traumatic* injuries and *nontraumatic* damage. Traumas are by far the most frequent cause of injury in adult rehabilitation populations. They result from damage caused by a traumatic event such as a motor vehicle accident, fall, or gunshot wound. Because of their higher incidence, management of traumatic injuries will be described in this chapter; however, the treatment principles discussed will have direct application to nontraumatic lesions as well.

Statistics from the NSCID indicate that accidents involving motor vehicles are the most frequent cause of traumatic SCI (36.6%), followed by acts of violence (27.9%), falls (21.4%), recreational sports injuries (6.5%), and other trauma (7.6%).

Nontraumatic damage in adult populations generally results from disease or pathological influence. Several examples of nontraumatic conditions that may damage the spinal cord are vascular malfunctions (arteriovenous malformation [AVM], thrombosis, embolus, or hemorrhage); vertebral **subluxations** secondary to rheumatoid arthritis or degenerative joint disease; infections such as syphilis or transverse myelitis; spinal neoplasms; syringomyelia; abscesses of the spinal cord; hysterical paralysis; and neurological diseases such as multiple sclerosis and amyotrophic lateral sclerosis. Statistics are not currently available that detail the incidence of nontraumatic cord damage. However, it is estimated that nontraumatic etiologies account for 30 percent of all spinal cord injuries.

Distribution by NSCID Variables

The NSCID has collected data on multiple patient variables. The most salient statistics are presented here. Of the patients for whom data were collected 81.9 percent were men, representing slightly over a 4:1 ratio of men and women. More than half of the population (56%) was between the ages of 16 and 30 years. Ethnic distributions indicate that whites represented 56.2 percent of the database, followed by African-Americans (28.7%), Hispanics (10.5%), Asians (2.1%), Native Americans (0.4%), and unknown ethnicity (0.4%).

Data were also collected on employment status, residence, marital status, and length of hospital stay. At the time of injury, 63.4 percent of the patients were employed. Postinjury employment status is slightly higher among individuals with paraplegia as compared to those with tetraplegia (preferred term to "quadriplegia").[3] Follow-up information indicates that at 8 years postinjury, 37 percent of individuals with paraplegia were employed as compared to 30 percent of those with tetraplegia. At time of discharge, the majority of patients (88.9%) returned to a private residence (most to their homes) and 4.3 percent were discharged to nursing homes. Because the majority of individuals with SCIs are young adults, more than half (53.7%) were single at the time of injury. The average length of hospital stay in an acute care unit was 15 days and the average stay in a rehabilitation unit was 44 days.

The financial impact of SCI is extremely high. The disability is characterized by lengthy hospitalization, medical complications, extensive follow-up care, and recurrent hospitalizations. The costs of medical care during the first year postinjury were $417,067 for high tetrapelgia (C1–C4), $269,324 for low tetraplegia (C5–C8) and $152,396 for paraplegia. Average medical costs of subsequent years were $74,707 for high tetraplegia (C1–C4), $30,602 for low tetraplegia (C5–C8) and $15,507 for paraplegia.

This brief presentation of demographic information provides some important general perspectives on characteristics of SCI. It is a relatively low-incidence disability affecting a predominantly young population and is associated with lengthy and costly care.

CLASSIFICATION OF SPINAL CORD INJURIES

Neurological Classification

Spinal cord injuries typically are divided into two broad functional categories: tetraplegia and paraplegia. **Tetraplegia** refers to partial or complete paralysis of all four extremities and trunk, including the respiratory muscles, and results from lesions of the cervical cord. **Paraplegia** refers to partial or complete paralysis of all or part of the trunk and both lower extremities, resulting from lesions of the thoracic or lumbar spinal cord or sacral roots.

Designation of Lesion Level

Several methods of identifying the specific level of lesion are used throughout the world.[3,4] The most commonly used method is to indicate the most distal uninvolved nerve root segment with normal function together with the skeletal level. The term *normal function* has a precise meaning used in this context.[5] The muscles innervated by the most distal nerve root segment must have at least a fair+ or 3+ grade on manual muscle testing. This grade generally indicates sufficient strength for functional use. For example, if the patient has an intact C7 nerve root segment (with no sensory or motor function below C7), the condition would be classified as a C7 *complete tetraplegia*. However, if spotty sensation and some muscle function (with less than a fair+ muscle grade) were evident below the C7 nerve root segment, the lesion would be classified as a C7 incomplete tetraplegia.

Oblique injuries to the cord present asymmetric sensory and/or motor function. These lesions are classified in the same manner. However, they require designating the most distal nerve root segment with normal function on each side of the patient's body. For example, the designation for an oblique lesion would be recorded as C6 complete on the right and C7 complete on the left. This designation may be abbreviated to read C6(R) complete and C7(L) complete.

In considering designation of spinal cord lesions it is useful to review briefly the anatomical relationship of the spinal cord and nerve roots to the vertebral bodies (Fig. 27-1). There are 31 pairs of

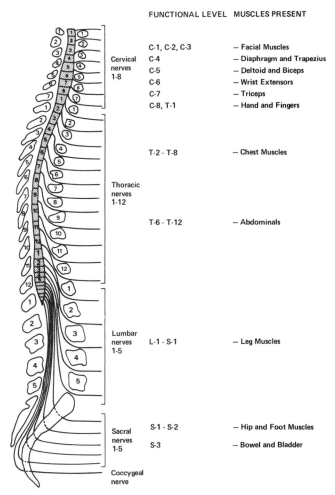

FUNCTIONAL LEVEL   MUSCLES PRESENT

Cervical nerves 1-8	C-1, C-2, C-3	— Facial Muscles
	C-4	— Diaphragm and Trapezius
	C-5	— Deltoid and Biceps
	C-6	— Wrist Extensors
	C-7	— Triceps
	C-8, T-1	— Hand and Fingers
Thoracic nerves 1-12	T-2 - T-8	— Chest Muscles
	T-6 - T-12	— Abdominals
Lumbar nerves 1-5	L-1 - S-1	— Leg Muscles
Sacral nerves 1-5	S-1 - S-2	— Hip and Foot Muscles
	S-3	— Bowel and Bladder
Coccygeal nerve		

Figure 27-1. Relationship between the spinal cord and nerve roots to vertebral bodies and innervation of major groups. (From Coogler,[5] p150, with permission.)

spinal nerves: 8 cervical, 12 thoracic, 5 lumbar, 5 sacral, and 1 coccygeal. The upper cervical nerves are relatively horizontal as they exit the intervertebral foramina. However, the remaining nerves exit in a downward direction and do not emerge at the corresponding vertebral level. During fetal development the cord fills the entire length of the vertebral canal, and the spinal nerves run in a horizontal direction. As the vertebral column elongates with growth, the spinal cord, which does not elongate, is drawn upward. The roots assume an increasingly oblique and downward direction, running in an almost vertical direction in the lumbar area, giving the appearance of a "horse's tail" (cauda equina).

COMPLETE LESIONS

In a **complete lesion** there is no sensory or motor function below the level of the lesion. It is caused by a complete transection (severing), severe compression, or extensive vascular impairment to the cord.

INCOMPLETE LESIONS

Incomplete lesions are characterized by preservation of some sensory or motor function below the

level of injury. This preservation of function indicates that some viable neural tissue is crossing the area of injury to more distal segments.[6] Incomplete lesions often result from **contusions** produced by pressure on the cord from displaced bone and/or soft tissues, or from swelling within the spinal canal. Some or even complete recovery from contusion is possible when the source of pressure is relieved. Incomplete lesions also may result from partial transection of the cord.

The clinical picture presented by incomplete lesions is unpredictable. There is a mixture of sensory and motor function below the level of lesion, with variable patterns of recovery. Early return of function is generally considered a good prognostic sign.

Despite the uncertainty associated with recovery of incomplete lesions, several syndromes have emerged with consistent clinical features. Information related to the anticipated sensory and motor functions of these syndromes is useful in establishing goals, outcomes, and plan of care. The area of cord damage of each syndrome is presented in Figure 27-2.

Brown-Sequard Syndrome

Brown-Sequard syndrome occurs from hemisection of the spinal cord (damage to one side) and is typically caused by stab wounds. Partial lesions occur more frequently; true hemisections are rare. The clinical features of this syndrome are asymmetrical. On the *ipsilateral* (same) side as the lesion, there is loss of sensation in the dermatome segment corresponding to the level of the lesion. Owing to lateral column damage, there are decreased reflexes, lack of superficial reflexes, clonus, and a positive Babinski sign. As a result of dorsal column damage, there is loss of proprioception, kinesthesia, and vibratory sense. On the side *contralateral* (opposite) to the lesion, damage to the spinothalamic tracts results in

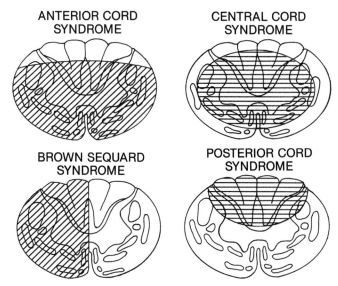

ANTERIOR CORD SYNDROME   CENTRAL CORD SYNDROME

BROWN SEQUARD SYNDROME   POSTERIOR CORD SYNDROME

Figure 27-2. Areas of spinal cord damage in incomplete cord syndromes. (From Rieser, et al,[6] p14, with permission.)

loss of sense of pain and temperature. This loss begins several dermatome segments below the level of injury. This discrepancy in levels occurs because the lateral spinothalamic tracts ascend two to four segments on the same side before crossing.[6-8]

Anterior Cord Syndrome

Anterior cord syndrome is frequently related to flexion injuries of the cervical region with resultant damage to the anterior portion of the cord and/or its vascular supply from the anterior spinal artery. There is typically compression of the anterior cord from fracture, dislocation, or cervical disk protrusion. This syndrome is characterized by loss of motor function (corticospinal tract damage) and loss of the sense of pain and temperature (spinothalamic tract damage) below the level of the lesion. Proprioception, kinesthesia, and vibratory sense are generally preserved, because they are mediated by the posterior columns with a separate vascular supply from the posterior spinal arteries.[6-9]

Central Cord Syndrome

Central cord syndrome most commonly occurs from hyperextension injuries to the cervical region. It also has been associated with congenital or degenerative narrowing of the spinal canal.[6] The resultant compressive forces give rise to hemorrhage and edema, producing damage to the most central aspects of the cord. There is characteristically more severe neurological involvement of the upper extremities (cervical tracts are more centrally located) than of the lower extremities (lumbar and sacral tracts are located more peripherally).[10,11]

Varying degrees of sensory impairment occur[12] but tend to be less severe than motor deficits. With complete preservation of sacral tracts, normal sexual, bowel, and bladder function will be retained.

Patients with central cord syndrome typically recover the ability to ambulate with some remaining distal arm weakness. Surgical intervention to relieve the source of compression has produced significant improvement in some patients.

Posterior Cord Syndrome

Posterior cord syndrome is an extremely rare syndrome resulting in deficits of function served by the posterior columns.[13] The clinical picture includes preservation of motor function, sense of pain, and light touch.[6] There is loss of proprioception and epicritic sensations (e.g., two-point discrimination, graphesthesia, stereognosis) below the level of lesion. A wide-based step gait pattern is typical. In the past, this syndrome was seen with tabes dorsalis, a condition found with late-stage syphilis.

Sacral Sparing

Sacral sparing refers to an incomplete lesion in which the most centrally located sacral tracts are spared. Varying levels of innervation from sacral segments remain intact. Clinical signs include perianal sensation, rectal sphincter contraction, cutaneous sensation in the "saddle area," and active contraction of the sacrally innervated toe flexors. These are important neurological findings and often the first signs that a cervical lesion is incomplete.[6,9]

Cauda Equina Injuries

The spinal cord tapers distally to form the conus medullaris at the lower border of the first lumbar vertebra. Although some anatomical variations exist, this is the typical termination point of the spinal cord. Below this level is the collection of long nerve roots known as the *cauda equina*. Complete transections in this area may occur. However, **cauda equina lesions** are frequently incomplete owing to the great number of nerve roots involved and the comparatively large surface area they encompass (i.e., it would be unlikely that an injury to this region would involve the entire surface area and all the nerve roots).

Cauda equina lesions are peripheral nerve **(lower motor neuron [LMN]) lesions.** injuries. As such, they have the same potential to regenerate as peripheral nerves elsewhere in the body. However, full return of innervation is not common because (1) there is a large distance between the lesion and the point of innervation, (2) axonal regeneration may not occur along the original distribution of the nerve, (3) axonal regeneration may be blocked by glial-collagen scarring, (4) the end organ may no longer be functioning once reinnervation occurs, and (5) the rate of regeneration slows and finally stops after about 1 year.

Root Escape

Peripheral nerve roots at or above the lesion site may also be damaged following SCI. As with other peripheral nerve injuries, the potential for regeneration of nerve roots exists, and some improved function may be evident. The term **root escape** refers to the preservation or return of function of nerve roots at, or near, the level of the lesion. Although it is frequently associated with incomplete cauda equina injuries, root escape may occur at any lesion level.

MECHANISMS OF INJURY

Various mechanisms, often in combination, produce injuries to the spinal cord. SCI most frequently occurs from indirect forces produced by movement of the head and trunk and less often from direct injury to a vertebra.[14] Common mechanisms operating in SCI include flexion, compression, hyperextension, and flexion-rotation. These forces result in either a fracture and/or **dislocation.** The intensity and combination of forces imposed have direct influence on the type and location of fracture(s), the amount of dislocation, and the extent of soft tissue damage.[15]

The spine demonstrates various degrees of susceptibility to injury. Some areas are inherently more vulnerable because of their high mobility and relative lack of stability as compared with other segments of the spine (e.g., the rigid thoracic region).[16] The areas of the spine that demonstrate the highest frequency of injury are between C5 and C7 in the cervical region and between T12 and L2 in the thoracolumbar region.

Table 27–1 presents a summary of the major mechanisms of injury involved in SCI.[14,15,17,18] Although these forces typically occur in combination, they are presented individually inasmuch as each has characteristic patterns of primary and associated injuries.

Two additional contributing mechanisms involved in SCI are shearing and distraction. **Shearing** occurs when a horizontal force is applied to the spine relative to the adjacent segment.[9] Shearing frequently disrupts ligaments and is associated with fracture dislocations of the thoracolumbar region.[14] **Distraction** involves a traction force and is the least common mechanism. It occurs when significant momentum of the head is created, as in whiplash injuries. This momentum creates a tensile force in the cervical spine as the head is pulled away from the body.[9,14]

CLINICAL MANIFESTATIONS

Spinal Shock

Immediately following SCI there is a period of areflexia called **spinal shock.** This period of transient reflex depression is not clearly understood. It is believed to result from the very abrupt withdrawal of connections between higher centers and the spinal cord.[6,7,19] It is characterized by absence of all reflex activity, flaccidity, and loss of sensation below the level of the lesion. It may last for several hours to several weeks, but typically subsides within 24 hours. Early resolution of spinal shock is an important prognostic sign. One of the first indicators that spinal shock is resolving is the presence of a positive **bulbocavernosus reflex (positive).** This test is part of the neurologist's examination. During a digital rectal examination, this reflex is elicited by pressure applied to the glans penis or glans clitoris or by intermittently "tugging" on an indwelling catheter. If positive, a reflex contraction of the anal sphincter around the examining digit will be evident.[20] A positive bulbocavernosus reflex indicates that spinal shock has terminated. This reflex may be present several weeks before deep tendon reflexes are apparent in the lower extremities. However, if this reflex is positive without some evidence of accompanying sensory or motor return (particularly in the perianal region), spinal shock has subsided, and it usually indicates the presence of a complete lesion.

Motor and Sensory Impairments

Following spinal cord injury there will be either complete or partial loss of muscle function below the level of the lesion. Disruption of the ascending sensory fibers following SCI results in impaired or absent sensation below the level of the lesion.

The clinical presentation of motor and sensory impairments depends on the specific features of the lesion. These include the neurological level, the completeness of the lesion, the symmetry of the lesion (transverse or oblique), and the presence or absence of sacral sparing or root escape.

Impaired Temperature Control

After damage to the spinal cord the hypothalamus can no longer control cutaneous blood flow or level

Table 27–1 MECHANISMS OF INJURY[14,15,17,18]

Force	Etiology	Associated Fractures	Potential Associated Injuries
Flexion	1. Head-on collision in which head strikes steering wheel or windshield. 2. Blow to back of head or trunk. 3. Most common mechanism of SCI.	1. Wedge fracture of anterior vertebral body (vertebral body compressed). 2. High percentage of injuries occur from C4 to C7 and from T12 to L2.	1. Tearing of posterior ligaments. 2. Fractures of posterior elements: spinous processes, laminae, or pedicles. 3. Disruption of disk. 4. Anterior dislocation of vertebral body.
Compression	1. Vertical or axial blow to head (diving, surfing, or falling objects). 2. Closely associated with flexion injuries.	1. Concave fracture of endplate. 2. Explosion or burst fracture (comminuted). 3. Teardrop fracture.	1. Bone fragments may lodge in cord. 2. Rupture of disk.
Hyperextension	1. Strong posterior force such as a rear-end collision. 2. Falls with chin hitting a stationary object (more commonly seen in elderly populations).	1. Fractures of posterior elements: spinous processes, laminae, and facets. 2. Avulsion fracture of anterior aspect of vertebrae.	1. Rupture of anterior longitudinal ligament. 2. Rupture of disk. 3. Associated with cervical lesions; only of minor influence in thoracolumbar injuries.
Flexion-rotation	Posterior to anterior force directed at rotated vertebral column (e.g., rear-end collision with passenger rotated toward driver).	Fracture of posterior pedicles, articular facets, and laminae (fracture is very unstable if posterior ligaments rupture).	1. Rupture of posterior and interspinous ligaments. 2. Subluxation or dislocation of facet joints. 3. In thoracic and lumbar regions, facets may "lock."

of sweating. This autonomic (sympathetic) dysfunction results in loss of internal thermoregulatory responses. The ability to shiver is lost; vasodilation does not occur in response to heat nor does vasoconstriction occur in response to cold. There is absence of thermoregulatory sweating, which eliminates the normal evaporative cooling effects of perspiration in warm environments. This lack of sweating is often associated with excessive compensatory **diaphoresis** above the level of lesion. Patients with incomplete lesions may also demonstrate "spotty" areas of localized sweating below the lesion level.[21]

Changes in thermal regulation result in body temperature being significantly influenced by the external environment. This is a more frequent problem with cervical lesions than with thoracic or lumbar involvement. Patients must rely heavily on sensory input from the head and neck regions to assist in determining appropriate environmental temperatures. Although some improvement in thermoregulatory responses occurs over time, patients with tetraplegia typically experience long-term impairment of body temperature regulation, especially in response to extreme environmental changes.[9]

Respiratory Impairment

Respiratory function varies considerably, depending on the level of lesion. With high spinal cord lesions between C1 and C3, phrenic nerve innervation and spontaneous respiration are significantly impaired or lost. An artificial ventilator or phrenic nerve stimulator is required to sustain life. In contrast, lumbar lesions present with full innervation of both primary (diaphragm) and secondary (neck, intercostal, and abdominal) respiratory muscles.

All patients with tetraplegia and those with high-level paraplegia demonstrate some compromise in respiratory function. The level of respiratory impairment is directly related to the lesion level, residual respiratory muscle function, and additional trauma sustained at time of injury, as well as premorbid respiratory status. Respiratory involvement represents a particularly serious and life-threatening feature of SCI. Pulmonary complications (especially bronchopneumonia and pulmonary embolism) are responsible for a high mortality during the early stages of tetraplegia.[22,23]

There is a progressively greater loss of respiratory function with increasingly higher lesion levels. Multiple respiratory changes occur that are related to both the inspiratory and expiratory phases of ventilation. The primary muscles of inspiration are the diaphragm and external intercostals. As the diaphragm contracts and descends, the intercostals normally elevate the ribs and increase the lateral anterior-posterior diameter of the thorax.[24] Paralysis of the intercostals results in decreased chest expansion and a lowered inspiratory volume. With progressively higher level lesions, increased involvement of the accessory muscles of respiration will be noted. These muscles assist with elevation of the ribs and include the sternocleidomastoid, trapezii, scaleni, pectoralis minor, and serratus anterior.

The primary muscles of expiration are the abdominals and internal intercostals. Normally, relaxed expiration is essentially a passive process that occurs through elastic recoil of the lungs and thorax. However, the abdominals and internal intercostals contribute several important functions related to movement of air out of the lungs. Loss of these muscles significantly decreases expiratory efficiency. When fully innervated, the abdominal muscles play an important role in maintaining intrathoracic pressure for effective respiration. They support the abdominal viscera [25,26] and assist in maintaining the position of the diaphragm. They also function to push the diaphragm upward during forced expiration. With paralysis of the abdominals this support is lost, causing the diaphragm to assume an unusually low position in the chest.[27] This lowered position and lack of abdominal pressure to move the diaphragm upward during forced expiration results in a decreased expiratory reserve volume. This subsequently decreases cough effectiveness and the ability to expel secretions.

Paralysis of the external obliques also influences expiration. Their normal function is to depress the ribs and compress the chest wall to assist with forceful expulsion of air.[25,26] With higher-level lesions this function becomes less efficient, with a further reduction in the patient's ability to cough and to expel secretions. These factors combine to make the patient with SCI particularly susceptible to retention of secretions, atelectasis, and pulmonary infections.[22]

Paralysis also results in the development of an altered breathing pattern.[24,28,29] This pattern (Fig. 27-3) is characterized by some flattening of the upper chest wall, decreased chest wall expansion, and a dominant epigastric rise during inspiration. With relaxation of the diaphragm, a negative intrathoracic pressure gradient moves air into the lungs.[24,28] Over time, this breathing pattern will lead to permanent postural changes.

Two additional factors may further impair the respiratory status of the patient: additional trauma sustained at the time of injury, and premorbid respiratory problems. Fractures (e.g., ribs, sternum, or extremities), lung contusions, or soft tissue damage will also compound respiratory problems. These secondary injuries are particularly problematic if long periods of immobility are required for healing or if pain inhibits full lung expansion. Premorbid respiratory problems, such as existing pulmonary disease, allergies, asthma, or a history of smoking, will further compromise respiratory function.

Spasticity

Spasticity results from release of intact reflex arcs from central nervous system control and is charac-

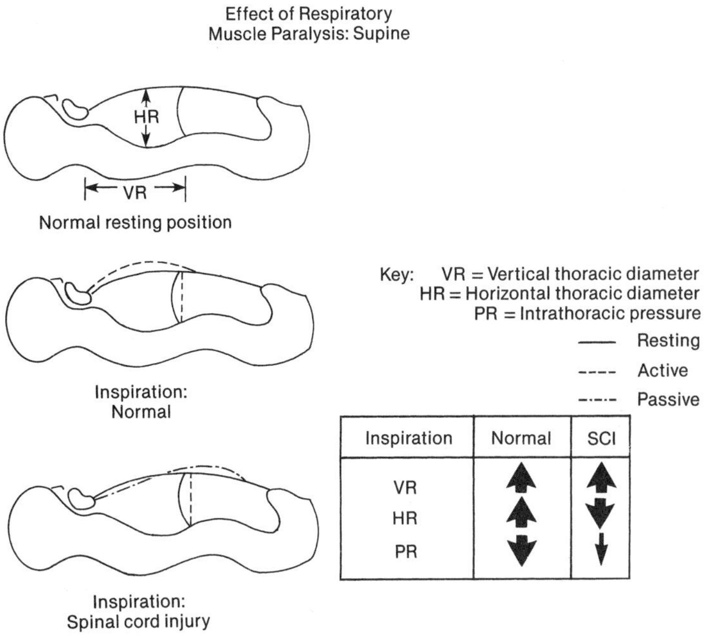

Effect of Respiratory
Muscle Paralysis: Supine

Normal resting position

Inspiration:
Normal

Inspiration:
Spinal cord injury

Key: VR = Vertical thoracic diameter
HR = Horizontal thoracic diameter
PR = Intrathoracic pressure
——— Resting
- - - - Active
-·-·- Passive

Inspiration	Normal	SCI
VR	↑	↑
HR	↑	↓
PR	↓	↓

Figure 27-3. Effect of paralysis on thoracic volume and breathing pattern. (From Alvarez, et al,[24] p 1738, with permission.)

terized by hypertonicity, hyperactive stretch reflexes, and clonus. It typically occurs below the level of lesion after spinal shock subsides. There is a gradual increase in spasticity during the first 6 months and a plateau is usually reached 1 year after injury. Spasticity is increased by multiple internal and external stimuli, including positional changes, cutaneous stimuli, environmental temperatures, tight clothing, bladder or kidney stones, fecal impactions, catheter blockage, urinary tract infections, decubitus ulcers, and emotional stress.[9,30]

Spasticity varies in the degree of severity. Patients with minimal to moderate involvement may learn to trigger the spasticity at appropriate times to assist in functional activities. However, strong spasticity interferes with many aspects of rehabilitation and can be a deterrent to independent function. In these situations spasticity is often managed first through drug therapy. Drugs typically used include muscle relaxants and spasmolytic agents such as diazepam (Valium),[13] baclofen (Lioresal),[31] and dantrolene sodium (Dantrium).[32] Pharmacological management is usually not completely successful in alleviating spasticity, and its benefits must be weighed against potentially adverse side effects (see Chapter 24). Additionally, patients often develop a tolerance to prolonged use of individual drugs.

Injected chemical agents also have been used to decrease spasticity. Generally, these are considered only if results obtained from pharmacological management are deemed inadequate. The two approaches used are **peripheral nerve blocks** and **intrathecal injections.** In nerve blocks, the chemical injection is used peripherally to selectively block transmission of the motor nerve to a spastic muscle and therefore to interrupt the intact reflex arc peripherally. These procedures provides a temporary reduction in spasticity and include (1) phenol

peripheral nerve blocks, and (2) phenol motor point blocks.[32]

Intrathecal (within the spinal canal) injections are used to interrupt the reflex arc mechanism and subsequently to reduce spasticity. Intrathecal approaches provide a more permanent abatement of spasticity. These procedures include intrathecal phenol or alcohol injections. Intrathecal injections are used only rarely because they interfere with bladder and sexual function.[32,33]

Surgical approaches also have been used to combat spasticity in more severe cases. They range from relatively simple orthopedic procedures to complex neurosurgery. Orthopedic surgical procedures used include **myotomy,** a sectioning or release of a muscle; **neurectomy,** a partial or complete severance of a nerve; or **tenotomy,** a sectioning of a tendon that allows subsequent lengthening (e.g., heel cords). Each of these procedures decreases spasticity by altering the contraction potential of the muscle.[32,33]

A number of more radical neurosurgical interventions are used to eliminate extremely severe spasticity. These destructive approaches (neural tissue is damaged) result in permanent and profound alterations in spasticity. These procedures are useful when spasticity is at an intolerable level and prohibits or significantly limits functional activities. Examples of these interventions include severance of nerve roots **(rhizotomy)** or of spinal cord nerve fibers **(myelotomy).**

Bladder and Bowel Dysfunction

BLADDER DYSFUNCTION

The effects of bladder dysfunction following SCI pose a serious medical complication requiring consistent and long-term management. Urinary tract infections (UTIs) are among the most frequent medical complication during the initial medical-rehabilitation period. During the stage of spinal shock, the urinary bladder is flaccid. All muscle tone and bladder reflexes are absent.[34] Medical considerations during this period are focused on establishing an effective system of drainage and prevention of urinary retention and infection.

The spinal integration center for **micturition** is the conus medullaris. Primary reflex control originates from the sacral segments of S2, S3, and S4. Following spinal shock, one of two types of bladder conditions will develop, depending on location of the lesion. Patients with lesions that occur within the spinal cord above the conus medullaris typically develop a *spastic* or reflex (automatic) bladder. Following a lesion of the conus medullaris or cauda equina, a *flaccid* or nonreflex (autonomous) bladder develops.[35]

A spastic or reflex (upper motor neuron [UMN]) bladder contracts and reflexively empties in response to a certain level of filling pressure. The reflex arc is intact. This reflex emptying may be triggered by manual stimulation techniques such as stroking, kneading, or tapping the suprapubic region[33] or thigh, and lower abdominal stroking, pinching, or hair pulling.[36]

A flaccid or nonreflex (lower motor neuron [LMN]) bladder is essentially flaccid because there is no reflex action of the detrusor muscle. This type of bladder can be emptied by increasing intra-abdominal pressure using a Valsalva maneuver or by manually compressing the lower abdomen using the **Crede maneuver.** Characteristics of spastic and flaccid urinary dysfunction are presented in Table 27–2.

Bladder Training Programs

The primary goal of bladder training programs is to allow the patient to be free of a catheter and to control bladder function. Because urinary incontinence has very strong psychosocial implications for the patient, a coordinated approach to this problem is particularly important. Knowledge of and participation in the bladder training program is an important consideration for the physical therapist.

The bladder training program most frequently used with a reflex bladder is *intermittent catheterization.* The purpose of this program is to establish reflex bladder emptying at regular and predictable intervals in response to a certain level of filling. Briefly, the program involves establishing a fluid intake pattern restricted to approximately 2000 mL/d. Fluid intake is monitored at 150 to 180 mL/h from morning until early evening. Intake is stopped late in the day to reduce the need for catheterization during the night. Initially, the patient is catheterized every 4 hours. Prior to catheterization, the patient attempts to void in combination with one or more of the manual stimulation techniques. The catheter is then inserted and residual volume drained. A record is maintained of voided and residual urine. As bladder emptying becomes more effective, residual volumes will decrease and time intervals between catheterizations can be expanded.[37]

A *timed voiding program* is another method of bladder training and is indicated for the autonomous or nonreflex bladder. This program involves

Table 27–2 CHARACTERISTICS OF SPASTIC AND FLACCID URINARY DYSFUNCTION

	Spastic (Automatic) Urinary Dysfunction (Upper Motor Neuron)	Flaccid (Autonomous) Urinary Dysfunction (Lower Motor Neuron)
Level of cord injury	Occurs above micturition reflex center (S2–S4) located within the conus medullaris.	Involves micturition reflex center (S2–S4) in the conus medullaris and/or sacral nerve roots in the cauda equina.
Level of innervation: 1. Local	Stretch receptors in bladder wall and afferent neuron intact.	Same as for UMN.
2. Spinal micturition reflex (S2–S4)	Micturition reflex intact. Parasympathetic innervation to detrusor muscle and bladder neck sphincter (internal) intact.	Micturition reflex center in conus medullaris and/or sacral nerve roots destroyed.
3. Sympathetic innervation cord segments T1 to T2	Reflexes may be intact depending on level of cord injury.	Same as for UMN.
4. Brain/higher centers • Motor	• Nerve pathways between brain and spinal micturition reflex center (S2–S4) interrupted; loss of inhibiting influences on spinal reflexes from higher centers.	• Loss of final common pathway for transmission of impulses between CNS and detrusor muscle and bladder sphincters (internal and external).
• Sensory	• Ascending sensory pathways interrupted; loss of sensation of bladder distention and urge to urinate.	• Same as for UMN.
Results of pathology	1. Loss of UMN innervation. 2. Intact micturition reflexes. 3. Spastic bladder dysfunction.	1. Loss of LMN innervation. 2. Loss of micturition reflexes. 3. Flaccid bladder dysfunction.
Prognosis for bladder control[a]	Bladder training is aimed at using micturition reflexes and "trigger" stimulus to establish planned reflex voiding.	Unable to establish reflex voiding; intermittent bladder catheterization may be best method for bladder management.

From Dolan,[35] p 629, with permission.
[a]Bladder training depends on many factors, such as level of injury, prior bladder habits, patient/family motivation, and teamwork.
CNS, central nervous system; LMN, lower motor neuron; UMN, upper motor neuron.

Table 27–3 CHARACTERISTICS OF SPASTIC AND FLACCID BOWEL DYSFUNCTION

	Spastic Bowel Dysfunction (Upper Motor Neuron)	Flaccid Bowel Dysfunction (Lower Motor Neuron)
Level of cord injury	Occurs above defecation reflex center (S2–S4) located within the conus medullaris.	Involves defecation reflex center (S2–S4) in the conus medullaris and/or sacral nerve roots in the equina.
Level of vertebral injury	Involves T11 to T12 vertebra or above.	Involves T12 vertebra or below.
Levels of innervation:		
1. Local	Intrinsic (myenteric plexus) intact; responsible for weak peristaltic activity, which is not of sufficient strength by itself to produce a large bowel movement.	Same as for UMN.
2. Spinal defecation reflex center S2 to S4	Defecation reflex intact; parasympathetic tone to descending and sigmoid colon, rectum, and internal anal sphincter intact.	Defecation reflex center in the conus medullaris and/or sacral nerve roots destroyed.
3. Brain/higher centers • Motor	• Nerve pathways between brain and spinal defecation reflex center (S2–S4) interrupted: loss of inhibitory influences on spinal reflexes from higher centers.	• Loss of final common pathway for transmission of impulses between CNS and descending and sigmoid colon, rectum, and anal sphincters.
• Sensory	• Ascending sensory pathways interrupted: loss of sensation of fullness in bowel and urge to defecate.	• Same as for UMN.
Results of pathology	1. Loss of UMN innervation. 2. Intact spinal defecation reflexes. 3. Spastic bowel dysfunction with spastic contraction of bowel and anal sphincters.	1. Loss of LMN innervation. 2. Loss of spinal defecation reflexes. 3. Flaccid bowel dysfunction.
Prognosis for bowel control[a]	With intact defecation reflexes, bowel training is aimed at using these reflexes to evacuate the bowel. Bowel and anal sphincters respond to rectal/anal stimulation, enabling a planned bowel regimen, which empties the rectum and prevents incontinence. Prognosis is excellent for good bowel control.	With loss of spinal defecation reflex activity and LMN innervation, the bowel and anal sphincters are flaccid. They do not respond to planned rectal or anal stimulation. Arrival of feces in the rectum results in incontinence. Bowel training is deployed to evacuate stool from rectum. Presence of stool in rectum precipitates incontinence. Prognosis is favorable for bowel control providing a routine of regular bowel evacuation removes the stimulus for bowel emptying.
Bowel incontinence	Rarely occurs with good bowel management. Incontinence is due to spastic contraction. Diet is a significant factor in effective bowel management.	Occasionally occurs even with good bowel management, due to flaccid sphincters. As with spastic bowel dysfunction, diet is a significant factor in effective bowel management.
Bowel training program	Regularly scheduled evacuation, usually every other day.	Evacuation necessary on a daily basis to keep rectum clear of feces and prevent incontinence.
Use of medications including suppositories and laxatives	Responsive to a combination of laxatives (milk of magnesia), stool softener (dioctyl sodium sulfosuccinate [docusate, Colace]), and suppositories (Dulcolax).	Response to medications less effective than with spastic bowel dysfunction.
Digital stimulation	Used to initiate a planned reflex bowel evacuation.	Nonresponsive to digital stimulation, manual removal of stool from rectum may be required.

From Dolan,[35] p 627, with permission.

[a]Successful bowel training depends on many factors, such as level of injury, prior bowel habits, patient/family motivation, teamwork.

CNS, central nervous system; LMN, lower motor neuron; UMN, upper motor neuron.

first establishing the patient's pattern of incontinence. The residual urine volume is then checked to ensure that it is within safe limits. Once the pattern of incontinence has been established, it is compared with the patterns of intake. This information provides the basis for establishing a new intake and voiding schedule. The bladder gradually becomes accustomed or "trained" to empty at regular, predictable intervals. As incontinence decreases, the schedule is readjusted to expand the intervals between voiding. Fluid intake is avoided late in the day to decrease the risk of **nocturia.** Stimulation techniques are also incorporated into this type of training program.

It should be noted that not all bladder training programs are successful. Some patients will require long-term use of either an external (condom) or indwelling catheter. For male patients, the condom catheter is preferred because it provides decreased risk of infection. For female patients, an indwelling catheter is currently the only option.

BOWEL DYSFUNCTION

As with the bladder, the neurogenic bowel conditions that develop after spinal shock subsides are of two types. In cord lesions above the conus medullaris there is a spastic or reflex bowel, and in conus medullaris or cauda equina lesions a flaccid or nonreflex bowel develops.[36] Table 27–3 presents the characteristics of each type of bowel dysfunction together with treatment implications.

Bowel Programs

Typically, reflex bowel management requires use of suppositories and digital stimulation techniques to initiate defecation. Digital stimulation involves manual stretch of the anal sphincter, either with a gloved finger or an orthotic digital stimulator. This stretch stimulates peristalsis of the colon and evacuation of the rectum (mediated by S2, S3, and S4).[32] Nonreflex bowel management relies heavily on straining with available musculature and manual evacuation techniques.

The major goal of a bowel program for the patient with a SCI is establishment of a regular pattern of evacuation. This is achieved through multiple interventions, including diet, fluid intake, stool softeners, suppositories, digital stimulation, and manual evacuation.

As with bladder programs, bowel management is an emotionally laden issue and an extremely high priority for most patients. Lack of bowel control may negate other rehabilitation efforts because it will seriously limit the patient's involvement.

Sexual Dysfunction

"Sexual information is as vital and as 'normal' a part of the rehabilitation process as is providing other information to enable the patient to better understand and adapt to his medical condition."[38] For many years physical disability was assumed to depress or to eliminate sex drives. This erroneous attitude fostered considerable neglect of sexual function as a component of the rehabilitation process.[39] Today, sexual disturbances are recognized as a complex rehabilitation issue. Characterized by physiological dysfunction, and sensory and motor impairment, these disturbances are often accompanied by social and psychological distress.[40,41] Greater numbers of SCI care centers now include a sexual counselor as a component team member. This individual may be a physician or a psychologist with a specialty in this area or a nonphysician specialist trained in the treatment of sexual dysfunction.[40] Many rehabilitation centers also offer structured programs to assist patients with sexual adjustment.[38,42] Although the format of these programs varies, common shared goals include (1) direct patient care including assessment, prognosis, treatment, and counseling; (2) education of the patient and his or her partner; and (3) preparation of staff members to deal with sexual concerns.

THE MALE RESPONSE

A gradually expanding body of literature is available on the male sexual response following SCI.[43-51] Sexual response is directly related to level and completeness of injury. As with bowel and bladder function, sexual capabilities are broadly divided between **upper motor neuron lesions [UMN]** (damage to the cord above the conus medullaris) and LMN lesions (damage to the conus medullaris or cauda equina).

Statistics related to sexual capacity provide important general information regarding anticipated function following a given type of injury. However, these statistics must be considered cautiously. Owing to the inherent methodological difficulties in collecting these types of data and the close relationship between sexual activity and self-image, some discrepancy may exist between reported and actual sexual function.[52]

Erectile Capacity

In a review of the literature on sexual response after SCI, Higgins[52] presented two consistent findings: (1) erectile capacity is greater in UMN lesions than in LMN lesions, and (2) erectile capacity is greater in incomplete lesions than in complete lesions.

There are two types of erections: reflexogenic and psychogenic. Reflexogenic erections occur in response to external physical stimulation of the genitals or perineum. An intact reflex arc is required (mediated through S2, S3, and S4). Psychogenic erections occur through cognitive activity such as erotic fantasy. They are mediated from the cerebral cortex either through the thoracolumbar or sacral cord centers.[53]

An early study by Comarr[54] examined erectile capability in 525 patients with UMN lesions. His findings indicated that 93 percent of the patients with complete lesions and 98 percent of those with incomplete lesions had reflexogenic erections. Data were also collected on 154 patients with LMN lesions. In the group with complete LMN lesions, 74 percent had no erections and 26 percent had erections only by psychogenic stimuli. With incomplete LMN lesions, 83 percent had erections, but all by psychogenic means. More recently, drug intervention has been used to improve erectile function. This option may be a consideration for some patients.

Ejaculation

There is a higher incidence of ejaculation with (1) LMN lesions than with UMN lesions, (2) lower-level versus higher-level cord lesions, and (3) incomplete as compared with complete lesions.[52,54] Historically, relatively few patients with SCI were able to sire children. This low level of fertility was associated with impaired spermatogenesis and an inability to ejaculate.[53] However, recent evidence suggests improved ejaculatory response and higher semen quality by use of vibratory stimulation.[43-45] The semen samples produced are used for intrauterine inseminations.

Orgasm

Orgasm and ejaculation are two separate events. Orgasm is a cognitive, psychogenic event, whereas ejaculation is a physical occurrence. Relatively little information is available related to the effects of SCI on orgasm. This again relates to inherent difficulties in collecting such data. Higgins[52] also suggests that the few studies that have been done have demonstrated serious methodological flaws. He identifies the major problems in these studies as a lack of criteria for defining orgasm, considering ejaculation and orgasm as identical events, and a lack of reported data on how subjects achieved orgasm. Currently, accurate data on the effects of SCI on male orgasm are not available.

THE FEMALE RESPONSE

Relatively little literature exists addressing the impact of SCI on sexual function in women. This may be a function of women remaining capable of sexual intercourse following SCI. It also may be related to the fact that fertility is unaffected, or, perhaps, because of the proportionately lower number of female patients.[55] Trieschmann[39] also believes that this relates to the traditionally passive sexual roles ascribed to women. Historically, sexual functions of women following SCI have been considered relatively unimpaired and given comparatively little attention. However, more recent additions to the literature indicates a growing interest in female sexual response following SCI.[56–61]

Female sexual responses also follow a pattern related to location of lesion. In patients with UMN lesions, the reflex arc will remain intact. Therefore, components of sexual arousal (vaginal lubrication, engorgement of the labia, and clitoral erection) will occur through reflexogenic stimulation, but psychogenic response will be lost. Conversely, with LMN lesions, psychogenic responses will be preserved and reflex responses lost.

Menstruation

The menstrual cycle typically is interrupted for a period of 1 to 3 months following injury. After this time normal menses return.

Fertility and Pregnancy

The potential for conception remains unimpaired. Pregnancy is possible under close medical supervision inasmuch as the patient is placed at high risk for impaired respiratory function. In addition, owing to impaired sensation the initiation of labor may not be perceived. Labor also may precipitate the onset of autonomic dysreflexia (see the following section on indirect impairments and complications). Consequently, patients are frequently hospitalized for a period of time prior to the expected delivery date to monitor cervical dilation.[55] Although uterine contractions are hormonally controlled and not affected by paralysis, patients with an inability to bear down during the final stages of delivery[55] or who experience prolonged or difficult labor may be candidates for cesarean section.[20]

A major consideration for the physical therapist regarding sexual dysfunction is that a patient will often direct questions to the individuals with whom he or she feels most comfortable. It is not uncommon for such a discussion to arise during a physical therapy session. These questions or issues should be addressed openly and honestly. In addition, the therapist must anticipate and be prepared for these situations by (1) obtaining accurate information about the patient's physiological state and anticipated sexual function, and (2) having knowledge of referral options and support services available to the patient for appropriate assessment and counseling.

Indirect Impairments and Complications

PRESSURE SORES

Pressure sores are ulcerations of soft tissue (skin or subcutaneous tissue) caused by unrelieved pressure and shearing forces. They are subject to infection, which can migrate to bone. Pressure sores are a serious medical complication, a major cause of delayed rehabilitation, and may even lead to death. Pressures sores are among the more frequent medical complications following SCI[63] and are an important factor in increasing duration and subsequently cost of hospital stay.

Impaired sensory function and the inability to make appropriate positional changes are the two most influential factors in the development of pressure sores. Other important factors are (1) loss of vasomotor control, which results in a lowering of tissue resistance to pressure; (2) spasticity, with resultant shearing forces between surfaces; (3) skin **maceration** from exposure to moisture (e.g., urine); (4) trauma, such as adhesive tape or sheet burns; (5) nutritional deficiencies (low serum protein and anemia will reduce tissue resistance to pressure); (6) poor general skin condition; and (7) secondary infections.[37,64] Another primary factor in the development of pressure sores is the intensity and duration of the pressure. The higher the intensity of pressure, the shorter the time required for anoxia of the skin and soft tissues to occur.

Pressure sores will develop over any bony prominence subjected to excessive pressure.[65,66] Among the more common sites of involvement are the sacrum, heels, trochanters, and ischium. Other areas susceptible to skin breakdown are the scapula, elbows, anterior iliac spines, knees, and malleoli.

By far the most important intervention for eliminating the potential development of pressure sores is prevention. This involves a coordinated approach, and it is a responsibility shared by each member of the rehabilitation team. Initially, the patient will be turned every 2 hours by the nursing staff on a 24-hour schedule. Skin condition should be monitored on a continual basis. If a reddened area occurs, the patient's position must be altered immediately to alleviate the pressure. As the rehabilitation program progresses, the patient gradually assumes responsibility for skin care. Preparation for assumption of this responsibility will include patient education about the potential risks of pressure sores, and instruction in skin inspection techniques and the use of pressure relief equipment and procedures.

AUTONOMIC DYSREFLEXIA

Autonomic dysreflexia (hyperreflexia) is a pathological autonomic reflex that typically occurs in lesions above T6 (above sympathetic splanchnic outflow). However, it has been reported in patients with injuries at T7 and T8.[67,68] Incidence of this problem varies. One study[69] found a 48 percent occurrence in a group of 213 patients. Rosen[70] estimates that as many as 85 percent of those with tetraplegia and high-level paraplegia experience this problem during the course of rehabilitation. Episodes of autonomic dysreflexia gradually subside over time and are relatively uncommon, but not rare, 3 years following injury.[70] It is seen in patients with both complete and incomplete lesions.[71]

This clinical syndrome produces an acute onset of autonomic activity from noxious stimuli below the level of the lesion. Afferent input from these stimuli reach the lower spinal cord (lower thoracic and sacral areas) and initiate a mass reflex response resulting in elevation of blood pressure. Normally, the impulses stimulate the receptors in the carotid sinus and aorta, which signal the vasomotor center to readjust peripheral resistance. Following SCI, however, impulses from the vasomotor center cannot pass the site of the lesion to counteract the hypertension by vasodilation.[70,72,73] This is a critical, emergency situation. Owing to the lack of inhibition from higher centers, hypertension will persist if not treated promptly. Death may result.

Initiating Stimuli

The most common cause of this pathological reflex is bladder distention (urinary retention). Other precipitating stimuli include rectal distention, pressure sores, urinary stones, bladder infections, noxious cutaneous stimuli, kidney malfunction, urethral or bladder irritation, and environmental temperature changes.[69] Episodes of autonomic dysreflexia also have been reported following passive stretching at the hip.[74]

Symptoms

The symptoms of autonomic dysreflexia include hypertension, bradycardia, headache (often severe and pounding), profuse sweating, increased spasticity, restlessness, vasoconstriction below the level of lesion, vasodilation (flushing) above the level of the lesion, constricted pupils, nasal congestion, piloerection (goose bumps), and blurred vision.[69,75]

Intervention

The onset of symptoms should be treated as a medical emergency. If lying flat, the patient should be brought to a sitting position, inasmuch as blood pressure will be lowered in this position. Because bladder distention is a primary cause of autonomic dysreflexia, the drainage system should be assessed immediately. If the patient is wearing a clamped catheter, it should be released. The drainage tubes also should be checked for internal or external blockage or twisting. The patient's body should be checked for irritating stimuli such as tight clothing, restricting catheter straps, or abdominal binders. If symptoms do not subside, or if the source of irritation cannot be located, medical and/or nursing assistance should be sought immediately. Additional measures may include bladder irrigation (a higher-level block may exist), removal and replacement with a new catheter, and assessment for bowel impaction. Drug therapy (antihypertensives) may be indicated to control these episodes if more conservative approaches are unsuccessful.

The attending physician, nursing staff, and other team members should always be notified of occurrences of autonomic dysreflexia. This will allow careful monitoring of the patient for several days following the episode and will alert others to the risk of future occurrences. The individual patient's symptoms, precipitating stimuli, and methods of relief should be documented.

POSTURAL HYPOTENSION

Postural hypotension (orthostatic hypotension) is a decrease in blood pressure that occurs when assuming an erect or vertical position (e.g., lying-to-sitting or sitting-to-standing. It is caused by a loss of sympathetic vasoconstriction control. The problem is enhanced by lack of muscle tone, causing peripheral venous and splanchnic bed pooling. Reduced blood cerebral flow and decreased venous return to the heart typically occurs, producing symptoms of lightheadedness, dizziness, or fainting.[32]

Inasmuch as many patients may be immobilized for several weeks, episodes of postural hypotension are a fairly common occurrence during early progression to a vertical position. They tend to occur more frequently with lesions of the cervical and upper thoracic regions. Patients will often describe the onset as feelings of "dizziness," "faintness," or impending "blackout." Although the exact mechanism is not clearly understood, the cardiovascular system, over time, gradually reestablishes sufficient vasomotor tone to allow assumption of the vertical position.[76]

A related problem is edema of the legs, ankles, and feet, which is usually symmetric and pitting in nature. It occurs secondary to the above problems and is complicated by decreased lymphatic return.[32]

To minimize these effects, the cardiovascular system should be allowed to adapt gradually by a slow progression to the vertical position. This frequently begins with elevation of the head of the bed and progresses to a reclining wheelchair with elevating leg rests and use of a tilt table. Vital signs should be monitored carefully, and the patient should always be moved very slowly. Use of compressive stockings and an abdominal binder will further minimize these effects. Pharmacological therapy may be indicated (e.g., ephedrine to increase blood pressure or low-dose diuretics to relieve persistent edema of legs, ankles, or feet).[32] As vasomotor stability returns, tolerance to the vertical position will gradually improve.

HETEROTOPIC (ECTOPIC) OSSIFICATION

Heterotopic ossification is osteogenesis in soft tissues below the level of the lesion.[77-79] The etiology of this abnormal bone growth is unknown. However, multiple theories have been proposed, including tissue hypoxia secondary to circulatory stasis,[80] abnormal calcium metabolism, local pressure, and microtrauma related to overly aggressive range of motion (ROM) exercises.[81]

Heterotopic ossification is always extra-articular and extracapsular.[82] It may develop in tendons, connective tissue between muscle, aponeurotic tissue, or the peripheral aspects of muscle.[77,81,82] It must be differentiated from myositis ossificans, which results from injury to a muscle and is characterized by bony deposits within muscle tissue. No relationships have been found between the development of heterotopic bone formation and level of injury, amount of exercise, or degree of spasticity or flaccidity.[80,83]

Heterotopic ossification typically occurs adjacent to large joints, with the hips and knees most commonly involved.[78] Other joints that have demonstrated involvement include the elbows,[77] shoulders, and spine.[78] Early symptoms of heterotopic ossification resemble those of thrombophlebitis, including swelling, decreased ROM, erythema, and local warmth near a joint.[84] Early onset is also characterized by elevated serum alkaline phosphatase levels and negative radiographic findings.[85] During later clinical stages, soft tissue swelling subsides and radiographic findings are positive.[85]

For many patients the development of heterotopic ossification will pose no significant functional limitations. However, a serious complication affecting 20 percent of patients is joint ankylosis, with the hip most commonly affected.[77]

Management of ectopic bone formation utilizes several approaches, including pharmacological therapy, physical therapy, and, with severe functional limitations, surgery. Pharmacological therapy (diphosphates) has been used to inhibit the formation of calcium phosphate and to prevent ectopic bone formation.[77] These agents, however, have no effect on mature ectopic bone. Physical therapy is important in maintaining ROM and preventing deformity. Early research discouraged the use of ROM, indicating that the exercise increased ectopic bone formation.[82] However, later studies have shown no increase in the formation of bone deposition with ROM exercises.[78,80,83] A logical approach to maintaining functional ROM appears to be a combination of pharmacological therapy with regular exercises during the early formation stages of ectopic development. Finally, surgery is used when extreme limitations in function impede rehabilitation. This generally involves resection of the ectopic bone.[77]

CONTRACTURES

Contractures develop secondary to prolonged shortening of structures across and around a joint, resulting in limitation in motion. Contractures initially produce alterations in muscle tissue but rapidly progress to involve capsular and pericapsular changes. Once the tissue changes have occurred, the process is irreversible. A combination of factors places the patient with SCI at particularly high risk for developing joint contractures. Lack of active muscle function eliminates the normal reciprocal stretching of a muscle group and surrounding structures as the opposing muscle contracts.[77] Spasticity often results in prolonged unopposed muscle shortening in a static position. Flaccidity may result in gravitational forces maintaining a relatively consistent joint position. In addition, faulty positioning, heterotopic ossification, edema, and imbalances in muscle pull (either active or spastic) contribute to the specific direction and location of contracture development.

Contractures are strongly influenced by the existing pattern of spasticity and the positioning methods used. The hip joint is particularly prone to flexion deformities and typically includes components of internal rotation and adduction. The shoulder may develop tightness in flexion or extension (depending on early positioning). Both patterns at the shoulder are associated with internal rotation and adduction. All joints of the body are at risk for contractures, including the elbows, wrist and fingers, knees, ankles, and toes.

The most important management consideration related to the potential development of contractures is prevention. A consistent and concurrent program of ROM exercises, positioning, and, if appropriate, splinting effectively maintains joint motion.

DEEP VENOUS THROMBOSIS

Deep venous thrombosis (DVT) results from development of a thrombus (abnormal blood clot) within a vessel. The occurrence of such a clot is a dangerous medical complication. It has the potential to break free of its attachment and float freely within the venous bloodstream. Such mobile clots are known as *emboli*. They are particularly likely to block pulmonary vessels (pulmonary emboli), which can result in death.[21]

The most important factor contributing to the development of DVT following SCI is loss of the normal "pumping" mechanism provided by active contraction of lower extremity musculature. This slows the flow of blood, allowing higher concentrations of procoagulants (e.g., thrombin) to develop in localized areas. This in turn results in a predisposition to thrombus formation. Normally, these procoagulants are rapidly mixed with large quantities of blood and removed in the liver.[21] The risks of DVT are heightened with age and prolonged pressure (e.g., extended contact against the bed or supporting surface). Prolonged pressure can damage the vessel wall and precipitate initiation of the clotting process. In addition, loss of vasomotor tone and immobility further enhance the potential development of DVT. Other contributing factors include immobility leading to venous stasis, sepsis, hypercoagulability, and trauma.[34,86,87] DVT most frequently occurs within the first 2 months following injury.

The formation of a thrombus results in inflammation (thrombophlebitis) with characteristic clinical features of local swelling, erythema, and heat. These signs are similar to those of early ectopic bone formation and long bone fractures.[77] Differential diagnosis is made on the basis of venous flow studies and venography.[77,88]

The clinical manifestations of DVT have been estimated to occur in approximately 15 percent of SCI patients.[88] However, one study reported an incidence as high as 40 percent.[89] Studies using iodine-125 fibrinogen scanning have yielded a much higher incidence. Fibrinogen scanning is sensitive to fibrin deposits and can detect the presence of an active thrombotic process in the absence of clinical manifestations.[90] Using this technique, incidence of DVT in patients with acute SCI has been reported at 90 percent in one group of 10 patients[91] and 100 percent in a group of 14 patients.[90]

Management of this secondary complication focuses on prevention. Prophylactic anticoagulant drug therapy is typically initiated following the acute onset of injury and routinely continued for 2 to 3 months[89,92,93] or for up to 6 months for patients at high risk.[94] Other preventative measures include (1) a turning program designed to avoid pressure over large vessels, (2) passive ROM exercises, (3) elastic support stockings,[34] and (4) positioning of the lower extremities to facilitate venous return.

PAIN

Pain is a common occurrence following SCI.[95,96] Several classification systems have been developed to describe this pain. These classifications are related to the source and type of pain as well as to the length of time since onset (acute versus chronic pain).

Traumatic Pain

Initially, pain experienced following acute traumatic injury is related to the extent and type of trauma sustained as well as to the structures involved. Pain may arise from fractures, ligamentous or soft tissue damage, muscle spasm, or early surgical interventions. This acute pain generally subsides with healing in 1 to 3 months. Typical management includes immobilization and use of analgesics.[32] Transcutaneous electrical nerve stimulation (TENS) also has been found effective in reducing this type of acute, postinjury pain.[97]

Nerve Root Pain

Pain or irritation may arise from damage to nerve roots at or near the site of cord damage. Pain can be caused by acute compression or tearing of the nerve roots,[98] or it may arise secondary to spinal instability, periradicular scar tissue and adhesion formation, or improper reduction.[32] Nerve root pain is often described as sharp, stabbing, burning, or shooting and typically follows a dermatomal pattern. It is most common in cauda equina injuries, in which a high distribution of nerve roots is present.[95]

Management of nerve root pain is a challenging clinical problem. Multiple approaches have been suggested, with varying degrees of success. Conservative management involves pharmacological therapy[98] and TENS. Surgical interventions for more severe, debilitating pain include nerve root sections (neurectomy) and posterior rhizotomies.[32]

Spinal Cord Dysesthesias

It is not uncommon for patients to experience many peculiar, often painful sensations (**dysesthesias SCI**) below the level of the lesion. The sensations tend to be diffuse and usually do not follow a dermatome distribution.[32] They occur in body parts that otherwise lack sensation and are often described by the patient as burning, numbness, pins and needles, or tingling feelings. Occasionally, they involve abnormal proprioceptive sensations, causing the individual to perceive a limb in other than its actual position. Dysesthesias have been described as "phantom" pains or sensations similar to those experienced following amputation.[99] The exact etiology of this pain is not well understood. However, it is theorized to be related to scarring at the distal end of the severed spinal cord.[32] These sensations are present following the acute onset of injury and typically subside over time. However, they tend to be more persistent and long-standing in cauda equina lesions.

Dysesthesia pain is particularly resistant to treatment. It is important that the complaints be acknowledged as real and that the patient be educated as to the legitimacy of the pain. Gentle handling of the patient's limbs and careful positioning frequently make the pain more tolerable. Pharmacological management using carbamazepine (Tegretol) and phenytoin (Dilantin) has been found effective in reducing dysesthesia pain.[98] Narcotic analgesics are usually discouraged because of the danger of addiction.[36] Other forms of treatment have not been found effective in managing this type of pain.[98]

Musculoskeletal Pain

Pain also may occur above the level of lesion and frequently involves the shoulder joint.[100,101] Pathological changes at the shoulder often are related to faulty positioning and/or inadequate ROM exercises, resulting in tightening of the joint capsule and surrounding soft tissue structures. In addition, the shoulder muscles are excessively challenged in their role as tonic stabilizers to substitute for lack of trunk innervation. This situation may be complicated by muscle imbalances around the joint, inflammation, or upper extremity fractures sustained at the time of injury.

Prevention of secondary shoulder involvement is critical, considering the importance of this joint in self-care and functional activities. Shoulder pain and limitation of ROM will significantly delay the rehabilitation process. The most important preventative measures include a regular program of ROM exercise and a positioning program designed to facilitate full motion at the shoulder. To achieve this latter goal, several useful additions to traditional positioning programs have been suggested for use during the acute phase.[100] The first involves use of arm boards, which can be slid under a mattress with pillows used to alter the height of the supporting surface. With the patient in a supine position, the side boards will allow positioning of the shoulders in 90 degrees of abduction with the elbows extended. A second suggestion, also with the patient in a supine position, is to place the arm above the patient's head for a short period of time. This will encourage external rotation and abduction beyond 90 degrees. The elbows should be in approximately 80 degrees of flexion. Finally, in sidelying, with the lower arm in 90 degrees of shoulder flexion, it is suggested that an axillary pillow be placed under the chest to help relieve pressure on the acromion process and head of the humerus. When the patient is in a sidelying position, the uppermost arm can be extended, abducted, and supported on a pillow.

OSTEOPOROSIS AND RENAL CALCULI

Changes in calcium metabolism following SCI lead to **osteoporosis** below the level of the lesion and development of renal calculi.[102] Normally, there is a dynamic balance between the bone resorption activity of osteoclasts and the role of osteoblasts in laying down new bone. Following SCI, there is a net loss of bone mass because the rate of resorption is greater than the rate of new bone formation.[77] Consequently, there is a greater susceptibility to fracture. As a result of this resorption there are large concentrations of calcium present in the urinary system (hypercalciuria), creating a predisposition to stone formation.

The highest incidence of bone mass changes and hypercalciuria occurs during the first 6 months following SCI.[103,104] After this period, changes gradually diminish and assume a constant low-normal level after approximately 1 year.[103,105]

The exact mechanism causing bone mass changes following paralysis is not clearly understood. However, immobility and lack of stress placed on the skeletal system through dynamic weight-bearing activities are well accepted as major contributing factors.

Treatment consists primarily of dietary management and early and continuing weight-bearing activities (e.g., tilt-table). Dietary considerations include calcium-restricted foods and vigorous hydration (especially increased amounts of water). Excessive intake of foods such as milk, ice cream, and other dairy products high in calcium is generally discouraged. High protein foods such as meats, whole-grain products, eggs, and vitamin-rich foods such as cranberries or dried fruit (e.g., prunes or plums) are encouraged.[40] In addition, the risk of calculi formation will be reduced by prevention of urinary tract infections and careful maintenance of bladder drainage to prevent urinary stasis.[106]

PROGNOSIS

The potential for recovery from SCI is directly related to the extent of damage to the spinal cord and/or nerve roots. Donovan and Bedbrook[106] have identified three primary influences on potential for recovery: (1) the degree of pathological changes imposed by the trauma, (2) the precautions taken to prevent further damage during rescue, and (3) prevention of additional compromise of neural tissue from hypoxia and hypotension during acute management.

Formulation of a prognosis is initiated only after spinal shock has subsided and is guided by whether or not the lesion is complete. Following spinal shock, a lesion is generally considered complete in the absence of any sensory or motor function below the level of cord damage. Early appearance of reflex activity in these instances is considered a poor prognostic indicator.[107] With complete lesions, no motor improvement is expected other than that which may occur from nerve root return.

With incomplete lesions, some evidence of sensory and/or motor function is noted below the level of the cord lesion after spinal shock subsides. Early signs of an incomplete lesion may be indicated by sacral sparing (perianal sensation, rectal sphincter tone, or active toe flexion). Incomplete lesions also may present with areas of spotty or scattered sensory and motor function throughout the body.

It is important to note that with most incomplete lesions improvement begins almost immediately following cessation of spinal shock. Many patients will have some progressive improvement of muscle return. It may be minimal or, less frequently, dramatic and usually becomes apparent during the first several months following injury. With a consistent progression of returning function (daily, weekly, or even monthly) further recovery can be expected at the same rate, or a slightly slower rate. Meticulous and frequent assessment of sensory and motor functions during this period will provide important information about the progression of recovery.

In time, the rate of recovery will decrease, and a plateau will be reached. When the plateau is reached and no new muscle activity is observed for several weeks or months, no additional recovery can be expected.

MANAGEMENT

The remainder of this chapter is divided into the acute and subacute phases of rehabilitation. The section on acute management addresses treatment interventions from the onset of injury until the fracture site is stable and upright activities can be initiated. The rehabilitation phase includes suggested treatment activities following initial orientation to the vertical position through preparation for discharge from the rehabilitation facility.

Acute Phase

EMERGENCY CARE

Ideally, management of SCI begins at the location of the accident. Techniques used in moving and managing the patient immediately following the trauma can influence prognosis significantly. Rescue personnel must be adept at questioning and assessing for signs of SCI before moving the individual. When a SCI is suspected, efforts should be made to avoid both active and passive movements of the spine.[106] Movement of the spine can be averted by strapping the patient to a spinal backboard or a full-body adjustable backboard, use of a supporting cervical collar, and assistance from multiple personnel in moving the patient to safety. These measures will assist in maintaining the spine in a neutral, anatomical position and will prevent further neurological damage.[106] Administration of high doses of steroids (e.g., methylprednisolone) for the first 48 hours after injury can improve potential for recovery of function.

On arrival at the emergency room, initial attention is focused on stabilizing the patient medically. A complete neurological examination is performed. Radiographic and imaging[108] studies, tomograms, and myelography assist in determining the extent of damage and plans for management. Attention is directed toward preventing progression of neurological impairment by restoration of vertebral alignment and early immobilization of the fracture site. A catheter typically is inserted, and secondary injuries are addressed. Unstable spinal fractures require early reduction and fixation. Symptoms of instability may include pain and tenderness at the fracture site, radiating pain, increasing neurological signs, and decreasing motor function.

FRACTURE STABILIZATION
Cervical Injuries

Immobilization of unstable cervical fractures is achieved via skeletal traction. Traction can be applied by use of tongs attached to the outer skull (Fig. 27-4) or by a halo device (Figs. 27-5 and 27-6).

Tongs

Several types of tongs are available (e.g., Crutchfield, Barton, Vinke, Gardner-Wells), each with a slightly different design. The tongs or calipers are inserted laterally on the outer table of the skull. Traction is accomplished by attachment of a traction rope to the skull fixation. With the patient in a supine position, this rope is threaded through a pulley or traction collar with weights attached distally. The weights hang freely without touching the floor. With the use of tongs as the method of skeletal traction the patient is generally immobilized for about 12 weeks until healing occurs. Today, however, tongs are used primarily as a temporary mode of skeletal traction with replacement using a halo device or for uncomplicated low cervical injuries.

Turning Frames and Beds

Several types of frames and beds are used for immobilization during the acute phase of care. Each has different design characteristics and functions.

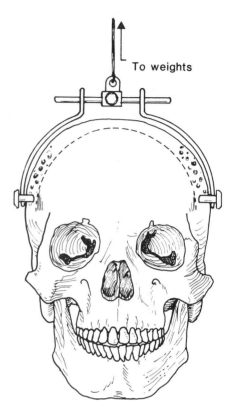

Figure 27-4. Cervical tongs. (From Judd, E (ed): Nursing Care of the Adult. FA Davis, Philadelphia, 1983, p 482, with permission.)

Among the most commonly used turning frame is the Stryker frame. It consists of an anterior and posterior frame attached to a turning base (Fig. 27-7). In turning from a supine position, the anterior

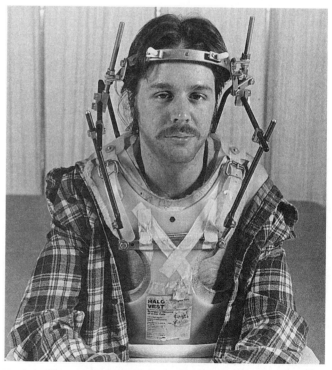

Figure 27-5. Halo device on an individual with a cervical cord lesion.

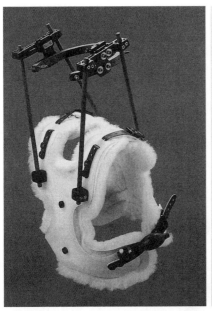
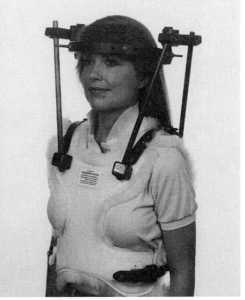

Figure 27-6. The Progress Mankind Technology (PMT) graphite halo system that is MRI compatible. (Courtesy PMT Corporation, Chanhassen, MN.)

frame is placed on top of the patient. A circular ring clamps in place to secure the two frames during turning. Safety straps provide additional security. Rotation to the prone position is accomplished by manually turning the two frames as a unit. The uppermost frame is then removed. Return to the supine position is accomplished in the same manner. The primary benefit of these devices is that they allow positional changes while maintaining anatomical alignment of the spine. Turning can be accomplished without interruption of the cervical traction. A disadvantage of turning frames is that positioning is limited to prone and supine. This is particularly problematic for patients with a low tolerance for the prone position (e.g., cardiac or respiratory involvement). In addition, these frames cannot accommodate obese patients and are unsuitable for unconscious patients. Although once the norm for

managing spinal fractures, frames are now used primarily as a temporary method of immobilization or for uncomplicated low cervical, thoracic, or lumbar injuries.

The Roto Rest Kinetic Treatment Table (Roto Rest Bed) is an electronically operated unit that provides continuous side-to-side rotation along its longitudinal axis (Fig. 27-8). Its basic components include an oscillating base frame and a series of bolsters, pads, and supports for patient positioning. The primary advantage of this system for patients with SCI is the ability to maintain spinal alignment with reduction of the secondary complications of bed rest. The continuous oscillation provides the important advantages of improved pulmonary and kidney drainage as well as assisting with prevention of pressure sores via continual redistribution of tissue pressure.

It should be noted that some patients cannot tolerate the continuous oscillation provided by this unit and develop motion sickness. These symptoms may be successfully treated with pharmacological intervention (e.g., dimenhydrinate [Dramamine]). If symptoms persist, it may be necessary to discontinue use of the bed. In addition, severe claustrophobia is generally considered a contraindication for use of this bed.

Historically, circular frame beds were also used for patients with SCI. These electrically powered units provided positional changes from supine to prone and reverse by a vertical (upright) turn. An anterior frame was placed on the patient before turning. This type of bed is no longer used for patients with acute SCI because of the excessive loading of the spine in a vertical position.[109]

Finally, in some facilities standard hospital beds are used. Any of a variety of special pressure-relieving mattresses (gel, sand, water, air, or foam)

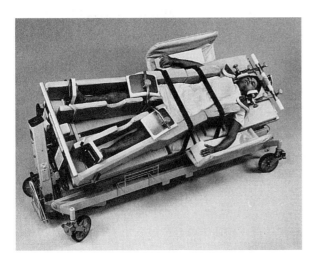

Figure 27-7. Stryker turning frame. (Courtesy Stryker Corporation, Kalamazoo, MI.)

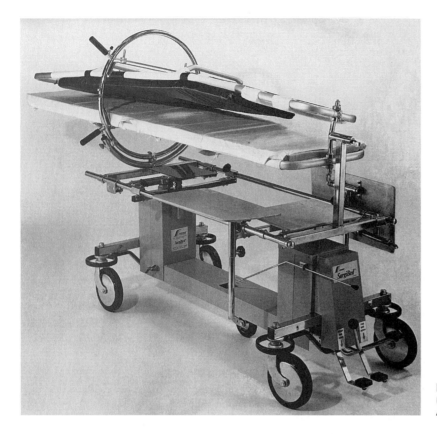

Figure 27-8. Roto Rest kinetic treatment table. (Roto Rest bed, courtesy of Kinetic Concepts, San Antonio, TX.)

are used for pressure relief. Positional changes are accomplished by log rolling.

Halo Devices

Halo devices are used commonly with much greater frequency to immobilize cervical fractures. They have replaced much of the earlier prolonged use of skeletal tongs and turning frames and radically altered management of cervical cord lesions. These traction devices (see Figs. 27-5 and 27-6) consist of a halo ring with four steel screws that attach directly to the outer skull. The halo is attached to a body jacket or vest by four vertical steel posts. Owing to their structural configuration these devices are contraindicated with severe respiratory involvement.

The introduction of halo devices has generally been considered a major advance in managing cervical fractures. They provide several important advantages over use of tongs and prolonged confinement to a bed or turning frame. These devices reduce the secondary complications of prolonged bed rest, permit earlier progression to upright activities (typically within a few weeks), allow earlier involvement in a rehabilitation program, and reduce the length and cost of hospital stay.[110] In addition, for patients without neurological involvement, discharge from the hospital may occur several days after application of the halo device. These patients are then followed closely on an outpatient basis.[111]

Skeletal traction devices are left in place until radiographic findings indicate stability has been achieved (approximately 12 weeks). Following re-

moval, a cervical orthosis is applied during a transitional period (approximately 4 to 6 weeks) until unrestricted movement is allowed. The sterno-occipital-mandibular immobilizer (SOMI) cervical orthosis, Philadelphia collar (Fig. 27-9), or custom-made plastic collars are frequently used during this period, with progression to a soft foam collar prior to resuming unsupported movement.

Thoracic and Lumbar Injuries

Fractures of the thoracic and lumbar area are typically managed by immobilization through bed rest or by application of a body cast or jacket. Bed rest is achieved by use of a turning frame or a standard bed, maintaining a log-roll technique for positional changes. The expanded use of spinal orthotics also has allowed for earlier mobility activities following thoracic and lumbar injuries. Plaster or plastic body jackets (Fig. 27-10) function to immobilize the spine and allow earlier involvement in a rehabilitation program. Body jackets are typically bivalved to allow for removal during bathing and skin inspection.

Surgical Intervention

Surgery may be indicated to restore bony anatomical alignment, prevent further damage to the spinal cord, or stabilize the fracture site. Compared with spontaneous healing times, surgical stabilization allows earlier initiation of rehabilitation activities.[106]

Surgical interventions for cervical fractures may include decompression (anterior or posterior) and fusion. Fusion is achieved by bone grafting and may

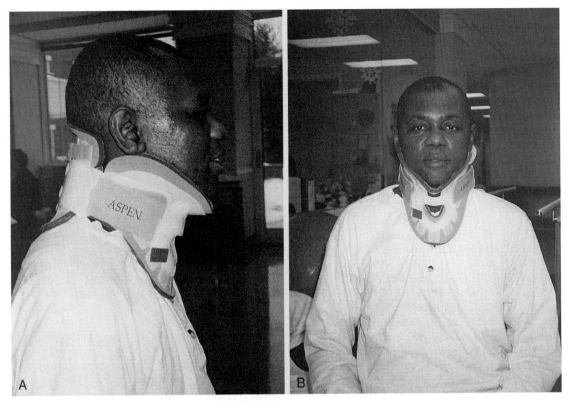

Figure 27-9. Lateral *(A)* and anterior *(B)* views of the Philadelphia collar.

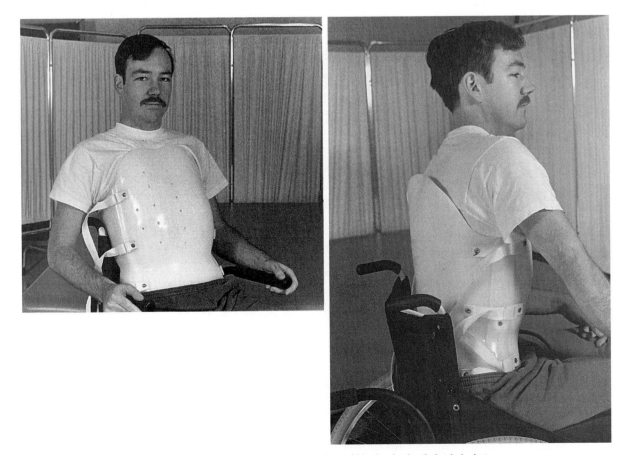

Figure 27-10. Anterior and lateral view of bivalved, plastic body jacket.

be combined with posterior wiring of the spinous processes.[112]

Frequently, surgery for thoracic and lumbar fractures requires use of an internal fixation device, which may be used in combination with bone grafts. The three most common devices used for achieving spinal realignment, stability, and internal fixation are Harrington distraction rods, Harrington compression rods, and Weiss compression springs.[113] Following thoracic or lumbar surgery, the patient is placed in a spinal orthosis (e.g., Knight-Taylor orthosis, Jewett hyperextension orthosis, or a custom-made, plastic, bivalved body jacket) for a minimum of 3 months.[113]

Physical Therapy Examination

A general assessment of the patient is indicated, including respiratory function, skin condition, sensation, tone, and muscle strength. Results will assist the therapist in determining the lesion level, identifying general functional expectations, and formulating appropriate treatment goals. As noted, the lesion level is considered to be the lowest segmental level in which muscle strength is present at a fair+ grade. During the acute stage, spinal instability often precludes a thorough physical therapy assessment. However, gross screening will provide important

Table 27–4 IMPAIRMENT SCALE

Asia Impairment Scale

- ☐ **A = Complete:** No motor or sensory function is preserved in the sacral segments S4 to S5.
- ☐ **B = Incomplete:** Sensory but not motor function is preserved below the neurological level and includes the sacral segments S4 to S5.
- ☐ **C = Incomplete:** Motor function is preserved below the neurological level, and more than half of key muscles below the neurological level have a muscle grade less than 3.
- ☐ **D = Incomplete:** Motor function is preserved below the neurological level, and at least half of key muscles below the neurological level have a muscle grade of 3 or more.
- ☐ **E = Normal:** motor and sensory function is normal.

Clinical Syndromes

- ☐ Central cord
- ☐ Brown-Sequard
- ☐ Anterior cord
- ☐ Conus medullaris
- ☐ Cauda equina

From American Spinal Cord Injury Association,[114] p 28, with permission.

initial data until the patient is cleared for further activity.

Useful tools for documenting results of the examination are the Impairment Scale (Table 27–4) and the Standard Neurological Classification of Spinal Cord Injury (Fig. 27-11) developed by the American Spinal Injury Association (ASIA). These tools im-

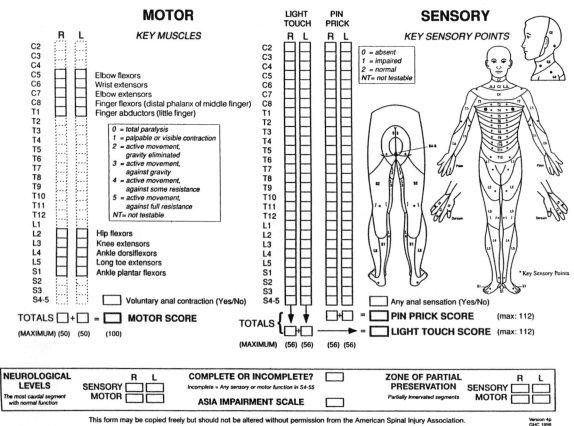

Figure 27-11. Motor and sensory examination form recommended by the ASIA. (From American Spinal Injury Association,[114] p 27, with permission.)

prove standardization of the examination process for patients with spinal cord injury. ASIA also endorses use of the Functional Independence Measure (FIM) (see Chapter 11) to assess the impact of spinal cord injury on daily function.[114]

1. *Respiratory assessment.* Details of respiratory status and function are essential. The areas listed below should be assessed:

   a. *Function of respiratory muscles.* Muscle strength and tone, and atrophy of the diaphragm, abdominals, and intercostals should be assessed; respiratory rate should be noted.

   b. *Chest expansion.* Circumferential measurements should be taken at the level of the axilla and xiphoid process using a cloth tape measure. Chest expansion is recorded as the difference in measurement between maximum exhalation and maximum inhalation. Normally, chest expansion is approximately 2.5 to 3 inches (6.4 to 7.6 cm) at the xiphoid process.[27]

   c. *Breathing pattern.* A determination should be made of muscles that are functioning and their contributions to respiration. This may be accomplished by manual palpation over the chest and abdominal region or by observation. Particular attention should be directed toward use of accessory neck muscles and alteration in breathing pattern when the patient is talking or moving.[24]

   d. *Cough.* Coughing allows the patient to remove secretions. Ineffective cough function will necessitate suctioning to avoid pulmonary complications. Alvarez et al.[24] have defined three cough classifications: (1) *functional*, strong enough to clear secretions; (2) *weak functional*, adequate force to clear upper respiratory tract secretions in small quantities; assistance is required to clear mucus secondary to infection; and (3) *nonfunctional*, unable to produce any cough force.

   e. *Vital capacity.* Initial measures may be taken with a hand-held spirometer.[24] Vital capacity measures also can be used as a baseline for defining respiratory muscle weakness.

2. *Skin assessment.* During the acute phase, meticulous and regular skin inspection is a shared responsibility of the patient and the entire subacute team. As management progresses into the rehabilitation phase, the patient will gradually assume greater responsibility for this activity. Patient education related to skin care is crucial and should be initiated early. Frequent position changes and skin inspection may be viewed by the patient as bothersome or distracting from sleep if there is not adequate awareness of the importance and purpose of these activities. Skin inspection combines both visual observation and palpation.[115] The patient's entire body should be observed regularly with particular attention to areas most susceptible to pressure (Table 27–5). Palpation is useful for identifying skin temperature changes that may be indicative of a hyperemic reaction. This is particularly important in assessing individuals with dark skin, because early skin responses to pressure may not be readily apparent. Skin reactions to excess pressure include redness, local warmth, local edema, and small open or cracked skin areas. Careful attention should be directed toward accidental skin abrasions or bruises, which increase the potential for skin breakdown.[115] If the patient is wearing a halo, vest, or other orthotic device, contact points between the body and the appliance must also be inspected.

3. *Sensory assessment.* A detailed assessment of superficial and deep sensations should be completed (see Chapter 6). Particular emphasis should be placed on pin prick and light touch responses (typically used to identify sensory level of lesion) as well as proprioceptive responses. It should be noted that the sensory level of injury may not correspond to the motor level of injury (i.e., incomplete lesions).

4. *Tone and deep tendon reflexes.* Muscle tone should be assessed (see Chapter 8) with reference to quality, muscle groups involved, and factors that appear to increase or to decrease tone. An assessment of deep tendon reflexes is indicated. Level of the lesion will influence the specific tendons selected for testing. The deep tendon reflexes most commonly assessed and their levels of innervation are the biceps (C6), triceps (C7), quadriceps (L3, L4), and gastrocnemius (S1).[55]

5. *Manual muscle test (MMT) and range of motion (ROM) assessment.* Standard techniques should be used for MMT[116] and ROM assessments.[117] Because mobility will be limited during the acute phase, deviations from standard positioning will be necessary and should be carefully documented. In cases of spinal instability, extreme caution should be used when performing gross muscle and ROM tests, because movements of this sort may place

Table 27–5 AREAS MOST SUSCEPTIBLE TO PRESSURE IN RECUMBENT POSITIONS

Supine	Prone	Sidelying
Occiput	Ears (head rotated)	Ears
Scapulae	—	Shoulders (lateral aspect)
Vertebrae	—	Greater trochanter
Elbows	Shoulders (anterior aspect)	Head of fibula
Sacrum		Knees (medial aspect from contact between knees)
Coccyx	Illiac crest	
Heels	Male genital region	Lateral malleolus
	Patella	Medial malleolus (contact between malleoli)
	Dorsum of feet	

undue stress on the fracture site. Discretion should be used in applying resistance around the shoulders in tetraplegia and around the lower trunk and hips in paraplegia.

6. *Functional assessment.* Accurate and specific determination of functional skills usually must be delayed until the patient is cleared for activity. Once activity is allowed, a more detailed assessment of function can be made (see Chapter 11).

7. *Sacral sparing.* Periodic checks should be made for the presence of sacral sparing, which may not have been evident on admission (e.g., perianal sensation, rectal sphincter tone, or active toe flexion).

Physical Therapy Intervention

During the acute phase of rehabilitation, emphasis is placed on respiratory management, prevention of secondary complications, maintaining ROM, and facilitating active movement in available musculature. Pending orthopedic clearance, limited strengthening activities also may be initiated during this early phase.

RESPIRATORY MANAGEMENT

Respiratory care will vary according to the level of injury and individual respiratory status. Primary goals of management include improved ventilation, increased effectiveness of cough, and prevention of chest tightness and ineffective substitute breathing patterns.[24] Depending on the individual patient the following treatment activities may be appropriate:

1. *Deep breathing exercises.* Diaphragmatic breathing should be encouraged. To facilitate diaphragmatic movement and increase vital capacity, the therapist can apply light pressure during both inspiration and expiration. Manual contacts can be made just below the sternum. This will assist the patient to concentrate on deep breathing patterns even in the absence of thoracic and abdominal sensation. To facilitate expiration, manual contacts are made over the thorax with the hands spread wide. This creates a compressive force on the thorax, resulting in a more forceful expiration followed by a more efficient inspiration.[33] Patients immobilized in traction devices or limited to recumbent positions may benefit from use of a mirror to provide visual feedback during these activities. Inflation hold and incentive spirometry are also useful adjuncts to deep breathing exercises.[118]

2. *Glossopharyngeal breathing.* This activity is often appropriate for patients with high-level cervical lesions. The technique utilizes accessory muscles of respiration to improve vital capacity. The patient is instructed to inspire small amounts of air repeatedly, using a "sipping" or "gulping" pattern, thus utilizing available facial and neck muscles. By using this technique, enough air is gradually inspired to improve chest expansion despite paralysis of the primary muscles of respiration.

3. *Airshift maneuver.* This technique provides the patient with an independent method of chest expansion. It is accomplished by closing the glottis after a maximum inhalation, relaxing the diaphragm, and allowing air to shift from the lower to upper thorax. Airshifts can increase chest expansion by 0.5 to 2 inches (1.3 to 5.1 cm).

4. *Strengthening exercises.* Progressive resistive exercises can be used to strengthen the diaphragm. This can be accomplished by manual contacts over the epigastric area below the xiphoid process or by use of weights. Strengthening exercises for innervated abdominal and accessory musculature are also indicated.

5. *Assisted coughing.* To assist with coughing and movement of secretions, manual contacts are placed over the epigastric area. The therapist pushes quickly in an inward and upward direction as the patient attempts to cough.[119]

6. *Abdominal support.* An abdominal corset or binder is indicated for patients whose abdomen protrudes, allowing the diaphragm to "sag" into a poor position for function. The corset will support the abdominal contents and improve the resting position of the diaphragm. In addition, abdominal supports provide the secondary benefits of maintaining intrathoracic pressure and decreasing postural hypotension.

7. *Stretching.* Mobility and compliance of the thoracic wall can be facilitated by manual stretching of pectoral and other chest wall muscles.

In addition to these respiratory approaches, intermittent positive pressure breathing may be utilized to assist in maintenance of lung compliance. Modified postural drainage and percussion techniques also may be indicated to assist with mobilizing and eliminating secretions.

RANGE OF MOTION AND POSITIONING

While the patient is immobilized in bed or on a turning frame, full ROM exercises should be completed daily except in those areas that are contraindicated or require selective stretching. With paraplegia, motion of the trunk and some motions of the hip are contraindicated. Generally, straight leg raising more than 60 degrees and hip flexion beyond 90 degrees (during combined hip and knee flexion) should be avoided. This will avert strain on the lower thoracic and lumbar spine. If possible, ROM exercises should be completed in both the prone and supine positions (prone positioning may be contraindicated for some patients owing to fracture and/or respiratory compromise in this position). In the prone position, attention should be directed toward shoulder and hip extension and knee flexion. With tetraplegia, motion of the head and neck is contraindicated pending orthopedic clearance. Stretching of the shoulders should be avoided during the acute period; however, the patient should be positioned out of the usual position of comfort, in which there is internal rotation, adduction and extension of the shoulders, elbow flexion, forearm pronation, and wrist flexion. Full ROM exercises are generally included for both lower extremities.

Patients with SCIs do not require full ROM in all joints. Some joints benefit from allowing tightness to develop in certain muscles to enhance function. For example, with tetraplegia, tightness of the lower trunk musculature will improve sitting posture by increasing trunk stability; tightness in the long finger flexors will provide an improved tenodesis grasp. Conversely, some muscles require a fully lengthened range. After the acute phase, the hamstrings will require stretching to achieve a straight leg raise of approximately 100 degrees. This ROM is required for many functional activities such as sitting, transfers, lower extremity dressing, and self-ROM exercises. This process of understretching some muscles and full stretching of others to improve function is referred to as **selective stretching.**

Positioning splints for the wrist, hands, and fingers are an important early consideration. Alignment of the fingers, thumb, and wrist must be maintained for functional activities or future dynamic splinting. For high-level lesions the wrist is positioned in neutral, the web space is maintained, and the fingers are flexed.[120] If the wrist extensors are functional (fair muscle grade), a C-bar or short-opponens splint is usually sufficient.

Ankle boots or splints are indicated to maintain alignment and to prevent heel cord tightness and pressure sores. Ankle boots designed to suspend the heel in space and distribute pressure evenly along the lower leg are available commercially (Fig. 27-12). Sandbags or towel rolls also may be required to maintain a position of neutral hip rotation.

Following orthopedic clearance, the patient typically is placed on a schedule to increase tolerance to the prone position. For patients wearing a halo device, one or two pillows under the chest will allow assumption of the prone position. The ankles should be positioned at a 90-degree angle. Tolerance to the prone position should be increased gradually until the patient is able to sleep all, or at least part, of the night in this position. This routine will assist with prevention of pressure sores on posterior aspects of the body and development of flexor tightness at the hips and knees. Proning schedules also are considered to promote improved bladder drainage.

SELECTIVE STRENGTHENING

During the course of rehabilitation, all remaining musculature will be strengthened maximally. However, during the acute phase certain muscles must be strengthened very cautiously to avoid stress at the fracture site. During the first few weeks following injury, application of resistance may be contraindicated to (1) musculature of the scapula and shoulders in tetraplegia, and (2) musculature of the hips and trunk in paraplegia.

An important consideration in planning exercise programs during the acute phase is to emphasize bilateral upper extremity activities because these will avoid asymmetric, rotational stresses on the spine. Several forms of strengthening exercises are appropriate during this early phase: bilateral manually resisted motions in straight planes, bilateral upper extremity proprioceptive neuromuscular facilitation (PNF) patterns, and progressive resistive exercises using cuff weights or dumbbells. Biofeedback training also may be a useful adjunct during early exercise programs. With tetraplegia, emphasis should be placed on strengthening the anterior deltoid, shoulder extensors, biceps, and lower trapezius. If present, the radial wrist extensors, triceps, and pectorals should also be emphasized because they will be of key importance in improving functional capacity. With paraplegia, all upper extremity musculature should be strengthened, with emphasis on shoulder depressors, triceps, and latissimus dorsi, which are required for transfers and ambulation.

Early involvement in functional activities should be stressed. In addition to their intrinsic value, many activities afford the important benefit of progressive strengthening. For example, self-feeding and involvement in limited personal care activities will assist with strengthening the shoulder and elbow flexors. Another example of a functional activity

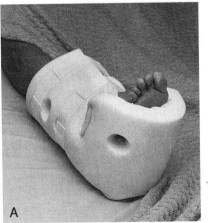
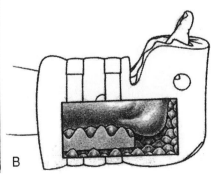

Figure 27-12. Ankle boot designed to distribute pressure along lower leg *(A)* and suspend the heel in space *(B)*. (Courtesy of DM Systems, Inc., Evanston, IL.)

A

B

(although not appropriate during the acute phase) with important strengthening benefits is wheelchair propulsion (deltoids, biceps, and shoulder rotators).

ORIENTATION TO THE VERTICAL POSITION

Once radiographic findings have established stability of the fracture site, or early fracture stabilization methods are complete, the patient is cleared for upright activities. As discussed, the patient typically will experience symptoms of postural hypotension if approach to management has required some period of immobility. A very gradual acclimation to upright postures is most effective. The use of an abdominal binder and elastic stockings will retard venous pooling. During early upright positioning, elastic wraps are often used in combination with (placed over) the elastic stockings.

Initially, upright activities can be initiated by elevating the head of the bed and progressing to a reclining wheelchair with elevating leg rests. Use of the tilt-table provides another option for orienting the patient to a vertical position. Vital signs should be monitored carefully and documented during this acclimation period.

Patients who have been immobilized in halo devices or undergone surgical spine stabilization will not be confined to recumbent positions for prolonged periods. For these patients, the same progression is used, although a more rapid advance to the vertical position can be anticipated.

Subacute Phase

FUNCTIONAL EXPECTATIONS

A SCI will require that specific functional goals be established as part of overall rehabilitation planning. Table 27–6 presents reasonable functional expectations, at various lesion levels, for a young, healthy patient with a complete lesion and unimpaired by secondary complications. This information may provide a useful guide in establishing realistic goals. However, it is important not to adhere too closely to established "norms" and, hence, to limit the patient by your own expectations. Goals should be established individually for each patient on the basis of assessment findings in accordance with the level and extent of injury.

The term **key muscles** is a common expression in the management of patients with SCI and is used in Table 27–6. Key muscles are those that add significantly to a patient's functional capability at each successive level of lesion. It is also important to note that the neurological level of innervation may vary slightly from source to source.

PHYSICAL THERAPY EXAMINATION

All the assessments completed during the acute phase will be continued at regular intervals during the subacute phase of rehabilitation. Inasmuch as greater patient mobility is now allowed, more complete testing of muscle strength, ROM, and

functional skills can be performed. A high level of skill in MMT is needed for the therapist to distinguish accurately between true voluntary contraction and movement associated with spasticity or substitution.

Once some wheelchair mobility has been achieved, assessment of cardiovascular endurance is indicated (see Chapter 16). The patient's age, sex, and cardiac history should be taken into account. Upper extremity stress testing[121] or telemetry monitoring during wheelchair propulsion may be indicated for patients who are suspected of having impaired cardiovascular adaptation to exercise.

PHYSICAL THERAPY INTERVENTION
Skin Inspection

During this phase of management, the patient will be instructed gradually to assume responsibility for skin inspection. This will involve practice in use of long-handled (Fig. 27-13) or adapted mirrors to allow inspection of areas not easily visible. Wall mirrors adjacent to the bed may assist in achieving independence with this activity. Patients with high-level lesions may be incapable of skin inspection. It is important that these patients be instructed in how to direct others to complete this assessment. Continued emphasis by the therapist should be placed on the importance of skin inspection and the rationale for pressure relief. Skin inspection must become a regular and lifelong component of the patient's daily routine.

Continuing Activities

During the subacute phase of management, many of the treatment activities initiated during the acute period will be continued. Emphasis will remain on respiratory management, ROM, and positioning. The patient also will be involved in a continuing and expanded program of resistive exercises for all muscles that remain innervated (e.g., PNF, progressive resistance exercise [PRE] using manual resistance, weights, wall pulleys, and sling suspension, and group exercise classes). Development of motor control and muscle reeducation techniques directed at appropriate muscles (depending on lesion level) are indicated. Emphasis is also placed on regaining postural control and balance by substituting upper body control and vision (for lost proprioception). This phase of treatment will also focus on improved cardiovascular response to exercise. This can effectively be accomplished by use of interval training using an upper extremity aerobic activity (e.g., upper extremity ergometer).[120]

Mat Programs

Mat activities constitute a major component of treatment during the rehabilitation phase. The sequence of activities typically progresses from achievement of stability within a posture and advances through controlled mobility to skill in functional use.[121] Early activities are bilateral and symmetrical. A progression is then made to weight

Table 27–6 FUNCTIONAL EXPECTATIONS FOR PATIENTS WITH SPINAL CORD INJURY[a]

Most Distal Nerve Root Segments Innervated and Key Muscles	Available Movements	Functional Capabilities	Equipment and Assistance Required
C1, C2, C3 Face and neck muscles (cranial innervation)	Talking Mastication Sipping Blowing	1. Total dependence in ADL	Respirator dependent: may use phrenic nerve stimulator during the day Full-time attendant required
		Activation of light switches, page turners, call buttons, electrical appliances, and speaker phones	Environmental control units
		2. Locomotion	Electric wheelchair (typical components include a high, electrically controlled reclining back, a seatbelt and trunk support); a portable respirator may be attached; microswitch or sip-and-puff controls may be used
C4 Diaphragm Trapezius	Respiration Scapular elevation	1. ADL a. Limited self-feeding	Mobile arm supports (possibly with powered elbow orthotic), powered flexor hinge hand splint Adapted eating equipment (long straws, built-up handles on utensils, plate guards, and so forth) Plexiglas lapboard
		b. Typing	Computer keyboard using head or mouth stick or sip-and-puff controls; another option is a rubber-tipped stick held in hand by a splint (in combination with mobile arm supports and powered splints)
		c. Page turning	Head or mouth stick Environmental control unit for powered page turner
		d. Activation of light switches, call buttons, electrical appliances, and speaker phones	Environmental control units
		2. Locomotion	Electric wheelchair with head, mouth, chin, breadth, or sip-and-puff controls
		3. Pressure relief	Electric tilt-in-space wheelchair
		4. Transfers and bed mobility	Dependent
		5. Skin inspection	Dependent
		6. Cough with glossopharyngeal breathing	Dependent
		7. Recreation a. Table games such as cards or checkers	Head or mouth stick Built-up playing pieces
		b. Painting and drawing	Full-time attendant required
C5 Biceps Brachialis Brachioradialis Deltoid Infraspinatus Rhomboid (major and minor) Supinator	Elbow flexion and supination Shoulder external rotation Shoulder abduction to 90 degrees Limited shoulder flexion	1. ADL: able to accomplish all activities of a C4 quadriplegic with less adaptive equipment and more skill	Assistance is required in setting up patient with necessary equipment; patient can then accomplish activity independently Mobile arm supports, deltoid aid
		a. Self-feeding	Adapted utensils and splinting
		b. Typing	Computer keyboard Hand splints Adapted typing sticks Some patients may require mobile arm supports or slings
		c. Page turning	Same as above
		d. Limited upper extremity dressing	Assistance required
		e. Limited self-care (i.e., washing, brushing teeth, and grooming)	Hand splints Adapted equipment (wash mitt, adapted toothbrush, and so forth)
		2. Locomotion	Manual wheelchair with plastic-coated handrim projections Electric wheelchair with joystick or adapted upper extremity controls
		3. Transfer activities	Overhead swivel bar Sliding board Dependent
		4. Skin inspection	Dependent
		5. Pressure relief	Independent with power tilt-in-space wheelchair
		6. Cough with manual pressure to diaphragm	Assistance required
		7. Driving	Van with hand controls; part-time attendant required

Continued

897

Table 27–6 FUNCTIONAL EXPECTATIONS FOR PATIENTS WITH SPINAL CORD INJURY[a] *Continued*

Most Distal Nerve Root Segments Innervated and Key Muscles	Available Movements	Functional Capabilities	Equipment and Assistance Required

C6
Extensor carpi radialis
Infraspinatus
Latissimus dorsi
Pectoralis major (clavicular portion)
Pronator teres
Serratus anterior
Teres minor
	Shoulder flexion, extension, internal rotation, and adduction
	Scapular abduction and upward rotation
	Forearm pronation
	Wrist extension (tenodesis grasp)
		1. ADL
		  a. Self-feeding
		
		  b. Dressing
		
		  c. Self-care
		
		  d. Bed mobility
		
		2. Locomotion
		
		3. Transfer activities
		4. Skin inspection and pressure relief
		5. Bowel and bladder care
		
		6. Cough with application of pressure to abdomen
		7. Driving
		
		8. Wheelchair sports
		9. Meal preparation
			Universal cuff
			Intertwine utensils in fingers
			Adapted utensils
			Utilizes momentum, button hooks, zipper pulls, or other clothing adaptations; dependent on momentum to extend limbs
			Cannot tie shoes
			
			Flexor hinge splint
			Universal cuff
			Adaptive equipment
			Independent with use of side rails on bed or overhead triangle
			Manual wheelchair with projection or friction surface hand rims; power wheelchair may be required for long distances
			Independent with sliding board on level surfaces
			Independent
			
			Can be independent with equipment depending on bowel and bladder routine
			Independent
			
			Automobile with hand controls and U-shaped cuff attached to steering wheel
			Usually requires assistance in getting wheelchair into car
			Limited participation (i.e., bowling, fishing)
			Can be independent with occasional light meals with adaptive equipment

C7
Extensor pollicus longus and brevis
Extrinsic finger extensors
Flexor carpi radialis
Triceps
	Elbow extension
	Wrist flexion
	Finger extension
		1. ADL
		  a. Self-feeding
		  b. Dressing
		
		  c. Self-care
		
		2. Locomotion
		3. Transfers
		4. Bowel and bladder care
		
		5. Manual cough
		6. Housekeeping
		
		7. Driving
			Independent
			Independent
			Button hook may be required
			
			Shower chair
			Adapted hand shower nozzle
			Adapted handles on bathroom items may be required
			Manual wheelchair with friction surface hand rims
			Independent (with or without sliding board)
			Independent with appropriate equipment (digital stimulator, suppositories, raised toilet seat, urinary drainage device, etc.)
			Independent
			Light kitchen activities
			Requires wheelchair-accessible kitchen and living environment
			Adapted kitchen tools
			Automobile with hand controls
			Able to get wheelchair in and out of car

C8 to T1 Extrinsic finger flexors Flexor carpi ulnaris Flexor pollicis longus and brevis Intrinsic finger flexor	Full innervation of upper extremity muscles including fine coordination and strong grasp	1. ADL 2. Locomotion 3. Housekeeping 4. Driving 5. Employment	Independent in all self-care and personal hygiene Some adaptive equipment may be required (e.g., tub seat, grab bars, etc.) Manual wheelchair with standard hand rims Independent in light housekeeping and meal preparation Some adaptive equipment may be required (e.g., reachers) Requires a wheelchair-accessible living environment Automobile with hand controls Able to work in a building free of architectural barriers

Table 27–6 FUNCTIONAL EXPECTATIONS FOR PATIENTS WITH SPINAL CORD INJURY[a] *Continued*

Most Distal Nerve Root Segments Innervated and Key Muscles	Available Movements	Functional Capabilities	Equipment and Assistance Required
T4 to T6 Top half of intercostals Long muscles of back (sacrospinalis and semispinalis)	Improved trunk control Increased respiratory reserve Pectoral girdle stabilized for lifting objects	1. ADL 2. Physiological standing (not practical for functional ambulation) 3. Housekeeping 4. Curb climbing in wheelchair 5. Wheelchair sports	Independent in all areas Standing table Bilateral knee-ankle orthoses with spinal attachment Some patients may be able to ambulate for short distances with assistance Independent with routine activities Requires a wheelchair-accessible living environment Able to negotiate curbs using a "wheelie" technique Full participation
T9 to T12 Lower abdominals All intercostals	Improved trunk control Increased endurance	1. Household ambulation 2. Locomotion	Bilateral knee-ankle orthoses and crutches or walker (high energy consumption for ambulation) Wheelchair used for energy conservation
L2, L3, L4 Gracilis Iliopsoas Quadratus lumborum Rectus femoris Sartorius	Hip flexion Hip adduction Knee extension	1. Functional ambulation 2. Locomotion	Bilateral knee-ankle orthoses and crutches Wheelchair used for convenience and energy conservation
L4, L5 Extensor digitorum Low back muscles Medial hamstrings (weak) Posterior tibialis Quadriceps Tibialis anterior	Strong hip flexion Strong knee extension Weak knee flexion Improved trunk control	1. Functional ambulation 2. Locomotion	Bilateral ankle-foot orthoses and crutches or canes Wheelchair used for convenience and energy conservation

[a]This table presents general functional expectations at various lesion levels. Each progressively lower segment includes the muscle from the previous levels. Although the key muscles listed frequently receive innervation from several nerve root segments, they are listed here at the neurological levels where they add to functional outcomes.

shifting and movement within the posture. A gradual emphasis is placed on improved timing and speed.

Mat activities are often individual components of more complex functional skills. They should be

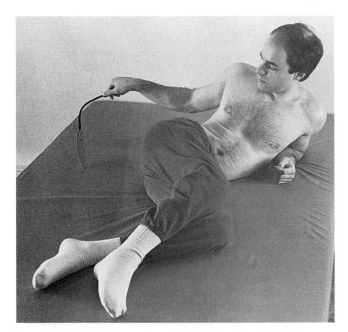

Figure 27-13. Skin inspection with use of long-handled mirror.

sequenced from easiest to most difficult so that the patient is performing activities within, or almost within, the sphere of mastery. As mastery of the various components of more complex and difficult activities is achieved, the patient should be asked to perform these tasks in the current living environment (i.e., hospital room, or eventually, home on weekends).

The therapist must determine the appropriate mat activities for each patient based on level of injury and medical status. It is important to note that complete mastery of an activity is not always necessary before moving on to the next. At some points in treatment, several components of the mat progression will be worked on concurrently.

Mat activities should be initiated as soon as the patient is cleared for activity. Progression through the sequence of mat activities develops improved strength and functional ROM, improves awareness of the new center of gravity, promotes postural stability, facilitates dynamic balance, and assists with determining the most efficient and functional methods for accomplishing specific tasks. It also provides the opportunity to develop functional patterns of movement (e.g., use of innervated musculature or momentum to move body parts that lack active movement).

The following section represents a sample progression of selected mat activities. The degree to which they can be performed independently and the time needed to learn them vary considerably with the level of lesion. Each component of the mat progression is presented with its functional implications and several suggested treatment activities to facilitate accomplishment of the activity. Chapter 13 and *Physical Rehabilitation Laboratory Manual: Focus on Functional Training*[121] will provide additional treatment suggestions.

Rolling

Rolling is of functional significance for improved bed mobility, preparation for independent positional changes in bed (for pressure relief) and lower extremity dressing. Rolling is a frequent starting point of mat programs for patients with SCI and provides an early lesson in developing functional patterns of movement. It requires the patient to learn to use the head, neck, and upper extremities, as well as momentum, to move the trunk and/or lower extremities. It is usually easiest to begin rolling activities from the supine position, working toward the prone position. If asymmetric involvement exists, rolling should be initiated with movement toward the weaker side.

The activity is initially taught on a mat. However, rolling must also be mastered on the surface of a bed similar to the one that the patient will use at home. To develop maximum independence, bed rails, ropes, or overhead devices should be avoided, if possible. In addition, the patient should achieve independent rolling when covered by sheets and blankets. To begin training and facilitate rolling, several approaches can be used.

1. Flexion of the head and neck with rotation may be used to assist movement from supine to prone positions.
2. Extension of the head and neck with rotation may be used to assist movement from prone to supine positions.
3. Bilateral, symmetrical upper extremity rocking with outstretched arms produces a pendular motion when moving from supine to prone positions. The patient rhythmically rocks the outstretched arms and head from side-to-side and then forcefully "tosses" them to the side to which the patient is rolling. The trunk and hips will follow (Fig. 27-14). Use of wrist cuff weights (2 to 3 lbs) may be used initially to increase kinesthetic awareness and momentum.
4. Crossing the ankles will also facilitate rolling (see Fig. 27-14). The therapist crosses the patient's ankles so that the upper limb is toward the direction of the roll (e.g., the right ankle would be crossed over the left when rolling toward the left). Rolling can be promoted further by flexing the hip and knee of the top lower extremity and placing it over the opposite limb (e.g., the hip and knee of the right lower extremity would be flexed and placed over the left when rolling toward the left).
5. In moving from the supine position to the prone position, pillows may be placed under one side of the pelvis (or scapula, if needed) to create initial rotation in the direction of the roll. The activity can be started with two pillows, progress to one, and then to rolling without the use of pillows. If difficulty is encountered in initiating the roll, the activity can be started from a sidelying position. To facilitate

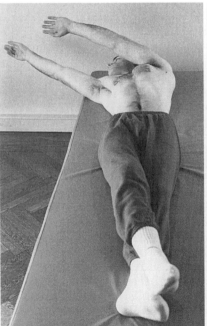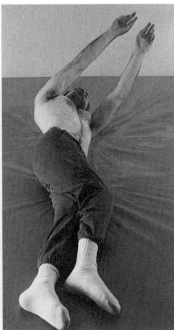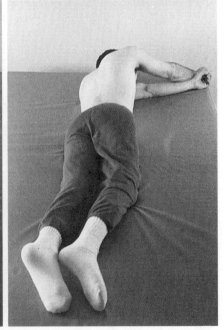

Figure 27-14. Rolling from supine position to prone position facilitated by upper extremity momentum and crossing of the ankles.

movement from prone to supine positions, pillows may be placed under one side of the chest and/or pelvis. Again, the number and height of pillows should be reduced gradually and eventually eliminated.

6. Several PNF patterns are useful during early rolling activities. The upper extremity patterns of D1 flexion, D2 extension, and reverse chop will facilitate rolling toward the prone position. The upper extremity lifting pattern will facilitate rolling toward the supine position from sidelying.

Prone-on-elbows Position

The functional implications of this activity are improved bed mobility and preparation for assuming the quadruped and sitting positions. This component of the mat progression facilitates head and neck control as well as proximal stability of the glenohumeral and scapular musculature via co-contraction. Scapular strengthening exercises also can be accomplished in this position. At first, the patient may require the therapist's assistance in assuming the prone-on-elbows position. To assume this position independently (from prone), the patient places the elbows close to the trunk and the hands near the shoulders and pushes the elbows down into the mat while lifting the head and upper trunk. From this position, one of two maneuvers can be used: (1) weight shifting from elbow to elbow will allow progressive movement of the elbows forward until they are under the shoulders; (2) or body weight can be shifted posteriorly until the elbows are under the shoulders.

The prone-on-elbows position must be used with caution, particularly following thoracic and lumbar injuries. Some patients may find it difficult to tolerate the increased lordotic curve imposed by this position.

1. Weight-bearing in the prone-on-elbows position will improve stability at the shoulders through increased joint approximation. Weight shifting assists with the development of controlled mobility and is usually easiest in a lateral direction with a progression to anterior or posterior movements.
2. Rhythmic stabilization may be used to increase stability of the head, neck, and scapula.
3. Manually applied approximation can be used to facilitate stabilization of proximal musculature.
4. Unilateral weight bearing on one elbow (static dynamic activity) can be achieved in the prone-on-elbows position by having the patient lift one arm. This further facilitates co-contraction in the weight-bearing limb.
5. Movement within this posture can be achieved by an on-elbows forward, backward, and side-to-side progression.
6. Strengthening of the serratus anterior and other scapular muscles can be achieved with prone-on-elbows push-ups. This is accomplished by having the patient push the elbows

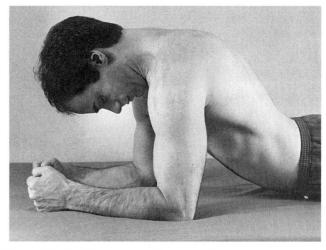

Figure 27-15. The prone-on-elbows position can be used for strengthening the serratus anterior and other scapular muscles.

down into the mat and tuck in the chin while lifting and rounding out the shoulders and upper thorax (Fig. 27-15). This is similar to the "cat/camel" maneuver used in the quadruped position. The patient lowers the chin and upper chest to the mat again by allowing the scapula to adduct.

Prone-on-hands Position (with Paraplegia)

The functional carryover of this position (Fig. 27-16) includes development of the initial hyperextension of the hips and low back for patients who will require this postural alignment during ambulation, and standing from a wheelchair or rising from the floor with crutches and bilateral knee-ankle-foot orthoses (KAFOs).

Some patients may have difficulty assuming this position initially, and a gradual acclimation may be indicated (strong pectoralis major and deltoid muscles are required to accomplish this activity). A gradual progression can be made by supporting the patient's upper trunk with a wide, firm bolster, wedge, or a sling suspension system. As the patient gradually becomes accustomed to the new position, the height of the support can be increased (if gradual acclimation is needed) and eventually removed.

Hand placement for the prone-on-hands position is similar to a standard push-up position except that the hands are slightly more lateral and the arms are externally rotated.

It should be noted that this position will not be appropriate for every patient with paraplegia owing to the excessive lordosis required to assume and to maintain the position.

1. Lateral weight shifting with weight transfer between hands will increase joint approximation.
2. Additional approximation force can be applied through manual contacts to facilitate tonic holding of proximal musculature further.
3. Scapular depression and prone push-ups may be utilized as strengthening exercises.

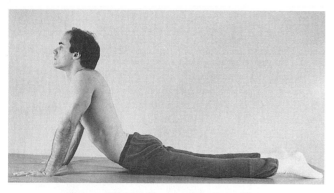

Figure 27-16. Prone-on-hands position.

Supine-on-elbows Position

The purpose of this activity is to assist with bed mobility and to prepare the patient to assume a long sitting position (Fig. 27-17). There are several approaches to assuming the supine-on-elbows position. If control of abdominal muscles is present, the patient may have sufficient strength to achieve the position by pushing the elbows into the mat and lifting into the position.

A more common technique is for the patient to "wedge" the hands under the hips or to hook the thumbs into pants pockets or belt loops. By contracting the biceps and/or wrist extensors, the patient can pull up partially into the posture. By shifting weight from side-to-side, the elbows can then be positioned under the shoulders.

Finally, some patients may find it easiest to assume this position from sidelying. The lower elbow is first positioned and pushed into the mat. The patient then rolls toward the supine position and quickly extends the upper arm, landing on the elbow as close to the shoulder as possible. By weight shifting, placement of the elbows can then be adjusted.

Much of the inherent benefit of this activity is achieved in learning to assume the posture and then move into long sittings. In addition to its direct functional significance, this activity is also an important strengthening exercise for shoulder extensors and scapular adductors.

1. Lateral weight shifting can be practiced in this position.
2. Side-to-side movement in this posture will

enhance the patient's ability to align the trunk over the lower extremities when in bed or in preparation for positional changes.

Pull-ups (with Tetraplegia)

The purpose of pull-ups is to strengthen the biceps and shoulder flexors in preparation for wheelchair propulsion. The patient is positioned in the supine position. The therapist assumes the high-kneeling position with one lower extremity on each side of the patient's hips. The therapist grasps the patient's supinated forearms just above the wrists. The patient pulls to sitting and then lowers back to the mat. Alternately, an overhead trapeze bar can be used for training.

Sitting

Both long (Fig. 27-18) and short (Fig. 27-19) sitting positions are essential for many activities of daily living, such as dressing, self-ROM, transfers, and wheelchair mobility. Good sitting balance and the ability to move within this posture are also critical prerequisite skills to standing.

Patients with tetraplegia require at least 100 degrees of straight-leg ROM to assume a long-sitting position. Without this available motion, hamstring tension will cause a posterior tilting of the pelvis. This will result in the patient's sitting on the sacrum, with resultant stretching of the lower back musculature.

It is important to note that sitting posture will vary considerably with lesion level. Patients with low thoracic lesions can be expected to sit with a relatively erect trunk. Individuals with low cervical and high thoracic lesions will maintain sitting balance by forward head displacement and trunk flexion. Patients with high cervical lesions will demonstrate poor sitting posture.

For patients with triceps and abdominal musculature (paraplegia), the sitting position can generally be assumed without difficulty. Patients with tetraplegia initially are taught to assume a stable sitting

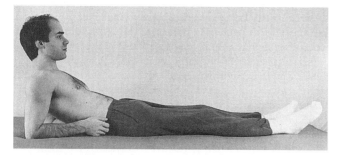

Figure 27-17. Supine-on-elbows position.

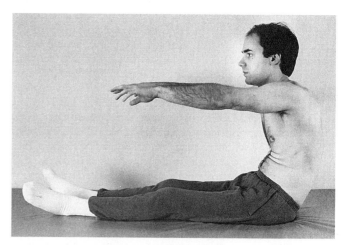

Figure 27-18. Individual with a T4 complete paraplegia in long-sitting position without upper extremity support.

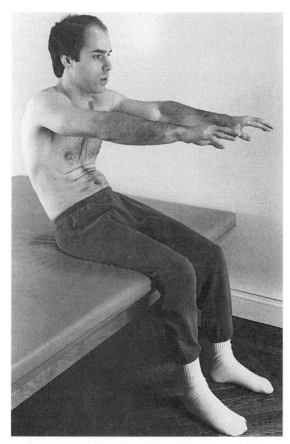

Figure 27-19. Individual with a T4 complete paraplegia in sitting position without upper extremity support.

position by placing the shoulders in hyperextension and external rotation, and the elbows and wrists in extension with the fingers flexed (flexion of the fingers is particularly important to avoid overstretching, which will interfere with a functional tenodesis grasp). Weight is then borne on the base of the hand. Patients without triceps function can be taught to lock the elbows mechanically, using shoulder girdle musculature. The patient first tosses the shoulder into hyperextension with the forearm supinated. Once the base of the hand makes contact with the mat, the shoulder is quickly elevated to extend the elbow, followed by rapid shoulder depression to maintain elbow extension. This technique will stabilize the arm in hyperextension and external rotation.

There are two basic approaches to instructing the patient to assume the sitting position. Starting in the supine-on-elbows position, the patient is instructed to shift weight from side to side. Once sufficient momentum is achieved, the patient tosses one arm behind and shifts the weight onto that extended arm. The opposite arm is then tossed behind into an extended position. From this point, the patient "walks" the arms forward until a stable sitting position is achieved.

From a prone-on-elbows position, the patient creeps sideward, using the elbows and forearms.

This will position the trunk in flexion and allow the patient to reach the lower extremities. The patient then hooks the uppermost forearm under the knee, pulls forward with this arm using the biceps, and then quickly tosses the opposite extremity behind. The upper extremity originally placed under the knee is then also thrown into an extended position. The patient then "walks" forward until a stable sitting position is achieved.

Numerous patients have developed their own variations on these basic techniques. Often patient-devised approaches may be the most appropriate for the individual and should be assessed in terms of safety, function, and energy expenditure. In addition, during the early stages of rehabilitation, adaptive equipment such as an overhead trapeze, rope ladders, or graduated loops hanging from over-bed frames may be used to facilitate movement into sitting.

Several suggestions that can be utilized in a sitting position are listed below.

1. Initial activities will focus on practice in maintaining the position. During early sitting, a mirror may provide important visual feedback.
2. Manual approximation force may be used at the shoulders to promote co-contraction.
3. A variety of PNF techniques may be used. Specifically, alternating isometrics and rhythmic stabilization are important in promoting early stability in this posture.
4. Balancing activities may be practiced in sitting. The base of support provided by the upper extremities can be gradually decreased, progress to single limb support, or, with some patients, be eliminated (see Figs. 27-18 and 27-19). The patient's limits of stability can be challenged progressively in each position. Activities such as ball throwing or tapping a balloon between the patient and therapist (with or without cuff weights) also may be incorporated into a progression of sitting activities.
5. Sitting push-ups are an important preliminary activity for transfers and ambulation. For tetraplegia, the patient is positioned with the shoulders in extension, the elbows locked, and the hands posterior to the hips. The patient leans forward and depresses the shoulders to clear the buttocks. Initially this activity may be facilitated by manual assistance from the therapist and/or by use of sandbags or small, hard bolsters to provide a firmer weight-bearing surface for the upper extremities (Fig. 27-20). For paraplegia, a progression can be achieved by initiating the activity with weight-bearing on the base of the hands placed directly on the mat and then using push-up blocks (Fig. 27-21) with graded increments in height.
6. Movement within this posture can be accomplished by using a sitting push-up in combination with momentum created by movement of

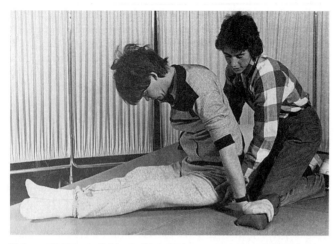

Figure 27-20. Individual with a C5 incomplete quadriplegia in long-sitting position. Push-ups are initially facilitated by manual assistance from the therapist with use of sandbags for weight-bearing. Note that hand placement maintains finger flexion during wrist extension to avoid stretching of the long finger flexors.

the head and upper body. This momentum is created by throwing the head and shoulders forcefully in the direction opposite to the desired direction of motion. For example, while performing a sitting push-up on the mat from a long sitting position. simultaneous rapid and forceful extension of the head and shoulders

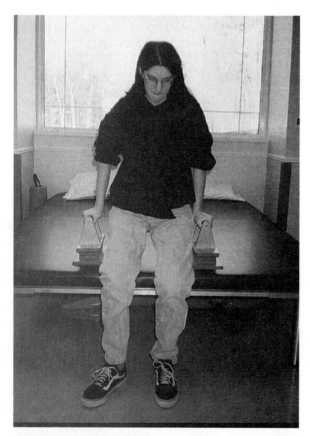

Figure 27-21. Individual with a complete lesion at T12 using push-up blocks in preparation for transfers and ambulation.

will move the lower extremities forward; movement in a posterior direction can be achieved by use of a sitting push-up with simultaneous rapid and forceful flexion of the head and trunk. This same progression of movement is used with the swing-to and swing-through gait patterns. Early mobility activities in both long and short sitting should emphasize adequate clearance of the buttocks for skin protection.

Quadruped Position

The functional implication of this all-fours position is its importance as a lead-up activity to ambulation. It is the first position in the mat sequence that allows weight-bearing through the hips and is useful for facilitating initial control of the available musculature of the lower trunk and hips.

Generally the patient is instructed to assume a quadruped position from the prone-on-elbows position. From this position the patient can "walk" backward on elbows, progressing to weight-bearing on hands, one at a time. Forceful flexion of the head, neck, and upper trunk while pushing into the mat with the elbows or hands will assist with elevating the pelvis. The patient continues to "walk" backward until the hips are positioned over the knees.

A second technique is to assume the quadruped posture from long sitting. In this approach the patient rotates the trunk to allow weight-bearing on the hands with the elbows extended. From this sidesitting position the patient then moves into the quadruped position by a combination of upper extremity and available trunk strength and momentum from the head and shoulders (moving opposite the direction of the hips).

Several suggested activities that can be utilized in the quadruped position are listed below.

1. Initial activities will involve practice in maintaining the position; rhythmic stabilization can be used to facilitate co-contraction.
2. Manual application of approximation force also can be used to facilitate co-contraction.
3. Weight shifting can be practiced in a forward, backward, and side-to-side direction.
4. Rocking through increments of range (forward, backward, side-to-side, and diagonally) will promote development of equilibrium responses.[102,103]
5. Alternately freeing one upper extremity from a weight-bearing position may be used in the quadruped position (Fig. 27-22). This static-dynamic control activity provides greater joint approximation forces on the supporting extremity and increased tonic holding of the available postural muscles (e.g., moving the dynamic limb in a diagonal pattern).
6. Movement within the quadruped position (creeping) has important implications for ambulation. Creeping can be used to improve strength (resisted forward progression), to facilitate dynamic balance reactions, and to improve coordination and timing.

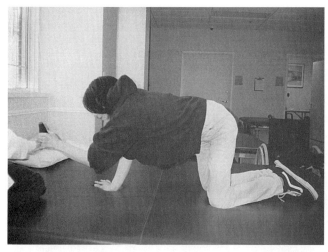

Figure 27-22. Static-dynamic activity. Freeing one upper extremity from a weight-bearing position will promote dynamic stability because of the reduction in the overall base of support and the shift of the center of gravity over the support limbs.

Kneeling Position

This position is particularly important for establishing functional patterns of trunk and pelvic control and for further promoting upright balance control. It is an important lead-up activity to ambulation using crutches and bilateral knee-ankle orthoses.

It is usually easiest to assist the patient into the kneeling position from the quadruped position. From the quadruped position, the patient moves or "walks" the hands backward until the knees further flex and the pelvis drops toward the heels. The patient will be "sitting" on the heels. From this position the patient may be assisted to kneeling by using the upper extremities to climb stall bars (wall ladder) while the therapist guides the pelvis. Another method is for the therapist to assume a heel-sitting position directly in front of the patient. The patient's upper extremities are supported on the therapist's shoulders while the therapist manually guides the pelvis. In time, the patient can be taught to assume a kneeling position using mat crutches (Fig. 27-23) or other support surface.

Several suggested activities that can be utilized during kneeling are listed below.

1. Initial activities will concentrate on maintaining the position using available musculature and postural alignment (hips fully extended with the pelvis slightly anterior to the knees).
2. The patient's balance may be challenged in this position. Balancing activities may progress from support with both upper extremities to support from only one.
3. A variety of mat crutch activities can be used in the kneeling position; examples include weight shifting anteriorly, posteriorly, and laterally, with emphasis on lower trunk and pelvic control; placing the crutches forward, backward, and to the side with weight shifts in each

direction, alternately raising one crutch at a time and returning it to the mat; hip hiking; instruction in gait pattern; and forward progression using crutches.

Transfers

Transfer training is generally initiated once the patient has achieved adequate sitting balance. It is a necessary prerequisite skill to many other functional activities, such as tub transfers, ambulation, and driving. Training is usually initiated on a firm mat surface and progresses to alternate surfaces such as a bed, toilet, bathtub, car, chair-to-floor (and reverse), and so forth. Patients with SCI most frequently use some variation of a sliding transfer (with or without the use of a sliding board) (Fig. 27-24) Some experimentation and problem solving between the patient and therapist are generally required to determine the most efficient and safest method for an individual patient. Patients using wheelchairs with tubular foot rests attached directly to the frame (nonremovable) typically transfer with the feet remaining on the tubular foot support (Fig. 27-25). This technique requires careful attention to balance strategies during transfer training.

As with all functional skills, the patient is instructed in the component parts of the activity (e.g., locking the brakes, removing the armrests, placing the sliding board) before the entire sequence is attempted.

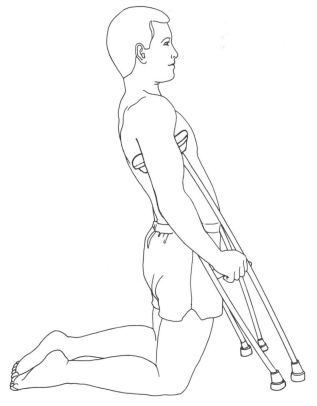

Figure 27-23. Kneeling position with use of mat crutches.

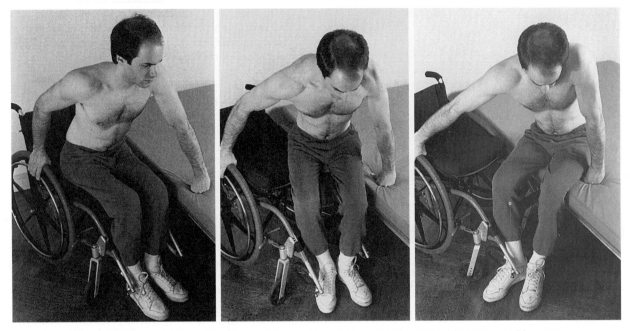

Figure 27-24. Individual with a T4 complete paraplegia transferring from wheelchair to mat without use of a sliding board.

Prescriptive Wheelchair

Most patients with SCI will use a wheelchair as the primary means of mobility. Even the patient with paraplegia who has mastered ambulation with crutches and orthoses will choose to use a wheelchair on many occasions because it provides a lower energy expenditure and greater speed and safety.

Because most patients will be using a wheelchair extensively, it should be custom-ordered (prescribed) for each individual. A wheelchair prescription will vary according to the level and extent of injury. More specific information is presented in

Chapter 32; however, some general considerations follow:

1. Seat depth should be as close as possible to 1 inch (2.5 cm) back from the popliteal space to allow an even weight distribution on the thighs and to prevent excessive pressure on the ischial tuberosities.
2. Floor-to-seat height is important. If a chair has a sling-type seat, a seat cushion will be required (some contoured, custom-designed seats eliminate the need for a seat cushion). The type and dimensions of the cushion or custom-seat must be known so that seat

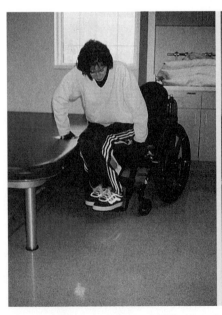
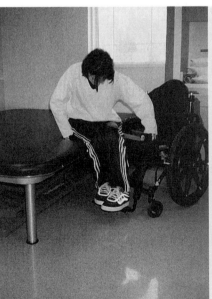
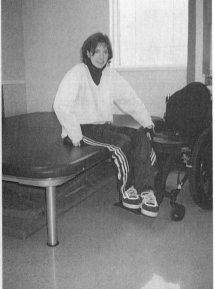

Figure 27-25. Transfer with feet remaining on permanently attached tubular foot supports.

height can be measured accurately, allowing adequate (2 in [5.1 cm]) clearance from the floor to the foot pedals, and can provide 90-degree angles at the knees.

3. Back height is also a consideration. If the patient will not be pushing the wheelchair, a high back may be desired for added comfort and stability. A patient with tetraplegia who will be pushing the wheelchair requires a back height that is below the inferior angle of the scapula so that the axilla is free of the handles during functional activities. Most patients with paraplegia prefer a lower back height, especially if they have intact abdominal muscles.

4. Seat width is variable. Wheelchairs come in narrow (16 in [40.6 cm]) or adult (18 in [46 cm]) sizes. The patient should be fitted in the narrowest chair possible as long as there is at least a hand's width between the hips and each side of the chair. The patient's previous weight should be considered, especially if there has been a significant loss since the initial injury, and potential exists to regain the weight. If orthoses are worn, they must also be included in the consideration of width.

5. Patients with lower extremity spasticity may require heel loops and/or toe loops on the footrests to keep the feet in place. A pelvic belt may be necessary for extensor spasms affecting the lower trunk and hips. Elevating footrests may be necessary if circulatory problems are present.

6. Removable armrests and detachable swing-away leg rests are important components of wheelchairs used by many patients with SCI. On some chairs (especially the newer models with tubular designs), the leg rests do not detach and the armrests are of a "flip-up" design. The suitability of these features must be considered with respect to the transfer capabilities and techniques used by the individual patient.

7. For individuals who plan to transfer into a car, a lightweight chair is an important

consideration. In addition, chairs designed without a below-seat crossbar further facilitate moving the chair into and out of a car. On these chairs the seat back folds down and the entire seating system lifts off. Each of the wheels can also be removed from the axle foundation. This design allows placement of the wheelchair into and out of the car as components rather than as one large unit.

8. Additional wheelchair accessories may be required to meet specific patient needs. Several features that warrant consideration include enlarged release mechanisms on the leg rests, a friction surface on the hand rims (rubber tubing wrapped around the hand rim is often effective), brake extensions, anti-tipping devices, and grade aids (which decrease backward movement of the chair while ascending inclined surfaces).

9. Electric wheelchairs are indicated for all patients with C4 lesions and above. Many patients with C5 level lesions also elect to use electric wheelchairs, particularly for long-distance travel. Tilt-in-space models are often prescribed. Controls are usually either joystick or puff-and-sip types. Hydraulic reclining units are available that allow patients with tetraplegia or high thoracic lesions to manage independent reclining and pressure relief.

10. Some patients may require more than one wheelchair. Many standard lightweight chairs currently available are suitable for sport and recreational activities. However, depending on the interests of the patient, a second chair specifically designed for a particular sport may be required (e.g., racing chairs).

Because patients with SCI are at high risk for skin breakdown, a wheelchair cushion will be required. A large variety of cushion styles are commercially available (see Chapter 32). The cushion should be comfortable, and provide a stable seating surface for functional use of the upper extremities. Figure 27-26 presents several styles of available seat cushions.

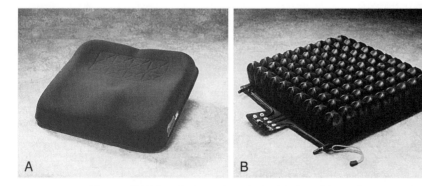
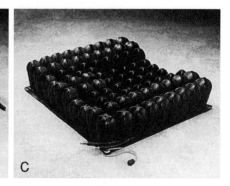

Figure 27-26. A large variety of wheelchair cushion styles are available. Shown here are *(A)* a contoured cushion, *(B)* high-profile air chamber cushion, and *(C)* a contoured air chamber cushion. (Courtesy of ROHO, Inc., Belleville, IL.)

Wheelchair Training

The patient should be taught how to operate all the specific parts of the wheelchair. Management of the brakes, arms, and pedals is crucial for all transfer activities. Many patients with limited hand function are able to propel the wheelchair by using the base of the hand against the hand rim. Some patients require assistive devices to aid in propulsion. Vertical or horizontal hand rim projections (Fig. 27-27) are useful for patients with poor hand function. The use of leather hand cuffs (or cycling gloves) will protect the skin and also will improve the patient's grip on the hand rims.

Wheelchair mobility activities should begin on level surfaces (including doorways and elevators) and progress to outdoor, uneven surfaces. Patients with sufficient upper extremity strength and upper trunk control also should be instructed in "wheelies," which involve balancing on the back wheels of the chair with the casters off the floor. Wheelies are required for independent curb climbing. Many facilities utilize canvas straps secured to the ceiling to assist with teaching this technique. The distal end of each strap has a C-clamp, which attaches to the push handle of the wheelchair. This allows safe practice by eliminating the danger of a posterior fall.

The patient should be instructed in pressure relief techniques from a sitting position. Ten to 15 seconds of pressure relief (or tissue redistribution) for every 5 to 10 minutes of sitting should become part of the patient's daily routine. Although many patients will develop their own techniques, several common approaches to these activities include (1) wheelchair push-ups (Fig. 27-28), (2) hooking an elbow or wrist around the push handle and leaning toward the opposite wheel (Fig. 27-29), and (3) hooking one elbow or wrist around the push handle and leaning forward (if triceps are available, hooking the elbow or wrist will be unnecessary).

Those patients who will be driving a car must learn how to fold and/or disassemble the wheelchair and slide it in and out of the car as well as learn

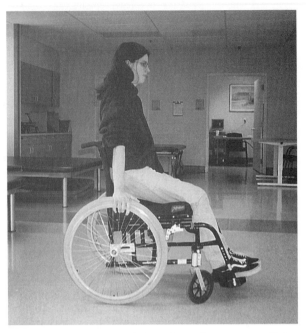

Figure 27-28. Wheelchair push-ups for pressure relief.

to drive with hand controls. Transfer techniques should be considered with respect to the type of car the patient will drive. Vans with self-contained ramps (Fig. 27-30) or lifting platforms are a great asset for patients with tetraplegia and can increase their functional independence significantly.

Ambulation: Patients with Paraplegia

After the patient has mastered bed, mat, and wheelchair activities, ambulation can be initiated. The goals of such training include (1) teaching

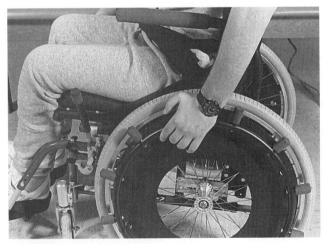

Figure 27-27. Hand rim projections assist with forward propulsion of wheelchair for patients with limited grip.

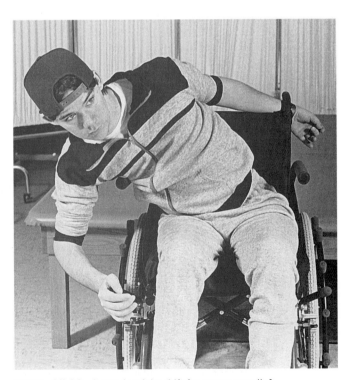

Figure 27-29. Lateral weight shift for pressure relief.

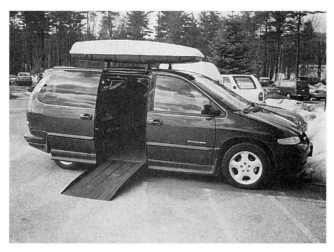

Figure 27-30. Ramp allows entry to van while individual remains seated in a wheelchair.

functional ambulation, or (2) increasing physiological standing tolerance. Standing tolerance can be enhanced by use of a tilt-table, standing platform, or standing frame (Fig. 27-31).

Initially, most patients expect that they will become functional ambulators. A number of factors will influence the success or failure in attaining this goal. Patients must possess adequate muscle strength, postural alignment, ROM, and sufficient cardiovascular endurance to be considered a candidate for ambulation. Patients who become func-

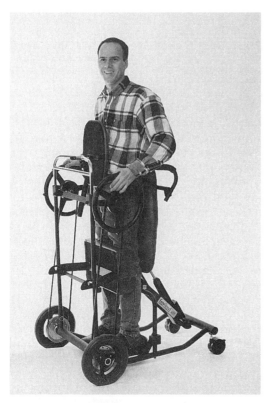

Figure 27-31. A standing frame provides mobility within environment. The posterior support can be moved slowly into a seat configuration to facilitate transfers. (Courtesy of Altimate Medical, Morton, MN.)

tional ambulators are those whose trunk muscles (abdominals and erector spinae) grade fair or better. This usually excludes patients with high thoracic lesions (T2–T8) who lack the ability to stabilize the trunk and pelvis and, in addition, who demonstrate poor respiratory reserve. Patients with incomplete lesions who demonstrate some residual strength in one or both hip flexors and/or quadriceps are more likely to achieve success in ambulating functionally.[122]

Inasmuch as spinal bracing is too restrictive, heavy, and impractical for functional ambulation, adequate ROM and postural alignment are crucial in achieving stability of the trunk. Full ROM in hip extension is essential in attaining balance in the upright position. The patient learns to lean into the anterior ligaments of the hip to stabilize the trunk or pelvis. The absence of knee flexion and plantarflexion contractures is also important in attaining upright standing balance.

Adequate cardiovascular endurance also is a criterion for functional ambulation.[123] Because the energy cost of ambulation for a patient with paraplegia is two to four times greater than normal walking, endurance becomes an important factor in determining success or failure as a functional ambulator. Although some training effects can be attained with a program of endurance training for the upper extremities, the patient's age, body weight, and history of cardiovascular disease or respiratory problems can restrict the amount that can be achieved. Other factors that may restrict ambulation include severe spasticity, loss of proprioception (particularly at the hips and knees), pain, and the presence of secondary complications such as decubitus ulcers, heterotopic bone formation at the hips, or deformity. In addition, the patient's motivation plays a key role in determining success or failure in ambulation. A highly motivated patient can learn to ambulate with limited residual function. However, these patients may eventually find that the energy cost of ambulation is too great.

Follow-up studies of long-term continuation of ambulation have not been extensive. Mikelberg and Reid[124] surveyed 60 individuals with SCI for whom orthotics had been prescribed. From this group, 60 percent used their wheelchairs as the primary means of mobility. Thirty-one percent completely discarded their orthoses. Those that did use their orthoses reserved them primarily for standing and exercise activities. Considering the high cost of orthoses and ambulatory training, the authors suggest careful individual consideration of each patient before orthoses are prescribed. They also suggest delaying decisions about ambulation; training might reasonably occur during later, follow-up care.

Orthotic Prescription

The orthotic prescription varies according to the lesion level. Usually only ankle and/or knee control bracing is necessary. Patients with low thoracic lesions, T9 to T12, will require KAFOs. Conventional KAFOs include bilateral metal uprights, posterior thigh and calf bands, an anterior knee flexion pad, drop-ring or bail locks, adjustable locked ankle joints, a heavy-duty stirrup, and a cushion heel. The ankle joints are usually locked in 5 to 10 degrees of dorsiflexion to assist hip extension at heel strike. Orthotic hip control is not necessary, because the braces allow the patient to balance weight over the feet with the hips hyperextended (Fig. 27-32). The center of gravity is kept posterior to the hip joints but anterior to the ankles.

The Scott-Craig orthosis[125] is another type of KAFO that is frequently prescribed for patients with paraplegia (see Chapter 31). These orthoses consist of standard double uprights, an offset knee joint providing improved biomechanical alignment, bail locks, a posterior thigh band, an anterior tibial band, adjustable ankle joint, and a sole plate that extends beyond the metatarsal heads. A modification of this orthosis (Fig. 27-33) includes a plastic solid ankle section in place of the metal ankle joint and sole plate. This change decreases overall weight of the orthosis, improves cosmesis, and eliminates the need for custom-made shoes.[126]

Another type of orthotic device available to patients with SCI is the reciprocating gait orthosis (RGO) (see Chapter 31). The RGO is composed of two plastic KAFOs that are joined by a molded pelvic

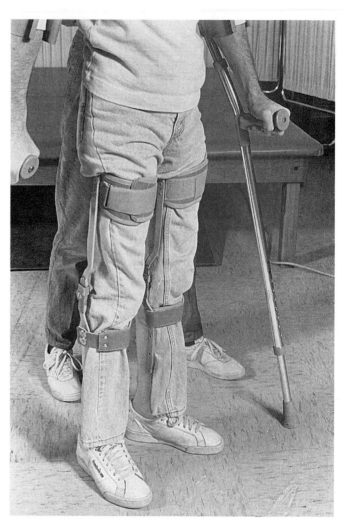

Figure 27-33. New England Regional Spinal Cord Injury Center (NERSCIC) orthosis (modification of the Craig-Scott orthosis). Note that patient is wearing orthoses over clothing for purposes of demonstration.

band with thoracic extensions. The RGO has a dual-cable system that runs posteriorly and attaches at the hip joints. These cable attachments transmit forces between lower extremities and provide reciprocal movement. Movement at the hip in one direction facilitates movement in the opposite direction on the contralateral hip. For example, as weight is shifted onto the left lower extremity the right is moved forward. The dual-cable system allows control of both flexion and extension. These cables function to "coordinate" action between the two extremities during ambulation. As the advancing leg is unloaded, it is assisted into flexion while the stance leg is simultaneously pushed into extension. Thus, the orthosis allows for unilateral leg advancement and a reciprocating gait pattern. With this orthosis, a two- or four-point gait pattern can be used in combination with crutches or a reciprocating walker. Movement to a seated position is accomplished by unlocking the drop lock at the knee joint.[127–129]

Pelvic bands and spinal attachments are rarely prescribed for use with conventional KAFOs. These

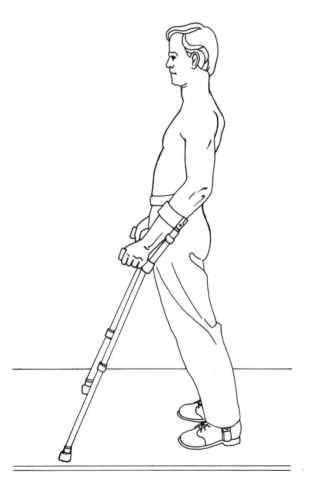

Figure 27-32. Standing alignment using bilateral knee-ankle-foot orthoses. Note that the upright position is maintained by leaning into the anterior Y ligaments, creating hyperextension at the hips.

attachments severely restrict dressing activities, movement from sitting-to-standing, and ambulation, by reducing trunk and pelvis flexibility and by adding extra weight (often as much as 4 lbs). Furthermore, the use of these components makes gait slow, laborious, and usually nonfunctional. Patients who would require these attachments (T2–T8 lesions) are usually not candidates for orthotic prescription. Instead, these patients can achieve physiological standing with the use of posterior splints, or standing frame.

Ankle-foot orthoses (AFOs) are often appropriate for patients with lower-level lesions (e.g., L3 and below). Either a conventional metal-upright or plastic AFO may be indicated. Patients with lesions of L3 and below often demonstrate a maximus-medius gait pattern. The absence of control of gluteal muscles and hamstrings result in a sharp posterior movement of the trunk at heel strike. Lateral trunk flexion also will be noted at midstance. Crutches or canes are typically prescribed to improve the patient's gait pattern.

The Vannini-Rizzoli orthosis is a stabilizing boot most frequently used for patients with paraplegia (see Chapter 31). It is composed of a plastic orthosis conformed to the shape of the leg which is then inserted into a leather boot. The ankle is held in approximately 15 degrees of plantarflexion shifting the patient's center of gravity anterior to the ankles. Standing requires that the hips and knees be held in extension with the trunk in lumbar lordosis. The plantarflexion angle at the ankle stabilizes the knee in standing. Ambulation is achieved by shifting the trunk from side-to-side and swinging the unweighted limb forward. The orthosis is used with crutches, a walker, or bilateral canes.[130,131]

Functional Electrical Stimulation

Functional electrical stimulation (FES) involves the use of electrical stimulation to elicit a muscle contraction that translates into a functional activity. In recent years, this approach has become increasingly promising for patients with SCI as a mechanism to improve function and maintain muscle mass and bone density. Most work in this area has focused on control of standing and stepping functions, exercise activities, and upper extremity activities of daily living (ADLs). It has also been used with cycle ergometry to improve endurance. The gait patterns achieved are somewhat unrefined and allow for only short-distance ambulation.[132–135]

Electrical impulses for FES are provided via surface electrodes, surgically implanted electrodes, or percutaneous electrodes.[135] The electrical stimulation is interfaced with a computer, which controls the timing and onset of stimulation. The majority of systems in use are controlled by an open loop system. That is, the stimulus intensity and order of stimulation is preprogrammed for the individual. The problem with this system is lack of stimulus gradation and frequent overstimulation of the targeted muscle. The current focus of research is directed toward a closed loop system in which movement is also initiated by the user but is modified without the user's input. For example, a movement could be modified without the user's knowledge by a feedback measure such as force or position.[135]

Although not yet in widespread clinical use, application of FES is expanding gradually. It has enabled some individuals to ambulate on level surfaces, stairs, and mild inclines, and to perform some upper extremity functional activities. Function has been further enhanced by combining FES with both upper and lower extremity orthoses. The RGO is frequently used in this capacity. FES appears to hold some future potential for achieving functional ambulation and improved upper extremity function for selected patients with SCI. However, the current high cost of FES training is generally prohibitive for most patients.

Gait Training

A swing-through type of gait pattern (Fig. 27-34) should be the ultimate goal for functional ambulators with KAFOs. In teaching this pattern, it is important to stress a smooth, even cadence. Crutches should be placed equidistant from both toes at toe-off and be equidistant from both heels at heel strike. It is important to establish an overall rhythm, as improved timing will result in improved energy efficiency and cosmesis. Relevant training activities include those described below.

1. *Putting on and removing orthoses.* The patient is first taught the correct way to apply the orthoses. The entire procedure is usually done in the supine or sitting position. The patient must be cautioned to check constantly for pressure areas, particularly after brace removal.

2. *Sit-to-stand activities.* These activities should be practiced in the parallel bars using a wheelchair. The patient must learn to slide to the edge of the chair and lock and unlock the orthoses. Initially the patient is taught to pull to standing, using the parallel bars (a progression is made to using the wheelchair armrests to push to standing). Once in an upright position, the patient pushes down on the hands and tilts the pelvis forward in front of the shoulders. Return to sitting is a reversal of this procedure.

3. *Trunk balancing.* The patient learns to balance the trunk in the hips-extended position, keeping the weight balanced over the feet, and learns to remove first one hand then both from the support. Placing hands forward and backward behind the hips while maintaining a stable position should also be practiced. Chapter 14 should be consulted for a more detailed description of suggestions for early parallel bar activities.

4. *Push-ups.* This includes lifting the body off the floor using shoulder depression, ducking the head to gain added height, and controlled lowering of the body.

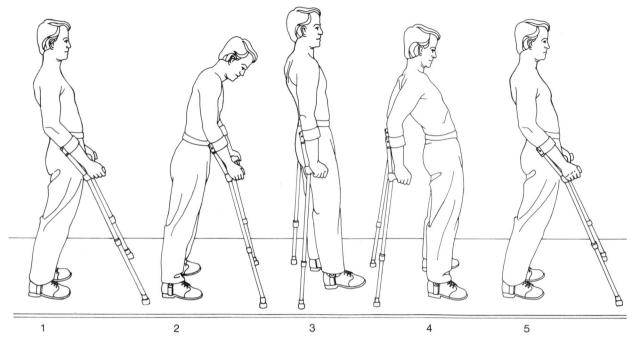

Figure 27-34. Swing-through gait pattern.

5. *Turning around.* This involves lifting and lowering the body in 90-degree turns and changing hands from one bar to another.
6. *Jack-knifing.* This entails controlling the pelvic position using upper extremity support and positioning the head and shoulders forward

ahead of the pelvis. This is an unstable position, and the patient must be taught recovery to overcome and/or to prevent this from happening during ambulation.
7. *Ambulation activities in the parallel bars.* Four- and two-point gaits require hip flexion or hip

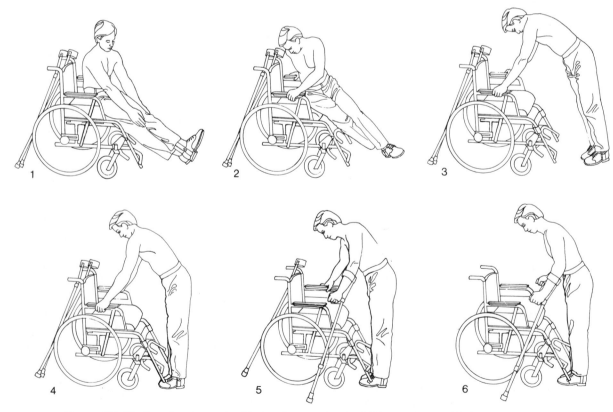

Figure 27-35. Standing from wheelchair using crutches and bilateral knee-ankle-foot orthoses. The reverse sequence is used to return to the chair.

hiking. Patients with high lesions may learn this movement using the secondary hip hikers (internal and external obliques and latissimus dorsi). Those with low lesions will have the quadratus lumborum intact. Trunk rotation on the swing side or lateral flexion toward the stance side will facilitate forward progression.

Swing-to and swing-through gaits require varying degrees of body elevation and push off. These gait patterns involve some jack-knifing and recovery. At push off, the head ducks to gain increased height, and at foot contact the head and back arch to help regain stability.

Forearm crutches are most often selected for patients with paraplegia. These crutches provide several advantages. They are lightweight; they allow use of the hand without the crutch becoming disengaged; they fit more easily into an automobile; and, most importantly, they improve function in ambulation and stair climbing by allowing unrestricted movement at the shoulders.

1. *Standing from the wheelchair with crutches.* To begin this activity the patient first places the crutches behind the chair, leaning against the push handle(s). To assume a standing position with crutches, the patient moves forward in the chair, locks both knee joints, crosses one leg over the other (Fig. 27-35), and then rotates the trunk and pelvis. Hand placements on the armrest are reversed and the patient pushes to standing by pivoting around to face the chair. The reverse of this technique is used to return to the chair.

2. *Crutch balancing.* Initially, the patient must learn to become secure in the tripod stance. This is best achieved by first balancing in the parallel bars or against a wall. Weight shifting, alternating lifting one crutch off the floor, and jack-knifing should be practiced.

3. *Ambulation activities.* Four-point, two-point, swing-to, and swing-through gaits should be practiced. They demonstrate a progression from a slow, steady gait pattern to a faster, more unstable one. A gradual emphasis should be placed on improved timing and speed.

4. *Travel activities.* The patient should become proficient in walking sideward and backward, turning, and walking through doorways. Changes in floor surface (e.g., carpeting, tile) and terrain (sidewalks and grass) may present

problems for the patient if they are not introduced during training. All patients will require proficiency in ambulation on level surfaces to master these more difficult activities successfully.

5. *Elevation activities.* The easiest pattern of ascent or descent of stairs is usually upstairs backward (Fig. 27-36) and downstairs forward (Fig. 27-37). Most patients will use a handrail; only the very exceptional patient can manage stairs without one. Once some degree of proficiency is attained, going upstairs forward and downstairs backward can be practiced as well. The use of graduated steps will help make the initial task of learning easier. The therapist needs to guard and to support the patient adequately. The use of a properly fitting guarding belt is essential. Curbs should be attempted last, because this is usually the most difficult elevation activity. Using graduated platforms or curbs will assist the patient in mastery of this task. A four-point gait pattern, going up backward and down forward is the slower, more stable method. Swinging both legs up together takes considerable balance and is for the more advanced ambulator.

6. *Falling.* Controlled falling and getting up from the floor are important considerations for patients expected to become functional ambulators.

LONG-RANGE PLANNING

An important aspect of long-range rehabilitation planning involves educating the patient in lifelong management of the disability. This will focus on community reintegration and methods of maintaining the optimal state of health and function achieved during rehabilitation. Consideration must be given to multiple issues, including housing, nutrition, transportation, finances, maintaining functional skills and level of physical fitness, employment or further education, and methods for involvement in desired social or recreational activities. Each of these issues must be addressed early in the course of rehabilitation in consultation with the patient, family, and appropriate team members. The patient also should be encouraged to contact and to explore the resources available through publications and re-

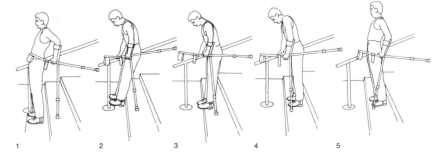

Figure 27-36. Ascending stairs backward. The crutch is placed on the step to which the patient is ascending. The head and trunk are forcefully flexed while depressing the shoulders and extending the elbows. This maneuver unweights the lower extremities and creates momentum for movement to the next higher step. Postural alignment is then regained.

1   2   3   4   5

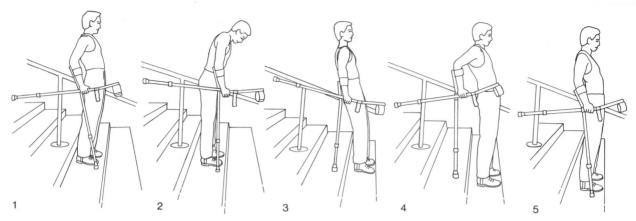

Figure 27-37. Descending stairs forward. To begin, the crutch remains on the step that the patient is leaving. Initial flexion of the head and trunk is immediately followed by forceful extension while depressing the shoulders and extending the elbow. This procedure unweights the lower extremities and creates momentum for the movement to the next lower step. The crutch is then lowered and postural alignment regained.

gional national chapters of The National Spinal Cord Injury Association. Several potential sources of information are listed below.

1. National Spinal Cord Injury Association
   8701 Georgia Ave., Suite 500
   Silver Springs, MD 20910
   web site: http://www.spinalcord.org
   SCI hotline: 800-526-3456
2. Periodicals such as *SCI Life*
   545 Concord Ave., Suite 29,
   Cambridge, MA 02138
3. *Spinal Network*
   P.O. Box 4162
   Boulder, CO 80306
4. *Paraplegia News*
   2111 East Highland, Suite 180
   Phoenix, AZ 85016
5. *Disability Rag*
   Circulation and Subscription Office
   P.O. Box 145
   Louisville, KY 40201
6. *Sports and Spokes*
   2111 East Highland, Suite 180
   Phoenix, AZ 85016
7. *New Mobility*
   c/o Miramar Communications Inc.
   P.O. Box 15518
   North Hollywood, CA 91615

The National Spinal Cord Injury Association's National Resource Directory will provide the patient with current information on a variety of topics such as research related to SCI, legislative activities, conferences, housing, transportation, new adaptive equipment, and sporting and recreational activities. Many cities have local chapters of The National

Spinal Cord Injury Association. The National Spinal Cord Injury Information Resource Center (NSCIRC) maintains a helpline (phone: 800-962-9629) that provides information on a variety of topics related to SCI. Membership in The National Spinal Cord Injury Association is also available to health care professionals. Finally, a coordinated plan must be developed for long-term periodic rehabilitation follow-up visits.

SUMMARY

This chapter has presented the principal clinical manifestations, indirect impairments, and secondary complications of traumatic SCI. Emphasis has been placed on physical therapy intervention during both the acute and subacute phases of rehabilitation. Anticipated goals and outcomes and treatment interventions have been addressed. Each must be tailored to meet the needs of an individual patient. This will be achieved through a process of careful assessment with specific attention to length of time since onset, lesion level, method(s) of fracture stabilization, premorbid interests, psychosocial factors, and presence of secondary complications.

Management of the patient with SCI is a complex and challenging task in which continuity of care is critical to achieving the overall goals of rehabilitation. Frequent and open communication among team members, patient, and family is vital to maintaining an organized and highly individualized approach to both rehabilitation and reintegration of the patient into the community.

QUESTIONS FOR REVIEW

1. Identify the clinical features of Brown-Sequard, anterior, central, and posterior cord syndromes.

2. Define spinal shock.
3. Describe the impairments associated with spinal cord injury. Your description should

address alterations that occur in each of the following areas:

    a. Motor function
    b. Sensory function
    c. Temperature control
    d. Respiratory function
    e. Muscle tone
    f. Bladder and bowel function
    g. Sexual function

4. What is autonomic dysreflexia? Describe the initiating stimuli and symptoms of this syndrome. What action would you take if a patient experienced an onset of symptoms during a physical therapy treatment?

5. What is heterotopic ossification? Describe the early symptoms. Where does it most commonly develop following SCI?

6. Describe the clinical features of deep venous thrombosis. Why are patients with SCI at risk for development of this secondary complication?

7. Suggest a positioning program to prevent limitations in ROM at the shoulders for a patient with tetraplegia during the acute phase of management.

8. Identify three primary factors affecting prognosis following spinal cord injury.

9. Describe the major advantages of halo devices as compared with tongs for immobilizing cervical fractures.

10. What is included in a physical therapy assessment during the acute phase of management? How might some of the standard assessment techniques have to be modified?

11. What is meant by the term *selective stretching*?

12. Identify the primary goals of respiratory care during the acute phase of management. Suggest potential treatment activities to meet these goals.

13. What forms of strengthening exercises are appropriate during the acute phase? Why are bilateral upper extremity activities emphasized?

14. Outline sample mat progressions for two patients, one with a C6 tetraplegia and one with a T12 paraplegia. Assume that both patients have complete lesions. Describe the specific mat sequence and activities you would include. Identify the functional significance of each. What type of progressive strengthening activities would you suggest for each patient as an adjunct to the mat program?

CASE STUDY

HISTORY: Patient is a 40 year-old male who was involved in a motor vehicle accident. Upon admission to a trauma center, he was found to have a fracture at the level of T4 with no motor or sensory function distal to T4 level. He was treated with a course of methylprednisolone and immobilized in a plastic body jacket. After a 3-week hospital stay, he was transferred to the local rehabilitation center. His status was as follows:

- Nonambulatory
- Trace MMT grades of hip flexors and external rotators, otherwise without active movement in both lower extremities (BLEs)
- Absent sensation below the nipple line
- Dependent in bed mobility, transfers, dressing, and bathing; some assist needed with feeding
- Incontinent of bowel and bladder
- Brisk knee and ankle jerk reflexes with bilateral ankle clonus and bilateral positive Babinski

He received a 6-week course of rehabilitation and was discharged home with the following functional status:

- Transfer activities: FIM level 5; supervision required for safety (uncontrollable spasms can throw him out of w/c)
- W/c mobility: FIM level 7
- Self-care:

Dressing: FIM level 3
Bathing: FIM level 3
Sphincter control: FIM level 2

Over the course of the next 7 months he remained at home with limited functional independence. He exhibited continued bowel and bladder incontinence, continuing paralysis and sensory loss below T4, severe spasticity in abdominals and BLEs, and severe extensor thrust which caused him to jack-knife out of w/c. His out of bed time was limited to 4 hours per day and he was unable to return to community mobility or work.

Recently he was referred for surgical implantation of an intrathecal baclofen pump. Following surgery an immediate decrease was noted in spasticity in the abdominals and BLEs. He is now referred for active rehabilitation to your facility.

PAST MEDICAL HISTORY: Unremarkable.

CURRENT MEDICAL MANAGEMENT

- Intrathecal baclofen (Lioresal)
- External catheter
- Bowel program: suppositories, digital stimulation techniques

SOCIAL HISTORY: He lives with his wife in a first floor apartment they recently moved to. He has a w/c accessible bathroom including shower. He is presently out of work but wants to return part time to his position as a computer programmer as soon as possible. His level of spasticity and extensor spasms had previously prevented this from serious consideration.

PHYSICAL THERAPY ASSESSMENT

Cognitive: alert, oriented × 3
Communication: WNL
Visual/Auditory: WNL
GI/GU: spastic bowel and bladder
Cardiopulmonary Status

- No apparent cardiac or respiratory dysfunction
- Level of deconditioning: unable to assess at the present time

Sensation: T6 level; reports diminished sensation below sternum

Pain
- Reports abdominal pain secondary to spasticity and spasms.
- Reports some discomfort in BLEs.

Skin Condition/Edema: WNL, no areas of breakdown noted.

ROM
- Bilateral hip flexion contractures: unable to measure secondary to spasticity
- Bilateral knee flexion contractures: L knee 20 to 120 degrees, R knee 30 to 110 degrees, (unable to fully extend knees due to spasm and pain)
- Bilateral ankle limitations: L ankle dorsiflexion to neutral only; with knee flexion, R ankle dorsiflexion 0 to 5 degrees

Posture
- Severe forward head with rounded shoulders
- Sits with posterior pelvic tilt
- Has difficulty maintaining upright sitting, tends to fall to left

Motor Control
Tone
- Moderate increase in tone BLEs (3 on the modified Ashworth scale)
- Moderate increase in trunk tone (3 on the modified Ashworth scale)
- Patient reports decreased spasticity since pump implantation; no additional episodes of jack-knifing out of w/c

Voluntary control/ strength:
- Loss of voluntary muscle control below T4 except for: Sitting, able to lift L heel off floor through ¼ ROM.

On powder board:
L poor (2/5) hip ext (full range)
L poor (2/5) knee ext (range limited by contracture)
R trace (1/5) hip ext
R trace (1/5) knee ext
R trace (1/5) hip and knee flex
Bilateral trace (1/5) gluteals: unable to bridge

Balance
Sitting
- Static control: independent in sitting, less than

1 minute with bilateral UE support; unable to maintain sitting without UE support
- Dynamic control: goes through minimal excursions with loss of balance (LOB) at end range; less than 30 percent of normal sway
- Standing: unable to stand

Gait: N/A

Functional Mobility (FIM)
Locomotion: level 7 (w/c independent in home, limited community mobility)
Transfers: level 7 (independent in lateral slide transfer with transfer board)

Self-Care
Dressing: level 4 (requires minimal assist to put on socks and shoes)
Bathing: level 5 (shower chair and set-up required)
Sphincter control: level 3

Endurance: Tolerated 45-minute examination with minimal fatigue

Equipment
- Wheelchair: Quickie design
- Pressure-relieving fluid/foam cushion

Patient is very motivated and cooperative. He wants to walk and regain lower extremity strength and return to work.

Case Study Guiding Questions

1. Identify/categorize this patient's problems in terms of
   a. Direct impairments
   b. Indirect impairments
   c. Composite impairments: combined effects of both direct and indirect impairments
   d. Functional limitations/disabilities
2. Identify three goals (remediation of impairments) and three outcomes (remediation of functional limitations/disability) for this patient.
3. Formulate five treatment interventions with one progression that could be used during the first 3 weeks of therapy. Provide a brief rationale that justifies your choice.
4. Identify relevant motor learning strategies appropriate for the initial physical therapy sessions with this patient.

REFERENCES

1. Cash, L: The status of spinal cord research: A reason to hope. SCI Life 10:12, 1999.
2. Spinal Cord Injury: Facts and Figures at a Glance. The National Spinal Cord Injury Statistical Center. University of Alabama, Birmingham, 1998.
3. International Standards for Neurological and Functional Classification of Spinal Injury. American Spinal Injury Association (ASIA) and International Medical Society of Paraplegia, Chicago, 1996.
4. Michaelis, LS: International inquiry on neurological terminology and prognosis in paraplegia and tetraplegia. Paraplegia 7:1, 1969.
5. Coogler, CE: Clinical decision making among neurologic patients: Spinal cord injury. In Wolf, SL (ed): Clinical Decision Making in Physical Therapy. FA Davis, Philadelphia, 1985, p 149.
6. Rieser, TV, et al: Orthopedic evaluation of spinal cord injury and management of vertebral fractures. In Adkins, HV (ed): Spinal Cord Injury. Churchill Livingstone, New York, 1985, p 1.
7. Gilman, S and Newman, SW: Manter and Gatz's Essentials of Clinical Neuroanatomy and Neurophysiology, ed 9. FA Davis, Philadelphia, 1996.
8. Lundy-Ekman, L: Neuroscience: Fundamentals for Rehabilitation. Saunders, Philadelphia, 1998.
9. Atrice, MB, et al: Traumatic spinal cord injury. In Umphred, DA (ed): Neurological Rehabilitation, ed 3. CV Mosby, St. Louis, 1995, p 484.
10. Levi, ADO, et al: Clinical syndromes associated with disproportionate weakness of the upper versus the lower extremities after cervical spinal cord injury. Neurosurgery 38:179, 1996.

11. Alexeeva, N: Central cord syndrome of cervical spinal cord injury: Widespread changes in muscle recruitment studied by voluntary contractions and transcranial magnetic stimulation. Exp Neurol 148:399, 1997.

12. Brodkey, JS, et al: The syndrome of acute central cervical spinal cord injury revisited. Surg Neurol 14:251, 1980.

13. Esses, SI: Textbook of Spinal Disorders. JB Lippincott, Philadelphia, 1995.

14. Rogers, LF: Fractures and dislocations of the spine. In Calenoff, L (ed): Radiology of Spinal Cord Injury. CV Mosby, St. Louis, 1981.

15. McKinnis, LN: Fundamentals of Orthopedic Radiology. FA Davis, Philadelphia, 1997.

16. Buchanan, LE: An overview. In Buchanan, LE, and Nawoczenski, DA (eds): Spinal Cord Injury: Concepts and Management Approaches. Williams & Wilkins, Baltimore, 1987, p 1.

17. Buchanan, LE: Emergency care. In Buchanan, LE, and Nawoczenski, DA (eds): Spinal Cord Injury: Concepts and Management Approaches. Williams & Wilkins, Baltimore, 1987, p 21.

18. English, E: Mechanisms of cervical spine injuries. In Tator, CH (ed): Early Management of Acute Spinal Cord Injury. Raven, New York, 1982, p 25.

19. Young, PA, and Young, PH: Basic Clinical Neuroanatomy. Williams & Wilkins, Baltimore, 1997.

20. Edibam, RC: Medical management. In Bedbrook, G (ed): The Care and Management of Spinal Cord Injuries. Springer-Verlag, New York, 1981, p 109.

21. Guyton, AC, and Hall, JE: Human Physiology and Mechanisms of Disease, ed 6. Saunders, Philadelphia, 1997.

22. Lemons, VR, and Wagner, FC: Respiratory complication after cervical spinal cord injury. Spine 19:2315, 1994.

23. Jackson, AB, and Groomes, TE: Incidence of respiratory complications following spinal cord injury. Arch Phys Med Rehabil 75:270, 1994.

24. Alvarez, SE, et al: Respiratory treatment of the adult patient with spinal cord injury. Phys Ther 61:1737, 1981.

25. Moore, KL: Clinically Oriented Anatomy, ed 3. Williams & Wilkins, Baltimore, 1992.

26. Smith, LK, et al: Brunnstrom's Clinical Kinesiology, ed 5. FA Davis, Philadelphia, 1996.

27. Nixon, V: Spinal Cord Injury: A Guide to Functional Outcomes in Physical Therapy Management. Aspen, Rockville, MD, 1985.

28. Wetzel, J: Respiratory evaluation and treatment. In Adkins, HV: Spinal Cord Injury. Churchill-Livingstone, New York, 1985, p 75.

29. Bach, JR, and Wang, TG: Pulmonary function and sleep disordered breathing in patients with traumatic tetraplegia: A longitudinal study. Arch Phys Med Rehabil 75:279, 1994.

30. Seidel, AC: Spinal cord injury. In Logigian, MK (ed): Adult Rehabilitation: A Team Approach for Therapists. Little, Brown, Boston, 1982, p 325.

31. Campbell, SK, et al: The effects of intrathecally administered baclofen on function in patients with spasticity. Phys Ther 75:352, 1995.

32. Rosen, JS: Rehabilitation process. In Calenoff, L (ed): Radiology of Spinal Cord Injury. CV Mosby, St. Louis, 1981, p 309.

33. Bromley, I: Tetraplegia and Paraplegia: A Guide for Physiotherapists, ed 3. Churchill-Livingstone, New York, 1985.

34. Buchanan, LE, and Ditunno, JF: Acute care: Medical/surgical management. In Buchanan, LE and Nawoczenski, DA (eds): Spinal Cord Injury: Concepts and Management Approaches. Williams & Wilkins, Baltimore, 1987, p 35.

35. Dolan, JT: Clinical management of the patient with a spinal disorder. In Ruppert, SD, Kernicki, JG, and Dolan, JT: Dolan's Critical Care Nursing: Clinical Management Through the Nursing Process, (ed 2). FA Davis, Philadelphia, 1991, p 613.

36. Cardenas, DD, et al: Manual stimulation of reflex voiding after spinal cord injury. Arch Phys Med Rehabil 66:459, 1985.

37. Zejdlik, CP: Maintaining urinary function. In Zejdlik, CP (ed): Management of Spinal Cord Injury, ed 2. Jones and Bartlett, Boston, 1992, p 353.

38. Comarr, AE, and Vigue, M: Sexual counseling among male and female patients with spinal cord and/or cauda equina injury, I. Am J Phys Med 57:107, 1978.

39. Trieschmann, RB: Spinal Injuries: Psychological, Social and Vocational Adjustment, ed 2. Demos Publications, New York, 1988.

40. Miller, S, et al: Sexual health care clinician in an acute spinal cord injury unit. Arch Phys Med Rehabil 62:315, 1981.

41. Weitzenkamp, DA, et al: Spouses of spinal cord injury survivors: The added impact of caregiving. Arch Phys Med Rehabil 78:822, 1997.

42. Dunn, KL: Sexuality education and the team approach. In Sipski, ML, and Alexander, CJ (eds): Sexual Function In People With Disabilities and Chronic Illness. Aspen, Gaithersburg, MD, 1997, p 381.

43. Brackett, NL, et al: An analysis of 653 trials of penile vibratory stimulation in men with spinal cord injury. J Urol 159:1931, 1998.

44. Pryor, JL, et al: Vibratory stimulation for treatment of anejaculation in quadriplegic men. Arch Phys Med Rehabil 76:59, 1995.

45. Brackett, NL, et al: Semen quality of spinal cord injured men is better when obtained by vibratory stimulation versus electroejaculation. J Urol 157:151, 1997.

46. Brackett, NL, et al: Sperm from spinal cord injured men lose motility faster than sperm from normal men: The effect is exacerbated at body compared to room temperature. J Urol 157:2150, 1997.

47. Brackett, NL, et al: Predictors of necrospermia in men with spinal cord injury. J Urol 159:844, 1998.

48. Kreuter, M, et al: Sexual adjustment and quality of relationships in spinal paraplegia: A controlled study. Arch Phys Med Rehabil 77:541, 1996.

49. Brackett, NL, et al: Male fertility following spinal cord injury: Facts and fiction. Phys Ther 76:1221, 1996.

50. Chao, R, and Clowers, DE: Experience with intracavernosal tri-mixture for the management of neurogenic erectile dysfunction. Arch Phys Med Rehabil 75:276, 1994.

51. Brackett, NL, et al: Andrology: Treatment by assisted conception of severe male factor infertility due to spinal cord injury or other neurologic impairment. J Assist Reprod Genet 12:210, 1995.

52. Higgins, GE: Sexual response in spinal cord injured adults: A review of the literature. Arch Sex Behav 8:173, 1979.

53. Gott, LJ: Anatomy and physiology of male sexual response and fertility as related to spinal cord injury. In Sha'ked, A (ed): Human Sexuality and Rehabilitation Medicine: Sexual Functioning Following Spinal Cord Injury. Williams & Wilkins, Baltimore, 1981, p 67.

54. Comarr, AE: Sexual function in patients with spinal cord injury. In Pierce, DS, and Nickel, VH (eds): The Total Care of Spinal Cord Injuries. Little, Brown, Boston, 1977, p 171.

55. Hanak, M, and Scott, A: Spinal Cord Injury: An Illustrated Guide for Health Care Professionals. Springer-Verlag, New York, 1983.

56. Baker, ER, and Cardenas, DD: Pregnancy in spinal cord injured women. Arch Phys Med Rehabil 77:501, 1996.

57. Cross, LL, et al: Pregnancy, labor and delivery post spinal cord injury. Paraplegia 30:890, 1992.

58. Baker, ER, et al: Risks associated with pregnancy in spinal cord-injured women. Obstet Gynecol 80:425, 1992.

59. Sipski, ML, and Alexander, CJ: Sexual activities, response and satisfaction in women pre- and post-spinal cord injury. Arch Phys Med Rehabil 74:1025, 1993.

60. Westgren, N, et al: Pregnancy and delivery in women with traumatic spinal cord injury in Sweden. Obstet Gynecol 81:926, 1993.

61. Sipski, ML, et al: Orgasm in women with spinal cord injuries: A laboratory-based assessment. Arch Phys Med Rehabil 76:1097, 1995.

62. Feyi-Waboso, PA: An audit of five years' experience of pregnancy in spinal cord damaged women: A regional unit's experience and a review of the literature. Paraplegia 30:631, 1992.

63. Levi, R, et al: The Stockholm spinal cord injury study: Medical problems in a regional SCI population. Paraplegia 33:308, 1995.
64. Nettina, SM: The Lippincott Manual of Nursing Practice, ed 6. Lippincott, Philadelphia, 1996.
65. Patterson, RP, et al: The impaired response of spinal cord injured individuals to repeated surface pressure loads. Arch Phys Med Rehabil 74:947, 1993.
66. Kernozek, TW, and Lewin, JE: Seat interface pressures of individuals with paraplegia: Influence of dynamic wheelchair locomotion compared with static seated measures. Arch Phys Med Rehabil 79:313, 1998.
67. Comarr, AE: Autonomic dysreflexia (hyperreflexia) J Am Paraplegia Soc 7:53, 1984.
68. Moeller, BA, and Scheinberg, D: Autonomic dysreflexia in injuries below the sixth thoracic segment. JAMA 224:1295, 1973.
69. Lindan, R, et al: Incidence and clinical features of autonomic dysreflexia in patients with spinal cord injury. Paraplegia 18:285, 1980.
70. Rosen, JS: Autonomic dysreflexia. In Calenoff, L (ed): Radiology of Spinal Cord Injury. CV Mosby, St. Louis, 1981, p 554.
71. Comar, AE, and Eltorai, I: Symposium on autonomic dysreflexia. J Spinal Cord Med 20:345, 1996.
72. Comarr, AE: Autonomic dysreflexia. In Pierce, DS and Nickel, VH (eds): The Total Care of Spinal Cord Injuries. Little, Brown, Boston, 1977, p 181.
73. Yeo, JD: Recent research in spinal cord injuries. In Bedbrook, G (ed): The Care and Management of Spinal Cord Injuries. Springer-Verlag, New York, 1981, p 285.
74. McGarry, J, et al: Autonomic hyperreflexia following passive stretching to the hip joint. Phys Ther 62:30, 1982.
75. Erickson, RP: Autonomic hyperreflexia: Pathophysiology and medical management. Arch Phys Med Rehabil 61:431, 1980.
76. Belson, P: Autonomic nervous system dysfunction in recent spinal cord injured patients: A physical therapist's perspective. In Eisenberg, MG, and Falconer, JA (eds): Treatment of the Spinal Cord Injured: An Interdisciplinary Perspective. Charles C Thomas, Springfield, MA, 1978, p 34.
77. Hendrix, RW: Soft tissue changes after spinal cord injury. In Calenoff, L (ed): Radiology of Spinal Cord Injury. CV Mosby, St. Louis, 1981, p 438.
78. Wharton, GW: Heterotopic ossification. Clin Orthop 112:142, 1975.
79. Lal, S, et al: Risk factors for heterotopic ossification in spinal cord injury. Arch Phys Med Rehabil 70:387, 1989.
80. Stover, SL, et al: Heterotopic ossification in spinal cord-injured patients. Arch Phys Med Rehabil 56:199, 1975.
81. Rossier, AB, et al: Current facts on para-osteo-arthropathy (POA). Paraplegia 11:36, 1973.
82. Damanski, M: Heterotopic ossification in paraplegia: A clinical study. J Bone Joint Surg Br 43-B:286, 1961.
83. Wharton, GW, and Morgan, TH: Ankylosis in the paralyzed patient. J Bone Joint Surg Am 52-A:105, 1970.
84. Cioschi, H, and Staas, WE: Follow-up care. In Buchanan, LE, and Nawoczenski, DA (eds): Spinal Cord Injury: Concepts and Management Approaches. Williams & Wilkins, Baltimore, 1987, p 219.
85. Nicholas, JJ: Ectopic bone formation in patients with spinal cord injury. Arch Phys Med Rehabil 54:354, 1973.
86. McCagg, C: Postoperative management and acute rehabilitation of patients with spinal cord injuries. Orthop Clin North Am 17:171, 1986.
87. Turpie, A: Thrombosis prevention and treatment in spinal cord injured patients. In Bloch, R, and Basbaum, M (eds): Management of Spinal Cord Injuries. Williams & Wilkins, Baltimore, 1986, p 212.
88. Neiman, HL: Venography in acute spinal cord injury. In Calenoff, L (ed): Radiology of Spinal Cord Injury. CV Mosby, St. Louis, 1981, p 298.
89. van Hove, E: Prevention of thrombophlebitis in spinal injury patients. Paraplegia 16:332, 1978.
90. Todd, JW: Deep venous thrombosis in acute spinal cord injury: A comparison of 1251 fibrinogen leg scanning, impedance plethysmography and venography. Paraplegia 14:50, 1976.
91. Brach, BB, et al: Venous thrombosis in acute spinal cord paralysis. J Trauma 17:289, 1977.
92. Green, D, et al: Prevention of thromboembolism in spinal cord injury: Role of low molecular weight heparin. Arch Phys Med Rehabil 75:290, 1994.
93. Merli, GJ, et al: Etiology, incidence and prevention of deep vein thrombosis in acute spinal cord injury. Arch Phys Med Rehabil 74:1993.
94. El Masri, WS, and Silver, JR: Prophylactic anticoagulant therapy in patients with spinal cord injury. Paraplegia 19:334, 1981.
95. Nepomuceno, C, et al: Pain in patients with spinal cord injury. Arch Phys Med Rehabil 60:605, 1979.
96. Yezierski, RP: Pain following spinal cord injury: The clinical problem and experimental studies. Pain 68:185, 1996.
97. Richardson, RR, et al: Transcutaneous electrical neurostimulation in musculoskeletal pain of acute spinal cord injuries. Spine 5:42, 1980.
98. Davis, R: Pain and suffering following spinal cord injury. Clin Orthop 112:76, 1975.
99. Bors, E: Phantom limbs of patients with spinal cord injury. Arch Neurol Psychiatry 66:610, 1951.
100. Scott, JA, and Donovan, WH: The prevention of shoulder pain and contracture in the acute tetraplegic patient. Paraplegia 19:313, 1981.
101. Ohry, A, et al: Shoulder complications as a cause of delay in rehabilitation of spinal cord injured patients: Case reports and review of the literature. Paraplegia 16:310, 1978.
102. Cole, J: The pathophysiology of the autonomic nervous system in spinal cord injury. In Illis, L (ed): Spinal Cord Dysfunction: Assessment, Oxford University Press, New York, 1988, p 201.
103. Claus-Walker, J, et al: Calcium excretion in quadriplegia. Arch Phys Med Rehabil 53:14, 1972.
104. Burr, RG: Urinary calculi composition in patients with spinal cord lesions. Arch Phys Med Rehabil 59:84, 1978.
105. Hancock, DA, et al: Bone and soft tissue changes in paraplegic patients. Paraplegia 17:267, 1979.
106. Donovan, WH, and Bedbrook, G: Comprehensive management of spinal cord injury. Ciba Clin Symp 34, 1982.
107. Holdsworth, F: Fractures, dislocations, and fracture-dislocations of the spine. J Bone Joint Surg Am 52:1534, 1970.
108. Marciello, MA, et al: Magnetic resonance imaging related to neurologic outcome in cervical spinal cord injury. Arch Phys Med Rehabil 74:940, 1993.
109. Bohlman, HH: Complications and pitfalls in the treatment of acute cervical spinal cord injuries. In Tator, CH (ed): Early Management of Acute Spinal Cord Injury. Raven, New York, 1982, p 373.
110. Tator, CH, et al: Halo devices for the treatment of acute cervical spinal cord injury. In Tator, CH (ed): Early Management of Acute Spinal Cord Injury. Raven, New York, 1982, p 231.
111. Edmonds, VE, and Tator, CH: Coordination of a halo program for an acute spinal cord injury unit. In Tator, CH (ed): Early Management of Acute Spinal Cord Injury. Raven, New York, 1982, p 263.
112. Cerullo, LJ: Surgical stabilization of spinal cord injury: Section A: Cervical spine. In Calenoff, L (ed): Radiology of Spinal Cord Injury. CV Mosby, St. Louis, 1982, p 202.
113. Meyer, PR: Surgical stabilization of spinal cord injury: Section B: Thoracic and lumbar spine. In Calenoff, L (ed): Radiology of Spinal Cord Injury. CV Mosby, St. Louis, 1981, p 202.
114. American Spinal Cord Injury Association: International Standards for Neurological and Functional Classification of Spinal Cord Injury, Chicago, 1996.
115. Zejdlik, CP: Maintaining protective functions of the skin. In Zejdlik, CP (ed): Management of Spinal Cord Injury. Jones and Bartlett, Boston, 1992, p 451.
116. Daniels, L, and Worthingham, C: Muscle Testing: Techniques of Manual Examination, ed 5. Saunders, Philadelphia, 1986.

117. Norkin, CC, and White, DJ: Measurement of Joint Motion: A Guide to Goniometry, ed 2. FA Davis, Philadelphia, 1995.

118. Clough, P, et al: Guidelines for routine respiratory care of patients with spinal cord injury: A clinical report. Phys Ther 66:1395, 1986.

119. Jaeger, RJ, et al: Cough in spinal cord injured patients: Comparison of three methods to produce cough. Arch Phys Med Rehabil 74:1358, 1993.

120. Lamont, LS, et al: A comparison of two arm exercises in patients with paraplegia. Cardiopulmonary Physical Therapy 7:3, 1996.

121. O'Sullivan, SB, and Schmitz, TJ: Physical Rehabilitation Laboratory Manual: Focus on Functional Training. FA Davis, Philadelphia, 1999.

122. Hussey, RW, and Stauffer, ES: Spinal cord injury: Requirements for ambulation. Arch Phys Med Rehabil 54:544, 1973.

123. Hirokawa, S, et al: Energy expenditure and fatigability in paraplegic ambulation using reciprocating gait orthosis and electric stimulation. Disabil Rehabil 18:115, 1996.

124. Mikelberg, R, and Reid, S: Spinal cord lesions and lower extremity bracing: An overview and follow-up study. Paraplegia 19:379, 1981.

125. Scott, BA: Engineering principles and fabrication techniques for the Scott-Craig long leg brace for paraplegics. Orthot Prosthet 25:14, 1971.

126. Lobley, S, et al: Orthotic design from the New England Regional Spinal Cord Injury Center: Suggestion from the field. Phys Ther 65:492, 1985.

127. Franceschini, M, et al: Reciprocating gait orthosis: A multicenter study of their use by spinal cord injured patients. Arch Phys Med 78:582, 1997.

128. Sykes, L, et al: The reciprocating gait orthosis: Long-term usage patterns. Arch Phys Med 76:779, 1995.

129. Bernardi, M, et al: The efficiency of walking of paraplegic patients using a reciprocating gait orthosis. Paraplegia 33:409, 1995.

130. Kent, HO: Vannini-Rizzoli stabilizing orthosis (boot): Preliminary report on a new ambulatory aid for spinal cord injury. Arch Phys Med 73:302, 1992.

131. Lyles, M, and Munday, J: Report on the evaluation of the Vannini-Rizzoli stabilizing limb orthosis. Journal of Rehabilitation Research 29:77, 1992.

132. Tinsley, SL: Rehab in SCI: From the laboratory to the clinic. PT Magazine 1:42, 1993.

133. Stein, RB, et al: Electrical systems for improving locomotion after incomplete spinal cord injury: An assessment. Arch Phys Med Rehabil 74:954, 1993.

134. Jacobs, PL, et al: Relationships of oxygen uptake, heart rate, and ratings of perceived exertion in persons with paraplegia during functional neuromuscular stimulation assisted ambulation. Spinal Cord 35:292, 1997.

135. Sipski, ML, and DeLisa, JA: Functional electrical stimulation in spinal cord injury rehabilitation: A review of the literature. NeuroRehabilitation 1:46, 1991.

SUPPLEMENTAL READINGS

Allison, GT, et al: Transfer movement strategies of individuals with spinal cord injuries. Disabil Rehabil 18:35, 1996.

Amodie-Storey, C, et al: Head position and its effect on pulmonary function in tetraplegia patients. Spinal Cord 34:602, 1996.

Athanasou, JA, et al: Vocational achievements following spinal cord injury in Australia. Disabil Rehabil 18:191, 1996.

Beekman, CE, et al: Energy cost of propulsion in standard and ultralight wheelchairs in people with spinal cord injuries. Phys Ther 70:146, 1997.

Bohannon, RW: Tilt table standing for reducing spasticity after spinal cord injury. Arch Phys Med Rehabil 74:1121, 1993.

Brownlee, S, and Williams, S: Physiotherapy in the respiratory care of patients with high spinal injury. Physiotherapy 73:148, 1987.

Buchanan, LE, and Nawoczenski, DA (eds): Spinal Cord Injury: Concepts and Management Approaches. Williams & Wilkins, Baltimore, 1987.

Calancie, B, et al: Involuntary stepping after chronic spinal cord injury: Evidence for a central rhythm generator for locomotion in man. Brain 117:1143, 1994.

Calancie, B, et al: Central nervous system plasticity after spinal cord injury in man: Interlimb reflexes and the influence of cutaneous stimulation. Electroencephalography and Clinical Neurophysiology 101:304, 1996.

Carpenter, C: The experience of spinal cord injury: The individual's perspective: Implications for rehabilitation practice. Phys Ther 74:614, 1994.

Carter, ER: Respiratory aspects of spinal cord injury. Paraplegia 25:262, 1987.

Dietz, V, et al: Locomotion in patients with spinal cord injuries. Phys Ther 77:508, 1997.

Eriksson, P: Aerobic power during maximal exercise in untrained and well-trained quadri- and paraplegics. Scand J Rehabil Med 20:141, 1988.

Fuhrer, MJ, et al: Pressure ulcers in community-resident persons with spinal cord injury: Prevalence and risk factors. Arch Phys Med Rehabil 74:1172, 1993.

Gardner, MB, et al: Partial body weight support with treadmill locomotion to improve gait after incomplete spinal cord injury: A single-subject experimental design. Phys Ther 78:361, 1998.

Guest, RS, et al: Evaluation of a training program for persons with SCI paraplegia using the Parastep[R]1 ambulation system: Part 4. Ambulation performance and anthropometric measures. Arch Phys Med Rehabil 78:804, 1997.

Gerhart, KA, et al: Long-term spinal cord injury: Functional changes over time. Arch Phys Med Rehabil 74:1030, 1993.

Holtzman, RNN, and Stein, BM (eds): Surgery of the Spinal Cord: Potential for Regeneration and Recovery. Springer-Verlag, New York, 1992.

Hornstein, S, and Ledsome, J: Ventilatory muscle training in acute quadriplegia. Physiotherapy Canada 38:145, 1986.

Jacobs, PL, et al: Evaluation of a training program for persons with SCI paraplegia using the Parastep[R]1 ambulation system: Part 2. Ambulation performance and anthropometric measures. Arch Phys Med Rehabil 78:794, 1997.

Jette, DU, and Jette, AM: Physical therapy and health outcomes in patients with spinal impairments. Phys Ther 76:930, 1996.

Klose, KJ, et al: Evaluation of a training program for persons with SCI paraplegia using the Parastep[R]1 ambulation system: Part 1. Ambulation performance and anthropometric measures. Arch Phys Med Rehabil 78:789, 1997.

Krause, JS, et al: Mortality after spinal cord injury: An 11-year prospective study. Arch Phys Med Rehabil 78:815, 1997.

Kralj, A, et al: Enhancement of gait restoration in spinal injured patients by functional electrical stimulation. Clin Orthop 233:34, 1988.

Lindan, R, et al: The team approach to urinary bladder management in SCI patients: A 26-year retrospective study. Paraplegia 28:314, 1990.

Lynch, SM, et al: Reliability of measurements obtained with a modified functional reach test in subjects with spinal cord injury. Phys Ther 78:128, 1998.

Marino, RJ, et al: Assessing selfcare status in quadriplegia: Comparison of the quadriplegia index of function (QIF) and the functional independence measure (FIM). International Medical Society of Paraplegia 31:225, 1993.

Marsolias, E, and Kobetic, R. Functional electrical stimulation for walking with paraplegia. J Bone Joint Surg Am 69:728, 1987.

Moakley, TJ: Informing spinal cord injured persons about their rights and expectations under the Americans with Disabilities Act. SCI Psychosocial Process 7:8, 1994.

Nash, MS, et al: Evaluation of a training program for persons with SCI paraplegia using the Parastep[R]1 ambulation system: Part 5. Ambulation performance and anthropometric measures. Arch Phys Med Rehabil 78:808, 1997.

Needham-Shropshire, BM, et al: Evaluation of a training program for persons with SCI paraplegia using the Parastep^R1 ambulation system: Part 3. Ambulation performance and anthropometric measures. Arch Phys Med Rehabil 78:799, 1997.

Needham-Shropshire, BM, et al: Manual muscle test score and force comparisons after cervical spinal cord injury. J Spinal Cord Med 20:324, 1997.

Needham-Shropshire, BM, et al: Improved motor function in tetraplegics following neuromuscular stimulation-assisted arm ergometry. J Spinal Cord Med 20:49, 1997.

Nussbaum, EL, et al: Comparison of ultrasound/ultraviolet-C and laser for treatment of pressure ulcers in patients with spinal cord injury. 74:812, 1994.

Nygaard, I, et al: Sexuality and reproduction in spinal cord injured women. Obstet Gynecol Surv 45:727, 1990.

Oakes, D: Benefits of an early admission to a comprehensive trauma center for patients with SCI. Arch Phys Med Rehabil 72:637, 1990.

O'Neil, L, and Seelye, R: Power wheelchair training for patients with marginal upper extremity function. Neurology Report 14:19, 1990.

Parke, B, and Penn, RD: Functional outcome after delivery of intrathecal baclofen. Arch Phys Med Rehabil 70:30, 1989.

Penn, RD, and Kroin, JS: Long-term intrathecal baclofen infusion for treatment of spasticity. Neurosurgery 66:181, 1987.

Phillips, CA: Functional electrical stimulation and lower extremity bracing for ambulation exercise of the spinal cord injured individual: A medically prescribed system. Phys Ther 60:842, 1989.

Quencer, RM, and Bunge, RP: The injured spinal cord: Imaging, histopathologic, clinical correlates, and basic science approaches to enhancing neural function after spinal cord injury. Spine 21:2064, 1996.

Rutchik, A, et al: Resistive inspiratory muscle training in subjects with chronic cervical spinal cord injury. Arch Phys Med Rehabil 79:293, 1998.

Saitoh, E, et al: Clinical experience with a new hip-knee-ankle-foot orthotic system using a medial single hip joint for paraplegic standing and walking. Am J Phys Med Rehabil 75:198, 1996.

Santosh, L, et al: Risk factors for heterotopic ossification in spinal cord injury. Arch Phys Med Rehabil 70:387, 1989.

Saxena, S, et al: An EMG-controlled grasping system for tetraplegics. J Rehabil Res Devel 32:17, 1995.

Segal, ME, et al: Interinstitutional agreement of individual functional independence measure (FIM) items measured at two sites on one sample of SCI patients. International Medical Society of Paraplegia 31:622, 1993.

Schindler, L, et al: Functional effect of bilateral tendon transfers on a person with C-5 quadriplegia. Am J Occup Ther 48:750, 1994.

Signorile, JF, et al: Increased muscle strength in paralyzed patients after spinal cord injury: Effect of beta-2 adrenergic agonist. Arch Phys Med Rehabil 76:55, 1996.

Somers, MF: Spinal Cord Injury: Functional Rehabilitation. Appleton & Lange, Norwalk, CT, 1992.

Tang, SFT, et al: Correlation of motor control in the supine position and assistive device used for ambulation in chronic incomplete spinal cord-injured persons. Am J Phys Med Rehabil 73:268, 1994.

Thomas, CK, et al: Motor unit forces and recruitment patterns after cervical spinal cord injury. Muscle Nerve 20:212, 1997.

Thomas, CK, et al: Muscle weakness, paralysis and atrophy after human cervical spinal cord injury. Exp Neurol 148:414, 1997.

Waters, RL, et al: Motor and sensory recovery following incomplete tetraplegia. Arch Phys Med Rehabil 75:306, 1994.

Waites, KB, et al: Epidemiology and risk factors for urinary tract infection following spinal cord injury. Arch Phys Med Rehabil 74:691, 1993.

Walker, J, and Shephard, RJ: Cardiac risk factors immediately following spinal injury. Arch Phys Med Rehabil 74:1129, 1993.

Williams, DO: Spinal cord injury under managed care. PT Magazine 4:34, 1996.

GLOSSARY

Anterior cord syndrome: Incomplete spinal cord lesion with primary damage in the anterior cord; loss of motor function, and sense of pain and temperature; preservation of proprioception, kinesthesia, and vibration below the level of the lesion.

Autonomic dysreflexia (hyperreflexia): A pathological autonomic reflex seen in patients with high-level spinal cord injuries. It is precipitated by a noxious stimulus below the level of the lesion and produces an acute onset of autonomic activity. It is considered an emergency situation; symptoms include hypertension, bradycardia, headache, and sweating.

Avulsion: Pulling or tearing of a piece of bone away from the main bone.

Brown-Sequard syndrome: Incomplete spinal cord lesion caused by hemisection of the cord; loss of motor function, proprioception, and kinesthesia on the side of the lesion; loss of sense of pain and temperature on the opposite side.

Bulbocavernosus reflex (positive): Pressure on the glans penis or glans clitoris that elicits a contraction of the external anal sphincter.

Burst (explosion) fracture: A comminuted vertebral fracture associated with pressure along the long axis of the vertebral column, also associated with flexion injuries, bone fragments are displaced centripetally.

Cauda equina lesion: Damage to peripheral nerve roots below the first lumbar vertebra; some regeneration is possible.

Central cord syndrome: Incomplete spinal cord lesion producing greater neurological involvement in upper extremities (cervical tracts more centrally located) than in the lower extremities (lumbar and sacral tracts more peripheral).

Complete lesion (SCI): No sensory or motor function below the level of lesion.

Compression fracture: A vertebral fracture resulting from pressure along the long axis of the vertebral column and closely associated with flexion injuries.

Contusion (SCI): Damage to the spinal cord produced by pressure from displaced bone and/or soft tissues or swelling within the spinal canal.

Crede maneuver: Technique for emptying urine from a flaccid bladder; repeated pressure is placed between the umbilicus and symphysis pubis in a downward direction; manual pressure is also placed directly over bladder to further facilitate removal of urine.

Deep vein thrombosis (DVT): Formation of a blood clot in the deep venous system; occurs most frequently in the lower extremities; clinical manifestations include warmth, pain, and swelling in the affected extremity.

Diaphoresis: Profuse sweating.

Dislocation: Displacement of a bone or vertebral body from its normal position.

Distraction: A traction force; separation of joint surfaces.

Dysesthesias (SCI): Bizarre, painful sensations experienced below the level of a lesion following spinal cord injury; often described as burning, numbness, pins and needles, or tingling sensations.

Heterotopic ossification: Abnormal bone growth in soft tissues, a potential secondary complication following spinal cord injury; occurs below the level of the lesion (*synonym*: ectopic bone formation).

Incomplete lesion (SCI): Some preservation of sensory or motor function below the level of the lesion.

Intrathecal injection: A central (within the spinal canal) chemical injection that interrupts the reflex arc; used to decrease severe spasticity.

Key muscles: Muscles that add significantly to a patient's functional capacity at each successive level of lesion.

Lower motor neuron (LMN) lesion: Motor dysfunction, associated wtih lesions of the anterior horn cell or peripheral nerve.

Maceration: Softening of a solid by exposure to water or other fluid; usually pertains to the skin.

Micturition: Voiding of urine (*synonym*: urination).

Myelotomy: Severance of nerve fibers of the spinal cord; used to reduce severe spasticity.

Myotomy: Surgical sectioning or release of a muscle; used to reduce spasticity.

Neurectomy: Partial or total excision or resection of a nerve; used to reduce severe spasticity.

Nocturia: Excessive urination during the night.

Osteoporosis: Abnormal loss of bone density.

Paraplegia: Partial or complete paralysis of all or part of the trunk and both lower extremities from lesions of the thoracic or lumbar spinal cord or sacral roots.

Peripheral nerve block: A local chemical injection used to block transmission of a motor nerve selectively; used to decrease spasticity.

Posterior cord syndrome: A rare incomplete lesion with primary damage to the posterior cord; preservation of motor function, sense of pain, and light touch, with loss of proprioception and epicritic sensations below the level of the lesion.

Postural hypotension (orthostatic hypotension): A decrease in blood pressure that occurs when assuming an erect or vertical posture; decreased venous return and cerebral blood flow produces symptoms of lightheadedness or fainting. This may occur normally and is typically severe following prolonged bed rest.

Pressure sore: Ulceration of soft tissue caused by unrelieved pressure and shearing forces (*synonym*: decubitus ulcer, bed sore).

Rhizotomy: Division or severance of a nerve root; used to reduce severe spasticity.

Root escape: Preservation of peripheral nerve roots at the level of a spinal cord injury.

Sacral sparing: An incomplete lesion in which some sacral innervation remains intact; complete loss of motor function and sensation in other areas below the level of the lesion.

Selective stretching: The process of under stretching some muscles and full stretching of others to enhance function.

Shearing: Application of a horizontal or parallel force relative to adjacent structures; opposite to the force that is normally present; associated with fracture dislocations of the thoracolumbar region.

Spinal shock: Period immediately following injury to the spinal cord, characterized by absence of all reflex activity, flaccidity, and a loss of sensation below the level of the lesion; generally subsides within 24 hours.

Subluxation: Incomplete or partial dislocation.

Teardrop fracture: A bursting type fracture of the cervical region that produces a characteristic anterior-inferior bone chip. The fragment resembles a "teardrop" on radiographs and is associated with flexion and compression forces.

Tenotomy: Surgical section of a nerve; used to reduce spasticity.

Tetraplegia (quadriplegia): Partial or complete paralysis of all four extremities and trunk, including the respiratory muscles from lesions of the cervical cord.

Upper motor neuron (UMN) lesion: Motor dysfunction associated with lesions of corticol, subcorticol or spinal cord structure.

APPENDIX

Suggested Answers to Case Study Guiding Questions

1. Identify/categorize this patient's problems in terms of:

ANSWER:

a. Direct impairments
- Decreased strength and sensation below T6
- Increased tone/muscle spasms BLEs and trunk
- Incontinent/spastic bowel and bladder

b. Indirect impairments
- Poor sitting posture
- Decreased ROM/contracture BLEs: left greater than right
- Pain associated with spasms: abdominals and BLEs

c. Composite impairments: combined effects of both direct and indirect impairments
- Impaired static/dynamic balance
- Decreased endurance

d. Functional limitations/disabilities
- Decreased ability to sit independently
- Dependent on w/c for mobility
- Unable to stand or ambulate
- Decreased ADLs, IADLs (community mobility)
- Unable to work

2. Identify three goals (remediation of impairments) and three outcomes (remediation of functional limitations/disability) for this patient.

ANSWER

Goal: Patient will demonstrate proper sitting alignment in w/c within 2 to 3 weeks of treatment.

Goal: Patient will increase tolerance in sitting on platform mat without UE support to 5 minutes within 2 to 3 weeks of treatment.

Goal: Patient will be independent in daily self-ranging techniques within 2 to 3 weeks of treatment.

Outcome: Patient is independent in w/c sitting with appropriate posture for 6 to 7 hours per day after 6 to 8 weeks of treatment.

Outcome: Patient is independent and safe in all transfers without adaptive equipment after 6 to 8 weeks of treatment.

Outcome: Patient is independent in unrestricted BUE activity to enable patient to perform desk top activities and return to work after 6 to 8 weeks of treatment.

3. Formulate five treatment interventions with one progression that could be used during the first 3 weeks of therapy. Provide a brief rationale that justifies your choice.

ANSWER

Intervention 1
- Sitting, holding with BUEs weight-bearing on ball on lap
- Alternating isometrics

- Progress to rhythmic stabilization technique
- Rationale: develops stability in sitting, control of residual trunk muscles.

Intervention 2
- Sitting, weight shifting side to side with BUEs extended and weight bearing
- Active movements
- Progression: increase range of movements and directions; weight shifting against light resistance (slow reversals); weight shifting without BUEs weight bearing
- Rationale: develops controlled mobility function in sitting, ability to move trunk without loss of stability.

Intervention 3
- Sitting, reaching movements of BUEs, forward and backward
- Active movements
- Progression: increase range and direction of movements
- Rationale: develops controlled mobility function (static-dynamic control) in sitting, ability to move extremities without loss of stability.

Intervention 4
- Kneeling, holding with BUEs weight-bearing in modified prone-on-elbows on large ball
- Active assisted movements
- Progression: weight shifting, slowly moving the ball side-to-side
- Rationale: develops stability in supported kneeling, trunk and hip extensor control; counteracts flexor spasms and contractures, postural hypotension responses to upright positioning.

Intervention 5
- Long sitting, push-ups using push-up blocks
- Active movements
- Progression: long-sitting push-ups without blocks progressing to short-sitting push-ups
- Rationale: develops strength of BUEs (shoulder depressors and triceps); promotes independence in transfers without use of transfer board.

4. Identify relevant motor learning strategies appropriate for the initial physical therapy sessions with this patient.

ANSWER: Patient will be assisted in initial development of motor skills (cognitive mapping) with demonstration and augmented feedback (verbal cueing, manual contacts). Movements will be assisted as necessary to ensure correct and safe performance. The functional purpose of each task will be highlighted to ensure carryover into real-life tasks. Initially distributed practice with frequent rest periods will be used to decrease the risk of fatigue. Verbal feedback (knowledge of results) will be given after every practice trial during initial practice sessions; as learning progresses feedback will be less frequent (fading feedback design) to allow for learner introspection and self-correction. Patients with spinal cord injury require independent decision making skills to deal with the constant environmental challenges. Training will progress from a closed environment (physical therapy clinic) to open environments (community and work). Focus on return to work skills is particularly important for this patient given his age and personal goals.

Chronic Pain 28

Barbara Headley

LEARNING OBJECTIVES

1. Explain the physiology of pain and the mechanisms that contribute to chronic pain.
2. Describe the clinical manifestations of chronic pain.
3. Describe the medical management of chronic pain.
4. Explain the assessment tools for identifying the factors contributing to a patient's pain experience.
5. Describe a treatment model for the patient with chronic pain.
6. Describe the contributions of the members of a multidisciplinary pain management team.
7. Analyze and interpret patient data, formulate realistic goals and outcomes, and develop a plan of care when presented with a clinical case study.

Patients with chronic pain present with multiple complaints and problems, and provide a unique challenge to the physical therapist. Because physical therapists often treat patients emerging from an acute pain stage into a chronic pain state, they must be able to recognize this changing state and plan treatment accordingly. Although patients with acute pain respond well to various therapeutic modalities, patients with chronic pain present with a complex of psychological, sociological, and emotional states that affect the manner in which they experience and report their physical pain. All components of the pain experience must be addressed, and a multidisciplinary treatment program must be considered. Restoration of function, not pain relief, is the primary physical therapy outcome with this patient population, and physical therapists play a primary role in the rehabilitation process.

HISTORICAL PERSPECTIVE

Throughout the ages, pain has had a variety of meanings to those experiencing it and those seeking to alleviate it. Our view of health, disease, and pain are a reflection of history. The introduction to the Hippocratic oath presupposes the sharing of concern for health and illness by man and the gods and goddesses:

I swear by Apollo the physician, by Asclepius, by Hygeia and Panacea and by all the gods and goddesses making them my witnesses, that I will fulfill according to my ability and judgement this oath and this covenant.[1]

In ancient history, cause and cure of pain were linked to religion and other nonphysical reasons. Ancient Egyptians believed that either the spirits of the dead or the religious influences of their gods were responsible for painful afflictions, which generally entered the body in darkness. In ancient India, the universality of the pain experience was attributed to unfulfilled desires. The ancient Chinese held that pain was a result of an imbalance of yin and yang, resulting in either excess or blocked chi.[2] Rebalancing the chi, or the flow of energy throughout the body, was believed necessary to restore physiological balance and health. In ancient Greece, Sibyls and Pythoness held virtually exclusive power for exorcising the demons that were thought to cause illness and pain.

Pain subsequently was removed from the realm of religion and placed into the realm of the emotions. Plato deduced that pain and pleasure, though opposite sensations, were linked together on a continuum, originating from the heart and representing passions of the soul. Aristotle, his student, held that the experience of pain was a hypersensitivity of every sensation and was caused by an excess of vital heat. Despite descriptions of pain related to inflammation by Celsus and Galens, the concept described by Aristotle prevailed for 23 centuries, attributing pain to a "passion of the soul."[2]

Discovery of physical reasons for pain resulting in significant changes in philosophy were not evident until after the Middle Ages and Renaissance. In 1628, Harvey discovered the circulation of blood. Dissection of human bodies was still largely forbidden because of the strong religious convictions that had predominated for centuries. As long as the heart was considered the center of the soul and mind, the church forbade the study of the human body. To remove such strong prohibition by the church, Descartes conceptualized the separation of the mind and body. He described the pineal body as the connecting point, the center of the brain. Descartes proposed that for a person to be conscious of something, the experience had to go through this center. The pineal body then was believed to be the point at which the physical transmission of information along the nervous system became transformed into conscious thoughts, feelings, and emotions.[2] Descartes considered nerves to be tubes containing a large number of fine threads that form the marrow of the nerves and connected a substance of the brain with nerve endings in the skin and other tissues. Pain, experienced in the brain, was sent to the periphery by a stimulus that traveled up this hollow tube (Fig. 28-1).[3]

Over the next several hundred years, rudimentary medicine grew. Complex discoveries of the nervous system and developing theories of the nature and mechanism of pain developed.

THEORIES OF PAIN

The method by which we explain the origin of pain greatly influences how we rationalize and formulate treatment plans. Since the time pain was considered a problem of injury or disease, rather than a problem related to religion or the soul, many theories concerning the mechanism of origin of pain have been developed. These theories evolved as scientific knowledge in general evolved. They represent the best logical integration of current available information. These theories also are instructive in understanding historical influences on how pain has been treated. For example, the *Specificity Theory*, which describes pain as a specific physical sensation, led to medical practice that "cut out" the pain, or the tissue from which the pain was believed to originate. Other theories, such as the *Fourth Theory of Pain*, suggest there is a one-to-one relationship between the intensity of the stimulus and pain experience. Such a theory suggests that two individuals experiencing the same problem (i.e., a fractured leg) would have exactly the same amount of pain and exactly the same response to that pain. This suggestion negates what we now know regarding the influence of cultural, environmental, and personality factors on how an individual experiences pain. When examining two patients who have, in our minds, the same pain problem, we often consider one patient's response as being what we would expect from that experience whereas another individual's response falls outside these expectations. Theories such as these continue to have a subtle impact on our perception of someone else's pain, and are worth exploring in detail. These theories are summarized in Table 28–1.

Livingston's theory of a *Central Summation of Impulses* has been expanded by many of the current theorists. Livingston proposed a "vicious cycle of reflexes" involving a chronic irritation of a peripheral sensory nerve with increased afferent impulses. This irritation resulted in abnormal activity in an internuncial pool of neurons in the lateral and anterior horn of the spinal cord, and in turn increased sympathetic reflex efferent activity, including increased heart rate, vasoconstriction, and muscle spasm. This heightened sympathetic activity was thought to produce further abnormal input, thereby creating a feedback loop that perpetuated the experience. The prolonged excitability of the internuncial pool is further maintained by fear and anxiety. Such pain was thought to no longer be triggering an alarm of imminent danger, but to have become itself the

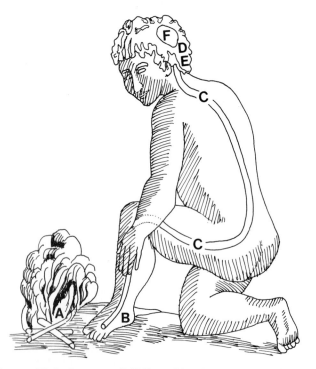

Figure 28-1. Descartes (1664) considered nerves to be tubes that contain a large number of fine threads, connecting the brain with the skin and other tissues. (From Melzack and Wall,[3] p 72, with permission.)

Table 28–1 HISTORICAL THEORIES OF PAIN

Theory	Date/Author	Summary
Intensive (summation) theory	1874/Erb	This theory, built on Aristotle's concept that pain resulted from excessive stimulation of the sense of touch, was described by several authors in the 1840s. Erb maintained that every sensory stimulus was capable of producing pain if it reached sufficient intensity. The theory was further developed by Goldscheider in 1894, who described both stimulus intensity and central summation as critical determinants of pain. It was implied that the summation occurred in the dorsal horn cells.
Specificity theory	1895/vonFrey	Based on the assumption that the free nerve endings are pain receptors and that the other three types of receptors are also specific to a sensory experience. The primary argument against this theory is that pain perception is not simply a function of the amount of physical damage alone; complex psychological components are part of the pain experience.
Strong's theory	1895/Strong	As president of the American Psychological Association, Strong believed that pain was an experience based on both the noxious stimulus and the psychic reaction or displeasure provoked by the sensation.
Pattern theories	1934/Nafe	Early pattern theories suggested that all cutaneous qualities are produced by spatial and temporal patterns of nerve impulses rather than by separate, modality-specific transmission routes.
Central summation theory	1943/Livingston	Proposal that the intense stimulation resulting from nerve and tissue damage activates fibers that project to internuncial neuron pools within the spinal cord. Abnormal reverberating circuits are created. Prolonged abnormal activity bombards cells in the spinal cord, and information is projected to the brain for pain perception.
The fourth theory of pain	1940s/Hardy, Wolff, and Goodell	Theory developed to further expand Strong's theory. It stated that pain was composed of two components: the perception of pain and the reaction one has to it. The reaction was described as a complex physiopsychological process involving cognitive functions of the individual, influenced by past experiences, culture, and various psychological factors that produce great variation in the "reaction pain threshold."
Sensory interaction theory	1959/Noordenbos	Description of two systems involving transmission of pain and other sensory information with a fast and slow system. The slow system, unmyelinated small diameter fibers, were presumed to conduct somatic and visceral afferents. The fast system, composed of large fibers, were said to inhibit transmission of the small fibers.
Gate control theory	1965/Melzack and Wall	Proposal that the neural mechanisms in the dorsal horns of the spinal cord act like a gate that can increase or decrease the flow of nerve impulses from peripheral fibers to the spinal cord cells that project to the brain. The somatic input is therefore subjected to the modulating influence of the gate before it evokes pain perception and response. It is suggested that large-fiber inputs tend to close the gate, whereas small-fiber inputs generally open it; descending controls from the brain also influence what is experienced.

pathology, residing within the nervous system. The pain pathways were thought to fire although no noxious stimuli were present. The transmission of the signal was thought to be faulty, so that when a very minor, non-noxious stimulus was present, the information was garbled and distorted causing the pain pathways to fire inappropriately.[5,6]

The **Gate Control Theory,** originally presented in 1965 by Melzack and Wall,[3] and modified in 1982, continues to be the dominant theory influencing our approach to pain management. A schematic diagram of the theory is shown in Figure 28-2. The substantia gelatinosa appears to be the site of the "gate," which controls access to the spinal cord. The noxious stimulus is projected to the spinal cord. Modification of the noxious stimulus occurs as a result of either excitatory or inhibitory influences within the spinal cord cells and by descending influences from the brain. The final product, or pain experience, is a complex highly individualized phenomenon that results in significant variability in the response observed.[7] Within the Gate Control Theory neurological connections and processes are explained.

Pain-sensitive nerves, called **nociceptive** afferents, supply skin, subcutaneous tissue, periosteum, joints, muscles, and viscera. Some nociceptors respond only to noxious stimuli. Polymodal nociceptive fibers, which are multifaceted pain receptors, respond to strong, long-lasting stimuli, including

mechanical, thermal, and chemical stimuli, which may not initially be perceived as noxious. Most primary afferents, after entering the spinal cord, terminate in the ipsilateral dorsal horn of the spinal cord, but some extend across to the contralateral horn. Once in the spinal cord, the small **C fibers** appear to travel in the lateral portion of the dorsal white matter, and the large **A fibers** travel more

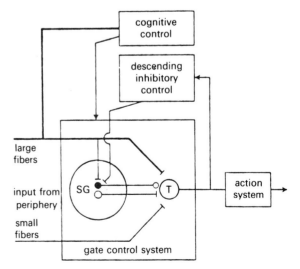

Figure 28-2. Melzack and Wall's 1983 revised gate control theory. (From Bonica,[2] p 10, with permission.)

medially in the dorsal column. Collateral branches are given off at the same and nearby levels. The A and C fibers ending in the substantia gelatinosa are subject to excitatory and inhibitory influences. These influences may significantly affect the final pain experience. Wide dynamic range receptors in lamina V also have a major impact on pain. These receptors respond to a variety of inputs from low-threshold and high-threshold mechanical, thermal, and chemical stimuli by way of afferent fibers with a full range of diameters. These wide dynamic range receptors affect the threshold of neurons that subsequently project into ascending tracts. The "gating" action, where the primary afferents enter the spinal cord, can either increase or decrease the amount of sensory information transmitted through this gate to the brain. The Gate Control Theory suggests that sensory information traveling on large A fibers (e.g., comfortable, non-noxious stimuli) tend to close the gate, while small-fiber inputs (C fibers) generally open it. Inhibitory systems come from higher centers via descending tracts, such as the reticulospinal (RST) and corticospinal (CST) tracts. The synaptic connections occurring as the information is transmitted to the brain also have an effect on the information through a variety of neurotransmitters. In clinical practice pain control interventions are based on producing stimuli carried on A fibers to block pain stimuli carried on C fibers.

Three ascending spinal tracts carry nociceptive information. These include the dorsal column medial lemniscus postsynaptic system (DCPS), the spinocervical tract (SCT), and the (lateral) neospinothalamic tract (nSTT). A nociceptive message ascending via one pathway may trigger different perceptions or responses to pain in contrast to the same message ascending via another pathway. When the system is carrying non-pain information such as proprioception or light touch sensations, it cannot transmit nociceptive stimuli. Another system, therefore, is used to transmit nociceptive information, assuring that the noxious input always has an available tract through which it can travel. It is hypothesized that slower conducting tracts, for example, the spinoreticular tract (SRT) and the anterior paleospinothalamic tract (pSTT) in particular, are likely to play a role in chronic, deeply unpleasant, diffuse pain. The stimulus characteristics of these tracts include response to innocuous stimuli, which may be perceived as noxious as the stimulus continues and thresholds are lowered. Stimulation of portions of the SRT provides the sensation of diffuse pain, while surgical lesions including portions of the SRT result in relief of chronic pain. The pSTT provokes suprasegmental responses, which may include the motivational drive and unpleasant effect that trigger the organism into action.[8]

The understanding of factors influencing nociceptive information has undergone modification. The complex sequence of behavior that characterizes pain is understood to be a composite of sensory, motivational, and cognitive processes that act on those brain areas that contribute to overt behavioral responses. These factors, described by Melzack,[7] led to an expansion of the Gate Control Theory to include the motivational dimension of pain. The rapidly conducting spinal tracts accounted for the majority of the sensory-discriminative dimension of pain. The slowly conducting spinal systems together with the reticular and limbic structures were responsible for much of the motivational drive and unpleasant affect characteristics of pain. In addition, neocortical or higher central nervous system (CNS) processes, such as evaluation of input in terms of past experience, exert control over activity in both the discriminative and motivational systems.

Neurotransmitters with specific receptor sites function in pain inhibition. Endorphin and opiate receptors are inhibitory influences in the perception or experience of pain. **Stimulation-produced analgesia (SPA)** from endorphin release and induced by brain stimulation and from opiate drug use appear to share common receptor sites and modes of action. Opiate analgesia, like SPA, is an active process of pain inhibition. Receptors for morphine, a synthetic copy of endogenous beta-endorphins, are abundant in central areas of pain control, including the periaqueductal gray matter, dorsal spinal cord, and limbic system.[9]

Patients with chronic pain have a lower level of endorphins in their cerebrospinal fluid as compared to healthy individuals. This depletion of endorphins is negatively correlated with pain tolerance. Bonica[5] and Sternbach[10] suggest that this depletion, in conjunction with depletions of serotonin, may account for many of the physiological and behavioral characteristics of patients with chronic pain, such as poor quality sleep, irritability, depression, and withdrawal. The motivational-affective dimension of pain has added an important component related to how an individual perceives pain.

Theories regarding the perpetuation of pain are further extensions of the Gate Control Theory. The **Pattern-Generating Theory** proposed by Melzack[7] suggests that perpetuation of pain results from sustained activity in the neuron pools, including the dorsal horn (i.e., the entire gate system) and the homologous interacting systems associated with the cranial nerves. With reduction in the inhibitory influences, there is an abnormal bursting activity, which goes on unchecked and allows recruitment of additional neurons into the abnormally firing pools. This leads to the spread of pain. This theory is helpful in that it emphasizes the independence of pain transmission from the original precipitating stimulus. Once the pattern-generating mechanisms become capable of producing patterns for pain, any input may act as a trigger. Such triggers may include gentle sensory input from distant areas, sympathetic activity, and/or changes in one's emotional stress level. The clinical support for this theory lies in the countless patients who continue to suffer severe phantom limb, neuralgia, and back pain after surgical removal of neuromas, discs, or following ablative surgeries such as rhizotomies, cordotomies, and even total spinal cord resection.[7]

The evolving theories of pain have had important implications for selection of treatment interventions. Early theories suggested that pain might be related to the spirits of the dead in certain religions. As pain took on more physical relations to the body, pain was considered a physical problem directly proportional to the pain, resulting in attempts to cut out the pain. The Gate Control Theory provided important concepts of pain modulation by internal and external systems, and treatment interventions were modified accordingly. As the motivational-affective and cognitive components of the pain experience were added, theories were expanded. The perpetuation of pain is now understood to include emotional, behavioral, and physiological components. Influenced by both the Gate Control Theory and Pattern-Generating Theory, the multidisciplinary team considers the multidimensional aspects of pain in planning appropriate interventions.

Pain Classification

Humans have difficulty with the definition of pain. Painful experience is so intimately associated with affective distress that behavior devoid of disagreeable emotional components may be questioned by some as to whether or not pain could be present. Autonomic as well as emotional responses, including motivation, affective, and cognitive functions, contribute to the pain experience. Interpretation of a painful stimulus is ascribed based on past and present experience.[11,12]

Acute Pain

Acute pain of a physical nature is a signal of real or impending tissue damage; it represents a signal of biological dysfunction. It appears concurrent with either tissue damage or stress and generally disappears with healing.[13,14] Acute pain is also a psychological experience interpreted within the context of one's experience, environment, and cultural background. The psychological responses to acute pain under specific conditions are summarized in Table 28–2. The degrees to which these psychological reactions to pain exist (i.e., the duration and the psychological adaptation responses to pain) differentiate acute from chronic pain. In the presence of acute pain, removal of the physical cause of the pain eliminates these psychological reactions to the pain. The patient is then able to return to a normal life-style without difficulty. In the presence of chronic pain, however, psychological reactions become problematic as they reflect adaptive responses. The responses persist even as the pathology of the original injury subsides. If some of these components are addressed early in treatment, the progression to a chronic pain state may be avoided.

Table 28–2 PSYCHOLOGICAL REACTIONS TO SPECIFIC CONDITIONS IN ACUTE PAIN SITUATIONS

Antecedent Conditions	Consequent Reactions
Lack of information (uncertainty)	Anxiety
Perceived loss of control	Helplessness, escape/avoidance
Social isolation	Anxiety, depression
Observation of another's pain behaviors	Increased pain behaviors

From Chapman, CR, and Turner, JA: Psychologic and Psychosocial Aspects of Acute Pain. Lea & Febiger, Philadelphia, 1990, p 128, with permission.

Chronic Pain

Although acute pain is related to injury or damage to tissue, **chronic pain** is said to be the pain that persists after healing is completed. The taxonomy of the International Association for the Study of Pain has stipulated an arbitrary time of 3 months post injury when pain, if still present, is considered chronic. This does not, in practice, reflect the different time frames needed for various types of tissue injury to heal. In reality, pain extending beyond the time of the repair of tissue damage might be less than 1 month or more than 6 months.[5] Although acute pain generates sympathetic response mechanisms such as anxiety, patients with chronic pain often display few autonomic responses. Rather, these patients display increased preoccupation with somatic symptoms, disrupted interpersonal relationships, and disturbances in sleep, appetite, or libido.[15] Chronic pain is not an entity but a process; its neurophysiological components are something of a mystery.[16] Every practitioner must remember that chronic pain is no less "real" just because it is no longer a response triggered by a specific noxious stimulus or injury. The patient experiences pain, and that experience alone is sufficient to establish the pain diagnosis. Mechanisms by which pain may be perpetuated independent of any external or peripheral stimulus are described below.

Central Pain

Central pain is pain that is associated with a central nervous system (CNS) lesion that is independent of peripheral injury or tissue damage. It is characterized by the type of "vicious cycle of reflexes" originally described by Livingston.[4] **Thalamic pain syndrome** was first described by Dejerine and Roussy in 1906. A prominent feature of this disorder is continuous pain, described as aching, boring, gnawing, burning, or crushing sensation and occurs in response to a lesion in the thalamas; symptoms are opposite to the side of injury. Autonomic and vasomotor dysfunction is common with this pain.[6] Patients with stroke may develop thalamic pain immediately, with lesions affecting that area of the brain. In other cases, an acute type of pain can become centrally maintained owing to such factors as those described in the Pattern-Generating Theory. These patients have a variable period during which, if accurate diagnosis can be made, intervention can eliminate the development of the central pain. Such patients often present with many or all of the characteristics of chronic pain, while continuing to experience a very definitive, physically driven pain.

Central pain phenomenon also can include both **causalgia** and **reflex sympathetic dystrophy (RSD)**. These are now categorized under the term **complex regional pain syndromes (CRPS)**. This complex disorder or group of disorders (i.e., a syndrome) may develop as a consequence of trauma affecting body part(s), with or without an obvious nerve lesion. CRPS consists of pain and related sensory abnormalities, abnormal blood flow and sweating, abnormalities in the motor system, and trophic changes in the structure of both superficial and deep tissues. These disturbances are typically restricted to one extremity, usually distal, and are variable in clinical expression, but may spread to other extremities.[17,18] A quote from the medical journals of S. Weir Mitchell,[19] a physician in the American Civil War, provides an eloquent description of this type of CRPS pain:

> *Its intensity varies from the most trivial burning to a state of torment. . . . Exposure to the air is avoided by the patient with a care which seems absurd, and most of the bad cases keep the hand constantly wet, finding relief in the moisture rather than in the coolness of the application. . . . As the pain increases, the general sympathy becomes more marked. The temper changes and grows irritable, and the face becomes anxious, and has a look of weariness and suffering . . . the rattling of a newspaper, a breath of air, the step of another across the ward, the vibrations caused by a military band, or the shock of the feet in walking, gives rise to an increase of pain.[19 p 221]*

There are generally three stages associated with RSD:[18,19]

1. *Acute (or early) stage:* The patient experiences constant burning or aching pain, **hyperalgesia, hyperesthesia, hyperpathia,** localized edema, muscle spasm, and accelerated hair and nail growth. Skin temperature is often higher than normal by 2° to 6°F and movement is guarded and limited.
2. **Dystrophic** *stage:* Characterized by increased hypersensitivity and burning pain, lowered skin temperature, cessation of hair and nail growth, **hyperhidrosis,** pale cyanotic skin color, muscle atrophy, spotty osteoporosis, and emotional changes, including seclusion and marked protection of the extremity.
3. *Atrophic stage:* Characterized by decreased hypersensitivity; normalization of blood flow and temperature; smooth, glossy skin; drawn, severe muscle atrophy; pericapsular fibrosis with diffuse osteoporosis; and personality

characteristics associated with a chronic pain syndrome.[18,19]

Chronic pain and central pain often are used synonymously. The controversy is first one of terminology then one of pathophysiology. The patient with chronic pain does not benefit from the modalities and interventions appropriate for acute pain. The chronicity of pain itself imposes additional components, including psychological, emotional, and sociological consequences. Some patients with chronic pain may experience all the characteristics of true central pain phenomenon.

Overt compensatory responses to pain, such as an antalgic gait or a guarded stance are key clinical factors to the chronicity of pain.[20] Dysfunctional movement adaptation results in abnormal shortening or lengthening of muscles and ligaments, creating **postural stress syndrome (PSS)**. As these adaptive movement patterns become habituated, **movement adaptation syndrome (MAS)** may become the source of the pain.[21] Patients are often told, when the original injury has healed, that they will "have to learn to live with their pain." These patients often make extraordinary progress with symptom reduction and increased function when the movement patterns are normalized. Failure to correct faulty postures and dysfunctional movement may contribute to the eventual development of true central pain.

CLINICAL MANIFESTATIONS

The clinical manifestations of a patient who is developing chronic pain, rather than recovering from acute pain, are initially subtle. When the physical therapist determines that response to acute care treatment is slow or negligible, it is important to begin exploration of a bigger picture, and not simply the site, mechanism, and manifestation of the injury. By asking open-ended questions and waiting for answers, the therapist might learn that the patient has several significant stressors; for example, the patient may mention a family crisis, or speak reluctantly of returning to work under a certain supervisor or co-worker. The pain also might appear to spread to areas distant from the original site of injury, confusing both the therapist and the patient.

Clinical Presentation

Leriche, in 1939, wrote eloquently of the ramifications of prolonged physical pain:

> *In a very short time it will convert the brightest spirit into a being haunted, driven upon himself, thinking only of his disease, selfishly indifferent to everything and everybody, and constantly obsessed by the dread of recurrent spasms of pain.[5]*

When pain has been experienced for several months, the patient will present for treatment with a composite of symptoms and complaints. The longer the pain persists, the greater the probability that the patient will become depressed, fearful, irritable, somatically preoccupied, and erratic in the search for relief.[12] As chronic pain persists, both the rehabilitation team and the patient often become uncertain as to the most appropriate course of treatment, and both parties may develop a sense of helplessness. The more disappointed the patient and the team members are with each other, the less direct are their interactions.[22]

A patient often will interpret questions about other areas of his or her life as threatening, especially if some form of compensation is being awarded. The patient may perceive questions about family, work environment, and other stressors as an attempt by the team to negate pain complaints and terminate benefits. Whereas, this information is easily gathered and addressed in the acute phase, patients may become angry and threatened about addressing such issues when the pain is chronic. It is as if, in the patient's mind, the rehabilitation team members have given up looking for the physical problem and are trying to find another reason for the pain. The patient with chronic pain is committed to the belief that the pain has a physical cause (i.e., the body has been damaged) and that the cause will be found within the health care system. To the patient who is **suffering,** it borders on absurdity to suggest that the experienced discomfort is not real.[23] This communication breakdown, in conjunction with the frustration of not finding the relief sought from the health care provider, exacerbates the lack of trust and increases patient difficulty when interacting within the health care system.[16]

Exclusive use of sensory formulations of pain neglect the major affective, cognitive, and behavioral components of the pain experience that are amenable to other forms of control. Discriminating between expressions of pain having origins in physical pathology versus psychological and social sources is a major challenge for the physical therapist.[12] A patient whose primary complaint is chronic low-back pain often complains of fatigue, sleep disturbance, change in appetite, and decline in libido. Each of these complaints is common in clinical depression. The patient often will persist in attributing all symptoms to a physical pain problem.[24]

Although many chronic pain conditions begin as a single treatable problem, with time the pain experience becomes enmeshed in a complex web of emotional, behavioral, and social interactions that defy simple solutions.[16] The social impact of the pain expression can be enormous, significantly influencing the role of the patient in the community, in the family, and among friends. What is crucial in the development of a treatment plan is the impact these changes have on the patient. A patient often undergoes an identity crisis because his or her role in society is no longer as clear. The patient no longer meets the criteria of either a healthy person with a job or a sick person. Owing to the lack of clarity about what status applies to patients with chronic pain, some adopt a position of disablement and assume the attitude that society has a responsibility to take care of them. Others with chronic pain see themselves as willing to pass as normal whenever possible, and wish that no such disablement be applied to their status even though they have restrictions on their activity, their role in society, and probably their role in the work force.

The dilemma for the patient with chronic pain is that the traditional medical model was strongly founded in a split between mind and body, and provided a role structure suited for those with acute rather than those with chronic pain. A model long overdue in its application to patients with chronic pain is one of greater collaboration between rehabilitation team and patient. For patients with chronic pain, who often maintain a much longer relationship with their rehabilitation team, the **collaborative health care model** supports more active involvement in decision making by the patient. This fosters a greater sense of control and empowerment, both critical for patients with chronic pain. Differences between the more traditional medical model and the collaborative model are shown in Table 28–3. The patient would have expected not to work under the traditional medical model. Patients may feel there is a great deal of pressure to work and are unclear why they should not be allowed to stay home until well. The benefits of working in pain and remaining more active rather than withdrawing into the isolation of home are unclear to many patients. A few patients, whose traditional expectations of adopting the sick role are not fulfilled, may feel caught in a world where "going through the motions" is good enough for everyone, except the patient still seeking relief from suffering. The identity crisis, which develops in some individuals when role conflict becomes chronic, may result in a loss of self-esteem and self-identity, and an overwhelming sense of shame.[25,26]

A Case Presentation

How an individual experiences pain, and how that pain is reported to another person depends not only on a complex interaction among numerous physiological, psychological, social and cultural variables, but also on past pain experiences and how those pain experiences have been handled by health care providers.[16] These variables may be appreciated best in examining a case study. A 25 year-old woman is referred to a physical therapist for evaluation following a skiing injury. The diagnosis is a torn plantar fascia of the right foot. The patient first is seen 2 weeks after the injury, and enters the physical therapy clinic on crutches. The physician requested initiation of weight-bearing but the patient finds this painful and difficult. During the initial examination, the therapist notes a loss of dorsiflexion of the right ankle; otherwise, range of motion (ROM) of the extremity is within normal limits. The strength of

Table 28–3 DIFFERENCES BETWEEN THE MEDICAL AND COLLABORATIVE MODEL OF HEALTH CARE

Medical Model	Collaborative Model
Assumption that illness requires a separate, well-defined status and role to reduce issues of secondary gain and that a physician must declare a person eligible for this role.	Assumption that individuals want to remain involved in their daily social situations as much as possible.
Patient-physician role relationship is not a spontaneous form of interaction, but a well-defined encounter whose object is the health of a single individual.	Patient-physician role relationship is less well-defined, the two parties discussing and agreeing to a course of action and accountability for changes agreed upon.
Goal of the encounter is to promote significant change for the better in the patient's health, using the imbalance of power of the physician-patient relationship.	Goal is to promote change for the better and/or increased adaptation skills of the patient by a collaborative approach.
1. Sick person is exempt from normal social roles, i.e., an acute sick role is adopted.	1. Patient is expected to maintain active social roles, both at work and at home in a compromise role, integrating healthy activity when possible.
2. Sick person is not responsible for his or her condition.	2. Patient is educated about how his or her behavior contributes to disease and how to develop self-management skills.
3. Sick person must recognize that illness is inherently undesirable and should try to get well.	3. Getting well occurs with active participation; encouraged to seek out options.
4. Sick person is expected to cooperate with physician, i.e., follow instructions.	4. Patient is an active team member, participating in treatment planning.
5. The physician's role is to return the sick person to his or her normal state of functioning.	5. Physician's role is to educate, assist in decision making regarding treatment, and facilitate self-responsibility for symptom control.

the right leg is normal, although attempts to test the dorsiflexors are limited by pain and decreased ROM. The right foot is slightly warmer than the left foot. Treatment interventions include whirlpool, active and passive ROM of the right ankle, and progressive weight-bearing. The physical therapy goals and outcomes include restoring full ROM and return to full weight-bearing without an assistive device. The therapist anticipates that 2 to 3 weeks will be sufficient to accomplish these outcomes.

At the end of 3 weeks, the therapist has not seen any significant progress and reports these findings to the physician. These physician sees the patient, agrees with the therapist's findings, and requests that the patient be pushed harder to become weight-bearing. The patient becomes more fearful, and reports that many common stimuli are now increasing the pain in the right foot. Vibrations, drafts, and sunlight are painful, and weight-bearing attempts elicit crying, refusal to cooperate, and anger.

The therapist notes progressive withdrawal, and decides to spend time listening to the patient, and encouraging conversation about home and family. The patient reports an inability to work, difficulty in living alone, and difficulty getting around in the apartment. She reports not having family close enough to help, and that friends are becoming less willing to spend time helping her. She reports that most of the day is spent alone, reading or trying to sleep. The patient is losing weight, and indicates that sleep intervention medication is ineffective. The pain medication provided to her has been used up, and the prescription cannot be refilled. When the therapist asks how much control she feels over the pain, the answer is "none." The therapist asks about childhood pain experiences, and how these incidences were dealt with by her family. The patient reports that she was encouraged to ignore pain, to "tough it out," and that her many sports injuries often were ignored. The pa-

tient recalls being able to cope with these earlier injuries and that pain was never much of a problem. The patient further reports wanting to stop coming to therapy because she feels it is not helping.

The therapist's documentation indicates that several problems are becoming evident with this patient:

- The pain is becoming worse, and the patient shows signs of early CRPS.
- The patient reports changes in sleep and eating patterns.
- There is a suggestion that the patient is becoming more isolated and withdrawn, possibly showing signs of depression.
- The patient reports that she feels no control over the pain and that this situation differs dramatically from past experiences with pain.

The therapist has identified several important problems with this patient, who is not recovering as first expected. An original minor injury is developing into early CRPS, and the original treatment plan is no longer considered sufficient. In a collaboration with the physician, decisions are made to (1) consult an anesthesiologist specializing in CRPS to assist in outlining future physical interventions, (2) request that the patient see a psychologist to determine the extent to which current coping skills can be enhanced to restore some sense of control, and (3) reevaluate the medication needs and prescribe medication to assist with sleep and address the anxiety the patient reports.

A multidisciplinary approach is needed and a team is formed to develop new treatment interventions. In general, the multidisciplinary **rehabilitation team** includes a physician, physical therapist, psychologist, social worker, vocational counselor, and others. The original injury is not a good predictor, at this point, of the level of disablement the patient will self-report or the level indicated by examination findings. The original injury is now one of many factors influencing current functional limitations and the patient is significantly more disabled than the original injury would predict. The challenge to the team is to determine what factors are creating the disablement and address the possible causes.

Current level of impairments and functional limitations must be determined. The pain arising from the acute injury is no longer the problem. Factors influencing the pain experience may include financial difficulties, marital problems, lack of education and training, work stress, and an overall failure of coping skills to manage the experience. Information revealed to only one team member must be shared with the other team members. These initial confidences may reflect either the team member's skill at addressing specific issues or the patient's expectations of who is the appropriate person to receive certain information. The patient, for example, who sees the physician as wanting only information directly related to symptoms might designate a physical therapist or psychologist as a person to whom other information can be revealed (Table 28–4).

Sociological Perspective

The **sick role** has been studied extensively by medical sociologists. There not only are expectations regarding the physical condition, but also social expectations to be followed. These expectations are reflective of the traditional medical model. As defined by Talcott Parson,[27] they fall into the four behavioral mandates:

- The sick person is exempt from "normal" social roles.
- The sick person is not responsible for the condition.
- The sick person should try to get well.
- The sick person should seek technically competent help and cooperate with the physician.[28]

The differences between the medical (traditional) and collaborative models are summarized in Table 28–3. The patient with chronic pain may be seen as assuming the "sick role" on an ongoing or permanent basis. The dependency and regression expected in the acute sick-role behavior is often expedient in allowing the physician to make diagnostic and treatment recommendations. These attributes in patients with chronic pain become part of the problem.

One's response to stress (or pain) is a product of the personal skills and abilities available to cope with the problem. Just as each individual possesses different coping skills, each also differs in the ability to manage problems effectively.[6] By identifying the coping skills the patient has acquired prior to the pain experience, one removes the patient's blame or lack of motivation as the primary issue. This allows for assessing what coping skills can be taught to enhance the ability to function and resume a normal role in society.

Pain is regarded in our society not as a natural part of life but as something that one expects to be rid of, and often something that reflects negatively on who that person perceives him- or herself as being. Pain may be experienced as a situation in which terrible things are happening. People in great pain feel that there is no certainty that pain will not worsen; there is no sense of control, only a sense of feeling helpless to take action.[28]

Behavioral Categories

Just as there are many factors that contribute to how a patient manifests the pain experience, there are many components within a presentation that health care providers can view as typical or atypical. This information will help guide how to respond to the patient, and how the plan of care is developed. Gildenberg and DeVaul[6] have defined four categories of patients with chronic pain that can be considered in understanding patient behavior and influences responsible for that behavior (Table 28–5).

Some behaviors, if identified by the therapist in the acute stages, may indicate that the problems presented are no longer the type amenable to acute therapy. Indications may include one or more of the following patient behaviors:

Table 28–4 DETERMINING PATIENT'S NEEDS

Initial Examination	Treatment	Reexamination
ROM: Right dorsiflexion limited to neutral	Active and active assistive ROM in whirlpool	ROM decreased; patient refuses to allow active assistive exercise; active exercise more painful
Strength: WNL; dorsiflexion could not be tested	Attempt to increase weight-bearing; strengthening to hip and knee non-weight-bearing using weights	Hip and knee strength stable, remains WNL; ankle and foot too painful to assess
Sensation: Normal above ankle, mildly hypersensitive on dorsal and plantar surfaces to light touch and pinprick	Use whirlpool to assist with normalizing sensation and ROM	Very critical of controlling water temperature; tolerance to turbines in whirlpool decreased; marked increase in sensitivity, i.e., very guarded of foot being touched
Stress loading: Weight-bearing only to 10 lbs after sympathetic block; ambulating non-weight-bearing with crutches	Stress loading techniques in water and not to increase weight-bearing tolerances	Has not tolerated stress loading protocol; measure only 2 lbs loading with much resistance due to pain
Skin: Foot slightly warmer to touch; skin shows some spotty redness		Foot significantly warmer, red, blotchy; skin appears more transparent

Table 28–5 CATEGORIES OF PATIENTS WITH CHRONIC PAIN

The need-to-suffer-patient	This patient represents only a small minority but is responsible for most of the frustration and disappointment associated with chronic pain management. Pain is a psychological necessity, and sickness is used to fill a life-long need to suffer.
The overwhelmed patient	This patient best fits the observation by Mechanic (see text) that an individual may not have the necessary coping skills to handle a given stressor.
The psychogenic patient	This patient is one that has been studied for years; presents with pre-existing psychological problems, inadequate defense mechanisms, or other trauma, which then makes it impossible for the patient to mobilize the necessary forces to deal with the current, chronic pain problem.
The assigned patient	The assigned patient is felt to have developed a chronic problem largely by the actions of primary health care provider. Identification of psychosocial stressor immediately after injury can have a significant impact on reducing the chronicity of the physical problem, but such issues are not often dealt with by the primary care physician or the physical therapist who sees the patient in the acute setting.

1. No longer discusses a return to work in relation to a specific time frame but rather in relation to a "cure."
2. Unwilling to discuss family situations.
3. Maintains that the injury has caused all his or her problems and that life was fine until then.
4. Directs excessive anger at a situation or an individual involved in the case (e.g., employer, physician, insurance representative).
5. Demonstrates an "I'll show them attitude."
6. Is less interested in his or her home program than before.
7. Expresses comfort with role reversals in the home.

Any of these behaviors may indicate the existence of a variety of complex problems in addition to the specific tissue damage. These behaviors are representative of a patient who, to some degree, is entering a crisis state. The pain is perceived as something senseless that has taken control of the patient's life.

MEDICAL MANAGEMENT

When someone experiences an injury or sudden onset of pain, the involvement of the physician is appropriate and often necessary. Initial examination may include taking a history, conducting tests, and dispersing medication. Specialty physicians may offer treatment interventions ranging from injections to surgery. In addition, physical therapy intervention often is appropriate. The medical management of pain is addressed below followed by rehabilitation management. A function of the collaborative model is to ensure that care is comprehensive rather than segregated. A primary function of the case manager is to ensure that treatment is comprehensive and multidisciplinary, thereby maximizing the treatment outcomes.

Pharmacological Intervention

The use of analgesics for acute pain management is common. Their function is not only to relieve pain but also the anxiety that accompanies the experience. In addition, nonsteroidal anti-inflammatory drugs (NSAIDs) and muscle relaxants may be pre-scribed. The function of these medications is to minimize tissue damage and to maximize tissue healing. Reducing patient anxiety and fear also reduces the sympathetic arousal level, allowing for increased blood flow and changes in pain perception. Prolonged use of any medication can be problematic, because adverse side effects may develop over time. Generally, nonaddictive medications may be taken for a longer time if side effects do not become a problem. Narcotic analgesics are often both physiologically and psychologically addicting, but research provides ample evidence that when the medication is properly adjusted to the pain level, psychological addiction is less likely.[29] Patients must be carefully screened and monitored, but may stay on narcotics for years, enabling them to reach a level of activity with significantly higher function.[30,31] Patients using properly managed narcotics sometimes will report they perceive the nociceptive component of their pain, but "it no longer bothers them," (i.e., there is less suffering associated with the pain experience). The use of narcotics designed to fill the same receptor sites as the endorphins made within the body results in a decreased production of endorphins. Endorphin depletion can occur with prolonged use of narcotics and, with such depletion, the need for the drug increases. New advances in pharmacology are enabling narcotic medication dosages to remain stable for long periods of time. The use of pumps to continuously infuse narcotic medication locally or systemically have been developed for immediate postoperative use as well as long-term pain management.

At the time the patient first seeks medical care, expectations are established based on the description of the problem. Studies by Fordyce et al.[32] have shown that patient expectations have a significant effect on the duration, intensity, and problems associated with the pain. In a prospective study with two groups, one group was given medication and specific expectations regarding the duration the medication would be needed, and that they would rapidly regain their level of function.[23] The other group was handled in a more traditional manner. These patients were encouraged to call for more medication if needed, and were given no specific time frames in which they could expect to recover. Not only did the first group return to function faster, but they sustained higher levels of function after a year. The demographics and injuries were the same; the expectations of both health care provider and patient were not.

As the injury becomes chronic, adjustments need to be made to the treatment regimen. Medications that were helpful in the acute phase are often no longer helpful when the pain becomes chronic. Data from pain clinics, often the last stop for patients seeking help within the medical model, indicate that the most important factor in increasing level of function and successfully managing the pain is the reduction of excessive use of multiple addictive medications.[6] Patients traditionally collect a wide array of drugs, including pain medications, muscle relaxants, anti-anxiety medication, and tranquilizers. Such medication is often prescribed initially in lieu of a psychological assessment. Chronic use of such medication may contribute to the withdrawn, depressed appearance of patients with pain.

Primary care physicians often have little experience in discussing with patients the advantages of a psychological intervention rather than prescribing anti-anxiety medications. Although the practice of using anti-anxiety medications rather than dealing with the psychological reasons for anxiety may be useful in the short term, this practice can be detrimental to the patient if it is continued over many months.

Role of Anesthesiology

Anesthesiologists may perform blocks, injections or other procedures for several reasons:
1. To determine the anatomical source of the pain.
2. To ascertain specific nociceptive pathways.
3. To differentiate between local and referred somatic pain.
4. To determine the role of the sympathetic nervous system in the pain experience.
5. To differentiate local pathology from reflex muscle spasm in such disorders as torticollis and the piriformis syndrome.

These procedures also may be used to block pain to determine the patient's response to the elimination of pain. By blocking afferent (nociceptive) or efferent (sympathetic) fibers for several hours, abnormal activity may not return when the blockade wears off. In addition, during that time rehabilitation is facilitated and more aggressive therapy can be performed that otherwise might not be tolerated. The restoration of normal movement patterns may enhance the perpetuation of relief after the block wears off. These procedures, which may be diagnostic and/or therapeutic in nature, are listed in Table 28–6.

When pathology cannot be corrected surgically and tissue health restored, occasional treatment using blocks or injections may improve function as well as quality of life. Stimulators can be implanted

Table 28–6 ANESTHESIOLOGIST'S INTERVENTIONS

Procedure	Diagnostic	Therapeutic
Facet block	Identify location of pain in facets rather than disks	Not repeated routinely but may be used in an occasional patient if long-term relief (months) obtained by interrupting reflex cycle
Epidural injection done with fluroscope	Considered best intervention when pain is one sided, i.e., lateral foramenal disc herniation; 1–3 steroid injections done when nerve root is pain generator to decrease swelling	In some patients, may be repeated every 1–2 years if symptoms relieved for several months
SI injection	Identify SI as source of pain; steroid injections to determine duration of pain relief	If SI is primary pain generator steroid injection may be repeated only when severe irritation/inflammation limits function up to maximum of 3 per year
Diskogram	Used prior to surgery when fusion considered; several disks are injected, including one normal to identify disks causing symptoms	New techniques include intradiscal steroid for annular tear or internal disk derangement
Nerve block	Identify nerve as pain generator; may include steroid use to decrease inflammation	May be repeated in some patients if significant relief is followed by return of significant pain
Piriformis/other muscle block	Identify pain generator; steroid injected to decrease muscle tone and decrease inflammation of nerve	Allows aggressive rehabilitation efforts to stretch muscle, decrease nerve entrapment, relieve pain; may need to be repeated for full therapeutic effect
Sympathetic blocks	Determine role of complex regional pain syndrome[a] in pain complaint	May be repeated 4–10 times to reverse complex regional pain syndrome cycle; done in conjunction with aggressive therapy and prior to sympathectomy
Dorsal column stimulator (considered for neuropathic pain)	Determine if pain can be controlled after all other conservative attempts have failed	May be implanted for long-term pain control
Indwelling pain pump (indicated for nociceptive pain)		May be used for long term pain control if surgery is not an option and pain cannot be altered. Evens out and provides better pain coverage than oral medications, physical therapy, injections, etc.

[a]Complex regional pain syndrome is newly developed terminology that includes reflex sympathetic dystrophy (RSD).

along the spinal cord, using the Gait Control Theory to block pain impulses from traveling to the brain where perception of pain occurs. This procedure, most commonly used for failed low back syndrome requires careful patient selection. It may be more successful than alternatives such as additional surgery for segmental stabilization, rhizotomies, and ganglionectomies.[33] The development of scar tissue, altered nociceptive feedback loops, and permanent tissue compromise from either the injury or surgery may be indications for pain management provided by the anesthesiologist. These interventions are generally accompanied by patient instruction in self-management, pain medication in some cases, and rehabilitation efforts.

Blocks may be used after surgery to reduce postoperative pain or used in the early stages of CRPS to reduce progression to full CRPS. Therapeutic blocks for CRPS interrupt the cycle of continuous pain transmission and allow treatment to mobilize and restore function. The effect of a block may extend beyond the duration of the drugs, allow for normalization of sensory feedback loops, and provide some relief from physical pain. Patients often are more able to work and function at a higher level with an increased sense of control over the pain. Patients may also be more willing to work on the psychosocial aspects of their lives that impact the pain experience.[34]

Ablative Neurosurgery

Techniques such as **rhizotomies** and **cordotomies** previously have been considered last-resort techniques. In many cases, the short-term results were excellent, but the long-term results were found to be poor; the pain found other tracts or neurons on which to travel, and the pain returned after variable time periods of several months to years.[35–37]

Permanent **sympathectomy** for any of the CRPS may be very successful. Usually, multiple sympathetic **nerve blocks** are performed first to determine the effectiveness of the blockade. If the block relieves pain but the duration of the relief does not increase with several blocks, a permanent sympathectomy might be very beneficial. This technique is more successful in the earlier stages of the disorder as compared to the later stages.

REHABILITATION MANAGEMENT

Assessment

The information collected during the examination must be thorough and identify all possible obstacles to successful treatment. From this information, the therapist is able to establish an appropriate plan of care. Physical therapy alone will not meet all the needs of patients with chronic pain. Referrals to other disciplines will be needed.

PATIENT INTERVIEW

Data should be gathered about past treatments, medications, and health care providers from the medical record and directly from the patient. The patient should be requested to identify what treatment was beneficial in the past, what was considered not helpful, and why. The patient should describe the original pain, its location, and the mechanism of onset. From this history, it is often possible to identify the initial injury and the various compensatory mechanisms that have evolved into dysfunctional responses.

As mentioned, an individual's response to pain is a product of unique life experiences. If one concedes that chronic pain is a stressor, then we can examine the methods by which someone may respond to pain with stress-coping mechanisms. Several responses have been outlined by Sternbach:[38]

1. *Adaptive response:* The individual may remain calm and optimistic and continue to function well despite adversity.
2. *Behavior disorder:* Addictive behavior, such as alcoholism or overuse of medications, may emerge; other forms of acting out may occur.
3. *Thought disorder:* Patients may respond by escaping into schizophrenic or paranoid disordered thinking.
4. *Affective disorder:* The sense of being overwhelmed may pervade, with the patient experiencing intolerable anxiety or depression.
5. *Somatoform disorder:* Physical dysfunction in excess of the original injury may develop, and symptoms such as nausea, dizziness, and fatigue emerge as a way to cope with the emotional distress.

These responses are likely to occur when significant stressors (e.g., concerns about job security, home, family relationships) are imposed in addition to the chronic pain. Chronic pain is unique in the degree to which the individual may become disabled as a result of the stressor, but the responses are similar to other major stressors. The high levels of **disability** often encountered with chronic pain have also been suggested to arise from other factors (e.g., the requirements for workers' compensation, recompense through litigation following motor vehicle accident, or classification of disability as defined by the Social Security Administration).

Having a stress checklist[39] is helpful to assist the therapist in determining the impact of pain on the person's life. This list often identifies problems in family relationships, financial problems, or problems with intimacy (see the Appendices in Chapter 2). The patient is likely, at this chronic stage in rehabilitation, to argue that these problems arose at the time of the injury and pain onset. What is important is the recognition that these problems also must be dealt with during treatment by appropriate professionals.

The patient should be asked to describe his or her perception of the cause of the continued pain. For example, patients may harbor fears of cancer and paralysis that, if alleviated, may significantly reduce symptom complaints. Patients should also be asked how improvement will be manifested. The answer should be related to improved function, not solely on the elimination of pain. The answer may help lead to a discussion of the patient's expected outcomes of treatment. Outcomes of physical therapy for patients with chronic pain should be functionally oriented, not dependent upon cessation of pain. To assess changes in function, a list of functional activities can be used that details tasks that the patient does, no longer does, or has never done. This information is often a revelation for patients who may not realize the extent to which they have limited their usual activities.

BODY DIAGRAMS

Patients are asked to complete **body diagrams** with various symbols to represent pain and other symptoms related to the complaints that precipitated seeking treatment. Body diagrams are a useful tool for understanding the location of pain. Comparison with earlier records from other facilities is also helpful. Body diagrams can be used in several ways. First, they can be used to determine whether the areas marked on the body diagram represent specific anatomical localization, or magnification of the pain with extensive marking outside of the lines of the body. These indicators may be scored, and the score used to determine whether extensive psychological testing is warranted.[40] Another use of pain drawings is to determine the extent to which compensatory movement patterns have developed. Particularly for patients with soft tissue injuries and myofascial pain syndrome, the development of satellite **trigger points,** altered movement strategies, and adaptive changes in the muscles and ligaments often have a significant impact on the body diagram. Figure 28-3 is a body diagram from a patient who was perceived as having significant functional overlay with emotional issues. Treatment was based on identifying and treating each component problem represented on the patient's body diagram. The diagram at discharge showed no complaints.

PSYCHOSOCIAL ASSESSMENT

The plethora of tests available for assessment of chronic pain is a testimony to the complexity of the problems. Patients can be asked to provide information in a structured format about the pain, but this does not ensure that the reporting reflects any more than an interpretation of the pain at a specific point in time. Changes in function become increasingly important as the disability from pain increases with no objective findings. Many factors are included in these tests and measures and provide valuable data to assist with establishing a diagnosis and prognosis,

determining a plan of care, and identifying the need for collaboration with other case providers.

The *Sickness Impact Profile (SIP)* is an instrument developed to measure health status and health-related dysfunction. This profile is not specific to patients with pain, although it has been used in evaluating patient populations with pain.[41] It covers physical and psychosocial factors, including information on home management and social interaction. See Chapter 11 for a more detailed description.

The *Multi-Dimensional Pain Inventory (MPI)* is an instrument designed to measure similar variables to the SIP, but is targeted to patients with chronic pain. One of three profiles emerges, with characteristic scales elevated within each profile. The MPI provides information in the area of support, perceived solicitous or punishing behavior by others, and levels of distress or lack of control.[42] A sample of the test is included in Appendix A. This test also can be used to evaluate patients with acute pain and who are seen for physical therapy. This inventory provides some indicators for early involvement of a multidisciplinary intervention.

The *McGill Pain Questionnaire* examines the various dimensions in which pain is perceived. The categories include sensory, affective, and evaluative descriptors.[43] A sample of a portion of this questionnaire is presented in Appendix B. This questionnaire addresses the quality and complexity of the patient's pain experience. However, several factors may influence the quality and level of detail provided by the patient. Some patients may feel past reporting has been misinterpreted by previous health care providers. They often express reluctance in filling out tests that might contribute, from their perspective, to mislabeling the nature of the presenting complaints.

Visual analog scales (VAS) also are important tools and can be used each session to assess present pain intensity. The patient is asked to rate his or her pain on a 1 to 10 scale, where 1 is equal to no pain and 10 is the worst possible pain. Some patients report that the pain never changes (i.e., they continue to rate their pain with the same number). These patients may fall within a category of patients who are unable to rate their pain unless it is absent; that is, either they perceive themselves as having pain or they do not. For this subgroup of patients, carefully planned instruction is indicated to teach them to discriminate between the various levels of pain. The numbers on these scales also may take on an unintended meaning. If, for example, a patient rates pain high at one therapy session, the patient might be allowed to skip exercise that day. That patient might then continue to associate any pain experience rated that high as a reason to stop all activity. Some practitioners using this scale have chosen to assign a meaning to the various numbers so that the ratings chosen by the patient are more meaningful. Visual analog scales also have been designed as pre- and post-treatment outcome measures, ranking a variety of activities and situations. A sample visual analog scale is presented in Appendix C.

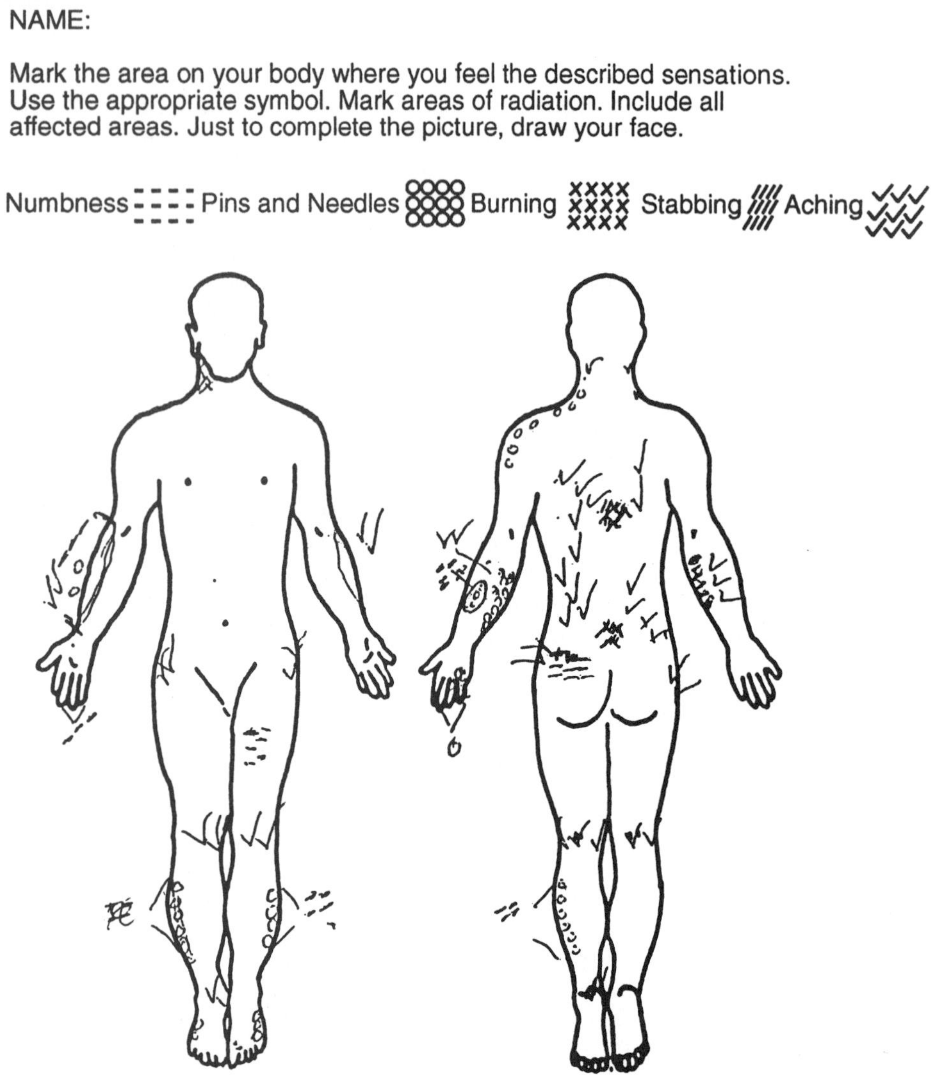

NAME:

Mark the area on your body where you feel the described sensations.
Use the appropriate symbol. Mark areas of radiation. Include all
affected areas. Just to complete the picture, draw your face.

Numbness ⚊⚊⚊ Pins and Needles ⊗⊗⊗ Burning ✕✕✕ Stabbing ⫽⫽ Aching 〰〰

Figure 28-3. Admission body diagram of a patient identified as having functional overlay; diagram used in developing a plan of care. The patient was asked to show where the pain was and what quality best described the pain.

The *Symptom Checklist-90 (SCL-90)* is a more detailed test than the MPI, but less involved and shorter than the *Minnesota Multiphasic Personality Inventory (MMPI)*. The SCL-90 contains nine symptom dimensions and a scale of distress. This test was not designed exclusively for use with patients with chronic pain.[44] The test provides useful information regarding patient perception of his or her situation in relation to distress behaviors such as anxiety, depression, and disordered thinking.

The MMPI is a psychological assessment. Many patients perceive it as having negative connotations. For example, the test is suggestive that health care providers do not believe the pain they are experiencing is real and that other reasons for the pain are being sought. In reality, the test does not seek to challenge the pain as not being real, but rather assesses the coping styles of the patient to the pain. The patterns of scale elevation that emerge from the MMPI assist the health care provider in understanding patients' response to pain, as well as how they are coping with and reporting their symptoms. Specific patterns have been derived for the popula-

tion of patients with chronic pain, such as the P-A-I-N cluster from among the MMPI scales described by Costello.[45] How a patient with chronic pain scores on the MMPI has been strongly correlated with how they respond to treatment. The MMPI also has proven useful in predicting a patient's response to major surgeries.[29,45,46]

There is ample research on the use of the MMPI with patients having chronic pain. Early research was directed at attempting to define a "pain-prone personality."[47,48] Evaluation of military men using the MMPI before injury failed to demonstrate any predisposing psychogenic factor that might predict which individuals would develop chronic pain following an injury.[18] A study by Sternbach and Timmermans[49] suggests that the profiles seen so commonly with patients having chronic problems may represent the effect of living with chronic pain. It is reasonable to infer that it is the marked decrease in pain that permits a return to previously normal levels of psychological functioning.[49]

The information obtained from these instruments assists in the development of an effective plan of care as well as helping to predict surgical outcomes.[50] Loeser[51] presents a graphic method of visualizing the complexity of chronic pain, and the multiple layers comprising the problem (Fig. 28-4).

It is imperative to keep in mind that individuals with chronic pain do have real pain. The incidence of true **malingering** (pretending to have pain when it does not exist) is extremely rare and all members of the team must be thorough in ruling out its possibility. This typically requires a psychological evaluation. Unless the diagnosis of malingering is correctly applied, the pain should be regarded as real even when objective measures cannot confirm its presence. The fact that objective testing has not made pain quantifiable is our failure, not our patient's. Accepting that patients who say they have chronic pain do actually have pain is the first step in establishing the rapport necessary to planning patient-centered interventions. Invalidation of a patient's symptoms by others is a common experience, and the patient must then devote more time to convincing the next health professional that the pain is real and that a physical reason for the pain exists. This attitude, along with the increased perceived need to have symptoms to justify the search for help and alleviation of suffering may lead to behavior considered **symptom magnification (SM)**. The patient displaying SM is a patient whose behavior is considered excessive and more severe than objective findings warrant. When one treatment intervention does not work, patients often find a reluctance to proceed with further treatment unless there is an increase in symptoms or problems. Thus, there develops an inadvertent tendency to magnify

symptoms so that the provider will be willing to support additional treatment.

Another disservice is to tell a patient "to learn to live with the pain." Some psychologists suggest that such a statement can be interpreted as life is not possible without pain.[52] Telling a patient who is overwhelmed and to some degree out of control with a symptom such as pain that there is nothing that can be done, and that he or she must accept living with the pain, may be unkind and unrealistic at a time when the patient's pain is mixed with suffering. The patient asking for help does not hear this message in terms of the pain but rather hears the gestalt of the experience. So, in effect, while the team member is saying that the pain will not change (i.e., the pathology that might be the cause of the pain cannot be repaired), the patient internalizes the statement with all the cognitive, affective, motivational, and emotional components associated with the pain. They hear that the amount of suffering they are currently experiencing along with the pain will not change. The team member must understand the patient's perspective of the gestalt and be willing to address the concerns, even if they are not verbally expressed. It is unlikely that the patient will make any attempt to seek clarification; what they hear, to them, sounds like a death sentence. The various components of the pain experience are represented in the outer circles of Loeser's Model (see Fig. 28-4). If the patient has developed the skills to cope with persistent pain, they have typically developed mechanisms of reducing their suffering and actively seek less treatment.

Patients of different cultures interpret pain differently, and attribute different meaning to pain that has become chronic. The practitioner must be sensitive to these differences.[53] Cultural differences often worsen the outcome of treatment intended to be helpful and may impose limitations in choosing treatment options. The practitioners must be aware of how their own biases alter their perception of the patient and what the patient reports. Any team member may have biases related to a particular method of communicating pain. Individual differences, such as the posture of the patient, can impact how seriously the problem is perceived by certain team members and what the projected outcome will be.[54]

PHYSICAL ASSESSMENT

The physical therapist is presented with a complex challenge when asked to assess patients with chronic pain. These patients may be dysfunctional in the psychological sense, as described in the previous section, and this may make physical assessment more difficult. Patients with chronic pain vary in the amount they communicate, from one extreme of wanting to tell you about everything that has happened since the onset of pain (characteristic of neuroticism), to saying almost nothing (characteristic of significant depression or lethargy).

When tests and measures are performed on patients with chronic pain, the complexity of the

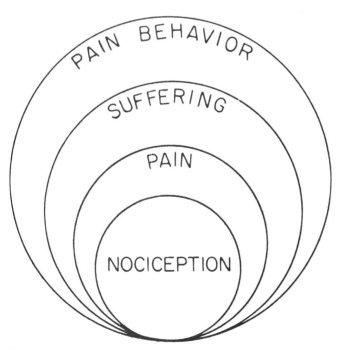

Figure 28-4. The four components of Loeser's concept of pain. (From Loeser,[51] with permission.)

problem becomes apparent. Multiple systems must be examined, and the tests and measures may vary, depending on the chronicity, scope, and type of complaints reported. Some common assessments and their application to the patient with chronic pain are presented in Table 28–7. The findings from the neurological examination may be normal and muscle strength testing is often within normal limits. Posture may appear outwardly within normal limits, although this is less common. Musculoskeletal examination may reveal asymmetrical posture. Typically, patients have little knowledge of the extent of the postural asymmetries until measured by a physical therapist.

Postural asymmetries often develop quickly after the injury, as the body seeks to protect the injured area. Tissue lengths adapt over time, and become part of the established, or habituated, movement pattern. The movement patterns of patients with chronic pain are frequently rigid and guarded to compensate first for the pain and later for balance disturbances that may arise from the postural asymmetries. Joints distant from the original injury eventually may be limited in ROM as these asymmetries become chronic.[21] Movement dysfunction becomes a perpetuating factor and may persist long after the initial pathology is resolved. With extensive postural and movement dysfunction, the patient may report virtually all movements to be painful. Movements also may be limited by fear as the patient experiences pain in areas distant from the initial injury. Testing ROM in standing and then in a prone position may result in a marked increase in joint excursion. Testing the same task in two different positions can assist the therapist in determining the influence of shortening of muscles or other soft tissue involved in the test movement. These discrepancies have been seen by some as support for the

patient attempting to "fake" limitations. In reality, they represent differences in movement related to movement strategies. This phenomenon of apparent changes in ROM and movement strategies can be demonstrated in normal, healthy subjects as well.

The use of equipment may allow objective documentation of impairments of endurance, muscle function, or balance. Cardiovascular fitness often is poor in these patients, and low endurance combined with rapid muscle fatigue may result in inconsistent testing. Surface electromyography (sEMG) is invaluable in assessing these patients, because it can identify movement strategies and the muscle firing patterns.[55–58] These components generally are not able to be monitored by the clinician, yet may be the most significant component in the adaptation to chronic pain.

In patients with chronic pain, the therapist may feel as if chasing an elusive perpetrator. A patient presenting with relatively new symptoms of temporomandibular disease (TMD), for example, may reveal older injuries that significantly impact the ability to treat the newer complaint. The presenting complaint of TMD may be a secondary problem arising from an old injury that became symptomatic as compensatory mechanisms failed. In such situations treatment directed at the presenting compliant (i.e., TMD pain) will not relieve symptoms. Evaluation of the symptoms in the context of possible old injuries and compensatory mechanisms will lead to a more satisfactory outcome. For example, a leg length discrepancy, either structural or functional, if left to impose its postural stresses, may lead to (1) altered pelvic alignment, (2) scoliosis, (3) altered head position, (4) changes in cervicocranial junction, (5) changes in neck muscle activity, (6) altered lower limb joint alignment, and (7) muscle imbalances, to name a few. The presence of subtle postural stress syndromes for years, with eventual adaptation failure, may be the reason for the presenting complaint of TMD.[59] Old injuries and adaptive postural changes are typically not disclosed unless the examiner makes the possible connections and asks those questions.

Central pain often is presumed present if a patient with pain appears to have had sufficient time for healing of the injured tissues. This relates to the rather arbitrary decision to label pain as chronic if it persists for 3 months beyond the injury. If healing is presumed completed, then pain is no longer seen as coming from the site of the injury, but is now a central pain phenomenon. Therefore, treatment of the injury site is considered no longer necessary. It is the responsibility of the physical therapist to determine if any adaptive changes of muscles or ligaments or any adhesions are contributing to the symptom complaints.

Patients with chronic pain can experience autonomic and central nervous system dysfunction such as myofascial pain syndrome, localized tissue problems, major movement strategy dysfunctions, and a sense that they are totally out of control (Fig. 28-5). Autonomic dysfunction often can be observed, at

Table 28–7 ASSESSMENT TOOLS

Tool, Skill Application	Use in Chronic Pain Evaluation
ROM, goniometry	Document changes in ROM as it relates to primary and secondary symptom complaints
Manual muscle testing	May be inconsistent; trigger points and pain may inhibit muscles during break testing as a reflex protective mechanism
Neurological exam	Generally normal; does not assess muscle dysfunction or soft tissue problems
Manual and soft tissue exam	Multiple adaptive changes in muscle length and tension; myofascial trigger points will often be prevalent
Aerobic testing	Patients may have significant habit of self-limiting activity; aerobic exercise without pain is not possible, so they avoid
Balance	Muscle dysfunction and postural stress syndrome, along with poor sense of body position, often contribute to poor balance
sEMG	Assess muscle dysfunction; provide objective documentation of symptom complaints, fatigue, physical tolerances, and functional limitations

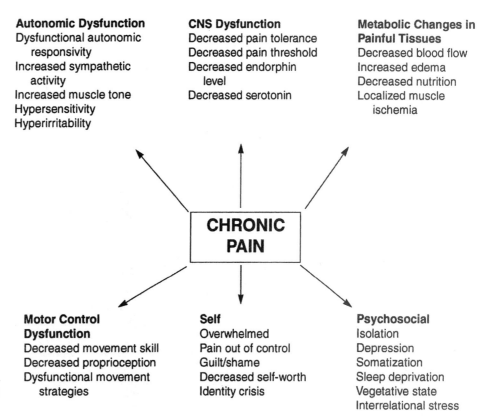

Autonomic Dysfunction
Dysfunctional autonomic
    responsivity
Increased sympathetic
    activity
Increased muscle tone
Hypersensitivity
Hyperirritability

CNS Dysfunction
Decreased pain tolerance
Decreased pain threshold
Decreased endorphin
    level
Decreased serotonin

**Metabolic Changes in
Painful Tissues**
Decreased blood flow
Increased edema
Decreased nutrition
Localized muscle
    ischemia

**CHRONIC
PAIN**

**Motor Control
Dysfunction**
Decreased movement skill
Decreased proprioception
Dysfunctional movement
    strategies

Self
Overwhelmed
Pain out of control
Guilt/shame
Decreased self-worth
Identity crisis

Psychosocial
Isolation
Depression
Somatization
Sleep deprivation
Vegetative state
Interrelational stress

Figure 28-5. The assessment components for the complex psychophysiological dimensions of chronic pain.

least in part, through multiple-channel biofeedback recordings. For example, a discrepancy might be seen between objective and subjective thermal information (Fig. 28-6). Other examples of autonomic dysfunction are altered response patterning of two different factors such as temperature and sweat gland activity. For these autonomic factors, the temperature of the hand should increase and the sweat gland activity, measured as electrodermal activity, should decrease when the person is achieving a greater degree of relaxation. With dysfunctional autonomic states, two parameters may both increase simultaneously.[60]

Interventions

Coordination of the information gained by each member of the rehabilitation team is necessary to ensure a comprehensive plan of care. An overview of goals and outcomes of physical therapy and interventions is presented in Figure 28-7, relative to the problems identified in Figure 28-5.

A problem arises when the team has identified a level of indirect **impairment** that does not correlate with a higher level of **functional disability.** The basic premise of the medical model is that symptoms are impairments and are an expression of anatomical, physiological, or biochemical abnormalities indicative of a disease process.[16] Patients with chronic pain often do not fit this model, because their level of disability far exceeds the known pathology and symptoms. The medical and legal issues become inseparable because the health care providers are asked to determine if someone should receive compensation, such as social security, for his or her pain, which may exist without sufficient objective pathological explanation. The overall objective is to restore homeostasis, or internal stability and equilibrium, to the extent that this can be accomplished. Full homeostasis may not be possible. The patient and the team must then come to terms with the fact that a cure is not the end outcome of physical therapy and that the patient will

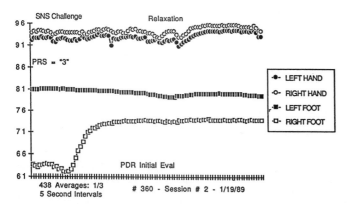

Figure 28-6. Patient with diagnosis of failed low-back syndrome subjectively experienced the left foot as cooler than the right foot; objective measurement demonstrated a 20°F difference, with the left foot warmer than the right foot. Thermal recordings from hands and feet were collected over a 20-minute time period and plotted. SNS 3D, sympathetic nervous system challenge; PRS 3D, pain rating scale; PDR 3D, physiological dysregulation evaluation.

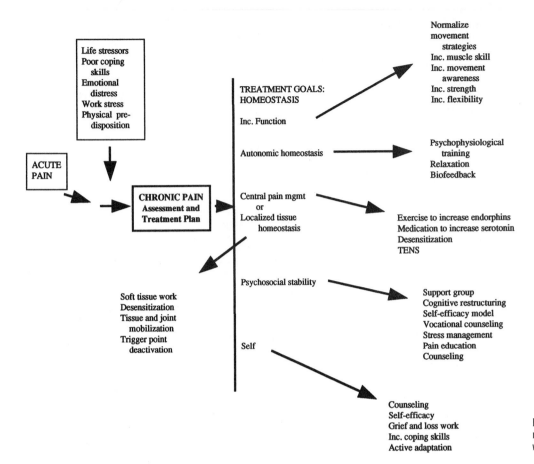

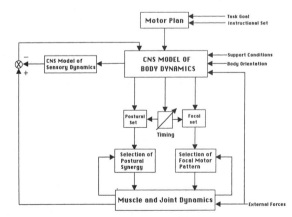

Figure 28-7. Use of the assessment model shown in Figure 28-5, with treatment interventions.

need to adjust to permanent functional limitations, disability, or continued pain. The confrontation of this adjustment issue may be responsible for moving patients across the nebulous line from acute to chronic pain or from practitioner to practitioner.

FUNCTIONAL RESTORATION

Patients with chronic pain adopt dysfunctional movement, postural, and psychological patterns. Habituated adaptation of movement and postures affects the motor strategies used as well as the length-tension relationship of muscle, tendon, and other soft tissues. The movement abnormalities include motor strategies, speed, coordination, and slowing of the reversal of antagonists. Over time, the sensory feedback from these dysfunctional patterns will convince the CNS that these altered patterns are normal. A model of the motor plan in governing coordination of posture and movement is shown in Figure 28-8.

Use of the term *functional restoration* implies normalization of aspects of function such as movement strategies, skilled muscle recruitment, muscle strength, and flexibility, resulting in an improvement at functional levels. sEMG is a useful tool for the normalization of motor control strategies.[61,62] The compensatory patterns that developed immediately after the injury may have been useful then to protect structures and reduce pain, but these same patterns can become the source of the pain after the original

injury has healed. Flor et al.[63] have described the difficulty that patients with chronic pain have in the discrimination of muscle tension. This problem was evident when the discrimination involved the affected, painful area and when the discrimination task involved nonaffected muscles. This research suggests that delay or inability to respond to changes in muscle tension, which may be psychological or postural in origin, may lead to significant changes in muscle function. Muscle recruitment imbalances (Fig. 28-9) can be assessed with sEMG, and the same modality used for treatment.

Figure 28-8. Sensory feedback mechanisms having an effect on altering posture and movement. (From Guymer,[98] p 58, with permission.)

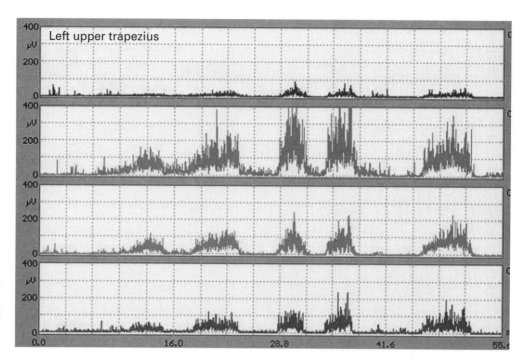

Figure 28-9. Patient was asked to shrug shoulders evenly; sEMG records asymmetry that may arise from proprioceptive or muscle firing dysfunction. LUTR 3D, left upper trapezius muscle site; RUTR 3D, right upper trapezius muscle site.

Over time, sEMG has become useful in understanding the effects of trigger points and myofascial pain syndrome. Not only can trigger points refer pain, as has been so well documented by Travell and Simon,[64,65] but trigger points can refer muscle spasm or inhibition[66,67] and other phenomena.[68] In reviewing the soft tissue problems of 45 patients with chronic low-back problems and assessing their muscle function with sEMG, Headley[69] showed that inhibition of the gluteal muscles by active trigger points palpated in the quadratus lumborum may play a role in the chronicity of low-back pain. Release of the inhibition by deactivation of the trigger points in the quadratus lumborum (Fig. 28-10) resulted in rapid increases in strength and function of the gluteal muscles. This phenomenon has been described by Rosomoff et al.[70] Mayer,[71] who also reports that low strength levels generally are not a sign of severely advanced muscle atrophy but rather of deficits from factors such as fear of reinjury, neuromuscular inhibition, and altered neural input to the muscle from higher centers (i.e., movement strategies).

Repetitive motion disorder, also known as **cumulative trauma disorder (CTD)** refers to a number of work-related syndromes seen by physical therapists. Muscle fatigue and overload are common characteristics in CTD and present unique challenges in the chronic pain population.

The pathophysiology of muscle fatigue has been outlined by Simons[72] and the effect of muscle fatigue leading to overload, as measured with sEMG, can be seen in Figure 28-11. These problems may not be observable clinically, and fatigue with overload often yields test results that suggest submaximal patient effort. This is another situation where the use of sEMG provides an advantage,

because it allows documentation of which muscles are being used to perform a task. Muscles recruited may be the prime movers, but also may be compensatory muscles that are poorly equipped to perform as the prime mover for any length of time.

CTD presents with the unique problems of repetition and static loading creating physiological stress to soft tissue that is progressive and somewhat predictable. A model of four stages of CTD developed by Headley[73] is presented in Table 28–8. The documentation of underlying muscle dysfunction and fatigue components using this model provides insight into problem identification, treatment planning, and outcome measurement. In the latter two stages of CTD, patients exhibit significant muscle fatigue that affects execution of a treatment plan and functional outcomes related to home and work tolerances.

Presence of severe, chronic muscle fatigue has significant implications for rehabilitation. Normal muscles, when worked to fatigue, can recover to the pre-exercise level in 5 to 20 minutes.[57] This is measured with sEMG, using spectral analysis (i.e., a distribution of the firing rates of the motor units, rather than amplitude). In patients with severe CTD, several minutes of work can overload a muscle, and recovery of its spectral value can take 45 to 90 minutes. When tested over several days, these patients often do not recover overnight, so they present for the second day of testing with lower spectral frequencies (more muscle fatigue) than they presented with the first day. These patients may report increasing difficulty with job performance over the course of a week, with pain higher at the end of the week than at the beginning. They may report spending the weekend resting to recover for the next work week.

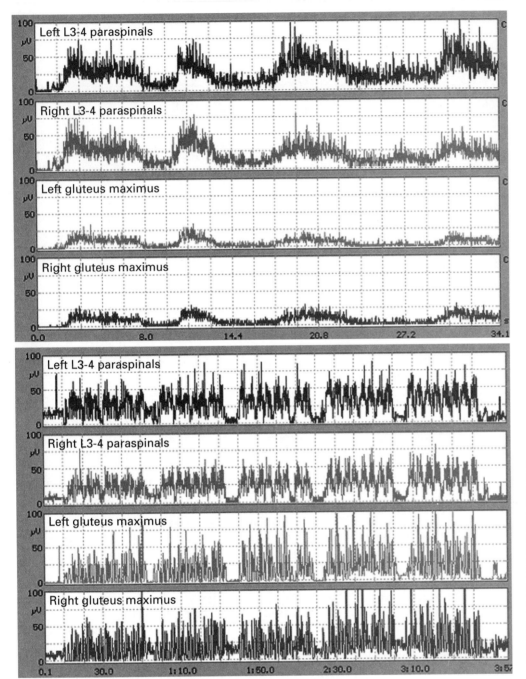

Figure 28-10. Poor amplitude in the gluteal muscles, associated with trigger points in the quadratus lumborum (*top*). Retesting of the same patient, with an increase in gluteal amplitude following deactivation of quadratus lumborum trigger points (*bottom*). With proper gluteal recruitment, the level of function of the patient has increased. Gluteal muscle site chosen was 3 inches below the middle of the iliac crest. LL5 3D, the left lumbar muscles adjacent to the fifth lumbar vertebra; RL5 3D, right lumbar muscles adjacent to the fifth lumbar vertebra; LGLT 3D, left gluteal muscles; RGLT 3D, right gluteal muscles.

Many patients with chronic pain initially cannot tolerate the type of exercise program used during acute rehabilitation. These patients have fundamental problems with movement. They may not be able to produce slow, smooth, controlled movements, even in body parts distant from the original injury. The misuse of muscles is significant, and may be more of a problem than actual loss of strength. Retraining these patients to move with slow, smooth, and controlled motions must precede any general strengthening program. Patients often cannot isolate a single joint movement, so retraining of this isolated joint movement is helpful as well. The first level of rehabilitation for these patients often is movement therapy. This can be based on Felden-

krais,[74] the Alexander Technique,[75] Tai Chi, or any other techniques which increase awareness of how movement is performed and how corrections can be made.

Attempts to strengthen these muscles invariably fail. The endurance to sustain an activity simply is not available. Muscles may fail to be recruited even when they are expected to perform as the prime mover. Or they are recruited during active movement, but as soon as slight resistance is added, the muscle shuts down as a protective mechanism (Fig. 28-12). When accessory muscles are required to do a task for long periods, these muscles become fatigued, with poor recovery as well, and other muscles are forced to take over. Patients with CTD

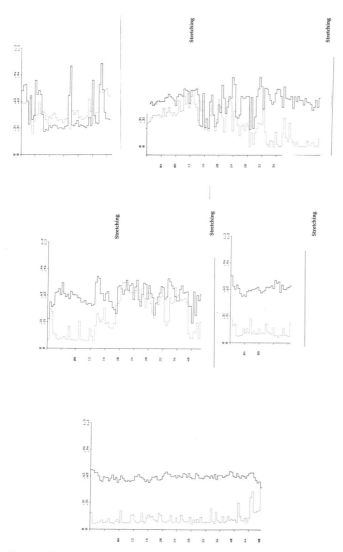

Figure 28-11. Patient monitored on upper trapezius muscles with sEMG at the work site for 4 hours. The right upper trapezius (*lighter line*) experiences rapid fatigue as compared with the left upper trapezius (*dark line*). The patient continues to perform the symmetrical task with the sEMG showing overload on the right side after the first hour, despite stretching breaks. (Each panel is 45 minutes in duration; patient was instructed to stretch every 20 to 25 minutes throughout the recording period.)

re-education and movement training before any strengthening program can be attempted.

Many patients present with a combination of recent dysfunction in addition to chronic changes, which have set the scene for the current problems. The entire system of postural stress and MAS should be considered to determine what factors are contributing to the current symptom complaints and loss of function. Progressive postural adaptation leads to exhaustion of the body's adaptive potential.[59] This may lead to a gradual increase in symptom complaints and functional deficits that make identification of the primary problem difficult and complex. Someone with years of chronic pain may not have a new injury, but simply present with a failure to continue movement adaptation.

Once muscle recruitment has been normalized and efficiency of the muscle restored, strengthening is appropriate. Strengthening can be done either with minimal equipment or with sophisticated computerized equipment. *The principle of specificity of training* indicates that muscle strengthening is specific to the mode of training.[76] A muscle strengthened isometrically at 45 degrees of flexion will use that increased strength within that narrow range of joint motion and more so when stressed isometrically. Functional strengthening of muscle is imperative, with monitoring of muscle activity to ensure that the muscle is working as expected during the functional tasks.

Exercise has important advantages in addition to strengthening muscles and restoring endurance. Both mental status and sleep have reportedly improved with exercise.[77] Various measurement tools have shown that depression is lessened and self-esteem increased with an increase in cardiovascular fitness. McCain[77] reports that the stages of sleep may be affected by exercise, with an increase in slow-wave sleep and a decrease in REM sleep.

EDUCATION

Increasingly, as the collaborative model is adopted and integrated, the patient bears greater responsibility for actively planning treatment and following through. An important focus of education is to facilitate patient problem-solving ability. Exercises should not be prescribed without the patient's thorough understanding of what each exercise is designed to accomplish, for example, which muscle is being stretched or strengthened. The patient must develop the skills to monitor and evaluate performance and determine changes in symptoms.

These expectations of self-responsibility remove patients from the passive sick role model and elevate them to the role of an active team member in maintaining their own health (see Table 28–3).

For a patient to change level of function, he or she must understand when symptoms reflect hurt as opposed to harm. It is critical for a patient with chronic pain to understand when injury or a change in pathology may occur. Patients may experience an increase in their pain after an activity, when muscles are sore but no physical damage has been done.

often present with a different movement strategy at several points during the same day. One set of compensatory patterns used to perform the required task is subsequently replaced with other compensatory patterns. Restoration of strength and endurance, once the muscles have reached this stage is long, costly (physiologically, emotionally, and financially), and not always successful.

The presence of trigger points, muscle spasm, and altered muscle tone are treated to enhance the work targeted at restoring normal length, contractility, and relaxation. Both physical and physiological changes can have a significant impact on the ability of the muscle to function normally, and restoration of muscle function may begin with soft tissue work directed at muscle, ligaments, and the fascial layers. Such work must then be followed by muscle

Table 28–8 STAGES OF CUMULATIVE TRAUMA DISORDERS: RELATED MUSCLE DYSFUNCTION

	Trigger Points	Muscle Dysfunction	Fatigue Characteristics[a]	Functional and Symptom Complaints
Stage 1	LTR, UTR	LTR ↓, UTR ↑, task-specific	Mild delay (2–3× normal) in recovery from fatigue	Pain between shoulder blades, UTR area; possible soreness when leaving work at end of day; no problem performing leisure activities, seldom recognized as an evolving CTD problem
Stage 2	LTR, UTR, levator, infraspinatus, SPS, scalene	LTR ↓, UTR ↓↑, scalene ↓, task-specific	Moderate delay (4–6× normal) in recovery from fatigue; fatigue failure is specific (i.e., limited to low load, static fibers)	Soreness that may persist to next morning; pain that might be eliminated only with rest; inability to do static tasks at home without pain but still able to perform other activities without symptoms
Stage 3	LTR, UTR, levator, infraspinatus, SPS, scalene, teres minor, posterior deltoid, FA flexors	LTR ↓, UTR ↓↑ scalene ↑, FA flexors ↓↑, dysfunction generalized to most tasks	Severe delay (8–12 h) in recovery from fatigue; fatigue failure more generalized, involving entire muscle(s)	Increasing fatigue during week; reported need for rest after work by midweek to continue working; use of weekend and holidays to recover; great difficulty maintaining a static work task
Stage 4	LTR, UTR, levator, infraspinatus, SPS, scalene, teres minor, posterior deltoid, FA flexors, FA extensors, SCM	LTR ↓, UTR ↓, scalene ↓, FA flexors ↓, FA extensors ↓↑, SCM ↓↑, generalized dysfunction	Profound delay (12–36 h) in recovery from fatigue; MF fails to show any recovery 1 full day after fatigue testing	Profound functional limitation in all daily activities; inability to do simple activities of daily living at home; poor prognosis for any work requiring static load on involved muscle groups

[a]Determined by surface electromyography and reflecting the power spectrum median frequency of LTR.

Note: This table reflects surface electromyography examinations of more than 200 patients who had a CTD, using electrode sites overlying the LTR, UTR, scalene, SCM, and FA flexors and extensors. Dynamic functional muscle testing is standardized, as is the isometric fatigue testing for spectral analysis, done before and after fatigue and after specified rest periods.

↑ = hyperactive; ↓ = inhibited; ↓↑ = either inhibited or hyperactive; LTR = lower trapezius; UTR = upper trapezius; CTD = cumulative trauma disorder; SPS = serratus posterosuperior, FA = forearm; SCM = sternocleidomastoid; MF = median frequency.

From Headley, BJ,[73] with permission.

Although this type of pain may hurt, there is no harm done; that is, there has been no physical damage to tissue. The increase in pain may cause distress until a patient learns to understand and problem-solve the difference between hurt and harm. This skill-building requires assistance to develop a sense of control over the pain, giving the patient confidence to manage flare-ups, and to modify the exercise program or activity level without seeking assistance. There are two strong indicators of the success of this model. The first is whether the patient has a support system that offers assistance when needed. The second relates to the patient's success in dealing with the anger and grief over the functional, economic, and social losses.

AUTONOMIC HOMEOSTASIS

The autonomic nervous system plays a significant role in the perpetuation of chronic pain states. Individuals differ in specificity of the autonomic nervous system. Specific situations may evoke different patterns in different people.[60,78] Some autonomic parameters may be overactive, others may be underreactive. Autonomic parameters often habituate as pain becomes more chronic.[79] A multi-modal assessment and treatment plan may be necessary, and can be implemented easily with new biofeedback technology. More than one autonomic parameter can be monitored (e.g., thermal and skin conductance, or blood pressure and heart rate) to allow for specificity training and normalization of autonomic nervous system activity.

Biofeedback can be a successful and natural method of allowing patients to develop insight into the role emotions can play in perpetuating dysfunction. Stress in patients with chronic pain may result in an increase in hyperirritability of muscles both at the site of the chronic pain and in distant muscle groups.[80] If the muscle activity is sustained, muscle fiber bundles can develop ischemia, energy depletion, and trigger points.[59] Development of self-management skills to decrease these effects has both physical and psychological benefits. Evidence of hyperirritability, or high resting levels of muscle tension, when shown to a patient, can result in rapid changes being made (Fig. 28-13). High resting activity in muscles may be specific to a particular functional position. Training designed to reduce muscle tension in novel and then functional positions can achieve good carryover to other positions.

CENTRAL PAIN MANAGEMENT

The central pain model presented by Melzack in the Pattern-Generating Theory suggests several methods of intervention from a rehabilitation perspective. This theory describes the alteration of the central, self-perpetuating feedback loop with either hyperstimulation or hypostimulation. Hypostimulation, a quieting of the nervous system, can be achieved in deep states of relaxation and environmental quieting. Hypostimulation can be induced to a greater degree when a nerve is blocked, temporarily interrupting pain pathways. The block is followed immediately by treatment interventions designed to restore normal movement and sensory input while the CNS cannot respond to these interventions with the unwanted hyperactivity that contributes to the central pain experience. Hyperstimulation can be achieved through rapid changes in an environment, such as what occurs using contrast baths by alternating hot and cold water. The spray techniques of spray-and-stretch described by Travell and Simons[64,65] may be used as a brief form of hyperstimulation. A hypercoolant is sprayed in quick strokes in one direction along the muscle fibers to alter neural input.

Several forms of intervention may assist in reversing the low endorphin levels often present in people with chronic pain. One approach is to use a hypostimulation model to treat the low endorphin levels arising from the maintenance of a state of chronic stress. This approach may include the use of deep relaxation and imagery.[5,81] **Relaxation training** may include autogenic training, open focus relaxation or music-enhanced relaxation. **Guided imagery** is a specific relaxation technique that may involve imagery chosen by the patient or chosen as a standardized sequence used by the therapist.

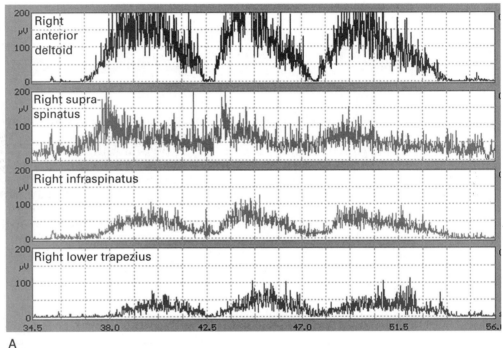

A

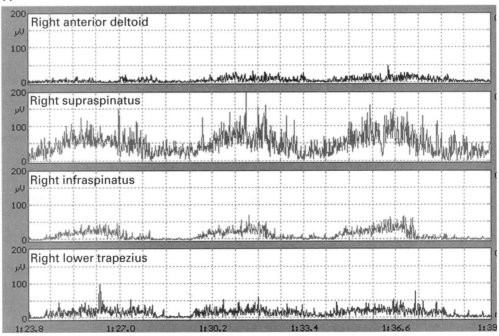

B

Figure 28-12. Patient was being tested during active external rotation of the right shoulder. The infraspinatus, a prime mover for this task, is performing with a peak amplitude of 122 uVts. (*A, top figure*). When the patient was given slight resistance, which should have resulted in an increase in infraspinatus activity, the amplitude decreased to a peak of 68 uVts. (*B, bottom*). Attempts to strengthen this prime mover would have resulted in compensatory activity and an increase in symptoms. (Scale = 0–200 uVts)

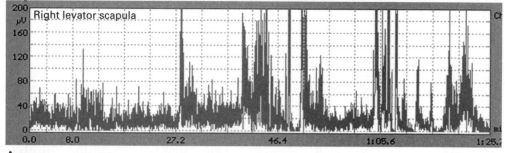

A

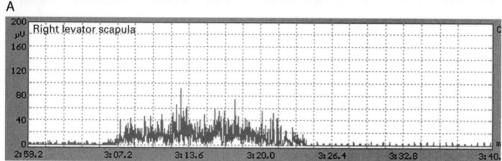

B

Figure 28-13. Patient had persistant pain in area of right upper trapezius and levator scapula. Monitoring of upper trapezius showed minimal dysfunction. Monitoring of levator scapula, however, showed unilateral hyperirritability while standing and sitting. In (*A*) the patient is standing, not making any attempt to change data being collected. In (*B*) patient has been working briefly with biofeedback to lower resting level of muscle tension with good success. (Scale = 0-200 uVts)

Relaxation training and guided imagery have been added to the multidisciplinary rehabilitation for patients with chronic pain in the last 15 years.[82] The rationale for use is to decrease muscle tension and anxiety by reducing the sympathetic arousal level.

The hypostimulation approach uses biofeedback training to assist in mitigating the effects of chronic stress.[83,84] Increased sympathetic tone may be a persistent problem, which in turn contributes to unbalanced or labored breathing patterns, chronic muscle tension and anxiety, and even a chronic low-grade level of panic. Biofeedback has a number of physiological measurement tools to monitor respiration, muscle tension, and sympathetic arousal for self-awareness training in altering these physiological responses. Reduction of this dysfunctional state, and return to a more homeostatic state, enhances normal neurochemistry.[60,78] A constant state of alertness (e.g., Why is this pain getting worse? When am I going to be normal? Why can't someone find out what's wrong?) contributes to the negative effects of chronic stress on the organism. Biedermann[85] and others[86] attribute the success of relaxation enhanced with biofeedback to an increased sense of control over the problem rather than to specific physiological changes.

The other approach of increasing endorphin levels is in the use of a hyperstimulation model such as exercise.[87] McCain[77] has reported that true modulation of pain sensitivity may depend on tissue levels of endogenous opioids (i.e., the body's endorphins), which are increased during exercise. Because serotonin levels are low in many patients with chronic pain, serotonergic antidepressants have been used for reduction of the clinical signs of decreased activity or motivation, social withdrawal, and appetite impairment associated with serotonin depletion.[88] These medications have the added benefit of helping the patient sleep.

Stress loading, another approach to hyperstimulation of a more localized nature, is a method of desensitization that has gained increased popularity in recent years. Stress loading involves very carefully graded increases in weight-bearing through the involved extremity. Stress loading may be accomplished in conjunction with sympathetic blocks to enhance patient cooperation and progression. This method can be done at home frequently throughout the day. Tasks duplicating activities such as scrubbing the floor may enhance not only joint compression but range of motion.[89–91]

Transcutaneous electrical stimulation (TENS) is another useful modality in pain management. The Gate Control Theory described by Melzack and Wall[3] is the theoretical basis for the use of TENS. A small electrical stimulation is provided either near or distant from the area of pain and alters the information sent to the CNS from the area of pain. The type of stimulation applied may differ with specific types of pain. Acute pain, which travels through fast ipsilateral corticospinal tracts from the Aα fiber groups, responds to a different stimulation pattern than the pain carried through the C fibers, which are slower and more diffuse in their path. The use of TENS has been found effective in a number of acute pain syndromes and helpful in the immediate postoperative period.[92,93] The efficacy of TENS with chronic pain is more difficult to determine, because long-term follow up is necessary. Choi and Tsay[94] reviewed a number of clinical studies of TENS with patients having chronic pain. They found an overall success rate of 60 percent initially, decreasing to 40 percent at 1 year and 30 percent at 2 years. Achterberg and Lawlis[95] cite a possible increase in endorphin production with TENS application, but emphasize the need to try various placements of the electrodes. Effective electrode placement may vary widely among patients. These authors report that the most successful placements often were those chosen by the patients themselves. The wide variance in electrode placement, combined with the options for waveforms used, complicate the ability to provide a straightforward protocol for TENS application.[94] Differences in stimulus frequencies alter neurophysiological effects. The wide variation of options now available with TENS units is reflective of the variety of approaches available in pain modulation. Appropriate use of TENS for any condition requires an understanding of the neurophysiology underlying pain modulation and a commitment to identifying a wide variety of electrode sites and stimulus characteristics. TENS was criticized when claims were made that it was capable of curing the cause of the pain. Literature is now clear that its role is one of altering the pain experience, not one of curing the pain.[96]

The most recent modality for altering pain perception is *cranial electrotherapy stimulation (CES)*. Using auricular electrode clips, current is said to have an effect on normalizing the erratic alpha wave activity seen in patients with chronic pain. The effects may be produced through direct effect on the parasympathetic autonomic nervous system or through direct action on the brain at the limbic system. Significant changes reported include anxiolytic relaxation responses such as smoothing and slowing on electroencephalograms, lowered electromyographic (EMG) activity, increased peripheral temperature, and reductions in blood pressure, pulse, respiration, and heart rate.[97]

SOFT TISSUE TREATMENT

Many types of soft tissue treatment, for example, pressure on myofascial trigger points, muscle energy techniques, **cross friction massage,** and **craniosacral therapy** can be used to reduce adhesions and restore tissue homeostasis. Such treatment also may have a positive benefit on the pain experience and functional level of activity. Muscle imbalances, existing for long periods or producing a multitude of dysfunctional patterns, have an influence on joint alignment and tissue length. Pain may result when the muscle imbalance imposes abnormal forces upon the joint for a long period. Grieve[98] emphasizes the need to treat the entire arthrokinetic system including the muscular imbalance, connective-tissue tightness or tethering, and localized soft tissue changes to reduce the abnormalities of movement. Homeostasis of tissue length, tissue tension, and muscle-firing patterns are as important to the overall well-being of the patient with chronic pain as is homeostasis of the autonomic nervous system.

Psychosocial Issues and Self Issues

The team members will address psychosocial issues and negative self-image. Although these may be seen as the primary focus of behavioral medicine, psychology, and social service, all team members must be involved to provide a consistent approach. Team members can enhance the development of self-responsibility and can address the fears and belief system that support disability.

Patients often have fears related to their role in the family, support system, and work. Chronic pain affects all aspects of life, often decreasing leisure activities, increasing social isolation, and causing role reversals. Patients frequently express a loss of control over not only the pain, but also life. Limited education increases the difficulty in seeing positive options for gainful employment in the future. The goals they had may now need significant modification. If they remain angry, these changes may be seen as someone else's fault and they continue to blame others. That anger spills over into marriage and relationships. When the pain seems out of control, they live with fears few others seem to understand. Fear of pain, as well as fear of activities that may cause pain, can be generalized to fear of movement **(kinesiophobia).** Scales have been developed to evaluate this phenomenon.[99]

A cognitive-behavioral model of fear of movement has been developed.[99] The study of this phenomenon has found that patients can be classified as "avoiders" or "confronters," those who avoid or confront tasks of increasing physical difficulty as documented on pen-and-paper testing. Those patients with chronic low-back pain who were classified as avoiders had a significant deficit in endurance of the lumbar paraspinal muscles when performing trunk extension and stabilization activities, when compared with those categorized as confronters.[100] The clinician must be thoughtful in exploration of causes for behavior and must examine physiological explanations before using labeling such as symptom magnification.

Common fears among patients with chronic pain include fear of movement, fear of the pain, and fear of lack of control. Such fears can have a significant impact on rehabilitation efforts. The psychobiology of changing a threat into a challenge has been well described by Rossi.[81] Whereas threats are associated with the release of catecholamines and cortisol into the bloodstream, a challenge is associated only with elevation of catecholamine levels. Rossi found that as the self-responsibility of subjects increased their levels of catecholamine levels decreased. Cognitive work to convert a negative stress or threat into a positive coping experience (i.e., a challenge) is associated with an altered perception of pain.

Pain viewed as a threat has numerous implications in rehabilitation. Often, in an attempt to increase the activity levels of patients with chronic pain, therapists have implemented a "no pain, no gain" strategy that ignores the complaints of the patients. This philosophy is used in work hardening programs. For example, patients who experience a knifelike, stabbing pain in the back, will be encouraged to continue to perform the task, with assurances that no harm is being done. However, the image the person has of the pain, especially when threatened, can have a significant impact on muscle recruitment patterns. In Figure 28-14, a subject was asked to perform a task that required the use of the muscles being monitored with sEMG. As the imagery of a "knife stabbing in the back" was introduced, muscle recruitment changed dramatically. Removal of the imagery allowed normalization of the muscle recruitment pattern. Both the functional level of activity and exercise and the patient's perception of pain are important. Using biofeedback techniques during imagery and cognitive restructuring, team members can assist patients and therapists in achieving more rapid gains in activity level.

Illness behavior is a psychosocial component of chronic pain that can be best addressed by the team as a whole, through recognition of what the behaviors represent and how positive coping skills can be implemented to reduce disability. By and large, most patients have coped with some adversity in the past. Exploring past stressors and methods of coping may shed light on how a program can be tailored to maximize the use of such skills. A patient who has a sense of being able to effect a change in his or her own life is said to have an *internal locus of control*. Such an individual has a strong conviction that what he or she does impacts the environment as well as life events.

When a strong internal locus of control is not present and the patient is more comfortable with concrete details, a program with a highly structured design will be helpful. Patients who need to come to decisions on their own will succeed in a program that presents them with material that allows them to effect own change. Other patients will easily accept the decisions of others. Some patients like to feel they are personally important and recognized every day, even in a group setting. To others, such individualized attention may have a negative impact. Every individual has a unique style of coping with life; understanding and enhancing the skills he or she has used well in the past increases the possibility of success in a pain management program.

Increasing the level of function is enhanced if patients have the confidence to proceed with the task, and if they actively make the choice to do so, as compared to feeling forced to do so. Teaching a patient to recognize the discomfort arising from the activation of a trigger point, for example, can be beneficial if he or she has developed problem-solving skills such as application of pressure or stretch. This allows the patient to eliminate the problem rather than having the pain increase. This problem solving becomes a positive coping mechanism.

Behavior modification techniques have become a vital component of pain management.[101,102] Fordyce introduced a program for elimination of chronic pain behaviors in the 1970s. Figures released by the University of Washington in Seattle, where Fordyce established his program, indicated that it was not uncommon for patients seen at this pain center to have undergone as many as 20 or more surgeries.[103] The focus of the new pain management programs

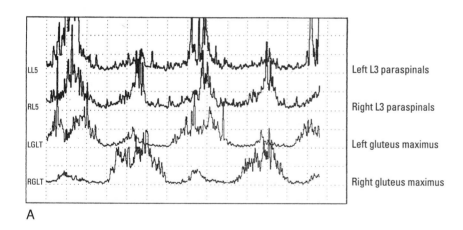

A

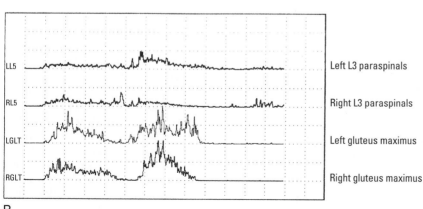

B

Figure 28-14. Subject performing task requiring use of L3 paraspinal and gluteal muscles. Subject has history of low back pain but was not experiencing any at the time of the testing. Amplitude of muscles before imagery (*A*). Recruitment changes after stabbing back pain imagery imposed (*B*). The subject's movement pattern did not change during the imagery, but the amplitude decreased to 20 percent of the pre-imagery values. With imagery reversing the pain experience, the amplitude return to normal levels.

was the modification of behavior and actions of both the patient and his or her family. Early pain programs focused on behaviors and resultant disability. Behaviors were categorized as those not occurring often enough and needing reinforcement, those that occurred too often and needing to be reduced in frequency, and those behaviors that were missing from the patient's repertoire that were needed. Behavior frequently was learned from the environment, comprised of either the family or others in pain. The program stressed modification of the behaviors to reduce disability. The model was an operant one in that the staff was encouraged to provide positive feedback for well behaviors and to ignore pain behaviors. The patient increased his or her level of activity by decreasing pain behaviors and learning, often for the first time in years, that the pain did not increase with an increase in activity.[103] Unnecessary surgeries were avoided and the success rate at least equaled that of those patients who continued to be treated with surgery.

Patient populations in these early programs differ from the population currently benefiting from chronic pain programs, as surgeons have learned that repeat surgeries often will not eliminate pain. Patients chosen for repeated spine fusions are now carefully selected based on clear findings of pathology and instability rather that just the continued presence of pain. Patients entering chronic pain programs now are more likely to be those with extensive soft tissue injuries or movement adaptation syndromes that have not been addressed, rather than those having central pain. These patients have experienced pain for long periods and often benefit from the multidisciplinary approach.

Cognitive-behavioral interventions are used to enhance coping skills and address covert pain behaviors amenable to operant treatment programs. Much of the illness behavior and the potential roadblocks to successful rehabilitation are a combination of inadequate coping skills, lack of education, and inappropriate labeling of sensation. All of these issues must be addressed during the active restoration phase of rehabilitation to ensure that techniques taught in counseling sessions are generalized.

Changes to the sense of self must be addressed. Some patients experience the very boundaries of their bodies changing as a result of the pain. The body image may be distorted when one area of the body is the only area of which one is conscious, because this sensory information overrides other sensory input and overwhelms the individual.[76] Children have eloquently demonstrated attacks to their body image through drawings of themselves during the rehabilitation phase.[104] A child burned on both legs and hospitalized for skin grafting, when asked to draw a picture of himself, drew his body without legs. Even when questioned by the therapist administering the test, the boy replied that the drawing represented "all of me." A patient who has been in an occupation that has significantly contributed to his or her sense of self has great difficulty in describing that self in the absence of that occupation.[105] Inherent in these changes are the losses incurred in function. The losses must be acknowledged, and grieving must be allowed.

Educational groups have several benefits for patients with chronic pain. First, if the information is used to reduce the threat of a patient's experience, psychobiological changes may occur. The neurotransmitters involved in the perception of pain may change as the sense of threat is reduced.[76] Second, because the sense of support is often crucial, a supportive environment can provide positive reinforcement. Third, the group reinforces the realization that patients are not alone in their pain, and that they have common issues and concerns. Group process alone often reduces the self-defeating cognitive thinking that has prohibited patients from asking questions to allay their anxiety because they are fearful they will be labeled as a "psych" case. Groups that focus on structured topics and dialogue are more beneficial than groups that allow patients to tell their stories repeatedly and to dwell on the failure of health care providers to help them.

SUMMARY

Chronic pain management provides unique opportunities and challenges for the physical therapist. Accurate identification of impairments, functional limitations, and disabilities can be extremely challenging. Additional challenges exist in selecting and implementing appropriate assessments and interventions to effect change. During the patient's acute stage, the role of the physical therapist is unique as the treating practitioner. Problems must be identified early and the patient referred to a multidisciplinary team for more effective intervention.

Chronic pain management also provides unique challenges in communication. Team members work with patients who expect a cure. The therapist must deal with those expectations. By approaching these patients as individuals who are overcome by the complexity of chronic stressors and as individuals who need tools to assist in dealing with those stressors, much of the stigma and blaming attitude can be eliminated. Patients are a vital component of the team; they must work with the rest of the team, as valued and active participants, to effect the highest level of functional change possible.

Identification of the component parts of the individual's complaints will assist the therapist in determining specific interventions. The overall outcomes of physical therapy include improved homeostasis, increased function, and self-responsibility.

Pain management is best when initiated early. During acute care, therapists can determine what the pain means to the patient and which coping skills might be lacking in managing it. Early identification of psychosocial factors often reduces chronicity. The use of such tools as sEMG may assist the clinician in identifying physical factors, which perpetuate pain symptoms.

Patients with chronic pain present with problems both unique and universal. Pain, one of the primary reasons for seeking health care, cannot be quantified or proven. The challenge to the therapist lies in altering a patient's perception of the experience and enhancing coping skills. The extent and costs of treatment can far exceed what would be expected from the known pathology or physical impairment. Yet, lack of pathology does not negate pain. Successful pain management takes the threat and the fearful mystery of pain and presents them to the patient as a challenge. It also provides the patient with the necessary skills needed to cope and manage pain.

QUESTIONS FOR REVIEW

1. On what basis should a physical therapist consider referring a patient (and to whom) to a chronic pain specialist?

2. Describe how the chronic pain from RSD differs from the chronic pain following a low back sprain.

3. List three ways sEMG may be helpful in assessing a patient with chronic pain.

4. List the members of the team who participate in the management of chronic pain. Describe the contributions of each.

5. What is the benefit of a self-responsibility model over one that stresses "no pain, no gain?"

CASE STUDY

PATIENT HISTORY: The patient is a 50 year-old female, seen for recurrence of her low back complaints 16 years after the original injury. Patient underwent a two-level fusion, L4 to S1 with internal fixation by Steffee plates 10 years prior to this episode of care. She originally returned to work 1 month after surgery. One year later the pain recurred, with subsequent surgical removal of the Steffee plates 18 months following the initial surgery. A pseudoarthrosis was found and a second fusion was carried out. Patient reported a return to work 3 days post surgery in a body cast. For the next 8 years, the patient reported intermittent flare-ups and low-level chronic pain, requiring daily self-management with stretching and trigger point work. Her activity level consisted of biking, hiking, cross-country skiing, and frequent travel. The patient worked without lost time, modifying her activity level and structure of her workload.

CURRENT PROBLEMS: Patient presents for treatment with debilitating pain limiting function and work. The patient began physical therapy, including manual therapy, stabilization training, and exercises, with some improvement. Rapid deterioration began 3 months into treatment that included the following changes from the initial examination:

1. Increased segmental instability L2 to S1, both anterior-posterior and posterior-anterior; increasing severity with lower levels.
2. Increased sacroiliac instability bilaterally with upslip right ilium anterior innominate and sacral torsion increased with increased activity level.
3. Hip flexor weakness bilaterally, MMT grade +2-3-/5 from 3/5.
4. Right foot dorsiflexor weakness, MMT grade +2/5 from 3-/5.
5. Increase neural tension sciatic nerve with dural tension. The right leg motion lacked 60 degrees from full extension when tested sitting and having knee extension done pas-

sively; on left leg knee extension lacked 35 degrees from neutral.
6. Increased falls requiring bilateral forearm crutches for safety compared to no assistive devices 3 months previously.
7. Increased difficulty walking and stair climbing. Gait pattern: no heel-toe gait on left, with foot placed flat or on ball of foot only; right hip externally rotated throughout gait and patient slides right lower limb through swing phase with increased hip hiking on right side.

Orthopedic examination determined that the second fusion 8 years prior has also been a pseudoarthrosis. A third fusion was performed, using both an anterior and posterior approach with titanium cages placed in the L3 to L4 and L4 to L5 disk spaces and Harrington rods placed bilaterally from L3 to S1 with screw fixation.

PAST MEDICAL HISTORY: Patient has had experience with chronic pain since age 9, when she reported onset of bilateral foot pain that was treated conservatively without a clear diagnosis. She had multiple sports-related injuries through high school. At age 9 she was involved in a motor vehicle accident in which she penetrated the windshield and suffered facial cuts and a concussion. Two years after college the patient developed reflex sympathetic dystrophy. This resolved over 18 months with a sympathectomy. She was out of work for 9 months. She returned to work without restrictions and worked 11 years before her initial low back injury. She has no other medical problems.

SOCIAL HISTORY: The patient is single and career oriented. She has been active in her professional career, traveling worldwide as a lecturer. She has been a participant in community volunteer organizations, sports, and hobbies. Her activity level has reflected her adaptation to prior injuries. She seldom revealed her problems with chronic pain or her low back surgeries unless asked. Patient is described by herself and others as "stoic" and a "survivor" with a high pain tolerance. She is a nonsmoker and does not drink alcohol.

PSYCHOLOGICAL ASSESSMENT: Her psychological assessment using the MMPI found a type "N" score that is characterized as follows (1) least likely to report "multiple pains;" (2) the lowest subjective estimate of pre- and postsurgical pain; (3) the least limitation of activity pretreatment; (4) the greatest reduction in pain as a result of treatment; (5) the shortest duration of vocational disability; and (6) the most physical improvement as a result of treatment.[45]

PHYSICAL THERAPY ASSESSMENT FINDINGS

1. Range of motion thoracic and lumbar spine during forward trunk flexion and extension from neutral decreased to 40 to 50 percent of normal. Lumbar corset is being used to compensate for instability at L3 through S1. Patient has secondary restrictions in diaphragmatic breathing excursion and postural dysfunction above unstable levels.
2. Ambulation increases pain symptoms in legs. Difficulty clearing right leg during swing phase of gait. When patient walks without assistive device she demonstrates bilateral Trendelenberg, hip abduction with attempted hip flexion, and decreased right dorsiflexion with compensatory locked-knee gait.
3. Strength in trunk decreased with testing of trunk extensors and abdominals to grade 2-3/5.
4. Hip range of motion decreased with extension, abduction and flexion to 75 to 80 percent of normal.
5. Increased neurological symptoms: reflexes (patellar and ankle bilaterally) absent; dural tightness: unable to obtain posture for stage one of slump test.

PROBLEM LIST

1. Patient reporting marked increase in falls during basic functional ADL and walking on level surfaces.

2. Segmental instability of lumbar segments has increased in spite of bracing and segmental stabilization exercises.

Outcomes/Goals

1. Outcome: Patient will be independent and safe in ambulation with no evidence of falls.
2. Goal: Patient will demonstrate decreased compensatory postural dysfunction in lower thoracic area and improved muscle activation in lumbar area.

Guiding Questions

1. This patient expresses a strong desire to avoid any outward sign of physical disability. The body-brace is totally hidden and according to the patient provides sufficient stability without using crutches or canes. How might you provide the patient with a rationale for using a more visible intervention to improve safety? What aids might you recommend?

2. Needle EMG studies demonstrate that no major nerve compression is evident. In light of negative EMG findings, how might you explain muscle weakness (right drop foot and bilateral hip flexor weakness) to the patient? How might you design a therapeutic exercise program?

3. What guidelines would you provide for exercise repetitions and frequency? Describe how the exercise program would be tailored to this patient in light of lumbar instability needing fusion as well as secondary SI instability?

4. The patient has already had two failed fusions. What factors would be important to assess in terms of her expectations and possible outcomes? What would be "red flags" that you might pass on as concerns to the primary physician and surgeon?

5. What factors would be indications to continue treatment until surgery or discontinue as no longer being beneficial? What considerations would indicate continued treatment benefit if surgery approval were delayed several months?

REFERENCES

1. Achterberg, J: Woman as Healer. Shambhala, Boston, 1990.
2. Bonica, JJ: History of Pain Concepts and Therapies. In Bonica, JJ (ed): The Management of Pain. Lea & Febiger, Philadelphia, 1990, p 2.
3. Melzack, R, and Wall, PD: Pain mechanisms: A new theory. Science 150:971, 1965.
4. Sternschein, MJ, et al: Causalgia. Arch Phys Med Rehabil 56:58, 1975.
5. Bonica, JJ: General Considerations of Chronic Pain. In Bonica, JJ, (ed): The Management of Pain. Lea & Febiger, Philadelphia, 1990, p 180.
6. Gildenberg, PL, and DeVaul, RA: The Chronic Pain Patient: Evaluation and Management. In Gildenberg, PL (ed): Pain and Headache. Karger, New York, 1985.
7. Melzack, R: Neurophysiological Foundations of Pain. In Sternbach, R (ed): The Psychology of Pain. Raven, New York, 1986, p 1.
8. Bonica, JJ: Anatomic and Physiologic Basis of Nociception and Pain. In Bonica, JJ (ed): The Management of Pain. Lea & Febiger, Philadelphia, 1990, p 28.
9. Bonica, JJ: Biochemistry and Modulation of Nociception and Pain. In Bonica, JJ (ed): The Management of Pain. Lea & Febiger, Philadelphia, 1990, p 95.
10. Sternbach, RA: Pain Patients. Traits and Treatment. Academic, New York, 1974.
11. Casey, KL: The neurophysiologic basis of pain. Postgrad Med J 53:58, 1973.
12. Craig, KD: Emotional Aspects of Pain. In Wall, P, and Melzack, R (ed): Textbook of Pain. Churchill Livingstone, Edinburgh, 1984, p 153.
13. Bonica, JJ: Definitions and Taxonomy of Pain. In Bonica, JJ (ed): The Management of Pain. Lea & Febiger, Philadelphia, 1990, p 18.
14. Wu, W, and Grzesiak, RC: Psychologic Aspects of Chronic Pain. In Wu, W-h, (ed): Pain Management. Assessment and Treatment of Chronic and Acute Syndromes. Human Sciences Press, New York, 1987, p 44.

15. Skevington, S: Social cognitions, personality and chronic pain. J Psychosomat Res 5:421, 1983.
16. Osterweis, M, et al (eds): Pain and Disability. National Academy Press, Washington, DC, 1987.
17. State of Colorado: Reflex Sympathetic Dystrophy/Complex Regional Pain Syndrome: Treatment Guidelines. Department of Labor and Employment, Division of Workers' Compensation, Denver, 1997.
18. Headley, BJ: Historical perspective of causalgia: Management of sympathetically maintained pain. Phys Ther 67: 1370, 1987.
19. Bonica, JJ: Causalgia and Other Reflex Sympathetic Dystrophies. In Bonica, JJ (ed): The Management of Pain. Lea & Febiger, Philadelphia, 1990, p 220.
20. Headley, BJ: EMG and postural dysfunction. Clinical Management 10:14, 1990.
21. Riegger-Krugh, C, and Keysor, JJ: Skeletal malalignments of the lower quarter: Correlated and compensatory motions and postures. JOSPT 23:164, 1996.
22. Aronoff, GM: The role of the pain center in the treatment for intractable suffering and disability resulting from chronic pain. Semin Neurol 3:377, 1983.
23. Fordyce, W: Learning Processes in Pain. In Sternbach, R (ed): The Psychology of Pain. Raven, New York, 1986, p 46.
24. Sternbach, RA, et al: Aspects of chronic low back pain. Psychosomatics 14:52, 1973.
25. Chapman, R: Psychological aspects of pain patient treatment. Arch Surg 112:767, 1977.
26. Alonzo, AA: An illness behavior paradigm: A conceptual exploration of a situational-adaptation perspective. Soc Sci Med 19:499, 1984.
27. Cockerham, WC: Medical Sociology, ed 3. Prentice-Hall, Englewood Cliffs, NJ, 1986.
28. LeShan, L: The World of the Patient in Severe Pain of Long Duration. In Garfield, CA (ed): Stress and Survival. The Emotional Realities of Life-Threatening Illness. CV Mosby Company, St. Louis, 1979, p 273.
29. Block, AR: Presurgical Psychological Screening in Chronic Pain Syndromes. J. Erlbaum, Mahwah, NJ, 1996.
30. Wen-hsien, W: Pain Management. Assessment and Treatment of Chronic and Acute Syndromes. Human Sciences Press, New York, 1987.
31. Benedetti, C, and Butler, SH: Systemic Analgesics. In Bonica, JJ (ed): The Management of Pain. Lea & Febiger, Philadelphia, 1990, p 1640.
32. Fordyce, WE, et al: Acute back pain: A control-group comparison of behavioral vs traditional management methods. J Behav Med 9:127, 1986.
33. North, RB, et al: A Prospective, Randomized Study of Spinal Cord Stimulation versus Reoperation for Failed Back Surgery Syndrome: Initial Results. In Proceedings of the 11th Meeting of the World Society for Stereotactic and Functional Neurosurgery, Ixtapa, Mexico, 1993.
34. Bonica, JJ, and Buckley, FP: Regional Analgesia with Local Anesthetics. In Bonice, JJ (ed): The Management of Pain. Lea & Febiger, Philadelphia, 1990, p 1883.
35. Hurt, R, and Ballantine, H: Stereotactic anterior cingulate lesions for persistent pain: A report on 68 cases. Clin Neurosurg 21:334, 1973.
36. Nashold, BJ: Current status of the DREZ operation. Neurosurgery 15:942, 1984.
37. Spiegel, E, and Wycis, H: Present status of stereoencephalotomies for pain relief. Confin Neurol 27:7, 1966.
38. Sternbach, RA: Psychophysiologic Pain Syndrome. In Bonica, JJ (ed): The Management of Pain. Lea & Febiger, Philadelphia, 1990, p 287.
39. Lieberman, M, et al: Psychosocial Adjustment to Physical Disability. In O'Sullivan, S, and Schmitz, T (ed): Physical Rehabilitation: Assessment and Treatment, ed 3. FA Davis, Philadelphia, 1994, p 9.
40. Ransford, A, et al: The pain drawing as an aid to the psychologic evaluation of patients with low-back pain. Spine 1:127, 1976.
41. Turner, JA, and Romano, JM: Psychologic and Psychosocial Evaluation. In Bonica, JJ (ed): The Management of Pain. Lea & Febiger, Philadelphia, 1990, p 595.
42. Kerns, RD, et al: The West Haven-Yale Multidimensional Pain Inventory. Pain 23:345, 1985.
43. Melzack, R: The McGill Pain Questionnaire: Major properties and scoring methods. Pain 1:277, 1975.
44. Derogatis, LR, et al: The SCL-90 and the MMPI: A step in the validation of a new self-report scale. Br J Psychiatry 128:280, 1976.
45. Costello, RM, et al: P-A-I-N: A four-cluster MMPI typology for chronic pain. Pain 30:199, 1987.
46. Tollison, CD, and Satterthwaite, JR: Multiple spine surgical failures: The value of adjunctive psychological assessment. Orthopaedic Review, 19:1073, 1990.
47. Cox, GB, et al: The MMPI and chronic pain: The diagnosis of psychogenic pain. J Behav Med 1:437, 1978.
48. Trief, PM, and Yuan, HA: The Use of the MMPI in a chronic back pain rehabilitation program. J Clin Psychol 39:46, 1983.
49. Sternbach, RA, and Timmermans, G: Personality changes associated with reduction of pain. Pain 1:177, 1975.
50. Turner, JA, et al: Utility of the MMPI pain assessment index in predicting outcome after lumbar surgery. J Clin Psychol 42:764, 1986.
51. Loeser, JD: Concepts of Pain. In Stanton-Hicks, M, and Boas, R (ed): Chronic Low Back Pain. Raven, New York, 1982.
52. Rossi, EL, and Cheek, DB: Mind-Body Therapy. Methods of Ideodynamic Healing in Hypnosis. WW Norton, New York, 1988.
53. Arluke, A, et al: Reexamining the sick-role concept: An empirical assessment. J Health Social Behavior, 20:30–36, 1979.
54. Young, LM, and Powell, B: The effects of obesity on the clinical judgements of mental health professionals. J Health Soc Behav 26:233, 1985.
55. Kasman, G: Use of Integrated Electromyography for the Assessment and Treatment of Musculoskeletal Pain: Guidelines for physical medicine practitioners. In Cram, J (ed): Clinical EMG for Surface Recordings, vol 2. Clinical Resources, Nevada City, 1990, p 255.
56. Khalil, T, et al: Electromyographic symmetry in patients with chronic low back pain and comparison to controls. Advances in Industrial Ergonomics and Safety III:483, 1991.
57. Seidel, H, et al: Electromyographic evaluation of back muscle fatigue with repeated sustained contractions of different strengths. Eur J Appl Physiol 56:592, 1987.
58. Sihvonen, T, et al: Electric behavior of low back muscles during lumbar pelvic rhythm in low back pain patients and healthy controls. Arch Phys Med Rehabil 72:1080, 1991.
59. Chaitow, L: Muscle Energy Techniques. Churchill-Livingstone, New York, 1996.
60. Schwartz, GE: Self-regulation of response patterning. Implications for psychophysiological research and therapy. Biofeedback and Self-Regulation 1:7, 1976.
61. Kasman, GS, et al: Clinical Applications in Surface Electromyography. Aspen, Gaithersburg, MD, 1998.
62. Headley, BJ: Habitual patterns can be assessed with surface EMG Advance for Physical Therapists. PT News Magazine, November 18, 1996.
63. Flor, H, et al: Discrimination of muscle tension in chronic pain patients and healthy controls. Biofeedback and Self-Regulation 17:165, 1992.
64. Travell, J, and Simons, D: Myofascial Pain and Dysfunction. The Trigger Point Manual, vol 1. Williams & Wilkins, Baltimore, 1983.
65. Travell, J, and Simons, D: Myofascial Pain and Dysfunction. The Trigger Point Manual, vol 2. Williams & Wilkins, Baltimore, 1992.
66. Headley, B: EMG and myofascial pain. Clinical Management 10:43, 1990.
67. Headley, BJ: Evaluation and treatment of Myofascial Pain Syndrome Utilizing Biofeedback. In Cram, JR (ed): Clinical EMG for Surface Recordings. Clinical Resources, Nevada City, 1990, p 235.
68. Simons, DG: Referred phenomena of myofascial trigger points. In Vecchiet, L, et al (eds): New Trends in Referred Pain and Hyperalgesia. Elsevier Science, Amsterdam, 1993, p 341.

69. Headley, B: Use of SEMG in Discerning Myofascial Pain Syndrome in the Quadratus Lumborum: A Syndrome Common to Low Back Pain. Presented at American Physical Therapy Association Conference, Denver, 1992.

70. Rosomoff, HL, et al: Myofascial findings in patients with "chronic intractable benign pain" of the back and neck. Pain Management 2:114, 1990.

71. Mayer, TG, and Gatchel, RJ: Functional Restoration for Spinal Disorders: The Sports Medicine Approach. Lea & Febiger, Philadelphia, 1988.

72. Simons, DG: Myofascial Pain Syndrome Due to Trigger Points. In Goodgold, J, (ed): Rehabilitation Medicine. CV Mosby Company, St. Louis, 1988, p 686.

73. Headley, BJ: Physiological Risk Factors. In Sanders, MJ, (ed): Management of Cumulative Trauma Disorders. Butterworth-Heinemann, Boston, 1997, p 107.

74. Feldenkrais, M: Awareness Through Movement: Health Exercises for Personal Growth. Harper & Row, New York, 1977.

75. Leibowitz, J, and Connington, B: The Alexander Technique. HarperCollins, New York, 1990.

76. Sale, D, and MacDougall, D: Specificity in strength training: A review for the coach and athlete. Can J Appl Sport Sci 6:87, 1981.

77. McCain, GA: Role of physical fitness training in the fibrositis/fibromyalgia syndrome. Am J Med 81(suppl 3A): 73, 1986.

78. Lacey, JI, and Lacey, BC: Verification and extension of the principle of autonomic response-stereotypy. Am J Psychol 71:50, 1958.

79. Sternbach, RA: Clinical Aspects of Pain. In Sternbach, R (ed): The Psychology of Pain. Raven, New York, 1986, p 124.

80. Flor, H, et al: Discrimination of muscle tension in chronic pain patients and healthy controls. Biofeedback and Self-Regulation 17:165, 1992.

81. Rossi, EL: The Psychobiology of Mind-Body Healing: New Concepts of Therapeutic Hypnosis. WW Norton, New York, 1986.

82. Hendler, N, et al: EMG biofeedback in patients with chronic pain. Dis Nervous System 7:505, 1977.

83. Large, RG, and Lamb, AM: Electromyographic (EMG) feedback in chronic musculoskeletal pain: A controlled study. Pain 17:167, 1983.

84. Peck, CL, and Draft, GH: Electromyographic biofeedback for pain related to muscle tension: A study of tension headache, back and jaw pain. Arch Surg 112:889, 1977.

85. Biedermann, HJ: Mechanism of biofeedback in the treatment of chronic back pain. Psychol Rep 53:1103, 1983.

86. Holroyd, KA, et al: Change mechanisms in EMG biofeedback training: Cognitive changes underlying improvements in tension headache. J Consult Clin Psychol 52:1039, 1984.

87. Achterberg, J: Shamanism and Modern Medicine. New Science Library, Boston, 1985.

88. Sternbach, RA: Effects of Altering Brain Serotonin Activity on Human Chronic Pain. In Bonica, JJ, and Albe-Fessard, D (eds): Advances in Pain Research and Therapy. Raven, New York, 1976, p 601.

89. Carlson, LK, and Watson, HK: Treatment of reflex sympathetic dystrophy using the stress-loading program. J Hand Ther 3:149, 1988.

90. Watson, HK, and Carlson, LK: Treatment of reflex sympathetic dystrophy of the hand with an active "stress loading" program. J Hand Surg 12A:779, 1987.

91. Watson, HK, and Carlson, LK: Stress loading treatment for reflex sympathetic dystrophy. Complications in Orthopedics 1:19, 1990.

92. Lampe, G: Transcutaneous electrical nerve stimulation. In O'Sullivan, SB, and Schmitz, TJ (eds): Physical Rehabilitation: Assessment and Treatment, ed 2. FA Davis, Philadelphia, 1988, p 647.

93. Sjolund, BH, et al: Transcutaneous and Implanted Electric Stimulation of Peripheral Nerves. In Bonica, JJ (ed): The Management of Pain. Lea & Febiger, Philadelphia, 1990, p 1852.

94. Choi, J, and Tsay, C: Technology of Transcutaneous Electrical Nerve Stimulation. In Wu, W (ed): Pain Management. Assessment and Treatment of Chronic and Acute Syndromes. Human Sciences Press, New York, 1987, p 137.

95. Achterberg, JA, and Lawlis, GF: Bridges of the Body-mind. Behavioral Approaches to Health Care. Institute for Personality and Ability Testing, Champaign, IL, 1980.

96. Carlos, J: Clinical electrotherapy: Physiology and basic concepts. PT Magazine, July 1998, p 62.

97. Smith, RB, et al: The use of cranial electrotherapy stimulation in the treatment of closed-head-injured patients. Brain Inj 8:357, 1994.

98. Grieve, GP: Common Vertebral Joint Problems, (ed 2) Churchill Livingstone, New York, 1988.

99. Biedermann, H, et al: Power Spectrum Analyses of Electromyographic Activity: Discriminators in the Differential Assessment of Patients with Chronic Low-back Pain. Spine 16:1179, 1991.

100. Vaeyen, JWS, et al: Fear of movement/(re)injury in chronic low back pain and its relation to behavioral performance. Pain 62:363, 1995.

101. Loeser, JD, et al: Interdisciplinary, Multimodal Management of Chronic Pain, vol 2. In Bonica, JJ (ed): The Management of Pain. Lea & Febiger, Philadelphia, 1990, p 2107.

102. Chapman, C, et al: Pain and Behavioral Medicine. A Cognitive-Behavioral Approach. Guilford Press, New York, 1983.

103. Fordyce, WE: Behavioral Methods for Chronic Pain and Illness. Mosby, St. Louis, 1976.

104. Headley, B: Effect of Burns on the Body Image of Children. Unpublished Masters Thesis, Boston University, 1974.

105. Headley, B: Am I a physical therapist? Physical Therapy Forum, 1987.

SUPPLEMENTAL READINGS

Basmajian, J, and DeLuca, C: Muscles Alive. Their Functions Revealed by Electromyography, ed 2. Williams & Wilkins, Baltimore, 1985.

Bonica, J (ed): The Management of Pain, vols 1 and 2, ed 2. Lea & Febiger, Philadelphia, 1990.

Caillet, R: Pain Mechanisms and Management. FA Davis, Philadelphia, 1993.

Soderberg, G (ed): Selected Topics in Surface Electromyography for Use in the Occupational Setting: Expert Perspectives. US Department of Health and Human Services, Publication nos. 91–100, March 1992.

Sternbach, R (ed): The Psychology of Pain, ed 2. New York, Raven, 1986.

Turk, D, et al: Pain and Behavioral Medicine. A Cognitive-Behavioral Perspective. New York, Guilford Press, 1983.

GLOSSARY

Acute pain: Pain provoked by noxious stimulation produced by injury and/or disease with unpleasant sensory and emotional experiences.

A fibers: Large diameter, myelinated nerve fibers that innervate muscles, tendons and joints; mechanoreceptors, fast conducting.

Body diagrams: Pictures of the body that patients are asked to fill in with the location and nature of their symptom complaints. May be used at initial examination and/or follow-up.

Causalgia: *See* reflex sympathetic dystrophy.

Central pain: Pain that is associated with a lesion of the central nervous system independent of peripheral injury or tissue damage.

C fibers: Small diameter, unmyelinated nerve fibers. Fibers innervating nociceptors, mechanoreceptors, and sympathetic postganglionic bodies; slow conducting.

Chronic pain: Pain that persists beyond the usual course of healing of an acute disease or beyond a reasonable time for an injury to heal.

Collaborative health care model: Evolved from hierarchical medical model, with expectations that the patient is active in decision making and treatment planning.

Complex regional pain syndrome (CRPS): A complex disorder or group of syndromes that include causalagia and reflex sympathetic dystrophy (RSD); symptoms include pain and related sensory abnormalities, abnormal blood flow and sweating; abnormal motor function and trophic changes.

Cordotomies: Surgical division of a tract of the spinal cord for relief of severe intractable pain.

Craniosacral therapy: A manual therapy involving extremely delicate touch and adjustments to restore craniosacral rhythm and reduce tissue adhesions.

Cross friction massage: Deep massage technique applied at right angles to tendon near attachment to bone.

Cumulative trauma disorder (CTD): A group of syndromes characterized by pain and discomfort that develop gradually in soft tissue structures; related to repeated stress or awkward movement of a body part (*synonym:* repetitive motion disorder).

Disability: Disadvantage for a given individual that limits or prevents the fulfillment of a role that is normal for that individual.

Dystrophic: Related to abnormal nutrition, growth, or health; a stage of reflex sympathetic dystrophy.

Functional disability: An inability to complete functional task within parameters typically considered reasonable or normal for that individual.

Gate Control Theory: A theory of pain, developed by Melzack and Wall,[3] that suggests pain can be blocked at various gate locations in the spinal cord.

Guided imagery: A structured relaxation session with imagery for relaxation.

Hyperalgesia: Increased response to a stimulus that is normally painful.

Hyperesthesia: Increased sensitivity of skin to stimulus.

Hyperpathia: Increased reaction to stimuli, especially when repetitive; increased threshold to stimuli.

Hyperhidrosis: Increased sweating response.

Impairment: Loss of abnormality of psychological, physiological, or anatomical structure or function.

Kinesiophobia: Fear of movement, often related to fear of re-injury.

Malingering: Pretending to have pain when it does not exist.

Movement adaptation syndrome (MAS): Habituation of compensatory movement patterns that may contribute to the persistence of pain.

Nerve block: Injection for temporary obstruction of function of a particular nerve; may be diagnostic or used for short term treatment of pain.

Nociceptive: System or receptor that is preferentially sensitive to a noxious stimulus or to a stimulus that would become noxious if prolonged.

Pattern-generating Theory: Suggests that perpetuation of pain results from sustained activity in the neuron pools. Lowered threshold to activation and activation of non-noxious stimuli may be contributing factors.

Postural stress syndrome (PSS): Abnormal shortening or lengthening of muscles and ligaments.

Reflex sympathetic dystrophy (RSD): Originally termed causalgia, now a CRPS with dysfunction of the autonomic nervous system.

Rehabilitation team: Multidisciplinary health care providers; may include physician, physical and occupational therapists, psychologists, social workers, and vocational counselors.

Relaxation training: Used to decrease sympathetic arousal, muscle tension, anxiety using imagery, autogenic training, or music.

Rhizotomies: Surgical cutting of anterior or posterior spinal nerve roots.

Sick role: Social expectations about both patient and health care providers' behavior; considered to be the role delineation of the traditional medical model.

Stimulation-produced analgesia (SPA): Use of mechanical means to block transmission of pain signal.

Stress loading: Carefully graded increase in weight-bearing forces through the involved extremities to normalize sensory feedback and reduce hypersensitivity.

Suffering: State of severe distress associated with events that threaten the intactness of the person. The state may or may not be associated with pain.

Symptom magnification (SM): Behavior is considered excessive and more severe than objective findings warrant.

Sympathectomy: Surgical severing of the sympathetic nervous system at either the cervical or lumbar ganglion.

Thalamic pain syndrome: Continuous pain, described as aching, boring, gnawing, burning, or crushing sensation, occurs in response to a lesion in the thalamus; symptoms are opposite to the side of injury. Autonomic and vasomotor dysfunction is common.

Trigger points: Palpable band or nodule within the muscle or connective tissue that refers pain, elicits a local twitch response when pressed, and is generally hypersensitive.

APPENDIX A

A sample of the Multidisciplinary Pain Inventory showing a dysfunctional profile. The solid line represents the patient's scores on each scale; the dotted line connects the mean scores for this profile against which the patient's answers are scored.

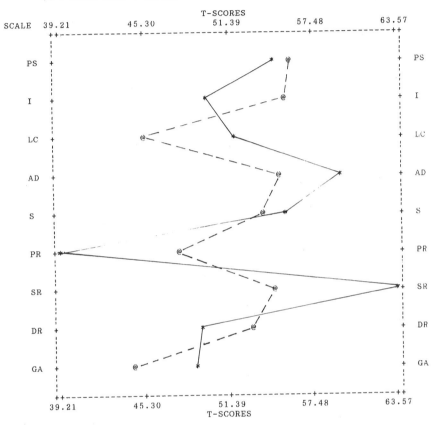

```
                    PLOT OF AXES II AND III T-SCORES
               PROFILE CLASSIFICATION: Dysfunctional
              (@ = GROUP MEAN T-SCORES   * = PATIENT T-SCORES   # = OVERLAP)

                                    T-SCORES
      SCALE   39.21        45.30      51.39       57.48        63.57
```

```
    FIGURE LEGEND:
       PS = PAIN SEVERITY          PR = PUNISHING RESPONSES
       I  = INTERFERENCE           SR = SOLICITOUS RESPONSES
       LC = LIFE CONTROL           DR = DISTRACTING RESPONSES
       AD = AFFECTIVE DISTRESS     GA = GENERAL ACTIVITY LEVEL
       S  = SUPPORT                     (MEAN OF ACTIVITY SCALES)
```

APPENDIX B

The McGill Pain Questionnaire asks patients to select the words that best describe how their pain feels. From their choices, scores are obtained in sensory, affective, evaluative, and miscellaneous categories.

McGill Pain Questionnaire

What does your pain feel like?

Some of the words below describe your present pain. Circle ONLY those words that best describe it. Leave out any category that is not suitable. Use only a single word in each appropriate category - the one that applies best.

Sensory: 1-8   Evaluative: 16
Affective: 9-15   Miscellaneous: 17-20

1	2	3	4
Flickering	Jumping	Pricking	Sharp
Quivering	Flashing	Boring	Cutting
Pulsing	Shooting	Drilling	Lacerating
Throbbing		Stabbing	
Beating		Lancinating	
Pounding			

5	6	7	8
Pinching	Tugging	Hot	Tingling
Pressing	Pulling	Burning	Itchy
Gnawing	Wrenching	Scalding	Smarting
Cramping		Searing	Stinging
Crushing			

9	10	11	12
Dull	Tender	Tiring	Sickening
Sore	Taut	Exhausting	Suffocating
Hurting	Rasping		
Aching	Splitting		
Heavy			

13	14	15	16
Fearful	Punishing	Wretched	Annoying
Frightful	Gruelling	Blinding	Troublesome
Terrifying	Cruel		Miserable
	Vicious		Intense
	Killing		Unbearable

17	18	19	20
Spreading	Tight	Cool	Nagging
Radiating	Numb	Cold	Nauseating
Penetrating	Drawing	Freezing	Agonizing
Piercing	Squeezing		Dreadful
	Tearing		Torturing

APPENDIX C

A sample visual analog scale developed by the author. Numerical scores can be obtained by measuring the placement of the mark along the line. Scores may be compared with repeat administration of the scale.

Pain Evaluation & Rehabilitation Center

Please mark an "X" along the line to show how your pain has effected your level of function.

1. At what level do you perceive your pain?
No Pain _____ Worst possible

2. At what level do you experience pain at night?
No Pain _____ Worst possible

3. Has the pain effected your level of activity?
No problem _____ Total change

4. How well does medication relieve your pain?
Complete relief _____ No relief

5. How stiff is your back/neck?
No stiffness _____ Totally stiff

6. Does your pain interfere with sitting?
No problem _____ Cannot sit

7. Is it painful for you to walk?
No pain _____ Cannot walk

8. Does your pain keep you from standing/sitting still?
No problem _____ Cannot do it

9. Does your pain interfere with your normal household chores?
No problem _____ Cannot do them

10. Does your pain effect your driving time in a car?
No problem _____ Cannot do it

11. Do you get relief from your pain by lying down?
Complete relief _____ No relief at all

12. How much have you had to change your job responsibilities?
No change _____ So much I can't work

13. How much control do you feel you have over the pain?
Total control _____ No control

14. How much control have you lost over other areas of your life due to the pain?
No control lost _____ Total loss of control

Name:_____ Date:_____

APPENDIX D

Suggested Answers to Case Study Guiding Questions

1. This patient expresses a strong desire to avoid any outward sign of physical disability. The body brace is totally hidden and according to the patient provides sufficient stability without using crutches or canes. How might you provide the patient with a rationale for using a more visible intervention to improve safety? What aids might you recommend?

ANSWER: Hiding an instability problem increases the risk of falls, especially in public, high traffic volume areas. You might suggest to the patient she (1) use an aid such as a cane to decrease fatigue and (2) use a cane in public to make people aware that she should not be bumped. Giving a patient a larger boundary for movement in a crowded area such as a mall can help in reducing the risk of falling. People will slow down, pay attention, and provide a greater space. All of these are important for not falling, which can make the lumbar instability worse and a good outcome more difficult.

2. Needle EMG studies demonstrate that no major nerve compression is evident. In light of negative EMG findings, how might you explain muscle weakness (right drop foot and bilateral hip flexor weakness) to the patient? How might you design a therapeutic exercise program?

ANSWER: Muscle weakness (or apparent weakness) in the absence of neurological damage may be due to rapid fatigue of the involved muscles or a learned motor behavior that no longer includes using a healthy muscle. The exercise program should be done in short exercise bouts, with low repetitions or unweighted to reduce fatigue. Using biofeedback or motor control retraining may be helpful in getting a muscle to work. Allowing the muscle to not work when it should be working increases compensation patterns and makes rehabilitation and return to normal movement more difficult.

3. What guidelines would you provide for exercise repetitions and frequency? Describe how the exercise program would be tailored to this patient in light of lumbar instability needing fusion as well as secondary SI instability?

ANSWER: Exercises should not produce severe fatigue or overload. This may delay muscle use for hours or even days if severe. In designing a strengthening program when the lumbar spine is unstable, all attempts should be make to provide external stability. This can be done using bracing, or by having the patient do the exercises lying supine rather than standing. Exercise should focus on recognizing proper movement patterns, isolating movements, and using the correct range during movement. If a hip capsule has tightened and limits motion, treatment should be directed toward increasing the flexibility of the capsule so that normal movement can be restored and practiced. Pool exercises are easier to perform, give some pain relief with movement, and allow for some strengthening. Teaching body awareness during movement and the sense of proper movement facilitates rehabilitation after surgery. The combination of lumbar and SI instability suggests muscle energy techniques will be limited.

4. The patient has already had two failed fusions. What factors would be important to assess in terms of her expectations and possible outcomes? What would be "red flags" that you might pass on as concerns to the primary physician and surgeon?

ANSWER: The patient's beliefs about why the first two fusions failed should be explored. The compliance of the patient should also be discussed to determine if compliance failure postoperatively may have jeopardized the surgical outcome. Does the patient understand the amount of time required for the fusion to become solid? How to protect the fused surgical area? What has the patient learned from friends and family about this surgery that might hinder compliance? What is the patient's belief system about surgery, the surgeon, and the outcome? Has the patient "learned to fail"? Is the patient willing to follow instructions, ask for help, and wait out the restrictions as long as necessary? Is the patient prepared to handle complications?

5. What factors would be indications to continue treatment until surgery or discontinue as no longer being beneficial? What considerations would indicate continued treatment benefit if surgery approval were delayed several months?

ANSWER: Stopping physical therapy because the patient is waiting for surgery may not take advantage of a valuable time to make changes. The patient has been using compensatory movement patterns for years. These movement patterns require changes in muscle, ligament, and joint capsule that may restrict normal movement after surgery. This, in turn, can add stress to the new surgical site. Working toward postural homeostasis before surgery can make the postsurgical rehabilitation move more quickly and keep the patient in the mode of being an active, involved participant. The more the patient feels part of the "team" before surgery, the more compliant she will be after the surgery. Continued therapy also maintains a higher activity level. Becoming a "couch potato" will not help the patient respond to the insult of surgery and can delay rehabilitation afterwards.

Assessment and **29** Intervention Strategies for Cognitive and Perceptual Dysfunction

Carolyn Unsworth
Chaye Lamm Warburg

LEARNING OBJECTIVES

1. Explain why it is essential for physical therapists to be familiar with the signs of cognitive and perceptual dysfunction.
2. Describe how cognitive and perceptual disturbances affect the ability of the patient to participate in rehabilitation.
3. Explain how a patient can be assisted to compensate for body scheme and/or body image disorders.
4. Describe how spatial relations problems can affect the patient's ability to follow directions.
5. Explain the effect of the various agnosias on the patient's ability to recognize stimuli in the environment.
6. Differentiate between ideomotor and ideational apraxia. Describe how a patient with apraxia might behave in response to different instructional sets commonly employed in rehabilitation.
7. Describe how the psychological and emotional status of a patient with cognitive and perceptual impairments may affect participation in rehabilitation.
8. Analyze and interpret patient data, formulate realistic goals and outcomes, and identify appropriate interventions when presented with a clinical case study.

Cognitive and perceptual deficits are among the chief causes of confusion about and lack of progress in patients who have sustained brain damage, even among those whose motor skills have returned.[1] Cognitive and perceptual problems are some of the most puzzling and disabling difficulties that a person can experience.[2] Problems with thinking, remembering, reasoning, and making sense of the world around us is fundamental to carrying out daily living activities. When individuals experience problems with these capacities, it can have a devastating effect on their lives and the lives of their family. These people may not be able to live alone, fulfill the responsibilities of paid employment, or sustain a family life and relationships.[2] Thus, effective treatment of many patients with brain damage depends on understanding perception and cognition.

The brain may be damaged through several mechanisms including infections such as encephalitis; anoxia as may occur following near drowning; cardiopulmonary arrest, or carbon monoxide poisoning; tumors that are benign or malignant; trauma resulting from motor vehicle accidents, falls, or violent incidents (e.g., sport, or gunshot); toxins such as alcohol or substance abuse; and vascular disease, which may produce an infarct or hemorrhagic stroke. The largest two groups of people who acquire cognitive and perceptual problems following brain damage are persons who experienced stroke and traumatic brain injury. The physical aspects of rehabilitation of these patient groups are addressed in Chapters 17 and 24, respectively.

The patient who has sustained an initial cerebral vascular accident (CVA) is thought to have focal or localized damage to discrete areas of the brain, often resulting in discrete cognitive or perceptual problems. In contrast, patients who have sustained a traumatic brain injury are presumed to have generalized brain damage resulting in cognitive impairment with generalized deficits in attention, memory, learning, and so forth, rather than specific difficulties in discrete cognitive or perceptual functions. However, elements of both perceptual and cognitive dysfunction may occur in brain damage owing to either CVA or trauma. The distinctions between the two groups of patients become particularly blurred when one considers the patient who has suffered multiple strokes; this patient may in fact present with combined elements of focal and generalized brain damage. Throughout this chapter, the patient with hemiplegia in whom brain damage has occurred as a result of a stroke will be the focus. The primary objective of this chapter is to introduce the reader to concepts relating to cognitive and perceptual dysfunction following brain damage.

An important focus for the physical therapist should be on understanding of how a particular cognitive or perceptual impairment might be manifested clinically, and how assessment and treatment of movement disorders might be adjusted to capitalize on the abilities and minimize the cognitive or perceptual limitations of the patient. Disorders in the cognitive or perceptual domain must be considered to accurately assess the patient's true residual abilities. Using sets of directions that would confuse a patient with apraxia during a specific assessment may paint a picture of a greater or different motor disability than that which actually exists. Often the first clue to a cognitive or perceptual problem appears during the initial sensorimotor assessment. Awareness of the possibility and nature of cognitive or perceptual deficits will signal the therapist to redirect the method of assessment, particularly the instructional sets and cues.

COGNITION AND PERCEPTION

The perceptual motor process is a chain of events through which the individual selects, integrates, and interprets stimuli from the body and the surrounding environment. Cognition can be conceived of as the method used by the central nervous system (CNS) to process information. Cognitive processes include knowing, understanding, awareness, judgement, and decision making.[1] The difficulty of separating perceptual and cognitive deficits is readily apparent, both in patient behavior and in contradictory conceptualizations of these two domains of function. For example, according to some authors, cognition is conceived of as a general term that includes perception, attention, thinking, and memory.[3] According to other authors, perception is an umbrella term that encompasses both cognition and visual perception as subcomponents.[3] At this time, there is insufficient research evidence to suggest which approach most accurately reflects the way we think about and perceive information. What is clear is that normally functioning perceptual and cognitive systems are a necessary key to successful interaction with the environment. Because the majority of work in this field does distinguish between cognition and perception[2] and because it is probably easier to learn about these processes individually, they are defined separately for the purposes of this chapter.

Cognitive and perceptual capacities are clearly prerequisites for learning[4] and rehabilitation is largely a learning process.[2] Thus, it is not surprising that patients with cognitive and perceptual disorders are limited in their ability to learn self-care and activities of daily living (ADL) skills; hence, as a group, they are more limited in their potential for achieving independence.[5] In any rehabilitation program geared toward achievement of maximum independence, there is a compelling need for therapists to learn to recognize behavior related to perceptual deficits. The therapist's modification of assessment and intervention approaches in light of these deficits will ensure that patients receive the full benefit of these services.

Cognition and Higher Order Cognition

Cognitive processes are generally defined as the abilities that enable us to "think," which includes the ability to concentrate or pay attention, remember, and learn. **Executive functions** are sometimes discussed under this heading as well. Executive functions include the capacity to plan, manipulate information, initiate and terminate activities, recognize errors, problem solve, and think abstractly. Commonly, executive functions are categorized as **higher order cognitive** functions[6] or metacognitive functions.[7,8]

Perception

Lezak[4] defines **perception** as the integration of sensory impressions into information that is psychologically meaningful. Thus, perception is the ability to select those stimuli that require attention and action, to integrate those stimuli with each other and with prior information, and finally to interpret them. The resulting awareness of objects and experiences within the environment enables the individual to make sense out of a complex and constantly changing internal and external sensory environment.[9]

The terms perception and **sensation** are often confused with each other. Sensation may be defined as the appreciation of stimuli through the organs of special sense (e.g., eyes, ears, nose, etc.), the peripheral cutaneous sensory system (e.g., temperature, taste, touch, etc.), or internal receptors (e.g., deep receptors in muscles and joints).[9] Perception cannot be viewed as independent of sensation. However, the quality of perception is far more complex than the recognition of the individual sensation.[9] Perceptual deficits do not lie in the sensory ability itself, but rather with the individual's ability to interpret the sensation accurately, and therefore respond appropriately.[2]

RESPONSIBILITIES OF THE PT AND OT

Occupational therapists are the members of the rehabilitation team who are specially trained to assess and treat cognitive and perceptual dysfunction in relation to functional adaptation. They are responsible for the selection and administration of an appropriate constellation of assessment tools, accurate interpretation of results, and formulation of an overall program for cognitive and perceptual rehabilitation. If appropriate, the occupational therapist may refer a patient to a neuropsychologist for specific intellectual assessment.

In the hospital setting, the physical therapist is often the first member of the rehabilitation team to see a patient with brain injury. The physical therapist must understand the nature of cognitive and perceptual dysfunction and recognize that individuals in certain diagnostic categories, such as those with stroke or traumatic head injury, are likely to behave in ways that indicate the presence of particular cognitive or perceptual problems.[10] When this occurs, the physical therapist should be aware that it is appropriate to refer the patient to occupational therapy for assessment and treatment.

The assessment tools described in this chapter are included to assist the reader in understanding the nature of the different cognitive and perceptual disabilities. They are not meant to be used as a substitute for an intensive assessment by a trained occupational therapist when it is deemed necessary.

An understanding of cognitive and perceptual dysfunction may go a long way toward alleviating much of the potential frustration that often accompanies treatment of a patient with brain damage, most of which is the result of inappropriate expectations on the part of the therapist, the patient, and the family. Furthermore, by collaborating with the occupational therapist, other members of the rehabilitation team, and the family, consistent treatment strategies may be developed and carried out, with obvious benefits to the patient.

CLINICAL INDICATORS

Cognitive and perceptual deficits ought to be ruled out as a cause of diminished functioning in all patients suffering from brain damage. Such problems are particularly likely culprits in cases in which the patient seems unable to participate fully in self-care tasks and has difficulty participating in physical therapy for reasons that cannot be accounted for by lack of motor ability, sensation, comprehension, or motivation. Cognitive and perceptual dysfunction resulting from acquired brain damage must be differentiated from premorbid cognitive perceptual deficits (from previous trauma, illness, congenital abnormality, or dementing process) and from the general confusion and emotional sequelae that often accompany stroke and brain injury.[4]

Often, patients with cognitive and perceptual difficulties may display the following characteristics: inability to do simple tasks independently or safely, difficulty in initiating or completing a task, difficulty in switching from one task to the next, and a diminished capacity to locate visually or to identify objects that seem obviously necessary for task completion. Additionally, they may be unable to follow simple one-stage instructions, despite apparently good comprehension. They may make the same mistakes over and over. Activities may take an inordinately long time to complete, or they may be done impulsively. Patients may hesitate many times, appear distracted and frustrated, and exhibit poor planning. They are frequently inattentive to one side of the body and extrapersonal space, and they may deny the presence or extent of their disability. These characteristics, all or some of which may be present, often make participation in daily living activities and therapy seem an insurmountable problem. These clinical features will be explained and expanded upon throughout the remainder of this chapter.

Two typical scenarios will be presented to give the reader a concrete idea of when to suspect perceptual dysfunction. The first case involves a patient with a right-hemisphere stroke who presents clinically with a left hemiparesis and good speech. Upon observation in the nursing unit, the patient appears to have functional strength in the unaffected right extremities and fair return on the affected left side. Yet the patient seems to have difficulty with simple range of motion (ROM) activities, even in the intact extremities, appearing confused and unable to move the arm up or down on command. The patient cannot seem to follow instructions for walking with a quad cane, constantly confuses the proper step sequence, and is unable to maneuver a wheelchair around the corner without crashing into the wall.

This patient should not be dismissed as uncooperative, intellectually inferior, or confused. In this instance, the patient is likely to be experiencing difficulty in spatial relations, right-left discrimination, and vertical disorientation, or perhaps left-sided neglect and apraxia. Further observation and assessment should reveal the precise cause of the difficulties.

The second case involves a patient with left-hemisphere damage and a resulting right hemiparesis and mild **aphasia.** The patient can respond reliably to "yes/no" questions and is able to follow simple one-stage commands such as, "Put the pencil on the table," or "Give me the cup." However, if asked to point to the arm, or asked to imitate the therapist's movements during an active ROM assessment even with the unaffected limbs, the patient does not respond and appears totally uncooperative. During therapy the same patient is on a mat table. The therapist explains and then demonstrates the proper techniques for rolling to one side. The patient does not move. However, a moment later when his wife arrives, the patient quickly initiates rolling in an attempt to sit up and to greet his wife. The astute therapist will realize that this patient may not be confused, stubborn, or uncooperative, as indeed he may appear. Rather, he may be suffering from a lack of awareness of body structure and relationship of body parts (somatagnosia), as evidenced by the assessment incident, and an inability to perform a task on command or to imitate gestures **(ideomotor apraxia),** as demonstrated in the rolling episode.

HOSPITALIZATION FOLLOWING BRAIN DAMAGE

The brain that has been damaged functions as a whole, just as it does in individuals without brain damage. When one part is damaged, the behavior observed is not merely the result of the brain operating precisely as in the intact individual minus the function of the area that was subject to anoxia. Rather, it is an outward manifestation of the reorganization of the entire CNS, at multiple levels, working to compensate for the loss.[11]

Because of the brain damage, the patient must cope with a nervous system operating without normal sensory input at all levels, both cortical and subcortical.[11] Normal responses to environmental stimuli are difficult to obtain when the input on which they have to act is deranged or incomplete. Recovery of function can be attributed to structural reorganization of the CNS into a new dynamic system widely dispersed within the cerebral cortex and lower segments.[12,13]

A significant contributor to the clinical picture of a patient after a CVA is the response to hospitalization. From a cognitive and perceptual perspective, when a patient is hospitalized (with or without brain damage), the inputs impinging on that patient's nervous system are radically different from the ones normally received. On the one hand, the environment is sensorially impoverished. There is no variation in temperature and lighting, and familiar background noises (e.g., familiar telephones, airplanes, dogs, and buses) are missing. On the other hand, an enormous array of unfamiliar noises are present: nurses talking, loudspeakers, and the whir of machines. Strange and different smells, and unfamiliar, unavoidable, and unpleasant sights abound. Often, because of motor impairment, the patient cannot move around to seek or to escape inputs; therefore, a multiplicity of sensory inputs bombards the nervous system. Even if orienting responses are preserved, there is a profound sense of loss of control. This sensory derangement compounds the problems faced by the patient with brain damage, because those very abilities that enable the individual to select, filter out, and integrate incoming sensations to organize the self for appropriate action often fail in this sensorially bizarre environment.

To gain insight into the experience of the patient under such circumstances, it is enlightening to browse through the biographical and autographical reports of some noted neurologists and neuropsychologists, themselves victims or relatives of victims of CVAs. Particularly instructive are the reports of Bach-y-Rita,[14] Brodal,[15] and Gardner.[16]

THEORETICAL FRAMEWORKS

The theoretical bases of five approaches to therapy will be examined in this section. The therapist will be guided in the selection of assessment and intervention approaches consistent with the theoretical model. It is important to note that these approaches are not mutually exclusive. Many therapists use a combination of approaches, guiding selection by their clinical expertise and the patient's response to the techniques. The functional approach offers a great deal of practical support for the physical therapist. Specific applications of these approaches will be presented following the description of individual cognitive and perceptual deficits in the final section of this chapter. Further information on a variety of theoretical approaches used by occupational therapists when working with patients who have cognitive and perceptual problems can be found in Katz[17] and Unsworth.[2]

The Transfer-of-Training Approach

The premise underlying the **transfer-of-training approach** is that practice in one task with particular perceptual requirements will enhance performance on other tasks with similar perceptual demands.[1,18,19] Thus, doing specifically selected perceptual exercises, such as pegboard activities, or parquetry blocks and puzzles will result in improving the perceptual skills required to perform those functional tasks. For example, Young et al.[20] demonstrated that training patients with left hemiplegia in block design, in addition to visual scanning and **visual cancellation tasks,** resulted in improvements in reading and writing, although no specific training in writing was offered. Because all tasks require the use of multiple perceptual skills it is difficult to ascertain precisely which perceptual skills are being trained during any one session.[21]

Research to date has not unequivocally demonstrated a generalization from perceptual-motor training to functional skills.[18,21] Neistadt[19] suggests that the patient's capacity to learn must be evaluated and that learning capacity is the key to a patient's ability to generalize material learned in one situation to others. If transfer of training does occur, then strategies to enhance this can be incorporated into other components of the treatment program such as those aimed at maintaining sitting or standing balance, weight-bearing exercises, or functional use of the affected extremities.

Sensory Integrative Approach

Ayres developed the theory of **sensory integration (SI)** in an effort to explain the relationship between neural functioning and the behavior of children with sensorimotor or learning problems.[22] The theory, strongly influenced by the neurobehavioral literature, describes normal sensory integrative development and functioning, defines patterns of sensory integrative dysfunction, and suggests treatment techniques.[22] Sensory integration can be defined as the organization of sensation for use.[23,24]

Integration of basic sensorimotor functions (tactile, proprioceptive, and vestibular) proceeds in a developmental sequence in the normal child within the context of goal-directed, meaningful activity. It is assumed that the production of an adaptive response facilitates sensory integration, which in turn enhances the ability to produce higher-level adaptive behaviors. Sensory integration is thought to occur at all levels of the nervous system.

The underlying assumption for treatment is that, by offering opportunities for controlled sensory input, the therapist can effect normal CNS processing of sensory information and thus elicit specific desired motor responses.[25] The performance of these adaptive responses, in turn, influences the way in which the brain organizes and processes sensation, thus enhancing the ability to learn.

Some of the treatment modalities employed include rubbing or icing to provide sensory input, resistance and weight-bearing to impart proprioceptive input, and the use of spinning to provide vestibular input. Following the controlled sensory input, an adaptive motor response is required by the patient to integrate the sensations provided by the therapist. In young children, the use of compensatory or **splinter skills** (skills acquired in a manner inconsistent with, or incapable of being integrated with, those already present) is avoided in favor of remediating underlying deficits. For more detailed information the reader is referred to the work of Ayres.[22-24]

Zoltan[1] argues that elderly patients, who comprise the majority of the stroke population, experience sensory integrative dysfunction similar to that of children with learning disabilities, and that this is because of the physiological changes associated with aging, along with environmentally induced sensory deprivation. The limitations in mobility caused by a stroke further prevent the patient from receiving and thus processing adequate sensory input.

The application of this theory to the adult post-stroke population, however, is open to serious debate. Fisher et al.[22] argue that the theory explains mild to moderate learning and behavioral problems that are the result of a central deficit in processing sensations that are specifically not associated with frank brain damage. Further, there are a number of problems with the application of this approach to adult populations, even if it is theoretically tenable.

The treatment process is ordinarily quite lengthy. In addition, specific assessment and treatment regimens have been developed for and standardized on children, who presumably have sufficiently plastic nervous systems to be influenced by this form of therapy. The neurophysiological literature is replete with examples of ability that would be completely lost in mature individuals with similar lesions.[26-28] Furthermore, a mature adult with diffuse cerebral damage may have other complicating medical concerns and deficits in mobility that actually contraindicate the use of the equipment that is essential to the treatment process.[22] It is likely that many of the treatment regimes described as sensory integration are best described as a sensorimotor approach, which utilizes handling or directed sensory stimulation to elicit a specific motor response.[22]

Neurodevelopmental Approach

From a neurodevelopmental treatment (NDT) approach, perception is facilitated during normal infant neuromotor development by the kinesthetic, proprioceptive, tactile, and vestibular feedback received through normal movement experience. The infant utilizes these sensations as a progression from early physiological flexion to movement against gravity for sitting, crawling, kneeling, standing, and initial walking. Sensorimotor development provides a sense of midline orientation, awareness of the two sides of the body, and total body awareness.[1]

For adults with neurological impairment, perception is considered integral to the handling techniques that provide the patient with sensory input and to the subsequent feedback accompanying correct movement during movement retraining. For example, weight-bearing activities enhance proprioception, and bilateral activities enhance total body awareness and diminish unilateral neglect.[1,29]

Functional Approach

Probably the most widely used approach in treating perceptual dysfunction is the **functional approach.**[29] The basic assumptions underlying the functional approach are that adults with brain trauma will have difficulty generalizing and learning from dissimilar tasks.[30] Direct repetitive practice of specific functional skills that are impaired is an efficient means of enhancing the patient's independence in those specific tasks. The proponents of this approach favor addressing the functional problem over and above the treatment of its underlying cause when working with an adult post-stroke population. For example, a patient with difficulty in depth and distance perception, who is therefore unable to navigate a flight of stairs, would be made aware of the deficit, provided with external cues to compensate for the perceptual disorder, and would repetitively practice adapted techniques for safe stair climbing. The more closely the therapeutic practice situation resembles the home situation in terms of stair depth and height, amount of traffic, lighting, and so forth, the less generalizing is required and the more success the patient is likely to have when he or she returns home. However, problems might still be displayed in depth and distance perception in other areas of daily function.

In the functional approach, therapy is viewed as a learning process that takes into consideration the unique strengths and limitations of the individual patient. It is composed of two complementary components: compensation and adaptation.[1] **Compensation** refers to the changes that need to be made in the patient's approach to tasks. **Adaptation** refers to the alterations that need to be made in the human and physical environment in order to facilitate relearning of skills.

To compensate for the disability, the patient first has to be made aware of deficiencies (**cognitive awareness**) and must then be taught how to circumvent them using intact sensations and perceptual skills. The patient should be instructed in specific techniques and assisted in developing successful functional habits. The patient will need to be taught to attend to cues from the environment to enhance skill performance. The therapist helps the patient identify and then call upon these new cues. For example, if the patient has a visual field cut, the therapist should explain that because of a visual problem, the patient is seeing only one half of the environment. The patient should then be shown how to turn the head to compensate for the deficit. Environmental scanning could be incorporated into general therapy sessions as well.

A few general suggestions when teaching compensatory techniques are:
1. Use simple directions.
2. Establish and carry out a routine.
3. Do each activity in a consistent manner.
4. Employ repetition as much as necessary.

Adaptation refers to the alteration not of the patient's strategy, but of the environment. For example, if the patient cannot differentiate between right and left, or tends to neglect the left side of the body, a piece of red tape on the left shoe during gait training will allow the patient to attend more easily to the left side and thus to follow the therapist's instructions more accurately. The therapist can use the functional approach to assist patients in improving specific motor skills related to treatment goals.

There are several inherent benefits to the functional approach. First, in the current managed care environment there is a limited amount of time for inpatient rehabilitation. Therefore, therapists need to concentrate on outcome-directed real-life functional activities because independent performance of these activities at home is the ultimate goal of therapeutic intervention. In addition, interventions directed toward specific functional outcomes are typically reimbursable.[31] Second, the activities are age appropriate, concrete, and clearly relevant to the patient's concerns. For this reason they tend to be the most motivating. Third, tasks can be incorporated into daily hospital routine. Dressing can be reinforced at bedside by the nursing staff, and eating skills can be reinforced at each mealtime.

The major limitation of this approach is that the methods learned in one task are not typically generalized to the performance of another task. The functional approach has been criticized as the teaching of splinter skills, in which the causes of the dysfunction are not addressed.

Cognitive Rehabilitation

Cognitive rehabilitation focuses on training individuals with brain injury to structure and organize information.[32] It addresses memory, high language disorders, and perceptual dysfunction under one umbrella.[33] Information processing, problem solving, awareness, judgement, and decision making are among the areas addressed. The therapist using a cognitive remediation approach might be concerned with the patient's perceptual style, including perceptual strategy, response to different types of cues, and rate and consistency of task performance.[34] Diller and Gordon[35] provide a review of the literature pertaining to intervention strategies for cognitive deficits.

Research has demonstrated that even in a non–brain-injured population, skills learned in one task do not automatically transfer to other tasks.[36] Hence, cognitive strategies can be used to facilitate the carryover of skills learned in therapy to functional activities. In her multicontext treatment approach to cognition, Toglia[36] proposes that learning can be conceptualized as a dynamic interplay between characteristics of the patient, characteristics of the task, and the environment in which it is performed (Fig. 29-1). This has also been termed a dynamic interactional approach.[37] Characteristics of the individual patient that might affect learning include information processing strategies, metacognition (including awareness of one's own performance) and prior experience, attitudes, and emotions. Task-related variables that are proposed to affect learning include the nature of the task itself (familiarity with the task, spatial arrangements, instruction set, and movement and postural requirements), and the criteria that are used to assess the learner's abilities. Environmental variables include the social and cultural environment in which treatment occurs, as well as the physical context.

The cognitive treatment approach proposes a number of treatment strategies that may be relevant to the practice of physical therapy. These treatment strategies include:[36]

1. Use of multiple environments in which to carry out the training activity to enhance transfer of learning.
2. Analyzing the characteristics of the task to establish criteria to determine if transfer of learning in fact took place.
3. Providing training to make the patient aware of abilities, the level of difficulty of the task, and promote self-assessment of performance.
4. Relating new information or skills to previously learned ones.

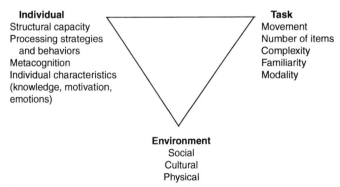

Figure 29-1. Dynamic interactional model of cognition. (From Toglia,[37] p 108, with permission.)

Although these treatment strategies are well known within the field of cognitive-perceptual rehabilitation, the efficacy of the techniques remains to be established with the poststroke population. For a comprehensive understanding and practical guidelines to the evaluation and treatment of patients with cognitive impairments from a dynamic perspective see Toglia[37] and Abreu.[38]

ASSESSMENT OF COGNITIVE AND PERCEPTUAL PROBLEMS

The use of systematic data collection provides the scientific basis for guiding intervention. Its importance cannot be overemphasized with respect to all facets of therapeutic intervention, including remediation of cognitive and perceptual dysfunction. **Task analysis** is the breakdown of an activity or task into its component parts together with a delineation of the specific motor, perceptual, and cognitive abilities necessary to perform each component. Task analysis is another tool that is critical to appropriate therapeutic intervention. For example, the strength, ROM, and balance abilities necessary to accomplish bed mobility and ambulation activities can be clearly defined by the physical therapist. However, the specific perceptual and cognitive requirements of each step needed to perform these two tasks may not be known. Without knowledge of the perceptual and cognitive requirements for successful completion of a task, the therapist cannot simplify the task for the patient and progressively upgrade it.

The Purpose of Assessment

The presence of cognitive and perceptual dysfunction must be confirmed if it is suspected to be interfering with the patient's ability to carry out functional activities.[1] Perceptual performance is positively correlated with ability to perform ADLs; however, it is often difficult to correlate specific perceptual deficits gleaned from testing with specific elements of functional ability and loss.[1,39] Thus, formal testing is indicated when there is a functional loss unexplained by motor deficit, sensory deficit, or deficient comprehension. It should be noted that not all areas of functional loss are typically detected within the hospital setting. It is not uncommon for the patient to perform adequately in self-care skills after therapy in the hospital but to fail on the same tasks in other environmental contexts, such as the home. Higher-level tasks, such as driving, banking, or planning a meal may only emerge as areas of difficulty once the patient is discharged home. When appropriate, the patient's competence in these areas should be considered within the context of an instrumental activities of daily living (IADL) assessment with the occupational therapist while the patient is still hospitalized.

The purpose of assessment is to determine which cognitive and perceptual abilities are intact and which are limited. Understanding the manner in which a particular deficit influences task performance will foster the application of a therapeutic strategy in which intact capabilities may be used to compensate for or to overcome deficits.[40]

Failure in the performance of a task may result from any number of processes underlying cognition and perception. For example, a patient's inability to complete a jigsaw puzzle may result from an inability to organize the pieces or problem solve where they go (disorder of executive function) or difficulty in attending to one half of the picture (unilateral neglect). The patient may be incapable of concentrating on the instructions (attention deficit), unable to know what the pieces are for **(ideational apraxia),** or unable to manipulate them (ideomotor apraxia). Although it is often difficult to implicate reliably one or another of these problem areas, the therapist must be aware of the different deficits that may produce similar patterns of behavior.[5,40]

A fascinating study conducted by Galski et al.[41] concerning the prediction of driving ability following brain injury (including stroke) in 35 patients underscores the critical nature of carefully selected perceptual and cognitive tests. In this study, 64 percent of actual behind-the-wheel driving performances were predicted by performance on a selected battery of neuropsychological tests that measured visual perception. Examination of individual test results uncovered the reasons for unsafe driving, enabling instructors to focus on remediating the specific deficits in preparation for safe driving.

Assessment is not an end in itself. Careful assessment paves the way for realistic and cost-effective intervention.[42] Continuous monitoring of the patient's cognitive and perceptual status will ensure the use of appropriate treatment regimens and their modification when necessary.

Factors Influencing Assessment

Psychological and emotional status play an important role in the patient's ability to cope with disability and with the testing situation. The therapist needs to be aware of behaviors that reflect a patient's psychological response to illness rather than particular cognitive or perceptual abilities. Psychological adjustment to disability depends on many factors, including age, vocational status, education, economic situation, attitude toward the reactions of others, family support, and feelings of competence prior to the onset of disease (see Chapter 2).[39,43,44]

When assessing psychological and emotional status the following should be noted: whether the patient is confused; the level of comprehension for verbal instructions (written and spoken); whether communication is enhanced through the use of visual cues and demonstration; the ability to recognize errors; the level of cooperation and initiative (whether the patient is realistic about capabilities

and goals); and emotional stability.[45] Disturbances of emotional response are evidenced by rapid and frequent mood changes and low frustration tolerance. Difficult tasks may cause a catastrophic reaction.[39]

The patient's ability to detect relevant cues from the environment or to discriminate between relevant and irrelevant stimuli (necessary for cognitive and perceptual competence) may be adversely influenced by poor judgement, fatigue, and prior expectations. Poor judgement is a major contributor to accidents in patients with hemiplegia. This is related in part to the diminished awareness by these patients as to their altered capabilities. The ambiguity of having one set of limbs that works normally and one set that is not functional may lead the patient to rely on solutions to the problems of daily living that are familiar but now inappropriate.[39]

Anxiety over capabilities may inhibit optimal performance during assessment and therapy. The patient's capacity to perform optimally on testing and to learn is enhanced if anxiety can be reduced.[39] Motivation is influenced by many factors, among them premorbid personality. It is of utmost importance for the therapist to structure the therapeutic environment so that the patient will be positively motivated to learn to the maximum ability.[39] To this end, therapeutic tasks should be structured to ensure success, thereby diminishing frustration.

Other factors that may limit a patient's performance on cognitive and perceptual assessments include reduced receptive and expressive communication skills, depression, and fatigue. Prior to assessment, the therapist should consider the patient's language skills, and confirm these observations with the speech-language pathologist. The therapist should also be aware of any medications the patient is taking and how these may affect performance. For example many medications produce drowsiness as a side effect, which would affect patient performance during assessment.[2] Following stroke, 30 to 50 percent[12] of people are said to experience depression, and these symptoms can easily be mistaken for cognitive or perceptual problems. Finally, a determination should be made of the patient's level of fatigue prior to any assessment procedure.

The patient's behavior should not be misinterpreted because of a cultural bias, such as a lack of experience in taking tests. Premorbid intellectual ability should be ascertained from an interview with family or friends, because intellectual abilities may affect performance on some of the assessments as well as affecting behavior in general. Premorbid memory should also be determined.

Finally, it is very important to conduct a sensory assessment prior to cognitive or perceptual testing to establish whether the patient has sufficient sensory abilities to proceed with testing (this includes visual screening as well). Distinguishing between sensory and cognitive or perceptual problems is explored in more detail in the next section of this chapter. Each of these problems may adversely influence performance and may also reduce the patient's performance in treatment and capacity to learn from treatment. The therapist should be aware of the potential for these problems arising, and seek to minimize their impact.

Distinguishing Between Sensory and Cognitive/Perceptual Problems

Cognitive and perceptual dysfunction must be differentiated from sensory loss, language impairment, hearing loss, motor loss (weakness, spasticity, incoordination), visual disturbances (poor eyesight, **hemianopsia**), disorientation, and lack of comprehension. The therapist must rule out pure sensory deficits prior to testing for cognitive and perceptual problems, otherwise the therapist may incorrectly attribute poor performance to perceptual problems and design treatment accordingly when in fact the problem has a sensory base and should be treated quite differently. The therapist should conduct an assessment of deep (proprioceptive) sensations (kinesthesia, position sense, vibration), superficial sensations (pain, temperature, light touch, and pressure), and combined cortical sensations (stereognosis, tactile localization two-point discrimination, barognosis, graphesthesia, and recognition of texture) using methods described in Chapter 6. The patient's hearing also requires assessment. For example, if the patient does not seem to understand what the therapist is saying, hearing problems should be ruled out before more extensive language and cognitive tests are conducted. The therapist may need to confirm with the family if the patient wears a hearing aid and ensure its availability during therapy. If in doubt, the therapist may need to request assessment by the speech-language pathologist or audiologist.

The therapist must also determine if the patient has any visual impairments because they can easily be mistaken for perceptual problems. Given the prevalence of sensory-based visual problems, the following section focuses on identification of these impairments and the importance of distinguishing between visual and perceptual origins for treatment purposes.

VISUAL DISTURBANCES

Although they have received relatively little attention in the literature,[47] visual impairments are one of the most common forms of sensory loss affecting the patient with hemiplegia.[46] The lesion resulting from a stroke may affect the eye, optic radiation, or visual cortex and subsequently the reception, transmission, and appreciation of any visual array. Visual impairments commonly encountered by patients with hemiplegia include poor eyesight, diplopia, **homonymous hemianopsia,** damage to the visual cortex, and retinal damage. Awareness of the presence of these deficits is important so as not to confuse them with visual perceptual deficiencies, and to ensure their consideration during treatment planning and therapeutic intervention.

The critical nature of the basic visual skills (i.e., acuity, oculomotor control, and intact visual fields) in forming a basis for higher level visual perception is highlighted by Warren[48,49] in a hierarchical model for the treatment and evaluation of visual perceptual dysfunction. In this developmental model, the basic visual skills enumerated above form the foundation for the next level of visual skills, which include visual attention, visual scanning, and pattern recognition. These skills, along with memory, are required to facilitate the highest level visual skill termed visual cognition.[48,49] This model has implications for the assessment and treatment of visual perceptual disorders in a bottom-up sequence (Fig. 29-2).[49]

Impairments of oculomotor control (control of eye movements) are a common occurrence following a CVA. Poor visual acuity is another frequent finding following stroke or brain injury, even in the absence of other visual problems.[46] Therefore, it is recommended that the patient receive a comprehensive eye examination and have his or her eyeglass prescription checked.

Diplopia, or double vision, is often present following brain damage. The patient sees two of the entire environment. Diplopia is usually the result of defective function of extraocular muscles in which both eyes are used but not in focus. Treatment usually consists of exercises for the eye muscles. In addition, the patient usually is instructed to wear a patch on alternate eyes until the condition clears. If the condition does not clear, the optometrist may recommend prisms.

Visual field deficit is probably the most common visual deficit affecting patients with hemiplegia[39] and occurs most frequently following damage to the middle cerebral artery near the internal capsule.[9] The diagnostic term for this deficit is homonymous hemianopsia. Studies indicate that the frequency of hemianopsia following a right-hemisphere stroke is around 17 percent.[12] In addition, there is a signifi-

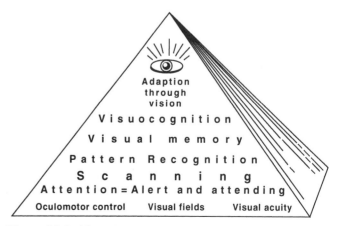

Figure 29-2. Hierarchy of visual perceptual skills in the central nervous system. (Drawing courtesy of Josphine C. Moore PhD, OTR. (From Warren,[48] p 43, with permission.)

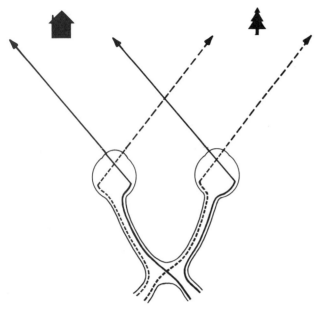

Figure 29-3. Normally functioning visual system; right and left visual fields. See text for explanation. (From Sharpless,[9] p 247, with permission.)

cant correlation between the presence of visual field deficits and visual neglect.[50] Most important, the presence of a visual field deficit is a significant prognostic sign, predicting both a higher death rate following stroke and poorer performance in ADLs, even following rehabilitation.[12,51]

Figure 29-3 demonstrates the normal functioning of the visual fields, in which the left side of the environment (the house) is perceived by the nasal retina of the left eye and the temporal retina of the right eye, and the right side of the environment (the tree) is perceived by the nasal retina of the right eye and the temporal retina of the left eye.[9]

The lesion producing homonymous hemianopsia interrupts inflow to the optic pathways on one side of the brain. This produces a loss of the outer half of the visual field from one eye and the inner half of the visual field of the other eye. The result is a loss of incoming information from half of the visual environment (left or right) contralateral to the side of the lesion. Thus, the loss of the left half of the visual field accompanies left hemiplegia and loss of the right visual field accompanies right hemiplegia. Figure 29-4[52] illustrates visual field deficits associated with a number of lesions to the visual system.

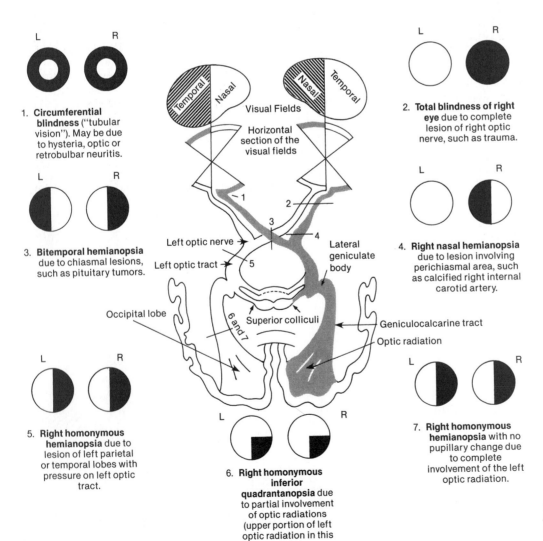

1. **Circumferential blindness** ("tubular vision"). May be due to hysteria, optic or retrobulbar neuritis.

2. **Total blindness of right eye** due to complete lesion of right optic nerve, such as trauma.

3. **Bitemporal hemianopsia** due to chiasmal lesions, such as pituitary tumors.

4. **Right nasal hemianopsia** due to lesion involving perichiasmal area, such as calcified right internal carotid artery.

5. **Right homonymous hemianopsia** due to lesion of left parietal or temporal lobes with pressure on left optic tract.

6. **Right homonymous inferior quadrantanopsia** due to partial involvement of optic radiations (upper portion of left optic radiation in this case).

7. **Right homonymous hemianopsia** with no pupillary change due to complete involvement of the left optic radiation.

Figure 29-4. Visual field deficits and associated lesions sites. (From Chusid,[2] p 114, with permission.)

The presence of a visual field cut may inhibit performance in many daily activities. The patient is usually unaware of the condition and does not automatically compensate by turning the head unless specifically instructed. One of the dangers in this condition is street crossing (Fig. 29-5).[53] Another example of the effects of a visual field cut is illustrated in Figure 29-6.[9] When presented with a tray of food, a patient with right homonymous hemianopsia may attend to the plate and fork on the left side and fail to see the knife, spoon, and cup on the right side of the plate. The patient might read only one half of the newspaper page, either to or from the midline.

Because of its prevalence, it is essential for the therapist to assess whether hemianopsia is present or not. A number of assessment tools are currently employed. In the confrontation method, the patient sits opposite the therapist and is instructed to maintain his or her gaze on the therapist's nose (Fig. 29-7).[54] The therapist slowly brings a target, such as a pen, into the patient's field of view alternately from the right or left. The patient is instructed to indicate when and where he or she sees the targets.

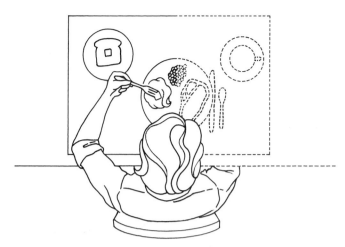

Figure 29-6. A table setting as it might appear to a patient with right homonymous hemianopsia following a stroke. The dotted lines indicate that she may be unable to locate her knife, spoon, cup, and so forth. (From Sharpless,[9] p 248, with permission.)

To help the patient compensate for the visual field deficit, the patient can first be made aware of the deficit and then be instructed to turn the head to the affected side. Patients usually require constant reminders at first, which may be tapered off with time and practice. Early in therapy, items (e.g., eating utensils, writing implements) should be placed where the patient is most apt to see them (on the intact side). They can be moved progressively to the midline and then to the affected side, when appropriate. The nursing staff should be made aware of the condition and be requested to place the patient's essential bedside needs such as telephone, tissues, and so forth within the intact visual field. The therapist initially should sit on the patient's intact side when instructing or giving demonstrations and should alternate this with the affected side so that the patient receives maximum stimulation. Of

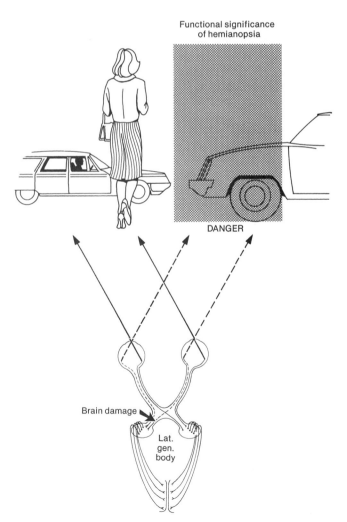

Figure 29-5. The functional significance of hemianopsia—it may lead to accidents. (From Tobis and Lowenthal,[53] p 78, with permission.)

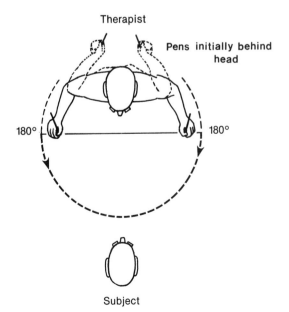

Figure 29-7. Method for assessing hemianopsia. See text for explanation. (Modified from Predretti[54] p 99, with permission.)

course, the patient will have to be reminded to turn the head at first. External cues can be employed as well. For reading, a red line can be drawn on the side of the page that is not seen. Red tape can be placed on the floor, mat, or parallel bars to attract the patient to scan to the side of the environment that is not seen. The patient should be taught to look for these cues. These external cues can be slowly tapered off over time. Patients can be instructed that they can devise their own cues to clue them into the unseen side of the environment in situations that have not been addressed per se in therapy. Exercises that require motor crossing of the midline can be used to reinforce visual crossing of the midline and turning of the head.[55,56]

Oculomotor dysfunction is the third potential area of deficit in basic visual skills that is common in patients who have had a stroke. Eye movements, which are controlled by the extraocular muscles, are used to detect, identify, and derive meaning from objects and the environment. They allow a person to become oriented to and explore the critical visual aspects of the environment.[11] Two types of eye movements are important to assess: (1) **visual fixation,** which allows the patient to maintain focus on an object as it is brought nearer or farther away; and (2) **ocular pursuits,** which enable the eyes to follow a moving object and visually scan the environment. Often the eyes will not follow a moving object visually, although the patient seems aware of the presence of that object and can locate it if asked. The patient is visually hypoactive. Oculomotor dysfunction often accompanies visual-perceptual dysfunction[57] and is frequently related to attention deficits.[58]

Visual scanning can be assessed as follows. Sit opposite the patient. Hold up a pencil with a colorful pencil topper 18 inches in front of the patient's eyes. Slowly move the topper horizontally, then vertically, then diagonally. Repeat each direction two to three times. Note the smoothness of eye movements, the presence of a midline jerk or jump, and whether the eyes move together.[1,57]

Aside from the visual sensory deficits outlined above, many patients suffer from visual-perceptual dysfunction. Damage to areas of the cortex upon which visual information converges with information from other senses may interfere with the recognition and interpretation of visual information, even though the visual stimuli may have arrived at the visual cortex uninterrupted. A total failure to appreciate incoming visual sensory information owing to a lesion in the cortex is referred to as **cortical blindness.**[57] There is no statistical correspondence between the presence of visual field cuts and the presence of visual-perceptual disorders.[47] Similarly, there is no correspondence between aphasia, age, and time since infarct, and measures of visual-perceptual dysfunction.[47] However, within the realm of visual-perceptual disorders, there is a significant difference between the performances of patients with right hemiplegia and those with left hemiplegia. Patients with left hemiplegia have frequently been found to perform more

poorly on measures of visual-perceptual dysfunction than patients with right hemiplegia. Thus, therapists should be aware of the possibility of visual-perceptual deficits, particularly in the population with left hemiplegia.

Standardized Cognitive and Perceptual Assessments

A standardized assessment is one that has a uniform procedure to administer and score the assessment, operational definitions for all terms, and possesses normative data[59] and information concerning its reliability and validity, which is essential for correct interpretation of results.[60] Results from standardized assessments of cognition and perception can be communicated to other therapists who will share an understanding of the patient's capacities or abilities. Standardized assessments can be administered both at admission and discharge to provide the therapist with a reliable and valid measure of the outcome of therapy.

When conducting a standardized assessment, the patient should be sitting comfortably and wearing glasses and/or a hearing aid if needed. Ideally the room should be quiet and free of distraction. The therapist should be positioned opposite or next to the patient. Age, gender, and hand dominance should be noted.[40] In addition, the performance of a patient who has had a stroke may vary from day to day; a single assessment session is, therefore, usually unreliable.[61] A number of short sessions scheduled on successive days are preferable. To enhance its practical value, perceptual testing must be done in conjunction with observation in self-care and ADL skills, where the patient's judgement and discriminative abilities with regard to real-life tasks can be determined. It is not uncommon for patients to test poorly for visual perceptual skills but to perform adequately in ADLs with minimal effort or assistance.[58]

The quality of the patient's response to the test media (e.g., how the task is approached, how and why the error is made) is as important to note as the success or failure in completing the assessment task. Some aspects of response in the testing situation or during ADLs can be referred to as the patient's individual *perceptual style*. Included under this rubric are the patient's perceptual strategy, response to various cues (such as auditory, visual, and tactile), rate of performance, and consistency of performance.[32]

Occupational therapists use a variety of standardized assessments to test for the presence of cognitive and perceptual impairments and resulting disabilities. When selecting a standardized assessment the therapist must consider many factors. The selection depends on what the therapist wants to learn about the patient, and what the assessment can potentially reveal.[2] In many cases a single assessment will not provide all the information required by a therapist to plan treatment, so several assessments may be administered (Table 29–1).[63-76] Several other global

Table 29-1 SUMMARY OF STANDARDIZED ASSESSMENTS

Assessment	Description
Arnadottir OT-ADL Neurobehavioral Evaluation (A-ONE)[5]	This assessment was developed to measure a patient's neurobehavior through daily living tasks (dressing, grooming, hygiene, transfer and mobility, feeding, and communication). Occupational therapists must undertake a 5-day training and certification course to qualify to administer this assessment. A wide variety of cognitive and perceptual impairments can be detected with this assessment.
Structured Observational Test Of Function (SOTOF)[62]	The SOTOF was designed to assess older persons' level of occupational performance and neuropsychological functioning following neurological damage of cortical origin.[63] The assessment consists of a screening assessment, neuropsychological checklist, and four ADL scales (eating from a bowl, pouring a drink and drinking, putting on an upper body garment, and washing and drying hands). After analyzing observational data, a wide variety of neuropsychological deficits are extrapolated.[62]
Allen Cognitive Level Test (ACL)[64,65]	The ACL is used as a screening tool to estimate a person's cognitive level. Although originally developed for use with clients who have psychiatric problems, this assessment is also used with people who have acquired brain damage, or experience a dementing illness such as Alzheimer's disease. Following an interview to gain information concerning the client's educational and work background, the client is observed performing the visuomotor task of leather lacing. It is assumed that the client's cognitive functioning is reflected through their motor actions.[2]
Chessington Occupational Therapy Neurological Assessment Battery (COTNAB)[66]	The COTNAB was designed to assess cognitive and perceptual deficits in clients aged 16 years and over following stroke or head injury. The battery consists of 12 tests divided into four sections assessing visual perception, constructional ability, sensory-motor ability, and ability to follow instructions. Further information about this assessment may be found in Stanley et al.[67] and Sloan et al.[68]
Loewenstein Occupational Therapy Cognitive Assessment (LOTCA)[69]	The LOTCA is a battery-style assessment lasting 35 to 40 minutes and composed of 20 subtests that assess four areas: orientation, visual and spatial perception, visuomotor organization, and thinking operations. The assessment was developed for use with people who have experienced stroke, traumatic brain injury, or tumor. Further information about this assessment is contained in Katz et al.[70]
The Behavioural Inattention Test (BIT)[71]	The BIT was developed to assess clients for the presence of unilateral visual neglect and to provide the therapist with information concerning how the neglect impacts the client's ability to perform everyday occupations.[72] The BIT consists of nine activity based subtests and six pen-and-paper subtests. Many of these test items have been used in the past in a nonstandardized way to examine for the presence of neglect.
Rivermead Perceptual Assessment Battery (RPAB)[73]	This assessment was designed to assess visual perceptual deficits in clients following head injury or stroke. The RPAB is a battery consisting of 16 performance tests that assess form discrimination, color constancy, sequencing, object completion, figure-ground discrimination, body image, inattention, and spatial awareness. The test can be completed in approximately 1 hour. For further information on the RPAB, the reader is referred to Jesshope et al.[74]
Rivermead Behavioural Memory Test (RBMT)[75]	This battery was designed to assess a person's everyday memory abilities. It offers the therapist an initial assessment of the client's memory function, an indication of appropriate areas for treatment, and enables the therapist to monitor memory skills throughout the treatment program. The RBMT can be administered in approximately 30 minutes by occupational therapists, speech-language pathologists, and psychologists. For further reading on the RBMT, the reader is referred to Cockburn et al.[75] and Wilson et al.[76]

assessments of function such as the Functional Life Scale,[77] the Riverdale Hospital Home and Community Skills Assessment,[78] and the Functional Independence Measure (Adult FIM SM)[79] also incorporate items that measure cognition and perception. For example, the FIM includes three cognition-related items: memory, problem solving, and social interaction. The assessments described in the section on specific cognitive and perceptual deficits are used widely in the clinic. Although some of the assessments presented are not standardized, they are still useful, particularly for examining the quality of response to the test stimuli.

INTERVENTION

Treatment Approaches

Five major approaches to cognitive and perceptual rehabilitation are commonly employed by occupational therapists. They are the transfer-of-training approach, the sensory integrative approach, the neurodevelopmental approach, the cognitive rehabilitation or retraining approach, and the functional approach. These approaches were described earlier in the chapter. Although research directly comparing the efficacy of the various approaches has been sparse, attempts have been made recently to empirically define and test the methodologies.[21,25,30,80] Issues to consider in examining the techniques are standardized measures of change in functional status and ADLs, length and frequency of feedback, group versus individual treatment, specific stimulus properties, format and frequency of feedback, and individual information processing styles.[21]

Neistadt[25,30] described these treatments dichotomously as either remedial or adaptive/compensatory. The remedial approach encompasses the sensory integrative approach, neurodevelopmental treatment, transfer-of-training approach, and the cognitive retraining model.[34] The functional approach is described as adaptive or compensatory. A description of the key components of these two main approaches is outlined below. A discussion on education is also provided because no intervention program would be complete without the provision of education to both the patient and the caregivers. Finally, a discussion is provided on integrating these three elements within a rehabilitation program.

REMEDIAL APPROACH

Remedial approaches focus on the patient's deficits and attempt to improve functional ability by retraining specific perceptual components of behavior.[25] The assumption uniting this set of tactics is that facilitation of, or training in, underlying skills will enhance the recovery or reorganization of deficient CNS functioning.[21,25] This, in turn, will automatically translate into improvement in functional skills. Remedial approaches are also referred to as bottom-up approaches. These approaches work from the bottom, which is the recovery of underlying skills, and assume that the patient will be able to generalize skills to occupational performance, which is at a higher level.[1,42]

ADAPTIVE/COMPENSATORY APPROACH

The adaptive or compensatory approach mandates direct training in the functional skills that are deficient. It does not assume automatic carryover from tasks that are not obviously similar to the functional task to be learned, and thus minimizes the need for generalization. In an adaptive or "top-down" approach, the therapist works with the patient on specific tasks that are required, or those that the patient wants to achieve. In other words, the therapist starts at the top, which is the desired outcome functional, rather than working with the patient on the underlying performance components. For a comparison of the assumptions underlying the remedial and adaptive approaches, see Table 29–2.

EDUCATION

Education for the patient, family, and friends is essential for continuity of care. The patient and family should understand why it is inadvisable or impossible for the patient to do some things safely or independently, and why other things must be done in a specific way. Explaining the reasons why the patient behaves in a particular way reduces the likelihood of inappropriate expectations from those without the background to know that brain damage affects not only how the patient moves but how he or she experiences and thus responds to the world.

Feedback is essential in the patient's own education. The patient's own feedback may be inaccurate owing to perceptual and cognitive dysfunctions. Thus, the individual may be unaware that a task has not been accomplished or that it has not been performed in the safest or most efficient manner. Feedback should be provided in the form of **knowledge of results (KR),** and **knowledge of performance (KP).** Knowledge of results is information regarding whether or not the patient attained the correct outcome. Knowledge of performance is

Table 29–2 COMMON ASSUMPTIONS OF ADAPTIVE AND REMEDIAL APPROACHES

Adaptive Approach	Remedial Approach
The adult brain has limited potential to repair and reorganize itself after injury.	The adult brain can repair and reorganize itself after injury.
Intact behaviors can be used to compensate for ones that are impaired.	This repair and reorganization is influenced by environmental stimuli.
Adaptive retraining can facilitate the substitution of intact behaviors for impaired ones.	Cognitive, perceptual and sensorimotor exercises can promote brain recovery and reorganization.
Adaptive ADLs provide training in functional behaviors.	Cognitive, perceptual, and sensorimotor exercises provide training in the cognitive and perceptual skills needed for those exercises.
Training in specific, essential activities of daily living tasks is necessary because adults with brain injury have difficulty generalizing learning.	Remedial training in cognitive and perceptual skills will be generalized across all activities requiring those skills.
Functional activities require cognitive and perceptual skills.	Functional activities require cognitive and perceptual skills.
Adaptation and compensation will lead to improved functional performance.	Cognitive and perceptual remediation will lead to improved functional performance.

information regarding the manner in which the task was accomplished.[81]

The form in which this feedback is delivered depends on the specific limitations and strengths of the patient. For example, the physical therapy goal for a patient with left hemiplegia and visual perceptual involvement might be to walk to the end of the parallel bars. KR would consist of a verbal confirmation by the therapist as to whether or not the patient reached the end of the parallel bars. KP might include comments by the therapist concerning the adequacy of the patient's visual scanning, positioning of the lower extremities, correct posture, and appropriate use of the upper limbs. For the patient with communication impairments the feedback would have to be visual. Tactile input also can be used effectively to cue patients with either right or left hemiplegia. A combination of inputs, using a number of sensory modalities, often facilitates patient success at a given task.

When involving the patient in education sessions, the patient must be addressed as a competent adult, and not patronized. He or she must be regarded as the principal participant in the rehabilitation process. In situations in which the perceptual deficit does not interfere with assimilation of information, the patient should have the major role in the decision making process regarding the goals of therapy.

Refocussing Intervention

Many clinicians commence an intervention program by adopting remedial strategies. In these circumstances, therapists are aiming to maximize recovery of function and educate their patients about the problems experienced and ways that can improve their function. However, some patients may not make much progress. In some cases the patient may have inadequate language skills to be able to work with the therapist, or may have limited insight to his or her problems and therefore will not work with the therapist. In other cases still, improvements simply do not seem to occur for a variety of reasons that the therapist may not be able to pinpoint. Finally, in the current climate of managed care, the therapist may not have very much time allocated to work with the patient using remedial techniques. The patient's discharge may be imminent, and yet he or she may not be independent or safe enough to be discharged. In all these cases, the therapist may switch from a remedial approach to a compensatory one.

When using a adaptive compensatory approach, the therapist will target education at the caregivers as well as the patient. Intervention strategies will focus on changing the environment or the strategy for task completion so that the patient can be safe and independent as quickly as possible. In many instances, therapists use a three-point approach to intervention where they educate patients and caregivers, commence the program using remedial techniques, and then switch to compensation techniques when the patient's improvements have plateaued and/or discharge is imminent.

The Impact of Managed Care

The introduction of managed care in the US heath system has many implications for treatment of patients with cognitive and perceptual deficits. The most striking of these is the reduction in time allocated for inpatient assessment and intervention.[31] Cognitive and perceptual problems are not readily visible and are therefore more easily overlooked than physical problems. Hence, pressure to discharge patients quickly, possibly before the full extent of cognitive and perceptual problems has been revealed means that patients may be discharged to potentially hazardous situations at home. Therapists need to do an initial screening of all patients with brain damage to determine potential problems as early as possible, and ensure that patients are discharged to a safe environment. Although inpatient rehabilitation time is reduced, there is more opportunity for outpatient services conducted in the clinic or in the patient's home.[82] The advantage of home care is that therapists have an opportunity to work with the patient in his or her own environment, and tailor therapy to the patient's current circumstances. Patients with cognitive and perceptual problems often perform better in their own familiar environments.

The major disadvantage of reduced inpatient treatment time for many patients, including those with cognitive and perceptual problems, is that a home discharge may not be safe after only 1 or 2 weeks of inpatient rehabilitation. The situation is complicated by having to discharge a patient who does not have family support to another type of institutional care (possibly a nursing home or skilled nursing facility) when in the long term this level of care is not necessary. It is distressing for patients who are confused owing to cognitive and perceptual problems to be moved, particularly when they may believe the move is permanent.

DISCHARGE PLANNING

Discharge planning commences as soon as the patient is admitted for rehabilitation.[83] The most important question to be answered during this stage is where the patient will live upon discharge. There are two major types of housing available to persons with disabilities: community-based accommodation and supported accommodation. Community-based accommodation includes private homes, retirement villages, and hotels or rooming houses. Supported accommodation may be defined as any accommodation that provides personal care and medical services on a consistent, continual, or per need basis, and includes nursing homes, skilled nursing facilities, assisted living centers, and sheltered or group housing.[84,85]

The key to discharge planning is to consider the match between the patient's skills and the demands of the environment, and then factor in the support systems available from a spouse, friends, or family to assist with tasks that the patient cannot manage.[85,86] This approach works well when patients and their families have insight and an understanding of the patient's problems. However, cognitive and perceptual problems are often not very visible and it may be difficult for the family and the patient to understand the functional impact of these deficits. For example, a patient may regain full motor function following a stroke, but experience ongoing difficulties with unilateral neglect. This problem is not readily apparent to the untrained onlooker. However, this patient cannot drive and may be in danger when simply crossing the road. These problems have major life-style implications for the patient.

Interventions that facilitate a patient's return to community-based housing usually center around enabling the patient to carry out ADLs in an acceptable and safe manner. If this cannot be achieved and the patient does not have a live-in caregiver, then supported housing such as a nursing home may be the only alternative. Research examining the discharge process for a sample of 62 patients following stroke revealed that the majority were reluctant to consider alternatives to returning home despite having significant self-care deficits.[86] Our housing is central to who we are as an individual and it is very difficult for patients, particularly those with limited insight, to understand and accept that they can no longer live in the community.

REVIEW OF COGNITIVE AND PERCEPTUAL DEFICITS

This section is divided into seven parts: disorders of attention, disorders of memory, disorders of executive function, disorders of body scheme and body image, spatial relations syndrome, agnosia, and apraxia (Table 29–3.) Each category encompasses a constellation of deficits, which are grouped together for ease of understanding. Information pertaining to each deficit will be organized identically:

1. Individual deficits are defined.
2. Clinical examples are offered.
3. An approximate lesion area is identified, although for some disorders controversy exists as to the actual area of the cortex involved in producing a specific perceptual deficit, and to its laterality. When a cerebral hemisphere is designated it refers to the majority of cases cited in the literature. Exceptions do occur.
4. Assessment methods in current use are described.
5. Suggestions are presented for the therapist to employ in treatment.

The value of dwelling on probable areas of cortical damage is controversial. The indication of cortical loci is an attempt to relate the study of neuroanatomy to actual patient behavior involving cognitive and perceptual dysfunction. An examination of

Table 29–3 SUMMARY OF COGNITIVE AND PERCEPTUAL IMPAIRMENTS

Area of Deficit	Specific Impairments
Cognition	Attention disorders
	Sustained attention
	Selective attention
	Divided attention
	Alternating attention
	Memory disorders
	Immediate recall and short-term memory
	Long-term memory
Higher order cognition	Executive functions
	Volition
	Planning
	Purposeful action
	Effective performance
Perception	Body scheme/body image disorders
	Unilateral neglect
	Anosognosia
	Somatoagnosia
	Right-left discrimination
	Finger agnosia
	Spatial relation disorder (complex perception)
	Figure-ground discrimination
	Form constancy
	Spatial relations
	Topographic disorientation
	Depth and distance perception
	Vertical disorientation
	Agnosias
	Visual object agnosia
	Auditory agnosia
	Tactile agnosia
	Apraxia
	Ideomotor apraxia
	Ideational apraxia
	Constructional apraxia

cortical loci will give the reader a sense of which cognitive and perceptual deficits are likely to be seen together.

As therapists, we are required to assist the patient to bridge the gap between maladaptive behavior and independent function in ADLs. Whether or not the area of the brain purported to produce a particular dysfunction appears damaged on a computed axial tomography (CAT) scan or other neurological or radiological test is not a key determinant of the rehabilitative approach to therapy. The patient's approach to task performance and the relative strengths or weaknesses of the patient (motorically, cognitively, and perceptually), which the therapist ascertains through thorough observation and assessment, are much more pertinent to the selection of appropriate therapeutic strategies than the locus of the lesion.

Assessment tools are described for each cognitive or perceptual disability to enhance the reader's awareness of the complexity of behavior ascribed to perceptual deficiencies. Familiarity with the tools used to assess cognitive or perceptual dysfunction can serve as an aid in communication between physical and occupational therapists engaged in the treatment of the same patient.

The following section also includes specific treatment suggestions from the sensorimotor, transfer of training, and functional approaches described. The treatment techniques most relevant are those dealing with the functional approach and adaptation of the environment. In these sections, examples are given of how to facilitate the patient's success within a treatment session. Information is provided on how the therapist might gear language, demonstrations, feedback, and the use of media and environment to the individual needs of the cognitively or perceptually impaired patient.

Attention Disorders

1. The inability of many patients with hemiplegia to maintain attention during therapy is a frequent complaint of therapists. **Attention** is the ability to select and attend to a specific stimulus while simultaneously suppressing extraneous stimuli.[87] A patient who is inattentive or distractible will have difficulty in processing and assimilating new information or techniques.[88] Often, patients who have suffered a CVA will have low arousal levels, and require a great deal of sensory input to be alerted to the environment. Low arousal thus must be considered as a cause for seeming inattention.

    Four different kinds of attention are generally discussed in the literature. These are sustained attention, focused or selective attention, alternating attention, and divided attention. **Sustained attention** is a capacity to attend to relevant information during activity. Sustained attention implies that a person can maintain a consistent response during a continuous activity. **Focused** or **selective attention** is the capacity to attend to a task despite environmental visual or auditory stimuli. **Alternating attention** is the capacity to move flexibly between tasks and respond appropriately to the demands of each task. **Divided attention** is the capacity to respond simultaneously to two or more tasks or stimuli when all stimuli are relevant.

2. Clinically, the patient with a disorder of sustained attention may report that he or she starts to watch a TV program and then "just drifts off." A patient who has to stop a dressing activity to talk to the therapist may be demonstrating difficulties with focused attention. Patients who are easily disturbed by music or other forms of background noise may also be experiencing problems with focused attention. Hence, a problem with focused attention is often referred to as *distractibility*. Divided attention is required when more than one response is required or more than one stimuli needs to be monitored.[89] Selective concentration is required when stimuli are required to be ignored.[90] Patients who have difficulty with divided and alternating attention may have great difficulties with more complex daily living activities such as cooking a meal or driving.

3. Multiple brain regions are thought to be responsible for producing attention. These include the reticular formation (which regulates arousal), the various sensory systems that bring and code relevant sensory information, and the limbic and frontal regions that underlie the drive and affective components of concentration.[90]

4. General screening assessments such as the Loewenstein Occupational Therapy Cognitive Assessment[69] or Chessington Occupational Therapy Neurological Assessment Battery (COTNAB)[66] include subtests that examine attentional abilities. To investigate problems of attention, neuropsychologists generally administer the Stroop Test,[91] the Paced Auditory Serial Attention Test (PASAT),[92] and the Trail Making Test.[93]

5. The purpose of therapy is to increase the patient's attention to appropriate stimuli, and disregard inappropriate stimuli.

   a. *Remedial approach:* Clinically, the ability to attend to a task has implications for the therapeutic process. Diller and Weinberg[94] suggest that to improve performance, the patient with left hemiplegia should be trained to scan the visual environment. A patient scanning too quickly should be advised to slow down. In the presence of right hemiplegia, the patient should be spoken to more slowly to afford an opportunity to process verbal information.[95] Additionally, patients with left hemiplegia should be encouraged to use verbalization to improve performance in visual tasks, and patients with right hemiplegia should be taught to use visualization techniques to facilitate attendance to verbal tasks.

   Some additional tools that may be used for the remediation of attentional deficits and distractibility are setting time or speed limits, amplification of critical stimuli, and making the crucial stimuli salient (noticeable) to the patient.[58] The environment can be graded by having the patient initially perform some aspects of therapy in a nondistracting setting (closed environment) and then slowly increasing potentially distracting elements, both visual and auditory, as patient tolerance improves.[96]

   b. *Adaptive approach:* For many patients, the inability to attend to significant stimuli is compounded by distraction due to extraneous stimuli in the environment. Often noise is the most distracting stimulus, causing irritability and diminished concentration. Ideally, distractible patients should be assessed in a noise-free, visually bland environment. For patients who have difficulty reading as a result of diminished concentration abilities, a card with a slit large enough for only one line to appear at a time can be placed over the page while the patient reads. The slit is enlarged as the patient is able to tolerate more extraneous stimuli.[1]

Memory Disorders

Memory can be defined as a "mental process that allows the individual to store experiences and perceptions for recall at a later time."[88] All memory is not localized in one particular place in the nervous system; rather, many and perhaps all regions of the brain may contain neurons with adequate plasticity for memory storage.[97] Memory comprises acquisition or learning, storage or retention, and retrieval or recall.[98] Learning is a crucial in rehabilitation. If the patient is unable to learn then time in rehabilitation may not be well spent. Hence, it is very important for the therapist to take steps to evaluate the patient's memory before commencing physical retraining programs. Three levels of memory will be examined: immediate recall, short-term memory, and long-term memory.

IMMEDIATE RECALL AND SHORT-TERM MEMORY

1. **Immediate recall** involves retention of information that has been stored for a few seconds. **Short-term memory** mediates retention of events or learning that has taken place within a few minutes, hours or days.[4]

2. A patient with immediate recall difficulties may not be able to remember the instructions given only seconds before by the therapist for what the patient is to do. A patient with a short-term memory problem may not come back to the therapy department, even though

the therapist asked him or her to return in an hour. Alternatively, the therapist may teach the patient a new transfer technique, and on the following day find that the patient has not retained any of the steps involved. Patients with severe short-term memory problems may not even be able to hold a simple conversation.[40]

3. Memory is a complex capacity involving many brain regions including four of the major structures of the cerebral cortex (the frontal, parietal, temporal, and occipital lobes) and the limbic system.[4,99]

4. The Rivermead Behavioural Memory Test (RBMT)[75] can be used. Alternatively the adequacy of memory functions can be assessed by having the patient recall lists or collections of objects that have just been presented (immediate recall) or by teaching the patient a new verbal or visual task and asking him or her to recall it a few hours or a day later (short-term memory). Frequently there is a loss of short-term memory following stroke, and this particularly interferes with the patient's ability to benefit from rehabilitation, especially from those activities involving the use of new and heretofore unfamiliar techniques.[39]

5. The purpose of memory retraining is to enable the patient to effectively encode and recall information so that learning can occur.
   a. *Remedial approach:* As good attention skills are vital for memory, the therapist must ensure that attention problems are addressed and improvements are noted before commencing work on memory retraining.[1] A primary focus of this approach is working with the patient to effectively encode information so it can be more easily retrieved when appropriate. This may include organizing material to be remembered, and making logical associations. A determination should be made of how the patient used to remember information and build on these past strategies. There is very little evidence to suggest that drills, computer games, or memory tests such as recalling a list of items that have been covered over have any effect on retraining memory. However, if the therapist assists the patient to develop memory strategies when playing these games, then these strategies can be generalized to everyday activities.
   b. *Compensatory approach:* The use of a diary or notebook system (memory log) can help many patients to manage their daily living activities. However, the patient needs to have sufficient memory to use this system. Environmental prompts such as a beeper or a wall calendar can be useful to assist patients to remember their routine, or to look at their diary. When external aids are used, the patient needs to be taught how to

use them. Guidelines for the use of such devices may be found in Zoltan.[1]

LONG-TERM MEMORY

1. **Long-term memory** consists of early experiences and information acquired over a period of years. Patients who do not have long-term memory are often described as having amnesia.

2. Patients who experience long-term memory problems may have difficulty recalling events from many years ago such as a child's birth, or work experiences. Long-term memory problems are common following brain injury and in Alzheimer's disease, but are not commonly seen following stroke.[40]

3. As described, memory is a complex capacity involving many brain regions. For a detailed discussion, the reader is referred to Fuster[99] and Lezak.[4]

4. The adequacy of memory functions can be assessed by having the patient recall personal historical events. The Rivermead Behavioral Memory Test (RBMT)[75] can be used to assess memory in a standardized way. It is advisable to question the patient's family as to premorbid memory, because many patients in the stroke-prone age group have already begun to experience declining memory as part of the aging process.

5. Treatment suggestions for assisting patients overcome long-term memory problems are similar to those outlined above for immediate recall and short-term memory. Further information on the management of memory problems may be found in Wilson and Moffat.[100]

Executive Functions

1. As defined by Lezak,[4p42] "executive functions consist of those capacities that enable a person to engage successfully in independent, purposive, self-serving behavior." Lezak goes on to describe executive functions as consisting of four overlapping components: volition, planning, purposive action, and effective performance.
   Volition is the capacity to determine what one needs and wants to do. It also encompasses a future realization of one's needs and wants. Volition encompasses goal planning and task initiation, self-awareness, awareness of the environment, and social awareness. *Planning* is ". . . the identification and organization of the steps and elements (e.g., skills, material, other persons) needed to carry out an intention or achieve a goal."[4p653] Planning involves weighing alternatives and making choices. *Purposive action* includes productivity and self-regulation, which encompasses the ability to initiate, maintain, switch, and stop complex

action sequences in an orderly manner to realize a goal. *Effective performance* is the capacity for quality control, including the ability to self-monitor and self-correct one's behavior. Because ineffective self-monitoring and difficulty with self-correction are the primary features of the performance of persons with problems with effective performance, patients may not even perceive their mistakes, whereas others may identify them but take no action to correct them.[10]

2. Although some patients with executive function disorders are unable to either formulate realistic goals or intentions (volition) or plan, others may be able to formulate goals and initiate goal-directed task performance, but owing to defective planning are not able to realize their goals. Patients with planning problems may say or intend one thing, but do another.[4] Patients who have difficulty with effective performance may not even perceive their mistakes, whereas others may identify them but do not take corrective action. Family and hospital staff may complain of the patient's apparent apathy, poor or unreliable judgment, inappropriate behavior, difficulty adapting to new situations, and/or lack of attention to the needs and feelings of others.

3. Executive functions have traditionally been associated with the frontal and prefrontal cortex,[6] but the current view is that these capacities are mediated by reciprocal connections with other cortical and subcortical regions via the dorsolateral prefrontal-subcortical circuit.[102]

4. Assessment of executive functions include the Executive Functions Assessment[103] and the Good Samaritan Hospital for Cognitive Rehabilitation's Executive Functions Behavioural Rating Scale.[104] Other specific assessments of initiation, self-monitoring, planning, problem solving, and abstraction may be found in Zoltan.[1]

5. The combination of impulsiveness, poor judgement, poor planning ability, and lack of foresight, which is particularly problematic in patients with left hemiplegia, does not bode well for independent functioning. These impairments may diminish somewhat with the passage of time.[9] Although some general remedial and adaptive treatment suggestions are described here, for more specific details refer to Zoltan[1] and Duran and Fisher.[101]

   a. *Remedial approach:* By providing structure, feedback, and routine, a person's performance can be enhanced (e.g., providing structure by giving the patient steps to follow, assisting the task to become routine by repeated practice, or providing immediate feedback about the patient's behavior and the effect it has on others). The therapist initially acts as the patient's frontal lobes, and gradually transfers these responsibilities to the patient. Unless the patient has some awareness of the problems, a remedial approach will not be particularly successful.[1]

   b. *Adaptive approach:* The therapist can assist the patient to compensate for poor abilities by utilizing other intact cognitive functions and/or modifying the environment. For example, the therapist might ask the patient to perform a task in a room with minimal distractions, or change the demands of the patient's work, home, or community to diminish the need to employ executive functions. A beeper or alarm clock may be used to assist a patient overcome poor initiation.

Body Scheme/Body Image Disorders

Body image is defined as a visual and mental image of one's body that includes feelings about one's body, especially in relation to health and disease.[1,105] The term **body scheme** refers to a postural model of the body, including the relationship of body parts to each other and the relationship of the body to the environment. Body awareness is derived from the integration of tactile, proprioceptive, and interoceptive sensations, in addition to the individual's subjective feelings about the body.[105] An awareness of body scheme is considered one of the essential foundations for the performance of all purposeful motor behavior.[105] According to Van Duesen,[105p118] body image is ". . . a dynamic synthesis of the body schema and those environmental inputs providing relevant emotional and conceptual components." The two terms, body image and body scheme, are often used interchangeably; therefore, when researching this topic, close attention should be paid to the particular definition put forth by the author. Specific disturbances of body image and body scheme are unilateral neglect, somatoagnosia, right-left discrimination, finger agnosia, and anosognosia.

UNILATERAL NEGLECT

1. **Unilateral neglect** is the inability to register and integrate stimuli and perceptions from one side of the body (body neglect) and the environment or **hemispace** (spatial neglect), which is not due to a sensory loss. Unilateral neglect usually, although not always, affects the left side of the body or hemispace, and for purposes of this discussion, we will assume that it is the left. If a patient has unilateral neglect, he or she seems to ignore the left side of the body and stimuli occurring in the left personal space. This may occur despite intact visual fields, or concomitantly with right or left homonymous hemianopsia; however, it is not caused by homonymous hemianopsia.[106] Fre-

quently the patient has sensory loss on the affected side, which compounds the problem. Although the patient with left-sided hemianopsia has actual loss of vision from the left visual field of both eyes, he or she may be aware of the problem and compensate automatically or learn to compensate by turning the head. The patient with visual neglect has intact vision but seems unaware of the problem and does not attempt to compensate spontaneously by turning the head. In extreme cases the patient appears totally indifferent to the left side of the body and environment, and may deny that the left extremities belong to him or her.[107] More time seems to be required in learning to compensate for this disability than with hemianopsia. There is great difficulty in integrating all stimuli from the left half of the body and personal space for use in ADLs. As with hemianopsia, the patient with visual unilateral neglect often avoids crossing the midline visually or motorically.[55,56] Current theories consider spatial neglect a disturbance of attention.[107] It is important for the therapist to be familiar with this disorder because it is a frequent clinical finding.[108] Neglect following right cerebral infarction occurs in 12 to 49 percent of patients.[12]

2. Clinically, the patient may ignore the left half of the body when dressing and forget to put on the left sleeve or left pants leg. Often a male patient will forget to shave the left half of his face. A woman may neglect to put makeup on the left side of her face.[109] The patient may neglect to eat from the left half of a plate and will start reading a newspaper from the middle of the line. Typically, the patient bumps into objects on the left side or tends to veer toward the right when walking or propelling a wheelchair.

3. It has been suggested that lesions involving the inferior-posterior regions of the right parietal lobe are significant determinants of neglect.[106,110]

4. *Assessment techniques:* A variety of techniques can be used because unilateral neglect may be manifested differently in individual patients, and no single task is adequate to identify the syndrome in all patients.

   a. The Behavioural Inattention Test (BIT)[71] can be used to assess unilateral neglect (see Table 29–1). In one of the subtests, the patient is asked to copy simple drawings. The drawings done by a patient with this deficit will have parts missing from the left half of the picture or be lacking in detail (Fig. 29-8).[111] In contrast, drawings by a patient suffering from constructional apraxia will have most parts present but not in correct relation to each other. In addition, many patients with constructional apraxia (usually those with left-hemisphere damage) will improve when copying a model,

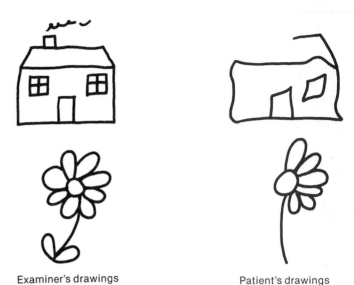

Examiner's drawings   Patient's drawings

Figure 29-8. Assessment for unilateral neglect. Therapist's drawing of a house and a flower (*left*). Impaired copying by a patient with unilateral neglect following a stroke (*right*). (From Zoltan et al.[111] p 61, with permission.)

but those with unilateral neglect (usually right-hemisphere damage) will not.

   b. The patient is asked to perform a personal ADL such as dressing, or an IADL such as baking cookies. The therapist observes performance, and observes changes in the patient's behavior in response to cueing.

5. The purpose of therapy is to increase awareness of the left side of the body and space.

   a. *Remedial approach:* Capitalizing on the rationale of the hemi-inattention theories, the following suggestions are proposed. Stimuli that are specialized for the right side of the brain, such as shapes and blocks, should be used to enhance right brain activation. At the same time, the presence of stimuli that are known to activate the left side of the brain, such as letters and numbers, should be minimized. Use of verbal instructions should be minimized. Simple verbal instructions should be used to encourage the patient to turn the head to the left to anchor his or her attention to that side of space.[107] In addition, research suggests that conducting motor activities with the left body side, such as simply clenching and unclenching the fist, can improve attention to the left body side and hemispace.[112]

   b. *Cognitive compensation* (based on Weinberg et al.[113]): The patient is taught to be aware of the deficit through the method of visual scanning. This technique is used to help the patient become aware of the imbalance in perception of the two sides of space. The patient practices turning toward the left and shifting the eyes to the left (visual scanning). With experience, the patient will begin to trust visual cues to guide action. For example, a patient does not shave properly on his left (affected) side. When asked to touch both sides of his face, or to look in the mirror, he will not notice that anything is amiss. However, after being trained to systematically scan the visual environment, starting with the left side of his face, the patient may notice the unshaven side in the mirror. At a later date, when asked to touch both sides of his face, he will confirm that one side is unshaven and take appropriate action.

A comprehensive and systematic training program for treatment of patients with right-brain damage (including the problem of left-sided neglect) has been developed over the past 15 years at the Department of Rehabilitation Medicine at New York University Medical Center in New York. For a detailed description of this program the reader is referred to Gordon et al.[109] and Weinberg et al.[113,114]

c. Using the functional approach, repeated practice is used in particular areas of difficulty in ADLs, such as transferring from a wheelchair or eating. Visuospatial deficits may interfere extensively with performance of ADLs. Training in functional tasks in the hospital may not generalize to performance of the same functional skills at home, and may need to be learned anew.

Stanton et al.[115] recommend the following steps. The activity should be broken down into small components. The patient should practice each one in sequence until a criterion level has been reached. The cues should then be tapered. Finally the activity should be arranged into larger components. Maintenance of ongoing records of progress will assist the therapist in guiding treatment appropriately. Verbal self-cueing should be encouraged in verbally intact patients. It is worthwhile to refer to the aforementioned article for further details concerning the systematic implementation of therapeutic procedures.

d. *Adapting the environment:* The patient is addressed and given demonstrations from the unaffected side. The nursing staff should place the patient's call button, telephone, and other essential items on the unaffected side. A bold red line may be drawn on the side of the page that is neglected.[105] A mirror may be placed in front of the patient while he or she is dressing or ambulating to draw attention to the neglected side.

e. Using the sensorimotor approach, the therapist stimulates the left side of the patient's body using a rough cloth, ice, or other material. The patient is reminded to watch what the therapist is doing. Next, the patient stimulates the affected side himself or herself while watching.[55]

f. In the transfer-of-training approach, the pa-

tient participates in tasks that make it necessary to look toward the affected side,[114] such as watching television. For example, the television can be placed initially at the midline and progressively moved toward the affected side. A brightly colored tape track may be placed along the floor and the patient may be instructed to walk or to guide the wheelchair along it.[1]

ANOSOGNOSIA

1. **Anosognosia** is a severe condition including denial and lack of awareness of the presence or severity of one's paralysis.[116] Anosognosia is defined as a lack of awareness, or denial, of a paretic extremity as belonging to the person, or a lack of insight concerning, or denial of, paralysis.[1] Presence of this disability may compromise rehabilitation potential greatly, because it limits the patient's ability to recognize the need for, and thus to use, compensatory techniques.

2. Typically, the patient maintains that there is nothing wrong and may disown the paralyzed limbs and refuse to accept responsibility for them. The patient may claim that the limb has a mind of its own or that it was left at home, or in a closet. It has been observed that patients experiencing anosognosia have a tendency to cover the paretic arm.[117]

3. The lesion is usually located in the nondominant parietal lobe,[118] in the region of the supramarginal gyrus.[52]

4. Anosognosia is assessed by talking to the patient. The patient is asked what happened to the arm or leg, whether he or she is paralyzed, how the limb feels, and why it cannot be moved. A patient with anosognosia may deny the paralysis, say that it is of no concern, and fabricate reasons why a limb does not move the way it should.

5. It is extremely difficult to compensate for this condition. Safety is of paramount importance in the treatment and discharge planning for patients suffering from anosognosia, because they typically do not acknowledge that they have a disability and will therefore refuse to be careful.[9]

SOMATOAGNOSIA

1. **Somatoagnosia,** or impairment in body scheme, is a lack of awareness of the body structure and the relationship of body parts to oneself or to others. Somatoagnosia is also referred to as autopagnosia or simply body agnosia.[119] Patients with this deficit may display difficulty following instructions that require distinguishing body parts and may be unable to imitate movements of the therapist.[61] Often patients report that the affected arm or leg feels unduly heavy.[55] Lack of proprioception may underlie or compound this disorder.[120]

2. Clinically, the patient may have difficulty performing transfer activities because he or she does not perceive the meaning of terms related to body parts, for example, "Pivot on your leg and reach for the armrest with your hand." Additionally a patient with a body scheme disorder will have difficulty dressing. Patients may have a hard time participating in exercises that require some body parts to be moved in relation to other body parts; for example, "Bring your arm across your chest and touch your shoulder."

3. The lesion site is the dominant parietal lobe[52] or posterior temporal lobe.[118] Thus, this disorder is seen primarily with right hemiplegia. However, impairment in body scheme may also occur with left hemiplegia.

4. Assessment techniques
   a. The patient is requested to point to body parts named by the therapist, on him- or herself, on the therapist, and on a picture or puzzle of a human figure. Zoltan[1] provides details of these assessment procedures. An example of verbal directives from these assessments include "Show me your feet. Show me your chin. Point to your back." The words "right" and "left" should not be used because they may lead to an inaccurate diagnosis in patients who have difficulty with right-left discrimination. Aphasia should be ruled out as a cause of poor performance.
   b. The patient is asked to imitate movements of the therapist. For example, the therapist touches his or her cheek, arm, leg, and so forth. A mirror-image response is acceptable.[1]
   c. The patient is requested to answer questions about the relationship of body parts. For example, "Are your knees below your head? Which is on top of your head, your hair or your feet?" For patients with aphasia, questions should be phrased to require a yes or no, or true or false response. Patients with intact function in this area should respond correctly most of the time and within a reasonable period of time. Those patients with receptive aphasia are particularly likely to do poorly on tests for somatagnosia.[119]

5. Treatment suggestions
   a. The sensorimotor approach attempts to associate sensory input with an adaptive motor response.[1] Facilitation of body awareness is accomplished through sensory stimulation to the body part affected. For example, the patient is asked to rub the appropriate body part with a rough cloth as the therapist names it or points to it.[55]
   b. With the transfer-of-training approach, the patient verbally identifies body parts, or points to pictures of them as the therapist touches them.[119]

RIGHT-LEFT DISCRIMINATION

1. A **right-left discrimination disorder** is the inability to identify the right and left sides of one's own body or of that of the examiner.[106] This includes the inability to execute movements in response to verbal commands that include the terms "right" and "left." Patients are often unable to imitate movements.[106]

2. Clinically, the patient cannot tell the therapist which is the right arm and which is the left. The right shoe cannot be discerned from the left shoe, and the patient is unable to follow instructions using the concept of right-left, such as "turn right at the corner." The patient cannot discriminate the right from the left side of the therapist.

3. The lesion site is the parietal lobe of either hemisphere.[106] A close relationship between aphasia (usually owing to left hemisphere damage) and deficits in right-left discrimination has been reported. In patients without aphasia (usually those with right hemisphere damage), a relationship has been reported between general mental impairment and right-left discrimination.[119]

4. The patient is asked to point to body parts on command: right ear, left foot, right arm, and so forth.[1] Six responses should be elicited on the patient's own body, on that of the therapist, and on a model or picture of the human body.[119] To rule out somatoagnosia, the patient should be tested first without the directional words.

5. Treatment techniques
   a. In giving instructions to the patient, the words "right" and "left" should be avoided. Instead, pointing or providing cues using distinguishing features of the limb are more effective (e.g., "the arm with the watch"). These guidelines are particularly salient for the therapist teaching locomotion or transfers, where confusing instructions may have dangerous consequences.
   b. *Adaptive environment:* The right side of all common objects such as shoes and clothing should be marked with red tape or seam binding.[121]

FINGER AGNOSIA

1. **Finger agnosia** can be defined as the inability to identify the fingers of one's own hands or of the hands of the examiner.[106] This includes difficulty in naming the fingers on command, identifying which finger was touched, and, by some definitions, mimicking finger movements. This deficit usually occurs bilaterally and is more common in the middle three fingers.[122] Finger agnosia correlates highly with poor dexterity in tasks that require movements of individual fingers in relation to each other,[1] such as buttoning, tying laces, and typing.

2. Finger agnosia may be the result of a lesion located in either parietal lobe,[123] in the region of the angular gyrus, or in the supramarginal gyrus.[118] It is often found in conjunction with an aphasic disorder,[119] or with general mental impairment.[106,119] Bilateral finger agnosia along with right-left discrimination problems, **agraphia,** and **acalculia** is termed **Gerstmann's syndrome.**[106] Gerstmann's syndrome usually is associated with a focal lesion of the dominant hemisphere in the region of the angular gyrus.[52]
3. A portion of Sauguet's test[1,119] is recommended.
   a. The patient is asked to name the fingers touched by the therapist, with the eyes open (five times) and if successful, with vision occluded (five times).
   b. The patient is asked to point to the fingers named by the therapist on the patient's own hands (10 times), on the therapist's hands (10 times), and on a schematic model (10 times).
   c. The patient is asked to point to the equivalent finger on a life-sized picture when each finger is touched by the therapist (Fig. 29-9).
   d. The patient is asked to imitate finger movements; for example, curl the index finger, touch the thumb to the middle finger.
4. Treatment suggestions
   a. To apply sensory integrative principles, the patient's discriminative tactile systems (touch and pressure) are stimulated. A rough cloth can be used to rub the dorsal surface of the affected arm, hand, and fingers, and the ventral surface of the affected fingers. Pressure can be applied to the ventral surface of the hand. For additional details the reader is referred to Zoltan.[1]
   b. To use the transfer-of-training approach, the patient is quizzed on finger identification.[1]

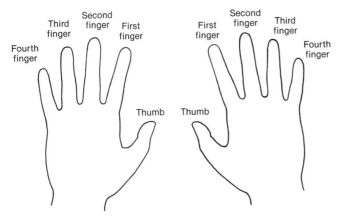

Figure 29-9. Hand chart for testing for finger agnosia (reduced from life size). (From Zoltan et al.[111] p 68, with permission.)

Spatial Relations Disorder (Complex Perception)

Spatial relations disorder encompasses a constellation of deficits that have in common a difficulty in perceiving the relationship between the self and two or more objects.[1] Research suggests that the right parietal lobe plays a primary role in space perception.[124] Thus a spatial relations deficit most frequently occurs in patients with right-sided lesions with resulting left hemiparesis.[118]

Spatial relations syndrome includes disorders of figure-ground discrimination, form discrimination, spatial relations, position in space, and topographical disorientation. Additional visuospatial deficits, such as depth and distance perception and vertical disorientation will also be discussed in this section. The apraxias are sometimes viewed as spatial relations problems.[1]

FIGURE-GROUND DISCRIMINATION
1. A disorder in visual figure-ground discrimination is the inability to visually distinguish a figure from the background in which it is embedded.[5] Functionally, it interferes with the patient's ability to locate important objects that are not prominent in a visual array. The patient has difficulty ignoring irrelevant visual stimuli and cannot select the appropriate cue to which to respond.[5] This may lead to distractibility, resulting in a shortened attention span,[125] frustration, and decreased independent and safe functioning.[61]
2. Clinically, the patient cannot locate items in a pocketbook or drawer, locate buttons on a shirt, or distinguish the armhole from the remainder of a solid-colored shirt. The patient may not be able to tell when one step ends and another begins on a flight of stairs, especially when descending.
3. Parieto-occipital lesions of the right hemisphere and less frequently the left hemisphere commonly produce this disorder.[126]
4. Assessment techniques
   a. Ayres Figure Ground Test (subtest of the Southern California Sensory Integration Tests):[127] The subject must distinguish the three objects in an embedded test picture, from a possible selection of six items (Fig. 29-10). This test was standardized on children but may be useful as a clinical tool in identifying perceptual disorders in adults with brain damage.[4] Normative data have been generated for normal adult males.[128]
   b. *Functional tests:* A white towel can be placed on a white sheet, and the patient is asked to find the towel. The patient can be asked to point out the sleeve, buttons, and collar of a white shirt, or to pick out a spoon from an unsorted array of eating utensils. It is necessary to rule out poor eyesight, hemianopsia, visual agnosia, and poor com-

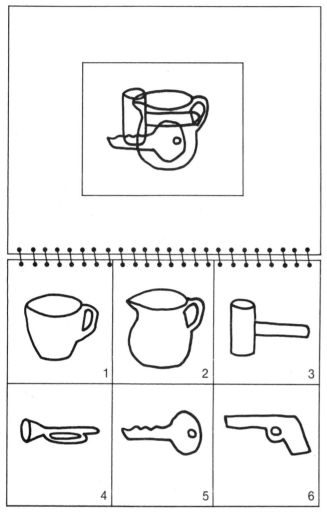

Figure 29-10. An example of the figure-ground perception test. (From Ayres,[127] Plate 2A, with permission.)

prehension to improve the validity of these assessment techniques.

5. Treatment techniques
   a. *Compensation through cognitive awareness:* The patient is taught to become aware of the existence and nature of the deficit. The patient should be cautioned to examine groups of objects slowly and systematically and should be instructed to use other, intact senses (e.g., touch) when searching for items such as clothing or silverware. When learning to lock a wheelchair, the patient should be advised to locate the brake levers by touch rather than by searching for them visually.
   b. *Adaptation and simplification of the environment:* Red tape may be placed over the Velcro strap of the shoe or orthosis to aid the patient in locating it. Few items should be placed in the patient's drawers or nightstand, and they should be replaced in the same location each time. Brightly colored tape can be used to mark the edges on stairs.
   c. With the functional approach, repeated

practice is used in each specific area of difficulty. The same procedure should be employed during each practice session, incorporating verbal cues and touch as adjuncts to vision.
   d. Using the transfer-of-training approach, the therapist should arrange for practice in visually locating objects in a simple array (such as three very different objects), and progress to more difficult ones (four or five dissimilar objects and three similar ones).

FORM DISCRIMINATION

1. Impairment in **form discrimination** is the inability to perceive or attend to subtle differences in form and shape. The patient is likely to confuse objects of similar shape or not to recognize an object placed in an unusual position.
2. Clinically, the patient may confuse a pen with a toothbrush, a vase with a water pitcher, a cane with a crutch, and so forth.
3. The lesion site is the parieto-temporo-occipital region (posterior **association areas**) of the nondominant lobe.[4]
4. *Assessment techniques:* A number of items similar in shape and different in size are gathered. The patient is asked to identify them. One set of items might be a pencil, pen, straw, toothbrush, watch, and the other might be a key, paper clip, coins, and a ring. Each object is presented several times in different positions (e.g., upside down). Visual object agnosia must be ruled out as a cause for poor performance by first presenting objects separately and asking the patient to identify them or to demonstrate how they are used.
5. Treatment suggestions
   a. With the transfer-of-training approach, the patient should practice describing, identifying, and demonstrating the usage of similarly shaped and sized objects. The patient should sort like objects and should be assisted to focus on differentiating cues.
   b. To achieve cognitive awareness and compensate for the disability, the patient must be made aware of the specific deficit. If the patient can read, frequently used and confused objects can be labeled. The patient should be encouraged to use vision, touch, and self-verbalization in combination when objects are confused.

SPATIAL RELATIONS

1. A **spatial relations deficit,** or spatial disorientation, is the inability to perceive the relationship of one object in space to another object, or to oneself. This may lead to, or compound, problems in constructional tasks and dressing.[5] Crossing the midline may be a problem for patients with spatial relations deficits.[55]
2. Clinically, the patient might find it difficult to place the cutlery, plate, and spoon in the proper

position when setting the table. The patient may be unable to tell the time from a clock because of difficulty in perceiving the relative positions of the hands (Fig. 29-11).[29] The patient may have difficulty learning to position his or her arms, legs, and trunk in relation to the wheelchair to prepare for transferring.

3. The lesion site is predominantly the inferior parietal lobe or parieto-occipital-temporal junction, usually of the right side.[5]

4. Assessment techniques
   a. The therapist draws a picture of a clock and then asks the patient to fill in the numbers and draw in the hands to designate a particular time. Responses indicative of impaired perception of spatial relations are illustrated in Figure 29-11. Patients with poor eye-hand coordination can be requested to place markers in the appropriate positions instead of drawing numbers.
   b. Two or three objects (such as matchsticks or pencils) are placed on a piece of paper in a particular pattern. The patient is asked to duplicate the pattern.
   c. To improve the validity of these assessments, unilateral neglect and hemianopsia should be ruled out as the causes of poor performance. If these deficits are present, the stimulus array should be positioned appropriately.

5. Treatment suggestions
   a. Using the transfer-of-training approach to improve the ability to orient to other objects, the patient can be given instructions on positioning himself or herself in relation to the therapist or another object; for example, "Sit next to me," "Go behind the table," "Step over the line." In addition, the therapist can set up a maze of furniture. Having the patient copy block or matchstick designs of increasing difficulty will increase awareness of the relationship between one object (block or matchstick) and the next.
   b. With the sensorimotor approach, if the patient avoids crossing the midline, activities that require crossing the midline both motorically and visually can be incorporated into other therapeutic activities. One specific activity is to have the patient hold a dowel with both hands. The therapist guides it from the uninvolved side to the

involved side. Later, the patient can progress to manipulating the dowel with only verbal or visual cues, and finally to guiding it independently. [55]

POSITION IN SPACE

1. **Position in space disorder** is the inability to perceive and to interpret spatial concepts such as up, down, under, over, in, out, in front of, and behind.

2. Clinically, if a patient is asked to raise the arm "above" the head during a ROM assessment or is asked to place the feet "on" the footrests, the patient may behave as if he or she does not know what to do.

3. The lesion is usually located in the nondominant parietal lobe.[118]

4. *Assessment techniques:* To assess function, two objects are used, such as a shoe and a shoebox. The patient is asked to place the shoe in different positions in relation to the shoebox; for example, in the box, on top of the box, or next to the box. Alternatively, the patient is presented with two objects and asked to describe their relationship. For example, a toothbrush can be placed in a cup, under a cup, and so forth, and the patient is then asked to indicate the location of the toothbrush.

   Another mode of assessment is to have the patient copy the therapist's manipulations with an identical set of objects. For example, the therapist hands the patient a comb and a brush. The therapist then takes an identical set and places them in a particular relationship to each other, such as the comb on top of the brush. The patient is requested to arrange his or her comb and brush in the same way. Success in this task may represent sufficient ability to use position in space functionally.

   Figure-ground difficulty, apraxia, incoordination, and lack of comprehension should be ruled out when performing these assessments. Objects should be positioned to avoid compounding of results with hemianopsia and unilateral spatial neglect.

5. Treatment suggestions
   a. To use the transfer-of-training approach, three or four identical objects are placed in the same orientation (wrist weights, combs, mugs, etc.). An additional object is placed in a different orientation. The patient is asked to identify the odd one, and then to place it in the same orientation as the other objects.
   b. The sensorimotor approach used for treatment of spatial relations is similar to that used for treatment of disorders of position in space.

TOPOGRAPHIC DISORIENTATION

1. Topographic disorientation refers to difficulty in understanding and remembering the relationship of one location to another.[1] As a result, the patient is unable to get from one

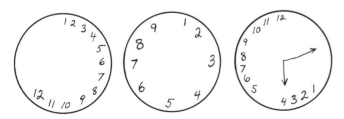

Figure 29-11. Responses to the draw-a-clock test, which may be indicative of defective perception of spatial relations. (From Pedretti,[29] p 109, with permission.)

place to another, with or without a map. This disorder is frequently seen in conjunction with other difficulties in spatial relations.[39]

2. Clinically, the patient cannot find the way from his or her room to the physical therapy clinic, despite being shown repeatedly. The patient cannot describe the spatial characteristics of familiar surroundings, such as the layout of his or her bedroom at home.[126]

3. Possible lesion sites are the inferior parietal lobe or occipital association cortex and the occipitotemporal cortex, particularly on the right side. Bilateral parietal lesions can produce this problem, as well as occasional left-sided parietal lesions.[126]

4. *Assessment techniques:* The patient is asked to describe or to draw a familiar route, such as the block on which he or she lives, the layout of his or her house, or a major neighborhood intersection.[126] The impaired patient will be unable to succeed in this task.

5. Treatment suggestions
   a. Using the transfer-of-training approach, the patient practices going from one place to another, following verbal instructions. Initially, simple routes should be used, and then more complicated ones.[1]
   b. Using the functional approach, important routes in the hospital or in the patient's home are repeatedly practiced.
   c. *Adaptions to the environment:* Frequently traveled routes can be marked with colored dots. The spaces between the dots are gradually increased and eventually eliminated as improvement takes place.[1] This is an example of taking a normally right-hemisphere task and (because there is right-sided damage) converting it into a left-hemisphere task. In this instance we take the spatial task of remembering routes (right-hemisphere task) and substitute sequential landmarks (sequencing is typically a left-hemisphere strength) to accomplish the goal of getting from place to place.
   d. To reinforce cognitive awareness, the patient should be instructed not to leave the clinic, room, or home unattended, because he or she may get lost.

DEPTH AND DISTANCE PERCEPTION

1. The patient with a disorder of depth and distance perception experiences inaccurate judgment of direction, distance, and depth. Spatial disorientation may be a contributing factor in faulty distance perception.

2. Clinically, the patient may have difficulty navigating stairs, may miss the chair when attempting to sit, or may continue pouring juice once a glass is filled.[1,125]

3. This may occur with a lesion in the posterior right hemisphere in the superior visual association cortices, bilateral or right-sided lesions.[126]

4. Assessment techniques
   a. For a functional assessment of distance perception, the patient is asked to take or to grasp an object that has been placed on a table. The object may be held in front of the patient, in the air, and the patient is again asked to grasp it. The impaired patient will overshoot or undershoot.[1]
   b. To assess depth perception functionally, the patient can be asked to fill a glass of water.[1] A patient with a depth perception deficit may continue pouring once the glass is filled.

5. Treatment suggestions
   a. The patient should be assisted in becoming aware of the deficit (cognitive awareness). Emphasis should be placed on the importance of walking carefully on uneven surfaces, particularly the stairs.
   b. With the transfer-of-training approach, the patient is requested to place the feet on designated spots during gait training.[55] Also, blocks can be arranged in piles 2 to 8 inches high. The patient is asked to touch the top of the piles with the foot. This is done to reestablish a sense of depth and distance.[55]
   c. With the functional approach, practice in compensating for disturbances in depth and distance perception occurs intrinsically in many ADLs, both those involving moving through space and those that involve manipulation.

VERTICAL DISORIENTATION

1. **Vertical disorientation** refers to a distorted perception of what is vertical. Displacement of the vertical position can contribute to disturbance of motor performance, both in posture and in gait. Early on in recovery most patients post-CVA demonstrate some impairment in the sense of verticality.[129] This is not influenced by the presence of homonymous hemianopsia.[61] Scores on one test for visual perception of the vertical position were found to correlate with differences in walking ability.[47]

2. An example of the way in which a person with distorted verticality views the world and the way this may affect posture is depicted in Figure 29-12.

3. The lesion site is in the nondominant parietal lobe.

4. *Assessment techniques:* The therapist holds a cane vertically and then turns it sideways to a horizontal plane. The patient is handed the cane and asked to turn it back to the original position. If the patient's perception of the vertical position is distorted, the cane will most likely be placed at an angle, representing the patient's conception of the world around him or herself.[130]

5. *Treatment suggestions:* The patient must be made aware of the disability. The patient

Degree of verticality

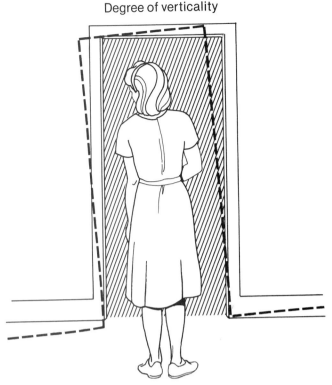

Figure 29-12. Vertical disorientation may contribute to disturbances of posture and gait. (From Tobis and Lowenthal,[53] p 37, with permission.)

should be instructed to compensate by using touch for proper self-orientation, especially when going through doorways, in and out of elevators, and on the stairs.

Agnosias (Simple Perception)

Agnosia is the inability to recognize or make sense of incoming information despite intact sensory capacities. Although this condition is relatively rare, it can affect any sensory modality (e.g., vision, audition, touch, taste) and anything (e.g., faces, sounds, colors, familiar or less familiar objects). Although there is an inability to recognize familiar objects using one or two of the sensory modalities, the ability to recognize the same object using other sensory modalities is usually present.[52] All types of agnosia represent an impairment in the sensory signal to the conceptual level.

VISUAL OBJECT AGNOSIA

1. **Visual object agnosia** is the most common form of agnosia.[4] It is defined as the inability to recognize familiar objects despite normal function of the eyes and optic tracts.[131] One remarkable aspect of this disorder is the readiness with which the patient can identify an object once it is handled (i.e., information is received from another sensory modality).[132] The patient may not recognize people, possessions, and common objects. Specific types of

visual agnosia and some clinical presentations are described below.

Simultanagnosia, also known as Balint's syndrome,[4] is the inability to perceive a visual stimulus as a whole. The patient perceives an entire array one part at a time. The lesion is usually in the dominant occipital lobe.

Prosopagnosia was traditionally considered to be the inability to recognize familiar faces. This phenomenon is now thought to be related to any visually ambiguous stimulus, the recognition of which depends on evoking a memory context, such as different species of birds or different makes of cars. Prosopagnosia is usually accompanied by visual field defects. Bilaterally symmetric occipital lesions are thought to be responsible for this deficit.[116,133]

Color agnosia is the inability to recognize colors; it is not color blindness. The patient is unable to name colors or to identify them on command, although the ability to name objects is retained.[116] Color agnosia is frequently associated with facial or other visual object agnosias.[4,126] It is usually the result of a dominant hemisphere lesion.[4] The simultaneous occurrence of left-sided hemianopsia, alexia, and color agnosia is a classic occipital lobe syndrome.[4]

2. The lesions associated with visual object agnosias are thought to occur in the occipito-temporo-parietal association areas of either hemisphere; these areas are responsible for the integration of visual stimuli with respect to memory.[52]

3. To assess this disorder, several common objects are placed in front of the patient. The patient is asked to name the objects, to point to an object named by the therapist, or to demonstrate its usage. It is important to rule out aphasia and apraxia, although this is not easily done. Details of other nonstandardized and standardized assessment procedures are provided in Zoltan.[1]

4. Treatment suggestions
   a. Using the transfer-of-training approach, drills can be used to practice discrimination between faces that are important to the patient (using photographs), in discrimination between colors, and common objects. The therapist should assist the patient in picking out salient visual cues for relating names to faces.
   b. With compensation techniques, the patient is instructed to use intact sensory modalities, such as touch or audition, to distinguish people and objects.

AUDITORY AGNOSIA

1. **Auditory agnosia** refers to the inability to recognize nonspeech sounds or to discriminate between them. This rarely occurs in the absence of other communication disorders.[4]

2. The patient with auditory agnosia cannot tell, for example, the difference between the ring of a doorbell and that of a telephone, or between a dog barking and thunder.
3. The lesion is located in the dominant temporal lobe.[4]
4. *Assessment techniques:* Assessment is usually carried out by a speech-language pathologist. The patient is asked to close the eyes and to identify the source of various sounds. The therapist rings a bell, honks a horn, rings a telephone, and so forth, and asks the patient to identify the sound (verbally or by pointing to a picture).
5. *Treatment suggestions:* Treatment generally consists of drilling the patient on sounds, but this has not been found to be particularly effective.[1]

TACTILE AGNOSIA OR ASTEREOGNOSIS

1. Tactile agnosia, or **astereognosis,** is the inability to recognize forms by handling them, although tactile, proprioceptive, and thermal sensations may be intact. This condition commonly causes difficulties in ADLs, inasmuch as many self-care activities that are normally done in the absence of constant visual monitoring require the manipulation of objects. If tactile agnosia is present in combination with unilateral neglect or sensory loss, performance in ADLs may be severely hampered.[61]
2. If a patient is handed an object (key, comb, safety pin) with vision occluded, the patient will fail to recognize it.
3. The lesion is in the parieto-temporo-occipital lobe (posterior association areas) of either hemisphere.[4]
4. *Assessment techniques:* The patient is asked to identify objects placed in the hand by examining them manually without visual cues.
5. Treatment suggestions
   a. With the transfer-of-training approach, the patient practices feeling various common objects, shapes, and textures with vision occluded. The patient is instructed to immediately look at the object for visual feedback and note special characteristics of the object.
   b. To achieve cognitive awareness, the patient is made aware of the deficit and is instructed in visual compensation.

Apraxia

Apraxia is a disorder of voluntary skilled learned movement. It is characterized by an inability to perform purposeful movements, which cannot be accounted for by inadequate strength, loss of coordination, impaired sensation, attentional difficulties, abnormal tone, movement disorders, intellectual deterioration, poor comprehension, or uncoopera-

tiveness.[134–136] Many patients with apraxia also present with aphasia, and the two disorders are sometimes difficult to distinguish.[4]

The two main forms of apraxia discussed in the literature are ideomotor and ideational apraxia. Ideomotor and ideational apraxias are generally thought to be the result of dominant hemisphere lesions and may be particularly difficult to assess in the patient with aphasia. Although aphasia and apraxia often occur together, there is not a strong correlation between the severity of the aphasia and the severity of the apraxia. Apraxia is a disorder of skilled movement and not a language disorder.[116] A third form of apraxia, **constructional apraxia,** is characterized by faulty spatial analysis and conceptualization of the task.

IDEOMOTOR APRAXIA

1. Ideomotor apraxia refers to a breakdown between concept and performance. There is a disconnection between the idea of a movement and its motor execution. It appears that the information cannot be transferred from the areas of the brain that conceptualize to the centers for motor execution. Thus the patient with ideomotor apraxia is able to carry out habitual tasks automatically and describe how they are done but is unable to imitate gestures or perform on command.[137,138] Patients with this form of apraxia often perseverate;[52] that is, they repeat an activity or a segment of a task over and over, even if it is no longer necessary or appropriate. This makes it difficult for them to finish one task and go on to the next. Patients with ideomotor apraxia appear most impaired when requested to perform tasks that require use of many implements and that have many steps. This form of apraxia can be demonstrated separately in the facial areas, upper extremity, lower extremity, and for total body movements.[139] Patients with apraxia are often observed to be clumsy in their actual handling of objects. Impairment is often suspected when observing the patient in ADLs or during a routine motor assessment.
2. Several examples of ideomotor apraxia follow. The patient is unable to "blow" on command. However, if presented with a bubble wand, the patient will spontaneously blow bubbles. The patient may fail to walk if requested to in a traditional manner. However, if a cup of coffee is placed on a table at the other end of the room and the patient is told, "Please have coffee," the patient is likely to traverse the room to get it.[120] A male patient is asked to comb his hair. He may be able to identify the comb and even tell you what it is used for; however, he will not actually use the comb appropriately when it is handed to him. Despite this observation in the clinic, his wife reports that he combs his hair spontaneously every morning.

A female patient is asked to squeeze a dynamometer. She appears not to know what to do with it, although her comprehension is adequate, the task has just been demonstrated, and it is clear that she has adequate strength.

3. Apraxia results most frequently from lesions in the left, dominant hemisphere. There is evidence that both frontal lesions and posterior parietal lesions can result in apraxia.[140]

4. Assessment techniques
   a. The Goodglass and Kaplan[139] test for apraxia is composed of universally known movements, such as blowing, brushing teeth, hammering, shaving, and so forth. It is based on what the authors consider a hierarchy of difficulty for patients with apraxia. First the patient is told, "Show me how you would bang a nail with a hammer." If the patient fails to do this or uses his or her fist as if it were a hammer, the patient is asked, "Pretend to hold the hammer." If the patient fails following this instruction, the therapist demonstrates the act and asks the patient to imitate it. The patient with apraxia typically will not improve after demonstration but will improve with use of the actual implements.[4] Ability to correct oneself on following verbal suggestions is considered not indicative of apraxia.
   b. The therapist sits opposite the patient. The patient is asked to imitate different postures or limb movements.[127] The patient with apraxia is unable to imitate postures. Additional apraxia tests may be found in Zoltan[1] or Butler.[141]

5. Treatment suggestions
   a. Anderson and Choy[55] suggest the modification of instructional sets as follows: Speak slowly and use the shortest possible sentences. One command should be given at a time, and the second command should not be given until the first task is completed. When teaching a new task, it should be broken down into its component parts. One component is taught at a time, physically guiding the patient through the task if necessary. It should be completed in precisely the same manner each time. When all the individual units are mastered, an attempt to combine them should be made. A great deal of repetition may be necessary.[61] Family members must be advised to use the exact approach found to be successful in the clinic. Performing activities in as normal an environment as possible is also helpful.
   b. Using the sensorimotor approach, multiple sensory inputs are used on the affected body parts to enhance the production of appropriate motor responses. The reader is referred to the work of Okoye[142] for additional details on this approach.

IDEATIONAL APRAXIA

1. Ideational apraxia is a failure in the conceptualization of the task. It is an inability to perform a purposeful motor act, either automatically or on command, because the patient no longer understands the overall concept of the act, cannot retain the idea of the task, or cannot formulate the motor patterns required. Often the patient can perform isolated components of a task but cannot combine them into a complete act. Furthermore, the patient cannot verbally describe the process of performing an activity, describe the function of objects, or use them appropriately.[143,144]

2. Ideational apraxia is typified by the following behavior: when presented in the clinic with a toothbrush and toothpaste and told to brush the teeth, the patient may put the tube of toothpaste in the mouth, or try to put toothpaste on the toothbrush without removing the cap. Furthermore, the patient may be unable to describe verbally how tooth brushing is done. Similar phenomena may be evident in all aspects of ADL (washing, meal preparation, and so forth) and so may limit the safety and potential independence of the patient.[5] It has been shown that patients with ideational apraxia who test poorly in the clinical situation appear more able to perform ADLs at the appropriate time and in a familiar setting.[142]

3. The lesion causing ideational apraxia is thought to be in the dominant parietal lobe. This deficit also may be seen in conjunction with diffuse brain damage, such as cerebral arteriosclerosis.[52]

4. *Assessment techniques:* The tests for ideational apraxia are essentially the same as those for ideomotor apraxia. The major difference to be expected in response is that the patient with ideomotor apraxia can perform a motor act spontaneously and automatically at the appropriate time, but the patient with ideational apraxia is unable to do so.

5. *Treatment suggestions:* The treatment techniques used are the same as those for ideomotor apraxia.

CONSTRUCTIONAL APRAXIA

1. Constructional apraxia is characterized by faulty spatial analysis and conceptualization of the task. Normal constructional skills encompass the capacity to understand the relationship of parts to a whole.[116] This ability is critical in activities such as drawing, dressing, building from a model, copying block designs, and the like. Performance of these complex tasks requires a combination of visual perception, motor planning, and motor performance.[25]

   Thus, constructional apraxia is most evident in the inability to produce two- or three-dimensional forms by drawing, constructing, or arranging blocks or objects spontaneously or on command.[116] It hampers the patient's ability to manipulate the environment effectively because of an inability to construct things from component parts. Although able to understand and identify the individual components, the patient cannot place them into a correct, meaningful relationship.

The presence of constructional apraxia is thought to be related to body scheme disorders, and often results in difficulty in dressing and diminished performance in other ADL skills.[1,145]

2. Constructional apraxia is demonstrated, for example, by a patient who understands all about sandwiches and what they are for but is unable to assemble one, even with all ingredients laid out in front of him or her.

3. Lesions are located in the posterior parietal lobe of either hemisphere.[146] Although it is widely believed that constructional apraxia is more common and more severe in patients with right-hemisphere lesions, controversy remains.[147]

4. Assessment techniques
   a. The patient is asked to copy a drawing of a house, a flower, or a clock face. Figure 29-13 depicts typical drawings of a house done by patients with left- and right-hemisphere lesions.
   b. The patient is requested to copy geometric designs (e.g., circle, square, or T shape).
   c. The patient is instructed to copy block bridges, matchstick designs, or pegboard configurations. Initially only three pieces are used and a progression is made to use more.

   Visuoconstructive difficulties found with right- and left-sided lesions demonstrate qualitative differences. In response to the assessment materials, patients with right-sided damage tend to draw on the diagonal and neglect the left side of the page.[4] They draw pieces of the picture without any coherent relationship to each other. Thus their drawings tend to be complex, yet unrecognizable.[4] They have immense diffi-

culty with copying or constructing anything in three dimensions, are not helped by the presence of a model or by landmarks in a picture, and do not generally improve with practice.[148]

In contrast, the drawings of patients with left-hemisphere damage are usually more recognizable.[149] They are characterized by great simplicity.[146] Patients with left-side lesions draw slowly and hesitatingly, are often unable to draw angles, and have general difficulty in execution.[146] In contrast to that of patients with right-hemisphere stroke, their performance often improves with the aid of a model,[149] the use of landmarks in drawing, and with repeated trials.[148] Short-term visual memory impairment is thought to be associated with constructional apraxia in patients with right-sided lesions.[124]

Verbal and comprehension difficulties, poor manual dexterity, and the presence of homonymous hemianopsia must be ruled out during assessment for this disorder.

5. With the transfer-of-training approach, the patient is asked to practice copying geometric designs, both by drawing and by building. Initially, simple patterns are used, progressing to the more complex.[1] Patients with left-hemisphere lesions may benefit from the use of landmarks and then their gradual withdrawal as skill improves.[148] The remedial approach has been criticized by Neistadt[25] for its use of pediatric materials, an underlying assumption that the sequence of recovery from brain injury follows the sequence of normal child development, and the use of treatment materials that closely resemble assessment tools.

SUMMARY

Cognition and perception, the processes by which an individual thinks, and selects, integrates, and interprets stimuli from the body and surrounding environment, are critical to the normal functioning of each human being. The patient with brain damage may be lacking in those abilities that allow one to make sense of and to respond appropriately to the outside world. It is essential for the physical therapist to be able to recognize when a patient is suffering from some type of perceptual dysfunction and to have the requisite tools to understand the causes of the behavior.

This chapter has attempted to provide an overview of cognitive and perceptual dysfunctions that may occur following brain damage, particularly those resulting from a stroke, and how such dysfunctions can affect the functioning of the patient, especially within the context of the rehabilitation setting. The importance of differentiating cognitive and perceptual dysfunction from problems related to lack of

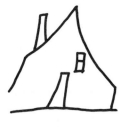

A   Left hemisphere lesion

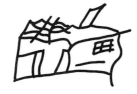

B   Right hemisphere lesion

Figure 29-13. Impaired responses to the draw-a-house test for constructional apraxia. Note the differences in response between the patient with a left hemisphere lesion (*A*) compared with a right (*B*) hemisphere lesion. (From Zoltan et al,[111] p 39, with permission.)

motor ability, inadequate sensation, poor language skills, and simple uncooperativeness has been emphasized. Although alluded to in a very abbreviated fashion, activity analysis and systematic data collection remain two of the most powerful tools at the disposal of the therapist attempting to develop a firm rationale for, and empirically to justify the efficacy of any treatment regimen selected. Treatment in the form of adaptation of the physical environment and instructional sets and the teaching of compensatory techniques has been singled out as the most effective avenue for intervention.

QUESTIONS FOR REVIEW

1. What general characteristics are displayed by patients with cognitive and perceptual difficulties during execution of a task?

2. Identify the underlying premise of the *transfer-of-training approach* to treatment.

3. What is the underlying assumption of the *sensory integrative approach* to treatment? Provide examples of the treatment modalities employed with this approach.

4. How is the performance of specific functional skills enhanced using the *functional approach* to treatment? What are the inherent benefits of using the functional approach?

5. Describe general suggestions for optimizing teaching/learning strategies when using compensatory techniques.

6. Identify the four treatment strategies included in the *cognitive approach* to treatment.

7. What potential influencing factors must be considered when evaluating a patient with cognitive and perceptual disabilities?

8. What assessment procedures will assist the therapist in distinguishing between sensory and cognitive or perceptual problems?

9. Distinguish the difference between feedback provided in the form of knowledge of results (KR) versus knowledge of performance (KP).

10. Identify and define the four different types of attention.

11. What is the purpose of memory retraining? Compare and contrast the focus of the *remedial approach* and the *compensatory approach* to memory retraining.

12. Define the following terms: unilateral neglect, somatoagnosia, right-left discrimination, finger agnosia, and anosognosia.

13. Identify four spatial relations disorders. What general clinical manifestation do these disorders have in common? Define each of the four disorders identified together with an example of how the disorder would influence patient performance of a task.

14. Provide examples of the functional implications of a disorder in *visual figure-ground discrimination*. What is the most common lesion site producing this disorder?

15. What is the characteristic feature of apraxia? Define the three types of apraxias. Provide examples of task performance characteristics associated with each type of apraxia.

CASE STUDY

The patient is a 72 year-old woman who has just been admitted to a rehabilitation facility following a stroke. The patient experienced a right parietal hemorrhagic stroke. A CT scan revealed a 4-cm hemorrhage that was subsequently drained. She will be able to stay in the rehabilitation facility for 20 days. Although the patient has some physical problems, the emphasis of this case study is on cognitive and perceptual tests and interventions. The occupational therapist and the physical therapist are collaboratively using a combination of cognitive retraining and the functional approach in therapy.

PAST MEDICAL HISTORY: Her past medical history includes insulin-dependent diabetes and mild rheumatoid arthritis in her right shoulder and both hands.

SOCIAL: Lives alone in her own home. Supportive friends and family, her two children and their families live nearby. Insured by a local HMO. Retired from police force. Enjoys gardening, reading, and watching television. Previously drove automatic transmission vehicle.

PHYSICAL THERAPY ASSESSMENT: Initially when the patient was approached from the left, she seemed to ignore the physical therapist and did not respond to greetings. However, when the therapist sat in the chair on the patient's right side, she seemed to have no problems talking to the therapist.

Range of Motion, Muscle Tone, and Balance Assessment: Examination revealed full ROM, reduced strength in the left arm and hand and some reduced dynamic standing balance reactions.

Sensation: The physical therapist assessed sensation and noted normal sensation in all areas (sharp/dull, light touch, temperature, proprioceptive sensations, cortical sensations) on the right side. However, the patient seemed to have difficulties on the left side and her performance in detecting stimuli seemed inconsistent. Because the physical therapist suspected cognitive and perceptual problems, a complete sensory assessment was deferred until the occupational therapist had more fully assessed the patient.

Functional Assessment: The physical therapist examined the patient's transfers and showed her a safer way to get in and out of bed.

FIM
- Transfer bed/chair/wheelchair: FIM level = 5
- Transfer tub: FIM level = 4
- Transfer toilet: FIM level = 5
- Locomotion: FIM level = 5

Personal Care FIM
- Eating: FIM level = 4
- Bathing: FIM level = 3
- Dressing upper body: FIM level = 5
- Dressing lower body: FIM level = 4
- Grooming: FIM level = 5
- Toilet: FIM level = 6

The physical therapist asked about her family and she was able to provide many details. However, she seemed puzzled about where she was and was concerned that she was not looking her best and needed to do her hair. The therapist suggested that she might like to brush her hair. Although the brush was on the table on the patient's right side, she said she did not have one. The physical therapist cued her to check her bedside table, but on checking she maintained she did not have a brush. At the end of the session (which lasted about 40 minutes) the therapist asked her to demonstrate the bed transfer technique again that she had been taught at the beginning of the session. She seemed confused and could not do what the physical therapist had taught her.

COGNITION AND PERCEPTION ASSESSMENT WITH THE OCCUPATIONAL THERAPIST: The occupational therapist conducted two standardized assessments: the Rivermead Behavioural Memory Test (RBMT)[75]

because the patient demonstrates memory problems, and the Arnadottir OT-ADL Neurobehavioral Evaluation (A-ONE)[5] to examine the impact of the patient's problems on her daily living activities. The occupational therapist also reasoned that further tests of the patient's IADLs including home and driving abilities would need to be conducted closer to her discharge.

Social Cognition FIM
- Communication: FIM level = 7
- Expression: FIM level = 7
- Memory: FIM level = 3
- Social interaction: FIM level = 6
- Problem solving: FIM level = 6

Guiding Questions

1. What are some of the difficulties the patient is having and what cognitive and perceptual problems might be causing these? Please note that there may be more than one possible impairment for the functional problems noted.

2. Develop a clinical asset and problem list.

3. Identify outcomes and goals appropriate for this patient.

4. Identify two treatment strategies to improve spontaneous use of RUE and decrease unilateral neglect.

5. Identify two treament strategies to improve her memory.

6. How can the success of the patient's rehabilitation program be measured?

REFERENCES

1. Zoltan, B: Vision, perception and cognition: A manual for evaluation and treatment of the neurologically impaired adult, ed 3 rev. Charles B. Slack, Thorofare, NJ, 1996.
2. Unsworth, C: Cognitive and perceptual dysfunction: A clinical reasoning approach to evaluation and intervention. FA Davis, Philadelphia, 1999.
3. Katz, N, et al: Lowenstein Occupational Therapy Cognitive Assessment (LOTCA) battery for brain injured patients: reliability and validity. Am J Occup Ther 43:184, 1989.
4. Lezak, MD: Neuropsychological assessment, ed 3. Oxford University Press, New York, 1995.
5. Árnadóttir, G: The brain and behavior: Assessing cortical dysfunction through activities of daily living. CV Mosby, St. Louis, 1990.
6. Glosser, G, and Goodglass, H: Disorders of executive control functions among aphasic and other brain-damaged patients. J Clin Exp Neuropsychol 12:485, 1990.
7. Katz, N, and Hartman-Maeir, A: Occupational performance and metacognition. Canadian J Occup Ther 64:53, 1997.
8. Winegardner, J: Executive functions. In Cohen, H (ed): Neuroscience for Rehabilitation. Lippincott, Philadelphia, 1993, p 346.
9. Sharpless, JW: Mossman's A Problem Oriented Approach to Stroke Rehabilitation, ed 2. Charles C Thomas, Springfield, IL, 1982.
10. Edwards, S: Neurological physiotherapy: A problem solving approach. Churchill Livingstone, New York, 1996.
11. Luria, AR: Higher Cortical Functions in Man. Basic Books, New York, 1966.
12. Pak, R, and Dombrovy, ML: Stroke. In Good, DC, and Couch, JR (eds): Handbook of Neurorehabilitation. Marcel Dekker, New York, 1994, p 461.
13. Meir, M, et al: Individual differences in neuropsychological

recovery: An overview. In Meier, M, et al (eds). Neuropsychological Rehabilitation. Churchill Livingstone, London, 1987, p 71.
14. Bach-y-Rita, P: Brain plasticity as a basis for therapeutic procedures. In Bach-y-Rita, P (ed): Recovery of Function: Theoretical Considerations for Brain Injury Rehabilitation. University Park Press, Baltimore, 1980, p 225.
15. Brodal, A: Self-observations and neuronanatomical considerations after a stroke. Brain 76:675, 1973.
16. Gardner, H: The Shattered Mind: The Person After Brain Damage. Alfred A Knopf, New York, 1975.
17. Katz, N (ed): Cognitive rehabilitation: Models for intervention in occupational therapy. Andover Medical, Boston, 1992.
18. Neistadt, ME: The neurobiology of learning: Implications for treatment of adults with brain injury. Am J Occup Ther 48:421, 1994.
19. Neistadt, ME: Assessing learning capabilities during cognitive and perceptual evaluations for adults with traumatic brain injury. Occupational Therapy in Health Care 9:3, 1995.
20. Young, GC, et al: Efficacy of pairing scanning training with block design training in the remediation of perceptual problems in left hemiplegics. J Clin Neuropsychol 42:312, 1983.
21. Neistadt, ME: Occupational therapy for adults with perceptual deficits. Am J Occup Ther 42:434, 1988.
22. Fisher, AG, et al: Sensory Integration: Theory and Practice. FA Davis, Philadelphia, 1991.
23. Ayres, JA: Sensory Integration and Learning Disorders. Western Psychological Service, Los Angeles, 1972.
24. Ayres, JA: Sensory Integration and the Child. Western Psychological Services, Los Angeles, 1980.

25. Neistadt, ME: A critical analysis of occupational therapy approaches for perceptual deficits in adults with brain injury. Am J Occup Ther 44:299, 1990.

26. Moore, J: Neuronanatomical considerations relating to recovery of function following brain injury. In Bach-y-Rita, P (ed): Recovery of Function: Theoretical Consideration for Brain Injury Rehabilitation. University Park Press, Baltimore, 1980, p 9.

27. Finger, S, and Stein, DG: Brain Damage and Recovery: Research and Clinical Perspectives. Academic Press, New York, 1982.

28. Braziz, PW, et al: Localization in Clinical Neurology, ed 2. Little, Brown, Boston, 1990.

29. Pedretti, LW, Zoltram, B and Wheatly, CJ: Evaluation and treatment of perceptual and perceptual motor deficits. In Pedretti, LW (ed): Occupational Therapy: Practical Skills for Physical Dysfunction, ed 4. CV Mosby, St. Louis, 1996, p 231.

30. Neistadt, ME: Occupational therapy treatment for constructional deficits. Am J Occup Ther 46:141, 1992.

31. Ellek, D: Managed competition: Maintaining health care within the private sector. Am J Occup Ther 49:468, 1995.

32. Toglia, J, and Abreu, BC: Cognitive Rehabilitation Supplement to Workshop: Management of Cognitive-Perceptual Dysfunction in the Brain-Damaged Adult. Sponsored by Braintree Hospital, Braintree, MA and Cognitive Rehabilitation Associates, New York, May, 1987.

33. Giantusos, R: What is cognitive rehabilitation? J Rehabil 46:36, 1980.

34. Abreu, BC, and Toglia, JP: Cognitive rehabilitation: A model for occupational therapy. Am J Occup Ther 41:439, 1987.

35. Diller, L, and Gordon, WA: Intervention strategies for cognitive deficits in brain-injured adults. J Consult Clin Psychol 49:822, 1981.

36. Toglia, JP: Generalization of treatment: A multicontext approach to cognitive perceptual impairment in adults with brain injury. Am J Occup Ther 45:505, 1991.

37. Toglia, JP: A dynamic interactional model to cognitive rehabilitation. In Katz, N (ed): Cognition and Occupational in Rehabilitation: Cognitive Models for Intervention in Occupational Therapy. The American Occupational Therapy Association, Inc., Bethesda, 1998, p 5.

38. Abreu, BC: The quadraphonic approach: Holistic rehabilitation for brain injury. In Katz, N (ed): Cognition and Occupation in Rehabilitation: Cognitive Models for Intervention in Occupational Therapy. The American Occupational Therapy Association, Inc., Bethesda, 1998, p 51.

39. Wilcock, AA: Occupational therapy approaches to stroke. Churchill Livingstone, Melbourne, 1986.

40. Grieve, J: Neuropsychology for occupational therapists: Assessment of perception and cognition. Blackwell Scientific, Oxford, 1993.

41. Galski, T, et al: Driving after cerebral damage: A model with implications for evaluation. Am J Occup Ther 46:324, 1992.

42. Trombly, CA: Occupational therapy for physical dysfunction, ed 4. Williams & Wilkins, Baltimore, 1995.

43. Gainotti, G: Emotional and psychosocial problems after brain injury. Neuropsychological Rehab 3:259, 1993.

44. Bronstein, KS, et al: Promoting stroke recovery. CV Mosby, St. Louis, 1991.

45. Meier, M, et al (eds): Neuropsychological Rehabilitation. Churchill Livingstone, London, 1987.

46. Sandin, KJ, and Mason, KD: Manual of stroke rehabilitation. Butterworth-Heinemann, Boston, 1996.

47. Van Ravensberg, CD, et al: Visual perception in hemiplegic patients. Arch Phys Med Rehabil 65:304, 1984.

48. Warren, M: A hierarchical model for evaluation and treatment of visual perceptual dysfunction in adult acquired brain injury, I. Am J Occup Ther 47:42, 1993.

49. Warren, M: A hierarchical model for evaluation and treatment of visual perceptual dysfunction in adult acquired brain injury, II. Am J Occup Ther 47:55, 1993.

50. Hier, DB, et al: Recovery of behavioral abnormalities after right hemisphere stroke. Neurology 33:345, 1983.

51. Haerer, AF: Visual field defects and the prognosis of stroke patients. Stroke 4:163, 1977.

52. Chusid, JG: Correlative Neuroanatomy and Functional Neurology, ed 19. Lange Medical Publications, Los Altos, CA, 1985.

53. Tobis, JS, and Lowenthal, M: Evaluation and Management of the Brain-Damaged Patient. Charles C Thomas, Springfield, IL, 1960.

54. Pedretti, LW: Evaluation of sensation, perception and cognition. In Pedretti, LW and Zoltan, B (eds): Occupational Therapy: Practice Skills for Physical Dysfunction, ed 2. CV Mosby, St. Louis, 1985, p 99.

55. Anderson, E, and Choy, E: Parietal lobe syndromes in hemiplegia: A program for treatment. Am J Occup Ther 24:13, 1970.

56. Stilwell, JM: The meaning of manual midline crossing. Sensory Integration Quarterly 21:1, 1994.

57. Efferson, L: Disorders of vision and visual perceptual dysfunction. In Umphred, DA (ed): Neurological rehabilitation, ed 3. CV Mosby, St. Louis, 1995, p 769.

58. Diller, L, and Weinberg, J: Differential aspects of attention in brain-damaged persons. Perceptual and Motor Skills 35:71, 1972.

59. Anastasi, A: Psychological testing, ed 6. Macmillan Publishing Co., New York, 1988.

60. de Clive-Lowe, S: Outcome measurement, cost-effectiveness and clinical audit: The importance of standardised assessment to occupational therapists in meeting these new demands. Br J Occup Ther 59: 357, 1996.

61. Wall, N: Stroke rehabilitation. In Logigian, MK (ed): Adult Rehabilitation: A Team Approach for Therapists. Little, Brown, Boston, 1982, p 225.

62. Laver, AJ, and Powell, GE: The Structured Observational Test of Function (SOTOF). NFER-NELSON, Windsor, England, 1995.

63. Laver, AJ: The structured observational test of function. Gerontology Special Interest Section Newsletter 17:1, 1994.

64. Allen, CK: Allen cognitive level test manual. S & S/ Worldwide, Colchester, 1990.

65. Allen, CK, et al: Occupational therapy treatment goals for the physically and cognitively disabled. American Occupational Therapy Association, Rockville, MD, 1992.

66. Tyerman, R, et al: COTNAB-Chessington Occupational Therapy Neurological Assessment Battery Introductory Manual. Nottingham Rehab Limited, Nottingham, 1986.

67. Stanley, M, et al: Chessington Occupational Therapy Neurological Assessment Battery: Comparison of performance of people aged 50–65 years with people aged 66 and over. Australian Occupational Therapy Journal 42:55, 1995.

68. Sloan, RL, et al: Routine screening of brain damaged patients: A comparison of the Rivermead Perceptual Assessment Battery and the Chessington Occupational Therapy Neurological Assessment Battery. Clin Rehab 5:265, 1991.

69. Itzkovich, M, et al: The Loewenstein Occupational Therapy Assessment (LOTCA) manual. Maddak Inc., Pequanock, NJ, 1990.

70. Katz, N, et al: Loewenstein occupational therapy cognitive assessment (LOTCA), battery for brain injured patients: Reliability and validity. Am J Occup Ther 43:184, 1989.

71. Wilson, B, et al: Behavioural Inattention Test. Thames Valley Test Company, Bury St Edmunds, 1987.

72. Wilson, B, et al: Development of a behavioural test of visuospatial neglect. Arch Phys Med Rehabil 68:98, 1987.

73. Whiting, S, et al: RPAB-Rivermead Perceptual Assessment Battery. NFER-NELSON, Windsor, 1985.

74. Jesshope, HJ, et al: The RPAB: Its application to stroke-patients and relationship with function. Clin Rehab 5:115, 1991.

75. Wilson, B, et al: RBMT-The Rivermead Behavioural Memory Test. Thames Valley Test Company, Bury St Edmunds, 1991.

76. Wilson, B, et al: Development and validation of a test battery for detecting and monitoring everyday memory problems. J Clin Exp Neuropsychol 11:885, 1989.

77. Sarno, JE, et al: The Functional Life Scale. Arch Phys Med Rehabil 54:214, 1973.

78. Brown, H: The standardisation of the Riverdale Hospital's Home and Community Skills Assessment. Canadian J Occup Ther 55:9, 1988.

79. Guide for the Uniform Data Set for Medical Rehabilitation (Adult FIM SM): Version 4.0. State Univ of New York at Buffalo, Buffalo, 1993.

80. Jongbloed, L, et al: Stroke rehabilitation: Sensory integrative treatment versus functional treatment. Am J Occup Ther 43:391, 1989.

81. Gentile, AM: A working model of skill acquisition with special reference to teaching. Quest Monograph 17:61, 1972.

82. Bailey, DM: Legislative and reimbursement influences on occupational therapy: Changing opportunities. In Neistadt, ME, and Crepeau, EB (eds): Willard and Spackman's Occupational Therapy, ed 9. Lippincott, Philadelphia, 1998, p 763.

83. McKeehan, KM: Conceptual framework for discharge planning. In McKeehan, KM (ed): Continuing Care: A Multidisciplinary Approach to Discharge Planning. CV Mosby, Toronto, 1981, p 3.

84. Unsworth, CA, and Thomas, SA: Information use in discharge accommodation recommendations for stroke patients. Clin Rehabil 7:181, 1993.

85. Unsworth, CA, et al: Rehabilitation team decisions concerning discharge housing for stroke patients. Arch Phys Med Rehabil 76:331, 1995.

86. Unsworth, CA: Clients' perceptions of discharge housing decisions following stroke rehabilitation. Am J Occup Ther 50:207, 1996.

87. Stringer, AY: A Guide to Adult Neurological Diagnosis. FA Davis, Philadelphia, 1996.

88. Strub, RL, and Black, FW: The Mental Status Examination in Neurology, ed 2. FA Davis, Philadelphia, 1985.

89. Mateer, CA, et al: Management of attention and memory disorders following traumatic brain injury. J Learning Disabilities 29:618, 1996.

90. van Zomeren, AH, and Brouwer, WH: The Clinical Neuropsychology of Attention. Oxford University Press, New York, 1994.

91. Stroop, JR: Studies of inference in serial verbal reactions. J Exp Psychology 18:643, 1935.

92. Gronwall, D: Paced auditory serial addition task: A measure of recovery from concussion. Perceptual and Motor Skills 44:367, 1977.

93. US Army: Army Individual Test Battery. Manual of directions and scoring. Adjutant General's Office, 1944.

94. Diller, L, and Weinberg, J: Evidence for accident prone behavior in hemiplegic patients. Arch Phys Med Rehabil 51:358, 1970.

95. Diller, L, and Weinberg, J: Differential aspects of attention in brain-damaged persons. Perceptual and Motor Skills 35:71, 1972.

96. Spencer, EA: Functional restoration. In Hopkins, HL, and Smith, HD (eds): Willard and Spackman's Occupational Therapy, ed 8. Lippincott, Philadelphia, 1993, p 605.

97. Kepferman, I: Learning and Memory. In Kandel, ER, et al (eds): Principles of Neuroscience, ed 3. Elsevier, New York, 1991, p 996.

98. Wickelgren, WA: Learning and memory. Prentice-Hall Inc, Englewood Cliffs, NJ, 1977.

99. Fuster, JM: Memory in the Cerebral Cortex: An Empirical Approach to Neural Networks in the Human and Nonhuman Primate. MIT Press, Cambridge, 1995.

100. Wilson, BA, and Moffat, N: Clinical Management of Memory Problems. Chapman & Hall, London, 1992.

101. Duran, L, and Fisher, AG: Evaluation and intervention with executive functions impairment. In Unsworth, CA: Cognitive and Perceptual Dysfunction: A Clinical Reasoning Approach to Evaluation and Intervention. FA Davis, Philadelphia, 1999, p 209.

102. Cummins, JL: Anatomic and behavioral aspects of frontal-subcortical circuits. In Grafman, J, et al (eds): Annals of the New York Academy of Sciences: Structure and Function of the Human Prefrontal Cortex, vol 769. New York Academy of Sciences, New York, 1995, p 1.

103. Pollens, R, et al: Beyond cognition: Executive functions in closed head injury. Cognitive Rehabilitation 65:23, 1988.

104. Sohlberg, MM, et al: Contemporary approaches to the management of executive control dysfunction. J Head Trauma Rehab 8:45, 1993.

105. Van Deusen, J: Body image and perceptual dysfunction in adults. Saunders, Philadelphia, 1993.

106. Benton, A, and Sivan, AB: Disturbances of the body schema. In Heilman, KM, and Valenstein, E (eds): Clinical Neuropsychology, ed 3. Oxford Univ Pr, New York, 1993, p 123.

107. Herman, EWM: Spatial neglect: New issues and their implications for occupational therapy practice. Am J Occup Ther 46:207, 1992.

108. Hier, DB, et al: Behavioral abnormalities after right hemisphere stroke. Neurology 33:337, 1983.

109. Gordon, WA, et al: Perceptual remediation in patients with right brain damage: A comprehensive program. Arch Phys Med Rehabil 66:353, 1985.

110. Vallar, G: The anatomical basis of spatial hemineglect in humans. In Robertson, IH, and Marshall, JC (eds): Unilateral Neglect: Clinical and Experimental Studies. Lawrence Erlbaum Associates Ltd., Hove, 1993, p 27.

111. Zoltan, B, et al: The Adult Stroke Patient: A Manual for Evaluation and Treatment of Perceptual and Cognitive Dysfunction, ed 2 rev. Charles B. Slack, Thorofare, NJ, 1986.

112. Robertson, IH, et al: Walking trajectory and hand movements in unilateral left neglect: A vestibular hypothesis. Neuropsychologia 32:1495, 1994.

113. Weinberg, J, et al: Training sensory awareness and spatial organization in people with right brain damage. Arch Phys Med Rehabil 60:491, 1979.

114. Weinberg, J, et al: Visual scanning training effect in reading-related tasks in acquired right brain damage. Arch Phys Med Rehabil 58:479, 1977.

115. Stanton, KM, et al: Wheelchair transfer training for right cerebral dysfunctions: An interdisciplinary approach. Arch Phys Med Rehabil 64:276, 1983.

116. Bradshaw, JL, and Mattingley, JB: Clinical Neuropsychology: Behavioral and Brain Science. Academic Press, San Diego, 1995.

117. Zankie, HT: Stroke Rehabilitation. Charles C Thomas, Springfield, IL, 1971.

118. McFie, J: The diagnostic significance of disorders of higher nervous activity. In Vinken, PJ and Bruyen, GW (eds): Handbook of Clinical Neurology, vol 4. Disorders of Speech, Perception, and Symbolic Behavior, New York, 1969, p 1.

119. Sauguet, J, et al: Disturbances of the body scheme in relation to language impairment and hemispheric locus of lesion. J Neurol Neurosurg Psychiatry 34:496, 1971.

120. Johnstone, M: Restoration of Motor Function in the Stroke Patient, ed 2. Churchill Livingstone, New York, 1983.

121. Burt, MM: Perceptual deficits in hemiplegia. Am J Nurs 70:1026, 1970.

122. Hecaen, H, et al: The syndrome of apractagnosia due to lesions of the minor vertebral hemisphere. Arch Neurol Psychiatry 75:400, 1956.

123. Gainotti, G: Emotional behaviour and hemispheric side of the lesion. Cortex 8:41, 1972.

124. Warrington, EK, and James, M: Disorders in visual perception in the patients with localized cerebral lesions. Neuropsychologia 5:253, 1967.

125. Halperin, E, and Cohen, BS: Perceptual-motor dysfunction. Stumbling block to rehabilitation. Md Med J 20:139, 1971.

126. Benton, A, and Tranel, D: Visuoperceptual, visuospatial, and visuoconstructive disorders. In Heilman, KM, and Valenstein, E (eds): Clinical Neuropsychology, ed 3. Oxford Univ Pr, New York, 1993, p 165.

127. Ayres, JA: Southern California Sensory Integration Tests. Western Psychological Services, Los Angeles, 1972.

128. Peterson, P, and Wikoff, RL: The performance of adult males on the Southern California figure-ground visual perception test. Am J Occup Ther 37:554, 1983.

129. Anderson, TP: Rehabilitation of patients with a completed stroke. In Kottke, FJ, and Ellwood, PM (eds): Krusen's Handbook of Physical Medicine and Rehabilitation, ed 4. Saunders, Philadelphia, 1990, p 666.

130. Jones, M: Approach to Occupational Therapy, ed 3. Butterworths, London, 1977.

131. Laver, AJ, and Unsworth, CA: Evaluation and intervention with simple perceptual impairment (agnosias). In Unsworth, CA (ed): Cognitive and Perceptual Dysfunction: A Clincial Reasoning Approach to Evaluation and Intervention. FA Davis, Philadelphia, 1999, p 299.

132. Wade, DT, et al: Stroke: A Critical Approach to Diagnosis. Treatment, and Management. Yearbook Medical, Chicago, 1986.

133. Damasio, AR, et al: Prosopagnosia: Anatomical basis and behavioral mechanism. Neurology 32:331, 1982.

134. Croce, R: A review of the neural basis of apractic disorders with implications for remediation. Adapted Physical Activity Quarterly 10:173, 1993.

135. Tate, R, and McDonald, S: What is apraxia? The clinician's dilemma. Neuropsychological Rehab 5:273, 1995.

136. Kirshner, H: The Apraxias. In Bradley, W, et al (eds): Neurology in Clinical Practice: Principles of Diagnosis and Management, vol 1. Butterworth-Heinmann, London, 1991, p 117.

137. Raade, AS, et al: The relationship between buccofacial and limb apraxia. Brain and Cognition 16:130, 1991.

138. Mozaz, M, et al: Apraxia in a patient with lesion located in right sub-cortical area: Analysis of errors. Cortex 26:651, 1990.

139. Goodglass, H, and Kaplan, E: The Assessment of Aphasia and Related Disorders, ed 2. Lea & Febiger, Philadelphia, 1983.

140. Halsband, U, et al: The role of the pre-motor and the supplementary motor area in the temporal control of movement in man. Brain 116:243, 1993.

141. Butler, J: Evaluation and intervention with apraxia. In Unsworth, CA: Cognitive and Perceptual Dysfunction: A Clincial Reasoning Approach to Evaluation and Intervention. FA Davis, Philadelphia, 1999, p 257.

142. Okoye, R: The apraxias. In Abreu, BC (ed): Physical Disabilities Manual. New York, 1981, p 241.

143. De Renzi, E, and Lucchelli, F: Ideational apraxia. Brain, Raven, New York, 111:1173, 1988.

144. Mayer, NH, et al: Buttering a hot cup of coffee: An approach to the study of errors of action in patients with brain damage. In Tupper, DE, and Cicerone, KD (eds): The Neuropsychology of Everyday Life: Assessment and Basic Competencies. Kluwer, London, 1990, p 259.

145. Neistadt, ME: The relationship between constructional and meal preparation skills. Arch Phys Med Rehabil 74:144, 1993.

146. McFie, J, and Zangwill, OL: Visual-constructive disabilities associated with lesions of the left cerebral hemisphere. Brain 83:243, 1960.

147. Fisher, B: Effect of trunk control and alignment on limb function. J Head Trauma Rehab 2:72, 1987.

148. Hecaen, H, and Assal, G: A comparison of constructive deficits following right and left hemisphere lesions. Neuropsychologia 8:289, 1970.

149. Piercy, M, et al: Constructional apraxia associated with unilateral cerebral lesions: Left and right sided cases compared. Brain 83:225, 1960.

150. Unsworth, CA: Reflections of the process of therapy in cognitive and perceptual dysfunction. In Unsworth, CA (ed): Cognitive and Perceptual Dysfunction: A Clinical Reasoning Approach to Evaluation and Intervention. FA Davis, Philadelphia, in press.

SUPPLEMENTAL READINGS

Carter, LT, et al: The relationship of cognitive skills performance to activities of daily living in stroke patients. Am J Occup Ther 42:449, 1988.

Cohen, H (ed): Neuroscience for Rehabilitation. Lippincott, Philadelphia, 1993.

Sacks, O: The Man who Mistook his Wife for a Hat. Harper & Row, New York, 1985.

Zoltan, B: Vision, Perception and Cognition, ed 3. Slack, Thorofare, NJ, 1996.

GLOSSARY

Acalculia: Difficulties in computation or the ability to perform numerical operations.

Adaptation: Alteration of the environment in order to compensate for perceptual dysfunction.

Agnosia: The inability to recognize familiar objects with one sensory modality, while retaining the ability to recognize the same object with other sensory modalities.

Agraphia: Disorders of writing not due to motor difficulties in letter formation.

Alternating attention: The capacity to move flexibly between tasks and respond appropriately to the demands of each task.

Anosognosia: A perceptual disability including denial, neglect, and lack of awareness of the presence or severity of one's paralysis.

Aphasia: Absence or impairment of the ability to communicate through speech, writing, or signs owing to dysfunctions of brain centers.

Apraxia: A disorder of voluntary learned movement that is characterized by an inability to perform purposeful movements and that cannot be accounted for by inadequate strength, loss of coordination, impaired sensation, attentional deficits, or lack of comprehension.

Association areas: Areas of the cerebral cortex that border on and are connected to the primary sensory areas; analyzes and synthesizes incoming isolated sensations into a whole or gestalt, so that complex environmental displays can be perceived and acted upon.

Astereognosis (tactile agnosia): The inability to recognize objects by handling them, although tactile, proprioceptive, and thermal sensations may be intact.

Attention: The ability to select and to attend to a specific stimulus while simultaneously suppressing extraneous stimuli.

Body image: A visual and mental image of one's body that includes feelings about one's body, especially in relation to health and disease.

Body scheme: A postural model of one's body, including the relationship of the body parts to each other and the relationship of the body to the environment.

Cognitive awareness (decreased): Inability to recognize a deficit or problem caused by neurological injury.

Cognitive processes: The abilities that enable us to 'think' which includes the ability to concentrate or pay attention, remember, and learn.

Cognitive rehabilitation: An approach to the remediation of cognitive-perceptual skills that focuses on how the individual acquires and uses knowledge, and seeks overall strategies for the brain-damaged patient to approach task performance.

Color agnosia: An inability to recognize colors.

Compensation: An approach to the treatment of the neurologically impaired individual that advocates use of intact abilities and alternate methods for solution to functional problems.

Constructional apraxia: Faulty spatial analysis and conceptualization of a task. It is most evident in the inability to produce two- or three-dimensional forms by drawing, constructing, or arranging blocks or objects, spontaneously or on command.

Cortical blindness: A total failure to appreciate incoming visual sensory information owing to a lesion in the cortex, rather than injury to the eyes.

Depth and distance perception: Judgement of the distance between objects and self, and the depth between objects and self.

Divided attention: The capacity to respond simultaneously to two or more tasks or stimuli when all stimuli are relevant.

Executive functions (higher order cognitive functions): Include the capacity to plan, manipulate information, initiate and terminate activities, recognize errors, problem solve and think abstractly.

Figure-ground discrimination: The ability to distinguish a figure from the background in which it is embedded.

Finger agnosia: The inability to identify the fingers on one's own hands or on the hands of the examiner, including difficulty in naming the fingers on command, identifying which finger was touched, and mimicking finger movements.

Focused attention: The capacity to attend to a task despite environmental visual or auditory stimuli.

Form discrimination: The ability to perceive or to attend to subtle differences in form and shape. The perceptually impaired patient is likely to confuse objects of similar shape or to fail to recognize an object placed in an unusual position.

Functional approach: An approach to the treatment of the neurologically impaired individuals that advocates practice in the specific functional tasks in which the patient is deficient, in order to enhance independence.

Gerstmann's syndrome: Bilateral finger agnosia with problems in right-left discrimination, agraphia, and acalculia is termed Gerstmann's syndrome.[106] Gerstmann's syndrome usually is associated with a focal lesion of the dominant hemisphere in the region of the angular gyrus.[52]

Hemianopsia: Inability to see half the field of vision in one or both eyes.

Hemispace: One half of the spatial field around the body. For example, the space surrounding the left body side including the person's back, front, and head.

Higher order cognition: Complex cognitive functions that include capacities such as planning, manipulating information, initiation and termination of activities, recognition of errors, problem solving, and abstract thinking.

Homonymous hemianopsia: Blindness in the outer half of the visual field of one eye and the inner half of the visual field of the other eye, producing an inability to receive information from either the right or the left half of the visual environment.

Ideational apraxia: An inability to perform a purposeful motor act, either automatically or upon command; an inability to retain the idea of the task and to formulate the necessary motor patterns. The patient no longer understands the overall concept of the act.

Ideomotor apraxia: The inability to perform a task on command and to imitate gestures, even though the patient understands the concept of the task; patient is able to carry out habitual tasks automatically.

Immediate recall: The ability to remember information that has been stored for a few seconds.

Knowledge of results (KR): Information concerning whether or not the patient attained the desired outcome.

Knowledge of performance (KP): Information concerning the manner in which the activity was accomplished.

Long-term memory: A compilation of early experiences and information acquired over a period of years.

Memory: A mental process that allows the individual to store experiences and perceptions for recall at a later time.

Ocular pursuit: The ability of the eyes to follow a moving object.

Perception: The process of selection, integration, and interpretation of stimuli from one's own body and the surrounding environment.

Position in space disorder: The inability to perceive and interpret spatial concepts such as up, down, under, over, in, out, in front of, and behind.

Prosopagnosia: An inability to recognize faces or other visually ambiguous stimuli as being familiar and distinct from one another.

Right-left discrimination disorder: The inability to identify the right and left sides of one's own body or that of the examiner.

Selective attention: The capacity to attend to a task despite environmental visual or auditory stimuli.

Sensation: A feeling or awareness that results from stimulation of the body's sensory receptors.

Sensory integration (SI): An approach to perceptual remediation that focuses on offering specific sensory stimulation and carefully controlling the subsequent motor output; influences the way in which the brain organizes and processes sensations.

Short-term memory: The retention of events or learning that has taken place within a few hours or days.

Simultanagnosia: The inability to perceive a visual stimulus as a whole; also known as Balint's syndrome.

Somatoagnosia: Impairment in body scheme; a lack of awareness of the body structure and the relationship of body parts of oneself or of others.

Spatial relations deficit: The inability to perceive the relationship of one object in space to another object or to oneself.

Spatial relations disorder: A constellation of deficits that have in common a difficulty in perceiving the relationship between objects in space, or the relationship between the self and two or more objects. Included are disorders of figure-ground discrimination, form discrimination, spatial relations, position in space perception, and topographic orientation.

Splinter skill: A trained or learned skill that is acquired in a manner inconsistent with, or incapable of being integrated with, skills the individual already possesses.

Sustained attention: A capacity to attend to relevant information; sustained attention implies that a person can maintain a consistent response during a continuous activity.

Task analysis: The breakdown of an activity or task into its component parts and a delineation of the specific motoric, perceptual, and cognitive abilities that are necessary to perform each component.

Topographical disorientation: Difficulty in understanding and remembering the relationship of one place to another.

Transfer-of-training approach: Remediation that focuses on practice in tasks with particular perceptual requirements; enhances performance in tasks with similar perceptual demands.

Unilateral neglect: The inability to register and to integrate visual stimuli and perceptions from one side of the environment (usually the left), not attributable to sensory-based problems. As a result, the patient ignores stimuli occurring in that side of personal space.

Vertical disorientation: A distorted perception of the upright (vertical) position.

Visual cancellation task: An activity where a person is required to locate and check (or mark) several target stimuli from an array. For example, a person may be asked to mark all examples of the letter 'a' on a page full of random letters.

Visual Fixation: The ability to maintain focus on an object as it is brought closer to and farther away from the eyes.

Visual object agnosia: The inability to recognize familiar objects despite normal function of the eyes and optic tracts.

APPENDIX A

Suggested Answers to Case Study Guiding Questions

1. What are some of the difficulties the patient is having and what cognitive and perceptual problems might be causing these? Please note that there may be more than one possible impairment for the functional problems noted.

ANSWER: Difficulties attending to information on her left could be due to a unilateral neglect or homonymous hemianopsia. Difficulty repeating the transfer technique after a 20-minute break could be short-term memory problems. It could be an apraxia, but this is unlikely because she had no difficulties performing the transfer when first taught. Difficulties locating her brush could be visual object agnosia.

2. Develop a clinical asset and problem list.

ANSWER: The occupational and physical therapists constructed the following asset and problem list:

Assets:
- Good communication skills (both expressive and receptive)
- Potential for full return of function in left upper extremity
- Potential to walk unaided
- Motivated and friendly

Problems:

Problems included difficulties in completing all basic and instrumental ADLs and engaging in leisure activities due to the following direct impairments:
- Reduced short-term memory
- Unilateral neglect
- Visual object agnosia
- Reduced standing dynamic balance
- Reduced strength and dexterity in her left arm and hand

These problems were compounded by morning pain and stiffness in her shoulder and hands due to arthritis.

3. Identify outcomes and goals appropriate for the patient.

ANSWER: The patient, the occupational and physical therapists met to discuss their outcomes and goals for therapy. They agreed that they would all work toward returning the patient home with some additional support from the community and her family as the outcome of therapy. Specifically, they listed the goals and outcomes of treatment they wanted to achieve as follows. For the patient to:
- Independently eat, bathe, dress, toilet and groom, (FIM = 6)
- Be able to prepare a light snack safely and independently
- Continue at least two of her former leisure interests

Achieving these treatment outcomes and goals relies on the patient overcoming her reduced short-term memory, unilateral neglect, and visual object agnosia.

4. Identify two treatment strategies to improve spontaneous use of right upper extremity neglect.

ANSWER:

Right UE Function: The occupational therapist, physical therapist, and the other rehabilitation team members constructed a therapy plan, that included 1 physical therapy and 2 occupational therapy sessions per day. The physical therapist worked on balance reactions using a balance board and the occupational therapist reinforced the gains made by doing functional activities in occupational therapy such as cooking snacks. Both the physical therapist and the occupational therapist worked with the patient to increase function in her right arm and hand. Progress was affected by the unilateral neglect, and the occupational therapist taught the physical therapist several techniques to ensure that she used the left arm and hand in therapeutic activities. The treatment aimed at cognitive and perceptual problems.

Unilateral Neglect: Using a remedial approach, the occupational therapist minimized the presence of stimuli that are known to activate the left side of the brain, such as letters and numbers, and kept verbal instructions to a minimum. In all personal and instrumental ADLs, the occupational therapist began the session by conducting motor activities with the left body side to both improve function in the arm and attention to the left body side and hemispace.[112]

5. Identify two treatment strategies to improve her memory.

ANSWER: In conjunction with therapy activities directed toward improved memory skills, the therapist must also consider the patient's attentional skills. The occupational therapist chose a distraction-free enviornment initially and worked on simple functional tasks such as making coffee, with inherent memory requirements such as remembering that the occupational therapist preferred coffee black with two sugars. The occupational therapist upgraded this activity so that the patient was making coffee for several other patients.

The use of a notebook system was introduced to assist the patient manage her daily routine. The physical therapist wrote instructions for the exercises for her to practice, and how often she should do these exercises. The whole therapy team reinforced the use of the notebook by constantly directing her to use it rather than repeatedly questioning staff.

6. How can the success of the rehabilitation program be measured?

ANSWER: The success of the therapy program can be measured in several ways, including

- Reassess the patient using standardized assessments (LOTCA and A-ONE) to determine if improvements have been made.
- Reexamine documented outcomes of therapy and goals to determine whether these have been met.
- Ask the patient if she feels she has improved.
- Ask the patient's family or friends if they see improvements.
- Assess if specific intervention strategies have generalized across to other activities.[150]

Neurogenic Disorders of Speech and Language

Martha Taylor Sarno

LEARNING OBJECTIVES

1. Explain the organization of language with respect to the role of phonological, lexical, syntactic, and semantic systems.
2. Gain an understanding of the role of the motor speech system in the speech production process.
3. Explain and characterize the classic aphasic syndromes.
4. Identify and explain the critical factors in the evaluation of the recovery and rehabilitation of aphasia.
5. Identify and describe general approaches to aphasia rehabilitation and some specific treatment methods.
6. Describe the primary types of dysarthria and rationales for dysarthria treatment.
7. Describe speech apraxia and its treatment.
8. Gain an understanding of neurogenic swallowing disorder.
9. Describe the goals and rationales for the use of augmentative communication systems.

Most human beings take the ability to produce and understand speech for granted and pay little attention to the nature and function of the processes involved in communication. Yet speech, like tool making, sets us apart from animals and is one of our most human behaviors. Even in primitive societies, humans have used the oral-motor speech code to share experiences, ideas, and feelings. Not all human communities have developed writing and reading systems.

The term **communication** encompasses all of the behaviors, including speech, that human beings use to transmit information. Speech is comprised of a delicate and rapid sequence of sensory and motor events requiring the coordinated activity of several parts of the body. The use of speech for communication involves many levels of human activity, including the fine motor coordination of components of the oral-motor system to the subtle shades of meaning that occur at the cognitive/semantic level. Gestures, pantomime, and other nonverbal **pragmatic language** behaviors, such as turn taking, are also essential elements of communication.

Among unimpaired speakers, speech behavior varies greatly, yet the oral-motor system is efficient for the exchange of even complicated information. The range of variability is so wide that individuals generally produce different sound waves with different characteristics even when producing the same word. But listeners do not rely solely on information derived from speech waves. We also depend on cues, which are components of what is referred to as **context.** Context includes aspects of a communicative exchange such as the purpose of the activity, the location of the exchange, the knowledge of the

The preparation of this chapter was supported in part by the National Institute of Deafness and Other Communication Disorders (NIDCD) grant RO1NS25367-01A1, of which the author is Principal Investigator, and the National Institute of Disability and Rehabilitation Research (NIDRR) grant G00830000.

participants, the roles of each participant, and the level of formality required by the situation.

The use of speech for communication contributes to our identity as human beings and to the perception of "self." As a result, disruptions in the ability to communicate, whether on the basis of structural abnormalities (e.g., cleft palate), neurological conditions (e.g., Parkinson's disease), or nonorganic conditions (e.g., nonorganic articulatory disorders) may impact on an individual's daily life in important ways. For some, the acquisition of a communication disorder may have sufficient impact to cause an individual to withdraw from the work force. In other cases, the disorder may not impede the individual's vocational life, but draw sufficient attention to itself that it interferes with socialization. For those whose communication disorders have persisted since childhood, the disorder may represent a significant vocational handicap. Communication disorders are complex, multifaceted behavioral impairments that compromise an aspect of human behavior that is closely associated with one's personhood and may negatively impact on all aspects of life.

This chapter addresses the neurogenic disorders of communication, a category of communication disorders represented by the majority of patients receiving speech-language pathology services in rehabilitation medicine programs. The most common of these disorders is **aphasia,** a language disorder, and **dysarthria,** a motor-speech disorder.

The field of speech-language pathology, which came into being in 1925 with the establishment of the American Speech-Language-Hearing Association (ASHA), is dedicated to the diagnosis and treatment of individuals with congenital or acquired disorders of speech and language. Communication disorders exact a large economic toll, costing the United States economy an estimated $30 billion a year in lost productivity, special education costs, and medical costs. The National Institute on Deafness and Other Communication Disorders (NIDCD) estimates the number of cases of language disorders at 6 to 8 million and of speech impairment at 10 million.[1] Approximately 28 million Americans have a hearing loss. Fifty-five percent of those with hearing impairments are over the age of 65.[2] More than 1.4 million children under the age of 18 have a hearing impairment.[1]

In the population over the age of 65, 10.8 percent have speech and language disorders, whereas among those under 45 years of age, 9.9 percent have speech and language disorders. The largest population of communication impaired are children with language disorders (43.7%) and **articulation disorders** (32.1%).[1] Aphasia affects approximately 15 percent of the adult speech-language impaired population.[3]

The field of speech pathology has grown rapidly. Affiliates (members and certificate holders) in the ASHA increased from 1623 to 35,000 between 1950 and 1980. Today, there are over 89,000 speech-language pathologists certified by ASHA, of whom more than 90 percent are female.[4] Speech-

language pathology is a Master's degree entry field and more than 85 percent of all states require licensure to practice. The ASHA awards the Certificate of Clinical Competence (CCC) to speech-language pathologists who meet specified academic and clinical experience requirements, which includes a Clinical Fellowship Year (CFY). Healthcare facilities account for about 40 percent of the settings in which speech-language pathologists are employed. However, only slightly more than 15 percent of certified speech-language pathologists work in hospital settings.[4,5] The CCC and licensure are usually required for hospital employment. The term *speech-language* pathologist is the official designation of professionals in the field who hold the CCC. The term *speech therapist*, although no longer considered professionally appropriate, is a term that is often used informally.

In order that the presence and degree of speech or language pathology manifested by a given person can be identified and measured, his or her performance must be compared with a standard of "normal." One may choose as the standard (1) the language common to the cultural community of unimpaired persons in which the patient lives, in which case an individual's verbal function would be compared with that of others in the same community of similar age, sex, education, and achievement, or (2) the patient's verbal behavior prior to the onset of illness or trauma. The latter will vary from individual to individual and is based on premorbid educational achievement, specific cultural characteristics, personality, and other factors. A patient is verbally impaired when he or she deviates in any parameter of language and/or speech processing from the "normal" communication behavior of the community in which he or she functioned premorbidly.

A "normal" standard is implied in the terms *impairment*, *disability*, and *handicap*. In 1980, the World Health Organization (WHO)[6] presented a classification schema that distinguished among the terms: **impairment** referring to the pathology itself (its location, measured size, etc.); **disability** is the consequences of an impairment and its impact on everyday personal, social, and vocational life; and **handicap** is the value the individual, family, and community place on the disability and the degree to which the individual is disadvantaged.

THE ORGANIZATION OF LANGUAGE

When an individual generates an idea that he or she wants to say, it is transformed into words and sentences by calling into play certain physiological and acoustic events. The message is converted into linguistic form at the listener's end. The listener, in turn, fits the auditory information into a sequence of words and sentences that are ultimately understood.

We refer to the system of symbols that are strung together into sentences expressing our thoughts and the understanding of those messages as *language*. In the first few years of life, infants and children gain a great deal of practice and experience in the use of language, until it becomes habitual and is used without conscious awareness.

Phonology refers to the study of the sound system of language. Words are made up of speech sounds or **phonemes,** which are generally classified as either **vowels** or **consonants.** Phonemes in and of themselves do not symbolize ideas or objects, but when put together they are the basic linguistic units that make words. Words comprise the **lexicon,** or vocabulary, of a language. In English, there are 16 vowels and 22 consonants, which are combined into larger units called **syllables.**

There are between one and two thousand syllables in English, which are usually comprised of a vowel as a central phoneme surrounded by one or more consonants. Most languages have their own rules about how phonemes may be combined into larger units. For example, in English, syllables never start with the *ng* phoneme. The most frequently used words in English are sequences of from two to five phonemes. Some have as many as 10 phonemes or as few as 1. Generally, however, the most frequently used words have few phonemes. New words are added to the English language every day, even though only a small number of phoneme combinations are possible. Although there are several hundred thousand English words, we use a repertoire of only about 5000 to 10,000 words 95 percent of the time.

The grammar, or **syntax,** of a language determines the sequence of words that are acceptable in the formation of sentences. In English, for example, it is possible to say "The black box is on the table," but the sequence "Box black table on the" is unacceptable. Another example is "The old radio played well," is syntactically correct but "Old the well played radio" is not. The sentence, "The boy walked to the store" is meaningful, but the sentence, "The book walked to the store" is not. The language system that refers to the meanings of words is called **semantics**.

In addition to the phonological (sounds), lexical (vocabulary), syntactical (grammar), and semantic (meaning) systems of a language, we also utilize **prosody** (stress and intonation) to help make distinctions between questions, statements, expressions of emotional feelings, shock, exclamations, and so forth.

SPEECH PRODUCTION

The speech organs consist of the lungs, trachea, larynx (which contains the vocal cords), pharynx, nose, and mouth. When considered together, these organs comprise a "tube" referred to as the **vocal tract,** which extends from the lungs to the lips. Vocal tract shape is varied by moving the tongue, lips, and any other parts of the tract. Changes in the configuration of the vocal tract act to modify the aero-

dynamic qualities of the air stream during speech (Fig. 30-1).

The primary function of the vocal organs relates to basic life-sustaining functions such as breathing and swallowing. These organs not only take on different roles for speech, but function differently when engaged in speech production. For example, breathing for life-sustaining purposes is far more rapid than for speech production. A full cycle inhalation/exhalation takes approximately 5 seconds, whereas during speech we control the breathing rate according to the demands of the words and sentences we are producing, sometimes reducing the rate of breathing to as little as 15 percent devoted to inhalation. This is dictated in part by the fact that, when speaking, we generally take in air sufficient to produce a complete thought and we exhale the air gradually during the production of the thought.

The steady stream of air exhaled from the lungs is the source of energy for speech production, which is made audible by the rapid vibration of the vocal cords. During speech we continuously alter the shape of the vocal tract by moving the tongue, lips, and other parts of the system. By moving the vocal

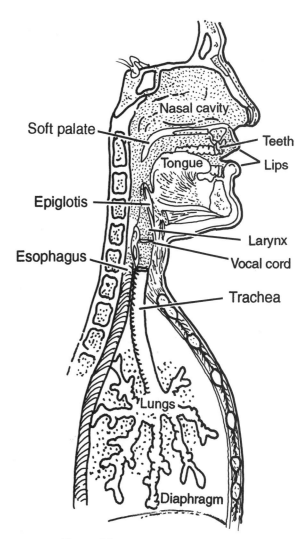

Figure 30-1. The human vocal organ.

tract, thereby modifying its acoustic properties, we are able to produce the different sounds. That is, by altering the shape of the vocal tract upon phonation, we transform the air stream into a resonance chamber (Figs. 30-2 and 30-3).

The *larynx* acts as a barrier to prevent food from entering the trachea and lungs by closing automatically during the act of swallowing, which is also helped by the action of the epiglottis. By opening and closing the flow of air from the lungs, the larynx acts as a valve between the lungs and the mouth. The laryngeal valve also acts to lock air into the lungs, which we do automatically when we perform heavy work with our upper extremities. The larynx is not a fixed, rigid organ but, because of its cartilaginous construction and corresponding connecting muscles and ligaments, it moves up and down during both swallowing and speaking.

The *vocal cords* extend on either side of the larynx from the Adam's apple at the front to the arytenoid cartilages at the back. We refer to the space between the vocal cords as the **glottis.** When the cords are pressed together, the passage of air is sealed off and the valve is shut. Because the cords are held together at the front where they articulate with the Adam's apple, the open glottis is V-shaped, opening only at the back. When we speak, we vibrate the vocal cords in a rhythmic fashion, opening and closing the air passage from the lungs to the oral/nasal cavities.

The frequency of sound produced by the vocal cords is directly related to their mass, tension, and length. We alter the tension and length of the vocal cords continuously while speaking. In normal speech, the range of vocal cord frequencies is from about 60 to 350 cps. Most people use a vocal cord frequency range that covers about one and a half octaves.

The **pharynx** is the area of the vocal tract connecting the larynx with the nose and mouth. We isolate the nasal cavity from the pharynx and back of the mouth by raising the soft palate. The most adjustable component of the vocal tract is the mouth, whose shape and size can be modified more than any other organ of the oral-motor system by changing the relative position of the palate, tongue, lips, and teeth. The lips are rounded, spread, or closed to alter the shape and length of the vocal tract or to stop airflow. The teeth and their relationship to the lips or tongue tip change the airflow. An important component of the teeth ridge is the *alveolus*, which is the area covered by the gums.

The term **articulation** refers to the articulating, or "meeting," of the various organs of the oral-pharyngeal cavity to produce the sounds of speech. Speech **intelligibility** refers to how a person "sounds" when speaking. A number of factors can influence judgements of intelligibility such as the presence or absence of visual cues or of extraneous movements (i.e., tremor). The precision of the production of consonant sounds is one of the primary factors that contributes to speech intelligibility. Consonants are described by specifying their place and manner of articulation and whether they are voiced

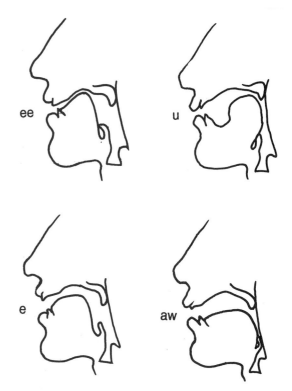

Figure 30-2. Outlines of the vocal tract during articulation of various vowels.

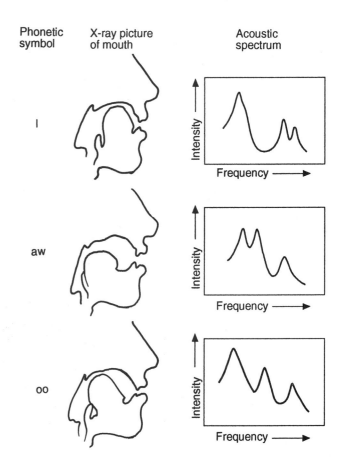

Figure 30-3. Vocal tract configuration and corresponding spectra for three different vowels. The peaks of the spectra represent vocal tract resonances. The vertical lines for individual harmonics are not shown.

or unvoiced (Table 30–1). The "places" of articulation are the lips (labial), teeth, gums (alveolar), palate, and glottis. The *manner of articulation* refers to the plosive, fricative, nasal, liquid, and semi-vowel categories.

Plosive sounds, sometimes referred to as "stop" sounds, are those produced by building up air pressure in the oral cavity and suddenly releasing it (e.g., *p, t*). The blockage can occur by pressing the lips together or by pressing the tongue against either the gums or soft palate. There are plosive consonants that are labial, alveolar, or velar.

Fricatives are produced by making the air turbulent (e.g., *f, v*). Most consonants are produced with the soft palate raised, thereby closing off the flow of air to the nasal cavity, except for the **nasals** (e.g., *m, n, ng*), which are made by lowering the soft palate and blocking the oral cavity somewhere along its length. **Liquids** are sounds made with the soft palate raised: /r/, /l/.

Semi-vowels refer to those sounds produced by maintaining the vocal tract in a vowel-like position, then changing the position rapidly for the vowel that follows (e.g., *w, y*).

Speech sounds are affected by their *context*, that is, the sounds that immediately precede or follow. A speech sound wave is a continuous event rather than a sequence of discrete segments. The identification of a speech sound depends on relating acoustic features of the sound wave at different points in time.

A standard reference for the quality of vowels is the eight cardinal vowels (Fig. 30-4). This schema of the positions of the tongue for the production of the vowels of the language help us to visualize the tongue's movements during speech. It is, in a sense, a map of the tongue positions for vowel production. Tongue placement is described by specifying the location of the main body of the tongue at its highest point. For example, for the vowel /i/ as in the word *beat*, the tongue tip is pointed in a high frontal configuration, whereas for the a as in the word *father* the highest point of the tongue is low and posterior in the oral cavity.

All vowel sounds and some consonant sounds are **voiced.** That is, the vocal cords vibrate during their production. When a sound is produced without

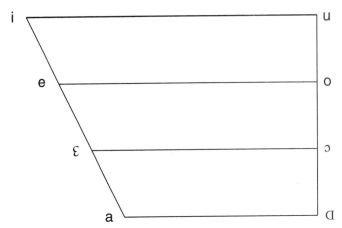

Figure 30-4. The cardinal vowels represented as a vowel quadrilateral. The cardinal vowels are extremely placed reference points for vowel articulation. Vowels on the same horizontal line were believed to have an equally high tongue height while vowels in the left-right position were assumed to be equally backed and fronted. (Adapted from Ladefoged, P: A Course in Phonetics. Harcourt Brace Jovanovich, New York, 1975, with permission.)

vocal cord vibration, we say that it is **unvoiced** (e.g., *p, s*). Table 30–1 shows that many consonant sounds are articulated in the same manner, and differ only with respect to voicing (e.g., *p-b; s-z; f-v; k-g*).

Speech behavior comprises a complex motor event that goes well beyond the skilled movements required of the oral-motor system. Yet we produce speech without thinking about it, even while simultaneously involved in other activities. However, to transform thought into speech takes some voluntary, conscious behavior that allows us to take information stored in memory and translate it into a coherent production of words and utterances that follow certain grammatical rules.

In addition to its linguistic aspects, neurogenic communication disorders often involve coexisting mild to severe cognitive deficits that may not only aggravate the communication disorder but make it difficult to differentiate cognitive from communication deficits. Although the communication disorder manifested in the patient with right brain damage will not be addressed in this chapter, it is an example of a disorder in which the cognitive component is a major issue.

The importance of the communication process and its underlying systems becomes apparent when we consider the two most common neurogenic communication disorders: aphasia and dysarthria. This chapter will focus primarily on aphasia and dysarthria and will also consider verbal apraxia, dysphagia, and the use of augmentative/alternate systems of communication.

APHASIA

In the past two decades the population age 65 and older has increased by 56 percent while the population under age 65 has grown by only 19 percent.[7] The proportion of persons over 65 is projected to

Table 30–1 CLASSIFICATION OF ENGLISH CONSONANTS BY PLACE AND MANNER OF ARTICULATION

Place of Articulation	Manner of Articulation				
	Plosive	Fricative	Semi-vowel	Liquids (including laterals)	Nasal
Labial	p b	—	w	—	m
Labiodental	—	f v	—	—	—
Dental	—	θ th	—	—	—
Alveolar	t d	s z	y	l r	n
Palatal	—	sh zh	—	—	—
Velar	k g	—	—	—	ng
Glottal	—	h	—	—	—

reach 21 to 22 percent of the total population by the year 2030.[8]

It is estimated that there are more than 1 million individuals with aphasia in the United States alone[9,10] and that there are approximately 84,000 new patients with aphasia in the United States each year, most of whom desire treatment.[11] The majority are over 65 years of age and acquired aphasia as a result of a stroke. A smaller number are the consequence of head trauma and neoplasms. Aphasia is also frequently present in the early stages of Alzheimer's disease. In 1969, the cost of speech-language rehabilitation for aphasia was estimated at $13.2 million per year,[12] and this number has probably tripled in the intervening years.

Classification and Nomenclature

In this chapter the term *aphasia* refers to the acquired communication disorder that is manifest in individuals who were previously capable of using language appropriately. It does not refer to those developmental language disorders that may be present in individuals who never developed normal language and for whom the ability to use language may never reach age-appropriate performance levels.

In acquired aphasia, central nervous system disease or trauma compromises certain structures in a focal rather than generalized fashion. The study of the neuroanatomical correlates of the aphasias has engaged neurologists since the late nineteenth century, and the correlation between aphasic syndromes and cerebral localization is relatively consistent. However, recent advances in neuroradiological technology have made aphasia localization a subject of increased research.

Aphasiologists generally agree that there are distinct major aphasic syndromes that adhere to specific profiles of impairment. This is not surprising, because the lesions that produce aphasia, particularly in the patient with cerebrovascular disease, tend to be located in brain loci that are especially vulnerable. It is not always possible, however, to classify patients according to these syndromes. Estimates of the proportion of cases that can be unambiguously classified range from 30 to 80 percent.[13]

The characteristics of an individual's speech production are used to determine aphasia classification. Speech output that is characterized as hesitant, awkward, interrupted, and produced with effort is referred to as *nonfluent aphasia* in contrast to speech output that is facile in articulation, produced at a normal rate, with preserved flow and melody, and is referred to as *fluent aphasia*. Fluency judgements are made during extended conversation with a patient and are defined as follows.

Fluent aphasia is characterized by impaired auditory comprehension and fluent speech that is of normal rate and melody. Fluent aphasia is usually associated with a lesion in the vicinity of the posterior portion of the first temporal gyrus of the left hemisphere. When fluent aphasia is severe, word and sound substitutions may be of such magnitude and frequency that speech may be rendered meaningless. Patients with fluent aphasia tend to have greatest difficulty in retrieving those words that are substantive (nouns and verbs). They also tend to have some degree of impaired awareness and are rarely physically disabled, because their lesions are located in the posterior portion of the brain, distant from motor areas. There are several types of syndromes subsumed under the fluent aphasia classification (Table 30–2).

Nonfluent aphasia is characterized by limited vocabulary, slow, hesitant speech, some awkward articulation, and restricted use of grammar in the presence of relatively preserved auditory comprehension. Nonfluent aphasia is associated with anterior lesions usually involving the third frontal convolution of the left hemisphere. Patients with nonfluent aphasia tend to express themselves in vocabulary that is substantive (nouns, verbs) and lack the ability to retrieve less substantive parts of speech (prepositions, conjunctions, pronouns). Patients with nonfluent aphasia tend to have good awareness of their deficit and usually have impaired motor function on the right side (right hemiplegia-paresis).

A severe aphasia with marked dysfunction across all language modalities and with severely limited residual use of all communication modes for oral-aural interactions is referred to as **global aphasia.** Global aphasia is not a type of aphasia but rather a designation of severity. The patient with global aphasia generally has extensive damage, which may be anywhere in the left hemisphere, and is sometimes bilateral.[14] Global aphasia has been cited as among the most common type of aphasia in patients referred for speech rehabilitation services.[15,16]

The most common category of fluent aphasia is *Wernicke's aphasia* (also referred to as sensory aphasia and/or receptive aphasia). Wernicke's aphasia is usually the result of a lesion in the posterior portion of the first temporal gyrus of the left hemisphere. It is characterized by impaired auditory comprehension and fluently articulated speech marked by word substitutions. Reading and writing are usually severely impaired as well. Although patients with Wernicke's aphasia may produce what seem like complete utterances and use complex verb tenses, they often add a word or phrase and "augment" speech production. They may also speak at a rate greater than normal. Although the production of speech sounds is generally precise, patients with Wernicke's aphasia may reverse phonemes and/or syllables (hopspipal/trevilision) and may produce *neologisms* (nonsense words).

Wernicke's aphasia may evolve into anomic aphasia in the course of recovery. *Anomic aphasia* is characterized by a significant word finding difficulty in the context of fluent, grammatically well-formed speech. Auditory comprehension is relatively preserved for most speaking situations. Speech output

Table 30-2 CLASSIFICATION BY APHASIA SYNDROMES

	Wernicke's Aphasia	Broca's Aphasia	Global Aphasia	Conduction Aphasia	Anomic Aphasia	Transcortical Motor Aphasia	Pure Word Deafness
Area of infarction	Posterior portion of temporal gyrus	Third frontal convolution	Third frontal convolution and posterior portion of superior temporal gyrus	Parietal operculum or posterior superior temporal gyrus	Angular gyrus	Supplementary motor areas	Both Heschl's gyri or connection between Heschl's gyrus and posterior superior temporal gyrus
Spontaneous speech	Fluent	Nonfluent	Nonfluent	Fluent or nonfluent	Fluent	Nonfluent	Fluent
Comprehension	Poor	Good	Poor	Good	Good	Good	Poor
Repetition	Poor	Poor (but may be better than spontaneous speech)	Poor	Very poor	Good	Excellent	Poor
Naming	Poor	Poor (but may be better than spontaneous speech)	Poor	Poor	Very poor	Poor	Good
Reading comprehension	Poor	Good	Poor	Good to poor	Good to poor	Good	Good
Writing	Poor	Poor	Poor	Poor	Good to poor	Poor	Good

may be somewhat vague and the patient may be facile in producing circumlocutions to skirt the lack of specificity of language use.

Broca's aphasia is a nonfluent type of aphasia also referred to as expressive aphasia, motor aphasia, and/or verbal aphasia. Broca's aphasia is the result of a lesion involving the third frontal convolution of the left hemisphere, the subcortical white matter, and extending posteriorly to the inferior portion of the motor strip (precentral gyrus). It is characterized by awkward articulation, restricted vocabulary, and restriction to simple grammatical forms in the presence of a relative preservation of auditory comprehension. Writing skills generally mirror the pattern of speech. Reading may be less impaired than speech and writing. The patient may be limited to one and two word productions for expression and find it impossible to combine words into sentences. Articulation may be awkward and effortful (see the section on Verbal Apraxia). Nonfluent Broca's aphasia is rarely found in aphasia after traumatic brain injury (TBI). Anomic disturbances predominate in aphasia secondary to TBI. In children, aphasia after TBI is generally characterized by a reduction of output with hesitancy, difficulty initiating speech, and sometimes mutism.[17]

Many measures of aphasia and related disorders have been developed for use in both clinical and research settings. In an inpatient setting, patients with aphasia are generally screened at bedside evaluation. The purpose of a bedside screening is to obtain a general idea of a patient's profile of deficits and preserved areas of language function as a basis for recommendations for more comprehensive test-ing and possible rehabilitation. Obviously, screening tests have limited value because they offer few details about the type and severity of aphasic deficits that lead to a syndrome classification. An important purpose of a comprehensive examination is to provide a baseline measure against which to gauge progress in the course of rehabilitation.

Aphasia Assessment

Comprehensive language tests designed to measure aphasic impairment generally contain specific domains of performance assessment. In addition to the general requirements for the construction of tests, such as reliability, standardization, and demonstrated validity, certain factors are considered important in the design of tests intended to identify and measure aphasia. These include range of item difficulty, use in measuring recovery, and ability to contribute to diagnostic classification.[18] Aphasia tests are generally based on assessments of linguistic task performance and at a minimum include tasks of visual confrontation *naming;* a spontaneous or conversational *speech sample* that is analyzed for fluency of output, effort, articulation, phrase length, prosody, word substitutions, and omissions; *repetition* of digits, single words, multisyllable words, and sentences of increasing length and complexity; *comprehension of spoken language* of single words, of sentences that require only yes-no responses, and pointing on command; *word retrieval* (word finding) measuring the ability to generate words beginning with a particular letter of the alphabet or in a particular semantic category (animals); *reading;* and *writing* from dictation and spontaneously. Some widely used aphasia measures include the *Boston Diagnostic Aphasia Examination* (*BDAE*),[13] the *Neurosensory Center Comprehensive Examination for Aphasia* (*NCCEA*),[19] and the *Western Aphasia Battery*.[20]

In addition to the measurement of performance on specific linguistic tasks, an aphasia assessment also requires supplementary measures of **functional communication** measures. This is necessary because an individual's actual use of language in everyday life may not correspond to the degree of pathology measured by specific language task performance. Functional communication measures are usually in the form of rating scales with high interrater reliability. The *Functional Communication Profile* (*FCP*),[21,22] *Communicative Activities of Daily Living* (*CADL*),[23] and the *Functional Assessment of Communication* (*ASHA-FACS*),[24] which have high interrater reliability, are widely used for this purpose.

Aphasia Rehabilitation

Language disturbances were recorded as early as 3500 BC[25] and attempts to "retrain" individuals with aphasia have been recorded throughout history. Some of the first documented cases of both natural recovery and intervention were the patients of Nicolo Massa and Francisco Arceo in 1558.[26]

In a landmark paper in the late nineteenth century, "Du siège de la faculté du langage articule,"[27] Paul Broca was one of the first to discuss the possibility of retraining in aphasia. Dr. Charles K. Mills was the first to address recovery and rehabilitation in aphasia in an English-language publication. He reported the training of a patient with post-stroke aphasia whom he and Donald Broadbent treated, using methods largely determined by the patient, who began by systematically repeating letters, words, and phrases.[28,29] Mills' observations and approach to aphasia rehabilitation, published over a century ago, are remarkably similar to much present-day practice and thought. Mills noted that not all patients benefit from retraining to the same degree and acknowledged that spontaneous recovery might have an influence on the course and extent of recovery.

The First World War and its brain injured combat survivors led to the establishment of treatment centers where patients with post-traumatic aphasia were treated, especially in Europe. Reports of aphasia rehabilitation experiences during and after the war in England and the United States were also published.[35,36] One of the most comprehensive descriptions of the systematic treatment of a large number of patients with brain injuries, of whom 90 to 100 were followed for a 10-year period, was provided by Kurt Goldstein in Frankfurt during the Second World War.[37]

Until World War II, reports of retraining civilians with post-stroke aphasia were rare. The aphasia literature was based almost exclusively on post-traumatic aphasia. In 1933, Singer and Low[38] reported the case of a 39 year-old woman who suffered an apparent vascular infarct after a full-term delivery and showed continuous language improvement with consistent training over a 10-year period.

In a landmark 5-year study supported by the Commonwealth Fund, Weisenburg and McBride[39] addressed the general topic of aphasia and commented on the effectiveness of reeducation. The study concerned 60 patients who were less than 60 years of age, a majority of whom had suffered strokes, and concluded that reeducation increased the rate of recovery, assisted in facilitating the use of compensatory means of communication, and improved morale. Their work also documented the psychotherapeutic benefits of treatment.

Aphasia and its concomitant neurological deficits in the patient with stroke were generally viewed as natural and necessary components of the aging process in the period before the World War II. The treatment of aphasia in the civilian population was not considered an option.

Many variables had an influence on making the treatment of aphasia the common practice that it is today. The advent of speech pathology as a health profession, the emergence of rehabilitation medicine as a medical specialty, the mass media explosion, a larger and more affluent middle class, an increase in the life span, the number of stroke and brain injury survivors, and public expectations of medicine in the age of technology are among them. The last has been particularly true in the industrialized world, where it is widely believed that there is a treatment for every human ill.

Journals devoted to brain/language issues have become indispensable information sources for aphasiologists (e.g., *Aphasiology, Brain and Language*, and *Cortex*). The Academy of Aphasia, a scholarly society dedicated to the study of aphasia, was established in 1962. The National Aphasia Association (NAA) was founded in the United States in 1987 for the purpose of providing information to the public about aphasia, advocating for the aphasic community, and encouraging the establishment of support groups called Aphasia Community Groups (ACGs).[40]

Several informational publications designed for use by the families and friends of patients with aphasia also appeared in the period following World War II.[41–47] One of these, "Understanding Aphasia,"[47] is still widely read and has been published in 11 languages.

CRITICAL FACTORS IN THE EVALUATION OF RECOVERY AND TREATMENT

If complete recovery from aphasia is to occur, it usually happens within a matter of hours or days following onset. Once aphasia has persisted for several weeks or months, a complete return to a premorbid state is usually the exception.

Most patients do not consider themselves recovered unless they have fully returned to previous levels of language performance.[48] When unrecovered patients are satisfied with their level of competence and consider themselves recovered, this is a psychological perception and should not be confused with an objective evaluation of communication abilities. The true test of aphasia rehabilitation outcome is the patient's perception of the quality of their lives. Measures of life function that include activity levels, socialization, mobility and community reintegration can be used for this purpose.[49]

It is desirable to distinguish between two separate recovery dimensions in aphasia: one that is objective and attempts to quantify the extent to which the patient has regained language abilities; and a second, which in humanistic terms may be more important, that measures the recovery of functional communication.

The concept of a functional dimension of communication behavior emerged logically from the experience of treating patients with aphasia in the rehabilitation medicine setting.[20,50] Historically, rehabilitation medicine has acknowledged that the ability of patients to function in their daily lives, the so-called activities of daily living (ADL), does not necessarily correlate with the extent of physical disability. Improvement in quantitative measures of language performance does not necessarily correlate with improvement in functional communication.[51]

STUDIES ON THE EFFICACY OF THERAPY IN THE PATIENT WITH POST-STROKE APHASIA

Many methodological problems have limited the number of studies that examine the efficacy of aphasia rehabilitation.[52–57] Nevertheless, treatment accountability issues are compelling and a focus of professional concern.

Studies that investigate treatment effects, specific techniques, and approaches have been reported since the late 1950s.[58] Vignolo,[59] Hagen,[60] and Basso et al.[61,62] have utilized untreated control and treated groups and shown a treatment effect. The work of Shewan and Kertesz[63] and Poeck et al.[64] with treated and untreated groups has also yielded positive treatment effects. Variables such as spontaneous recovery,[65–67] age,[68] duration and treatment intensity,[55] and specific treatment techniques[69,70] have been studied. Although studies to date have varied methodologically and by research focus, the results provide strong indication for positive treatment effects. Meta-analyses of efficacy studies have been reported for 45 studies published between 1946 and 1988 and for 55 studies that support better clinical outcome for patients who received early, intensive treatment.[71,72]

RECOVERY

In the period immediately following onset, some degree of natural recovery takes place in the majority of patients with or without intervention. There is, however, a lack of consensus about the duration of the **spontaneous recovery** period.[73–75] Culton[76] reported rapid spontaneous language recovery in the first month following the onset of aphasia. A number of studies have concluded that the greatest improvement occurs in the first 2 to 3 months post-onset.[59,61,65,76,78] Butfield and Zangwill,[79] Sands et al.,[80] and Vignolo[59] found that the recovery rate dropped significantly after 6 months. Others have reported that spontaneous recovery does not occur after 1 year,[61,76] and Sarno and Levita[81] reported that the greater change took place within a 3-month than a 6-month post-onset period in a sample of patients with severe aphasia seen up to 6 months post-stroke.

In a survey of 850 patients following acute (first month post) stroke patients, aphasia was present in 177 patients during the acute phase. In the 4 to 12 weeks following the stroke, aphasia improved in 74 percent of the patients and cleared in 44 percent.[11]

Basso's review of this topic[82] concluded that factors such as age, gender, and handedness do not affect recovery from aphasia.

In the healthy aged, language performance declines significantly between the seventh and eighth decades,[83,84] comprehension performance begins to decline in the sixth decade and continues through the eighth decade.[85–87] Although age has been reported as significant[59,80,88] many do not support this view.[62,82,89–92] The wide discrepancy regarding the influence of age in the aphasia recovery literature may relate to differences in sampling and methodology. Gender does not appear to have an important influence on outcome.[82,93,94]

It is generally agreed that post-traumatic aphasia has a better prognosis than aphasia secondary to vascular lesions.[59,79] In fact, some cases of aphasia secondary to TBI have been reported to recover completely.[65,95] The finding that traumatic aphasia carries a better prognosis than vascular aphasia may be influenced by the fact that patients involved in traumatic events are generally neurologically healthy whereas patients who have had strokes may have widespread vascular involvement.[82]

Both type and severity of aphasia appear to carry predictive value, with global aphasia having the poorest prognosis.[62,96–98] Basso reported that when patients with fluent and nonfluent aphasias of the same severity were compared, there were no differences in degree of recovery. In 881 consecutive acute stroke admissions to a community-based hospital, it was possible to make valid prognoses within 1 to 4 weeks after stroke depending on the initial severity of aphasia.[82]

The majority of investigators report that patients with severe aphasia do not recover as well as those with mild aphasia.[65,80,96,98] Sarno and Levita[97] found that people with fluent aphasia reached the highest level of functional communication, whereas patients with nonfluent and global aphasia made smaller gains in the 8- to 52-week post-stroke period. Global aphasia sometimes evolves to severe Broca's aphasia when there is significantly improved comprehension. Broca's aphasia may become anomic aphasia, and Wernicke's aphasia may evolve to anomic or conduction aphasia.[65,98–100] When patients with aphasia recover a great deal of language function they are usually left with residual anomia.

Patients whose computed tomography (CT) scans show large dominant hemisphere lesions, many small lesions, or bilateral lesions are less likely to recover than those with smaller or fewer lesions.[48,96] Lesions in Wernicke's area or those that extend more posteriorly tend to lead to severe and persistent aphasia. The neuroradiological correlates of aphasia recovery have been addressed by many investigators.[78,101,102] Yarnell et al.[48] reported little prognostic value in angiographic and radioscintigram findings. Similarly, CT scans did not help in predicting who might profit from language retraining in a Norwegian study.[74]

Comprehension tends to recover to a greater degree than expression.[16,59,77,103–105] Educational level or occupational status before illness does not always correlate with recovery; however, Sarno and Levita[81] reported that aphasic individuals who were employed at the time of stroke recovered more than those who were unemployed.

The presence of depression, anxiety, and paranoia have been cited as negative factors in recovery.[106–108] Premorbid personality traits have been identified as important prognostic factors. Eisenson and Herrmann[109–111] felt that patients with outgoing personalities had a better prognosis than those with introverted, dependent, or rigid personalities.

It is the general consensus that language gains in aphasia take place earlier rather than later, and that time since onset is an important recovery variable.[97,112–115]

Psychosocial and Related Factors

Psychological factors such as depression, anxiety, premorbid personality, fatigue, and paranoia are often cited as elements that have an adverse effect on recovery and communication. The social isolation experienced by people with aphasia and their families has a profound impact on their quality of life.[57] The effect of aphasia on the individual's sense of "self" is often extremely negative, leading to a loss of self-esteem and feelings of helplessness. The opportunity for "healing conversation," so essential to individuals who have suffered losses, is often unavailable to those with aphasia. Deep depression is frequently the result of this combination. The influence of these psychosocial variables is usually negative and is believed to be considerable.

Approaches to the Treatment of Aphasia

Literally hundreds of specific treatment techniques are cited in the aphasia rehabilitation literature. Aphasia therapy is rarely the same in any two treatment settings. The lack of therapeutic uniformity has undoubtedly impeded carefully controlled studies on the effects of language retraining.[43] Most methods derive essentially from traditional pedagogic practices, relying heavily on repetition.[116]

The primary assumption in aphasia rehabilitation is that language in the brain is not "erased," but that retrieval of its individual units has been impaired. Approaches to aphasia therapy have generally followed one of two models: a *substitute skill model* or a *direct treatment model*, both of which are based on the assumption that the processes that subserve normal performance need to be understood if rehabilitation is to succeed.[117] An example of the *substitute skill model* can be found in deaf individuals, some of whom use speech reading, a visual input rather than an auditory input, as an aid to comprehend spoken language. If a *direct treatment model* is followed, specific exercises individually designed to ameliorate specific linguistic deficits are the basis of treatment.

In general, treatment methods can be categorized as those that are largely indirect stimulation-facilitation and those that are essentially direct structured-pedagogic.[43,95,106,113,116,118] The two principles that underlie most treatment methods reflect contrasting views of aphasia as either impaired access to language or a "loss" of language. The stimulation methods generally follow an impaired access theory and pedagogic approaches are based on a theory of aphasia as a language loss.

In practice, however, much of aphasia therapy addresses the "performance" aspect of language in which repeated practice and "teaching" strategies are assumed to help restore impaired skills through a "task-oriented" approach (i.e., naming practice). One of the commonly used techniques involves self-cueing and repetition exercises that manipulate components of grammar and vocabulary. Another approach involves "stimulating" the patient to use residual language by encouraging conversation in a permissive setting where a patient's responses are unconditionally accepted and topics are of personal interest.[119]

Visual communication therapy (VIC)[120] is an experimental technique designed for global aphasia. VIC employs an index card system of arbitrary symbols representing syntactic and lexical components that patients learn to manipulate so as to (a) respond to a command and (b) express needs, wishes, or other emotions. The system attempts to circumvent the use of natural oral language, which is severely impaired and often unavailable to the patient with global aphasia. An adaptation and application of the VIC system called Computer-Aided Visual Communication system, (C-VIC) was developed by Steele et al.[121–124] Weinrich et al.[125] demonstrated that C-VIC training can lead to improved spoken language.

Investigators conclude that the evidence supports the view that some patients who have severe aphasia can master the basics of an artificial language and that some of the cognitive operations entailed in natural language are preserved despite severity.

Visual Action Therapy (VAT) developed at the Boston Veterans Administration Medical Center by Helm-Estabrooks et al. is designed to train people with global aphasia to use symbolic gestures representing visually absent objects.[126,127] The tasks leading to this goal include associating pictured forms with specific objects, manipulating real objects appropriately, and finally producing symbolic gestures that represent the objects used (e.g., cup, hammer, razor).

In an attempt to utilize systematized gestural language to facilitate oral production, American Indian sign language has been modified in a method that combines common gestural sign with oral speech production (Amerind) for selected cases.[128–130]

In the *functional communication treatment (FCT)* method developed by Aten et al.,[131] emphasis is placed on restoration of communication in the broadest sense. Therapy is designed to improve information processing in the activities necessary to conducting ADLs, social interactions, and self-expression of both physical and psychological needs.[132]

Promoting Aphasics' Communicative Effectiveness (PACE),[133] a technique intended to reshape structured interaction between clinicians and patients into more natural communicative exchanges, includes several pragmatic components common to natural conversation.

In addition to these methods, some investigators have reported the use of drawing as a potential means of communication.[134–137] Others describe interactive approaches to aphasia rehabilitation. These approaches include: the *communication partners* approach of Lyon,[134–136] a treatment plan designed to enhance communication and well-being in settings where the person with aphasia and the caregiver live; the *supported conversation* approach introduced by Kagan,[138,139] in which volunteers are trained as conversation partners to facilitate conversation in the person with aphasia by using all available modalities, thereby revealing the individual's competence and permitting a communicative interaction; and the social model of aphasia rehabilitation introduced by Simmons-Mackie[140] and Simmons-Mackie and Damico,[141,142] which focuses on the fulfillment of social needs and the encouragement of a greater conversational burden on the part of communication partners. Partners are trained to facilitate interaction by modifying some of their interactive behavior.

The unfortunate reality is that once the condition of aphasia has stabilized, very few patients recover normal communication function, with or without speech therapy. Accordingly, aphasia rehabilitation should be viewed as a process of patient management in the broadest sense of the term. That is, the task is primarily one of helping the patient and his or her intimates adjust to the alterations and limitations imposed by the disability. Effective aphasia rehabilitation management requires the participation of a variety of disciplines, including medicine, psychology, physical therapy, occupational therapy, social work, vocational counseling, and, most critically, aphasia therapy.

The Patient with Aphasia

It has been observed that the variability of patients' psychological reactions is rarely determined by the type or location of their lesions but is an expression of the whole life experience of the person who has had a stroke.[49,82,108,143]

In a study of patients with aphasia participating in a group psychotherapy program, Friedman[144] investigated the nature of psychological regression with impaired reality testing in aphasia. Beyond the communication difficulties posed by aphasia, he observed that patients remained psychologically isolated. They did not maintain a consistent level of group participation and expressed intense feelings that they were very different from those of other people. Both withdrawal and projection were apparent as each patient acted in isolation and yet complained of this characteristic in others.

The selective and discriminating use of speech therapy to stimulate and support the patient through the various stages of recovery is an effective management tool.[75,145,146] Experienced aphasia therapists recognize that while working on aphasic deficits, they are simultaneously dealing psychotherapeutically with a readjusting personality.[108] Speech therapy, therefore, serves different purposes at different points along the way. Sometimes it allows patients to "borrow time," as Baretz and Stephenson[147] have aptly stated. Occasionally depression lifts after speech therapy has been initiated, reflecting the supportive and nurturing nature of the therapeutic relationship rather than an objective improvement in recovery of speech-language.[143]

Aphasia rehabilitation can be viewed as a dynamic process consisting of a series of stages like the stages of mourning described by Kübler-Ross,[148] through which the majority of patients evolve. Some, of course, never emerge from a state of severe depression.[149] Kübler-Ross[148] and other authors have suggested that the stages through which someone with aphasia passes could be characterized as attempts to overcome the sense of loss, which includes denial, rage, and bargaining, awareness of the loss, and acceptance of the loss.

By directly addressing a patient's linguistic deficits and channeling attention and energies toward constructive ends, speech therapy may produce a noticeable reduction in depression. Therapy tasks in this instance act as an equivalent for work, which has long been recognized as an antidote for depression.

There is a great tendency to overestimate the capacity of individuals with aphasia to return to work, particularly if the verbal deficits are mild. Premature attempts to return to work can have a negative psychological impact. Professional rehabilitation counselors are best equipped to explore and evaluate a patient's vocational potential and carry out the long and arduous process of evaluating work performance and job requirements.

Experienced aphasia clinicians stress the importance of the patient's family in the rehabilitation process. Some of the potentially negative reactions of the family include overprotectiveness, hostility, anger, unrealistic expectations, overzealousness, lack of knowledge of the dimensions of the disorder, and inability to cope with practical difficulties. The apparently natural tendency of family members to minimize the patient's communication impairment, particularly in the early stages of recovery, requires understanding and tactful management.[108]

The quality of premorbid relationships generally tends to be intensified after a catastrophic event; those that were problematic may deteriorate further, whereas the bond between a loving couple may become stronger. The reversal of roles, changes in levels of dependency, and a changed economic situation, so often a consequence of chronic disability, can have a critical negative impact on the patient and his or her family.

In a positive family milieu, patients are encouraged to develop regular daily routines as close to premorbid patterns as possible and are treated as contributing members of the family. Patients need to be allowed some sense of control. Including the patient in rehabilitation planning helps to restore feelings of self-worth. In this regard, the emphasis on function rather than complete recovery, pointing out success rather than performance failure, adds to a patient's sense of self. It is essential to listen to patients, particularly to their expressions of loss. Commiseration is often more comforting than optimistic prognostic statements.

Group speech therapy, stroke clubs, and other social groups are frequently used resources that can be effective tools in the management of some patients with chronic aphasia. The National Aphasia Association (NAA) was founded in the United States in 1987, following the lead of existing organizations established in Finland in 1971, Germany in 1978, the United Kingdom in 1980, and Sweden in 1981. Knowledge that one is not alone often helps to reduce depression and loneliness.[75,106]

Group therapy with peers also provides a comfortable atmosphere in which patients can meet new friends and share feelings, although not all individuals with aphasia find it beneficial. A positive effect seems related to level of comprehension, time since onset, and personality factors. Although group therapy generally plays an important role in aphasia rehabilitation, it should be noted that much of its effectiveness depends on the skill and experience of the group leader.[150,161]

In our present state of knowledge, aphasia rehabilitation remains eclectic and specifically tailored to the individual patient. Fundamental to this therapeutic philosophy is the acknowledgement and appreciation of the uniqueness of the individual. No two persons with aphasia are exactly alike in pathology, personality, linguistic deficits, reactions to catastrophic illness, life experience, spiritual values, or a host of other factors. The influence of these factors carries different weight and strength at different stages of recovery and they are all related to recovery outcome.

Experience suggests that, except for severely depressed individuals with aphasia, patients generally produce everything they are capable of producing. Therapists must not allow their expectations to contaminate the therapeutic interaction; this is not uncommon and is usually motivated by laudatory aspirations—therapists want to see their patients improve—but is nonetheless counterproductive. Patients with involvement of subcortical areas may have low levels of activation, a purely physiological process independent of psychological motivation. The distinction between these two processes must be understood.

Many ethical-moral dilemmas face those who manage the rehabilitation of patients with aphasia. One of the principal issues is a result of the necessity to select those individuals who will receive treatment. Rehabilitation medicine services are not only scarce in many situations, but they are also not considered to be a right or entitlement. Services are usually provided on a selective basis to those individuals believed to have the potential to benefit. This process assumes that we know who can benefit.[9,152,154,155] Many who are experienced in aphasia rehabilitation management hold the view that all people should be given a trial treatment period to determine their candidacy for further treatment and that trials should be provided at different points in the recovery course. Goal setting, the patient's right to self-determination, and the criteria appropriate in determining the termination of therapy are also important ethical issues.[108,155]

DYSARTHRIA

The term dysarthria refers to an impairment of speech production resulting from damage to the central or peripheral nervous system, which causes weakness, paralysis, or incoordination of the motor-speech system. Any one or all of the components of the motor-speech system (respiration, phonation, articulation, resonance, and prosody) may by compromised by neural damage. The type and degree of dysarthria depends on the underlying etiology, degree of neuropathology, coexistence of other disabilities, and the individual response of the patient to the condition. It is not unusual for dysarthria to coexist with aphasia in patients who have suffered cerebrovascular accidents or traumatic brain injury. The severity of dysarthria may range from the production of occasional imprecisely articulated consonant sounds to speech that is rendered totally unintelligible by the degree of impairment to the underlying systems. When patients are totally unintelligible as the result of severe motor-speech system impairment, they exhibit **anarthria.**

The incidence of dysarthria in the population of individuals with neurogenic disorders is approximately 46 percent,[156] representing a significant proportion of the patients with communication impairments seen in medical settings.

Dysarthria is generally reflected in deficits occurring in multiple motor-speech systems, but may sometimes occur in a single system (i.e., an impairment of soft palate movement resulting in hypernasality). It is most notably prevalent in cerebral palsy, traumatic brain injury, cerebrovascular accidents, demyelinating diseases (e.g., multiple sclerosis) Parkinson's disease, amyotrophic lateral sclerosis, and neoplasm.

There are five primary types of dysarthria: *spastic, flaccid, ataxic, hypokinetic,* and *hyperkinetic.* When two or more types coexist, the term **mixed dysarthria** is used. Coexisting physical disabilities are present in a majority of patients who manifest dysarthria.

Classification and Nomenclature

Spastic dysarthria is characterized by imprecise articulation, slow labored articulation, hypernasality, harsh to strained phonation, and monotonous pitch. Syllables may be given equal stress and inflection. There is often reduced control of exhalation, with shallow inhalations and slow breaths. Spastic dysarthria is the result of bilateral pyramidal system damage involving the corticobulbar tracts (upper motor neurons). The pathology may cause weakness and paresis of the face and tongue musculature on the side opposite to the lesion. There is a high incidence of spastic dysarthria among those with cerebral palsy.[156]

Flaccid dysarthria is characterized by slow/labored articulation, hypernasality, and hoarse, breathy phonation. Phrases may be short, inhalation is shallow, and the control of exhalation may be reduced. There is often a reduction in the variation of pitch and loudness with audible inspirations. Most of these deviant speech characteristics are related to muscular weakness and reduced muscle tone, which affect the speech, accuracy, and range of speech movements.

Ataxic dysarthria is characterized by disturbances of timing, speech, movement, range, and control and coordination of the muscles of speech and respiration. Speech is imprecise, slow, and irregular. There may be intermittent periods of explosive inflection, syllable stress, and loudness patterns. Phonemes may be prolonged; pitch and loudness are monotonous. The lesions producing ataxic dysarthria are bilateral, generalized lesions involving the deep midline nuclei and pathways of the cerebellum. Patients with multiple sclerosis often manifest ataxic dysarthia.

Hypokinetic dysarthria is characterized by variable articulatory precision, slow rate of speech, harsh, hoarse voice quality, excessive and overly long pauses, prolonged syllables and reduced pho-

nation. Patients with Parkinson's or parkinsonian-like symptoms often manifest hypokinetic dysarthria, which is caused by lesions of the substantia nigra.

Hyperkinetic dysarthria is characterized by variable articulatory precision, vocal harshness, prolonged sounds and intervals between words, monotonous pitch, and loudness. Patients with Huntington's disease manifest hyperkinetic dysarthria, which is caused by lesions of the basal ganglia and/or their extrapyramidal projections.

Dysarthria Rehabilitation

Dysarthria rehabilitation must be individually designed and account for the profile of impairment as well as the variability of its disabling effects. The performance of components of the motor-speech system does not necessarily result in changes in the disabling effects of the dysarthria;[157] that is, the intelligibility of speech. Goals that relate to the level of disability rather than normal speech are generally more realistic because they do not focus on normalcy, which is usually an unachievable goal, or improvement in the performance of a single component of the motor speech system, which may not, in the overall picture, be functionally important. There is relatively little data-based information available on the long-term prognosis for patients with dysarthria.

The focus of dysarthria rehabilitation is sometimes based on an approach to treatment that stresses compensatory skills. These techniques tend to encourage the patient to minimize the overall disability by using strategies that may actually deviate from normal (i.e., slowing down the rate of speech production to increase intelligibility of consonant production).

The primary objective of dysarthria rehabilitation is to improve the intelligibility of speech, which can be negatively affected if the speaker is in a dark, noisy place. Patients and communication partners must be trained to seek the most optimal situations for communication interactions. Although exercises are generally administered that intend to increase the precision, strength, and coordination of movements of the motor-speech system and the coordinated action of various components of the system, the general focus of dysarthria rehabilitation is phonetic, because it is articulatory precision that contributes most to overall intelligibility. Clearly, as a patient's overall physical coordination and precision of movement are increased, there are corresponding improvements noted in the control of the motor-speech system, and hence improved speech intelligibility.

VERBAL APRAXIA

Some patients with nonfluent (Broca's) aphasia present with articulatory difficulty that manifests as imprecise and awkward articulation, distortion of phoneme production, and some literal *paraphasic* (sound substitution) errors in the absence of impaired strength or coordination of the motor speech system. This characteristic, which may be so severe that the patient is barely intelligible, can appear to be independent of difficulty in language processing and is referred to as **verbal apraxia** (or speech dyspraxia, apraxia of speech, cortical dysarthria, phonetic disintegration). Unlike dysarthric speakers, apraxic speakers do not generally have deficits in performing nonspeech movements of the oral musculature. The possible independence of this deficit from the language disorder of Broca's aphasia remains controversial.

Dyspraxia Rehabilitation

The disorder of articulation referred to as speech dyspraxia seldom, if ever, is manifest in the absence of a coexisting Broca's aphasia, however mild. The speech dyspraxia component of this multifaceted communication disorder appears to be especially amenable to direct therapeutic intervention using approaches adapted primarily from traditional articulation therapy techniques, including stress and intonation drills. These approaches, designed to improve phonetic placement accuracy, typically depend on imitation, stress, and progressive approximation, which are drilled using kinesthetic, visual, and auditory cues. Generally, the stimuli used as the bases for these exercises are selected in a presumed order of difficulty, beginning with nonoral imitation, followed by sounds, words, phrases, and finally utterances.

Treatment techniques for speech dyspraxia have been described by many clinicians.[158–166] Dworkin et al.[167] reported an effective treatment regimen in a study of a single subject. Various rhythmic techniques in which the patient generates the rhythm have also been reported as facilitory methods to increase articulation accuracy.[96,168] In contrast, Shane and Darley[169] found that articulation precision tended to deteriorate under externally imposed rhythmic stimulation. Melodic intonation therapy has also been employed as a facilitory technique in the treatment of the patient with speech dyspraxia.

The long-term nature of recovery of phonemic production in patients with verbal apraxia was confirmed in a study of a patient with Broca's aphasia who received speech therapy for 10 years. The errors that prevailed in the first poststroke year were compared with performance at 10 years. The features of place and manner of production had improved; although voicing and addition errors persisted, omission errors were virtually eliminated.[170]

DYSPHAGIA

The swallowing process is comprised of a complex number of neuromuscular events. Normal swallow-ing requires that an individual be able to move food or liquid from the mouth *(oral swallow phase)*, through the pharynx *(pharyngeal swallow phase)*, and into the esophagus. In the oral swallow phase food is collected in the oral cavity in a single mass, or bolus, which is then passed into the pharynx and propelled under pressure into the esophagus. During the oral swallow phase the bolus is first held on the floor of the mouth and then propelled by the tongue from the front to the back of the oral cavity. As the bolus moves over the back of the tongue into the pharynx, the pharynx is activated to propel it into the esophagus. The entrance to the airway closes, bottom up, from the vocal folds to the epiglottis moving downward to prevent food from entering the trachea during this process.

Dysphagia is defined as a condition in which an individual has had an interruption in either eating function or the maintenance of nutrition and hydration.[171] Many patients with neurogenic communication disorders also manifest deficits in swallowing (dysphagia). Thirty to 40 percent of individuals who have suffered strokes may have swallowing deficits ranging from mild to severe.[172–175] In some cases dysphagia is only present in the acute phase with rapid recovery of swallowing function taking place in the first 3 weeks post-stroke.[176] Swallowing deficits in poststroke patients are often due to a combination of weakness and incoordination of the oral, pharyngeal and laryngeal musculature, resulting in inefficient propulsion of a food bolus or liquid through the pharynx and into the esophagus. Oral or pharyngeal transit times may be slow. Reduced closure of the vocal cords or elevation of the larynx may result in material being misdirected into the airway (aspiration). Dysphagia is also often present in patients with Parkinson's disease, Huntington's disease, the dystonias and dyskinesias, amyotrophic lateral sclerosis, multiple sclerosis, neoplasm, dementia, Alzheimer's disease, and other degenerative neurological conditions, as well as cerebral palsy.

A dysphagia evaluation usually begins with a clinical assessment at bedside and is followed by more objective, instrumental assessments if indicated. The pharyngeal aspects of swallowing and the rapid complex neuromuscular activity involved can sometimes make simple observation insufficient for an assessment. The most frequently used physiological measurement used in a dysphagia evaluation is the modified barium swallow because it provides a moving and pictorial radiographic view of the greatest number of components of the oral and pharyngeal aspects of swallowing. Another useful assessment procedure is videoendoscopy. In most settings the swallowing evaluation is carried out by the swallowing therapist who is most often a speech-language pathologist.[176]

Dysphagia Rehabilitation

Dysphagia rehabilitation is designed to improve swallowing efficiency for nutritional purposes and to increase swallowing safety. This can be accomplished by compensatory strategies and/or techniques that are designed to change swallow physiology and reduce the risk of aspiration. Compensatory strategies include postural changes that affect the way food passes through the mouth and pharynx, dietary management, and placing food in the mouth in optimal positions. Postural techniques may also be introduced to reduce the possibility of aspiration.[150] Specific exercises to increase the coordination, range of motion, strength, and sensory input of the muscles involved in the pharyngeal swallow, such as laryngeal elevation and tongue base approximation to the posterior pharyngeal wall, also may be employed.[177]

The physical therapist can play an important role in positioning the patient for the most efficient swallow, and providing treatment to reduce muscle spasticity, improve muscle strength and coordination, and prevent primitive reflex patterns from interfering with swallowing.[178]

ALTERNATIVE/AUGMENTATIVE COMMUNICATION SYSTEMS AND DEVICES

New technology, especially synthetic speech and microcomputers, has been adapted for use as **augmentative communication devices.** These devices provide a compensatory means of communication and are used as a facilitory technique to enhance or substitute for impaired speech (aphasia, dysarthria). Since the advent of microcomputers, they have been adapted for use in the treatment of aphasia.

Microcomputers were the basis for an approach that Seron et al.[179] found effective in treating patients with writing disorders associated with aphasia. With continued exposure to training, improvement in accuracy and recognition time in reading commonly used words,[180] and improvement in auditory comprehension were noted in a patient with aphasia who, when followed up at a later date, showed additional gains.[181,182] Computer-generated phonemic cues were effective in improving naming in five patients with Broca's aphasia.[183] An augmentative system was developed for a patient with Broca's aphasia;[184] a word retrieval facilitation program was developed for individuals with aphasia;[185] and Steele et al.[123] and Weinrich et al.[186] replicated and extended the findings of Gardner et al.[120] and Baker et al.[187] by training those with aphasia to use a computerized version of the VIC system.

If an individual who is unable to make him- or herself understood has residual writing/spelling skills, aids that utilize the alphabet can provide a means of communication (e.g., an alphabet board). A communication book may consist of pictures or words arranged according to topics (e.g., foods, family members) in a notebook for easy access. The same type of material has also been adapted for computerized access in the form of portable or table-top devices. Augmentative and alternative communication aids can be divided into high-tech and low-tech categories. Typewriters, telephones, communication books, and other similar devices are in the low-tech category, requiring only batteries or electricity. The high-tech category includes specially adapted computers and switching systems.

Thus far, only a small proportion of the aphasia population has benefited from alternative and **augmentative communication devices.** A larger number of persons with motor-speech impairments (e.g., those with cerebral palsy) have been able to increase their communicative effectiveness with technical aids. The complex interaction of the language, motor-speech system, and cognition in aphasia pose a challenge to current and future technology.[188]

THE PHYSICAL THERAPIST AND THE PATIENT WITH COMMUNICATION IMPAIRMENT

Physical therapists often work in settings where they may be the first to become aware of a patient's communication disorder, and should refer such patients to a speech-language pathologist for evaluation. The physical therapist can contribute to the patient's improvement in communication function in two important ways: by providing physiological support for speech functions, and by stimulating and facilitating communication through successful, fulfilling interaction with the patient. In either case, the physical therapist will want to work closely with the speech-language pathologist to ensure that they agree as to the treatment goals, and that their respective roles are not in conflict.

The provision of physiological support for speech functions is especially relevant to the patient with pathology of the oral-motor system (e.g., dysarthria). The physical therapist will want to explore the influence of physiological support on the patient's speech in determining a comprehensive plan of care. Proper posture, for example, can help to inhibit reflexes that may trigger primitive movements. When patient's speech function is influenced by overflow movements, stabilization techniques may be indicated.

Control of respiration is essential to the improvement of vocalization and the phrasing of speech. The muscles of respiration can be strengthened along with exercises designed to increase head control, stability, and sitting balance. Proper posture and eye contact enhance the possibility that speech will be audible and clear.

When a patient with a communication impairment is prescribed a communication board, the physical therapist contributes by determining a patient's sitting balance and tolerance, upper extremity motor control, and the best method for responding (e.g., pointing).

Muscle-strengthening exercises to increase the speech and range of motion of the tongue, lips, and general facial musculature and to improve coordination of the oral-motor system also increase the probability of intelligible speech and help the patient with dysarthria and dysphagia. Postural techniques are especially important for patients with dysphagia, who require individually tailored treatment programs designed to facilitate swallowing and prevent aspiration.

Because communication is a social activity, the physical therapy setting is a natural context for social interaction. The setting can be supportive by providing an atmosphere that is conducive to conversation and allows the patient to engage in a successful verbal interaction.

Patients who are neurologically compromised often have difficulty processing information in a distracting setting. Excessive noise, competing voices, and the presence of other multiple stimuli can make communication particularly difficult. When possible, the physical therapist should strive to work with patients who are communicatively impaired in a setting that is free of these distractions (closed environment). Patients with communication disabilities do best when they are positioned in such a way that face-to-face communication is possible, including the visualization of gestures and facial expressions. For this reason, room lighting needs to be sufficient.

The physical therapist can be confused and frustrated by patients who manifest neurogenic speech-language disorders, especially those with aphasia. The individual nature of each aphasia argues for a close working relationship between physical therapist and speech-language pathologist. It is desirable that the physical therapist discuss individual cases with the speech-language pathologist requesting guidelines on the most effective communication strategies.

One of the greatest difficulties in addressing the needs of patients with acquired aphasia has to do with assessing and accounting for patient's level of auditory comprehension. Virtually all patients with aphasia have some degree of difficulty in comprehending spoken language. Physical therapists need to become skilled at recognizing and dealing with auditory comprehension deficits because they can be a major deterrent to successful rehabilitation.

Misconceptions of the auditory comprehension level of a patient with aphasia can range from the assumption that a patient understands everything to the assumption that the patient comprehends nothing and must be excluded from conversation. A guiding principle to keep in mind is that auditory comprehension can vary greatly, depending on the context and complexity of the task at hand. Switching topics quickly, speaking too quickly, background noises, talking while a patient is engaged in physical activity, and conversing with more than one person at a time can impede the individual's ability to process information in the auditory mode. Sentences should be short and simple and the patient should be given sufficient time to process the information and formulate a response. Questions that require elaborate answers, such as "Tell me about your vacation" or "What do you think about the latest news?" are generally difficult for patients with aphasia to answer. It is best to ask questions that can be answered with "yes," "no," or another single word.

Physical assistive cues to comprehension such as gestures, facial expression, and voice inflection can facilitate and enhance a patient's understanding. It is important for the physical therapist to know that patients with aphasia often find it easier to respond to whole body or axial commands ("stand up," "sit down") than distal commands ("point," "pick up").

It can be tempting to try to remedy a laborious communication situation by "talking down" to a patient with aphasia as if speaking to a child, or raising one's voice as if speaking to someone with impaired hearing. The best strategy is to endeavor to speak a little more slowly, using language that is not too complex, and remaining consistent in giving instructions. This can be particularly important in the physical therapy setting, where verbal commands are a fundamental element in the patient-therapist interaction. At times it may be necessary to repeat a sentence to be understood.

It is almost universal that rehabilitation team members overestimate the degree to which a person with aphasia understands spoken language. Physical therapists, when possible, should turn to the speech-language pathologist for an indication of the patient's preserved auditory comprehension. It may be necessary to rephrase questions and supplement with body language to ensure comprehension.

The use of accompanying visual cues, such as gestures and facial expressions, can be extremely helpful for some patients. Others may understand best if a message is supplemented by written cues. Sometimes one can assist by asking questions that can be answered by *yes* or *no* in a "twenty questions" format. When someone with aphasia is having trouble expressing him- or herself, it usually helps to allow them extra time to speak. If the patient becomes visibly frustrated, it is desirable to remain calm and suggest that the patient wait and try again later.

In carrying out physical therapy techniques, patients with aphasia can be encouraged to produce single-word, repetitive speech that coincides with physical movements as a means of providing supplemental speech practice. Activities such as counting movements in series 1 to 10, and using words like up/down, left/right, and so forth while performing physical movements are examples. The physical therapist, however, should always remain sensitive to the possibility of making speech demands that are beyond a patient's level of preserved communicative skill.

SUMMARY

Ever since World War II, speech-language pathologists have played an important role on the rehabilitation medicine team in the management of patients with neurogenic speech-language disorders, especially aphasia and dysarthria. For the physical therapist, an understanding of normal and pathological communication behaviors cannot only make this population of patients more interesting to work with, but can also enhance the quality of treatment provided for them.

Communication using speech is a complex, species-specific behavior that consists of the coordinated interaction of cognitive, motor, sensory, psychological, and social skills. The neurogenic disorders of speech and language, specifically aphasia and dysarthria, dominate the population of communication impaired patients in the rehabilitation medicine setting. Viewed as a group, patients with neurogenic communication disorders comprise a relatively severely impaired segment of the disabled population.

The impact of neurogenic speech-language disorders on the self, family, community life, and vocational options makes these disorders especially challenging. The close relationship of one's verbal characteristics to personality and identity may cause even the mildest neurogenic communication disorder to affect the psychosocial domain. Current research is investigating the interaction of linguistic, cognitive, and psychosocial variables and their influence on the outcome of recovery and rehabilitation.

QUESTIONS FOR REVIEW

1. Define aphasia.
2. Describe the differences that distinguish nonfluent from fluent aphasic syndromes and give clinical examples.
3. Discuss the components of a comprehensive language test designed to measure aphasic impairment.
4. Describe some critical factors that influence recovery from aphasia.
5. Describe the psychological sequelae that may have a negative effect on the outcome of aphasia rehabilitation.
6. Define dysarthria.
7. What neurological conditions are generally associated with dysphagia?
8. Describe augmentative communication systems and some specific techniques /devices that may enhance the treatment of aphasia.

CASE STUDY

The patient is a 62 year-old man who teaches high school. He sustained a right hemiplegia and difficulty communicating as the result of a hemorrhagic stroke, which occurred 8 months ago. At this time, except for dressing, he is ADL independent and ambulates with a cane.

At 1 month post-stroke, the patient was limited to yes-no responses and a vocabulary ranging from 30 to 50 nouns and verbs as well as everyday greetings (hello, goodbye). In the course of a communicative interaction he often resorted to writing a letter or word or gesturing to help in his communication efforts. He appeared to understand most of what was said especially when the topic was familiar. He received rehabilitation services during the acute poststroke phase while hospitalized and received 20 sessions of speech-language pathology services as an outpatient.

At 8 months poststroke the patient's communication disorder is marked by a slow, hesitant production of one and two word utterances, easily produced automatic speech (i.e., everyday greetings), difficulty expressing complex information, awkward and labored articulation, which causes occasional articulatory imprecision, impaired writing, and some difficulty reading lengthy or complex material. Although the majority of his speaking vocabulary consists of nouns and verbs, adverbs and adjectives are now used with greater frequency. There is a persistent lack of conjunctions, articles, and prepositions in speech, which causes him to have impaired grammar. The patient has no apparent difficulty understanding spoken language except when it is rapid, complex, and/or unfamiliar.

Both the patient and his caregiver report that the frequency of social interactions in his current life have been curtailed dramatically. He continues to see close family members on a regular basis but he rarely sees friends and work companions. They report that he is frustrated and depressed over this and feels isolated from the community much of the time. They also indicate that there has been a gradual but noticeable increase in his speaking vocabulary, ability to write, and reading skill. He has recently joined a local stroke group where he hopes to meet others with similar communication difficulties.

Guiding Questions

1. A team conference is scheduled for the patient the day after you assume treatment responsibilities for the patient. What types of information would you obtain in consultation with the speech-language pathologist?
2. What communication strategies are generally useful with patients who have sustained a stroke?
3. What approach might you use if the patient became frustrated trying to express himself during a physical therapy treatment?
4. As a physical therapist what might you do to decrease the patient's sense of isolation and enhance his emotional well-being?
5. In what ways can physical therapy treatment sessions serve to reinforce communication behavior?

REFERENCES

1. American Speech-Language-Hearing Association (ASHA): Personal communication, December 1992.
2. National Institute on Deafness and other Communication Disorders. National Strategic Research Plan for Hearing and Hearing Impairments. Bethesda, MD, 1996.
3. Slater, SC: Portrait of the professions. 1992 Omnibus Survey. ASHA 34:61, 1992.
4. ASHA Demographic Profile of ASHA members and affiliations for period January–June 1998. Rockville, MD, 1998.
5. Shewan, CM, and Slater, SC: ASHA Data: ASHA's speech-language pathologists and audiologists across the United States. ASHA, 64, November 1992.
6. World Health Organization (WHO): International classification of impairment, disabilities and handicap. World Health Organization, Geneva, Switzerland, 1980.
7. US Department of Health and Human Services: Aging America: Trends and projections, 1987–88 Edition. Government Printing Office, Washington, DC, 1988.
8. Spencer, G: Projections of the population of the United States by age, sex, and race: 1983 to 2080. Current Population Reports, Series P-25, No. 952. US Bureau of the Census, Washington, DC, 1984.
9. National Institutes of Health (NIH): Aphasia: Hope through research. NIH Publication No. 80-391. Bethesda, MD, 1979.
10. National Institute on Deafness and other Communication Disorders. NIDCD Fact Sheet: Aphasia. NIH Publication No. 97-4257. Bethesda, MD, 1997.
11. Brust, JC, et al: Aphasia in acute stroke. Stroke 7:167, 1976.
12. National Institutes of Health (NIH): Decade of research: Answers through scientific research. The National Advisory Neurological and Communicative Disorders and Stroke Council. The National Institutes of Health, Bethesda, MD, 1989.
13. Goodglass, H, and Kaplan, E: The Assessment of Aphasia and Related Disorders, ed 2. Lea & Febiger, Philadelphia, 1983.
14. Damasio, A: Signs of aphasia. In Sarno, MT (ed): Acquired Aphasia, ed 3. Academic, New York, 1998, p 25.
15. Sarno, MT: A survey of 100 aphasic Medicare patients in a speech pathology program. J Am Geriatr Soc 18:471, 1970.
16. Prins, R, et al: Recovery from aphasia: Spontaneous speech versus language comprehension. Brain Lang 6:192, 1978.
17. Levin, HS: Linguistic recovery aphasia closed head-injury. Brain Lang 12:360, 1981.
18. Spreen, O, and Risser, A: Assessment of aphasia. In Sarno, MT (ed): Acquired Aphasia, ed 3. Academic, New York, 1998, p 71.
19. Spreen, O, and Benton, AL: Neurosensory Center Comprehensive Examination for Aphasia, ed 2. University of Victoria, Department of Psychology, Neuropsychology Laboratory, Victoria, BC, 1977.
20. Kertesz, A: Western Aphasia Battery. Grune & Stratton, New York, 1982.
21. Sarno, MT: A measurement of functional communication in aphasia. Arch Phys Med Rehabil 46:107, 1965.
22. Sarno, MT: The Functional Communication Profile: Manual of Directions (Rehabilitation Monograph No. 42). New York University Medical Center, Rusk Institute of Rehabilitation Medicine, New York, 1969.
23. Holland, AL: Communicative Abilities in Daily Living. University Park Press, Baltimore, 1980.
24. Frattali, CM, et al: Functional Assessment of Communication Skills for Adults: Administration and Scoring Manual. American Speech & Hearing Association, Rockville, MD, 1995.
25. Benton, AL: Contributions to aphasia before Broca. Cortex 1:314, 1964.
26. Benton, AL, and Joynt, RJ: Early descriptions of aphasia. Arch Neurol 3:109, 1960.
27. Broca, P: Du siege de la faculte du language articule. Bulletinde la Societe d'Anthropologie 6:377, 1885.
28. Broadbent, D: A case of peculiar affection of speech, with commentary. Brain 1:484, 1879.
29. Mills, CK: Treatment of aphasia by training. JAMA 43:1940, 1904.
30. Poppelreuter, W: Ueber psychische ausfall sercheinungen nach hirverletzungen. Munchener Medizinische Wochenschrift 62:489, 1915.
31. Isserlin, M: Die pathologische physiologie der sprache. Ergebnisse der Physiologie, Biologischene Chemie und Experimentellen Pharmakologie 29:129, 1929.
32. Frazier, C, and Ingham, S: A review of the effects of gunshot wounds of the head. Arch Neurol Psych 3:17, 1920.
33. Gopfert, H: Beitrage zur Frage der Restitution nach Hirnverletzung. Zeitschrift fur die Gesamte Neurologie und Psychiatrie 75:411, 1922.
34. Franz, S: Studies in re-education: The aphasics. J Comp Psychol 4:349, 1924.
35. Head, H: Aphasia and Kindred Disorders of Speech, vols 1 and 2. Cambridge Univ Pr., London, 1926.
36. Nielsen, J: Agnosia, Apraxia, Aphasia: Their Value in Cerebral Localization. Hoeber, New York, 1946.
37. Goldstein, K: After Effects of Brain Injuries in War: Their Evaluation and Treatment. Grune & Stratton, New York, 1942.
38. Singer, H, and Low, A: The brain in a case of motor aphasia in which improvement occurred with training. Arch Neurol Psychiatry 29:162, 1933.
39. Weisenburg, T, and McBride, K: Aphasia: A Clinical and Psychological Study. Commonwealth Fund, New York, 1935.
40. Klein, K: Community-based resources for persons with aphasia and their families. Topics in Stroke Rehabilitation 2:18, 1996.
41. American Heart Association: Aphasia and the family. Author, Publication EM 359, Dallas, 1969.
42. Backus, O, et al: Aphasia in Adults. Univ of Michigan Pr., Ann Arbor, 1947.
43. Sarno, MT: Language therapy. In Burr, HG (ed): The Aphasic Adult: Evaluation and Rehabilitation, Proceedings of the Short Course in Aphasia. Wayside Press, Charlottesville, VA, 1964.
44. Boone, D: An Adult Has Aphasia: For the Family, ed 2. Danville, IL, Interstate Printers and Publishers, 1984.
45. Sarno, JE, and Sarno, MT: Stroke: A Guide for Patients and Their Families, ed 3. McGraw-Hill, New York, 1991.
46. Simonson, J: According to the aphasic adult. Univ of Texas (Southwestern) Medical School, Dallas, 1971.
47. Sarno, MT: Understanding Aphasia: A Guide for Family and Friends. Monograph #2. Rusk Institute of Rehabilitation Medicine, New York University Medical Center, New York, 1958.
48. Yarnell, P, et al: Aphasia outcome in stroke: A clinical neuroradiological correlation. Stroke 7:514, 1976.
49. Sarno, MT: Quality of life in aphasia in the first poststroke year. Aphasiology 11:665, 1997.
50. Sarno, MT: The functional assessment of verbal impairment. In Grimby, G (ed): Recent Advances in Rehabilitation Medicine. Almquist & Wiksell, Stockholm, 1983, p 75. (Also published as Suppl Scand J Rehabil 1983.)
51. Sarno, JE, et al: The functional life scale. Arch Phys Med Rehabil 54:214, 1973.
52. Darley, F: The efficacy of language rehabilitation in aphasia. J Speech Hear Disord 37:3, 1972.
53. Prins, R, et al: Efficacy of two different types of speech therapy for aphasic stroke patients. Applied Psycholinguistics 10:85, 1989.
54. Wertz, RT, et al: VA cooperative study on aphasia: A comparison of individual and group treatment. J Speech Hear Disord 24:580, 1981.
55. Wertz, RT, et al: Comparison of clinic, home, and deferred language treatment for aphasia: A VA cooperative study. Arch Neurol 43:653, 1986.
56. Wertz, RT: Language treatment for aphasia is efficacious, but for whom? Topics Lang Disord 8:1, 1987.
57. Sarno, MT: Recovery and rehabilitation in aphasia. In

Sarno, MT (ed): Acquired Aphasia, ed 2. Academic, San Diego, 1991.

58. Marks, M, et al: Rehabilitation of the aphasic patient: A survey of three years experience in a rehabilitation setting. Neurology 7:837, 1957.

59. Vignolo, LA: Evolution of aphasia and language rehabilitation: A retrospective exploratory study. Cortex 1:344, 1964.

60. Hagen, C: Communication abilities in hemiplegia: Effect of speech therapy. Arch Phys Med Rehabil 54:545, 1973.

61. Basso, A, et al: Etude controlee de la reeducation du language dans l'aphasie: Comparaison entre aphasiques traites et non-traites. Revue Neurologique (Paris) 131:607, 1975.

62. Basso, A, et al: Influence of rehabilitation on language skills in aphasic patients. Arch Neurol 36:190, 1979.

63. Shewan, C, and Kertesz, A: Effects of speech and language treatment on recovery from aphasia. Brain Lang 23:272, 1984.

64. Poeck, K, et al: Outcome of intensive language treatment in aphasia. J Speech Hear Disord 54:471, 1989.

65. Kertesz, A, and McCabe, P: Recovery patterns and prognosis in aphasia. Brain Lang 100:1, 1977.

66. Levita, E: Effects of speech therapy on aphasics' responses to the Functional Communication Profile. Percept Mot Skills 47:151, 1978.

67. Shewan, CM: Expressive language recovery in aphasia using the Shewan Spontaneous Language Analysis (SSLA) System. J Comm Disord 17:175, 1988.

68. Wertz, RT, and Dronkers, N: Effects of age on aphasia. Paper presented at the American Speech-Language-Hearing Association Research Symposium on Communication Sciences and Disorders and Aging, Washington, DC, 1988.

69. Helm-Estabrooks, N, and Ramsberger, G: Treatment of agrammatism in long-term Broca's aphasia. Br J Disord Commun 21:39, 1986.

70. Glindemann, R, et al: The efficacy of modelling in PACE-therapy. Aphasiology 5:425, 1991.

71. Whurr, R, et al: A meta-analysis of studies carried out between 1946 and 1988 concerned with the efficacy of speech and language therapy treatment for aphasic patients. European Journal of Communication 27:1, 1992.

72. Robey, RR: The efficacy of treatment for aphasic persons: A meta-analysis. Brain Lang 47:172, 1998.

73. Darley, F: Language rehabilitation: Presentation 8. In Benton, A (ed): Behavioral Change in Cerebrovascular Disease. Harper, New York, 1970.

74. Reinvang, I, and Engvik, E: Language recovery in aphasia from 3–6 months after stroke. In Sarno, MT, and Hook, O (eds): Aphasia: Assessment and Treatment. Almquist & Wiksell, Stockholm; Masson, New York, 1980.

75. Sarno, MT: Review of research in aphasia: Recovery and rehabilitation. In Sarno, MT, and Hook, O (eds), Aphasia: Assessment and Treatment. Almquist & Wiksell, Stockholm, 1980.

76. Culton, G: Spontaneous recovery from aphasia. J Speech Hear Res 12:825, 1969.

77. Lomas, A, and Kertesz, A: Patterns of spontaneous recovery in aphasic groups: A study of adult stroke patients. Brain Lang 5:388, 1978.

78. Demeurisse, G, et al: Quantitative study of the rate of recovery from aphasia due to ischemic stroke. Stroke 11:455, 1980.

79. Butfield, E, and Zangwill, O: Re-education in aphasia: A review of 70 cases. J Neurol Neurosurg Psychiatry 9:75, 1946.

80. Sands, E, et al: Long term assessment of language function in aphasia due to stroke. Arch Phys Med Rehabil 50:203, 1969.

81. Sarno, MT, and Levita, E: Natural course of recovery in severe aphasia. Arch Phys Med Rehabil 52:175, 1971.

82. Basso, A: Prognostic factors in aphasia. Aphasiology 6:337, 1992.

83. Nicholas, M, et al: Empty speech in Alzheimer's disease and fluent aphasia. J Speech Hear Res 28:405, 1985.

84. Bayles, KA, and Kaszniak, AW: Communication and Cognition in Normal Aging and Dementia. Little, Brown, Boston, 1987.

85. Obler, LK, et al: On comprehension across the adult life span. Cortex 21:273, 1985.

86. Bloom, R, et al: Impact of emotional content on discourse production in patients with unilateral brain damage. Brain Lang 42:153, 1992.

87. Nicholas, M, et al: Aging, Language, and Language Disorders. In Sarno, MT (ed): Acquired Aphasia, ed 3. Academic, San Diego, 1998.

88. Holland, AL, et al: Predictors of language restriction following stroke: A multivariate analyses. J Speech Hearing Res 31:232, 1989.

89. Kertesz, A: Recovery from aphasia. In Kese, FC (ed): Advances in Neurology, 42. Raven, New York, 1984.

90. Wertz, RT, and Dronkers, NF: Effects of age on aphasia. Paper presented at the American Speech-Language-Hearing Association Research Symposium on Communication Disorders and Aging, Washington, DC, 1988.

91. Pedersen, M, et al: Aphasia in acute stroke: Incidence, determinants, and recovery. Annals of Recovery 38:659, 1995.

92. Sarno, MT: Preliminary findings: Age, linguistic evolution and quality of life in recovery from aphasia. Scand J Rehabil Med Suppl 26:43, 1992.

93. Sarno, MT, et al: Gender and recovery from aphasia after stroke. J Nerv Ment Dis 173:605, 1985.

94. Borod, J, et al: Long term language recovery in left handed aphasic patients. Aphasiology 78:301, 1990.

95. Kertesz, A: Aphasia and Associated Disorders: Taxonomy, Localization and Recovery. Grune & Stratton, New York, 1979.

96. Schuell, H, et al: Aphasia in Adults. Harper, New York, 1964.

97. Sarno, MT, and Levita, E: Recovery in treated aphasia in the first year post-stroke. Stroke 10:663, 1979.

98. Selnes, OA, et al: Recovery of single-word comprehension CT scan correlates. Brain Lang 21:72, 1984.

99. Pashek, GV, and Holland, AL: Evolution of aphasia in the first year post onset. Cortex 24:411, 1988.

100. Kertesz, A: Evolution of aphasic syndromes. Topics in Language Disorders 1:15, 1981.

101. Kaplan, E, et al: Boston Naming Test, ed 2. Lea & Febiger, Philadelphia, 1983.

102. Goldenberg, G, and Scott, J: Influence of size and site of cerebral lesions on spontaneous recovery of aphasia and success of language therapy. Brain Lang 47:684, 1994.

103. Kenin, M, and Swisher, L: A study of pattern of recovery in aphasia. Cortex 8:56, 1972.

104. Lebrun, Y: Recovery in polyglot aphasics. In Lebrun, Y, and Hoops, R (eds): Recovery in Aphasics. Neurolinguistics, vol 4. Swets and Zeitlinger BV, Amsterdam, 1976.

105. Basso, A, et al: Sex differences in recovery from aphasia. Cortex 18:469, 1982.

106. Benson, DF: Aphasia, Alexia, and Agraphia. Churchill Livingston, New York, 1979.

107. Damasio, AR: Aphasia. N Engl J Med 336:531, 1992.

108. Sarno, MT: Aphasia rehabilitation: Psychosocial and ethical considerations. Aphasiology 7:321, 1993.

109. Eisenson, J: Adult Aphasia: Assessment and Treatment. Prentice-Hall, Englewood Cliffs, NJ, 1973.

110. Herrmann, M, et al: The impact of aphasia on the patient and family in the first year post-stroke. Topics in Stroke Rehabilitation 2:5, 1995.

111. Eisenson, J: Aphasia: A point of view as to the nature of the disorder and factors that determine prognosis and recovery. International Journal of Neurology 4:287, 1964.

112. Marshall, RC, and Phillipps, DS: Prognosis for improved verbal communication in aphasic stroke patients. Arch Phys Med Rehabil 4:597, 1983.

113. Darley, FL, et al: Motor Speech Disorders. Saunders, Philadelphia, 1975.

114. Sarno, MT: Aphasia rehabilitation. In Dickson, S (ed): Communication Disorders: Remedial Principles and Practices. Scott, Foresman, Glenview, IL, 1974.

115. Sarno, MT: Disorders of communication in stroke. In Licht, S (ed): Stroke and Its Rehabilitation. Williams & Wilkins, Baltimore, 1975, p 380.

116. Sarno, MT: Language rehabilitation outcome in the elderly aphasic patient. In Obler, LK, and Albert. ML (eds): Language and Communication in the Elderly: Clinical, Therapeutic and Experimental Issues. DC Heath, Lexington, MA, 1980, p 191.

117. Goodglass, H: Neurolinguistic principles and aphasia therapy. In Meier, M, et al (ed): Neuropsychological Rehabilitation. Guilford, New York, 1987.

118. Burns, MS, and Halper, AS: Speech/Language Treatment of the Aphasias: An Integrated Clinical Approach. Aspen, Rockville, MD, 1988.

119. Sarno, MT: Management of aphasia. In Bornstein, RA, and Brown, GG (eds): Neurobehavioral Aspects of Cerebrovascular Disease. Oxford Univ Pr, New York, 1990.

120. Gardner, H, et al: Visual communication in aphasia. Neuropsychologia 14:275, 1976.

121. Weinrich, MP, et al: Implementation of a visual communicative system for aphasic patients on a microcomputer. Ann Neurol 18:148, 1985.

122. Steele, RD, et al: Evaluating performance of severely aphasic patients on a computer-aided visual communication system. In Brookshire, RH (ed): Clinical Aphasiology: Conference Proceedings. BRK Publications, Minneapolis, 1987.

123. Steele, RD et al: Computer-based visual communication in aphasia. Neuropsychologia, 27:409, 1999.

124. Weinrich, MP: Computerized visual communication (C-VIC) therapy. Paper presented at the Academy of Aphasia, Phoenix, Arizona, 1987.

125. Weinrich, M, et al: Training on an iconic communication system for severe aphasia can improve natural language production. Aphasiology 9:343, 1995.

126. Helm, N, and Benson, DF: Visual action therapy for global aphasia. Presentation at the 16th Annual Meeting of the Academy of Aphasia, Chicago, 1978.

127. Helm-Estabrooks, N, et al: Visual action therapy for aphasia. J Speech Hear Disord 47:385, 1982.

128. Skelly, M, et al: American Indian sign (AMERIND) as a facilitator of verbalization for the oral verbal apraxic. J Speech Hear Disord 39:445, 1974.

129. Rao, P, and Horner, J: Gesture as a deblocking modality in a severe aphasic patient. In Brookshire, RH (ed): Clinical Aphasiology: Conference Proceedings. BRK Publications, Minneapolis, 1978.

130. Rao, P, et al: The use of American-Indian Code by severe aphasic adults. In Burns, M, and Andrews, J (eds): Neuropathologies of Speech and Language Diagnosis and Treatment: Selected Papers. Institute for Continuing Education, Evanston, IL, 1980.

131. Aten, JL, et al: The efficacy of functional communication therapy for chronic aphasic patients. J Speech Hear Disord 47:93, 1982.

132. Aten, JL: Function communication treatment. In Chapey, R (ed): Language Intervention Strategies in Adult Aphasia, ed 2. Williams & Wilkins, Baltimore, 1986.

133. Wilcox, M, and Davis, G: Promoting aphasics' communicative effectiveness. Paper presented to the American Speech-Language-Hearing Association, San Francisco, 1978.

134. Lyon, JG: Drawing: Its value as a communication aid for adults with aphasia. Aphasiology 9:33, 1995.

135. Lyon, JG: Coping with Aphasia. Singular Publishing Group, San Diego, CA, 1997.

136. Lyon, JG: Communication use and participation in life for adults with aphasia in natural settings: The scope of the problem. American Journal of Speech-Language Pathology 1:7, 1992.

137. Rao, PR: Drawing and gesture as communication options in a person with severe aphasia. Topics in Stroke Rehabilitation 2:49, 1995.

138. Kagan, A, and Gailey, GF: Functional is not enough: Training conversation partners for aphasic adults. In Holland, A, and Forbes, MM (eds): Aphasia Treatment:

139. Kagan, A: Revealing the competence of aphasic adults through conversation: A challenge to health professionals. Topics in Stroke Rehabilitation 2:15, 1995.

140. Simmons-Mackie, N: An ethnographic investigation of compensatory strategies in aphasia. Unpublished doctoral dissertation. Louisiana State Univ, Baton Rouge, 1993.

141. Simmons-Mackie, N, and Damico, J: Communication competence in aphasia: Evidence from compensatory strategies. In Lemme, ML (ed): Clinical Aphasiology, vol 23. Pro-Ed, Austin, 1995, p 3.

142. Simmons-Mackie, N, and Damico, J: Reformulating the definition of compensatory strategies in aphasia. Aphasiology 11:761, 1997.

143. Ullman, M: Behavioral Changes in Patients Following Strokes. Thomas, Springfield, IL, 1962.

144. Friedman, M: On the nature of regression. Arch Gen Psychiatry 3:17, 1961.

145. Brumfitt, S, and Clarke, P: An application of psychotherapeutic techniques to the management of aphasia. Paper presented at Summer Conference: Aphasia Therapy. Cardiff, England, July 19, 1980.

146. Tanner, D: Loss and grief: Implications for the speech-language pathologist and audiologist. J Am Speech Hear Assoc 22:916, 1980.

147. Baretz, R, and Stephenson, G: Unrealistic patient. NYS J Med 76:54, 1976.

148. Kübler-Ross, E: On Death and Dying. MacMillan, New York, 1969.

149. Espmark, S: Stroke before fifty: A follow-up study of vocational and psychological adjustment. Scand J Rehab Med (Suppl) 2:1, 1973.

150. Kearns, KJ: Group therapy for aphasia: Theoretical and practical considerations. In Chapey, R (ed): Language Intervention Strategies in Adult Aphasia, ed 2. Baltimore, Williams & Wilkins, 1986.

151. Bollinger, R, et al: A study of group communication intervention with chronic aphasic persons. Aphasiology 7:301, 1993.

152. Caplan, AL, et al: Ethical and policy issues in rehabilitation medicine. A Hastings Center Report, Briarcliff Manor, NY. Special Supplement, 1987.

153. Hass, J, et al: Case studies in ethics and rehabilitation. The Hastings Center, Briarcliff Manor, NY, 1988.

154. Sarno, MT: The case of Mr. M: The selection and treatment of aphasic patients. Case studies in ethics and rehabilitation medicine. The Hastings Center, Briarcliff Manor, NY, 1988, p 24.

155. Sarno, MT: The silent minority: The patient with aphasia. Hemphill Lecture. Rehabilitation Institute of Chicago, Chicago, 1986.

156. Duffy, JR: Motor Speech Disorders: Substrates, Differential Diagnosis, and Management. Mosby, St. Louis, 1995.

157. Yorkston, KM, et al (eds): Clinical Management of Dysarthric Speakers. Little, Brown, Boston, 1988.

158. Deal, J, and Florance, C: Modification of the eight-step continuum for treatment of apraxia of speech in adults. J Speech Hear Disord 43:89, 1978.

159. Halpern, H: Therapy for agnosia, apraxia, and dysarthria. In Chapey, R (ed): Language Intervention Strategies in Adult Aphasia. Williams & Wilkins, Baltimore, 1981.

160. Rosenbek, JC: Treating apraxia of speech. In Johns, DF (ed): Clinical Management of Neurogenic Communication Disorders. Little, Brown, Boston, 1978.

161. Rosenbek, JC, et al: A treatment for apraxia of speech in adults. J Speech Hear Disord 38:462, 1973.

162. Wiedel, IMH: The basic foundation approach for decreasing aphasia and verbal apraxia in adults (BFA). In Brookshire, RH (ed): Clinical Aphasiology: Conference Proceedings. BRK Publications, Minneapolis, 1976.

163. Rosenbek, JC: Advances in the evaluation and treatment of speech apraxia. In Rose, FC (ed): Advances in Neurology. Progress in Aphasiology, vol 42. Raven, New York, 1984, p 327.

World Perspectives. Singular Publishing Group, San Diego, CA, 1993.

164. Wertz, RT, et al: Apraxia of Speech in Adults: The Disorder and Its Management. Grune & Stratton, New York, 1984.

165. Wertz, RT: Language disorders in adults: State of the clinical art. In Holland, AL (ed): Language Disorders in Adults. College Hill, San Diego, 1984.

166. Rubow, R, et al: Vibrotactile stimulation for intersystemic reorganization in the treatment of apraxia of speech. Arch Phys Med Rehabil 63:97, 1982.

167. Dworkin, JP, et al: Dyspraxia of speech: The effectiveness of a treatment regimen. J Speech Hear Disord 53:289, 1988.

168. Rosenbek, JC, et al: Treatment of developmental apraxia of speech: A case study. Language, Speech and Hearing Services in the Schools 5:13, 1974.

169. Shane, H, and Darley, FL: The effect of auditory rhythmic stimulation on articulatory accuracy in apraxia of speech. Cortex 14:444, 1978.

170. Sands, E, et al: Progressive changes in articulatory patterns in verbal apraxia: A longitudinal case study. Brain Lang 6:97, 1978.

171. Buchholz, D: Editorial: What is dysphagia? Dysphagia11:23, 1996.

172. Groher, MD, and Bukutman, R: The presence of swallowing disorders in two teaching hospitals. Dysphagia 1:3, 1986.

173. Veis, S, and Logemann, J: The nature of swallowing disorders in CVA patients. Arch Phys Med Rehabil 66:372, 1985.

174. Wade, DT, and Hewer, RL: Motor loss and swallowing difficulty after stroke: Frequency, recovery, and prognosis. Acta Neurologica Scandinavia 76:50, 1987.

175. Cherney, LR: Dysphagia in adults with neurologic disorders: An Overview. In Cherney, LR (ed): Clinical Management of Dysphagia in Adults and Children. Aspen, Gaithersburg, MD, 1994.

176. Logemann, JA: Evaluation and Treatment of Swallowing Disorders, ed 2. Pro-Ed, Austin, 1998.

177. Logemann, JA, and Kahrilas, P: Relearning to swallow post CVA: Application of maneuvers and indirect biofeedback: A case study. Neurology 40:1136, 1990.

178. Groher, ME: Dysphagia: Diagnosis and Management, ed 3. Butterworth-Heinemann, Boston, 1997.

179. Seron, X, et al: A computer-based therapy for the treatment of aphasic subjects with writing disorders. J Speech Hear Disord 45:45, 1980.

180. Katz, RC, and Nagy, V: A computerized approach for improving word recognition in chronic aphasic patients. In Brookshire, RH (ed): Clinical Aphasiology: Conference proceedings. BRK Publishers, Minneapolis, 1983.

181. Mills, RH: Microcomputerized auditory comprehension training. In Brookshire, RH (ed): Clinical Aphasiology: Conference Proceedings. BRK Publications, Minneapolis, 1982.

182. Mills, RH, and Hoffer, P: Computers and caring: An integrative approach to the treatment of aphasia and head injury. In Marshall, RC (ed): Case Studies in Aphasia Rehabilitation. University Park Press, Baltimore, 1985.

183. Bruce, C, and Howard, D: Computer-generated phonemic cues: An effective aid for naming in aphasia. Br J Disord Commun 22:191, 1987.

184. Garrett, K, et al: A comprehensive augmentative communication system for an adult with Broca's aphasia. Augmentative and Alternative Communication 5:55, 1989.

185. Hunnicutt, S: Access: A lexical access program. Proceedings of RESNA 12th Annual Conference, New Orleans, LA, 1989, p 284.

186. Weinrich, MP, et al: Processing of visual syntax in a globally aphasic patient. Brain Lang 36:391, 1989.

187. Baker, E, et al: Can linguistic competence be dissociated from natural language functions? Nature 254:609, 1975.

SUPPLEMENTAL READINGS

Albert, ML, and Helm-Estabrooks, N: Manual of Aphasia Therapy. Pro-Ed, Austin, 1991.

Chapey, R: Language Intervention Strategies in Adult Aphasia, ed 2. Williams & Wilkins, Baltimore, 1994.

Code, C (ed): The Characteristics of Aphasia. Taylor & Francis, London, 1989.

Goldstein, K: Language and Language Disturbances. Grune & Stratton, New York, 1948.

Levin, H, et al: Neurobehavioral consequences of closed head injury. Oxford Univ Pr, New York, 1982.

Obler, LK, and Albert, ML (eds): Language and Communication in the Elderly. D.C. Heath, Lexington, MA, 1980.

Ponzio, J, et al (eds): Living with Aphasia. Singh Publishers, San Francisco, 1993.

Reinvang, I: Aphasia and Brain Organization. Plenum, New York, 1985.

Sarno, MT (ed): Acquired Aphasia, ed 3. Academic Press, New York, 1998.

Sarno, MT (ed): Acquired Aphasia, ed 3. Academic, San Diego, 1998.

Sarno, MT: Quality of life in aphasia in the first poststroke year. Aphasiology 11:665, 1997.

GLOSSARY

Anarthria: Unintelligible speech resulting from a brain lesion, particularly in the brain stem, causing severe impairment of the motor-speech system. *See also* dysarthria.

Aphasia: Communication disorder caused by brain damage and characterized by an impairment of language comprehension, formulation, and use; excludes disorders associated with primary sensory deficits, general mental deterioration, or psychiatric disorders. Partial impairment is often referred to as *dysphasia*.

Fluent aphasia: A type of aphasia in which speech flows smoothly, with a variety of grammatical constructions and preserved melody of speech; paraphasias and circumlocutions may be present. Auditory comprehension is impaired. Wernicke's aphasia and anomic conduction aphasia are the most common types of fluent aphasia.

Nonfluent aphasia: A type of aphasia in which the flow of speech is slow and hesitant, vocabulary is limited, and syntax is impaired. Articulation may be labored. Broca's aphasia is the most frequently occurring type of nonfluent aphasia.

Global aphasia: Severe aphasia characterized by marked impairments of the production and comprehension of language; all sensory modalities may be impaired. The individual may be unable to use any expressive speech and may use some gestures or pantomime instead. Gestural language may also be impaired. Responses are not necessarily relevant to context.

Apraxia: *See* verbal apraxia.

Articulation: In speech, vocal tract movements for speech and sound production; involves accuracy in placement of the articulators (lips, tongue, velum, or pharynx), timing, direction of movements, speed of response, and neural integration of all events.

Articulation disorder: Omission or incorrect production of speech sounds owing to faulty placement, timing, direction, pressure, speed, or interaction of the lips, teeth, tongue, velum, or pharynx.

Augmentative communication device: A device used by a person impaired by a communication disorder that provides a compensatory means of communication or enhances the individual's residual communication skills. Examples include manual and electronic communication boards.

Communication: Any means by which an individual relates experiences, ideas, knowledge, and feelings to another; includes speech, sign language, body language, gestures, writing; the process by which meanings are exchanged between individuals through a system of symbols.

Consonants: Speech sounds made with (voiced) or without (unvoiced) vocal fold vibration, by certain successive movements of the vocal tract, including the interaction of the articulators (lips, tongue, teeth, velum), which modify, interrupt, or obstruct the exhaled air stream.

> **Fricatives:** A category of speech sounds using friction formed by directing the breath stream with adequate pressure against one or more surfaces, principally, the hard palate, gum ridge behind the upper teeth, and lips. The breath stream is continuously flowing but restricted (e.g., /f/, /v/).

> **Nasals:** A category of speech sounds resulting from the closing of the oral cavity, preventing air from escaping through the mouth, with a lowered position of the velum or soft palate and a free passage of air through the nose; usually voiced but may lose its voicing in combination with voiceless consonants (e.g., /n/, /m/, /ng/).

> **Liquids:** A category of speech sounds made with the soft palate raised (e.g., /l/, /r/).

> **Plosive sounds:** A category of speech sounds produced when the impounded air pressure in the portion of the vocal tract behind the constriction is released through the oral cavity (e.g., /t/ in shor*t*). Plosive sounds are often referred to as "stop" sounds.

> **Semi-vowels:** A category of speech sounds produced by keeping the vocal tract briefly in the vowel-like position, and then changing to the position required for the following vowel in the syllable. Semi-vowel sounds are usually followed by a vowel in whatever syllable they are used (e.g., /w/, /y/, /r/).

Context: Aspects of communicative exchange, such as its purpose, environment, location, knowledge of the participants and their various roles, and the level of formality required by the situation.

Disability: The consequences of an impairment and its impact on everyday personal, social, and vocational life.

Dysarthria: Term for a category of motor speech disorders caused by impairment in parts of the central or peripheral nervous system that mediate speech production. Respiration, articulation, phonation, resonance, and/or prosody may be affected; volitional and automatic actions (e.g., chewing and swallowing) and movement of the jaw and tongue may also be deviant. It excludes apraxia of speech and functional or central language disorders.

> **Ataxic dysarthria:** Dysarthria associated with damage to the cerebellar system that is characterized by speech errors relating primarily to timing, which results in giving equal stress to each syllable. Articulation problems are typically characterized by intermittent errors ranging from mild to severe; vocal quality is harsh, with monotonous pitch and volume; prosody may range from reduced to unnatural stress.

> **Flaccid dysarthria:** Dysarthria associated with disorders of the lower motor neurons that is characterized by mild to marked hypernasality, coupled with nasal emission; continuous breathiness may be present during phonation, with audible inspiration of air; consonant production is imprecise.

> **Mixed dysarthria:** When two or more types of dysarthria coexist, the term mixed dysarthria is used.

> **Spastic dysarthria:** Dysarthria associated with a bilateral upper motor lesion and characterized by imprecise articulation, monotonous pitch and loudness, and poor prosody; muscles are stiff and move sluggishly through a limited range; speech is labored and words may be prolonged; it is often accompanied by facial distortions and short phrasing.

Dysphagia: A swallowing disorder.

Dysphasia: *See* aphasia.

Functional communication: An individual's communicative effectiveness in everyday life; specifically, the ability to communicate needs, desires, and reactions.

Glottis: Vocal apparatus of the larynx, consisting of the true vocal folds and the opening between them.

Handicap: The value that an individual, family, and community place on a disability and the degree to which an individual is disadvantaged because of it.

Impairment: Refers to the pathology itself, including its location and measured size.

Intelligibility: Degree of clarity with which one's utterances are understood by the average listener; influenced by articulation, rate, fluency, vocal quality, and intensity.

Lexicon: (1) The vocabulary or list of all the words in a language. (2) The repertoire of linguistic signs, words, and morphemes in a given language.

Pharynx: Irregular tubular space, considered part of the respiratory and alimentary tracts, which extends from the nasal cavities to the esophagus and is also continuous with the eustachian tubes, mouth, and larynx; in its lower two thirds, it is capable of considerable change of dimension from front to back and from side-to-side, a factor that contributes to the act of swallowing and influences vocal resonance. It is considered the principal resonator of the human voice.

Phoneme: A sound; the basic linguistic units with which words are formed.

Phonology: Study of the sound system of a language.

Pragmatic language: Those nonverbal components of communication that influence the transmission of information (e.g., initiating, turn-taking, maintaining a topic).

Prosody: The melody of speech, determined primarily by modifications of pitch, quality, strength, and duration which are perceived primarily as stress and intonational patterns.

Semantics: Study of meaning in language which includes the relationships of language, thought, and behavior.

Spontaneous recovery: In aphasia, the return, complete or incomplete, of impaired communication skills, usually in the first few months post onset.

Syllables: Units of speech consisting of a vowel for a central phoneme which may stand alone or be surrounded by one or more consonants (e.g., I, in, me, men).

Syntax: The internal structure of language, including the order in which the parts of speech of a language can occur and these relationships among the elements in an utterance. Sometimes referred to as grammar.

Unvoiced (sounds): Denotes sounds produced without vibration of the vocal folds.

Verbal apraxia: Impairment of volitional articulatory movement secondary to cortical, dominant hemisphere lesion manifested in imprecise and awkward articulation, distortion of phoneme production without commensurate pathology to the motor-speech system. Sometimes referred to as speech dyspraxia, apraxia of speech, cortical dysarthria, or phonetic disintegration.

Vocal tract: That part of the speech mechanism above the level of the vocal folds capable of modifying speech sounds generated by the vocal folds, including the pharyngeal, oral, and nasal cavities.

Voiced (sounds): Sounds produced with simultaneous vibration of the vocal folds; includes all vowels, semi-vowels, diphthongs, and voiced consonants.

Vowel: Voiced speech sound resulting from the unrestricted passage of the air stream through the mouth or nasal cavity without audible friction or stoppage. It is described in terms of (a) relative position of the tongue in the mouth; (b) relative height of the tongue in the mouth; and (c) relative shape of the lips.

APPENDIX

Suggested Answers to Case Study Guiding Questions

1. A team conference is scheduled for the patient the day after you assume treatment responsibilities for the patient. What types of information would you obtain in consultation with the speech-language pathologist?

ANSWER
- Information on the patient's preserved auditory comprehension.
- Suggestions for use of a standardized approach among team members to ensure optimum patient comprehension (e.g., how to phrase questions, the most effective method of providing directions, use of body language, and so forth).

2. What communication strategies are generally useful with patients who have sustained a stroke?

ANSWER
- The use of visual cues (such as gestures and facial expressions)
- Supplementing messages with written cues
- Formulation of questions that can be answered with a single-word response
- Allowing extra time for the patient to respond verbally

3. What approach might you use if the patient became frustrated trying to express himself during a physical therapy treatment?

ANSWER: Remain calm and suggest that the patient wait and try again later.

4. As a physical therapist what might you do to decrease the patient's sense of isolation and enhance his emotional well-being?

ANSWER
- Address familiar subjects.
- Allow the patient to talk about his disability and how he feels.
- Let the patient know that you are aware of his emotional distress.

5. In what ways can physical therapy sessions serve to reinforce communication behavior?

ANSWER
- By avoiding variations in verbal commands and (keeping commands consistent) auditory comprehension may be reinforced.
- By engaging the patient in conversation on familiar topics, the patient has an opportunity to use residual communication skills.
- By not correcting the patient's attempt to communicate, supporting his attempts, and accepting less than perfect communication the patient gains confidence in communication.

Orthotic Assessment and Management **31**

Joan E. Edelstein

LEARNING OBJECTIVES

1. Relate the major parts of the shoe to the requirements of individuals fitted with lower-limb orthoses.
2. Compare the characteristics, advantages, and disadvantages of plastics, metals, and other materials used in orthoses.
3. Describe the main components of foot, ankle-foot, knee-ankle-foot, hip-knee-ankle-foot, trunk-hip-knee-ankle-foot, and trunk orthoses.
4. Describe the orthotic options available for patients with paraplegia.
5. Identify the principal features of lower-limb and trunk orthoses that are assessed during the examination process.
6. Describe the physical therapist's role in management of patients fitted with lower-limb and trunk orthoses.
7. Analyze and interpret patient data, formulate realistic goals and outcomes, and develop a plan of care when presented with a clinical case study.

An orthosis is an external appliance worn to restrict or assist motion or to transfer load from one area to another. The older term, brace, can be used synonymously. A splint connotes an orthosis intended for temporary use. Alternative designations, such as walking irons and calipers, give insight into orthotic materials and designs. An orthotist is the health care professional who designs, fabricates, and fits orthoses. *Orthotic* is an adjective, although some use the word as a noun. Archaeological evidence indicates that orthoses have been used at least since the fifth Egyptian dynasty (2750 to 2625 BC). The term orthosis appears to have been coined soon after World War II.

This chapter presents contemporary orthoses for the lower limb and the trunk, and includes descriptions of the most frequently prescribed orthoses, together with key elements in training patients in their use. The focus is on orthotic design characteristics, their biomechanical rationale, merits of specific materials, and criteria for judging the adequacy of orthotic fit, function, and construction.

TERMINOLOGY

Generic terminology is superseding the traditional use of eponyms. Naming orthoses by the joints they encompass and the type of motion control facilitates communication among clinicians and consumers. Thus, *foot orthoses* (FO) are appliances applied to the foot and placed inside or outside the shoe, such as metatarsal pads and heel lifts. *Ankle-foot orthoses* (AFO) encompass the shoe and terminate at some point below the knee. The term replaces the older nomenclature, short leg brace and below-knee orthosis. The *knee-ankle-foot orthosis* (KAFO) extends from the shoe to the thigh; the term is preferable to long leg brace or above-knee orthosis. A *hip-knee-ankle-foot orthosis* (HKAFO) is a KAFO with a pelvic band that surrounds the lower trunk. A *trunk-hip-knee-ankle-foot orthosis* (THKAFO) covers the thorax as well as the lower limbs. A *knee orthosis* (KO) and a *hip orthosis* (HO) are other applications of the same terminology system.

TYPES OF ORTHOSES

Characteristics and functions of the principal FOs, AFOs, KAFOs, HKAFOs, and THKAFOs, and trunk orthoses, together with the clinically important attributes of shoes, will be described. Although physical therapists also encounter KOs, HOs, and orthoses for special purposes, such as management of Legg Calve Perthes' disease, these orthoses are not included because they are used less frequently than the appliances that appear in this chapter.

LOWER-LIMB ORTHOSES

Lower-limb orthoses range from shoes used for clinical purposes to THKAFOs.

Shoes

The shoe is the foundation for most lower-limb orthoses. Each part of the shoe contributes to the efficacy of orthotic management and offers many options for selection.[1,2] Shoes transfer body weight to the ground and protect the wearer from the bearing surface and the weather. The ideal shoe should distribute bearing forces so as to preserve optimum comfort, function, and appearance of the foot. For the individual with an orthopedic disorder, footwear serves two additional purposes: (1) it reduces pressure on sensitive deformed structures by redistributing weight toward pain-free areas; and (2) it serves as the foundation for AFOs and more extensive bracing. Unless the shoe is correctly fitted and appropriately modified, the alignment of the orthosis will not provide the designed pattern of weight bearing. The major parts of the shoe are the upper, sole, heel, reinforcements, and the last (Fig. 31-1). These fea-

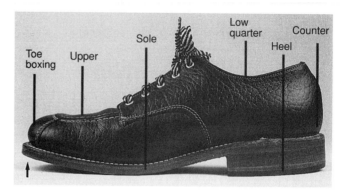

Figure 31-1. Low quarter Blucher shoe.

tures are found in both the traditional leather shoe and the contemporary athletic sneaker.

UPPER

The portion of the shoe over the dorsum of the foot is the *upper* (Fig. 31-2). It consists of an anterior component called the *vamp* and the posterior part, the *quarter*. If the shoe is to be used with an AFO having an insert as its distal attachment, then the vamp should extend to the proximal portion of the dorsum to secure the shoe and the rest of the orthosis high onto the foot. The vamp contains the lace stays, which have eyelets for shoelaces. Laces provide more precise adjustment over the entire opening than do pressure closures. The latter, however, enable some individuals with manual impairment to manage the shoe more easily. For most orthotic purposes, a *Blucher* lace stay is preferable; it is distinguished by the separation between the anterior margin of the lace stay and the vamp. The alternate design is the *Bal, or Balmoral*, lace stay, in which the lace stay is continuous with the vamp. The Blucher opening permits substantial adjustability, an important feature for the patient with edema. It also offers a large inlet into the shoe, so that one can determine that paralyzed toes lie flat within the shoe.

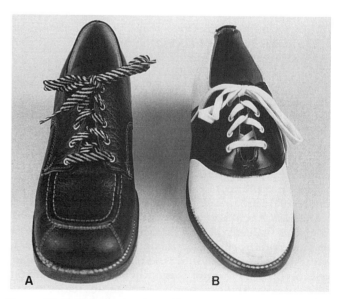

Figure 31-2. Low quarter shoes: (*A*) Blucher and (*B*) Bal (Balmoral).

An extra depth shoe is one having an upper contoured with additional vertical space. The shoe is manufactured with a second inner sole that can be removed to accommodate an insert or thick surgical dressing.

Quarter height is another consideration in shoe prescription. The low-quarter terminates below the malleoli and is satisfactory for most orthotic purposes. This style does not restrict foot or ankle motion and is faster to don. If the patient will be wearing a plastic orthosis molded about the ankle, it should not be necessary to go to the additional expense of providing a high-quarter shoe for ankle support. A high-quarter shoe, covering the malleoli, is indicated to cover the foot having rigid pes equinus. It is also appropriate to augment foot stability in the absence of an AFO. The high-quarter shoe, however, is more difficult to don and more expensive than a comparable low-quarter one.

SOLE

The *sole* is the bottom portion of the shoe. For use with a riveted metal attachment between shoe and orthosis, the sole should have two parts, the outer and the inner sole, both made of leather. Between the two lies a metal reinforcement that receives the rivets. This type of shoe, however, is heavier than an athletic shoe with a single sole. Leather soles absorb little impact shock and provide minimal traction.

Regardless of material, the outer sole should not contact the floor at the distal end; the slight rise of the sole is known as *toe spring* (Fig. 31-3), which allows a rocker effect at late stance. If a lift is added to the sole to compensate for leg length discrepancy, the lift should be beveled to achieve toe spring.

HEEL

The *heel* is the portion of the shoe adjacent to the outer sole, under the anatomical heel. A broad, low heel provides greatest stability and distributes force between the back and front of the foot. For adults, a 1 inch (2.5 cm) heel tilts the center of gravity slightly forward to aid transition through stance phase, but does not disturb normal knee and hip alignment significantly. A higher heel places the ankle in its extreme plantarflexion range and forces the tibia forward. The wearer compensates either by retaining slight knee and hip flexion or by extending the

knee and exaggerating lumbar lordosis. The high heel transmits more stress to the metatarsals. Nevertheless, transferring load anteriorly may be desirable if the patient has heel pain. The higher heel also reduces tension on the Achilles tendon and other posterior structures and accommodates rigid **pes equinus.** Although most heels are made of firm material with a rubber plantar surface, a low resilient heel is indicated to permit slight plantarflexion if the ankle cannot move because of orthotic or anatomical limitation.

REINFORCEMENTS

Reinforcements located at strategic points preserve the shape of the shoe. *Toe boxing* in the vamp protects the toes from stubbing and vertical trauma; it should be high enough to accommodate hammer toes or similar deformity. The *shank* piece is a longitudinal plate that reinforces the sole between the anterior border of the heel and the widest part of the sole at the metatarsal heads. A corrugated steel shank is necessary if an orthotic attachment is to be riveted to the shoe. The **counter** stiffens the quarter and generally terminates at the anterior border of the heel. The patient with **pes valgus,** however, should have a shoe with a long medial counter that provides reinforcement along the medial border of the foot to the head of the first metatarsal, thus resisting the tendency of the foot to collapse medially.

Because reinforcements are not visible in the finished shoe, it is important that the physical therapist become familiar with details of construction of the shoes that are being considered for orthotic wearers.

LAST

The **last** is the model over which the shoe is made. The last, whether of traditional wood, custom-made plaster, or computer-generated design, remains with the manufacturer; the shoe shape duplicates the last's contour. A given shoe size may be achieved with many lasts, each transmitting different forces to the foot. Consequently, the physical therapist should ascertain that the shoe shape fits the foot satisfactorily, rather than relying on a particular shoe size. The patient with a markedly deformed foot requires a shoe made over a special last, either factory- or custom-made.

Foot Orthoses

Foot orthoses are appliances that apply forces to the foot. These may be an **insert** placed in the shoe, an internal modification affixed inside the shoe, or an external modification attached to the sole or heel of the shoe. They can enhance function by relieving pain and improving the wearer's transition during stance phase. Pain may be lessened by transferring weight-bearing stresses to pressure-tolerant sites, and by protecting painful areas from contact with the shoe and with adjacent portions of the foot.

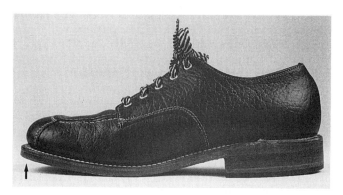

Figure 31-3. Toe spring of anterior portion of sole.

Shoes also may improve gait by modifications to equalize foot and leg lengths on both limbs and by altering the rollover point in late stance. Comfort and mobility can be improved by correcting alignment of a flexible segment, or by accommodating fixed deformity by altering the contour of the shoe. In many instances, a particular therapeutic aim can be achieved by various devices.

INTERNAL MODIFICATIONS

Generally, the closer the modification is to the foot, the more effective it is. Consequently, inserts and internal modifications are widely used. Biomechanically, both are identical. The insert permits the patient to transfer the orthosis from shoe to shoe, if the shoes have the same heel height; otherwise, a rigid insert may rock in the shoe. Most inserts terminate anteriorly, just behind the metatarsal heads; thus, they may slip forward, particularly if the shoe has a relatively high heel. Some inserts extend the full length of the sole, preventing slippage, but occupying the often limited space in the anterior portion of the shoe. Internal modifications are fixed to the shoe's interior, guaranteeing the desired placement, but limiting the patient to the single pair of modified shoes. Both inserts and internal modifications reduce shoe volume, so proper shoe fit must be judged with these components in place.

Inserts made of soft materials, such as the **viscoelastic** plastics (e.g., PPT, Sorbothane, and Viscolas), reduce shear and impact shock, thus protecting painful or sensitive feet.[3] Inserts are also constructed of semirigid or rigid plastics, rubber, or metal, often with a resilient overlay. A heel-spur insert orthosis (Fig. 31-4), for example, may be made of viscoelastic plastic or rubber. In either case, the orthosis will slope anteriorly to reduce load on the painful heel. In addition, the orthosis will have a concave relief to minimize pressure on the tender area.

Longitudinal arch supports are intended to prevent depression of the subtalar joint and flattening of the arch (**pes planus**). The orthosis may include a

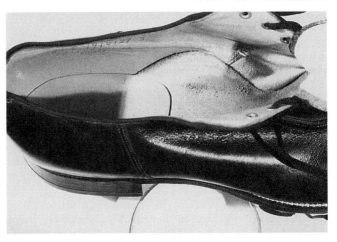

Figure 31-5. Leather scaphoid pad glued to the inside of the shoe.

wedge (post) to alter foot alignment. The minimum support is a rubber **scaphoid pad** (Fig. 31-5) positioned at the medial border of the insole with the apex between the sustentaculum tali and the navicular tuberosity.[4-6] Flexible flat foot can be realigned with a semirigid plastic **University of California Biomechanics Laboratory (UCBL) insert** (Fig. 31-6). It is molded over a plaster model of the foot, taken with the foot in maximum correction. It encompasses the heel and midfoot, applying medialward force to the calcaneus, and lateral and upward force to the medial portion of the midfoot.[7] Inserts are used successfully by runners, who benefit from improved foot alignment.[8]

The **metatarsal pad** (Fig. 31-7) is a convexity that may be incorporated in an insert or may be a resilient domed component glued to the inner sole so that its apex is under the metatarsal shafts. The pad transfers stress from the metatarsal heads to the metatarsal shafts.

Occasionally, modifications are sandwiched between the inner and outer soles; for example, the patient with marked arthritic changes in the front of the foot probably will be more comfortable if the shoe has a long steel spring between the soles to eliminate motion at the painful joints. The same effect can be achieved with a rigid insert.

EXTERNAL MODIFICATIONS

An external modification ensures that the patient wears the appropriate shoes and does not reduce shoe volume, but will erode as the patient walks and is somewhat conspicuous. In addition, the client is limited to wearing the modified shoe, rather than being able to choose from a wide selection of shoes.

A *heel wedge* (Fig. 31-8) is a frequently prescribed external modification. It alters alignment of the calcaneus. A medial heel wedge, by applying laterally directed force, can aid in realigning flexible **pes valgus** or can accommodate rigid **pes varus** by filling the void between the sole and the floor on the medial side. A medial wedge is incorporated in a **Thomas heel,** intended for flexible pes valgus. The anterior border of the Thomas heel extends forward

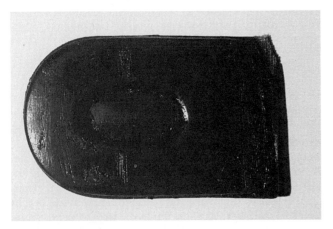

Figure 31-4. Plastic heel spur pad, inferior aspect. Note the depression for spur.

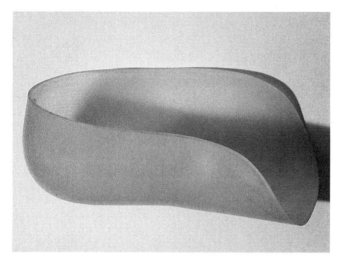

Figure 31-6. University of California Biomechanics Laboratory (UCBL) insert.

on the medial side to augment the effect of the medial wedge in supporting the longitudinal arch. A *cushion heel* is made of resilient material to absorb shock at heel contact. Because it provides slight plantarflexion, the cushion heel is indicated when the patient wears an orthosis with a rigid ankle. Sole wedges alter medial-lateral metatarsal alignment. A lateral wedge shifts weight bearing to the medial side of the front of the foot. It compensates for fixed forefoot valgus, allowing the entire front of the foot to contact the floor.

A **metatarsal bar** (Fig. 31-9) is a flat strip of leather or other firm material placed posterior to the metatarsal heads. At late stance, the bar transfers stress from the metatarsophalangeal joints to the metatarsal shafts. A **rocker bar** is a convex strip affixed to the sole proximal to the metatarsal heads. It reduces the distance the wearer must travel during stance phase, improving late stance,[9,10] as well as shifting load from the metatarsophalangeal joints to the metatarsal shafts.

The patient with leg length discrepancy of more than ½ inch (1 cm) will walk better with a shoe lift

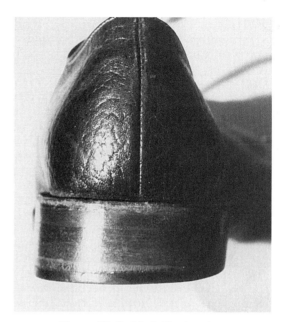

Figure 31-8. Medial heel wedge.

made of cork or lightweight plastic. Approximately ⅜ inch (0.8 cm) of the elevation can be accommodated inside a low-quarter shoe at the heel.

Ankle-Foot Orthoses

The AFO is composed of a foundation, ankle control, foot control, and a superstructure.

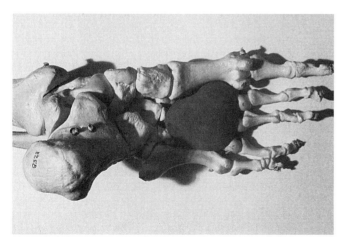

Figure 31-7. Rubber metatarsal tab. Whether used as an internal modification or as part of an insert, the pad should be oriented as shown on the skeleton.

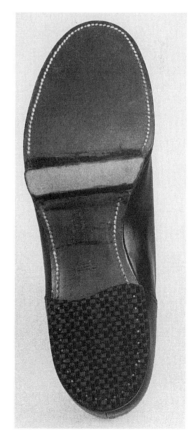

Figure 31-9. Leather outer sole with metatarsal bar.

FOUNDATION

The foundation of the orthosis consists of the shoe and a plastic or metal component.

Foot Plate

An insert or foot plate foundation (Fig. 31-10) is often used; it provides the best control of the foot, because internal modifications can be incorporated. To use an insert, the shoe must close high on the dorsum of the foot to retain the orthosis. The foot plate facilitates donning the orthosis because the shoe can be separated from the rest of the brace. The insert also permits interchanging shoes, assuming that all shoes have been made on the same last, so that the orthosis can exert the intended effect on the lower limb. Less expensive shoes, such as sneakers, can also be worn, because the foundation does not need to be riveted to the shoe. The orthosis with an insert is relatively lightweight because the insert is usually made of a thermoplastic material, such as polyethylene or polypropylene. These materials are heated, then molded over a plaster model of the patient's limb. The orthotist modifies the model, removing some plaster in areas where the orthosis is to apply substantial pressure, and adding plaster where pressure relief is required.

A foot plate foundation is inappropriate if the patient cannot be relied on to wear the orthosis with

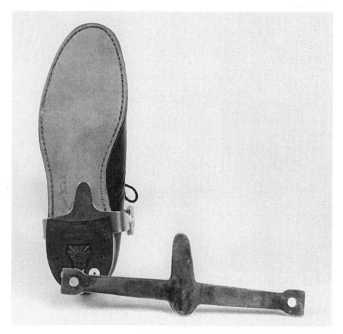

Figure 31-11. Solid stirrup.

a shoe of proper heel height. If the orthosis is placed in a shoe with too low a heel, the uprights would incline posteriorly, increasing the tendency of the wearer's knee to extend.[11] Conversely, if the orthosis is worn with a higher heeled shoe, the patient might experience knee instability. The insert reduces interior shoe volume, and thus must be used with suitably spacious shoes. Custom-molded foot plates may be more expensive than other types of foundations. If the orthosis is to be used by a very obese or exceptionally active individual, a plastic foot plate may not provide adequate support. Some insurance programs insist that the shoe be physically attached to the remainder of the brace in order that the cost of the shoes be reimbursed.

Stirrup

The traditional foundation for the AFO is a steel **stirrup,** a U-shaped fixture, the center portion of which is riveted to the shoe through the shank. The arms of the stirrup join the brace uprights at the level of the anatomical ankle, providing congruency between orthotic and anatomical joints. The **solid stirrup** (Fig. 31-11) is a one-piece attachment that provides maximum stability of the orthosis on the shoe. The **split stirrup** (Fig. 31-12) has three segments. The central portion has a transverse rectangular opening on each side. Medial and lateral angled side pieces fit into the openings. The split stirrup simplifies donning the orthosis because the wearer can detach the uprights from the shoe. If a central piece is riveted to other shoes, then shoes can be interchanged. The extremely active client may dislodge a side piece from its receptacle unintentionally. The split stirrup is bulkier and heavier than a solid stirrup or foot plate.

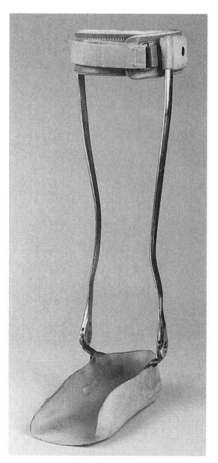

Figure 31-10. AFO with plastic shoe insert.

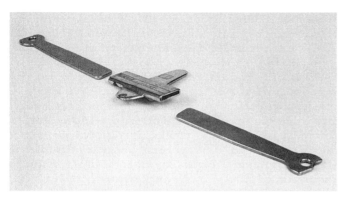

Figure 31-12. Split stirrup.

ANKLE CONTROL

Most AFOs are prescribed to control ankle motion by limiting plantarflexion and/or dorsiflexion, or by assisting motion. The patient with dorsiflexor weakness or paralysis risks dragging the toe during swing phase. Dorsiflexion assistance can be provided by a **posterior leaf spring** that arises from a plastic insert (Fig. 31-13). The upright is bent backward slightly during early stance. When the patient progresses into swing phase, the plastic recoils to lift the foot. Thin, narrow plastic permits relatively greater motion. Motion assistance can also be achieved with a steel dorsiflexion spring assist (Klenzak joint) (Fig. 31-14) incorporated into each stirrup. The coil spring is compressed in stance and rebounds during swing. The tightness of the coil can be adjusted, but the orthosis is noticeably bulkier than the posterior leaf spring model. Both types of spring assists will yield slightly into plantarflexion at heel contact, affording the wearer protection against inadvertent knee flexion.

The alternate approach to prevent toe drag is plantarflexion resistance, which prevents the foot from plantarflexing so that the patient with drop foot will not catch the toe and stumble during swing phase. A *plastic overlap joint* in a hinged solid ankle AFO or a metal *posterior stop* (Fig. 31-15) can be incorporated in the stirrup. The posterior stop tends to impose a flexion force at the knee during early stance and prevents the lax knee from hyperextending.

An *anterior stop* limits dorsiflexion, aiding the individual with paralysis of the triceps surae to achieve late stance. A flexible alternative is a plastic anterior spring extending from the mid dorsum of the foot to the proximal margin of the orthosis.[12]

A *limited motion stop* is a metal joint that resists both plantarflexion and dorsiflexion. **Bichannel adjustable ankle locks (BiCAALs)** (Fig. 31-16) consist of a pair of joints, each of which has an anterior and a posterior spring. Ordinarily, the springs are replaced by metal pins, the lengths of which determine the amount of motion and thus the alignment of the orthosis. The plastic **solid ankle-**

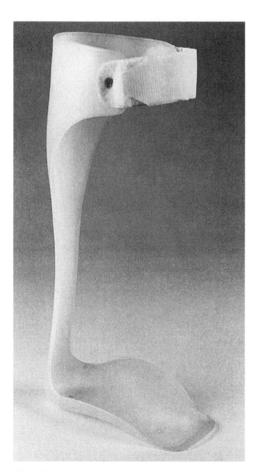

Figure 31-13. Plastic foot plate on posterior leaf spring AFO.

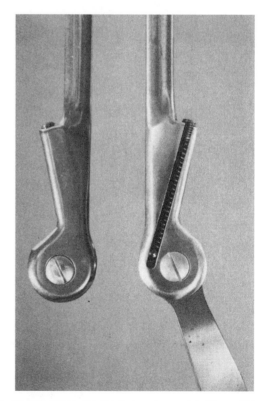

Figure 31-14. Steel dorsiflexion spring assist. (From Fishman, S, et al: Lower-limb orthoses. In American Academy of Orthopaedic Surgeons: Atlas of Orthotics, ed 2. Mosby, St. Louis, 1985, p 203, with permission.)

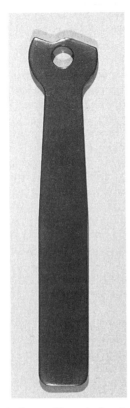

Figure 31-15. Steel stirrup with posterior stop at its proximal end. Stop is to the left.

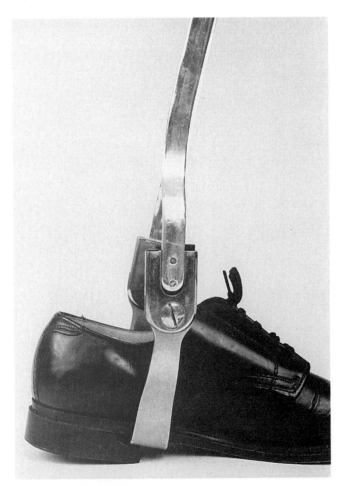

Figure 31-16. BiCAAL joints.

foot orthosis (Fig. 31-17) also limits all foot and ankle motion. Its trimline is anterior to the malleoli. To compensate for lack of plantarflexion in early stance, the shoe used with the solid ankle-foot orthosis or the orthosis with a limited motion stop should have a resilient heel. Similarly, to facilitate early rollover in late stance, the shoe sole should have a rocker bar. The solid ankle orthosis may be divided transversely at the ankle, with the two sections hinged. The **hinged solid ankle-foot orthosis** provides slight sagittal motion, fostering achievement of the foot-flat position in early stance. The joint at the hinge may be a plastic overlap or a plastic rod. A versatile option is a pair of metal hinges that can be adjusted to alter the excursion of ankle motion.

FOOT CONTROL

Medial-lateral motion can be controlled with a solid ankle AFO. The rigidity of the orthosis can be increased by using thicker or stiffer plastic, corrugating the plastic, forming the edges with a rolled contour, or embedding carbon fiber reinforcements. A solid ankle AFO or a hinged solid ankle AFO also controls frontal and transverse plane foot motion. Less effective is a metal and leather orthosis to which a leather valgus (varus) correction strap (Fig. 31-18) is attached. The *valgus correction strap* is sewn to the medial portion of the shoe upper near the sole, and buckles around the lateral upright, exerting a laterally directed force to restrain pronation. The *varus correction strap* has opposite attach-

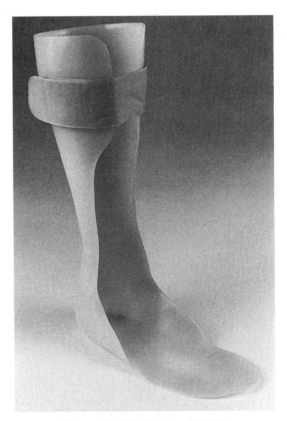

Figure 31-17. Plastic solid AFO.

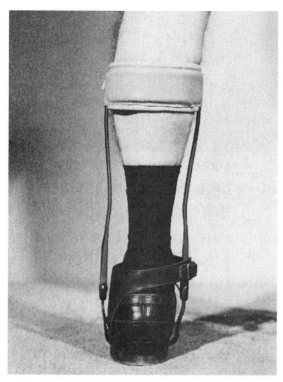

Figure 31-18. Valgus correction strap incorporated in metal and leather AFO. (From Fishman, S, et al: Lower-limb orthoses. In American Academy of Orthopaedic Surgeons: Atlas of Orthotics, ed 2. Mosby, St. Louis, 1985, p 200, with permission.)

ments and force application. Either strap, although adjustable, complicates donning.

SUPERSTRUCTURE

The proximal portion of the orthosis, the superstructure, consists of uprights, and a shell, band, or brim. Plastic AFOs usually have a single upright or shell. The solid ankle and hinged solid ankle AFOs have a posterior shell extending from the medial to the lateral midline of the leg, thus providing excellent medial-lateral control and a broad surface to minimize pressure. The posterior leaf spring AFO has a single posterior upright and thus does not contribute to frontal or transverse plane control. The *spiral AFO* (Fig. 31-19) is a design made of nylon acrylic or polypropylene, in which the single upright spirals from the medial aspect of the foot plate around the leg, terminating medially in a proximal band.[13] The spiral orthosis controls, but does not eliminate, motion in all planes. Orthoses with plastic shells or uprights are molded over a cast of the patient's leg and are designed to fit snugly for maximal control and minimal conspicuousness. Such AFOs are contraindicated for the individual whose ankle and leg volume fluctuates markedly, because the orthoses cannot be adjusted readily.

Metal and leather orthoses usually have medial and lateral uprights to maximize structural stability. Occasionally, a single side upright will suffice when a less conspicuous orthosis is required and the wearer is not expected to exert undue force. Aluminum uprights are of lighter weight than steel; to increase the rigidity of the orthosis, a broader bar of aluminum can be used. Carbon graphite uprights weigh appreciably less than aluminum and rival the strength of steel; however, orthoses made of the newer material are more expensive.

Most orthoses have a posterior *calf band* made of plastic or leather-upholstered metal. The band has an anterior buckled or pressure closure strap (Fig. 31-20). The farther the band is from the ankle joint, the more effective the leverage of the orthosis; however, the band must not impinge on the peroneal nerve. An anterior band that is part of a solid ankle AFO imposes posteriorly directed force near the knee, enabling the AFO to resist knee flexion.[14] Such an orthosis is sometimes known as a **floor reaction orthosis.** In fact, all orthoses are influenced by the floor reaction when the wearer stands or is in the stance phase of gait. If the AFO is to reduce the amount of weight transmitted through the foot, it may have a **patellar-tendon-bearing brim** (Fig. 31-21), resembling a transtibial (below-knee) prosthetic socket. The plastic brim has a slight indentation over the patellar ligament (tendon), and is hinged to facilitate donning. The brim must be used with a plastic solid ankle or a metal limited-motion ankle joint.

Tone-reducing orthoses are plastic AFOs designed for children with spastic cerebral palsy and adults with spastic hemiplegia. The foot plate and broad upright are designed to modify reflex hypertonicity by applying constant pressure to the plantar-

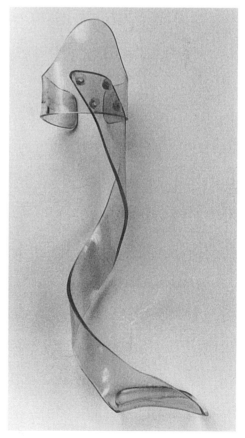

Figure 31-19. Spiral AFO.

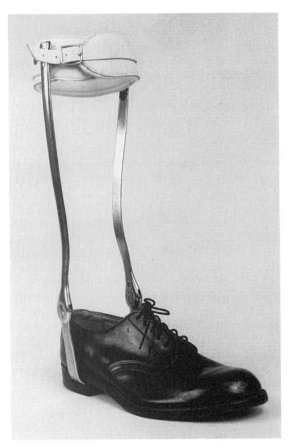

Figure 31-20. AFO with stirrup attachment, limited motion ankle joints, bilateral uprights, and upholstered metal calf band.

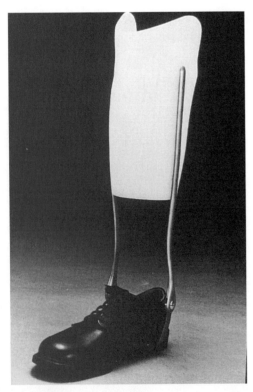

Figure 31-21. AFO with stirrup, hinged ankle joint, steel uprights, and plastic patellar-tendon-bearing brim.

flexors and invertors. They are particularly useful for individuals who have moderate spasticity with varus instability, but do not have fixed deformity. They control the tendency of the foot to assume an equinovarus posture; in addition, some versions have a foot plate that maintains the toes in an extended or hyperextended position, thus assisting children who have spasticity to walk with better foot and knee control. Similar versions have proved successful with adults who have sustained cerebral vascular accident.[15,16] Before a custom-made plastic orthosis is ordered, however, the patient should be assessed in a tone-reducing cast that subjects the limb to the same pressures as will the orthosis.

Knee-Ankle-Foot Orthoses

Individuals with more extensive paralysis or limb deformity may benefit from KAFOs, which consist of a shoe, foundation, ankle control, knee control, and superstructure. KAFOs often include a foot control. The shoe, foundation, ankle control, and foot control of the KAFO may be selected from the components already described. Donning a plastic and metal KAFO is appreciably faster than putting on a metal and leather orthosis.[17]

KNEE CONTROL

The simplest knee joint is a hinge. Because most KAFOs include a pair of uprights, the orthosis has a pair of knee hinges that provide medial-lateral and hyperextension restriction while permitting knee flexion.

The **offset joint** (Fig. 31-22) is a hinge placed posterior to the midline of the leg. The patient's weight line falls anterior to the offset joint, stabilizing the knee in extension during the early stance phase of gait when the wearer is on a level surface. The offset joint does not hamper knee flexion during swing or sitting. The joint may, however, flex inadvertently when the wearer walks on ramps. The joint is contraindicated in the presence of knee flexion contracture.

The most common knee control is the *drop ring lock* (Fig. 31-23). When the client stands with the knee fully extended, the ring drops, preventing the uprights from bending. Both medial and lateral joints should be locked for maximum stability. A pair of drop ring locks is thus inconvenient, unless each upright is equipped with a spring-loaded **retention button.** The button permits the wearer to unlock one upright, then attend to the other one without having the first lock drop. The buttons also enable the physical therapist to give the patient a trial period of walking with the knee joints unlocked.

The **pawl lock** with **bail** release (Fig. 31-24) also provides simultaneous locking of both uprights. The pawl is a spring-loaded projection that fits into a notched disk. The patient unlocks the brace by pulling upward on the posterior bail. Some people are agile enough to be able to nudge the bail by pressing it against a chair. The bail is bulky and may

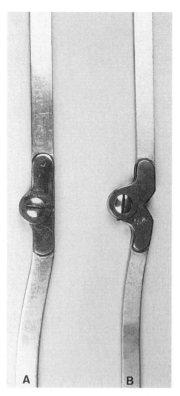

Figure 31-22. Knee joint-offset hinge.

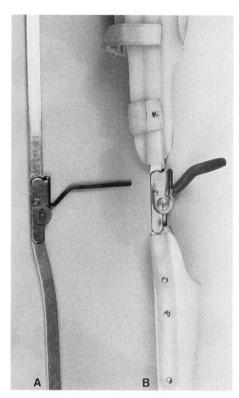

Figure 31-24. Pawl lock: basic component *(A)* and pawl lock installed in KAFO with bail shaped to curve posteriorly *(B)*.

release the locks unexpectedly if the wearer is jostled against a rigid object.

The offset joint and the basic drop ring and pawl locks are contraindicated in the presence of knee flexion contracture. If one cannot achieve full passive knee extension, an adjustable knee joint (Fig.

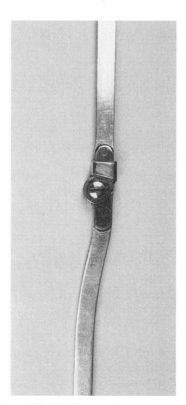

Figure 31-23. Hinge with drop ring lock.

31-25) is required. Such joints have a drop ring lock for stability in the partially flexed attitude.

Sagittal stability is augmented by a kneecap (Fig. 31-26) or anterior band or strap (Fig. 31-27) that completes the three-point pressure system necessary for stability. The cap or band applies a posteriorly directed force to complement the anteriorly directed forces from the back of the shoe and the thigh band. The leather kneecap is the traditional component. It has four straps buckled to both uprights above and below the knee and applies a posteriorly directed force to oppose any tendency of the knee to flex. The kneecap requires the patient to buckle two straps when donning the orthosis. When the straps are tight enough to stabilize the knee, the pad is likely to restrict flexion when the wearer sits. A more practical alternative is a rigid anterior band, either a pretibial band or a suprapatellar band, both of which apply posteriorly directed force,[18] but do not interfere with sitting and are easier to don. The bands generally are molded of plastic and are not readily adjustable. The prepatellar band rests over the bony proximal portion of the leg and requires careful contouring to be comfortable. The suprapatellar band fits over the fleshy anterodistal thigh.

Frontal plane control may be achieved with plastic calf shells shaped to apply corrective force for **genu valgum** or **genu varum.** To reduce genu valgum, the medial portion of the shell extends proximally in order to apply laterally directed force at the knee. The semirigid shell is more effective than a valgum correction strap, which is a kneecap with a fifth strap designed to be buckled around the lateral

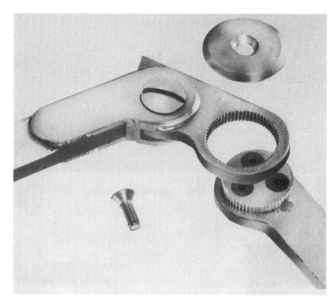

Figure 31-25. Serrated knee lock. Note the location of the knee hinge and the serrated disk, (From Fishman, S, et al: Lower-limb orthoses. In American Academy of Orthopaedic Surgeons: Atlas of Orthotics, ed 2. Mosby, St. Louis, 1985, p 213, with permission.)

upright. The opposite force application is indicated for the patient who has genu varum. The shell does not require time in donning and applies force over a broad area without impinging on the popliteal fossa.

When control in the transverse plane, as well as the frontal and sagittal planes, is required, the *Oregon Orthotic System* incorporating rigid plastic AFOs or KAFOs may be effective. The AFO version includes a foot plate, BiCAAL ankle joints, bilateral

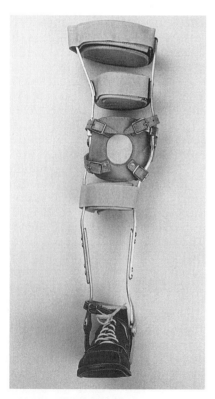

Figure 31-26. KAFO with knee cap.

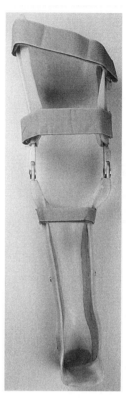

Figure 31-27. KAFO with Velcro webbing anterior prepatellar and supracondylar bands.

uprights, and an anterior band over the proximal leg. The KAFO model adds thigh uprights and thigh bands. The orthoses are aligned to establish triplanar control at the foot, ankle, and knee joints by strategic placement of the ankle and knee joint axes.

SUPERSTRUCTURE

Thigh bands provide structural stability to the orthosis. If the distal portion of the limb cannot tolerate full weight bearing, then the proximal thigh band may be shaped to form a weight-bearing brim. Either the quadrilateral or the ischial containment design can be used. To eliminate all weight bearing through the entire leg, the orthosis must include a weight-bearing brim, a locked knee joint, and a **patten** bottom. The patten is a distal extension that keeps the shoe on the braced side off the floor. To maintain a level pelvis, the patient must also wear a lift on the opposite shoe; the height of the lift should equal the height of the patten.

Hip-Knee-Ankle-Foot Orthoses

Addition of a pelvic band and hip joints converts the KAFO to an HKAFO.

HIP JOINT

The usual hip joint is a metal hinge (Fig. 31-28) that connects the lateral upright of the KAFO to a pelvic band. The joint prevents abduction and adduction, as well as hip rotation. If the patient requires only control of hip rotation, a simpler alterna-

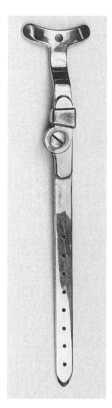

Figure 31-28. Hip joint with drop ring lock.

tive to the hip joint and pelvic band is a webbing strap. To reduce internal rotation, the strap resembles a prosthetic Silesian bandage. To reduce external rotation, the strap joins the lateral uprights

of the KAFOs and passes anteriorly at the level of the groin. If flexion control is required, a drop ring lock is added to the hip joint. A two-position lock stabilizes the patient in hip extension for standing and walking, and at 90 degrees of hip flexion for sitting.

PELVIC BAND

An upholstered metal band (Fig. 31-29) will anchor the HKAFO to the trunk. The band is designed to lodge between the greater trochanter and the iliac crest on each side. HKAFOs are not used very often because they are much more awkward to don than KAFOs, and, if the hip joints are locked, they restrict gait to the swing-to or swing-through pattern. The pelvic band is likely to be uncomfortable when the wearer sits.

Trunk-Hip-Knee-Ankle-Foot Orthoses

Patients who require more stability than provided by HKAFOs may be fitted with THKAFOs (Fig. 31-30), which incorporate a lumbosacral orthosis attached to KAFOs. The pelvic band of the trunk orthosis serves as the pelvic band used on HKAFOs. Because the THKAFO is very difficult to don and is heavy and cumbersome, it is seldom worn after the client is discharged from the rehabilitation program. Alternative orthoses providing standing stability, with or without provision for walking, are available for individuals with paraplegia.

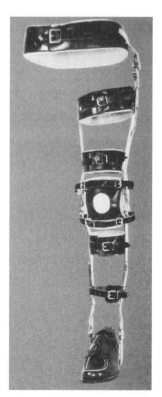

Figure 31-29. HKAFO with stirrup; steel uprights; hinged ankle, knee, and hip-joints; drop ring locks at the knee and hip; and pelvic band.

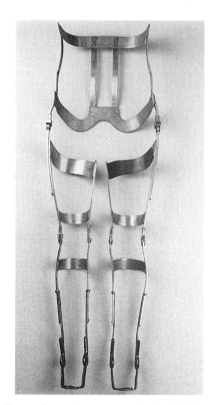

Figure 31-30. THKAFO without upholstery.

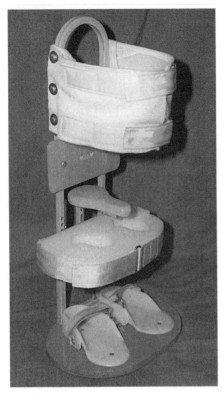

Figure 31-31. Standing frame. (Courtesy of Variety Village, Electro Limb Production Centre, Scarborough [Toronto], Ontario, Canada.)

Orthotic Options for Patients with Paraplegia

Orthoses are often prescribed for patients with spina bifida, spinal cord injury, or other disorders that result in paraplegia. The functional goals for such people include standing to maintain skeletal, renal, respiratory, circulatory, and gastrointestinal function and some form of ambulation.[19,20] Upright posture also affords the individual important psychological benefits.

MASS-PRODUCED ORTHOSES

Several appliances are readily available for children with spina bifida or other disorders resulting in paraplegia. The appliances provide the youngster with considerable function and are less expensive and easier to don than custom-made orthoses.

Standing Frame and Swivel Walker

Designed for children, the **standing frame** (Fig. 31-31) consists of a broad base, posterior nonarticulated uprights extending from a flat base to a midtorso chest band, and a posterior thoracolumbar band. Anterior leg bands contribute to stability. The child wears ordinary shoes without any special attachments. The shoes are strapped to the base of the frame.

A similar orthosis is the **swivel walker,** which is made in both child and adult sizes.[21] The major difference is the base, which has two distal plates that rock slightly to enable a swiveling gait.

The mass-produced frame and walker are less expensive than custom-made orthoses. They permit the wearer to stand without crutch support, freeing the hands for play or vocational activities. With either device, the user can move from place to place by rotating the upper torso to shift weight, causing the frame to rock and rotate alternately on one edge then the other.

Parapodium

The **parapodium** (Fig. 31-32) differs from the standing frame by virtue of joints that permit the wearer to sit. The base is flat. The stabilizing points on the standing frame, swivel walker, and the parapodium are the same. One version of parapodium has a provision for keeping the knees locked while the child unlocks the hips for leaning forward to pick up objects from the floor.[22] Crutchless ambulation in the parapodium is achieved by using the same technique as with the standing frame. For walking longer distances, the youngster uses crutches or a walker in the swing-to or swing-through pattern. Both the standing frame and the parapodium are worn on the outside of trousers, which school-age children eventually find cosmetically objectionable.

CUSTOM-MADE ORTHOSES

Whereas the mass-produced devices afford considerable function to their users, many individuals seek more streamlined orthoses. Custom-made AFOs, KAFOs, and THKAFOs provide sufficient rigidity, either by metal joints or anatomical alignment, to enable selected patients to stand. Ambulation requires crutches or similar aids, together with

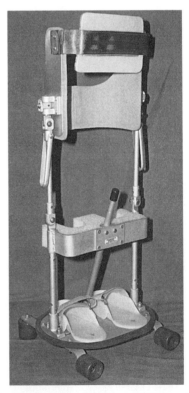

Figure 31-32. Parapodium. (Courtesy of Variety Village, Electro Limb Production Centre, Scarborough [Toronto], Ontario, Canada.)

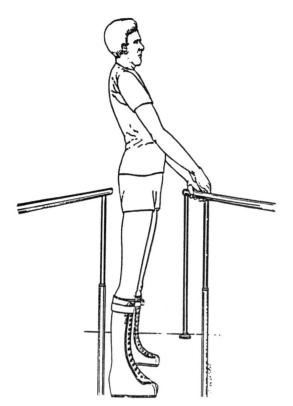

Figure 31-33. Standing balance with lumbar lordosis using stabilizing boots set in approximately 15 degrees of plantarflexion. (From Kent,[23] p 304, with permission.)

well-coordinated use of the upper trunk and upper limbs. Some patients may not realize the extent of the physical conditioning program required to prepare them for ambulation. Consequently, a trial period is advisable using mass-produced, adjustable, temporary orthoses.

Stabilizing Boots

AFOs designed for adults with paraplegia include a pair of plastic orthoses molded to conform to the patient's legs and feet (Fig. 31-33). The foot plate is angled at approximately 15 degrees plantarflexion to shift the wearer's center of gravity anterior to the ankles.[23,24] The plastic component is inserted into leather boots with flat soles. The legs are thus inclined posteriorly to keep the knees extended. The patient maintains standing stability by leaning backward, with the iliofemoral ligaments resisting a backward fall. Crutches, a walker, or a pair of canes are needed for two- or four-point gait. Ambulation requires shifting the upper torso diagonally forward to allow one leg to swing ahead. The orthoses are easy to don and do not restrict sitting. The candidate must not have any hip or knee flexion contractures, and must be able to extend the hips and lumbar trunk fully.

Craig-Scott KAFOs

A pair of **Craig-Scott KAFOs** (Fig. 31-34) is often prescribed for adults with paraplegia. The original design of each orthosis included a shoe reinforced

with transverse and longitudinal plates, BiCAAL ankle joints set in slight dorsiflexion, a pretibial band, a pawl lock with bail release, and a single thigh band.[25] An alternate version substitutes a plastic solid ankle section for the reinforced shoe and metal ankle joints.[26] The orthosis enables the patient to stand with sufficient backward lean so as to prevent untoward hip or trunk flexion. The gait pattern usually is swing-to or swing-through, with the aid of crutches or a walker. Although the orthoses do not restrict hip motion, the patient with thoracic spinal injury cannot flex the hips voluntarily, and the orthosis has no mechanism to aid single-leg progression. Some individuals perform a two- or four-point gait by shifting the trunk enough to allow the leg to swing forward in a pendular manner.

A new version of Craig-Scott KAFOs is the *Walkabout orthosis*, which consists of a pair of KAFOs with a hinge mechanism joining the medial uprights of the two orthoses. The mechanism permits hip flexion and extension, but restricts abduction, adduction, and rotation.[27,28]

Reciprocating Gait Orthosis

Both children and adults can be fitted with a **reciprocating gait orthosis (RGO)** (Fig. 31-35), a THKAFO in which the hips are joined by one or two metal cables.[29–33] The knees are stabilized with knee locks, offset knee joints, or pretibial bands, and the feet are encased in solid ankle orthoses. The latest version has no thigh shells. To walk, the wearer uses a four-stage procedure: (1) shift weight to the right

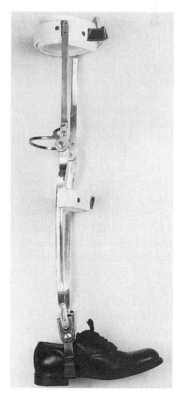

Figure 31-34. Craig-Scott KAFO.

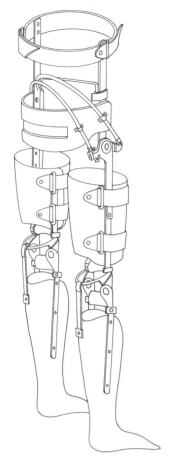

Figure 31-35. Reciprocating gait orthosis. (From *LSU* Reciprocating Gait Orthosis: A Pictorial Description and Application Manual. Durr-Fillauer Medical, Chattanooga, TN, 1983, p 14, with permission.)

leg, (2) tuck the pelvis by extending the upper thorax, (3) press on the crutches, and (4) allow the left leg to swing through. The procedure is reversed for the next step. The steel cable(s) prevent inadvertent hip flexion on the supporting leg. Reciprocal four- or two-point gait is stable, because one foot is always on the floor, but the pace is slow. For sitting, the wearer releases the cable(s) to enable the hips to flex.[34,35]

ParaWalker

The **ParaWalker**[36] is a THKAFO that has exceptionally sturdy hip joints; these limit the excursion of hip flexion and resist hip abduction and adduction as the wearer shifts weight from side-to-side during ambulation. The shoes fit into loops on flat foot plates. The gait maneuver is the same as used with the RGO.

Functional Electrical Stimulation

Orthoses may be combined with functional electrical stimulation (FES) to enable selected patients to achieve household, or in rare cases, community ambulation.[37] This technique involves the use of electrical current to produce muscular contractions. Typically, stimulation is provided to the quadriceps and gluteus maximus. If the ankles are not supported by AFOs, then the system also includes surface elec-

trodes over the peroneal nerves to initiate dorsiflexion, as well as reflex hip flexion. The candidate should have full passive mobility in all joints and should be able to use a control system that regulates the timing and amount of current needed to transfer from the chair to the standing position and to walk in various directions. FES is occasionally used to foster lower-limb exercise, thereby maintaining muscle bulk and reducing the risk of pressure ulcers.

TRUNK ORTHOSES

Trunk orthoses may be used in association with lower-limb orthoses or may be worn to reduce the disability caused by low-back pain, neck sprain, scoliosis, or other skeletal or neuromuscular disorders. Although the traditional name for an orthosis that encompasses the torso is *spinal orthosis,* in fact, such an appliance does not contact the spine directly. By supporting the trunk, the orthosis assists in controlling spinal motion; however, forces that the orthosis exerts are modified by the skin, subcutaneous tissue, and musculature that surround the vertebral column, and, in the case of higher orthoses, by the thoracic cage. Patients with spinal cord injury benefit from trunk orthoses in two ways: (1) the orthoses impart control of motion of the lumbar region, with or without thoracic control, and (2) they compress the abdomen to improve respiration. Individuals with cervical lesions may need to wear an orthosis that restrains neck motion until stability is achieved by surgery or other means. A special group of trunk orthoses has been designed for children and adolescents with scoliosis.

Corset

If abdominal compression is the sole goal, a **corset** (Fig. 31-36) will suffice. It is a fabric orthosis that has no horizontal rigid structures, although frequently it has vertical rigid reinforcements. The corset may cover only the lumbar and sacral regions, or may extend superiorly as a thoracolumbosacral corset. The primary effect of a corset is to increase intra-abdominal pressure.

Some individuals with low-back disorders find that corsets relieve pain.[38,39] The increase in intra-abdominal pressure reduces stress on posterior spinal musculature, thus diminishing the load on the lumbar intervertebral disks. Although temporary reduction of abdominal and erector spinae muscular activity is therapeutic, long-term reliance on a corset can promote muscular atrophy and contracture, as well as psychological dependence on the appliance.

Rigid Orthoses

Most lumbosacral and thoracolumbosacral orthoses include a corset or a fabric abdominal front to compress the abdomen. Rigid orthoses are distinguished by the presence of horizontal, as well as vertical, rigid plastic or metal components. Motion limitation is accomplished by a series of three-point pressure systems, in which force in one direction is counteracted by two forces in the opposite direction.

LUMBOSACRAL FLEXION, EXTENSION, LATERAL CONTROL ORTHOSIS

A typical example of a rigid trunk orthosis is the lumbosacral flexion, extension, lateral control (LS FEL) orthosis (Fig. 31-37), also known as a **Knight spinal orthosis.** This appliance includes a pelvic band, which should provide firm anchorage over the midsection of the buttocks, and a thoracic band, intended to lie horizontally over the lower thorax without impinging on the scapulae. The bands, which may be foam-lined rigid plastic or leather-upholstered metal, are joined by a pair of posterior uprights, which lie on either side of the vertebral spines, and a pair of lateral uprights placed at the lateral midline of the torso. A corset or abdominal front completes the LS FEL orthosis. The orthosis restrains flexion by a three-point system consisting of posteriorly directed force from the top and bottom of the abdominal front or corset and an anteriorly directed force from the midportion of the posterior uprights. Extension is controlled by posteriorly directed force from the midsection of the abdominal front or corset and anteriorly directed force from the thoracic and pelvic bands.[40] The lateral uprights resist lateral flexion.[41]

A plastic lumbosacral jacket restricts motion in all directions, and is effective in the management of selected patients who complain of low-back pain.[42] An alternate version combining the jacket with the LS FEL has been shown to be effective at controlling spondylolisthesis.[43]

THORACOLUMBOSACRAL FLEXION, EXTENSION CONTROL ORTHOSIS

Also called a **Taylor brace,** the thoracolumbosacral flexion, extension control (TLS FE) orthosis

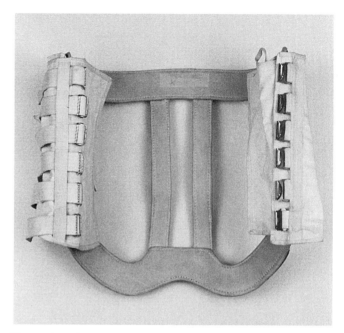

Figure 31-37. Lumbosacral flexion-extension-lateral control orthosis.

consists of a pelvic band, posterior uprights terminating at midscapular level, an abdominal front or corset, and axillary straps attached to an interscapular band. This orthosis reduces flexion by a three-point system consisting of posteriorly directed force from the axillary straps and the bottom of the abdominal front or corset, and anteriorly directed force from the midportion of the posterior uprights. Extension resistance is provided by posteriorly directed force from the midsection of the abdominal front or corset and anteriorly directed force from the pelvic and interscapular bands. Addition of lateral uprights converts the orthosis to a TLS FEL orthosis (Fig. 31-38). A plastic thoracolumbosacral jacket limits trunk motion in the frontal, sagittal, and transverse planes, and provides maximum support.

Cervical Orthoses

Cervical orthoses are classified according to design characteristics.[44–46] Minimal motion control is provided by *collars* (Fig. 31-39) that encircle the neck with fabric, resilient material, or rigid plastic. A few collars encompass the chin and posterior head (Fig. 31-40) for slightly greater restraint. For moderate control, a **four-post orthosis** (Fig. 31-41) is used. Usually it has two anterior adjustable posts joining a sternal plate to a mandibular plate and two posterior uprights connecting a thoracic plate to an occipital plate. The sternal plate is strapped to the thoracic plate and the occipital plate is strapped to the mandibular plate.

Maximum orthotic control of the neck may be achieved either with a Minerva[47] or a **halo**[48,49] orthosis (Fig. 31-42). The **Minerva orthosis** is a noninvasive appliance that has a rigid plastic posterior section extending from the head to the midtrunk; the superior portion is held in place by a

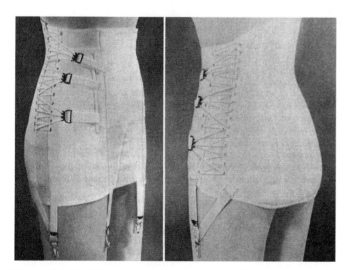

Figure 31-36. Women's model of a canvas lumbosacral corset. (Camp International, 1991, BISSELL Healthcare Corporation.)

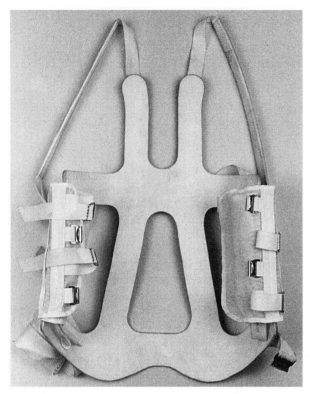

Figure 31-38. Thoracolumbosacral flexion-extension-lateral control orthosis.

forehead band. The halo orthosis has a circular band of metal that is fixed to the skull by four tiny screws. Uprights connect the halo to a thoracic orthosis.

Scoliosis Orthoses

Children and adolescents with thoracic, thoracolumbar, or lumbar scolioses or kyphoses may be fitted with a TLS orthosis that applies forces to realign the vertebral column and thoracic cage. Although substantial improvement is evident when the

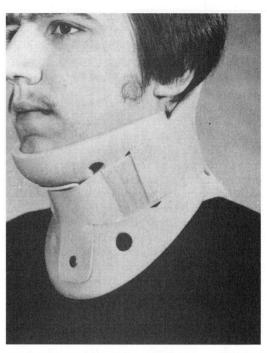

Figure 31-40. Philadelphia collar. (Camp International 1991, BISSELL Healthcare Corporation.)

orthosis is worn, long-term follow up indicates that the major achievement is that the orthosis prevents the curve from increasing beyond its original contour.[50–52] The **Milwaukee orthosis**[53] (Fig. 31-43) is often prescribed. The orthosis consists of a frame composed of a pelvic girdle, two posterior uprights, an anterior upright, and a superior ring. Unlike the original Milwaukee orthosis, the current version fea-

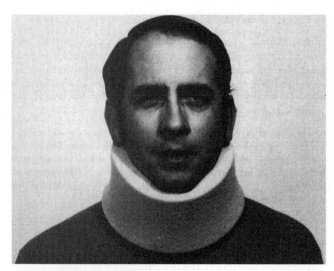

Figure 31-39. Soft foam rubber collar. (Camp International 1991, BISSELL Healthcare Corporation.)

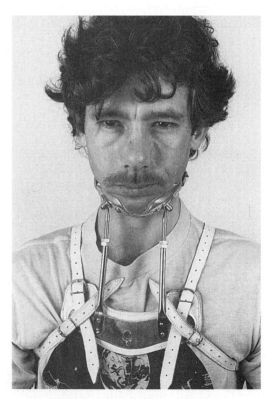

Figure 31-41. Four-poster cervical orthosis.

extend as high as the Milwaukee orthosis; its foundation is a mass-produced plastic module that the orthotist alters to meet the needs of the individual patient. The **Wilmington orthosis**[56] is another design that is in current use. It consists of a custom-made thoracolumbosacral jacket intended to guide the trunk to straighter alignment. These and most other scoliosis orthoses are most effective on patients who have immature spines and moderate vertebral curves in the midthoracic or more inferior portions of the trunk. The classic protocol required the youngster to wear the orthosis 23 hours each day; however, part-time wearing is almost as effective in terms of maintaining trunk alignment and is better tolerated by adolescent patients.[57] Another approach to scoliosis management requires the patient to wear an orthosis only at night when the effects of gravity are minimized. One example is the **Charleston bending brace,**[58] which provides overcorrection of the spinal curve.

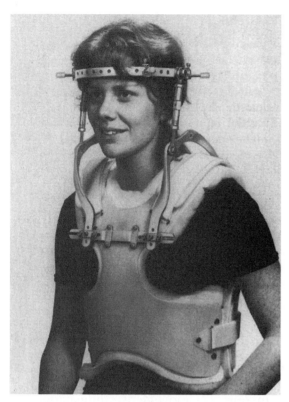

Figure 31-42. Halo-vest orthosis. (Courtesy Durr-Fillauer Medical, Chattanooga, TN.)

ORTHOTIC MAINTENANCE

To obtain the best service from orthoses, the patient should observe basic routine inspection and care procedures. Written instructions help reinforce the recommendations of the orthotist and therapist.

tures a superior ring that lies on the upper chest and can be hidden by most clothing. Various pads are strapped to the frame to apply corrective forces. The **Boston orthosis**[54,55] (Fig. 31-44) usually does not

Shoes

Whether or not the shoe is attached directly to the orthosis, it is important that footwear be kept in

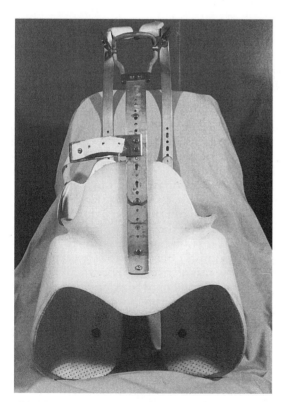

Figure 31-43. Anterior view of the plastic and metal Milwaukee orthosis.

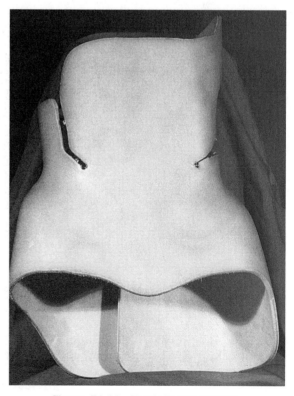

Figure 31-44. Plastic Boston orthosis.

good condition, with replacement of the sole and heel as soon as moderate wear is evident. The replacements should include whatever wedges, bars, or elevations were originally prescribed. The patient who tends to strike on the toe may need metal toe plates to preserve the sole. Shoes that are outgrown or distorted will not afford the wearer optimal function from the orthosis. If a stirrup is attached to the shoe, the patient should inspect the rivets to make certain that none have separated; if they have, the shoe should be returned to the orthotist for repair.

Clean hose without holes or repairs should be worn. In addition, long hosiery or cotton leggings shield the leg from pressure at the edges of the brace uprights, bands, and shells.

Shells, Bands, and Straps

Plastic bands and shells should be wiped with a damp cloth to remove any surface soil. It is inadvisable to try to hasten drying by using a hair dryer or other heat source that might soften the plastic. The patient should check the plastic periodically for any cracking; if any is noted, the orthosis should be brought to the orthotist for immediate repair. Pressure straps eventually become infiltrated with lint, which interferes with the hook and loop closing action; the straps should be inspected to determine when they should be replaced. Leather bands require periodic cleaning and can be washed with mild saddle soap. If the original leather deteriorates to the point that portions of the underlying metal are exposed, new leatherwork is required. Leather straps eventually become brittle and may break. A loss of flexibility indicates that it is time to replace the straps, before they break.

Uprights

In a plastic and metal KAFO for a child, the metal upright is screwed or riveted to the plastic shell. The orthosis can be lengthened by removing the fasteners and inserting them in new holes drilled farther up on the calf shell and farther down on the thigh shell. In a metal and leather AFO or KAFO for a child, the uprights are overlapped and secured with screws. The screws tend to work loose, reducing the stability of the orthosis. This problem should be reported to the orthotist. The orthosis is lengthened by removing all screws, setting the uprights at the appropriate distance, and reinserting the screws.

Joints and Locks

Metal components should be kept away from sand, liquids, and other foreign substances. If the joints do not articulate smoothly or become noisy or if the locks do not engage properly, then cleaning and lubrication may remedy the problem. Otherwise, professional attention is required.

PHYSICAL THERAPY MANAGEMENT

Physical therapists participate in management of the wearer of an orthosis (1) prior to orthotic prescription, (2) at orthotic prescription, (3) upon delivery of the orthosis, and (4) during training to facilitate proper use and care of the orthosis. In the ideal situation, the therapist is a member of an orthotic clinic team, working directly with the physician and orthotist to develop the orthotic prescription and assess the patient and orthosis before and after training. The physical therapist is also responsible for training the patient. Whether or not the hospital or rehabilitation center has a clinic team, the physical therapist is expected to accomplish the following:

1. Perform the preorthotic assessment.
2. Contribute to the orthotic prescription (analyze potential of orthotic components to remediate impairment, functional limitation, or disability).[59]
3. Assess the prescribed orthosis through analysis of (1) effects and benefits in terms of improved function, (2) movement while patient wears the device, (3) practicality and ease of use, (4) alignment and fit, and (5) safety during use of device.[59]
4. Facilitate orthotic acceptance.
5. Train the patient to don, use, and maintain the orthosis.

Preprescription Assessment

Matching the patient's biomechanical requirements to the appropriate orthosis requires careful assessment.

JOINT MOBILITY

A thorough goniometric examination, including both active and passive ranges of motion, is a prerequisite to orthotic prescription. If the patient has a fixed foot deformity, either the shoe will have to be modified to accommodate the foot, or an insert will have to be fabricated. In either instance, the goal is to achieve comfortable contact of the entire plantar surface of the foot on the inner sole of the shoe. Knee flexion contracture necessitates prescription of accommodative joints, because the regular drop ring and pawl locks can be used only with a knee that can be brought to the fully extended position. Hip flexion contracture precludes the prescription of orthoses that depend on alignment for stability, such as the offset knee joint, stabilizing boots, or Craig-Scott KAFOs.

LIMB LENGTH

The therapist should ascertain whether there is a discrepancy in leg length. If the patient can stand, one can check the pelvis to determine if it is level. For the recumbent individual, one can measure each lower extremity from the anterior superior iliac spine to the medial malleolus. With a difference of more than ½ inch (1 cm) there should be compensation by a shoe elevation. For the patient with weakness in one limb, a ½-inch (1-cm) lift on the contralateral shoe will aid clearance of the paralyzed leg during swing phase.

MOTOR FUNCTION

The manual muscle test should be augmented by an assessment of functional activities to determine what substitutions the patient is able to make to accomplish standing and walking. Although the muscle test may reveal marked weakness, if the patient can manage without an orthosis, it is unlikely that it will be accepted. For example, the person with dorsiflexor paralysis who can ambulate by exaggerating hip flexion during swing phase may not agree to an AFO with a posterior stop. An important consideration in assessment of motor function is that traditional manual muscle tests are inappropriate in the presence of marked spasticity. In such instances, functional tests of motor performance are essential.

SENSATION

The clinician should record the extent of any sensory loss. Intimately fitted plastic orthoses are satisfactory for individuals with sensory loss if the edges of the orthosis are smooth and the orthosis does not pinch the patient's flesh. Proprioceptive loss may indicate the need for orthotic stabilization, such as a solid ankle AFO to control a Charcot neuropathic ankle. Patients should be taught to regularly inspect the skin (including presence of volume changes) and instructed to bring any changes to the attention of the physical therapist for assessment.

UPPER LIMBS

Although the patient is being considered as a candidate for lower-limb or trunk orthoses, the therapist must determine the mobility and motor power of the upper limbs. Significant weakness, stiffness, or deformity will interfere with donning the orthosis. Substitution of pressure closures for leather buckles may suffice. If the individual cannot ambulate without canes or crutches, the therapist should determine whether standard aids will be satisfactory or whether modification of the hand pieces is required. If the upper limbs are very weak, the patient will not be able to use the lower-limb orthoses for walking. Alternate standing arrangements may be preferable, such as the use of a standing frame, standing table, or standing wheelchair to provide weight-bearing stress.

PSYCHOLOGICAL STATUS

Realistic orthotic prescription requires ascertaining that the patient is willing to wear the orthotic device. The patient with a recent spinal cord injury may still deny the permanence of paralysis and thus be against wearing orthoses that are visible reminders of disability. The adolescent with spina bifida may prefer to sit unbraced in a wheelchair rather than struggle with donning orthoses and walking slowly, in a manner very different from the individual's peers. The patient with spinal cord injury must be prepared to work vigorously to increase upper limb and trunk strength and aerobic capacity. The person who has sustained a cerebral vascular accident resulting in severe perceptual deficiency may not be able to walk, even with orthotic assistance, because the environment now seems unfamiliar. An orthosis for prevention of deformity may be prescribed, rather than one that is designed to aid gait.

The therapist should determine the extent to which the patient is likely to comply with instructions pertaining to orthotic use and care. For example, if it is doubtful that the individual will wear appropriate shoes with an insert orthosis, then the prescription should specify stirrup attachment to suitable shoes.

Orthotic Prescription

Lower-limb orthoses benefit individuals with a wide variety of musculoskeletal and neurological disorders. The particular diagnosis is less important in formulating the prescription than consideration of the patient's impairments and functional limitations. Prognosis also influences prescription. The person who is likely to recover partial or full function should have an orthosis that can be adjusted to accommodate the changing status. An individual with recent hemiplegia, for example, may exhibit marked spasticity, indicating a need for a limitation in motion at the ankle. As the person regains voluntary control and spasticity decreases, the ankle can be adjusted to permit more movement.

Life-style has a bearing on orthotic selection. A very active patient requires an orthosis made of exceptionally sturdy materials. Split stirrups, for example, may not be appropriate because they can spring loose from the receptacle on the shoe if excessive medial-lateral stress is applied. The patient's concern with appearance is another practical consideration; it may dictate use of a shoe insert so that reasonably fashionable shoes may be worn. Similarly, plastic shells are less bulky than metal uprights and calf bands, and do not present a shiny metal appearance. Although most people want the orthosis to be as inconspicuous as possible, some children and adults opt for bright colors, which can be achieved with various plastics.

ANKLE-FOOT ORTHOSES

The primary candidates for AFOs are those with peripheral neuropathy, especially peroneal lesions, and hemiplegia. Those with foot drag can be fitted with an AFO with a posterior stop; this design, however, tends to cause the knee to flex excessively in early stance when controlled plantarflexion is normally achieved. In the absence of plantarflexion, the patient may flex the knee to effect a foot-flat position. The alternative is a resilient shoe heel, or an AFO with a plastic posterior leaf spring or a metal dorsiflexion spring assist, both of which permit controlled plantarflexion early in stance to prevent knee stress.

Orthotic management of a patient with hemiplegia depends on the extent of spasticity and paralysis. If the motor loss is confined to poor dorsiflexion, the posterior leaf spring AFO suffices. An even simpler and less expensive option is a ½-inch (1-cm) lift on the heel and sole of the contralateral shoe to provide clearance for the paretic limb during swing phase. Those with medial-lateral and sagittal plane instability require an AFO with limited-motion ankle joints or a plastic spiral AFO. With pain or severe instability, a solid ankle AFO is required. In the presence of severe spasticity, a spring assist for joint motion is contraindicated because the spring action may serve to increase spasticity.

KNEE-ANKLE-FOOT AND OTHER LOWER-LIMB ORTHOSES

A KAFO may be used to compensate for paralysis of the entire leg. The physical therapist should assess the patient with a temporary orthosis to proceed more confidently with prescription of an expensive, custom-made orthosis. Several versions of temporary orthoses are manufactured and prove exceedingly useful in demonstrating whether the patient is likely to benefit from orthotic knee control.

Stabilizing AFOs, Craig-Scott KAFOs, HKAFOs, the reciprocating gait orthosis, and the ParaWalker are options for patients with paraplegia. For the child, the orthotic program should start with a simple standing frame and progress to the parapodium before involving the child in the greater expense and donning difficulty of form-fitting bracing. Children and adults may begin with a swivel walker or lightweight modular frames.

TRUNK ORTHOSES

A corset may be adequate to increase intra-abdominal pressure and thereby reduce the discomfort of low-back pain. Where greater motion restriction is indicated, such as for the individual with trunk paralysis, the LS FEL, TLS FE, or TLS FEL orthosis will provide substantial support. Plastic lumbosacral or thoracolumbosacral jackets offer maximum support. Cervical orthoses, whether collars or post devices, restrain motion and remind the wearer not to move the head in an abrupt manner. Collars also retain body heat, which may prove therapeutic. For maximum neck control, a Minerva or halo orthosis is required.

An array of orthoses have been designed for management of patients with scoliosis. These include the Milwaukee orthosis, which is the most extensive, as well as the Boston and Wilmington orthoses, which do not terminate quite so high on the trunk.

Orthotic Assessment

Assessment is an essential element of orthotic management. The physical therapist should be certain that the orthosis fits and functions properly before attempting to train the patient to use it. Analysis may be conducted under the aegis of a formal orthotic clinic team. If so, when the orthosis is delivered, the team should assess the adequacy of the orthosis as pass, provisional pass, or fail. *Pass* indicates that the orthosis is altogether satisfactory and the patient is ready for training. *Provisional pass* means that minor faults exist, generally having to do with the cosmetic finishing of the appliance; the patient can wear the orthosis in the training program without harmful effect. *Failure* signifies that the orthosis has a major defect that would interfere with training; for example, shoes that are too tight for the patient. The problem must be resolved before training can begin. If the orthosis is not prescribed by a clinic team, then the physical therapist should use the assessment procedure to assure that the orthosis meets the patient's needs. Final assessment is performed at the conclusion of training to reassess the fit and function of the orthosis and the patient's skill in using it.

LOWER-LIMB ORTHOTIC STATIC ASSESSMENT

Assessment involves both static *assessment* of the orthosis on the patient while standing and sitting, as well as examination of the device off the individual. *Dynamic assessment* refers to analysis of the wearer's gait.

The orthosis is assessed as the wearer stands and sits. The patient's skin and the construction of the orthosis are checked with the orthosis off the patient. The orthosis should be compared with the prescription. Departures from the original specifications must be approved by the individual(s) who developed the prescription.

The patient should stand in parallel bars, or other secure environment, and should attempt to bear equal weight on both feet. The shoe should fit satisfactorily, particularly in length, width, and snugness of the counters. Whether or not wedges or lifts have been added to the shoe, the sole and heel should rest flat on the floor, except for the distal portion, which should curve upward slightly to aid in late stance. The ankle joint should be at the distal tip of the medial malleolus to be congruent with the anatomical ankle and avoid vertical motion of the orthosis on the leg during gait.

The calf band should terminate below the fibular head to avoid impingement on the peroneal nerve. If a patellar-tendon-bearing brim is used, it should have a concave relief to limit pressure on the fibular head. This component does not eliminate distal weight-bearing; however, one should judge to see that the shoe heel is somewhat unloaded. This can be estimated by placing a ribbon in the shoe before the patient dons the shoe. One end of the ribbon hangs out the back of the shoe. When the patient stands with the shoe and orthosis on, the therapist should be able to pull the ribbon out of the shoe. The calf shell, band, or patellar-tendon-bearing brim should not intrude on the popliteal fossa so that the patient has difficulty flexing the knee when sitting. Donning ease is affected by the type of closure of both the shoe and band.

The mechanical knee joints should be congruent with the anatomical knee; for the adult, the usual placement is approximately three-quarters of an inch (2 cm) above the medial tibial plateau. The knee lock should function properly, because use of a lock is often the major reason for wearing a KAFO. The medial upright should terminate approximately 1½ inches (4 cm) below the perineum. The calf and distal thigh shells or bands should be equidistant so that when the orthosis is flexed, as in sitting, the plastic or metal parts will contact one another, rather than pinch the back of the wearer's leg.

If the KAFO has a quadrilateral brim to reduce weight-bearing through the bony skeleton, the brim should have adequate provision for the sensitive adductor longus tendon and should provide a sufficient seat for the ischial tuberosity.

The pelvic joint is set slightly above and anterior to the greater trochanter to compensate for the usual angulation of the femoral neck; setting the joint anterior to the trochanter takes into account the medial rotation of the femur. The pelvic band should conform to the contours of the wearer's torso, without edge pressure.

When the brace is off, the therapist should inspect the patient's skin to detect any irritations attributable to the orthosis. One should move the joints slowly to check range of motion. *Binding* refers to tilting of the distal portion of the joint in relation to the proximal member so as to interfere with movement. If the medial and lateral stops do not contact their respective stops at the same time, the stop that contacts first will erode rapidly and may contribute to twisting of the orthosis.

DYNAMIC ASSESSMENT

The gait pattern exhibited by the person who wears an orthosis reflects both the contribution of the wearer's physique and the orthotic motion control and assistance. Table 31–1 relates orthotic and anatomical causes of the most commonly observed gait deviations. It should be noted that observational gait analysis is a moderately reliable assessment; sagittal plane deviations are easier to judge than are those that occur in the frontal or transverse plane.[60]

During early stance the patient may exhibit foot slap, striking with toes first, or flat-foot contact, indicating inability to restrain plantarflexion or failure of the orthosis to support the foot and ankle. Excessive medial or lateral contact may indicate that the orthosis does not track the way the patient's limb does. Knee hyperextension or excessive flexion indicates that the orthosis is not applying adequate control. A posterior stop on the AFO should prevent the lax knee from hyperextending. If the patient wears a KAFO and has knee hyperextension, the stops in the knee joint are set improperly or have eroded, or the calf and thigh shells or bands are too deep. Anterior and posterior trunk bending are seen at early stance when the patient attempts to control a weak knee or hip. If the quadriceps are weak, the patient will bend forward. The person who fears that the knee may collapse may benefit from an AFO with a solid ankle and an anterior band, or a KAFO with a knee lock. If the gluteus maximus is weak, the individual is apt to lean backward. Lordosis indicates hip flexion contracture or a KAFO that does not fit properly. Lateral trunk bending in early stance phase may result from hip abductor weakness or hip instability; however, uncompensated shortness of the limb will also give rise to this problem, as will a medial upright on a KAFO that is too high, or an abducted pelvic joint on an HKAFO. A wide walking base may be the patient's compensation for a medial upright or shell that impinges into the perineum.

The client may have difficulty during late stance either delaying weight transfer or being unable to transfer weight over the paralyzed foot. The problem can be mitigated with an anterior stop and a rocker bar. One should be certain that the trimlines of the solid ankle AFO or the stops on the stirrup function properly.

During swing phase the patient must be able to clear the floor with the braced leg. Hip hiking occurs when the hip flexors are weak, as well as when the limb is functionally longer than the contralateral limb. Increased length may be produced by a faulty posterior stop that no longer limits plantarflexion, or by a locked knee joint. The problem should be anticipated and, for the unilateral KAFO wearer, can be prevented by adding a ½-inch (1-cm) lift to the contralateral shoe. Internal or external hip rotation may be caused by motor imbalance between medial and lateral musculature; the orthotic causes relate to malalignment of the brace. Similarly, excessive medial or lateral foot contact may indicate that the orthosis does not track the way the patient's limb does. A walking base that is abnormally wide can be caused by a limb that is longer than that on the opposite side. Vaulting refers to exaggerated plantarflexion on the contralateral limb during swing phase of the affected side. Vaulting occurs because the braced leg is functionally too long, possibly because the posterior ankle stop has eroded or a knee lock is used. The less agile patient may obtain foot clearance by hip hiking, that is, elevating the pelvis on the swing side.

TRUNK ORTHOSIS STATIC ASSESSMENT

Lumbosacral and thoracolumbosacral orthoses usually include thoracic and pelvic bands, which should fit flat against the trunk without edge pressure. Uprights should not press against bony prominences, particularly when the patient sits. The abdominal front should extend from just below the xiphoid process to just above the pubic symphysis.

Table 31–1 ORTHOTIC GAIT ANALYSIS

Deviation	Orthotic Causes	Anatomical Causes
Early Stance		
1. Foot slap: forefront slaps the ground	Inadequate dorsiflexion assist Inadequate plantarflexion stop	Weak dorsiflexors
2. Toes first: tiptoe posture may or may not be maintained throughout stance	Inadequate heel lift Inadequate dorsiflexion assist Inadequate plantarflexion stop Inadequate relief of heel pain	Short leg Pes equinus Extensor spasticity Heel pain
3. Flat foot contact: entire foot contacts ground initially	Inadequate traction from sole Requires walking aid, e.g., cane Inadequate dorsiflexion stop	Poor balance Pes calcaneus
4. Excessive medial (lateral) foot contact: medial (lateral) border contacts floor	Transverse plane malalignment	Weak invertors (evertors) Pes valgus (varus) Genu valgum (varum)
5. Excessive knee flexion: knee collapses when foot contacts ground	Inadequate knee lock Inadequate dorsiflexion stop Plantarflexion stop Inadequate contralateral shoe lift	Weak quadriceps Short contralateral leg Knee pain Knee and/or hip flexion contracture Flexor synergy Pes calcaneus
6. Hyperextended knee: knee hyperextends as weight is transferred to leg	Genu recurvatum inadequately controlled by plantarflexion stop Excessively concave calf band Pes equinus uncompensated by contralateral shoe lift Inadequate knee lock	Weak quadriceps Lax knee ligaments Extensor synergy Pes equinus Short contralateral leg Contralateral knee and/or hip flexion contracture
7. Anterior trunk bending: patient leans forward as weight is transferred to leg	Inadequate knee lock	Weak quadriceps Hip flexion contracture Knee flexion contracture
8. Posterior trunk bending: patient leans backward as weight is transferred to leg	Inadequate hip lock Knee lock	Weak gluteus maximus Knee ankylosis
9. Lateral trunk bending: patient leans toward stance leg as weight is transferred to leg	Excessive height of medial upright of KAFO Excessive abduction of hip joint of HKAFO Insufficient shoe lift Requires walking aid, e.g., cane	Weak gluteus medius Abduction contracture Dislocated hip Hip pain Poor balance Short leg
10. Wide walking base: heel centers more than 4 in (10 cm) apart	Excessive height of medial upright of KAFO Excessive abduction of hip joint of HKAFO Insufficient lift on contralateral shoe Knee lock Requires walking aid, e.g., cane	Abduction contracture Poor balance Short contralateral leg
11. Internal (external) rotation: limb internally (externally) rotated	Uprights incorrectly aligned in transverse plane Requires orthotic control, e.g., rotation control straps, pelvic band	Internal (external) hip rotators spastic External (internal) hip rotators weak Anteversion (retroversion) Weak quadriceps: external rotation
Late Stance		
1. Inadequate transition: delayed or absent transfer of weight over the forefoot	Plantarflexion stop Inadequate dorsiflexion stop	Weak plantarflexors Achilles tendon sprain or rupture Pes calcaneus Forefoot pain
Swing		
1. Toe drag: toes maintain contact with ground	Inadequate dorsiflexion assist Inadequate plantarflexion stop	Weak dorsiflexors Plantarflexor spasticity Pes equinus Weak hip flexors
2. Circumduction: leg swings outward in a semicircular arc	Knee lock Inadequate dorsiflexion assist Inadequate plantarflexion stop	Weak hip flexors Extensor synergy Knee and/or ankle ankylosis Weak dorsiflexors Pes equinus
3. Hip hiking: leg elevated at pelvis to enable the limb to swing forward	Knee lock Inadequate dorsiflexion assist Inadequate plantarflexion stop	Short contralateral leg Contralateral knee and/or hip flexion contracture Weak hip flexors Extensor synergy Knee and/or ankle ankylosis Weak dorsiflexors Pes equinus
4. Vaulting: exaggerated plantarflexion of contralateral leg to enable the limb to swing forward	Knee lock Inadequate dorsiflexion assist Inadequate plantarflexion stop	Weak hip flexors Extensor spasticity Pes equinus Short contralateral leg Contralateral knee and/or hip flexion contracture Knee and/or ankle ankylosis Weak dorsiflexors

The cervical orthosis should hold the head in the best tolerated position. Rigid components, such as a mandibular plate, occipital plate, sternal plate, or thoracic plate should be shaped to apply maximum area to the body segment.

Facilitating Orthotic Acceptance

Clinic team management is valuable in fostering acceptance of the orthosis by the patient. The team also enables clinicians to join efforts to help the client achieve the maximum benefit from orthotic rehabilitation. Bringing the new wearer of an orthosis in contact with other users in the physical therapy department can help the new patient recognize that orthotic use is not a strange occurrence. Peer support groups for patients and their families are helpful for sharing concerns and anxieties, and reaching workable solutions to common problems. Support groups usually are organized for people having particular disabilities, such as paraplegia or hemiplegia; many clients will have orthoses as part of their rehabilitation. The physical therapist can guide some meetings of the group. The therapist works most closely with the patient, usually on a daily basis, and thus is able to identify those individuals whose response to disability is sufficiently aberrant as to require psychological attention.

Orthotic Training

Orthoses are designed to provide the individual with a maximum of function with a minimum of discomfort and effort. No single training program suits every orthosis wearer because of the wide range of disorders for which orthotic management is indicated. To the extent possible, however, the physical therapist should instruct the patient in the correct manner of donning the orthosis, developing standing balance, walking safely, and performing other ambulatory activities.

Optimal performance depends on the favorable interaction of many factors. Foremost is the extent of skeletal and neuromuscular involvement. The mobility, strength, and coordination of all body segments, especially in the lower limbs and trunk, are important, as are the individual's muscle tone, cardiovascular and pulmonary health, body weight, psychological status, and chronological age. The quality of the orthosis also influences the client's achievements.

Most orthosis wearers have chronic conditions, such as rheumatoid arthritis, or permanent sequelae from trauma, such as paraplegia following spinal cord injury. Orthotic management enhances function without necessarily influencing the underlying pathology. Training prepares the patient for lifelong activity with an orthosis. Persons with reversible disorders, such as peroneal nerve injury, often benefit from temporary use of an orthosis. Such individuals should learn proper use of the orthosis to prevent secondary disorders and should receive reassessment so that the orthosis may be altered as the condition changes. Patients with progressive disorders, such as muscular dystrophy and multiple sclerosis, require vigilant reassessment so that the extent of physical deterioration may be reflected in orthotic changes, as well as continual training to cope with altered functional abilities. For all situations, a carefully devised exercise and activity program should enable the patient to manage efficiently for maximum independence.

DONNING ORTHOSES

Regardless of type of orthosis, the patient should wear clean, properly fitting hose. The AFO with shoe insert is most easily donned by applying the orthosis to the foot and leg, prior to placing the braced limb in the shoe. If the AFO has a split stirrup, the shoe should be donned first; then the orthosis should be fitted into the box caliper on the shoe. If the AFO has a solid stirrup, the patient will have to insert the foot into the shoe, then fasten the calf band.

The same general procedures are useful with KAFOs. The patient may find donning easier if the brace is applied while lying on a bed or a mat table. If the KAFO is donned while the patient sits, the therapist should check the tightness of the kneecap, if this component is part of the orthosis. A kneecap that is comfortable for sitting will probably be too loose for effective knee control when the wearer stands. Donning HKAFOs and THKAFOs is much more arduous. The beginner should lie on a mat table alongside the orthosis. By rolling to one side, the patient should be able to pull the brace under the legs so as to permit lying in it. Then the patient dons the shoes and fastens the various straps.

Lumbosacral and thoracolumbosacral corsets and rigid orthoses should be donned while the patient is supine to achieve maximum compression of the abdomen. The orthosis should be fastened from the bottom upward.

STANDING BALANCE

The problem of standing safely is most difficult for the individual who wears a pair of KAFOs or more extensive bracing. In ordinary standing, all weight passes through the feet, whereas when standing and walking with orthoses and crutches, the patient must learn to distribute weight partly on the hands and partly on the feet. The line of gravity falls within a tripod bounded by the hands and feet. The tripod is a compromise between leaning too far forward on the hands, to increase stability at the price of fatiguing the arms, and leaning too far backward, which reduces arm strain but makes balance precarious. As balance improves, the patient uses the hands only for balance, rather than for substantial weight-bearing.

The person who wears bilateral KAFOs will need crutches or other aids for independent gait. A prerequisite for crutch ambulation is the ability to shift weight. Shifting weight to the heels takes pressure off the hands so they can be moved. Using parallel bars, the beginner shifts all weight to the feet and raises and lowers one hand, then the other hand. The goal is to be able to lift both hands simultaneously, as may be done with crutches when performing a drag-to or similar gait. Once the patient is able to shift weight from the feet to the hands and back to the feet confidently, the same exercise should be done with crutches. Advanced skills, such as moving the hands and eventually the crutches, behind the body, should be practiced. Those who will walk in reciprocal fashion, alternating footsteps, need to practice diagonal weight shifting.

GAIT TRAINING

The various crutch gaits differ in the sequence of crutch and footsteps. Patterns vary in speed, safety, and amount of energy required. The patient should learn as many gaits as possible, so as to modify walking in crowds, over long distances, and in situations in which speed is desired. In addition to walking forward, the client needs to be able to walk sideward, turn corners, and maneuver on different surfaces, such as rugs, gravel, grass, and through doors. A repertoire of gaits permits the client to adjust to environmental requirements.

Gait selection depends on the individual's functional ability, including:
1. *Step ability:* Can the patient take steps with either or both lower limbs?
2. *Weight-bearing and balance ability:* Can the patient bear weight and remain balanced on one or both lower limbs?
3. *Upper-limb power:* Can the patient push the body off the floor by pressing down on the hands?

Reciprocal Gaits

The four- and two-point gaits require that one move the lower limbs alternately by hip flexion or pelvic elevation. The patient shifts weight as each limb is moved. The four-point sequence is (1) right hand, (2) left foot, (3) left hand, and (4) right foot. The two-point sequence requires greater balance and coordination, but is a faster mode of walking: (1) right hand and left leg; (2) left hand and right leg. The patterns also are useful when one is confronted with crowds or slippery surfaces. These gaits are suited to persons who lack the coordination and balance needed for simultaneous gaits.

Simultaneous Gaits

If both lower limbs are moved simultaneously, the patient places considerable stress on the upper limbs. The series includes the drag-to, swing-to, and swing-through patterns. Although the swing-through gait can be performed rapidly, simultaneous gaits generally are slow and very fatiguing, because the upper limbs are poorly adapted for ambulatory function; a sizable amount of nonfunc-

tioning bodily structure must be controlled by a smaller muscular apparatus. The weight of the orthoses, and in the case of a patient with spinal cord lesion, absence of peripheral sensation, aggravate the problem of using a simultaneous gait pattern.

The drag-to gait is the most elementary of the group, but it is very slow. The sequence is (1) advance both hands, then (2) push on the crutches enough to drag the feet forward. The feet do not pass ahead of the hands. The swing-to pattern is more rapid, because the patient swings rather than drags the lower limbs. Swinging is accomplished by extending the elbows and depressing the shoulder girdle to elevate the trunk and lower limbs. The swing-through gait is the most advanced pattern, requiring much balance, strength, and coordination of the upper limbs, because the patient swings the legs beyond the hands, or crutch tips. The sequence is (1) advance both hands, (2) swing both legs to a point in front of the hands to reverse the basic tripod position, and (3) advance both hands to the starting position. The swing-through gait requires extensive preliminary training, including push-ups to strengthen the arms. The gait is rapid but requires more floor space than the other patterns, to permit alternate swinging of legs and crutches. Detailed instructions in gait training are provided in Chapters 14 and 27.

The ultimate test of walking proficiency is the ability to conduct a conversation while ambulating, an activity pattern that indicates some degree of automatic functioning. Practice in the clinical setting should be extended to walking on varied terrain, indoors and outdoors.

ACTIVITIES

The patient should learn as many ADLs as the physical condition permits. Daily life often involves negotiating stairs, curbs, and ramps, as well as transferring from the chair to the upright position, and into an automobile. Instruction in driving a suitably equipped automobile is an important part of rehabilitation. Not all individuals who wear orthoses achieve the full range of ambulatory activities, yet they benefit from partial independence in accomplishing tasks, at least from the psychological and physiological values attendant to ambulation.

Final Assessment and Follow-up Care

Prior to discharge, the orthosis wearer and the brace should be reassessed to make certain that fit, function, appearance, and use are acceptable. The patient should return to the hospital or rehabilitation center at regular intervals so that the clinic team can monitor the individual's function and the orthosis, and can spot incipient abrasions or other signs of misfit or disrepair. The follow-up visit also enables the physical therapist to reinforce skills taught in the intensive program and address any new problems the patient may present.

Functional Capacities

The patient's ambulatory ability and capacity for other physical activities reflect both orthotic and anatomical factors. Energy measurement is a valuable guide to functional capacity. Energy cost is calculated from the amount of oxygen consumed as the subject performs. Consumption may be determined either per unit of distance traversed or per unit of time. One tends to select a walking speed that requires the least energy per unit of distance. If the energy cost is too high, the patient will realize that ambulation is not a practical mode of locomotion. Sometimes, high energy cost is tolerable for short distances, as in household ambulation. Community ambulation, however, demands sustained effort for longer distances, plus the ability to maneuver over curbs and other irregularities in the walking surface. Many energy studies have been conducted with the two largest groups of individuals who wear orthoses, namely those with paraplegia and those with hemiplegia.

PARAPLEGIA

The level of spinal cord damage is a critical determinant of functional capacity. Investigators generally conclude that functional ambulation is not feasible for those with lesions above the T11 segment of the spinal cord. Subjects consume more energy and walk more slowly with the Walkabout as compared with the reciprocating gait orthosis.[28] Children wearing the reciprocating gait orthosis while performing the swing-through crutch gait have approximately the same energy expenditure as when propelling a wheelchair.[61] Adults with thoracic injuries consume nine times the energy expended by nondisabled individuals per meter, while those with lumbar lesions require triple the normal amount of oxygen, when walking at self-selected speeds. Those with high-level paraplegia use three times their own basal oxygen rate ambulating with Craig-Scott KAFOs; they choose a very slow walking pace. Subjects with lesions between T11 and L2 wearing bilateral KAFOs select walking speeds less than half that of nondisabled persons, with oxygen uptake six times normal. Wheelchair propulsion by the same group increases oxygen uptake less than 10 percent more than normal, at a considerably faster speed.[62,63] The very high energy cost may be accounted for by the fact that the lower-limb paralysis requires that the individual move by upper limb and thoracic action, usually in a swing-to or swing-through gait. This pattern is extremely strenuous, taxing nondisabled adults by at least 75 percent more energy than normal walking.

Of less significance in determining functional capacity is the type of orthosis. Restraining both plantarflexion and dorsiflexion, as provided by Craig-Scott KAFOs, reduces energy demand very slightly. Ankle restraint, however, makes no appreciable difference in the energy required to negotiate stairs and ramps. Performance is somewhat more efficient with molded plastic KAFOs, which weigh slightly less than traditional metal and leather braces. Most subjects fitted with both the ParaWalker and the reciprocating gait orthosis preferred the latter primarily because of its appearance and perception of stability.[35]

One should not lose sight of the principal purpose of ambulation, namely to get from one place to another, rather than to execute an exhausting physical stunt. The near universal abandonment of orthoses by individuals with thoracic spinal cord injury upon discharge from the rehabilitation center attests to the fact that most decide that accomplishing vocational and recreational tasks is more important than struggling with brace donning and energy costly ambulation.

HEMIPLEGIA

Although the increased energy demand occasioned by hemiplegic ambulation is not nearly as dramatic as that for paraplegic gait, the cost should be considered in planning reasonable goals. Energy cost rises in proportion to the amount of spasticity. The increase ranges from no appreciable difference for persons with hemiplegia to a 100 percent increase for relatively inexperienced walkers. On average, comfortable gait is approximately half the speed of that for nondisabled individuals.

The type of orthosis does not appear to make much difference in functional capacity, although patients with hemiplegia perform more efficiently with some form of AFO than without any bracing. Investigation of the factors that influence energy expenditure, especially physical status, help the clinician plan the most appropriate rehabilitation program and forecast long-term performance.

SUMMARY

This chapter has focused on lower-limb and trunk orthoses. The most frequently prescribed orthoses and orthotic components have been presented. In addition, the responsibilities of the physical therapist in orthotic management have been emphasized.

Ideally, an orthosis is prescribed by an orthotic clinic team composed of a physician, physical therapist, and orthotist. The prescription should be based on a thorough assessment, with particular attention to the specific factors discussed in this chapter. Input from the patient and all team members during the decision making process is critical. This approach will ensure an optimum match between the patient's biomechanical and psychological requirements and an appropriate orthosis capable of performing its intended function. Once the orthosis has been prescribed, it should be evaluated to ensure satisfactory fit, function, and construction, and the patient should have the benefit of a suitable training program for donning the orthosis and using it effectively.

QUESTIONS FOR REVIEW

1. Describe the major parts of the shoe. What is the advantage of the Blucher opening? A low quarter?

2. Specify the purpose and placement of a metatarsal bar.

3. What are the advantages and disadvantages of the shoe insert as compared with the solid stirrup?

4. Indicate the clinical use of a posterior leg band, an anterior leg band, and a patellar-tendon-bearing brim.

5. How do tone-inhibiting AFOs improve the patient's function?

6. What orthotic knee joint is indicated for the patient with knee flexion contracture?

7. How do stabilizing AFOs or Craig-Scott KAFOs support a client with paraplegia?

8. What orthoses permit the child with paraplegia to stand without the aid of crutches?

9. Describe the three-point system in a lumbosacral, flexion, extension control orthosis that controls flexion.

10. Outline a maintenance program for a plastic and metal KAFO with solid ankle and pawl lock.

11. What facts should be assessed prior to formulating an orthotic prescription?

12. What features of the AFO are considered in static assessment?

13. Delineate the training program for a person with paraplegia who has been fitted with bilateral KAFOs.

14. Compare and contrast the orthotic options for a patient with hemiplegia.

15. What are the anatomical and orthotic causes of vaulting?

CASE STUDY

PATIENT HISTORY AND CURRENT PROBLEM: The patient is a 55 year-old woman who had poliomyelitis at the age of 3. She sustained complete paralysis of the right lower limb and left foot and ankle. During childhood she wore bilateral knee-ankle-foot (KAFO) orthoses and ambulated with a four-point gait with the aid of a pair of axillary crutches. When she was 18 she had a left ankle and subtalar fusion. She was fitted with a right KAFO, which included a stirrup foundation, posterior ankle stop, drop ring knee lock, knee pad, and leather-covered calf and thigh bands. For the next 30 years she wore the same brace, and had the leather and shoe replaced whenever they became worn. She used a cane in the left hand when she walked outdoors. She returned to the rehabilitation department today complaining of pain in the knee and fatigue. She also said that her brace tears her stockings at the knee. She is curious about new orthotic developments.

PAST MEDICAL HISTORY: Except for the poliomyelitis, she enjoyed good health although her endurance was always less than that of her friends.

SOCIAL HISTORY: She is a reference librarian who lives with her husband. She enjoys visiting her grandchildren, attending the theater, and participating in political campaigns.

PHYSICAL THERAPY ASSESSMENT FINDINGS

Review of Systems

Cognitive Status: Alert, oriented, memory intact.

Endurance: Limited, primarily restricted by discomfort in her right knee. She can walk for three city blocks before having to rest.

Vision: Intact with corrective lens.

Blood Pressure: 136/74.

Respiratory Rate: WFL.

RANGE OF MOTION GONIOMETRIC ASSESSMENT (DEGREES)

		Right	Left
Hip	Flexion	WFL	WFL
	Extension	WFL	WFL
	Abduction	WFL	WFL
	Adduction	WFL	WFL
	External rotation	WFL	WFL
	Internal rotation	WFL	WFL
Knee	Flexion	WFL	WFL
	Extension	25° hyperextension	WFL
Ankle	Dorsiflexion	0–5°	0° (no motion)
	Plantarflexion	0–40°	0° (no motion)
	Inversion	0–10°	0° (no motion)
	Eversion	0–5°	0° (no motion)

Sensation

- All modalities WFL bilaterally in both limbs
- Sensation in both upper limbs WFL

STRENGTH

MANUAL MUSCLE TEST (MMT) GRADES

	Right	Left
Hip Flexion	P–	G
Extension	0	G
Abduction	0	G
Adduction	0	G
External rotation	0	G
Internal rotation	0	F+
Knee		
Flexion	0	G–
Extension	0	F+
Foot/ankle		
Dorsiflexion	0	N/A
Plantarflexion	0	N/A
Inversion	0	N/A
Eversion	0	N/A
Upper limb strength	WFL	

N/A, not applicable owing to fusion; WFL, within functional limits.

Orthotic Assessment: Uprights malaligned permitting 20 degrees knee hyperextension. Posterior ankle stop worn, permitting 10 degrees plantarflexion. Leather on calf and thigh bands is worn.

Balance

Standing

Static: Good; able to maintain static position for unlimited period

Dynamic: Good on level surface. Not tested on ramp; patient reports that balance on ramps is precarious

Sitting: WFL

Gait: Patient walks slowly with a right KAFO with considerable lateral trunk bending to the right. Trunk bending reduces when she uses a cane in the left hand. She reports that she has great difficulty ascending and descending ramps.

Additional Findings Include:

- Overall decrease in speed of movement
- Broad walking base
- Circumducts right leg
- Right knee hyperextends within the orthosis
- Right ankle plantarflexion limited by orthosis
- Left foot and ankle fused in neutral position

Functional Status

- Transfers, sit-to-stand: FIM level = seven
- Independent in all BADL (FIM level = 7); floor-to-stand transfer FIM level = six
- Independent in approximately 85 percent of IADL (limitations imposed by pain, fatigue, and low ambulatory tolerance)

PATIENT DESIRED OUTCOME AND GOALS

- Walk without knee pain
- Improve endurance
- Improve appearance
- Reduce frequency of torn stockings in the vicinity of the knee

Guiding Questions

1. Formulate a clinical problem list.
2. Formulate a patient asset list.
3. Establish functional outcomes and goals of physical therapy.
4. Formulate a physical therapy plan of care.

REFERENCES

1. Edelstein, JE: Foot care for the aging. Phys Ther 68:1882, 1988.
2. Janisse, DJ: The shoe in rehabilitation of the foot and ankle. In Sammarco, GJ (ed): Rehabilitation of the Foot and Ankle. Mosby Yearbook, St. Louis, 1995.
3. Shiba, N, et al: Shock-absorbing effect of shoe insert materials commonly used in management of lower extremity disorders. Clin Orthop 310:130, 1995.
4. Bennett, P, et al: Analysis of the effects of custom moulded foot orthotics. Gait & Posture 3:183, 1994.
5. Kogler, GF, et al: Biomechanics of longitudinal arch support mechanisms in foot orthoses and their effect on plantar aponeurosis strain. Clin Biomech 11:243, 1996.
6. McCulloch, MU, et al: The effect of foot orthotics and gait velocity on lower limb kinematics and temporal events of stance. J Orthop Sports Phys Ther 17:69, 1993.
7. Leung, AKL, et al: Biomechanical gait evaluation of the immediate effect of orthotic treatment for flexible flat foot. Prosthet Orthot Int 22:25, 1998.
8. Gross, ML, et al: Effectiveness of orthotic shoe inserts in the long-distance runner. Am J Sports Med 19:409, 1991.
9. Postema, K, et al: Primary metatarsalgia: The influence of a custom moulded insole and a rockerbar on plantar pressure. Prosthet Orthot Int 22:35, 1998.
10. Richardson, JK: Rocker-soled shoes and walking distance in patients with calf claudication. Arch Phys Med Rehabil 72:554, 1991.
11. Cook, TM, and Cozzens, B: The effects of heel height and ankle-foot-orthosis configuration on weight line location: A demonstration of principles. Orthot Prosthet 30:43, 1976.
12. Yamamoto, S, et al: Comparative study of mechanical characteristics of plastic AFOs. J Prosthet Orthot 5:59, 1993.
13. Armesto, DG, et al: Orthotics design with advanced materials and methods: A pilot study. Rehabilitation Research and Development Reports, Department of Veterans Affairs, Baltimore, 1997, p 215.
14. Yang, GW, et al: Floor reaction orthosis: Clinical experience. Orthot Prosthet 40:33, 1986.
15. Dieli, J, et al: Effect of dynamic AFOs on hemiplegic adults. J Prosthet Orthot 9:82, 1997.
16. Lohman, M, and Goldstein, H: Alternative strategies in tone-reducing AFO design. J Prosthet Orthot 5:1, 1993.
17. Krebs, DE, et al: Comparison of plastic/metal and leather/metal knee-ankle-foot orthoses. Am J Phys Med Rehabil 67:175, 1988.
18. Lehmann, JF, et al: Knee-ankle-foot orthoses for paresis and paralysis. Phys Med Rehabil Clin N Am 3:161, 1992.
19. Lotta, S, et al: Restoration of gait with orthoses in thoracic paraplegia: A multicentric investigation. Paraplegia 32:608, 1994.
20. Ogilvie, C, et al: The physiological benefits of paraplegic orthotically aided walking. Paraplegia 31:111, 1993.
21. Stallard, J, et al: The ORLAU VCG (variable center of gravity) swivel walker for muscular dystrophy patients. Prosthet Orthot Int 16:46, 1992.
22. Gram, M: Using the Parapodium: A Manual of Training Techniques. Eterna Press, Rochester, 1984.
23. Kent, HO: Vannini-Rizzoli stabilizing orthosis (boot): Preliminary report on a new ambulatory aid for spinal cord injury. Arch Phys Med Rehabil 73:302, 1992.
24. Lyles, M, and Munday, J: Report on the evaluation of the Vannini-Rizzoli stabilizing limb orthosis. J Rehabil Res Dev 29:77, 1992.
25. Scott, BA: Engineering principles and fabrication techniques for the Scott-Craig long leg brace for paraplegics. Orthot Prosthet 25:14, 1971.
26. Lobley, S: Orthotic design from the New England Regional Spinal Cord Injury Center. Phys Ther 65:492, 1985.
27. Saitoh, E, et al: Clinical experience with a new hip-knee-foot orthotic system using a medial single hip joint for paraplegic standing and walking. Am J Phys Med Rehabil 75:198, 1996.
28. Harvey, LA, et al: Functional outcomes attained by T9-T12 paraplegic patients with the Walkabout and the Isocentric reciprocal gait orthoses. Arch Phys Med Rehabil 78:706, 1997.
29. Guidera, KJ, et al: Use of the reciprocating gait orthosis in myelodysplasia. J Pediatr Orthop 6:341, 1993.
30. Bernardi, M, et al: The efficiency of walking of paraplegic patients using a reciprocating gait orthosis. Paraplegia 33:409, 1995.
31. Franceschini, M, et al: Reciprocating gait orthoses: A multicenter study of their use by spinal cord injured patients. Arch Phys Med Rehabil 78:582, 1997.
32. Sykes, L, et al: The reciprocating gait orthosis: Long-term usage patterns. Arch Phys Med Rehabil 76:779, 1995.

33. Winchester, PK, et al: A comparison of paraplegic gait performance using two types of reciprocating gait orthoses. Prosthet Orthot Int 17:101, 1993.

34. Baardman, G, et al: The influence of the reciprocal hip joint link in the Advanced Reciprocating Gait Orthosis on standing performance in paraplegia. Prosthet Orthot Int 21:210, 1997.

35. Whittle, MW, et al: A comparative trial of two walking systems for paralysed people. Paraplegia 29:97, 1991.

36. Summers, BN, et al: A clinical review of the adult hip guidance orthosis (ParaWalker) in traumatic paraplegics. Paraplegia 26:19, 1988.

37. Solomonow, M, et al: Reciprocating gait orthosis powered with electrical muscle stimulation (RGO II): Performance evaluation of 70 paraplegics. Part I: Orthopedics 20:315, 1997, and Part II: Orthopedics 20:411, 1997.

38. Alaranta, H, and Hurri, H: Compliance and subjective relief by corset treatment in chronic low back pain. Scand J Rehabil Med 20:133, 1988.

39. Stillo, JV, et al: Low-back orthoses. Phys Med Rehabil Clin N Am 3:57, 1992.

40. Spratt, KF, et al: Efficacy of flexion and extension treatments incorporating braces for lower-back pain patients with retro-displacement, spondylolisthesis, or normal sagittal translation. Spine 18:1839, 1993.

41. Tuong, NH, et al: Three-dimensional evaluation of lumbar orthosis effects on spinal behavior. J Rehabil Res Dev 35:34, 1998.

42. Micheli, LJ: The use of the modified Boston brace system (B.O.B.) for back pain: Clinical indications. Orthot Prosthet 39:41, 1985.

43. Smith, KM: A preliminary report on a new design of a spinal orthosis for spondylolytic patients: Review of the literature and initiation for future study of a new design. J Prosthet Orthot 10:45, 1998.

44. Fisher, SV: Cervical orthotics. Phys Med Rehabil Clin N Am 3:29, 1992.

45. Lunsford, T, et al: The effectiveness of four contemporary cervical orthoses in restricting cervical motion. J Prosthet Orthot 6:93, 1994.

46. Sandler, AJ, et al: The effectiveness of several cervical orthoses: An in vivo comparison of the mechanical stability provided by several widely used models. Spine 21:1624, 1996.

47. Sharpe, KP, et al: Evaluation of the effectiveness of the Minerva cervicothoracic orthosis. Spine 20:1475, 1995.

48. Wang, GJ, et al: The effect of halo-vest length on stability of the cervical spine: A study in normal subjects. J Bone Joint Surg [Am] 70A:357, 1988.

49. Pringle, RG: Review article: Halo versus Minerva: Which orthosis? Paraplegia 28:281, 1990.

50. King, HA: Orthotic management of idiopathic scoliosis. Phys Med Rehabil Clin N Am 3:45, 1992.

51. Nachemson, AL, and Peterson, LE: Effectiveness of treatment with a brace in girls who had adolescent idiopathic scoliosis: A prospective, controlled study based on data from the brace study of the Scoliosis Research Society. J Bone Joint Surg 77-A:815, 1995.

52. Rowe, DE, et al: A meta-analysis of the efficacy of non-operative treatments for idiopathic scoliosis. J Bone Joint Surg 79-A:664, 1997.

53. Lonstein, JE, and Winter, RB: The Milwaukee brace for the treatment of idiopathic scoliosis: A review of 1020 patients. J Bone Joint Surg 76-A:1207, 1994.

54. Olafsson, Y, et al: Boston brace in the treatment of idiopathic scoliosis. J Pediatr Orthop 15:524, 1995.

55. Patwardhan, AG, et al: Biomechanical comparison of the Milwaukee brace and the TLSO for treatment of idiopathic scoliosis. J Prosthet Orthot 8:115, 1996.

56. Allington, NJ, and Bowen, JR: Adolescent idiopathic scoliosis: Treatment with the Wilmington brace: A comparison of full-time and part-time use. J Bone Joint Surg 78-A:1056, 1996.

57. Roach, CJ, and Andrish, JT: Preliminary results of part-time bracing for the management of idiopathic scoliosis. J Prosthet Orthot 10:71, 1998.

58. Katz, DE, et al: A comparison between the Boston brace and the Charleston bending brace in adolescent idiopathic scoliosis. Spine 22:1302, 1997.

59. American Physical Therapy Association: Guide to Physical Therapist Practice. APTA, Alexandria, VA, 1999.

60. Krebs, DE, et al: Reliability of observational kinematic gait analysis. Phys Ther 65:1027, 1985.

61. Reister, JA, and Eilert RE: Hip disorders. In Goldberg, B, and Hsu J: Atlas of Orthoses: Rehabilitation Principles and Application of Orthotic and Assistive Devices, ed 3. CV Mosby, St. Louis, 1996, p 509.

62. Bowker, P, et al: Energetics of paraplegic walking. J Biomed Eng 14:34, 1992.

63. Cerny, K, et al: Walking and wheelchair energetics in persons with paraplegia. Phys Ther 60:1133, 1980.

SUPPLEMENTAL READINGS

Aisen, ML: Orthotics in Neurologic Rehabilitation. Demos, New York, 1992.

Bowker, P, et al (eds): Biomechanical Basis of Orthotic Management. Butterworth-Heinemann, Oxford, 1993.

Bunch, WH, and Patwardhan, AG: Scoliosis: Making Clinical Decisions. CV Mosby, St. Louis, 1989.

Goldberg, B, and Hsu J: Atlas of Orthoses: Rehabilitation Principles and Application of Orthotic and Assistive Devices, ed 3. CV Mosby, St. Louis, 1996.

McKee, P, and Morgan, L: Orthotics in Rehabilitation: Splinting the Hand and Body. FA Davis, Philadelphia, 1998.

Nawoczenski, DA, and Epler, ME: Orthotics in Functional Rehabilitation of the Lower Limb. Saunders, Philadelphia, 1997.

Redford, JB, et al: Orthotics: Clinical Practice and Rehabilitation Technology. Churchill Livingstone, New York, 1995.

Rose, GK: Orthotics: Principles and Practice. William Heinemann, London, 1986.

Smidt, GL (ed): Gait in Rehabilitation. Churchill Livingstone, New York, 1990.

Wu, KK: Foot Orthoses: Principles and Clinical Applications. Williams & Wilkins, Baltimore, 1990.

GLOSSARY

Bail: Posteriorly protruding semicircular handle of a pair of knee locks, usually pawl locks. Moving the bail upward releases the locks.

Bichannel adjustable ankle lock (BiCAAL): Ankle joint having posterior and anterior receptacles with springs that can be compressed to assist motion or can be replaced by pins to alter the alignment of the joint and thus the uprights attached to the joint.

Boston orthosis: Thoracolumbosacral orthosis intended for correction of scoliosis; its foundation is a mass-produced plastic module which is custom altered.

Charleston bending brace: Thoracolumbosacral orthosis intended for nocturnal correction of scoliosis; its foundation is a custom-made plastic jacket curved in the direction opposite to the curve.

Corset: Lumbosacral or thoracolumbosacral fabric orthosis that may have vertical reinforcements, but does not have rigid horizontal components.

Counter: Shoe component consisting of stiff material placed in the posterior aspect of the shoe to reinforce the quarter and increase stability of the back of the shoe.

Craig-Scott KAFO: KAFO intended for persons with paraplegia and invented by Bruce Scott, an orthotist at the Craig Rehabilitation Center, Denver, Colorado. Each of the pair of orthoses consists of a reinforced shoe, stirrup, BiCAAL ankle joints, anterior leg band, pawl locks with bail release, and a single thigh band. A solid ankle may be substituted for the reinforced shoe, stirrup, and BiCAAL ankle joints.

Four-post orthosis: A cervical orthosis with two anterior adjustable posts attached to sternal and mandibular plates and two posterior adjustable posts attached to thoracic and occipital plates; straps connect the sternal and thoracic plates; provides *moderate control of cervical motions.*

Floor reaction orthosis: Any lower-limb orthosis; the term is usually applied to an AFO that has an anterior band and a solid ankle.

Genu valgrum: A deformity in which the lower extremities curve inward with knees close together; knock knees.

Genu varum: A deformity in which the lower extremities curve outward with knees far apart; bow legs.

Halo: Cervical orthosis that includes a metal ring secured to the skull, four vertical posts, and a thoracic vest.

Insert: Removable component placed in the shoe, extending from the posterior margin of the inner sole to a point immediately posterior to the point corresponding to the metatarsophalangeal joints, or farther anterior.

   University of California Biomechanics Laboratory (UCBL) insert: Custom-made plastic insert intended to maintain correction of a flexible pes valgus; it includes a wall covering the medial, posterior, and lateral margins of the foot; the wall is continuous with a plantar plate.

Knight spinal orthosis: Lumbosacral flexion, extension, lateral control orthosis.

Last: Foot-shaped form over which a shoe is made.

Metatarsal bar: Strip of firm material attached transversely to the outer sole immediately posterior to a point corresponding to the metatarsophalangeal joints; intended to relieve weight-bearing on those joints.

Metatarsal pad: Resilient dome-shaped material placed on the inner sole or in an insert, with the apex immediately posterior to one or more metatarsophalangeal joints; intended to relieve weight-bearing on those joints.

Milwaukee orthosis: Thoracolumbosacral orthosis intended for correction of scoliosis that consists of a frame composed of a pelvic girdle, one anterior and two posterior uprights, and a thoracic ring, to which various corrective pads may be strapped.

Minerva orthosis: Cervical orthosis consisting of a rigid posterior section extending from the head to the thorax, and an anterior section extending from the mandible to the thorax. The orthosis is held in place by a forehead band.

Offset joint: Knee joint in which the axis is located posterior to the midline of the leg; intended to increase knee stability.

Parapodium: Mass-produced frame intended to enable children to stand and sit. Consists of a base connected to a thoracolumbar band by lateral uprights that are hinged and locked at the knees and hips. Chest and anterior leg bands stabilize the device.

ParaWalker: THKAFO originally known as the hip guidance orthosis. Includes sturdy hip joints that permit a limited flexion excursion, but block frontal and transverse plane motion; also includes foot plates to which shoes are strapped.

Patellar-tendon-bearing brim: Plastic proximal portion of an AFO, intended to support part of the client's weight proximally, especially on the patellar ligament (tendon).

Patten: Distal termination of a KAFO intended to relieve the braced limb of all weight-bearing.

Pawl lock: Knee lock consisting of a proximal segment having a pivoted bar that lodges in a notch on the distal segment.

Pes planus: A flattening of the longitudinal arch of the foot; flat foot.

Pes equinus: A foot deformity in which the heel is elevated and the foot is maintained in plantarflexion.

Pes valgus (talipes valgus): A foot deformity in which the heel and foot are turned outward.

Pes varus (talipes varus): A foot deformity in which the heel and foot are turned inward.

Posterior leaf spring: Plastic AFO that has a posterior upright continuous with an insert; intended to assist dorsiflexion. The upright does not extend anteriorly beyond the malleoli.

Reciprocating gait orthosis RGO: THKAFO intended for patients with paraplegia. Consists of a pair of KAFOs to which is attached a mechanism having steel cables passing from the right to the left proximal margin of the thigh shell. The mechanism is secured to the torso with a thoracic strap.

Retention button: Spring-loaded projection on a drop ring knee lock.

Rocker bar: A convex strip affixed to the sole proximal to the metatarsal heads.

Scaphoid pad: Resilient dome-shaped material placed at the junction of the inner sole and medial quarter of the shoe, with the apex located between the navicular tuberosity and the sustentaculum tali of the calcaneus; intended to support the longitudinal arch.

Solid ankle-foot orthosis: Plastic AFO that has a posterior shell continuous with an insert. The shell extends anteriorly beyond the malleoli.

Hinged solid ankle-foot orthosis: Plastic orthosis with similar trimlines that has a transverse separation between the shell and the insert to provide sagittal plane motion.

Stabilizing boot: Also known as the Vannini-Rizzoli boot. AFO that includes an inner plastic foot plate and shell that maintains the foot in plantarflexion. The plastic component is worn in a flat-bottomed boot. This orthosis is intended for clients with paraplegia.

Standing frame: Mass-produced THKAFO that supports the wearer with a nonarticulated posterior frame equipped with a thoracolumbar pad, and an anterior chest band and knee band. The base of the frame is flat and has loops to secure the shoes.

Stirrup: Steel U-shaped shoe attachment that connects the uprights to the shoe.

Solid stirrup: One-piece attachment, the central portion of which is riveted to the shoe shank; the shoe cannot be detached from the uprights.

Split stirrup: Three-piece attachment, the central portion of which is riveted to the shoe shank; the shoe can be detached from the uprights.

Swivel walker: Mass-produced THKAFO that supports the wearer with a nonarticulated posterior frame equipped with a thoracolumbar pad, and an anterior chest band and knee band. The base of the frame has two plates that pivot slightly enabling the wearer to achieve a swiveling gait.

Taylor brace: Thoracolumbosacral flexion extension control orthosis.

Thomas heel: Heel designed in the nineteenth century by Hugh Owen Thomas in which the anterior margin is curved, such that its medial border extends anteriorly, usually with a slight medial wedge; intended to support flexible pes valgus.

Tone-reducing orthosis: AFOs designed to inhibit spasticity by maintaining a neutral foot position; some tone-reducing orthoses position the toes in hyperextension and have pads that apply constant pressure to the Achilles tendon.

Viscoelastic: Having both viscous and elastic properties; exhibited by various polyurethane plastics, such as Sorbothane, Viscolas, and PPT, which are used in shoe inserts to absorb shock.

Wilmington orthosis: Thoracolumbosacral orthosis intended for correction of scoliosis; its foundation is a custom-made plastic jacket.

APPENDIX A

Lower-Limb Orthotic Evaluation

1. Is the orthosis as prescribed?
2. Can the client don the orthosis easily?

Standing

3. Is the shoe satisfactory and does it fit properly?
4. Are the sole and heel of the shoe flat on the floor?
5. If a shoe insert is used, is there minimal rocking between insert and shoe?

Ankle

6. Do the mechanical ankle joints coincide with the anatomical ankle?
7. Is there adequate clearance between the anatomical ankle and the mechanical ankle joints?
8. Does the valgus or varus correction strap control the foot position?

Knee

9. Does the mechanical knee joints coincide with the anatomical knee (¾″ (7.62 cm) above medial tibial plateau)?
10. Is there adequate clearance between the anatomical knee and the mechanical knee joint?
11. Is the knee lock secure and easy to operate?

Shells, Bands, Cuffs, and Uprights

12. Do the shells, bands, cuffs, and uprights conform to the contours of the leg and thigh?
13. Is there adequate clearance between the top of the calf shell or band and the head of the fibula?
14. Is there adequate clearance between the orthosis and the perineum?
15. Is the orthosis below the greater trochanter but at least ≈1″ (2.5 cm) higher than the medial shell or upright?
16. Are the uprights at the midline of the leg and thigh?
17. Do the shells, bands, and cuffs conform to the contours of the leg and thigh?
18. Is any flesh roll above the shell or band minimal?
19. Are the bottom of the thigh shell or distal thigh band and the top of the calf shell or band equidistant from the knee?

20. In a child's orthosis, is there adequate provision for lengthening the orthosis?

Weight-Relieving Components

21. In a patellar-tendon-bearing brim, is there adequate relief for the head of the fibula?
22. With a quadrilateral brim, is the client free from excessive pressure in the anteromedial and medial aspect of the brim?
23. With a quadrilateral brim, does the ischial tuberosity rest on the ischial seat?
24. With a patellar-tendon-bearing or proximal thigh brim, is there adequate reduction in weight-bearing through the orthosis?

Hip

25. Is the center of the pelvic joint slightly above and ahead of greater trochanter?
26. Is the hip lock secure and easy to operate?
27. Does the pelvic band fit the torso accurately?

Stability

28. Does the orthosis provide adequate stability to the client?

Sitting

29. Can the patient sit comfortably with hips and knees flexed 90 degrees?
30. Can the patient lean forward to touch the shoes?

Walking

31. Is the patient's performance in level walking satisfactory?
32. Is the patient's performance on stairs and ramps satisfactory?
33. Is the orthosis sufficiently rigid?
34. Does the varus or valgus correction strap provide adequate support?
35. Does the orthosis operate quietly?
36. Does the patient consider the orthosis satisfactory as to comfort, function, and appearance?

Orthosis off the Patient

37. Is the skin free of abrasions or other discolorations attributable to the orthosis?
38. Is the construction satisfactory?
39. Do all components function satisfactorily?

APPENDIX B

Trunk Orthotic Evaluation

1. Is the orthosis as prescribed?
2. Can the client don the orthosis easily?

Standing

Pelvic Band

3. Does the pelvic band lie flat on the trunk below the posterior superior iliac spines?
4. Does the pelvic band pass between the trochanters and iliac crests?

Thoracic Band

5. Does the thoracic band lie flat on the trunk below the scapulae?
6. Does the thoracic band lie horizontally on the trunk?

Uprights

7. Do the posterior uprights avoid pressure on bony prominences, such as the vertebral spines or scapulae?

8. Do the lateral uprights extend along the lateral midlines of the trunk?

Abdominal Front

9. Is the abdominal front of adequate size?

Cervical Orthosis

10. Is the head in the prescribed position?
11. Do all rigid components fit properly?

Sitting

12. Can the patient sit comfortably with the hips and knees flex 90 degrees?
13. Does the patient consider the orthosis satisfactory as to comfort, function, and appearance?

Orthosis off the Patient

14. Is the skin free of abrasions or other discolorations attributable to the orthosis?
15. Is the construction satisfactory?
16. Do all components function satisfactorily?

APPENDIX C

Suggested Answers to Case Study Guiding Questions

1. Formulate a clinical problem list.
ANSWER
1. Orthotic knee joint malaligned in hyperextension
2. Orthotic ankle joint malaligned in plantarflexion
3. Leather on orthosis is worn
4. Asymmetrical gait
5. Poor walking endurance
6. Difficulty walking on ramps
7. Paralysis of right lower limb
8. Fusion of left ankle and foot

2. Formulate a patient asset list.
ANSWER
1. Active life-style
2. Motivated; interested in a new orthotic design.

3. Establish functional outcomes and goals of physical therapy.
ANSWER
A. Functional outcomes of physical therapy:
1. Independenced in all functional activities with new orthosis.
2. Tolerance to positions and activities is increased.
3. Safety is improved.
4. Deformity is prevented.

B. Goals of treatment: short-term goals
1. Provide new orthosis, preferably ankle-foot orthosis with plastic insert foundation, BiCAAL ankle joint, aluminum uprights, and plastic calf band.
2. Increase aerobic endurance.

4. Formulate a physical therapy plan of care.
ANSWER
- Make appointment for patient with the orthotist and physician to formulate prescription for new orthosis. AFO with ankle joint locked in neutral position should reduce tendency of knee to hyperextend. AFO would eliminate clothing wear in the vicinity of the knee. If AFO fails to control knee hyperextension, then patient will require a KAFO, preferably with plastic foot plate, BiCAAL ankle, plastic covered uprights, plastic calf and thigh bands. She may not require a knee lock.
- Cybex exercise for left quadriceps.
- Stationary bicycle for aerobic conditioning.
- Home program to include Theraband resistance exercises for left quadriceps and gluteus maximus.

The Prescriptive Wheelchair: An Orthotic Device

Adrienne Falk Bergen

LEARNING OBJECTIVES

1. Identify the postural support components of a wheelchair seating system.
2. Identify the components that make up a wheeled mobility base.
3. Describe the components of the patient examination process.
4. Describe the measurements required for correct fitting of a prescriptive wheelchair.
5. Understand the function and indications for common wheelchair features and postural support components.
6. Recognize the functional implications of a properly prescribed wheelchair for environmental access.
7. Analyze and interpret patient data and identify appropriate prescriptive elements when presented with a clinical case study.

Physical therapists are often called on to prescribe a wheelchair. A properly prescribed wheelchair can be a useful device in reintegrating a person with a disability into the community, whereas a poorly prescribed one can actually exacerbate the problems associated with functional limitations and disability. This chapter presents a systematic approach to determining the appropriate components of a prescriptive wheelchair. First, attention is directed toward the seating system required to provide the proper support for the individual user. Second, the features available to create a proper mobility base for the seating system are described. The seating system and mobility base combine to create a prescriptive wheelchair, a seated environment from which the patient can achieve maximum function.

A wheelchair is truly a mobility orthosis. An *orthosis* is a device used to provide support or to straighten or to correct a deformity. It is typically a brace made of metal or plastic that increases or maintains a person's level of function. If properly prescribed, a wheelchair will provide sufficient support to help deter the effect of deforming forces or weakened structures on function of the system. In simpler terms, it should support the user as needed to allow maximum function. Inasmuch as it is on wheels, the system can be called a *mobility orthosis*, providing appropriate support to allow maximum functional mobility.

Like a well-made orthosis, the wheelchair should fit correctly. It should be reasonably cosmetic to the user. It should also be as lightweight and yet as strong as possible. It can be obtained from a stock supply when appropriate, but most often individual modifications for the patient's special needs are required.

Like a well-made orthosis, the wheelchair should be prescribed by qualified professionals. The entire team should make the decision concerning a prescriptive wheelchair. It is important that all those concerned with the person's present and future function be a part of this team. This includes the wheelchair user, therapists, family members, caregivers, nurses, physicians, vocational counselors, and a qualified rehabilitation technology supplier. To ensure that the most suitable device is obtained, the team must have a clear idea of who will be using it, what functional level is expected, and where the chair will be used. Once the chair is supplied, the team is responsible for adjusting and fitting the final device, as well as teaching the patient how to use and maintain the device to ensure optimal long-term performance.

A prescriptive wheelchair is a combination of a postural support system and a mobility base that are joined to create a dynamic seated environment (Fig. 32-1). The **postural support system** is made up of the surfaces that contact the user's body directly. This includes the seat, back, and foot supports as well as any additional components needed to maintain postural alignment. Maintenance of postural alignment may require such additions as a head support; lateral supports for the trunk, hips, and knees; medial support for the knees; and upper extremity support surfaces, as well as straps or bands (such as anterior chest and pelvic controls) needed to keep the user interfaced with the support surfaces. The **mobility base** consists of the tubular frame, armrests, foot supports, and wheels. Once the decisions are made about the type of support system needed, the team must then decide what type of mobility base best suits the user's functional level and environmental needs. For some patients, caregiver needs are of paramount importance. Clear information will be needed to ensure that the postural support system and the mobility base interface prop-

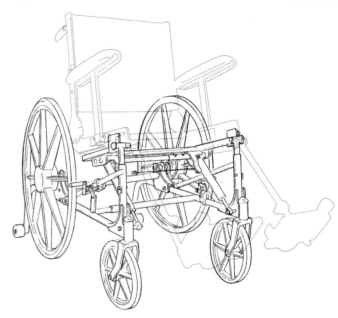

Figure 32-1. A prescriptive wheelchair consists of the postural support system and a mobility base.

erly. For users who utilize more than one mobility base (e.g., power and manual), the most cost-effective approach is to have one support system interface with all the mobility bases. This is not always practical, and sometimes it is best to have the individual use the full-support system in the chair used most frequently, and forgo optimal postural support in the backup system to facilitate transport for short trips.

PLANNING THE SYSTEM

Creating a dynamic seating environment involves three steps: (1) assessment and evaluation, (2) determining goals and outcomes, and (3) planning the intervention. This process will allow appropriate recommendations and product choices. As noted, the overall outcome is to create a dynamic seating environment that is a comfortable base from which the user can attain a maximal functional level. Before the physical assessment is begun, information must be gathered from the entire team regarding their expectations. A great deal can be learned at this point about what the various team members hope the system will be able to do for the patient. It is extremely important to bring all the obvious and hidden issues out into full view before the process is begun. Patients, family members, or caregivers may assume that the wheelchair and seating system can achieve unrealistic goals (normalize posture, provide total pain relief, facilitate independent transfers). When these hidden goals are not met, these individuals are often so disappointed that they cannot see the other benefits of the system.

THE EXAMINATION PROCESS

It is important to take time at the beginning of the examination process to explain to the patient and caregivers what will be happening, what information will be gathered, and why the information is important. Everyone should be made to feel that their input is necessary and valuable. Time should be allocated during data collection for comments or questions from the patient, caregivers, and other team members. Prior to each stage of the process the patient should be asked if it is acceptable to proceed. For example, "I would like to put my hands on your pelvis, is that okay?" It is important to move slowly and speak calmly, because quick movements or loud speech may increase anxiety. In some patients this may increase muscle tone, interfering with data collection. It is important to explain what is being observed or measured so that patients and caregivers can understand comments that may be made between team members, and so that they can fully comprehend the team's findings and the subsequent recommendations.

Information must be gathered from the entire team to determine the person's present level of function and the targeted goals and outcomes. Complete information about physical, psychosocial, and cognitive perceptual areas are imperative to the process. The tests and measures should be completed by the appropriate professionals and submitted to the wheelchair team for review. The team must be totally informed about the patient's medical and surgical history and plans, neurological status, postural control, musculoskeletal status, sensory status, functional skill level, cognitive-behavioral status, and communication level. Accurate information about the patient's home, work, educational, and recreational environments must be considered, along with the method the patient will use to transport the wheelchair. Funding sources should be identified so that the team is aware of any possible problems and advanced planning can begin.

Physical Examination

Although it may be time consuming, it is absolutely critical that the physical examination be complete and accurate, because changes may be difficult to make later. Accurate recording provides a permanent record of why certain decisions were made. During the ordering or manufacturing process, additional decisions concerning modifications may be needed. If accurate measurements are on file, decisions can often be made without recalling the person to the clinic.

The purpose of the physical examination is to learn as much as possible about the person's range of available movement and about how movement of one body part affects tone, comfort, position, control, and performance in other body segments. The goal is to preserve spinal alignment whenever possible, maintaining the natural lumbar curve whenever

it can be produced. The person should be examined in a gravity-minimized position (supine or side lying), as well as a gravity-dependent position (sitting), whenever possible. To create a properly fitted system, range of motion measurements are required. Accurate measurements are also needed of under thigh length; leg length; distance from the seat to the lower scapula, midscapula, and shoulder; distance from hanging elbow-to-seat surface; and width across the hips, shoulders, and from outside the knee to outside the opposite knee.

Examination of Function Using Existing Equipment

A great deal can be learned by observing the patient in his or her existing wheelchair. The patient should be in the best or most commonly assumed position, with supports and straps in place. Questions should include how the patient and or caregiver feels the device is working, has it always worked like this, or has its function decreased over time. If it worked well initially, but does not work well now, is this because of patient change (weight gain or loss, growth, functional gain or loss) or equipment change (broken or missing parts, decreased reliability)? Information can be gathered during this portion of the examination about the patient's and caregiver's attitudes and technology savvy, as well as their physical use of the equipment. During the initial visit team members should observe the existing equipment, the patient, the caregivers and their physical and psychosocial interactions.

During this period, the team should gather data about the patient's postural alignment at the head, shoulders, trunk, pelvis, and lower extremities using both visual observation and hands-on assessment. Pelvic alignment is examined by palpation along the pelvis crests, and on the anterior superior iliac spines (ASIS). The position of the pelvis (e.g., rotation, posterior or anterior tilt) should be carefully documented.

With the patient's shirt removed or at least lifted to nipple level, trunk posture can be observed directly. A combination of visual observation and palpation will allow determination of alignment (abdominal wrinkles usually mean a rounded spine). In the presence of abnormal alignment, the therapist should determine (1) if alignment can be corrected using gentle pressure, and (2) what factors may be interfering with good postural alignment.

The patient should be requested to transfer (or be transferred) onto a mat table. Observation of the specific transfer method used will avoid creating a new system that interferes with this function.

Examination in the Supine Position

Examination may require more than one examiner. The patient should be positioned supine on a firm surface (a mat or carpeted floor works well; a bed may not be firm enough). Range of motion of pelvic movements and hip flexion as they relate to spinal and pelvic alignment should be determined. The purpose is to assess the maximum range of motion available before attempts are made to alter positioning. The lower extremities must be well supported by the examiner, with the knees flexed 95 to 100 degrees or as much as is needed to eliminate the influence of the hamstring muscle group (Fig. 32-2). Care should be taken to neutralize pelvic tilt if at all possible. This may require tone reduction techniques for patients with spasticity. The examiner palpates the anterior superior iliac crests of the pelvis. If gross range of motion limitations such as abduction and/or adduction contractures are present, the lower extremities should be allowed to assume whatever posture is needed to provide good pelvic alignment.

With the lower extremities positioned as needed, both hips can then be flexed at the same time to obtain a gross estimate of range of motion. This can be followed by more detailed examination of each limb individually. Range of motion measurements should include hip flexion, abduction, adduction, and internal and external rotation as well as their affect on pelvic position and general body alignment. If the pelvis is asymmetric when the knees are pointed upright, this may indicate limited range of hip abduction or adduction. In some cases it will be necessary to allow the lower extremities to rotate off to one side **(windblown position),** be widely abducted, and/or internally or externally rotated, to achieve good pelvic alignment and minimize any negative effect on spinal alignment. If movement through hip range of motion, and/or opening of the knee angle (introducing hamstring influence) in one or both lower extremities negatively affects pelvic alignment and the lumbar curve, decisions must be made about eliminating this influence in the seating unit. If spasticity is problematic, the team may consider recommending therapeutic interventions such as chemical blocks, oral medications, or surgery.

Once range of motion is documented, a linear measurement of seat depth should be determined. From a supine position, the examiner should support the limb(s) in an optimal position and neutralize the pelvis. A second person measures the undersurface of the thigh from the popliteal fossa to the support surface. This should be done for each lower extremity individually, obtaining a left and right measurement of seat depth (Fig. 32-3). If the lower extremities are abducted or in a windblown position, the examiner must use caution to measure a line perpendicular to the support surface, and not along the line the limbs assume.

Examination in the Seated Position

Once examination in the supine position is completed, the patient should be placed in a supported sitting position with the knees flexed to 100 degrees

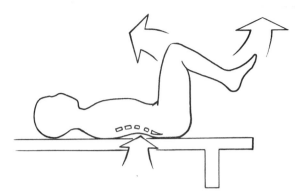

Figure 32-2. The examiner must monitor the lumbar curve as the hips are flexed and the knees extended.

or more to eliminate the influence of the hamstring muscle group. Accommodation must be made for any limitations documented in the supine position. If support is needed, one examiner can be positioned in front of the person and another behind, offering support (Fig. 32-4). The examiner in front should now assess pelvic position and mobility with the hips in flexion. Pressure is used at the front of the knees and counterbalanced by manipulation of the pelvis to achieve a neutral posture with good lumbar and trunk alignment. The examiner determines the degree of flexibility and the influence of gravity on posture. Initial ideas can be formulated about where control may be needed to achieve postural goals.

In the supported sitting position the examiner should remeasure (Fig. 32-5Asit) the sitting depth from behind the buttocks to the popliteal fossa. This may differ from the supine measurement, and careful assessment should reveal whether the difference is secondary to correctable postural difficulties or simply variable flesh distribution in sitting versus supine. Leg measurement (Fig. 32-5B), from the popliteal fossa to the heel with customary footwear in place, will be needed to determine footrest length on the wheelchair. The sitting knee flexion angle is found in Fig. 32-5C. Measurement of back height should be taken from the sitting surface to the

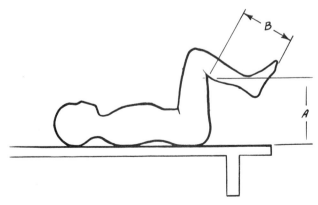

Figure 32-3. In the supine position with the hips and knees flexed the examiner can measure the undersurface of the thigh from the popliteal fossa to a firm support surface (A) and the length from the popliteal fossa to the heel (B).

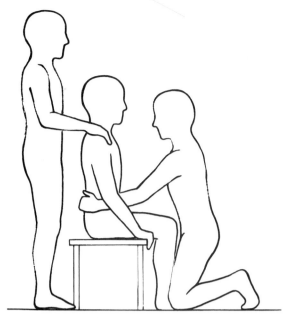

Figure 32-4. Measurements in sitting must be taken with the patient sitting on a surface with a thin top. This will allow the knees to flex as needed.

posterior superior pelvic crests (Fig. 32-5D), lower scapula (Fig. 32-5E), midscapula, and to the top of the shoulder (Fig. 32-5F), occiput (Fig. 32-5G), and crown of the head (Fig. 32-5H). These measure-

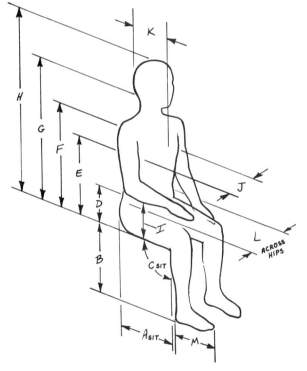

Figure 32-5. The following measurements are added to those taken in the supine position. (A) Sit (right and left side): behind hips to popliteal fossa. (B) Right and left side: popliteal fossa/heel. (C) Knee flexion angle. (D) Sitting surface/pelvic crest. (E) Sitting surface/lower scapula. (F) Sitting surface/shoulder. (G) Sitting surface/occiput. (H) Sitting surface/crown of head. (I) Sitting surface/hanging elbow. (J) Width across trunk. (K) Depth of trunk. (L) Width across hips. (M) Heel/toe.

ments will provide a detailed record should decisions regarding wheelchair back height be needed once the assessment is completed. Measurement of the "hanging elbow" (Fig. 32-5I) is needed to determine proper armrest height. With the person in a corrected sitting position, the upper extremity is positioned at the side of the body with 90 degrees of elbow flexion, and the shoulder in a neutral position. A measurement is taken from the bottom of the elbow to the sitting surface.

During this seated assessment, measurements should be taken across the shoulders, trunk (Fig. 32-5J), hips (Fig. 32-5K), and knees for decisions regarding support accessories, as well as width of the seating system and the mobility base. A measurement of trunk depth (Fig. 32-5L) and foot length (Fig. 32-5M) should also be taken. To ensure accurate recommendations it is important to consider orthoses, clothing, and recent weight loss or gain, as well as the patient's potential for growth when recording these measurements.

DETERMINING GOALS AND OUTCOMES

Information from the entire team must be compiled and evaluated to determine the person's present level of function and the targeted goals and outcomes. It is important that all goals and projected outcomes be discussed adequately to avoid system failure owing to poor planning, poor communication, and/or unrealistic expectations from any of the team members. It may be necessary to compromise and set priorities if all of the goals cannot be met.

A well-planned seating system may be able to normalize tone, decrease pathological reflex activity, improve postural symmetry, enhance range of movement, maintain and/or improve skin condition, increase comfort and sitting tolerance, decrease fatigue, and improve function of the autonomic nervous system.[1] In addition, the base of the seating system can provide the user with changes in orientation in space (recline and tilt, both manual and power activated). A properly prescribed mobility base will provide the user with access to the environment outside the home, whether alone or with a caregiver. It should be effective for accomplishing all daily goals at home, school, work, and recreation and, where necessary, assist the caregiver with patient management.

When setting priorities it is important that clinical team members do not override the patient with their professional opinions. Clinical teams may not be fully aware of the barriers facing the individual using a wheelchair in the outside environment. Clinicians may observe a patient ambulating in the clinic and feel that with added practice he or she could ambulate full time. This clinician will often recommend crutches and a simple manual wheelchair. In the real environment, the patient may need to traverse long distances to independently shop, attend community activities, and function at school or work. Walking to these activities would require extraordinary effort. Propelling a standard manual wheelchair may not offer very much additional assistance. A motorized scooter may be more effective as a supplement for environmental mobility.

INTERVENTION

Once all of the information is evaluated, the team plans the intervention. The postural goal is to achieve good trunk position, because all function, both central (control, alignment, internal organ function) and distal (gross and fine motor control in the head and upper extremities), is based on the position and control in the trunk and limb girdles. The mobility goal is to provide efficient ease of movement from the user's and caregiver's perspectives. The system outcome is to provide comfort and maximal functional independence. The intervention consists of prescription of the seating system and the mobility base.

The data can now be used to determine whether the patient is functioning at his or her highest potential, or whether additional support would be helpful in freeing distal body parts to improve function.[2] The consequences of poor posture on skin condition, respiratory function, speech, and general functioning should also be considered. It is usually helpful at this point to simulate various interventions. This can be accomplished using a simulator chair, which has various adjustments for surface dimensions (e.g., seat depth, back height, calf length), as well as angles between seat and back, seat and calf, and calf and foot, as well as tilt-in-space and postural supports.[3] If one is not available, the team can sample various available chairs and/or support systems set up in different configurations. The mode of propulsion, method of transfer, and interaction with the environment can be observed. Performance in each of these areas will be influenced by the individual's strength, posture, and tone, and can be modified by support system intervention. Proper intervention may enhance function (e.g., respiratory or motor), whereas improper intervention (e.g., insufficient support, poorly placed wheels, or excessive chair width) may interfere with function.

In choosing chair properties, careful attention must be given to possible secondary problems that may be created. For example, if the intervention includes a high seat cushion for pressure relief, will the user be able to get under tables and desks, transfer, or reach the wheels for self-propulsion? If the recommendation includes a custom support system, will the weight preclude easy self-propulsion or caregiver management? Will the bulk make automobile transport difficult or impossible? Attention to these issues can produce modifications that will create workable systems; inattention can produce impaired function and disability.

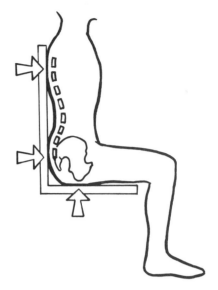

Figure 32-6. Patients seated on planar surfaces may show increased pressures over bony prominences.

POSTURAL SUPPORT SYSTEM

The components of the system that will directly affect comfort and maintenance of posture are the seat surface, back surface, pelvic belt, and upper extremity and foot supports. These areas should be addressed together as the postural support system. Increased contact between the user and the support surfaces increases comfort and control, and decreases pressure over bony prominences.[3–10] The continuum of available support surfaces runs from firm **planar surfaces** (wood, firm foam) (Fig. 32-6), through deformable surfaces (knit-covered foam) (Figs. 32-7, 32-8), and **contoured surfaces** (Fig. 32-9), up to and including **custom-molded surfaces** (Fig. 32-10).

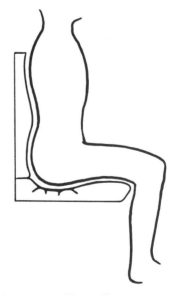

Figure 32-7. Some types of foam will contour as a response to body weight.

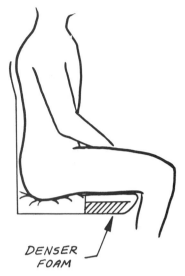

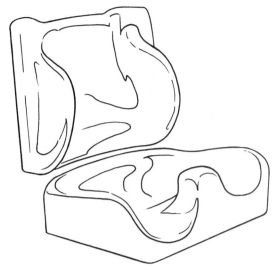

Figure 32-8. Varying the firmness of the foams can create a more contoured seat.

Figure 32-10. Custom-molded cushions match the patient's body contours.

Angular relationships between the surfaces at the hip and knee joints (seat and back surfaces, seat and calf surfaces) must be determined by the range of motion measures obtained in the physical examination. This information will allow the planned intervention to accommodate limitations in range of motion, assure proper alignment of body segments, and minimize pressure distal to the joint. The user's comfort level is affected by changes of orientation in space (fixed or dynamic) affect the user's comfort level, pressure over skin surfaces, fatigue, and ability to work in gravity-minimized and gravity-influenced positions. Attention to these features will help ensure the success of the seating intervention.

undersurface of the thigh and the seating surface will enhance sitting ability by providing a stable base of support on which to mount upper body function.[4-7] In some cases, the front of the seat can actually extend into the popliteal fossa, provided that the front edge is well padded and contoured to provide relief for hamstring tendons, calf bulk, and/or bracing. This surface many require specialized foam in one or varying firmnesses, or a specific contour. The patient also may require a special cushion for comfort, control, and/or pressure relief. Cushions are generally made of foam, gel, liquid, pockets of air, or a combination of these elements (Table 32–1).

Text continued on p 1072

Seat Surface

Many wheelchairs come with a *sling seat*. This type of surface reinforces a poor pelvic position because the hips tend to slide forward, creating a posterior pelvic tilt. The thighs typically move toward adduction and internal rotation, and the patient tends to sit asymmetrically (Fig. 32-11). Most wheelchair users can benefit from a firm sitting surface (Fig. 32-12). Total contact between the

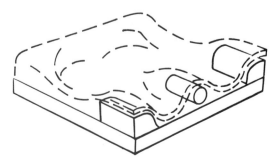

Figure 32-9. Firmer foam shapes can be placed under a more flexible foam to create a contoured cushion.

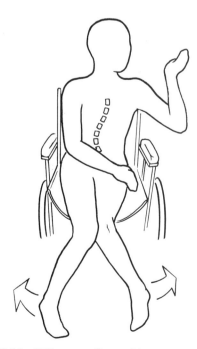

Figure 32-11. Sitting on a sling seat increases asymmetries.

Table 32–1 FEATURES OF THE WHEELCHAIR POSTURAL SUPPORT SYSTEM

	Characteristics	Postural Control Provided (at impairment level)
Seat Supports		
Solid insert	• Padded insert board; reinforcement board inside cushion cover; contoured or flat insert board between cushion and wheelchair upholstery. • Can be used with any cushion, custom or pre-made, for comfort or pressure relief. • Velcro interface to upholstery. • Spans seat rails or mounts to upholstery between seat rails. • Works best with cushions that have zip-off cover to allow use of wide strips of Velcro interfacing to hold cushion securely. • Addition of extra Velcro sewn to upholstery and underside of insert or cover will hold better during sliding transfers.	• Creates stable, level base of support. • Decreases tendency toward adduction and internal rotation of lower extremities, posterior pelvic tilt, and slipping forward on the seat. • Improves pelvic position. • Encourages level pelvis, neutral pelvic tilt, symmetrical spinal alignment.
Solid hook-on seat	• Seat upholstery is removed and solid seat is installed using hardware to hook to seat rails. • Hardware can be fixed level with seat rails or dropped lower than seat rails. • Angle and height adjustable; allows changing position of seat surface on frame of new or existing frame. • Can be integrated into cushion, or provide platform for cushion with Velcro interface.	• Improves pelvic position. • Creates stable, level base of support. • Decreases tendency toward adduction and internal rotation of lower extremities, posterior pelvic tilt, and slipping forward on the seat. • Encourages level pelvis; promotes neutral pelvic tilt; and symmetrical spinal alignment. • Raising anterior portion of seat can help keep patient back on wheelchair seat. • Raising posterior aspect of seat can facilitate trunk co-contraction.
Seat Cushions		
Comfort cushion (planar/contoured)	• Usually planar, but may have slight generic contour. • Varying degrees of firmness available for different comfort levels. • Can be made of layered foam to mix firmness for postural control and to accommodate limited range of motion (e.g., more flexion in one hip as compared to the other can be accommodated by different firmnesses, or by actually cutting the foam into different shapes).	• Increases comfort; facilitates level pelvis; promotes a neutral pelvic position. • Provides surface to create stable base of support.
Pressure-relieving foam (contoured, custom contoured)	• Based on principle that increased surface contact results in improved pressure distribution/relief. • Custom or pre-made contour depends on need to accommodate individual postural asymmetries. • Varying degrees of firmness available for different comfort levels. • Can be made of layered foam to mix firmnesses for postural control and to accommodate limited range of motion. • Generic shapes work best with symmetrical individuals.	• Shaped to control postural alignment. • Increases comfort; facilitates level pelvis; promotes a neutral pelvic position. • Provides surface to create stable base of support. • Custom-made contour more effective when accommodating asymmetries.
Pressure-relieving fluid or fluid/foam combination	• Based on principle that increased surface contact results in improved pressure distribution/relief; generic contour or planar surface with fluid filled sack. • Bony prominences are immersed in the fluid, increasing surface contact. • Some types have positioning components to accommodate for postural asymmetries and provide improved postural control. • Combination units allow the foam base to be cut to accommodate limited range of motion. • Generic contoured shapes work best with symmetrical individuals. • Firm under base provides stable support for proper seating alignment.	• Provides surface to create stable base of support. • Some arc-shaped or have add-on pieces to control postural alignment. • Increases comfort; facilitates level pelvis; promotes a neutral pelvic position. • Increases sitting tolerance for patients who sit with oblique pelvis. • Provides appropriate support for pelvis to promote level shoulders and erect head.

Functional Assistance Provided (at functional limitation/disability level)	Advantages	Disadvantages
Seat Cushions (*Continued*) • Good base on which to promote trunk extension and upper body stability. • Enhances distal function (head and upper extremities).	• Low cost. • Adds minimal weight to frame. • Removes easily for chair folding. • Wheelchair can still be used if solid insert is lost or forgotten.	• Increases seat height. • Can shift on seat and produce asymmetrical sitting surface.
• Good base on which to promote trunk extension and upper body stability. • Enhances distal function (head and upper extremities). • With forward slope, allows increased range of movement in upper extremities for reach and wheel approach.	• Can change slope of seat without tilt-in-space chair. • Wheelchair cannot be used if seat support is missing; ensures use at all times. • Dropped style can reduce effect of thick seat cushion on seat height. • Does not shift during transfers. • Seat angles can be changed to accommodate limited range of motion.	• More difficult to remove for folding than Velcro interface. • Adds weight to frame.
• Appropriate for patients with minimal seating needs. • Does not interfere with side transfers.	• Inexpensive. • Lightweight. • Patient can sit anywhere on cushion without discomfort. • Totally flat cushions with one firmness throughout can be rotated to decrease spot wear.	• No pressure relief. • Minimal support. • Minimal postural control.
• Appropriate for patients with moderate to significant seating needs. • Assists with controlling posture and/or accommodating pelvic asymmetries to allow level shoulders and more erect head position. • Increases sitting time; decreases problems with pressure over boney prominences; improves postural stability that results in increased upper body function.	• Increased surface contact creating improved pressure distribution. • Accommodates moderate to severe postural asymmetry. • Easier for caregivers to position and reposition patient. • Low maintenance.	• More expensive. • May interfere with side transfers. • Patient may feel (locked in) because movement on cushion surface restricted.
• Appropriate for patients with moderate to significant seating needs. • Assists with controlling posture and/or accommodating pelvic asymmetries to allow level shoulders and more erect head position. • Results in increased sitting time; decreased problems with pressure over boney prominences; improved postural stability; and increased upper body function. • Gel medium usually increases stability at the pelvis; the pelvis sinks in and is "held" by the foam, essentially broadening the base of the support area.	• Increases surface area, contact creates improved pressure distribution. • Accommodates moderate to severe postural asymmetry. • Increases stability at the pelvis. • Easier for caregivers to position and preposition patient.	• More expensive. • Some maintenance required. • Heavier than foam or air. • Patient may feel (locked in) because movement on cushion surface is restricted.

(Continued)

Table 32–1 FEATURES OF THE WHEELCHAIR POSTURAL SUPPORT SYSTEM *(Continued)*

	Characteristics	Postural Control Provided (at impairment level)
Seat Cushions *(Continued)* Pressure-relieving air	• Appears planar, but responds to patient weight. • Patient is immersed in the cushion based on regulation of the amount of air. • Based on principle that increased surface contact results in improved pressure distribution/relief; bony prominences are floating. • Usually the best pressure relief of any cushion.	• Does not provide a very stable base of support; some users find it too unstable. • Individuals with decreased trunk stability tend to keep arms closer to the body for stability, decreasing upper extremity reach distance. • Segmented cushions are available allowing more air into selected segments to increase firmness; firmer cells may improve postural control; segmented cushions are less pressure relieving because the air cannot flow from one segment of the cushion to the other. • Some postural accommodation can be provided by placing foam pieces under the cushion, allowing use of the more pressure relieving single valve (single segment) style; when electing to do this pressure must be monitored carefully.
Back Supports Pita back	• Solid board (padded or unpadded) that slips into a pocket in the back upholstery. • Provides mild to moderate level of support. • Useful for patients who need a slight reminder to sit upright.	• Assists patients who need a reminder to sit with trunk extension. • Assists with maintaining a neutral pelvis and an upright sitting posture.
Solid insert	• Maintains pelvic alignment when correctly interfaced with seat surface (based on range of motion assessment to determine available hip flexion). • If attached to the upholstery by Velcro, or hung between the back canes, it provides moderate support and will not decrease seat surface depth on the chair. • If hung or belted in front of the back canes, will decrease seat surface depth. • Will assume the angle of the back canes unless braced across the top. • Special foaming can be used to accommodate back contour or provide some postural control.	• Maintains pelvic alignment when interfaced with seat surface; enhances upright sitting, trunk, and head alignment. • Provides some lateral control if shaped foaming is used.
Solid hook-on back	• Very stable back support that can be aligned and angled as needed to create appropriate seat/back angle; accommodates for limited range of motion. • Can hold planar, contoured or molded back, or air flotation cushion for pressure relief. • Can be manufactured or custom-made. • Allows for provision of maximum support when needed. • Mounts using permanent or removable hardware; with use of permanent hardware can actually strengthen frame.	• Enhances upright sitting; accommodates for limited range of motion; accommodates for any degree of deformity; provides support as needed. • Maintains client in position deemed appropriate based on assessment findings.
Specialized Support Components Head/neck support	• Provides support for patients with fair, poor, or absent head control. • Mounting hardware can be fixed, removable and/or flip back; hardware can be adjusted in one, two, or multiple planes.	• Posterior, lateral, and anterior head or neck controllers available. • Promotes maintenance of a neutral cervical spine and head position. • Eliminates lateral flexion and rotation which, when not controlled, can disturb trunk and pelvic alignment.
Lateral trunk supports	• Indicated in the presence of weak or spastic trunk muscles. • Can be straight or contoured for more control. • Mounting hardware can be fixed or swing-away for transfers.	• Improves trunk stability and alignment (within available range); improves pelvic alignment. • Controls lateral trunk flexion.
Anterior chest support	• Assists with maintenance of upright trunk posture and control of shoulder position. • Can be minimally supportive or maximally supportive depending on configuration straps, padded straps, butterfly, and bib.	• Supports trunk along anterior surface of trunk and shoulders; eliminates forward lean. • May influence and discourage shoulder protraction.

Functional Assistance Provided (at functional limitation/disability level)	Advantages	Disadvantages
• Imperative for patients with moderate to significant pressure-relieving needs. • Results in increased sitting time; decreased problems with pressure over bony prominences.	• Very lightweight. • Accommodates moderate to severe postural asymmetry. • Increases surface contact for improved pressure distribution.	• More expensive. • Base provided may be too unstable for some users; unstable base may make transfers difficult. • Continuous maintenance required.
• Provides enough support to encourage trunk extension.	• Lightweight. • Slips in and out easily for folding.	• Only provides slight degree of support. • Wheelchair can be used without this back support. • It can be lost or left behind when the chair is folded. • May not be stable in chair.
• Enhances trunk control to allow improved distal function.	• Removes easily for folding. • Assists with postural control. • Adds minimal weight to chair.	• Wheelchair can be used without this back support. • It can be lost or left behind when the chair is folded.
• Provides support to enhance movement control of the upper extremities and head. • Increases surface area, contact provides improved comfort and pressure relief. • Maintains trunk alignment to enhance pelvic positioning.	• Solid support structure. • Resists extensor thrusting. • Accepts planar, contoured, or molded surfaces. • Wheelchair cannot be used without this back support in place. • Allows attachment of additional supports such as headrests which work best when back structure is solid and stable.	• Increases weight of wheelchair. • Requires manipulation of hardware to remove and fold wheelchair.
• Supports the head to assist with respiration, visual interaction with environment, feeding and swallowing. • Improves safety during transport on level surfaces and when patient is transported seated in wheelchair placed in a motor vehicle.	• Provides support and improves alignment. • Improves safety during transport.	• May interfere with head movement. • May trigger extensor thrust. • May cause skin problems in areas of high pressure.
• Improves trunk control; facilitates upper extremity movement and distal control. • Improves respiration, feeding, and swallowing.	• Improves stability and alignment. • Improves head alignment and control. • Enhances safety during movement through space.	• May interfere with trunk movement. • Increases weight of the system. • May interfere with attempts to self-propel with upper extremities.
• Trunk support may improve respiration, feeding, and swallowing. • Stabilizes trunk to allow improved upper extremity function and head control. • Shoulder control promotes better head posture.	• Supports trunk in upright position. • Stabilizes trunk to free arms and head for movement. • Improves head position for respiration, feeding, swallowing and visual interaction with environment.	• Restricts trunk movement. • Overuse limits patient's opportunity to improve trunk control.

(Continued)

Table 32–1 FEATURES OF THE WHEELCHAIR POSTURAL SUPPORT SYSTEM *(Continued)*

	Characteristics	Postural Control Provided (at impairment level)
Specialized Support Components *(Continued)*		
Lateral hip guides	• Improves pelvic alignment on seat. • Assists with maintaining pelvic position on contoured seat.	• Improves weight distribution in pelvis. • Improves pelvic positioning; enhances alignment of upper and lower body segments; contributes to alignment of entire body. • Assists with maintenance of pelvic alignment which reduces asymmetries in trunk and lower extremities.
Lateral knee guides	• May be built into the cushion contours, or fabricated from separate pieces of padded wood or plastic attached to the seat or armrest of the wheelchair; should extend to the end of the knee if maximal control is required.	• Helps to maintain lower extremity alignment; reduces increased abduction and external rotation (e.g., patients who tend to fall into abduction, push into abduction, or whose legs do not come into neutral). • Improves neutral alignment of lower extremities; assists with maintenance of pelvic position. • Maintains lower extremity alignment with use of anterior knee block.
Medial knee block	• May be built into the cushion contours, or be a separate removable or flip-down block. • For maximal control, the medial knee block should be positioned at the distal portion of limb, between condyles. • The support should never be used to stabilize the pelvis on the seat by pressing into the groin; it also should not be used to stop the user from sliding off the front of the seat.	• Prevents lower extremities from moving into adduction. • If wide enough, may decrease hypertonus. • Maintains lower extremity alignment; when used with windblown posture, medial knee block can prevent pelvis from continuing to rotate forward, use of wider blocks will keep the greater trochanter properly seated in the hip joint.
Anterior knee block	• Increases pelvic stability; most powerful way to maintain proper pelvic position on the seat (if hips are subluxed, dislocated, or not properly formed, approval from an orthopedist should be obtained).	• Maintains pelvic alignment; maintains pelvis in neutral tilt; prevents pelvis from moving forward on the seat surface. • Assists with maintenance of lower extremity alignment when used with medial and lateral knee controllers.

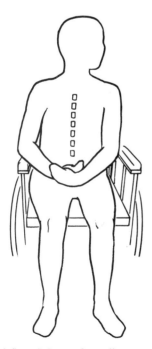

Figure 32-12. A firm sitting surface offers a good support base.

The depth of the seat should be measured carefully, because an overly deep seat will encourage a posterior pelvic tilt and a resultant tendency toward **kyphotic posturing.** A seat that is too shallow will not provide enough support, making maintenance of lower extremity alignment more difficult.

For persons with neuromuscular problems (e.g., multiple sclerosis, muscular dystrophy, cerebral palsy, traumatic head injury), the seat may require lateral hip, or **medial** or **lateral knee positioners** to maintain alignment of the lower extremities. The chair must be prepared for these additions before being upholstered. The seat also may require a change in orientation, or increased contour, to affect tone at the hips. This can be done with varying foam firmnesses, contouring, hardware changes, or properties built into the chosen mobility base.

Back Surface

Individuals using a wheelchair who have fair to good trunk control usually require only back support to the midscapula. Many prefer it lower.

Functional Assistance Provided (at functional limitation/disability level)	Advantages	Disadvantages
• Allows patient to achieve or tolerate better alignment. • Increases sitting time.	• Improves and maintains alignment. • Improves symmetrical weight-bearing through pelvis.	• May interfere with transfers if not removable. • Patient may feel "locked in" on seat. • Increases weight of the system.
• Improves pelvic position, promotes improved trunk position and upper extremity function. • Maintains neutral alignment of lower extremities; reduces forward sliding of pelvis on seat.	• Maintains lower extremity alignment. • May help to elongate adductors. • Assists with maintenance of pelvic position on the seat.	• If high enough to provide control, may interfere with transfers unless removable. • Adds weight to the seating system.
• Helps to maintain a broad, stable base of support; this base improves alignment of upper body.	• Maintains lower extremity alignment. • Reduces extensor tone. • Provides broader base of support.	• May interfere with transfers. • Increases weight of the seat.
• Helps to maintain a broad, stable base of support with neutral pelvic alignment; this base will promote improved alignment and functional use of upper body. • When used in conjunction with forward sloped seat may facilitate trunk co-contraction, extension, and improved upper extremity range of movement.	• Maintains lower extremity alignment. • Reduces extensor tone. • Provides broader base of support. • Increases stability.	• May impose too much pressure at the hips and over the patellas. • Patient may feel too restricted.

However, although some lower back supports work well in the short run, they may cause problems over longer periods of use, with users experiencing fatigue and back pain. For persons who have poor trunk control and those who tend to push into extension, the back height should be to the shoulders (approximately to the level of the acromium process). This is especially critical if any type of anterior shoulder support is to be used. This higher back may make it more difficult for caregivers to adjust the person's posture, but the added control offered will decrease the need for frequent postural adjustments.

Many individuals will not be provided adequate support from the standard fabric back that comes with a wheelchair. Some wheelchair backs are available with reinforcing straps that can be adjusted to provide contoured support. This type of support may be sufficient for some patients. Others will require a solid panel or insert placed into a pocket in the upholstery, strapped or attached by Velcro to the front of the upholstery, or installed on hardware instead of upholstery. The insert is fabricated from a firm base such as very firm foam, wood, plastic, or Triwall cardboard padded with foam. If placed in front of the upholstery, the foam can vary in thickness and firmness allowing more or less control at the pelvis or across the scapular and shoulder areas. The team must assess the patient's response to a back insert and vary the surface consistency, shape, and/or angle to the seat surface according to postural needs and comfort level. A very firm foam may work well for individuals with low central tone by encouraging more extension, but those with prominent bony protuberances may not tolerate this type of surface. Others may achieve good extension following alignment, but lose lateral stability requiring additional lateral contour and/or lateral supports.

Pelvic Positioner

A belt or more rigid pelvic positioner may be needed for safety and for assistance with postural control.[8] When using a belt, attention must be given to style, size, direction of pull, and placement to achieve maximum effectiveness.[9] Generally, the belt should form a 45-degree angle with the sitting surface (Fig. 32-13).[10] For some people, a 90-degree angle of pull may be more effective in providing postural control and alignment, while leaving the pelvis free for anterior or posterior movement (Fig. 32-14). Padding is recommended if the belt is pulled tightly to influence or maintain pelvic alignment.

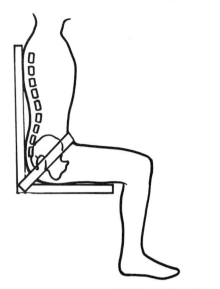

Figure 32-13. A belt crossing the pelvic-femoral junction works well for most patients.

Upper Extremity Supports

Wheelchair armrests have many important functions. They provide assistance for pushing up to standing, a support surface for arms and upper extremity support surfaces such as lap boards, a mechanism for relief of ischial pressure (sitting push ups), and some small amount of lateral stability. Attention should be directed to the height of the armrests, and the length and size of the support surface. It may be necessary for the patient to use the armrests to support the upper extremities and thus to decrease pull on the shoulders and trunk. This approach is often used for individuals with significant weakness, such as those with higher-level spinal cord injuries or muscular dystrophy. Individuals who lean on their armrests for postural

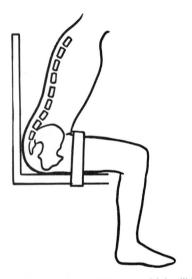

Figure 32-14. A belt placed over the upper thigh will free the pelvis for natural anterior tilting.

assistance will have decreased functional use of the upper extremities.

For many individuals, the armrests will be used to mount an **upper extremity support surface (UESS)** such as a tray or trough. These surfaces provide several important functions. They can be used to achieve symmetric positioning of the upper extremities, maintain corrected alignment of the glenohumeral joint and scapula, and serve as a work or communication surface. They also can act as an adjunct to the postural control system by supporting the weight of the upper limbs and decreasing pull on the shoulders and trunk. Additionally, in special cases, high (elevated) UESSs can be used to inhibit tone around the shoulders and neck. In extreme cases, the upper extremities of individuals with athetosis may be purposely anchored beneath the UESS to decrease interference from involuntary movement when using a head pointer or during feeding activities. Some individuals with involuntary movements find that stabilizing their upper extremities under the UESS, or with a combination of side walls and straps on the top of the UESS, allows them to isolate head and oral movements for feeding, switch access, and so forth.

Foot Supports

Style and position are important considerations when selecting wheelchair foot support systems. Placement of the foot support system will directly affect the position of the entire lower body, affecting tone and posture in the trunk, head, and arms. Good hip flexion will help keep the pelvis well positioned on the sitting surface. Good foot support height and style are required for maintenance of this position. Foot supports that are too low will result in lower knees, placing the hips in a more open angle and encouraging forward sliding of the pelvis. Foot supports that are too high may unload the thighs, placing increased weight on the ischial tuberosities. Elevating leg rests even in their lowered position may place excessive stretch on tight hamstrings, pulling the pelvis into a posterior tilt (Fig. 32-15). Any limitation of motion imposed by the hamstrings will directly influence the choice of foot positioners. To achieve maximum comfortable hip flexion, it may be necessary to flex the knees more than 90 degrees, requiring special intervention on the foot supports. Decisions regarding straps and foot positioners must be made early, based on range of motion assessment, to ensure clearance for placement on the final unit.

THE WHEELED MOBILITY BASE

The wheeled base forms the mobility structure for the seating system. Mobility bases include dependent systems, independent systems activated manually, and independent systems activated under battery power.

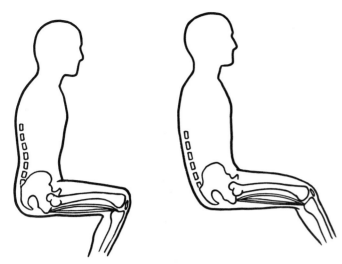

Figure 32-15. Overstretching tight hamstring muscles will pull the pelvis into a posterior pelvic tilt.

Dependent systems include strollers, pushchairs, and many of the elaborate postural support systems used with individuals with severe physical and mental impairments. These systems may have small wheels that are not intended for self-propulsion. When considering a dependent mobility system, it is important to determine the function of the unit. Is this a primary mobility system or a backup for the person who has a powered mobility unit? If the ability to use any independent movement system exists, (i.e., using one arm, one leg, or even eye blink, breath, or tongue movement) the person should be considered for either a manual or powered wheelchair as the primary mobility system. Sophisticated technology now allows even the most severely physically impaired individual to achieve independent mobility. If at all possible, even very young children (12 months or older) and the elderly should be provided with a means of independent mobility that allows them to extend beyond the boundary of their physical limitation. Research supports the beneficial impact of independent functioning on all aspects of cognitive and psychosocial well-being.[11–14]

When preparing the specifications for a wheeled mobility base, many features must be carefully considered. There are dozens of bases available, each with subtly different features. The team will be challenged in their effort to make the correct match between user and product (Fig. 32-16).

The Seat

SEAT DEPTH

Correct seat depth is particularly important to achieve maximum postural support and control. Wheelchairs are readily available from manufacturers in various seat depths. The depth measurements given in the catalog usually correspond to the depth of the upholstery itself from the back to the front edge. Depending on the manufacturer, the uphol-

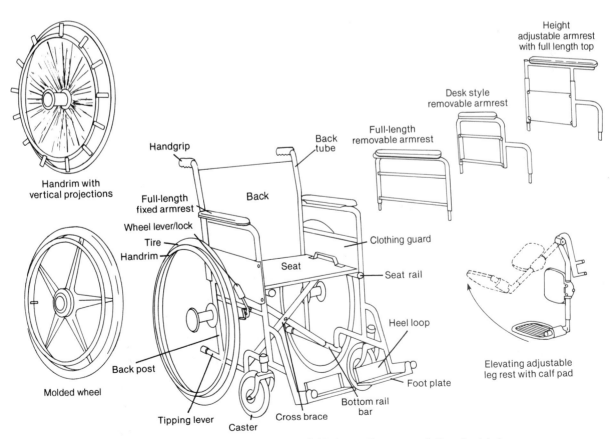

Figure 32-16. Multiple options are available in creating a prescriptive wheelchair.

stery depth may be equal to, less than, or greater than that of the metal seat rail. The team must be aware of different manufacturers' features. If the patient does not fit a listed size, modifications can be made by use of a back insert, by frame construction, or by upholstery modifications. Most seat depth modifications can be made on a new or existing wheelchair.

BACK INSERT

A back insert can be used to alter the overall depth of the sitting surface. This back insert, or cushion, can be ordered with any specified overall thickness, and usually consists of a piece of wood or plastic and foam padding. Inserts can be placed in front of the wheelchair's upholstery, or the upholstery can be removed and the back insert can be mounted with specialized hardware (Fig. 32-17). When ordering back inserts it is imperative to know the manufacturer's standard thickness and type of foam. With most styles of wheelchairs one can specify whether the insert is to be positioned between the back tubes or in front of them. This choice will affect the impact of the back insert on overall available sitting surface. If the upholstery is to remain in place, it is important to note whether it is mounted in front of the back tubes, between the back tubes, or half and half, inasmuch as this will directly affect the placement of the back insert. It is also critical to note whether the back tube has a bend, which will affect the vertical orientation of the back insert. Putting the insert in front of the back tubes will push the user forward, and may affect the patient's ability to reach the wheels for self-propulsion.

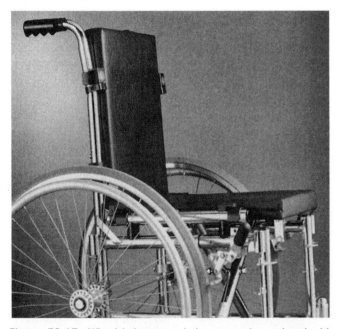

Figure 32-17. Wheelchair seat upholstery can be replaced with firm inserts held to the frame by specialized hardware. Usually the seat, or a cushion with a seat board inside, can safely extend approximately 2 inches (5 cm) beyond the end of the seat rail.

FRAME CONSTRUCTION

Seat depth also can be modified (increased or decreased) by frame construction. Modifications by construction should be considered with short and wide individuals, very tall persons, or long-legged individuals who have slowed or completed their growth cycle. An important factor to consider is that lengthening the chair frame will increase the turning radius and may prevent the user from maneuvering the chair in small spaces. A few manufacturers supply seat extension kits or special rear frame designs that extend the seat rail a few inches without changing the overall length of the frame. Seat rail extension kits work well on many frames, but on others they may extend over the top of the footrest and prevent removal of the footrest when the wheelchair is in the open position.

UPHOLSTERY MODIFICATIONS

Wheelchair seat depth may also be altered by upholstery changes. This can be achieved symmetrically if leg length is equal, or asymmetrically if leg length is unequal. Seat depth can be increased or decreased within specific dimensions set by the manufacturer. Generally, a seat insert or a seat cushion with a board inside its cover can be extended 1 to 2 inches (2.54 to 5.08 cm) beyond the front end of the seat rail without creating an unstable sitting surface (see Fig. 32-17). The seat upholstery, insert, or cushion can be cut back several inches to shorten the seat surface. Inserts can be fabricated with growth tails that fit between the back tubes as unused sitting surface; more seat depth can be exposed by pulling the seat forward along the seat rail as needed. The effects on foot placement of any of these modifications must be assessed. Subsequent foot plate adjustments may be required.

Working on the upholstery of the chair requires detailed knowledge of what each manufacturer considers standard. For instance, is upholstery depth as listed in the catalog the same as seat rail length, 1 inch (2.54 cm) shorter, or 1 inch (2.54 cm) longer? If the chair is offered with a seating system, are the measurements supplied taken from the seating system or the wheelchair frame? Are standard foot plates a large or small size, and how close are they to the front end of the frame? Can they be ordered closer to the frame to minimize effect on overall length, so that the seat can be deepened without affecting turning radius? Careful assessment of various wheelchairs will reveal differences in available parts and interfaces depending on wheelchair style and manufacturer.

SEAT WIDTH

The width of the seat, as well as the overall width of the wheelchair, is important to functional use. Special considerations will be needed for individuals who wear orthoses, require **control blocks** at the hip, wear bulky clothing, or experience weight fluctuations. The natural tendency is to increase the width of the seat. Such a solution must be approached cautiously, however, inasmuch as this will also increase the overall width of the chair and may create difficulty for those needing to reach the wheels for self-propulsion or for those who must maneuver in tight places. The overall outside width of the chair should be as narrow as possible for optimal function. Excessive width makes the chair difficult to maneuver through doorways and in small areas. It is also more difficult to propel the chair if the user must widely abduct his or her arms to reach the wheels. This wide abduction requires the patient to use available muscular strength around the shoulder girdle for stability and posture, leaving less to use for functional push (Figs. 32-18 and 32-19). The goal is to create a chair that fits as close to the user's body as possible. This will make the chair easy to wheel and maneuver. It also will make the chair seem, visually, more congruent with the user's body lines.

Seat width can be changed in several ways. Widening can be accomplished by (1) use of fixed offset or removable arms, (2) construction design of a new chair, and (3) changing the cross braces on an existing chair. Seat narrowing can be achieved by upholstery or by construction modifications. Narrowing a chair by upholstery essentially creates a "growing" chair out of any size chair. The chair is simply folded a bit. A limiter strap and/or narrower upholstery is mounted, preventing full-width opening. This will raise the seat height. This should not be done on chairs where the top seat rail must clip to the bottom rail for stability. Other width modifications include various hand rim and armrest options, internal mounting of the wheel axle plate on some ultra light wheelchairs, and wheelchair narrowing devices (which can be used to move the chair through a narrow space for a short distance). Narrowing devices are useful only for individuals who have sufficient coordination to rock the chair forward and back while turning the crank handle of the device. The device will not work with solid seat inserts, or with reclining wheelchairs that have spreader bars to reinforce the back. If there is enough room to use the wheelchair-narrowing device comfortably, perhaps the wheelchair should have been narrower in the first place.

SEAT HEIGHT

The height of the wheelchair seat is important for optimal independent functioning in foot-assisted, self-propulsion transfers (especially reentering the chair using a standing or stand pivot approach), approaching working surfaces, interacting with peers, and transferring into a van via lift or ramp. Seat height must be assessed with respect to the entire chair, inasmuch as it may alter the user's position relative to the armrests, back height, wheel locks, wheels, and footrests. Seat height can be al-

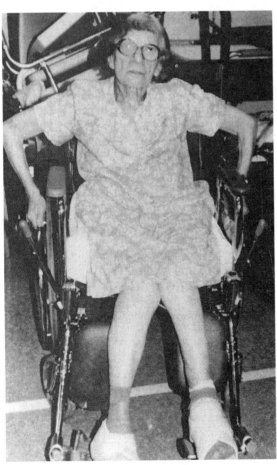

Figure 32-18. A wheelchair that is too wide will make wheel propulsion more difficult for the patient.

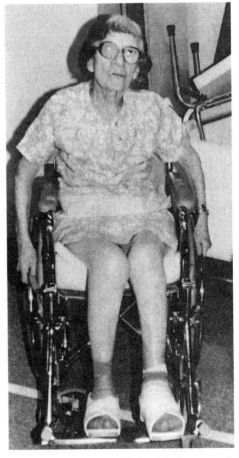

Figure 32-19. A narrower wheelchair with the armpads turned to the inside allows easier wheel propulsion.

tered by one or more methods, including (1) altering the frame construction when ordering the chair, (2) changing the wheel size, (3) altering the rear axle and front caster placement on frames that allow this, (4) altering the thickness of the seat inserts or cushions, (5) removing the seat upholstery, and (6) using solid hook-out seat boards with varying depth hardware to raise or drop the seat on the frame.

SEAT SURFACE

A firm sitting surface will provide a more symmetric sitting base. The firm surface will provide a more stable base of support for the upper body, usually resulting in improved function. A firm sitting surface can be achieved in a variety of ways, with or without specialized cushions (see Table 32–1).

Prior to deciding on a nonstandard seat surface, the team should inspect what the manufacturer considers a standard seat. Some manufacturers use extremely taut fabric for their seat slings (notably some of the ultra light wheelchairs). In combination with a firm foam cushion, no other support may be needed. Others use a fabric design that allows the sling component to be adjusted. This works adequately for some users, allowing them to adjust the tension as the sling becomes slack with extended use. Some manufacturers of nonfolding and motorized wheelchairs replace the seat upholstery with a solid metal or plastic pan, allowing a cushion to be attached to the surface with Velcro.

If a firmer seat is needed, there are several ways this can be achieved (Fig. 32-20). The simplest is to incorporate a homemade or commercially fabricated board into the foam cushion that comes with the chair. An off-the-chair foam cushion that comes with a removable cover can be purchased separately from the chair. It is possible that this lightweight unit may slide about in the chair, producing an asymmetric sitting surface. Many cushions do have special nonslip fabric or Velcro strips on the underside that discourage slippage. It may be helpful for some patients to have extra Velcro attached to the seat upholstery and to the bottom of a zip-on cushion cover to avoid cushion shift during transfers. Some manufacturers offer cushion rigidness.

This is usually a plastic panel attached by Velcro between the seat upholstery and the underside of the cushion. These work well with many patients, but may also slip out of place and provide asymmetrical seating.

A second option for a firm seat is to order the wheelchair with a standard hammock seat and a solid seat insert on top. This type of insert adds slight additional weight to the wheelchair system. The insert is usually made of foam and wood, and is covered with vinyl to match the chair. The standard thickness and firmness of the foam varies with each manufacturer. The individual rehabilitation technology supplier will provide information on standard foam characteristics so that alterations can be made as needed. Custom thicknesses and firmnesses are available if requested, either directly from the primary manufacturer or from a manufacturer of wheelchair component parts. The solid seat insert has several drawbacks. The insert may slip about in the seat, especially when the armrests are spaced away from the seat, creating an asymmetric sitting surface with one side on the seat rail and the other on the upholstery only. The insert must be removed to fold the chair.

Another option for firm seating is a solid folding seat. This type of seat is an integral part of the frame. It is permanently hinged to one seat rail, folding up when the chair is folded and dropping down into place as it is opened. When the chair is folded, this style of seat alters the shape of the chair. It is important to determine whether this shape will fit into the patient's car. When this folding seat is in the opened position, it rests between the seat rails, leaving the rails exposed. If it is 1 inch (2.54 cm) thick overall, its top surface will be level with the seat rails. If it is fabricated with thicker foam, the solid folding seat surface will be above the seat rails. In a 16-inch (40.64 cm) wide wheelchair, for instance, there will be 14 inches (35.56 cm) of upholstered and padded seating surface and 1 inch (2.54 cm) of rail exposed on each side. Some users find this uncomfortable if they are using the full seat width as a sitting surface. The advantage of a solid folding seat is that it cannot get lost, or be eliminated from the seating system for

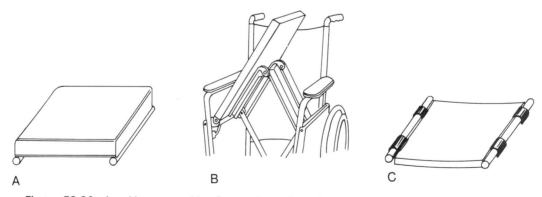

Figure 32-20. A cushion can provide a firm seating surface with a solid internal board (A), a solid folding seat (B), or a solid hook-on seat (C).

convenience. Some manufacturers provide hardware for solid folding seats that adds strength to the frame but will also add 7 to 10 pounds to the weight of the chair. Other manufacturer's wheelchairs have a simpler mechanism, adding neither weight nor additional strength to the frame of the chair.

A fourth option for providing a solid seating surface is the solid hook-on seat. This is a separate seat board that has hook-type hardware along both sides. These hooks clip onto the seat rail, securing the seat in the chair. The seat can hook on at the level of the seat rails, or below or above them. With this variability, and with the different thicknesses of foam available for the insert and/or separate seat cushions, it is possible to change the height of the sitting surface without altering the frame. When the seat is removed to fold the chair, there is no sitting surface on the chair frame and there is no extra hardware. The hook-on seat does not add weight to the folded frame, but will add weight to the open frame. Care should be taken in providing this alternative to users who drive, because the wheelchair's seat upholstery is frequently used as a handle for pulling the chair into the car. In addition to the standard bent hooks, the solid hook-on seat can be equipped with specialized hardware that allows the seat surface to be angled. Many styles of hardware are available from different manufacturers. Several wheelchair manufacturers include angle-adjustable seats in their catalogs.

The Back

To determine the height of the back, the degree of back support needed to achieve optimal function must be ascertained. The wheelchair back can be ordered to specification. Until the person's medical status is stable, consideration should be given to ordering add-on or removable parts, such as a headrest extension, a sectional-height back that can be removed and replaced later with lower upholstery and back tubes, or an adjustable-height back. The additional back height may make the chair too large to fit into a car, or may not allow adequate clearance for entering a van. In such cases, or in cases in which a custom chair is not possible or an existing chair is in good condition, a removable back insert in a custom height might suffice.

When increasing or decreasing the back height, attention should be directed to the level of the push handles. On many chairs these can be mounted at a height most useful for the caregivers. An extra reinforcement cap of upholstery may provide additional strength to the upper edge of the upholstery. A few wheelchairs are upholstered with the top edge of the back upholstery wrapped around the front of the back tubes; on other chairs, the upholstery forms a sleeve around the back tubes.

On standard wheelchairs, the back tubes rise straight to midback level and then angle backward. When a user leans on these for support, they tend to facilitate shoulder retraction and back extension. Patients often need this leeway to feel comfortable. If a solid back insert is used, the user may push the top edge until it rests on the tubes, forcing the bottom edge to push the pelvis forward on the wheelchair seat. If this problem is anticipated, it is possible to order the chair with straight tubes instead of the standard angled ones. It is also possible to brace the insert to maintain the designated angle for good posture. For active individuals who require clearances for a full upper extremity movement to access the wheels efficiently, it may be necessary to use a H-back with a rounded contour, or a scapula cut-out. This type of back will provide good support along the spine while freeing scapula, shoulder, and humerus for wheel access and push. In addition to back height, many wheelchairs offer angle adjustable back canes, allowing the chair to be set up with a more open or closed seat/back angle. Again, this can be achieved with a back insert on angle adjustable hardware if only a small amount of adjustment range is required. It should be noted that back inserts add extra weight to the chair for pushing and must be removed for folding

The Pelvic Positioner

The pelvic belt is one of the simplest features on a prescription wheelchair. Most clinicians know that the pelvic belt should cross the pelvis at a 45-degree angle to the sitting surface, and many understand that the closure style is often critical. There is more than this involved, however, in deciding on a proper pelvic belt. The style of closure is important in facilitating independent use. Many patients can manage only Velcro, whereas others can manage only buckles. If the user is not able to use the belt independently, and/or significant postural control is required, the style of belt is limited. Some Velcro closure belts are not strong enough for use by persons with severe extensor spasm. For these, and for others who require a great deal of control, a Velcro and D-ring style closure belt, or a belt with a cinching-style buckle arrangement, is the most suitable. Cinching-style buckles similar to those on automobile seat belts are available in push-button and flipper styles. The critical feature desired on all styles is that, once the initial contact has been made with the fastener, the belt can be adjusted further to increase tightness.

The direction and angle of pull of the belt is important. For example, if one hip tends to pull forward consistently, it may be useful to have the belt tighten by pulling it down toward that hip. The angle of pull to the seating surface should normally be 45 degrees. Some patients respond well to belts that form a 90-degree angle with the sitting surface. This pull discourages patients who tend to "stand" in their wheelchairs as a result of tone increases. This 90-degree placement also leaves the pelvis free for anterior tilting, an assist for those patients who can use this mobility for added function. Mounting the belt to the seat rail is common. Caution should be used with patients who push into excessive extension. This type of belt placement may cause the wheelchair to fold as the rider pushes upward on the belt. In such situations, a custom-made piece of hardware may be needed to mount the belt at a specific point on the lower wheelchair rail (Fig. 32-21).

The width of the belt and size of the buckle will affect the level of control offered. The belt and buckle must be correctly proportioned to the user's body. Small children should have belts 1 inch (2.54 cm) wide; larger children, belts 1.5 inches (3.81 cm) wide; and adults, belts 2 inches (5.08 cm) wide. The buckles should be comfortable. Plastic buckles may be more comfortable for some users. Padding may increase comfort and allow for tighter control.

The Lower Extremity Support

The footrest (swing-away) and legrest (elevating and swing-away) lengths are determined by measuring the leg length from the popliteal fossa to the heel and subtracting 1 inch. The corresponding measurement on the wheelchair is called the **minimum footboard extension** (MinFBX). This measurement is the distance from the seat rail to the foot plate. If separate cushions or an insert with or without special foam thickness has been added, or if the seat itself must be angled, the MinFBX measurement must be modified accordingly when the chair is ordered from the manufacturer. For example, if the distance from the popliteal fossa to the heel is 16 inches (40.64 cm), and the patient is to sit on a cushion 2 inches (5.08 cm) thick, a MinFBX of approximately 14 inches (35.56 cm) will be needed if the seat is firm, or 15 inches (38.1 cm) if the seat is of soft foam.

Optimal foot placement may be difficult to achieve in the presence of postural control problems or abnormal tone. Proper sitting posture for maximum control may call for a 90-degree knee flexion angle with a neutral ankle position. Many times this knee-foot alignment is imperative for maintaining total body alignment, especially for people with tightness in the hamstring muscle group. For small individuals this is rather simple. When dealing with larger patients it may be necessary to (1) raise them on cushions, (2) order special, smaller casters (with or without special-length stem bolts or forks), (3) use

a special extended, or flared wheelchair frame, or (4) order a chair with the large fixed wheels in the front to allow the knees to be flexed to 90 degrees without the feet interfering with caster movement.

There are several styles of foot support: a one-piece footboard, tubular foot supports, or two individual foot plates. These supports can be mounted directly to the frame, on clip-off hangers, on swing-away hangers, or on elevating hangers. The style of hardware the particular manufacturer uses will change the orientation of the foot support to the frame of the chair and to the user's body. Swing-away hangers, for example, may place the foot plates parallel to the floor, or at an angle, and may locate them close to the chair frame or as much as 3 to 4 inches anterior to the front upright. Many manufacturers offer hangers as standard options at various angles (90, 70, 75, 60, and 65 degrees being the most common), and still others will make custom hangers on request. Angle adjustable hangers that allow seat/calf board adjustment from 60 to 180 degrees are also available. Rotational hanger brackets (also called spica clamps) can be adjusted to properly support lower extremities that are abducted or adducted when the patient is properly seated. These can be ordered on the original wheelchair, or as a later addition.

The mounting hardware should be chosen for function as well as posture. For individuals with edema, detachable elevating legrests may be required. For patients with increased hamstring tone or tightness (as in cerebral palsy, multiple sclerosis, or muscular dystrophy), elevating legrests are usually not recommended because opening the knee angle will stretch the hamstrings and may pull the pelvis out of alignment. Detachable swing-away footrests do not elevate, but do swing away to assist in transfers and in a better approach to the front of the wheelchair. When ordering front-rigging styles, consideration must be given to both present and future function so that the user will be able to continue to improve within the chair and not have a chair that actually exacerbates problems of management.

The size of the foot plate surface can vary. A few manufacturers offer three different sizes; others offer only one or two. The ultra light wheelchairs are often available with open or filled-in foot plates. The foot plate should accommodate the length of the foot, as well as the width of orthoses or oversized shoes. Narrowing a chair for a better fit around the hips and better hand placement on the rims also decreases the available space between the front tubes for the foot plates. Some of the flip-up style foot plates have additional hardware, which further limits the available space in this area.

Calf straps or pads can be used to help keep the feet on the foot plates. Heel loops and/or ankle straps may be needed to control the feet on the foot plate. Heel loops are available in webbing, vinyl, and plastic in various heights. Although plastic and extra high heel loops offer more control, they can prevent the foot plates from being flipped up, interfering with some transfer styles. Ankle straps control the

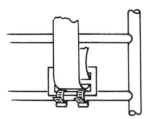

Figure 32-21. Specialized hardware can be used to clamp a lapbelt to the wheelchair rail.

heel position on the foot plate. The straps should make a 45-degree angle with the foot plate surface, causing weight to be placed into the heel. These straps can be simple Velcro, Velcro with D rings, or straps with buckles. Crossed ankle straps or figure-of-eight strapping also can be effective. A few users also may benefit from toe loops (or straps). Toe loops are generally fabricated from leather webbing and attach in a half-circle pattern to the anterior portion of the foot plate. Many toe loops are solid; others have Velcro or buckle openings. Toe loops are used to help control severe involuntary movements or spasticity (especially extensor spasms).

The Upper Extremity Support

Nonremovable armrests offer no specific benefits for an individual using a wheelchair unless it is likely that removable armrests will be lost. They are often ordered in an attempt to reduce the overall width of the chair. This can be achieved with wrap-around or space saver armrests that are removable and allow for transfers, sitting without armrests, use of special adapted inserts, changing from fixed-height to adjustable-height armrests, and so forth. Although adjustable and wraparound armrest styles may be more costly on the initial frame, they provide for a more flexible system that can be altered as the patient's functional needs change.

Wraparound armrests reduce the overall outside width of the chair by 1.5 inches (3.81 cm) because they allow the wheels to be mounted closer to the frame. This is accomplished by structural placement of the posterior upright of the armrest behind (wrapped around) the back tube (Fig. 32-22). This narrows the chair for easier maneuverability and places the wheels closer for better hand approach. Removal and repositioning of this style armrest may be difficult for some individuals, and a careful assessment is needed.

Height-adjustable armrests (Fig. 32-23) are important for children, especially those whose chair frames have been ordered with built-in growth allowance. This type of adjustability also is useful for users who need more or less support depending on the time of day or activity. For example, they can be raised to assist in sit-to-stand transfers and lowered for every day wheelchair use. They also permit placement of an upper extremity support surface without extensive custom modifications.

Full-length arm pads give more room for an UESS to be secured. They also afford the user a larger surface to grasp for push ups and transfers. Standard full-length armrests, however, may prevent the user from getting close to tables or work surfaces. Shorter-length, desk arms can be ordered to allow for this function. Alternately, full-length height-adjustable armrests allow the user to remove the armrest top or to raise it above the table surface; the front jog feature can then be used in a manner similar to a desk arm, while providing the longer top surface of a full-length pad.

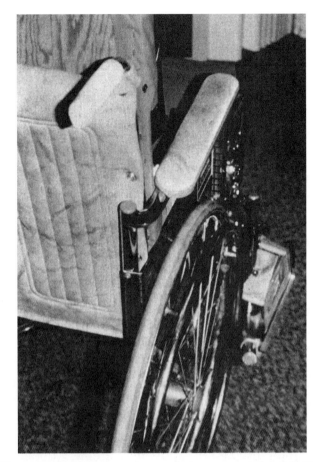

Figure 32-22. Wraparound or space-saver armrests insert behind the wheelchair's back tube.

Many of the wheelchairs in use today have non-traditional armrest styles. Some armrests are tubular, with rounded tops rather than flat armrest pads. Several of these styles have only one point of mounting on the chair (Figure 32-24). Although they may appear unstable, most of these work well for weight-bearing (e.g., for pressure relief or depression transfers). A few of the newer styles flip up but do not remove, and others swing out to the side. Some have

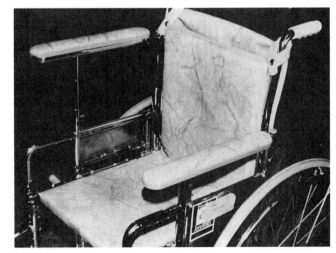

Figure 32-23. Height adjustable arms are available in desk or full length. They allow variable arm heights with a simple adjustment.

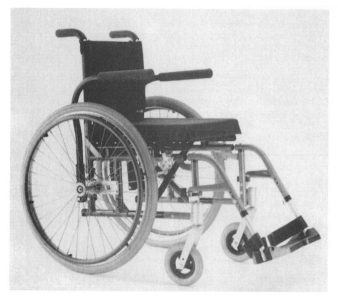

Figure 32-24. Traditional wheelchairs have the large wheel in the rear and a smaller wheel, or caster, in the front. (Photo courtesy of Quickie Designs.)

clothing guards, and others do not. It is important to examine all available options with function in mind to be certain which product will best suit the consumer's need.

When ordering a specific armrest style, the height of the armrest from the seat rail should be checked. After comparing this to the measurement obtained for the hanging elbow, a custom-ordered armrest height may be required. Wheelchair armrest height is determined by adding 1 inch (2.54 cm) to the hanging-elbow measure. Armrests that are too high will cause shoulder elevation, and those that are too short may encourage leaning. Those spaced too far apart may interfere with the person's ability to wheel the chair.

Wheels, Hand Rims, and Tires

Wheels are available in 12-, 16-, 20-, 22-, 24-, and 26-inch (30.48-, 40.64-, 50.8-, 55.88-, 60.96-, and 66.04-cm) diameters and are available through wheelchair manufacturers, as well as through specialty companies. They are available with standard or heavy-duty spokes (Figure 32-24), and in spokeless or molded styles (Figure 32-35). The spokeless styles are growing in popularity because they are easier to maintain, but they do add some extra weight to the frame. When quick-release axles are available as an option, they may be desirable because removing the rear wheels can reduce the folded chair size as well as reduce the weight of the chair by 8 pounds, making it more readily lifted or stored.

Wheel size and location are critical to the patient's ability to self-propel.[15–17] The rule of thumb is to achieve hand to wheel-crest touch with the elbow in at least 30 degrees of flexion. This will allow the user to produce an efficient stroke. Individuals with im-

paired strength or power may require a greater angle at stroke initiation and will tend to lean forward or to the side to increase the elbow angle and achieve a stronger push. Generally, the 24-inch (60.96-cm) wheel is adequate. This size may need to be specially ordered on small chairs. Although these large wheels often look strange on small chairs, they can add significantly to function because of their proximity to the user's hands. Patients who are weak or poorly coordinated may be able to self-propel if a choice of axle position allows for a personalized wheel placement. This is often a justification for ordering an ultra light wheelchair with a multiposition axle plate.

For patients who are unable to manage dual-wheel propulsion, one-arm drive systems are available (Fig. 32-25). These units use a double hand rim on one wheel to drive both wheels. Operation can be confusing and difficult to coordinate for those with limited cognitive or perceptual ability. Patients with increased tone may demonstrate spastic overflow and asymmetry when using one hand to propel the chair. When supplying this type of chair, attempts should be made to use one of the units with a very lightweight frame, multiple axle positions, and precision wheel bearings, which decrease rolling resistance.

Separate metal hand rims are standard on most wheels. They can be spaced further from the wheel if requested, but this will add width to the chair. Some users have difficulty propelling the wheelchair because of poor hand control or a weak grip. A leather glove or coated hand rim will add friction between the hand and rim, making wheeling easier. At higher speeds the friction on an ungloved hand may be uncomfortable when trying to slow or stop the wheelchair. Special hand rims can be ordered in increased diameter, with sponge coatings, and with knobs or projections.

Tires affect performance in both forward and

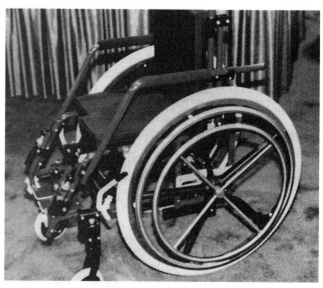

Figure 32-25. A double hand rim on one side allows the user to drive a one-arm drive wheelchair with one hand.

turning movements, because they interface with the environmental surface. The goal is minimal resistance between the tire and the floor surface. This allows the user to achieve the maximum result from each push. This is especially critical for patients who are weak or uncoordinated, and for those who are using the chair in athletic competition. Standard hard rubber tires are useful for most individuals. They are durable and easily maintained. Their narrow footprint offers minimal resistance to wheeling on most surfaces. Pneumatic (air-filled) tires are standard on some models (Fig. 32-24) and are available as a special order on others. These require more maintenance but provide a smoother ride and improved traction in some instances. Special high-pressure pneumatics offer the minimal resistance of the narrow, hard tire with the ride and performance of a pneumatic. In most pneumatic tires, zero pressure tubes or flat-proof liners can be substituted for the tube to create a flat-proof tire with the appearance of a pneumatic. The ride with these liners is not as smooth, and in some cases the life of the tire may be shortened.

The Frame

Most people who use wheelchairs utilize outdoor frames (Fig. 32-24). This means that the large wheels are in the back and the casters are in the front. Chairs with large wheels in the front (Fig. 32-26) are sometimes ordered for individuals with severe knee flexion contractures, for those whose upper extremity range of motion is limited, and for children who do better if they see the wheels. Although access to the wheels may be easier with the indoor model, overall maneuverability may be more difficult, and transfers may present a problem. Use of these chairs outdoors is difficult because it is almost impossible to pull them up curbs or steps. Front-wheel drive and outdoor power wheelchairs have their larger wheel in the front. They are usually powerful enough to climb small curbs, but the wheel configuration precludes a caregiver's pulling them up larger curbs and steps.

Chair frames are available in rigid or folding styles. Most rigid frames offer fold-down backs and removable wheels to allow some breakdown for stowage in vehicles. Rigid frames are tighter, and each of the user's pushes is translated more efficiently into chair motion. However, on uneven terrain the user of a rigid frame may be uncomfortable, because the frame transfers rather than absorbs shock. Rigid frames are the lightest available, with some weighing 20 pounds or less with the wheels in place (Fig. 32-27).

Chair frames are available in heavy-duty, standard, lightweight, active-duty lightweight, and ultra-lightweight construction. Patients and their caregivers who are functioning in the community should be offered the lightest, strongest possible frame feasible. The lighter frames are easier for the user to propel and easier for caregivers to manage. For

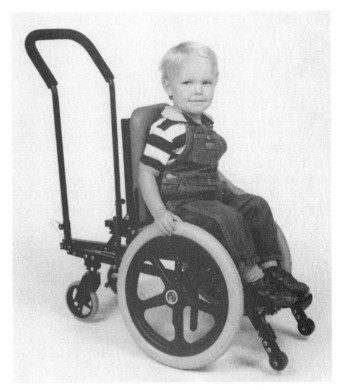

Figure 32-26. Wheelchairs with large front wheels and small rear casters may be easier for some patients to push, but are more difficult to use outdoors. (Photo courtesy of Mulholland Positioning Systems.)

individuals in institutions, or when caregivers do not have to lift and carry the unit, the issue of weight may be secondary to the issue of price. To justify the added expense of an active-duty lightweight or ultra-lightweight chair, explanation for its necessity must be provided to the third-party payer as a medical need.

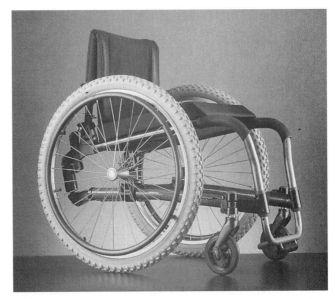

Figure 32-27. Lightweight rigid frame chair with adjustable dual-slider suspension system, seat back angle, adjustable wheel base, and footrest lengths. (Photo courtesy of Everest & Jennings.)

Accessories

Many accessories are available to personalize the chair for functional and aesthetic reasons. Crutch holders, anti-tippers, utility bags, and upper extremity support surfaces all serve a functional purpose. A choice of frame and upholstery color, usually at no extra cost, will help to personalize the chair. Making the perfect match between consumer and product will require a careful determination of the user's needs and a matching of these to the product features. Something as simple as the style of arm lock or the type of push handle may have important long-term functional or care-giving implications.

SPECIALIZED WHEELCHAIRS

Positioning

Patients with poor postural control, abnormal tone, muscle shortening, or skeletal deformities often require wheelchairs that offer varied positioning possibilities. A frame may be needed that offers a fixed or adjustable posterior tilt-in-space orientation (Fig. 32-28). This frame may need to be combined with a reclinable back or an angle-adjustable seating surface or both. Some chairs allow caregivers to change the seat position, whereas others afford the rider this control. Some offer components for positioning, such as head and torso supports. Several manufacturers offer systems that include positioning components on a mobility base. Others do not offer the components and it is necessary to interface more than one manufacturer's products to have a complete chair (see Table 32–1).

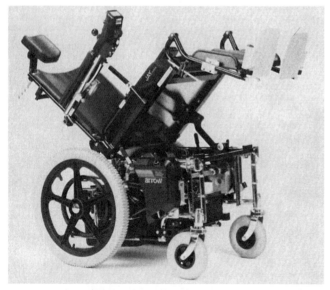

Figure 32-28. Wheelchairs that tilt through space with all their angles preset are called tilt-in-space wheelchairs. They are available in manual and motorized models. (Photo courtesy of La Bac.)

Power

A powered mobility system (Fig. 32-29) consists of a base or frame, a seat, and electronics (batteries, motors, control module, and driver control). A powered mobility system should be considered when a person cannot independently access his or her environment. Some wheelchair riders are marginal self-propellers in manual wheelchairs. They are able to move around indoors comfortably, and on level surfaces outdoors, but cannot move around in the community environment without unduly stressing muscles and joints, creating postural problems, and/or imposing cardiovascular strain. The long-term overuse injury of muscles and joints and the possibility of skeletal deformity must be discussed with the patient and caregiver as part of the examination process. Patients must face the possibility that they may create problems significant enough to impede function in critical areas such as transfers and activities of daily living.[19–21]

An assessment of the patient's full environment (micro [in the home] and macro [outside the home]) must be made to determine if powered mobility will be helpful and usable. Architectural barriers such as steps might preclude the use of powered mobility or require that the patient have both a powered and manual system for use at different times. In addition, attention should be given to how the chair will be transported, and the level of technology tolerance of both the consumer and caregiver. For patients whose condition is changing, a long-term plan must be established to guide decision making when choosing products. When considering powered mobility for children (from approximately 18 months of age) and adults who may have cognitive impairments, the rule of thumb is that the driver is aware of safety for themselves and others. In most cases the ability to stop and to judge when to stop, is more difficult to teach than driving itself. Awareness, reliable movement, and good response time are all important factors in wheelchair use. Some patients who can drive using a joystick cannot release it quickly enough, and might be safer using a different control site and/or a different type of controller.

The base or frame of the powered chair and the seat portion are the mechanical parts of the chair. As in all other areas there are advantages and disadvantages to the various systems available. Frame-style wheelchairs were the norm in previous years. In this type of chair the seat and base are one continuous structure. Many of these can be folded like a traditional manual wheelchair once the batteries (and their support frame if necessary) are removed. This type of system has some flexibility and may offer a more shock-absorbing ride. They offer more room underneath the seat for positioning of a ventilator and extra batteries if needed. However, because there are more flexing or moving parts there may be more breakage.

A base style frame is usually a one-size-fits-all wheeled component that accepts different seating

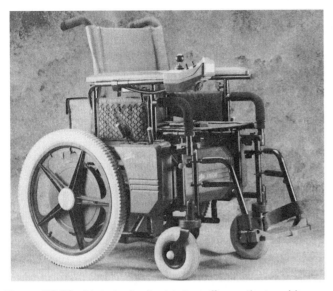

Figure 32-29. Motorized wheelchairs offer patients with poor coordination, weakness or paralysis, an opportunity to move around in their environment. (Photo courtesy of Invacare Corp.)

units. This allows positioning of wider seating units without affecting the base width proportionally as with frame-style chairs. Most manufacturers use the same base even with extra-wide seats, but may require the use of wider tires and casters. Therefore, for most adult users a base style chair will be narrower. This type of chair usually has a lower seat height, accepts larger batteries, and more easily accepts power seat components. They are usually extremely stable, making it more difficult for caregivers to assist with tilting the chair to mount curbs.

Belt-driven chairs are becoming rarer. These chairs perform best over firm surfaces, but some of the energy produced by the motors is lost in the belt and slippage before going to the wheel. Direct drive systems allow all of the energy to pass directly from the motor into the wheel. They are quieter, can have more torque when needed, and can use smaller, wider wheels for stability and an overall narrower footprint. Direct drive wheels can have rear, middle, or front placement. Although rear-wheel placement is more common, mid- and front-wheel drive chairs have a smaller turning radius and may allow for a tighter knee position to accommodate tight hamstrings and shorten the overall length of the systems. Mid-wheel drive chairs perform well outdoors, but may produce a "rocking chair" effect on acceleration and deceleration, which may be problematic for users with postural instability, or startle responses.

Power seat functions (e.g., power recline, power tilt, power elevating legrests, power seat elevator, and power stand-up) are extremely important for individuals using a powered wheelchair who are prone to pressure ulcers or orthostatic hypotension, those with poor endurance for upright sitting, as well as those with painful conditions that require frequent change of position. They are available in many combinations, with a few chairs offering all

of the features in one system. Addition of these features makes the chairs heavier and more difficult to maintain.

Motorized two-, three-, and four-wheeled vehicles and wheelchairs are available in many styles with varying degrees of portability, power, and electronic sophistication. In all cases it would be ideal if a proportional drive system could be used. **Proportional drives** respond to pressure like an automobile accelerator; the more pressure, the more speed. Because the speed and degree of acceleration are controlled by the rider's movement of the joystick, this type of system gives the user the greatest degree of control.

With the advent of microprocessor-controlled wheelchairs, the performance parameters of the joystick can be altered to adapt to the user's ability. Such systems allow individuals with severe spasticity and those who are extremely weak to achieve wheelchair mobility with a proportional system. Alternate access spots for users who cannot use their hands should be considered. This might include the head, foot, chin, tongue, or extensions of body parts, and using pointers or similar adapted accessors.

For patients who cannot use a proportional controller the team may want to consider using a microswitching system. A **microswitching system** is an all-or-none drive system. The speed is preset. The operator applies any degree of pressure, and as soon as the switch (mechanical or electrical) is activated the system runs at the preset speed. Individual switches are provided for the four directions (forward, reverse, right, left), and a series of individual movements are required to maneuver in tight spaces. Individual switches can be operated through a puff-n-sip tube, they can be arranged around a joystick in a control box, or they can be placed anywhere around the body to allow the user to drive the chair. For example, there might be two switches on an UESS for gross pressing with the hand, and additional switches at the head, knees, or feet to allow mobility in all four directions. For patients with less than four or five movements, chairs with dual- and single-switch accessing systems are available; however, such systems make the chair progressively more tedious to operate.

Sports and Recreation

Many users are active in recreational and competitive sports, some of which are done from the wheelchair. These patients may need more than one wheelchair: a "street" or "everyday" chair, and a finely tuned competition chair or recreational chair (Fig. 32-24, Fig. 32-30). It is even possible to have a chair personally built for the user from a computer design based on the user's body parameters and the specific use the chair will have. For some sports such as archery, discus, shot put, and precision javelin, a more stable chair is an advantage. A wide wheel camber can achieve this even on a lightweight frame. For basketball, tennis, and dancing the chair's responsiveness is critical. Competition chairs (Fig. 32-31) are usually of rigid construction, and made of very strong lightweight materials (the newest units are made of carbon). Wheel and caster placement, tires, axles, and bearings can make a radical difference in chair performance when matched with the user's body weight and configuration. Users who participate in more than one activity may want a chair with a great deal of adjustability to allow parameter changes for various activities or multiple chairs, if possible.

Individuals who use their wheelchairs on off-road challenging trails will require knobby tires, because the tread of normal wheelchair tires will tend to get stuck in softer ground (Fig. 32-30). Those who compete in road racing will need competition chairs that have taken many of their design features from racing bicycles: narrow, hard tires; frames made of lightweight alloys or carbon; low seats for minimum air resistance; and small pushrims for higher gearing. Racers usually sit in a tucked position, with approximately 120 degrees of hip flexion and knees and legs strapped together to present a very sleek line and minimal wind resistance as the unit (wheelchair and user) moves quickly along the track. For tennis and dance the chair is trimmed down to its sleekest configuration with all accessories, even wheel locks, removed. Wheel hubs and spoke configurations are designed to hold a tennis ball during competition. The backs are as low as possible to leave the user's upper body free for movement (Fig. 32-31).

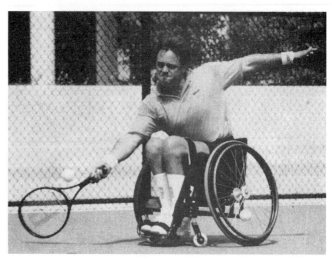

Figure 32-31. Wheelchairs that are designed for sports have special features specific to the intended use of the chair. (Photo courtesy of Quickie Designs.)

WHEELCHAIR TRAINING STRATEGIES

Many individuals using a wheelchair for the first time will require a training period. During this time the patient will learn how to propel the chair in all directions (i.e., using both arms, one or two arms in combination with one or two legs, or one arm using a dual-wheel drive system). He or she must also learn how to operate the wheel locks, foot supports, and armrests, and to use the mechanisms safely without tipping forward or sideways out of the chair seat. He or she will learn how to transfer in and out of the chair with the least possible assistance. Some users will always require maximal assistance for transfer activities, but others will be able to achieve functional independence. Chair features such as removable or swing-away arm and foot supports, and lowered seat heights are important features for independence. For patients who perform standing transfers (independent or assisted), special attention should be given to the user's ability to get out of or back into the chair, because the seat height may prove problematic. Most chairs with a cushion allow a user to slide forward and come to standing. Some patients (e.g., the patient with bilateral transfemoral amputation) may benefit from adjustable height armrests. The armrests are raised during sit-to-stand transfers.

Although sidewalk cutouts are now mandated in many areas, patients who are capable of independent community mobility benefit from learning to **wheelies** to negotiate existing curbs. The chair is balanced on the rear wheels while the front casters are elevated and then propelled forward to mount the curb. Patients who drive need to practice transfers from the wheelchair to the car seat. The wheelchair is then pulled into the vehicle either behind the seat, or across his or her body into the passenger seat. Either method is very dependent on the chair's folded size and weight, the user's upper body skill and strength, and the internal configura-

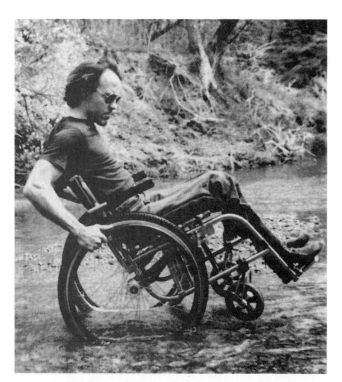

Figure 32-30. There are many specialized wheelchairs available that allow patients full access to their environment. (Photo courtesy of Iron Horse Productions.)

tion of the car. Active patients also need to practice controlled falls out of the wheelchair and floor-to-wheelchair transfers that can be utilized in the event of falls.

Power chair training is slightly different, and usually concentrates primarily on driving skill and safety. The initial challenge is to locate a reliable access site and method (e.g., hand control with a joystick, head control with individual switches). Training then involves working with the user on consistent responses (especially to "stop" commands, or the recognized need to stop based on the user's awareness), and accurate maneuverability. Although switch activation can be judged using a computer program, actual road time is necessary for training and assessment to be sure how the driver will respond to a variety of situations, distractions, and obstacles.

Some rehabilitation facilities have large fleets of sample chairs that can be used with patients for assessment and training. If this option is not available, a qualified supplier in the area should be located.

THE ROLE OF THE CERTIFIED REHABILITATION TECHNOLOGY SUPPLIER

Traditional home care and/or durable medical equipment companies are well qualified to accept prescriptive information over the phone. They keep standard-sized items in stock, and can get them to the user quickly, often within 24 hours. More specialized equipment usually requires input to the team from a certified rehabilitation technology supplier (CRTS). He or she is a specialist and can work with the team to design a system that fits the patient's unique needs. Once the team's goals are explained to the supplier, he or she will be able to provide a list of available products that match the user's needs. The CRTS will be able to explain the pros and cons prices of various options to everyone involved. It may be advisable for the user to actually try several chairs before a decision is made. The supplier can work with the team to arrange this opportunity.

Once a system has been selected, the clinical team's recommendations (including physical, psychosocial, and cognitive factors if applicable) are compiled into a *letter of medical necessity*. The letter of medical need (with physician and clinic team member signatures), a physician's prescription, and price estimate are then forwarded to the third-party payer(s). The justification package should explain the medical need for each feature requested, along with an expected outcome from the intervention.

Providing measurable functional outcomes is essential to help the payer make an informed decision.

The CRTS should keep all of the team members apprised as the process moves along from submission through approval, ordering, and receiving of the chair and its components. Once the system is complete, the supplier must deliver it as instructed by the prescriber (to the clinic, school, or home of the user). At delivery those involved with formulating the prescription should have an opportunity to inspect the system and be sure that it meets the specifications, as well as to observe and assist as the supplier makes final adjustments. The process may require more than one or two visits for complex systems that require interim fittings.

On final delivery, the CRTS explains to the user and/or caregivers how to use the chair, including use of all safety features (straps, wheel locks, anti-tippers), assembly and disassembly for folding, and normal maintenance (including battery maintenance on power wheelchairs and scooters). Once the chair is delivered, the user and/or caregivers should carefully read any manuals provided and mail in all warranty and registration materials. The user and/or caregivers are responsible for all normal cleaning and maintenance. The supplier and the company he or she works for should be located close enough to the user to provide emergency repairs as needed. Warranty repairs are the responsibility of the supplier who provided the chair (most warranties cover the cost of labor for 12 months following purchase and then labor costs become the responsibility of the owner).

SUMMARY

A systematic approach to prescribing a wheelchair has been presented. The individual components of both the postural support and the wheeled mobility base have been described. The primary outcome in developing any prescriptive wheelchair is maximum function and independence. It must be the result of a thorough evaluation using a problem-solving approach, with attention to the specific factors discussed in this chapter. Input from the user and all team members during the decision making phase is critical. This process will result in an optimally designed chair capable of achieving its intended purpose. This problem-solving approach, with open communication among team members, rehabilitation technology supplier, and manufacturer will ensure that each prescriptive wheelchair will meet the needs of the individual.

QUESTIONS FOR REVIEW

1. Explain what information or data is gathered during each of the following portions of the examination process.
   a. Physical examination
   b. Examination of function using existing equipment
   c. Examination in the supine position
   d. Examination in the seated position

2. Describe the following seating components and provide two indications for their use.
  a. Firm seat
  b. Firm back
  c. Lapboard
  d. Lapbelt

3. Describe the following wheelchair components; compare and contrast their functional benefits.
  a. Detachable swing-away footrests/elevating legrests
  b. Fixed-height armrests/adjustable-height armrests
  c. Single-axle placement/multiple-axle placement
  d. Proportional drive/microswitching system

4. When measuring seat depth, what two positions would you place the patient in and why?

5. Identify landmarks and measurements needed to help determine the size of the following parts of a wheeled mobility system:
  a. Seat width
  b. Seat depth
  c. Seat back height
  d. Armrest height
  e. Minimum footrest extension (MinFBX)

6. Compare and contrast the characteristic features, postural control provided, as well as the advantages and disadvantages of:
  a. Wheelchair seats: (1) solid insert, and (2) solid hook-on seat
  b. Wheelchair seat cushions: (1) comfort cushion (planar/contoured), (2) pressure relieving foam (contoured, custom contoured), (3) pressure-relieving fluid or fluid/foam combination; and (4) pressure-relieving air
  c. Back supports: (1) pita back, (2) solid insert, and (3) solid hook-on back

CASE STUDY

The patient is a 24 year-old male who suffered a traumatic brain injury when he was 15 years old. He presents in a tilt-in-space manual wheelchair with a high back, back insert, planar seat with a loose gel pad covering it, anterior chest support and padded lap belt. He sits poorly in the chair and caregivers report that he consistently slips down on the seat, curves his trunk to the side and keeps his head flexed forward and to the side. He is dependent in feeding and transfers. He makes eye contact occasionally and can indicate yes/no with a hand movement. The immediate goal of his team and caregivers is to improve postural alignment and then, in the future, determine a site where he can consistently access a switch that will allow use of a computer for communication, learning, and recreational activities.

When seated in the chair his head is down and laterally flexed to the left. His trunk is shortened on the left with the shoulder depressed; the pelvis is in an oblique position with the left side raised. The pelvis is tilted posteriorly with both lower extremities abducted. His hips are shifted toward the left. The seat/back angle of the chair is set at 90 degrees. The knees are positioned at 90 degrees and the feet do not remain in position on the foot plates. The upper extremities rest on an upper extremity support surface.

A supine examination revealed that the patient's head, trunk, and pelvis can be neutrally aligned. There is some pelvic mobility, and the hips can be flexed to 75 degrees before the pelvis begins to rotate backward. There is limited hip adduction and internal rotation, but both lower extremities can achieve neutral position. The hamstrings are moderately tight, but should not interfere with sitting. There are no red or scarred areas over bony prominences despite a marked pelvic obliquity in sitting.

Using a simulator chair, the patient sat with a seat/back angle of 105 degrees. Lateral trunk, hip, and knee supports were placed to help keep him centered on the sitting surface. The lateral knee supports were very effective in preventing the abduction pattern typically assumed. A head/neck support was used posteriorly and laterally. An additional support pad was placed at the left temple to address the lateral flexion. A forehead strap was suggested to assist with upright head positioning, but was uncomfortable and rejected by the patient. The patient answered yes/no questions while postural response to the support and angle changes were observed. He was able to remain symmetrically seated with the pelvis well positioned on the seat surface for approximately 45 minutes, with the chair in 10 degrees of posterior tilt.

Guiding Questions

1. What components would you recommend be added to the patient's tilt-in-space wheelchair to improve postural alignment for each of the following areas? Identify the postural control and functional assistance that will be provided by each of your recommendations.
  a. Head and neck
  b. Trunk
  c. Hip
  d. Knee

2. The patient already has an anterior chest support. What function does this component provide?

3. What recommendations would you make to address the problem of foot positioning on the foot plates?

4. What type of seat cushion would you recommend for this patient? Provide a rationale for your selection.

REFERENCES

1. Troy, BS, et al: An analysis of work postures of manual wheelchair users in the office environment. J Rehabil Res Dev 34:151, 1997.
2. Curtis, KA, et al: Functional reach in wheelchair users: The effects of trunk and lower extremity stabilization. Arch Phys Med Rehabil 76:360, 1995.
3. Saftler, F, et al: Use of a positioning chair in conjunction with proper seating principles for a seating evaluation. Proceedings from ICCART, 1988.
4. Sprigle, S, et al: Reduction of sitting pressures with custom contoured cushions. J Rehabil Res Dev 27:135, 1990.
5. Sprigle, S, et al: Factors affecting seat contour characteristics. J Rehabil Res Dev 27:127, 1990.
6. Hobson, D: Comparative effects of posture and pressure distribution at the body-seat interface. Proceedings of the 12th Annual Conference of RESNA (Rehabilitation Engineering and Assistive Technology Society of North America), New Orleans, LA, June 25–30, 1989. RESNA Press, Washington, DC, 1989.
7. Sprigle, S, and Chung, K: The use of contoured foam to reduce seat interface pressures. Proceedings of the 12th Annual Conference of RESNA, New Orleans, LA, June 25–30, 1989. RESNA Press, Washington, DC, 1989.
8. Bergen, AF: A seat belt is a seat belt is a. . . . Assistive Technology 1:7, 1989.
9. Margolis, S, et al: The sub-ASIS bar: An effective approach to pelvic stabilization in seated position. Proceedings of the 8th Annual Conference of RESNA, Memphis, TN, June 24–28, 1985. RESNA Press, Washington, DC, 1985.
10. Bergen, AF, et al: Positioning for Function: Wheelchairs and Other Assistive Technologies. Valhalla Rehab, Valhalla, NY, 1990.
11. Butler, C: Effects of powered mobility on self-initiated behaviors of very young children with locomotor disability. Dev Med Child Neurol 28:325, 1986.
12. Butler, C, et al: Powered mobility for very young disabled children. Dev Med Child Neurol 25:472, 1983.
13. Lotto, W, and Milner, M: Evaluations and Development of Powered Mobility Aids for 2–5 Year Olds with Neuromuscular Disorders. Ontario Crippled Child Centre, Toronto, Ontario, 1983.
14. Trefler, E, et al: Selected Readings on Powered Mobility for Children and Adults with Severe Physical Disabilities. RESNA Press, Washington, DC, 1986.
15. Vaeger, H, et al: The effect of rear wheel camber in manual wheelchair propulsion. J Rehabil Res Dev 26:37, 1989.
16. Van der Woude, L, et al: Seat height in handrim wheelchair propulsion. J Rehabil Res Dev 26:31, 1989.
17. Brubaker, C: Wheelchair prescription: An analysis of factors that affect mobility and performance. J Rehabil Res Dev 23:19, 1986.
18. van der Linden, ML, et al: The effect of wheelchair handrim tube diameter on propulsion efficiency and force application. IEEE Trans Rehabil Eng 4:123, 1996.
19. Jackson, DL, et al: Electrodiagnostic study of carpal tunnel syndrome in wheelchair basketball players. Clin J Sport Med 6:27, 1996.
20. Lal, S: Premature degenerative shoulder changes in spinal cord injury patients. Spinal Cord 36:186, 1998.
21. Dozono, D, et al: Peripheral neuropathies in the upper extremities of paraplegic wheelchair marathon racers. Paraplegia 33:208, 1995.
22. Beaumont-White, S, and Ham, RO: Powered wheelchairs: Are we enabling or disabling? Prosthet Orthot Int 21:62, 1997.

SUPPLEMENTAL READINGS

Axelson, P, et al: A Guide to Wheelchair Selection. Paralyzed Veterans of America, Washington, DC 1994.

Bertocci, GE, et al: Development of transportable wheelchair design criteria using computer crash simulation. IEEE Trans Rehabil Eng 4:171, 1996.

Brienza, DM, and Angelo, J: A force feedback joystick and control algorithm for wheelchair obstacle avoidance. Disabil Rehabil 18:123, 1996.

Brienza, DM, et al: Seat cushion design for elderly wheelchair users based on minimization of sift tissue deformation using stiffness and pressure measurements. IEEE Trans Rehabil Eng 4:320, 1996.

Brubaker, C: Wheelchair prescription: An analysis of factors that affect mobility and performance. J Rehabil Res Dev 223:19, 1986.

Butler, C: Effects of powered mobility on self-initiated behaviors of very young children with locomotor disability. Dev Med Child Neurol 28:325, 1986.

Cook, AM, and Hussey, SM: Assistive Technologies: Principles and Practice. Mosby, St. Louis, 1995.

Cooper, RA, et al: Braking electric-powered wheelchairs: Effect of braking method, seatbelt, and legrests. Arch Phys Med Rehabil 79:1244, 1998.

Cooper, RA, et al: Performance of selected lightweight wheelchairs on ANSI/RESNA tests. Arch Phys Med Rehabil 78:1138, 1997.

Enders, A, and Hall, M (eds): Assistive Technology Source Book, RESNA Press, Washington, DC, 1990.

Engstrom, B: Ergonomics Wheelchairs and Positioning. Posturalis, Hasselby, Sweden, 1993.

Furumasu, J (ed): Pediatric Powered Mobility: Developmental Perspectives, Technical Issues, Clinical Approaches. RESNA, Arlington, VA, 1997.

Gaal, RP, et al: Wheelchair rider injuries: Causes and consequences for wheelchair design and selection. J Rehabil Res Dev 34:58, 1997.

Hedman, G (ed): Seating Systems: The Therapists and Rehabilitation Engineering Team. Physical Therapy and Occupational Therapy in Pediatrics. American Physical Therapy Association 10:11, 1990.

Kernozek, TW, and Lewin, JE: Seat interface pressures of individuals with paraplegia: Influence of dynamic wheelchair locomotion compared with static seated measurements. Arch Phys Med Rehabil 79:313, 1998.

Kirby, RL, et al: Wheelchair stability and maneuverability: Effect of varying the horizontal and vertical position of a rear-antitip device. Arch Phys Med Rehabil 75:525, 1994.

Kirby, RL, et al: Wheelchair safety: Effect of locking or grasping the rear wheels during a rear tip. Arch Phys Med Rehabil 77:1266, 1996.

Papaioannou, G, et al: A methodological approach towards the design of a highly innovative wheelchair with enhanced safety, manoeuvrability and comfort. Technology and Health Care 7:39, 1999.

Parent, F, et al: The flexible contour backrest: A new design concept for wheelchairs. Asst Technol 10:94, 1998.

Padula, W: A Behavioral Vision Approach for Persons with Physical Disabilities. Optometric Extension Program, Santa Ana, CA, 1988.

Presperin, J: Seating systems: The therapist and rehabilitation engineering team. J Phys Ther Occup Ther Pediatrics Spring, 1990.

Rosenthal, MJ, et al: A wheelchair cushion designed to redistribute sites of sitting pressure. Arch Phys Med Rehabil 77:278, 1996.

Trefler, E. (ed): Seating and Mobility for Persons with Physical Disabilities. Therapy Skill Builders, Tucson, AZ, 1993.

Yoder, JD, et al: Initial results in the development of a guidance system for a powered wheelchair. IEEE Trans Rehabil Eng 4:143, 1996.

Zacharkow, D: Wheelchair Posture and Pressure Sores. Charles C Thomas, Springfield, IL, 1984.

Zacharkow, D: Posture: Sitting, Standing, Chair Design and Exercise. Charles C Thomas, Springfield, IL, 1988.

Zollars, JA: Special Seating: An Illustrated Guide. Otto Bock, Minneapolis, MN, 1996.

GLOSSARY

Contoured surface: Custom-molded seating surface created by carving foam, building up the surface with pads and blocks, or preforming, based on research about human contours.

Control blocks (blocking): Use of upholstered supports or pads attached to the seating system to enhance postural alignment.

Custom-molded surfaces: Seated environment created from a casted shape taken of the person's body contours. Foam is carved or poured to create an exact duplicate of the person's shape.

Kyphotic posturing (kyphosis): Excessive convex curvature of the thoracic spine as viewed laterally.

Lateral knee positioner (adductor cushion): An upholstered block or pad placed on the lateral aspect of the wheelchair seating surface; used to control excessive adduction of the lower extremities.

Medial knee positioner (abductor pommel): An upholstered block or wedge placed on the front of the wheelchair seating surface; used to maintain abduction of the lower extremities.

Microswitching system: Power wheelchair activation system that produces an all-or-none response; the switch is preset to respond to a specific degree of pressure; when the right amount of pressure is applied the switch activates the system at a preset speed.

Minimum footboard extension (MIN FBX): Measurement of leg length from the popliteal fossa to the heel and subtracting 1 inch (2.5 cms).

Mobility base: A wheelchair support and movement system; consists of the tubular frame, the legrests and armrests, foot supports, and wheels.

Planar surface: A seated environment created from the interfacing of flat support surfaces arranged as needed to create postural alignment and/or stability.

Postural support system: A wheelchair seating, support, and postural alignment system; consists of the seat surface, seat back, and any additional components such as a torso support, lateral and medial knee cushions, and/or pelvic belt needed to maintain alignment.

Proportional drive: Power wheelchair activation system that is joystick-controlled and responds to movement through an arc. The further the joystick is moved the faster the chair moves.

Upper extremity support surface (UESS): A support surface such as a tray or trough mounted to the arm rest.

Wheelie: A wheelchair maneuver to negotiate curbs; the chair is balanced on the rear wheels while the front casters are elevated and then propelled forward to mount the curb.

Windblown position: Positioning of the lower extremities to the side with one limb adducted and the other abducted.

APPENDIX

Suggested Answers to Case Study Guiding Questions

1. What components would you recommend be added to the patient's tilt-in-space wheelchair to improve postural alignment for each of the following areas? Identify the postural control and functional assistance that will be provided by each of your recommendations.

ANSWER

a. Head and neck
Recommendation: Head/neck support with lateral controller.
Postural control provided:
- Promotes maintenance of a neutral cervical spine and head position.
- Eliminates forward and lateral flexion.

Functional assistance provided:
- Supports the head to assist with respiration, visual interaction with environment, feeding, and swallowing.
- Improves safety during transport on level surfaces and in a motor vehicle.

b. Trunk
Recommendation: Lateral trunk supports.
Postural control provided:
- Improves trunk stability and alignment; improves pelvic alignment.
- Controls lateral trunk flexion.

Functional assistance provided:
- Improved trunk control facilitates upper extremity positioning.
- Improves respiration, feeding, and swallowing.

c. Hip
Recommendation: Lateral hip guides.
Postural control provided:
- Improved weight distribution on pelvis.
- Improved pelvic positioning.
- Assists with maintenance of pelvic alignment.

Functional assistance provided:
- Allows patient to achieve or tolerate better alignment.
- Increased sitting time.

d. Knee
Recommendation: Lateral knee guides.
Postural control provided:
- Helps maintain lower extremity alignment; reduces increased abduction.

- Improves neutral alignment of lower extremities; assists with maintenance of pelvic position.
- Maintains lower extremity alignment.

Functional assistance provided:
- Improved pelvic position.
- Maintenance of neutral alignment of lower extremities.

2. The patient already has an anterior chest support. What function does this component provide?

ANSWER
- Supports trunk along anterior surface of trunk and shoulders; eliminates forward lean.
- Assists with maintenance of upright trunk posture.
- Improves head position for respiration, feeding, swallowing, and visual interaction with environment.
- Shoulder control promotes better head posture.

3. What recommendations would you make to address the problem of foot positioning on the foot plates?

ANSWER: The addition of heel loops and ankle straps would provide the needed control to maintain foot alignment on the foot plate.

4. What type of seat cushion would you recommend for this patient? Provide a rationale for your selection.

ANSWER: Recommendation: Custom-contoured pressure relieving foam seat cushion.
Rationale:
- Custom contour allows accommodation of individual postural asymmetries.
- Can be shaped to control postural alignment; promotes a neutral pelvic tilt.
- Provides a stable base of support; increased surface contact creates improved pressure distribution.
- May increase sitting time and improve postural stability.
- Improves caregiver ability to position and reposition patient.

Timothy L. Fagerson
David E. Krebs

LEARNING OBJECTIVES

1. Describe the purposes of biofeedback techniques.
2. Describe the motor learning principles underlying biofeedback techniques.
3. Describe the technical requirements and limitations of biofeedback equipment.
4. Identify differences in electromyographic (EMG) biofeedback techniques used for spastic versus paretic muscle groups.
5. Describe the application of kinematic and kinetic biofeedback techniques to gait training.
6. Illustrate application of biofeedback with a series of individual patient problems and guiding questions to facilitate learning.

Feedback and practice are considered to be among the most important variables in the process of motor learning.[1] Biofeedback is a specialized form of feedback that provides information directly to a patient about internal biological mechanisms via a somewhat sophisticated electronic device. To quote John Basmajian[2] p 1 (the "father" of EMG biofeedback), **biofeedback** is "the technique of using equipment (usually electronic) to reveal to human beings some of their internal physiological events, normal and abnormal, in the form of visual and auditory signals in order to teach them to manipulate these otherwise involuntary or unfelt events by manipulating the displayed signals." Traditionally the biofeedback signal has been auditory or visual. Tactile feedback devices (e.g., vibration) have recently been developed, and if there were a need, smell and taste biofeedback could also be devised. In physical rehabilitation, biofeedback can be used to inform the patient about movement, muscle activity, whole body balance, force, joint displacement, skin temperature, heart rate, blood pressure, and more.

Strictly speaking, biofeedback is feedback for the patient. The same device that provides the patient with biofeedback can also, however, provide the rehabilitation professional with very important monitoring feedback to help in evaluation, decision making, and patient education (e.g., as a monitor of muscle activity or weight-bearing load).[3] Figure 33-1 provides a conceptual framework for the role of biofeedback (regardless of type) in the rehabilitation process.

Biofeedback is probably used more in the field of psychology than in physical rehabilitation. This is reflected in the name of the largest organization for professionals involved or interested in this area: the *Association of Applied Psychophysiology and Biofeedback* (AAPB). In 1997, the journal for this organization recently (in 1997) underwent a name change from *Biofeedback and Self-Regulation* to *Applied Psychophysiology and Biofeedback*.

Muscle activity or EMG biofeedback is most frequently employed in clinical physical therapy settings, so this chapter will focus primarily on EMG

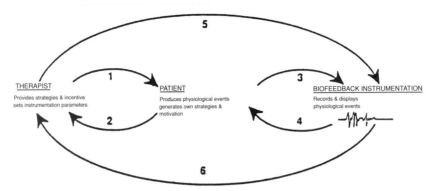

Figure 33-1. Middaugh's conceptual framework for biofeedback therapy. Note that there are three basic components in the biofeedback process: the therapist, the patient, and the biofeedback machine. The therapist evaluates, sets instrumentation parameters, develops intervention strategies, and instructs the patient. The biofeedback instrumentation records the patient-generated physiological events, processes them, and displays the information. The patient attempts to manipulate the biofeedback signal, thereby altering the physiological mechanism being measured and, it is hoped, effecting therapeutic benefit. (From Middaugh, SJ: Presidential address: On clinical efficacy: Why biofeedback does—and does not—work. Biofeedback & Self-Regulation 15:204, 1990, with permission.)

biofeedback. Joint position and force feedback will be considered less comprehensively.

GENERAL PRINCIPLES

The goal of biofeedback in physical therapy is to improve motor performance by facilitating motor learning. To use biofeedback correctly and effectively, therapists must understand the principles of motor learning and the technical limitations of biofeedback machines.

Motor Learning

Excellent reviews of motor control are available to the student, many of them substantial and comprehensive (e.g., Schmidt[1], Shumway-Cook and Woollacott[4]), so the field will be considered here only briefly. The motor control literature, however, has few unifying theories, and the limited work that has been done on abnormal populations tends to contradict the remaining areas of agreement. Thus, although it is accepted that motor control requires information from the external world as well as **proprioception**,[5]* how that information is processed is presently unknown. Therefore, attempts to dogmatically view biofeedback as a substitute for proprioceptive pathways reflect, at best, a naïve misunderstanding of the extremely sophisticated human control systems that have evolved.

A behavioral positive reinforcement or "reward" model is usually employed with biofeedback techniques. Simply stated, when patients generate appropriate motor behaviors, they are positively rein-

forced. The audio and visual feedback stimuli, and other nonverbal information, are usually much faster and more accurate than the therapist's comments. Unlike other interventions, the benefits of accomplishing small changes in motor behavior in the desired direction can be reinforced, which should speed the rehabilitation process. In behavioral learning terminology, the therapist uses the biofeedback signal to shape the motor behavior by reinforcing the patient's successive approximations to the goal behavior or functional outcome.[6]

When the patient succeeds in controlling the signal, the therapist must relate it to the underlying motor behavior and then reestablish the expected outcomes. Reinforcing already-learned behaviors is, of course, futile, so the machine's threshold should be monitored frequently, increasing the task's difficulty as motor skills progress.

Schmidt[1p246] defined **motor learning** as "a set of processes associated with practice or experience leading to relatively permanent changes in the capability for responding." It is permanent change in the ability to perform or respond that truly defines learning. Four primary factors influencing motor learning have been identified: (1) stage of the learner, (2) type of task, (3) feedback, and (4) practice.[7] Feedback and practice are considered to be the most important.[1,6,8]

Feedback can be intrinsic or extrinsic. Intrinsic feedback is the body's internal feedback mechanism, which uses visual, auditory, vestibular, and proprioceptive mechanisms. Extrinsic feedback is any feedback derived from an external source (e.g., a biofeedback signal or physical therapists' comments) that augments intrinsic feedback. Two types of extrinsic feedback can be given: **knowledge of results (KR)** and **knowledge of performance (KP).** KR is feedback given after performance of a task and is related to the overall result of the task (e.g., whether or not 25% partial weight-bearing gait was maintained). KP is feedback given during or after performance of a task and is related to how the task was performed (e.g., "Place the foot of your

---

*"Proprioception" is the internal feedback process that uses muscle and skeletal mechanoreceptors for controlling movement.[5]

operated leg directly between the two crutches"). Biofeedback given continuously during performance of a task is KP feedback (e.g., concurrent EMG feedback). Biofeedback given about the outcome of the task is KR feedback (e.g., a limb load monitor beeping when too much load is applied). Refer to Chapter 13 for more detail on motor control and motor learning.

PHYSIOLOGICAL FEEDBACK

The fastest cortical feedback circuits (i.e., those that can take into account changes in environmental conditions) have at least 100- to 200-millisecond latencies.[9] For example, a pianist performing a "run" cannot possibly rely on visual or auditory feedback during the run. If a mistake is made, several notes will be played before the performer is even aware that a mistake has occurred. For the run to be played correctly on the next attempt requires pre-planning of the motor event. This pre-planning is called feedforward or **open-loop control.**

Ambulation also requires a series of pre-planned motor events. If a disruption occurs, feedback of the "mistake" can only be acted upon and built into the plan for *ensuing* steps. Normal walking cadence is about 1 cycle per second. Ankle dorsiflexors, for example, must resist foot-slap from heel strike to foot-flat for about 60 msec. Therapists attempting to encourage normal gait in patients with hemiplegia by using feedback from dorsiflexor EMG should not, therefore, request the patient to correct inadequate dorsiflexor motor unit activity *within* each gait cycle. At best, patients will use that information during the next gait cycle, but the information is merely that EMG activity was inadequate during the past gait cycle. The therapist and patient must determine the correct neurophysiological strategy to increase dorsiflexor motor unit activity in anticipation of ensuing heel strikes.

BIOFEEDBACK IN REHABILITATION

When using biofeedback, the patient must (1) understand the relationship of the electronic signal to the desired functional task, (2) practice controlling the biofeedback signal, and (3) perform the functional task until it is mastered and the patient no longer needs the biofeedback. Biofeedback techniques thus require, at least at first, that patients utilize in **closed-loop control** (Fig. 33-2), using continuous external feedback (Fig. 33-3), until motor skills develop sufficiently so that "open loop" control (where intermittent or no feedback is used) can be accomplished.*

Winstein[7] and others[10–12] have shown that a combination of open- and closed-loop learning, called *scheduled feedback*, can be more effective than clas-

---

*The reader should be aware that the oversimplified dichotomy of open- and closed-loop control is included here for its heuristic value, not because it is a physiologically validated motor control paradigm.

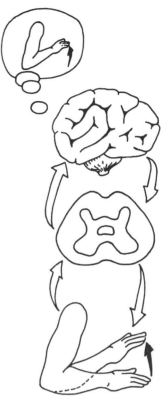

Figure 33-2. Schematic representation of closed-loop motor learning theory.

sic closed-loop biofeedback. In scheduled feedback paradigms, subjects practice the task initially with feedback following each trial, then spend increasingly long practice periods without feedback following each trial. Apparently, scheduled feedback encourages subjects to rely on normal, internal feedback mechanisms and decreases their dependence on relatively unnatural continuous biofeedback.

Conventional neuromuscular re-education is based heavily on providing patients with helpful comments (feedback) to assist their recovery of previously acquired skills. The therapist's job, often, is to focus the patient's attention on the underlying motor programs and biomechanical schema required to recoup those skills (i.e., KP). Following a meniscectomy, if the patient cannot straight leg raise, for example, then gait rehabilitation will be impeded, and the therapist will then usually prescribe quadriceps-setting exercise. Biofeedback-assisted quadriceps setting might improve that patient's information processing and result in more rapid rehabilitation by augmenting knee joint or quadriceps proprioception with electronic feedback, supplementing the normal feedback inhibited by the meniscectomy.[13,14] As shown schematically in Figure 33-4, when a patient's normal proprioception and other physiological mechanisms are disrupted, normal movement control and relearning of motor skills is restricted.

Most biofeedback techniques, and in fact much of the instruction given to patients by physical therapists, is KP feedback. Although KP feedback is

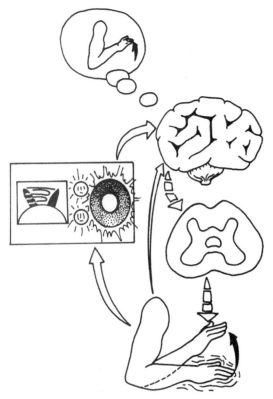

Figure 33-3. Abnormal feedback loop impedes normal movement control.

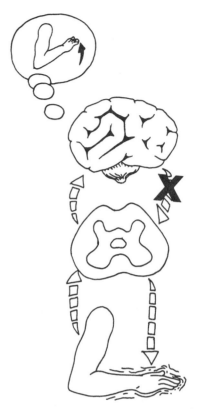

Figure 33-4. Abnormal feedback loop augmented by biofeedback signal.

important, research comparing KP feedback with KR feedback has found KR feedback to be superior in terms of retention of the learned task.[15]

Recent applications of biofeedback have been directed at muscle imbalances and the fine-tuning of motor control. The focus, for example, with the quadriceps, might be a balanced vastus medialis oblique:vastus lateralis (VMO:VL) ratio and not merely gross strength (Fig. 33-5).[16]

Biofeedback is simply one technique that therapists may employ to help convey their message about motor programs and biomechanical schemata to the patient. Biofeedback can assist the rehabilitation process by:

1. Providing a clear treatment outcome or goal for the patient to accomplish.
2. Permitting the therapist and patient to experiment with various strategies (processes) that generate motor patterns to achieve the desired outcome or goal.
3. Reinforcing appropriate motor behavior.
4. Providing a process-oriented, timely, and accurate KP or KR of the patient's efforts.

By attending to the biofeedback signal, the patient can "close the loop" (Fig. 33-3). Some patients become more motivated when biofeedback is employed because they know the machine will not be falsely encouraging. Both the therapist and the patient must therefore understand the meaning of the feedback signal, and appropriate goals must be set.

The therapist must explain what the machine's signals mean to the patient, and what consti-

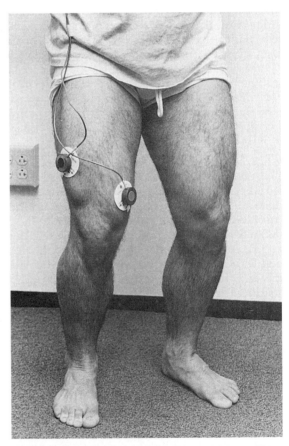

Figure 33-5. EMG biofeedback electrode set-up for VMO:VL training during ⅓ knee bends. (Courtesy of NeuroDyne Medical Corp., Newton, MA.)

tutes "success." The machine should be set to give auditory or visual feedback that corresponds to the motor behavior desired. For example, if spastic antagonist muscles are monitored, the patient should be instructed to decrease the EMG activity; the biofeedback device is set to flash a light to signal accomplishment of this outcome. Alternatively, an **electrogoniometer** (el-gon) might be employed that changes the pitch of a buzzer as the joint is moved in the proper direction.

In summary, biofeedback techniques are used to augment the patient's sensory feedback mechanisms through precise information about body processes that might otherwise be inaccessible. Positive reinforcement is the operative learning model.

Technical Limitations

The unique aspect of biofeedback is the source of the information obtained (i.e., otherwise undetectable physiological mechanisms). The feedback, however, must be relevant, accurate, and rapid to enhance motor learning. If any of these three elements is missing, traditional verbal feedback may be just as useful, and is certainly more convenient.

RELEVANCY

Useful information is pertinent to the desired motor outcome: neither too much nor too little information is given, and the information is immediately applicable to the behavior. Although therapists may verbally describe the location of agonist and antagonist muscles, and even make attempts to describe the feelings patients should experience if the muscles are used appropriately, there is no way to communicate which motor units to activate. EMG biofeedback can provide relevant information regarding motor unit activity, which patients do not otherwise have available.

ACCURACY

Many therapists prefer to work with devices that directly measure force or joint range of motion (ROM). These therapists feel that EMG signals are neither sufficiently informative nor sufficiently sophisticated to constitute true process feedback, and that EMG does not adequately reflect actual outcome (e.g., limb displacement or torque) to provide accurate KR. To maximize the utility of biofeedback, one must be certain that the type of device and the way it is attached provide truthful, accurate information.

SPEED OF INFORMATION

Feedback must be timely to be useful. While feedback is employed, the movements are necessarily closed loop, as described.

In addition to **endogenous,** physiological latencies, most EMG biofeedback instruments have built-in integrators or averagers that further slow the signal output. Moreover, all EMG processors delay electrical events during signal amplification and conversion to the audio speaker and visual meter, because of inherent delays from the electrical circuits. Most commercial EMG feedback instruments introduce 50- to 100-msec delays before the signal can even reach the ears and eyes of patients, and further delays ensue within the patient's neural circuits.

In summary, information to be fed back to patients must be accurate, relevant, and timely to be of therapeutic use. Therapists must choose the instrument or device that provides the most meaningful information to patients. Commercially available EMG instruments, for example, can provide timely feedback if the motor behavior being monitored is at least 0.5 seconds in duration. Thus, for feedback during a 5-second isometric contraction, adequate time may be available for patients to adjust the motor program and change the motor strategy being employed. During most functional activities, therefore, the feedback acts as an *error signal* (or if the task is performed correctly, a *reference of correctness*[17]) to provide knowledge of results, which is used in planning future movements.

BIOFEEDBACK LITERATURE

Since the peak in publications in the early 1980s, there has been a gradual decline of published articles in the PsychLit and Medline databases on biofeedback.[18] This may reflect the pragmatic trend that biofeedback should no longer be viewed as *the* treatment but part of a broader intervention package. This trend has most likely evolved from the failure of many studies to find a significant difference when comparing biofeedback with another approach. This is often, however, related to flaws in the design of the research and unrealistic expectations as to what biofeedback can achieve.[19]

Well over 10,000 professional articles[2] have addressed biofeedback, more than 300 of which directly were related to physical rehabilitation.[20] Indeed, a literature search on the use of EMG biofeedback in rehabilitation of patients after stroke identified 124 citations for the years 1966 to 1991 on the subject of biofeedback and stroke alone.[21]

The AAPB provides a list of diagnoses for which appropriate research has demonstrated that biofeedback is an established, nonexperimental treatment. This list includes anxiety disorders, asthma, attention deficit hyperactivity disorder, diabetes, headache (migraine and tension), hypertension, incontinence (fecal and urinary), insomnia, mild brain injury, motion sickness, myofascial pain, Raynaud's disorder, neuromuscular rehabilitation, rheumatoid arthritis pain, and temporomandibular joint syndrome.

Although it is beyond the scope of this chapter to examine the validity of this list of diagnoses for which it is claimed that biofeedback is effective, the supplemental readings for this chapter have been chosen to illustrate the wide range of contemporary applications of biofeedback in physical rehabilitation. Additionally, if the reader has access to the Internet, excellent World Wide Web sites are maintained by the AAPB and the Biofeedback Society of Europe (BSE).

USING EMG FEEDBACK FOR NEUROMUSCULAR RE-EDUCATION

A surface EMG device could be as useful for skeletal muscle activity as electrocardiography (ECG) is for the heart. The basic EMG biofeedback device includes one ground and two surface electrodes, an amplifier, an audio speaker, and a video display. The EMG signal (which is on the order of millionths of a volt, or microvolts) is transmitted from the muscle through the skin, through the electrode paste, through the electrodes, through the wires, and then to the amplifier. The equipment is quite complex and for skilled use a good understanding of the EMG signal's characteristics is required.

In this section, the origins of the EMG signal will be briefly reviewed and its progress followed from the patient (starting with the intention to move) through the monitoring instrumentation, and back to the patient for error correction. See also Chapter 9.

Muscle Physiology: Origin if the EMG Signal

After the central nervous system signals its intention to move and the signal travels down the spinal cord, the anterior horn cell discharges. The motor nerve then depolarizes, conducting its electrical current toward the muscle at 40 to 60 m/sec. Because a *motor unit* is, by definition, the anterior horn cell, its nerve, and all the muscle fibers it innervates, the amount of muscle that is activated depends on the size of the motor unit field (i.e., the number of muscle fibers innervated by each anterior horn cell and its axon).

After all motor nerve terminal branches have discharged, the action potential hits the neuromuscular junction. The distal-most end of the nerve contains acetylcholine, which diffuses across the synaptic cleft. The acetylcholine receptors cause a second action potential to occur, this time in the sarcolemma, or jacket, surrounding the muscle fiber (Greek, *sarcos* = flesh, and *lemma* = sheath). The sarcolemnal depolarization, or action potential, conducts more slowly than the nerve action potential propagation. The EMG device registers this sarcolemnal depolarization; it does not register muscle tension. After the electrical excitation travels through the muscle, the action potential reaches a storage area for calcium ions. Only after the electrical depolarization reaches this storage area and causes calcium to be released does the mechanical event, muscle contraction, occur. The muscle's electrical action potential normally, although not always, results in tension (force) production by the muscle.[22,23]

In EMG feedback, surface electrodes are most often used. Surface electrodes summate all potentials beneath their surfaces. Therefore, an increase in observed EMG activity may result from more muscle cells discharging, or from changes in electrode placement. The surface electrodes' summation masks the precise source of the signal. EMG activity may be from a muscle immediately below the electrodes or from a distant source. Furthermore, the EMG signal will increase whether patients are developing increased activation of small motor units more rapidly and synchronously, or whether a greater number of units are being recruited.

It should be understood from the preceding paragraphs that measuring a muscles' electrical activity, as is done with EMG, is *not* the same as measuring muscle tension. The important point for understanding biofeedback is that the EMG signal arises prior to, and occasionally independent of, muscle mechanical activity, so blind reliance on EMG output can be deceiving.

EMG Biofeedback Equipment and Technical Specifications

The EMG biofeedback device is at heart a very sensitive **voltmeter** with a speaker and meter attached. Like any differential voltmeter, EMG instruments can sense electrical signals only if one pole experiences a different voltage than the other: one pole of the instrument must be negative with respect to the other pole to register any activity. After the electrical signal is detected, most biofeedback instruments condition the signals so that positive and negative impulses are *rectified* (the machine finds the signal's absolute amplitude); then the device *smooths* (filters) the signal prior to display in order to decrease the normal fluctuations present in the muscle's electrical output (see Chapter 9 for further details on signal conditioning). Thus, although the muscle's electrical event occurs before its mechanical contraction, by the time the EMG machine produces the feedback signal, the mechanical event is over. The quality of the machine, and therefore its output, are chiefly governed by the electrodes used, input **impedance, common mode rejection ratio (CMRR),** bandwidth, gain, noise level, and ability to cope with non-EMG artifacts. These features should be considered when choosing between different instruments, and certainly before purchasing an EMG device. This information is listed under specifications with the literature on a particular device.

ELECTRODES
EMG activity can be detected using needle, fine-wire, or surface electrodes. Although a needle or fine-wire electrode is more specific in its ability to detect activity in a single muscle, its recordings are not as reproducible as surface electrodes. Placement of fine-wire electrodes is an invasive procedure, and

these electrodes are not as reflective of a whole muscle's activity (and therefore function) as are surface electrodes.

Surface electrodes (active or passive) are usually metal discs or bars, 0.5 to 1 centimeters in diameter. It is generally agreed that active electrodes are preferred to passive electrodes. An active electrode has the electronics needed to amplify the signal from the muscle within its housing. Amplifying the signal at the skin surface negates the significance of any artifact that is picked up while the signal travels to the biofeedback machine. In other words, the signal leaving the electrode will now have a large voltage so that any artifact picked up after this time is relatively insignificant.

The closer the electrodes are to one another, the more confidence the therapist has that the signal is coming from the target muscle. Wider electrode spacing yields greater signal amplitude (more apparent voltage), but today's electronic amplifiers do not need assistance from widely spaced electrodes. For the same reason, if the signal amplitude recordings are made to help chronicle the patient's progress, the therapist should also document the electrode locations and separation distance.

Most authorities agree that a fixed (e.g., 1 cm) interelectrode distance is preferred. Fixed-distance active electrodes are usually 1-centimeter diameter disks or 1-centimeter long bars with a 2- or 3-centimeter interelectrode distance. If a wider interelectrode distance or larger electrode size is required, electrodes can be attached to the preamplifier via short leads; this still allows one to reap the benefits of signal amplification close to the source.[24]

Choice of electrode size is essentially a decision based on the quality of the equipment to be used. In general, smaller electrodes are better; they are less likely to transmit volume-conducted artifact, and they permit a wider choice of electrode sites because few sites are too small to seat them well. However, impedance varies inversely with electrode size, so unless the amplifier has high input impedance, small electrodes may induce signal artifacts. Different types of surface electrodes are shown in Figure 33-6.

There are many ways to attach electrodes to the skin: self-adhesive collars on most modern electrodes, adhesive tape, rubber or elastic bands, nonelastic hook-and-loop fasteners, spring-loaded clips, adhesive electrode paste, or any combination thereof. The goal is to ensure that the electrodes remain securely attached to the skin. Electrode paste is a gel that reduces the resistance between the electrodes and the skin. Many modern biofeedback units do not require the use of electrode paste or gel (so-called *dry electrodes*) because they have very high input impedance (more on impedance later in this section) or they use active electrodes. Those that do, however, require the user to carefully apply the paste so that it just covers the electrode. Not only is excess paste sloppy, but it also affects the apparent amplitude of the EMG signal, perhaps even short-circuiting the two electrodes. Electrodes should be placed parallel

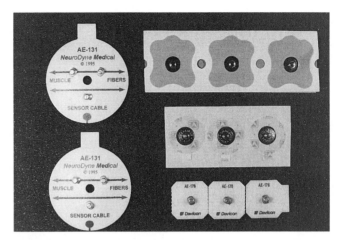

Figure 33-6. A selection of different sizes and shapes of electrodes. (Courtesy of NeuroDyne Medical Corp., Newton, MA.)

to the muscle fibers just off center of the muscle belly (most motor end-points are found at the center of the muscle belly). Straddling the motor point should be avoided with EMG biofeedback.

INPUT IMPEDANCE

Ohm's Law indicates that resistance (impedance) is inversely related to voltage. At the muscle fiber level, muscle action potentials have a magnitude of several thousandths of a volt. The summated current passes through the resistive subcutaneous tissues and skin, reducing the voltage sometimes by 100-fold. Therefore, EMG signals from body areas with above-average amounts of adipose tissue will appear less than normal, even if the signals at the muscle fiber level are equivalent to that from other muscles with less intervening tissue. In fact, all intervening tissues, including bone and atrophic, necrotic, or especially oily skin, resist the muscles' electrical signals. Because skin resistance varies but internal resistance from fat and other tissues probably remains constant, only skin resistance is typically a concern.

If the EMG machine's impedance is much greater than skin impedance, skin resistance becomes trivial in comparison, and the biofeedback signal reflects more valid muscle EMG activity. As a rule of thumb, EMG instruments should have at least 1000 times as much input impedance as that measured between the two active electrodes. Skin impedance can be as high as 10,000 ohms; EMG machines with only a few megOhms of input impedance require skin preparation, whereas machines with input impedance in the order of hundreds of megOhms or gigaOhms do not require skin preparation (dry electrodes). One can easily measure skin electrode impedance by attaching an **ohmmeter** to the surface electrodes after they are attached to the skin. Generally, a standard, careful skin preparation to remove dead surface skin and excess oil will decrease resistance to 1000 ohms or less, a level that can be accommodated by contemporary instruments with high (at least 100 megOhms) input impedance.

Electrode size also alters the effective resistance seen by the amplifier. Larger electrodes have lower resistances. The greatest resistance occurs with needle electrodes, because their surface area is so small. Changing electrodes may cause an ostensible change in the EMG signal, and the therapist must realize that this is an artifact.

COMMON MODE REJECTION RATIO

Contemporary EMG instruments (Fig. 33-7) almost always use a differential amplifier, comparing the voltage at one active electrode to the other active electrode. The ground electrode in a good EMG machine may be placed almost anywhere on the patient. If the voltage travels down the muscle and arrives at both electrodes simultaneously, no difference between the electrodes is registered and the instrument would reflect no change in activity. Therefore, therapists must choose electrode placements that maximize the likelihood that EMG signals will first reach one active electrode and later reach the other active electrode.

The advantage of the differential recording system is its rejection of extraneous voltages (Fig. 33-8). Although we may not be aware of it, patients' skin receives a great many voltages, such as from lights, motors, and other appliances that produce currents that travel through the air and can affect the recordings on the skin. Other muscles (e.g., the heart) also produce voltages. If the electricity from these other sources reaches the two active electrodes simultaneously, a differential amplifier with a high CMRR will reject those artifactual signals.

The voltage from lights and other exogenous generators nearly always reach the two skin electrodes simultaneously, so room current (60 Hz) interference, is often minimal. Myocardial activity, however, is often a problem when electrodes are on the chest or upper back, near the heart. The presence of a regularly alternating signal in the feedback signal, unrelated to the muscle(s) being monitored, indicates that the electrodes should be replaced perpen-

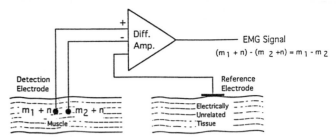

Figure 33-8. A schematic of the differential amplifier configuration. The EMG signal is represented by 'm' and the noise signals by 'n.' (From CJ De Luca: Surface electromyography: Detection and recording, with permission. Available online from: www.Delsys.com, 1997.)

dicular to the progression of the ECG wave, so that the ECG signal arrives at both electrodes concurrently. Alternatively, a bandwidth filter (see the section on bandwidth) of 100 to 200 hertz can cancel myocardial artifact, but this reduces EMG signal in this range as well.

Electronic common mode rejection is not perfect. If a signal of 60 hertz interferes with a therapy session, the room lights should be turned off or determine if a nearby whirlpool or diathermy machine is the culprit. An ungrounded appliance operating from the same electrical circuit as the EMG feedback instrument will occasionally interfere with EMG recordings. If the EMG instrument cannot operate by batteries, then disconnect the ungrounded appliance, or install an outlet for the EMG that is isolated from other appliances.

As with input impedance, higher is better. CMRRs should be at least 100 decibels. If the muscles being monitored are especially weak and generate only a few microvolts, then large amplifier gains are required; large gains, unfortunately, also amplify the artifacts. Therefore, high CMRR is especially desirable when using biofeedback for the low myoelectric signals common in neuromuscular re-education.

BANDWIDTH

Bandwidth is the difference between the lowest and highest frequency detected by an EMG instrument. Consider the difference between the treble (high-frequency) and bass (low-frequency) pitch settings of a stereo player's tone control. Some stereos have a broader frequency range (more bass, usually) than others. Similarly, EMG amplifiers vary in their frequency bandwidth.

Although most of the power at surface kinesiological EMG recordings is between 20 and 300 hertz, instrument responsiveness (bandwidth) relates not only to the frequency of the monitored signal but also to how quickly the signal changes. Therefore, monitoring rapid, transient movements like piano runs, requires up to a 500-hertz bandwidth.

NOISE LEVEL

Noise is any unwanted electrical signal that is detected with the desired signal. In general, the lower the noise is, the better. If the noise level of the

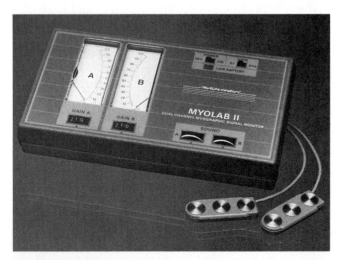

Figure 33-7. Electrode/preamplifier combination in a commercially available biofeedback instrument for neuromuscular reeducation. (Courtesy of Motion Control, Salt Lake City, UT.)

device is, say, 5 microvolts, a muscle contraction of 4 microvolts would be lost within the machine. Modern devices, using high-quality electronic components, typically generate acceptable noise levels of 2 microvolts or less. The noise level is usually described as *specificity* or *resolution* on a machine's specification sheet.

GAIN

Gain is the ability of a biofeedback machine to amplify an input signal (i.e., the amplifier's sensitivity). Surface EMG (sEMG) requires an amplifier with a high gain in order to display the small voltage detected from a muscle into a perceptible visual or auditory output signal.

OTHER ARTIFACTS

Artifacts or false readings can be traced to many sources, but the most common artifacts in EMG biofeedback are volume conduction and movement.

Volume-conducted artifact results when signals from nearby muscles are inadvertently sampled by the surface electrodes. The easiest solution is to bring the active electrodes closer to one another. The therapist might also palpate the suspected muscle during the movement, but one should be aware that tendons and muscle bellies become palpably tense from simply being passively stretched. A better solution is to use a second set of electrodes to monitor the offending muscle's activity on another channel.[25]

For example, when treating a patient with hemiplegia to increase elbow extension by increasing triceps EMG amplitude, the therapist should realize that spastic elbow flexors may be contracting. Although the EMG signal may appear to increase, the elbow still does not extend. The increase in EMG registered by the biofeedback device in this case might result from spastic biceps muscle activity, which, in turn, explains why the elbow does not extend. The solution, therefore, would be to attempt first to relax the biceps brachii, then to facilitate triceps motor activity using the EMG biofeedback.

Patients with paretic muscles caused by lower motor neuron disorders sometimes use similarly incorrect strategies. Because paretic muscles (e.g., those resulting from peroneal palsy) have too few active motor units, the low EMG signals must be amplified greatly, perhaps by using an EMG scale of 0 to 10 microvolts. By using the biofeedback machine at such high gains, therapists can discern practically any amount of motor unit activity. Unfortunately, patients often try to please their therapists and to show themselves that "there is life in my muscle," so they clench their teeth and co-contract throughout the limb. In so doing, they are successful in increasing the response of the biofeedback instrument, but in this case, biofeedback reinforces functionally inappropriate motor behavior. Therefore, it is the therapist's responsibility to ensure that the feedback is valid.

Many patients are referred to physical therapists with an expertise in biofeedback because, according to the referring clinician, "The patient can increase the muscle's EMG, but can't achieve any functional gains." The problem is virtually always volume-conduction EMG artifact. As indicated earlier, multichannel biofeedback is employed to monitor all the muscles in the limb to allow an understanding of the strategy the patient is employing to increase the EMG signal. The goal of therapy becomes inhibition of the antagonists and facilitation of the agonists. Some patients require as many as three or more sessions to reverse the effects of previous biofeedback (which was in fact artifact feedback!).

Movement artifacts are one of the most vexing problems in EMG biofeedback. Particularly where muscles are weak and amplification per force is high, movement artifacts, whose greatest power is below 20 hertz, can be easily mistaken for EMG signals. Whenever movement occurs, the cables move and signals are fed back, even if the muscles are not generating electrical activity. Of course, a high CMRR can decrease this problem, but the best solution is to eliminate the cables altogether by putting the preamplifier at the electrode site (Fig. 33-9).

Table 33–1 gives examples of specification sheets from two different biofeedback machines.

Therapeutic Intervention

In the most general terms, EMG feedback can be used only to help the patient increase or decrease muscle activity. Thus, for weak muscles, the goal is usually to increase the EMG signal (*uptrain*), and for overactive muscles the goal is to decrease the EMG signal (*downtrain*). Note that the etiology of the weakness or overactivity is not mentioned. Biofeedback techniques to date make no distinction among the various diagnostic categories. Biofeedback applications distinguish only between weakness or overactivity (i.e., *functional* classifications). As a result, a typical treatment session should include (1) patient

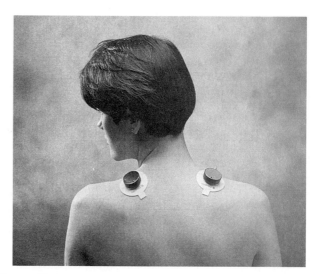

Figure 33-9. Electrode placement of a preamplifier on each upper trapezius for "down-training" (relaxation) of these muscles. (Courtesy of NeuroDyne Medical Corp., Newton, MA.)

Table 33–1 SPECIFICATION VALUES FOR TWO DIFFERENT EMG BIOFEEDBACK DEVICES

	Device A	Device B
Input impedance	100 megOhms	1,000,000 megOhms
Sensitivity	1.1 microvolts RMS	<0.08 microvolts/RMS
Bandwidth	95–500 Hz	20–500 Hz
CMRR	85 dB	180 dB
Calibrated range (gain)	1.1–2250 microvolts	0.08–2000 micro-volts RMS
Electrode type	Passive, single channel	Active, dual channel
Settings	Basic	Multiple
Accessory options	None	Multiple
Approximate cost	$300	$3,000

functional assessment, (2) problem identification and establishing expected outcomes and goals of treatment, and (3) therapeutic intervention.

Patient functional assessment is performed in the usual way: tests and measurements are conducted to determine the status of motor, psychological, and other relevant factors. The therapist should be especially observant of cooperation and attention because they are critical to successful implementation of biofeedback techniques.

After determining the functional deficit, the therapist performs a kinesiological assessment to identify the muscle(s) that require(s) intervention (problem identification). The EMG device can be connected to further enhance the information gathered at this time, which can be particularly helpful in identifying outcomes and goals of initial treatment sessions. If the therapist's kinesiological assessment is correct, then therapeutic interventions to augment control of the muscle group(s) should lead directly to enhanced function (a physical therapy outcome). Data from functional assessments and other appropriate tests and measures allows the therapist to delinate goals and outcomes and establish a plan of care incorporating biofeedback.

Therapeutic interventions in EMG feedback typically require the therapist to:

1. Select the muscle(s) to be monitored.
2. Prepare the skin at the surface electrode site with alcohol or other skin abrasive.
3. Prepare the electrodes and apply them to the skin.
4. Determine the maximum and minimum EMG readings *without* patient feedback, to determine baseline readings. At this time, be sure that the signal reaching the patient is artifact-free and valid.
5. Together with the patient, set the goals for the session and ensure patient understanding. Typically, outcome setting at each session requires the audio and visual thresholds to be set. Treatment can be progressed after roughly two-thirds or more of the biofeedback trials are successful (*two-thirds criterion*).
6. Teach the patient to manipulate the controls of the machinery to elicit the maximal amount of

patient participation in the intervention. The more responsibility the patient assumes for the treatment, the greater the chances of a successful intervention.

7. Use facilitation or other neuromuscular re-education techniques. In so doing, both the therapist and the patient react to the EMG feedback to monitor their success.
8. Remove and clean the device and the patient's skin after the session's end.

The initial session is structured to permit the therapist to understand the motor dysfunction, and to permit the patient to understand the equipment. Therefore, simple tasks are given to the patient, and following mastery, more difficult tasks are given. After explaining to the patient the purpose of biofeedback techniques and after choosing the appropriate muscle, the therapist will demonstrate what the patient should make the biofeedback device do by placing the electrodes on the patient's sound, contralateral limb. If both limbs are affected, the therapist may use his or her own limb for the demonstration.

For use in subsequent treatments, the therapist can mark the patient's skin, tracing the electrode locations for replication on ensuing days. Alternately, the therapist can specify in the treatment record the electrode locations according to anatomical markers on that patient: a mole, blemish, or any other permanent skin marker is optimal. The closer the reference point to the electrode site the easier the replication will be at the next visit.

PATIENT CONSIDERATIONS

After the equipment is in place and the therapist is satisfied that the feedback signal is accurate, the patient should be taught to master the movement. Generally, the therapist should begin by requesting a simple isometric contraction, setting the amplification gains so the patient achieves the criterion for feedback (the audio or video threshold) on about two of three contractions. Thus, the gains are set quite high for weak muscles and low for overactive muscles.

Use of imagery, proprioceptive neuromuscular facilitation (PNF), ice, vibration, indeed even electrical stimulation, in conjunction with biofeedback can enhance the patient's motor performance—so long as the adjunctive treatment (e.g., melting ice) does not induce artifactual feedback. Among the most useful techniques is to have the patient imagine the motor activity, and while the electrodes monitor the muscle and the therapist gives verbal reinforcement and manual assistance such as tapping, tendon pressure, or putting the muscle on stretch, the patient attempts to perform that activity.[26]

EXAMPLE

Consider the typical patient with hemiplegia having classic foot-drop gait. Initial sessions should concentrate on recruiting more dorsiflexor activity (and/or less plantarflexor spasticity, if present) until the patient can reliably isolate dorsiflexion. Positional differences are important. Most patients will be able to dorsiflex most easily in sitting, with the knee at about 45 to 75 degrees flexion and the foot flat on the floor. The difficulty of the task should be increased incrementally. The patient should be required to dorsiflex with the knee flexed to 90 degrees and then with the knee in progressively less flexion until dorsiflexion is possible in sitting with the knee at full extension. The patient should now be able to dorsiflex while standing, so the next task is to introduce this skill during walking. As indicated previously, dorsiflexion must be rapid to be helpful in clearing the foot, so the patient should be trained from the outset to contract the dorsiflexors explosively while keeping the plantarflexors relatively quiet.

To help relax spastic muscles, the EMG device can be used to monitor muscle activity during slow, passive stretch. The challenge of keeping the spastic muscle relatively quiet can be increased by more rapid stretch. Finally, a progression should be made to active-assisted movement, and then to independent movement. The patient must keep the EMG levels below a certain threshold, say 20 microvolts at first. As the patient improves his or her ability to control spastic muscle activity during passive or active stretch, the task difficulty should be increased incrementally by lowering the detection threshold to, say 17 or 15 microvolts.

During gait training, the patient should walk with the dorsiflexor EMG feedback acting as an error signal, guided by the therapist's feedback indicated which strategies have been successful in eliciting the appropriate motor activity. The therapist should, of course, continue to treat the patient, including the "non-affected limb," whether or not these muscles participated directly in the feedback session.

Note that little clinical research has been done to delineate the usefulness of providing EMG feedback for spasticity, so the above example should be considered only as a guide. Furthermore, there is no agreement among gait analysis experts on what constitutes normal EMG activity for a given muscle group[27,28] nor even of the best way to analyze and present the EMG signal.[29] Therefore, use and interpretation of EMG biofeedback signals for gait training, in general, should be undertaken with circumspection. The therapist should not rely on the EMG signal alone for signs of functional progress, particularly for patients with spastic muscles.

Patients with paretic or weak muscles present a different challenge. The challenge is to recruit more motor units or to use the motor units more effectively, rather than to find strategies for controlling the muscle or its antagonist. Patients with weak muscles whose manual muscle test (MMT) values are F+ (3+/5) or less, are good candidates for EMG feedback. If some resistance can be accommodated (i.e., G– [4–/5] or greater MMT value) then resistive exercises should be given. Biofeedback can enhance muscle control, but no research to date has shown that EMG feedback plus resistive exercises are better

than the latter alone. Experimental research has, however, shown that EMG feedback plus isometric quad-setting is substantially more effective than the quad-setting exercises alone, in increasing muscle power following knee arthrotomy.[13]

GENERAL RELAXATION

Relaxation therapy techniques sometimes combine EMG feedback with Jacobson's progressive relaxation, Schultz's autogenic imagery, and other psychological techniques.[30] In these sessions, the EMG is typically monitored from frontalis or forearm muscle sites. The patient sits quietly while passively attempting to decrease the EMG signal, attending to the psychological and behavioral correlates of relaxation.[31] Very deep relaxation can be induced, so nonpsychologists must be wary of their comments and actions around patients whose defenses are so relaxed.

Relaxation sessions may also include finger temperature, skin impedance, blood pressure, or heart rate feedback. Particularly with respect to skin temperature feedback, the therapist's knowledge of physiology is an important determinant of whether or not the patient's experience can be successful. Temperature biofeedback has been a first-line treatment for Raynaud's disease for two decades.[32] Of considerable importance is the therapist's support of the patient's goals and outcomes, empathy and compassion. The techniques that have been demonstrated are as important as technical capabilities in relaxation therapies.[33]

Patients who find it difficult to relax, or those with stress-related disorders, may benefit from relaxation biofeedback techniques. Occasionally, patients with spasticity recalcitrant to the interventions described may benefit from general relaxation. In general, most individuals have relatively little information about tension-related muscle activity. Some patients literally do not realize that when they clench their fists, grind their teeth, or otherwise tense their muscles, they are increasing their muscle tension. These patients find it quite difficult to relax their spastic muscles because they do not know how to relax their normal muscles!

No matter the diagnosis, the biofeedback technique treatment approach is similar: (1) select a muscle whose EMG signal is relevant to the functional activity, (2) have the patient practice controlling the signal, and (3) withdraw the feedback as function is gained.

KINEMATIC (JOINT MOTION) FEEDBACK

Joint motions are commonly measured by using a goniometer. An *electrogoniometer (el-gon)* (Fig. 33-10) is an electronic version of the manual goniometer that employs a **potentiometer** (i.e., a variable resistor, or **rheostat**) attached to the movable and stationary arms. The arms move just as they do in a conventional goniometer and they correspond to the position of the limb segments.[34]

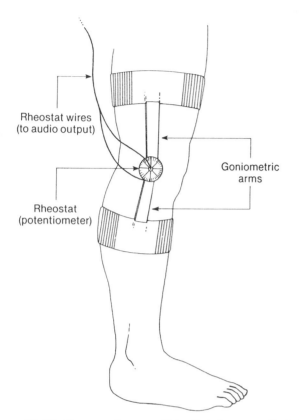

Figure 33-10. Electrogoniometer. Note that its arms attach to patient's limb segments.

Rheostats are commonly used as the volume control knob on stereos or as room light dimmers. Rotating the rheostat changes its resistance, which in turn increases or decreases the current from the feedback device's signal. If a volume control knob or room light dimmer were connected to an el-gon on a knee, for example, each step would cause the audio signal or lights to fluctuate.

It is important to be sure that the feedback is linearly related to joint motion. For the same reason that a 20-degree turn of a stereo's volume control knob should always result in the same audio volume change, so should a 20-degree knee flexion always result in the same change in electrogoniometer feedback. The voltage through the electrogoniometer is provided by a battery; joint movement causes the rheostat's pitch or volume to change proportionately.[35,36]

Clinical Applications

As with all biofeedback techniques, the therapist should first demonstrate the desired behavior by attaching the electrogoniometer to the patient's uninvolved limb or to the therapist's corresponding limb segments.[37] The other principles of biofeedback techniques also apply to **kinematic feedback,** such as positive reinforcement and the two-thirds criterion for success. The therapist should begin by setting the error signal range to be quite forgiving during early stages of training and then increase the task's difficulty incrementally as mastery is achieved.[38] The baseline position on the el-gon is generally set for silence (no feedback), but movement in the desired direction is reinforced with sound.

Children with orthopedic disorders can be especially easy to treat, by making the volume of the TV or radio contingent on movement in the proper direction. For example, louder volume could be used to indicate increased knee flexion, and the child's postsurgical recovery can be hastened by allowing cartoons to be watched and heard as long as knee flexion is above a criterion level.

Stiff-legged (insufficient knee flexion) gait of hemiplegia has been successfully treated by el-gon biofeedback. Subjects with hemiplegia learned to reduce knee stance phase hyperextension and to increase swing phase flexion.[39]

Patients with trans-femoral (above-knee) amputations need to learn to keep their prosthetic knee extended during stance. Fernie et al.[40] and Wooldridge et al.[41] described the use of an el-gon to facilitate this learning by providing audio feedback that indicated when the knee was safe for weight-bearing.

The therapist must, however, have a good working knowledge of normal **kinematics** and of the kinematics expected of patients with a particular diagnosis (Fig. 33-11). It is, for example, inappropriate to ask a patient with hemiplegia to dorsiflex beyond neutral during the swing phase, or to ask a patient with trans-femoral (above-knee) amputation to employ normal knee kinematics during prosthetic stance phase (Fig. 33-12).[42]

The same logic applies to orthotic rehabilitation. Orthoses are frequently prescribed to support or restrict joint motions quite distant from the device itself. For example, setting the orthotic ankle joint in slight plantarflexion encourages knee extension during stance. Patients using such devices should not be expected to attain normal knee motions, and kinematic biofeedback should not be used to encourage flexion when such ground reaction orthoses are being employed.

Construction

DeBacher[36] provides detailed instructions on the use and construction of electrogoniometers. Therapists can easily and inexpensively fabricate a simple el-gon. The electrical parts are available from the local electronics store, and the remainder consists essentially of a manual goniometer.[35] The potentiometer should have at least 90 percent linearity, but almost all commercially available rheostats today satisfy that requirement. Finally, note that most isokinetic devices have a built-in electrogoniometer. Asking the patient to monitor the printed goniometric channel is often a good method of encouraging joint mobility through kinematic biofeedback techniques.

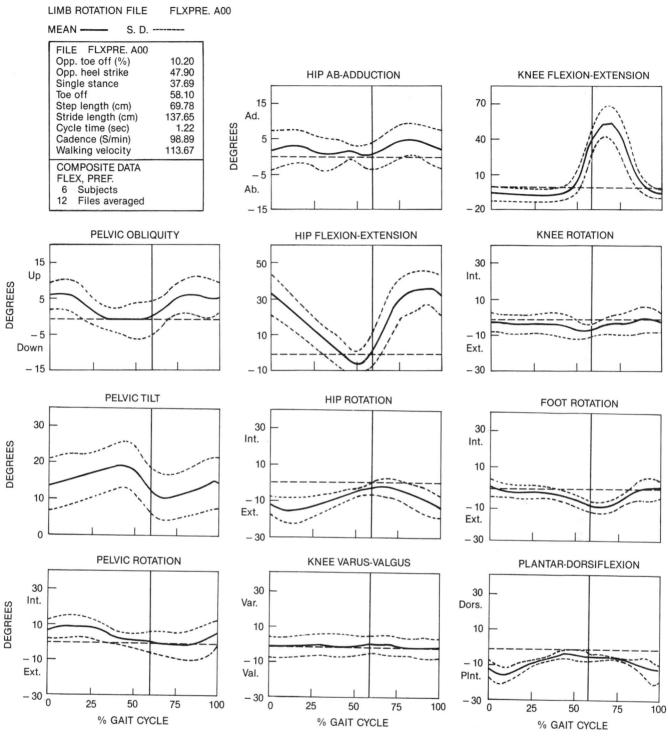

Figure 33-11. Normal adult kinematics. Solid line is average joint angle; dashed line represents mean plus or minus 1 standard deviation. Note particularly the dorsiflexion angle. (Data collected at Newington Children's Hospital Gait Analysis Laboratory, Newington, CT.)

STANDING BALANCE FEEDBACK

Somewhere between kinematic and **kinetic** feedback lies standing balance or **posturography feedback.** Balance feedback has become increasingly popular as therapists are asked to treat elderly patients and others at risk of falling. Posturography feedback devices usually consist of force-measuring scales on which the subject is requested to stand as still as possible. Although they are typically marketed as measuring center of gravity or center of mass sway, balance platforms such as Balance Master™ only measure the *center of pressure (COP)* under the feet. COP displacement is loosely associated with whole body center of mass (COM) sway such that the COP acts to push the COM back or

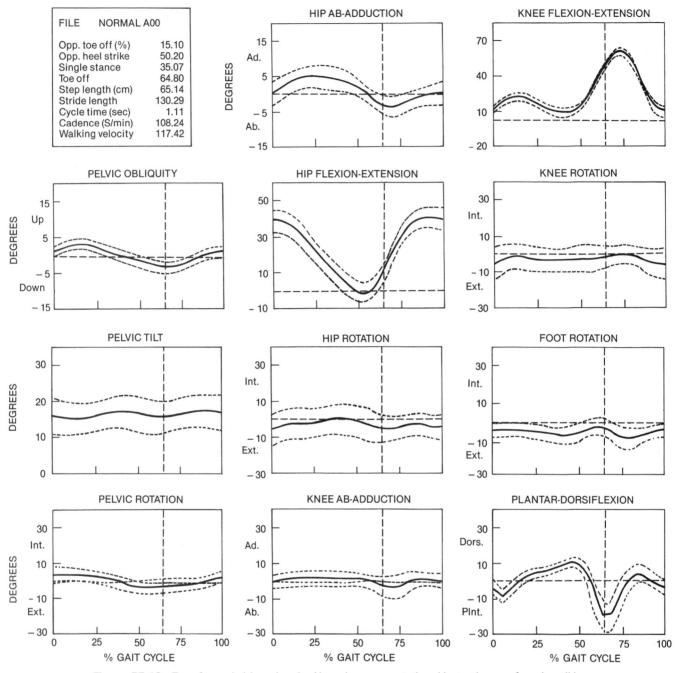

FILE	NORMAL A00
Opp. toe off (%)	15.10
Opp. heel strike	50.20
Single stance	35.07
Toe off	64.80
Step length (cm)	65.14
Stride length	130.29
Cycle time (sec)	1.11
Cadence (S/min)	108.24
Walking velocity	117.42

Figure 33-12. Transfemoral (above-knee). Above-knee amputation kinematics, preferred walking speed. Note that the knee remains fully extended throughout the stance. (Data collected at Newington Children's Hospital Gait Analysis Laboratory, Newington, CT.)

forward.[43] Hence, COP excursion always exceeds COM sway if any movement is occurring.

Biofeedback of postural sway (whether the COP, COM, or other variables are actually measured) in patients with balance impairment is becoming widespread in clinical use.[44] It seems reasonable that subjects who sway excessively should be taught to decrease their sway using balance feedback, but research results to date are equivocal. Balance control in the past has been defined as the ability to maintain an upright position by attaining equilib-

rium of the forces of gravity, muscles, and inertia acting on the body's COG, thus maintaining the ground reaction forces' COP within the base of support (Fig. 33-13).[45] For example, Shumway-Cook et al.[46] determined that standing balance feedback improved balance control (measured by COP) in 14 subjects with hemiplegia following cerebrovascular accident (CVA). Winstein et al.,[47] however, reported that although a controlled trial of standing balance training improves static standing measures, no specific improvement in locomotor parameters could be demonstrated. Indeed, three decades ago Sheldon[48] found that older subjects can be confused by sway biofeedback, and may perform better with their eyes closed than while receiving postural sway biofeedback.

One limitation of using the COP to measure postural sway is that COP motion maintains a close relationship to COG motion only during relatively normal ankle strategy motions, where the subject moves like a pendulum, or a rigid body, about his or her ankles.[49] When upper body motion becomes significant as in a hip strategy, or when postural sway cannot be assumed to stem from ankle motion alone, the COP:COG relationship becomes distorted such that the COP does not adequately reflect the COM sway.[50]

A second limitation is that during dynamic activities, such as locomotion, the body's mass *must* be displaced outside its support base (Fig. 33-14). This fundamental difference between static and dynamic stability may account for the reported poor ability of static balance tests to explain or predict locomotor instability, such as falling, among elders.[51] Most falls occur during dynamic body displacements, such as walking, climbing stairs, or arising from a seated position.[52] For individuals with impaired balance, the relationship between the results of standing posturography balance training and dynamic stability (e.g., gait, stair climbing, sit-to-stand transfers) is not definitive. The lack of information persists despite the growing clinical use of standing posturography to assess and treat patients with balance disorders as well as the elderly.[53] For individuals with vestibular impairments, posturography does not predict functional performance cross-sectionally,[54] nor does it correlate with change in gait and functional performance longitudinally.[55]

Clearly, balance rehabilitation is becoming in-

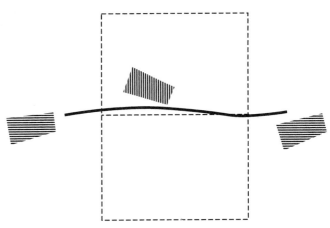

Figure 33-14. Top view of subject walking. The sinusoidal line shows the route taken by the center of gravity (COG) (see Fig. 33-12). Note the COG never comes within the foot perimeter and so cannot be within the base of support during single limb support (midstance).

creasingly more important, but it is not yet clear how significant a role biofeedback will play. An update on the use of force platform biofeedback for balance training after stroke concludes that current research supports a role for this method in patients with postural asymmetry or decreased limits of stability, but that further research is needed.[44]

In summary, available literature supports the assertion that elderly subjects at risk for falling, and those with neurological disorders including parkinsonism and hemiplegia, improve their standing balance as a result of standing balance training. Insufficient data exist to assert that standing balance biofeedback confers any benefit upon dynamic locomotor control or other functional mobility skills. Better conceptual definitions of static and dynamic balance are needed,[19] as well as more empirical research.

KINETIC (DYNAMIC FORCE) FEEDBACK

Kinetic feedback or dynamic force feedback renders information regarding the amount or rate of loading through the limbs. As in other types of biofeedback, an audio or visual feedback signal is used. In kinetic feedback, the goal is usually one of informing the patient that weight-bearing is correct, excessive, or insufficient.

Force feedback requires the therapist to be familiar with the same general motor learning strategies (the time sequence, positive reinforcement, and the two-thirds criterion) as discussed under EMG and kinematic biofeedback. Understanding the expected outcomes with kinetic feedback and the equipment limitations is also required.

Types of Kinetic Feedback Devices

The most familiar type of kinetic feedback is a bathroom scale, which can be used to habituate

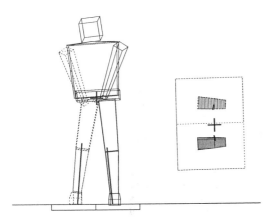

Figure 33-13. During stable, quiet standing, the whole body center of gravity (COG, dark plus sign [+] shown between feet) remains within the base of support, as bounded by the feet (right). Individual center of pressure (CP) positions from each foot can be combined to create a whole-body CP. A front view of a whole-body model of the same subject in the same quiet standing task (left). The ground reaction vectors (heavy lines from each foot) have, by definition, the CP as their point of application at the ground. Here again, the whole body COG is shown as a dark plus sign (+) at waist height.

patients to the weight-bearing requirements of their fracture, prosthesis, or orthosis during static standing. The bathroom scale, however, is not useful for dynamic force feedback in part because it will register artifactually high forces during the loading phase, as in the stance phase of gait. Another familiar, but little-appreciated kinetic feedback device, is the force reading from isokinetic devices such as the Cybex machine.

FOOTSWITCHES

A simple footswitch can be used for kinetic feedback. It is easily fabricated in the physical therapy clinic. A buzzer and a battery connected to a footswitch can warn the patient not to weight bear on a fractured limb, or help to encourage heel-strike gait from a patient with hemiplegia or cerebral palsy. When the metal parts of the footswitch contact during the stance phase, the buzzer sounds, thus giving audible biofeedback. Two footswitches could be used bilaterally to provide stance time symmetry biofeedback. Of course, the weight-bearing force is unknowable using this simple system, but footswitches have the benefit of convenience.

Another advantage of footswitches is that they can be used to record the patient's progress in achieving heel contact by attaching them to a strip chart recorder. This technique was previously used in gait laboratories before more sophisticated methods were devised.

LIMB LOAD MONITOR

A **limb load monitor** (LLM) is most frequently used to provide kinetic feedback in the clinic, because it gives feedback concerning the *amount* of weight born on a limb.[56] LLMs generally have a strain gauge built into an insole or the sole of a sandal. The strain gauge works by decreasing its electrical resistance as the force on the foot increases.[57] Less resistance, in turn, permits more electricity to reach the audio speaker, which beeps faster or at a higher pitch as greater loads are applied.

The feedback threshold is set according to the amount of weight required to be applied on the limb. For example, if nonweight-bearing is required, the therapist might set the audio signal to respond as soon as 2 pounds or more is sensed by the LLM. When weight bearing exceeds the threshold, an audible tone warns the patient and informs the therapist that the protocol is being violated.[58]

In other applications, the therapist may want to encourage weight bearing. Patients with amputation, hemiplegia, and other weight-bearing disorders can use the LLM to inform them when they have achieved the criterion weight-bearing set by the therapist.[59] Again, modest goals are set initially, and then increased incrementally as success is achieved consistently. When the patient achieves full weight bearing on the limb, feedback is withdrawn and the patient attempts to maintain the treatment effect without supervision. The LLM can then be used to monitor the patient's success surreptitiously.

Technical Limitations

Only the vertical ground reaction component is registered by LLMs. Before and after, torsional, and horizontal sheer forces are not monitored separately in present devices. Therefore, LLMs may feed back invalid signals, especially if the patient uses a pathological gait pattern, as is typically true of lower limb disability. The greatest danger of artifact occurs during heel-strike, particularly during fast walking. Until technology improves, the prudent therapist will employ limb-load feedback only as an indication of gross errors in timing and weight bearing.

The therapist should also understand that forces and pressures experienced at a joint such as the hip are a product not only of ground reaction forces, but also of muscle forces. A LLM provides only part of the picture with information on ground reaction loads. Thus, using the hip joint example, applying knowledge of in vivo hip forces or acetabular contact pressures (measurements of the resultant loads experienced) should be considered in clinical decision making.[60]

Clinical Applications

Gait training itself is fatiguing, but even more so with the addition of kinetic feedback where the patient is asked to cope with another cognitive demand. The patient must not only exercise, but also concentrate on the feedback signal. The therapist must therefore provide frequent rest periods, and occasionally reassess the patient's progress to ensure that treatment goals are accomplished. Fatigue may interfere with learning in biofeedback as it does in other types of neuromuscular reeducation.

The therapist will usually start a treatment session by reviewing the goals for that day with the patient. If it is the patient's first exposure to balance biofeedback or the LLM, the therapist will demonstrate the task using his or her own limb, and then will demonstrate on the patient's uninvolved limb.

The first session usually consists of static weight shifting. Next, the patient practices walking in place, usually between the parallel bars. If the patient cannot understand the LLM feedback, the therapist can use bathroom scales combined with the LLM to show the LLM feedback's relationship to a familiar load monitor.[61]

After consistently successful static performance, the patient is asked to walk in place while generating the appropriate biofeedback signal. Weight shifting and balance should be encouraged by stance and swing-phase biofeedback. After roughly two-thirds or more of the trials are successful, short-distance ambulation with biofeedback should be assessed.

After several sessions, the patient's progress should be reassessed. Are the therapy goals appropriate? Is biofeedback enhancing or interfering with progress in other areas of therapy? Review sessions should occasionally be provided, including static weight shifting and dynamic gait activities to ensure that the basic skills are not forgotten.

Most importantly, assess the patient's performance without biofeedback. Normal gait is a smooth, automatic, and subconsciously controlled activity; that goal should remain preeminent. In contrast, biofeedback compels voluntary attention to the tasks to be practiced. Hesitation or slow gait may indicate excessive reliance on the biofeedback, which in fact detracts from normal gait. Some therapists have patients with reasonable cognitive levels recite the pledge of allegiance, or perform mental arithmetic, to allay excessive cognitive control and elicit more automatic control.

To develop normal locomotor skills, the therapist must encourage normal walking speed. Many patients with hemiplegia, for example, can look fairly normal while using biofeedback during slow walking, but when asked to walk at a normal pace, about 1 cycle per second, their control deteriorates. Biofeedback is only a tool; the therapist retains responsibility for the correct timing and speed of movement training.

In summary, effective kinematic and kinetic biofeedback depends on setting appropriate outcomes for the patient to achieve. Patients with hemiplegia should generally be encouraged to flex the affected knee during stance, but patients with transfemoral amputations should not. The patient's diagnosis and prosthetic/orthotic appliances will manifest differences in gait requirements, which modify treatment goals and functional expectations. Any therapeutic technique, including biofeedback, should achieve the most efficient gait possible, consistent with safety and stability.

NEW CONCEPTS AND AREAS FOR FURTHER RESEARCH

The necessity for continued research in biofeedback cannot be overemphasized. An important aspect of biofeedback techniques is that they place responsibility for healthy behavior directly with the patient. The paradigm of therapist or doctor as healer is no longer valid if the patient assumes the role of healer. However, self-regulation techniques such as biofeedback need to be subjected to the scrutiny of critical thinkers and tested empirically through clinical research.

Perhaps the chief impediment to giving patients more direct control of their rehabilitation is our current inability to understand all the rules and mechanisms governing human orthopedic and neurological recovery. We can hardly translate to layman's terms that which scientists do not understand. The challenge to the therapist, then, is to better understand the rules of human behavior. Biofeedback techniques can be used to monitor physiological and to help patients gain access to

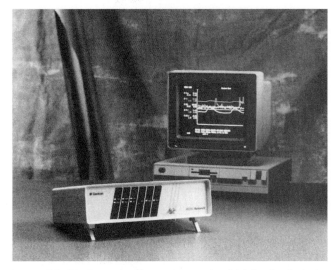

Figure 33-15. Example of computer-assisted biofeedback device. (Courtesy of NeuroDyne Medical Corp., Newton, MA.)

these results otherwise unfelt components of recovery.

One recent area of interest is adaptation of computers to rehabilitation. The addition of microcomputers to biofeedback-assisted therapy may improve information processing (Fig. 33-15). Storing normal movement templates in the microcomputer and subsequently requesting patients to approximate those movement patterns has been widely purported to be effective in teaching neuromuscular skills. However, excessive information can overwhelm patients and therapists with its sheer volume.

Perhaps the most pressing deficiency in the rehabilitation biofeedback literature is the lack of controlled studies involving patients. Most of the evidence that supports the utility of biofeedback techniques is based on normal subjects or small samples of patients.

SUMMARY

This chapter has dealt with biofeedback as the therapeutic tool that provides physiological information directly back to the patient.

It is abundantly clear that electronic advances should be applied clinically to the advantage of disabled populations. The therapist must assume the responsibility for exploring its potential and validating biofeedback techniques through clinical research, particularly on patient populations.

In the 1990s, biofeedback became a very important adjunct modality, mostly as a means of monitoring muscles; however, it is not considered a treatment per se.[62] Middaugh[63p207] states: "How can we justify working with muscles and *not* use EMG monitoring? How we can we teach relaxation and *not* monitor physiological change? I see a future in which it will be malpractice *not* to monitor and measure the physiological responses we are working with."

QUESTIONS FOR REVIEW

1. What is the primary psychological/motor learning model employed in biofeedback?

2. What event during muscle activation does EMG biofeedback record?

3. What is the most likely source of an artifactual, rhythmically repeating EMG interference when the EMG electrodes are on the patient's back?

4. Why is input impedance important to therapists using EMG feedback?

5. What is an el-gon? How can it be made in the clinic?

6. What type of biofeedback, kinetic or kinematic, is represented by a bathroom scale?

CASE STUDY

Case Study 1

A 73 year-old man is referred to physical therapy for attempt to wean him from an AFO, which he has been wearing for the last year since a right CVA (left hemiparesis). A left foot drop is the only significant residual that remains, and his physician believes that because there is some dorsiflexion power, a physical therapy intervention trial is warranted. On examination, you note that passive left ankle dorsiflexion (with patient sitting, foot on floor, knee flexed 45 degrees) is –5 degrees (i.e., 5 degrees short of neutral [0 degrees]) and active dorsiflexion in this position brings the ankle to –10 degrees (2+/5 MMT grade). During gait, heel strike is absent on the lower left extremity. On the right side both passive and active dorsiflexion is to 0–5 degrees.

Guiding Questions

1. Explain whether the dorsiflexion weakness is likely to be a direct, indirect, or composite impairment.

2. In addition to dorsiflexion weakness, what other impairment is likely contributing to his inability to heel strike during gait? Is this a direct, indirect, or composite impairment? How will you address it?

3. What role might biofeedback have in the management of this patient?

4. To create a change in motor learning, what feedback strategies should be employed?

Case Study 2

You have been treating a 25 year-old woman with anterior knee pain for 3 weeks, and she is not experiencing the degree of improvement you were hoping for. In addition to other interventions, you have been encouraging the patient to recruit vastus medialis oblique (VMO) prior to and more strongly than vastus lateralis (VL) during isometric contraction of the quadriceps. You have *not* been using biofeedback.

Guiding Questions

1. How do you know that there is a VMO:VL imbalance? If there is, how do you know that the patient is selectively recruiting VMO during isometric quad sets?

2. (a) What advantage does biofeedback provide to VMO rehabilitation? (b) What concerns might you have?

3. What strategies should be employed in using biofeedback for treating a VMO:VL imbalance?

Case Study 3

A 50 year-old woman is status post-open reduction internal fixation (ORIF) of a left acetabular fracture. The orthopedic surgeon has emphasized that he wants the patient touch-weight bearing (TWB) on the left leg. When you clarify what the surgeon's operational definition for TWB is, he states "not more than 10 pounds."

Guiding Questions

1. How can you ensure that the patient does not exceed 10-pound loads through the operated limb: (a) in static standing; (b) during gait?

2. What advantage is there to constant feedback during gait?

3. What advantage is there to intermittent feedback during gait?

4. What additional cause of hip joint loading besides ground reaction load are you concerned with?

REFERENCES

1. Schmidt, RA, and Lee, TD: Motor Control and Learning: A Behavioral Emphasis, ed 3. Human Kinetics Publishers, Champagne, IL, 1999.
2. Basmajian, JV: Introduction: Principles and background. In Basmajian, JV (ed): Biofeedback: Principles and Practice for Clinicians, ed 3. Williams & Wilkins, Baltimore, 1989, p 1.
3. Middaugh, SJ: Biofeedback instruments are teaching tools that guide motor learning. Biofeedback: The Newsmagazine of the AAPB 24:10, 1996.
4. Shumway-Cook, A, and Woollacott, MH: Motor Control: Theory and Practical Applications. Williams & Wilkins, Baltimore, 1995.
5. Seaman, DR: Proprioceptor: An obsolete, inaccurate word. J Manipulative Physiol Ther 20:279, 1997.
6. Mulder, T, and Hulstyn, W: Sensory feedback therapy and theoretical knowledge of motor control and learning. Am J Phys Med 63:226, 1984.
7. Poole, JL: Application of motor learning principles in occupational therapy. Am J Occup Ther 45:531, 1991.
8. Winstein, CJ: Knowledge of results and motor learning implications for physical therapy. Phys Ther 71:140, 1991.
9. Brooks, VB: The normal basis of motor control. Oxford Univ Pr, New York, 1986, p 114.

10. Dunn, TG, et al: The learning process in biofeedback: Is it feed-forward or feedback? Biofeedback & Self-Regulation 11:143, 1986.

11. Schmidt, RA, et al: Summary knowledge of results for skill acquisition: Support for the guidance hypothesis. J Exp Psychol Learn Mem Cogn 15:352, 1989.

12. Segreto, J: The role of EMG awareness in EMG biofeedback learning. Biofeedback & Self-Regulation 20:155, 1995.

13. Krebs, DE: Clinical electromyographic feedback following meniscectomy: A multiple regression experimental analysis. Phys Ther 61:1017, 1981.

14. Krebs, DE, et al: Knee joint angle: Its relationship to quadriceps femoris activity in normal and postarthrotomy limbs. Arch Phys Med Rehabil 64:441, 1983.

15. Vander Linden, DW, et al: The effect of frequency of kinetic feedback on learning an isometric force production task in nondisabled subjects. Phys Ther 73:79, 1993.

16. Ingersoll, CD, and Knight, KL: Patellar location changes following EMG biofeedback or progressive resistive exercises. Med Sci Sports Exerc 23:1122, 1991.

17. Kasman, GS, et al: Clinical Applications in Surface Electromyography: Chronic Musculoskeletal Pain. Aspen, Gaithersburg, MD, 1998.

18. Andrasik, F: Twenty-five years of progress: Twenty-five more? Biofeedback & Self-Regulation 19:311, 1994.

19. Krebs DE. Biofeedback in therapeutic exercise. In: Basmajian, JV, and Wolf, SL, (eds): Therapeutic Exercise, ed 5. Williams & Wilkins, Baltimore, 1990, p 109.

20. Wolf, SL: Biofeedback. In Downey, JA, et al (eds): The Physiological Basis of Rehabilitation Medicine, ed 2. Butterworth-Heinemann, Woburn, MA, 1994.

21. Schleenbaker, RE, and Mainous, AG: Electromyographic biofeedback for neuromuscular reeducation in the hemiplegic stroke patient: A meta-analysis. Arch Phys Med Rehabil 74:1301, 1993.

22. Lenman, JAE: Quantitative electromyographic changes associated with muscular weakness. J Neurol Neurosurg Psychiatry 22:306, 1959.

23. Lippold, OCJ: Relation between integrated action potentials in human muscle and its isometric tension. J Physiol 117:492, 1952.

24. Cram, JR, et al: Introduction to surface electromyography. Aspen, Gaithersburg, MD, 1998.

25. Wolf, SL: Essential considerations in the use of EMG biofeedback. Phys Ther 58:25, 1978.

26. Cataldo, ME, et al: Experimental analysis of EMG feedback in treating cerebral palsy. J Behav Med 1:311, 1978.

27. Shiavi, R, et al: Variability of electromyographic patterns for level-surface walking through a range of self-selected speeds. Bull Prosthet Res 10:5, 1981.

28. Winter, DA: Pathologic gait diagnosis with computer-averaged electromyographic profiles. Arch Phys Med Rehabil 65:393, 1984.

29. Yang, JF, and Winter, DA: Electromyographic amplitude normalization methods: Improving their sensitivity as diagnostic tools in gait analysis. Arch Phys Med Rehabil 65:517, 1984.

30. Stoyva, JM: Autogenic training and biofeedback combined: A reliable method for the induction of general relaxation. In Basmajian, JV (ed): Biofeedback: Principles and Practice for Clinicians, ed 3. Williams & Wilkins, Baltimore, 1989, p 169.

31. Collins, GA, et al: Comparative analysis of paraspinal and frontalis EMG, heart rate and skin conductance in chronic low back pain patients and normals to various postures and stress. Scand J Rehabil Med 14:39, 1982.

32. Sedlacek, K: Biofeedback for Raynaud's Disease. Psychosomatics 20:537, 1979.

33. Stroebel, CF, and Glueck, BC: Biofeedback treatment in medicine and psychiatry: An ultimate placebo? Seminars in Psychiatry 5:379, 1973.

34. Binder, SA: Assessing the effectiveness of positional feedback to treat an ataxic patient: Application of a single-subject design. Phys Ther 61:735, 1981.

35. Gilbert, JA, et al: Technical note: Auditory feedback of knee angle for amputees. Prosthet Orthot Int 6:103, 1982.

36. DeBacher, G: Feedback goniometers for rehabilitation. In Basmajian, JV (ed): Biofeedback: Principles and Practice for Clinicians, ed 3. Williams & Wilkins, Baltimore, 1989.

37. Koheil, R, and Mandel, AR: Joint position biofeedback facilitation of physical therapy in gait training. Am J Phys Med 59:288, 1980.

38. Colborne, CR, and Olney SJ: Feedback of joint angle and EMG in gait of able-bodied subjects. Arch Phys Med Rehabil 71:478, 1990.

39. Morris, ME, et al: Electrogoniometric feedback: Its effect on genu recurvatum in stroke. Arch Phys Med Rehabil 73:1147, 1992.

40. Fernie, G, et al: Biofeedback training of knee control in the above-knee amputee. Am J Phys Med 57:161, 1978.

41. Wooldridge, CP, et al: Biofeedback training of knee joint position of the cerebral palsied child. Physiother Can 28:138, 1976.

42. Krebs, DE: Effect of Variations in Residuum Environment and Walking Rate on Residual Limb Muscle Activity of Selected Above-Knee Amputees. Dissertation, University Microfilms International, Ann Arbor, MI, 1986.

43. Murray, MP, et al: Normal postural stability and steadiness: Quantitative assessment. J Bone Joint Surg 57A:510, 1975.

44. Nichols, DS: Balance retraining after stroke using force platform biofeedback. Phys Ther 77:553, 1997.

45. Horak FB: Clinical measurement of postural control in adults. Phys Ther 67:1881, 1987.

46. Shumway-Cook, A, et al: Postural sway biofeedback: Its effect on reestablishing stance stability in hemiplegic patients. Arch Phys Med Rehabil 69:395, 1988.

47. Winstein, CJ, et al: Standing balance training: Effect on balance and locomotion in hemiparetic adults. Arch Phys Med Rehabil 70:755, 1989.

48. Sheldon, JH: The effect of age on the control of sway. Gerontology Clinics 5:129, 1963.

49. Nashner, LM, and McCollum, G: The organization of human postural movements: A formal basis and experimental synthesis. Behav Brain Sci 8:135, 1985.

50. Benda, BJ, et al: Biomechanical relationship between center of gravity and center of pressure during standing. IEEE Trans Rehab Eng 2:3, 1994.

51. Fernie, GR, et al: The relationship of postural sway in standing to the incidence of falls in geriatric subjects. Age Ageing 11:11, 1982.

52. Tinetti, ME, et al: Risk factors for falls among elderly persons living in the community. N Engl J Med 319:1701, 1988.

53. Peterka, RJ, and Black, FO: Age-related changes in human posture control: Sensory organization tests. J Vestib Res 1:73, 1990.

54. Evans, MK, and Krebs, DE: Posturography does not test vestibulospinal function. Otolaryngol Head Neck Surg 120:164, 1999.

55. O'Neill, DE, et al: Posturography changes do not predict functional performance changes. Am J Otol 19:797, 1998.

56. Gapsis, JJ, et al: Limb load monitor: Evaluation of a sensory feedback device for controlled weight-bearing. Arch Phys Med Rehabil 63:38, 1982.

57. Wolf, SL, and Binder-Macleod, SA: Use of the Krusen limb load monitor to quantify temporal and loading measurements of gait. Phys Ther 62:976, 1982.

58. Wannstedt, GT, and Herman, RM: Use of augmented sensory feedback to achieve symmetrical standing. Phys Ther 58:553, 1978.

59. Kegel, B, and Moore, AJ: Load cell: A device to monitor weight-bearing for lower extremity amputees. Phys Ther 57:652, 1977.

60. Fagerson, TL: Post-operative physical therapy. In Fagerson, TL (ed): The Hip Handbook. Butterworth-Heinemann, Woburn, MA, 1998, p. 282.

61. Peper, E, and Robertson, J: Biofeedback use of common objects: The bathroom scale in physical therapy. Biofeedback & Self-Regulation 1:237, 1976.

62. Fogel, E, and Kasman, G (eds): Special Issue: Physical medicine and rehabilitation. Biofeedback: Newsmagazine of the AAPB 24:4, 1996.

63. Middaugh, SJ: On clinical efficacy: Why biofeedback does—and does not—work. Biofeedback & Self-Regulation 15:204, 1990.

SUPPLEMENTAL READINGS

Allison, L: The role of biofeedback in balance retraining. Biofeedback: Newsmagazine of the AAPB 24:16, 1996.

Arena, JG, et al: A comparison of frontal electromyographic biofeedback training, trapezius electromyographic biofeedback training, and progressive muscle relaxation therapy in the treatment of tension headache. Headache 35:411, 1995.

Asfour, SS, et al: Biofeedback in back muscle strengthening. Spine 15:510, 1990.

Barlow, JD: Biofeedback in the treatment of fecal incontinence. European Jour of Gastroenterology & Hepatology 9:431, 1997.

Barton, L: Uses of surface EMG for neuromuscular evaluation and training in patients with neurological impairments. Biofeedback: Newsmagazine of the AAPB 24:12, 1996.

Basmajian, JV, et al: Biofeedback treatment of foot-drop after stroke compared with standard rehabilitation technique: Effects on voluntary control and strength. Arch Phys Med Rehabil 56:231, 1975.

Beckham, JC, et al: Biofeedback as a means to alter electromyographic activity in a total knee replacement patient. Biofeedback & Self-Regulation 16:23, 1991.

Behr, D, and Krebs, DE: The role of biofeedback in the reeducation of patients with musculoskeletal disorders. Phys Ther Practice 2:20, 1993.

Blanchard, EB: Biofeedback and its role in the treatment of pain. In NIH technology assessment conference on integration of behavioral and relaxation approaches into the treatment of chronic pain and insomnia, October 16–18, 1995, Bethesda.

Blanchard, EB: Biofeedback treatments of essential hypertension. Biofeedback & Self-Regulation 15:209, 1990.

Brach, JS, et al: Facial neuromuscular retraining for oral synkinesis. Plast Reconstr Surg 99:1922, 1997.

Brown, DM, et al: Feedback goniometers for hand rehabilitation. Am J Occup Ther 33:458, 1979.

Brucker, BS, and Bulaeva, NV: Biofeedback effect on electromyography responses in patients with spinal cord injury. Arch Phys Med Rehabil 77:133, 1996.

Bugio, KL, et al: The role of biofeedback in Kegel exercise training for stress urinary incontinence. Am J Obstet Gynecol 154:58, 1986.

Colborne, GR, et al: Feedback of triceps surae EMG in gait of children with cerebral palsy: A controlled study. Arch Phys Med Rehabil 75:40, 1994.

de Kruif, YP, and van Wegen, EEH: Pelvic floor muscle exercise therapy with myofeedback for women with stress urinary incontinence. Physiotherapy 82:107, 1996.

De Weerdt, W, and Harrison, MA: The efficacy of electromyographic feedback for stroke patients: A critical review of the main literature. Physiotherapy 72:108, 1986.

Delk, KK, et al: The effects of biofeedback assisted breathing retraining on lung function in patients with cystic fibrosis. Chest 105:23, 1994.

Freedman, RR: Physiological mechanisms of temperature biofeedback. Biofeedback and Self-Regulation 16:95, 1991.

Gallego, J, et al: Learned activation of thoracic inspiratory muscles in tetraplegics. Am J Phys Med Rehabil 72:312, 1993.

Gentile, AM: A working model of skill acquisition with application to teaching. Quest 17:3, 1972.

Glanz, M, et al: Biofeedback therapy in post-stroke rehabilitation: A meta-analysis of the randomized controlled trials. Arch Phys Med Rehabil 76:508, 1995.

Goodman, M: An hypothesis explaining the successful treatment of psoriasis with thermal biofeedback: A case report. Biofeedback & Self-Regulation 19:347, 1994.

Huckabee, ML: sEMG biofeedback: An adjunct to swallowing therapy. Biofeedback: Newsmagazine of the AAPB 24:20, 1996.

Hurd, WW, et al: Comparison of actual and simulated EMG biofeedback in the treatment of hemiplegic patients. Am J Phys Med 59:73, 1980.

Jahanshahi, M, et al: EMG biofeedback treatment of torticollis: A controlled outcome study. Biofeedback & Self-Regulation 16:413, 1991.

James, R: Biofeedback treatment for cerebral palsy in children and adolescents: A review. Pediatric Exercise Science 4:198, 1992.

Klose, KJ, et al: An assessment of the contribution of electromyographic biofeedback as an adjunct therapy in the physical training of spinal cord injured persons. Archives of Phys Med & Rehab 74:453, 1993.

Kyberd, PJ, et al: A clinical experience with a hierarchically controlled myoelectric hand prosthesis with vibro-tactile feedback. Prosthet Orthot Int 17:56, 1993.

LeVeau, BF, and Rogers, C: Selective training of the vastus medialis muscle using EMG biofeedback. Phys Ther 60:1410, 1980.

Levitt, R, et al: EMG feedback-assisted postoperative rehabilitation of minor arthroscopic knee surgeries. J Sports Med Phys Fitness 35:218, 1995.

Mannarino, M: The present and future roles of biofeedback in successful aging. Biofeedback and Self-Regulation 16:391, 1991.

Mass, R, et al: Biofeedback-induced voluntary reduction of respiratory resistance in severe bronchial asthma. Behavior Research & Therapy 34:815, 1996.

McGrady, A: Good news-bad press: Applied psychophysiology in cardiovascular disorders. Biofeedback and Self-Regulation 21:335, 1996.

Moreland, J, and Thomson, MA: Efficiency of electromyographic biofeedback compared with conventional physical therapy for upper-extremity function in patients following stroke: A research overview and meta-analysis. Phys Ther 74:534, 1994.

Plummer, M: Pelvic floor muscle disorders. Biofeedback: Newsmagazine of the AAPB 24:24, 1996.

Saunders, JT, et al: Thermal biofeedback in the treatment of intermittent claudication in diabetes: A case study. Biofeedback & Self-Regulation 19:337, 1994.

Sczepanski, TL, et al: Effect of contraction type, angular velocity, and arc of motion on VMO:VL EMG ratio. J Orthop Sports Phys Ther 14:256, 1991.

Sherman, RA, and Arena, JG: Biofeedback for assessment and treatment of low back pain. In Basmajian, JV, and Nyberg, R, (eds): Rational Manual Therapies. Williams & Wilkins, Baltimore, 1993.

Souza, DR, and Gross, MT: Comparison of vastus medialis obliques:vastus lateralis muscle integrated electromyographic ratios between healthy subjects and patients with patellofemoral pain. Phys Ther 71:310, 1991.

Swinnen, SP, et al: Information feedback for skill acquisition: Instantaneous knowledge of results degrades learning. J Exp Psychol 16:706, 1990.

Tremain, L: Orthopedics and sports medicine: Surface EMG applications for the knee and shoulder. Biofeedback: Newsmagazine of the AAPB 24:14, 1996.

Winstein, CJ, et al: Effects of summary knowledge of results on the acquisition and retention of partial-weight-bearing during gait. Phys Ther Practice 2:40, 1993.

Winstein, CJ, et al: Learning a partial-weight-bearing skill: Effectiveness of two forms of feedback. Phys Ther 76:985, 1996.

Winstein, CJ, and Schmidt, RA: Reduced frequency of knowledge of results enhances motor skill learning. J Exp Psychol 16:677, 1990.

Wolf, SL, and Binder-MacLeod, SA: Electromyographic biofeedback applications to the hemiplegic patient: Changes in lower extremity neuromuscular and functional status. Phys Ther 63:1404, 1983.

Wolf, SL, and Binder-MacLeod, SA: Electromyographic biofeedback applications to the hemiplegic patient: Changes in upper extremity neuromuscular and functional status. Phys Ther 63:1393, 1983.

Wolf, SL, et al: Concurrent assessment of muscle activity (CAMA): A procedural approach to assess treatment goals. Phys Ther 66:218, 1986.

Wong, AM, et al: Clinical trial of a cervical traction modality with electromyographic biofeedback. Am J Phys Med Rehabil 76:19, 1997.

Young, MS: Electromyographic biofeedback use in the treatment of voluntary posterior dislocation of the shoulder: A case study. J Orthop Sports Phys Ther 20:171, 1994.

GLOSSARY

Artifact: A voltage signal generated by a source other than the one of interest.

Bandwidth: The difference between the lowest and highest frequency detected by an EMG instrument.

Biofeedback: "A technique to reveal to human beings some of their internal physiological events, normal and abnormal, in the form of visual and auditory signals in order to teach them to manipulate these otherwise involuntary or unfelt events by manipulating the displayed signals."[2p1]

Closed loop control: A control system that uses feedback and error-detected processes.

Common mode rejection ratio (CMRR): A proportion expressing an amplifier's ability to reject unwanted noise while amplifying the wanted signal.

Electrogoniometer: A rheostat, or variable resistor, with extended attachments for limb segments. Joint rotation changes the electrogoniometer's resistance to a current passing to a recorder or speaker for kinesiological recording or biofeedback, respectively.

Endogenous: Produced or caused by factors within a cell or organism.

Gain: The ability of a biofeedback instrument to amplify an input signal.

Impedance: The property of a substance that offers resistance to current flow in an alternating current.

Kinematics: The description of the movement and displacement of objects (usually limb segments) in motion without reference to the forces that cause the motion.

Kinetic feedback (dynamic force feedback): Feedback regarding the amount or rate of loading through the limbs.

Kinetics: The description of the forces applied to objects (usually limb segments) in motion.

Knowledge of performance (KP): Feedback related to performance of a task.

Knowledge of results (KR): Feedback related to the overall result (outcome) of a task.

Limb load monitor: A device to measure and report the forces experienced by the lower limbs during walking or other weight-bearing activities.

Motor learning: "A set of processes associated with practice or experience leading to relatively permanent changes in the capability for responding."[1p246]

Noise: An unwanted electrical signal that is detected along with the desired signal.

Ohmmeter: A device that measures electrical resistance; measured in ohms.

Ohm's law: The strength of an electrical current is equal to the voltage divided by the resistance.

Open loop control: A control system that uses preprogrammed instructions to an effector; does not use feedback information and error-detection processes.

Posturography feedback: Standing (or sitting) balance feedback. Usually involves a computerized force-plate system.

Potentiometer: An instrument used to measure voltage.

Proprioception: The internal feedback process that uses muscle and skeletal mechanorecptors for controlling movement.[5]

Rheostat: A mechanism for regulating the resistance in an electrical circuit; controls the amount of electrical current entering a circuit; variable resistor.

Voltmeter: An instrument for measuring electromotive force (in volts).

APPENDIX

Suggested Answers to Case Study Guiding Questions

Case Study 1

1. Explain whether the dorsiflexion weakness is likely to be a direct, indirect, or composite impairment.

ANSWER: Weakness of left ankle dorsiflexion occurred and, for the most part, is maintained as a direct consequence of the neurological insult. The dorsiflexors have weakened further from disuse (an indirect effect of the lesion). Therefore, because of combined direct and indirect effects, the left ankle dorsiflexion weakness is a composite impairment.

2. In addition to dorsiflexion weakness, what other impairment is likely contributing to his inability to heel strike during gait? Is this a direct, indirect, or composite impairment? How will you address it?

ANSWER: Contracture of the triceps surae muscle is limiting passive ankle dorsiflexion and preventing heel strike. This is an indirect impairment that occurred secondary to the neurologic lesion. Although the AFO will have helped, triceps surae will have shortened because the ankle is rarely being moved into dorsiflexion. A program of stretching exercises in weight-bearing would be advocated for this problem.

3. What role might biofeedback have in the management of this patient?

ANSWER: Surface EMG (sEMG) biofeedback will be a very useful adjunct to therapy. Electrodes can be used on the tibialis anterior and peroneus longus to encourage increased activation of these muscles (*uptraining*). The internal feedback mechanism of how it feels to use these muscles may have been lost, and the biofeedback signal provides an external compensation. Increased tone in the triceps surae muscle may be limiting the dorsiflexion ability and therefore teaching relaxation of this muscle should also be included (*downtraining*). Combining recruitment of the tibialis anterior with relaxation of the triceps surae can then be done simultaneously using a dual channel biofeedback machine.

4. To create a change in motor learning, what feedback strategies should be employed?

ANSWER: Continuous biofeedback should be used initially to give the patient knowledge of performance (KP) feedback. However, once the patient has achieved the ability to recruit the tibialis anterior and peroneus longus selectively, and to relax the triceps surae selectively, the feedback should be removed for progressively longer and longer periods so that the patient can develop his own intrinsic feedback mechanism and hopefully retain the motor skill.

This same principle should be applied not only in static practice, but also during gait and other functional activities to encourage transfer of what is learned to dynamic tasks.

Case Study 2

1. How do you know that there is a VMO:VL imbalance? If there is, how do you know that the patient is selectively recruiting VMO during isometric quad sets?

ANSWER: With palpation and observation alone it would be very difficult to tell if there is: (a) a VMO:VL imbalance; and (b) whether VMO is being selectively recruited during quad sets.

2. (a) What advantage does biofeedback provide to VMO rehabilitation? (b) What concerns might you have?

ANSWER: (a) Essentially, surface EMG provides more sensitive and more specific information about muscle activity (than palpation and observation) and at a rapid speed. (b) When comparing activity between VMO and VL, caution should be exercised, because a technical error (e.g., improper electrode placement) could result in serious misinformation. Even if electrode placement were correct, comparing VMO and VL activity should be based more on timing of contraction (e.g., trying to recruit VMO before VL) and duration of an isometric hold (e.g., VMO may fatigue much more quickly than VL) than on quantity (raw microvolts) of activity. Stating that a significant difference in amount of EMG activity has occurred (both within and between treatment sessions) should be made only if the difference is large (e.g., >25 microvolts difference) or if a dichotomous situation exists (e.g., someone who can fire VMO while keeping VL relaxed).

3. What strategies should be employed in using biofeedback for treating a VMO:VL imbalance?

ANSWER: If VMO is under-recruited and VL is over-recruited, as would be the likely scenario, the strategy would be to encourage less activity in VL and more activity in VMO. Initially this could involve selectively *downtraining* VL and selectively *uptraining* VMO. Then VL and VMO feedback could be given simultaneously using a dual-channel machine. When attempting to recruit VMO, too strong a contraction of VL will be discouraged to avoid co-contraction of all the muscles in the quadriceps group. Initially treatment will involve isometrics at different points in a range (0, 30, 60, 90), progressing to open- and closed-chain isotonic exercises, and, most importantly, progressing to functional activities such as gait, stairs, and individual recreational preferences.

Case Study 3

1. How can you ensure that the patient does not exceed 10-pound loads through the operated limb: (a) in static standing; (b) during gait?

ANSWER: (a) In static standing, a weighing scale could be used to teach the patient what it feels like to bear 10 pounds of load, and instructing the patient not to exceed that load. (b) During gait, an educated guess on the part of the patient and the physical therapist is all there is to go on unless an instrumented feedback device is used. A limb load monitor could be placed in the patient's shoe and set to give an audio signal (beep) if the patient exceeds 10 pounds during gait or other weight-bearing activities.

2. What advantage is there to constant feedback during gait?

ANSWER: Constant feedback ensures less error during performance, provided the feedback is maintained.

3. What advantage is there to intermittent feedback during gait?

ANSWER: Intermittent feedback has been shown to enable retention of skill (true learning). Unless you plan to have the patient use an LLM at all times, scheduled feedback should be incorporated in training. Initially constant feedback should be given to ensure that the skill can be correctly learned, but then it should be given after say 5 trials, then 10 trials, then 20 trials, to enable the patient to develop an internal reference for correctness.

4. What additional cause of hip joint loading besides ground reaction load are you concerned with?

ANSWER: During normal FWB, hip muscle contraction actually generates greater hip forces and pressures than ground reaction load. The rationale for TWB is that theoretically it minimizes ground reaction loads and minimizes muscle co-contraction by having the foot only lightly touch down. A LLM provides information only about ground-reaction load. Knowledge of *in vivo* loads at the hip during exercises and functional activities should also be included in clinical decision making and patient education.

Index

Note: Illustrations are indicated by (*f*); tables are indicated by (*t*).